? premature for
ant branch iliac?

July - OB -
Aug -
Sept - Gyn - Brye
Oct -
Nov - EI/ - Sherott
Dec -
Jan - Onco - Disaia
Feb - Urogyn
March - MFM - creasy nosnick
April -
May - Urogyn
June - genetics
July - Path
Aug -
Sept -
Oct -

OBSTETRICS
NORMAL AND PROBLEM PREGNANCIES

Second Edition

OBSTETRICS
NORMAL AND PROBLEM PREGNANCIES

Second Edition

Edited by

Steven G. Gabbe, M.D.
Professor and Chairman
Department of Obstetrics and Gynecology, Ohio State University
College of Medicine, Columbus, Ohio

Jennifer R. Niebyl, M.D.
Professor and Head
Department of Obstetrics and Gynecology, University of
Iowa College of Medicine, Iowa City, Iowa

Joe Leigh Simpson, M.D.
Faculty Professor and Chairman
Department of Obstetrics and Gynecology, University of Tennessee, Memphis
College of Medicine, Memphis, Tennessee

With contributions by

Garland D. Anderson
George J. Annas
Thomas J. Benedetti
Richard L. Berkowitz
John Bissonnette
Watson A. Bowes, Jr.
D. Ware Branch
John E. Buster
Sandra A. Carson
Robert C. Cefalo
Frank A. Chervenak

David H. Chestnut
Usha Chitkara
Dwight P. Cruikshank
Alan H. DeCherney
Richard Depp
Sherman Elias
Roger K. Freeman
Anna-Riitta Fuchs
Fritz Fuchs
Charles P. Gibbs
Stanley F. Gould

John H. Grossman III
Patricia M. Hays
Nelson B. Isada
Timothy R. B. Johnson
David C. Lagrew, Jr.
Mark B. Landon
William C. Mabie
Denise M. Main
Elliott K. Main
Mary Ellen Mortensen
Godfrey P. Oakley, Jr.

William F. O'Brien
Tim H. Parmley II
Roy H. Petrie
Adam A. Rosenberg
Philip Samuels
James R. Scott
John W. Seeds
David B. Seifer
Lowell E. Sever
Baha M. Sibai
Phillip G. Stubblefield
Marlene A. Walker

Illustrated by Mickey Senkarik, M.S., A.M.I.

CHURCHILL LIVINGSTONE
New York, Edinburgh, London, Madrid, Melbourne, Tokyo

Library of Congress Cataloging-in-Publication Data

Obstetrics : normal and problem pregnancies / edited by Steven G.
 Gabbe, Jennifer R. Niebyl, Joe Leigh Simpson ; with contributions by
Garland D. Anderson ... [et al.] ; illustrated by Mickey Senkarik. -
 - 2nd ed.
      p. cm.
   Includes bibliographical references and index.
   ISBN 0-443-08714-8
   1. Obstetrics. I. Gabbe, Steven G.   II. Niebyl, Jennifer R.
III. Simpson, Joe Leigh, date.   IV. Anderson, Garland D.
   [DNLM: 1. Obstetrics. 2. Pregnancy. 3. Pregnancy Complications.
WQ 100 0165]
RG524.03 1991
618.2—dc20
DNLM/DLC
for Library of Congress   91-15900
                                                          CIP

Distributed in the United Kingdom by Churchill Livingstone, Robert Stevenson
House, 1–3 Baxter's Place, Leith Walk, Edinburgh EH1 3AF, and by associated
companies, branches, and representatives throughout the world.

Accurate indications, adverse reactions, and dosage schedules for drugs are provided in this book, but it is possible that they may change. The reader is urged to
review the package information data of the manufacturers of the medications mentioned.

The Publishers have made every effort to trace the copyright holders for borrowed
material. If they have inadvertently overlooked any, they will be pleased to make
the necessary arrangements at the first opportunity.

Acquisitions Editor: *Toni M. Tracy*
Copy Editor: *Kathleen P. Lyons*
Production Designer: *Marci Jordan*
Production Supervisor: *Christina Hippeli*

Printed in the United States of America

First published in 1991   7 6 5 4

To our children
Adam, Amanda, Daniel, and Erica
Peter and Tim
Scott and Reid

and to our professor, Fritz Fuchs,
whose academic children we all are

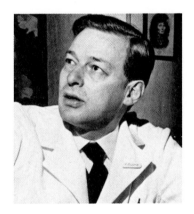

CONTRIBUTORS

Garland D. Anderson, M.D.
Professor and Chairman, Department of Obstetrics and Gynecology, University of Texas Medical Branch at Galveston, Galveston, Texas

George J. Annas, J.D., M.P.H.
Edward Utley Professor, Department of Health Law, Boston University Schools of Medicine and Public Health, Boston, Massachusetts

Thomas J. Benedetti, M.D.
Professor and Director, Division of Perinatal Medicine, Department of Obstetrics and Gynecology, University of Washington School of Medicine, Seattle, Washington

Richard L. Berkowitz, M.D.
Professor and Chairman, Department of Obstetrics, Gynecology, and Reproductive Science, Mount Sinai School of Medicine of the City University of New York, New York, New York

John Bissonnette, M.D.
Professor, Departments of Obstetrics and Gynecology and Cell Biology and Anatomy, Oregon Health Sciences University School of Medicine, Portland, Oregon

Watson A. Bowes, Jr., M.D.
Professor, Department of Obstetrics and Gynecology, University of North Carolina at Chapel Hill School of Medicine, Chapel Hill, North Carolina

D. Ware Branch, M.D.
Assistant Professor, Department of Obstetrics and Gynecology, University of Utah School of Medicine, Salt Lake City, Utah

John E. Buster, M.D.
Professor and Director, Division of Reproductive Endocrinology and Infertility, Department of Obstetrics and Gynecology, University of Tennessee, Memphis, College of Medicine, Memphis, Tennessee

Sandra A. Carson, M.D.
Associate Professor, Division of Reproductive Endocrinology and Infertility, Department of Obstetrics and Gynecology, University of Tennessee, Memphis, College of Medicine, Memphis, Tennessee

Robert C. Cefalo, M.D., Ph.D.
Professor and Director, Division of Maternal-Fetal Medicine, Department of Obstetrics and Gynecology, University of North Carolina at Chapel Hill School of Medicine, Chapel Hill, North Carolina

Frank A. Chervenak, M.D.
Director of Obstetrics, Department of Obstetrics and Gynecology, The New York Hospital-Cornell Medical Center, New York, New York

David H. Chestnut, M.D.
Professor, Departments of Anesthesia and Obstetrics and Gynecology, University of Iowa College of Medicine; Director of Obstetric Anesthesia, University of Iowa Hospitals and Clinics, Iowa City, Iowa

Usha Chitkara, M.D.
Associate Professor, Department of Obstetrics, Gynecology, and Reproductive Science, Mount Sinai School of Medicine of the City University of New York, New York, New York

Dwight P. Cruikshank, M.D.
Professor and Chairman, Department of Obstetrics and Gynecology, Medical College of Wisconsin, Milwaukee, Wisconsin

Alan H. DeCherney, M.D.
John Slade Ely Professor, Department of Obstetrics and Gynecology, Yale University School of Medicine, New Haven, Connecticut

Richard Depp, M.D.
Professor and Chairman, Department of Obstetrics and Gynecology, Jefferson Medical College of Thomas Jefferson University, Philadelphia, Pennsylvania

Sherman Elias, M.D.
Director, Division of Reproductive Genetics, Department of Obstetrics and Gynecology, University of Tennessee, Memphis, College of Medicine, Memphis, Tennessee

Roger K. Freeman, M.D.
Professor, Department of Obstetrics and Gynecology, University of California, Irvine, College of Medicine, Irvine, California; Director, Women's Services, Long Beach Memorial Medical Center, Long Beach, California

Anna-Riitta Fuchs, D.Sc.
Professor, Department of Obstetrics and Gynecology, and Professor of Reproductive Biology, Department of Physiology and Biophysics, Cornell University Medical College, New York, New York

Fritz Fuchs, M.D., Ph.D.
Professor Emeritus, Department of Obstetrics and Gynecology, Cornell University Medical College, New York, New York

Steven G. Gabbe, M.D.
Professor and Chairman, Department of Obstetrics and Gynecology, Ohio State University College of Medicine, Columbus, Ohio

Charles P. Gibbs, M.D.
Professor and Chairman, Department of Anesthesia, University of Colorado School of Medicine, Denver, Colorado

Stanley F. Gould, M.D.
Chief, Department of Obstetrics and Gynecology, Waltham Weston Hospital, Waltham, Massachusetts

John H. Grossman III, M.D., Ph.D
Professor and Director, Division of Maternal-Fetal Medicine, Departments of Obstetrics and Gynecology and Microbiology, George Washington University School of Medicine and Health Sciences, Washington, D.C.

Patricia M. Hays, M.D.
Assistant Professor, Department of Obstetrics and Gynecology, Virginia Commonwealth University Medical College of Virginia School of Medicine, Richmond, Virginia

Nelson B. Isada, M.D.
Fellow, Division of Reproductive Genetics, Department of Obstetrics and Gynecology, Wayne State University School of Medicine, Detroit, Michigan

Timothy R. B. Johnson, M.D.
Associate Professor and Director, Division of Maternal-Fetal Medicine, Departments of Pediatrics and Gynecology and Obstetrics, The Johns Hopkins University School of Medicine; Joint Appointment, Department of Maternal-Child Health, The Johns Hopkins University School of Hygiene and Public Health, Baltimore, Maryland

David C. Lagrew, Jr., M.D.
Assistant Professor, Department of Obstetrics and Gynecology, University of California, Irvine, College of Medicine, Irvine, California; Medical Director, Women's Hospital, Saddleback Memorial Medical Center, Laguna Hills, California

Mark B. Landon, M.D.
Assistant Professor, Division of Maternal-Fetal Medicine, Department of Obstetrics and Gynecology, Ohio State University College of Medicine, Columbus, Ohio

William C. Mabie, M.D.
Associate Professor, Division of Maternal-Fetal Medicine, Department of Obstetrics and Gynecology, University of Tennessee, Memphis, College of Medicine, Memphis, Tennessee

Denise M. Main, M.D.
Assistant Professor, Department of Obstetrics, Gynecology, and Reproductive Sciences, University of California, San Francisco, School of Medicine; Director, Prenatal Diagnosis, Department of Obstetrics and Gynecology, Children's Hospital of San Francisco, San Francisco, California

Elliott K. Main, M.D.
Assistant Professor, Department of Obstetrics, Gynecology, and Reproductive Sciences, University of California, San Francisco, School of Medicine; Associate Chief, Perinatal Services, Children's Hospital of San Francisco and Pacific Presbyterian Medical Center, San Francisco, California

Mary Ellen Mortensen, M.D.
Assistant Professor of Clinical Pediatrics, Division of Clinical Pharmacology/Toxicology, Department of Pediatrics, Ohio State University College of Medicine; Medical Director, Central Ohio Poison Center, Children's Hospital, Columbus, Ohio

Jennifer R. Niebyl, M.D.
Professor and Head, Department of Obstetrics and Gynecology, University of Iowa College of Medicine, Iowa City, Iowa

Godfrey P. Oakley, Jr., M.D.
Director, Division of Birth Defects and Developmental Disabilities, Center for Environmental Health and Injury Control, Centers for Disease Control, Public Health Service, U.S. Department of Health and Human Services, Atlanta, Georgia

William F. O'Brien, M.D.
Professor and Director, Division of Obstetrics, Department of Obstetrics and Gynecology, University of South Florida College of Medicine, Tampa, Florida

Tim H. Parmley II, M.D.
Professor, Departments of Pathology and Obstetrics and Gynecology, University of Arkansas College of Medicine, Little Rock, Arkansas

Roy H. Petrie, M.D., Sc.D.
Professor and Director, Division of Maternal-Fetal Medicine, Department of Obstetrics and Gynecology, Washington University School of Medicine, St. Louis, Missouri

Adam A. Rosenberg, M.D.
Associate Professor, Section of Neonatology, Department of Pediatrics, University of Colorado School of Medicine; Medical Director, Education and Research, Division of Neonatology, Department of Pediatrics, The Children's Hospital, Denver, Colorado

Philip Samuels, M.D.
Assistant Professor, Department of Obstetrics and Gynecology, University of Pennsylvania School of Medicine; Staff Physician, Department of Obstetrics and Gynecology, Hospital of the University of Pennsylvania, Philadelphia, Pennsylvania

James R. Scott, M.D.
Professor and Chairman, Department of Obstetrics and Gynecology, University of Utah School of Medicine, Salt Lake City, Utah

John W. Seeds, M.D.
Professor and Director, Division of Maternal-Fetal Medicine, Department of Obstetrics and Gynecology, University of Arizona College of Medicine, Tucson, Arizona

David B. Seifer, M.D.
Assistant Professor, Department of Obstetrics and Gynecology, Division of Gynecologic Endocrinology, Women and Infants' Hospital, Brown University Program in Medicine, Providence, Rhode Island

Lowell E. Sever, Ph.D.
Assistant Director for Science, Division of Birth Defects and Developmental Disabilities, Center for Environmental Health and Injury Control, Centers for Disease Control, Public Health Service, U.S. Department of Health and Human Services, Atlanta, Georgia

Baha M. Sibai, M.D.
Faculty Professor and Chief, Division of Maternal-Fetal Medicine, Department of Obstetrics and Gynecology, University of Tennessee, Memphis, College of Medicine, Memphis, Tennessee

Joe Leigh Simpson, M.D.
Faculty Professor and Chairman, Department of Obstetrics and Gynecology, University of Tennessee, Memphis, College of Medicine, Memphis, Tennessee

Phillip G. Stubblefield, M.D.
Professor, Department of Obstetrics and Gynecology, University of Vermont College of Medicine, Burlington, Vermont; Chief, Department of Obstetrics and Gynecology, Maine Medical Center, Portland, Maine

Marlene A. Walker, R.N.
Nurse Practitioner, Department of Obstetrics and Gynecology, The Johns Hopkins Hospital, Baltimore, Maryland

PREFACE TO THE SECOND EDITION

Change can be unsettling. For those of us who practice obstetrics, change brings with it the responsibility to learn more about the physiology of pregnancy and the pathophysiology of obstetric disorders and, more importantly, the opportunity to apply this information to improving perinatal outcome.

Since the publication of the first edition of *Obstetrics: Normal and Problem Pregnancies*, both the knowledge base and the practice of obstetrics have changed considerably. For this reason, readers familiar with our first book will note several important modifications in the second edition. Each chapter has been carefully reviewed and rewritten to assure the most up-to-date information. Chapters have been added on ultrasound assessment of fetal anatomy and growth and on critical care. The various medical complications of pregnancy are addressed in separate chapters so that the desired information may be more easily located. Discussions on prenatal genetic diagnosis, acquired immune deficiency syndrome, prepregnancy counseling, and the ethical dilemmas that result from new technologies have been greatly expanded. Many of these changes reflect the constructive feedback we have received from our readers.

As editors, we greatly appreciate the efforts and expertise of our collaborators throughout the United States. Their contributions to this book will help each of us meet the challenges of our changing field.

We are especially indebted to the guidance and support of Toni M. Tracy who, despite her responsibilities as President of Churchill Livingstone Inc., played a major role in this edition. We are pleased that Mickey Senkarik has again contributed illustrations for this textbook. Her original artwork in our first edition received the Association of Medical Illustrators Award of Excellence in 1987. Last, but certainly not least, we greatly appreciate the secretarial support provided by Sally Bourne, Nancy Schaapveld, and Gaye Inman.

Yes, change is unsettling, but with an understanding of these changes comes the excitement of mastering new information and using it to better the health care of pregnant women and their children. Here, then, is the second edition of *Obstetrics: Normal and Problem Pregnancies*.

Steven G. Gabbe, M.D.
Jennifer R. Niebyl, M.D.
Joe Leigh Simpson, M.D.

PREFACE TO THE FIRST EDITION

This book is written for a new generation of obstetricians and gynecologists. Today's obstetrician must not only be able to plot and interpret a labor curve and deliver a breech presentation but also must assess fetal heart rate tracings and scalp pH data. While doing so, he or she must also consider the legal and ethical ramifications for these actions. In the past decade, the practice of obstetrics has been altered by a technologic explosion. Antepartum and intrapartum fetal monitoring, diagnostic ultrasound, and a host of advances in prenatal genetic diagnosis have enabled obstetricians to identify and understand some of the most important disease processes. This information has already led to significant improvements in maternal and perinatal outcome. Yet, the practice of obstetrics and the applications of this technology must be built on a firm base of knowledge in anatomy, embryology, physiology, pathology, genetics, and teratology.

Obstetrics: Normal and Problem Pregnancies has been written to meet these needs. The first sections of the book provide the essential foundation for the practice of obstetrics. The reader can then proceed to discussions of the problems encountered in clinical practice and finally progress to the chapters devoted to high-risk obstetrics. Where does the information necessary to be a specialist end and that needed to be a subspecialist begin? This boundary is difficult to define. It is hoped that *Obstetrics: Normal and Problem Pregnancies* will serve as a reference source for the general practice of obstetrics and provide the necessary base of information for those in fellowship programs in maternal-fetal medicine.

The contributors to this book represent the vanguard in their areas of expertise. Each chapter has been written to stand on its own and, in general, can be read in one evening. As editors, we are most indebted to our collaborators for their excellent contributions and their willingness to create a new book with a new approach.

Our book could not have been written without the help of many special people. Toni M. Tracy, Editor-in-Chief at Churchill Livingstone, and Linda Panzarella, Sponsoring Editor, successfully guided us through this enormous but rewarding project. Lynne Herndon got us off to a good start. Mickey Senkarik prepared all of the original artwork for the book and, in doing so, showed her unique artistic skills and understanding. Dr. Gerald Lazarus, Chairman of the Department of Dermatology, Dr. Marshall Mintz of the Department of Radiology, and Dr. James Wheeler of the Department of Pathology, all at the Hospital of the University of Pennsylvania, provided guidance in the selection of illustrations for the chapters on infectious diseases, placental development, and antepartum fetal evaluation. Also, all of us owe so much to the secretarial support provided by Michele Simons and C. Winston Wisehart.

This is the first edition of *Obstetrics: Normal and Problem Pregnancies.* Now a neonate, it has completed its months and years of gestation. Hopefully, it will help those embarking on careers in obstetrics to enjoy the specialty as much as we have. We look forward to hearing comments, both positive and negative, from our readers.

Steven G. Gabbe
Jennifer R. Niebyl
Joe Leigh Simpson

CONTENTS

SECTION 1: Anatomy and Physiology

1. Anatomy   3
   Stanley F. Gould

2. The Placenta   39
   Tim H. Parmley II

3. Placental Endocrinology and Diagnosis of Pregnancy   59
   John E. Buster and Sandra A. Carson

4. Placental and Fetal Physiology   93
   John Bissonnette

5. Maternal Physiology in Pregnancy   125
   Dwight P. Cruikshank and Patricia M. Hays

6. Physiology of Parturition   147
   Anna-Riitta Fuchs and Fritz Fuchs

7. Physiology and Endocrinology of Lactation   175
   Anna-Riitta Fuchs

SECTION 2: Prenatal Care

8. Preconception and Prenatal Care   209
   *Timothy R. B. Johnson, Marlene A. Walker,
   and Jennifer R. Niebyl*

9. Teratology and the Epidemiology of Birth Defects   233
   *Mary Ellen Mortensen, Lowell E. Sever,
   and Godfrey P. Oakley, Jr.*

10. Genetic Counseling and Prenatal Diagnosis   269
     Joe Leigh Simpson

11. Drugs in Pregnancy and Lactation   299
     Jennifer R. Niebyl

12. Obstetric Ultrasound: Assessment of Fetal Growth
     and Anatomy   329
     Frank A. Chervenak and Steven G. Gabbe

13. Antepartum Fetal Evaluation   377
     Steven G. Gabbe

SECTION 3: Intrapartum Care

14. Labor and Delivery   427
     William F. O'Brien and Robert C. Cefalo

15. Intrapartum Fetal Evaluation   457
     Roy H. Petrie

16. Obstetric Anesthesia   493
     David H. Chestnut and Charles P. Gibbs

17. Malpresentations   539
     John W. Seeds

18. Obstetric Hemorrhage   573
     Thomas J. Benedetti

19. Critical Care Obstetrics   607
     William C. Mabie

20. Cesarean Delivery and Other Surgical Procedures   635
     Richard Depp

SECTION 4: Postpartum Care

21. The Neonate   697
     Adam A. Rosenberg

22. Postpartum Care   753
     Watson A. Bowes, Jr.

Section 5: Complicated Pregnancies

23. Fetal Wastage   783
    Joe Leigh Simpson

24. Ectopic Pregnancy   809
    Alan H. DeCherney and David B. Seifer

25. Preterm Birth   829
    Denise M. Main and Elliott K. Main

26. Multiple Gestations   881
    Usha Chitkara and Richard L. Berkowitz

27. Intrauterine Growth Retardation   923
    Steven G. Gabbe

28. Prolonged Pregnancy   945
    Roger K. Freeman and David C. Lagrew, Jr.

29. Isoimmunization in Pregnancy   957
    D. Ware Branch and James R. Scott

SECTION 6: Pregnancy and Co-existing Disease

30. Hypertension   993
    Baha M. Sibai and Garland D. Anderson

31. Cardiac and Pulmonary Disease   1057
    Mark B. Landon and Philip Samuels

32. Renal Disease   1085
    Philip Samuels

33. Diabetes Mellitus and Other Endocrine Diseases   1097
    Mark B. Landon

34. Hematologic Diseases   1137
    Philip Samuels

35. Collagen Vascular Diseases   1151
    Philip Samuels

36. Hepatic and Gastrointestinal Disorders   1169
    Philip Samuels and Mark B. Landon

37. Neurologic Disorders   1183
    Philip Samuels

38.   Malignant Diseases   1199
          Mark B. Landon

39.   Dermatologic Disorders   1215
          Mark B. Landon

40.   Perinatal Infections   1223
          Nelson B. Isada and John H. Grossman III

SECTION 7: Pregnancy Termination

41.   Pregnancy Termination   1303
          Phillip G. Stubblefield

SECTION 8: Legal and Ethical Issues in Perinatology

42.   Legal and Ethical Issues in Perinatology   1333
          George J. Annas and Sherman Elias

Index   1351

SECTION 1
Anatomy and Physiology

Chapter 1

Anatomy

Stanley F. Gould

THE BONY PELVIS

The pelvis is the lowermost extension of the abdominal cavity; it is surrounded by a bony girdle consisting of the sacrum and coccyx posteriorly and of the two hip bones (os coxae or innominate bones) laterally. The two hip bones curve anteriorly and are connected at the symphysis pubis but are separated posteriorly by the sacrum and coccyx (Fig. 1.1). The innominate bone is composed of three bones—the ilium, ischium, and pubis—which are separate in the immature skeleton but which become fused by cartilage in the adult. In the sitting position, most of the weight of the trunk is supported by the ischium (ischial tuberosities), whereas when erect the weight of the trunk and viscera contained within are transmitted by the pelvis to the lower limbs.

The ilium forms the broad upper portion of the bony pelvis. It extends downward and forms the upper part of the hip articulation. The upper margin is curved and forms the iliac crest, while its anterior and posterior limits form two projections termed the anterosuperior iliac spine and posterosuperior iliac spine. Numerous muscular attachments are derived from the lateral surface of the ilium. These muscles include the external and internal obliques, transversus abdominis, quadratus lumborum, erector spinae, sartorius, rectus femoris, gluteus maximus, gluteus medius, and gluteus minimus. The medial surface of the ilium is divided into a superior and inferior portion by the arcuate line. The superior portion is termed the iliac fossa to which is attached the iliacus muscle. The inferior portion forms a more flattened surface continuous with the medial portions of the ischium and pubis. It is this inferior portion of the ilium and fused portions of the ischium and pubis that form the "true" or minor pelvis, while that portion of the ilium above the arcuate line is called the "false" or major pelvis.

The ischium consists of a body and ramus, each portion of which forms the posterior aspect of the obturator foramen. The ischial tuberosity is a heavy projection of the lower part of the body of the ischium, while the ischial spine is a sharp projection of the posterior aspect of the body of the ischium. The ischial spine and ischial tuberosity are separated by the lesser sciatic notch. Superior to the level of the ischial spine, the ischium forms a portion of the greater sciatic notch. The muscles of the levator ani and the coccygeus muscle derive, either in whole or in part, attachment from the medial surface of the ischium. The lateral aspect of the ischium provides attachments for the hamstrings, adductors, quadratus femoris, obturator externus, and gracilis muscles. The ischium also provides attachments to two important ligaments, the sacrospinous and sacrotuberous ligaments (Fig. 1.2).

The pubis consists of a body, a superior ramus, and an inferior ramus. The body is flattened anteriorly.

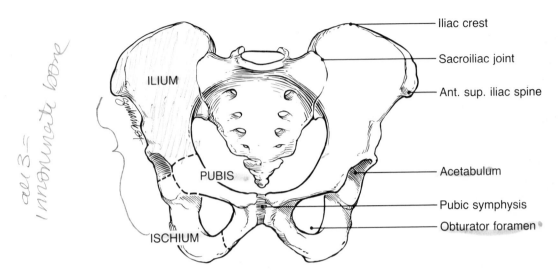

Fig. 1.1 Major components of the bony pelvis, frontal view. This is a superior view of the female pelvis. The plane of the pelvic brim faces forward and forms an angle of about 60 degrees to the horizontal. Features that most clearly distinguish the female from male pelvis include subpubic angle, width of the sciatic notch, and distance from pubic symphysis and anterior edge of the acetabulum.

The most medial end of the body of the pubis is covered with hyaline cartilage and meets its counterpart medially by uniting with a fibrocartilaginous joint called the pubis symphysis. The inner surface of the pubic body forms the anterior wall of the pelvic cavity and provides the anterior attachment for the levator ani. The superior and inferior rami form much of the boundaries of the obturator foramen.

At birth the three bones of the os coxae are separated by hyaline cartilage; the iliac crest and ischial

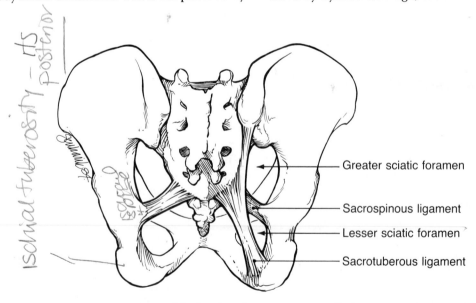

Fig. 1.2 Major ligaments and notches of the female pelvis, posterior view. During pregnancy, temporary changes take place in the ligaments that permit both movement of the joints and enlargement of the pelvic cavity. This becomes important during parturition.

tuberosities are cartilaginous. Because growth occurs by addition of bone to the surfaces adjacent to the cartilage, the hip bone appears to grow interstitially. At around age 7 to 9 years, the pubis and ischium fuse inferior to the obturator foramina, whereas fusion of the ilium, ischium, and pubis superiorly does not occur until puberty. Even after the menarche, growth continues at the iliac crest, pubic symphysis, and ischial spines. This growth ceases in young adult life. It is not until about age 25 years, however, that the main mass of the hip bone is finally fused with these cartilaginous portions of the iliac crest, pubic symphysis, and ischial tuberosity.

The opening of the "true" or minor pelvis is termed the inlet and is formed posteriorly by the upper anterior margin of the first sacral vertebra and anterior margin of the sacrum (promontory), laterally by the arcuate line of the ilium, and anteriorly by the pubic crest along the anterosuperior border of the body of the pubis. The pelvic cavity is surrounded by the ischium and pubis and by the ilium below the level of the arcuate line. The outlet of the "true" pelvis is bounded by the inferior margin of the symphysis pubis, the ischiopubic rami, the sacrotuberous ligaments, and the coccyx.

In the standing, anatomic position, the plane of the pelvic inlet forms approximately a 60-degree angle with the horizontal. In the same position, the outlet forms an angle of approximately 10 degrees. In this position the anterosuperior iliac spines are in the same vertical plane as the pubic crests.

MUSCLES AND FASCIA OF THE PELVIS

Because the pelvis is a curved basin, it is difficult to delineate the various walls clearly. There is no question, however, in determining those elements that form the floor of the pelvis. The posterior wall consists of the sacrum and coccyx, with their associated muscles, the piriformis and coccygeus. The lateral walls are formed by the ischium and ilium, with the obturator internus forming the superior portion of

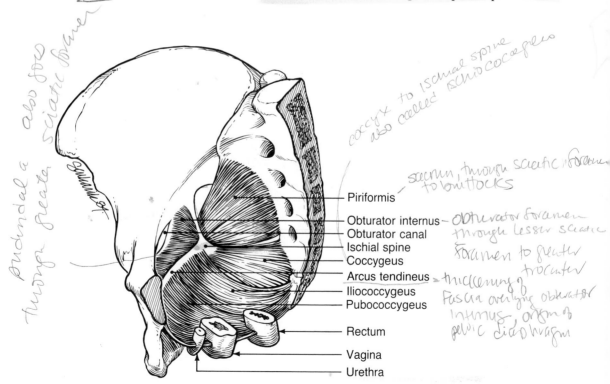

- Piriformis
- Obturator internus
- Obturator canal
- Ischial spine
- Coccygeus
- Arcus tendineus
- Iliococcygeus
- Pubococcygeus
- Rectum
- Vagina
- Urethra

Fig. 1.3 Muscles of the pelvic diaphragm, oblique view. The pelvic diaphragm forms a muscular floor for the support of the pelvic organs. Note the placement of the urethra, uterus, and rectum as they pierce the floor of the pelvic diaphragm.

the lateral wall and the levator ani forming the inferior limit of the lateral wall. The anterior surface is formed by the anterior aspect of the obturator internus muscle, by a portion of the pubic symphysis and pubes, and by the most anterior portion of the levator ani, which arises from the pubis bones. The floor of the pelvis is formed by the pelvic diaphragm or levator ani muscle.

Figure 1.3 shows the musculature of the pelvic wall as seen in sagittal section. The obturator internus arises from the pelvic surface of the obturator foramen and from the inner surface of the obturator membrane. It passes around the lesser sciatic notch and inserts in the greater trochanter. It forms a major portion of the lateral wall of the pelvis and ischiorectal fossa but is actually classified as a muscle of the buttocks. This muscle is covered by a heavy fascia (obturator fascia) that gives rise to the origin of the pelvic diaphragm, termed the arcus tendineus of the levator ani muscle. The other major muscle of the lateral pelvic wall is the piriformis, which arises primarily from the sacrum and through which course the sacral plexus and arteries to the buttocks. Like the obturator internus, the piriformis is a muscle of

the buttocks, almost completely filling the greater sciatic foramen and inserting into the buttocks.

The coccygeus, also termed the ischiococcygeus, forms the most posterior portion of the pelvic diaphragm. It arises from the ischial spine and inserts onto the sacrum and coccyx. This muscle lies immediately anterior to the sacrospinous ligament.

Support for the pelvic viscera is largely maintained by the levator ani. This tripartite muscle forms most of the pelvic diaphragm (Figs. 1.4 and 1.5). It consists of several components—the iliococcygeus, pubococcygeus, and puborectalis muscles. Not only does the levator ani form the major supporting structure for the pelvic viscera, but it provides the elasticity of the pelvic floor. It is pierced by the urinary, vaginal, and rectal canals.

The iliococcygeus is the most broad and posterior portion of the levator ani, which arises from the ischial spines and arcus tendineus. It inserts into the side and tip of the coccyx, while its more anterior fibers fuse in the midline with fibers from its counterpart on the opposite side. This fusion occurs between the anus and coccyx and is termed the anococcygeal ligament. The iliococcygeus is considered the most

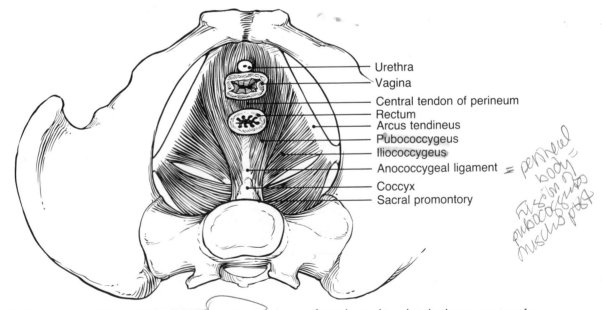

Urethra
Vagina
Central tendon of perineum
Rectum
Arcus tendineus
Pubococcygeus
Iliococcygeus
Anococcygeal ligament
Coccyx
Sacral promontory

Fig. 1.4 Muscles of the pelvic diaphragm, superior view. As seen from above, the pelvic diaphragm consists of a number of different muscles and ligaments. The spaces between these muscles transmit a number of vessels and nerves as they leave the pelvis. Note the relationship of the central tendon of the perineum to the rectum and uterus.

variable portion of the levator ani; it may be highly developed in some women or largely fibrous in others.

The pubococcygeus is the more anterior portion of the levator ani, arising from the posterior surface of the pubis and arcus tendineus. Its medial fibers are directed posteriorly, while the more lateral aspects of the muscle course both posteriorly and medially. The dorsal vein of the clitoris is found between the muscles of the two sides. The more medial fibers of the pubococcygeus sweep around the vagina and urethra and insert into the perineal body. There is no true hiatus between the two pubococcygeus muscles, as fibers are actually attached to the urethra, vagina, and rectum.

The third portion of the levator ani is formed by the puborectalis muscle. Although smaller in breadth than the pubococcygeus, this muscle is the most massive portion of the pelvic diaphragm. It arises in continuity with the most anterior portions of the pubococcygeus but actually lies inferior to and is derived from the inferior surface of pubes. It courses posteriorly, but, unlike the pubococcygeus, which inserts into the anococcygeal ligament and perineal body, it fuses with fibers of the opposite side below the anococcygeal ligament and forms a heavy muscular sling behind the rectum.

The levator ani is innervated by the third and fourth sacral nerves, with an overlapping distribution between these two roots. The most anterior portion of the diaphragm is innervated by the pudendal nerve (S2 to S4). The levator ani forms the most significant supporting structure for the uterus. The pubococcygeus muscles provide support for the bladder; the puborectalis muscle is intricately involved in maintaining anal continence.

Each muscle within the pelvis, those forming the lateral and posterior walls as well as the floor, are invested in a fascial sheath derived from the transversalis fascia of the more superior abdominal wall. This fascia is actually fused to the periosteum at the pelvic brim but continues without interruption across the pelvis. Although specific division of this fascia is artificial, it is useful to think of the pelvic fascia in terms of a parietal fascia covering the muscles of the lateral walls, of a visceral (endopelvic) fascia covering the pelvic viscera, and of a fascia of the superior and inferior surfaces of the pelvic diaphragm (Fig. 1.6).

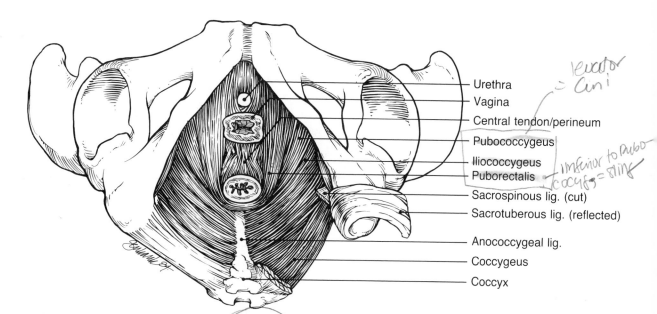

— Urethra
— Vagina
— Central tendon/perineum
— Pubococcygeus
— Iliococcygeus
— Puborectalis
— Sacrospinous lig. (cut)
— Sacrotuberous lig. (reflected)
— Anococcygeal lig.
— Coccygeus
— Coccyx

Fig. 1.5 Muscles of the pelvic diaphragm, inferior view. As seen from below, the pelvic diaphragm is bilaterally symmetric, with the perineal body (central tendon) and the anococcygeal ligament forming a strong median raphe. Note the relationship of the vaginal and urethral canals to the inferior rami of the pubic bone.

The parietal or parietal–diaphragmatic fascia is defined as that fascia lying over the piriformis and obturator internus muscles. The obturator fascia is the chief component of the parietal fascia, originating in the arcuate line of pubis and ilium. It is thick and consists of two parts: a thin outer layer, considered the fascia of the obturator internus, and a thick inner layer, considered the tendon of origin of the levator ani. This tendon of origin actually splits into three layers: an outer layer that follows the obturator internus into the ischiorectal fossa and an inner layer that splits into two layers that follow the surfaces of the levator ani, forming the superior and inferior fascias of the pelvic diaphragm. The visceral or endopelvic fascias are condensations of connective tissue around the pelvic organs, which blend inferiorly with the fascia of the superior aspect of the pelvic diaphragm. It is this fascia that forms the "ligaments" of the pelvic viscera (uterosacral and cardinal), which are really perivascular condensations of subperitoneal tissue derived from the visceral pelvic fascia rather than true ligaments. Damage to these condensations of connective tissue and to their muscles of origin (levator ani) during parturition is of paramount concern in the development of pelvic relaxation and the development of cystocele, rectocele, and uterine procidentia.

THE PERINEUM

The term *perineum* has a wide circle of connotations; it is defined one way by the anatomist and another by the obstetrician/gynecologist. From an anatomic viewpoint, the perineum is the area between the thighs that extends from coccyx to pubis—the inferior aspect of the pelvic outlet. Thus the lower or perineal surface of the levator ani forms the superior or upper boundary of the perineum, with the anal and urogenital canals piercing the levator ani and traversing the expanse of the perineum. Because the urogenital and anal canals traverse the perineum, the perineum may be divided into two distinct parts. These parts are roughly triangular in shape and are separated by a line drawn between and slightly anterior to the two ischial tuberosities. Division of the perineum in this way gives rise to an anterior or urogenital triangle and to a posterior or anal triangle (see

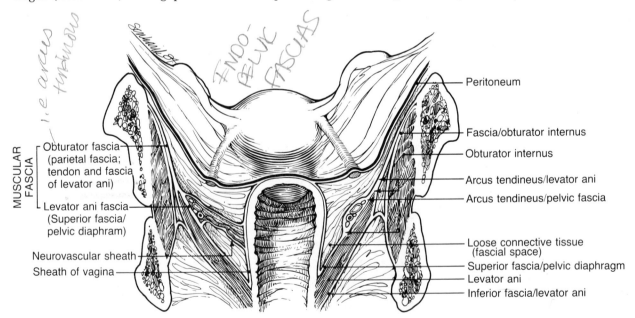

Fig. 1.6 Fascial and peritoneal relationships of the pelvic diaphragm. In this frontal view of the pelvis, note the levator ani as it slopes downward and medially, surrounding the vagina. The loose connective tissue beneath the pelvic peritoneum is variable in thickness, depending on the general adiposity of the individual. Note also the continuity of the different fascias as they merge to form the neurovascular sheaths.

(handwritten annotations in top margin: "lower surface levator ani fascia", "Deep or external or inferior perineal fascia", "Scarpas = Colles", "campers", "skin", "Fascial layers of perineum")

Fig. 1.8, inset). The urogenital triangle is the more complex, as it is further subdivided by the presence of another fibromuscular septum that extends across the anterior portion of the pelvic outlet below the levator ani. This septum is the urogenital diaphragm. Both triangles or regions share in common the levator ani as their superior boundary, and each triangle has a common sagittal midline attachment for its respective musculature. This common midline muscular attachment, which is roughly bisected by the interischial line described above, forms a fibromuscular mass called the central tendon of the perineum or perineal body. It is this fibromuscular structure that the obstetrician/gynecologist often refers to as the perineum.

Regardless of its name, the central tendon of the perinum is interposed between the most anterior surface of the anal canal and the posterior surface of the vagina, anchoring the anterior surface of the anal canal and posterior surface of the vagina. Thus expansion of the anal and vaginal canals occurs in a more lateral plane.

In both the urogenital and anal triangles, the most external or inferior boundaries of the perineum consist of the skin and superficial perineal fascia. This fascia is a continuation of the superficial fascia of the abdominal wall and follows the description of the fascia as seen superiorly: a superficial and more fatty layer, known as the fascia of Camper, and a deeper, more fibrous layer, termed Scarpa's fascia. Unlike the well-developed layers seen in the abdomen, however, the superficial perineal fascia is far less well segregated into these two distinct layers. The outer, more fatty portion of the superficial fascia in the perineum has no specific name. This fatty portion of the superficial fascia is more highly developed around the vulva and gives form to the labia majora but contributes little to the substance of the labia minora. It is continuous with the superficial fatty fascia of the thigh and blends posteriorly with the fat of the ischiorectal fossa. The more fibrous and deeper portion of the superficial perineal fascia, especially in the urogenital triangle, is also known as Colles' fascia. Deep to Colles' fascia there is another fascial layer, which is attached laterally to the ischiopubic rami and posteriorly to the posterior border of the urogenital diaphragm. This fascia is named the deep, inferior, or external perineal fascia and forms the true, most infe-

rior boundary of the "spaces" of the perineum. Because the fascia of the female perineum is not significant in preventing urinary extravasation (as is true in the male), relatively little attention has been paid to this layer. Nevertheless, it is important to note that infection can spread unimpeded throughout the superficial layers of the perineum in the female.

External Genitalia

The labia majora are prominent folds of skin containing a well-developed fat pad derived from the fatty portion of the superficial fascia of the perineum. These folds are homologous to the scrotum of the male and surround a midline cleft containing the labia minora and vestibule. This cleft is termed the pudendal cleft. The labia majora are fused both anteriorly and posteriorly into the anterior and posterior commissures.

The labia minora are smaller, thinner tissue folds that lie within the pudendal cleft and medial to the labia majora. These folds immediately surround the vestibule of the vagina into which the vaginal and urethral orifices open. They are connected anteriorly and posteriorly as the anterior and posterior fourchette. The anterior fourchette is actually divided into two parts, where the lateral portion of the labia minora fuse to form the prepuce of the clitoris just anterior to the glans clitoridis, while the medial parts unite to form the frenulum of the clitoris.

The space between the labia minora is termed the vaginal vestibule. The vaginal orifice lies in the posterior portion of the vestibule. On either side of the vaginal orifice are the openings of the ducts of the greater vestibular glands (Bartholin's glands). These lie slightly anterior to the commissure. On either side of the urethral meatus lies the opening to the paraurethral or Skene's glands. Between the urethral and vaginal orifices, and within the vestibule, are the duct openings to the lesser vestibular glands.

The clitoris is the homologue of the male penis; it lies just posterior to the pubic symphysis above the anterior commissure. It is composed of a body and glans. The body is formed by the union of the two corpora cavernosa, but, unlike the male, where the corpus spongiosum surrounds the urethra, the corpus spongiosum in the female is represented only by a slender thread of erectile tissue. The body of the clitoris is approximately 2.5 cm long and is covered by a

(handwritten margin notes at right: "majora", "susc tissues", "commissura", "minora", "fuse to", "prepuce")

(handwritten note at bottom right: "c. cavernosa", "c. spongiosa (vestigial)", "urethra")

small mass of erectile tissue called the glans clitoridis. The homologue of the glans is the glans penis, which is provided with numerous sensory nerve endings. The prepuce and frenulum of the clitoris are derived from the labia minora.

Urogenital Triangle

The urogenital triangle is divided into two distinct spaces: the superficial space and the deep perineal space. Each space contains its own muscles, vessels, and nerves, but, as a rule, both are poorly developed in the female as compared with the urogenital triangle in the male.

The superficial perineal space contains three sets or pairs of muscles: the ischiocavernosae, bulboca-

vernosae (bulbospongiosae), and superficial transverse perinei (Fig. 1.7). Also included within this space are the greater vestibular glands (Bartholin's glands) and the vestibular bulbs. The superficial perineal space is bounded inferiorly by the deep perineal fascia. The superior boundary is the inferior fascia of the deep perineal space (Fig. 1.8).

The superficial transverse perinei muscles arise from the anterior portion of the ischial tuberosities and run transversely across the perineum, inserting in the central tendon. Many of the fibers of insertion merge imperceptibly with the external anal sphincter and the bulbocavernosus. The muscle is generally quite small and variably developed, but it can usually be seen during an episiotomy as distinct cross sections

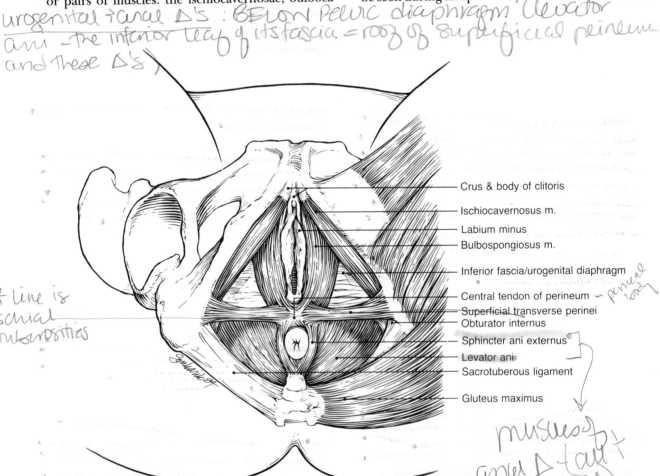

Fig. 1.7 Muscles of the superficial perineal space, from below. As viewed with the patient in dorsal lithotomy position, the muscles of the superficial perineal space of the urogenital triangle and the muscles of the anal triangle all converge in the midline.

of muscle surrounded by a discrete circumferential fascia. It is important to recognize this muscle at the time of episiotomy repair, if the perineum is to be reopposed in the proper planes.

The ischiocavernosus muscles are associated with the crus of the clitoris; they arise from the medial surface of the ischial tuberosities, traverse the medial surface of the pubic rami, and insert into the pubic arch on each side of the crus of the clitoris.

The bulbospongiosus muscles (bulbocavernosus), also termed the sphincter vaginae, arise posteriorly from the central tendon of the perineum. These muscles form the most medial boundaries of the superficial perineal spaces and are separated from each other by the vestibule of the vagina. They insert into the dorsum of the clitoris and into the inferior fascia of the urogenital diaphragm. Their origin shows continuity with the central tendon of the perineum.

The vestibular bulbs are the female homologue of the erectile components of the penile bulb in the male. They lie on either side of the vestibule under cover of the bulbospongiosus muscles. While they represent the bulb of the penis, they are completely separated from each other by the vestibule and are far less vascular than their male counterpart. During sexual arousal, the vestibular bulbs become more or less engorged. Immediately behind the vestibular bulb, although usually under cover by the bulbospongio-

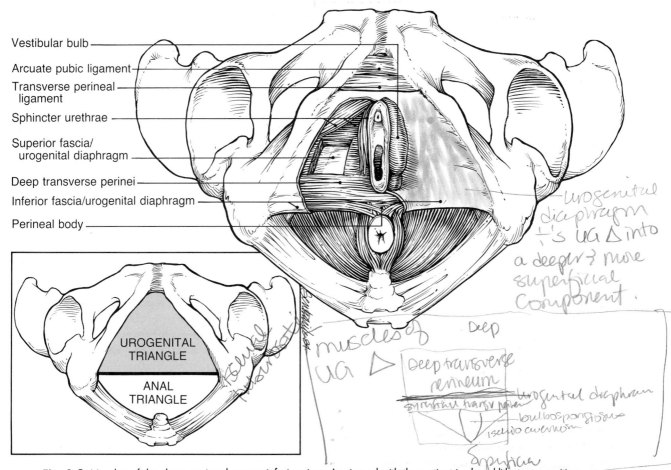

Vestibular bulb

Arcuate pubic ligament

Transverse perineal ligament

Sphincter urethrae

Superior fascia/ urogenital diaphragm

Deep transverse perinei

Inferior fascia/urogenital diaphragm

Perineal body

UROGENITAL TRIANGLE

ANAL TRIANGLE

Fig. 1.8 Muscles of the deep perineal space, inferior view. As viewed with the patient in dorsal lithotomy position, the deep perineal space consists of far less well-developed muscles than the superficial perineal space. Note that the vestibular bulb lies within the superficial perineal space. Inset: Division of the perineum into a urogenital (anterior) triangle and an anal (posterior) triangle.

sus, is found the greater vestibular gland. This gland is the homologue of the bulbourethral gland, which has a long slender duct that opens into the vaginal vestibule.

The deep perineal space, also called the perineal membrane or triangular ligament, is regarded as a closed compartment that contains the urogenital diaphragm. It is limited inferiorly by the inferior fascia of the urogenital diaphragm. It is bounded superiorly by the superior fascia of the urogenital diaphragm and laterally by the insertion of the inferior and superior fascia to the ischiopubic rami. The muscles contained within this space include the deep perineal musculature, specifically the sphincter urethrae and deep transverse perineal muscles. The diaphragm is poorly developed in the female, as it is perforated by both the urethra and the vagina (Fig. 1.8).

The sphincter urethrae arises from the rami of the ischium and pubis; it sends medially directed fibers toward the urethra. These fibers variably surround the distal urethra as well as the anterior portion of the vagina. The more posterior portion of the muscle sends transverse fibers across the deep perineal space, inserting into the sides of the vagina.

The deep transverse perinei are composed of transverse muscle fibers at the posterior border of the sphincter urethrae, inserting into the central tendon of the perineum. Unlike the male, the deep transverse perinei muscles play little or no role in maintaining female urinary continence.

Anal Triangle

The anal triangle is the simpler of the two regions of the perineum and is identical in both sexes. It is traversed by the terminal portion of the anal canal and by the surrounding muscles forming the external anal sphincter. The ischiorectal fossa is the most significant space within this portion of the triangle; it lies lateral and posterior to the terminal portion of the anal canal.

Figure 1.9 depicts a frontal section through the ischiorectal fossa and the anal triangle. The ischiorectal fossa is seen as a potential space lying between the skin and levator ani and on each side of the anal canal. The fossa connects posteriorly with the fossa on the opposite side, thus making the two fossae continuous in the form of a horseshoe. Each fossa is bounded laterally by the obturator internus muscle and its fascia, while the medial walls are formed by the sloping inferior surface of the levator ani as it descends and surrounds the anal canal. Posterior to the anal canal, no medial wall exists; the levator ani forms the superior boundary of the ischiorectal fossa. The lateral walls and superior margin meet sharply at the origin of the levator ani from the obturator fascia.

The ischiorectal fossa is not confined to the anal triangle but extends both posteriorly beneath the lower edge of the gluteus maximus as far as the sacrotuberous ligament and anteriorly above the superior fascia of the urogenital diaphragm to the inferior surface of the levator ani (Fig. 1.10). The ischiorectal fossa is horseshoe shaped, as the most anterior portions of the respective fossae are prohibited from meeting in the midline by the central tendon of the perineum and the midline structures of the urogenital system.

The ischiorectal fossa is fat filled and is thus classified as a potential space. Connective tissue septa derived from the fascia lining the lateral walls of the fossa as well as from Colles' fascia penetrate this fossal fat pad and provide support and shape to the adipose tissue. The presence of fat within the fossa permits distention of the anal canal during defecation and of the vaginal canal during the second stage of labor. This capacity for distention can also lead to significant accumulations of blood or pus of as much as 1 L of fluid. The ischiorectal fossa is therefore a prime target in concealed postpartum hemorrhage. Ischiorectal fossa abscesses may push the levator ani superiorly and into contact with the wall of the lower portion of the rectum. These abscesses may cross to the other side of the pelvis, point, and drain through the anal canal or, more infrequently, rupture through the levator ani and produce severe intraperitoneal or retroperitoneal abdominal infection.

The fascia of the ischiorectal fossa consists of the tough fascia lining the obturator internus (obturator fascia) and of the inferior fascia of the levator ani. Along the lateral wall of the ischiorectal fossa, the fascia splits, forming the fascia lunata. This fascia, in combination with the obturator fascia, forms a canal that carries the pudendal nerve and internal pudendal vessels. This canal is termed the pudendal canal, or Alcock's canal (Fig. 1.9).

The voluntary muscular sphincter, which accounts for fecal continence, is known as the external anal sphincter; it is located within the anal triangle. This tripartite structure surrounds the anal canal and rectum from the inferior surface of the levator ani to the anal verge. Its total length is approximately 2 cm. The sphincter is composed of the joint effort of three muscles (Fig. 1.11): the subcutaneous, superficial, and deep components of the external anal sphincter. While there is no clear subdivision between these parts, their identification is possible in vivo. It is imperative that this anatomy be accurately restored should laceration or surgical incision occur at the time of parturition.

Immediately deep to the perianal skin are found two sets of muscle fibers, which run in a posterior to anterior direction in the anal triangle. These muscles originate in the coccyx and are often attached to the overlying skin. They run toward the perineal body and diverge, running around the sides of the anal canal and inserting into the central tendon of the perineum. These two sets of fibers lie one on top of the other and are termed the superficial and deep portions of the external anal sphincter. Surrounding the anal canal and running circumferentially around it is the third component of the external sphincter, the subcutaneous component.

Between the two bundles of the longitudinally directed superficial anal sphincter and posterior to the subcutaneous circumferential fibers is a triangular space termed Minor's triangle. This triangle is often the site of exit for anal fistulae. It is through this subsphincteric potential space that infection often gains entrance into the ischiorectal fossa.

Nerve Supply to the Perineum

The cutaneous nerve supply to the perineum is derived from a number of different nerves. Local or regional anesthesia for surgical intervention demands a thorough understanding of the distribution

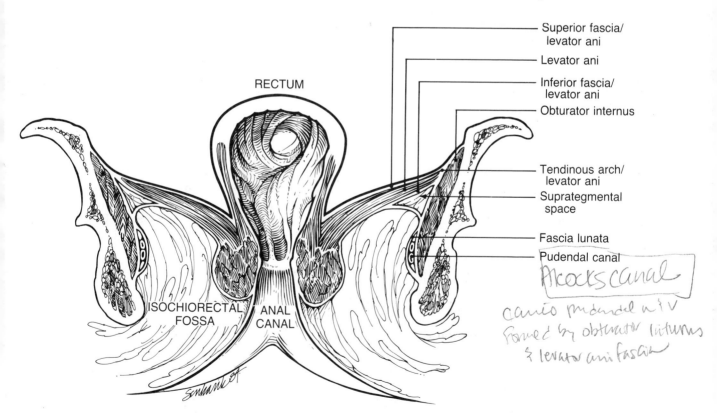

Fig. 1.9 Ischiorectal fossa, frontal section. The ischiorectal fossa surrounds the rectum and vagina and forms most of the potential space within the posterior triangle of the perineum. Note the pudendal canal on the lateral wall of each fossa. The fascia of the levator ani merges with the visceral sheath of the rectum and vagina to lend support.

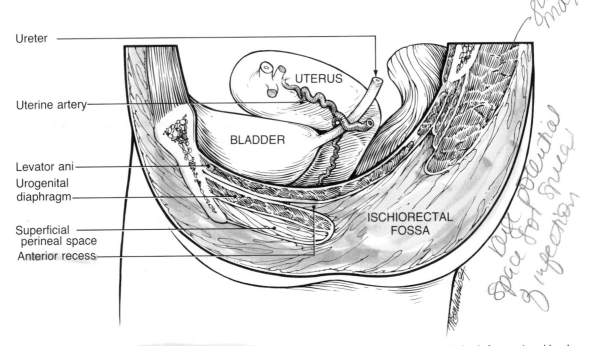

gluteus maximus

best potential space for spread of infection

Fig. 1.10 Ischiorectal fossa and urogenital diaphragm, sagittal section. The ischiorectal fossa extends both forward and backward from the anal triangle. Note how the urogenital diaphragm subdivides the urogenital triangle, with the anterior recess of the ischiorectal fossa superior to it. The subcutaneous fat between the inferior aspect of the superficial perineal space and the skin varies from patient to patient.

of these nerves. The major nerves supplying the skin of the perineum are the pudendal nerve (S2 to S4), coccygeal and last sacral nerve, perineal branch of posterior femoral cutaneous nerve, ilioinguinal nerve (L1), and the genitofemoral nerve (L1,2) (Fig. 1.12). The area most laterally in the perineum is supplied by the posterior femoral cutaneous nerves. These nerves supply the perineal skin lateral to the anus and in-

clude the most posterior and lateral portions of the labia majora. The skin directly posterior to the anus, directly over the tip of the coccyx, is supplied by the cutaneous twigs of the coccygeal and by the fourth and fifth sacral nerves. The mons pubis and most anterior portions of the labia majora (except the clitoris) are supplied by the ilioinguinal and genitofemoral nerves derived from the lumbar plexus. These nerves

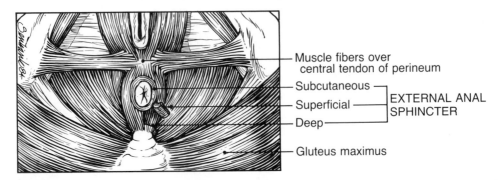

Fig. 1.11 External anal sphincter as viewed with the patient in dorsal lithotomy position. The external anal sphincter is composed of three muscles that arise from the coccyx and converge into the central tendon of the perineum. Midline or mediolateral episiotomy may damage this sphincter; proper reapproximation is essential for fecal continence.

descend from the anterior abdominal wall to supply this region of the perineum.

With the exception of the above-named regions, most of the perineum is supplied by the branches of the pudendal nerve. This nerve is both motor and sensory to the perineum. The posterior two-thirds of the circumanal skin is supplied by the inferior rectal (hemorrhoidal or anal) branches of the pudendal nerve, while the anterior one-third of the perianal skin, most of the vulva, and most of the clitoris are supplied by the labial nerves and dorsal nerve of the clitoris. As significant overlap in distribution occurs with these nerves, one cannot rely on singular nerve block to provide complete anesthesia in this region. Consequently, pudendal block may not always provide the degree of anesthesia desired, as the vulva may well be dually supplied.

The pudendal nerve is the only large nerve in the anal portion of the perineum; it traverses the area, giving off branches (inferior rectal nerves) as it courses toward the urogenital triangle (Fig. 1.13).

These nerves mainly innervate the external anal sphincter. The external anal sphincter may also be innervated by perineal branches of the fourth sacral nerve. The pudendal nerve leaves the pelvis below the piriformis muscle, courses through the buttocks, where it crosses the ischial spine, and then passes through the lesser sciatic foramen. After entering the most posterior and lateral aspect of the perineum, it enters the pudendal canal and is joined by the internal pudendal vessels (Fig. 1.14). The nerve runs within the pudendal canal and quickly gives off the inferior rectal branches, which run medially and anteriorly toward the anal sphincter and perianal skin.

As the pudendal nerve continues beyond the origin of the inferior rectal nerves, it gives origin to the perineal nerve and dorsal nerve to the clitoris. These nerves continue within the pudendal canal in an anterior and medial direction. The perineal nerve then divides into superficial and deep branches just posterior to the posterior border of the urogenital diaphragm. At this point, branches course medially

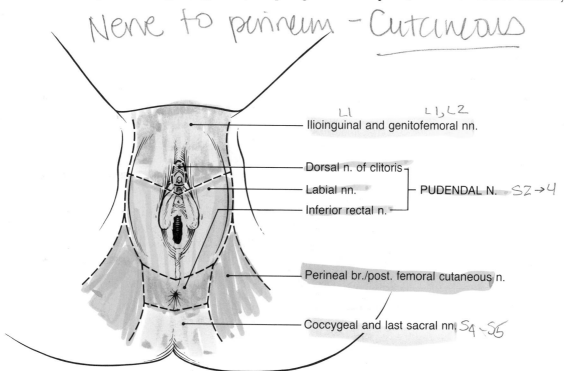

Fig. 1.12 Cutaneous nerve supply to the perineum. While most cutaneous innervation to the perineum comes from the pudendal nerve, important regions are supplied by other sources. Thus pudendal block only anesthetizes a portion of the perineal surface. The exact limits of each specific nerve supply are variable, with significant overlap observed in a number of patients.

across the urogenital diaphragm and form the posterior labial branches, which supply the posterior, lateral, and anteroinferior portions of the vulva (Fig. 1.13). The superficial branches of the labial nerves supply the muscles of the superficial perineal space, while the deep branches supply the musculature of the urogenital diaphragm.

The terminal portion of the pudendal nerve is the dorsal nerve to the clitoris (Fig. 1.14). At the anterior end of the pudendal canal, this nerve pierces the upper surface of the urogenital diaphragm and runs within the deep perineal space. It then penetrates the inferior fascia of the urogenital diaphragm and provides innervation to the clitoris.

Vascular Supply to the Perineum

The internal pudendal artery is the major blood supply to the perineum; its branching pattern mimics that of the pudendal nerve, to which it runs almost parallel. The internal pudendal is the terminal branch of the internal iliac (hypogastric) artery and leaves the

pelvis through the greater sciatic foramen between the piriformis and coccygeal muscles. It accompanies the pudendal nerve across the ischial spine but lies lateral to the nerve and then enters the pudendal canal (Fig. 1.14). Almost immediately, the artery forms the inferior rectal arteries, which, with their corresponding nerves, course through the ischiorectal fossa, supplying the external anal sphincter and perianal skin (Fig. 1.13). After branching into the inferior rectal arteries, the internal pudendal artery gives off a transverse perineal branch that follows the superficial transverse perineal muscle. The artery continues anteriorly, following the pudendal nerve, and divides into posterior labial branches, which supply the muscles of superficial and deep perineal spaces. The artery terminates as the dorsal artery to the clitoris, which enters the perineum through the ischiorectal fossa, penetrating the superior fascia of the urogenital diaphragm and supplying the anterior portion of the sphincter urethrae. It finally pierces the inferior fascia and supplies the clitoris.

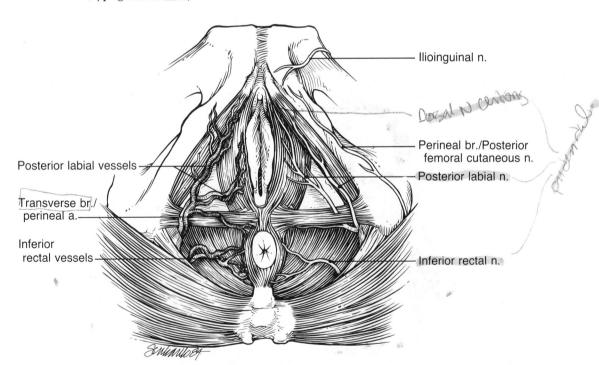

Fig. 1.13 Superficial perineal blood supply and nerves. As viewed with the patient in dorsal lithotomy position, the vessels and nerves to the superficial perineal space follow each other. The vasculature is markedly engorged during pregnancy, and there may be significant bleeding from these vessels because of laceration, trauma, or episiotomy. Note the transverse branch of the perineal artery. This vessel is often encountered during routine midline or mediolateral episiotomy.

∴ all ext genitalia
nn L1-S5 mostly pudendal, some ilioing, genitofem
  p fem cut & coccygeal
a int iliac → pudendal
v int iliac → pudendal   ∵ p clitoral → plexus @ bladder
Anatomy 17

The veins of the perineum follow the divisions of the artery and drain into the internal iliac vein. The only significant exception is the dorsal vein to the clitoris, which passes entirely into the pelvis, joining the vesicle plexus of veins. This anatomic consideration should be included in an evaluation of the spread of malignancy or infection involving the clitoris.

THE INTERNAL GENITAL ORGANS

The pelvic viscera include organs specific to the genital tract as well as a number of organs that are present in both sexes and that represent portions of the urinary and gastrointestinal systems. The organs of the female genital tract include the ovaries, fallopian tubes, uterus and cervix, and vagina. With the exception of the vagina, these organs are superior to the levator ani and are encased in whole or in part by the peritoneum, which is specialized to form specific quasimesenteric structures termed *ligaments*. The organs of the urinary system present within the pelvis include the bladder and lower parts of the ureters as well as a portion of the urethra. Organs representing the gastrointestinal tract include the lower end of the sigmoid colon, rectum, and loops of small intestine (Fig. 1.15).

Ovaries

The ovaries are the female gonads. These two organs are small, flattened, ovoid structures measuring about $4 \times 2 \times 1$ cm. Each ovary is described as having an upper and a lower pole, an anterior and a posterior border, and a medial and a lateral surface. The anterior border is also known as the mesovarian border; it is through this aspect that the vessels and nerves enter and leave the ovaries.

The ovaries are located within the true pelvis, lying against the lateral pelvic wall just inferior to the bifurcation of the common iliac artery. They lie within a fossa termed the ovarian fossa, which is situated in the angle formed by the iliac vessels above, and by a ridge of peritoneum posteriorly, which is formed by the ureter as it passes the bifurcation of the common iliac

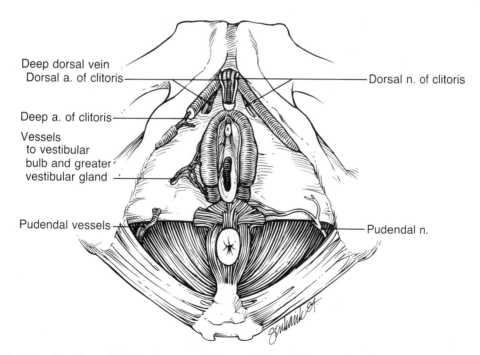

Deep dorsal vein
Dorsal a. of clitoris
Deep a. of clitoris
Vessels to vestibular bulb and greater vestibular gland
Pudendal vessels
Dorsal n. of clitoris
Pudendal n.

Fig. 1.14 Vessels and nerves of the deep perineal space. The vasculature and innervation to the deep perineal space enters the anterior triangle from superior to inferior, in contrast to the superficial perineal space vessels and nerves. Note that the blood supply and innervation to the vestibular bulb and greater vestibular gland (Bartholin's gland) are derived from the deep perineal vessels and nerves.

artery (Fig. 1.15). The ovary lies posterior to a peritoneal reflection termed the broad ligament. The medial surface of the organ is covered in part by the fimbriated end of the fallopian tube.

Each ovary is suspended from the posterior layer of the broad ligament by a peritoneal reflection called the mesovarium. The vascular supply and innervation to the organ course through the mesovarium (Fig. 1.16). The surface of the ovary is covered by a modified peritoneum called the germinal epithelium, which is continuous with the mesovarium. A peritoneal "ligament" that attaches the upper pole of the ovary to the lateral pelvic wall is termed the infundibulopelvic or suspensory ligament of the ovary. The lower pole of the ovary is attached to the lateral wall of the uterus. This attachment is termed the ovarian ligament proper.

The greatest surface of the ovary, the lateral surface, is free and is often in contact with loops of small bowel within the pelvis. During pregnancy, the ovary not only enlarges but also leaves the pelvis as it follows the growing uterus into the upper abdomen. Immediately after parturition, the ovaries may be found at the level of the pelvic brim. They return to the true pelvis by the end of the puerperium.

Fallopian Tubes

The uterine, or fallopian, tubes represent the unfused portion of the paired paramesonephric (müllerian) ducts. Thus the lateral end of each fallopian tube is free and opens into the peritoneal cavity. The medial end of each tube joins with that portion of the paramesonephric duct that fuses to form the uterus, thereby opening into the endometrial cavity. Each tube is divided into four segments that can be distinguished on the basis of luminal diameter and histology. The area of the fallopian tube traversing the myometrium of the uterus and opening into the

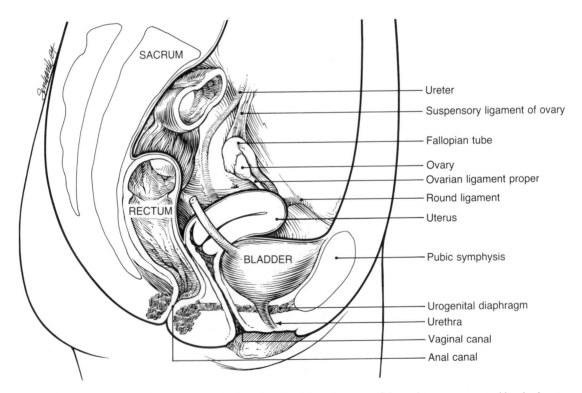

Fig. 1.15 Major organs of the pelvis, sagittal section. The internal organs of the pelvis are supported by the levator ani. Note how the anteverted, anteflexed uterus gains further support from both the urinary bladder and rectum. The ureter crosses the lateral aspect of the uterus at the level of the internal os on its way to the bladder. The actual position of the ovary and fimbriated end of the tube is quite variable.

① ② | ③ ④

①Interstitial ②Isthmic ③ampulla ④fimbria

endometrial cavity is termed the interstitial or intramural portion. This section has a large muscular coat that merges imperceptibly with the adjacent and continuous myometrium. Moving laterally, the next region is termed the isthmus. Here the lumen enlarges and the muscular coat thins. Lateral to the isthmus is the ampulla, which has the widest luminal diameter and in which fertilization occurs. The most lateral end of the fallopian tube is the fimbrial end, a flared or funnel-like opening into the pelvic portion of the peritoneal cavity.

The fallopian tube is attached to the posterior aspect of the broad ligament by its own mesentery, called the mesosalpinx (Fig. 1.16). The mesosalpinx is reflected onto the hilus of the ovary as the mesovarium. Each fallopian tube is approximately 10 cm in length, but the specific location within the pelvis will vary according to the phases of the menstrual cycle, as the fimbriated end of the tube is somewhat free to sweep the posterior aspect of the pelvis "in search" of the ovulated ovum.

Uterus

The uterus is the internal genital organ of nidation, formed by the fusion of the distal regions of both paramesonephric ducts. As such, the uterus is simply a continuation of the embryonic duct system, but it is highly modified by acquiring a substantial smooth

muscle coat and by the development of a highly differentiated and complex mucosa called the endometrium.

The uterus is a highly muscular, thick-walled, pear-shaped organ situated between the bladder and the rectum (Fig. 1.15). It is attached to the lateral pelvic side walls by a highly modified peritoneal mesentery, the broad ligaments, that both helps support the organ and serves as a supportive substrate for the vasculature and nervous innervation to the organ; it also subdivides the pelvis into different compartments. The uterus is slightly flattened in its anteroposterior axis. It opens into the vagina inferiorly and is continuous with the fallopian tubes superiorly. The junction of the uterus with the vagina is termed the cervix.

The uterus is divided into a number of different anatomic regions that serve crucial functions during gestation and parturition (Fig. 1.17). The dome of the uterus is the fundus, which is superior to the ostia of the fallopian tubes. The majority of the uterus is called the body or corpus. It is usually inclined somewhat anteriorly and forward. The junction between the cervix and the corpus is called the isthmus. This section was once termed the internal os, because it is in this region that the histology abruptly changes between the simple columnar, mucus-secreting epithelium of the endocervix to the classic stratified mucosa

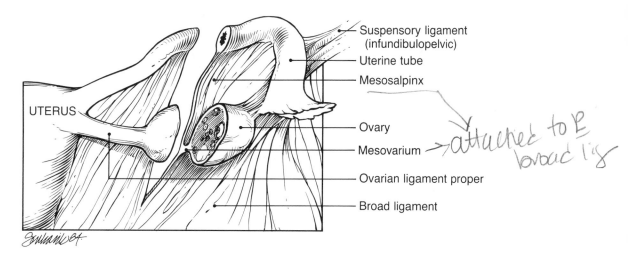

Fig. 1.16 Anatomy of the fallopian tube and ovary, posterior view. Note that the ovary and tube are suspended by mesenteries derived as specialized portions of the broad ligament. It is through the mesovarium and mesosalpinx that the vasculature and nerves enter these respective organs.

Labels on figure:
- Suspensory ligament (infundibulopelvic)
- Uterine tube
- Mesosalpinx
- Ovary
- Mesovarium → attached to broad lig
- Ovarian ligament proper
- Broad ligament
- UTERUS

of the endometrium. In the nonpregnant uterus, the isthmus appears to merge imperceptibly with the cervix; on gross examination, it may be very difficult to observe. During pregnancy, however, specifically beginning around week 12, the isthmus enlarges and is added to the uterine corpus. During labor, this region thins and enlarges substantially and is termed the lower uterine segment. Scars produced by a low transverse cesarean section are no longer apparent following the puerperium, because the lower uterine segment again becomes part of the cervix.

The uterus is covered by peritoneum on its anterior and posterior surfaces. The peritoneum on the posterior aspect of the uterus is carried past the cervix to the upper portion of the vagina, where it is reflected superiorly onto the anterior surface of the rectum. This reflection forms the rectouterine pouch, or pouch of Douglas. This pouch has also been termed the posterior cul-de-sac (Fig. 1.18). The peritoneum along the anterior surface of the uterus is reflected onto the bladder. This reflection forms the vesicouterine pouch, or anterior cul-de-sac, and the reflection begins at about the level of the uterine isthmus.

Thus surgical incision into the lower uterine segment during a cesarean section is actually retroperitoneal and lies inferior to the reflection of the anterior uterine peritoneum, forming the vesicouterine pouch. The connective tissue adjacent to this peritoneal reflection becomes edematous during pregnancy, facilitating dissection at the time of surgery.

The broad ligament, the mesentery that suspends the uterus within the pelvis, is bilaminar, with an anteroposterior layer, covering the uterus, tubes, and a portion of the ovary (Fig. 1.19). The mesosalpinx and mesovarium are only a portion of the broad ligament (see Fig. 1.16). The portion of the broad ligament below the origin of the mesovarium is more accurately termed the mesometrium. The infundibulopelvic or suspensory ligament of the ovary is an extension of this broad ligament; the ovarian ligament proper lies within the anterior and posterior leaves of the broad ligament.

A highly specialized remnant of the gubernaculum of the fetal gonad, the round ligament, is also contained within the leaves of the broad ligament. This ligament attaches to the anterolateral aspect of the

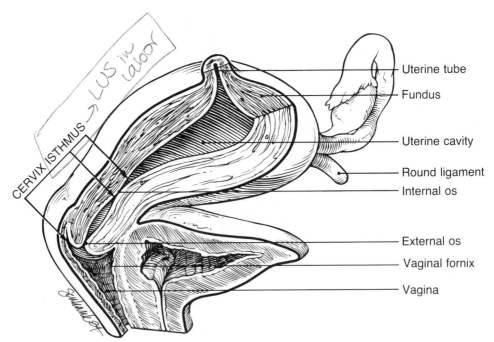

Fig. 1.17 Anatomic regions of the uterus, lateral view. The uterus is composed of cervix, isthmus, corpus, and fundus. The regions of the uterus grow at different rates during pregnancy. Thus the distance from cornual fallopian tube and fundus increases markedly with increasing gestation. Note that the peritoneal reflection of the bladder occurs at the level of the uterine isthmus.

uterus, traverses the broad ligament in its anteroinferior plane, and eventually enters the inguinal canal to insert into the labium majus. The ligament is termed the round ligament (Figs. 1.19 and 1.20). As the round ligament enters the inguinal canal, it may be accompanied by a peritoneal diverticulum termed the processus vaginalis, or canal of Nuck.

At the attachment of the broad ligament to the fundus of the uterus, the anterior and posterior layers are rather closely applied. As the broad ligament courses laterally and inferiorly, the anterior leaf expands forward and the posterior leaf diverges backward. Thus the broad ligament may be considered a quasipyramid with a broad attachment inferiorly. The base of this "triangle" resides near the pelvic floor (Fig. 1.19). Within this interligamentous space are found the uterine vasculature and ureters.

Perivascular connective tissue derived from the lateral pelvic walls lies between the leaves of the broad ligaments and swings medially to attach to the base of the uterus. This connective tissue is thickened at the base of the broad ligament and forms two ligaments known as the uterosacral and cardinal (or lateral cervical) ligaments (Fig. 1.20). The uterosacral ligaments are attached at their anterior ends to the lateral aspect of the cervix. They sweep posteriorly around the rectum and insert into the region of the second, third, and fourth foramina of the sacrum. As such, these ligaments form the rectouterine folds and thus limit the lateral aspect of the rectouterine pouch. The medial aspect of these ligaments is quite distinct, while the lateral aspect of the uterosacral ligaments merges with the cardinal ligaments.

The cardinal ligaments are situated at the base of the broad ligament and represent the condensed perivascular connective tissue anterior to the uterosacral ligaments. Thus this perivascular connective tissue is continuous with the connective tissue of the parametrium, and no distinct differentiation between these two anatomic structures can be noted. It is through their continuity with the superior fascia of the levator ani that the vagina and uterus are attached to the pelvic diaphragm. Many names have been given to these ligaments, including Mackenrodt's ligaments, the transverse cervical ligaments, the lateral pelvic ligaments, the cervicopelvic ligaments, the vascular or hypogastric sheath, and the parametrium.

Certain anatomic relationships involving the cardinal ligaments are of sufficient import to bear mention. The uterine artery is located toward the upper border of the cardinal ligament and runs at a right angle to it. At the point at which the uterine artery

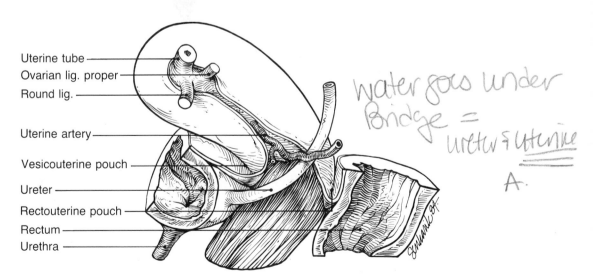

Uterine tube
Ovarian lig. proper
Round lig.

Uterine artery

Vesicouterine pouch

Ureter

Rectouterine pouch

Rectum

Urethra

Fig. 1.18 Anatomic relationships of the uterus, lateral view. The broad ligament contains the uterus and forms an anterior and posterior covering. The triangular space along the lateral uterine wall lies between the leaves of the broad ligament. Note the relationship of the round ligament, tube, and ovarian ligament proper, as well as the relationship of the ureter to the uterine artery.

makes an abrupt medial turn to course into the uterus (Fig. 1.21), the ureter may be found behind and beneath the artery. This relationship is of critical importance during surgical procedures that interrupt or violate the broad ligament in the region of the cardinal ligament. Care must be taken to avoid damaging the ureter at this point. Throughout much of its course within the pelvis, the ureter lies in direct relationship to the cardinal ligament.

Both the levator ani and the ligaments of the uterus have been given credit for providing the major support of the uterus within the pelvis. The uterosacral ligaments have been regarded as holding the cervix back toward the rectum, thereby keeping the uterus in an anteverted position. Their true role in providing support for the uterus is tenuous at best. Similarly, the cardinal ligaments have been vested with the function of uterine support, but because they are anatomically continuous with the superior fascia of the levator ani muscle, it would seem more reasonable to ascribe the major supportive role to the pelvic diaphragm. The normal levator ani forms a relatively flat floor for the pelvis; the weight of the uterus is thus transmitted to the posterior aspect of the levator. As the levator becomes weakened by parturition or other trauma, it becomes more concave. Thus the weight of the uterus is directed more toward the genital hiatus than toward the posterior aspect of the pelvic diaphragm. The resultant shift in weight distribution would cause more and more funneling of the levator and end in uterine and/or vaginal descensus.

Vagina

The vagina is the canal that connects the internal genital duct system with the labia. It extends from the vestibule of the perineum upward and backward to the cervix uteri. That region of the vagina immediately surrounding the cervix as it projects into the

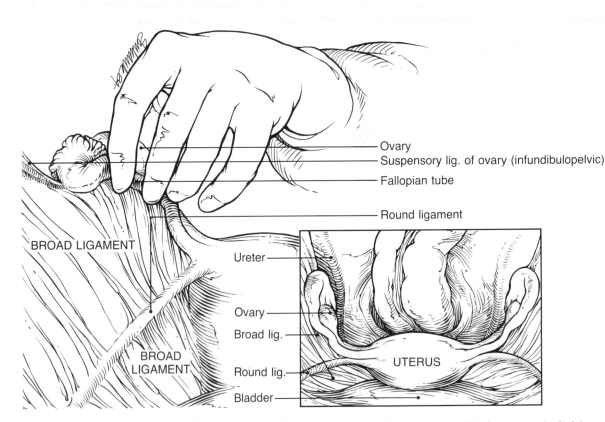

Fig. 1.19 Broad ligament and contained organs, frontal view. The round ligament runs within the anterior leaf of the broad ligament and inserts through the inguinal canal to the labium majus. Inset: The relationships as seen from an anterosuperior perspective. Note the rectovaginal pouch as seen from above and anteriorly.

vagina is considered the vaginal vault, with the anterior and posterior divisions of this space and of the surrounding walls referred to as the vaginal fornices.

The vagina is a fibromuscular tube, the anterior wall of which is in close contact with the posterior surface of the bladder. The posterior vaginal wall is in contact with the anterior wall of the rectum and the rectouterine pouch. The vagina is wider in its uppermost regions, with the lower end being the narrowest. In the empty condition, the anterior and posterior walls of the vagina are normally in contact with each other (Figs. 1.6 and 1.15).

The fascial sheath around the vagina merges with the fascia of the cardinal ligaments. Thus the support of the vagina is largely due to the superior fascia of the levator ani. A thin visceral fascia also surrounds the vagina. This sheath contains the vaginal plexus of veins. Between this visceral sheath and the visceral sheath of the bladder is a relatively loose and essentially bloodless cleavage plane. This plane permits dissection of the vaginal mucosa from the overlying bladder during anterior colporrhaphy. This is not true around the urethra, where these sheaths are firmly fused together; also, because the urethra is attached to the pubic arch, the vagina gains support

from this attachment. Additional support for the vagina is derived from the urogenital diaphragm, through which the vagina traverses.

VASCULAR AND NERVOUS SUPPLY TO THE PELVIS AND PELVIC ORGANS

Major Vessels of the Pelvis

The vascular supply of the pelvis and internal pelvic organs is derived from three sources: the internal iliac, middle sacral, and superior rectal (hemorrhoidal) arteries (Fig. 1.22).

The internal iliac artery, often called the hypogastric artery, is one of the terminal branches of the common iliac artery, it arises approximately at the level of the lumbosacral articulation. It is smaller than the external iliac and lies somewhat medial and posterior to it. The artery passes downward into the pelvis, where it crosses the common, or external, iliac vein. The common iliac vein lies lateral to the internal iliac artery. Of significant import is the relationship of the ureter to this vessel; the ureter lies more superficially, either medial or slightly anterior to the artery.

At about the level of the piriformis muscle, the

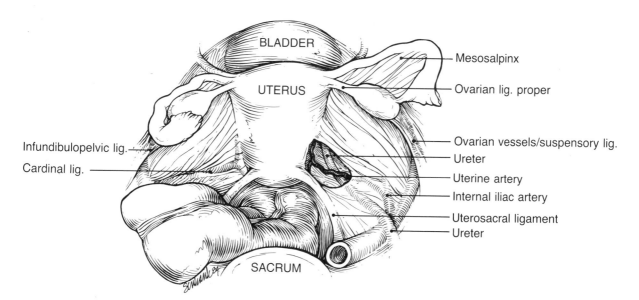

Fig. 1.20 Organs of the pelvis, posterior view. The rectouterine pouch is demarcated by the uterosacral ligaments. This is often termed the posterior cul-de-sac, and its depth is variable from patient to patient. A section of the posterior leaf of the broad ligament has been removed to show the relationship of the uterine artery to the ureter. Intraligamentous tumors, infection, endometriosis, or previous surgery can often alter this relationship.

internal iliac artery divides into anterior and posterior divisions or trunks (Fig. 1.22). This division into anterior and posterior trunks, as well as the further branching of these trunks, can be quite variable. Somewhere between its derivation and the origin of the anterior and posterior trunks, the internal iliac artery will give off a branch to supply the pelvic portion of the ureter lying in relationship to the internal iliac artery.

The posterior trunk of the internal iliac artery gives rise to three major vessels: the iliolumbar, lateral sacral, and superior gluteal arteries (Fig. 1.22). The iliolumbar artery passes superiorly and laterally, deep to the obturator nerve and external iliac vessels, dividing into a lumbar and an iliac branch. The lumbar branch supplies the psoas major and quadratus lumborum muscles. The iliac branch runs across the iliacus muscle and supplies both that muscle and the ilium. The lateral sacral artery supplies contents of the vertebral column. This artery may form two or more branches, more commonly a superior and an inferior branch, which may be found along the ventral surface of the sacrum. The superior gluteal artery is derived most commonly from the posterior trunk. It leaves the pelvis through the greater sciatic foramen above the level of the piriformis, between the lumbosacral trunk and the first sacral nerve or between the first and second sacral nerves. This vessel is somatic in distribution, as are all the branches of the posterior trunk, and supplies the blood flow to the

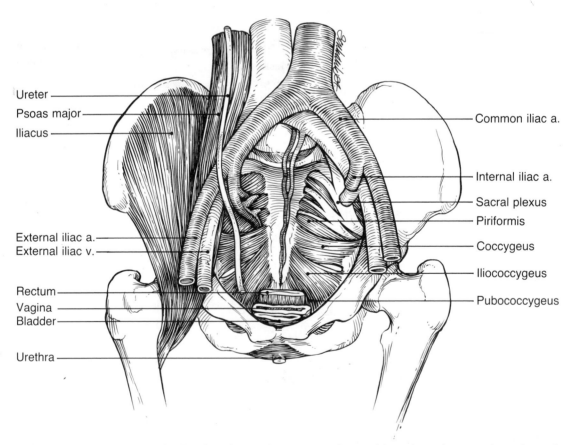

Fig. 1.21 Major vessels of the pelvis, frontal view. The major vasculature of the pelvis is shown in relationship to the pelvic diaphragm. Note the proximity of the ureter to the internal iliac (hypogastric) artery. Ligation of the hypogastric artery may jeopardize the ureter unless care is taken. Note the anterior and posterior trunks of the internal iliac artery.

muscles of the buttocks. Anastomoses between the iliolumbar and superior gluteal vessels are not uncommon.

The anterior trunk of the internal iliac artery is the main visceral vasculature supply to the organs of the pelvis. The pattern of branching of the anterior trunk is so variable that as many as nine different major branching patterns with 49 different subtypes of branchings have been described. The major branches derived from the anterior trunk include the umbilical, vesicle, middle rectal, uterine, vaginal, obturator, internal pudendal, and inferior gluteal arteries (Fig. 1.22). It should be noted that the obturator, internal pudendal, and inferior gluteal vessels are somatic in distribution.

The internal pudendal artery is considered by many to be the terminal branch of the anterior division of the internal iliac artery. It often shares a common origin with the inferior gluteal artery. This branch passes downward along the ventral surface of the sacral plexus and exits the pelvis through the greater sciatic foramen. The internal pudendal is often smaller in caliber than the inferior gluteal artery and lies lateral to it. After leaving the pelvis, the inferior gluteal artery passes between the branches of the sacral plexus, supplying the gluteus maximus muscle, while the internal pudendal artery curves around the sacrospinous ligament (ischial spine), entering the ischiorectal fossa.

The middle sacral artery and vein (Fig. 1.21) are found in the midline of the pelvis. The artery is a direct branch of the aorta and passes down the front

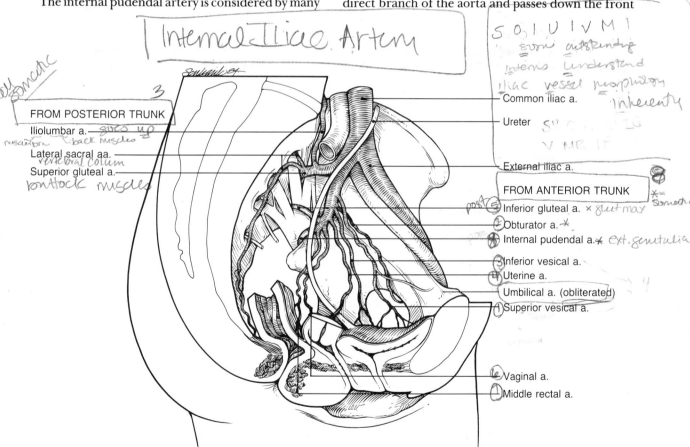

Fig. 1.22 Major vessels of the pelvis, lateral view. The major subdivisions of the anterior and posterior trunks are highly variable, and no singular branching pattern accounts for most patients. Note the relationship of the vessels to the sacral plexus. The uterus has been amputated at the level of the isthmus to permit a better view of the branching patterns of the anterior trunk.

of the sacrum. It anastomoses with branches of the lateral sacral arteries. This vessel is important not only as a source of collateral supply to the pelvis but also because it is easily damaged during such procedures as presacral neurectomy or sacrospinous vault fixation. The remainder of the vasculature will be discussed in relation to the organs supplied.

Blood Supply to the Ovary

The ovary receives a dual blood supply derived from two major vessels, the internal iliac artery and the aorta. The ovarian artery that provides the superior blood supply is a direct branch of the abdominal aorta. This artery descends to the pelvic brim and passes through the infundibulopelvic ligament (suspensory ligament), where it enters the mesovarium (Fig. 1.23). Here the artery anastomoses with the second major blood supply, the ovarian branch of the uterine artery. The ovarian artery becomes markedly enlarged during pregnancy and is thought by some to provide a major supply of blood to the fundus of the gravid uterus. It may also be of significant hemodynamic importance in the blood supply to the placenta. Surrounding each ovarian artery is a complex plexus of veins that drain into the vena cava on the right and into the renal vein on the left. This venous plexus likewise becomes significantly hypertrophied and engorged during pregnancy and is often the site of thrombus formation when intraperitoneal sepsis is present. Care must be exercised when performing a cesarean section or tubal ligation at the time of cesarean section, as these veins are easily torn and can be the source of severe and profuse bleeding. It should also be remembered that the infundibulopelvic ligament is extraperitoneal. Therefore, when large amounts of blood are lost into the infundibulopelvic ligament, hemodynamic compromise can result despite the absence of free intraperitoneal blood.

The ovarian branch of the uterine artery (Fig. 1.23) is the most superior, lateral, and the terminal branch

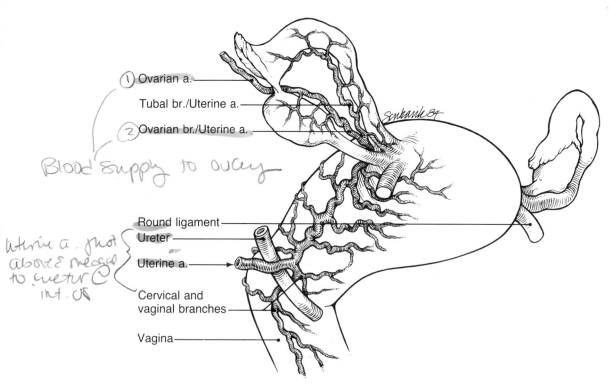

Ovarian a.

Tubal br./Uterine a.

Ovarian br./Uterine a.

Round ligament

Ureter

Uterine a.

Cervical and vaginal branches

Vagina

Fig. 1.23 Blood supply to the uterus, tube, and ovary. The vasculature supply to the major pelvic organs is derived from the internal iliac (uterine) artery and the ovarian artery. Note the anastomotic plexuses of vessels along the lateral aspect of the uterus at the region of the cornu. Descending branches from the uterine artery supply the cervix and vagina.

of the uterine artery. It extends laterally in the broad ligament to reach the mesovarium, where it enters the ovarian hilus and anastomoses with the ovarian artery.

Blood Supply to the Fallopian Tube

The main blood supply to the fallopian tube is derived from the ovarian branch of the uterine artery (Fig. 1.23), called the tubal branch. This branch may actually originate separately from the uterine artery and remain in the upper aspect of the broad ligament (mesosalpinx), where it will supply the tube. Alternatively, it may arise from a common point of origin with the ovarian branch of the uterine artery or from the most proximal end of the ovarian branch. Like the vasculature to the ovary, this artery and its vein become markedly engorged during pregnancy and must be carefully avoided when performing tubal ligation.

Blood Supply to the Uterus

The uterus receives its blood supply from two major vessels: the uterine and ovarian arteries. In the nonpregnant state, the uterine artery is most important, but during pregnancy the vascular supply is derived from both uterine and ovarian arteries.

The origin of the uterine artery off the internal iliac artery is quite variable; for this reason, attempts at isolation and ligation during episodes of life-threatening postpartum hemorrhage are often fruitless if not dangerous. It often appears as an independent vessel from the internal iliac artery but has been described as arising from the inferior gluteal, internal pudendal, umbilical, and obturator arteries.

Once formed, the artery courses medially and anteriorly along the lateral pelvic wall (Fig. 1.23) in very close relationship to the ureter. As it reaches a position just lateral to the internal os of the cervix, the uterine artery makes an abrupt medial turn at the base of the cardinal ligament. At this point, the uterine artery is just in front of and slightly above the ureter (Figs. 1.22 and 1.23). Here the uterine artery will give rise to small branches supplying the ureter.

As the uterine artery approaches the cervix, it bifurcates into major subdivisions: the ascending and descending trunks of the uterine artery. The ascending branch is the largest subdivision; it supplies the body and fundus of the uterus. The descending branch descends and supplies cervical and often vaginal branches. The descending branch may on occasion provide branches to the urinary bladder. As the branches course within the substance of the uterus, the caliber of vessels rapidly diminishes. It is for this reason that incisions in the midline of the myometrium will produce less bleeding than will incisions that transversely incise the smooth muscle.

The uterine vein receives most of the venous effluent from the uterus and vagina and forms a complicated plexus above and below the uterine artery as it enters the uterus. These veins run laterally within the broad ligament to form one or two trunks that drain into the internal iliac vein. The connective tissue around these veins forms a major portion of the cardinal ligament.

Blood Supply to the Vagina

The vagina is supplied by the vaginal artery. This artery is most often a branch of the internal iliac artery, either directly from a common trunk with the uterine artery or directly from the uterine artery itself (Fig. 1.24). It may, however, arise from the internal pudendal artery. Reports of its derivation from the inferior gluteal artery may also be found. This vaginal artery supplies the upper portions of the vagina, while the lower portion of the vagina receives blood through branches from the internal pudendal and middle rectal arteries. These arteries anastomose with the vaginal artery, thus allowing for a collateral blood supply from various visceral and somatic blood vessels (Fig. 1.25).

The above-named vessels anastomose within the vaginal walls, and their anterior and posterior branches may join with each other on the anterior and posterior surfaces of the vagina. These vessels formed by the anastomoses on the anterior and posterior walls form unpaired arteries known as the azygos arteries of the vagina. In addition to the vagina, the vaginal arteries supply the fundus of the bladder and, according to some authorities, are the equivalent of the inferior vesical arteries of the male.

The veins of the vagina form a dense plexus within the walls and along the visceral sheath of the vagina. Blood drains into both the uterine and vesical venous plexuses. The venous drainage below the pelvic diaphragm drains chiefly into the pudendal veins.

Lymphatics of the Pelvis and Pelvic Organs

With a few notable exceptions, most lymphatic drainage from the pelvic viscera drains into the iliac plexus of nodes. The major node association is the internal iliac nodes from which lymph enters the periaortic or lumbar plexus of nodes (Fig. 1.25). The internal iliac nodes are subdivided into various groups, including the gluteal and obturator nodes, but their division is somewhat artificial. Lymphatic drainage directly into the superior rectal nodes or the inguinal nodes may occur as well.

Lymphatic drainage of the ovary and fallopian tube occurs directly into the lymph nodes about the aorta and vena cava, bypassing the iliac cluster of nodes. The lymphatic effluent from the uterus drains predominantly through either the periaortic nodes (fundus and upper body of the uterus) or laterally in the lower portion of the broad ligament to the internal and external iliac nodes along the lateral pelvic

wall (lower part of body). Some of the drainage from the fundus travels along the round ligament through the inguinal canals to end in the superficial inguinal nodes. The lymphatics of the cervix follow those of the vagina.

The lymphatic effluent of the vagina follows two directions. Most lymph drains upward and laterally, emptying into the internal iliac nodes or following the vaginal arteries to these nodes. It has been estimated that 75 to 80 percent of the vaginal effluent follows this course. The lowermost portion of the vagina drains downward to the vulva, thereby entering the superficial inguinal node chain.

Collateral Circulation to the Pelvis

A highly developed architecture for collateral circulation has developed within the pelvis. This collateral circulation is efficient and permits almost instantaneous interruption of a major blood supply without producing significant ischemia.

The visceral branches off the internal iliac arteries anastomose with their counterparts on the opposite

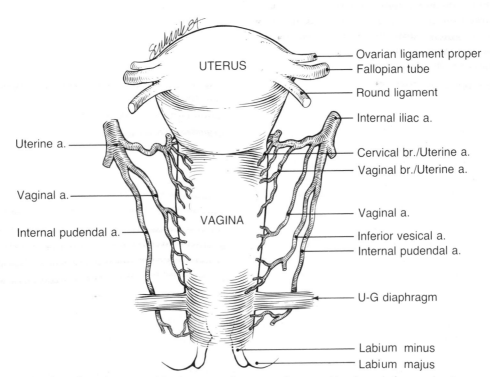

Fig. 1.24 Blood supply to the vagina. Like the uterus, the vagina derives its blood supply from two major sources: the uterine and pudendal arteries. The internal pudendal artery supplies the vagina from inferior to superior. The vaginal artery, often a branch from the uterine artery, and the uterine artery itself supply the superior portion of the vagina.

side, permitting collateral circulation between the two sides of the pelvis. However, such significant collateral circulation exists between the somatic and visceral branches to enable bilateral hypogastric (internal iliac) artery ligation to be carried out without cessation of blood flow to the pelvic organs. These parietal anastomotic bridges include connections between the gluteal arteries and the femoral circumflex arteries, anastomoses between the obturator artery and medial femoral circumflex artery, and anastomoses between iliac and lumbar branches of the iliolumbar artery and lumbar branches from the aorta. Anastomoses between the internal and external pudendal arteries are found in the perineum. Other important anastomoses include connections between the lateral and middle sacral arteries, connections between the middle and superior rectal (hemorrhoidal) vessels, and anastomoses between vessels of the bladder and anterior abdominal wall.

Nerves of the Pelvis

The nerves and their plexuses within the pelvis are found along the lateral pelvic walls. From there they extend to the viscera through the special ligaments of the organs. The major plexuses include the sacral plexus and the pelvic portion of the autonomic plexus. The lumbar plexus is represented by the obturator nerve, which traverses the pelvis to reach the obturator canal. The major nerves of the pelvis are diagrammed in Figure 1.26.

The sacral plexus is formed on the anterior surface of the piriformis muscle; it lies between the muscle

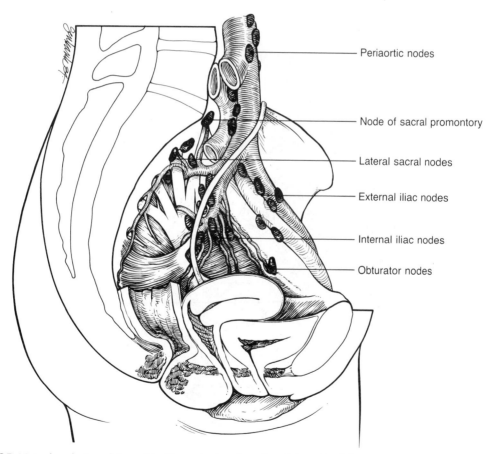

— Periaortic nodes

— Node of sacral promontory

— Lateral sacral nodes

— External iliac nodes

— Internal iliac nodes

— Obturator nodes

Fig. 1.25 Major lymphatics of the pelvis. The major lymph nodes of the pelvis follow the major vessels. Each group of nodes receives contributions from multiple organs. The groupings are somewhat artificial, and no distinct separation of individual node groups is often noted. Knowledge of these node groupings is important when dealing with malignant disease within the pelvis.

and the extraperitoneal pelvic connective tissue, which is often termed the presacral fascia. The uppermost contribution to the sacral plexus is the lumbosacral trunk, which is composed of trunks from L4 and L5. The lumbosacral trunk is joined at the upper edge of the piriformis by the sacral portion of the plexus, which consists of the anterior rami of S1 to 3, and sometimes S4. The major branches of this plexus, which are almost impossible to identify in vivo without extensive dissection, include the superior gluteal nerve and the sciatic, inferior gluteal, posterior femoral cutaneous, and pudendal nerves. The pudendal nerve is considered the most caudal portion of the sacral plexus and represents S2, S3, and S4.

The sympathetic nervous system of the pelvis is derived from three major areas. These contributions include the sacral sympathetic trunks, the superior rectal (hemorrhoidal) plexus, and the hypogastric plexus. The sacral sympathetic trunks represent the continuation of the lumbar sympathetic trunks, which consist of a number of ganglia united by inferiorly and superiorly running fibers. These trunks lie medial to the sacral foramina but frequently communicate with each other across the front of the sacrum and coccyx. Although they may represent an additional afferent pathway that bypasses the superior hypogastric plexus, their functional significance is doubtful.

The superior rectal plexus is a continuation of the inferior mesenteric plexus and probably consists only of sympathetic fibers with connections to the hypogastric nerves. As with the sacral sympathetic plexus, it is not crucial to the pelvic viscera.

The superior hypogastric plexus or presacral nerve

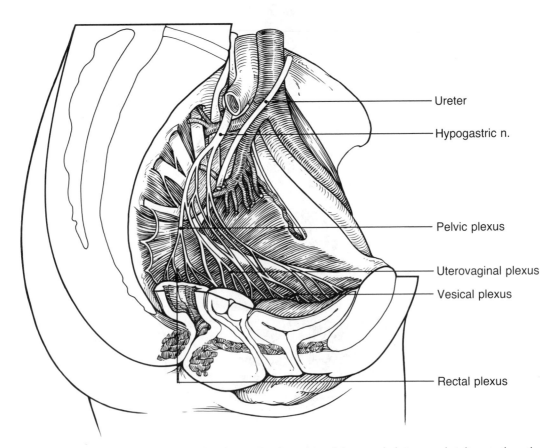

Ureter

Hypogastric n.

Pelvic plexus

Uterovaginal plexus

Vesical plexus

Rectal plexus

Fig. 1.26 Major nerves of the pelvis, lateral view. Few branches of the sacral plexus may be discerned, as these nerves leave the pelvis even as the branches are forming. Most of the pelvic plexus lies medial to the vasculature.

is the unpaired continuation of the lower end of the aortic plexus and is the major continuation of the sympathetic system. Located at about the level of the sacral promontory or slightly below, it divides into two plexuses or trunks that run along the lateral pelvic wall. These paired subdivisions have been termed the hypogastric nerves. Immediately lateral and to the right of the plexus is the right ureter, which traverses the lower aspect of the plexus. The ureter may be accidentally drawn into the operative field during a presacral neurectomy by medial displacement of the peritoneum covering the plexus.

The hypogastric nerves end in the pelvic plexus, an expanded network of fibers and ganglia on each side of the pelvic wall formed by the hypogastric nerves

and pelvic splanchnic nerves. This pelvic plexus has also been termed the inferior hypogastric plexus; it contains sympathetic, parasympathetic, and afferent fibers from the definitive pelvic viscera. This plexus gives off the rectal plexus and then continues forward in the rectouterine fold, giving off the uterovaginal plexus, which courses medially and forward, joining the uterine vessels (Figs. 1.26 and 1.27). The plexus then continues forward and downward, passing along the posterior surface and then the base of the cardinal ligament until it reaches the bladder.

The nervous innervation to the ovary is primarily derived from the abdomen, where branches of the renal plexus and upper part of the aortic plexus are found around the ovarian artery. Thus transsection

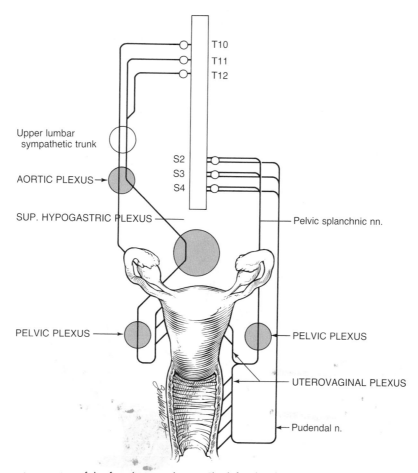

Fig. 1.27 Afferent innervation of the female genital tract. The left side of this diagram demonstrates the sympathetic nervous system. Fibers entering the spinal cord are illustrated on the right. Note that the major afferent pain fibers for the uterus, tubes, and ovaries enter the cord at T10, T11, and T12.

of the infundibulopelvic ligament interrupts the ovarian innervation while permitting the ovary to maintain a vascular supply through the ovarian branch of the uterine artery. Afferent fibers from the ovary enter the spinal cord at T10 (Fig. 1.27).

The nerves to the uterus and vagina form a dense plexus, termed the uterovaginal plexus. It is derived from the pelvic plexus and consists of a mixture of sympathetic and afferent fibers. Parasympathetic fibers may also be represented. The plexus passes medially toward the cervix in the upper part of the cardinal ligament and meshes around the uterine vasculature within the cardinal ligament. This uterine plexus has often been referred to as Frankenhauser's ganglion (Fig. 1.27). At the level of the cervix, the plexus penetrates the walls and accompanies the vessels. A portion of the lowermost region of the plexus is directed toward the vagina and is designated the vaginal plexus.

The afferent supply from the uterine body and fundus travel with the hypogastric nerves and enter the spinal cord at T11 and T12. Pain fibers from the cervix run through the sacral nerves.

While the upper end of the vagina is supplied by simple extension of the uterovaginal plexus, the lower end of the vagina is innervated by the pudendal nerve. The exact line of demarcation between these two distributions is ill defined, but that region of the vagina closer to the perineum sends afferent fibers to S2, S3, and S4.

THE HYPOTHALAMUS AND PITUITARY GLAND

The pituitary gland is a small, ovoid body measuring about $1.5 \times 1 \times 0.75$ cm. Located in the sella turcica of the sphenoid bone, it is covered by a connective tissue sheath that separates it from the bone. The stalk of the pituitary pierces a diaphragm-like fold called the diaphragma sellae and enters the hypothalamus above. The gland is firmly attached to the dura inferiorly and is closely related to the cavernous si-

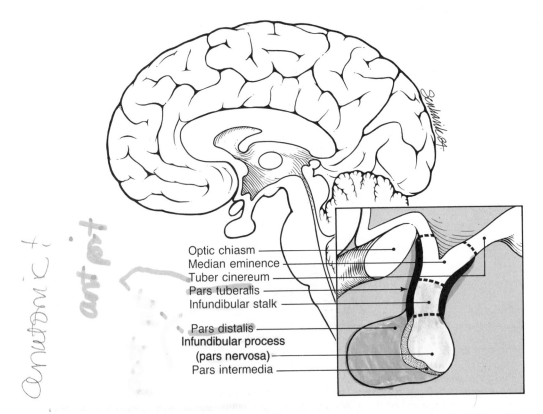

Optic chiasm
Median eminence
Tuber cinereum
Pars tuberalis
Infundibular stalk

Pars distalis
Infundibular process
(pars nervosa)
Pars intermedia

Fig. 1.28 General anatomy of the hypothalamus and the pituitary, sagittal section. Each lobe of the pituitary is responsible for a variety of hormones. The gland enlarges during pregnancy and may infrequently cause visual disturbances attributable to the relationship of the gland to the optic chiasm.

nuses. The weight of the gland is approximately 0.75 to 1.0 g.

The gland is composed of two embryologically distinct entities: the neurohypophysis and the adenohypophysis. It may also be divided into the anterior, the intermediate, and the posterior lobes. The posterior lobe is originally derived from neurectoderm derived from the infundibulum of the hypothalamus. To this is added a contribution from the oral ectoderm of Rathke's pouch, which forms the intermediate lobe, or pars intermedia. Although derived from oral ectoderm, the pars intermedia is anatomically incorporated into the posterior lobe. Thus the divisions of the posterior lobe include the pars nervosa, median eminence, infundibular stalk (all derived from neural ectoderm), and the pars intermedia derived from Rathke's pouch. The anterior lobe is formed exclusively from oral ectoderm and consists of the pars distalis and pars tuberalis (Fig. 1.28).

The terms adenohypophysis and neurohypophysis relate more to the functional relationships of secretory glandular activity than to the true anatomy. Thus the adenohypophysis secretes hormones when stimulated by releasing hormones produced in the hypo-thalamus and transported to the adenohypophysis through a specialized portal blood system. The neurohypophysis contains axons derived from nuclei in the hypothalamus that transport specific hormones to the neurohypophysis. These hormones are stored and released by inhibiting or releasing substances. The neurohypophysis includes the pars nervosa, median eminence, and infundibular stalk. The adenohypophysis includes the pars tuberalis, pars distalis, and pars intermedia.

Blood Supply

The pituitary is supplied by the superior hypophyseal arteries, which arise from the internal carotids and by the inferior hypophyseal arteries, which are also derived from the internal carotids (Fig. 1.29). The superior hypophyseal arteries supply the anterior lobe by way of a hypophyseal portal system. The inferior hypophyseal arteries serve mainly as the blood supply to the neurohypophysis.

Although there are several superior hypophyseal arteries, two main vessels can usually be identified on each side. These vessels are known as the anterior and posterior branches of the superior hypophyseal ar-

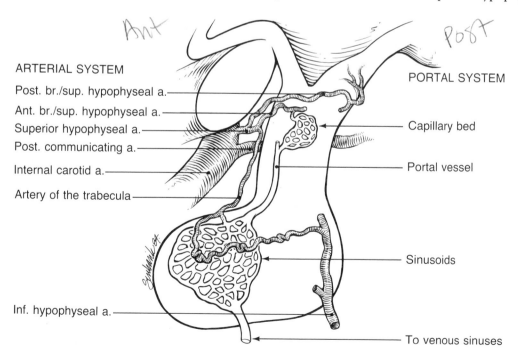

ARTERIAL SYSTEM

Post. br./sup. hypophyseal a.

Ant. br./sup. hypophyseal a.

Superior hypophyseal a.

Post. communicating a.

Internal carotid a.

Artery of the trabecula

Inf. hypophyseal a.

PORTAL SYSTEM

Capillary bed

Portal vessel

Sinusoids

To venous sinuses

Fig. 1.29 Blood supply to the pituitary and hypothalamus. The pituitary blood supply is derived from the internal carotid. A highly specialized portal system supplies the anterior and middle lobes of the pituitary. These eventually drain to the venous sinuses. The interposition of two capillary beds before deposition of blood in the venous sinuses makes this the hypophyseal–pituitary portal bed.

teries. The anterior branch of the superior hypophyseal artery enters the anterior portion of the infundibular stalk, while the posterior branch enters the posterior portion of the stalk. Within the infundibular stalk, arborizations from both vessels ascend to supply the median eminence. Other vessels from the anterior branch of the superior hypophyseal arteries descend in front of the neural stalk and enter the anterior lobe. These vessels are termed lobar or trabecular arteries. These arteries then form a characteristic pattern of looped sinusoidal capillaries that drain into venules. The venules in turn unite to form long descending veins, which lead to a second series of capillaries in the pars distalis. This hypophyseal portal system establishes a pathway that permits neurosecretory material released from the nuclei around the median eminence to pass into the pars distalis.

The posterior or neural lobe receives its blood supply from the inferior hypophyseal arteries, which form an arterial circle near the junction of the anterior and posterior lobes. Interlobar arteries that anastomose with branches of the superior hypophyseal arteries may be found in this region. The arterioles then form a capillary network that receives the neurosecretory product conveyed to the neural lobe from the hypothalamus.

Innervation of the Pituitary

Innervation to the pituitary consists chiefly of the hypothalamohypophyseal tracts (Fig. 1.30). These tracts are bundles of nonmyelinated nerve fibers that extend into the neurohypophysis from two major nuclei of the hypothalamus: the supraoptic and paraventricular nuclei. These tracts carry neurosecretory substances to the cells of the posterior lobe. The adenohypophysis is devoid of innervation other than vasomotor fibers that accompany the vasculature.

The secretory substances released into the bloodstream of the neurohypophysis are produced in the cell bodies of the neurons residing in the supraoptic and paraventricular nuclei of the hypothalamus. Most of these fibers terminate in the neural lobe, although a few do terminate in the pars tuberalis and pars intermedia. Neurosecretory products are stored in the pars nervosa. When released, these hormones pass through specialized, highly fenestrated capillary walls to enter the lumina of the capillaries. If the stalk of the pituitary is experimentally transected, large amounts of neurosecretory product will accumulate in the axons of the cells proximal to the incision.

ANATOMIC ADAPTATIONS DURING AGING AND PREGNANCY

The female genital tract undergoes considerable change during pregnancy and the puerperium. These changes indicate that these organs are highly plastic in their anatomic structure and can adapt to both chronic and acute stimuli with remarkable ease. Anatomic changes that occur during aging and pregnancy underscore the fact that these are target organs for the sex steroids and that much of their adaptation can be directly attributed to the changing hormonal milieu associated with puberty, pregnancy, and menopause.

Uterus

The uterus is a target organ for estrogen and progesterone; both steroid hormones play a decisive role in the remodeling that occurs during the different phases of the woman's life. Because the uterus is composed predominantly of smooth muscle and the myometrial cell contains both estrogen and progesterone receptors, it is not surprising that the anatomy as well as the physiology of the uterus will change depending on the hormonal status of the woman.

At birth, the uterus is composed of a relatively large cervix in comparison with the corpus and fundus. With the advent of the hormonal changes of puberty, the rising levels of estradiol initiate considerable growth and enlargement in the myometrial smooth muscle cells of the corpus and fundus. Although growth of the cervix occurs as well, it is outstripped by the growth of the corpus and fundus, with the resultant uterine change being a markedly lower cervix to corpus ratio. Before puberty, the cervix occupies approximately 66 percent of the total uterine mass; after puberty and with the menarche, the cervix and corpus–fundus are approximately equal in size. This differential response in two seemingly identical smooth muscle cell populations is not unexpected, because the estrogen receptor of the cervix does not appear to be modulated with the same degree of sensitivity as are the steroid receptors of the corporeal and fundal myometrium. Should the woman become

At puberty Cx = 66% size of uterus, Cx has fewer well developed
E₂ ∴ doesn't grow as much as uterus does. c̄ menarche;
∂ partum (p̄ puerperium) ut = 67% size of uterus, Cx ↓ to 33%)

Anatomy **35**

pregnant and subsequently parous, the nonpregnant parous uterus actually shows a reversal of the cervix to corpus ratio seen at birth. In this instance, the corpus–fundus accounts for two-thirds of the uterine size, while the cervix is reduced to approximately one-third the total uterine mass (Fig. 1.31).

The nonpregnant parous uterus weighs approximately 70 g. During pregnancy, both hypertrophy and hyperplasia of the myometrial smooth muscle occur. This is due not only to the action of the steroid hormones but also to the marked distention of the uterus with the developing fetus. The body of the uterus at term weighs approximately 1,100 g, which represents an almost 20-fold increase in mass. Similarly, the individual myometrial cell, through cellular hypertrophy, enlarges almost 100-fold to approximately 500 μm in length at term.

Not only does the myometrium itself increase in cellular density and size during pregnancy, but there is a concomitant increase in the collagenous connective tissue and intercellular ground substance. Blood vessels, lymphatics, and nerves increase in number, length, and size; these changes occur as early as the first trimester.

During the first few months of pregnancy, the thickness of the myometrium in the corpus and fundus actually increases. However, the increased distention of the uterine cavity, because of the growing fetus, placenta, and amniotic fluid, causes the uterine wall to become remarkably thin by term. This thinning should not be confused with the softening that occurs because of the increasing levels of progesterone.

While the changes in the uterine cervix are not as dramatic as those of the uterine corpus and fundus, they are nevertheless highly significant. It is known that the cervix is composed primarily of collagenous connective tissue with a relatively small amount of

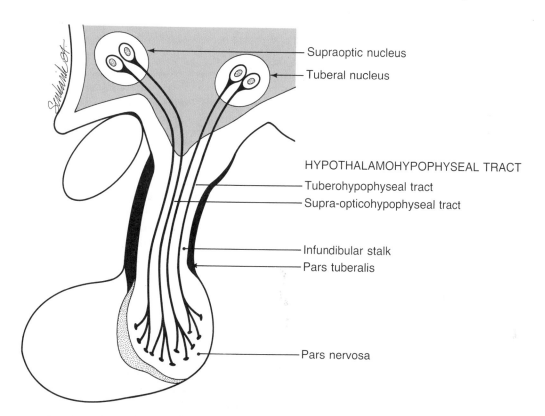

Fig. 1.30 Nerve pathways within the hypothalamus and pituitary. The major nerve tracts consist of the hypothalamo-hypophyseal tracts. These are derived from the supraoptic and tuberal nuclei and descend to the posterior lobe through the tuberohypophyseal and supraopticohypophyseal tracts.

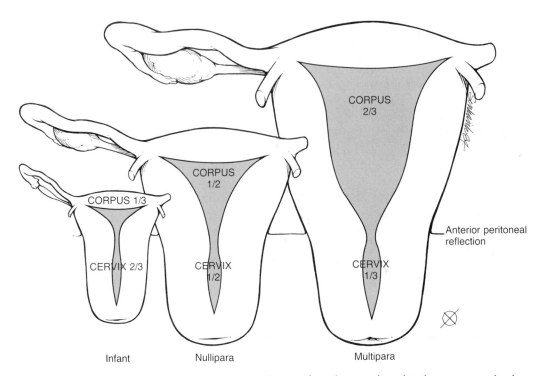

Fig. 1.31 Changes in the uterus with age. As the young girl moves from the prepubertal to the postmenarcheal state, and after she becomes parous, marked changes occur in the ratio of the different regions of the uterus. Growth occurs primarily in the corpus and the fundus, although the cervix continues to grow as well. After menopause, the uterus regresses to a state more closely allied to that of the premenarcheal anatomy.

smooth muscle. Significant biochemical changes occur in the connective tissue that result in increased water content (see Ch. 6). This combined with a significant increase in vascularity accounts for the softening and cyanosis that characterize the cervix of the gravid woman. The endocervical glands, under the influence of progesterone, secrete a thickened mucus that forms a cervical plug. Other changes in endocervical glandular histology include a relative basal cell hyperplasia caused by the increased levels of circulating estrogen. This is an interesting observation, considering the fact that, unlike the myometrium, whose estrogen and progesterone receptors modulate with fluctuating levels of estradiol and progesterone, the steroid receptors of the cervix do not appear to change substantially in either quantity or distribution.

The changes in the anatomic regions of the uterus

bear repetition here. During the antenatal period, a rather striking change occurs in the uterine wall, which becomes more pronounced during labor. Before the advent of pregnancy, the uterine isthmus is a small almost nonexistent region of the uterus that lies between the cervix and the corpus. Under the influence of the steroid hormones of pregnancy and the distention of the growing products of conception, this isthmic region becomes demarcated from the cervix inferiorly and from the corpus superiorly (Fig. 1.32). As pregnancy progresses, the isthmus becomes increasingly prominent, with a thinner and thinner wall. This development of the isthmus culminates during labor and is known as the lower uterine segment. This segment is very thin and contains little smooth muscle. As such, its contractility is markedly different from that of the corpus or fundus. Immediately after delivery, this stretched and thinned isth-

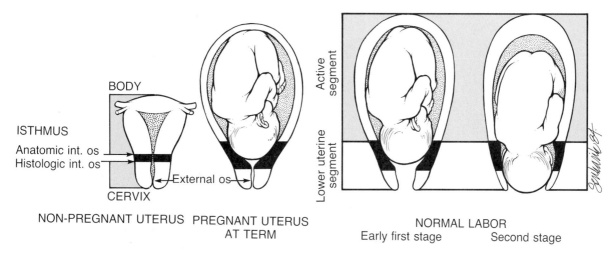

ISTHMUS
BODY
Anatomic int. os
Histologic int. os
External os
CERVIX

Active segment
Lower uterine segment

NON-PREGNANT UTERUS   PREGNANT UTERUS
AT TERM

NORMAL LABOR
Early first stage   Second stage

Fig. 1.32 Changes in the uterus caused by pregnancy and parturition. The hormonal changes of pregnancy as well as the dynamic forces of labor cause the development of the lower uterine segment from the vestigial uterine isthmus. After parturition, these changes regress dramatically. Low transverse cesarean section incisions are performed through this thinned isthmic region, known as the lower uterine segment.

mus appears as a floppy region of myometrium immediately superior to the internal cervical os. By the end of the puerperium, the isthmus has become reincorporated into the cervical–corpus junction and is no longer visible.

SUGGESTED READINGS

Embryology

Sadler TW: Langman's Medical Embryology. 5th Ed. Williams & Wilkins, Baltimore, 1985

Gross Anatomy

Gardner E, Gray DJ, O'Rahilly R: 3rd Ed. WB Saunders, Philadelphia, 1969

Grant JCB: An Atlas of Anatomy. 6th Ed. Williams & Wilkins, Baltimore, 1972

Hamilton WJ: Textbook of Human Anatomy. CV Mosby, St Louis, 1976

Hollinshead WH: Anatomy for Surgeons. 3rd Ed. Vol. 3. Harper & Row, New York, 1985

Snell RS: Clinical Anatomy for Medical Students. 2nd Ed. Little, Brown, Boston, 1981

Warwick R, Williams PL: Gray's Anatomy. WB Saunders, Philadelphia, 1973

Histology

Copenhaver WM, Bunge RP, Bunge MB: Bailey's Textbook of Histology. Williams & Wilkins, Baltimore, 1971

Weiss L, Greep RO: Histology. 4th Ed. McGraw-Hill, New York, 1977

Chapter 2

The Placenta

Tim H. Parmley II

ORIGIN OF THE TROPHOECTODERM

The placenta is derived, in part, from the surface epithelium of the blastocyst, the trophoectoderm.[1,2] This tissue has its origin in the phenomenon of compaction, which takes place at the eight-cell stage in the cleaving morula. At the beginning of the eight-cell stage, all the blastomeres are spherical. Although a portion of each is a part of the surface of the morula, each blastomere lacks any internal or surface asymmetry that suggests basal, apical, or lateral polarization. Before the eight-cell stage ends, however, the blastomeres flatten against each other so that each cell increases its area of contact with its neighbors. That portion of each blastomere that is most distant from the surface of the morula differentiates into a basal-type surface and forms intercellular junctions with adjacent blastomeres. That portion of each blastomere on the surface of the morula differentiates into an apical surface with microvilli. The lateral surfaces of each cell also form intercellular junctions. The internal organization of each blastomere mirrors these external changes, and before the onset of cleavage each cell has become a typical epithelial cell with basal–apical polarization.

Subsequent cleavage results in one of three outcomes for a cell. If both daughter cells have an area of contact with the surface, they will polarize and differentiate into epithelium–trophoectoderm. If one or both of them do not possess surface contact but are totally surrounded by other cells, then that cell becomes a portion of the inner cell mass and does not achieve epithelial differentiation. Thus the morula is divided into two cell populations—the surface epithelium or trophoectoderm and the inner cell mass.

IMPLANTATION

After the formation of the blastocyst and loss of the zona pellucida, the blastocyst expands. This is associated with flattening of the surface epithelium, which becomes mesothelial. However, as soon as implantation occurs, those trophoblastic cells in contact with endometrium become cuboidal—the cytotrophoblast. As the blastocyst becomes buried, the cytotrophoblast eventually surrounds the entire structure. However, the cytotrophoblast ceases to be in contact with the endometrium, because it produces a multinucleated syncytium, the syncytiotrophoblast, as an integral part of the implanting and invading mechanism. This syncytium thus lies between the cytotrophoblast and the maternal tissues (Fig. 2.1). The cells of the syncytium are markedly vacuolated, and, possibly through the coalescence of these vacuoles, the syncytium comes to contain an internal labyrinth of communicating lacunar spaces (Fig. 2.2). Mitotic figures are confined to the cytotrophoblast. Thus the

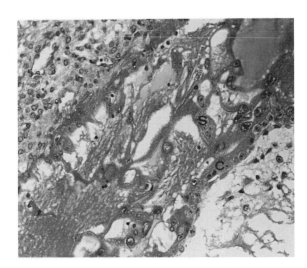

Fig. 2.1 A single cell layer of cytotrophoblast separates the extraembryonic mesoderm (lower right) from the syncytium (center). Maternal tissue is shown in the upper left-hand corner. Lacunar spaces within the syncytium are filled with maternal blood.

cytotrophoblast acts as a germinal epithelial layer to the overlying syncytiotrophoblastic epithelium. It is, however, an oversimplification to look at the cytotrophoblast as a germinal layer producing only syncytium. As will become apparent in this chapter, there are several different forms of trophoblast, and all of them seem to develop from the cytotrophoblast. Thus there is much more heterogeneity in the population of cells that result from cytotrophoblastic proliferation than is generally appreciated. Trophoblastic cells in the basal plate contain more human placental lactogen (hPL) and less human chorionic gonadotropin (hCG) than trophoblastic cells on the exchange surfaces of the placenta.[3] Also the trophoblast of the chorion laeve lacks some hormones produced by trophoblastic cells in the basal plate.[4]

The syncytium appears to burrow into the endometrium, altering both the local and the generalized decidual reaction. The latter alteration, termed *gestational hyperplasia* by Hertig,[5] consists of the persistence of glandular secretion and generalized edema in association with the developing decidua. In the cycling endometrium, Noyes et al.[6] described a sequence of peak secretion on days 20 and 21, peak edema on day 22, and peak decidua on day 27. Hertig[5] thought that if implantation occurred, secretion

and edema reappeared after day 24 and were present subsequently with peak decidualization. More locally, the implantation produces an increase in the amount of edema and pushes glands that are at the edge of the site laterally so that they deviate away from the base of the conceptus.

Capillaries and glands in the direct path of the invading trophoblast are entered (Fig. 2.2). No information is available about the nature of the fluid flows that result in the early implantation, but, on the basis of histologic considerations, it seems that both glandular secretion and maternal capillary blood enter the labyrinth of lacunar spaces in the syncytium, passively circulate, and then escape into the outflow limb of the same capillaries.[7] No pulsatile circulation exists. By and large these capillaries are entered by the syncytium so that the blood flow into and out of the labyrinth occurs without free hemorrhage; however, occasionally some blood is lost into adjacent gland lumina around the periphery of the implantation site. This phenomenon may account for so-called implantation bleeding. Variation in this process may also be responsible for many first-trimester abortions. The fluid accumulation beneath and around the early implantation that has been noted to precede some abor-

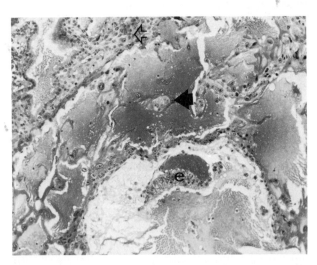

Fig. 2.2 A bilaminar embryo sits within the blastocystic space (mid-bottom). Maternal tissue is shown in the upper left-hand corner. A maternal capillary has been entered by the trophoblast (open arrow). A few cytotrophoblastic cells are beginning to proliferate within the syncytium above the chorionic membrane (closed arrow).

tions may be blood collections that separate trophoblast and decidua.[8]

DEVELOPMENT OF THE CYTOTROPHOBLASTIC SHELL

Soon the inner cell mass is separated from the internal surface of the cytotrophoblast by the development of an extraembryonic mesoderm that lines the entire inner surface of the blastocyst. Thus a chorionic membrane consisting of mesoderm and trophoblast surrounds the entire conceptus. During the last 2 or 3 days of the second week and the first few days of the third week of embryonic life, remarkable differentiation will take place in this chorionic membrane. The cytotrophoblast focally proliferates and forms columns of trophoblast, which, accompanied by the underlying extraembryonic mesoderm, protrude into the area of the syncytium, resulting in radial columns that project out from the blastocyst (Fig. 2.3). Initially, these columns consist only of cytotrophoblast. Shortly after their formation they are supported by the underlying mesoderm, and subsequently they develop vasculature. They eventually extend through the entire thickness of the syncytial labyrinth and reach the maternal tissue. At this point they become anchoring villi.

The proliferating cytotrophoblast on the tip of these anchoring villi extends entirely through the syncytium and comes into direct contact with the maternal tissues. It then extends laterally from the tip of each villus and, by joining that from adjacent villi, forms a continuous shell around the entire conceptus — the cytotrophoblastic shell (Figs. 2.3 and 2.4). Now, instead of syncytium, it is cytotrophoblast that is in direct contact with the maternal tissues. It should be noted that while cytotrophoblastic shell is the term that has been used to describe this proliferation, the cells are in fact a type of differentiated trophoblast that forms a portion of the basal plate and possibly the trophoblast of the chorion laeve. The contact between maternal tissues and the cytotrophoblastic shell becomes less direct as a layer of fibrinoid, Nitabuch's layer, is deposited between the shell and the maternal tissues. A layer of necrosis develops in the decidua beneath the implantation site. This necrosis is physiologic. Contained within the cytotrophoblastic shell are isolated giant cells that appear to

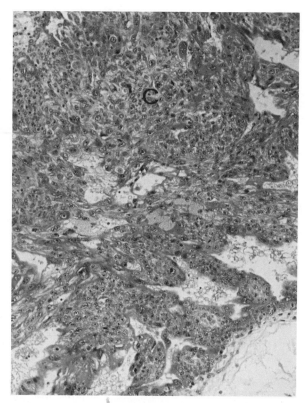

Fig. 2.3 The cytotrophoblast extends all the way from the chorionic membrane (lower right) through the syncytial layer to coalesce into a cytotrophoblastic shell (upper left).

represent in situ differentiation of some of the cytotrophoblastic cells. These are an example of a differentiated form of trophoblast that develops from the cytotrophoblast. Additionally, ultrastructural studies suggest that the cytotrophoblast of the shell is more differentiated than the layer of cytotrophoblast immediately adjacent to the villus stroma.[7] Only the most basal cells of the chorionic epithelium continue to lack differentiation. Both mononuclear and multinuclear cells of the shell contain hPL.[3]

Both glands and veins continue to communicate with the internal labyrinth through clefts in the cytotrophoblastic shell. The internal labyrinth is now properly called an intervillous space. Coiled arteries may be seen to open into the clefts in the cytotrophoblastic shell in the fourth week of embryonic life. According to Hamilton and Boyd,[7] the orifice of these arteries is nearly always partially obstructed by cytotrophoblast in the lumen of the vessel.

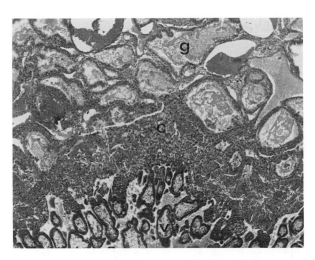

Fig. 2.4 Maternal hypersecretory glands (top). Immediately beneath them the cytotrophoblastic shell forms an arch over the intervillous space. The villi now contain a mesodermal core and scattered capillaries.

EXTRAPLACENTAL TROPHOBLAST

Isolated trophoblastic cells, again intermediate trophoblastic cells, also infiltrate the maternal tissues beyond the cytotrophoblastic shell. This infiltration takes at least two forms. In the first, the cytotrophoblastic cells invade the walls of the spiral arterioles that approach the cytotrophoblastic shell (Fig. 2.5). This results in the destruction of these walls and their replacement by a fibrinoid material, which presumably explains the inability of the terminal portion of the spiral arterioles serving the placental bed to respond to maternal "fight or flight."[9] Obviously, this is adaptive, as the physiologic response would be to constrict the spiral arterioles, thus shunting intervillous space blood flow to the skeletal muscle. Distressingly, cytotrophoblast also behaves this way at ectopic implantation sites. One assumes that this behavior is exhibited by a specific subpopulation of trophoblastic cells that are an additional form of mature trophoblast derived from undifferentiated cytotrophoblast. Failure of the trophoblast to invade the spiral arterioles properly has been suggested to be the primary cause of toxemia.[10]

The destruction of the walls of the spiral arterioles by trophoblast has histologic consequences that persist for at least months after the cessation of preg-

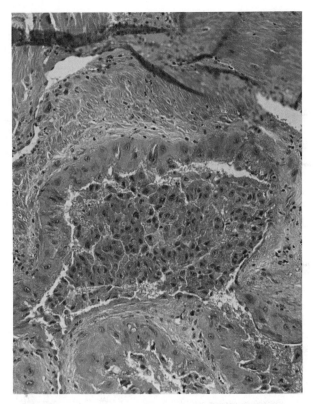

Fig. 2.5 Trophoblastic cells have infiltrated the wall of this spiral arteriole and occupy its lumen.

nancy. At first the trophoblastic cells are readily apparent, but gradually they die and become ghost cells embedded in fibrinoid. By the time the pregnancy has concluded, the spiral arterioles may have dense hyaline walls. Moreover, this change may extend into the myometrium such that large coiled vessels consisting only of hyaline may be seen beneath an old implantation site in either the endometrium or myometrium, occasionally being the only clue to a preceding pregnancy.

Another manifestation of trophoblastic cell infiltration is seen in the maternal decidua and myometrium, immediately beneath the implantation site. These tissues become infiltrated with cells that after maturation are isolated trophoblastic giant cells (Fig. 2.6). There is little destruction of maternal tissue. This infiltrative picture has given rise to the term syncytial endometritis (or myometritis). These cells are also intermediate trophoblastic cells and contain

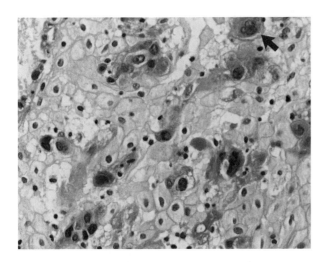

Fig. 2.6 Mononuclear and multinuclear trophoblastic cells infiltrated the decidua beneath this implantation site.

hPL and other hormones.[3] The biologic function of this maternal invasion is unknown, but if viable trophoblast is required to maintain pregnancy, the local production of hPL and progesterone by this population of trophoblast cells may promote local uterine quiescence at the site of placental attachment. Cells in this population also produce placental-type growth hormone, suggesting additional physiologic functions.[4]

Occasionally, the process of maternal infiltration is so spectacular that a gross tumor, termed a placental site tumor, forms. Rarely does this lesion demonstrate a malignant course.[11] It is possible to distinguish placental site tumor from choriocarcinoma on the basis of the former presumably being monocellular in character. Each cell remains distinct and separate even when multinucleated, rather than forming a syncytium, and there is minimal nuclear atypia. If syncytiotrophoblast is present, the diagnosis of choriocarcinoma should be suspected.

Therefore, the result of development up to this point is that the conceptus is completely surrounded by the cytotrophoblastic shell and by Nitabuch's layer, and beyond Nitabuch's layer isolated trophoblastic cells have infiltrated the implantation site. The outer layer of the trophoblastic shell is continuous along the anchoring villi, with the inner layer of cytotrophoblast that immediately surrounds the concep-

tus, and is in contact with the extraembryonic mesoderm. Between the inner and outer layers of cytotrophoblast is the intervillous space lined by syncytiotrophoblast. The anchoring villi contain extraembryonic mesoderm which during the fourth week of embryonic life will develop vasculature that subsequently contains nucleated fetal red cells.

DEVELOPMENT OF THE CHORION FRONDOSUM

Further development of the chorionic membrane depends on whether it maintains contact with the maternal tissue. Initially, the implanting blastocyst burrows into the endometrium and becomes entirely buried beneath the endometrial surface, and all of the chorionic membrane is in contact with maternal tissue and thus maternal blood supply. However, the conceptus secondarily bulges above the endometrial surface again as growth takes place. Eventually, most of the conceptus lies above the surface of the endometrium. Presumably that portion receiving no blood supply becomes the chorion laeve. Only minor villous projections are left over it by the third month of gestation. No vasculature develops in the mesoderm of the chorion laeve, but the trophoblast does engage in growth to produce a population of both mononuclear and multinuclear cells that forms a layer of trophoblast covering the external surface of the bulging membranous sack. As the conceptus grows and the endometrial cavity is obliterated by the apposition of the chorion laeve and the maternal endometrium, this trophoblastic cell layer lies in direct apposition to the maternal decidua. The layer remains hormonally active, producing, among other things, progesterone.

Meanwhile, that portion of the chorionic membrane that remains attached to the endometrium becomes the placental "cake." It is possible that malformations of the placenta, such as succenturiate lobes, are the result of additional blood supply obtained from adjacent surfaces. Torpin[12] has shown that in succenturiate or accessory lobes the placental implantation site is such as to suggest that a portion of the surface of the chorionic membrane, in addition to that at the primary implantation site, probably came into immediate contact with the endometrium, thus promptly achieving a blood supply.

The growth of the placental cake consists of the

extension of the cytotrophoblastic shell and the proliferation of more and more complex branching villi
in the intervillous space. The cytotrophoblastic shell
not only expands laterally, but also penetrates deeper
and deeper into the maternal tissues. As it does so, the
shell penetrates the maternal tissues more extensively
between the anchoring villi than at the site of these
villi. The result is that the growing placenta forms
projecting lobes between anchoring villi. The anchoring villi become septae as the maternal tissue is
excavated elsewhere by the lobes. That is, septae do
not specifically develop, but rather are simply the
column of maternal tissue remaining when the decidua between the septae is excavated by the expanding placental lobes. According to Hamilton and
Boyd,[7] 10 to 38 placental lobes result from this process. These do not correspond, however, to the presumed functional units, the cotyledons. Where the
anchoring villi attach to the septae, the cytotrophoblastic shell persists as a thick layer, but it is markedly
thinned to absent elsewhere. The cells in the remaining shell are an intermediate-type trophoblast containing hPL and placental-type growth hormone.

The fetal cotyledons, or trunci chorii, arise from
the fetal side of the intervillous space. Initially, only
sprouts of syncytium project into the intervillous
space from the lining syncytium, but soon the cytotrophoblast begins to proliferate, resulting in a projection from the chorion into the intervillous space.
Soon this cytotrophoblastic projection has a mesodermal core. The trunci chorii thus formed may split
many times as they grow toward the maternal side of
the intervillous space. Although there is debate about
the details, villous growth is oriented with respect to
the maternal arterioles, and villi also penetrate into
the venous orifices (Fig. 2.7).[13] Although estimates
vary, there are several hundred of these structures
around the entire conceptus initially but only about
50 in the term placenta, albeit with large variation
among individuals.

Total placental growth, which is initially very rapid,
decreases after mid-gestation and becomes hard to
detect at term; however, there is much controversy
about both the absolute nature and the significance
of these changes. Data of Teasdale[14] suggest absence
of placental growth after 36 weeks in the functionally
important parts of the placenta, confirming DNA results of Winnick et al.[15] but these observations in the

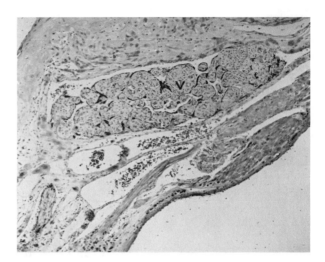

Fig. 2.7 Villi extending into a maternal vein within the decidua
beneath the implantation site.

face of ongoing fetal growth after 36 weeks suggest
that other factors are also at work.

IMPLANTATION ANOMALIES

A variety of placental abnormalities may result from
variation in the developmental process just described. Torpin[12] has suggested that placentas marginata and circumvallata occur with increasing degrees of deep initial implantation. An hourglass-like
structure results when the placenta enlarges beneath
the endometrial surface, and the sac containing the
embryo enlarges above it. The endometrium that
forms the waist between these two bulges is compressed between them as the pregnancy grows and is
obliterated, leaving only an acellular membrane.
These malformations are only significant when they
are extensive enough to result in reduced vascular
supply.

Implantation in which the inner cell mass is not
immediately adjacent to the endometrium may give
rise to twinning or to velamentous insertion. Hsu[16]
has produced evidence in mice showing that, when
the inner cell mass is opposite the implantation pole
of the blastocyst, the mass splits and twinning results.
On the other hand, if the mass is not immediately
adjacent to the implantation pole but near it, only a
singleton results. In either case, it is the blood supply
that determines where the placenta persists and thus

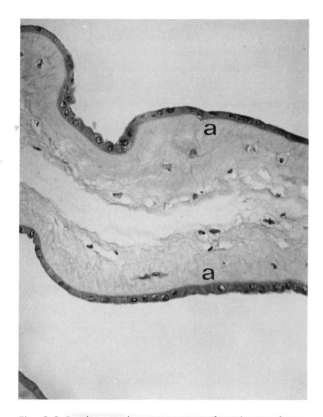

Fig. 2.8 Dividing membrane consisting of two layers of amnion opposed to each other.

[handwritten: Monochorionic = Monozygotic]

netically dissimilar blood cells and the very rare occurrence of human chimerism.

The examination of the dividing membranes between two twins is of increasing clinical importance. The most definitive biologic evidence that twins are monozygotic is finding divided membranes containing no chorionic tissue. Degeneration of previously existing chorionic tissue in such membranes has not been identified; therefore, absence is presumed to mean that the entire gestation is monochorial and therefore monozygotic. Clinically, such a membrane consists of two translucent layers that are easily pulled apart. No vasculature can be identified by inspection. Histologically, two layers of extraembryonic mesoderm are opposed. A single cell layer of amniotic epithelium lies on the opposite surfaces of both (Fig. 2.8).

In contrast, dividing membranes containing chori-

whether velamentous insertion will occur. Among the effects of monozygotic twinning on placentation are the vascular communications between the placentas of monozygotic twins and dividing membranes that lack chorions.

Strong and Corney[17] discuss the subject of vascular connections extensively. If all types of vascular communications are included, most monochorial twin placentas contain them. Communications may occur between major vessels or at the level of villous capillaries. Careful injection techniques are required to demonstrate their true extent. When the fetal transfusion syndrome occurs, the donor portion of the placenta may contain enlarged edematous villi with constricted vascular channels and immature red cells. In contrast, dichorial placentas almost never contain vascular communications; however, exceptions exist, and these present the potential for the mixing of ge-

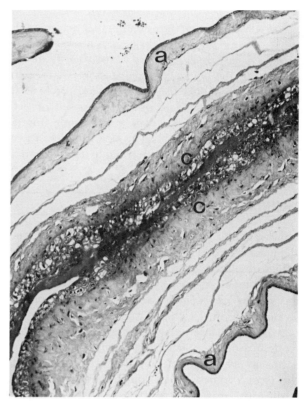

Fig. 2.9 Dividing membrane consisting of two amnions and chorions opposed to each other. The two chorions are almost fused and in some cases may be mistaken for one.

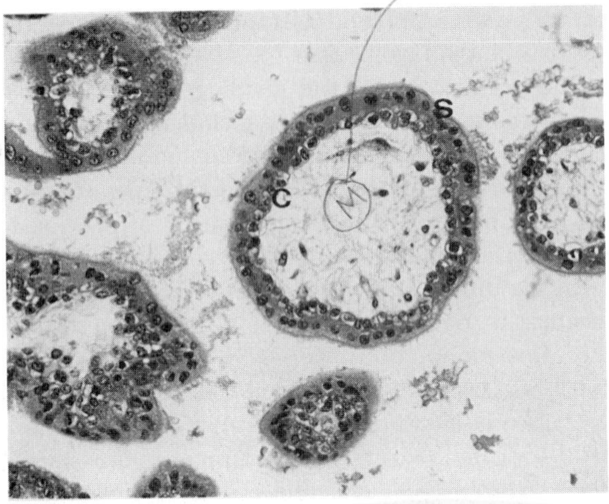

mesodermal tissue = stroma & vessels

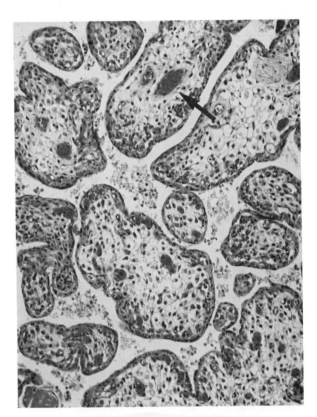

Fig. 2.10 First-trimester villi having a cellular stroma with few capillaries. The trophoblastic epithelium consists of two cell layers. The outer one is syncytium, and the inner one is cytotrophoblast.

onic tissue signify that the gestation may be the result either of preimplantation division of a single zygote or of dizygosity; membranes do not provide definitive evidence on this point. These membranes will contain vessels and when pulled apart will divide into at least three layers. The middle one is composed of two chorions, of course, but these may become fused. Histologically the chorions may look like one or two layers, depending on how thoroughly the fusion has occurred (Fig. 2.9).

PLACENTAL MATURATION

Concomitantly with total growth, maturational changes occur that result in the transformation of the immature placenta into one containing fine terminal villi maximally adapted to exchange. In the first trimester the villi contain a well-developed cellular stroma with only scattered capillaries. The trophoblast is two-cell layers in thickness, with the basal cytotrophoblastic layer being continuous. The syncytium forms an overlying surface cell layer (Fig. 2.10). In the second trimester, villi contain large amounts of stroma with scattered capillaries. The trophoblast is well developed around the villous stems, with both cytotrophoblast and syncytiotrophoblast represented (Fig. 2.11). The subsequent course is one of gradual,

apparent disappearance of the cytotrophoblast and thinning of the syncytium. In absolute terms, however, the cytotrophoblast persists until term and may even proliferate.

As a result of this development, at term the terminal villi consist largely of fetal capillaries with little or no stroma beyond that required for support and trophoblast, which is markedly altered. Cytotrophoblast is not commonly seen with the light microscope, and the remaining syncytium is sufficiently thin that in some areas, referred to as epithelial plates, electron microscopy is required to confirm its presence (Fig. 2.12). Comparative studies suggest that the development of these epithelial plates is a specific differentiation and not artifactual.[13] This particularly thin membrane may be adapted for specialized types of exchange between the maternal and fetal vascular compartments. In any case, the sum changes certainly

Fig. 2.11 Second-trimester villi are much larger and more cellular, but they still contain only small scattered capillaries. The trophoblast is not as clearly two-cell layered as in the first trimester, but large cytotrophoblastic cells are still apparent.

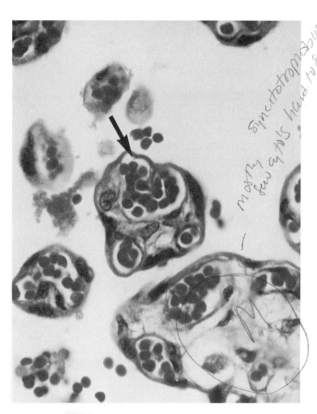

Fig. 2.12 Term villi consisting almost totally of capillaries with very little supporting stroma. The trophoblast is alternately thick and thin over the surface.

syncytotrophoblast, mostly gaps hard to see

appear to be ones that would result in increased diffusion capacity.

Although the foregoing description of placental growth and maturation describes events as occurring in a standard sequential manner, placental growth and development in fact persist until term and vary from place to place in the placenta. There is a marked diminution in growth and proliferative activity after the second trimester, but activity is not totally gone. This is reflected in the histology. The periphery of the placenta is the least active at term.

During the second and third trimesters, a variety of changes take place in the placenta that at first glance seem pathologic. First and most routine of these is the deposition of fibrin around the villi, with infarction of isolated villi. This process is sufficiently ubiquitous to be considered physiologic, but there are certainly cases in which deposition appears to be excessive. Deposition occurs most routinely both in the periph-

ery of the so-called placental cake and beneath the chorionic plate, as well as in the chorion laeve. It has always been assumed that fibrin deposition is the primary process and that death of the underlying trophoblast is secondary. It is conceivable that the opposite is true and that trophoblastic cell death in the chorion laeve and placental periphery results in fibrin deposition.

The most dramatic examples of fibrin deposition result in infarction of the entire fetal surface and are associated with intrauterine growth retardation and fetal death in utero. Calcium deposition in the degenerating tissue is also associated with fibrin. It has not been possible to correlate this calcification with any known physiologic or pathologic process.[18]

Much larger wedge-shaped infarctions of the placenta also occur. The base of the rough triangle is on the basal plate, and the apex reaches almost to the chorionic plate. These structures are the result of compromise of a single maternal spiral arteriole. They are more common in maternal vascular disease, such as toxemia, and are of interest because the lesions illustrate the area over which the flow from the artery in question was physiologically important (Fig. 2.13).

With increasing gestational age, syncytial knots become more common in the placental trophoblast. These knots are collections of small condensed nuclei in syncytial cells that histologically look degenerative but that in fact are not really understood. They resemble the pyknotic nuclei of advanced squamous epithelial cell maturation. Also associated with advancing gestational age is the development of fetal capillary leaks, with resulting fetomaternal hemorrhage. As the frequency of these fetomaternal bleeds increases as term approaches and passes, so does the incidence of the histology that such bleeding produces. When fetal blood escapes into the maternal circulation, a laminated thrombus results—an intervillous thrombus (Fig. 2.14). The presence of fetal red cells within these thrombi suggests their nature. Their observation has been correlated with the clinical occurrence of Rh sensitization in susceptible individuals.[18]

Because all of these pathologic changes look degenerative, it has for many years been fashionable to speak of placental "aging." Actually, no firm biologic definition of aging exists. Consequently, it is impossible to determine if the placenta meets the definition.

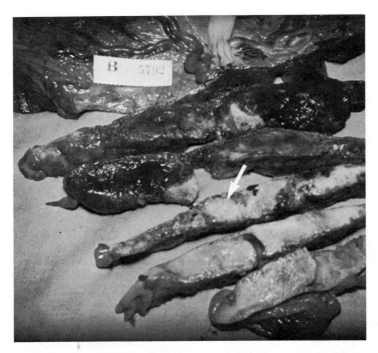

Fig. 2.13 Term placenta revealing extensive infarction (arrow) and calcification. (Courtesy of Dr. James Wheeler, Department of Surgical Pathology, Hospital of the University of Pennsylvania, Philadelphia, PA.)

Although there is some evidence that placental function decreases near term, there is also other evidence that it does not. Thus changes cannot necessarily be described as senescent. The role of decreasing placental function in some prolonged pregnancies remains an area to be assessed.[19]

THE POTENTIAL ROLE OF TROPHOBLASTIC CELL DEATH

A tissue does not have to be old or senescent to participate in a process that leads to the spontaneous or "physiologic" death of some of its cells. The potential importance of the spontaneous death of a given cell population is that this phenomenon characterizes a variety of biologic "clocks." The corpus luteum is an example. If a portion of the chorionic trophoblast is responsible for maintaining pregnancy, then its near-term death might terminate gestation.

Trophoblastic epithelium is initially composed largely of cytotrophoblast, undifferentiated and proliferating. High rates of proliferation persist into the second trimester but subsequently decline.[20] This is associated with a decrease in the amount of visible cytotrophoblast and an increase in the absolute and relative amounts of differentiated trophoblast. As differentiated cells usually have defined life spans, one or more of the differentiated forms of trophoblast could conceivably be the basis of a biologic clock.[21]

The maturation of the trophoblast is less well studied in the chorion laeve than in the chorion frondosum. Multinucleated cells are present in the second trimester but are gone by term. The trophoblastic cell layer begins to thin from the late second trimester onward. This tissue loss is characterized by the accumulation of lipofuscin and apoptosis.

In every respiring cell, oxygen-free radicals result in the peroxidation of lipids with the resulting formation of insoluble fluorescent pigments called *lipofuscin*. A fixed postmitotic cell will accumulate these pigments in proportion to its chronologic age. Lipofuscin appears in the trophoblast as early as 32 weeks of gestation.[22] It is much more prevalent in the trophoblast of the chorion laeve than in the chorion frondosum, and in many animal species below primates

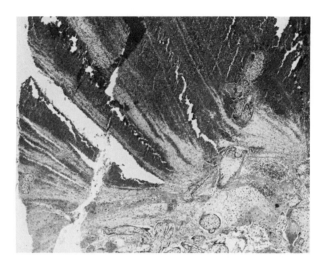

Fig. 2.14 Laminated thrombus occupying a space between villi (and thus is intervillous).

it is sufficiently voluminous as to be seen in hematoxylin– and eosin–stained sections with the light microscope. In primates, visualizing lipofuscin more commonly requires the electron microscope (Fig. 2.15). Its presence in both the membranes and the placenta proper in areas of fibrin deposition raises the possibility that fibrin deposition is not primary but secondary to trophoblastic cell death.

Apoptosis is the histologic manifestation of spontaneous cell death and characterizes the loss of the trophoblast in the chorion laeve as term approaches.[23] Initially the dying cells in the chorion laeve are replaced by fibrin, but eventually this too disappears. Increasingly after 36 weeks, maternal decidua is in direct contact with mesoderm of the chorionic membrane. Thus the trophoblast of the chorion laeve goes through a process of growth and maturation that results in its spontaneous death as term is approached. If the trophoblast of the chorion laeve is responsible for maintaining gestation, then its life span might constitute the clock that determines the length of gestation.

This idea would be consistent with much of the current thinking about the physiology of parturition. Rising amniotic fluid levels of cortisol after 30 weeks might induce differentiation in the chorion and thus promote cell death.[24] Such a role for fetal adrenal steroids would also be consistent not only with the observation that the placenta of the anencephalic is histologically immature, but also with the observation that the final organ size of primate fetuses exposed to prenatal steroids is small.[25,26] If adrenal steroids contribute to the regulation of the rate at which an undifferentiated cell population becomes differentiated, steroids would diminish the final size of an organ by prematurely differentiating an otherwise proliferating cell population.

PLACENTAL INFLAMMATION

Apart from the ubiquitous changes described in the discussion of maturation, the most common pathologic observation in the term placenta is inflammation. When infectious agents produce infections in the fetal compartment of an intact pregnancy, the most common placental manifestation is villitis (Fig. 2.16): villi that are swollen and infiltrated with acute or chronic inflammatory cells. The trophoblast may or may not be denuded. When fibrin deposition around the villus produces acute infarction, an inflammatory infiltrate may also occur, but this distinction is usually obvious. The infarcted villus will be small and surrounded by fibrin. A list of organisms that may produce villitis would contain all types of infectious agents. Syphilis, rubella, and toxoplasmosis are examples. In general, the histology of these infections is not unique. Toxoplasmosis may show encysted organisms within the membranes. Sander[27] described a hemorrhagic inflammatory lesion that he speculates may be viral, immunologic, or toxic but that in any case is associated with significant fetal morbidity and mortality.

Tuberculosis has been described in the placenta, and congenital cases in newborns are known; however, in most cases this represents an endometrial infection with involvement of the placenta by contiguity, and this is also the case for most of the infections described associated with intrauterine devices.

The most frequent inflammatory response seen in the placenta is that associated with chorioamnionitis (Fig. 2.17). Moreover, the pathology of this disorder contributes significantly to its understanding. That the pattern of inflammatory cell migration is always toward the amniotic sac indicates pathogenesis. Even more informative is the observation that if only one of

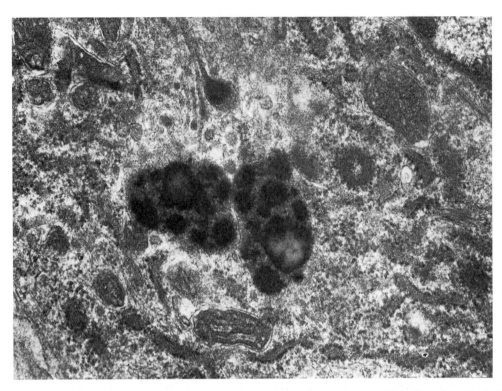

Fig. 2.15 Typical lipofuscin in the trophoblast of the chorion frondosum at term. (X 57,380) (Courtesy of Nola Walker and Daniel Roberts, MD, Department of Obstetrics and Gynecology, University of Kansas School of Medicine, Wichita, Wichita, KS.)

a set of twins is involved, it is always the most dependent one.[28]

The fetal response to chorioamnionitis is seen in both the chorionic plate of the placental body and the umbilical cord. In either site, fetal leukocytes first accumulate on the luminal edge of fetal vessels on the side closest to the amniotic sac. They then migrate through the vascular wall toward the sac, producing a pattern of infiltrate that moves through only one side of the vessel. (In the umbilical cord, this pattern is altered if the process has been present for several days.) Then the infiltrate becomes circumvascular. More prolonged inflammation in the presence of accessory vessels in the cord may result in granulation tissue. Accessory vessels, otherwise unimportant structures, are presumably remnants of the yolk sac vasculature.

Within the membranes, chorioamnionitis manifests itself as a maternal polymorphonuclear inflammatory reaction. In its earliest stages infiltration ex-tends into the trophoblastic epithelium of the chorion, concentrates there, and destroys this cell population. The reaction then moves into the mesoderm that separates the chorionic epithelium and the amniotic epithelium. The infiltrate tends to stop at the level of the dense acellular layer, which lies immediately beneath the amniotic epithelium. When chorioamnionitis is more severe, microabscess formation occurs. Situated immediately beneath the epithelium, these abscesses rupture into the sac, thus producing a focal ulcer on the fetal surface of the membrane. In the most severe cases, total loss of the amnionic epithelium occurs. Although in this last situation it is unusual for there to be no clinical infection, less severe examples of chorioamnionitis are routinely seen in the absence of maternal or fetal infection. This is particularly the case when the placenta is a premature one. Up to 50 percent of the placentas delivered at 28 weeks demonstrate chorioamnionitis. Absence of clinical infection in many of these cases

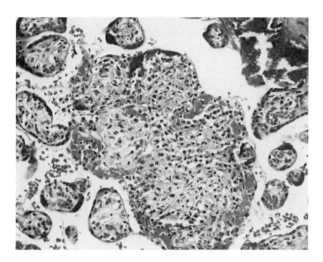

Fig. 2.16 Necrotic clumped villi infiltrated with inflammatory cells.

has led to the suggestion that they represent a sterile inflammatory reaction. It is possible that this is sometimes correct, but in many cases there is either focal or diffuse basophilia, which when stained with Brown-Hopps stain demonstrates the presence of bacteria. Thus it is possible that bacterial infection of the membranes is present much more commonly than is bacterial infection of the mother or infant. Presumably, if delivery occurs promptly, maternal and fetal defense mechanisms are adequate.

In any case, a maternal inflammatory infiltrate destroys the chorionic trophoblast as soon as the infiltrate enters the fetal compartment either in the chorion laeve or in the chorionic plate. Therefore, regardless of whether it is sterile, such an infiltrate might be associated with premature labor if the trophoblastic epithelium is important in the maintenance of gestation. Furthermore, if the infiltrate is due to infection, then the early destruction of this tissue might be responsible for inducing labor so early in the clinical course of chorioamnionitis that infection does not become apparent.

In the placental body, the maternal response to chorioamnionitis consists of margination of large numbers of chronic and acute inflammatory cells immediately beneath the chorionic plate and their subsequent migration through the mesoderm toward the amniotic surface. This may be extensive and may be associated with an adjoining fetal response to the same infection, so that maternal leukocytes and fetal leukocytes are migrating in the same direction through the same mesodermal layer. It would, of course, be fascinating to know about the interaction between these two genetically dissimilar populations.

PLACENTAL TUMORS

Tumors occur in the placenta as in other tissues. Chorioangiomas, benign hemangiomas of the fetal vasculature, are most common, with an incidence around 1 percent, depending on the care taken in detection[29] (Fig. 2.18). In the overwhelming majority of cases, chorioangiomas are clinically insignificant, but large ones (i.e., greater than 5 cm in diameter), may be associated with acutely developing polyhydramnios and premature labor.[18]

Malignant trophoblastic tumors may develop from any type of conception. Rarely does choriocarcinoma develop in the normal placenta associated with a term pregnancy (Fig. 2.19). When this occurs, it is particularly likely to go unnoticed and to be advanced before its malignant behavior finally comes to attention. Choriocarcinoma also rarely develops from placental site tumors.[11] Tumors themselves develop from the trophoblast that invades the implantation site. Most

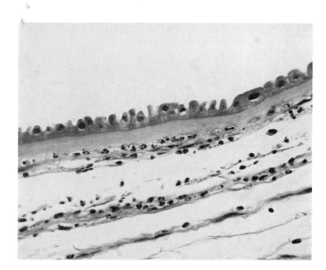

Fig. 2.17 Acute and chronic inflammatory cells infiltrate the mesoderm beneath this amniotic epithelium. Inflammatory cells stop immediately beneath the acellular layer that supports the amniotic epithelium.

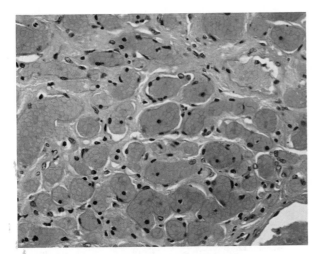

Fig. 2.18 Densely packed mass of capillaries supported by a thin inapparent stroma is typical of chorioangioma.

often choriocarcinoma follows a hydatidiform mole (Fig. 2.20).

Moles usually arise from one of two sources.[30] In some cases they are the result of the fertilization of an ovum by two sperm. The nucleus of the ovum is either absent or inactive, and subsequent growth is the result of the combination of two sets of paternal genomes. Such moles may be XY or XX. More commonly, moles result from the fertilization of a similar ovum by one haploid sperm that then reproduces

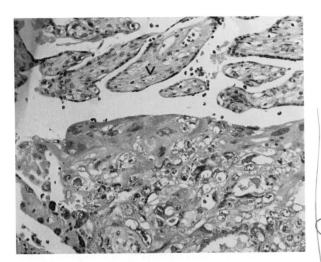

Fig. 2.19 Normal villi in choriocarcinoma in a normal placenta. The choriocarcinoma has typical features of this malignancy, with both syncytial and cytotrophoblastic cells and no organization.

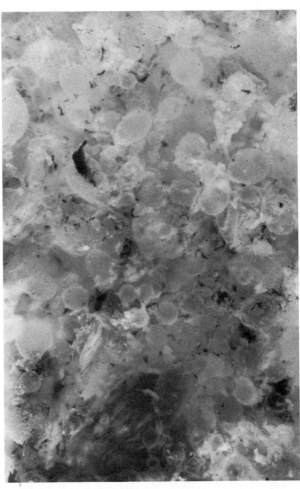

Fig. 2.20 Hydatidiform mole demonstrating the typical grape-like vesicals. (Courtesy of Dr. James Wheeler, Department of Surgical Pathology, Hospital of the University of Pennsylvania, Philadelphia, PA.)

itself. Only one set of paternal chromosomes is thus involved, and such moles are XX. No YY moles have as yet been identified.[31,32] These genetic observations are underscored by those of Surani,[33] who demonstrated that extraembryonic components of the conceptus require paternal genes for their successful development, whereas embryonic components are less dependent on paternal genes.[33]

The partial mole is a syndrome of anomalies associated with a triploid chromosomal complement. Most commonly two of these are of paternal origin and one of maternal origin.[34] This entity only rarely leads to persistent trophoblast. Thus, partial moles are not properly considered in the same biologic cate-

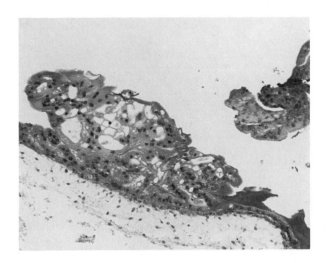

Fig. 2.21 Typical portion of the wall of dilated edematous villi of a hydatidiform mole. A central cystic cavity is shown (lower left). Cellular stroma has been pushed against the trophoblastic membrane, which consists of both cytotrophoblastic and syncytial cells. There is a marked persistence of lacunar space development in this trophoblast, representing significant immaturity.

gory as true hydatidiform moles. Confusion arises because the villi of partial moles are also swollen and edematous and superficially resemble those of the hydatidiform mole (Figs. 2.21 and 2.22). However, there is no trophoblastic proliferation per se, and other histologic differences exist. The triploid syndrome is often associated with a fetus that may or may not demonstrate various anomalies, including neural tube defects, retarded limb development, facial dysplasia, and subectodermal hemorrhage.[35,36]

In describing gestational trophoblastic neoplasia, it is customary to divide the usual spectrum into hydatidiform moles, invasive moles, and choriocarcinoma. Although we shall adhere to this description, it is important to realize that each of these entities may represent only a point in time in the life history of a single disease. Furthermore, this obviously ignores those examples of choriocarcinoma that arise in settings other than hydatidiform moles.

Known epidemiologic risk factors for hydatidiform moles include extremes of age in the reproductive years, which usually means adolescence or women over 40 years, low socioeconomic status, and prior reproductive loss, particularly prior gestational trophoblastic neoplasia.[37,38] For this reason, incidence figures vary widely. A commonly quoted one for North America is that hydatidiform moles occur

once in one thousand pregnancies. A study in an abortion clinic suggests a higher figure.[39] Grimes[37] has called attention to the inherent difficulties in interpreting these figures. The highest incidences are reported from Southeast Asia.

Hydatidiform moles tend to present as threatened or incomplete abortions, with the triploidy syndrome more commonly presenting as a missed abortion. True moles frequently demonstrate rapid uterine growth, theca–lutein cysts (Fig. 2.23), and toxemia and in some cases are complicated by hyperthyroidism.[40] The latter is the result of thyroid-stimulating hormone–like activity exhibited by high levels of hCG.[41] Hydatidiform moles are conveniently diagnosed by detecting a "snow storm" pattern on ultrasonography[42–44] (Fig. 2.24).

It is the physiologic function of the trophoblast to transport substances from the maternal to the fetal compartments, and even malignant trophoblasts do this. This fact, plus the absence of a vascular system within the villi, results in the hydropic enlargement of the villi in hydatidiform moles. Although swollen villi are a dramatic finding to both the clinician and the pathologist, they are not disease itself. This is an important diagnostic point, as swollen villi occur under a variety of circumstances and, in the absence of abnormal trophoblastic proliferation, are not at risk for producing a subsequent malignant clinical course. There are, however, relatively unique histologic fea-

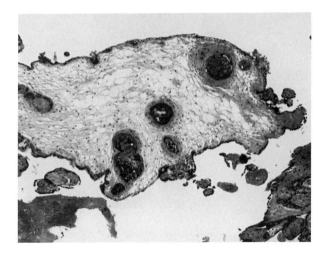

Fig. 2.22 Large villus from a triploid conception that is swollen but cellular. The trophoblast is abnormal in that infolding produces the appearance of trophoblastic islands within the villus, but it is cytologically normal.

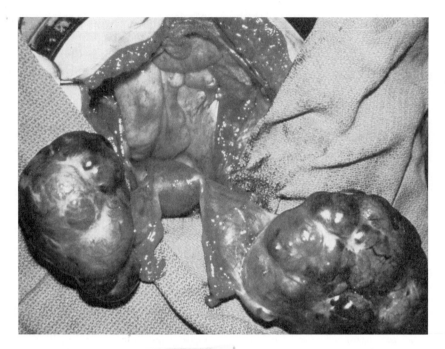

Fig. 2.23 Bilateral theca–lutein cysts associated with hydatidiform mole.

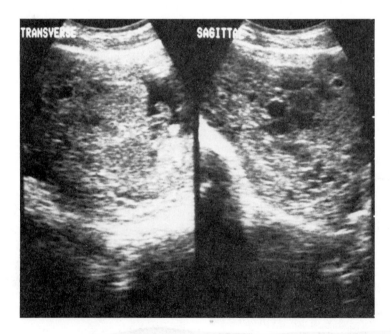

Fig. 2.24 Transverse and sagittal views. Ultrasound demonstrating the "snow storm" pattern associated with hydatidiform mole.

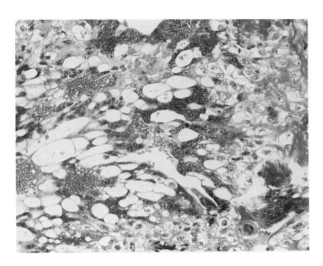

Fig. 2.25 Typical choriocarcinoma with both cytotrophoblastic and syncytial proliferation, both intermixed and lacking in organization. In addition, there is marked cytologic atypicality.

tures to this hydropic degeneration that make it possible to separate it from some other types. These features consist of fluid accumulation within the center of the villus, with lateral displacement of the mesoderm so that a central cistern develops.[35] This is often in contrast to the syndrome of triploidy described earlier. In this latter entity usually the entire villus is swollen with edema fluid, but the cells are uniformly distributed throughout the villous core. It is also in contrast to some, but not all, forms of degeneration.

The most distinctive histologic feature of trophoblastic neoplasia is, of course, related to the trophoblast. Although areas of normal trophoblast may be found in hydatidiform moles, at least focally the pattern of trophoblastic proliferation is dramatically atypical and differs from the normal pattern described in normal placentation in several specific ways. It lacks organization. The proliferative pattern does not result in a large sheet of proliferating cytotrophoblast surrounded at its periphery by the differentiated syncytial epithelium. Instead, the pattern consists of large masses of cytotrophoblastic cells, intermediate-type cells, and differentiated syncytial giant cells all intermixed in an indiscriminate way. Proliferation takes place not only at the tips of anchoring villi, but also at multiple sites around the villi, or it may involve the entire circumference. The lacunar development of the very early trophoblast may

persist until the second trimester in hydatidiform moles. Lastly, there is dramatic individual cell atypicality. The invasion of the decidua by normal trophoblast appears malignant, and for this reason it has not always been appreciated that malignant trophoblast is, nevertheless, considerably more atypical than normal trophoblast when the two are directly compared. Both atypical mitoses and other forms of cytologic atypicality are present.

Only about 10 percent of hydatidiform moles will ultimately pursue a malignant course, although current therapeutic regimens involve treating about 20 percent to avoid inappropriate delay for the problematic 10 percent. Consequently, it is current to speak of benign and malignant moles based on this knowledge. Despite attempts to do so, it has been difficult using histology to predict which course a given mole will follow. An alternative interpretation of this information is that all moles are malignant and that whether they pursue a clinically malignant course is dependent on other factors. In fact, the histology is more consistent with such a view.

Invasive moles do not appear histologically to be more malignant than hydatidiform moles, but instead to be cases in which villi have been carried into the myometrium by invading trophoblast and in some cases deported. Furthermore, the trophoblast in choriocarcinoma is not very histologically different than the atypical portion of the trophoblast of hydatidiform moles, although it is present in a pure form (Fig. 2.25)—either villi have been lost or their mesodermal cores have been invaded and replaced by the tumor. Choriocarcinoma at local or metastatic sites is often associated with dramatic destruction of tissue and significant, if not massive, hemorrhage (Fig. 2.26). This may be out of all proportion to the amount of tumor present. It is not uncommon to find a large pool of blood contained within a cystic space in the tissue involved, with only a thin shell of tumor lining the inner surface of the cyst (Fig. 2.27).

Deportation and metastases of choriocarcinoma are routine, with the lung being the primary site; however, one of the characteristic features of this disease is its ability to metastasize anywhere early (Fig. 2.28). The metastases may be the presenting symptom, in fact, and gestational trophoblastic neoplasia may present first as subarachnoid hemorrhage, a coin-sized lesion in the chest, or a subcutaneous nodule on

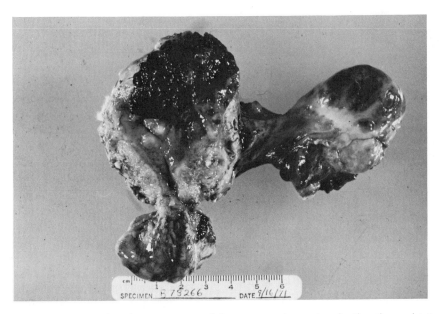

Fig. 2.26 Choriocarcinoma invading the myometrium of the uterus and associated with a theca–lutein cyst of the ovary. (Courtesy of Dr. James Wheeler, Department of Surgical Pathology, Hospital of the University of Pennsylvania, Philadelphia, PA.)

the shoulder. It is not too unusual for intrauterine choriocarcinoma to perforate the myometrium, producing intraperitoneal bleeding and presenting as an ectopic gestation.

When choriocarcinoma occurs after a full-term pregnancy, in some cases it can be shown to have been present in the placenta and to have grown prior to the delivery. This may explain why these cases tend to respond less well to therapy than cases detected as part of the follow-up of hydatidiform mole, as most of the prognostic factors that predict poor outcome in this disease can be understood in terms of the volume of tumor. In general, choriocarcinoma detected more than 4 months after the preceding pregnancy, with titers of β-hCG greater than 40,000 mIU/ml of serum, or with liver or brain metastases require multiagent chemotherapy and do not have 100 percent cure rates.[45]

CLINICAL EXAMINATION OF THE PLACENTA

At delivery, it is useful for the clinician to examine the placenta in some detail and to record the findings. The umbilical cord should be inspected for the presence of three vessels, true knots, and cysts or abnormalities of the surface. Excessively long cords are associated with true knots and with single or multiple entanglements of the fetus and cord. Excessively short cords are occasionally associated with acute fetal distress. Fetal heart rate abnormalities produced by cord compression are occasionally explained by these observations.

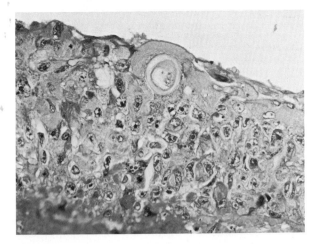

Fig. 2.27 Although the cytologic atypicality in this example of choriocarcinoma is quite dramatic, the bimodal cell type is less apparent. This thin layer of malignant trophoblast lined a large blood-filled space.

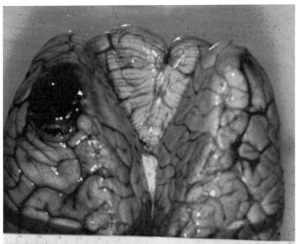

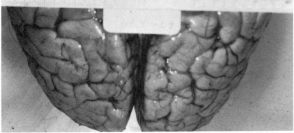

Fig. 2.28 Metastasis to the brain produced by choriocarcinoma. (Courtesy of Dr. James Wheeler, Department of Surgical Pathology, Hospital of the University of Pennsylvania, Philadelphia, PA.)

The membranes should be inspected for defects, clarity, and thickening. Amnion nodosum produces thick, whitish plaques on the fetal surface, and infection thickens the membranes and makes them opaque. Dividing membranes between multiple gestational sacs may be manually dissected to determine how many layers are present, but layers should not be disrupted in such a way as to interfere with microscopic confirmation.

The fetal surface of the placental cake should be inspected for chorionic cysts, fibrin plaques, vascular thromboses, or calcification. The maternal surface of the placenta should be inspected for completeness. Red or whitish nodules are plaques that may represent tumors, infarcts, or intervillous thrombi. Abruptions are detected by the presence of dark, adherent clot on the maternal surface. If old, there may be a depression in this surface. If the placenta is to be examined in the pathology laboratory, detailed analysis should be left to that facility. If no such analysis is

planned, the placenta may be cut in slices and the cut surfaces examined for tumors, infarcts, or thrombi. Placental weights are sufficiently problematic that some authors do not recommend obtaining them.[28] Both membranes and cords should be trimmed from the cake if the placenta is weighed. A fascinating, but not always convenient, observation can often be obtained by placing the freshly delivered placenta and membranes in a sink filled with water. Filling the sac and floating the whole in this manner illustrates the position the placenta occupied in utero.[12]

REFERENCES

1. Fleming TP, Johnson MH: From egg to epithelium. Annu Rev Cell Biol 4:459, 1988
2. Johnson MH, Maro B: Time and space in the mouse early embryo. p. 35. In Rosasant J, Pedersen RA (eds): Experimental Approaches to Mammalian Embryonic Development. Cambridge University Press, New York, 1986
3. Kurman RJ, Young RH, Norris HJ et al: Immuno-cytochemical localization of placental lactogen and chorionic gonadotrophin in the normal placenta and trophoblastic tumors, with emphasis on intermediate trophoblast and the placenta site trophoblastic tumor. Int J Gynecol Pathol 3:101, 1984
4. Jara CS, Salud AT, Bryant-Greenwood GD et al: Immunocytochemical localization of the human growth hormone variant in the human placenta. J Chem Endocrinol Metab 69:1069, 1989
5. Hertig AT: Gestational hyperplasia of endometrium. Lab Invest 13:1153, 1964
6. Noyes RW, Hertig AT, Rock J: Dating the endometria. Fertil Steril 1:3, 1950
7. Hamilton WJ, Boyd JD: Development of the human placenta. In Barnes PJ, Newton M (eds): Scientific Foundations of Obstetrics and Gynecology. FA Davis, Philadelphia, 1970
8. Dickey RP: Evaluation and management of threatened and habitual first trimester abortions. In Osofasky HJ (ed): Advances in Clinical Obstetrics and Gynecology. Vol. 2. Williams & Wilkins, Baltimore, 1984
9. Greiss F: Uterine and placental blood flow. In Sciarra JD (ed): Gynecology and Obstetrics. Vol. 3. Harper & Row, Hagerstown, MD, 1982
10. Robertson WB, Brosens I, Dixon HG: Uteroplacental vascular pathology. Eur J Obstet Gynecol Reprod Biol 5:47, 1975
11. Scully RE, Young RH: Trophoblastic pseudotumor, a reappraisal. Am J Surg Pathol 5:75, 1981
12. Torpin R: The Human Placenta. Charles C Thomas, Springfield, IL, 1969

13. Ludwig KS: The morphologic structure of the placenta in relation to its exchange function. p. 13. In Longo LD, Bartels H (eds): Respiratory Gas Exchange and Blood Flow in the Placenta. Publ. No. 73-361. DHEW, Washington, DC, 1972

14. Teasdale F: Gestational changes in the functional structure of the human placenta in relation to fetal growth: a morphometric study. Am J Obstet Gynecol 137:560, 1980

15. Winnick M, Coscia A, Noble A: Cellular growth in human placenta. I. Normal placenta growth. Pediatrics 39:248, 1967

16. Hsu YC: Monozygotic twin formation in mouse embryos in vitro. Science 209:605, 1980

17. Strong SJ, Corney G: The Placenta in Twin Pregnancy. Pergamon, New York, 1967

18. Fox H: Pathology of the placenta. p. 204. In Bennington JL (ed): Major Problems in Pathology. Vol. 7. WB Saunders, Philadelphia, 1978

19. Fox H: Placenta as a model for organ aging. p. 351. In Beaconfield P, Villee C (eds): Placenta, a neglected experimental animal. Pergamon Press, New York, 1979

20. Weinberg PC, Cameron IL, Parmley TH, et al: Gestational age and placental cellular replication. Obstet Gynecol 36:692, 1970

21. Walton J: The role of limited cell replicative capacity in pathologic age change: a review. Mech Aging Dev 19:217, 1982

22. Parmley TH, Gupta PK, Walker MA: "Aging" pigments in term human placenta. Am J Obstet Gynecol 139:760, 1981

23. Parmley TH: Spontaneous cell death in the chorion laeve. Am J Obstet Gynecol 162:1576, 1990

24. Murphy BEP: Conjugated glucocorticoids in amniotic fluid and fetal lung natural. J Clin Endocrinol Metabol 17:212, 1978

25. Batson JL, Winn K, Dubin NH, Parmley TH: Placental immaturity associated with anencephaly. Obstet Gynecol 65:846, 1985

26. Beck JC, Johnson JWC: Maternal administration of gluco-corticoids. Clin Obstet Gynecol 23:93, 1980

27. Sander CH: Hemorrhagic endovasculitis and hemorrhagic villitis of the placenta. Arch Pathol Lab Med 104:371, 1980

28. Bernirschke K, Driscoll SG: The pathology of the human placenta. p. 340. In Handbuch der speziellen pathologischen anatomie und histologie. Vol. 7. Springer-Verlag, New York, 1967

29. Dao AH, Rogers CW, Wong SW: Chorioangioma of the placenta: report of 2 cases with ultrasound study in 1. Obstet Gynecol 57:465, 1981

30. Surti U, Szulman AE, O'Brien S: Dispermic origin and clinical outcome of three complete hydatidiform moles with 46,XY karyotype. Am J Obstet Gynecol 144:84, 1982

31. Kajii T, Ohama K: Androgenetic origin of hydatidiform mole. Nature 268:633, 1977

32. Yamashita K, Wake N, Araki T et al: Human lymphocyte antigen expression in hydatidiform mole: androgenesis following fertilization by a haploid sperm. Am J Obstet Gynecol 135:597, 1979

33. Surani MAH: Evidences and consequences of difference between maternal and paternal genomes during embryogenesis in the mouse. p. 401. In Rossant J, Pedersen RA (eds): Experimental Approaches in Mammalian Embryonic Development. Cambridge University Press, New York, 1986

34. Vejerslev LO, Fisher RA, Surti U, Walke N: Cytogenetically unusual cases and their implications for the present classification. Am J Obstet Gynecol 157:180, 1987

35. Czernobilsky B, Barash A, Lancet M: Partial moles: a clinicopathology study of 25 cases. Obstet Gynecol 59:75, 1982

36. Harris MJ, Poland BJ, Dill FJ: Triploidy in 40 human spontaneous abortuses: assessment of phenotype in embryos. Obstet Gynecol 57:600, 1981

37. Grimes DA: Epidemiology of gestational trophoblastic disease. Am J Obstet Gynecol 150:309, 1984

38. Bandy LC, Clarke-Pearson DL, Hammond CB: Malignant potential of gestational trophoblastic disease at the extreme ages of reproductive life. Obstet Gynecol 64:395, 1984

39. Cohen BA, Burkman RI, Rosenhein NB et al: Gestational trophoblastic disease within an elective abortion population. Am J Obstet Gynecol 135:452, 1979

40. Montz FJ, Schlaerth JB, Morrow CP: The natural history of theca lutein cysts. Obstet Gynecol 72:247, 1988

41. Fradkin JE, Eastman RC, Lesniak MA, Roth J: Specificity spillover at the hormone receptor—exploring its role in human disease. N Engl J Med 320:640, 1989

42. Campbell V, Magrina JF, Capen CV, Masterson BJ: Gestational trophoblastic neoplasia: a review of new concepts. J Kansas Med Soc 84:61, 1983

43. Goldstein DP, Berkowitz RS: Gestational Trophoblastic Neoplasms. p. 152. WB Saunders, Philadelphia, 1982

44. Hammond CB, Weed JC, Barnard DE, Tyrey L: Gestational trophoblastic neoplasia. Cancer 31:322, 1981

45. Surwit EA, Alberts DS, Christian CD, Graham VE: Poor prognosis for gestational trophoblastic disease: an update. Obstet Gynecol 64:21, 1984

Chapter 3

Placental Endocrinology and Diagnosis of Pregnancy

John E. Buster and Sandra A. Carson

The evolutionary advent of viviparity necessitated changes in the maternal metabolic, hormonal, and immunologic systems. To compensate for the increased and altered demands of an intracorporeal pregnancy, nature designed a new organ—the placenta—and a series of proteins specific for and secreted only during pregnancy. These proteins, aided by alterations in the already stimulated steroids, allow invasion of a half-foreign tissue into the maternal system that not only tolerates but actively nourishes and protects the growing fetus. The changes in the hormonal milieu also offer clinical signs used in the diagnosis and monitoring of pregnancy and are the focus of this chapter.

FETAL PLACENTAL PEPTIDES

Ontogeny of Placental Peptide Production

From the moment of conception, proteins are released into the maternal system by the newly formed conceptus, presumably to alter the maternal immune, metabolic, and hormonal responses to the advancing gestation. The production and secretion of these proteins mirror the demands that each developmental stage of gestation brings.

The Preimplantation Conceptus

Peptides unique to pregnancy are present in the maternal circulation as early as conception. Presumably released from the fertilized ovum by sperm penetra-

tion, platelet-activating factor (PAF) is detectable almost immediately after fertilization.[1,2] In turn, PAF releases a maternal immunosuppressive protein from the maternal ovary: early pregnancy factor (EPF). EPF is detectable in maternal serum within 48 hours of conception.[3,4] Approximately 80 hours after follicular rupture, the conceptus leaves the tubal ampulla and enters the isthmus; after only 10 hours more, the conceptus enters the uterus.[5,6] Arriving with as few as 2 to 10 cells, the conceptus floats freely in the endometrial cavity from before 90 to up to 150 hours after conception.[5,6]

By 4.5 days, the embryo becomes a blastocyst.[7] Secretion of proteins into the maternal circulation by the blastocyst may occur but is limited by the absence of vascular communication. In vitro the human blastocyst secretes human chorionic gonadotropin (hCG) into culture media as early as 6 days after conception.[8] It is not detectable, however, in the maternal serum by present assays until 9 to 11 days.[9] This coincides with the time at which implantation is anatomically complete.[10,11]

The Implanted Conceptus

Blastomeres destined to form the placenta can be identified as trophectoderm lining the periphery of the blastocyst 5 days postconception (Fig. 3.1). By the tenth day, invading trophoblasts have formed two distinct layers: an inner layer composed of individual, well-defined, and rapidly proliferating cells, the cyto-

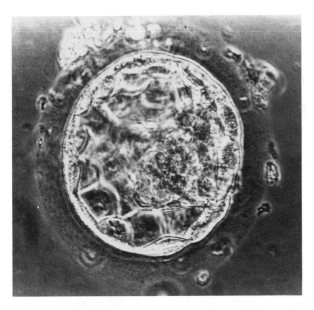

Fig. 3.1 The human preimplantation blastocyst 5 days after conception. The inner cell mass, the cells destined to form embryonic structures, is seen at between 3 and 6 o'clock. Trophectoderm comprises the remainder. (From Buster et al.,[6] with permission.)

trophoblasts, and an outer and thicker layer comprising a continuous mass of cell plasma containing multiple nuclei with indistinct cell borders, the syncytiotrophoblast (Fig. 3.2). The syncytiotrophoblasts make up the placental surface of the fetomaternal interface.[12]

Cytotrophoblasts stain immunohistochemically for hypothalamic-like peptides: corticotropin-releasing hormone (CRH), gonadotropin-releasing hormone (GnRH), somatostatin (SRIF), and thyrotropin-releasing hormone (TRH) (Table 3.1).[13-25] The juxtaposed syncytiotrophoblasts stain immunohistochemically for corresponding pituitary-like peptides: adrenocorticotrophic hormone (ACTH), hCG (analogous to pituitary luteinizing hormone [LH]), human chorionic somatomammotropin (hCS, analogous to human growth hormone), prolactin (PRL), and (probably) chorionic thyrotropin (hCT) (Table 3.1).[17-24] This anatomic arrangement suggests that these two layers mirror the hypothalamic–pituitary axis but in a paracrine relationship, with cytotrophoblasts stimulating syncytiotrophoblasts to secrete their respective hormones.[13-25] Syncytiotrophoblasts are the princi-

pal site of steroid and protein hormone biosynthesis. This cell layer contains abundant rough endoplasmic reticulum, Golgi complexes, and mitochondria, the subcellular machinery that synthesize hormones (Fig. 3.3).[12,20] Prohormones are assembled from maternal amino acids within the rough endoplasmic reticulum of the syncytiotrophoblast. Assembled into early secretory granules by the Golgi complex, these prohormones traverse the plasma membrane as mature granules.[12,20] The mature granules are solubilized in the maternal blood stream as circulating hormones (Fig. 3.3).[12,20] In summary, the syncytiotrophoblasts secrete hCG, hCS, ACTH, hCT, pregnancy-associated plasma protein A (PAPP-A) and placental protein 5 (PP5).[17-25]

The fetus also produces pregnancy-specific proteins. At the end of the first trimester, α-fetoprotein (AFP) is secreted into the maternal circulation. Its concentrations rise into the second trimester.[26]

The Mature Placenta

Throughout the second and third trimesters, the placenta adapts its structure to reflect its function. As fetomaternal exchange overwhelms hormone secretory functions, the relative numbers of trophoblasts decrease.[18] The villi near term (Fig. 3.4) consist largely of fetal capillaries with little or no stroma beyond that required for anatomic integrity. Cytotrophoblasts are sparse, and the remaining syncytium is thin, scarcely visible by light microscopy. In contrast to the early villus, in which the trophoblasts are present in abundance with a continuous basal cytotrophoblast layer and an overlying surface syncytium, the membranous interface between fetal and maternal circulation is extremely thin.[12] This villous structure of the term placenta facilitates specialized transport of compounds across the fetomaternal interface.[12]

Physiology of Fetoplacental Peptides

The sequential unfolding of placental protein secretion is characteristic for each protein, presumably reflecting the requirement of its function.

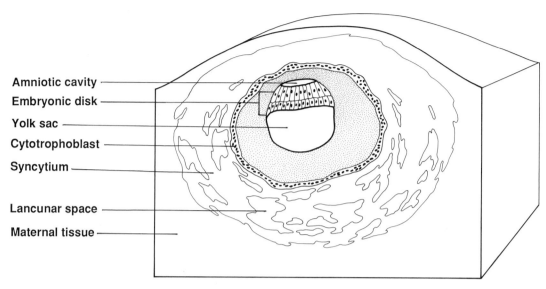

Amniotic cavity
Embryonic disk
Yolk sac
Cytotrophoblast
Syncytium

Lancunar space
Maternal tissue

Fig. 3.2 Postimplantation embryo and placental structures at approximately 9 days. Cytotrophoblasts are seen as a single layer within the rectangle. They abut against the syncytiotrophoblast, which in turn surround the maternal blood-filled lacunar spaces. The embryo has evolved as a simple embryonic disc in association with a very large yolk sac and developing amniotic cavity.

Table 3.1 Cytochemical Distribution of Placental Hypothalamic- and Pituitary-Like Peptides

Peptide	Abbreviation	Cytotrophoblast	Syncytiotrophoblast	Decidua	References
Hypothalamic analogues					
Corticotropin-releasing hormone	CRH	+			14,53,44
Gonadotropin-releasing hormone	GnRH	+			15
Thyrotropin-releasing hormone	TRH	+			13,16,63
Somatostatin	SRIF	+			25
Pituitary analogues					
Adrenocorticotropic hormone	ACTH		+		17
Human chorionic gonadotropin[a]	hCG		+		18,21,22
Human chorionic thyrotropin	hCT		?		19
Human chorionic somatomammotropin	hCS		+		21,22
Prolactin	PRL		+	+	24

The localization of hypothalamic-like peptides to the cytotrophoblast layer juxtaposed to the pituitary-like hormones in the syncytiotrophoblast layer suggests a paracrine interrelationship that is analogous to the hypothalamic–pituitary axis. No such analogue has been defined for prolactin.

[a] hCG is analogous to pituitary LH.

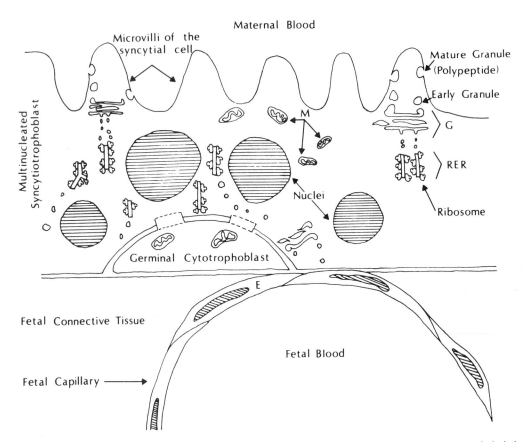

Fig. 3.3 The human placenta at term diagrammed as a cross-sectional electron microscopic view. E, endothelial cell; G, Golgi complex; M, mitochondria; RER, rough endoplasmic reticulum. (Modified from Osathanondh and Tulchinsky,[137] with permission.)

EPF

Molecular Structure of EPF

Recently isolated and purified from human pregnancy serum, EPF is a pregnancy-associated immunosuppressive protein with a molecular mass of 21,500 daltons.[27] There is not a specific radioimmunoassay for EPF. It is detected in a bioassay by its abilities to bind to lymphocytes in vitro and to amplify quantitatively the inhibition of rosette formation between lymphocytes and heterologous (sheep) red blood cells caused by antilymphocyte serum (Fig. 3.5).[4,28] This assay is lengthy, tedious, and subject to great variance.

Origin of EPF

EPF is produced by the maternal ovaries after stimulation by PAF, which is released from the conceptus at fertilization.[1,2] It is believed that PAF is already in the ovum and that sperm entry triggers its release. EPF is also produced by the preimplanted blastocyst and may have a local endometrial function. Because embryonic EPF probably does not reach the circulation until implantation, removal of the ovaries in experimental animals shortly after conception, but before implantation, results in immediate disappearance of ovarian EPF from the circulation.[4]

EPF Variation During Pregnancy

EPF may be the first serologic sign of fertilization. In early human studies, EPF was detected after intercourse in 18 of 28 ovulatory cycles, suggesting a fertilization rate of 67 percent. Embryonic loss was high (78 percent), because EPF disappeared from the circulation before the onset of menstruation in 14 of 18 of these cases.[29] In the remaining 4 cases, EPF remained detectable beyond 14 days, and a viable em-

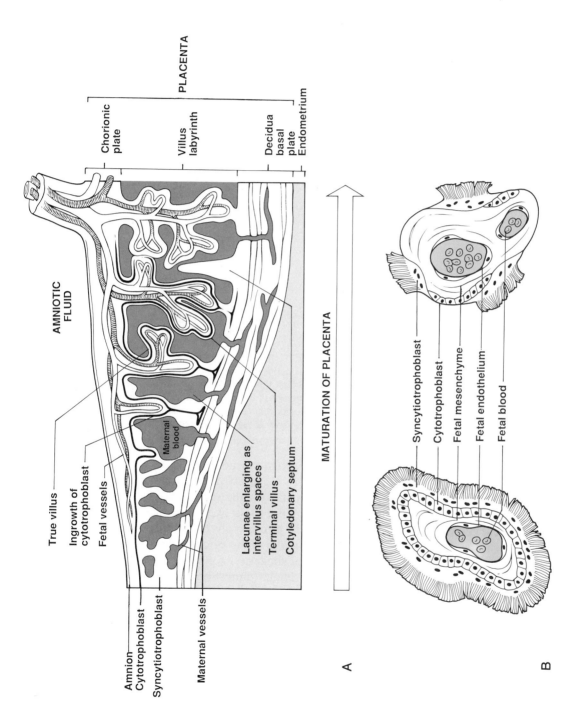

Fig. 3.4 (A) Gross morphology of the human placenta. Gestation advances from left to right. Placental mass increases, but hormonally active and invasive trophoblasts comprise a lesser percentage of the total mass as the placenta matures and evolves as an organ of transfer. (B) Anatomic structure of early and late terminal villi. These are transverse sections through terminal villi from early (left) and term (right) pregnancy. Cytotrophoblastic cells become infrequent with placental maturity, and increasing fibrin deposits occur by term gestation as placental function adapts more to transfer functions and relatively less to hormone production. Fetal capillary endothelium is the only structure separating maternal and fetal circulations. (Modified from Healy,[138] with permission.)

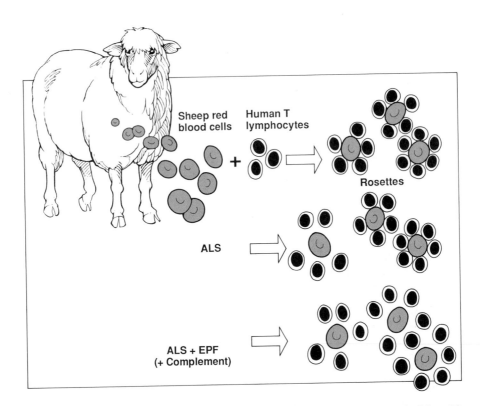

Fig. 3.5 Detection of early pregnancy factor by the rosette inhibition test (RIT). Approximately 80 to 90 percent of human T lymphocytes will bind spontaneously in vitro to sheep erythrocytes to form rosettes. Rosette formation is inhibited by antilymphocyte serum (ALS). Pregnancy serum contains a factor that reduces the amount of ALS required to produce inhibition by binding to the receptors on the red cells. This factor is the "early pregnancy factor."

bryo was later confirmed.[29] EPF appears within 48 hours after successful embryo transfer in in vitro fertilization patients. It disappears within 24 hours following induced abortion[4] and is undetectable in many spontaneous abortions and ectopic pregnancies.[4]

EPF Function in Pregnancy

EPF is believed to prevent rejection of an antigenically foreign embryo. Binding to a specific lymphocyte population, EPF recruits suppressor cells, which in turn release soluble suppressor factors that are believed to protect the pregnancy.[4]

hCG

Molecular Structure of hCG

hCG is a glycoprotein hormone with a structure similar to that of the pituitary glycoprotein hormones, follicle-stimulating hormone (FSH), LH, and thyroid-stimulating hormone (TSH). As are the other gly-coprotein hormones, hCG is composed of two non-identical, noncovalent subunits (Fig. 3.6).[12–14,18,20] The hCG α-subunit consists of 92 amino acids whose sequence is essentially identical to that of α-subunits of the pituitary glycoprotein hormones. Thus it is the β-subunit of these hormones that, despite some structural similarity, confers specific biologic activity on the intact (dimer) hormones. The β-subunits differ primarily at the COOH terminus; the β-subunit of hCG has a 30-amino acid tailpiece that is not present in the hLH β-subunit. Assuming an average carbohydrate content of 30 percent, the molecular mass of dimer hCG is approximately 36,700 daltons; the α-subunit contributes 14,500 and the β-subunit 22,200 daltons.[12,13,20]

hCG Variation During Pregnancy

Rising hCG production from hatching human blastocysts has been documented in vitro 6 days after fertilization.[8] There is no significant free α-hCG or β-hCG

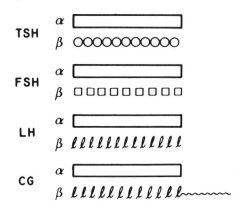

Fig. 3.6 Structural homology of human chorionic gonadotropin (hCG) and the three pituitary glycoprotein hormones LH, FSH, and TSH. The α-chain of hCG is biochemically and immunologically similar to the α-chain of the three pituitary glycoproteins. hCG and LH are structurally similar to one another except for a structurally distinct "tailpiece" at the terminus of the β-side chain of hCG. (Courtesy of Dr. Glenn Braunstein, Cedar Sinai Medical Center, Los Angeles, CA.)

subunit secretion in vitro at this time.[8] In vivo, hCG is secreted episodically and is detectable in maternal serum 9 to 11 days after conception.[9,30] Figure 3.7A depicts maternal levels of dimer hCG, α-hCG subunit, and β-hCG subunits (Fig. 3.7B) from 3 to 40 weeks gestational age.[18] At 4 weeks gestation, mean doubling times of dimer hCG are 2.2 (± 0.8 SD) days falling to 3.5 (±1.2 SD) days at 9 weeks.[18] The peak median level is 108,800 mIU/ml at 10 weeks.[18] Between 12 and 16 weeks, median dimer hCG decreases rapidly, with a mean halving time of 2.5 (±1.1 SD) days to become 25 percent of first-trimester peak values. Levels continue to fall from 16 to 22 weeks, at a slower mean halving rate of 4.1 (±1.8 SD) days to become 10.7 percent of peak first-trimester median hCG.[18] During the third trimester there is a gradual but statistically significant rise in mean hCG from 22 weeks until term.[18]

β-hCG subunit levels parallel dimer hCG levels during pregnancy (Fig. 3.7B). α-hCG, not detectable until about 6 weeks, rises in a sigmoid curve to reach peak levels at 36 weeks (Fig. 3.7B). Levels of α-hCG subunit are 2,000-fold to 150-fold less than dimer hCG, approximately, at 6 and 35 weeks, respectively[18] (Fig. 3.7C).

hCG production has a dose-dependent relationship to placental GnRH.[24] In an in vitro trophoblast

perfusion system, hCG is released in 11- to 22-minute pulses, where the pulse frequency and amplitude are entrained to the release of GnRH.[31] Thus in vitro GnRH augments hCG pulse frequency and amplitude, with the most marked responses observed in second-trimester placentas.[32] hCG production is stimulated by glucocorticoids and suppressed by dehydroepiandrosterone sulfate (DHEAS).[33] cAMP analogues augment secretion of hCG and α-hCG in vitro.[33,34]

Origin of hCG

hCG and its mRNA, localized respectively by histochemistry and in situ hybridization, is present in the outer syncytial layer and in some cytotrophoblastic cells that are developmentally intermediate.[18,21,22] α-hCG subunits are localized to the cytotrophoblasts with none in the syncytial layer.[18,21] The release of hCG in vivo has been correlated to the respective trophoblast layer microscopic widths from weeks 4 through 20 and to placental weights from 20 to 38 weeks (Tables 3.2 and 3.3).[18] Between 3 and 9 weeks gestation, rapidly rising dimer hCG coincides with proliferation of immature trophoblastic villi and an extensive syncytial layer.[18] Between 10 and 18 weeks gestation, declining hCG is associated with a relative reduction in syncytiotrophoblasts and cytotrophoblasts (Fig. 3.4). From 20 weeks until term, a gradual increase in dimer hCG corresponds with a gradual increase in placental weight and presumably villus volume.[18]

In summary, rising hCG coincides with histology that reflects a rapidly proliferating and invasive placenta. Falling hCG, associated with a relative reduction in cytotrophoblasts and syncytium, coincides with a morphologic transformation that reflects increasingly on the placenta as an organ of transfer.[18]

Function of hCG

hCG is luteotrophic.[35] It coregulates and stimulates both adrenal and placental steroidogenesis.[36] It also stimulates the fetal testes to secrete increasing testosterone to induce internal virilization.[37] It is immunosuppressive and may be involved in maternal lymphocyte function.[38] Finally, hCG possesses thyrotrophic activity.[39]

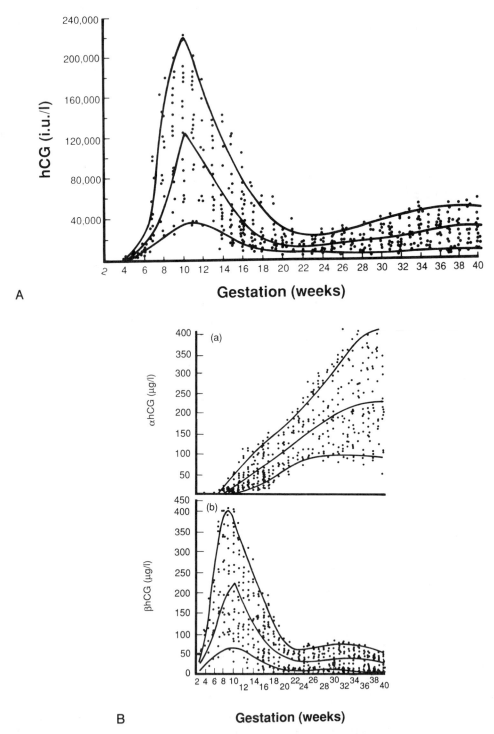

Fig. 3.7 (A) Dimer hCG levels (mlU/ml) in 500 serum samples collected between 3 and 40 weeks gestation (LMP) from 55 patients. The 5, 50, and 95 percentiles are shown. (B) Serum α-hCG (a) subunit and β-hCG (b) subunit levels measured directly without correcting for hCG cross-reaction, with 5, 50, and 95 percentiles. (*Figure continues.*)

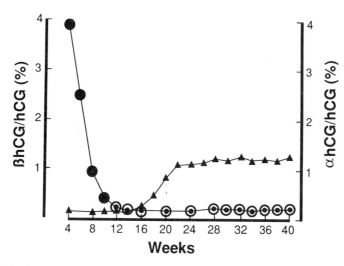

C   **Weeks**

Fig. 3.7 *(Continued)* (C) The mean percentage α-hCG/dimer (▲), β-hCG/dimer (●) hCG ratios between 3 and 40 weeks gestational age. (From Hay,[18] with permission.)

Table 3.2 Microscopic Widths of Placental Syncytium and Cytotrophoblast Layers Compared With hCG Titers at Gestational Ages 4 Through 20 Weeks

Gestation (Weeks)	Median hCG Titers (IU/L)	Syncytiotrophoblasts + Cytotrophoblasts (μm)		Syncytium (μm)		Average Ratio Syn. + Cyt.	No. of Placentas
		Mean	Range	Mean	Range	Syn.	
4	1885	15	(5–37)	13	(5–35)	1.1	3
6	12,870	17	(5–35)	11	(4–27)	1.6	5
8	56,010	25	(6–42)	7	(3–14)	3.6	7
10	108,800	21	(6–37)	5	(2–13)	4.2	5
12	99,260	13	(4–30)	5	(2–8)	2.6	3
14	52,760	10	(4–25)	4	(2–7)	2.5	2
16	35,810	7	(2–18)	4	(2–7)	1.7	2
18	22,630	6	(2–12)	4	(2–7)	1.5	1
20	16,110	4	(2–12)	3	(2–5)	1.3	2

Between 4 and 9 weeks gestation, an increasing ratio of cytotrophoblast to syncytiotrophoblast widths corresponds to rising hCG titers. After 8 to 10 weeks gestation, declining numbers of cytotrophoblasts in villi and the formation of the mature placenta coincide with falling dimer hCG, rising α-hCG, and barely decreased β-hCG subunit levels. (Modified from Hay,[18] with permission.)

hCS

Molecular Structure of hCS

hCS is a single-chain polypeptide with two intramolecular disulfide bridges. Its molecular mass is 22,308 daltons. Of the 191 amino acids, 167 (85 percent) are identical to human pituitary growth hormone and human pituitary prolactin (Fig. 3.8).[40,41] Accordingly,

hCS shares biologic properties with both growth hormone and prolactin.[42–44]

hCS Variation During Pregnancy

First detectable during the fifth gestational week, hCS concentrations rise throughout pregnancy but maintain a constant microgram/gram placental weight relationship.[43] Serum concentrations of hCS

Table 3.3 Comparison of Median Dimer hCG Titers and Placental Weight in Late Pregnancy From 20 to 38 Weeks Gestational Age

Gestation (Weeks)	No. of Patients	Median hCG Titers (IU/L)	Placental Weight (g)	
			Median	Range
20	11	15,110	110	(70–180)
22	10	11,670	130	(80–190)
24	12	14,100	150	(80–220)
26	12	17,730	190	(85–280)
28	12	18,210	240	(90–410)
30	12	22,030	260	(130–510)
32	14	20,200	280	(100–560)
34	15	22,900	300	(110–600)
36	15	25,900	320	(110–650)
38	13	21,400	320	(110–620)

Between 20 and 35 weeks, a secondary twofold increase in hCG titers coincides with a similar increase in average placental weight. (From Hay,[18] with permission.)

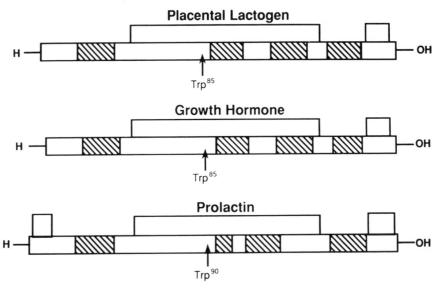

Fig. 3.8 Diagram of basic structural properties of human chorionic somatomammotropin (hCS), human growth hormone (hGH), and ovine prolactin (PRL). The bars represent the peptide chains, with the amino terminal to the left and the carboxyl terminal to the right. The shaded portions of each bar represent the recognizable areas, suggesting replicating sequences. The lines above the bars diagrammatically represent the position of disulfide bridges. (Modified from Niall et al.,[139] with permission.)

peak during the third trimester, with normal ranges from 3.3 to 25 μg/ml at that time (Fig. 3.9).[43–45] hCS is suppressed by maternal fasting and stimulating glucose intake.[44,45] hCS regulatory mechanisms are otherwise poorly understood.[41–45]

Origin of hCS

hCS is produced in the placental syncytiotrophoblasts as demonstrated by in situ mRNA hybridization and histochemical studies.[21–23]

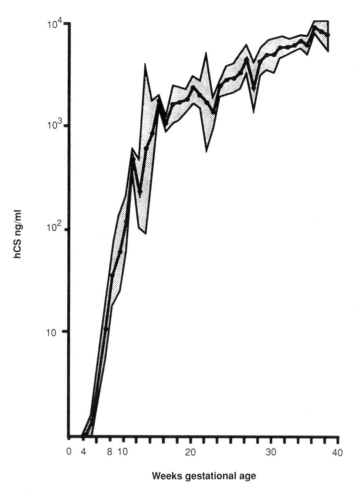

Fig. 3.9 Weekly concentrations of hCS (ng/ml) in maternal plasma throughout pregnancy. Solid dots represent the geometric mean, and the lines represent 95 percent confidence interval widths. LMP, last menstrual period. (From Braunstein et al.,[43] with permission.)

Function of hCS

Because hCS is produced in such an abundance by the placenta, intuitively its function would seem important. Thus it is surprising that women lacking the hCS gene and consequently having no hCS have pregnancies with entirely normal outcome.[46] hCS has weak somatotropic activity and stimulates somatomedin production in both pregnant and nonpregnant women.[47] In experimental animals, hCS has lactogenic activity.[48] hCS is stimulated by maternal intake of glucose and inhibits the insulin effect, in part causing the diabetogenic effect of pregnancy.[44,45,47,49,50]

AFP

Molecular Structure of AFP

AFP is a glycoprotein with a molecular mass of approximately 69,000.[51]

AFP Variation During Pregnancy

Detectable early in the first trimester, fetal plasma AFP peaks between 10 and 13 weeks gestational age and then declines exponentially from 14 to 32 weeks (Fig. 3.10).[26,52] The rapid fall in fetal plasma AFP concentration reflects increasing fetal blood volume

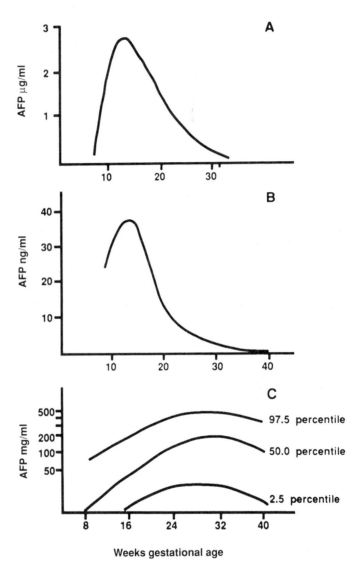

Fig. 3.10 Normal median concentrations of AFP in (A) fetal serum, (B) amniotic fluid, and (C) maternal serum. Maternal serum is shown with 2.5 and 97.5 percentile limits. (From Habib,[52] with permission.)

and a related decline in synthesis by fetal tissues. In contrast, amniotic fluid AFP (AFAFP) is detectable early in the first trimester, peaks between 12 and 14 weeks gestation, and then steadily declines to term (Fig. 3.10).[26,52] The concentration gradient between fetal plasma AFP and AFAFP is about 150- to 200-fold. Accordingly, if tiny amounts of fetal blood contaminate the amniotic fluid specimen, AFAFP will be spuriously elevated.[26] Detectable as early as 7 weeks gestation, maternal serum AFP (MSAFP) reaches peak concentrations between 28 and 32 weeks. Increasing placental permeability to fetal plasma proteins occurring with advancing gestation results in an apparent paradoxical rise in MSAFP, with decreased AFAFP and falling fetal serum AFP.[26,52]

Origin of AFP

AFP is believed to be synthesized principally in the yolk sac, gastrointestinal tract, and fetal liver.[53] It enters the fetal urine in abundance and is readily detected in the amniotic fluid.[26,53]

Function of AFP

AFP, structurally similar to albumin, may control fetal intravascular volume by osmoregulation.[26,52] It may also be involved in maintenance of the pregnancy immune privilege, as suggested by studies showing suppression of mitogen-induced lymphocyte proliferation.[54] AFAFP and MSAFP measurements are clinically important, because they are elevated in association with neural tube defects.[55] MSAFP is abnormally low in association with Down syndrome.[56] Clinical use of AFP in detecting neural tube defects and Down syndrome is considered in detail in Chapter 10.

Hypothalamic-Like Peptides: CRH, GnRH, and TRH

As discussed previously, the hypothalamic peptides (CRH, GnRH, SRIF, and TRH) have been histochemically localized to the cytotrophoblastic layer.[13,14-25] Likewise, the pituitary-like hormones (ACTH, hCG, hCS, and hCT) have been histochemically localized to the adjacent syncytiotrophoblastic layer.[17-19] This juxtaposition has raised the possibility that these two layers comprise a paracrine analogue of the hypothalamic–pituitary axis. Accordingly, the hypothalamic peptides and their corresponding pituitary hormone analogues are reviewed together. Unlike the hypothalamic–pituitary hormones, the end-organ feedback is not inhibitory in all cases, and placental proteins released may in some case involve positive feedback relationships with fetal steroids.

CRH and ACTH

Molecular Structures of Placental CRH and ACTH.
Hypothalamic CRH is a well-characterized peptide.[57] Placental CRH appears to be structurally similar to hypothalamic CRH.[58] The former shows immunoreactivity similar to hypothalamic CRH and is therefore readily measured by radioimmunoassay in amniotic fluid, fetal plasma, and maternal plasma.[59] Likewise, biologically active placental ACTH appears to be structurally similar to the putative pituitary ACTH 1-39 peptide.[57,59]

Normal CRH and ACTH Variation During Pregnancy.
CRH immunoreactivity has been measured in maternal plasma, fetal plasma, and amniotic fluid.[60,61] Ma-

ternal CRH levels increase sharply beginning week 20 of gestation, reaching the highest concentrations at term (Fig. 3.11).[60] Although concentrations in umbilical plasma are lower than in maternal plasma, there is a highly significant correlation between maternal and umbilical plasma CRH.[60] In amniotic fluid, there is an approximately threefold rise between the second and third trimesters.[61]

Origins of Placental CRH and ACTH.
Pro-CRH mRNA is present in the cytotrophoblast.[62] CRH activity, highest during the first trimester, diminishes toward term.[14,59] Also, there is intense CRH immunoreactivity in the fetal membranes and decidua.[14,59] Interestingly, both hypothalamic and placental CRH are products of the same gene, located on the long arm of chromosome 8.[62] Again, in parallel to the hypothalamic–pituitary axis, placental ACTH activity is localized histochemically to the syncytiotrophoblasts.[17]

Function of Placental CRH and ACTH.
A dose-dependent stimulation of placental ACTH by placental CRH mirrors that of the corresponding hypothalamic–pituitary peptides.[63] However, a paradoxical relationship exists between these placental peptides and their end-organ product, cortisol (Fig. 3.12). Glucocorticoids augment placental CRH and ACTH secretion.[63] After release into both the maternal and fetal circulations, placental CRH may stimulate the maternal and fetal pituitary as well as the placenta to secrete ACTH.[63,64] ACTH, from the maternal and fetal adrenal cortex, as well as from the placenta, in turn stimulates more glucocorticoid secretion (Fig. 3.12). Teliologically, this positive feedback mechanism allows an increase in glucocorticoid secretion in times of stress over and above the amount necessary if the mother was not pregnant.

Placental CRH and ACTH probably participate with the fetal hypothalamus and pituitary in the surge of fetal glucocorticoids associated with the late third trimester.

GnRH, hCG, and Inhibin

Molecular Structures of Placental GnRH, hCG (LH), and Inhibin.
Placental GnRH is biologically and immunologically similar to the hypothalamic decapeptide GnRH.[15,65] The molecular structure of hCG is described previously (see p. 64). Inhibin is a heterodi-

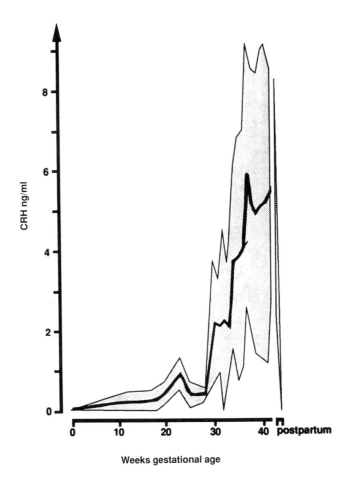

Fig. 3.11 Maternal serum concentrations of immunoreactive CRH in 256 individual pregnant women in relation to gestational age and at postpartum (mean ± SD). (From Stalla et al.,[60] with permission.)

meric glycoprotein with α- and β-subunits secreted by the adult ovary.[66,67]

GnRH, hCG, and Inhibin Variation During Pregnancy. GnRH activity in the syncytiotrophoblasts peaks at about 8 weeks gestation and decreases with advancing gestational age.[32] These changes in GnRH activity parallel those changes in placental hCG in both the placenta and the maternal circulation.[32] Inhibin levels have been studied only in term placental trophoblast cultures.[67]

Origins of Placental GnRH, hCG, and Inhibin. GnRH activity has been localized to cytotrophoblastic cells along the outer surface layer of the syncytiotrophoblast.[32] hCG is present in the syncytiotrophoblast layer, as described previously.[18] Inhibin-like immuno-

reactivity has been localized to the cytotrophoblast layer.[67] Although the amino acid sequence of human inhibin has been documented from cDNA sequences, only the α-chain RNA has been definitively identified in term placenta cDNA libraries.[66,67]

Function of Placental GnRH, hCG, and Inhibin. Placental GnRH stimulates release of hCG through a dose-dependent paracrine mechanism.[31] In tissue culture derived from first-trimester placenta, GnRH exerts little augmentation of hCG, because hCG production is already close to maximum.[32] In mid-trimester, however, GnRH markedly augments hCG release. This effect again diminishes in the term placenta.[32] As mentioned previously, in a superfusion system, pulsatile GnRH analogue significantly in-

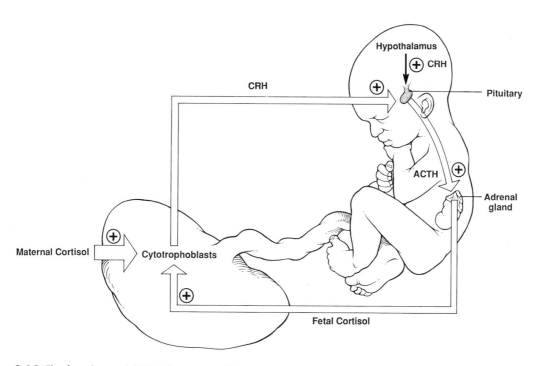

Fig. 3.12 The fetoplacental CRH–glucocorticoid positive feedback hypothesis. CRH, secreted by the placental trophoblast, enters the fetal circulation via the umbilical vein and stimulates (+) fetal ACTH release from the fetal pituitary. Fetal ACTH stimulates secretion of fetal adrenal cortisol, which enters the placental circulation via the umbilical artery. Cortisol further stimulates placental CRH secretion, thereby completing the positive feedback loop. Fetal CRH, secreted from the fetal hypothalamus, may independently stimulate fetal ACTH release, and placental and fetal hypothalamic CRH may be directly stimulated by environmental stresses. In addition, placental ACTH may stimulate the fetal adrenal directly. (Modified from Robinson et al.,[63] with permission.)

creases pulse amplitude and frequency of hCG secretion.[31] Placental inhibin may also function through a paracrine mechanism to inhibit GnRH release and, secondarily, hCG release.

TRH and hCT

TRH has been detected in the cytotrophoblast layer, but the molecule appears to be chromatographically different from synthetic TRH, a tripeptide.[68] Conversely, hCT is structurally similar to pituitary TSH α-subunit but has no demonstrated thyrotropic activity.[19] The placental content of hCT is very small.[19] hCG also has thyrotropic activity.[69] The significance of placental TRH/thyrotropin in fetal and maternal thyroid economy is not well understood.

Other Pregnancy-Related Peptides

Beside the chorionic glycoproteins, which are analogous to pituitary glycoprotein present in the non-pregnant state, the placenta secretes a host of proteins with no known analogue in the nonpregnant state.[70] One group of these proteins was first identified by producing an antiserum to serum drawn in term pregnancy. Antiserum was then used to isolate and identify the PAPP-A through -D. A second group was isolated by extraction of proteins from placental tissue that was later purified and characterized as pregnancy-specific β_1-glycoprotein (Schwanger-schaftsspeziffische protein 1 [SP1]).

Pregnancy-Specific β_1-Glycoprotein (SP1)

A glycoprotein circulating in heterogeneous forms, the predominant circulating species has a molecular mass of about 100,000 daltons. Secreted from trophoblastic cells, SP1 is detected 18 to 23 days post-ovulation.[71,72] SP1 rises exponentially, with an approximate doubling time of 2 to 3 days. Peak concentrations of 100 to 200 mg/L are reached at term. SP1 is a potent immunosuppressive of lymphocyte proliferation and therefore may prevent rejection of the conceptus.[73]

PAPP-A

PAPP-A is the largest of the pregnancy-related glycoproteins, with a molecular mass of 750,000 daltons. PAPP-A may actually originate from the maternal liver. It may thus be a response to pregnancy. With a mean detection time of 33 days postovulation, PAPP-A rises exponentially with a 3-day doubling time and continues to rise until term.[74] As a functional analogue of α_2-globulin, PAPP-A may play an immunosuppressive role during pregnancy.[75]

Placental Protein 5

A glycoprotein with a molecular mass of 36,000 daltons, placental protein 5 (PP5) is believed to be produced in the syncytiotrophoblasts. With a mean detection time of 42 days postovulation, PP5 increases until term.[76] Because PP5 has antithrombin and antiplasmic activities, it is believed to be a natural blood coagulation inhibitor active at the implantation site.[77]

FETOPLACENTAL STEROIDS

Ontogeny of Fetoplacental Steroid Production

The novel pregnancy peptides are in part responsible for the altered steroid milieu in pregnancy. In addition to stimulation of maternal hormones, the fetus and placenta produce and secrete steroids into the maternal circulation. The multiple sources of steroid production may replace each other in the event of a single system failure; however, it is more difficult to confirm contributions by, for example, the fetus or placenta as separate from that of the corpus luteum. The changes in maternal hormone concentrations are integrally related to metabolic and immunologic changes vital to intracorporeal gestation.

The Preimplantation Conceptus

Estradiol and progesterone, secreted by the conceptus and its cumulus, are detectable well before implantation in tissue culture media.[78] Human in vitro fertilization experiments demonstrate that early preimplantation concepti secrete approximately 50 ng of progesterone per day and approximately 100 pg of estradiol per day.[78]

There is little information on the regulation of steroid production by the preimplantation conceptus. Mechanical removal of the corona cells is associated with cessation of secretion, whereas return of the corona cells in coculture restores steroid secretion.[78] It is therefore likely that steroid production is negligible by the time the conceptus reaches the endometrial cavity, given that cumulus has been mechanically denuded during transport in the oviduct. Once implantation occurs and secretion of trophoblastic hCG and other pregnancy-related peptides is established, steroid production by the conceptus resumes.[78]

The Corpus Luteum

Although estradiol, progesterone, androstenedione, and 17α-hydroxyprogesterone are secreted by the human corpus luteum, progesterone is the secretory product of greatest importance.[79] Progesterone alone, if administered after luteectomy in early pregnancy, will prevent an otherwise certain abortion.[80] Corpus luteum steroid production is regulated by a complex interplay of steroid precursors and pituitary hormones (Fig. 3.13). Low-density lipoprotein (LDL) cholesterol is the principal precursor regulating corpus luteum progesterone production.[81] Progesterone secretion is maximal in corpora luteum obtained during the midluteal phase of the menstrual cycle. Corpus luteum hCG (LH) receptors, at their greatest concentration during the midluteal phase, stimulate LDL-binding sites on the corpus luteum, which in turn increase progesterone production (Fig. 3-13).[81]

In addition to LDL, FSH and LH, via their respective receptors, regulate progesterone secretion.[81] After binding to its receptor, FSH activates adenyl cyclase and cAMP to stimulate aromatase activity in the granulosa cell of the preovulatory follicle.[81] The granulosa cell then converts androstenedione from the theca and stromal cells into estradiol. Similarly, LH acts through cAMP to increase LDL receptors in the corpus luteum cell membrane, which in turn permits more LDL entry into the cell for conversion to progesterone.[81]

The Decidua

Cortisol is secreted by decidual tissues, much of it converted from circulating cortisone. In concert with hCG and progesterone, decidual cortisol probably

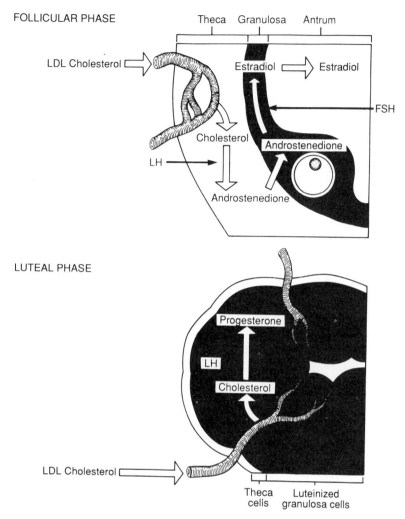

FOLLICULAR PHASE

LUTEAL PHASE

Fig. 3.13 Anatomic relationships governing the secretion of progesterone by the corpus luteum. An anatomic rearrangement of blood supply directly exposes LDL cholesterol to the luteinized cells, resulting in increased secretion of progesterone. (Modified from Carr et al.,[81] with permission.)

suppresses the maternal immune rejection response, further conferring immunologic privilege to the implanted conceptus.[82] The decidua probably converts and secretes other steroids, but this has not been extensively studied.

The Fetus and Placenta

The fetal adrenal cortex and placenta, serving as incomplete but complementary steroidogenic organs, function in concert to become the principal site of steroid production as gestation advances. After the seventh week of gestation, the corpus luteum wanes as the dominant steroid-secreting organ. Thereafter,

pregnancy will continue even if the corpus luteum is excised,[79-81] for in its stead is the beginning of the fetoplacental unit. At this time of gestation, pituitary basophilic cells are producing significant amounts of fetal ACTH and stimulating the fetal adrenal cortex, whose cells have been amassed for 4 weeks, awaiting trophic stimulation to synthesize its steroids.[82] This corresponds to the time in gestation when estriol is first detectable in the maternal circulation. The intricate interdependence of the fetal adrenal cortex and placenta allow these two relatively small organs to exchange, metabolize, and secrete more steroids than any other human endocrine tissue.

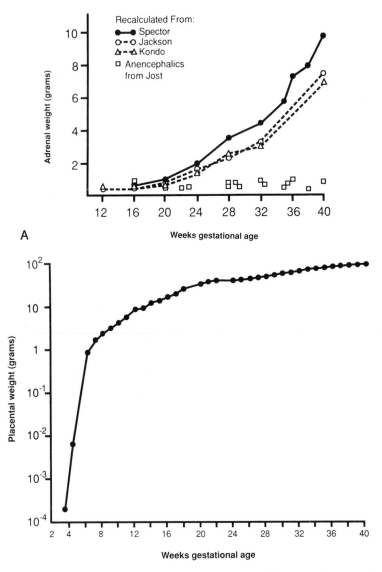

Fig. 3.14 (A) Growth of the fetal adrenal cortex. Total fetal adrenal mass is shown as a function of gestational age. Rapid increase in growth velocity occurs between 32 and 36 weeks gestation. In anencephalic pregnancies, adrenal mass does not increase after the second trimester. Data plotted from three separate reports.[85–87] (B) Growth of the placenta. Placental mass increases exponentially during the first trimester, with a gradual fall off in growth velocity at term. (From Buster,[88] with permission.)

The interdependence of these two organs is necessary, because the fetal adrenal cortex and placenta both contain incomplete but complementary steroidogenic enzyme systems. By constantly exchanging steroid precursors, together they produce the steroid profile characterizing normal pregnancy. As one might expect, nature has also evolved an organ that exists only in pregnancy to handle this unique function—the fetal zone of the adrenal cortex.[83,84] This zone comprises 80 percent of the fetal cortical mass and grows with increasing steroid requirements of pregnancy. Between 32 and 36 weeks (Fig. 3.14), a marked increase in fetal adrenal cortex growth velocity reflects the acceleration of fetal maturational pro-

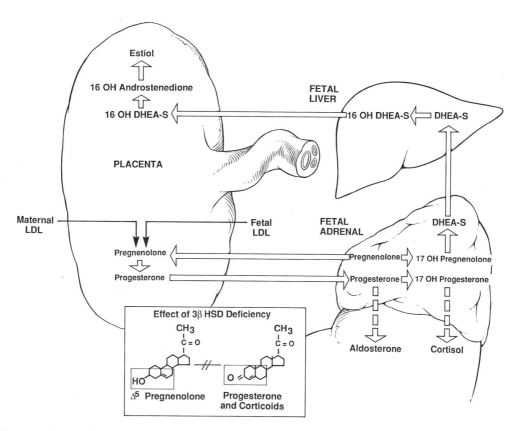

Fig. 3.15 Exchange of circulating steroid intermediates between adrenal fetal zone and placenta. Enzyme deficiencies of the fetal zone are offset by enzyme activities of the placenta, enabling the two organs to work as a mutual cooperative to produce an extensive profile of steroids not otherwise possible. The fetal adrenal cortex is functionally ucbdeficient in 3β-hydroxysteroid dehydrogenase, the enzyme that converts pregnenolone to progesterone and DHEA to androstenedione. The placenta contains 3β-hydroxysteroid dehydrogenase in abundance and can make this conversion. The placenta is deficient, however, in 17α-hydroxylase and cannot make corticoids.

cesses just before parturition.[85-88] This fetal zone then rapidly involutes postpartum.[84]

The anatomic distribution of key steroidogenic enzymes involved in the production of circulating intrauterine steroids is presented in Figure 3.15. The fetal adrenal cortex is functionally deficient in 3β-hydroxysteroid dehydrogenase, the enzyme that converts pregnenolone and DHEA to progesterone and androstenedione, respectively.[88,89] Therefore, the fetus cannot make progesterone or androstenedione, the immediate precursor to the sex steroids. The placenta, however, has an abundance of 3β-hydroxysteroid dehydrogenase. Therefore, the fetal adrenal cortex extracts LDL from the fetal circulation and converts it to pregnenolone sulfate and DHEAS.[88-91]

Pregnenolone sulfate is delivered through the umbilical artery to the placenta. The placenta converts pregnenolone to progesterone and returns the latter to the fetus for synthesis into mineralocorticoids and glucocorticoids. Interestingly, the placenta contains a relative lack of 17α-hydroxylase.[89] Teleologically, this deficiency may exist to prevent placental metabolism of progesterone, which is the destined precursor of fetal adrenal cortex corticosteroids.[89] The placenta also has the enzymatic capability to extract LDL cholesterol and to convert it into progesterone without relying on the fetal adrenal cortex.

The other fetal steroid precursor, DHEAS is first delivered to the fetal liver, where it is 16α-hydroxylated into 16α-hydroxydehydroepiandrosterone sul-

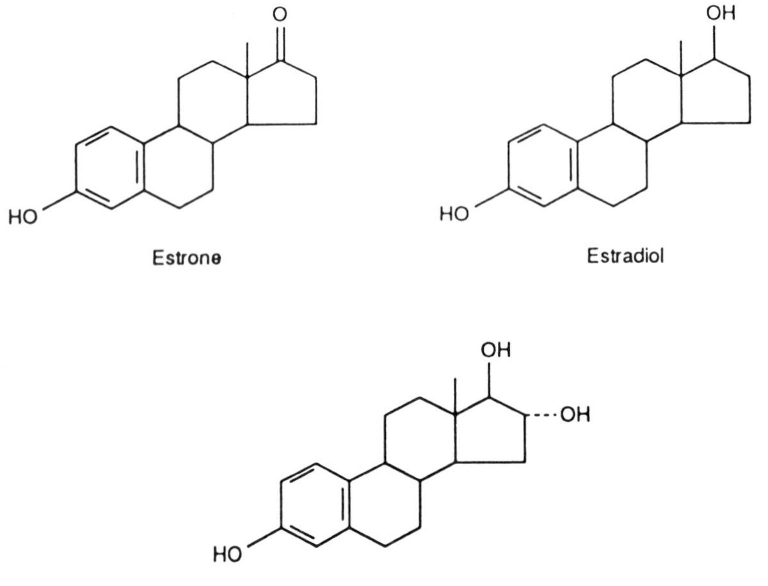

Fig. 3.16 Molecular structures of the estrogens. The basic 18-carbon estrane nucleus, shared by estrone, estradiol, and estriol, is modified for each by differences in the number and arrangement of hydroxyl groups.

fate (16α-OH DHEAS) before it is converted in the placenta first to 16α-hydroxyandrostenedione and then further aromatized into estriol.[89] The estrogens are then secreted into the maternal and fetal circulations.[89]

Besides the obvious functional interdependence of these two organs, the placenta also acts as a structural stimulator of the fetal adrenal cortex. In the first 20 weeks of gestation, placental hCG and progesterone play important roles in fetal adrenal cortex maintenance and regulation.[92] hCG stimulates fetal adrenal cortex production of DHEAS in vitro and in vivo.[93] Atrophy of the fetal zone after delivery may be in part due to removal of the trophic effect of hCG, although hCG appears to be less important after week 20 of gestation.[92,93] Indeed, the fetal adrenal cortex acquires increasing sensitivity to circulating ACTH, with advancing gestational age during the second half of gestation being primarily influenced by ACTH.[93-95] In addition, prolactin receptors have also been demonstrated in the adrenal cortex, and prolactin may therefore act in association with ACTH and hCG to regulate fetal adrenal cortex steroid production.[96,97] Accordingly, prolactin augments

ACTH-stimulated adrenal androgen production both in vivo and in vitro in the fetal baboon.[98]

Physiology of Fetoplacental Steroids

Fetoplacental estrogens, progestins, and corticoids are secreted abundantly into both fetal and maternal circulations. This section reviews molecular structures, normal variations, origins, and functions of the principal estrogens, progestins, and corticoids produced during pregnancy.

Estrogens: Estrone, Estradiol, and Estriol

Molecular Structures of Estrogens

Estrone, estradiol, and estriol share the same basic 18-carbon estrone nucleus but differ in the numbers and arrangements of hydroxyl groups (Fig. 3.16). That estriol has three hydroxyl groups allows it to be readily conjugated and excreted. This property makes estriol an ideal metabolite. In pregnancy, however, estriol is made in large amounts by the placenta and is secreted into the maternal circulation.

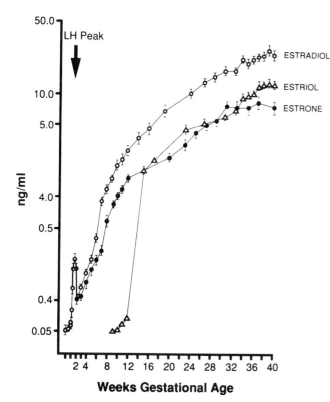

Fig. 3.17 Mean concentrations (± SEM) of estrone, estradiol, and estriol from conception to term. Unconjugated estriol is first detectable at about 9 weeks gestational age. Gestational ages are calculated from the last menstrual flow. (Modified from Buster et al.,[140] with permission.)

Estrogen Variation During Pregnancy

Maternal estrone concentrations are less than 0.1 ng/ml during the follicular phase and can reach 0.3 ng/ml during the luteal phase of a normal menstrual cycle.[7] After conception, estrone concentrations remain at luteal phase levels through 6 to 10 weeks. Subsequently there is a gradual increase to a range of approximately 2 to 30 ng/ml at term (Fig. 3.17).[99]

Maternal estradiol concentrations are less than 0.1 ng/ml during the follicular phase and reach 0.4 ng/ml during the luteal phase of normal menstrual cycles. After conception, estradiol increases gradually to a range of 6 to 30 ng/ml at term (Fig. 3.17).[99]

Maternal estriol levels are less than 0.01 ng/ml in nonpregnant women and reach 0.05 ng/ml at 9 weeks gestation. Estriol concentrations then increase gradu-

ally to approximately 10 to 30 ng/ml at term. Estriol concentrations increase sharply at 35 to 36 weeks, with the highest concentrations at 37 to 39 weeks.[99] This pattern probably reflects the final surge of intra-uterine steroidogenesis during the last weeks of prenatal life (Fig. 3.17).[99]

Origin of Estrogens

During the first 4 to 6 weeks of pregnancy, estrone originates primarily from maternal sources (ovaries, adrenal cortex, and peripheral conversion). After the first trimester, the placenta is the major source of circulating estrone, which is synthesized from maternal and fetal DHEAS.[89,100]

Estradiol originates almost exclusively from the maternal ovaries for the first 5 to 6 weeks. After this time, the placenta secretes increasing quantities of estradiol, which it synthesizes from conversion of circulating maternal and fetal DHEAS.[89,100]

Estriol originates from the placenta and is produced principally by placental conversion of fetal 16 α-OH DHEAS, which in turn is derived from fetal adrenal DHEAS.[89,100,101] Continued production of estriol is therefore dependent on the presence of a living fetus with intact adrenal cortex function.[102]

Function of Estrogens During Pregnancy

Estrogens stimulate the endometrium. The endometrium contains receptors for both estradiol and progesterone.[103] By the arrival of the preimplantation conceptus in the uterus, estradiol and progesterone have both stimulated the endometrium toward the full secretory structure that permits implantation and normal embryonic development.[104]

Estrogens augment uterine blood flow.[105] Because the uteroplacental bed is exposed to massive amounts of estriol, estriol may be primarily responsible for augmented uterine blood flow during pregnancy. It is excreted rapidly and thus exerts minimal peripheral effects.[105] Estriol may provide an important route of elimination for the estrogen precursors of pregnancy. High levels of more potent steroids must be eliminated after they play their role in the fetus but before they exert a similar effect in the mother. The maternal system tolerates higher levels of estriol than it does the more potent estrogens.

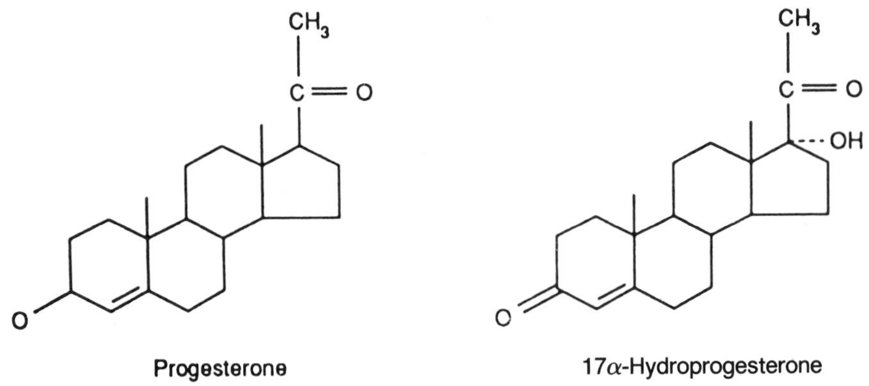

Fig. 3.18 Molecular structure of progestogens. The basic 21-carbon pregnene structure is shared in common by progesterone and 17α-hydroxyprogesterone. They differ in the number and arrangements in the hydroxyl groups.

Progestogens: Progesterone and 17α-Hydroxyprogesterone

Molecular Structures of Progestogens

Progesterone and 17α-hydroxyprogesterone share the same basic 21-carbon pregnene nucleus but differ in the numbers and arrangements of their hydroxyl groups (Fig. 3.18). Progesterone, the most biologically active progestin, is also higher in concentration than 17α-hydroxyprogesterone in the maternal circulation.[79,100] 17α-hydroxyprogesterone is probably a metabolic intermediate to progesterone and the corticosteroids.

Progestogen Variation During Pregnancy

Progesterone concentrations are less than 1 ng/ml during the follicular phase of the normal menstrual cycle. Progesterone concentrations rise to 1 to 2 ng/ml on the day of the LH peak, increase sharply, and plateau at 10 to 35 ng/ml over subsequent days. The luteal concentrations change little from conception through week 10; they then rise to reach 100 to 300 ng/ml at term (Fig. 3.19).[79,100]

17α-Hydroxyprogesterone concentrations are less than 0.5 ng/ml during the follicular phase of normal menstrual cycles. In conceptual cycles, 17α-hydroxyprogesterone concentration rises to about 1 ng/ml on the day of the LH peak, falls slightly for about 1 day, rises again over the subsequent 4 to 5 days to a level of 1 to 2 ng/ml, and then increases gradually to a mean of approximately 2 ng/ml (luteal phase levels) at the end of the 12 weeks. This level remains relatively stable until gestational week 32, when it abruptly rises, reaching a mean concentration of approximately 7.0 ng/ml at 37 weeks.[79,100] This abrupt rise is correlated with the terminal third-trimester surge of fetal corticosteroids initiated at this time (Fig. 3.19).[88,106]

Origin of Progestogens

Progesterone originates almost entirely from the corpus luteum before 5 to 6 weeks gestational age. At 7 weeks, the placenta begins production, and after 12 weeks it is the major source of progesterone.[79,89] The placenta contains all of the enzyme systems necessary to produce progesterone from circulating maternal LDL cholesterol and is only minimally dependent on fetal steroidogenesis for regulation of progesterone production.[79,89]

17α-Hydroxyprogesterone originates predominantly from the corpus luteum during the first trimester of pregnancy. The ovaries continue to be a significant source of 17α-hydroxyprogesterone until the third trimester. From about 32 weeks until term, however, the placenta secretes increasing amounts of 17α-hydroxyprogesterone, which is converted from 17α-hydroxy-Δ5-pregnenolone sulfate extracted from the fetal circulation.[79,88,89]

Function of Progestogens in Pregnancy

Progesterone affects maternal tubal motility, endometrial maturation, and uterine blood flow.[103,105] The preimplantation corona cells of the conceptus secrete progesterone and estradiol long before implantation.[78,107] Progesterone, secreted by the conceptus as

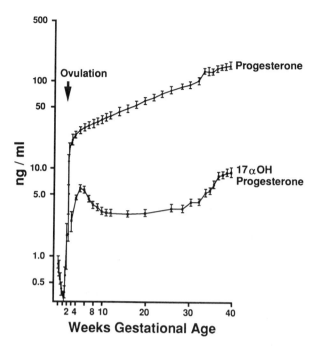

Fig. 3.19 Mean concentrations (± SEM) of progesterone and 17α-hydroxyprogesterone from conception until term. Data are compiled from several reports. 17α-Hydroxyprogesterone shows a marked rise in concentrations beginning at 32 weeks until term. Gestational ages are calculated from the last menstrual flow. (Modified from Buster et al.,[141] with permission.)

it is carried to the uterus, is believed to relax uterotubal musculature. Progesterone receptors are concentrated in the mucosal layer of the distal one-third of the fallopian tube, the site where ova and sperm are most likely to meet.[108] Estradiol secreted by the con-

ceptus may balance the effects of progesterone to maintain the desired level of tubal motility and tone.[107,108]

Progesterone is involved with implantation. It inhibits T-lymphocyte-mediated tissue rejection in concert with hCG and decidual cortisol.[109] Inhibition of rejection may confer immunologic privilege to the implanted conceptus and developing placenta. Thus high intervillous concentrations of progesterone are of major importance in blocking the rejection of foreign proteins.[109] Progesterone retards uterine blood flow.[110] It reverses the effects of estrogen by depleting cytoplasmic estrogen receptors.[111] Progesterone and estrogen thus appear to balance one another in the maintenance of normal blood flow to the implantation site.[110,111]

Adrenocorticoids: Cortisol and Cortisone

Molecular Structure of Adrenocorticoids

The adrenocorticoids, despite having the same 21-carbon pregnane structure as progesterone, differ markedly in their biologic activity because of the additional hydroxyl and ketone groups (Fig. 3.20).

Corticoid Variation During Pregnancy

Fetal plasma and amniotic fluid cortisol and cortisol sulfate concentrations increase considerably with advancing gestational age, particularly with the approach of parturition.[106,112,113] These increased concentrations are believed to reflect increasing corticoid production principally from the fetal adre-

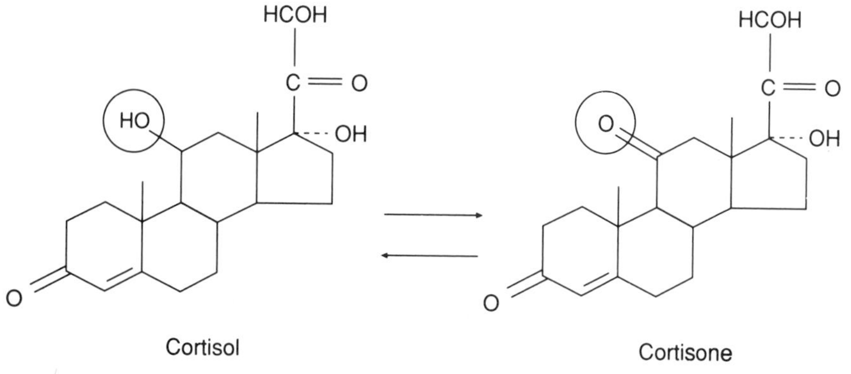

Fig. 3.20 Molecular structure of the corticoids. Cortisol and cortisone differ from progesterone in the number and arrangements of hydroxyl groups.

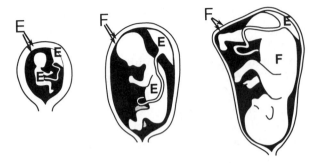

Fig. 3.21 Mechanism of intrauterine cortisol (F) modulation. Target organ cells autoregulate F interaction with corticoid receptors by diverting F (cortisol) to E (cortisone) through 11 β-hydroxysteroid dehydrogenase interconversion. Net conversion shifts toward F approaching term, but this varies with the organs studied. (From James et al.,[142] with permission.)

nal cortex but also from peripheral conversion of cortisone to cortisol.[82]

Maternal corticoid concentrations are elevated throughout gestation in part because of increased circulating cortisol-binding globulin (CBG). There is also a significant increase in free maternal cortisol. Maternal cortisol is resistant to exogenous corticoid suppression, presumably because of the effects of placental paracrine CRH and ACTH.[64]

Origin of Corticoids

The concentrations of circulating adrenocorticoids are determined by fetal adrenal secretion, peripheral steroid interconversions of cortisone to cortisol, and transplacental transfer of cortisol from the maternal circulation. Interconversions of cortisol to cortisone and cortisone to cortisol take place in the placenta, fetal lung, pancreas, gastrointestinal tract, spleen, kidney, and skin. Increasing corticoid concentrations found in the fetal circulation and in amniotic fluid approaching term thus represent effects of both increased cortisone to cortisol conversion and increased fetal adrenal corticoid secretion[82,112,113] (Fig. 3.21).

Although maternal glucocorticoids are derived predominantly from the maternal adrenal, circulating fetal adrenocorticoids are from three sources: fetal adrenal secretion, transplacental transfer of cortisol from the maternal circulation, and peripheral con-

version of cortisone to cortisol.[82] The conversion of cortisol to cortisone and vice versa takes place in the placenta, fetal lung, pancreas, gastrointestinal tract, spleen, kidneys, and skin. Increasing corticoid concentrations are found in the fetal circulation. As term approaches, the fetal adrenal cortex increases its corticoid secretion, more cortisone being converted to cortisol.[82,112,113] Thus amniotic fluid and fetal corticoid circulation increases dramatically (Fig. 3.21).

Function of Corticoids in Pregnancy

It is not surprising that the function of corticoids is a vital part of fetal maturation, as nature has assembled a variety of sources that in aggregate produce a dramatic increase in corticoid concentration.[106,114] Should one source fail, others can replace these hormones, which are responsible for the induction of enzymes in many organ systems.

Cortisol stimulates pulmonary surfactant production.[115] In association with thyroxine, prolactin, and estrogens, it stimulates choline phosphotransferase at about 34 to 36 gestational weeks to produce diplamitoyl lecithin, the principal surface-active phospholipid.[114–116] This increases the lecithin/sphingomyelin (L/S) ratio.

Mirroring the L/S ratio, the relative concentrations of liver glycogen increase with advancing gestation, with glycogen deposition controlled by cortisol.[117] Glycogen availability in the newborn is critical to its extrauterine adaptation. During the first 24 hours of life, continued blood glucose delivery to the brain is dependent on liver glycogen stores.[114]

Cortisol induces the adrenal medullary enzyme phenylethanolomine-N-methyltransferase, which converts norepinephrine to epinephrine. Thus, with advancing gestation, more epinephrine than norepinephrine is produced.[118]

Cortisol also induces duodenal alkaline phosphatase activity, which coincides with a sharp decrease in the ability of the gut to absorb antibodies. It also induces the multiple hepatic enzymes necessary for carbohydrate, protein, and fat metabolism. In experimental animals, cortisol is related to maturation of the hypothalamic–pituitary–adrenal axis, to CNS growth, and to hypothalamic rhythmicity.[114]

PREGNANCY DIAGNOSIS AND MONITORING

The novel hormones secreted only in pregnancy may be used for diagnosing and measuring deviations from normal. A variety of assay techniques with varying sensitivities are available to detect and measure these hormones.

hCG

Intact hCG

hCG and both subunits α-hCG and β-hCG rise predominantly during the first trimester. It is the intact hCG, however, that is measured to diagnose a pregnancy, although most assays depend on binding to the β-subunit of the intact molecule. hCG is detectable 9 to 11 days following ovulation, doubling every 1.3 to 2 days until its concentration reaches 100 mIU/ml at the time of the first missed menses.[9,18] Doubling slows to approximately every 2 to 3 days until 8 weeks gestation.[18] Deviation from this normal pattern suggests that the pregnancy is either ectopic in site or about to abort spontaneously. Thus, if hCG fails to rise 66 percent in 2 days, ancillary procedures are then necessary to differentiate the two possibilities.[119]

hCG levels can also be abnormally elevated. Multiple gestation and gestational trophoblastic neoplasia are the most likely causes; however, ovarian tumors such as embryonal cell carcinoma can also secrete hCG.[120]

hCG Subunits

Although the binding sites on the intact β-subunits are important in detecting the intact molecule, the measurement of the β-subunit alone is not clinically helpful during pregnancy. Unlike the hCG β-subunit, which rises in parallel to intact hCG, the α-subunit is first detectable at gestational week 6 and rises in sigmoid fashion to peak at gestational week 36.[18] In general, α-hCG is of little value for clinical interpretation although concentrations are elevated by persistent gestational trophoblastic neoplasia and are significantly lower in insulin-dependent diabetic women during first and second trimesters than in normal controls.[121,122]

Pregnancy Tests

The choice of pregnancy tests from the wide variety available (Table 3.4) depends on use of the test.[123] For example, in the emergency room, detection of ectopic pregnancy requires a test with a higher sensitivity than that used in an office to diagnose a normal pregnancy.

Radioimmunoassay

The radioimmunoassay (RIA) is the conventional clinical laboratory technique for measuring hCG.[123,124] hCG is labeled with a radioactive substance and is displaced from binding sites on an antibody directed against it by unlabeled hCG in the patient's serum. If no antibody is displaced, then there is no hCG in the patient's serum. If all is displaced then the patient's serum contains a high quantity of hCG. Therefore, one can make a quantitative measurement, useful in determining doubling times for management of ectopic pregnancy, spontaneous abortion, or gestational trophoblastic neoplasia. Although very precise, the RIA has limited sensitivity and requires hours to perform.[123,124] Thus RIAs are being replaced by the technically simpler immunoradiomimetic assay (IRMA).

IRMA

IRMA hCG assays require only about 30 minutes to complete and are highly sensitive to low concentrations of hCG.[125] IRMAs use a radioactive antibody to detect directly the hCG in the patient's serum. Briefly, anti-hCG antibodies are bound to a test tube, the patient's serum is added, and a second labeled antibody binds to the hCG–antibody complex already on the tube. The amount of labeled antibody bound to the tube is proportional to the amount of hCG in the patient's serum. The hCG molecule is thus "sandwiched" between two antibodies.[125] This "sandwich" assay is also the principle underlying the nonradioactive enzyme-linked immunosorbent assay (ELISA).

ELISA

ELISAs do not use radioisotopes.[126] The principle is the same as that of IRMA; however, instead of using a radiolabeled second antibody, the second antibody is

Table 3.4 Commercial Assays Available for Detection and Measurements of hCG

Technique	Radioactive Tracer Required	Sensitivity (mIU/ml)	Completion Time (Minutes)	Gestational Age When Positive (Weeks)	Tests Available
RIA	Yes	5	4 hours	3–4	Many products available
IRMA	Yes	150	30	4	Neocept
		1,500	2	5	Prognosis
ELISA	No	25	80	3.5	Model
		<50	15	4	Sensichrome, Quest
		<50	5	4	Confidot, Test Pack, Icon
		175	20	4–5	Preganstick
		200	4	4–5	Ventrascreen
FIA	No	1.0	2–3 hours	3.5	None commercially available

The ELISA and FIA assays do not require radioactive tracers.

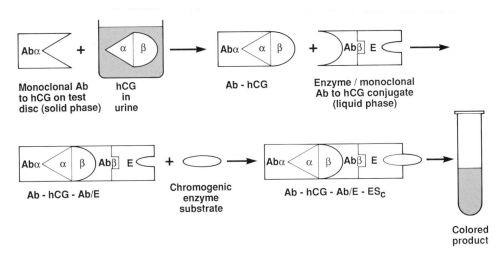

Fig. 3.22 Principle of enzyme-linked immunoassay (ELISA). In hCG ELISA, two antibodies are allowed to interact separately with the α- and β-subunits of the hCG molecule to form a sandwich around the entire hCG molecule. In ELISA, the first antibody, bound to the wall of the test tube, binds with α-subunit hCG. A second antibody binds with the β-subunit. Patient serum containing hCG is then added to the polystyrene tube with the immobilized anti α-hCG and allowed to incubate so that binding takes place. The anti-β-hCG, bound to an enzyme label, is added, and an additional incubation takes place. The sandwich, consisting of the polystyrene-bound anti-α-hCG, the hCG molecule, and the enzyme-labeled anti-β-hCG, is formed. After each incubation, the tube is washed with removal of unbound enzyme. The labeled antibody forms a blue color quantitatively in an enzyme-catalyzed colorimetric reaction. These results are determined visually by comparing the intensity of the blue color developed in a specimen to that of a positive reference. hCG, human chorionic gonadotropin α- and β-subunits; Ab_{α}, monoclonal antibody to the α-subunit of hCG; Ab_{β}, monoclonal antibody to the β-subunit of hCG. (Modified from Fletcher,[143] with permission.)

Table 3.5 Detection Time for Embryologic Structures by Vaginal Ultrasound

Embryonic/Fetal Structure	Gestational Age at Detection
Gestational sac	4 weeks 1–3 days
Yolk sac	5 weeks
Fetal heartbeats	5 weeks 6 days
Limb buds	8 weeks
Head	8 weeks
Ventricles	8 weeks 2–4 days
Choroid plexus	9 weeks
Hand, fingers	12 weeks

(Modified from Timor-Tritsch and Rottem,[133] with permission.)

labeled with a substance that can be detected by a color change after binding (Fig. 3.22). Although not as precise as IRMA, ELISA is sensitive and quick, making it ideal for early pregnancy diagnosis. ELISA assays can detect hCG at concentrations as low as 10 mIU/ml, allowing diagnosis up to 5 days before the first missed menses.[126]

Fluoroimmunoassay

The newest clinical laboratory method for hCG testing is the fluoroimmunoassay (FIA).[127] This technique is another "sandwich" assay in which the second antibody is labeled with a fluorescent label. Proportional to the amount of hCG in the test serum, the fluorescence emitted allows for detection of concentrations as low as 1 mIU/ml. The technique takes 2 to 3 hours, uses no radioactivity, and is highly precise. The FIA could replace all tests currently used to detect and follow hCG concentrations.

EPF

Even the highly sensitive FIAs can detect pregnancy only after hCG produced by the pregnancy is secreted into the maternal bloodstream after implantation.[9] Thus detection cannot be made until 9 to 11 days after conception.[9] Pregnancy diagnosis before this time may be possible through measurement of EPF, which seems to be detectable 24 to 48 hours after fertilization and cannot be detected 24 hours after delivery or termination of an ectopic or intrauterine pregnancy.[4]

Detection of EPF currently depends on a cumbersome biologic assay, the rosette inhibition test.[4,28] EPF inhibits binding of lymphocytes labeled with antibody to their antigen on sheep red blood cells.[4,28] If EPF is present, red cells form fewer rosettes than if EPF were not present (Fig. 3.5). The tediousness of the assay makes it very difficult to perform and interpret and has even led some to doubt whether EPF truly exists as a separate pregnancy-related protein.[28] However, EPF has recently been isolated, identified, and sequenced. Therefore, an RIA or related assay surely will become available for EPF measurement.[27]

Diagnosis of conception before implantation will open possibilities for contraception, for preimplantation genetics through uterine lavage, and for more accurate dating of intrauterine pregnancies. A posi-

Table 3.6 Appearance of Key Embryologic Structures in Association With Rising hCG Titers

Ultrasound Findings	Days from LMP	β-hCG (mIU/ml)	
		First IRP	Second International Standard
Sac	34.8 ± 2.2	1,398 ± 155	914 ± 106
Fetal pole	40.3 ± 3.4[a]	5,113 ± 298[a]	3,783 ± 683
Fetal heart motion	46.9 ± 6.0[a]	17,208 ± 3,772[a]	13,178 ± 2,898[a]

Failure to identify these structures in the uterus as hCG rises above these levels suggests ectopic pregnancy.

[a] $p < 0.05$ when compared with sac.

Abbreviations: IRP, international reference preparation.

(From Fossum et al.,[134] with permission.)

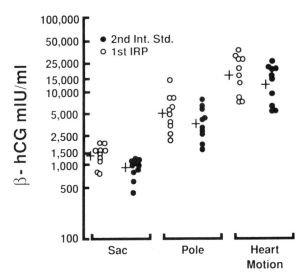

Fig. 3.23 Range of β-hCG titers (IRP) and predicted developmental landmarks detected by vaginal ultrasound. (Modified from Fossum et al.,[134] with permission.)

tive EPF result with a negative hCG result will pinpoint the date of conception within 5 days.

Progesterone

Progesterone concentrations in the first trimester of pregnancy may be helpful in determining fetal viability. A single progesterone measurement of 5 ng/ml or less rules out a viable intrauterine pregnancy[128]; a level of 25 ng/ml or more excludes 98 percent of ectopic pregnancies.[129] A progesterone value of 5 ng/ml or less allows the physician to perform a dilatation and curettage without fear of interfering with a viable pregnancy.[128] If villi are found, the patient is unlikely to have an ectopic pregnancy.[128]

RIAs are available that measure progesterone. They usually require 3 to 4 hours to perform.[130] FIAs are also available to measure progesterone, and they offer the advantage of avoiding radioactivity.[131]

Ultrasound and Hormone Measurements

Combined with hCG and progesterone measurements, ultrasound is helpful in determining the viability and location of a pregnancy (Tables 3.5 and 3.6).[132] Transvaginal ultrasound allows detection of an intrauterine pregnancy as early as 4.5 weeks from the last menstrual period,[133] when the gestational sac

measures 4 to 5 mm. At gestational week 5, the yolk sac becomes visible; at the end of the fifth week, all intrauterine pregnancies are detectable by transvaginal ultrasound (Table 3.5).[134] Fetal cardiac activity is detected just before gestational week 6.[133] In a well-timed pregnancy, these ultrasonographic milestones are useful to detect deviations from the norm. Table 3.6 correlates key embryologic structures with hCG levels.[134] When combined with serum measurements of hCG, detection of embryonic structure is vital in diagnosing ectopic gestation and impending spontaneous abortion.[132,134,135]

All patients with a healthy intrauterine pregnancy whose hCG level is 6,500 mIU/ml have a gestational sac visible by transabdominal ultrasound.[135] Similarly, transvaginal ultrasound visualizes all intrauterine pregnancies when the hCG level exceeds 2,400 mIU/ml (Fig. 3.23).[134] When hCG levels exceed these concentrations and no intrauterine pregnancy is detected by ultrasound, either a curettage or a laparoscopy must be employed to diagnose an ectopic pregnancy.[132] Conversely, a heartbeat detected at 8 gestational weeks assures a patient that her chance of continuing her pregnancy is 98 percent.[136]

CONCLUSIONS

No biologic events can exceed the events considered in this chapter in the long-term importance to human development. Endocrine factors always play important roles in the orchestration and outcome of these events. It is a privilege to detect, measure, observe, and occasionally assist nature in the nourishment and protection of the growing fetus in the otherwise invisible confines of the uterus.

REFERENCES

1. Cavanagh AC, Morton H, Rolfe BE et al: Ovum factor: a first signal of pregnancy? Am J Reprod Immunol 2:97, 1982
2. Shaw FD, Morton H: The immunological approach to pregnancy diagnosis: a review. Vet Rec 106:268, 1980
3. Morton H, Hegh V, Clunie GJ: Studies of the rosette

inhibition test in pregnant mice: evidence of immuno-suppression? Proc R Soc Lond [Biol] 193:413, 1976

4. Morton H, Rolfe BE, Cavanagh AC: Ovum factor and early pregnancy factor. Curr Top Dev Biol 23:73, 1987

5. Croxatto HB, Ortiz ME, Diaz S et al: Studies on the duration of egg transport by the human oviduct. II. Ovum location at various times following luteinizing hormone peak. Am J Obstet Gynecol 132:629, 1978

6. Buster JE, Bustillo M, Rodi IA et al: Biological and morphologic development of donated human ova recovered by nonsurgical uterine lavage. Am J Obstet Gynecol 153:211, 1985

7. Edwards RG: Causes of early embryonic loss in human pregnancy. Hum Reprod 1:185, 1986

8. Hay DL, Lopata A: Chorionic gonadotropin secretion by human embryos in vitro. J Clin Endocrinol Metab 67:1322, 1988

9. Kosasa, T, Levesque L, Goldstein DP, Taymor ML: Early detection of implantation using a radioimmunoassay specific for human chorionic gonadotropin. J Clin Endocrinol Metab 36:622, 1973

10. Enders A: Embryo implantation with emphasis on the rhesus monkey and the human. Reproduction 5:163, 1981

11. Edwards R: Conception in the Human Female. Academic Press, San Diego, 1980

12. Schlafke S, Enders A: Cellular basis of the interaction between trophoblast and uterus at implantation. Biol Reprod 12:41, 1975

13. Chard T: Proteins of the human placenta: some general concepts. p. 6. In Grudzinskas JG, Teisner BL, Sepala M (eds): Pregnancy Proteins: Biology Chemistry and Clinical Application. Academic Press, San Diego, 1982

14. Saijonmaa O, Laatikainen T, Wahlstrom T: Corticotrophin-releasing factor in human placenta: localization, concentration and release in vitro. Placenta 9:373, 1988

15. Khodr GS, Siler-Khodr TM: Placental luteinizing hormone-releasing factor and its synthesis. Science 207:315, 1980

16. Shambaugh G III, Kubek M, Wilber JF: Thyrotropin-releasing hormone activity in the human placenta. J Clin Endocrinol Metab 48:483, 1979

17. Al-Timimi A, Fox H: Immunohistochemical localization of follicle-stimulating hormone, luteinizing hormone, growth hormone, adrenocorticotropic hormone and prolactin in the human placenta. Placenta 7:163, 1986

18. Hay DL: Placental histology and the production of human choriogonadotropin and its subunits in pregnancy. Brit Obstet Gynaecol 95:1268, 1988

19. Harada A, Hershman JM: Extraction of human chorionic thyrotropin (hCT) from term placentas: failure to recover thyrotropic activity. J Clin Endocrinol Metab 47:681, 1978

20. Steiner DF: Peptide hormone precursors: biosynthesis, processing, and significance. p. 49. In Parsons JA (ed): Peptide Hormones. University Park Press, Baltimore, 1976

21. Hoshina M, Hussa R, Pattillo R et al: The role of trophoblast differentiation in the control of the hCG and hPL genes. Adv Exp Med Biol 176:299, 1984

22. Hoshina M, Boime I, Mochizuki M: Cytological localization of hPL, hCG, and mRNA in chorionic tissue using in situ hybridization. Acta Obstet Gynaecol Jpn 36:397, 1984

23. Kurman RJ, Young RH, Norris HJ et al: Immunocytochemical localization of placental lactogen and chorionic gonadotropin in the normal placenta and trophoblastic tumors, with emphasis on intermediate trophoblast and the placental site trophoblastic tumor. Int J Gynecol Pathol 3:101, 1984

24. Kasai K, Shik SS, Yoshida Y: Production and localization of human prolactin in placenta and decidua in early and at term normal pregnancy. Nippon Naibunpi Gakkai-Zasshi 56:1574, 1980

25. Watkins WB, Yen SS: Somatostatin in cytotrophoblast of the immature human placenta: localization by immunoperoxidase cytochemistry. J. Clin Endocrinol Metab 50:969, 1980

26. Milunsky A: The prenatal diagnosis of neural tube and other congenital defects. p. 452. In Milunsky A (ed): Genetic Disorders and the Fetus. Plenum, New York, 1986

27. Mehta AR, Eessalu TE, Aggarwal BB: Purification and characterization of early pregnancy factor from human pregnancy sera. J Biol Chem 264:2266, 1989

28. Chard T, Grudzinskas JG: Early pregnancy factor. Biol Res Pregnancy Perinatol 8:53, 1987

29. Mesrogli M, Schneider J, Maas DH: Early pregnancy factor as a marker for the earliest stages of pregnancy in infertile women. Human Reprod 3:113, 1988

30. Owens OM, Ryan KJ, Tulchinsky D: Episodic secretion of human chorionic gonadotropin in early pregnancy. J Clin Endocrinol Metab 53:1307, 1981

31. Barnea ER, Kaplan M: Spontaneous, gonadotropin-releasing hormone-induced, and progesterone-inhibited pulsatile secretion of human chorionic gonadotropin in the first trimester placenta in vitro. J Clin Endocrinol Metab 69:215, 1989

32. Siler-Khodr TM, Khodr GS, Valenzuela G: Gonadotropin-releasing hormone effects on placental hormones during gestation. I. Alpha-human chorionic gonadotropin, human chorionic gonadotropin and human chorionic somatomammotropin. Biol Reprod 34:245, 1986

33. Haning RV Jr, Choi L, Kiggens AJ et al: Effects of dibutyryl adenosine 3', 5'-monophosphate, luteinizing hormone-releasing hormone, and aromatase inhibitor on simultaneous outputs of progesterone, 17 beta-estradiol, and human chorionic gonadotropin by term placental explants. J Clin Endocrinol Metab 55:213, 1982

34. Kato Y, Braunstein GD: Discordant secretion of placental protein hormones in differentiating trophoblasts in vitro. J Clin Endocrinol Metab 68:814, 1989

35. Hanson FW, Powell JE, Stevens VC: Effects of hCG and human pituitary LH on steroid secretion and functional life of the human corpus luteum. J Clin Endocrinol Metab 32:211, 1971

36. Seron-Ferre M, Lawrence CC, Jaffee RB: Role of hCG in the regulation of the fetal zone of the human fetal adrenal gland. J Clin Endocrinol Metab 46:834, 1978

37. Huhtaniemi IT, Korenbrot CC, Jaffe RB: hCG binding and stimulation of testosterone biosynthesis in the human fetal testis. J Clin Endocrinol Metab 44:963, 1977

38. Adcock EW III, Teasdale F, August CS et al: Human chorionic gonadotropin: its possible role in maternal lymphocyte suppression. Science 181:845, 1973

39. Nisula BC, Ketelslegers JM: Thyroid stimulating activity and chorionic gonadotropin. J Clin Invest 54:494, 1974

40. Josimovich JB: Human placental lactogen. p. 191. In Fuchs F, Klopper A (eds): Endocrinology of Pregnancy. Harper & Row, New York, 1977

41. Gordon YB, Chard T: The specific proteins of the human placenta—some new hypotheses. p. 1. In Klopper A, Chard T (eds): Human Placental Proteins. Springer-Verlag, Amsterdam, 1979

42. Grumbach MM, Kaplan SL: Clinical investigation. p. 382. In Peelie A, Muller EE (eds): Second International Symposium on Growth Hormone. Excerpta Medica, Amsterdam, 1971

43. Braunstein GD, Rasor JL, Wade ME: Interrelationships of human chorionic gonadotropin, human placental lactogen, and pregnancy specific beta-1 glycoprotein throughout normal human gestation. Am J Obstet Gynecol 138:1205, 1980

44. Kim YJ, Felig P: Plasma human chorionic somatomammotropin levels during starvation in midpregnancy. J Clin Endocrinol Metab 32:864, 1971

45. Belleville F, Lasbennes A, Nabet P et al: hCS regulation in cultured placenta: action of glucose. Acta Endocrinol (Copenh) 92:336, 1979

46. Simon P, Decoster C, Brocas H et al: Absence of human chorionic somatomammotropin during pregnancy associated with two types of gene deletion. Hum Genet 74:235, 1986

47. Sara V, Hall K: Somatomedins and the fetus. Clin Obstet Gynecol 23:765, 1980

48. Samaan N, Yen SCC, Gonzales D: Metabolic effects of placental lactogen (hPL) in man. J Clin Endocrinol Metab 28:485, 1968

49. Williams C, Coltart TM: Adipose tissue metabolism in pregnancy: the lipolytic activity of human placental lactogen. Br J Obstet Gynaecol 85:43, 1978

50. Grumbach MM, Kaplan SL, Sciarra JJ et al: Chorionic growth hormone-prolactin: secretion, disposition, biologic activity in man, and postulated function as the "growth hormone" of the second half of pregnancy. Ann NY Acad Sci 148:501, 1968

51. Alpert E, Drysdale JW, Isselbacher KJ et al: Human fetoprotein: isolation, characterization, and demonstration of microheterogeneity. J Biol Chem 247:3792, 1972

52. Habib ZA: Maternal serum alpha-feto-protein: its value in antenatal diagnosis of genetic disease and in obstetrical-gynaecological care. Acta Obstet Gynecol Scand 61(suppl):1, 1977

53. Gitlin D, Perricelli A, Gitlin GM: Synthesis of fetoprotein by liver, yolk sac, and gastrointestinal tract of the human conceptus. Cancer Res 32:979, 1972

54. Murgita RA, Tomasi TB Jr: Suppression of the immune response by alpha-fetoprotein on the primary and secondary antibody response. J Exp Med 141:269, 1975

55. Ferguson-Smith MA, May HM, Vince JD et al: Avoidance of anencephalic and spina bifida births by maternal serum-alphafetoprotein screening. Lancet 1:330, 1978

56. Wald N, Cuckle H: AFP and age screening for Down's syndrome. Am J Med Genet 31:197, 1988

57. Chrousos GP, Calabrese JR, Avgerinos P et al: Corticotropin releasing factor: basic studies and clinical applications. Prog Neuropsychopharmacol Biol Psychiatry 9:349, 1985

58. Stalla GK, Hartwimmer J, von-Werder K et al: Ovine (o) and human (h) corticotropin releasing factor (CRF) in man: CRF-stimulation and CRF-immunoreactivity. Acta Endocrinol (Copenh) 106:289, 1984

59. Miyake A, Sakumoto T, Aono T et al: Changes in luteinizing hormone-releasing hormone in human placenta throughout pregnancy. Obstet Gynecol 60:444, 1982

60. Stalla GK, Bost H, Stalla J et al: Human corticotropin-

releasing hormone during pregnancy. Gynecol Endocrinol 3:1, 1989

61. Laatikainen TJ, Raisanen IJ, Salminen KR: Corticotropin-releasing hormone in amniotic fluid during gestation and labor and in relation to fetal lung maturation. Am J Obstet Gynecol 159:891, 1988

62. Shibahara S, Morimoto Y, Furutani Y et al: Isolation and sequence analysis of the human corticotropin-releasing factor precursor gene. EMBO J 2:775, 1983

63. Robinson BG, Emanuel RL, Frim DM et al: Glucocorticoid stimulates expression of corticotropin-releasing hormone gene in human placenta. Proc Natl Acad Sci USA 85:5244, 1988

64. Jones SA, Brooks AN, Challis JR: Steroids modulate corticotropin-releasing hormone production in human fetal membranes and placenta. J Clin Endocrinol Metab 68:825, 1989

65. Seeburg PH, Adelman JP: Characterization of cDNA for precursor of human luteinizing hormone releasing hormone. Nature 311:666, 1984

66. Mason AJ, Hayflick JS, Ling N et al: Complementary DNA sequences of ovarian follicular fluid inhibin show precursor stucture and homology with transforming growth factor-beta. Nature 318:659, 1986

67. Petraglia F, Sawchenko P, Lim AT et al: Localization, secretion, and action of inhibin in human placenta. Science 237:187, 1987

68. Youngblood WW, Humm J, Kizer S: Thyrotropin-releasing hormone-like bioactivity in placenta: evidence for the existence of substances other than Pyroglu-His-Pro-NH2 (TRH) capable of stimulating pituitary thyrotropin release. Endocrinology 106:541, 1980

69. Taliadouros GS, Canfield RE, Nisula BC: Thyroid-stimulating activity of chorionic gonadotropin and luteinizing hormone. J Clin Endocrinol Metab 47:855, 1978

70. Sinosich MJ, Grudzinskas JG, Saunders DM: Placental proteins in the diagnosis and evaluation of the "elusive" early pregnancy. Obstet Gynecol Surv 40:273:1985

71. Lenton EA, Grudzinskas JG, Gordon YB et al: Pregnancy specific β_1-glycoprotein and chorionic gonadotropin in early human pregnancy. Acta Obstet Gynecol Scand 60:489, 1981

72. Smith DH, Sinosich MJ, Saunders DM: Pregnancy specific β_1-glycoprotein and chorionic gonadotropin levels following conception. J Reprod Med 26:555, 1981

73. Tatarinov YS: Trophoblast-specific beta-glycoprotein as a marker for pregnancy and malignancies. Gynecol Obstet Invest 9:65, 1978

74. Sinosich MJ, Teisner B, Folkersen J et al: Radioimmu-

noassay for pregnancy associated plasma protein. Clin Chem 28:50, 1982

75. Bischof P, DuBerg S, Schindler A: The immunology of the human placenta and proteins. Placenta 4(Suppl):93, 1982

76. Obiekwe B, Pendlebury DJ, Gordon YB et al: The radioimmunoassay of placental protein 5 and circulating levels in maternal blood in the third trimester of normal pregnancy. Clin Chim Acta 95:509, 1979

77. Salem HT, Seppala M, Chard T: The effect of thrombin on serum placental protein 5 (PP5): is PP5 the naturally occurring antithrombin III of the human placenta? Placenta 2:205, 1981

78. Shutt PA, Lopata A: The secretion of hormones during the culture of human preimplantation embryos with corona cells. Fertil Steril 35:413, 1981

79. Tulchinsky D, Hobel CJ: Plasma human chorionic gonadotropin, estrone, estradiol, estriol, progesterone, and 17-hydroxyprogesterone in human pregnancy. III. Early normal pregnancy. Am J Obstet Gynecol 117:884, 1973

80. Csapo AI, Pulkkinen MO, Wiest WG: Effects of luteectomy and progesterone replacement therapy in early pregnancy patients. Am J Obstet Gynecol 115:759, 1973

81. Carr BR, MacDonald PC, Simpson ER: The role of lipoproteins in the regulation of progesterone secretion by the human corpus luteum. Fertil Steril 38:303, 1982

82. Baker BL, Jaffe RB: The genesis of cell types in the adenohypophysis of the human fetus as observed with immunocytochemistry. Am J Anat 143:137, 1975

83. Murphy BEP: Cortisol economy in the human fetus. p. 509. In James VHT, Serio M, Gusti G et al (eds): The Endocrine Function of the Human Adrenal Cortex. Academic Press, 1978

84. Johannison E: The foetal adrenal cortex in the human. Acta Endocrinol 58:130, 1968

85. Jost A: The fetal adrenal cortex. p. 426. In Greep RO, Astwood WB (eds): Handbook of Physiology. Vol 6, Endocrinology. American Physiology Society, Washington, DC, 1975

86. Kondo S: Developmental studies on the Japanese human adrenals. I. Ponderal growth. Bull Exp Biol 9:51, 1959

87. Spector WS (ed): Handbook of Biological Data. WB Saunders, Philadelphia, 1956

88. Buster J: Fetal adrenal cortex. Clin Obstet Gynecol 23:803, 1980

89. Dicztalusy E: Steroid metabolism in the feto-placental unit. In Pecile A, Finzi C (eds): The Feto-Placental Unit. Excerpta Medica, Amsterdam, 1969

90. Simpson ER, Carr BR, Parker CR et al: The role of

serum lipoproteins in steroidogenesis by the human fetal adrenal cortex. J Clin Endocrinol Metab 49:146, 1979

91. Carr BR, Porter JC, MacDonald PC et al: Metabolism of low density lipoprotein by human fetal adrenal tissue. Endocrinology 107:1034, 1980

92. Bloch E: Fetal adrenal cortex: Function and steroidogenesis. In McKerns KW (ed): Biochemical Endocrinology, Vol 2, Functions of the Adrenal Cortex. Appleton-Century-Crofts, East Norwalk, CT, 1968

93. Seron-Ferre M, Lawrence CC, Siliteri PK et al: Steroid production by definitive and fetal zones of the human fetal adrenal gland. J Clin Endocrinol Metab 47:603, 1978

94. Winters AG, Oliver C, MacDonald JC et al: Plasma ACTH levels in the human fetus and neonate as related to age and parturition. J Clin Endocrinol Metab 39:269, 1974

95. Walsh SW, Norman RL, Novy MJ: In utero regulation of rhesus monkey fetal adrenals: effects of dexamethasone, adrenocorticotropin, thyrotropin-releasing hormone, prolactin, human chorionic gonadotropin, and α-melanocyte stimulating hormone on fetal and maternal plasma steroids. Endocrinology 104:1805, 1979

96. Katikineni M, Davies TF, Catt KJ: Regulation of adrenal and testicular prolactin receptors by adrenocorticotropin and luteinizing hormone. Endocrinology 108:2367, 1981

97. Winters AJ, Colston C, MacDonald PC et al: Fetal plasma prolactin levels. J Clin Endocrinol Metab 41:626, 1975

98. Pepe GJ, Waddell BJ, Albrecht ED: The effects of adrenocorticotropin and prolactin on adrenal dehydroepiandrosterone secretion in the baboon fetus. Endocrinology 122:646, 1988

99. Buster JE: Estrogen metabolism. p. 1. In Speroff L, Simpson JL (eds): Reproductive Endocrinology, Infertility, and Genetics. Harper & Row, Hagerstown, MD, 1980

100. Tulchinsky D, Hobel CJ: Plasma human chorionic gonadotropin, estrone, estradiol, estriol, progesterone and 17 hydroxyprogesterone in human pregnancy. Am J Obstet Gynecol 117:884, 1973

101. Klopper A, Masson G, Campbell D et al: Estriol in plasma: a compartmental study. Am J Obstet Gynecol 117:21, 1973

102. Tulchinsky D, Hobel CJ, Korenman SG: A radioligand assay to plasma unconjugated estriol in normal and abnormal pregnancies. Am J Obstet Gynecol 111:311, 1971

103. Kreitmann-Gimbal B, Bayad F, Nixon WE et al: Patterns of estrogen and progesterone receptors in monkey endometrium during the normal menstrual cycle. Steroids 35:47, 1980

104. Johannisson E, Parker RA, Landgren BM et al: Morphometric analysis of the human endometrium in relation to peripheral hormone levels. Fertil Steril 38:564, 1982

105. Resnik R, Killam AP, Battaglia FC et al: The stimulation of uterine blood flow by various estrogens. Endocrinology 94:1192, 1974

106. Fencl MD, Stillman RJ, Cohen J et al: Direct evidence of sudden rise in fetal corticoids late in human gestation. Nature 287:225, 1980

107. Laufer N, Decherney AH, Haseltine FP et al: Steroid secretion by the human egg–corona cumulus complex in culture. J Clin Endocrinol Metab 58:1153, 1984

108. Punnonen R, Lukola A: Binding of estrogen and progestin in the human fallopian tube. Fertil Steril 36:610, 1981

109. Siiteri PK, Febres F, Clemens LE et al: Progesterone and maintenance of pregnancy: is progesterone nature's immunosuppressant? Ann NY Acad Sci 286:3384, 1977

110. Resnik R, Brink GW, Plumer MH: The effect of progesterone on estrogen-induced uterine blood flow. Am J Obstet Gynecol 128:251, 1977

111. Hsueh AJW, Peck EJ, Clark JH: Progesterone antagonism of the estrogen receptor and estrogen-induced uterine growth. Nature 254:337, 1975

112. Murphy BEP: Human fetal serum cortisol levels related to gestational age: evidence of a midgestational fall and a steep late gestational rise, independent of sex or mode of delivery. Am J Obstet Gynecol 144:276, 1982

113. Murphy BEP: Cortisol and cortisone in human fetal development. J Steroid Biochem 11:509, 1979

114. Liggins GC: Endocrinology of the feto-maternal unit. p. 138. In Shearman RP (ed): Human Reproductive Physiology. Blackwell Scientific Publications, Oxford, 1972

115. Kitterman JA, Liggins GC, Campos GA et al: Prepartum maturation of the lung in fetal sheep: relation to cortisol. J Appl Physiol 51:384, 1981

116. Colacicco G, Ray AK, Basu MK et al: Cultured lung cells: interplay effects of beta-mimetics, prostaglandins and corticosteroids in the biosynthesis of dipalmitoyl lecithin. J Biosci 34:101, 1979

117. Fowden AL, Comline RS, Silver M: The effects of cortisol on the concentration of glycogen in different tissues in the chronically catheterized fetal pig. J Exp Physiol 70:23, 1985

118. Cheung CY: Enhancement of adrenomedullary catecholamine release by adrenal cortex in fetus. Am J Physiol 247:E693, 1984

119. Kadar N, Taylor KJ, Rosenfield AT et al: Combined use of serum hCG and sonography in the diagnosis of ectopic pregnancy. AJR 141:609, 1983

120. Dawood MY, Saxena BB, Landesman R: Human chorionic gonadotropin and its subunits in hydatidiform mole and choriocarcinoma. Obstet Gynecol 50:172, 1977

121. Quigley MM, Tyrey L, Hammond CB: Utility of assay of alpha subunit of human chorionic gonadotropin in management of gestational, trophoblastic malignancies. Am J Obstet Gynecol 138:545, 1980

122. Braunstein GD, Mills JL, Reed GF et al: Comparison of serum placental protein hormone levels in diabetic and normal pregnancy. J Clin Endocrinol Metab 68:3, 1989

123. Hussa R, Cole LA: New horizons in hCG detection. Adv Exp Med Biol 176:217, 1984

124. Rasor JL, Braunstein GD: A rapid modification of the beta-hCG radioimmunoassay: use as an aid in the diagnosis of ectopic pregnancy. Obstet Gynecol 50:553, 1977

125. Hales CN, Woodhead JS: Labelled antibodies and their use in the immunoradiomimetic assay. Methods Enzymol 70:334, 1980

126. Joshi UM, Roy R, Sheth AR et al: A simple and sensitive color test for the detection of human chorionic gonadotropin. Obstet Gynecol 57:252, 1981

127. Steenman UH, Alfthan H, Myllynen L et al: Ultrarapid and highly sensitive time-resolved fluoroimmunometric assay for chorionic gonadotropin. Lancet 2:647, 1983

128. Stovall TG, Ling FW, Buster JE: Serum progesterone-directed endometrial curettage in the diagnosis of ectopic pregnancy without laparoscopy. Abstract P153, American Fertility Society, San Francisco, CA, 1989

129. Stovall TG, Ling FW, Cope BJ et al: Preventing ruptured ectopic pregnancy with a single serum progesterone. Am J Obstet Gynecol 160:1425, 1989

130. Ratcliffe WA, Corrie JE, Dalziel AH et al: Direct ^{125}I-radioligand assays for serum progesterone compared with assays involving extraction of serum. Clin Chem 28:1314, 1982

131. Ius A, Ferrara L, Meroni G et al: Evaluation of time-resolved fluoroimmunoassay with Eu-labelled protein-A for serum progesterone. J Steroid Biochem 33:101, 1989

132. Stoval TG, Kellerman AL, Ling FW, et al: Emergency department diagnosis of ectopic pregnancy. Emerg Med 19:1098, 1990

133. Timor-Tritsch IE, Rottem S (eds): Transvaginal Sonography. New York, Elsevier Science, 1988

134. Fossum GT, Davajan V, Kletzky OA: Early detection of pregnancy with transvaginal ultrasound. Fertil Steril 49:789, 1988

135. Kadar N, DeVore G, Romero R: Discriminatory hCG zone: its use in the sonographic evaluation for ectopic pregnancy. Obstet Gynecol 58:156, 1981

136. Simpson JL, Mills JL, Holmes LB et al: Low fetal loss rates after ultrasound-proved viability in early pregnancy. JAMA 258:2555, 1987

137. Osathanondh R, Tulchinsky D: Placental polypeptide hormones. p. 18. In Tulchinsky D, Ryan KJ (eds): Maternal–Fetal Endocrinology. WB Saunders, Philadelphia, 1980

138. Healy DL: Placental endocrinology. p. 24. In Gold JJ, Josimovich JB (eds): Gynecologic Endocrinology. 4th Ed. Plenum, New York, 1987

139. Niall HD, Hogan ML, Sauer R et al: Sequences of pituitary and placental lactogenic and growth hormones: evolution from a primordial peptide by gene reduplication. Proc Natl Acad Sci USA 68:866, 1971

140. Buster JE, Chang RJ, Preston DL et al: Interrelationships of circulating maternal steroid concentrations in third trimester pregnancies. II. C18 and C19 steroids: estradiol, estriol, dehydroepiandrosterone, dehydroepiandrosterone sulfate, Δ^5-andostenediol, Δ^4-andostenedione, testosterone, and dihydrotestosterone. J Clin Endocrinol Metab 48:139, 1979

141. Buster JE, Chang RJ, Preston DL et al: Interrelationships of circulating maternal steroid concentrations in third trimester pregnancies: C21 steroids: progesterone, 16α-hydroxyprogesterone, 17α-hydroxyprogesterone, 20α-dihydroxyprogesterone, Δ^5-pregnenolone sulfate, and serum 17α-hydroxy Δ^5-pregnenolone. J Clin Endocrinol Metab 48:33, 1979

142. James VHT, Serio M, Gusti G et al (eds): The Endocrine Function of the Human Adrenal Cortex. pp. 509–545. Academic Press, San Diego, 1978

143. Fletcher JL Jr: Update on pregnancy testing. Prim Care 13:667, 1986

Chapter 4

Placental and Fetal Physiology

John Bissonnette

Much of what is known in fetal and placental physiology comes from observations of mammals other than humans. This chapter contains information obtained from these studies in laboratory animals; in most instances, however, the species from which the data are obtained is not detailed. An effort has been made to include only those observations that would reasonably apply to the human fetus and placenta. The reader is referred to the references to verify from which species the observations originate.

PLACENTAL PHYSIOLOGY

Growth and Metabolism

It is incorrect to regard the placenta simply as an organ designed for the transport of substrates and respiratory gases between the mother and fetus. As detailed in Chapter 3, the placenta is an active site of steroid and peptide hormone synthesis. In addition, such transport systems as Na^+,K^+-ATPase require energy. From 22 to 36 weeks gestation there is a four- to fivefold increase in the number of trophoblast nuclei[1] so that cell growth also places a metabolic demand on the placenta. Thus fetal oxygen and nutrient supply may not only depend on their respective concentrations in maternal blood and the transport characteristics of the placenta, but also to a significant extent may be influenced by placental metabolism.

The oxygen consumption of the placenta is at least 10 ml/min/kg.[2-4] If one considers the total amount of oxygen that leaves the maternal circulation from uterine artery to uterine vein, approximately one-half is consumed by the placenta.[3] The remainder is for fetal oxygen consumption. On a weight basis the placenta has a much higher oxygen consumption than the fetus as a whole, and its metabolic rate has been compared with that of the brain.[3]

Glucose is the principal substrate for oxidative metabolism by placental tissue.[3,5] Of the total amount of glucose that leaves the maternal compartment to nourish the uterus and its contents, as much as 70 percent may be consumed by the placenta.[3,6,7] This statement refers to glucose uptake on a net basis, considering the mother as the sole supplier of sugar and the placenta and fetus as recipients who will partition glucose between them. With isotope-labeled glucose in animal studies it has been shown that a significant fraction of the glucose that the placenta takes up comes from the fetal umbilical circulation.[8] The glucose taken up by placental tissues is not all utilized for oxidative metabolism. As much as one-third of it may be converted to the three-carbon sugar lactate.[3,9] It is important to note that this does not imply that placental tissues function under conditions of anaerobic metabolism. Lactate production[4,5] is a normal feature of the placenta and takes place in the presence of high oxygen utilization rates. The factors (either extrinsic, such as maternal or fetal hormones, or intrinsic, such as the production of placental hormones) that influence short-term changes in placental oxygen and glucose consumption are at present incompletely understood. There is no definitive evidence that insulin in the maternal circulation increases the consumption of glucose by the placenta.[10]

The regulation of placental growth is also an area that is incompletely understood. The number of trophoblast nuclei increases to a greater extent than does the number of fetal placental capillary endothelial nuclei[1] during the period of 22 to 36 weeks of gestation. However, whether trophoblast proliferation is the primary growth event or whether these cells follow endothelial growth in a secondary manner is not known. A number of clinical observations suggest that a decrease in tissue oxygen content may lead to an increase in placental growth. These include maternal anemia,[11-13] fetal anemia associated with erythrocyte isoimmunization, and the hydrops fetalis variety of α-thalassemia in which the fetus has Bart's hemoglobin.[4] This form of hemoglobin has such a high affinity for oxygen that the blood remains saturated even at low oxygen tensions such that little oxygen is unloaded at the tissues.

The placenta has receptors for a number of peptide hormones that have been demonstrated to stimulate cell growth in vitro.[14] The association of a large placenta with diabetes in pregnancy is recognized. In addition to its short-term actions on transport processes and metabolism, insulin has mitogenic activity in some tissues. However, this effect is only seen at unphysiologically high concentrations. In addition to the insulin receptor,[15-19] which has been purified from human placenta,[20] the placenta contains receptors for insulin-like growth factor I (IGF-I) and insulin-like growth factor II (IGF-II). These two receptors are distinct from each other, and in turn they are distinct from the insulin receptor.[21-23] The IGF-II receptor is identical to the mannose-6-phosphate receptor, which binds lysosomal hydrolases within the cell.[24] IGF-I and IGF-II are polypeptides that have molecular weights and tertiary structures with a high degree of homology to human proinsulin.[25] They circulate bound to a carrier protein (which does not bind proinsulin) and are 50 times as potent as insulin in stimulating indices of cell growth in a number of tissues (for review, see ref. 25). The extent of the physiologic role for IGF-I and IGF-II in placental growth remains to be defined. Human placenta also contains epidermal growth factor receptors.[26,27] Epidermal growth factor increases RNA and DNA syntheses and cell multiplication in a wide variety of cell types.[14] The observation that specific epidermal growth factor binding is increased in term placentas compared with that at 8 to 18 weeks of gestation has led to the suggestion that it may play a role in the regulation of placental growth.[27]

Recent investigations have revealed the presence of a placental growth hormone for which there is both genetic[28] and immunologic[29,30] evidence that distinguish this variant from pituitary growth hormone. Placental growth hormone appears to be secreted primarily into the maternal rather than into the fetal circulation. Its role in the regulation of placental growth and metabolism is incompletely understood.

Placental Transfer

General Considerations

The movement of molecules from the maternal intervillous space to the interior of the fetal capillary takes place across a number of cellular structures. These are outlined in Figure 4.1. The first step is transport across the microvillous plasma membrane of the syncytiotrophoblast. Because there are no lateral intercellular spaces in the syncytiotrophoblast, all solutes first interact with the placenta at this plasma membrane. The interior of the syncytiotrophoblast may present a second step in the transport process, for example, separation of a molecule from the microvillous plasma membrane receptor with which it was internalized. The basal (or fetal) plasma membrane of the syncytiotrophoblast represents the third site of potential substrate membrane interaction. Because the cytotrophoblast cell layer is discontinuous in later gestation, it should not play a rate-limiting role in transport from mother to fetus. By virtue of the anionic sites on the glycoproteins that make up the basal lamina,[31] this layer has the potential of influencing movement of large charged molecules. The fetal capillary endothelial cell imposes two plasma membrane surfaces between the extracellular space of the villi and fetal blood. However, these cells also have lateral intercellular spaces so that transport may take place by a paracellular pathway.

Transfer of any solute from mother to fetus will be governed by the concentration gradient that exists

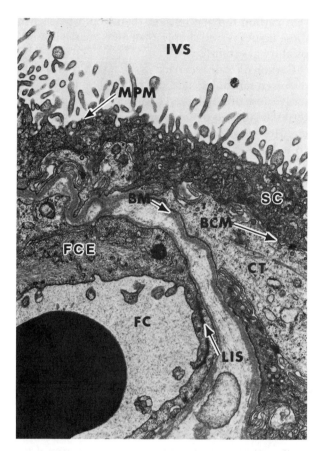

Fig. 4.1 Electron micrograph of human placenta demonstrating the cellular and extracellular components with which solutes most interact in moving from the maternal intervillous space (IVS) to the lumen of the fetal capillary (FC). MPM, microvillous plasma membrane of the syncytiotrophoblast; SC, syncytiotrophoblast; BCM, basal cell membrane of the syncytiotrophoblast; BM, basement membrane; CT, cytotrophoblast cell; FCE, fetal capillary endothelial cell; LIS, lateral intercellular space of fetal endothelial cell. (Courtesy of Kent L. Thornburg, Ph.D., Department of Physiology, Oregon Health Sciences University, Portland, OR.)

across the cell membranes and the interaction between the solute as it moves from plasma water through the lipid bilayers and lateral intercellular spaces of the placenta. For solutes that do not have specialized mechanisms for transport, the most important factors that govern their permeability is their size and their lipid solubility. Up to a molecular weight (MW) of at least 5,000, placental permeability is proportional to the free diffusion of a molecule in water.[32] This means that for solutes up to this size there are no restriction sites such as pores that hinder

permeability. For lipid insoluble molecules, size is an important determinant. For example, urea (MW = 60) is at least 1,000 times more permeable than inulin (MW = 5,000).[32] In the case of small solutes (MW < 200), their respective lipid solubilities have an important effect on placental permeability. Ethanol, which is 500 times more soluble in a lipid environment than is urea, a molecule of similar size, is 10 times more permeable.[33] For solutes that have very high permeabilities, such as ethanol, equilibrium is easily reached between the maternal intervillous space and the fetal capillary. Placental permeability for these solutes is therefore not rate limiting in governing maternal to fetal transfer.[34] Blood flow in the intervillous space and in the umbilical circulation become the important factors in regulating transfer for these small lipid soluble solutes.

Transfer of Individual Solutes

Respiratory Gases

The permeability characteristics of an organ that exchanges respiratory gases are obtained by measuring the diffusing capacity. Placental diffusing capacity is defined as the amount (in milliliters) of the respiratory gas in question that diffuses across the entire organ per unit of time (minute), per unit gas tension difference (mmHg) between maternal and fetal blood.[35] In animals, the amount of respiratory gas transferred can readily be measured as the product of umbilical blood flow and the oxygen content difference between umbilical vein and umbilical artery. However, the average partial pressure difference between maternal and fetal blood for oxygen and carbon dioxide can only be estimated by examining their respective tensions in maternal uterine artery and vein and in fetal umbilical artery and vein. If one assumes oxygen tension undergoes a linear decrease from its value in the uterine artery to reach that in the uterine vein, the average maternal oxygen tension will be significantly different than if one postulates that this decrease was exponential. For this reason, carbon monoxide has been used to measure placental diffusing capacity.[35] Carbon monoxide is similar to oxygen in size and lipid solubility. Therefore, it will have permeability characteristics in the placenta that are similar to oxygen. Because carbon monoxide is bound to hemoglobin more than 200 times more tightly than is oxygen, there is very little change in its partial pressure between uterine artery and vein or between umbilical artery and vein. Thus an accurate measurement of the transplacental carbon monoxide partial pressure difference can be made and from this the actual diffusing capacity of the organ determined. Placental diffusing capacity has been measured for a number of animals, including primates (for a summary, see ref. 36). It has also been estimated indirectly in humans.[37] These measurements indicate that the efficiency of the placenta as an organ of respiratory gas exchange is such that oxygen and carbon dioxide tensions will come to equilibrium at the maternal intervillous space and fetal capillary. In contrast to the estimates made with carbon monoxide, animal studies in which fetal oxygen consumption is either increased[38] or decreased[39] show widening and narrowing of the oxygen tension gradient across the placenta. This would indicate that there is a significant diffusional component for oxygen transfer from mother to fetus.[39]

The conclusions reached from the magnitude of the placental diffusing capacity (but not those obtained from changes in fetal oxygen consumption) are at variance with the observation that oxygen tension in the umbilical vein and uterine vein[40,41] and between the umbilical vein and intervillous[42] space show a difference of close to 10 mmHg. In addition, despite the fact that carbon dioxide is much more soluble than oxygen in water and tissues and therefore will diffuse more readily, it also shows a small (3 mmHg) difference from umbilical vein to umbilical artery.[43] Some of the P_{O_2} differences could be explained by uneven distributions of maternal to fetal blood flows in individual areas of the placenta analogous to uneven ventilation perfusion ratios in the lung. However, this alone would not explain the difference observed for carbon dioxide. Blood in either or both of the uterine and the umbilical circulations that is completely shunted away from an area that allows exchange with the other circulation would contribute to this difference in respiratory gas tension between maternal and fetal blood. Probably the most important contribution to this difference is made by the high metabolic rate of the placental tissues themselves. Thus oxygen consumption and carbon dioxide production by the trophoblast cells result in lower umbilical vein oxygen tension and a higher uterine vein carbon dioxide tension than would be seen if these tissues served simply as an inert barrier for respiratory gas transfer.

Carbon dioxide is carried in the fetal blood both as dissolved carbon dioxide and as bicarbonate. The latter because of its charged nature would not be transferred from fetus to mother as readily as carbon dioxide. However, it appears that carbon dioxide diffuses from fetus to mother in its molecular form and that bicarbonate does not contribute significantly to the elimination of fetal carbon dioxide.[44] Thus the placental exchange of respiratory gases is such that diffusion is not rate limiting, and the important variables for fetal oxygen uptake and carbon dioxide excretion will reside in uterine and umbilical blood flows and in the carrying capacities of maternal and fetal bloods for oxygen and carbon dioxide.

Glucose

The permeability of the placenta as a whole for D-glucose is at least 50 times what would be predicted from its size and lipid solubility.[45] This indicates that a specialized mechanism for transfer must exist in the cell membranes that separate the intervillous space from fetal capillary blood. The integral membrane proteins that facilitate the translocation of sugars and other molecules from the exterior to the interior of cells are termed transporters. The glucose transporter at the brush border surface of the adult kidney[46] and intestine is sodium dependent; that is, the entry of D-glucose is coupled to sodium, and, because there is a constant inwardly directed sodium gradient maintained by the sodium–potassium pump (Na^+,K^+-ATPase) at the basolateral cell membrane, glucose can accumulate inside the cell in concentrations that exceed that in the luminal fluid. The syncytiotrophoblast microvillous membrane glucose transporter is not sodium dependent,[47-49] and one would not expect glucose concentrations in placental cells to exceed those in the maternal intervillous space.

In a number of cell types, including human adipocytes,[50] insulin over the range of concentrations seen postprandially (10 to 250 $\mu U/ml$) can cause a threefold increase in the transport of D-glucose. The placental microvillous membrane transporter is not insulin sensitive.[47,51] The human placental glucose transporter has been characterized as an integral membrane protein[52] and identified as an approximately 55,000 MW component of the microvillous membrane.[53,54] Glucose transporters are a family of genes four of which have been well characterized.[55] Two of these are expressed abundantly in the human placenta.[56,57] As with any facilitated transport system, the placental D-glucose transporter can be saturated at high substrate concentrations. The microvillous membrane transporter reaches one-half its maximum ability to translocate glucose from the intervillous space at sugar levels of approximately 5 mM (90 mg/dl).[58] This means that glucose transfer from mother to fetus will not proceed in a linear manner as maternal glucose levels rise, but the transfer rates are less at high glucose concentration. This effect is reflected in fetal blood glucose levels following maternal sugar loading.[59]

Amino Acids

Like monosaccharides, amino acids enter the syncytiotrophoblast by means of transport-specific membrane proteins. In contrast to the glucose transporter, amino acid uptake is not the property of a single plasma membrane protein. While the amino acid placental transport systems have not been assigned to specific components of the microvillous membrane, as is the case for D-glucose, studies with nonmetabolizable analogues, in which the ability of various amino acids to inhibit the analogue competitively is examined, have demonstrated the existence of three systems for neutral and basic amino acids.[60,61] The acidic amino acids glutamate and aspartate are poorly transported from mother to fetus.[62–64] Glutamate, which shows a net loss to the placental from the umbilical circulation,[65] is taken up at the fetal surface and converted into glutamine.[66]

Table 4.1 outlines the three transport systems available for uptake of amino acids by trophoblast cells. It shows that the systems are not exclusive and that there are a number of amino acids transported by more than one system. Table 4.1 also summarizes the presence or absence of regulatory mechanisms that characterize the systems. Amino acids are present in higher concentrations in fetal cord blood than in maternal blood. The ability to transport against a concentration gradient takes place in two steps. Amino acids are concentrated in the trophoblast cells, and then they proceed down their concentration gradients into fetal blood. Many of the amino acids are

transported by a sodium-dependent system. Amino acid entry is coupled to sodium in a cotransport system located at the microvillous membrane that faces the maternal intervillous space.[67,68] As long as an inwardly directed sodium gradient exists, amino acid concentration in the trophoblast cells will exceed that in maternal blood. The sodium gradient is maintained by Na^+,K^+-ATPase located on the basal or fetal side of the syncytiotrophoblast.[69] Inhibition of Na^+,K^+-ATPase activity causes an increase in intracellular sodium, which in turn results in a decrease in amino acid uptake.[69]

Trophoblast cells have two mechanisms of regulating the uptake of amino acids that use the A system. Incubation of cells in the absence of amino acids results in a marked increase in their ability to take up amino acids.[70–72] This preincubation increase in transport capacity is due to an increased maximum rate of transport coupled with an increased affinity for the carrier.[70] The effect depends on protein synthesis and on aerobic metabolism by the trophoblast cells.[71] In addition, an increase in concentration of amino acid within the trophoblast is capable of suppressing uptake. This regulatory mechanism, which is termed transinhibition, is specific for the A system.[73] Transinhibition is not dependent on protein synthesis and is due to the intercellular substrate interacting with the transport system.[73] This regulatory mechanism would tend to maintain trophoblast cell levels of these amino acids constant during fluctuations in maternal plasma concentrations.

Lipids

Because of their hydrophobic nature, free fatty acids are relatively insoluble in plasma and circulate bound to albumin. They are transferred across the placenta but at relatively low rates[74,75] such that it has been estimated that placental transfer is not sufficient to account for the accumulation of fetal fatty acids in late pregnancy.[74] Transfer of fatty acids involves dissociation from maternal protein and association with fetal plasma proteins as two steps that are added to permeability across the placental membranes. These protein-binding steps are more important in determining the transfer of free fatty acids from mother to fetus than are their interactions with the lipid layers of the placenta.[76,77] Placental transfer of fatty acids increases logarithmically with a decrease in chain

Table 4.1 Placental Neutral Amino Acid Transport Systems

Transport	A	L	ASSC
Representative amino acids	Glycine, proline, alanine, serine, threonine, glutamine	Isoleucine, valine, phenylalanine, alanine, serine, threonine, glutamine	Alanine, serine, threonine, glutamine
Sodium dependency	+	−	+
Uptake increased by preincubation	+	−	+
Transinhibition	+	−	−

(Data from Enders et al,[61] Smith et al,[70] Smith and Depper,[71] Longo et al,[72] and Steel et al.[73])

length from C16 to C8, and then transfer declines somewhat for C6 and C4. This latter effect is due to a fall off in lipid solubility of the shorter chain molecules.[77] Placental uptake of cholesterol is discussed in the section on receptor-mediated endocytosis.

Water and Ions

The transfer of water from mother to fetus is determined by the filtration coefficient for water of the placenta (defined as the ratio of water flow and hydrostatic pressure in the absence of any solute), by the hydrostatic pressure difference between the intervillous space and the fetal capillaries, and by the osmotic pressure difference between fetal and maternal blood. The filtration coefficient for water across the placenta is such that it would not be rate limiting for the amount of water the fetus gains during growth.[78] The osmotic pressure forces exerted by a solute on water movement only achieve their theoretic value if the solute in question is impermeable to the membrane. Sodium and chloride, the principal plasma solutes, are relatively permeable across the placenta[79] and would not be expected to play an important role.[80] Osmotic gradients do not appear to be significant between maternal and fetal blood,[81] and when they are imposed with small solutes they do not persist because of the movement of water in one direction and the solute in the other.[82] Colloid osmotic pressure differences have to be included in the calculation of hydrostatic pressure differences across the placenta. It has been shown that colloid osmotic pressure differences can result in significant water movement,[83] and these forces together with hydrostatic pressure forces are probably the main determinants of water fluxes.

In comparison to other epithelia, the specialized mechanisms for ion transport in the placenta are incompletely understood. The mechanisms for sodium transport in syncytiotrophoblast membranes that have been characterized are outlined in Figure 4.2. The maternal facing microvillous membrane contains an amino acid cotransporter[68]; a sodium–phosphate cotransporter in which two sodium ions are transported with each phosphate radical[84] and a sodium–hydrogen ion antiport in which a proton is extruded while a sodium ion enters the cell.[85] In addition, a membrane potential with the inside negative (-30 mV) would promote sodium entry from the intervillous space.[86] The fetal-directed basal side of the cell contains the Na^+,K^+-ATPase.[69] The integration of these various mechanisms for sodium transport from mother to fetus is not completely understood, but it is increased by β-adrenergic stimulation.[87] The β-adrenergic receptors are located on the basal or fetal side of the cell.[88]

The microvillous or maternal-facing trophoblast membrane has a chloride–bicarbonate exchanger whereby one chloride ion enters the cell with the efflux of one bicarbonate radical.[89,90] This system accounts for about one-half of the chloride transport across this plasma membrane.[90]

Calcium

Ionized calcium levels are higher in fetal than in maternal blood.[81,91] The basal membrane of the syncytiotrophoblast has an ATP-dependent Ca^{2+} transport system.[92] This system has a high affinity for calcium and as such is capable of interacting with calcium at the nanomolar concentrations found within the trophoblast cells. It is stimulated by the calcium-de-

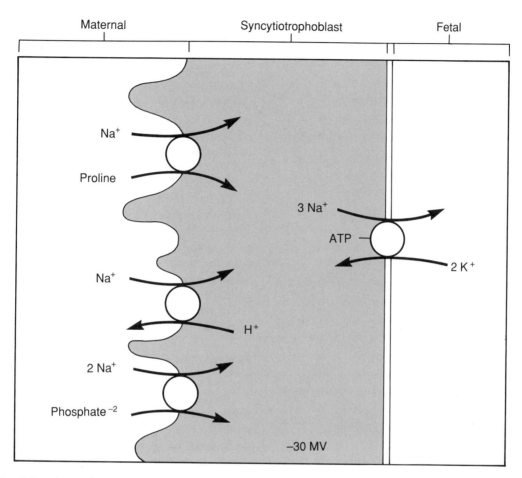

Fig. 4.2 Pathways for sodium entry into syncytiotrophoblast and exit to the fetal circulation. (Data from Boyd and Lund,[68] Whitsett and Wallick,[69] Lajeunesse and Brunette,[84] Balkovetz et al,[85] and Bara et al.[86])

pendent regulatory protein calmodulin.[92] Transport of calcium across the entire placenta is increased by 1,25-dihydroxycholecalciferol.[93] A calcium-binding protein has been extracted from the placenta.[94] This protein has been purified to chromatographic and electrophoretic homogeneity and has an MW of 150,000. It is made up of two subunits of equal size. The placental calcium-binding protein appears to differ from the human intestinal calcium-binding protein.[94] This protein in the placenta may be an important regulator of maternal to fetal calcium transport.

Receptor-Mediated Endocytosis

The microvillous plasma membrane of the syncytiotrophoblast contains receptors for insulin,[15–19] immunoglobulin G (IgG),[95] transferrin,[96] and low-density lipoprotein (LDL).[97] Each of these receptors is specific for its respective peptide. However, after the ligand binds to the receptor, there is a similarity in the mechanism by which the protein–receptor complex enters the cell and is further processed. While all the precise steps for each of these four protein–receptor complexes has not been worked out in the trophoblast, general principles can be drawn from what is known in other cell types.[98–101] Following binding of ligand to receptor, the receptors aggregate on the cell surface. They then collect in specialized membrane structures termed coated pits (Fig. 4.3). These coated pits, which contain the protein clathrin at their cytosolic bases, are invaginated, pinch off, and enter the cell. LDL receptors are usually found in coated pits even in the absence of bound LDL particles. They also enter the cell whether or not they have bound

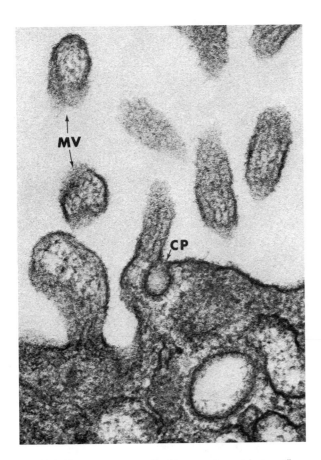

Fig. 4.3 Electron micrograph of human placental microvillous plasma membrane demonstrating presence of a coated pit (CP). Note the presence of cytoskeletal components extending into the microvillous space (MV). (Courtesy of Kent L. Thornburg, Ph.D., Department of Physiology, Oregon Health Sciences University, Portland, OR.)

ligand. The plasma membrane segment that has been pinched off is called a coated vesicle. The coated vesicles shed their clathrin coats and fuse with one another to form endosomes. The endosomes move deeper into the cytoplasm, and under the influence of their acidic environment the ligand is separated from its receptor.

The fates of ligand and receptor differ with respect to the four complexes under consideration. Insulin is degraded by lysosomal enzymes, and maternal insulin does not appear in the fetal circulation. The insulin receptor is probably recycled to the cell surface. Cholesterol that entered with the LDL receptor may be used for synthesis in the trophoblast, and some also appears in the fetal blood.[102] The IgG complexed to its receptor possibly remains intact for exocytosis at the basal side of the trophoblast in a manner analogous to secretion of immunoglobulin by other cell types. IgG is the only maternal immunoglobulin that crosses to the fetus. Ferrotransferrin, which carries two ferric ions per molecule, is unique in that it does not separate from the transferrin receptor in the acid environment of the prelysosomal vesicle. Rather, it is the iron that becomes dissociated and then binds to ferritin, an iron-storing protein in the cytoplasmic fluid. Iron is then picked up at the basal side of the cell by fetal apotransferrin. The apotransferrin–receptor complex that had entered at the maternal surface is then recycled. In the neutral pH environment of the cell surface, apotransferrin dissociates from the transferrin receptor, which is then free to bind ferrotransferrin. At neutral pH the iron that contains ferrotransferrin binds avidly to the transferrin receptor, while that without (apotransferrin) does not.

Placental Blood Flow

Because the transport characteristics of the placenta are such that respiratory gases and many solutes may reach equal concentration between the maternal intervillous space blood and that in the fetal capillaries, the rates of blood flow in these two circulations are important determinants of fetal oxygen and nutrient supply. It should be noted, however, that the arteriovenous difference in the uterine circulation (and venoarterial difference in the umbilical circulation) widens during periods of lowered blood flow so that oxygen consumption remains unchanged over a fairly wide range of blood flows.[103] Uterine and umbilical blood flows can each be significantly reduced before a fall in fetal oxygen consumption takes place.[104,105]

Uterine Blood Flow

Regulation of uterine blood flow can be considered under two categories. The first of these concerns the factors that produce the steady increase in blood flow that parallels fetal growth over the last half of pregnancy.[106] Because the diffusing capacity of the placenta increases during this time period,[107,108] it is reasonable to conclude that there is a growth of the intervillous space volume so that an increase in blood flow can take place without an increase in vascular resistance. Morphometric analysis demonstrates that intervillous space volume almost triples between weeks 22 and 36 of gestation.[1] The factors that control this long-term regulation of uterine blood flow are poorly understood. The metabolic demands of the placenta and fetus are no doubt involved in this process, but the signals that direct the changes are not known. Estrogen is an important dilator of the non-pregnant uterine circulation[109–111] and may well be involved in the long-term changes seen in pregnancy. The increase in blood flow is due to a direct action of estrogen on the uterine vasculature and is associated with protein synthesis at the translational level.[111] The magnitude of blood flow to the pregnant uterus in late gestation in women at rest is not known. From studies performed under anesthesia it seems reasonable to conclude that it is at least 750 ml/min,[112,113] that is, between 10 percent and 15 percent of maternal cardiac output.

Uterine blood flow is also subject to regulatory influences on a short-term basis. Blood flow is directly related to the pressure difference that exists between the uterine artery and the uterine veins; that is, either a fall in uterine artery pressure[114–116] or a rise in uterine vein pressure[116] results in a proportional fall in blood flow. During uterine contractions this relationship between pressures in the uterine artery and vein and blood flow no longer holds. Because intrauterine pressures are directly transmitted to the intervillous space,[117] the pressure governing blood flow becomes uterine artery pressure minus intervillous space pressure for the situation in which intervillous space pressure exceeds the pressure in the uterine veins. The higher the pressure in the intervillous space the lower the blood flow to the placenta.[118] There is histochemical evidence for the presence of adrenergic nerves near blood vessels in both the placental and the myoendometrial portions of the uterine circulation.[119] Both epinephrine[120] and norepinephrine[121] cause a reduction in uterine blood flow that is more pronounced in the myoendometrial bed than in the placenta. The effect can be completely inhibited by blocking α-adrenergic receptors.[122] Respiratory gases are important regulators of blood flow in a number of organs. However, there is no indication that either oxygen or carbon dioxide is responsible for short-term changes in uterine blood flow (data reviewed in ref. 123). The precise roles of a number of vasoactive substances, including angiotensin II and the prostaglandins, in modulating uterine blood

flow are not known (for reviews, see refs. 123 and 124).

Umbilical Blood Flow

The blood flow to the umbilical circulation represents approximately 40 percent of the combined output of both fetal ventricles.[125,126] Over the last one-third of gestation the blood flow in the fetal placental circulation remains constant when normalized to fetal weight[125]; that is, in absolute terms there is a significant increase in umbilical blood flow as the fetus grows.[127] The increase is most probably associated with an increase in the number of villous capillaries, but the factors that regulate this change are not known.

Short-term changes in umbilical blood flow are primarily regulated by the perfusion pressure. The relationship between flow and perfusion pressure in the umbilical circulation is linear.[116,128] Even small (2 to 3 mmHg) increases in umbilical vein pressure result in a proportional decrease in umbilical blood flow.[116,128] Because both umbilical artery and vein are completely enclosed in the amniotic cavity, all pressure changes that result from an increase in uterine tone are transmitted equally to these vessels. Therefore, perfusion pressure, the difference between umbilical artery and umbilical vein, will remain the same, and there will be no change in umbilical blood flow. Blood flow to the placenta remains constant over a wide range of oxygen tensions in the umbilical arteries.[129–132] Because hypoxemia is associated with an increase in fetal arterial blood pressure, the failure to achieve any increase in umbilical blood flow indicates an increase in the resistance of the placenta. This may not be a direct effect, as both epinephrine and norepinephrine are increased during hypoxemia. (The effects of other vasoactive substances on the umbilical circulation are reviewed in ref. 124.)

Immunologic Properties of the Placenta

The syncytiotrophoblast in intimate contact with maternal blood in the intervillous space and the amniochorion in contact with maternal decidua represent the fetal tissues that are most prone to immunologic reactions from maternal factors. The rejection of tissue grafts is under genetic control, and the genes responsible for this phenomenon are termed histocompatibility genes. Their products at the cell surface—major histocompatibility antigens—are integral to the hosts recognition of self and nonself. Neither β_2-microglobulin (which is tightly associated with human lymphocyte antigen [HLA] antigens) nor the HLA antigens A, B, C, DR, or DC can be demonstrated on the surface of syncytiotrophoblast.[133,134] However, the cytotrophoblasts that erode into the maternal spiral arterioles express an incomplete or truncated form of class I HLA antigens (reviewed in ref. 135). The chorionic sac in the first trimester has been shown to have HLA-A, -B, and -C antigens, but they are localized to nonvillous trophoblast of the cytotrophoblast cell columns and cytotrophoblastic shell.[136] In addition, HLA antigens can be demonstrated on fetal stromal cells such as fibroblasts and fetal endothelial cells within the placental villi.[137] While the normal syncytiotrophoblast at the hemochorial interface within the interstitial space lacks major HLA antigens, the observation that transformed trophoblast in vitro can manifest these antigens suggests that the genetic information is present in normal tissue in vivo but that it is suppressed.[137] Neither the A, B, or H blood group antigens[138] nor H-Y antigens[133] are thought to be present on the syncytiotrophoblast surface. The presence of antigens in the cells of the fetal stroma and endothelia of placental villi may also have consequences with respect to maintenance of the fetus. It has been suggested[139] that this area acts as an immunologic sink to bind maternal antibodies so that they do not reach the fetus itself. In this regard it is noted that the $Rh_o(D)$ antigen that does reach the fetus is not found in the placenta.[139]

The syncytiotrophoblast does, however, manifest unique antigens. These have been termed trophoblast antigens and trophoblast–lymphocyte cross-reactive antigens.[137] The two groups are distinguished by the fact that the latter are absorbed by leukocytes. These trophoblast antigens are structural components of the plasma membrane and are distinct from soluble proteins produced by the placenta.[140] The trophoblast–lymphocyte cross-reactive antigens are thought to be important for the induction of immunologic blocking factors in maternal serum during the second and third trimesters of normal pregnancy.[141] Antibodies against these antigens are thought to be important regulators of trophoblast

growth.[135] The absence of trophoblast antigens that the mother's immune system can recognize as nonself is thought to be related to a failure to produce these blocking factors, which in turn results in abortion.[135,137,142–144] Local immunoregulatory responses in the decidua that suppress lymphocyte activation play an important role in lack of rejection of the trophoblast but may also contribute to infection, which can occur at this site but not systematically.[145] In addition to the placenta, both the mother and the fetus make important contributions to the immunologic maintenance of pregnancy. (These are reviewed in refs. 135 and 146.)

Amniotic Fluid Volume

Amniotic fluid volume increases from a mean of 250 ml at 16 weeks gestation to close to 800 ml at about 22 weeks. Although there is considerable variability, the average volume remains stable to 39 weeks and then declines to about 500 ml at term.[147] The steady-state volume of fluid in the amniotic cavity at any point in time will represent a balance between the two sources that contribute bulk water (fetal urine and fetal alveolar fluid) and the two sources that remove bulk water (fetal swallowing and the amniotic chorionic interface with the maternal uterine wall). This analysis includes only the direct sources of amniotic fluid volume. The area of exchange for water transfer at the intervillous space and fetal villous capillaries is much greater than that present at the amniotic chorionic uterine interface. Thus water exchange across the placenta that could then influence fetal urine output may be an indirect but important factor in the regulation of amniotic fluid volumes. Although the ability to exchange water across the amnion is less than 1 percent of that of the placenta because the osmotic gradient at this interface is 30 times that at the placenta, this may be an important site for bulk amniotic fluid volume regulation.[148]

The fetal lung secretes fluid at a rate of 300 to 400 ml/day.[149] While the osmolarity of this fluid is similar to that of fetal plasma,[150] the chloride concentration is much higher, and this is balanced by a much lower bicarbonate concentration. Chloride is actively transferred from alveolar capillaries to lung lumen,[151] and, because the alveolar epithelium restricts passive ion movements, water transport follows that of chloride. The secretion of lung liquid over the last one-third of gestation is constant when normalized to fetal weight but decreases when expressed as a ratio of lung liquid volume. The decrease in secretion rate normalized to lung volume takes place at a time when the pulmonary epithelium is changing from columnar to cuboidal.[151] Fetal urine output can vary from 400 ml/day to a value three times that much.[152,153] Between 20 and 40 weeks gestation fetal urine production is increased about 10-fold.[153] The urine is hypotonic,[154] and it is the low osmolarity of fetal urine that results in amniotic fluid being hypotonic[154] with respect to maternal and fetal plasma. When the fetus is overhydrated the excess volume appears in the amniotic fluid as opposed to transplacental passage into the mother.[155] The regulation of fetal urine production is discussed further in the section on the fetal kidney.

Removal of fluid from the amniotic cavity is probably due primarily to fetal swallowing, which may account for volumes up to 1,500 ml/day.[156] Fluid swallowed by the fetus is made up of a mixture of amniotic and tracheal fluids.[157] Moderate increases in fetal plasma osmolality result in an increase in the number of swallowing episodes and volume swallowed studied over a short time period (minutes).[158] Because amniotic fluid is hypotonic with respect to maternal plasma, there is a potential for bulk water removal at the amniotic–chorionic interface. It has been estimated that up to 80 ml/day could be removed at this site.[159] Clearly, fetal swallowing is a more important site of bulk amniotic fluid removal.

FETAL PHYSIOLOGY

Growth and Metabolism

Substrates

The caloric requirements of the growing fetus can be considered under two categories. The first is metabolism, which results in the production of heat; the second is the synthesis and accretion of new tissue. Metabolism represents the energy necessary to sustain the existing organism and that needed to lay down new tissue. The metabolic rate is reflected by the oxygen consumption of the fetus and is of the order of 8 ml/kg/min. The requirements for new tissue will depend on the rate of growth and the type of tissue that is being acquired. The newborn infant has a body composition that is 16 percent fat.[160] Based on body composition and growth rates during the third trimester, it has been estimated that the fetus is taking on about 82 g (dry weight) of fat per week between 36 weeks and term.[161] At 26 weeks there is little fat content in the fetus, and the rate of acquisition increases gradually up to 32 weeks, when a rapid rate begins. In contrast, the nonfat acquisition by the fetus is linear from 32 to 39 weeks, when it flattens out. Also the rate of increase in nonfat is only about one-half that of fat in late gestation, about 43 g (dry weight) per week. With these rates of fat and nonfat tissue accretion, it has been estimated[161,162] that the fetus requires about 12 kcal/kg/day at 26 weeks made up of 7 kcal nonfat and 5 kcal fat. The nonfat requirements during the remainder of the third trimester vary between 7 and 14 kcal/kg/day, being maximal between 31 and 34 weeks. Fat acquisition with its steeper rise during this period increases to 35 kcal/kg/day by 36 weeks, when it plateaus. Thus the total caloric requirement for tissue acquisition in the last 4 weeks of gestation is about 40 kcal/kg/day. To this must be added the metabolic consumption of fetal substrates necessary to sustain the 8 ml/kg of oxygen that is consumed each minute. Because there is at present no definite evidence that fatty acids partake in oxidative metabolism, the caloric requirement of fetal oxygen consumption may be estimated by assuming that protein and carbohydrate are the substrates. Based on a figure of 4.9 kcal/L of oxygen, this works out to 56 kcal/kg/day. Thus the total caloric requirement for a 3.0-kg fetus in late gestation would be about 290 kcal/day. Of the total fetal oxygen consumed, it has been estimated that 20 percent is the metabolic requirement for acquiring new tissue and the remainder is to sustain the tissue that is present.[163]

The exact partitionings of substrates for oxidative metabolism and tissue accretion in the fetus are not known. However, a number of facts have been established. Glucose by itself cannot account for fetal oxidative metabolism. This is derived from the observed umbilical vein to umbilical artery concentration differences for glucose and oxygen.[164] If one assumes that all glucose is metabolized aerobically, then for glucose to act as the only substrate 6 mol would be taken up for each mole of oxygen. In fact, only 4.8 mol of glucose per mole of oxygen are taken up.[164] Added to this are the observations that the fetus has the necessary enzymes for conversion of carbohydrate to lipid[165] and that direct measurements of glucose oxidation indicate that only two-thirds appear as carbon dioxide.[166] Thus we must conclude that, in addition to glucose, the fetus uses other substrates for oxidative metabolism. Under normal conditions, the glucose utilized by the fetus is all derived from the placenta; that is, there is no significant endogenous glucose production.[167]

Amino acids are used by the fetus not only for the synthesis of proteins, but also as substrates for metabolism, resulting in the production of urea and carbon dioxide. Fetal plasma urea is higher than that in the mother, and the fetal urea production rate, which is greater than that in adults,[168] indicates that a considerable portion of the amino acids taken up by the umbilical circulation are used for aerobic metabolism. It has been shown that a number of amino acids are taken up by the fetus at rates that exceed their accretion into fetal tissues.[169] As discussed in the section on amino acid transport by the placenta, glutamate is an exception. There is evidence for placental–hepatic cycling of certain amino acids. Glycine shows a net flux from the placenta and then is taken up by the fetal liver, whereas serine, which has little or no uptake from the placenta, is released from the liver.[170,171] In fetal sheep lactate is taken up by the umbilical circulation and oxidized to carbon dioxide.[166] The role of lactate in human fetal metabolism is not presently known.

Hormones

Fetal hormones may influence fetal growth by acting on the intermediary metabolism of substrates or by acting as mitogenic agents for cell proliferation. Growth hormone is important for postnatal growth at which time its effects are mediated by the IGFs.[172] While the liver is a significant location for the synthesis of IGF-I, it has also been shown that this growth-promoting factor is present in many tissues.[173] This suggests that tissue concentration may be more important than plasma levels and that growth hormone may be a regulator by means of localized IGF-I release. IGF-II is significant for fetal growth, as shown in animal studies in which genetic manipulations resulting in only one allele and decreased mRNA for IGF-II results in small offspring. In the intra-uterine period growth hormone does not appear to play the major role in growth that it does postnatally.[174-178] The fetal thyroid is also not important for overall fetal growth, but it is important for the development of the central nervous system.[174,175]

The importance of insulin for fetal growth is suggested from the increase in fetal weight and increase in heart and liver weights in infants of diabetic mothers.[179] Less commonly observed but equally dramatic are the low birth weights associated with a lack of fetal insulin.[175] Fetal body weight increases can be achieved with elevated insulin levels that are within physiologic limits.[180] An increase in endogenous fetal insulin is associated with a significant increase in glucose uptake by the fetus.[181,182] In addition, the fetus responds to elevations in blood glucose with insulin secretion, although the rapid phase of insulin release is not seen.[183] At the plasma levels with which insulin causes an increase in fetal growth,[180] it would not be expected to act as a mitogen.[184] However, at these concentrations it could increase the binding of IGF-II[185] to its receptors and thus indirectly lead to cell proliferation. Fetal liver cells contain separate receptors for insulin and for IGF-II by the end of the first trimester.[186] The number of insulin receptors per gram of hepatic tissue triples by 28 weeks gestation while those for IGF-II are constant.[186] These observations on the concentration of IGF-II and insulin receptors suggest that the role of insulin may be more important in the later stages of pregnancy, a suggestion that is consistent with the growth patterns of infants of diabetic mothers.[187,188] Experimentally induced hypoinsulinemia results in decreased fetal growth and a 30 percent fall in glucose utilization by the fetus in utero.[189-191] It has also been shown that plasma levels of both IGF-I and IGF-II increase in fetal blood beginning at 32 to 34 weeks gestation.[192] The control of IGFs in fetal life is not understood. Based on the observation that placental lactogen stimulates IGF-II synthesis by embryo fibroblasts in vitro, it has been suggested that this hormone may be important for growth in utero.[193] Placental lactogen receptors are present in human fetal liver and muscle in the second trimester, and hepatic binding capacity correlates with body weight.[194] This has to be balanced against the clinical observation that undetectable levels of placental lactogen in maternal or cord blood have been associated with a normal birth weight.[195] However, subsequent studies have suggested that variants of placental lactogen are present in these cases.

The effect of endogenous insulin secretion on fetal glucose consumption has been mentioned above. As in the adult, fetal insulin secretion is modulated by the autonomic nervous system. β-Adrenergic activation results in insulin secretion, whereas α-adrenergic activation is responsible for the low basal rates at which insulin is secreted.[196,197] Glucagon is present in the fetus, and its secretion is modulated by the β-adrenergic system.[196] However, the glycemic response to glucagon is blunted in the fetus probably because of relative lack of hepatic receptors.[198]

In addition to the IGFs, other growth factors may be involved in the growth of specific fetal organs. Epidermal growth factor appears to have a role in lung growth and in growth and differentiation of the secondary palate.[199] The normal development of the sympathetic adrenergic system is dependent on nerve growth factor.[199]

Circulation

Anatomy

An understanding of fetal cardiovascular physiology requires familiarity with the peculiarities of the fetal circulatory anatomy. This is best traced from the entry of oxygenated blood in the umbilical vein (Fig. 4.4). The umbilical vein gives off branches to the left lobe of the liver; it then gives rise to the origin of the ductus venosus and to a major branch to the right that joins the portal vein to supply the right lobe of the liver. Approximately one-half of the umbilical blood flow courses through the ductus venosus.[200] Total umbilical blood flow has been estimated to range from 70 to 130 ml/min/kg fetal weight[201] during the last 10 weeks of pregnancy. Blood from the left hepatic vein, which has a higher oxygen content relative to that of the right hepatic vein, joins the inferior vena cava and forms a stream that is preferentially directed across the foramen ovale (Figs. 4.4 and 4.5). This results in umbilical vein blood with its higher oxygen content entering the left ventricle and supplying the carotid circulation. The right lobe of the

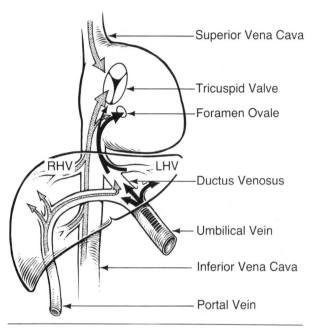

Fig. 4.4 Anatomy of the umbilical and hepatic circulation. RHV, right hepatic vein; LHV, left hepatic vein. (From Rudolph,[200] with permission.)

liver receives its blood supply from the portal vein (only a small fraction of portal vein blood passes through the ductus venosus) and the ductus venosus so that the blood in the right hepatic vein is less oxygenated than its counterpart on the left.[200] After joining the inferior vena cava, right hepatic vein flow is in the most part transmitted through the tricuspid valve (Fig. 4.4) for ejection by the right ventricle (Fig. 4.5). The blood from the superior vena cava also primarily passes through the tricuspid valve to the right ventricle. The major portion of the flow in the pulmonary artery courses through the ductus arteriosus and descends the aorta (Fig. 4.5); only about 5 percent to 10 percent of the combined output of both ventricles goes to the lung.[202] The flow across the ductus arteriosus is achieved by a 2 to 3 mmHg higher mean arterial pressure in the pulmonary artery compared with the abdominal aorta and represents about 50 percent of the biventricular output.[202] Flow across the foramen ovale is approximately one-third of combined cardiac output.[202]

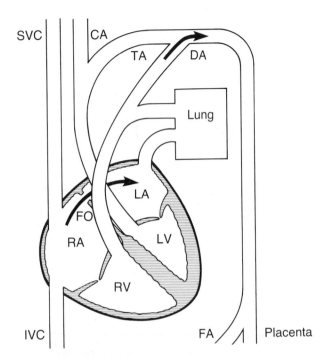

Fig. 4.5 Anatomy of fetal heart and central shunts. SVC, superior vena cava; CA, carotid artery; TA, thoracic aorta; DA, ductus arteriosus; RA, right atrium; FO, foramen ovale; LA, left atrium; RV, right ventricle; LV, left ventricle; IVC, inferior vena cava; FA, femoral artery. (From Anderson et al.,[202] with permission.)

Heart

The output of the fetus's left ventricle has been estimated at about 120 ml/min/kg body weight.[126] If left ventricular output is 40 percent of the combined biventricular output,[202] then total fetal cardiac output would be about 300 ml/min/kg. The distribution of the cardiac output to fetal organs is given in Table 4.2. It should be pointed out that the distribution to the fetal liver is only that portion that is supplied by the hepatic artery. In fact, the fetal liver receives about 25 percent of the total venous return to the heart, but its blood flow is derived principally from the umbilical vein and to a lesser extent from the portal vein.[204] The output of each of the fetal heart ventricles will depend on the contractility, the extent of lengthening of the chamber's sarcomeres, the pressure in the pulmonary artery and aorta, and the heart rate. Figure 4.6 depicts the relationship between mean right atrial pressure (the index often

Table 4.2 Distribution of Fetal Cardiac Ouput

Organ	Percentage of Biventricular Cardiac Output
Placenta	40
Brain	13
Heart	3.5
Lung	7
Liver	2.5 (hepatic artery)
Gastrointestinal tract	5
Adrenal glands	0.5
Kidney	2.5
Spleen	1
Body	25

(Data from Rudolph and Heymann[125] and Paton et al.[203])

used for ventricular volume at the end of diastole) and stroke volume. It can be seen that there is a steep ascending limb representing the length–active tension relation for cardiac muscle in the right ventricle.[205] However, because fetal right atrial pressure under normal conditions resides at the break point in this ascending limb, an increase in this pressure would not lead to an increase in stroke volume. Thus the Starling mechanism does not contribute to an increase in output of the right heart of the fetus in utero. However, a decrease in venous return leading to a fall in right atrial pressure would cause a decrease in stroke volume. The right ventricle is very sensitive to afterload, and there is a linear inverse relationship between stroke volume and pulmonary artery pressure.[205] Thus the fall in pulmonary artery pressure that takes place at birth would result in a significant increase in output from the right heart. Compared with its counterpart on the left, the right ventricle in the fetus has a greater anteroposterior dimension resulting in a greater volume and greater circumferential radius of curvature. This anatomic difference results in an increased ratio of radius to wall thickness for the right ventricle, producing increased wall stress in systole and a decrease in stroke volume when there is an increase in afterload.[206] The left ventricle has a relationship between atrial pressure and stroke volume similar to that shown in Figure 4.6 for the right ventricle. In addition, the break point occurs near the normal value for left atrial pressure, although there is a small amount of preload reserve.[207]

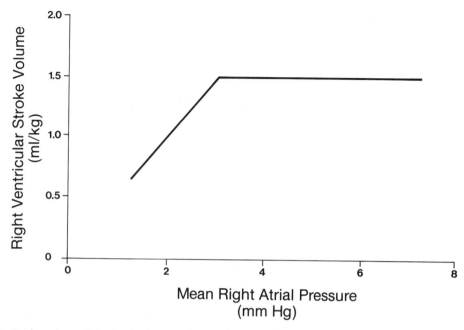

Fig. 4.6 Stroke volume of the fetal right ventricle as a function of mean right atrial pressure. (From Thornburg and Morton,[205] with permission.)

In contrast to the right ventricle, the left side of the fetal heart is not sensitive to increases in aortic blood pressure, and the postnatal increases in systemic blood pressure would not be expected to affect its stroke volume. The fetal heart in late gestation has β-adrenergic receptors in a concentration similar to that of the adult.[208] The fetal heart is stimulated by catecholamines, which may increase stroke volume by as much as 50 percent.[209] Blood flow to the myocardium reflects the greater stroke volume of the right side in that right ventricular free wall and septal blood flows are higher than those of the left ventricle.[210] Lactate and glucose constitute the major substrates used for oxidative metabolism of the fetal heart. In contrast to the adult heart, free fatty acids are not metabolized in significant amounts by the myocardium in utero.[211] This may be a function of substrate availability, as palmitate can be oxidized by fetal heart muscle,[212] although to a lesser extent than that in the neonate.

Fetal heart rate falls during the last half of gestation. This observation is particularly pronounced during the period from 20 to 30 weeks. If analysis is confined to episodes of low heart period variation, then the fall in mean heart rate continues from 30 weeks to term. However, if all heart rate data are analyzed, the value for mean heart rate is stable at 142 bpm over the last 10 weeks of gestation.[213] There is also significant change over 24 hours in mean fetal heart rate with a trough between 200 and 600 hours and a peak between 800 and 1000 hours.[214] The majority of fetal heart rate accelerations occur simultaneous with limb movement as a result of central neuronal brain stem output. A smaller number occur as a consequence of movement possibly because of decreased venous return and reflex tachycardia.[215]

In general, over a heart rate range of 120 to 180 bpm right and left ventricular stroke volumes decrease with an increase in heart rate such that fetal cardiac output remains constant.[216-218] The major effect of this inverse relationship between heart rate and stroke volume is an alteration in end diastolic dimension. If end diastolic dimension is kept constant, there is no fall in stroke volume and cardiac output goes up.[217,218]

Autonomic Regulation

The sympathetic and parasympathetic systems have important roles in the regulation of heart rate, cardiac contractility, and vascular tone. Their regulatory roles come into play by means of reflex stimulation of peripheral baroreceptors and chemoreceptors as well as central mechanisms. In the fetus the sympathetic system is developed early in fetal life, whereas the parasympathetic system develops somewhat later.[219–221] Nevertheless, in the third trimester parasympathetic tone is involved in the regulation of the fetal heart rate, and the tachycardia in response to atropine is well recognized.[222] The variability in R–R interval from one heart cycle to the next and the variability in basal heart rate seen over periods of a few minutes are caused in part by the opposing influences of the sympathetic and parasympathetic stimuli to the fetal heart. However, even when these are removed there is a residual variability.[222]

The fetal sympathetic innervation is not essential for maintenance of the resting blood pressure level as long as circulating catecholamines are present.[223] Nevertheless, fine cardiovascular control of blood pressure and fetal heart rate requires an intact sympathetic system, as the endocrine responses are too slow to maintain reflex vascular control effectively.[224] Moreover, in the circulatory response to hypoxia the normal increase in vascular resistance of the peripheral, renal, and splanchnic beds[129,131] and the associated increase in blood pressure are not seen without functional adrenergic innervation.[225,226] The fall in pulmonary blood flow and increase in myocardial, adrenal, and brain blood flow seen with hypoxia are preserved in the absence of sympathetic innervation, indicating that local regulation of blood flow is important in these organs.

Receptors located in the carotid body and arch of the aorta respond to pressor or respiratory gas stimulation with afferent modulation of heart rate and vascular tone. The fetus has baroreceptor activity, but the heart rate response in terms of degree of lengthening of the heart period per mmHg rise in blood pressure is blunted when compared with that of the adult.[227,228] During the last one-third of gestation, the sensitivity of the fetal baroreceptor effect on lengthening the heart period more than doubles.[227] The efferent limb of this reflex, which results in slowing of the heart rate, is through the parasympathetic system. The set point for fetal heart rate does not depend on intact baroreceptors. However, in the absence of functional arterial baroreceptors there is a marked increase in the variability of the fetal heart rate.[229]

The same observation has been made for fetal blood pressure, and it is evident that arterial baroreceptors exert a buffering effect on the variation in fetal blood pressure that takes place during fetal movement or breathing movements.[229,230] The baroreceptors may also modulate the increase in average fetal blood pressure that takes place in late gestation.[230] Peripheral arterial chemoreceptors are also important components for fetal reflex responses in that the initial bradycardia that takes place with hypoxia is not seen without functional chemoreceptors.[231] Chemoreceptors may also contribute to resting vascular tone in the peripheral circulation such that their absence is associated with a greater flow to the fetal body that takes place at the same mean arterial pressure.[229]

Hormonal Regulation

Arginine vasopressin is present in the fetal neurohypophysis by midgestation. Plasma levels increase in response to hypoxemia and fetal blood loss.[232] Infusions of vasopressin that raise fetal concentrations to the level seen during hypoxemia result in a decrease in blood flow to the gastrointestines and periphery whereas those to myocardium and brain increase. This is similar to the response seen with hypoxemia. However, the decrease in renal and pulmonary blood flows and the increase in blood flow characteristic of hypoxemia are not seen with vasopressin infusions.[233]

Angiotensin II levels in fetal plasma are also increased in response to small changes in blood volume and to hypoxemia.[232] In contrast to vasopressin, when angiotensin II is infused into the fetus to mimic the levels seen with fetal stress, a number of different responses are seen. Fetal heart rate is increased after an initial reflex bradycardia, and this appears to be a direct effect on the heart[234]; with vasopressin a bradycardia is seen. Both hormones cause an increase in fetal blood pressure similar to that seen with hypoxemia. However, angiotensin II does not cause a reduction in blood flow to the periphery, although it may be that the circulation to muscle, skin, and bone is always under maximum response to this hormone and further increases fail to augment the resting tone.[234] Renal blood flow is decreased with angiotensin II infusions and there is an increase in resistance of the umbilical circulation, while the absolute level of placental blood flow remains the same. Pulmonary blood flow increases because of release of vasodilatory substances within the pulmonary circulation. Adrenocorticotropic hormone (ACTH) and the catecholamines will be discussed in the section on fetal adrenal glands.

Hemoglobin

The partial pressure of oxygen in fetal arterial blood is in the range of 20 to 25 mmHg. Yet the fetus exists in a state of aerobic metabolism with no evidence of metabolic acidosis. One of the mechanisms that provides for adequate tissue oxygenation in the face of a hypoxemia relative to the adult is the higher cardiac output and organ blood flow. Another mechanism is the difference in the oxygen-carrying characteristics of fetal hemoglobin. The fetus has a higher hemoglobin concentration, averaging about 18 g/dl, than the adult. Fetal whole blood differs from that of the adult in the relationship between its oxygen saturation and the partial pressure of oxygen. The fetal oxygen dissociation curve lies to the left of that of the adult. That is, for any given oxygen tension fetal blood will have a higher oxygen saturation (see Fig. 4.7). Adult blood is

50 percent saturated with oxygen at a partial pressure of 26.5 mmHg. At this partial pressure fetal whole blood is 70 percent saturated, and the oxygen tension must fall to 20 mmHg before fetal whole blood reaches 50 percent saturation.[235]

The basis for the increased oxygen affinity of fetal whole blood resides in the interaction of fetal hemoglobin with the intracellular organic phosphate 2,3-diphosphoglycerate (2,3-DPG). The fetal hemoglobin (HgbF) tetramere is composed of two α-chains (identical to adult) and two γ-chains. The latter differs from the β-chain of adult hemoglobin (HgbA) in 39 of the 146 amino acid residues. Among these differences, that at β-143 is of particular importance. In adult hemoglobin histidine occupies this position, which is located at the entrance to the central cavity of the hemoglobin tetramere. By virtue of its positively charged imidazole group, histidine can form a bond with 2,3-DPG, which has about 3.5 negative charges at physiologic pH. 2,3-DPG binds to deoxyhemoglobin and stabilizes the tetramere in its reduced form. If adult or fetal hemoglobin is removed from the erythrocyte and stripped of its organic phosphates, then there is little difference in oxygen affinity for the soluble hemoglobins. However, when equal amounts of 2,3-DPG are added to the hemoglobins, the oxygen affinity of HgbA decreases (dissociation curve shifts to the right) to a greater extent than that of HgbF. The difference in 2,3-DPG's ability to bind to the respective hemoglobin is due in considerable part to the presence of serine at position 143 in the γ-chain of HgbF. Serine is nonionized and does not interact with 2,3-DPG to the extent that histidine would.[236] Thus HgbF on its own has an oxygen affinity similar to that of HgbA. However, inside their respective erythrocytes, where there is a similar concentration of 2,3-DPG, the HgbF interacts to a lesser extent with the organic phosphate than does HgbF, and this results in a higher oxygen affinity.

The proportion of HgbF to HgbA changes in the last one-third of pregnancy. At 26 weeks the fetus has virtually 100 percent HgbF. There is a gradual linear decrease so that at 40 weeks gestation there is about 70 percent HgbF and 30 percent HgbA.[237] This switch in synthesis from fetal to adult, which involves a change from γ- to β-globulin synthesis, takes place in erythroid progenitor cells.[238] These progenitor cells in turn are committed to the formation of nucleated

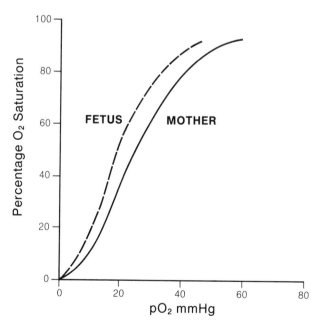

Fig. 4.7 Oxyhemoglobin dissociation curves of maternal and fetal human blood at pH 7.4 and 37°C. (Adapted from Hellegers and Schruefer,[235] with permission.)

erythroid cells from pro- to orthochromatic erythroblasts.

There is considerable understanding of the nature of human globin genes which is important for insights into the nature of such fetal hemoglobin disorders as the thalassemias and sickle cell anemia. The α-genes are on chromosome 16, and they are duplicated; that is, in the normal fetus there would be four gene loci. The genes for the remaining globins are located on chromosome 11 and consist of G_γ, A_γ, δ, and β. The two types of γ gene differ only in that one codes for glycine at position 136 and the other for alanine. The synthesis of hemoglobin A is dictated by the α- and β-genes, that of HgbF by α- and γ-genes, and that of HgbA by α- and δ-genes. There is evidence that sequences in the δ-region are responsible for the relative expression of the γ-gene such that there is persistence of fetal hemoglobin when these are absent.[239]

Kidney

Although the placenta does provide for fetal water and ionic homeostasis, the formation of urine by the fetal kidney in utero is important for amniotic fluid balance. Glomerular filtration rate (GFR) expressed as an absolute value increases during the third trimester. However, the rate of increase exactly parallels the increase in weight of the fetal kidney so that there is no change in GFR per gram of kidney weight.[240] Because the number of glomeruli become fixed at about 36 weeks,[241] the final stages of increase in GFR must be due to such factors as increases in surface area for filtration in each glomerulus, effective filtration pressure, and capillary filtration coefficient. Filtration in the glomerulus is related to hydrostatic pressure. There is a small increase in fetal blood pressure in the third trimester; however, the filtration fraction (defined as the GFR divided by renal plasma flow) remains constant.[240] Renal blood flow per gram of kidney weight does not increase in late gestation. The increase in filtration fraction that takes place in the newborn is of a magnitude similar to the increase in arterial pressure. This suggests that the relatively low GFR and filtration fraction of the intrauterine kidney are in part related to the lower hydrostatic pressure within the glomerulus.[240,242] Sodium and chloride reabsorption by the renal tubules increases in late gestation. There is some uncertainty whether the reabsorption rates change in parallel to the increases in GFR; nevertheless, there appears to be no large degree of tubuloglomerular imbalance in the third-trimester fetus.[242,243]

Relative to the newborn, fetal urine is hypotonic. Free water clearance is the index that relates actual urine flow to urine flow expected if urine osmolarity were equal to that of plasma. Solute-free water clearance, which is the difference between urine flow rate and osmolar clearance, is positive in the fetus. Although it does not become negative (indicative of a hypertonic urine), free water clearance may decrease in late pregnancy.[244] Because the collecting ducts have an arginine vasopressin response in the second trimester,[245] diminished urine-concentrating ability is not due to absolute lack of end-organ receptors. Nevertheless, there is evidence that the response of the fetal kidney to vasopressin is less than the adult in that a higher plasma concentration of this hormone is necessary before urine osmolarity reaches that of blood plasma.[246] In addition, the low rate of urea clearance and the relative short length of Henle's loop in the fetal kidney are thought to diminish the ability of the inner medula to reabsorb free water. Atrial natriuretic peptide granules are present in fetal hearts, and the plasma levels of this hormone are higher in the fetus than in the adult.[247] The fetus responds to volume expansion with an increase in atrial natriuretic peptide.[248] The actions of atrial natriuretic peptide in the fetus are primarily directed at volume homeostasis, with an increase in renal sodium excretion and a decrease in plasma volume. There is only a minor effect in lowering blood pressure.[247]

The fetus does not show the ability to develop a gradient between urine pH and that of plasma to the extent seen in the adult. This is due to the limited ability of the fetal kidney to excrete titratable acid and ammonia. In addition, renal bicarbonate excretion reaches its threshold (defined as the excretion of a determined amount of bicarbonate per unit GFR) at fetal plasma bicarbonate levels that are lower than in the adult. That is, despite the fact that fetal $Paco_2$ is higher than in the adult, the fetus shows a tendency to aklalinize its urine at a relatively low plasma bicarbonate level.[249] The ability to reabsorb glucose is well developed in the fetal renal tubule. When expressed as a function of their relative GFRs, the maximum ability of the fetal kidney to reabsorb glucose exceeds that of the adult.[250]

Gastrointestinal System

Gastrointestinal Tract

Because amniotic fluid contains significant concentrations of glucose, lactate, and amino acids, fetal swallowing has the potential to act as a source of nutrient uptake. However, direct measurement has shown that at the concentrations of these substrates that are present during normal conditions in utero there is no net uptake by the fetal intestines. In fact, the fetal gastrointestinal tract consumes small amounts of glucose, lactate, and amino acids.[251]

Blood flow to the fetal intestine does not increase during moderate levels of hypoxemia. The artery to mesenteric vein difference in oxygen content is also unchanged so that at a constant blood flow intestinal oxygen consumption can remain the same during moderate hypoxemia. However, with a more pronounced degree of hypoxemia fetal intestinal oxygen consumption falls as a result of a fall in blood flow and a failure of the oxygen content difference across the intestine to widen. This results in a metabolic acidosis in the blood draining the mesenteric system.[252]

Liver

The metabolic pathways for bilirubin and bile salts have not reached adult levels even in the full-term infant. Near term, the placenta is still the major route for bilirubin elimination. Less than 10 percent of an administered bilirubin load is excreted in the fetal biliary tree over a 10-hour period, and about 20 percent would remain in the fetal plasma.[253] In term infants, the pool size (normalized to body surface area) of cholate is only one-third that of the adult, and the synthetic rate from precursor is only one-half that of the adult. In premature infants, cholic acid pool size is even smaller, equalling less than one-half that of term infants, and synthesis is only one-third that at term. Indeed, in premature infants, intraluminal duodenal bile acid concentrations are near or below the level required to form lipid micelles.[253]

The fetal liver receives most of its blood supply from the umbilical vein. The left lobe is primarily supplied from this source, while the right lobe receives a blood supply from the portal vein as well. Under normal conditions, the fetal liver accounts for about 20 percent of the total fetal oxygen consumption.[254] The amount of glucose taken up by the fetal liver appears to be balanced by that released so that there is no net glucose removal under normal conditions.[254] During episodes of hypoxemia there is a significant release of glucose from the fetal liver, which is a major contribution to the hyperglycemia characteristic of short-term fetal hypoxemia.[197] This release of endogenous glucose from the fetal liver appears to be mediated in part by α-adrenergic stimulation in that it can be eliminated by an α-adrenergic blocker.[197] During hypoxia severe enough to cause a fall in fetal oxygen consumption there is a pronounced fall in right hepatic lobe oxygen uptake that exceeds that of the fetus as a whole. In contrast, oxygen uptake by the left lobe of the liver is unchanged.[254]

Adrenal and Thyroid Systems

Adrenal Glands

The fetal pituitary secretes ACTH in response to such stresses as hypoxemia, and there is an associated increase in cortisol.[255] Cortisol in turn has the ability to inhibit ACTH responses to stress.[256] Fetal ACTH, as with its adult counterpart, is derived from pro-opiomelanocortin, a precursor peptide that when cleaved gives rise to a number of hormones. This precursor is to be distinguished from preproenkephalin, a separate gene product that gives rise to met- and leu-enkephalin. The amount of the products from pro-opiomelanocortin in the fetal pituitary are different than those in the adult. In the fetus, there are large amounts of corticotropin-like intermediate lobe peptide (CLIP) and α-melanocyte–stimulating hormone (α-MSH). ACTH is also present in appreciable amounts, and the ratio of CLIP plus α-MSH to ACTH decreases in the fetus from the end of the first trimester to term.[257] With increasing gestational age there is a progressive increase in fetal cortisol levels secondary to maturation of the hypothalamic–pituitary axis. Arginine vasopressin serves as the major corticotropin-releasing factor in early gestation, and later corticotropin-releasing hormone is important. Cortisol has major positive effects on development in the pituitary (increasing the population of adult-type corticotrops) and the adrenal gland (increasing ACTH receptors).[258]

The fetal adrenal gland is an order of magnitude larger than that of the adult when compared proportionately with their respective body weights. Underneath the adrenal capsule lies the definitive zone. Cortisol is the major product of this zone, and, as previously mentioned, its output is stimulated by ACTH. Human chorionic gonadotropin (hCG) does not appear to regulate fetal adrenal cortisol secretion.[259,260] The major portion of the fetal adrenal glands is made up of the fetal zone, which constitutes 85 percent of the organ at birth. Dehydroepiandrosterone sulfate (DHEAS) is the major product of the fetal zone. In mid-pregnancy both ACTH and hCG serve as tropic agents for DHEAS secretion.[259,260] Corticosterone sulfate is secreted in only small amounts by the maternal adrenal glands, and it crosses the placenta from fetus to the maternal compartment without any metabolic conversion.[261] As such it serves as an excellent index of fetal adrenal corticosteroid activity. After the 30 weeks gestation corticosteroid sulfate levels rise in amniotic fluid,[262] and a late third-trimester increase is also seen in maternal plasma.[263] Together these observations indicate an increase in fetal adrenal cortisol production in late gestation. This cortisol rise apparently is not associated with an increase in fetal plasma ACTH. Two explanations are currently advanced for the dissociation between ACTH and cortisol in the third-trimester fetus[261]: (1) The large-molecular-weight peptides that are precursors of ACTH may suppress ACTH action on the adrenal system, which is then allowed to express its full potential as the concentration of these precursors falls. (2) The fetal adrenal definitive zone may become more responsive so that at the same ACTH level more cortisol is secreted. LDL-bound cholesterol (see section on receptor-mediated endocytosis above) is the major source of steroid precursor in the fetal adrenal system.[264] The fetal adrenal secretion of DHEAS and cortisol shows a diurnal pattern, with the evening being greater than the morning. This pattern arises from the maternal diurnal secretion of cortisol (morning greater and evening). The fetal pituitary–adrenal axis is passively influenced by the maternal corticoid steroids that cross the placenta and exert their influences on the fetus with an appreciable lag phase.[259]

Fetal plasma norepinephrine levels are higher than those of epinephrine.[265,266] Both catecholamines increase in fetal plasma after about 5 minutes of hypoxemia, and the concentration of norepinephrine always exceeds that of epinephrine.[266] Direct measurement of the adrenal gland secretory rates shows that under basal conditions norepinephrine is secreted at greater rates than is epinephrine. This relationship presists during a hypoxemic stimulus.[267] In response to hypoxemia norepinephrine secretion from the adrenal gland rises rapidly and then declines after about 5 minutes of persistent hypoxemia. The secretory rate, however, always remains above the basal rate. Epinephrine secretion begins more gradually and persists during 30 minutes of hypoxemia, suggesting that there are independent basic mechanisms for adrenal secretion of the two catecholamines.[267] The fetal plasma levels reflect these secretory rates.[266] Fetal blood pressure elevation during hypoxemia correlates with increases in norepinephrine levels, but the response plateaus so that no further hypertension is seen with continued increases in norepinephrine.[266]

Thyroid

Triiodothyronine (T3) is only minimally transferred across the placenta, and thyroid-stimulating hormone (TSH) is impermeable.[268] However, thyroxine (T4) of maternal origin is seen in appreciable levels in infants with congenital hypothyroidism.[269] By week 12 of gestation, thyrotropin-releasing hormone (TRH) is present in the fetal hypothalamus. During the remainder of the intrauterine period there is a progressive increase in TRH secretion and/or pituitary sensitivity to TRH. There is evidence that the fetal pancreas also contributes to the relatively high levels of TRH seen in the fetus.[268] Also during week 12, TSH is detectable in the fetal pituitary and can be measured in fetal serum. While T4 is measureable in fetal blood at 12 weeks, thyroid function remains low until about 20 weeks. T4 levels increase gradually from 20 weeks to term in response to a significant increase in TSH between 20 and 24 weeks, which then slowly drops off until delivery. Fetal liver T4 metabolism is immature and T3 levels are very low until week 30. In contrast, reverse T3 levels are high and decrease steadily in the last 10 weeks of gestation.

Central Nervous System

Among the many functions of the central nervous system there are two, fetal body movements and fetal breathing movements, that occupy an important place in clinical obstetrics. In the third trimester, the fetus exhibits periodic cycles that are often termed, respectively, active or reactive and quiet or nonreactive. The active cycle is characterized by clustering of gross fetal body movements, a high variability in the fetal heart period, accelerations of the fetal heart (often followed by a deceleration), and fetal breathing movements. The quiet cycle is noted by absence of fetal body movements and a low variability in the fetal heart period.[270,271] Fetal heart period variability in this context refers to deviations about the model heart rate period averaged over short (seconds) periods[272] and is to be distinguished from beat to beat variability. In the last 6 weeks of gestation approximately two-thirds of the time the infant is in the active state. The average duration of quiet periods ranges from 15 to 23 minutes (for review, see Table IV in ref. 272).

The fetal electrocorticogram shows two predominant patterns. Low-voltage electrocortical activity is associated with bursts of rapid eye movements and with fetal breathing movements.[273] As occurs with rapid eye movement sleep in the adult, there is inhibition of skeletal muscle movement that is most pronounced in those muscle groups having a high percentage of spindles. The diaphragm, which is relatively free of spindles, is not affected. The amount of time that the fetus spends moving during low-voltage electrocortical activity is much less than during high-voltage electrocortical activity.[274] Short-term hypoxia results in an inhibition of fetal body movements.[274] Polysynaptic reflexes elicited by stimulation of afferents from limb muscles are relatively suppressed when the fetus is in the low-voltage state.[275] Hypoxemia results in an inhibition of reflex limb movements, and the inhibitory neural activity arises in the midbrain area.[275]

Fetal breathing in utero is of a rapid and irregular nature. It is not associated with any significant movement of fluid into the lung.[273] The central respiratory chemoreceptors in the fetus located in the medulla are stimulated by carbon dioxide,[276,277] and central hydrogen ion concentrations must remain in the physiologic range to maintain fetal breathing. That is, central (medullary cerebrospinal fluid) acidosis stimulates respiratory incidence and depth, and alkalosis results in apnea.[278] Hypoxemia results in a marked decrease in breathing by the fetus in utero, and this may be due to an inhibitory input from centers above the medulla.[279]

The fetal brain uses glucose as its principal substrate for oxidative metabolism under normal conditions.[280] During low-voltage electrocortical activity there is an increase in cerebral blood flow and oxygen consumption relative to that seen in high-voltage[281] activity and a lactate efflux is present, whereas during high-voltage activity the fetal brain shows a net uptake of lactate.[282] Cerebral circulation in the fetus is sensitive to changes in arterial oxygen content. The marked increase in cerebral blood flow that occurs with hypoxemia is such that cerebral oxygen consumption is maintained without any widening of the oxygen content difference between artery and vein across the brain.[283] Carbon dioxide also causes cerebral vasodilatation, but the response to hypercarbia is less than that in the adult.[284]

Gonads and Genital Differentiation*

Primordial germ cells originate in the endoderm of the yolk sac and, during the eighth week of embryonic life, migrate to the genital ridge to form the indifferent gonad. 46,XY and 46,XX gonads are indistinguishable at this stage. Indifferent gonads develop into testes if the embryo or, more specifically, the gonadal stroma is 46,XY. This process begins about 43 days after conception. The testes are morphologically identifiable 7 to 8 weeks after conception (9 to 10 weeks gestation).[285]

Analysis of patients with structural abnormalities of the Y chromosome has long localized the region responsible for testicular determinant(s) to the short arm of the Y chromosome.[286] However, the manner by which the Y chromosome causes testicular differentiation is still not clear. H-Y antigen[287] is no longer considered necessary for testicular differentiation, although it may still play a pivotal role in spermatogene-

---

* Section prepared by Joe Leigh Simpson, M.D.

sis.[288] For several years a 160 kb sequence coding for a DNA zinc-binding protein, called zinc finger Y (ZFY), was considered the gene product of a unique Y testicular determinant[289]; however, recent exceptions have been found that invalidate this claim.[290,291] Whether the Y chromosome truly has a unique DNA sequence coding for a structural testis-determining factor is even beginning to be doubted. Indeed, other mechanisms of sex determination can be hypothesized, for example, presence or absence of gonadal determinants on the X and Y chromosomes differing in number between sexes solely as a result of X inactivation occurring in females but not males.[292,293] The existence of autosomal loci integral for normal testicular differentiation is consistent with this idea.[294]

In the absence of a Y chromosome, the indifferent gonad develops into an ovary. Transformation into fetal ovaries begins at 50 to 55 days of embryonic development. Initial ovarian differentiation may or may not require genes analogous to those on the Y chromosome. Actually, oocytes differentiate in 45,X embryos,[285,295] only to undergo atresia at a rate more

rapid than that expected in normal 46,XX embryos. Determinants for ovarian maintenance can be localized to specific regions of the X chromosome (see refs. 293 and 296 for further details). In addition, autosomal genes must also remain intact for successful oogenesis.

Independent of gonadal differentiation is the process of ductal and external genital development, processes that depend on the presence or absence of certain hormones. Pivotal to the process is the development of the fetal testes, which secrete two hormones (Fig. 4.8). Fetal Leydig cells produce testosterone. Testosterone stabilizes the wolffian ducts, thereby permitting differentiation of vasa deferentia, epididymides, and seminal vesicles. After conversion by 5α-reductase to dihydrotestosterone, the previously indifferent external genitalia become virilized.[297] Fetal Sertoli cells produce a second compound, antimüllerian hormone (AMH), a glycoprotein that diffuses locally to cause regression of müllerian derivatives, uterus, and fallopian tubes.[298,299] In the absence of testosterone and AMH,

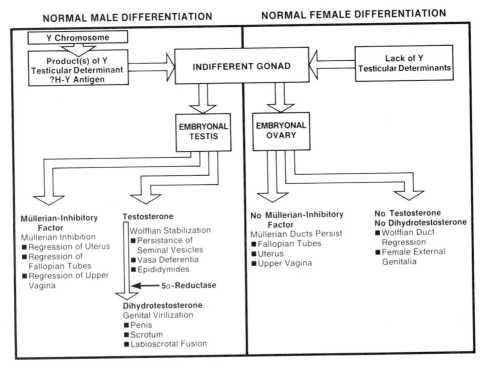

Fig. 4.8 Schematic diagram of normal male and female differentiation.

external genitalia develop in a female fashion. The müllerian ducts form the uterus and fallopian tubes, and the wolffian ducts regress. Such changes occur in normal XX embryos as well as in XY embryos castrated before testicular differentiation.

Late genital and ductal differentiation is also governed by genetic processes, as evidenced by various genetic syndromes.[294] However, their precise nature is uncertain. In females, polygenic/multifactorial factors appear operative in müllerian aplasia and incomplete müllerian fusion, implying that normal müllerian differentiation is similarly governed.[300] Moreover, Mendelian mutations are responsible for syndromes in which incomplete müllerian fusion and other uterine anomalies occur.[300] It may be assumed that autosomal genes must remain intact for normal genital differentiation. In males, similar conclusions are probably surely valid for ductal development.

REFERENCES

1. Teasdale F: Gestational changes in the functional structure of the human placenta in relation to fetal growth: a morphometric study. Am J Obstet Gynecol 137:560, 1980

2. Challier J-C, Schneider H, Dancis J: In vitro perfusion of human placenta. V. Oxygen consumption. Am J Obstet Gynecol 126:261, 1976

3. Meschia G, Battaglia FC, Hay WW Jr, Sparks JW: Utilization of substrates by the ovine placenta in vivo. Fed Proc 39:245, 1980

4. Hauguel S, Challier J-C, Cedard L, Olive G: Metabolism of the human placenta perfused in vitro: glucose transfer and utilization, O_2 consumption, lactate and ammonia production. Pediatr Res 17:729, 1983

5. Holzman I, Philipps AF, Battaglia FC: Glucose metabolism, lactate and ammonia production by the human placenta in vitro. Pediatr Res 13:117, 1979

6. Simmons MA, Battaglia FC, Meschia G: Placental transfer of glucose. J Dev Physiol 1:227, 1979

7. Hay WW Jr, Sparks JW, Wilkening RB et al: Partition of maternal glucose production between conceptus and maternal tissues in sheep. Am J Physiol 245:E347, 1983

8. Hay WW Jr, Sparks JW, Battaglia FC, Meschia G: Maternal–fetal glucose exchange: necessity of a three-pool model. Am J Physiol 246 (Endocrinol Metab 9):E523, 1984

9. Sparks JW, Hay WW Jr, Bonds D et al: Simultaneous measurements of lactate turnover rate and umbilical lactate uptake in the fetal lamb. J Clin Invest 70:179, 1982

10. Hay WW Jr, Sparks JW, Gilbert M et al: Effect of insulin on glucose uptake by the maternal hindlimb and uterus, and by the fetus in conscious pregnant sheep. J Endocrinol 100:119, 1984

11. Beischer NA, Holsman M, Kitchen WH: Relation of various forms of anemia to placental weight. Am J Obstet Gynecol 101:80, 1968

12. Beischer NA, Sivasamboo R, Vohras S et al: Placental hypertrophy in severe pregnancy anaemia. J Obstet Gynaecol Br Commonw 77:398, 1970

13. Agboola A: Placental changes in patients with a low haematocrit. Br J Obstet Gynaecol 82:225, 1975

14. Gospodarowicz D: Growth factors and their action in vivo and in vitro. J Pathol 141:201, 1983

15. Posner BI: Insulin receptors in human and animal placental tissue. Diabetes 23:209, 1974

16. Nelson DM, Smith RM, Jarett L: Nonuniform distribution and grouping of insulin receptors on the surface of human placental syncytiotrophoblast. Diabetes 27:530, 1978

17. Whitsett JA, Lenard JL: Characteristics of the microvillous brush border of human placenta: insulin receptor localization in brush border membranes. Endocrinology 103:1458, 1978

18. Steel RB, Mosley JD, Smith CH: Insulin and placenta: degradation and stabilization, binding to microvillous membrane receptors, and amino acid uptake. Am J Obstet Gynecol 135:522, 1979

19. Deal CL, Guyda HJ: Insulin receptors of human term placental cells and choriocarcinoma (JEG-3) cells: characteristics and regulation. Endocrinology 112:1512, 1983

20. Harrison LC, Itin A: Purification of the insulin receptor from human placenta by chromatography on immobilized wheat germ and receptor antibody. J Biol Chem 255:12066, 1980

21. Daughaday WH, Mariz IK, Trivedi B: A preferential binding site for insulin-like growth factor II in human and rat placental membranes. J Clin Endocrinol Metab 53:282, 1981

22. Bhaumick B, Bala RM, Hollenberg MD: Somatomedin receptor of human placenta: solubilization, photolabeling, partial purification, and comparison with insulin receptor. Proc Natl Acad Sci USA 78:4279, 1981

23. Armstrong DG, Hollenberg MD, Bhaumick B, Bala RM: Comparative studies on human placental insulin and basic somatomedin receptors. J Cell Biochem 20:283, 1982

24. MacDonald RG, Pfeffer SR, Coussens L et al: A single receptor binds both insulin-like growth factor II and mannose-6-phosphate. Science 239:1134, 1988

25. Zapf J, Rinderknecht E, Humbel RE, Froesch ER: Nonsuppressible insulin-like activity (NSILA) from human serum: recent accomplishments and their physiologic implications. Metab Clin Exp 27:1803, 1978

26. Richards RC, Beardmore JM, Brown PJ et al: Epidermal growth factor receptors on isolated human placental syncytiotrophoblast plasma membrane. Placenta 4:133, 1983

27. Lai WH, Guyda HJ: Characterization and regulation of epidermal growth factor receptors in human placental cell cultures. J Clin Endocrinol Metab 58:344, 1984

28. Cooke NE, Ray J, Emery JG, Liebhaber SA: Two distinct species of human growth hormone-variant mRNA in the human placenta predict the expression of novel growth hormone proteins. J Biol Cem 263:9001, 1988

29. Eriksson L, Frankenne F, Eden S et al: Growth hormone secretion during termination of pregnancy. Acta Obstet Gynecol Scand 67:549, 1988

30. Frankenne F, Closset J, Gomez F: The physiology of growth hormones (GHs) in pregnant women and partial characterization of the placental GH variant. J Clin Endocrinol Metab 66:1171, 1988

31. King BF: Distribution and characterization of the anionic sites in trophoblast and capillary basal lamina of human placental villi. Anat Rec 212:63, 1985

32. Thornburg KL, Faber JJ: Transfer of hydrophilic molecules by placenta and yolk sac of the guinea pig. Am J Physiol 233:C111, 1977

33. Bissonnette JM, Cronan JZ, Richards LL, Wickham WK: Placental transfer of water and nonelectrolytes during a single circulatory passage. Am J Physiol 236:C47, 1979

34. Meschia G, Battaglia FC, Bruns PD: Theoretical and experimental study of transplacental diffusion. J Appl Physiol 22:1171, 1967

35. Longo LD, Power GG, Forster RE II: Respiratory function of the placenta as determined with carbon monoxide in sheep and dogs. J Clin Invest 46:812, 1967

36. Bissonnette JM, Longo LD, Novy MJ et al: Placental diffusing capacity and its relation to fetal growth. J Dev Physiol 1:351, 1979

37. Delivoria-Papadopoulos M, Coburn RF, Forster RE II: The placental diffusing capacity for carbon monoxide in pregnant women at term. p. 259. In Longo LD, Bartles H (eds): Respiratory Gas Exchange and Blood Flow in the Placenta. DHEW, Bethesda, MD, 1972

38. Rurak DW, Gruber NC: Increased oxygen consumption associated with breathing activity in fetal lambs. J Appl Physiol 54:701, 1983

39. Wilkening RB, Boyle DW, Meschia G: Fetal neuromuscular blockade: effect on oxygen demand and placental transport. Am J Physiol 257:H734, 1989

40. Rooth G, Sjostedt S: The placental transfer of gases and fixed acids. Arch Dis Child 37:366, 1962

41. Stenger V, Eitzman D, Andersen T et al: Observations on the placental exchange of the respiratory gases in pregnant women in cesarean section. Am J Obstet Gynecol 88:45, 1964

42. Sjostedt S, Rooth G, Caligara F: The oxygen tension of the blood in the umbilical cord and intervillous space. Arch Dis Child 35:529, 1960

43. Wulf H: Der Gasaustausch in der reifen Plazenta des Menschen. Z Geburtshilfe Gynakol 158:117, 1962

44. Longo LD, Delivoria-Papadolpoulos M, Foster RE II: Placental CO_2 transfer after fetal carbonic anhydrase inhibition. Am J Physiol 226:703, 1974

45. Bissonnette JM: Studies in vivo of glucose transfer across the guinea-pig placenta. p. 155. In Young M, Boyd RDH, Longo LD, Telegdy G (eds): Placental Transfer: Methods and Interpretations. WB Saunders, Philadelphia, 1981

46. Turner RJ, Silverman M: Sugar uptake into brush border vesicles from normal human kidney. Proc Natl Acad Sci USA 74:2825, 1977

47. Johnson LW, Smith CH: Monosaccharide transport across microvillous membrane of human placenta. Am J Physiol 238:C160, 1980

48. Bissonnette JM, Black JA, Wickham WK, Acott KM: Glucose uptake into plasma membrane vesicles from the maternal surface of human placenta. J Membr Biol 58:75, 1981

49. Rice PA, Rourke JE, Nesbitt REL Jr: In vitro perfusion studies of the human placenta. VI. Evidence against active glucose transport. Am J Obstet Gynecol 133:649, 1979

50. Ciaraldi TP, Kolterman OE, Siegel JA, Olefsky JM: Insulin-stimulated glucose transport in human adipocytes. Am J Physiol 236:E621, 1979

51. Bissonnette JM, Ingermann RL, Thornburg KL: Placental sugar transport. p. 65. In Yudilevich DL, Mann GE (eds): Carrier-mediated transport of solutes from blood to tissue. Pitman, London, 1985

52. Bissonnette JM, Black JA, Thornburg KL et al: Reconstitution of D-glucose transporter from human placental microvillous plasma membranes. Am J Physiol 242:C166, 1982

53. Johnson LW, Smith CH: Identification of the glucose transport protein of the microvillous membrane of human placenta by photoaffinity labeling. Biochem Biophys Res Commun 109:408, 1982

54. Ingermann RL, Bissonnette JM, Koch PL: D-glucose-sensitive and -insensitive cytochalasin B binding pro-

teins from microvillous plasma membranes of human placenta: identification of the D-glucose transporter. Biochim Biophys Acta 730:57, 1983

55. Pilch PF: Glucose transporters: what's in a name? Endocrinology 126:3, 1990

56. Fukumoto H, Seino S, Imura H et al: Characterization and expression of human HepG2/erythrocyte glucose-transporter gene. Diabetes 37:657, 1988

57. Kayano T, Fukumuto H, Eddy RL et al: Evidence for a family of human glucose transporter-like proteins. J Biol Chem 263:15245, 1988

58. Ingermann RL, Bissonnette JM: Effect of temperature on kinetics of hexose uptake by human placental plasma membrane vesicles. Biochim Biophys Acta 734:329, 1983

59. Cordero L Jr, Yeh S-Y, Grunt JA, Anderson GG: Hypertonic glucose infusion during labor. Am J Obstet Gynecol 407:295, 1970

60. Christensen HN: Biological Transport. 2nd Ed. p. 175. WA Benjamin, Reading, MA, 1975

61. Enders RH, Judd RM, Donohue TM, Smith CH: Placental amino acid uptake. III. Transport systems for neutral amino acids. Am J Physiol 230:706, 1976

62. Stegink LD, Pitkin RM, Reynolds WA et al: Placental transfer of glutamate and its metabolites in the primate. Am J Obstet Gynecol 122:170, 1975

63. Stegink LD, Pitkin RM, Reynolds WA et al: Placental transfer of aspartate and its metabolites in the primate. Metabolism 28:669, 1979

64. Schneider H, Mohlen K-H, Dancis J: Transfer of amino acids across the in vitro perfused human placenta. Pediatr Res 13:236, 1979

65. Hayashi S, Sanada K, Sagawa N et al: Umbilical vein–artery differences of plasma amino acids in the last trimester of human pregnancy. Biol Neonate 34:11, 1978

66. Schneider H, Mohler K-H, Challier T-C, Dancis J: Transfer of glutamic acid across the human placenta perfused "in vitro." Br J Obstet Gynaecol 86:299, 1979

67. Ruzycki SM, Kelly LK, Smith CH: Placental amino acid uptake. IV. Transport by microvillous membrane vesicles. Am J Physiol 234:C27, 1978

68. Boyd CAR, Lund EK: L-proline transport by brush border membrane vesicles prepared from human placenta. J Physiol (Lond) 315:9, 1981

69. Whitsett JA, Wallick ET: [³H]oubain binding and Na⁺-K⁺-ATPase activity in human placenta. Am J Physiol 238:E38, 1980

70. Smith CH, Adcock EW III, Teasdale F et al: Placental amino acid uptake: tissue preparation, kinetics and preincubation effect. Am J Physiol 224:558, 1973

71. Smith CH, Depper R: Placental amino acid uptake. II.

Tissue preincubation, fluid distribution and mechanisms of regulation. Pediatr Res 8:697, 1974

72. Longo LD, Yuen P, Gusseck DJ: Anaerobic glycogen-dependent transport of amino acids by the placenta. Nature 243:531, 1973

73. Steel RB, Smith CH, Kelly LK: Placental amino acid uptake. VI. Regulation by intracellular substrate. Am J Physiol 243:C46, 1982

74. Dancis J, Jansen V, Kayden HJ et al: Transfer across perfused human placenta. II. Free fatty acids. Pediatr Res 7:192, 1973

75. Booth C, Elphick MC, Hentrickse W, Hull D: Investigation of [¹⁴C]linoleic acid conversion into [¹⁴C]arachidonic acid and placental transfer of linoleic and palmitic acids across the perfused human placenta. J Dev Physiol 3:177, 1981

76. Dancis J, Jansen V, Kayden HJ et al: Transfer across perfused human placenta. III. Effect of chain length on transfer of free fatty acids. Pediatr Res 8:796, 1974

77. Dancis J, Jansen V, Levitz M: Transfer across perfused human placenta. IV. Effect of protein binding on free fatty acids. Pediatr Res 10:5, 1976

78. Faber JJ, Thornburg KL: Fetal homeostasis in relation to placental water exchange. Ann Rech Vet 8:353, 1977

79. Dancis J, Kammerman BS, Jansen V et al: Transfer of urea, sodium, and chloride across the perfused human placenta. Am J Obstet Gynecol 141:677, 1981

80. Faber JJ, Thornburg KL: Placental Physiology. p. 95. Raven, New York, 1983

81. Faber JJ, Thornburg KL: The forces that drive inert solutes and water across the epitheliochorial placentae of the sheep and the goat and the haemochorial placentae of the rabbit and the guinea pig. p. 203. In Young M, Boyd RDH, Longo LD, Teleydy G (eds): Placental Transfer: Methods and Interpretations. WB Saunders, Philadelphia, 1981

82. Battaglia FC, Prystowski H, Smisson C et al: The effect of the administration of fluids intravenously to mothers upon the concentrations of water and electrolytes in plasma of human fetuses. Pediatrics 25:2, 1960

83. Anderson DF, Faber JJ: Water flux due to colloid osmotic pressures across the haemochorial placenta of the guinea pig. J Physiol (Lond) 332:521, 1982

84. Lajeunesse D, Brunette MG: Sodium gradient-dependent phosphate transport in placental brush border membrane vesicles. Placenta 9:117, 1988

85. Balkovetz DF, Leibach FH, Mahesh VB et al: Na⁺–H⁺ exchanges of human placental brush-border membrane: identification and characterization. Am J Physiol 251:C852, 1986

86. Bara M, Challier JC, Guit-Bara A: Membrane potential and input resistance in syncytiotrophoblast of human term placenta in vitro. Placenta 9:139, 1988

87. Sibley CB, Ward BS, Glazier JD et al: Electrical activity and sodium transfer across in vitro pig placenta. Am J Physiol 250:R474, 1986

88. Bahouth SW, Kelly LK, Smith CH et al: Identification of a novel MR = 76-kDa form of beta-adrenergic receptors. Biochem Biophys Res Commun 141:411, 1986

89. Shennan DB, Davis B, Boyd CAR: Chloride transport in human placental microvillous membrane vesicles. I. Evidence for anion exchange. Pflugers Arch 406:60, 1986

90. Illsley NP, Glaubensklee C, Davis B, Verkman AS: Chloride transport across placental microvillous membranes measured by fluorescence. Am J Physiol 255:C789, 1988

91. Care AD, Ross R, Pickard DW et al: Calcium homeostasis in the fetal pig. J Dev Physiol 4:85, 1982

92. Fisher GJ, Kelly LK, Smith CH: ATP-dependent calcium transport across basal plasma membranes of human placental trophoblast. Am J Physiol 252:C38, 1987

93. Durand D, Barlet JP, Braithwaite GD: The influence of 1,25-dihydroxycholecalciferol on the mineral content of foetal guinea pigs. Reprod Nutr Dev 23:235, 1983

94. Tuan RS: Identification and characterization of a calcium-binding protein from human placenta. Placenta 3:145, 1982

95. Johnson PM, Brown PJ: Fc receptors in the human placenta. Placenta 2:355, 1981

96. Loh TT, Higuchi DA, van Bockxmeer FM et al: Transferrin receptors on the human placental microvillous membrane. J Clin Invest 65:1182, 1980

97. Wild AE: Trophoblast cell surface receptors. p. 471. In Loke YW, Whyte A (eds): Biology of the Trophoblast. Elsevier Biomedical, London, 1983

98. Goldstein JL, Anderson RGW, Brown MS: Coated pits, coated vesicles and receptor-mediated endocytosis. Nature 279:679, 1979

99. Brown MS, Anderson RGW, Goldstein JL: Recycling receptors: the round trip itinerary of migrant membrane proteins. Cell 32:663, 1983

100. Pastan IH, Willingham MC: Journey to the center of the cell: role of the receptosome. Science 214:504, 1981

101. Dautry-Varsat A, Cierchanover A, Lodish HF: pH and the recycling of transferrin during receptor-mediated endocytosis. Proc Natl Acad Sci USA 80:2258, 1983

102. Lin DS, Pitkin RM, Connor WE: Placental transfer of cholesterol into the human fetus. Am J Obstet Gynecol 128:735, 1977

103. Clapp JF III: The relationship between blood flow and oxygen uptake in the uterine and umbilical circulations. Am J Obstet Gynecol 132:410, 1978

104. Wilkening RB, Meschia G: Fetal oxygen uptake, oxygenation, and acid–base balance as a function of uterine blood flow. Am J Physiol 244 (Heart Circ Physiol 13):H749, 1983

105. Itskovitz J, LaGamma EF, Rudolph LAM: The effect of reducing umbilical blood flow on fetal oxygenation. Am J Obstet Gynecol 145:813, 1983

106. Rosenfeld CR, Morriss FH Jr, Makowski ET et al: Circulatory changes in the reproductive tissues of ewes during pregnancy. Gynecol Invest 5:252, 1974

107. Longo LD, Ching KS: Placental diffusing capacity for carbon monoxide and oxygen in unanesthetized sheep. J Appl Physiol Respir Environ Exercise Physiol 43:885, 1977

108. Bissonnette JM, Wickham WK: Placental diffusing capacity for carbon monoxide in unanesthetized guinea pigs. Respir Physiol 31:161, 1977

109. Greiss FC Jr, Anderson SG: Effect of ovarian hormones on the uterine vascular bed. Am J Obstet Gynecol 107:829, 1972

110. Huckabee WE, Crenshaw C, Curet LB et al: The effect of exogenous oestrogen on the blood flow and oxygen consumption of the non-pregnant ewe. Q J Exp Physiol 55:16, 1970

111. Killam AP, Rosenfeld CR, Battaglia FC et al: Effect of estrogen on the uterine blood flow of oophorectomized ewes. Am J Obstet Gynecol 115:1045, 1973

112. Assali NS, Douglas RA, Baird WW et al: Measurement of uterine blood flow and uterine metabolism. Am J Obstet Gynecol 66:248, 1953

113. Metcalfe J, Romney SL, Ramsey LH et al: Estimation of uterine blood flow in normal human pregnancy at term. J Clin Invest 34:1632, 1955

114. Greiss FC Jr: Pressure–flow relationship in the gravid uterine vascular bed. Am J Obstet Gynecol 96:41, 1966

115. Greiss FC Jr, Anderson SG, King LC: Uterine pressure–flow relationships during early gestation. Am J Obstet Gynecol 126:799, 1976

116. Berman W Jr, Goodlin RC, Heymann MA, Rudolph AM: Relationships between pressure and flow in the umbilical and uterine circulations of the sheep. Circ Res 38:262, 1976

117. Hendricks CH, Quilligan EJ, Tyler CW, Tucker GJ: Pressure relationships between the intervillous space and the amniotic fluid in human term pregnancy. Am J Obstet Gynecol 77:1028, 1959

118. Novy MJ, Thomas CL, Lees MH: Uterine contractility and regional blood flow responses to oxytocin and

prostaglandin E_2 in pregnant rhesus monkeys. Am J Obstet Gynecol 122:419, 1975

119. Zuspan FP, O'Shaughnessy RW, Vinsel J, Zuspan M: Adrenergic innervation of uterine vasculature in human term pregnancy. Am J Obstet Gynecol 130:678, 1981

120. Rosenfeld CR, Barton MD, Meschia G: Effects of epinephrine on distribution of blood flow in the pregnant ewe. Am J Obstet Gynecol 124:156, 1976

121. Rosenfeld CR, West J: Circulatory response to systemic infusion of norepinephrine in the pregnant ewe. Am J Obstet Gynecol 127:376, 1977

122. Greiss FC Jr: Differential reactivity of the myoendometrial and placental vasculatures: adrenergic responses. Am J Obstet Gynecol 112:20, 1972

123. Meschia G: Circulation to female reproductive organs. p. 241. In Shepherd JT, Abboud FM (eds): Handbook of Physiology—The Cardiovascular System. III. Peripheral Circulation and Organ Blood Flow. American Physiological Society, Bethesda, MD, 1983

124. Rankin JHG, McLaughlin MK: The regulation of the placental blood flows. J Dev Physiol 1:3, 1979

125. Rudolph AM, Heymann MA: Circulatory changes during growth in the fetal lamb. Circ Res 26:289, 1970

126. Wladimiroff JW, McGhie J: Ultrasonic assessment of cardiovascular geometry and function in the human fetus. Br J Obstet Gynecol 88:870, 1981

127. Makowski EL, Meschia G, Droegemueller W, Battaglia FC: Measurement of umbilical arterial blood flow to the sheep placenta and fetus in utero. Circ Res 23:623, 1968

128. Thornburg KL, Bissonnette JM, Faber JJ: Absence of fetal placental waterfall phenomenon in chronically prepared fetal lambs. Am J Physiol 230:886, 1976

129. Cohn HE, Sacks EJ, Heymann MA, Rudolph AM: Cardiovascular responses to hypoxemia and acidemia in fetal lambs. Am J Obstet Gynecol 120:817, 1974

130. Parer JT: Fetal oxygen uptake and umbilical circulation during maternal hypoxia in the chronically catheterized sheep. p. 231. In Longo LD, Reneau DD (eds): Fetal and Newborn Cardiovascular Physiology. Vol. 2. Garland STPM, New York, 1978

131. Peeters LLH, Sheldon RE, Jones MD Jr et al: Blood flow to fetal organs as a function of arterial oxygen content. Am J Obstet Gynecol 135:637, 1979

132. Cohn HE, Piasecki GJ, Jackson BT: The effect of fetal heart rate on cardiovascular function during hypoxemia. Am J Obstet Gynecol 138:1190, 1980

133. Galbraith RM, Kantor RRS, Ferra GB et al: Differential anatomical expression of transplantation antigens within the normal human placental chorionic villus. Am J Reprod Immunol 1:331, 1981

134. Sunderland CA, Naiem M, Mason DY et al: The expression of major histocompatibility antigens by human chorionic villi. J Reprod Immunol 3:323, 1981

135. Beer AE: Immunologic aspects of normal pregnancy and recurrent spontaneous abortion. Semin Reprod Endocrinol 6:163, 1988

136. Sunderland CA, Redman CWG, Stirrat GM: HLA A, B, C antigens are expressed on nonvillous trophoblast of the early human placenta. J Immunol 127:2614, 1981

137. Faulk WP, Hsi B-L: Immunology of human trophoblast membrane antigens. p. 535. In Loke YW, Whyte A (eds): Biology of Trophoblast. Elsevier, New York, 1983

138. Szulman AE: The ABH blood groups and development. Curr Top Dev Biol 14:127, 1980

139. Faulk WP: Immunobiology of human extraembryonic membranes. p. 253. In Wegman TG, Gill TJ (eds): Immunology of Reproduction. Oxford, New York, 1983

140. Klopper A: The new placental proteins. Placenta 1:77, 1980

141. Rocklin RE, Kitzmiller JL, Farvoy MR: Maternal fetal relation. II. Further characterization of an immunologic blocking factor that develops during pregnancy. Clin Immunol Immunopath 22:305, 1982

142. Beer AE, Quebbeman JF, Ayers JW, Haines RF: Major histocompatibility antigens, maternal and paternal immune responses and chronic habitual abortion in humans. Am J Obstet Gynecol 141:987, 1981

143. Komlos L, Zamir R, Joshua H, Halbrecht I: Common HLA antigens in couples with repeated abortions. Clin Immunol Immunopath 7:330, 1977

144. Taylor C, Faulk WP: Prevention of recurrent abortions with leukocyte transfusions. Lancet 2:68, 1980

145. Redline RW, Lu CY: Role of local immunosuppression in murine fetoplacental listerosis. J Clin Invest 79:1234, 1987

146. Jacoby DR, Olding LB, Oldstone MD: Immunologic regulation of fetal–maternal balance. Adv Immunol 35:157, 1984

147. Brace RA, Wolf EJ: Normal amniotic fluid volume changes throughout pregnancy. Am J Obstet Gynecol 161:382, 1989

148. Anderson DF, Faber JJ, Parks CM: Extraplacental transfer of waters in the sheep. J Physiol (Lond) 406:75, 1988

149. Mescher EJ, Platzker ACG, Ballard PL et al: Ontogeny of tracheal fluid, pulmonary surfactant, and plasma corticoids in the fetal lamb. J Appl Physiol 39:1017, 1975

150. Adamson TM, Boyd RDH, Platt HS, Strang LB: Com-

position of alveolar liquid in the foetal lamb. J Physiol (Lond) 204:159, 1969

151. Olver RE, Schneeberger EE, Walters DV: Epithelial solute permeability, ion transport and tight junction morphology in the developing lung of the fetal lamb. J Physiol (Lond) 315:395, 1981

152. Gresham EL, Rankin JHG, Makowski EL et al: An evaluation of renal function in a chronic sheep preparation. J Clin Invest 51:149, 1975

153. Rabinowitz R, Peters MT, Uyas S et al: Measurement of fetal urine production in normal pregnancy by real-time ultrasonography. Am J Obstet Gynecol 161:1264, 1989

154. Canning JF, Boyd RDH: Mineral and water exchange between mother and fetus. p. 481. In Beard RW, Nathanielsz PW (eds): Fetal Physiology and Medicine. 2nd Ed. Marcel Dekker, New York, 1984

155. Brace RA: Amniotic fluid volume and its relationship to fetal fluid balance: review of experimental data. Semin Perinatol 10:103, 1986

156. Abramovich DR, Gordon A, Jandial L, Page KR: Fetal swallowing and voiding in relation to hydramnios. Obstet Gynecol 54:15, 1979

157. Harding R, Bocking AD, Sigger JN, Wickham PJD: Composition and volume of fluid swallowed by fetal sheep. Q J Exp Physiol 69:487, 1984

158. Ross MG, Sherman DJ, Ervin MG et al: Stimuli for fetal swallowing: systemic factors. Am J Obstet Gynecol 161:1559, 1984

159. Abramovich DR, Page KR, Jandial L: Bulk flows through human fetal membranes. Gynecol Invest 7:157, 1976

160. Widdowson EH, Spray CM: Chemical development in utero. Arch Dis Child 26:205, 1951

161. Sparks JW, Girard JR, Battaglia FC: An estimate of the calorie requirements of the human fetus. Biol Neonate 38:113, 1980

162. Battaglia FC: The comparative physiology of fetal nutrition. Am J Obstet Gynecol 148:850, 1984

163. Clapp JF III, Szeto HH, Larrow R et al: Fetal metabolic response to experimental placental vascular damage. Am J Obstet Gynecol 140:446, 1981

164. Morris FH Jr, Makowski EL, Meschia G, Battaglia FC: The glucose/oxygen quotient of the term human fetus. Biol Neonate 25:44, 1975

165. Warshaw JB: Fatty acid metabolism during development. Semin Perinatol 3:131, 1979

166. Hay WW, Myers SA, Sparks JW et al: Glucose and lactate oxidation rates in the fetal lamb. Proc Soc Exp Biol Med 173:553, 1983

167. Kalhan SC, D'Angelo LJ, Savin SM, Adam PAJ: Glucose production in pregnant women at term gestation:

168. sources of glucose for human fetus. J Clin Invest 63:388, 1979

169. Gresham EL, Simons PS, Battaglia FC: Maternal–fetal urea concentration differences in man: metabolic significance. J Pediatr 79:809, 1971

169. Lemons JA, Schreiner RL: Amino acid metabolism in the ovine fetus. Am J Physiol 244 (Endocrinol Metab 7):E459, 1983

170. Battaglia FC: An update of fetal and placental metabolism: carbohydrates and amino acids. Biol Neonate 55:347, 1989

171. Marconi AM, Battaglia FC, Meschia G, Sparks JW: A comparison of amino acid arteriovenous differences across the liver and placenta of the fetal lamb. Am J Physiol 257:E909, 1989

172. Schoenle E, Zopf J, Humbel RE, Groesch ER: Insulin-like growth factor I stimulates growth in hypophysectomized rats. Nature 296:252, 1982

173. D'Ercole AJ, Stiles AD, Underwood LE: Tissue concentration of somatomedin C: further evidence for multiple sites of synthesis and paracrine or autocrine mechanism of action. Proc Natl Acad Sci USA 81:935, 1984

173a. DeChiara TM, Efstratiadis A, Robertson EJ: A growth-deficiency phenotype in heterozygous mice carrying an insulin-like growth factor 11 gene disrupted by targeting. Nature 345:78, 1990

174. Jost A: Fetal hormones and fetal growth. Contrib Gynecol Obstet 5:1, 1979

175. Gluckman PD, Liggins GC: Regulation of fetal growth. p. 511. In Beard RW, Nathanielsz PW (eds): Fetal Physiology and Medicine. Marcel Dekker, New York, 1984

176. Gluckman PD: Functional maturation of the neuroendocrine system in the perinatal period: studies of the somatotrophic axis in the ovine fetus. J Dev Physiol 6:301, 1984

177. Palmiter RD, Norstedt G, Gelinas RE et al: Metallothionein–human GH fusion genes stimulate growth of mice. Science 222:809, 1983

178. Browne CA, Thorburn CA: Endocrine control of fetal growth. Biol Neonate 55:331, 1989

179. Hill DE: Fetal effects of insulin. Obstet Gynecol Ann 11:133, 1982

180. Susa JB, Neave C, Sehgal P et al: Chronic hyperinsulinemia in the fetal rhesus monkey: effects of physiologic hyperinsulinemia on fetal growth and composition. Diabetes 33:656, 1984

181. Philips AF, Dubin JW, Raye JR: Fetal metabolic responses to endogenous insulin release. Am J Obstet Gynecol 139:441, 1981

182. Hay WW, Meznarich HK, Sparks JW et al: Effect of

insulin on glucose uptake in near-term fetal lambs. Proc Soc Exp Biol Med 178:557, 1985

183. Philipps AF, Carson BS, Meschia G, Battaglia FC: Insulin secretion in fetal and newborn sheep. Am J Physiol 235 (Endocrinol Metab Gastrointest Physiol 4):E467, 1978

184. King GL, Kahn CR, Rechler MM, Nissley SP: Direct demonstration of separate receptors for growth and metabolic activities of insulin and multiplication-stimulating activity (an insulin-like growth factor) using antibodies to the insulin receptor. J Clin Invest 66:130, 1980

185. Oppenheimer CL, Pessin JE, Massague J et al: Insulin action rapidly modulates the apparent affinity of the insulin-like growth factor II receptor. J Biol Chem 258:4824, 1983

186. Sara VR, Hall K, Misaki M et al: Ontogenesis of somatomedin and insulin receptors in the human fetus. J Clin Invest 71:1084, 1983

187. Cardell BS: The infants of diabetic mothers: a morphological study. J Obstet Gynaecol Br Common 60:834, 1953

188. Siddiqi TA, Miodoonik M, Mimouni F et al: Biphasic intrauterine growth in insulin-dependent diabetic pregnancies. J Amer Coll Nutr 8:225, 1989

189. Fowden AL, Comline RS: The effects of pancreatectomy on the sheep fetus in utero. Q J Exp Physiol 69:319, 1984

190. Fowden AL, Hay WW Jr: The effects of pancreatectomy on the rates of glucose utilization, oxidation and production in the sheep fetus. Q J Exp Physiol 73:973, 1988

191. Fowden AL: The role of insulin in fetal growth. J Dev Physiol 12:173, 1989

192. Bennett A, Wilson DM, Liu F et al: Levels of insulin-like growth factor I and II in human cord blood. J Clin Endocrinol Metab 57:609, 1983

193. Adams SO, Nissley SP, Handwerger S, Rechler MM: Developmental patterns of insulin-like growth factor I and II synthesis and regulation in rat fibroblasts. Nature 302:150, 1983

194. Hill DJ, Freemark M, Strain AJ et al: Placental lactogen and growth hormone receptors in human fetal tissues: relationship to fetal plasma, human placental lactogen concentrations and fetal growth. J Clin Endocrinol Metab 66:1283, 1988

195. Nielsen PU, Pedersen H, Kampmann E-M: Absence of human placental lactogen in an otherwise uneventful pregnancy. Am J Obstet Gynecol 135:322, 1979

196. Sperling MA, Christensen RA, Ganguli S, Anand R: Adrenergic modulation of pancreatic hormone secretion in utero: studies in fetal sheep. Pediatr Res 14:203, 1980

197. Jones CT, Ritchie JWK, Walker D: The effects of hypoxia on glucose turnover in the fetal sheep. J Dev Physiol 5:223, 1983

198. Devaskar SU, Ganguli S, Styer D et al: Glucagon and glucose dynamics in sheep: evidence for glucagon resistance in the fetus. Am J Physiol 246 (Endocrinol Metab 9):E256, 1984

199. Gospodarowicz D: Epidermal and nerve growth factors in mammalian development. Annu Rev Physiol 43:251, 1981

200. Rudolph AM: Hepatic and ductus venosus blood flows during fetal life. Hepatology 3:254, 1983

201. Jouppila P, Kirkinen P, Eik-Nes S, Koivula A: Fetal and intervillous blood flow measurements in late pregnancy. p. 226. In Kurjak A, Kratochwil A (eds): Recent Advances in Ultrasound Diagnosis. Excerpta Medica, Amsterdam, 1981

202. Anderson DF, Bissonnette JM, Faber JJ, Thornburg KL: Central shunt flows and pressures in the mature fetal lamb. Am J Physiol 241:H60, 1981

203. Paton JB, Fisher DE, Peterson EN et al: Cardiac output and organ blood flows in the baboon fetus. Biol Neonate 22:50, 1973

204. Edelstone DI, Rudolph AM, Heymann MA: Liver and ductus venosus blood flows in fetal lambs in utero. Circ Res 42:426, 1978

205. Thornburg KL, Morton MJ: Filling and arterial pressures as determinants of RV stroke volume in the sheep fetus. Am J Physiol 244:H656, 1983

206. Pinson CW, Morton MJ, Thornburg KL: An anatomic basis for right ventricular dominance and arterial pressure sensitivity. J Dev Physiol 9:253, 1987

207. Thornburg KL, Morton MJ: Filling and arterial pressures as determinants of left ventricular stroke volume in fetal lambs. Am J Physiol 251:H961, 1986

208. Cheng JB, Goldfien A, Cornett LE, Roberts JM: Identification of β-adrenergic receptors using [^{3}H]dihydroalprenolol in fetal sheep heart: direct evidence of qualitative similarity to the receptors in adult sheep heart. Pediatr Res 15:1083, 1981

209. Andersen PAW, Manning A, Glick KL, Crenshaw CC Jr: Biophysics of the developing heart. III. A comparison of the left ventricular dynamics of the fetal and neonatal heart. Am J Obstet Gynecol 143:195, 1982

210. Fisher DJ, Heymann MA, Rudolph AM: Regional myocardial blood flow and oxygen delivery in fetal, newborn and adult sheep. Am J Physiol 243:H729, 1982

211. Fisher DJ, Heymann MA, Rudolph AM: Myocardial oxygen and carbohydrate consumption in fetal lambs in utero and in adult sheep. Am J Physiol 238:H399, 1980

212. Werner JC, Sicard RE, Schuler HG: Palmitate oxidation by isolated working fetal and newborn hearts. Am J Physiol 256:E315, 1989

213. Visser GHA, Dawes GS, Redman CWG: Numerical analysis of the normal human antenatal fetal heart rate. Br J Obstet Gynecol 88:792, 1981

214. Patrick J, Campbell K, Carmichael L, Probert C: Influence of maternal heart rate and gross fetal body movements on the daily pattern of fetal heart rate near term. Am J Obstet Gynecol 144:533, 1982

215. Bocking AD, Harding R, Wickham PJ: Relationship between accelerations and decelerations in heart rate and skeletal muscle activity in fetal sheep. J Dev Physiol 7:47, 1985

216. Kenny J, Plappert T, Doublet P et al: Effects of heart rate on ventricular size, stroke volume, and output in the normal human fetus: a prospective Doppler echocardiographic study. Circulation 76:52, 1987

217. Anderson PAW, Glick KL, Killam AP, Mainwaring RD: The effect of heart rate on in utero left ventricular output in the fetal sheep. J Physiol (Lond) 372:557, 1986

218. Anderson PAW, Killam AP, Mainwaring RD, Oakely AK: In utero right ventricular output in the fetal lamb: the effect of heart rate. J Physiol (London) 387:297, 1987

219. Nuwayhid B, Brinkman CR III, Su C et al: Development of autonomic control of fetal circulation. Am J Physiol 228:337, 1975

220. Assali NS, Brinkman CR III, Woods JR Jr et al: Development of neurohumoral control of fetal, neonatal, and adult cardiovascular functions. Am J Obstet Gynecol 129:748, 1977

221. Walker AM, Cannata J, Dowling MH et al: Sympathetic and parasympathetic control of heart rate in unanesthetized fetal and newborn lambs. Biol Neonate 33:145, 1978

222. Dalton KJ, Dawes GS, Patrick JE: The autonomic nervous system and fetal heart rate variability. Am J Obstet Gynecol 146:456, 1983

223. Tabsh K, Nuwayhid B, Murad S et al: Circulatory effects of chemical sympathectomy in fetal, neonatal and adult sheep. Am J Physiol 243:H113, 1982

224. Jones CT, Roeback MM, Walker DW et al: Cardiovascular, metabolic and endocrine effects of chemical sympathectomy and of adrenal demedulation in fetal sheep. J Dev Physiol 9:347, 1987

225. Iwamoto HS, Rudolph AM, Miskin BL, Keil LC: Circulatory and humoral responses of sympathectomized fetal sheep to hypoxemia. Am J Physiol 245:H767, 1983

226. Schuijers JA, Walker DW, Browne CA, Thorburn GD: Effect of hypoxemia on plasma catecholamines in intact and immunosympathectomized fetal lambs. Am J Physiol 251:R893, 1986

227. Shinebourne EA, Vapaavouri EK, Williams RL et al: Development of baroreflex activity in unanesthetized fetal and neonatal lambs. Circ Res 31:710, 1972

228. Dawes GS, Johnston BM, Walker DW: Relationship of arterial pressure and heart rate in fetal, newborn and adult sheep. J Physiol (Lond) 309:405, 1980

229. Itskovitz J, LaGamma EF, Rudolph AM: Baroreflex control of the circulation in chronically instrumented fetal lambs. Circ Res 52:589, 1983

230. Yardley RW, Bowes G, Wilkinson M et al: Increased arterial pressure variability after arterial baroreceptor denervation in fetal lambs. Circ Res 52:580, 1983

231. Rudolph AM: The fetal circulation and its response to stress. J Dev Physiol 6:11, 1984

232. Rudolph AM: Homeostasis of the fetal circulation and the part played by hormones. Ann Rech Vet 8:405, 1977

233. Iwamoto HS, Rudolph AM, Keil LC, Heymann MA: Hemodynamic responses of the sheep fetus to vasopressin infusion. Circ Res 44:430, 1979

234. Iwamoto HS, Rudolph AM: Effects of angiotensin II on the blood flow and its distribution in fetal lambs. Circ Res 48:183, 1981

235. Hellegers AE, Schruefer JJP: Normograms and empirical equations relating oxygen tension, percentage saturation, and pH in maternal and fetal blood. Am J Obstet Gynecol 81:377, 1961

236. Bunn HF, Jandl JH: Control of hemoglobin function within the red cell. N Engl J Med 282:1414, 1970

237. Bard H, Makowski EL, Meschia G, Battaglia FC: The relative rates of synthesis of hemoglobins A and F in immature red cells of newborn infants. Pediatrics 45:766, 1970

238. Alter BP, Jackson BT, Lipton JM et al: Control of the simian fetal hemoglobin switch at the progenitor cell level. J Clin Invest 67:458, 1981

239. Bank A, Mears JG, Ramirez F: Disorders of human hemoglobin. Science 207:486, 1980

240. Robillard JE, Weismann DN, Herin P: Ontogeny of single glomerular perfusion rate in fetal and newborn lambs. Pediatr Res 15:1248, 1981

241. Potter EL: Development of the human glomerulus. Arch Pathol 80:241, 1965

242. Lumbers ER: A brief review of fetal renal function. J Dev Physiol 6:1, 1984

243. Robillard JE, Sessions C, Kennedy RL et al: Interrelationship between glomerular filtration rate and renal transport of sodium and chloride during fetal life. Am J Obstet Gynecol 128:727, 1977

244. Robillard JE, Matson JR, Sessions C, Smith FG Jr: Developmental aspects of renal tubular reabsorption of water in the lamb fetus. Pediatr Res 13:1172, 1979

245. Abramow M, Dratwa M: Effect of vasopressin on the isolated human collecting duct. Nature 250:292, 1974

246. Robillard JE, Weitzman RE: Developmental aspects of the fetal renal response to exogenous arginine vasopressin. Am J Physiol 238:F407, 1980

247. Smith FG, Sata T, Vasille VA, Robillard JE: Atrial natriuretic factor during fetal and postnatal life: a review. J Dev Physiol 12:55, 1989

248. Robillard JE, Weiner C: Atrial natriuretic factor in the human fetus: effect of volume expansion. J Pediatr 113:552, 1988

249. Robillard JE, Sessions C, Burmeister L, Smith FG Jr: Influence of fetal extracellular volume contraction on renal reabsorption of bicarbonate in fetal lambs. Pediatr Res 11:649, 1977

250. Robillard JE, Sessions C, Kennedy RL, Smith FG Jr: Maturation of the glucose transport process by the fetal kidney. Pediatr Res 12:680, 1978

251. Charlton VE, Reis BL, Lofgren DJ: Consumption of carbohydrates, amino acids and oxygen across the intestinal circulation in the fetal sheep. J Dev Physiol 1:329, 1979

252. Edelstone DI, Holzman IR: Fetal intestinal oxygen consumption at various levels of oxygenation. Am J Physiol 242:H50, 1982

253. Lester R, Jackson BT, Smallwood RA et al: Fetal and neonatal hepatic function. II. Birth Defects 12:307, 1976

254. Bristow J, Rudolph AM, Itskovitz J, Barnes R: Hepatic oxygen and glucose metabolism in the fetal lamb. J Clin Invest 71:1047, 1983

255. Jones CT, Ritchie JWK: The effects of adrenergic blockage on fetal response to hypoxia. J Dev Physiol 5:211, 1983

256. Wood CE, Rudolph AM: Negative feedback regulation of adrenocorticotropin secretion by cortisol in ovine fetuses. Endocrinology 112:1930, 1983

257. Silman RE, Chard T, Lowry PJ et al: Human foetal pituitary peptides and parturition. Nature 260:716, 1976

258. Challis JRG, Brooks AN: Maturation and activation of hypothalamic pituitary adrenal function in fetal sheep. Endocrine Rev 10:182, 1989

259. Challis JRG, Mitchell BF: Endocrinology of pregnancy and parturition. p 106. In Warshaw JB (ed): The Biological Basis of Reproductive and Developmental Medicine. Elsevier, New York, 1983

260. Jaffe RB, Seron-Ferre M, Crickard K et al: Regulation and function of the primate fetal adrenal gland and gonad. Recent Prog Hormone Res 37:43, 1981

261. Challis JRG, Mitchell BR, Lye SJ: Activitation of fetal adrenal function. J Dev Physiol 6:93, 1984

262. Murphy BEP: Conjugated glucocorticoids in amniotic fluid and fetal lung maturation. J Clin Endocrinol Metab 17:212, 1978

263. Fencl M de M, Sillman RJ, Cohen J, Tulchinsky D: Direct evidence of sudden rise in fetal corticoids late in human gestation. Nature 287:225, 1980

264. Carr BR, Parker CR, Milewich L et al: The role of low density, high density and very low density lipoproteins in steroidogenesis by the human fetal adrenal gland. Endocrinology 106:1854, 1980

265. Nylund L, Langercrantz H, Lunell N-O: Catecholamines in fetal blood during birth in man. J Dev Physiol 1:427, 1979

266. Cohen WR, Piasecki GJ, Jackson BT: Plasma catecholamines during hypoxemia in fetal lamb. Am J Physiol 243:R520, 1982

267. Cohen WR, Piasecki GJ, Cohn HE et al: Adrenal secretion of catecholamines during hypoxemia in fetal lambs. Endocrinology 114:383, 1984

268. Fisher DA: Maternal–fetal thyroid function in pregnancy. Clin Perinatol 10:615, 1983

269. Vulsma T, Gons MH, DeVijlder JSM: Maternal–fetal transfer of thyroxine in congenital hypothyroidism due to a total organification defect or thyroid agenesis. N Engl J Med 321:13, 1989

270. Timor-Tritsch IE, Dierker LJ, Hertz RE et al: Studies of antepartum behavioral state in the human fetus at term. Am J Obstet Gynecol 132:524, 1978

271. Martin CB Jr: Behavioral states in the human fetus. J Reprod Med 26:425, 1981

272. Visser GHA, Goodman JDS, Levine DH, Dawes GS: Diurnal and other cyclic variations in human fetal heart rate near term. Am J Obstet Gynecol 142:535, 1982

273. Dawes GS, Fox HE, Leduc BM et al: Respiratory movements and rapid eye movement sleep in the foetal lamb. J Physiol (Lond) 220:119, 1972

274. Natale R, Clewlow F, Dawes GS: Measurement of fetal forelimb movements in the lamb in utero. Am J Obstet Gynecol 140:545, 1981

275. Blanco CE, Dawes GS, Walker DW: Effect of hypoxia on polysynaptic hindlimb reflexes of unanesthetized fetal and newborn lambs. J Physiol (Lond) 339:453, 1983

276. Bowes G, Wilkinson MH, Dowling M et al: Hypercapnic stimulation of respiratory activity in unanesthetized fetal sheep in utero. J Appl Physiol Respir Environ Exercise Physiol 50:701, 1981

277. Connors G, House C, Carmichal L et al: Control of fetal breathing in human fetus between 24 and 34 weeks gestation. Am J Obstet Gynecol 160:932, 1989

278. Hohimer AR, Bissonnette JM, Richardson BS, Machida CM: Central chemical regulation of breathing movements in fetal lambs. Respir Physiol 52:99, 1983

279. Dawes GS, Gardner WN, Johnston BM, Walker DW: Breathing activity in fetal lambs: the effect of brain stem section. J Physiol (Lond) 335:535, 1983

280. Jones MD Jr, Burd LI, Makowski EL et al: Cerebral metabolism in sheep: a comparative study of the adult, the lamb and the fetus. Am J Physiol 229:235, 1975

281. Richardson BS, Patrick JE, Abduljabbar H: Cerebral oxidative metabolism in the fetal lamb: relationship to electrocortical state. Am J Obstet 153:426, 1985

282. Chao CR, Hohimer AR, Bissonnette JM: The effect of electrocortical state on cerebral carbohydrate metabolism in fetal sheep. Dev Brain Res 49:1, 1989

283. Jones MD Jr, Sheldon RE, Peeters LL et al: Fetal cerebral oxygen consumption at different levels of oxygenation. J Appl Physiol Respir Environ Exercise Physiol 43:1080, 1977

284. Rosenberg AA, Jones MD Jr, Traystman RJ et al: Response of cerebral blood flow to changes in PCO_2 in fetal newborn and adult sheep. Am J Physiol 242 (Heart Circ Physiol 11):H862, 1982

285. Jirasek JE: Principles of reproductive embryology. p. 52. In Simpson JL (ed): Disorders of Sexual Differentiation: Etiology and Clinical Delineation. Academic, New York, 1976

286. Simpson JL: Disorders of Sexual Differentiation: Etiology and Clinical Delineation. Academic, New York, 1976

287. Wachtel SS: H-Y Antigen and Biology of Sex Determination. Grune & Stratton, New York, 1983

288. Simpson E, McLaren A, Chandler P et al: Expression of H-Y antigen by female mice carrying SXR. Transplantation 37:17, 1984

289. Page DC, Mosher R, Simpson E et al: The sex determining region of the human Y chromosome encodes a finger protein. Cell 51:1091, 1987

290. Palmer MS, Sinclair AH, Berta P et al: Genetic evidence that ZFY is not the testis-determining factor. Nature 342:937, 1989

291. Koopman P, Gubbay J, Collignon J et al: ZFY gene expression patterns are not compatible with a primary role in mouse sex determination. Nature 342:940, 1989

292. Chandra HS: Is human X chromosome inactivation a sex determining device? Proc Natl Acad Sci USA 82:6947, 1985

293. Simpson JL: Phenotypic–karyotypic correlations of gonadal determinants: current status and relationship to molecular studies. p. 224. In Sperling K, Vogel F (eds): Human Genetics: Proceedings of the 7th International Congress on Human Genetics (Berlin 1986). Springer-Verlag, Heidelberg, 1987

294. Simpson JL: Disorders of gonads and internal reproductive ducts. In Emery AEH, Rimoin DL (eds): Principles of Practice of Medical Genetics. 2nd Ed. Churchill Livingstone, Edinburgh, 1990

295. Singh RP, Carr DH: The anatomy and histology of XO human embryos and fetuses. Anat Rec 155:369, 1966

296. Simpson JL, Rebar RW: Normal and abnormal sexual differentiation and development. p. 710. In Becker KL (ed): Principles and Practice of Endocrinology and Metabolism. JB Lippincott, Philadelphia, 1990

297. Siiteri PK, Wilson JD: Testosterone formation and metabolism during male sexual differentiation in the human embryo. J Clin Endocrinol Metab 38:113, 1974

298. Cates RL, Mattaliano RJ, Hession C et al: Isolation of bovine and human genes for müllerian inhibiting substance and expression of human gene in animal cells. Cell 45:685, 1986

299. Cohen-Haguenauer O, Picard JY, Mattei MG et al: Mapping of the gene for anti-müllerian hormone to the short arm of human chromosome 19. Cytogenet Cell Genet 44:2, 1987

300. Simpson JL, Golbus MS: Genetics in Obstetrics and Gynecology. 2nd Ed. WB Saunders, Philadelphia (in press)

Chapter 5

Maternal Physiology in Pregnancy

Dwight P. Cruikshank and Patricia M. Hays

Many organs undergo physiologic changes during pregnancy. Understanding these changes is important in determining what is normal or abnormal in a pregnant woman.

ALIMENTARY TRACT

Appetite

Most women experience an increase in appetite beginning early in the first trimester and persisting throughout pregnancy. In the absence of nausea or "morning sickness," women eating according to appetite will increase their daily food intake by about 200 kcal by the end of the first trimester.[1] The recommended dietary allowance (RDA) calls for an additional 300 kcal/day during pregnancy,[2] although a greater increase may be necessary for adolescents, who are still growing themselves, and for women with high levels of physical activity.

There is extensive folklore about dietary cravings and aversions during pregnancy. Many of these are undoubtedly due to the individual woman's perception of which foods aggravate or ameliorate such symptoms as nausea and heartburn. The sense of taste may be blunted in some pregnant women, leading to an increased desire for highly seasoned food. Pica is not rare among pregnant women, and a history of such should be sought in those with poor weight gain or refractory anemia. Among rural Southern black women the most common forms of pica involve consumption of clay or starch (either laundry or cornstarch), while in the United Kingdom the most common craving is for coal. Soap, toothpaste, and ice pica are also reported, and we have cared for one patient who consumed coffee grounds and another who ate newspaper during pregnancy.

Mouth

The pH of saliva is probably unchanged during pregnancy. Some studies purport to show a decline, and others a rise, in salivary pH; all studies suffer from methodologic deficiencies in that the saliva was not collected anaerobically to prevent escape of CO_2 with a resultant change in pH.

Likewise, the production of saliva is probably unchanged in pregnancy. Kallander and Sonesson[3] catheterized the submandibular glands of pregnant women and found secretion rates of 0.10 ml/min compared with 0.15 ml/min in nonpregnant subjects. Ptyalism is an unusual complication of pregnancy, most often occurring in women suffering from nausea, associated with the loss of 1 to 2 L of saliva per day. It may be helped by decreased ingestion of starchy foods. Most authorities believe that ptyalism actually represents inability of the nauseated woman to swallow normal amounts of saliva rather than being a true increase in production of saliva.

There is no evidence that pregnancy causes or accelerates the course of dental caries. The gums, however, usually become edematous and soft and may bleed after tooth brushing. At times a tumorous gingivitis can occur during pregnancy, presenting as violaceous pedunculated lesions at the gum line that may bleed profusely. Called epulis gravidarum, these are the same lesions dentists refer to as pyogenic granulomas. They usually regress 1 to 2 months after delivery; if not, or if they bleed excessively during pregnancy, they should be excised.

Stomach

The tone and motility of the stomach are decreased during pregnancy, probably because of the smooth muscle – relaxing effects of progesterone. Decreased levels of motilin, a gut hormone that stimulates smooth muscle, have also been noted.[4] During pregnancy, the half-time of stomach emptying after a 750-ml watery test meal is 17.8 minutes compared with 11.2 minutes in the nonpregnant state. Furthermore, the volume remaining in the stomach 30 minutes after such a meal is 186 ml in the nonpregnant state, 275 ml during pregnancy, and 393 ml during labor.[5] Because the sensation of nausea does not occur without gastric relaxation, the decreased tone of the stomach may be part of the cause of nausea in pregnancy. In addition, the sphincter at the gastroesophageal junction shows reduced tone so that increases in intra-abdominal pressure lead to acid reflux into the esophagus, with resultant heartburn.

The reduced incidence and lessened symptoms of peptic ulcer disease during pregnancy are generally ascribed to reduced gastric acid secretion throughout pregnancy. Gastric acid secretion in the first and second trimesters probably is reduced below nonpregnant values, but in the third trimester it is significantly greater than in nonpregnant subjects both during fasting and after histamine stimulation.[6,7] The improvement in ulcer disease seen during pregnancy is probably related as well to delayed gastric emptying, increased gastric mucous secretion (normal in pregnancy), and a protective effect of prostaglandins on the gastric mucosa.

Small Bowel

The motility of the small bowel is reduced during pregnancy; transit time from stomach to cecum averages 58 ± 12 hours in the second trimester compared

with 52 ± 10 hours in the nonpregnant state.[8] Absorption of nutrients from the small bowel, with the exception of iron, is unchanged during pregnancy. Furthermore, the enhanced absorption of iron is not due to any alteration of small bowel function, but is rather a response to increased iron needs operating through the same mechanisms as in nonpregnant women.

Colon

Constipation is a common problem during pregnancy, resulting from several factors. These include mechanical obstruction by the uterus, reduced motility because of smooth muscle relaxation, and increased water absorption from the colon. Parry et al.[9] demonstrated a 59 percent increase in colonic water absorption and a 45 percent increase in sodium absorption during pregnancy, an effect perhaps caused in part by increased aldosterone levels.

Portal venous pressure is increased during pregnancy, leading to dilatation wherever there are portosystemic venous anastomoses. Dilatation of such vessels around the gastroesophageal junction is of no consequence unless the woman has preexisting esophageal varices, but similar dilatation of the hemorrhoidal veins leads to the common complaint of hemorrhoids.

Gallbladder

The function of the gallbladder is markedly altered during pregnancy. In the second and third trimesters, fasting and residual volumes are twice as great as in nonpregnant controls, and the rate at which the gallbladder empties is much slower.[10]

Data on the composition of bile during human pregnancy are conflicting and scanty, but in pregnant nonhuman primates[11] biliary cholesterol saturation is increased and the proportion of chenodeoxycholic acid is decreased. As both predispose to gallstone formation, it seems that pregnancy does increase the likelihood of gallstone formation. The effect of more than one pregnancy appears to be additive.

Liver

Unlike the livers of many animals, the human liver does not enlarge during pregnancy.[12] Furthermore, despite a marked increase in cardiac output, hepatic blood flow is unchanged[13] or is only slightly increased so that the proportion of cardiac output flowing to the liver is decreased about 35 percent. The histology of the liver is unchanged by normal pregnancy.

SIGNS OF NORMAL PREGNANCY THAT MAY MIMIC LIVER DISEASE

Spider angiomata

Palmar erythema

Reduced serum albumin concentration

Elevated serum alkaline phosphatase activity

Elevated serum cholesterol concentration

Many of the clinical and laboratory signs usually associated with liver disease are present in normal pregnancy. Spider angiomata and palmar erythema, caused by elevated estrogen levels, are normal and disappear soon after delivery. Serum albumin levels fall progressively during pregnancy and at term are 30 percent lower than nonpregnant values, averaging about 3.0 g/dl. Serum alkaline phosphatase activity rises progressively so that by term levels are two to four times those found in nonpregnant subjects. Most of the increase is due to placental production of the heat-stable isoenzyme, although there is probably some increase from hepatic sources as well, because nonpregnant women taking exogenous sex steroids also have somewhat increased alkaline phosphatase levels.[14] Serum cholesterol levels are elevated twofold by the end of pregnancy, as are those of most other lipids.

The serum concentrations of many proteins produced by the liver increase during pregnancy in response to estrogen. Fibrinogen levels are increased 50 percent by the end of the second trimester. The levels of ceruloplasmin and the binding proteins for corticosteroids, sex steroids, thyroid hormones, and vitamin D are also increased.

Serum levels of bilirubin, aspartate aminotransferase (AST, formerly SGOT), alanine aminotransferase (ALT, formerly SGPT) and 5'-nucleotidase are unchanged in normal pregnancy, as is the prothrombin time. Whether the serum γ-glutamyltranspeptidase (GGT) is changed in normal pregnancy is controversial; some investigators note normal values throughout pregnancy,[15] while others report a rise in the third trimester.[16]

Nausea and Vomiting of Pregnancy

Nausea and vomiting, or "morning sickness," complicate up to 70 percent of pregnancies.[17] Typical onset is between 4 and 8 weeks gestation, continuing to about 14 to 16 weeks. Although the symptoms often are quite distressing, morning sickness seldom leads to evidence of disturbed nutritional status such as weight loss, ketonemia, or electrolyte disturbances. The cause is not well understood, although relaxation of the smooth muscle of the stomach probably plays a role. There is some evidence that elevated levels of steroid hormones and human chorionic gonadotropin (hCG) may be involved. However, there does not appear to be good correlation between maternal serum hCG levels and the degree of nausea and vomiting either in patients with normal pregnancies or in those with hydatidiform moles.[18] Interestingly, nonmolar pregnancies complicated by nausea and vomiting often have a more favorable outcome than do those without.[19,20]

Treatment is largely supportive, consisting of reassurance, psychological support, avoidance of foods found to trigger nausea, and frequent small meals. Until June 1983, the best pharmacologic treatment of this condition was a combination of doxylamine succinate, 10 mg, and pyridoxine, 10 mg (Bendectin, Merrell Dow).[21-25] Although Bendectin is no longer manufactured, doxylamine succinate and pyridoxine both remain available as over-the-counter preparations (see Ch. 11).

Hyperemesis gravidarum, a more pernicious form of nausea and vomiting associated with weight loss, ketonemia, electrolyte imbalance, dehydration, and possible hepatic and renal damage, often persists throughout pregnancy. For these patients, one must rule out underlying diseases such as pyelonephritis, pancreatitis, cholecystitis, and hepatitis. Hospitalization with parenteral replacement of fluids, electrolytes, and calories is often necessary. We have found a continuous low-dose infusion of promethazine (Phenergan) helpful in this situation. To each liter of intravenous fluid, 10 to 25 mg promethazine

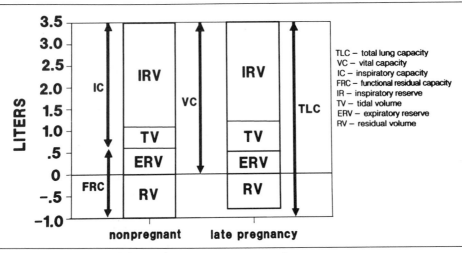

Fig. 5.1 Lung volumes in nonpregnant and pregnant women.

is added, and the patient is given 5 to 6 L/day. The patient should be kept NPO and continued on parenteral therapy for at least 48 hours after all vomiting has ceased to prevent rapid reappearance of symptoms.

RESPIRATORY SYSTEM

Upper Respiratory Tract

During pregnancy, the mucosa of the nasopharynx becomes hyperemic and edematous, with hypersecretion of mucus. These changes often lead to marked nasal stuffiness, and epistaxis is common. Polyposis of the nose and nasal sinuses develops in some patients and then regresses after delivery. Because of all these changes, many patients complain of a chronic cold during pregnancy. The temptation to use nasal decongestant sprays should be avoided, because chronic use may lead to atrophic mucosal changes.

Mechanical Changes

The configuration of the thoracic cage changes early in pregnancy, much earlier than can be accounted for by mechanical pressure from the enlarging uterus. The subcostal angle increases from 68 to 103 degrees,

the transverse diameter of the chest increases 2 cm, and the chest circumference increases 5 to 7 cm.[26] As pregnancy progresses, the level of the diaphragm is pushed up 4 cm; diaphragmatic excursion is not impeded by the enlarging uterus, but instead actually increases 1 to 2 cm. The old idea that diaphragmatic breathing is lessened in pregnancy is false; in fact, it is more diaphragmatic than costal, and all of the increased tidal volume seen in pregnancy can be accounted for by increased rib cage volume displacement.[27]

Lung Volume and Pulmonary Function

The most important change in lung volume during pregnancy is a 30 to 40 percent increase in tidal volume (VT), which occurs at the expense of the expiratory reserve volume (ERV) (Fig. 5.1 and Table 5.1). Thus ERV falls approximately 20 percent (range 8 to 40 percent), while vital capacity and inspiratory reserve volume remain essentially unchanged. Because respiratory rate is unchanged, the 30 to 40 percent increase in VT is responsible for the entire 30 to 40 percent increase observed in minute ventilation.

The elevation of the diaphragm decreases the volume of the lungs in the resting state, thereby reducing total lung volume by 5 percent and residual volume (RV) by 20 percent. Since both ERV and RV are decreased approximately 20 percent, it follows that

Table 5.1 Lung Volumes and Capacities in Pregnancy

	Definition	Change in Pregnancy
Respiratory rate (RR)	Number of breaths per minute	Unchanged
Vital capacity (Vc)	Maximum amount of air that can be forcibly expired after maximum inspiration (IC + ERV)	Unchanged
Inspiratory capacity (IC)	Maximum amount of air that can be inspired from resting expiratory level (Vt + IRV)	Increased 5%
Tidal volume (Vt)	Amount of air inspired and expired with normal breath	Increased 30 to 40%
Inspiratory reserve volume (IRV)	Maximum amount of air that can be inspired at end of normal inspiration	Unchanged
Functional residual capacity (FRC)	Amount of air in lungs at resting expiratory level (ERV + RV)	Decreased 20%
Expiratory reserve volume (ERV)	Maximum amount of air that can be expired from resting expiratory level	Decreased 20%
Residual volume (RV)	Amount of air in lungs after maximum expiration	Decreased 20%
Total lung capacity (TLC)	Total amount of air in lungs at maximal inspiration (Vc + RV)	Decreased 5%

the sum of these two volumes, the FRC, is reduced by 20 percent as well.

The forced expiratory volume in 1 second (FEV_1) and the ratio of FEV_1 to forced vital capacity are both unchanged in pregnancy, suggesting that large airway function is unimpaired.[28] In fact, many studies demonstrate a reduction in airway resistance during pregnancy.[28]

Studies of small airway mechanics during pregnancy are limited. Most studies suggest, however, that small airway closure may occur above FRC or closer to FRC than in the nonpregnant state because of decreases in ERV and FRC in the face of unchanged closing volumes.[29,30] However, normal maximal expiratory flow-volume curves are obtained in pregnancy,[30] indicating that there is not significant small airway dysfunction.

Gas Exchange

Minute ventilation increases 30 to 40 percent by late pregnancy, although oxygen consumption increases only 15 to 20 percent.[31] This leads to increased alveolar (PAO_2) and arterial (PaO_2) PO_2 levels.[32] Normal PaO_2 levels in late pregnancy are 104 to 108 mmHg. That the PaO_2 level does not further increase is probably due to the decreased FRC in late pregnancy lead-

ing to small airway closure. A more significant result of the increased minute ventilation of pregnancy is a fall in $PACO_2$ and $PaCO_2$ levels. In the second half of pregnancy, normal $PaCO_2$ levels are 27 to 32 mmHg compared with 40 mmHg in the nonpregnant state. This change is important, for it increases the CO_2 gradient between fetus and mother and facilitates transfer of CO_2 from the fetus to the mother. Maternal arterial pH (pHa) is maintained at normal levels (7.40 to 7.45) during pregnancy, because the decreased $PaCO_2$ is compensated for by increased renal excretion of bicarbonate. Thus, during pregnancy, normal serum bicarbonate concentrations are 18 to 31 mEq/L, significantly below nonpregnant levels.

The increased minute ventilation of pregnancy, caused by increased Vt, appears to be a result of increased progesterone levels. Although most studies suggest that progesterone increases the sensitivity of the respiratory center to CO_2,[33] there is some evidence that progesterone may act as a primary respiratory center stimulant.[34]

Dyspnea of Pregnancy

The sensation of dyspnea is a common complaint during pregnancy, occurring in 60 to 70 percent of normal subjects and usually beginning in the late first or early second trimester. It is probably due to a combination of factors, including reduced $Paco_2$ levels and an awareness of the increased V_T of normal pregnancy.

SKIN

Vascular Changes

The elevated estrogen levels of pregnancy cause the frequent appearance of spider angiomata and palmar erythema.[35] Vascular spiders, red elevations with tiny vessels branching out from a central body, occur in 67 percent of white women and in 10 percent of black women. They are most common on the face, upper chest, and arms and regress completely after delivery. Diffuse or blotchy palmar erythema, identical to that seen in hepatic cirrhosis, occurs in 60 percent of pregnant subjects and regresses after delivery.

Connective Tissue

Striae gravidarum develop in approximately 50 percent of pregnant women. Initially pink or purple, they develop on the breasts, lower abdomen, and upper thighs; they eventually become white or silvery, but never completely disappear. The development of striae is not due to excessive weight gain, as they can become severe in women gaining as little as 10 to 15 lb, while others who gain enormously escape unscathed. The presence of striae appears to be solely due to the normal stretching of the skin in women whose connective tissue is genetically predisposed; unfortunately, no prophylactic skin treatment has proved effective in preventing them.

Sweat Glands

Eccrine sweating and the excretion rate of sebum are increased in normal pregnancy, while apocrine function appears to be decreased.

Pigmentation

Elevated levels of estrogen, progesterone, and α-melanocyte–stimulating hormone (α-MSH), a polypeptide similar to adrenocorticotropic hormone (ACTH), during pregnancy lead to hyperpigmentation in many women. This is usually most marked on the nipples and areolae, umbilicus, axillae, perineum,

and in the midline of the lower abdomen, where the linea alba becomes the linea nigra.

Pregnancy-induced elevated levels of sex steroids, but apparently not α-MSH, also lead to the "mask of pregnancy" in many women. This condition was formerly referred to as chloasma, but the term melasma is now preferred. This blotchy, irregular hyperpigmentation of the forehead, cheeks, nose, and upper lip may also be seen in some women taking oral contraceptives. Both melasma and the other pigment changes described above occur more frequently in brunettes than in blondes, and, although they fade after delivery, they may never disappear completely.

Pigmented nevi seem to be stimulated by pregnancy. Preexisting nevi may darken, enlarge, and show increased junctional activity on histologic examination, and new nevi may form. After pregnancy they tend to regress, and the junctional activity lessens. Nonetheless, excision of very rapidly changing nevi in pregnancy remains a prudent course.

Hair

The anagen, or growth, phase of normal scalp hair lasts 2 to 6 years, after which it enters the telogen, or resting, phase. After about 3 months of telogen, the old hair strand is lost and a new one grows to replace it. Normally 15 to 20 percent of hairs are in telogen at any one time, but in late pregnancy this falls to 10 percent or less. Then, after delivery, the number of hairs entering telogen increases remarkably so that by 2 months postpartum 30 percent are in that phase. It is normal, therefore, to see a marked increase in scalp hair loss 2 to 4 months after delivery. The often frantic patient should be reassured of the normality of this phenomenon — these hairs will all regrow within 6 to 12 months.

Masculinization of the skin, with facial hirsutism and perhaps acne, occurs rarely during pregnancy. In most cases, no cause can be found, and the patient should be reassured that the changes will regress after delivery. Occasionally, pelvic examination or ultrasound imaging will reveal large ovarian tumors in such women. These usually are luteomas of pregnancy, which represent exaggerated luteinization of normal ovaries rather than true neoplasms. The tumors regress after pregnancy so that surgical intervention during gestation is not indicated.

URINARY SYSTEM

Anatomic Changes

The kidneys enlarge during pregnancy, their length as measured by intravenous pyelography increasing about 1 cm. This increase in size (and weight) is due to increased renal vascular and interstitial volume. The right kidney tends to enlarge more than the left. Pelvicalyceal dilatation by term averages 15 mm (range 5 to 25 mm) on the right and 5 mm (range 3 to 8 mm) on the left.[36]

The well-known dilatation of the ureters and renal pelves begins by the second month of pregnancy and becomes maximal by the middle of the second trimester, when ureteric diameter may be as much as 2 cm, and the volume of urine in each ureter 20 to 50 ml. The right ureter is almost invariably more dilated than the left, and the dilatation usually cannot be demonstrated below the pelvic brim. These findings have led some[37] to argue that the dilatation is entirely due to mechanical compression of the ureters by the enlarging uterus and the ovarian venous plexus. It would seem that mechanical factors are the most important cause of this dilatation, but the early onset of ureteral enlargement supports the hypothesis that smooth muscle relaxation caused by progesterone plays a role as well. However, at least one group of investigators[38] has in fact demonstrated increased ureteric tone during pregnancy; thus it seems that the role of progesterone is as yet unsettled.

The consequences of ureterocalyceal dilatation are obvious and include (1) increased incidence of pyelonephritis among gravidas with asymptomatic bacteriuria, (2) difficulty in interpreting urinary radiographs and in diagnosing urinary tract obstruction during pregnancy, and (3) interference with studies of renal blood flow, glomerular filtration, and tubular function, which, because of urinary stasis, must be done at high rates of urine flow.

Renal Hemodynamics

Renal plasma flow increases markedly and quite early in pregnancy. Dunlop[39] showed convincingly that effective renal plasma flow (ERPF) is increased 75 percent over nonpregnant levels, to a mean value of 840 ml/min, by 16 weeks gestation (see Table 5.2). This increase is maintained until the late third trimester, when a small but significant decline in ERPF occurs. The late-pregnancy fall in ERPF has been well demonstrated in subjects studied serially, in both the sitting[39] and left lateral recumbent[40] positions.

Like ERPF, glomerular filtration rate (GFR) measured by inulin clearance increases early in pregnancy, with increases demonstrated by 5 to 7 weeks; by the end of the first trimester, GFR is 50 percent higher than in the nonpregnant state. This increase is maintained until the end of pregnancy; there is no late-pregnancy fall in GFR as there is in ERPF.

Because the ERPF increases 75 percent and the GFR 50 percent early in pregnancy, the filtration fraction falls significantly from nonpregnant levels until the late third trimester. At that time, when the ERPF falls but the GFR does not, the filtration fraction returns to nonpregnant values of 20 to 21 percent.

Clinically, GFR is not determined by measuring the clearance of infused inulin (inulin is filtered by the glomerulus and is neither reabsorbed nor secreted by the tubules), but rather by measuring endogenous creatinine clearance. This test gives a less precise measure of GFR than does inulin clearance, because creatinine is secreted by the tubules to a variable extent as well as being filtered by the glomerulus. Therefore, endogenous creatinine clearance is usually higher than the actual GFR. The endogenous creatinine clearance is greatly increased in pregnancy, and values of 150 to 200 ml/min are normal. As with GFR, the increase in creatinine clearance begins by 5 to 7 weeks gestation, is maximal by the end of the first trimester, and in normal subjects is maintained at maximal levels until after delivery.

Blood Levels of Nitrogenous Metabolites

As a result of the increased GFR during pregnancy, serum levels of urea and creatinine decline. The blood urea nitrogen (BUN) level falls about 25 percent in early pregnancy to levels of 8 to 9 mg/dl by the end of the first trimester; these levels are maintained until delivery. Serum creatinine values likewise fall from a nonpregnant level of approximately 0.8 mg/dl to levels of 0.7 mg/dl by the end of the first trimester and to 0.5 to 0.6 mg/dl by term.

Serum uric acid levels decline in early pregnancy,

Table 5.2 Serial Changes in Renal Hemodynamics

	Nonpregnant[a]	Seated Position (N = 25)[a]			Left Lateral Recumbent Position (N = 17)[b]	
		16 wk	26 wk	36 wk	29 wk	37 wk
Effective renal plasma flow (ml/min)	480 ±72	840 ±145	891 ±279	771 ±175	748 ±85	677 ±82
Glomerular filtration rate (ml/min)	99 ±18	149 ±17	152 ±18	150 ±32	145 ±19	138 ±22
Filtration fraction	0.21	0.18	0.18	0.20	0.19	0.21

[a] Data from Dunlop.[39]

[b] Data from Equimokhai et al.[40]

reaching a nadir by 24 weeks, at which time levels of 2.0 to 3.0 mg/dl are normal. After 24 weeks, uric acid levels begin to rise again[41] so that by the end of pregnancy the serum urate levels in most gravidas are essentially the same as in the nonpregnant state. This rise in serum urate levels appears to be due to increased renal tubular reabsorption of urate during the third trimester, the reason for which is unknown. It is known that patients with preeclampsia have elevated plasma urate concentrations; because urate levels normally rise during late pregnancy, however, it is necessary to know a given subject's nonpregnant urate level before one can use third-trimester values in the clinical setting.[41]

Salt and Water Metabolism

Plasma osmolality begins to decline by 2 weeks after conception; by the fifth week of pregnancy, it is 10 mOsm/kg H_2O below normal nonpregnant values of 280 to 290 mOsm/kg H_2O. The fall is mainly due to a reduction in the serum concentration of sodium and associated anions. Thus, by early in gestation, plasma osmolality has fallen to 270 to 280 mOsm/kg, similar to the fall seen if a nonpregnant subject quickly drinks 1 liter of water. Although the pregnant woman's response to either water loading or dehydration is either normal or enhanced, she does not respond to her lowered osmolality by a water diuresis. This suggests a resetting of the osmoreceptor system at a lower level during pregnancy.

Sodium metabolism is delicately balanced in nor-

mal pregnancy to permit a net accumulation of about 900 to 1,000 mEq sodium in the fetus, placenta, and maternal intravascular and interstitial fluids. The factors that tend to promote sodium loss during pregnancy include the 50 percent increase in GFR, which increases the filtered load of sodium by 50 percent. Furthermore, the elevated levels of progesterone promote natriuresis. To overcome these effects, the renal tubules must increase their reabsorption of sodium remarkably; in fact, the increase in tubular sodium reabsorption represents the largest renal readjustment that occurs during pregnancy.

Sodium reabsorption is promoted by the hormones aldosterone, estrogen, and deoxycorticosterone, all of which are increased in pregnancy. In fact, the rise in aldosterone production during pregnancy is most likely the key factor that prevents sodium diuresis from occurring despite the elevation in GFR and serum progesterone levels. Plasma aldosterone levels are 200 to 700 ng/L during late pregnancy compared with 100 to 200 ng/L in the nonpregnant state.[37] During normal pregnancy there is a diurnal variation to aldosterone secretion, with the peak (acrophase) at 10 A.M. to noon.[42]

Remarkable changes occur during pregnancy in the renin–angiotensin system. Plasma renin activity in pregnancy is 5 to 10 times the nonpregnant level. Likewise, renin substrate (angiotensinogen) and angiotensin levels are increased four- to fivefold. Although the normal pregnant woman has a very reduced sensitivity to the hypertensive effects of angiotensin, the elevated levels in pregnancy lead to increased aldosterone production and preservation of sodium homeostasis. Atrial natriuretic peptide levels double by the third trimester of normal pregnancy, to a mean of 98 pg/ml from nonpregnant levels of about 44 pg/ml.[42] This is probably due to increased plasma volume leading to some atrial dilatation.

Excretion of Nutrients

Glucose excretion increases in almost all pregnant women. Normal glucose excretion in the nonpregnant state is less than 100 mg/day, but 90 percent of gravidas with a completely normal blood glucose level excrete 1 to 10 g glucose per day during pregnancy.[43] The major reason for the rise in glucose excretion is the 50 percent increase in GFR, presenting a much increased filtered load of glucose to the tubules. There may also be a change in the reabsorptive capacity of the proximal tubules themselves, but the old concept of a maximum tubular reabsorptive capacity for glucose (TmG) is almost certainly erroneous.[43,44] Two important consequences of increased glucose excretion during pregnancy are (1) inability to utilize urine glucose measurements in the management of the pregnant woman with diabetes mellitus because these values do not correlate with blood glucose levels and (2) increased susceptibility of pregnant women to urinary tract infections (UTI).

This susceptibility to UTI may also be enhanced by the normal increase in amino acid excretion during gestation. Hytten and Cheyne[45] found three distinct patterns of amino acid excretion during pregnancy. Excretions of glycine, histidine, threonine, serine, and alanine double by 16 weeks gestation and are four to five times nonpregnant levels by term. Excretions of lysine, cystine, taurine, phenylalanine, valine, leucine, and tyrosine double by 16 weeks but then remain at this level or fall slightly as term approaches. Excretions of glutamic acid, methionine, ornithine, asparagine, and isoleucine do not rise during pregnancy, and the excretion of arginine actually falls.

No increase in protein loss in the urine occurs during normal pregnancy,[37] the nonpregnant range of 100 to 300 mg/24 hr being equally valid in pregnancy. Urinary excretions of folate and vitamin B_{12} are increased in pregnancy, contributing to the decline in serum levels of these vitamins seen in normal gestation.

CARDIOVASCULAR SYSTEM

Cardiac Output

Maternal cardiac output increases about 30 to 50 percent during pregnancy,[46] with the mean increase being about 33 percent, from a nonpregnant level of 4.5 L/min to a pregnancy maximum of approximately 6.0 L/min.[47] According to Hytten and Lind,[47] cardiac output is maximal by 10 weeks gestation. Other investigators[48] state that the rise in cardiac output is most rapid during the first trimester but that smaller increments continue to a peak at about 20 to 24 weeks. There is almost universal agreement now that cardiac output remains maximal until delivery, the previously described terminal decline being an artifact of testing in the supine position.

Cardiac output is the product of heart rate and stroke volume, both of which increase during normal pregnancy. The earliest increases in cardiac output appear to be due to an increase in stroke volume, which increases 5 to 10 ml, to levels of 70 to 75 ml per stroke. As pregnancy progresses, there is a gradual increase in maternal heart rate so that by the beginning of the third trimester it has increased 15 to 20 bpm over nonpregnant levels. At this time, stroke volume declines to near-nonpregnant levels,[49] and the increased heart rate is responsible for maintaining the elevated cardiac output.

Cardiac output in pregnancy is dependent on maternal position, being lower when the gravida lies supine. In the supine position, the enlarged uterus compresses the inferior vena cava, reducing venous return to the heart and in turn cardiac output. In fact, in late pregnancy there is probably complete occlusion of the inferior vena cava in the supine position,[50,51] with venous return from the lower extremities occurring through the dilated paravertebral collateral circulation. The effect of the supine position on cardiac output is most marked in late pregnancy; at 38 to 40 weeks, turning from the side to the back is associated with a 25 to 30 percent fall in cardiac output.[48] Although there does not seem to be an effect of the supine position on maternal cardiac output before 24 weeks gestation, between 24 to 28 weeks turning from the side to the back reduces cardiac output 8 percent, and between 28 to 32 weeks the associated drop is 14 percent.

Most pregnant women do not become hypotensive when lying supine, because the fall in cardiac output is compensated by a rise in peripheral vascular resistance. However, 1 to 10 percent of subjects manifest the supine hypotensive syndrome, with a fall in blood pressure associated with symptoms such as dizziness, lightheadedness, nausea, and even syncope. Some[48] have proposed that such individuals have less well-developed paravertebral collateral circulation and perhaps a tendency toward vasovagal attacks as well.

The distribution of maternal cardiac output changes as pregnancy progresses. In the first trimester (as in the nonpregnant state), the uterus receives 2 to 3 percent of the cardiac output and the breasts less than 1 percent. By term the uterus receives 17 percent of cardiac output and the breasts 2 percent, mostly at the expense of a reduction of the fraction of the cardiac output going to the splanchnic bed and skeletal muscle. The absolute blood flow to these latter areas is not reduced, however, because of the increase in cardiac output. The percentage of cardiac output going to the kidneys (20 percent), skin (10 percent), brain (10 percent), and coronary arteries (5 percent) is the same throughout pregnancy as when not pregnant.[52]

Arterial Blood Pressure

Blood pressure is highest when the pregnant woman is seated, somewhat lower when she lies supine, and lowest when she lies on her side. Furthermore, there is a 10 to 12 mmHg difference in blood pressure between the superior and inferior arms in the lateral recumbent position, the superior arm having the lower pressure. Clearly, consistency is important when measuring blood pressure serially throughout gestation.

Peripheral vascular resistance falls during pregnancy. The most obvious cause for this is the smooth muscle–relaxing effect of elevated progesterone levels, although heat production by the fetus may be responsible for some of the vasodilatation, especially in heat-losing areas of the skin. The reduction in resistance results in a progressive fall in systemic arterial blood pressure during the first 24 weeks of pregnancy, the systolic pressure falling an average of 5 to 10 mmHg and the diastolic pressure falling 10 to 15 mmHg.[53] Thus there is a slight increase in pulse pressure by 24 weeks gestation. After 24 weeks, systolic and diastolic pressures gradually rise, returning to nonpregnant levels by term. It is abnormal for arterial pressure during pregnancy to be greater than nonpregnant values.

Venous Pressure

Venous pressure in the upper extremities remains unchanged in pregnancy,[47] but there is a progressive rise in the lower extremities. Femoral venous pressure rises from values near 10 cmH_2O at 10 weeks gestation to 25 cmH_2O near term[54] and is 2 to 3 cmH_2O higher on the side on which the placenta is implanted.[55] Central venous pressures are unchanged in pregnancy, averaging 10 cmH_2O in the third trimester.[56]

Left Ventricular Function

The preinjection period is the interval between the electrical stimulation of the left ventricle and the onset of blood flow through the aortic valve. Data regarding this interval in pregnancy are inconsistent, although most investigators find a prolongation in the third trimester.[48] Likewise, variable changes have been reported throughout gestation in the left ventricular ejection time (LVET), but there is agreement that in late pregnancy the LVET is shortened.[48]

Echocardiographic studies[40] have demonstrated that, despite increases in left ventricular dimensions and volume during pregnancy, most parameters of left ventricular function are the same as in the nonpregnant state. These include ejection fraction, rate of internal diameter shortening, percentage of fractional shortening, and ventricular wall thickness. Thus myocardial function is well preserved during gestation.

Central Hemodynamic Assessment

Clark et al.[57] studied 10 carefully selected normal patients at 36 to 38 weeks gestation and again at 11 to 13 weeks postpartum with arterial lines and Swan-Ganz catheterization to characterize the central hemodynamics of pregnancy (Table 5.3). During late pregnancy they found statistically significant increases in cardiac output and heart rate, accompa-

Table 5.3 Central Hemodynamic Assessment

	Nonpregnant	Pregnant
Cardiac output (L/min)	4.3	6.2
Heart rate (bpm)	71	83
Systemic vascular resistance (dyne · cm · sec^{-5})	1530	1210
Pulmonary vascular resistance (dyne · cm · sec^{-5})	119	78
Colloid oncotic pressure (mmHg)	21	18
Mean arterial pressure (mmHg)	86 (NS)	90
Pulmonary capillary wedge pressure (mmHg)	6.3 (NS)	7.5
Central venous pressure (mmHg)	3.7 (NS)	3.6
Left ventricular stroke work index (g · M · M^{-2})	41 (NS)	48

(From Clark et al,[57] with permission.)

nied by significant decreases in systemic vascular resistance (SVR) and pulmonary vascular resistance (PVR) and colloid oncotic pressure. There were no significant changes in mean arterial pressure, pulmonary capillary wedge pressure (PCWP), central venous pressure, or left ventricular stroke work index during normal pregnancy.

They postulated that the higher stroke volume of pregnancy is not associated with increased end diastolic pressure (PCWP) because of ventricular dilatation. As a result of the marked fall in SVR and PVR, PCWP does not go up despite the increased blood volume. Their finding of a significantly decreased gradient between colloid oncotic pressure and PCWP explains why pregnant women have a greater propensity to pulmonary edema with changes in capillary permeability or cardiac preload.

Normal Changes That Mimic Heart Disease

Reduction in exercise tolerance is common during pregnancy, as is the sensation of tiredness. The normal hyperventilation of pregnancy may be mistaken as dyspnea by the woman and other observers.

Edema of the ankles is an almost universal finding in late pregnancy because of increased venous pressure in the legs, obstruction of lymphatic flow, and reduced plasma colloid osmotic pressure. After 20 weeks gestation, the jugular veins are usually somewhat distended, and their pulsations are more obvious. The higher position of the diaphragm during pregnancy makes the heart lie in a more horizontal plane, thereby displacing the point of maximal impulse on the chest wall laterally.

At the end of the first trimester, both components of the first heart sound become louder, and there is exaggerated splitting. The second heart sound usually remains normal until the third trimester, when it becomes louder with persistent expiratory splitting. Up to 90 percent of normal pregnant women demonstrate a third heart sound or S3 gallop after midpregnancy.[58,59] Rarely a fourth heart sound may be auscultated in early pregnancy; phonocardiography detects such sounds in 10 to 15 percent of gravidas during the first half of pregnancy. Systolic ejection murmurs along the left sternal border occur in 96 percent of pregnant subjects[56] and are thought to be due to increased flow across the aortic and pulmonic valves. Diastolic murmurs are probably never normal in pregnancy, and their presence warrants evaluation by a cardiologist. A continuous murmur in the second, third, or fourth intercostal space, which may be heard bilaterally, is common in late pregnancy and early puerperium. Called the "mammary souffle," it is thought to be the result of increased flow through the vessels supplying the breasts.

Straightening of the left heart border is due to change in the position of the heart and prominence of the pulmonary conus. This, in addition to the more horizontal position of the heart caused by elevation of the diaphragm, give the appearance of cardiomegaly, but this is more apparent than real. The cardiothoracic ratio is unchanged in normal pregnancy.

SIGNS AND SYMPTOMS OF NORMAL PREGNANCY THAT MAY MIMIC HEART DISEASE

Symptoms
    Reduced exercise tolerance
    Dyspnea

Signs
    Peripheral edema
    Distended neck veins
    Point of maximal impulse displaced to left

Auscultation
    Increased splitting of first and second heart
        sounds
    Third heart sound (S3 gallop)
    Systolic ejection murmur along left sternal border
    Continuous murmurs

Chest x-ray
    Straightening of left heart border
    Heart position more horizontal
    Increased vascular markings in lungs

Electrocardiogram
    Left axis deviation
    Nonspecific ST-T wave changes

Effects of Labor and the Immediate Puerperium

Hemodynamic measurements during labor, including periods between contractions, demonstrate a cumulative rise in cardiac output of about 40 percent above late-pregnancy levels. Much of this increase appears to be due to pain and apprehension, however, because patients with caudal or epidural anesthesia demonstrate a much smaller rise.[60,61] The increased cardiac work of labor is not completely abolished by pain relief, because each contraction squeezes 300 to 500 ml blood out of the uterus into the circulation,[62] leading to increased venous return to the heart and a subsequent increase in cardiac output of 10 to 15 percent. Mean arterial blood pressure rises 10 mmHg during a contraction, although much of this increase is abolished by adequate pain relief.

The immediate puerperium is associated with a 10 to 20 percent increase in cardiac output[63] caused by release of the obstruction of venous return to the heart because the uterus is smaller and because of the rapid mobilization of extracellular fluid. The rise in cardiac output is accompanied by a reflex bradycardia, which means that the stroke volume is greatly increased. The bradycardia and increased stroke volume may persist for 1 to 2 weeks after delivery. These normal puerperal changes may be altered by excessive blood loss.

THE BREASTS

The breasts begin to change early in pregnancy; tenderness, tingling sensations, and a feeling of heaviness often occur within 4 weeks of the last menstrual period. The breasts rapidly enlarge in the first 8 weeks mostly because of vascular engorgement. Thereafter, the breasts enlarge progressively throughout pregnancy because of both ductal growth stimulated by estrogen and alveolar hypertrophy stimulated by progesterone. Little if any of the increase in breast size is attributable to the deposition of fat. The degree of breast enlargement is quite variable, ranging from 0 to 800 ml per breast, with an average value of about 200 ml per breast.[64] Therefore, total breast tissue increases an average of about 400 ml during pregnancy.

The nipples enlarge and become more mobile during pregnancy. The average increase in diameter is 2.0 to 2.5 mm, increasing from 9.5 to 11.5 mm in primigravidas and from 10.0 to 12.5 mm in parous women. Likewise, the areolae enlarge and become more deeply pigmented. The mean increase in the size of the areolae is 16 mm, from a nonpregnant size of 34 to 36 mm to about 50 to 52 mm in the early puerperium. Montgomery's glands (follicles, tubercles), small elevations throughout the areolae, enlarge and become more prominent. These are probably hypertrophic sebaceous glands, although histochemical studies suggest that they could be rudimentary mammary glands.[65]

In the latter half of pregnancy colostrum, a thick yellow fluid, may leak or be expressed from the nipples. This normal finding is more common in parous women.

The interaction of numerous hormones, including

estrogen, progesterone, prolactin, human placental lactogen (hPL), cortisol, and insulin are all necessary during pregnancy to prepare the breast for milk production. The profound drop in estrogen and progesterone levels after delivery seems to be the initiating stimulus for lactation.

THE SKELETON

Postural Changes

Progressively increasing anterior convexity of the lumbar spine (lordosis) occurs during pregnancy. This compensatory mechanism keeps the woman's center of gravity over the legs, because the enlarging uterus would otherwise shift the center of gravity quite anteriorly. The unfortunate side effect of this necessary alteration is low back pain, an almost universal complaint during pregnancy.

The ligaments of the pubic symphysis and sacroiliac joints loosen during pregnancy, probably secondary to the effects of the hormone relaxin.[66] Marked widening of the pubic symphysis occurs by 28 to 32 weeks gestation, when its width has increased 3.0 to 4.0 mm,[67] from a nonpregnant mean of 4.10 mm in nulliparas and 4.60 in multiparas up to 7.70 to 7.90 mm. This mobility of the pelvic joints facilitates vaginal delivery but can lead to pelvic discomfort in late pregnancy. Relaxation of the joints coupled with the increased lordosis and protuberant abdomen also lead to unsteadiness of gait; trauma from falls is more common during pregnancy than at any other time in adult life.[68] Sturdy, supporting shoes should be recommended.

Calcium Metabolism

Maternal total serum calcium concentration declines throughout pregnancy until 34 to 36 weeks, after which there is a slight rise. At term, mean calcium levels are 4.52 ± 0.18 mEq/L, approximately 0.25 mEq/L below nonpregnant levels.[69] The decline in total calcium concentration parallels and is due to the fall in maternal serum albumin concentration; however, maternal serum ionized calcium (Ca^{2+}) concentration is constant throughout pregnancy and unchanged from nonpregnant values.

Maternal ionized calcium levels remain unaltered despite several pregnancy-specific changes that should lower them; these include increased extracellular fluid volume, increased GFR, elevated estrogen levels, and transfer of calcium to the fetus. That maternal ionized calcium levels are unchanged is attributable to the marked increase in maternal parathyroid hormone (PTH) levels during pregnancy; during the second half of pregnancy, maternal PTH levels increase progressively to about 135 percent of nonpregnant values at term.[70] The effect of this "physiologic hyperparathyroidism" is to maintain serum Ca^{2+} levels by increasing absorption from the gut and decreasing renal losses of calcium. Despite elevated levels of PTH in pregnancy, the skeleton is well maintained; studies of bone density demonstrate no loss because of current or past pregnancies.[71,72] This preservation of the skeleton may be due to the action of calcitonin, which counteracts the effects of PTH on the skeleton while permitting the effects of PTH on the gut and kidney to continue. Although the data are conflicting, calcitonin levels are either unchanged[70] or elevated[73] during normal pregnancy.

The rate of bone turnover and remodeling increases throughout pregnancy; thus at term it is twice as great as in nonpregnant subjects. The rate of turnover of the exchangeable calcium pool increases by 20 percent.

HEMATOLOGIC CHANGES

Plasma Volume and Red Blood Cell Mass

In normal pregnancy, maternal plasma volume begins to increase at about 10 weeks gestation. Thereafter, it increases progressively until 30 to 34 weeks, after which time it plateaus. The mean increase in plasma volume by 30 to 34 weeks is 50 percent, although increases of 20 to 100 percent may be found in normal pregnancies.[74] Patients with multiple gestations have a greater increase in plasma volume than do those with singletons. Likewise, larger babies are associated with a great expansion of maternal plasma volume, but it is not clear whether this is cause or effect.

Erythrocyte volume also begins to increase at about 10 weeks gestation and thereafter increases progressively until term. The plateau seen in plasma volume

Table 5.4 Hemoglobin Values in Pregnancy

Weeks Gestation	Mean Hemoglobin (g/dl)	Fifth Percentile Hemoglobin (g/dl)
12	12.2	11.0
16	11.8	10.6
20	11.6	10.5
24	11.6	10.5
28	11.8	10.7
32	12.1	11.0
36	12.5	11.4
40	12.9	11.9

(From US Department of Health and Human Services.[76])

after 30 to 34 weeks is not observed in red blood cell (RBC) volume. Without iron supplementation, RBC mass increases about 18 percent by term, from a mean nonpregnant level of 1,400 ml up to 1,650 ml at term. Women whose diet is supplemented with iron show a greater RBC volume increment, increasing about 400 to 450 ml, or 30 percent, by term.[75]

Because plasma volume increases 50 percent on the average while RBC volume increases only 18 to 30 percent, the hematocrit drops during a normal pregnancy. This so-called physiologic anemia of pregnancy reaches its nadir at 30 to 34 weeks. Thereafter, the hematocrit may rise somewhat, because RBC volume expansion continues but that of plasma volume does not.

The mean and fifth percentile hemoglobin concentrations of normal iron-supplemented pregnant women are listed in Table 5.4.[76] For patients living at altitudes below 3,000 feet, the fifth percentile value should be considered the cutoff for the diagnosis of anemia. For patients living at higher altitudes, this volume should be increased by 0.2 g/dl for every 1,000 feet above 3,000 and by 0.3 g/dl for every 1,000 feet above 7,000.

There are many reasons for the increased blood volume of pregnancy. Clearly, it protects the mother from the possibility of hemorrhage at the time of delivery. Furthermore, the increased plasma volume serves to dissipate fetal heat production and provide increased renal filtration, while the increased RBC mass is necessary to increase oxygen transport to meet the needs of the fetus.

Vaginal delivery of a singleton infant at term results in a mean blood loss of 500 ml, whereas an uncomplicated cesarean birth results in a mean maternal blood loss of about 1,000 ml.[77-79] The average blood loss at cesarean hysterectomy is 1,500 ml, whereas the vaginal delivery of twins results in a maternal blood loss of about 1,000 ml. In the normal situation, almost all the blood loss associated with delivery occurs within the first hour. Thereafter, only about 80 ml of blood is lost over the next 3 days.[77]

Leukocytes and Platelets

The peripheral white blood cell (WBC) count rises progressively during pregnancy. During the first trimester, the mean WBC count is 9,500/mm^3, with a normal range of 3,000 to 15,000/mm^3; during the second and third trimesters, the mean is 10,500/mm^3, with a range of 6,000 to 16,000/mm^3.[77] During labor, the count may rise to 20,000 to 30,000/mm^3, after which it gradually returns to nonpregnant levels by the end of the first week of the puerperium. The increase in WBC count during pregnancy and delivery is largely due to increased numbers of circulating neutrophil polymorphonuclear cells (granulocytes). In the last trimester and during labor, the peripheral smear of normal subjects may even demonstrate occasional myelocytes and metamyelocytes.

Investigations of platelet counts in pregnancy done before the availability of automated cell counters yielded conflicting results, with various workers reporting a decline, a rise, or no change in the platelet count during normal pregnancy. Most recent studies demonstrate a progressive decline in platelet count throughout pregnancy, although the healthy gravida's count will remain within the normal range for nonpregnant subjects.[80-82] Fay et al.[83] studied 2,114 pregnant women and reported a progressive fall from a mean platelet count of 275,000/mm^3 at less than 20 weeks to a mean of 260,000/mm^3 at more than 35 weeks, the drop being significant after 32 weeks. These investigators also demonstrated a progressive rise in mean platelet size (volume) after 28 weeks gestation, indicating younger platelets; they concluded that the fall in platelet count in normal pregnancy is due to increased destruction in the periphery, a concept supported by the somewhat shorter average platelet life span in pregnancy (9.2 days) compared with the nonpregnant state (9.7 days).[84]

The Coagulation Mechanism

Pregnancy has long been called a hypercoagulable state, and indeed levels of fibrinogen (Factor I) increase during pregnancy to the range of 400 to 500 mg/dl. Furthermore, plasma levels of Factors VII through X rise progressively during pregnancy. By contrast, levels of prothrombin (Factor II) and Factors V and XII remain unchanged during pregnancy, while the platelet count and levels of Factors XI and XIII decline somewhat.[75,85]

Bleeding time and clotting time are unchanged during normal pregnancy, however. The "hypercoagulability" attributed to pregnancy does not seem to be due to changes in these parameters but rather to the perceived increase in the incidence of thromboembolism during pregnancy. The greatest increased risk of such complications is in the puerperium. If one assumes that the risk of thromboembolism in the nonpregnant state is 1.0, then during gestation this rises to 1.8, and during the puerperium to 5.5, demonstrating the importance of stasis and vessel wall injury in the genesis of thrombi.

Iron Metabolism in Pregnancy

Iron is absorbed from the duodenum only in the ferrous (divalent) state, its form in iron supplements. Ferric (trivalent) iron from vegetable food sources must be converted to the divalent state before it can be absorbed. If body iron stores are sufficient, only about 10 percent of ingested iron is absorbed, most of which remains in the mucosal cells of the duodenum until sloughing leads to excretion in the feces. Under conditions of increased iron needs, the fraction absorbed increases. The normal pregnant woman absorbs about 20 percent of ingested iron, while the iron-deficient gravida may absorb as much as 40 percent. Under these circumstances, iron is released from the mucosal cell into the circulation, where it is carried, bound to transferrin, to the liver, spleen, and bone marrow. In those sites it is freed from transferrin and is either incorporated into

hemoglobin or myoglobin or stored as ferritin and hemosiderin.

The iron requirements of pregnancy are about 1,000 mg. This includes 500 mg used to increase the maternal RBC mass, 300 mg transported to the fetus, and 200 mg to compensate for normal daily iron losses by the mother (mainly from cells sloughed into the bowel). Thus the normal pregnant woman needs to absorb an average of about 3.5 mg/day of iron. In actuality, the iron requirements of pregnancy are not constant, but increase remarkably during the third trimester. The fetus receives almost all the iron transported to it during the last 12 weeks of pregnancy.

In the past it was controversial as to whether nonanemic pregnant women should receive routine iron supplementation. Most American obstetricians favored the practice, while those in Britain and Europe generally considered it unnecessary. With the availability of serum ferritin levels as a reflection of iron stores, it has become apparent that the unsupplemented patient, although not anemic, is significantly iron deficient at term.[86,87] Table 5.5, adapted from the work of Romslo et al.,[87] demonstrates that women who are not anemic at the beginning of pregnancy and who do not receive iron supplementation have a significant drop in hemoglobin concentration, serum iron, and serum ferritin levels by term, whereas such changes do not occur in women supplemented with iron.

It is important to remember that the purpose of iron supplementation during pregnancy is not to raise or even to maintain the maternal hemoglobin concentration, and it is not to prevent iron deficiency in the fetus. Iron is actively transported to the fetus by the placenta against a high concentration gradient, and fetal hemoglobin levels do not correlate with maternal levels.[88] Maternal iron deficiency does not appear to lead to reduced fetal iron stores,[89] although this last point is still debated by some. Rather, the purpose of maternal supplementation is to prevent iron deficiency in the mother. It has been estimated that women who are iron sufficient at the beginning of pregnancy and who are not iron supplemented need about 2 years after delivery to replenish their iron stores from dietary sources. Because many women have a shorter interval than this between pregnancies and because many do not have an ideal

Table 5.5 Effect of Iron Supplementation During Pregnancy

	Iron Treated	Placebo Treated
Hemoglobin (g/dl)		
10 to 12 weeks	12.8	12.4
37 to 40 weeks	12.6	11.3[a]
Serum iron (μmol/L)		
10 to 12 weeks	19.2	20.4
37 to 40 weeks	21.9	9.5[a]
Serum ferritin (μg/L)		
10 to 12 weeks	28.0	27.0
37 to 40 weeks	24.0	6.0[a]
Serum iron-binding capacity (μm/dl)		
10 to 12 weeks	58.1	64.1
37 to 40 weeks	75.4[a]	92.3[a]

[a] Significant change between first trimester (10 to 12 weeks) and term (37 to 40 weeks).
(Adapted from Romslo et al,[87] with permission.)

diet, iron supplementation is recommended on a routine basis.

ENDOCRINE AND METABOLIC CHANGES

Thyroid

Despite alterations in thyroid morphology and histology and in laboratory indices of thyroid function, the normal pregnant woman is euthyroid. These changes are primarily due to the estrogen-induced increase in the thyroxine (T4)-binding globulin (TBG) concentration and to the decrease in the size of the circulating pool of extrathyroidal iodide resulting from increased renal clearance of iodide. These alterations cause the thyroid to enlarge and to synthesize and secrete thyroid hormone actively.

During pregnancy, the thyroid gland increases in size but not as much as was commonly believed. Ultrasound studies show a 13 percent increase in the size of the gland during pregnancy, which is not enough to be detected by physical examination.[90] Histologically, there is increased vascularity and the follicles are larger with abundant colloid and frequent vacuolization. The depth of the follicular epithelium is increased, and papillary infolding may be seen, indicative of follicular hyperplasia.

Authorities generally agree that the fundamental hypothalamic–pituitary–thyroid relationships re-main intact during pregnancy, although there are conflicting reports regarding the responsiveness of this axis. Although one study demonstrated a greater release of thyroid-stimulating hormone (TSH) in response to thyrotropin-releasing hormone (TRH) as pregnancy advanced,[91] most investigators have failed to confirm this finding.[92] The thyroidal uptake of iodide also appears to be normally responsive to thyroid hormone suppression and to TSH stimulation during pregnancy.[93]

Conflicting reports exist regarding the serum concentration of TSH during pregnancy. Some investigators have reported that TSH values do not change,[94] whereas others have reported a modest rise during the early trimesters.[95] With more sensitive assays, recent work suggests that serum TSH concentrations are in fact decreased during the early weeks of gestation and then rise to prepregnancy levels by the end of the first trimester.[96]

As a result of the estrogen-induced increase in TBG, increases in the concentration of thyroid hormones, total T4 (TT4), and total triiodothyronine (TT3) occur as early as the second month of pregnancy, rising sharply to a plateau that is maintained until after delivery. The concentration of TT4 increases from 5 to 12 μg/dl in nonpregnant euthyroid women to 9 to 16 μg/dl during pregnancy. Despite the elevation in the concentrations of TT4 and TT3, the concentrations of active hormones free T4 (FT4) and free T3 (FT3) are unchanged during normal pregnancy and are within the normal range for non-pregnant female controls.[96]

Before the availability of FT4 determinations, the FT4 index (FTI), a calculated value derived from the serum TT4 and resin T3 uptake (RT3U) determinations, was used as an indirect approximation of FT4 concentration. During pregnancy, however, the FTI correlates poorly with the FT4 concentration measured directly. This lack of correlation has been attributed to the inability of the RT3U to determine accurately the thyroid-binding capacity at high concentrations of TBG.[97] Therefore, during pregnancy the FTI is not directly proportional to the FT4 and may be seriously misleading. Determination of FT4 concentration by equilibrium dialysis, although complex and expensive, is the only method that compensates for alterations in TBG, making it the most reliable method of evaluating thyroid function in pregnancy.[98] As a result of these methodologic problems, the ratio of TT4 to TBG has been proposed as a reasonable substitution when the accuracy of the particular FT4 assay being used is affected by high TBG levels.[97]

At physiologic maternal blood levels, little if any transplacental passage of thyroid hormones T4 and T3 occur.[99] Maternal TSH does not cross the placenta, but the thyroid-stimulating immunoglobulins and TRH cross readily.

Adrenal Glands

Although the combined weight of the adrenal glands does not increase significantly in pregnancy, expansion of the zona fasciculata, which primarily produces glucocorticoids, does occur. The plasma concentration of corticosteroid-binding globulin (CBG) increases significantly from values of 33 mg/dl in nonpregnant patients to a plateau of 70 mg/dl by the sixth month of pregnancy. This increase reflects enhanced hepatic synthesis, induced by the increased estrogen level associated with pregnancy.[100] This estrogen-mediated increase in CBG results in elevated plasma cortisol concentration. The concentration of total plasma cortisol shows a twofold increase in the first trimester. By the end of the third trimester, the level is three times higher than the nonpregnant value.[101] No change in the affinity of cortisol to CBG

is apparent. Thus the percentage distribution of cortisol among CBG-bound, albumin-bound, and the free compartments is unchanged during pregnancy.[101]

Only the fraction of cortisol that is not bound to CBG is metabolically active. Unlike thyroid hormone, the concentration of free plasma cortisol is elevated during pregnancy, increasing progressively from the first trimester until term, when levels are approximately 2.5 times higher than in the nonpregnant state.[101] The elevated free plasma cortisol concentration overlaps with values reported in Cushing syndrome, but the diurnal variation is preserved during pregnancy.[102] The increase in free cortisol during pregnancy is a result of a combination of increased production[102] and delayed plasma clearance.

Marked elevations in the maternal plasma concentration of deoxycorticosterone (DOC) are present by mid-gestation, reaching peak levels during the last trimester of pregnancy. In contrast to the nonpregnant state, plasma DOC levels during pregnancy do not respond either to ACTH stimulation or to dexamethasone suppression.[103] These findings suggest that an autonomous source of DOC, specifically the fetoplacental unit, may be responsible for the increased maternal plasma concentration of DOC, especially in late pregnancy.

Dehydroepiandrosterone sulfate (DHEAS) levels are decreased in pregnancy because of a marked rise in the metabolic clearance rate of this steroid.[104] Most studies have found a modest decline in circulating levels of dehydroepiandrosterone (DHEA) as well. Maternal plasma levels of testosterone and androstenedione are slightly elevated during pregnancy, testosterone because of the estrogen-induced increase in sex hormone–binding protein and androstenedione because of an apparent small increase in its production rate.[104]

Pancreas and Fuel Metabolism

Pregnancy is characterized by hypertrophy and hyperplasia of the β-cells (insulin-producing cells) centrally located within the islets of Langerhans in the maternal pancreas. During normal pregnancy, maternal fasting is characterized by accelerated starvation. The fasting blood glucose level after a 12- to 14-hour fast is 15 to 20 mg/dl lower than that observed in the nonpregnant state.[105] This reduction in plasma glucose is evident even before 12 to 14 hours and is further exaggerated as the fasting period extends beyond 12 hours. This exaggerated response is largely due to the constant drain on maternal glucose by the fetoplacental unit. The relative maternal hypoglycemia probably results in a decline in the fasting levels of insulin,[106,107] although some have reported unchanged[108] or increased[109] maternal fasting insulin levels. An exaggerated starvation ketosis is observed, with elevated blood levels of β-hydroxybutyric acid and acetoacetic acid after an overnight fast.[105] In summary, maternal hypoglycemia, hypoinsulinemia, and hyperketonemia characterize the maternal response to starvation.

By contrast, hyperglycemia, hyperinsulinemia, hypertriglyceridemia, and reduced tissue sensitivity to insulin characterize the maternal response to feeding. Despite postprandial hyperinsulinemia, the blood glucose response to the same carbohydrate load is greater during pregnancy than in the nonpregnant state,[110] indicating that there is peripheral resistance to the action of insulin, the so-called diabetogenic effect of pregnancy. In fact, tissue sensitivity to the effects of insulin may be reduced as much as 80 percent during normal pregnancy.[111]

The factors responsible for this diabetogenic effect include a variety of hormones secreted by the placenta, especially hPL. Carbohydrate metabolism is significantly altered by hPL. This hormone reduces the effectiveness of insulin by decreasing the sensitivity of peripheral tissues and of the liver to the effects of insulin. hPL secretion is proportional to the total placental mass; thus insulin resistance increases as pregnancy advances, particularly during the second half of pregnancy. Elevated free cortisol concentrations may also contribute to the postprandial hyperglycemia characteristic of pregnancy.

The fetus is primarily dependent on glucose for its fuel requirements. The concentration of fetal plasma glucose is about 20 mg/dl less than maternal values. The rate of glucose delivery from the mother to the fetus is more rapid than can be accounted for by simple diffusion. This transfer occurs by facilitated diffusion, a carrier-mediated but not energy-dependent mechanism, resulting in the same fetal blood levels that would be achieved by simple diffusion, but at a faster rate. Maternal glucose levels are critically important in providing adequate glucose transfer to the fetus. However, hyperglycemia may alter embryogenesis. The fetus does not depend on maternal insulin for its utilization of glucose. In fact, maternal insulin and glucagon do not cross the placenta. Fetal insulin is present at 9 to 11 weeks gestation and has a critical role in fetal growth.

Amino acids are actively transported by the placenta from the mother to the fetus, where they are used for protein synthesis and as an energy source. Free fatty acids are transferred from mother to fetus to a limited extent, providing only those essential fatty acids required for tissue synthesis. Ketones, however, freely diffuse across the placenta from mother to fetus and may in fact be hazardous to fetal health.

Pituitary Gland

The pituitary gland enlarges in normal pregnancy, principally because of proliferation of chromophobe cells in the anterior pituitary. Gonzalez et al.[112] recently studied pituitary size by magnetic resonance imaging in 32 normal gravidas and 20 nonpregnant controls. The mean pituitary volume in nonpregnant women was 300 ± 60 mm^3 compared with 437 ± 90 mm^3 by 12 weeks gestation (a 45 percent increase) and 708 ± 12 mm^3 at term (a 136 percent increase). They were unable to visualize the posterior pituitary in any third-trimester patient and speculated that it was compressed by growth of the anterior pituitary. The pituitary stalk remained in the midline in all patients.

THE EYE

The two consistent and significant ocular changes during pregnancy are increased thickness of the cornea and decreased intraocular pressure. The corneas increase in thickness by about 3 percent, from a nonpregnant mean of 534 μm to a pregnant mean of 551 μm. This change is due to fluid retention, is apparent by 10 weeks gestation, and regresses by the sixth week of the puerperium.[113] It is probably the reason for the contact lens intolerance reported by some women during gestation. Intraocular pressure falls by about 10 percent during pregnancy, from

16.1 mmHg in the nonpregnant state to 14.7 mmHg during pregnancy.[113]

REFERENCES

1. Hytten FE, Lind T: Indices of alimentary function. p. 13. In Hytten FE, Lind T (eds): Diagnostic Indices in Pregnancy. Documenta Geigy, Basel, 1973
2. Miller DF, Voris L: Chronologic change in the recommended dietary allowances. J Am Diet Assoc 54:2, 1969
3. Kallander S, Sonesson B: Studies on saliva in menstruating, pregnant and post-menopausal women. Acta Endocrinol (Copenh) 48:329, 1965
4. Christofides ND, Ghatei MA, Bloom SR et al: Decreased plasma motilin concentrations in pregnancy. Br Med J 285:1453, 1982
5. Davison JS, Davison MC, Hay DM: Gastric emptying time in late pregnancy and labour. J Obstet Gynaecol Br Commonw 77:37, 1970
6. Murray FA, Eishine JP, Fielding J: Gastric secretion in pregnancy. J Obstet Gynaecol Br Emp 64:373, 1957
7. Hunt JN, Murray FA: Gastric function in pregnancy. J Obstet Gynaecol Br Emp 65:78, 1958
8. Parry E, Shields R, Turnbull AC: Transit time in the small intestine in pregnancy. J Obstet Gynaecol Br Commonw 77:900, 1970
9. Parry E, Shields R, Turnball AC: The effect of pregnancy on the colonic absorption of sodium, potassium and water. J Obstet Gynaecol Br Commonw 77:616, 1970
10. Braverman DZ, Johnson ML, Kern F: Effects of pregnancy and contraceptive steroids on gallbladder function. N Engl J Med 302:363, 1980
11. Deitrick JE, McSherry CK, Javitt NB: Bile salt kinetics in the pregnant baboon. A new model for the study of gallbladder function. Gastroenterology 65:536, 1973
12. Combes B, Adams RH: Disorders of the liver in pregnancy. p. 297. In Assali NS (ed): Pathophysiology of Gestation. Academic Press, San Diego, 1971
13. Munnell EW, Taylor HC: Liver blood flow in pregnancy—hepatic vein catheterization. J Clin Invest 26:952, 1947
14. Song CS, Kappas A: The influence of estrogens, progestins and pregnancy on the liver. Vitam Horm 26:147, 1968
15. Walker FB, Hobilt DL, Cunningham FG: Gamma glutamyl transpeptidase in normal pregnancies. Obstet Gynecol 43:745, 1974
16. Cerutti R, Ferrari S, Grella P: Behavior of serum enzymes in pregnancy. Clin Exp Obstet Gynecol 3:22, 1976
17. Jarnfelt-Samsioe A, Samsioe G, Veliner G-M: Nausea and vomiting in pregnancy—a contribution to its epidemiology. Gynecol Obstet Invest 16:221, 1983
18. Soules MR, Hughes CL, Garcia JA et al: Nausea and vomiting of pregnancy. Role of human chorionic gonadotropin and 17-hydroxyprogesterone. Obstet Gynecol 55:696, 1980
19. Yerushalmy J, Milkovich L: Evaluation of the teratogenic effect of meclizine in man. Am J Obstet Gynecol 93:553, 1965
20. Medalie JH: Relationship between nausea and/or vomiting in early pregnancy and abortion. Lancet 2:117, 1957
21. Geiger CJ, Fahrenbach DM, Healey FJ: Bendectin in the treatment of nausea and vomiting in pregnancy. Obstet Gynecol 14:688, 1959
22. US Department of Health and Human Services: Indications for Bendectin narrowed. FDA Drug Bull 11:1, 1981
23. Kolata GB: How safe is Bendectin? Science 20:518, 1980
24. Cordero JF, Oakley GP, Greenberg F et al: Is Bendectin a teratogen? JAMA 245:2307, 1981
25. Shapiro S, Heinonen OP, Siskind V et al: Antenatal exposure to Bendectin in relation to congenital malformations, perinatal mortality rate, birth weight, and intelligence quotient score. Am J Obstet Gynecol 128:480, 1977
26. Thompson KJ, Cohen ME: Studies on the circulation in pregnancy. II. Vital capacity observations in normal pregnant women. Surg Gynecol Obstet 66:591, 1938
27. Gilroy RJ, Mangura BT, Lavietes MH: Rib cage and abdominal volume displacement during breathing in pregnancy. Am Rev Respir Dis 137:668, 1988
28. Weinberger SE, Weiss ST, Cohen WR et al: Pregnancy and the lung. Am Rev Respir Dis 121:559, 1980
29. Holdcroft A, Bevan DR, O'Sullivan JC et al: Airway closure and pregnancy. Anaesthesia 32:517, 1977
30. Baldwin GR, Moorthi DS, Whelton JA et al: New lung functions and pregnancy. Am J Obstet Gynecol 127:235, 1977
31. Hytten FE, Leitch I: The Physiology of Human Pregnancy. 2nd Ed. Blackwell, Oxford, 1971
32. Boutourline-Young H, Boutourline-Young E: Alveolar carbon dioxide levels in pregnant, parturient, and lactating subjects. J Obstet Gynecol Br Emp 63:509, 1956
33. Lyons HA, Antonio R: The sensitivity of the respiratory center in pregnancy and after the administration

of progesterone. Trans Assoc Am Physicians 72:173, 1959

34. Skatrud JB, Dempsey JA, Kaiser DG: Ventilatory response to medioxyprogesterone acetate in normal subjects: time course and mechanisms. J Appl Physiol Respir Environ Exercise Physiol 44:939, 1978

35. Bean WB, Cogswell R, Dexter M et al: Vascular changes of the skin in pregnancy. Vascular spiders and palmar erythema. Surg Gynecol Obstet 88:739, 1949

36. Fried A, Woodring JH, Thompson TJ: Hydronephrosis of pregnancy. J Ultrasound Med 2:225, 1983

37. Hytten FE, Lind T: Indices of renal function. p. 18. In Hytten FE, Lind T (eds): Diagnostic Indices in Pregnancy. Documenta Geigy, Basel, 1973

38. Rubi RA, Sala NL: Ureteral function in pregnant women. III. Effect of different positions and of fetal delivery upon ureteral tonus. Am J Obstet Gynecol 101:230, 1968

39. Dunlop W: Serial changes in renal haemodynamics during normal human pregnancy. Br J Obstet Gynaecol 88:1, 1981

40. Equimokhai M, Davison JM, Philips PR, Dunlop W: Non-postural serial changes in renal function during the third trimester of normal human pregnancy. Br J Obstet Gynaecol 88:465, 1981

41. Lind T, Godfrey KA, Otun H: Changes in serum uric acid concentrations during normal pregnancy. Br J Obstet Gynaecol 91:128, 1984

42. Miyamoto S, Shimokawa H, Sumioki H et al: Circadian rhythm of plasma atrial natriuretic peptide, aldosterone, and blood pressure during the third trimester in normal and preeclamptic pregnancies. Am J Obstet Gynecol 158:393, 1988

43. Davison JM, Hytten FE: The effect of pregnancy on the renal handling of glucose. J Obstet Gynaecol Br Commonw 82:374, 1975

44. Kurtzman NA, Pillay VKG: Renal absorption of glucose in health and disease. Arch Intern Med 131:901, 1973

45. Hytten FE, Cheyne GA: The aminoaciduria of pregnancy. J Obstet Gynaecol Br Commonw 79:424, 1972

46. Katz R, Karliner JS, Resnik R: Effects of a natural volume overload state (pregnancy) on left ventricular performance in normal human subjects. Circulation 58:434, 1978

47. Hytten FE, Lind T: Indices of cardiovascular function. p. 30. In Hytten FE, Lind T (eds): Diagnostic Indices in Pregnancy. Documenta Geigy, Basel, 1973

48. Elkayam U, Gleicher N: Cardiovascular physiology of pregnancy. p. 5. In Elkayam U, Gleicher N (eds): Cardiac Problems in Pregnancy. Diagnosis and Management of Maternal and Fetal Disease. Alan R. Liss, New York, 1982

49. Ueland K, Novy MJ, Peterson EN et al: Maternal cardiovascular dynamics. IV. The influence of gestational age on the maternal cardiovascular response to posture and exercise. Am J Obstet Gynecol 104:856, 1969

50. Kerr MG: The mechanical effects of the gravid uterus in late pregnancy. J Obstet Gynaecol Br Commonw 72:513, 1965

51. Kerr MG, Scott DB, Samuel E: Studies of the inferior vena cava in late pregnancy. Br Med J 1:532, 1964

52. McAnolty JH, Metcalfe J, Ueland K: Heart disease and pregnancy. p. 1383. In Hurst JN (ed): The Heart. 6th Ed. McGraw-Hill, New York, 1985

53. MacGillivray I, Rose GA, Rowe B: Blood pressure survey in pregnancy. Clin Sci 37:395, 1969

54. McLennan CE: Antecubital and femoral venous pressure in normal and toxemia pregnancy. Am J Obstet Gynecol 45:568, 1943

55. Bickers W: The placenta: a modified arterio-venous fistula. South Med J 35:593, 1942

56. O'Driscoll K, McCarthy JR: Abruptio placentae and central venous pressures. J Obstet Gynaecol Br Commonw 73:923, 1966

57. Clark SL, Cotton DB, Lee W et al: Central hemodynamic assessment of normal term pregnancy. Am J Obstet Gynecol 161:1439, 1989

58. O'Rourke RA, Ewy GA, Marcus FI: Cardiac auscultation in pregnancy. Med Ann DC 39:92, 1970

59. Cutforth R, MacDonald MB: Heart sounds and murmurs in pregnancy. Am Heart J 71:741, 1966

60. Kerr MG: Cardiovascular dynamics in pregnancy and labour. Br Med Bull 24:19, 1968

61. Henricks CH, Quilligan EJ: Cardiac output during labor. Am J Obstet Gynecol 71:953, 1956

62. Ueland K, Hansen JM: Maternal cardiovascular dynamics. III. Labor and delivery under local and caudal analgesia. Am J Obstet Gynecol 103:8, 1969

63. Metcalfe J: The maternal heart in the postpartum period. Am J Cardiol 12:439, 1963

64. Hytten FE, Leitch I: Preparations for breast feeding. p. 234. In Hytten FE, Leitch I (eds): The Physiology of Human Pregnancy. Blackwell, Oxford, 1971

65. Giacometti L, Montagna W: The nipple and the areola of the human female breast. Anat Rec 144:191, 1962

66. Hall K: Relaxin. J Reprod Fertil 1:368, 1960

67. Abramson D, Roberts SM, Wilson PD: Relaxation of the pelvic joints in pregnancy. Surg Gynecol Obstet 58:595, 1934

68. Fort AJ, Harlin RS: Pregnancy outcome after non-ca-

tastrophic maternal trauma during pregnancy. Obstet Gynecol 35:912, 1970

69. Pitkin RM, Gebhardt MP: Serum calcium concentrations in human pregnancy. Am J Obstet Gynecol 127:775, 1977

70. Pitkin RM, Reynolds WA, Williams GA, Hargis GK: Calcium metabolism in normal pregnancy: a longitudinal study. Am J Obstet Gynecol 133:781, 1979

71. Walker ARP, Richardson B, Walker F: The influence of numerous pregnancies and lactations on bone dimensions in South African Bantu and caucasian women. Clin Sci 42:189, 1972

72. Christianson C, Rodero P, Heinild B: Unchanged total body calcium in normal human pregnancy. Acta Obstet Gynecol Scand 55:141, 1976

73. Samaan NA, Anderson GD, Adam-Mayne ME: Immunoreactive calcitonin in mother, child, and adult. Am J Obstet Gynecol 121:622, 1975

74. Pritchard JA: Changes in blood volume during pregnancy and delivery. Anesthesiology 26:393, 1965

75. Hytten FE, Lind T: Volume and composition of the blood. p. 36. In Hytten FE, Lind T (eds): Diagnostic Indices in Pregnancy. Documenta Geigy, Basel, 1973

76. US Department of Health and Human Services: MMWR 38:400, 1989

77. Pritchard JA, Baldwin RM, Dickey JC et al: Blood volume changes in pregnancy and the puerperium. II. Red blood cell loss and changes in apparent blood volume during and following vaginal delivery, cesarean section, and cesarean section plus total hysterectomy. Am J Obstet Gynecol 84:1271, 1962

78. DeLeeuw NKM, Lowenstein L, Tucker EC et al: Correlation of red cell loss at delivery with changes in red cell mass. Am J Obstet Gynecol 100:1092, 1968

79. Euland K: Maternal cardiovascular dynamics. VII. Intrapartum blood volume changes. Am J Obstet Gynecol 126:671, 1976

80. Pitkin RM, Whitte DC: Platelet and leukocyte counts in normal pregnancy. JAMA 242:2696, 1979

81. Sejeny SA, Eastham RD, Baker SR: Platelet counts during normal pregnancy. J Clin Pathol 28:812, 1975

82. O'Brien JR: Platelet counts in normal pregnancy. J Clin Pathol 29:174, 1976

83. Fay RA, Hughes AO, Farron NT: Platelets in pregnancy: hyperdestruction in pregnancy. Obstet Gynecol 61:238, 1983

84. Wallenberg HCS, VanKessel PH: Platelet lifespan in normal pregnancy as determined by a nonradioisotope technique. Br J Obstet Gynaecol 85:33, 1978

85. Laros RK, Alger LS: Thromboembolism and pregnancy. Clin Obstet Gynecol 22:871, 1979

86. Taylor DJ, Mallen C, McDougall N, Lind T: Effect of iron supplementation on serum ferritin levels during and after pregnancy. Br J Obstet Gynaecol 89:1011, 1982

87. Romslo I, Haram K, Sagen N, Augensen K: Iron requirement in normal pregnancy as assessed by serum ferritin, serum transferrin saturation, and erythrocyte protoporphyrin determinations. Br J Obstet Gynaecol 90:101, 1983

88. McFee JG: Iron metabolism and iron deficiency during pregnancy. Clin Obstet Gynecol 22:799, 1979

89. Van Eijk HG, Kroos MJ, Hoogendoorn GA et al: Serum ferritin and iron stores during pregnancy. Clin Chim Acta 83:81, 1978

90. Nelson M, Wickus GC, Caplan RH, Beguin EA: Thyroid gland size in pregnancy: an ultrasound and clinical study. J Reprod Med 32:888, 1987

91. Burrow FN, Polackwich R, Donabedian R: The hypothalamic–pituitary–thyroid axis in normal pregnancy. p. 1. In Fisher DA, Burrow GN (eds): Perinatal Thyroid Physiology and Disease. Raven, New York, 1975

92. Kannan V, Sinha MD, Deri PK, Pastogi GK: Plasma thyrotropin and its response to thyrotropin releasing hormone in pregnancy. Obstet Gynecol 42:547, 1973

93. Pochin EE: The iodine uptake of the human thyroid throughout the menstrual cycle and in pregnancy. Clin Sci 11:441, 1952

94. Fisher DA, Hobel CJ, Gazara R, Pierce CA: Thyroid function in the preterm fetus. Pediatrics 46:208, 1970

95. Malkasian GD, Mayberry WE: Serum total and free thyroxine in normal and pregnant women, neonates and women receiving progestogens. Am J Obstet Gynecol 108:1234, 1971

96. Harada A, Hershman JM, Reed AW et al: Comparison of thyroid stimulators and thyroid hormone concentrations in the sera of pregnant women. J Clin Endocrinol Metab 48:793, 1979

97. Burr WA, Evans SE, Lee J et al: The ratio of thyroxine to thyroxine-binding globulin in assessment of thyroid function. Clin Endocrinol (Oxf) 11:333, 1979

98. Chopra IJ, Van Herle AJ, Chua Teco GN et al: Serum free thyroxine in thyroidal and nonthyroidal illnesses: a comparison of measurements by radioimmunoassay, equilibrium dialysis, and free thyroxine index. J Clin Endocrinol Metab 51:135, 1980

99. Fisher DA, Lehman H, Lackey D: Placental transport of thyroxine. J Clin Endocrinol Metab 24:393, 1964

100. Doc RP, Fernandez R, Seal US: Measurement of corticosteroid-binging globulin in man. J Clin Endocrinol Metab 24:1029, 1964

101. Rosenthal HE, Slaunwhite WR Jr, Sandberg AA: Transcortin: a corticosteroid-binding protein of plasma. X. Cortisol and progesterone interplay and unbound levels of these steroids in pregnancy. J Clin Endocrinol Metab 29:352, 1969

102. Nolten WE, Lindheimer MD, Rueckert PA et al: Diurnal patterns and regulation of cortisol secretion in pregnancy. J Clin Endocrinol Metab 51:466, 1980

103. Nolten WE, Lindheimer MD, Oparil S et al: Desoxycorticosterone in normal pregnancy. I. Sequential studies of the secretory patterns of desoxycorticosterone, aldosterone, and cortisol. Am J Obstet Gynecol 132:414, 1978

104. Belisle S, Osathanondh R, Tulchinsky D: The effect of constant infusion of unlabelled dehydroepiandrosterone sulfate on maternal plasma androgens and estrogens. J Clin Endocrinol Metab 45:544, 1977

105. Felig P, Lynch V: Starvation in human pregnancy: hypoglycemia, hypoinsulinemia, and hyperketonemia. Science 170:990, 1970

106. Tyson JE, Austin KL, Farinholt JW, Fiedler AJ: Endocrine metabolic response to acute starvation in human gestation. Am J Obstet Gynecol 125:1073, 1976

107. Felig P: Maternal and fetal fuel homeostasis in human pregnancy. Am J Clin Nutr 26:998, 1973

108. Taylor GO, Modie JA, Agbedana EO: Serum free fatty acids, insulin and blood glucose in pregnancy. Br J Obstet Gynaecol 85:592, 1978

109. Bleicher SJ, O'Sullivan JB, Freinkel N: Carbohydrate metabolism in pregnancy. V. The interrelations of glucose, insulin, and free fatty acids in late pregnancy and postpartum. N Engl J Med 271:866, 1964

110. O'Sullivan JB, Mahan CM: Criteria for the oral glucose tolerance test in pregnancy. Diabetes 13:278, 1964

111. Fisher PM, Sutherland HW, Bewsher PD: Insulin response to glucose infusion in normal human pregnancy. Diabetologia 19:15, 1980

112. Gonzalez JG, Elizondo G, Saldivar D et al: Pituitary gland growth during normal pregnancy: an in vivo study using magnetic resonance imaging. Am J Med 85:217, 1988

113. Weinreb RN, Lu A, Beeson C: Maternal corneal thickness during pregnancy. Am J Ophthalmol 105:258, 1988

Chapter 6

Physiology of Parturition

Anna-Riitta Fuchs and Fritz Fuchs

Successful transition from intrauterine to extrauterine life requires that the fetus be mature enough to adapt to the vastly different conditions outside the womb. The fetus is therefore vitally dependent on the timing of its birth, as evidenced by the fact that perinatal mortality is lowest at normal term and increases both before and after term. The mother also has a vital interest in the timing of parturition, because her capacity to accommodate the fetus is limited and she must be able to expel it without endangering her life and the integrity of her reproductive organs.

Various species have developed different mechanisms for the orderly termination of pregnancy. In some, including rabbits, rodents, dogs, and cats, the maternal organism has the dominant role. In others, such as the ewe, cow, mare, and goat, the fetus has the overriding influence on the timing of parturition. In primates both organisms exert joint control, and the fetal and maternal signals must therefore be integrated. How this is achieved is still incompletely understood. The maternal endocrine adaptations to pregnancy and parturition are well known, whereas the fetal signals are still best understood only in various animal models, particularly the sheep.[1] While animal studies are helpful because of the great species variations, they do not permit conclusions with regard to the physiology of parturition in humans.

The uterine transition from the state of pregnancy with sporadic contractions to the state of parturition with frequent rhythmic contractions is gradual and often cannot be indicated with precision. All parts of the uterus undergo preparation for parturition and interact in the regulation of myometrial function either in a classic endocrine fashion with humoral mediators (placenta, fetal and maternal endocrine glands) or in a paracrine fashion with direct organ-to-organ communication (myometrium, decidua, and fetal membranes).

The following discussion covers the factors involved in this transition. First, however, the function of the various parts of the uterus and the biomedical basis for myometrial contractions are described.

STRUCTURE AND FUNCTION OF THE HUMAN UTERUS

The uterus consists of a corpus and a cervix, different with regard to structure and function but both having important roles in parturition. The corpus has three tissue layers, the endometrium (or decidua), the myometrium, and the serosa. The cervix also consists of three layers, the endocervical epithelial layer, the fibromuscular layer, and the squamous epithelial layer covering the vaginal portion. The anatomy of the uterus and its vascular supply and innervation are described in Chapter 2, but some relevant functional aspects are mentioned here.

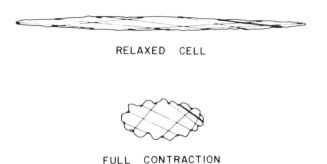

RELAXED CELL

FULL CONTRACTION

Fig. 6.1 Diagrammatic representation of a smooth muscle cell in the relaxed and contracted states, which shows the attachment of the contractile units to the cell surface. The densities along the cell membrane represent dense bodies and the lines between them the contractile units. One of the contractile units has been widened to emphasize the difference between the two contractile states. (From Fay and Delise,[132] with permission.)

Structural Aspects

Myometrium

The human myometrium is composed of smooth muscle cells in a matrix consisting mainly of collagen and glycosaminoglycans. The muscle cells are arranged in a network of intricately interwoven bundles, most of which follow a spiral course. Because the human uterus is formed through fusion of the lower ends of the two müllerian tracts, two sets of spirals can be traced, forming angles with each other.[2] Some of the spirals continue into the cervix, where they thin out rapidly. This pattern not only provides an exceptionally strong uterine wall but also permits three-dimensional expansion without compromising wall strength.

Myometrium, like all muscle cells, consists of thick and thin filaments. It also contains intermediate filaments and dense bodies, which serve as attachment sites for the contractile filaments made up of a structural protein, α-actinin. The organization of filaments in smooth muscle has been the subject of controversy, but is believed to be as shown in Figure 6.1. This model accounts for the fact that smooth muscle contraction can result in a degree of shortening that is one order of magnitude greater than in skeletal muscle.

Growth of the uterus during gestation takes place both by cell division and by hypertrophy of individual cells. The growth is induced not only by the preg-

nancy hormones estrogen and progesterone but also by the stimulus of distension as well. The uterus has a high degree of plasticity and can, if expanded gradually, greatly increase its volume without any increase in intrauterine tension. Acute polyhydramnios is an excellent example of this process.

Muscle cells are arranged in bundles, but there are few cellular contacts between the individual cells until the end of pregnancy, at least in laboratory animals (Fig. 6.2). The smooth muscle cells are surrounded by an intricate network of connective tissue elements; they are frequently connected end to end or attached side by side by fibrillar components of connective tissue. In late pregnancy, cellular contact zones, the so-called gap junctions (nexus), appear between adjacent smooth muscle cells.[3-5] In early labor, both the number and area of the gap junctions is increased. Still, considerable overlap has been found between nonlaboring and laboring patients.[5] Gap junctions are areas of specialized, intimate contacts between cells of the same type. They represent sites of communication, permitting rapid transmission of electrical impulses and chemical signals from one cell to the next. This electrical coupling facilitates synchronization of the contractions of individual cells, which is required for the propagated activity of the organ. The lack of gap junctions during most of gestation suppresses the spread of excitation, causing contractions to remain local and limiting propagation. In the rat uterus, the formation of gap junctions in the myometrium is stimulated by estrogens and prostaglandins and inhibited by progesterone and prostaglandin synthetase inhibitors.[6] Their formation is also promoted by distension,[7] which may be a factor in the human as well, where their regulation is still poorly understood.

Decidua

The decidua is derived from the endometrium of the nonpregnant uterus, which undergoes characteristic structural changes after implantation. The stromal cells enlarge and increase in number, resulting in thickening of the subepithelial layer. The glands and blood vessels also respond with increased growth. Subsequently, the decidua develops into a basal part beneath the placenta (decidua basalis), a capsular part covering the conceptus (decidua capsularis), and a parietal portion covering the inner surface of the myometrium (decidua vera). By week 22, the capsular

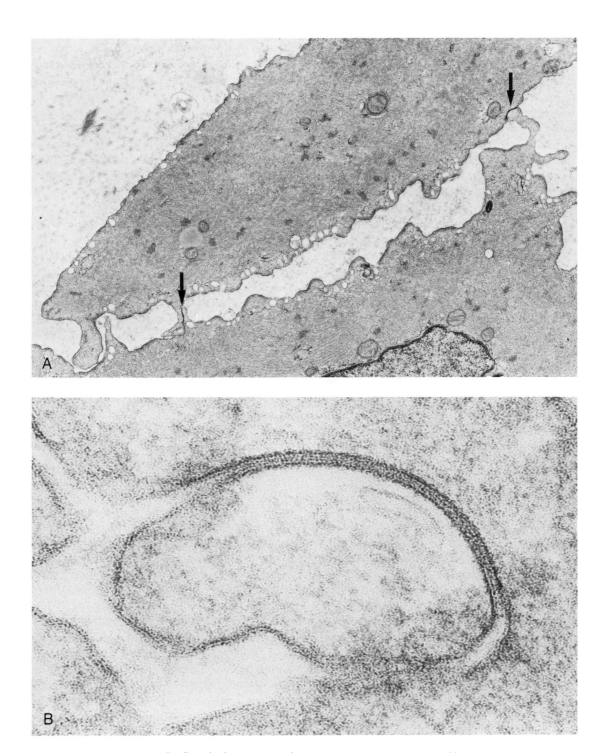

Fig. 6.2 (A) Two myometrial cells in the late pregnant human myometrium are connected by gap junctions (arrows) (×20,000). (B) Gap junction in larger magnification (×255,000), showing the close apposition of the cell membranes of the two cells, with a gap of about 2 to 3 nm between them. (Courtesy of Garfield RE, M.D., McMasters University, Hamilton, Ontario, Canada.)

layer has disappeared because of a reduced blood supply; the parietal decidua is then in direct contact with the fetal membranes, providing their closest vascular supply. A progressive degeneration of the endothelium takes place during pregnancy, but a thin layer remains in certain portions until term.[8]

Anatomically, the basal decidua separates the placenta from the myometrium and provides space not only for the coiling of the spiral arteries that supply each cotyledon but also for the large venous lakes that drain blood from the intervillous space. The parietal decidua separating the conceptus and the myometrium is richly vascularized and at term contains some epithelial cells and several layers of the characteristic decidual cells of the stroma. Ultrastructurally the cells of the decidua basalis and decidua parietalis differ, the former having a more developed Golgi apparatus and endoplasmic reticulum.[8] Gap junctions are found between processes of the same cells but not between different cells. The functional significance of these junctions is unknown. Many macrophages are found between the decidual cells at term, both before and after labor.[9]

Decidua plays an important part in the establishment of pregnancy by providing conditions that make implantation and early support of the embryo possible. It is also believed to form an immunologic barrier between the invading trophoblast and the myometrium and has receptors for immunoglobins. Recent studies have demonstrated that at least two different types of decidual cells have the capacity to metabolize steroid hormones and produce peptide hormones and other pregnancy-specific proteins.[10] These cells secrete large amounts of prolactin[11] and possibly relaxin,[12] and they are the site of highly active prostaglandin synthesis at the time of parturition.[13] The function of decidual prolactin has not been clarified, but it may be involved in the regulation of the permeability of the fetal membranes. In addition to prolactin, a role for vasopressin in this regulation has been suggested. Decidual cells possess receptors for ovarian hormones, glucocorticoids, immunoglobulins, and peptide hormones such as prolactin, oxytocin, and vasopressin.

Cervix and Cervical Ripening

The uterine cervix is structured to protect the fetus during its development by remaining firmly closed and by providing resistance to pressure from above created by the upright maternal position and, in the last trimester, by Braxton-Hicks contractions, which then occur with increasing frequency (Fig. 6.3B). While two-thirds or more of the myometrium is composed of smooth muscle cells, the muscular component tapers off in the cervix, constituting 25, 16, and 6 percent, respectively, in the upper, middle, and lower segments of the cervix. The muscular fibers are continuations of the spiral bundles from the corpus. The main components of the cervix are collagen fibers and a ground substance rich in glycosaminoglycans, which provides the firm consistency of the cervix during pregnancy.

Collagen is synthesized in the connective tissue cells and laid down as fibers in the ground substance. The structural unit, tropocollagen, is a helix of three collagen chains of approximately 100,000 daltons each. The formation of the triple helix is intracellular; after extrusion of the helix, it is cleaved into its final length by peptidases. Cross-links between the chains increase the tensile strength of the cervical tissue. Contributing to the consistency of the cervix is the composition of glycosaminoglycans in the ground substance.

Biochemical changes in the cervix, which we call cervical ripening, take place gradually over the last few weeks of gestation, proving that the process of parturition begins days or weeks before the onset of labor. The collagen chains fracture, and the fragments are solubilized by proteolytic enzymes. The glycosaminoglycans dermatan and chondroitin are replaced by the more hydrophilic hyaluronic acid, increasing the water content of the ground substance. These processes change the consistency of the cervix, which thereby becomes soft and distensible, and its compliance to stretch increases.[14,15] For the clinical assessment of cervical changes, various scoring systems have been developed; the most widely used is that of Bishop.[16] The Bishop score often begins to increase at a slow rate by the middle of gestation (Fig. 6.3).[17]

Cervical ripening is undoubtedly under hormonal control. In the rat it is promoted by relaxin and estrogens and is inhibited by progesterone. The same is probably true in humans, but, in the absence of consistent changes in the concentrations of estradiol and progesterone in the maternal circulation, one would have to analyze the concentrations of these steroids and their receptors in cervical tissue for verification.

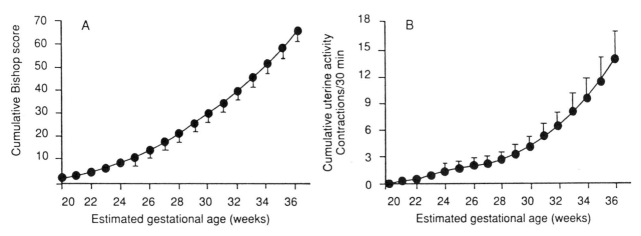

Fig. 6.3 (A) Cumulative Bishop score and estimated gestational age in a group of 13 women assessed at weekly or biweekly intervals. (B) Cumulative uterine activity and estimated gestational age in the same group of 13 women described in A. Patients were monitored for 45 minutes before cervical assessment at each visit. Uterine activity recorded as contractions per 30 minutes. Values are means ± SE; the number of subjects at each point varied between 6 and 13. Changes in the slopes indicate a change in the score or uterine activity. There was an increase in Bishop scores from week 23 onward and an increase in uterine activity from week 28 of gestation onward. (Modified from Catalano et al.,[17] with permission.)

Nakayama and co-workers[18] found ripened cervical tissue to contain higher concentrations of free estrone, conjugated estradiol, estriol, and dehydroepiandrosterone, with further increases noted during labor. Studies with the progesterone antagonist RU486 or other similar compounds indicate that these antagonists have a marked ripening effect on the cervix when administered to monkeys, rats, and guinea pigs.[19,20] Because these antagonists effect a functional withdrawal of progesterone, these experiments provide strong evidence for the inhibitory action of progesterone on cervical ripening. Interestingly, labor did not occur spontaneously in any of the animals treated with these progesterone antagonists, but proceeded normally after administration of oxytocin.[19,20]

Cervical ripening can be accelerated by both mechanical and pharmacologic factors. In classic obstetrics, the metreurynter, a pear-shaped inflatable bag inserted through the cervix and subjected to prolonged traction, was used. Later, laminaria rods that dilate the cervix by swelling with the uptake of water and recently rods of a synthetic, hygroscopic polyvinyl alcohol sponge impregnated with magnesium sulfate were employed. The dilatation of the cervix caused by the slow swelling of the rods seems to act

both mechanically and by acceleration of chemical changes, such as increased hydration of the tissues. Administration of dehydroepiandrosterone, either systemically or locally in substantial doses, has been widely used in Japan for pharmacologic ripening of the cervix.[21] Most successful has been the local application of prostaglandins, particularly PGE_2; $PGF_{2\alpha}$ is less effective. In Europe, this method, introduced by British obstetricians,[22] has become the method of choice for induction of labor in high-risk pregnant patients with an unripe cervix.

As little as 0.4 mg PGE_2 injected into the cervical canal in a viscous gel, with a second dose 8 to 12 hours later if necessary, will induce labor in about one-half of such patients and facilitate induction with oxytocin or amniotomy, or both, in the remaining patients.[23] It is also very useful in patients with preterm rupture of membranes and an unripe cervix. The action of PGE_2 is not mediated by uterine contractions. Cervical ripening proceeds even if uterine contractions induced by the application of PGE_2 are abolished by prior administration of a tocolytic agent.[24] Prostaglandins may therefore have direct actions on cervical connective tissue.[25] The fact that relatively small doses of PGE_2 can accomplish rapid changes in the cervix suggests that endogenous PGE is involved in the physio-

Table 6.1 Prostaglandin Concentrations in Cervical Mucus[a]

Gestation, weeks:	8–13	14–82	35–40
PGE[b]	2.8 ± 0.7	13.7 ± 4.2	10.6 ± 3.5
PGF[b]	4.6 ± 1.7	16.0 ± 9.1	23.1 ± 9.1
N	14	11	23

[a] Within a few hours after intercourse, prostaglandin levels in cervical mucus were increased.
[b] Values are ng/mg, mean $\pm$ SE.
(From Toth et al.,[26] with permission.)

logic mechanism of cervical ripening. The PGE content of cervical mucus rises significantly in the second trimester, indicating that cervical PGE production increases during the slow gradual cervical ripening that begins around weeks 20 to 23 (Fig. 6.3A). The PGE_2 content of the cervical mucus then remains relatively unaltered until term (Table 6.1).[26]

Relaxin effectively produces cervical ripening in many animal species and appears to be essential in this process because immunoneutralization of relaxin results in a prolonged and difficult parturition.[27] Human relaxin has not been available for in vivo experiments, but successful cervical ripening in pregnant women using porcine relaxin has been reported.[28]

The increased compliance to stretch that results from the ripening process does not in itself cause effacement and dilatation. As the cervix ripens, cervical tissue is gradually pulled upward and effaced by incorporation into the lower segment of the corpus. It must be assumed that both effacement and dilatation are accomplished by the activity of the muscular component of the cervix and uterus. Thus Braxton-Hicks contractions have an important role in the preparation of the birth canal in the prelabor phase of parturition.

Vascular Supply

The greatly enlarged uterine arteries provide the blood for the uterine tissues as well as for the conceptus, and the uterine veins drain both the uterus and the intervillous space. The vascular connections with the ovaries and the vagina are insignificant, although the latter can become quite large in cervical pregnan-

cies and placenta previa. About 70 percent of total uterine blood flow goes to the placenta near term. The uteroplacental vascular bed is a low-resistance system that causes a significant decrease in the total uterine vascular resistance and facilitates the marked increase in uterine blood flow during pregnancy.[29]

Innervation

Uterine contractility is autonomous in the sense that the uterus can contract without an external nerve supply. However, even denervation does not rule out nervous influences, because the uterus itself contains adrenergic ganglionic cells that can be visualized by special fluorescent staining methods.[30] Although autonomous nerves reach the uterus from the presacral ganglia, these seem to contain mainly pain neurons. The uterine vascular bed has mainly a sympathetic innervation; both α- and β-receptors have been identified in the uterine blood vessels.

Adrenergic innervation of the uterus is under hormonal control; the content of neurotransmitters increases under the influence of estrogen but decreases under the influence of progesterone. A dramatic decrease occurs during pregnancy, especially in the body of the uterus,[31,32] which at term appears to be devoid of adrenergic innervation.

The uterus is also innervated by peptidergic nerves. Substance P and vasoactive intestinal polypeptide (VIP) have been identified by immunohistochemical methods.[33] VIP fibers are particularly numerous in the cervical region, vagina, and tubal isthmus. VIP has a strong relaxing effect on both the isthmus and the cervical sphincters. Like the adrenergic neurotransmitters, VIP fibers in the uterine body are markedly reduced during pregnancy, whereas their number in the cervix and vagina is less affected.

Biochemical Aspects

Contractile Proteins

The contractile protein in the myometrium, as in all smooth and striated muscles, is actomyosin, formed by interaction of actin and myosin. Human myometrium contains from 1 to 5 mg of myosin and from 16 to 60 mg of actin per gram of tissue, with a ratio of actin to myosin of about 14 : 1, which corresponds to the ratio of thin to thick filaments observed in myometrial cells. In addition, tropomyosin (molecular

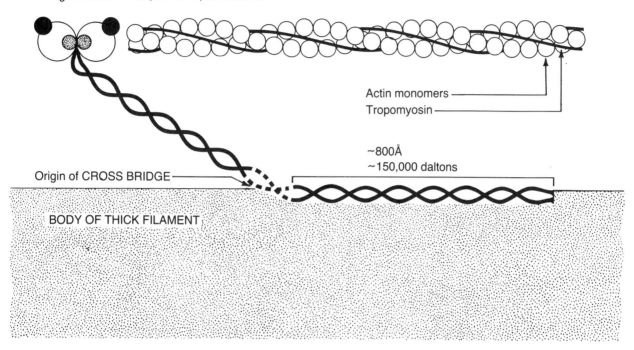

GLOBULAR HEAD
2 Identical units each containing:
■ 1 site for ATP hydrolysis and actin binding
■ 2 light chains of ~20,000 & 17,000 daltons

Actin monomers
Tropomyosin

~800Å
~150,000 daltons

Origin of CROSS BRIDGE

BODY OF THICK FILAMENT

Fig. 6.4 Diagrammatic representation of the myosin molecule, which is a hexamer consisting of one pair of heavy chains and two pairs of light chains. The molecule is very asymmetric, the carboxyl-terminal portion of the heavy chain being a fibrous, almost completely α-helically coiled structure that forms the thick filament. The amino-terminal portion is globular in shape and is associated with the light chains, although their precise position is unknown. The globular head binds to actin and exhibits ATPase activity. The light chain of MW 20,000 contains the phosphorylation site. The hinge region between head and tail is thought to be very flexible. (From Hartshorne and Gorecka,[133] with permission.)

weight [MW] 36,000) and a presumed structural protein, skeletin (MW 55,000), can be identified in protein extracts of human myometrium; α-actinin has been identified in the dense bodies. No difference in the concentration of actin and myosin is found between nonpregnant and pregnant myometria; the myosin purified from either source has an identical peptide pattern and ATPase activity.[34]

Myosin forms the thick filaments, which are about 16 nm thick and 2.2 mm long, and have a molecular weight of about 500,000. They consist of a helical tail and a globular head, formed by two heavy chains (MW 200,000 each). The head contains the ATPase enzymatic activity and the site for combination with actin. Two pairs of light chains of myosin of 20,000 and 27,000 MW, respectively, are attached to each globu-

lar head (MW approximately 240,000) (Fig. 6.4). The light chains are the sites of phosphorylation and calcium binding.

Actin is a much smaller molecule, about MW 42,000. In physiologic solutions, this protein polymerizes to form thin filaments about 6 nm in diameter that are much longer than the thick filaments. As in skeletal muscle, helically arranged strands of actin alternate with thin strands of tropomyosin (Fig. 6.4). Actomyosin is formed when actin activates the magnesium-dependent myosin ATPase, which provides the energy for the attachment of the globular head of myosin to the actin filament, forming cross-bridges between thick and thin filaments. After attachment, the angle of the cross-bridges changes, causing the filaments to slide past each other, thereby generating

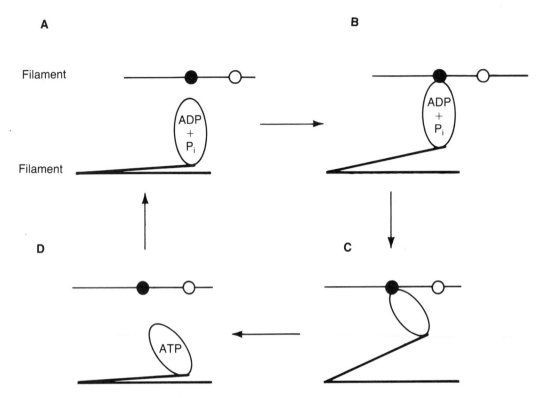

Fig. 6.5 A four-step, four-state model of cross-bridge formation, derived from studies on skeletal muscle, showing mechanical states with corresponding predominant biochemical species. (A) The myosin cross-bridge, with hydrolysis products of ATP still bound to it, is not yet attahced to actin. (B) Cross-bridge attaches to actin at approximately 90 degrees. (C) Cross-bridge–actin angle changes to 45 degrees, pulling the filaments past each other while the cleaved nucleotide products dissociate from myosin. (D) ATP binds to the myosin cross-link, causing the myosin cross-bridge to dissociate from actin filaments. Subsequent hydrolysis of ATP leaves the cross-bridge in its original state (A) ready to bind up to the next available actin monomer. (From Haselgrove,[134] with permission.)

the contractile force. Detachment of the cross-bridges results in relaxation (Fig. 6.5).

Regulatory Proteins

The interaction of actin and myosin is a complex biochemical process regulated by calcium ions, the calcium-binding protein calmodulin, cAMP, and enzymes concerned with the phosphorylation and dephosphorylation of the myosin light chain. In the uterus, as in most other smooth muscles, myosin can react with actin and form actomyosin only when it is phosphorylated. Phosphorylation of the MW 20,000 light chain is mediated by an enzyme, myosin light-chain kinase (MLCK).[35] Thus MLCK is the key enzyme. The action of MLCK is in turn dependent on calcium ions and on the calcium-dependent regulatory protein calmodulin. Calmodulin forms a complex with calcium when intracellular calcium rises from 10^{-7} to 10^{-6} M.[34] The kinase is activated by binding to the calcium–calmodulin complex; only the unphosphorylated form of MLCK can bind this complex with high affinity.

MLCK is inactivated by its own phosphorylation; this process is mediated by a cAMP-dependent protein kinase. When MLCK is inactivated, a phosphatase will dephosphorylate the actomyosin, breaking the cross-bridges and inducing relaxation. The levels of cAMP depend in turn on the relative activities of two enzymes: adenylate cyclase, which catalyzes the synthesis of cAMP, and phosphodiesterase, which causes cAMP breakdown. An outline of the regulation of myometrial cell contraction by phosphorylation and intracellular calcium is depicted in Figure 6.6.

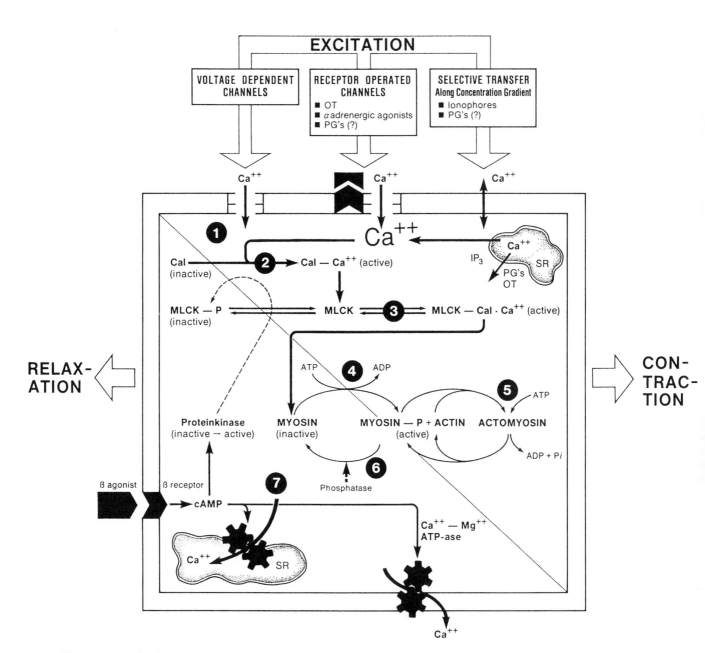

Fig. 6.6 The role of myosin light-chain (MLC) phosphorylation and calcium in uterine smooth muscle contraction. The diagonal separates the contracted state from relaxation. The numbers indicate the sequence of events thought to occur postexcitation: (1) intracellular calcium rises; (2) calmodulin binds to calcium to form an active complex; (3) the calmodulin–calcium complex interacts with myosin light-chain kinase (MLCK) to form an active complex; (4) this complex phosphorylates myosin, permitting activation of myosin ATPase activity by actin and (5) the formation of the acto-myosin complex; (6) when the calcium level is reduced, MLCK is inactivated, phosphatase dephosphorylates myosin, and the muscle relaxes. (7) Calcium can enter the cell through voltage-dependent or receptor-operated channels. Activation of β-receptors results in a reduction of intracellular calcium through two possible mechanisms, both dependent on cAMP: (A) cAMP-dependent protein kinase is activated and phosphorylates MLCK, rendering it inactive, and (B) calcium is extruded from the cell by a cell membrane-associated, cAMP-activated calcium ATPase. Calcium can also be taken up and released by sarcoplasmic vesicles through a calcium-stimulated Mg-ATPase. Other organelles, particularly mitochondria, can also take up and release calcium. (Adapted from Braunwald,[135] with permission.)

Excitability of the Myometrial Cells

A key factor in the excitability of the contraction–relaxation process is the membrane potential, which is dependent on fluxes of ions—in particular, sodium, potassium, calcium, and chloride. These fluxes depend on the permeability of the cell membranes to each species of ions and the intrinsic metabolic processes that maintain ionic gradients across the cell membrane, including those that bind or liberate ions. The membrane potential determines the excitability of the cell.

Depolarization and subsequent repolarization provide the action potential. The normal excitation of uterine muscle is tetanic, which means that the individual contraction is induced by a burst of rapid, repetitive potentials. The force of the contraction depends on the frequency of the tetanic potentials and on the number of filaments involved. When gap junctions are present, the propagation of action potentials from cell to cell is facilitated. Random asynchronous cell contractions can maintain a baseline tonus in the uterus, but simultaneous contractions of a majority of the cells are required for the development of significant increase in tension and the expulsive force. Synchronous contractions of the entire myometrium remain isometric as long as the membranes are intact and the cervix is closed, thus maintaining a constant intrauterine volume. Braxton-Hicks contractions may represent coincidental contractions of a large number of cells.

Excitation – Contraction Coupling

Calcium ion is vital not only for the contractile process in myometrial cells but also for transmitting the signal of excitation from the cell membrane to the contractile machinery inside the cell.[36] The level of intracellular free calcium is normally very low, less than 10^{-7}. It is controlled by specialized intracellular vesicles that sequester calcium avidly and by MgATPase-dependent calcium extrusion pumps or by $Na^+ - Ca^{2+}$ exchange mechanisms. The level of free Ca^{2+} can be raised by influx of calcium through cell membranes along a concentration gradient, through voltage-dependent Ca^{2+} channels, or through receptor-operated calcium channels. Calcium can also be released from intracellular stores, a process that re-

quires the participation of second messengers (Fig. 6.6).

Myometrial cells have a sparse sarcoplasmic reticulum and thus depend largely on the influx of extracellular calcium to raise their intracellular free calcium levels. This property is the basis for the effectiveness of calcium channel blockers as tocolytic agents.

Mechanisms of Action of Oxytocin and Tocolytic Agents

All oxytocic agents exert their action by mobilizing calcium. The main endogenous oxytocic agents are the α-adrenergic agonists, the neurohypophyseal hormones, and the prostaglandins. Some biogenic amines (serotonin), other peptides (substance P, eloidosin), and leukotrienes can have an oxytocic action, but their importance for the in vivo regulation of human uterine function has not been established.

Tocolytic agonists cause relaxation by decreasing intracellular free calcium in a variety of ways. Calcium channel blockers decrease intracellular calcium by inhibiting influx from the extracellular space.[36] The β-adrenergic compounds act through receptors that are coupled to adenylate cyclase and utilize cAMP as a second messenger. In the myometrial cells cAMP lowers intracellular free calcium by two mechanisms. It activates the uptake of Ca^{2+} into intracellular vesicles, and it activates a protein kinase that phosphorylates MLCK, causing its inactivation and subsequent dissociation of the actomyosin complex.

Oxytocin antagonists block the effects of oxytocin initiated by receptor binding, including the opening of receptor-operated Ca^{2+} channels.

Signal Transduction in Nonexcitable Cells and Arachidonic Acid Mobilization

All cells need a system whereby they can regulate cell function and coordinate organ function. Cells therefore possess various mechanisms for signal transduction. Cell membrane lipids and calcium have emerged as important participants in signal transduction in tissues that lack the capacity to elicit action potentials. Nonexcitable cells do not have voltage-dependent calcium channels, but they possess various cell membrane receptors that are coupled to the mobilization of calcium from intracellular stores. Occupation of these receptors by agonists activates phospholipase C

(PLC), a membrane-bound enzyme that hydrolyzes phospholipids. The hydrolysis of membrane phospholipids by PLC can yield several second messengers, including inositol triphosphate (IP₃) and diacylglycerol (Fig. 6.7).[37,38] IP₃ is water soluble and is released into the cytoplasm, where it reacts with calcium-storing vesicles to release free Ca^{2+}. The reaction is extremely rapid and contains an amplification step, each IP₃ molecule releasing at least 20 Ca^{2+} ions. The reaction can also be rapidly extinguished. The other moiety of the phosphatidylinositol molecule hydrolyzed by PLC, diacylglycerol, is simultaneously split off. As a lipid it remains in the membrane, where it can activate protein kinase C, which has multifunctional catalytic activity and elicits a variety of cellular responses, including the liberation of arachidonic acid.[39]

Formation of diacylglycerol will not only activate protein kinase C but also can lead directly to the mobilization of free arachidonic acid. Diacylglycerol contains the esterified arachidonic acid group of phosphatidylinositol in position 3 and therefore is a substrate for diacylglycerol lipase. This enzyme splits off the acyl group from position 2, and the subsequent action of a monoacylglycerol lipase yields free arachidonic acid. Decidual cells have the highest concentration of diacylglycerol lipase of all uterine tissues. Fetal membranes and placenta also contain these lipases.[40]

Calcium-mobilizing agonists can also cause the liberation of free arachidonic acid by the activation of phospholipase A₂, which is a Ca^{2+}-dependent enzyme. Phospholipase A₂ is the most widely distributed enzyme involved in the liberation of arachidonic acid. Its substrates are phospholipids that have arachidonic acid in the number 2 position, such as phosphatidylethanolamine and phosphatidylcholine. All intrauterine tissues have high concentrations of these phospholipids, with amnion cells having the highest concentration of phosphatidylcholine.[41] Figure 6.7

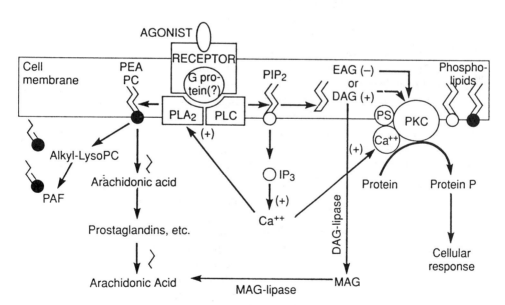

Fig. 6.7 Cellular signal transduction pathways involving calcium ions (Ca^{2+}) and lipid biomodulators. In response to receptor-mediated cell stimuli, phospholipase C (PLC) is activated to yield diacylglycerol (DAG) or 1-alkyl-2-acylglycerol (EAG), which activate and inhibit phosphokinase C (PKC), respectively. If PLC acts on phosphatidylinositol diphosphate (PIP₂), the resulting triphosphoinositol molecules (IP₃) increase cytosolic calcium. An increase in cytosolic free Ca^{2+} activates phospholipase A₂ (PLA₂), which releases arachidonic acid from phosphatidylcholine and phosphatidylethanolamine as precursors for prostaglandins, leukotrienes, and so forth. If the substrate is 1-alkyl-2-acylphosphatidylcholine, reacylation with acetyl-coenzyme A produces platelet-activating factor (PAF). Phosphatidylserine (PS) and Ca^{2+} are required, together with DAG, to activate PKC, which in turn leads to various cellular responses.

shows a schematic representation of signal transduction and mobilization of free arachidonic acid by calcium-mobilizing agonists.

PHYSIOLOGY OF LABOR

Neural Mechanisms

There is ample evidence that the function of the uterus during parturition is controlled by humoral and not by neural factors. As noted above, the content of uterine neurotransmitters is regulated by the ovarian hormones, with estrogen increasing and progesterone decreasing the uterine content of norepinephrine. After an initial increase in early pregnancy, the histochemically demonstrable catecholamines virtually disappear from the corpus, while the cervix and vagina retain their neurotransmitter content.[30,31] It is therefore unlikely that neural activity has much influence on myometrial function during parturition.

Does cervical innervation have a role in the ripening of the cervix and the initiation of labor? The dense sympathomimetic and VIPergic innervation of the cervix maintained throughout pregnancy could conceivably be of importance for cervical ripening.[32,33] The remarkable release of prostaglandins in response to cervical manipulation and stripping of the membranes[42] could perhaps be mediated by nervous activity, because catecholamines can release PGE_2 from nerve endings. The cervix and vagina have been implicated in the reflex release of oxytocin during labor, but the existence of the so-called Ferguson reflex has not been demonstrated in the human or in all animal species studied.[43]

Humoral Factors

The humoral factors affecting myometrial function comprise the steroid hormones, the oxytocic hormones, and the relaxing hormones.

Steroids

The steroid hormones estrogen and progesterone have no direct effect on contractility but exert a regulatory influence through their action on protein synthesis and the synthesis of cell surface receptors, phospholipids, and other lipids that are determinants of membrane structure and the precursors for prostaglandin synthesis. In contrast to most animal species, human parturition is not associated with significant changes in the levels of the major steroid hormones or in the ratio of estrogenic to progestational hormones.[44] However, marked diurnal variations in steroid levels have been observed in the rhesus monkey[45] and may occur in pregnant women. In monkeys these variations coincide with diurnal variations in uterine contractility.[46] In late pregnancy diurnal variations in uterine activity have also been observed, and the timing of the onset of parturition has a significant diurnal distribution.[47] It is likely that these circadian variations are causally related to changes in uterine contractility. Their possible relationship to diurnal variations in maternal and fetal steroid secretion remains to be established.

In several animal species fetal glucocorticoids, secreted in increasing amounts near term, direct placental or luteal steroid synthesis to estrogens instead of progesterone and thereby initiate labor. In the human, fetal glucocorticoids do not produce such effects, and their role in the initiation of human parturition, if any, is likely to be indirect via maturational changes in the fetus.

Relaxing Hormones

Catecholamines

Endogenous catecholamines exert their actions through α- and β-receptors, both of which are present in pregnant human myometrium.[48] Estrogens stimulate α-receptor formation. This process is inhibited by progesterone, which enhances β-receptor dominance. There are numerous β-receptors in the pregnant uterus, and their activation leads to myometrial relaxation, as noted earlier. Epinephrine is the main endogenous β-agonist. During pregnancy β-blockers have no significant effect on uterine contractility. Therefore, endogenous β-agonists seem to have little impact on myometrial function. During labor a considerable increase in maternal epinephrine secretion occurs that may play some role in uterine relaxation between contractions and in the maintenance of low vascular tone in uterine vessels.

Fetal catecholamines are excreted into the amniotic fluid in increased amounts during labor.[49] They may have an effect on the fetal membranes, which do have binding sites for β-adrenergic agonists.[41] Epinephrine stimulates $PGF_{2\alpha}$ release from the estrous rat uterus[50] and may have a similar effect on $PGF_{2\alpha}$ release from amniotic cells.

Relaxin

Relaxin is an ovarian polypeptide related structurally to insulin. It is produced in women by the corpus luteum of pregnancy[51] and is also found in the decidua[12] and placenta.[52] In many species relaxin has an important role in parturition through its effect on the pelvic ligaments. It also causes an inhibition of spontaneous uterine contractions in many species.[53] Relaxin is also believed to play a role in the remodeling of myometrial and cervical connective tissue and cervical ripening during pregnancy.[28] Its importance in human parturition is unclear, because human relaxin has not been available for in vivo experiments. Except for a small peak in early pregnancy, relaxin is found in the plasma of pregnant women throughout gestation without significant variations.[51]

Oxytocic Hormones

The main endogenous oxytocic agents are the α-adrenergic neurotransmitters, the neurohypophyseal hormones, and PGE and PGF. In addition, a variety of other compounds that are oxytocic can be formed from arachidonic acid besides PGE and $PGF_{2\alpha}$ (Fig. 6.8). Thromboxane A synthesized in platelets and placenta is the most potent oxytocic of the prostanoids.[54] It is not formed by the myometrium, however, and because of its rapid metabolism is unlikely to reach the myometrium from the circulation or amniotic fluid. Arachidonic acid metabolites formed by the lipo-oxygenase pathway (the hydroperoxyeicosatetranoic acids [HPETEs] and their hydroxy analogs [HETEs]) as well as the leukotrienes have been implicated in the mechanism of preterm labor, but only 5-HETE has a direct effect on myometrial contractions.[55,56] These compounds may affect uterine function indirectly.

Initiation of Labor

Withdrawal of Inhibitors or Release of Stimulators?

It was long believed that uterine quiescence during pregnancy was maintained by progesterone and that the uterus would contract spontaneously upon the withdrawal of progesterone.[57,58] Evidence for with-

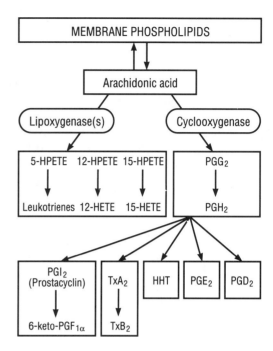

Fig. 6.8 Formation of eicosanoids from arachidonic acid by two enzymatic pathways, cyclo-oxygenase and lipo-oxygenase(s). Hydroperoxyeicosatetranoic acids (HPETEs) are formed by the incorporation of one mole of oxygen; the HPETEs are reduced to their hydroxy analogs (HETEs). The 5-HPETE can be converted to leukotrienes. The prostanoids are produced by the cyclo-oxygenase pathway. Nonenzymatic decomposition of arachidonic acid also occurs and can lead to species that affect cell function (e.g., as chemotactic factors).

drawal of progesterone at the end of human pregnancy has been elusive. Even in species in which progesterone withdrawal is a prerequisite for parturition, a fall in progesterone levels plays a permissive rather than a direct role in myometrial contractility.[59] Withdrawal of progesterone allows estrogenic effects such as the formation of cell membrane receptors and mobilization of arachidonic acid metabolism to dominate. Recently it has become possible by experimental means to produce progesterone withdrawal without affecting the production of other steroids. While administration of progesterone antagonists to monkeys and guinea pigs during late pregnancy produced spontaneous contractions and cervical effacement, labor was not initiated unless oxytocin was administered.[19,20] These data confirm our earlier hypothesis that participation of oxytocic hormones is essential for labor to proceed.[44,59,60]

Controversy exists, however, regarding the relative importance of the oxytocic hormones. Some investigators have set aside the idea that oxytocin is physiologically functional in the events that lead to spontaneous labor.[61] They propose that an increase in the release of $PGE_{2\alpha}$ from the amnion is the event that initiates parturition in women and that prostaglandins are the sole force that drives the laboring uterus. The following observations cannot, however, be explained by this theory.

1. The onset of labor can be delayed and labor can be stopped in its early stages either by agents that inhibit oxytocin release (ethanol)[62] or by agents that inhibit prostaglandin synthesis (indomethacin, aspirin).[63,64]
2. The levels of PGE and PGF in the amniotic fluid are not higher at the onset of labor than are levels observed in late pregnancy. They rise in the course of labor.[65,66]
3. Plasma oxytocin levels are increased in early labor and precede the rise in plasma $PGF_{2\alpha}$ metabolite levels, which occurs in the course of active labor.[67-69]
4. The uterine responsiveness to oxytocin undergoes a remarkable change during pregnancy and reaches a maximum at term, the optimal time of birth.[70] By contrast, the uterine responsiveness to prostaglandins undergoes only minor alterations during the course of pregnancy.[71]
5. Labor at term can be induced with oxytocin in doses that result in plasma oxytocin levels in the physiologic range[67]; by contrast, induction of labor with prostaglandins results in plasma levels that far exceed the physiologic range whether administered intravenously or intraamniotically.[69,73,74]

We propose that initiation of labor depends on oxytocin as the maternal signal and on oxytocin, vasopressin, epidermal growth factor, platelet-activating factor, and perhaps other compounds as the fetal signal; these signals are integrated in the decidua parietalis and transmitted to the myometrium using prostaglandins as a second messenger.

Regulation of Oxytocin Release and Action

Plasma Levels

It is important to recognize that oxytocin is so potent that the effective concentrations stimulating the uterus at term are in the picomolar range. For comparison, the concentrations of PGE and PGF are in the nanomolar range. The great potency of oxytocin makes the measurement of its plasma levels difficult. These studies are further hindered by the presence in pregnancy plasma of an enzyme, oxytocinase, that will rapidly inactivate oxytocin after the sample is withdrawn. Moreover, the secretory pattern of oxytocin appears to be pulsatile, which makes frequent sampling necessary for an accurate estimation of oxytocin secretion rates.

Mean plasma levels of oxytocin are relatively constant during pregnancy, with individual fluctuations suggestive of sporadic release.[75] During the first stage of labor, mean oxytocin levels in samples collected at 1- to 2-hour intervals were raised over values in nonlaboring women.[67] During induction of labor, infusion rates of 1 to 6 mU/min resulted in plasma levels that were similar to those observed during the first stage of spontaneous labor.[72]

In samples collected at 1-minute intervals for 30 minutes, a pulsatile oxytocin secretion pattern was confirmed.[68] Before the onset of labor, the pulse frequency in 10 women was 1.3 per minute. In the first stage of labor, before cervical dilatation of 4 cm, the pulse frequency was three to four times greater ($p < 0.001$), and in the second stage a further threefold increase ($p < 0.01$) was observed. In the third stage, the pulse frequency fell by about 60 percent, but remained greater than before labor. Injections of 2 to 8 mU of oxytocin intravenously produced levels similar to the spontaneous pulses. This study, performed with a highly specific and sensitive antibody,[76] proves conclusively that oxytocin secretion in pregnant women occurs in a pulsatile manner and is increased throughout the course of labor. The pulsatile administration of oxytocin has been found to be more effective than a continuous infusion in stimulating uterine contractions.[77] It reduces significantly the amount of oxytocin required for induction of labor or augmentation of dysfunctional labor.[78]

The fetus also secretes oxytocin. The concentration of oxytocin in the umbilical artery is about twice as high as in the umbilical vein, which has about the same concentration as maternal venous blood.[79,80] Oxytocin is a relatively small molecule (MW 1,000) and is able to pass through the placenta. If the amount of oxytocin corresponding to the arteriovenous difference in the umbilical cord were passed to the mother, it would be equivalent to an infusion of 2 to 3 mU/min. This quantity would almost double the amount of oxytocin reaching the uterus from the maternal circulation.

The placenta contains at least two aminopeptidases that are capable of degrading oxytocin and vasopressin.[81] Oxytocin nevertheless is able to traverse the placenta. An injection of oxytocin on the maternal side reverses the arteriovenous difference in the umbilical cord.[33] A substantial amount of immunoreactive oxytocin that is still bioactive can be extracted from the human placenta after spontaneous vaginal delivery, indicating that degradation of oxytocin in the placenta is not as important as was previously believed.[52] Oxytocin is not the only substrate for the placental aminopeptidases that may be saturated by other aminopeptides present in higher concentrations than oxytocin.

Oxytocin Receptor Concentrations

High-affinity, low-capacity oxytocin receptors are found in the uterus of premenopausal nonpregnant women in low concentrations.[82] Receptors are present in both myometrium and endometrium. During pregnancy the concentrations in both tissues rise dramatically; at 13 to 17 weeks they are about sixfold higher than the nonpregnant levels, and at the end of pregnancy they are about 80- to 100-fold higher.[60,83] The highest concentrations of receptors are found in early labor, when levels are two to three times higher than those at term prior to labor (Fig. 6.9). In preterm labor, the levels are nearly as high as in term labor and are again two to three times higher than levels in women at the same stage of gestation who are not in labor. The distribution of oxytocin receptors in the fundus, corpus, and upper part of the lower segment is rather uniform, but receptor concentrations taper

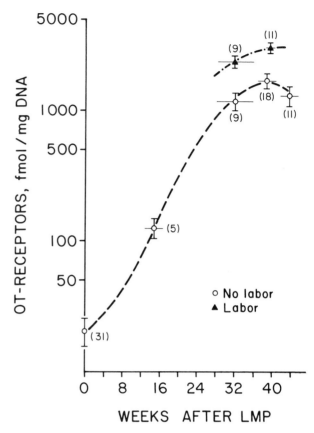

Fig. 6.9 Oxytocin receptor concentrations in human myometrium during pregnancy (O) and during preterm and term labor (▲). Note the logarithmic scale on the abscissa. Values are log-normal means; bars indicate SE. (From Fuchs and Fuchs,[44] with permission.)

off significantly in the lower part of the lower segment and are extremely low in cervical tissue (Fig. 6.10).

The rise in myometrial receptor concentrations increases the response to oxytocin by two mechanisms: (1) by lowering the threshold for stimulation of contractions by oxytocin and (2) by increasing the number of contractile units recruited to contract simultaneously, thereby causing the tension developed by a given oxytocin concentration to rise. It is well documented that the uterine responsiveness to oxytocin increases throughout pregnancy[64] in parallel to the receptor concentrations. It has been a matter of controversy whether the responsiveness increases fur-

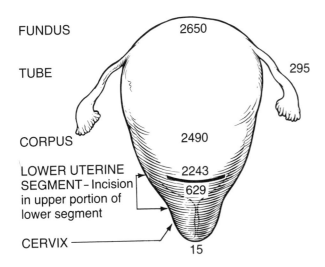

FUNDUS   2650

TUBE   295

CORPUS   2490

LOWER UTERINE
SEGMENT – Incision
in upper portion of
lower segment   2243 / 629

CERVIX   15

Fig. 6.10 Distribution of oxytocin receptors in a pregnant human uterus, removed in preterm labor at 34 weeks. (Adapted from Fuchs et al.,[83] with permission.)

ther in the last weeks before the onset of labor. Results from serial daily measurements indicate that there is a significant rise in oxytocin sensitivity during the last 5 to 7 days before the onset of spontaneous labor.[84] The threshold level falls, reaching normally circulating oxytocin concentrations, and labor begins. These events are schematically depicted in Figure 6.11.

In late pregnancy, Braxton-Hicks contractions occur with increasing frequency. They are abolished by intake of ethanol, as are those of false labor.[62] They are therefore responses to the sporadic pulses of oxytocin that are secreted before term.

What controls oxytocin receptor concentrations in the human uterus? The answer is still shrouded in uncertainty. In experimental animals, estrogens induce and progesterone inhibits the formation of oxytocin receptors.[85–87] The action of progesterone is mediated by suppression of estrogen receptors.[88] Distention acts synergistically with estrogen to increase oxytocin receptor density.[89] Estrogens probably have the same effect in humans, but the action of progesterone is clearly different, because oxytocin receptor levels increase in parallel with progesterone. Distention may be responsible for the increase in oxytocin receptors during the last days of pregnancy, because myometrial growth lags behind the growth of the conceptus and the uterine walls become increas-

ingly distended by the growing fetus. Distention may also be the cause of the preterm rise in oxytocin receptor concentrations in a multiple pregnancy.

Vasopressin

Vasopressin is more potent than oxytocin in nonpregnant women. It retains its potency during pregnancy, although the sensitivity to vasopressin increases less than that to oxytocin.[90] Vasopressin receptors are present in nonpregnant[91] and pregnant[92] uteri, the concentrations increasing in both myometrium and decidua during pregnancy. Vasopressin is bound with higher affinity to nonpregnant uteri than is oxytocin, but in pregnancy the affinities are similar.

Maternal plasma levels of vasopressin remain low during pregnancy and labor, but the levels are increased considerably in patients who are carriers of familial nephrogenic diabetes insipidus. The duration of labor in such patients is reported to be shorter than normal.[93] Vasopressin infusions have been used in the past to induce labor. High concentrations of vasopressin are found in cord blood, with a remarkably high arteriovenous difference.[80,94] Fetal hypoxia is a powerful stimulus for vasopressin release,[95] and cord blood levels are particularly high after fetal distress. Although uterine sensitivity to vasopressin is somewhat lower than its sensitivity to oxytocin, a high vasopressin level in the umbilical artery could add considerable oxytocin potency to that of fetal oxytocin. A significant amount of vasopressin is found in the amniotic fluid[95] and may diffuse through the membranes to reach the myometrium.

Both oxytocin and vasopressin stimulate PLC and induce the hydrolysis of phosphatidylinositol in the decidua.[96] Both peptides can thereby mobilize free arachidonic acid and stimulate prostaglandin synthesis.[60]

Regulation of Prostanoid Release and Action

Oxytocic Potencies

Several of the natural prostaglandins, including PGE_1, PGE_2, and $PGF_{2\alpha}$, are oxytocic.[73] Thromboxane, with the greatest oxytocic activity in vivo, is about 100 times as potent as $PGF_{2\alpha}$.[54] Prostacyclin (PGI_2) is a powerful vasodilator and relaxes various smooth

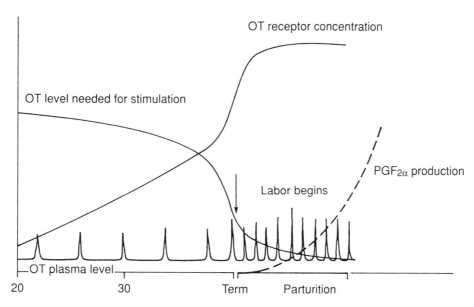

Fig. 6.11 Diagrammatic representation of the concentration of myometrial oxytocin, the level of oxytocin needed to elicit contractions, and maternal plasma oxytocin levels at the end of gestation and during labor. Oxytocin is secreted in pulses of low frequency. During labor, pulse frequency increases. Fetal secretion of oxytocin can be considerable and may contribute to the oxytocin level reaching the myometrium. $PGF_{2\alpha}$ production does not increase significantly until labor is in progress and then increases progressively throughout the third stage of labor. OT, oxytocin.

muscles, including human myometrial strips, in vitro. However, it has no effect on the contractility of the human uterus in vivo when administered intravenously or into the uterine lumen.[54] In pregnant rat uteri, PGI_2 has a transient oxytocic effect of its own and potentiates the action of oxytocin.[97] The role of PGI_2 in the regulation of uterine contractility in pregnant women remains unclear.

PGE_2 is about 10 times as potent as $PGF_{2\alpha}$ in the human uterus, but it has a dual action not shared with $PGF_{2\alpha}$. Besides its excitatory effect, PGE_2 also stimulates cAMP accumulation, which causes relaxation and leads to desensitization of the uterus to the oxytocic actions of PGE_2.[98] $PGF_{2\alpha}$ is the main prostanoid released during labor. $PGF_{2\alpha}$ has a similar action on the myometrium as oxytocin. It raises intracellular free calcium both by opening calcium channels and by the release of calcium from intracellular vesicles. More importantly, $PGF_{2\alpha}$ can increase the excitability of myometrial cells at concentrations lower than those required to produce contraction. This action enhances the properties of other oxytocics[99] and could explain the remarkable sensitization to oxytocin that occurs in the course of human labor.

Prostaglandin E and $F_{2\alpha}$ Receptors

PGE_2 receptor concentrations in human myometrium are, in contrast to those of oxytocin, highest in nonpregnant women and significantly lower in pregnant women.[100,101] $PGF_{2\alpha}$ binds to the same receptors as does PGE_2, but with an affinity that is 10 times lower. Separate receptors for $PGF_{2\alpha}$ may be present in the pregnant uterus.

Prostanoid Concentrations in Uterine Tissues

All uterine tissues are capable of synthesizing prostaglandins from endogenous precursors.[13,40,60,65] The prostanoids produced by different tissues in vitro vary. Our understanding of the factors that direct the metabolism of arachidonic acid in different tissues in vivo is fragmentary. There is, however, general consensus that the *amnion* produces almost exclusively PGE_2, with little $PGF_{2\alpha}$ and PGI_2, and has limited metabolic capacity to inactivate these prostanoids.[65,102] The large amounts of $PGF_{2\alpha}$ that accumulate in amniotic fluid during labor may therefore be derived from other sources, possibly the umbilical cord, chorion, decidua,[103] and fetal urine.

Chorion produces both PGE_2 and $PGF_{2\alpha}$ but has an active 15-ketodehydrogenase and 13,14-reductase system that converts both prostanoids to inactive metabolites.[65,102] The transfer across the membranes from fetus to mother decreases during labor.[104] It is therefore doubtful that a large proportion of the prostanoids produced by the amnion can pass through the chorion intact. Induction of abortion by intra-amniotic instillation of PGE_2 or $PGF_{2\alpha}$ requires doses that far exceed those produced during spontaneous labor (milligram rather than microgram quantities).

Decidua parietalis (vera) produces PGE_2, $PGF_{2\alpha}$, and PGI_2. It has the 15-ketodehydrogenase and 13,14-reductase enzyme complex but has considerably less activity than the chorion.[65,102] PGE_2 is metabolized more avidly than is $PGF_{2\alpha}$, because PGE_2 is the preferred substrate for this enzyme. Furthermore, 9-ketoreductase activity has been demonstrated in human decidua. This enzyme converts PGE_2 to $PGF_{2\alpha}$. Its activity is enhanced by oxytocin.[105] Decidua therefore releases predominantly $PGF_{2\alpha}$ and is considered to be the principal source of uterine $PGF_{2\alpha}$.

Myometrium produces almost exclusively prostacyclin.[106] It is synthesized in both the vascular compartment and the myometrium. The concentrations of the endoperoxide and prostacyclin synthase increase about threefold during pregnancy, but no changes occur during the last trimester or in relation to labor.[106]

The *placenta*[13,107] and umbilical cord[103] have a great capacity to produce PGE_2, thromboxane A_2, and lesser amounts of PGI_2. However, thromboxane A_2 production in the intact organ is blocked by an endogenous inhibitor.[107]

Mobilization of Arachidonic Acid During Labor

The cell membranes are the main source of the esterified arachidonic acid that serves as a precursor for prostanoid synthesis. Phospholipids are a major constituent of cell membranes. Arachidonic acid constitutes from 9 to 26 percent of the fatty acids in the phospholipids of all intrauterine tissues.[40,41] Arachidonic acid is released from membrane phospholipids by phospholipase A_2 (PLA_2) cleavage at the 2 position of phospholipids. PLC hydrolyzes the inositol phosphate bond of phosphatidylinositol, which contains arachidonic acid in the 3 position. The release of arachidonic acid by PLC requires the subsequent action of diacylglycerol lipase and monoglycerol lipase (Fig. 6.7). Decidua has the highest concentration of these lipases, while term amnion has the highest concentration of PLC and PLA_2.[41]

Free arachidonic acid can be converted to prostanoids or to other eicosanoids along the pathways shown schematically in Figure 6.8. Not all arachidonic acid liberated by the action of the various lipases is converted to prostanoids or to lipo-oxygenase products. A considerable part is rapidly reesterified by acyltransferases or, like other fatty acids, is metabolized to produce energy. Prostanoid production depends on the balance of all of these enzymatic activities.

No significant alterations have been detected in the phospholipid composition or lipase activities in relation to parturition, with the exception of PLC and PLA_2 concentrations in amnion, which are increased at term.[41] The content of arachidonic acid is lower and the concentrations of PGE_2 and $PGF_{2\alpha}$ are higher in amnion obtained after spontaneous vaginal delivery, suggesting that the mobilization of arachidonic acid from this tissue is increased during labor.[40,41] Liberation of arachidonic acid is usually the rate-limiting step in prostanoid synthesis. Because free arachidonic acid accumulates in amniotic fluid[61] during labor, its conversion to prostanoids must be limited. As noted earlier, the tissue concentrations of prostanoids and the production rates measured in vitro do not necessarily reflect the situation in vivo, but merely indicate the capacity of the tissues to metabolize arachidonic acid.

Plasma Levels. Plasma levels of the prostanoids themselves are poor indicators of production rates because of their rapid metabolism in the lungs, kidney, and liver. The measurement of stable metabolite levels has been helpful, particularly for $PGF_{2\alpha}$, whereas the corresponding metabolite for PGE_2 is unstable. Technical difficulties regarding assay specificity have made measurements of plasma levels of 6-keto-$PGF_{1\alpha}$, the nonenzymatic hydrolysis product of PGI_2, of questionable value.

The levels of the main metabolite of $PGF_{2\alpha}$, 15-keto-13,14-dehydro-$PGF_{2\alpha}$ (PGFM), in maternal plasma increase slightly during pregnancy, reflecting

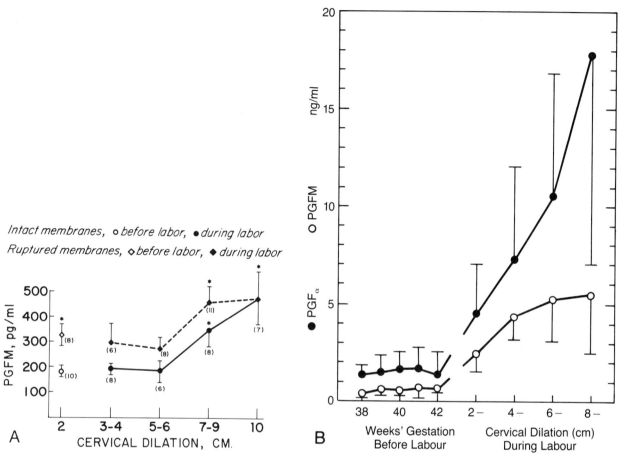

Intact membranes, o *before labor,* ● *during labor*

Ruptured membranes, ◇ *before labor,* ◆ *during labor*

Fig. 6.12 (A) Plasma prostaglandin F metabolite levels in parturient women, measured in serial samples taken during the first stage of labor and arranged according to the cervical dilatation. Values for women with intact membranes (—) are shown separately from those with ruptured membranes (– – –). Prelabor values in women with premature rupture of membranes (◇) and intact membranes (O). (From Fuchs et al.,[67] with permission.) (B) PGF$_{2\alpha}$ (●) and its metabolite (O) levels in amniotic fluid in late gestation and during labor. Values are for samples obtained at amniotomy in individual patients (not serial samples). (From Keirse,[65] with permission.)

the growth of the uterus. There is general agreement that, during the active phase of labor, a rapid and progressive increase in plasma PGFM occurs, but no significant changes have been observed before or during early labor (Fig. 6.12A).[67,69,109] Maximal levels occur after delivery of the baby, at the time of placental separation.[108–110] The concentrations of PGFM then fall rapidly, suggesting that the peak production during the third stage originates in the placental or fetal membranes. However, levels remain significantly increased at least 1 hour after delivery of placenta and fetal membranes, indicating that the decidua is also a major source of uterine PGF$_{2\alpha}$ during labor (Fig. 6.13).

Conflicting results with regard to the PGE$_2$ metabolite (PGEM) have been reported, reflecting the instability of the compound and technical difficulties that have not yet been resolved.[111,112]

Urinary Excretion. Stable urinary metabolite level is a useful measure of overall prostanoid production. The synthesis of PGE$_2$ and PGF$_{2\alpha}$ in men and nonpregnant women has been estimated to be in the range of 10 to 50 μg/24 g. During pregnancy the

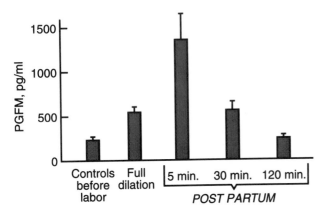

Fig. 6.13 Plasma levels of $PGF_{2\alpha}$ metabolite (PGFM) in parturient women measured in serial samples obtained at full dilatation and after delivery. Control levels were measured before the onset of labor. (Adapted from Fuchs et al.,[109] with permission.)

excretion of the metabolites of $PGF_{2\alpha}$ increases slightly.[113] The excretion of PGI_2 and thromboxane A_2 metabolites rises considerably in the second trimester with a nonsignificant increase in the third trimester.[114,115] At term, no significant increase is detected before the onset of labor, but excretion is higher on the day of delivery. In the second trimester, the excretion of prostacyclin metabolites increases proportionately more than that of thromboxane A_2 metabolites, which supports the concept of relative dominance of PGI_2 over thromboxane A_2 in normal pregnancies.[116]

Amniotic Fluid Levels. Neither amnion cells nor amniotic fluid can inactivate prostanoids. Therefore, amniotic fluid concentrations reflect production by the amnion and umbilical cord. Most investigators have found low prostanoid levels in human amniotic fluid before the onset of labor, provided that the membranes are intact and the cervix or internal os is not manipulated. During spontaneous and induced labor, a significant and progressive increase occurs (Fig. 6.12B). Stripping of the membranes, amniotomy, digital examination of the cervix, and spontaneous rupture of the membranes result in a rapid increase in prostanoid production that is reflected in both maternal plasma and amniotic fluid concentrations.[42,65,67,117] The mechanism of arachidonic acid metabolism activation by these procedures is not known. Puncture of the amniotic sac through the abdominal wall does not have the same effect, indicating that the cervical pole of the fetal membranes and the area of the internal os of the cervix are more susceptible to traumatic release of prostanoids.

Initiation of Prostanoid Production at Parturition. Because all intrauterine tissues have the capacity to generate prostaglandins throughout most of gestation, the release during labor is not regulated by substrate availability or de novo synthesis of the key enzymes. From the relatively low and constant total production of prostanoids during the third trimester, one can deduce that the activity of the phospholipases or prostaglandin synthetases is held at bay by some endogenous inhibitors. The increased production during labor could ensue as a result of (1) withdrawal of inhibitory substances or (2) increase in stimulators of synthesis.

Withdrawal of Endogenous Inhibitors. Several likely compounds have been identified. Placenta contains a cytosolic inhibitor of thromboxane synthesis.[107] Several PLA_2 inhibitors have also been identified. The major group consists of lipocortins, which are induced by glucocorticoids and are believed to be the basis for the antiinflammatory action of glucocorticoids.[118] Lipocortins have been isolated from several organs, including the placenta. While glucocorticoids have been shown to inhibit prostanoid production in myometrial cells, their action in decidual or chorioamnion cells is controversial.[61] Wilson and Liggins[119] have recently isolated a protein, gravidin, from amniotic fluid, chorion, and decidua that is an inhibitor of decidual cell PLA_2. It was reported to be active during pregnancy but seems to lose its activity in labor. If this finding is confirmed, gravidin could be a factor in the regulation of arachidonic acid mobilization at the onset of labor. The presence of other inhibitory compounds in the amniotic fluid that disappear at term has been reported.[120] However, when tested with slices of human uterine tissue instead of a model system derived from sheep seminal vesicles, amniotic fluid from mid or late pregnancy had no inhibitory activity.[121] Pregnancy serum contains an inhibitory substance, but no alteration in its concentration occurs at term and during labor.[122] Uteroglobin in rabbits has inhibitory activity, and a protein secreted by ovine or bovine conceptuses limits uterine $PGF_{2\alpha}$ release. It is unknown whether any of the pregnancy-specific placental or decidual proteins found in humans have such inhibitory activity. Thus far there is no conclusive evidence from these studies that a withdrawal of an inhibitory substance initiates prostanoid production during labor, although gravidin appears to be a promising candidate.

Endogenous Stimulators of Prostanoid Synthesis. Oxytocin was the first endogenous compound shown to stimulate PGE_2 and $PGF_{2\alpha}$ synthesis in decidua and amnion, and, because the fetus secretes oxytocin, it was proposed as a fetal signal for parturition in women.[60] The stimulatory action of oxytocin has been confirmed by several authors. Oxytocin activates PLC in human decidua, thereby increasing $PGF_{2\alpha}$ production.[96] Oxytocin has also been shown to be effective in vivo.[44] Other compounds have since been identified that stimulate prostanoid production in cultured amnion cells. Epidermal growth factor and platelet-activating factor have considerable activity and are found in amniotic fluid.[41,61] Their relevance for in vivo production of $PGF_{2\alpha}$ has not yet been demonstrated. Any one of these compounds is therefore a potential fetal signal for increased prostaglandin production, and others will probably be found with similar action. Considering the importance of this event, it is very likely that the fetus would utilize multiple signals to accomplish the task!

Another possibility is that prostanoid production is initiated by a shift in the balance of the inhibitory and stimulatory substances. Such a shift need not be very large at first, because once labor is in progress the production of prostanoids appears to be self-perpetuating. $PGF_{2\alpha}$ may stimulate its own release,[123] or myometrial contractions and intrauterine pressure changes may bring about sustained $PGF_{2\alpha}$ release. The latter proposition is supported by the finding in the rat uterus that all oxytocic agents stimulated and all tocolytic agents inhibited the production of PGI_2, the principal prostanoid produced by myometrium.[97]

Uterine Function During Labor

Having considered the functions of the various anatomic parts of the uterus at the cellular level, we now discuss the integrated function of the uterus as an organ during parturition. Essentially, this function is to develop sufficient expulsive force to propel the fetus through the birth canal against a varying degree of resistance. The work load is considerable and requires much energy. The uterine contractions must be intermittent to permit sufficient oxygen to be delivered to the fetus between contractions, and their force must progressively increase to enable the soft parts of the birth canal to stretch gradually. Oxytocin in low concentration produces rhythmic intrauterine pressure cycles with complete relaxation between contractions. High concentrations of oxytocin produce tonic contractures.

Many attempts have been made to quantitate uterine activity in labor. The pioneers in uterine physiology, Alvarez and Caldeyro-Barcia[124] devised the Montevideo unit to combine two variables: the amplitude and the frequency of the contraction. An alternative is the measurement of the active contraction area, described by Bourne and Burn[125] as early as 1927, that incorporates three variables: frequency, active pressure, and duration of contractions. With modern electronic equipment for intrauterine pressure recording, the active contraction area is easy to measure by integrating the pressure above the baseline with time and is expressed in units of kiloPascal-seconds.

As reported by Steer et al.,[126] the active contraction area correlates better than any other measure with the rate of cervical dilatation in the active phase of labor. The mean value for uterine activity over the whole first stage of labor was found to be 1,100 kiloPascal-seconds (kPas) per 15 minutes, with an SD of 333 kPas/15 min in 22 consecutive patients in spontaneous labor. During the period of dilatation from 4 to 10 cm, the active contraction area increased from about 800 to 1,200 kPas/15 min, a 50 percent increase that occurred primarily between 7 and 9 cm of dilatation.

The rate of cervical dilatation achieved with a certain amount of uterine activity depends on the resistance of the cervix. Below 430 kPas/15 min, significant progress in labor is unlikely to occur, but even above 500 kPas/15 min some women will exhibit slow rates of cervical dilatation because of increased cervical resistance. Augmentation of uterine activity in the presence of slow progress in cervical dilatation is not always advisable, especially if preaugmentation uterine activity is in the normal range. In these cases, hyperstimulation might occur. The fact that the nul-

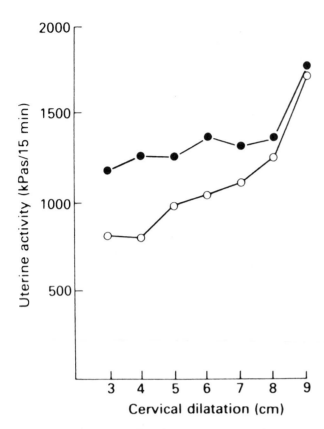

Fig. 6.14 Comparison of median uterine activity values in nulliparas (●) and multiparas (O) at each centimeter of cervical dilatation. (From Arulkumaran et al.,[127] with permission.)

liparous cervix is more resistant than the multiparous cervix explains the difference in the average duration of labor in nulliparas and multiparas. According to Arulkumaran et al.,[127] less uterine work is required to dilate the cervix in multiparas than in nulliparas (Fig. 6.14), whereas in the study of Steer et al.[126] there was no difference. However, the rate of cervical dilatation also depends on whether the expulsive forces are acting on the cervix. This may not be the case in certain forms of dystocia.

Friedman[128] has been influential in describing the temporal patterns of cervical dilatation and in developing standard curves for nulliparous and multiparous women with which individual cases can be compared. An even better index of the efficiency of labor would be a combination of cumulative uterine activity and cervical dilatation with time.

Correlation of uterine activity with the total amount of oxytocic agents acting on the uterus is impossible, because we cannot measure the amount of oxytocin and vasopressin reaching the myometrium from the fetus or the amount of prostaglandins generated within the uterus. During stimulation of the uterus with exogenous oxytocin, it is possible to correlate uterine activity with the amount of oxytocin administered. Systems actually have been constructed that automatically regulate the infusion rate to provide a constant uterine activity. Amico et al.[129] and Seitchik et al.[130] have studied the amounts of oxytocin delivered and the blood concentrations obtained in cases of hypokinetic labor. Infusion rates of 1 to 5 mU/min were sufficient to give adequate activity in all but 1 of the 11 experimental subjects and the concentration of oxytocin obtained was of the same order of magnitude as found in spontaneous labor, an observation that agrees with our own studies in oxytocin-induced labors.[69] The finding that uterine activity measured in kPas/15 min remains relatively stable at cervical dilatations up to 4 to 6 cm and then increases is compatible with the idea that oxytocin is the main driving force in the early part of labor, when mean levels of oxytocin remain rather constant. At cervical dilatations over 4 to 6 cm, PGF generation increases rapidly, potentiating oxytocin-induced activity and perhaps becoming the major myometrial stimulant.[67,69,70]

That it should be necessary to give an average dose of 75 mU/min to induce labor and obtain an activity of 1,500 kPas/15 min in cases with an unripe cervix, as claimed by one group of investigators,[131] is unlikely and possibly dangerous. There is no doubt, however, that the dosage of oxytocin required to produce a certain level of uterine activity can vary considerably and is dependent on uterine sensitivity to oxytocin, which again can be correlated with the concentration of oxytocin receptors.

A MODEL FOR HUMAN PARTURITION

The preparation of the uterus for parturition begins in the third trimester, and the initiation of labor is often a gradual process. It involves the following steps.

1. Growth and remodeling of the cervix occurs under the influence of placental hormones and

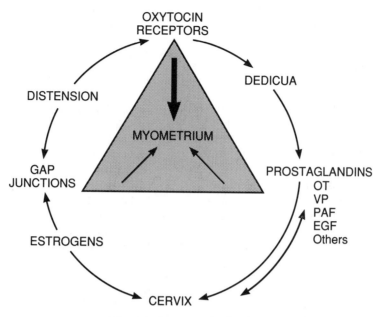

Fig. 6.15 Diagrammatic representation of the main factors involved in the control of uterine activity in pregnant women at term and during spontaneous labor. (From Fuchs,[136] with permission.)

relaxin throughout gestation. The process accelerates during the last trimester, when pressure on the cervix from above increases and brings about PGE_2 production at a slow rate. PGE_2 acts synergistically with relaxin and placental estrogens to promote cervical remodeling.

2. Placental hormones and uterine distention bring about an increase in oxytocin and vasopressin receptor concentrations that proceeds at a rate that accelerates in the second half of pregnancy.

3. Oxytocin is secreted in pulses of low frequency throughout gestation. In the third trimester the receptor concentrations have reached a point at which these pulses and the pulses released episodically in response to a variety of stimuli (from vagal afferents, food, stress, nipple stimulation, and so forth) elicit sporadic contractions that accelerate the progress of step 1.

4. Near term, distention of the uterus accelerates, and a crucial point is reached that causes oxytocin receptor concentrations to double or triple. Distention also increases gap junction formation between myometrial cells, more units are recruited to contract in response to the oxy-

tocin pulses, more tension is generated, and the intrauterine pressure developed at each contraction increases as the progress of step 1 is further accelerated.

5. By mechanisms not yet fully understood, the frequency of oxytocin pulses increases, perhaps as a result of reflexes arising in the densely innervated cervical region that is under growing pressure from above. Contractions are thus elicited with increasing frequency. The decidua begins to respond to oxytocin with the release of $PGF_{2\alpha}$ which diffuses into the inner layers of the myometrium, where the action of oxytocin is enhanced.

6. Concomitantly with step 4, maturational changes take place in the conceptus that result in the excretion from various organs of substances (e.g., epidermal growth factor, platelet-activating factor) that have the potential to stimulate arachidonic acid mobilization from uterine tissue phospholipids. Intermittent contractions cause transient hypoxic episodes that stimulate the release of stress hormones, oxytocin, vasopressin, and adrenocorticotropic hormone. These substances are in direct con-

tact with the amnion, but may also reach the decidua through canaliculi in the amnion. The presence of endogenous inhibitors may prevent their action at first, but eventually the stimulatory substances predominate and the production rate of prostaglandins increases.

7. Prostaglandin release from the chorioamnion increases during contractions, especially from the area in apposition with the internal os of the cervix, which is under the greatest strain. Large amounts are released into the amniotic fluid, but, as concentrations rise, the amounts diffusing into the decidua and further into the myometrium also increase. The responses to oxytocin are further enhanced, and the progress of labor becomes self-perpetuating. A diagrammatic representation of this model is shown in Figure 6.15.

REFERENCES

1. Liggins GC: Initiation of parturition. Br Med Bull 35:145, 1979

2. Goerttler K: Die Architektur der Muskelwand des menschlichen Uterus und ihre funktionelle Bedeutung. Gegenbaurs Morphol Jahrb 65:45, 1931

3. Garfield RE, Sims SM, Kannan MS, Daniel EE: Possible role of gap junctions in activation of myometrium during parturition. Am J Physiol 235:C168, 1978

4. Garfield RE, Hayashi RH: Appearance of gap junctions in the myometrium of women during labor. Am J Obstet Gynecol 140:254, 1981

5. Fuchs A-R, Helmer H, Fuchs F, Garfield RE: Oxytocin receptors and gap junctions in human pregnant and parturient myometrium. Am J Obstet Gynecol (submitted) 1990

6. Garfield RE, Kannan MS, Daniel EE: Gap junction formation in myometrium: control by estrogens, progesterone and prostaglandins. Am J Physiol 238:C81, 1980

7. Wathes DC, Porter DG: Effect of uterine distension and estrogen treatment on gap junction formation in the myometrium of the rat. J Reprod Fertil 65:497, 1982

8. Wynn RM: Histology and ultrastructure of the human endometrium. p. 341. In Wynn RM (ed): Biology of the Uterus. 2nd Ed. Plenum Press, New York, 1977

9. Nehemiah JC, Schnitzer JA, Schulman H, Novikoff AB: Human chorionic trophoblast, decidual cells and macrophages: a histochemical and electron microscopic study. Am J Obstet Gynecol 140:261, 1981

10. Bischof P: Three pregnancy proteins (PP-12, PP-14 and PAPP-A): their biological and clinical relevance. Am J Perinatol 6:110, 1989

11. Riddick DH, Kusnick WF: Decidua: a possible source of amniotic fluid prolactin. Am J Obstet Gynecol 127:187, 1977

12. Sakburn V, Ali SM, Greenwood FS, Bryant Greenwood GD: Human relaxin in the amnion chorion decidua parietalis, basal plate and placental trophoblast by immunocytochemistry and Northern analysis. J Am Endocrinol Metab 70:508, 1990

13. Willman EA, Collins WP: The concentrations of prostagladin E$_1$ and prostaglandin F$_{2-\alpha}$ in tissues within the foetoplacental unit after spontaneous or induced labor. Br J Obstet Gynaecol 83:786, 1976

14. Danforth DN, Buckingham JC, Raddick JW: Connective tissue changes incident of cervical effacement. Am J Obstet Gynecol 80:939, 1960

15. Naftolin F, Stubblefield PS (eds): Dilation of the Uterine Cervix: Connective Tissue Biology and Clinical Management. Raven Press, New York, 1980

16. Bishop EH: Pelvic scoring for elective induction. Obstet Gynecol 24:266, 1964

17. Catalano PM, Ashikaga T, Mann LI: Cervical change and uterine activity as predictors of preterm delivery. Am J Perinatol 6:185, 1989

18. Nakayama T, Tahara K, Yanaihara T et al: Ripening human cervix: steroid concentrations and proline hydroxylase activity in cervical tissue. Program of the Tenth World Congress on Obstetric Gynecology, San Francisco, October 17, 1982

19. Wolf JP, Sinosich M, Anderson TL et al: Progesterone antagonist (RU 486) for cervical dilatation, labor induction and delivery in monkeys: effectiveness in combination with oxytocin. Am J Obstet Gynecol 160:45, 1989

20. Elger W, Fährenrich M, Beier S et al: Endometrial and myometrial effects of progesterone antagonists in pregnant guinea pigs. Am J Obstet Gynecol 157:1065, 1987

21. Ishikawa M, Shimizu T: Dehydroepiandrosterone sulfate and induction of labor. Am J Perinatol 6:173, 1989

22. Calder AA: Pharmacological management of the unripe cervix in the human. p. 317. In Naftolin F, Stubblefield PS (eds): Dilatation of the Uterine Cervix: Connective Tissue. Biology and Clinical Management. Raven Press, New York, 1980

23. Goeschen K, Saling E: Induktion der Zervixreife mit

Oxytocin versus PGF$_2$-alpha-Infusion versus -PGE$_2$ Gel intrazervikal bei Risikoschwangeren mit unreifer Zervix. Geburtshilfe Frauenheilkd 42:810, 1982

24. Goeschen K, Fuchs A-R, Fuchs F et al: Effect of beta-mimetic tocolysis on cervical ripening and plasma prostaglandin F$_{2-\alpha}$ metabolite levels after endocervical application of prostaglandin E$_2$. Obstet Gynecol 65:166, 1985

25. Uldbjerg N, Ekman G, Malmström A, Ulmsten U: Biochemical changes in human cervical connective tissue after local application of prostaglandin E$_2$. Gynecol Obstet Invest 15:291, 1983

26. Toth M, Rehnström J, Fuchs A-R: Prostaglandins E and F in cervical mucus of pregnant women. Am J Perinatol 6:145, 1989

27. Lao Guico-Lamm M, Sherwood OD: Monoclonal antibody specific for rat relaxin II. Passive immunization with monoclonal antibodies throughout the second half of pregnancy disrupts birth in intact rats. Endocrinology 123:2479, 1988

28. MacLennan AH, Green RC, Grant P, Nicolson R: Ripening of the human cervix and induction of labor with intracervical purified porcine relaxin. Obstet Gynecol 68:598, 1986

29. Assali NS: Dynamics of the uteroplacental circulation in health and disease. Am J Perinatol 6:105, 1989

30. Owman CH, Rosengren E, Sjöberg NO: Adrenergic innervation of the human female reproductive organs: a histochemical and chemical investigation. Obstet Gynecol 30:763, 1967

31. Sjöberg NO: Considerations of the cause for the disappearance of adrenergic transmitter in uterine nerves during pregnancy. Acta Physiol Scand 72:510, 1968

32. Sjöberg NO: Increase in transmitter content of adrenergic nerves in the reproductive tract of female rabbits after oestrogen treatment. Acta Endocrinol (Copenh) 57:405, 1968

33. Owman CH, Alm P, Sjöberg NO, Stiernqvist M: Structural, biochemical, and pharmacological aspects of the uterine autonomous innervation and its remodeling during pregnancy. p. 6. In Huszar G (ed): The Physiology and Biochemistry of the Uterus in Pregnancy. CRC Press, Boca Raton, FL, 1986

34. Cavaillé F, Legér JJ: Characterization and comparison of the contractile proteins from human gravid and nongravid myometrium. Gynecol Obstet Invest 16:341, 1983

35. Huszar G: Physiology of myometrial contractility and cervical dilation. p. 21. In Fuchs F, Stubblefield PS (eds): Preterm Birth: Causes, Prevention and Management. Macmillan, New York, 1984

36. Fleckenstein A, Tritthart H, Fleckenstein B et al: Selective inhibition of myocardial contractility by competitive calcium antagonists. Naunyn Schmiedebergs Arch Pharmacol 264:3, 1969

37. Michell RH, Kirk GJ, Jones LM et al: The stimulation of inositol lipid metabolism that accompanies calcium mobilization in stimulated cells: defined characteristics and unanswered questions. Philos Trans R Lond [Biol] 296:123, 1981

38. Berridge MJ, Irvine RF: Inositol triphosphate, a novel second messenger in cellular signal transduction. Nature 312:315, 1984

39. Nishizuka Y: The role of protein kinase C in cell surface signal transduction and tumor promotion. Nature 308:693, 1984

40. MacDonald PC, Porter JC, Schwarz BE, Johnson JN: Initiation of parturition in the human female. Semin Perinatol 2:273, 1978

41. Bleasdale JE, Johnston JM: Prostaglandins and human parturition: regulation of arachidonic acid mobilization. Rev Perinatol Med 5:151, 1984

42. Mitchell MD, Flint APF, Bibby J et al: Rapid increases in plasma prostaglandin concentrations after vaginal examination and amniotomy. Br Med J 2:1183, 1977

43. Fuchs A-R, Olsen P, Petersen K: Effect of distension of uterus and vagina on uterine motility and oxytocin release in puerperal rabbits. Acta Endocrinol 50:239, 1965

44. Fuchs A-R, Fuchs F: Endocrinology of human parturition: a review. Br J Obstet Gynaecol 91:948, 1984

45. Ducsay CA, McNutt CM: Circadian uterine activity in the pregnant rhesus macaque: do prostaglandins play a role? Biol Reprod 38:988, 1989

46. Walsh SW, Ducsay CA, Novy MJ: Circadian hormonal interactions among the mother, fetus and amniotic fluid. Am J Obstet Gynecol 150:745, 1984

47. Cooperstock M, England JE, Wolfe RA: Circadian incidence of labor onset hour in preterm birth and chorioamnionitis. Obstet Gynecol 70:1, 1987

48. Roberts JS, Insel PA, Goldfien A: Regulation of myometrial adrenoreceptors and adrenergic response by sex steroids. Mol Pharmacol 20:52, 1981

49. Philippe M: Fetal catecholamines. Am J Obstet Gynecol 146:840, 1983

50. Ishikawa M, Fuchs A-R: Effects of epinephrine and oxytocin on the release of prostaglandin F from the rat uterus. Prostaglandins 15:89, 1978

51. Weis GE, O'Byrne EM, Hochman JA et al: Secretion of progesterone and relaxin by the human corpus luteum at mid-pregnancy and at term. Obstet Gynecol 50:679, 1977

52. Fields PA, Eldridge RK, Fuchs A-R et al: Human placental and bovine luteal oxytocin. Endocrinology 112:1544, 1983

53. Porter DG: The myometrium and the relaxin enigma. Anim Reprod Sci 2:77, 1979

54. Wilhelmsson L, Wikland M, Wiqvist N: PGF$_2$, TxA$_2$, and PGI$_2$ have potent and differentiated actions on human uterine contractility. Prostaglandins 21:277, 1981

55. Bennett PR, Elder MG, Myatt L: The effects of lipooxygenase metabolites of arachidonic acid on human myometrial contractility. Prostaglandins 33:837, 1987

56. Lopez Bernal A, Canette Soler R, Turnbull AC: Are leukotrienes involved in human uterine contractility? Br J Obstet Gynaecol 96:568, 1989

57. Csapo AI: Defense mechanism of pregnancy. Ciba Found Study Group 9:3, 1961

58. Knaus HH: Der Eintritt der Geburt. Zentralbl Gynäkol 90:77, 1968

59. Fuchs A-R: Hormonal control of myometrial function. Acta Endocrinol (Copenh) 89(Suppl 221):9, 1978

60. Fuchs A-R, Fuchs F, Husslein P et al: Oxytocin receptors in the human uterus during pregnancy and parturition: a dual role for oxytocin in the initiation of labor. Science 215:1396, 1982

61. Casey ML, MacDonald PC: The initiation of labor in women: regulation of phospholipid and arachidonic acid metabolism and of prostaglandin production. Semin Perinatol 10:270, 1986

62. Fuchs A-R, Fuchs F: Ethanol for prevention of preterm birth. Semin Perinatol 5:236, 1981

63. Lewis RB, Schulman JD: Influence of acetylsalicylic acid, an inhibitor of PG synthesis, on the duration of human gestation and labor. Lancet 2:1159, 1973

64. Gamissans O, Balasch J: Prostaglandin synthetase inhibitors in the treatment of preterm labor. p. 223. In Fuchs F, Stubblefield PG (eds): Preterm Birth: Causes, Prevention, Management. Macmillan, New York, 1984

65. Keirse MJNC: Endogenous prostaglandins in human parturition. p. 101. In Keirse MJNC, Anderson ABM, Gravenhorst JB (eds): Human Parturition. Boerhave Series for Postgraduate Medical Education. Vol. 15. Leiden University Press, Leiden, 1979

66. Dray F, Frydman R: Primary prostaglandins in amniotic fluid in pregnancy and spontaneous labor. Am J Obstet Gynecol 126:13, 1976

67. Fuchs A-R, Goeschen K, Husslein P et al: Oxytocin and the initiation of human parturition. III. Plasma concentrations of oxytocin and 13,14-dihydro-15-keto-prostaglandin F2-α in spontaneous and oxytocin-induced labor at term. Am J Obstet Gynecol 147:497, 1983

68. Fuchs A-R, Romero R, Parra M et al: Pulsatile release of oxytocin: significant increase in spontaneous labor. Am J Obstet Gynecol (submitted) 1990

69. Ghodgaonkar RB, Dubin NH, Blake DA, King TM: The 13,14-dihydro-15-keto-prostaglandin concentrations in human plasma and amniotic fluid. Am J Obstet Gynecol 134:265, 1979

70. Dubin NH, Johnson JWC, Calhouin S et al: Plasma prostaglandin in pregnant women with term and preterm deliveries. Obstet Gynecol 57:203, 1981

71. Caldeyro-Barcia R, Sereno JA: The response of human uterus to oxytocin throughout pregnancy. p. 177. In Caldeyro-Barcia R, Heller H (eds): Oxytocin. Pergamon Press, London, 1959

72. Fuchs A-R: The role of oxytocin in parturition. p. 163. In Huszar G (ed): Biochemistry of the Human Uterus. CRC Press, Boca Raton, FL, 1986

73. Karim SMM (ed): Prostaglandins and Reproduction. University Park Press, Baltimore, 1975

74. Rasmussen AB, Johannesen P, Allen J et al: Plasma prostaglandinF2α and 13,14-dihydro-15-keto-prostaglandinF2α levels in women during induction of labor with iv infusion of PGF2α in relation to uterine contractions. J Perinatol 13:15, 1985

75. Dawood MY, Raghavan KS, Pociask C, Fuchs F: Oxytocin in human pregnancy and parturition. Obstet Gynecol 51:138, 1978

76. Morris M, Stevens SW, Adams MR: Plasma oxytocin during pregnancy and lactation in the cynomolgus monkey. Biol Reprod 23:782, 1980

77. Randolph GW, Fuchs A-R: Pulsatile administration enhances the effect and reduces the dose of oxytocin required for induction of labor. Am J Perinatol 6:159, 1989

78. Dawood MY: Evolving concepts of oxytocin for induction of labor. Am J Perinatol 6:167, 1989

79. Dawood MY, Wang CF, Gupta R, Fuchs F: Fetal contribution to oxytocin in human labor. Obstet Gynecol 52:205, 1978

80. Chard T, Boyd NRH, Edwards CRW, Hudson CN: The release of oxytocin and vasopressin by the human fetus during labor. Nature 234:352, 1971

81. Lampelo S, Vanha-Perttula T: Fractionation and characterization of cystine aminopeptidase (oxytocinase) and arylamidase of the human placenta. J Reprod Fertil 56:285, 1979

82. Fuchs A-R, Fuchs F, Soloff MS: Oxytocin receptors in nonpregnant human uterus. J Clin Endocrinol Metab 60:37, 1985

83. Fuchs A-R, Fuchs F, Husslein P et al: Oxytocin receptors in the human uterus during pregnancy and parturition. Am J Obstet Gynecol 150:734, 1984

84. Kofler E, Husslein P, Langer M et al: Die Bedeutung der Oxytocinempfindlichkeit für den spontanen Wehenbeginn beim Menschen. Geburtshilfe Frauenheilkd 43:533, 1983

85. Soloff MS: Uterine receptor for oxytocin: effects of estrogen. Biochem Biophys Res Commun 65:205, 1975

86. Nissenson R, Flouret G, Hechter O: Opposing effects of estradiol and progesterone on oxytocin receptors in rabbit uterus. Proc Natl Acad Sci USA 75:2044, 1978

87. Fuchs A-R, Periyasami S, Alexandrova M, Soloff MS: Correlation between oxytocin receptor concentrations and responsiveness to oxytocin in pregnant rat myometrium: effect of ovarian steroids. Endocrinology 113:742, 1983

88. Clark JW, Peck EJ: Female Sex Steroids: Receptors and Functions. Monographs on Endocrinology. Berlin, Springer-Verlag, 1979

89. Fuchs A-R, Periyasamy S, Soloff MS: Systemic and local regulation of oxytocin receptors in the rat uterus. Can J Biochem Cell Biol 61:614, 1983

90. Embrey MP, Moir CJ: A comparison of the oxytocic effects of synthetic vasopressin and oxytocin. J Obstet Gynaecol Br Commonw 74:648, 1967

91. Guillon G, Balestre MN, Roberts JM, Bottari SP: Oxytocin and vasopressin: distinct receptors in myometrium. 64:1129, 1987

92. Ivanišević M, Behrens O, Helmer H, Fuchs A-R: Vasopressin receptors in human pregnant myometrium and decidua: interactions with oxytocin and vasopressin agonists and antagonists. Am J Obstet Gynecol 161:1639, 1989

93. Taslimi MM, Billedeaux LA, Ruiz AG, Herrick SN: Short labor in carriers of nephrogenic diabetes insipidus. Am J Gynecol Health 4:11, 1990

94. Pohjavuori M, Fyhrquist F: Hemodynamic significance of vasopressin in the newborn infant. J Pediatr Res 18:835, 1984

95. Stark RI, Daniel SS, Hussain MK et al: Vasopressin concentration in amniotic fluid as an index of fetal hypoxia: mechanism of release in sheep. Pediatr Res 18:835, 1984

96. Schrey MP, Reed AM, Steer PJ: Oxytocin and arginine vasopressin stimulate inositol phosphate production in human gestational myometrium and decidua cells. Biosci Rep 6:613, 1986

97. Williams KI: Prostaglandin synthesis and uterine contractility. p. 282. In Bottari S, Thomas JP, Vokaer A, Vokaer R (eds): Uterine Contractility. Masson, New York, 1984

98. Krall JE, Barrett JD, Jamgotduan N, Korenman SG: Interaction of PGE_2 and β-adrenergic catecholamines in the regulation of uterine smooth muscle motility and adenylatecyclase in the rat. J Endocrinol 102:329, 1984

99. Coleman HA, Parkington H: Induction of prolonged excitability in myometrium of pregnant guinea pig by $PGF2\alpha$. J Physiol (Lond) 399:33, 1988

100. Bauknecht T, Krake B, Rechenbach U et al: Distribution of PGE and $PGF2\alpha$ receptors in human myometrium. Acta Endocrinol (Copenh) 98:446, 1981

101. Giannopoulos G, Jackson K, Kredentser J: Prostaglandin E and $F_{2\alpha}$ receptors in human myometrium during the menstrual cycle and in pregnancy and labor. Am J Obstet Gynecol 153:904, 1985

102. Cheung PYC, Challis JRG: Prostaglandin E_2 metabolism in human fetal membranes. Am J Obstet Gynecol 161:1580, 1989

103. McCoshen JA, Tulloch HV, Johnson KA: Umbilical cord is the major source of prostaglandin E_2 in the gestational sac during term labor. Am J Obstet Gynecol 160:973, 1989

104. McCoshen JA, Johnson KA, Ghodkaongkar RB: PGE_2 release on the fetal and maternal sides of the amnion and chorion–decidua before and after term labor. Am J Obstet Gynecol 156:173, 1987

105. Schlegel W, Kruger S, Korte K: Purification of PGE_2-9-oxoreductase from human decidua vera. FEBS Lett 171:141, 1984

106. Moonen P, Klok G, Keirse MJNC: Increase in concentrations of prostaglandin endoperoxide synthase and prostacyclin synthase in human myometrium in late pregnancy. Prostaglandins 28:309, 1984

107. Dembelé-Duchesne MJ, Thaler-Dao H, Chairo C, Crastes de Paulet A: Some new prospects in the mechanism of control of arachidonate metabolism in human placenta and membranes. Prostaglandins 22:979, 1981

108. Granström E, Kindahl H, Swahn ML: Profiles of prostaglandin metabolites in the human circulation: identification of late appearing, long-lived products. Biochim Biophys Acta 713:46, 1982

109. Fuchs A-R, Husslein P, Sumulong L, Fuchs F: The origin of circulating 13,14-dihydro-15-keto-$PGF_{2\alpha}$ during delivery. Prostaglandins 24:715, 1982

110. Noort WA, Van Bulck B, Vereecken A et al: Changes in plasma levels of $PGF_{2\alpha}$ and PGI_2 metabolites at and after delivery at term. Prostaglandins 37:3, 1989

111. Husslein P, Sinzinger H: Concentration of 13,14-dihydro-15-keto-prostaglandin E_2 in the maternal pe-

ripheral plasma during labour of spontaneous onset. Br J Obstet Gynaecol 91:228, 1984

112. Brennecke SP, Castle BM, Demers LM, Turnbull AC: Endogenous PGE_2 metabolite levels in the human during pregnancy as detected by a novel radioimmunoassay. Br J Obstet Gynaecol 92:345, 1985

113. Hamberg M: Quantitative studies on prostaglandin synthesis in man. III. Excretion of the major urinary metabolite of $PGF_{1\alpha}$ and $F_{2\alpha}$ during pregnancy. Life Sci 14:247, 1974

114. Noort WA: Prostanoid Excretion in Human Term and Preterm Gestation. Thesis. p. 188. University of Leiden, Leiden, The Netherlands, 1989

115. Noort WA, DeZwart FA, Keirse MJNC: Changes in urinary 6-keto-$PGF_{1\alpha}$ excretion during pregnancy and labor. Prostaglandins 35:573, 1988

116. Walsh SW: Preeclampsia: an imbalance in placental prostacyclin and thromboxane production. Am J Obstet Gynecol 152:335, 1985

117. Husslein P, Kofler E, Rasmussen AB et al: Oxytocin and the initiation of human parturition. IV. Plasma concentrations of oxytocin and 13,14-dihydro-15-keto $PGF_{2\alpha}$ during induction of labor by artificial rupture of membranes. Am J Obstet Gynecol 140:261, 1981

118. Hirata F: The regulation of lipomodulin, a phospholipase inhibitory protein, in rabbit neutrophils by phosphorylation. J Biol Chem 256:7730, 1981

119. Wilson T, Liggins GC: Purification and characterization of a uterine phospholipase inhibitor that loses activity after labor onset in women. Am J Obstet Gynecol 160:602, 1989

120. Saeed SA, Strickland DM, Young DM et al: Inhibition of prostaglandin synthesis by human amniotic fluid: acute reduction in inhibitory activity of amniotic fluid obtained during labor. J Clin Endocrinol Metab 55:801, 1982

121. Rehnstrom J, Ishikawa M, Fuchs F, Fuchs A-R: Stimulation of myometrial and decidual prostaglandin production by amniotic fluid from term but not mid-trimester pregnancies. Prostaglandins 26:973, 1984

122. Brennecke SP, Bryce RL, Turnbull AC: The prostaglandin synthase inhibiting ability of maternal plasma and the onset of human labour. Eur J Obstet Gynecol Reprod 14:81, 1982

123. Morita I, Nakayama Y, Murota S: Characterization of the stimulatory effects of $PGF_{2\alpha}$ on the release of arachidonic acid. Prostaglandins 18:507, 1979

124. Alvarez H, Caldeyro-Barcia R: Contractility of the human uterus recorded by new methods. Surg Gynecol Obstet 91:1, 1950

125. Bourne AW, Burn JH: The dosage and action of pituitary extract and the ergot alkaloid on the uterus in labour, with a note on the action of adrenalin. J Obstet Gynaecol Br Emp 34:249, 1927

126. Steer PJ, Carter MC, Beard RW: Normal levels of active contraction area in spontaneous labor. Br J Obstet Gynaecol 91:211, 1984

127. Arulkumaran S, Gibb DMF, Lun KC et al: The effect of parity on uterine activity in labour. Br J Obstet Gynaecol 91:843, 1984

128. Friedman EA: Labor: Clinical Evaluation and Management. 2nd ed. Appleton-Century-Crofts, East Norwalk, CT, 1978

129. Amico JA, Seitchik J, Robinson AG: Studies of oxytocin in plasma of women during hypocontractile labor. J Clin Endocrinol Metab 58:274, 1984

130. Seitchik J, Amico J, Robinson AG, Castillo M: Oxytocin augmentation of dysfunctional labor. IV. Oxytocin pharmacokinetics. Am J Obstet Gynecol 150:225, 1984

131. Jagani N, Schulman H, Fleischer A: Role of the cervix in the induction of labor. Obstet Gynecol 59:21, 1982

132. Fay FS, Delise CM: Contraction of isolated smooth muscle cells—structural changes. Proc Natl Acad Sci USA 70:641, 1973

133. Hartshorne DJ, Gorecka A: Biochemistry of the contractile proteins of smooth muscle. p. 93. In Bohr DF, Somlyo AP, Sparkes HV Jr (eds): Handbook of Physiology. Vol. II. American Physiological Society, Bethesda, MD, 1980

134. Haselgrove J: Structure of vertebrate skeletal muscle. p. 144. In Peachey LD, Adrian RH (eds): Handbook of Physiology. Section 10. American Physiological Society, Bethesda, MD, 1983

135. Braunwald E: Mechanism of action of calcium-channel blocking drugs. N Engl J Med 307:1618, 1982

136. Fuchs A-R: Oxytocin and oxytocin receptors: maternal signals for parturition. p. 177. In Garfield RE (ed): Uterine Contractility. Serono Symposia USA, Norwell, MA, 1990

Chapter 7

Physiology and Endocrinology of Lactation

Anna-Riitta Fuchs

PHYSIOLOGIC SIGNIFICANCE OF BREAST-FEEDING

The mammary gland plays an essential role in the reproduction of most mammals. Failure to lactate means failure to reproduce, because the young are too immature to ward off the invasion of environmental microbial agents and to feed on foreign food stuffs. At birth, the mammary gland takes over some of the functions fulfilled by the placenta during intrauterine life. It provides the neonate with a ready source of easily digested nutrients and with a variety of immunologic factors that protect against infection. The period of lactation provides a gradual transition from a total dependence on the maternal organism to an independent existence.

The long evolutionary developmental process of the mammary gland has resulted in considerable differences in the composition of milk in various species, the secretions of the gland being uniquely adapted to the special needs of each species at the particular developmental stage at which the young are born. Milk from one species does not, as a rule, allow young from another species to survive. Technologic advances during the last century have made it possible to prepare formulas based on cow's milk or soy proteins that can provide acceptable substitutes for breast milk. Many mothers have found the use of such substitutes so convenient that breast-feeding has drastically declined around the world. Where the standards

of living and hygiene are high, bottle-feeding has had less impact, but in developing countries the consequences have often been disastrous. In the past 10 to 15 years there has been a marked increase in the motivation to breast-feed, particularly among well-educated and affluent women in the United States and Europe. Unfortunately, large groups of disadvantaged mothers, both in the United States and abroad, whose infants would most benefit from breast-feeding, are least likely to initiate it.

For the infant, the physical benefits of breast-feeding include significant protection against infection, particularly diarrhea and upper respiratory tract and ear infections. Breast-feeding also affords protection against atopic disease, particularly when maintained for at least 6 months,[1] and intestinal parasitic disease.[2] Many components of human milk are necessary for optimal development of the brain and other organs.[3] Several studies suggest that breast-fed infants have better somatic growth and physiologic development than those who are bottle-fed.[4-6]

Although the debate on the relative merits of breast-feeding and bottle-feeding continues, the benefits of breast-feeding appear to be so well established that physicians should encourage prospective mothers to breast-feed. Patients should be provided with sufficient information to permit a decision to breast-feed or bottle-feed to be made on a rational basis.

The decision whether to breast-feed is influenced

by many complex social and psychological factors. It is usually made long before the birth of the baby, and therefore the prenatal care provider should discuss the benefits and perceived disadvantages of breast-feeding with the expectant mother during her prenatal care and provide information and support. It is important to realize that in today's urban settings most mothers lack the social support system provided in earlier times by female relatives who themselves had breast-fed. The environment of the less privileged mothers tends to provide many negative and few positive inducements for breast-feeding, which should be taken into consideration when counseling such women about breast-feeding. Hospital practices in the early postpartum period also have a significant effect on the subsequent infant feeding mode.[7] Unfortunately, in many institutions the routine practices still have a strong negative impact on breast-feeding.[8] Proper lactation counseling should be an essential part of every maternity ward.

THE MAMMARY GLAND AND ITS SECRETORY FUNCTION

The mammary gland undergoes remarkable proliferation and differentiation during pregnancy. After parturition, the mammary gland begins to synthesize and secrete specific carbohydrates, proteins, and fats and selectively transfers minerals from plasma to milk in quantities sufficient to satisfy all the nutritional needs of the growing infant. In addition, it takes over an immunologic function, providing the infant with maternal antibodies until its own immune system is established. After weaning, the various functions of the mammary gland cease. The gland then regresses and returns to its resting state.

Morphology of the Breast and the Mammary Gland

Gross Anatomy

The adult breast consists of glandular tissue or parenchyma embedded in stroma made up of connective tissue and adipose tissue. The stroma carries the blood vessels, nerves, and lymphatic vessels. In the resting state, the glandular tissue occupies only a small fraction of the total volume of the breast. The stromal elements give the mature breast its size and shape.

The glandular tissue is termed a compound tubular alveolar gland. It consists of an arborized duct system that drains clusters of sac-like structures called alveoli or acini. These alveoli form the basic unit of the secretory system (Fig. 7.1). Each alveolus is surrounded by a mesh of myoepithelial cells and by a capillary network. The alveoli (0.2 mm in diameter) are arranged in lobuli with 10 to 100 alveoli per lobule. Twenty to 40 lobules form lobes, each of which is drained by a single lactiferous duct. There are 15 to 20 lactiferous ducts in the human breast. They converge toward the areola, beneath which they form the lactiferous sinuses that serve as small reservoirs of milk. Each lobe is separated by septa of connective tissue that merge imperceptibly with the fascia covering the anterior wall of the thorax.

The nipple is a condensation of epithelial tissue through which the lactiferous ducts pass to orifices at the surface. It is surrounded by a specialized pigmented skin, the areola, which contains sweat glands and sebaceous glands (glands of Montgomery) that hypertrophy during pregnancy and serve to lubricate and protect the nipple during lactation.

The mammary gland, being cutaneous in origin, shares with the contiguous skin its blood supply and innervation. The innervation of the nipple and the areola is abundant, with close connection between autonomic and sensory nerves. However, the remainder of the breast is very sparsely innervated, and the mammary myoepithelial cells themselves are without innervation. Free sensory endings are distributed in the peripheral skin of the breast as well as in the areola and nipple, whereas tactile corpuscles are located mainly in the dermis of the areola and nipple. This probably contributes to the great sensitivity of these areas to tactile stimuli. The sensory innervation of the peripheral skin appears to be influenced by the endocrine milieu. Thus the tactile sensitivity as determined by a two-point discrimination test increases significantly in pregnant women within 24 hours of parturition. Cyclic variations can also be discerned during the menstrual cycle.[9]

The innervation of the nipple and areola plays a vital role in lactation, mediating the reflex activation of the neurohumoral reflexes responsible for the removal of milk from the gland and the release of prolactin essential for the maintenance of lactation. The

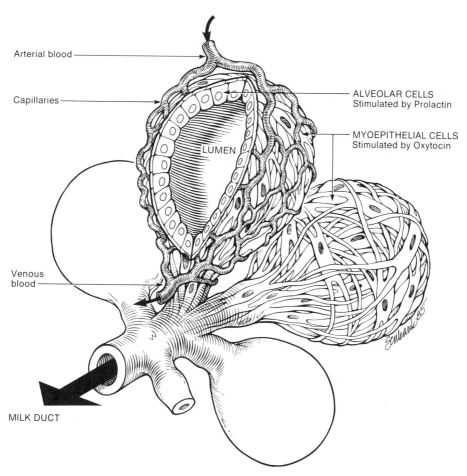

Arterial blood

Capillaries

ALVEOLAR CELLS
Stimulated by Prolactin

MYOEPITHELIAL CELLS
Stimulated by Oxytocin

LUMEN

Venous
blood

MILK DUCT

Fig. 7.1 Diagram of a cluster of alveoli, the basic units of the mammary gland. (Adapted from Cowie,[130] with permission.)

intraglandular innervation of the blood vessels may influence mammary blood flow and thus indirectly milk secretion.[10]

Microscopic Features of the Alveolar Cell

In the resting stage, the tubuloalveolar system is sparse, consisting of mostly ductal elements that are widely dispersed in the stroma. Two layers of epithelial cells line the alveoli, which are virtually indistinguishable from the simple cuboidal cells lining the ducts.[11] Myoepithelial cells, also small and cuboidal, form a distinct layer beneath the epithelial cells. Few mitoses are seen in the resting stage. In the mammogenic phase of early pregnancy, many of the epithelial

stem cells will divide but will maintain their undifferentiated appearance.[12]

The fully differentiated secretory epithelium of the lactating gland consists of a single layer of alveolar cells that are columnar and tall when the alveolar lumen is empty and that become flattened when the luman is full (Fig. 7.2). The cells have all the characteristics of secretory cells. Each alveolar cell is firmly attached to its neighbors by tight junctional complexes at the apical end. Many leukocytes that send processes toward the apex of the alveolar cells are found between the alveolar cells. During pregnancy, some of the junctional complexes are open, or "leaky," permitting accumulation of cells, plasma

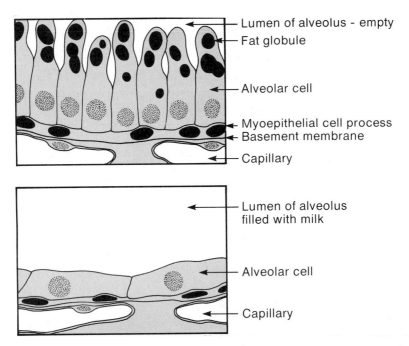

Fig. 7.2 Cells in the wall of an alveolus (A) just after milking and (B) just before milking. As the alveolus fills with milk, its walls are stretched and the shape of the cells is greatly altered. (Adapted from Cowie,[130] with permission.)

proteins, and sodium chloride in the lumen. During lactation, the junctions are tight.[13–16]

Mechanisms of Secretion

Ultrastructural studies of the alveolar cells combined with biochemical analyses have helped to clarify the pathways for the synthesis and secretion of milk components. Different pathways operate in parallel to transfer precursors into the alveolar cells and to transfer milk constituents from the cells to the alveolar lumina (Fig. 7.3).[15,17–21]

Exocytosis

Proteins and carbohydrates are secreted by a process known as exocytosis, whereby the membranes of the secretory vesicles fuse with the apical plasma membrane to expel their contents without the loss of membrane proteins. The proteins are synthesized in the endoplasmic reticulum and further processed and sorted in the Golgi apparatus, where calcium and phosphate combine with the milk protein casein to form aggregates, which are then packaged into secretory vesicles.

Lactose is also synthesized in the Golgi apparatus by lactose synthetase, an enzyme consisting of two parts: a protein, galactosyltransferase, bound to the Golgi membrane, and a soluble protein, α-lactalbumin, which also constitutes one of the secretory milk proteins. The Golgi membrane is impermeable to lactose. As lactose accumulates, water and ions are drawn osmotically into the Golgi system and into the alveolar lumen. At the apical end, lactose is packaged together with milk proteins into secretory vesicles from which they are released into the lumen by exocytosis.

Milk Fat Secretion

Lipids are secreted by an apocrine process in which the plasma membrane surrounds the droplets and is pinched off at the apex. Small amounts of cytoplasmic constituents are usually enclosed within the membrane, providing a source of enzymes and lipases. The fatty acids in human milk are mostly long chain (over C16) and originate from both dietary fat and adipose

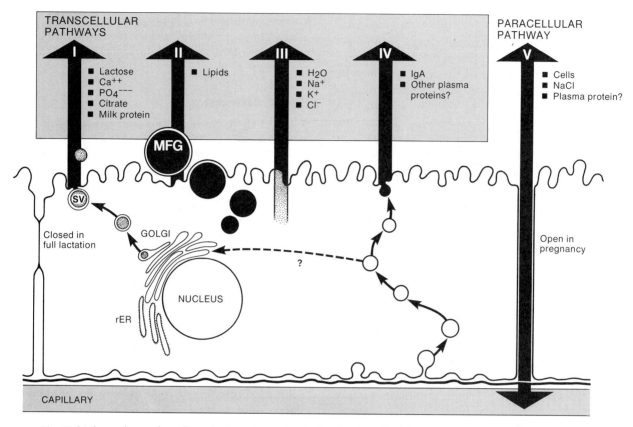

Fig. 7.3 The pathways for milk synthesis and secretion in the alveolar cell. (I) Exocytosis of milk protein and lactose in Golgi secretory vesicles. (II) Milk fat secretion in a plasma membrane–enclosed milk fat globule. (III) Diffusion of water and ions across the apical membrane. (IV) Pinocytosis–exocytosis of immunoglobulins. (V) The paracellular pathway for leukocytes and plasma components. SV, secretory vesicle; RER, rough endoplasmic reticulum; BM, basement membrane; MFG, milk fat globule. (Adapted from Neville et al.,[21] with permission.)

tissue, whereas shorter chain saturated fatty acids are synthesized de novo by the gland.

Diffusion

Monovalent cations and water are transported by diffusion. The apical cell membrane and the Golgi apparatus are freely permeable to monovalent ions and water. Water moves from the cell across these membranes in response to the osmotic gradient created by lactose, which accounts for about two-thirds of the osmotically active solutes in human milk. Sodium, potassium, and chloride concentrations are considerably lower in milk than in the cytoplasm and contribute about one-sixth the total osmolarity of milk. The movement of these ions through the apical membrane is limited by some as yet unknown mechanism so that equilibrium is attained at concentrations in milk that are lower than those in the cell.

Pinocytosis – Exocytosis

Immunoglobulins are transported through the alveolar cells by a receptor-mediated transcellular route.[22,23] The most abundant immunoglobulin found in human milk is secretory immunoglobulin A (IgA), the major part of which is synthesized locally by plasma cells present in the breast.[24] Small amounts of IgG, IgE, and IgM are also secreted into colostrum and milk. Colostrum represents the alveolar secretions before the production of milk.

Paracellular Pathway

Cellular elements, found in milk in great numbers, reach the lumen by a paracellular pathway.[19,25,26] During pregnancy, many of the tight junctions between cells appear to be open or leaky, accounting for the high concentration of cellular material and plasma components in the colostrum.[27] In the early puerperium, the concentration of cells is about 1 to 2×10^6 cells/ml, most of which are leukocytes (neutrophils, macrophages, and lymphocytes). The concentration of cells is reduced markedly during the first month of lactation. At that time, many of the cells are sloughed epithelial cells, although large numbers of leukocytes are found in mature milk. It is not clear how paracellular transport operates during established lactation, when all junctions between cells appear to be tight. Apparently, the permeability of the junctional complexes can be regulated by factors present in alveolar secretions.

DEVELOPMENT OF THE MAMMARY GLAND

The mammary gland develops in four distinct stages: (1) during embryonic and fetal life, (2) at puberty, (3) during pregnancy, and (4) in the early puerperium. Regression or atrophy may be considered a fifth stage, seen after weaning or after the menopause.

Embryonic Development

The mammary gland can be identified from about the fifth gestational week onward. Epithelial cells are derived from the ectoderm, which penetrates the underlying mesenchyme, the source of blood vessels, connective tissue, and lymphatic elements. By week 20, the anlage for the lactiferous ducts (mammary bud) has invaded the mesodermal connective tissue, growing deeper and deeper with advancing gestation. Cells destined to become the myoepithelial cells are present as highly differentiated ectodermal cells localized around and along the developing ductal elements. The nipple and areola arise rather late in gestation. Thus, at birth, a rudimentary mammary gland is present, consisting of a nipple and a primitive duct system.[28,29]

Failure of proper proliferation of the mesenchyme

underlying the mammary primordium results in a relatively common finding, inversion of the nipple. This condition often improves spontaneously during pregnancy.

Pubertal Development

From birth to puberty, the breast undergoes only isometric growth. Pubertal development, thelarche, normally begins between ages 8 and 14 years and is usually complete in about 4 years. At first, proliferation and branching of the duct system takes place, followed by the formation of the terminal bud system from which the alveoli and lobuli will later develop. In addition, a rapid deposition of fat and connective tissue in the stroma gives the mature breast its size and form. In nonpregnant adult women, no further glandular development takes place unless pregnancy intervenes. The gland remains in an inactive, resting state. The volume of the breast varies during the menstrual cycle, increasing by 15 to 30 cm³ on the average in the premenstrual phase and returning to its initial volume during menstruation.[30] This change is mainly due to enhanced water retention in the stroma and infiltration of connective tissue with lymphoid and plasma cells. Slight enlargement of the alveolar luminal diameter may occur with appearance of intra-alveolar secretory material. These changes are reversed in the postmenstrual phase. The size of the breast is smallest on days 4 to 7 of the cycle.[31]

Mammogenic Changes During Pregnancy

With the establishment of a functional trophoblast, hormonal changes occur, rapidly producing a spectacular cellular proliferation of both ductal and alveolar elements, sometimes called the proliferative or active stage of mammogenesis. This can be observed within 3 to 4 weeks of conception. In its earliest stages, ductal sprouting predominates, whereas from the third month on lobuloalveolar multiplication dominates. There is a progressive increase in the size of the lobules throughout pregnancy, initially through cellular hyperplasia and later by hypertrophy. Stromal elements progressively diminish, and at the end of gestation only thin septa of connective tissue separate the well-developed lobes of glandular tissue (Fig. 7.4).[10,12]

Around mid-gestation, the proliferation of the al-

FIRST TRIMESTER

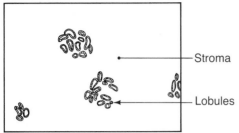

Stroma

Lobules

SECOND TRIMESTER

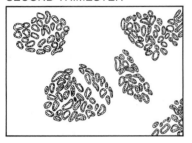

THIRD TRIMESTER

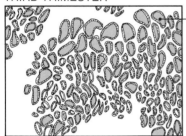

Alveolus contains many lipid droplets and some secretory material

Fig. 7.4 Mammary gland development during pregnancy, illustrated by sections of the mammary gland of pregnant women. In early pregnancy the stroma is the dominant component, containing only scattered ducts. By mid-pregnancy the lobules of alveoli form lobes that are separated by stromal tissues. Secretion is present in some alveolar cells. In the last trimester the lobules of the alveoli are almost fully developed, with cells full of secretory material and the stromal tissue reduced to bands separating lobules and thicker strands between lobes.

veolar epithelium gradually ceases. During the second half of gestation, mitosis of alveolar cells is rarely seen. Instead, the alveolar stem cells differentiate and begin to assume secretory characteristics. The alveoli are now lined with a single layer of epithelial cells, an appearance retained throughout late gestation and lactation. The cells are still simple, cuboidal or low columnar, with sparse secretory-type microvilli on their apical surface. Increasing amounts of rough endoplasmic reticulum and Golgi apparatus are seen, but the number of organelles remains relatively low. The myoepithelial cells hypertrophy, become flattened, and develop attenuated cytoplasmic processes that form an open network around the epithelial cells. The glandular hypertrophy is associated with a conspicuous infiltration of the connective tissue and epithelium by a variety of leukocytes.[32] In late gestation, the alveoli begin to fill with a proteinaceous material composed of desquamated epithelial cells and a variety of leukocytes. During pregnancy, no fat or protein appears to be released from the alveolar cells into the lumina, although pronounced accumulation of fat droplets and proteinaceous material is seen inside the cells during the last trimester.

Postpartum Development

After parturition, the fourth stage of development takes place, marked by a rapid increase in cell size and in the number of secretory organelles. The final differentiation of the mammary gland is completed during a few days. Within 48 hours the cells become tall, with abundant rough endoplasmic reticulum, well-developed Golgi, and numerous microvilli at their apical cell surface.[12-14,16] The alveoli distend with milk, and, as they do, the epithelial cells become flattened and distorted. Unless the breast is emptied, necrotic changes quickly occur in the alveolar epithelium.[15]

Mammary blood flow rises markedly during pregnancy and increases further in early lactation. It appears to be closely correlated with the rate of milk secretion. In cows and goats, about 400 to 500 L of blood flow through the gland for each liter of milk produced. The mammary blood flow can be regulated by changes in cardiac output as well as by local factors that influence vasomotor tone.[33]

ENDOCRINE CONTROL OF MAMMARY GLAND FUNCTION

The function of the mammary gland depends entirely on hormonal factors. Ovarian or placental steroids, anterior pituitary hormones or placental polypeptide hormones, adrenal steroids, as well as insulin and thyroxine participate in mammary gland development and secretory function. The endocrine control of mammary gland function is probably one of the most complex in the body. Not only are multiple hormones involved, but they must act in proper sequence as well.

The initiation and maintenance of milk production depend on several processes, all of which are controlled by specific hormonal complexes: (1) mammogenesis, or the development of the mammary gland; (2) lactogenesis, or the initiation of milk secretion; (3) galactopoiesis, or the maintenance of established milk secretion; and (4) galactokinesis, or the removal of milk from the gland. Involution also plays a role in the maintenance of milk secretion because of the rapidity with which degenerative changes can occur in the mammary gland.

Mammogenic Hormones

The endocrine control of mammary gland development has been studied extensively in both small laboratory animals and ruminants, in which milk production is of commercial interest. Using hypophysectomized immature mice and rats, as well as animals subjected to hypophysectomy, ovariectomy, and

---

MAMMOGENIC COMPLEX OF HORMONES

Ductal growth

    Estrogen

    Growth hormone

    Glucocorticoids

Lobuloalveolar growth

    Estrogen

    Growth hormone

    Glucocorticoids

    Prolactin

    Progesterone

---

adrenalectomy and given various hormonal replacement regimens, the minimal hormone milieu required for lactation has been established.[34,35]

Our knowledge about the mammogenic hormones in humans is limited and derived mostly from patients with genetic abnormalities in gonadal and pituitary function. Although species' differences do exist, especially in regard to the galactopoietic hormones, the findings in laboratory animals are probably applicable to human breast development and function as well.

Ovarian hormones are clearly important, because they initiate breast development in agonadal patients or in animals ovariectomized before puberty. However, they are without effect in the absence of the pituitary gland. The sex steroids may therefore have an indirect action mediated by the anterior pituitary gland. Estrogen stimulates prolactin release and also sensitizes the mammary gland to the action of prolactin.[36]

The role of growth hormone in women has not been firmly established, since normal mammary development has been reported in the congenital absence of growth hormone. Factors produced locally and in the liver, such as epidermal growth factor, somatomedin, and a specific mammary gland growth factor, promote mammogenesis. Some of these factors are induced by estrogen.

Breast stroma, particularly adipose tissue, appears to play an active role in the development of glandular tissue. Interactions between alveolar, ductal, and stromal cells may be necessary for normal growth. Adipose tissue from mammary glands supports the growth of mammary cells in culture and prevents individual ducts from fusing.[37,38] Because the mammary fat pad accumulates estrogen and possesses estrogen receptors, it may play a more active role in mammogenesis than previously suspected.[39]

Lactogenic Hormones

Lactogenesis (the onset of milk secretion) is usually measured by the output of milk sugar or by the most abundant milk protein, casein. The lactogenic complex of hormones was determined in experiments similar to those in which the minimal requirements for mammogenesis were established.[10,34,35]

REQUIREMENTS FOR LACTOGENESIS

Fully developed mammary gland

Prolactin

Glucocorticoids

Insulin

Thyroid hormones

Possibly growth hormone

Withdrawal of estrogen and progesterone

In pregnant women, placental lactogen can substitute for pituitary prolactin and growth hormone. The metabolic hormones insulin and thyroxine are themselves without lactogenic effect but play a permissive role in this process.[40] Thyroid hormones selectively enhance the secretion of lactalbumin.[41] Prerequisites for lactogenesis are a fully developed mammary gland and the withdrawal of estrogen and progesterone. While the sex steroids and prolactin have a synergistic effect on mammogenesis, they inhibit the lactogenic effects of prolactin.

Galactokinetic Hormones

Milk accumulating in the lumina of the alveoli cannot flow passively into the ducts. It must be squeezed out by the contraction of the surrounding myoepithelial cells. These cells compress the alveoli and force the milk into the duct system, resulting in milk ejection. Oxytocin is the most powerful galactokinetic hormone. It is now well established that oxytocin is the physiologic stimulus that activates the myoepithelial cells and permits milk removal from the gland.[42] Vasopressin has about one-fifth to one-hundredth the potency of oxytocin in the human breast.[43]

The myoepithelial cells, like myometrial cells, have specific receptors for oxytocin.[44] In the rat mammary gland, the concentration of oxytocin receptors increases gradually during pregnancy, with a more marked increase after parturition. There is some dis-

agreement about the changes in the oxytocin sensitivity of the mammary myoepithelium during pregnancy. However, all investigators agree that, after delivery, a marked increase occurs, reaching a plateau on the fifth to sixth day of the puerperium.[45–47]

Milk Ejection and the Suckling Stimulus

The release of oxytocin from the neurohypophysis is under neural control, and, during lactation, the stimulus is provided by the suckling of the infant. The sensory nerve endings that mediate the afferent path of this neuroendocrine reflex lie beneath the areola and the nipple. The neurons that secrete oxytocin are located in the hypothalamus, concentrated mainly in the paraventricular and supraoptic nuclei. Long axons from these neurons extend into the posterior pituitary gland, where the nerve terminals are located, abutting on a rich capillary network. The pathways of this neuroendocrine reflex are illustrated in Figure 7.5.

Oxytocin release is essential for milk removal. If local anesthesia is applied on the sensory nerve endings under the areola[42] or if the release of oxytocin is inhibited by high doses of ethyl alcohol, the young will be unable to obtain milk.[48,49] Only that fraction of milk that is stored in the lactiferous sinuses under the areola can be extracted by mechanical forces. Women suffering from diabetes insipidus are often able to breast-feed their babies, because this disorder does not affect the oxytocin-producing neurons. Oxytocin and vasopressin are produced in separate neurons; therefore, oxytocin secretion is usually intact in patients who are unable to synthesize vasopressin.

Adequate milk ejection is essential for successful lactation. First, it makes the alveolar luminal milk available for the infant, and, second, the removal of milk from the alveoli is necessary for the continuation of milk secretion. The flattened alveolar cells of distended alveoli cease their secretory activity and quickly begin to undergo degenerative changes.[15] Frequent suckling and adequate milk ejection therefore promote the production of milk. It is important to instruct the young mother in the right technique for breast-feeding so that her baby can provide an adequate stimulus. In the early puerperium, oxytocin treatment (e.g., buccal tablets) has been found to be

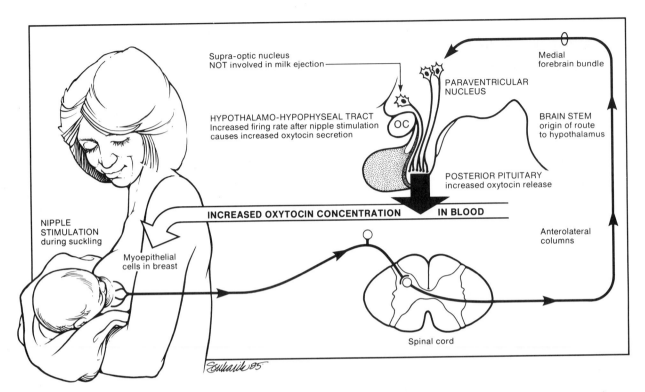

Fig. 7.5 The somatosensory pathways for the suckling-induced reflex release of oxytocin. (Adapted from Johnson and Everitt,[131] with permission.)

helpful in women with very engorged breasts, probably because the distention of the breast makes it difficult for the newborn to apply proper pressure at the base of the nipple when suckling.

During the nursing period oxytocin is released over several minutes, causing rhythmic intramammary pressure changes, as shown by recordings from one breast while the baby is suckling on the other breast.[47] Plasma oxytocin levels rise rapidly after the onset of suckling, usually remain elevated while the infant is nursing, and then drop[50] (Fig. 7.6). In advanced lactation the increment in oxytocin levels in response to suckling increases.[51] This increase is seen only in mothers who exclusively breast-feed and not in mothers who provide supplemental feeding[52] (Fig. 7.7). This indicates that an infant who is accustomed to the bottle becomes a less effective sucker at the breast and reflects the fact that feeding at the breast requires different coordination and movement of tongue and lips than feeding at the bottle.

In women, the reflex release of oxytocin often becomes conditioned. It is experienced as milk "let down" during the preparation for nursing the infant, playing with the infant, or even thinking about it. After prolonged breast-feeding, many mothers learn to decondition this reflex.

Oxytocin released during suckling also reaches the uterus, which it stimulates to contract.[49] The contractions are strong in the early puerperium and may be of significance for the expulsion of lochia and for the involution of the uterus.

Galactopoietic Hormones

In lactating women, prolactin appears to be the single most important galactopoietic hormone, because selective inhibition of prolactin secretion by bromocriptine inhibits lactation.[53,54] Ovarian hormones are not required for the maintenance of established milk production and have little effect on established lacta-

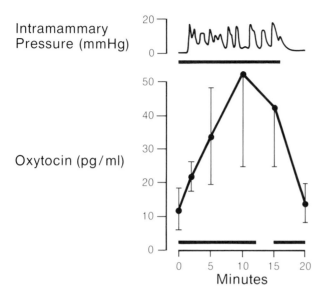

Intramammary Pressure (mmHg)

Oxytocin (pg/ml)

Minutes

Fig. 7.6 Milk ejection and plasma levels of oxytocin in women during breast-feeding. (Top) Recording of intramammary pressure from the contralateral breast during the nursing of the baby for 15 minutes (event bar). (Bottom) Plasma oxytocin levels (±SEM) in 12 women during breast-feeding (event bar) on days 3 to 5 postpartum. (Data from Dawood et al.[50] and Lincoln.[132])

tion. Glucocorticoids and metabolic hormones are necessary for continuous milk secretion but need not be present in concentrations higher than those in the nonpregnant state.

The Suckling Stimulus and Prolactin Release

Prolactin, the main lactogenic and galactopoietic hormone in women, is secreted in increasing amounts during pregnancy. During parturition, a further increase, probably stress related, is observed.[55] In pregnancy, high estradiol levels are responsible for the rise in plasma prolactin, as estrogens stimulate the synthesis and release of prolactin from the pituitary lactotrophs. After delivery of the placenta, plasma estrogens decline; as a consequence, plasma prolactin levels also decline in both lactating and nonlactating women (Fig. 7.8).

A stimulus other than estrogen is required for the maintenance of prolactin levels. Selye et al.[56] were the first to realize that suckling provides the stimulus that supports lactation. It has become clear that suckling by the young initiates both the milk ejection reflex and a reflex that releases prolactin (Fig. 7.9).

Prolactin release is controlled by hypothalamic do-

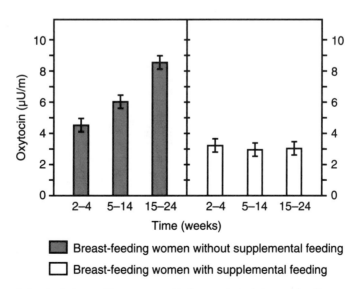

Time (weeks)

■ Breast-feeding women without supplemental feeding

□ Breast-feeding women with supplemental feeding

Fig. 7.7 Plasma oxytocin levels during suckling measured in four exclusively breast-feeding women (hatched columns) and in four women giving supplemental food (open columns) in early, middle, and late lactation. Values are mean ± SEM of averages for five measurements performed with 3-minute intervals at each suckling episode. (From Johnston et al.,[52] with permission.)

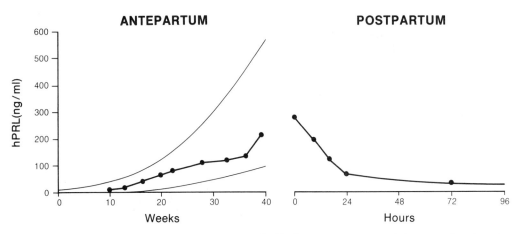

Fig. 7.8 Plasma levels of prolactin in women increase markedly during pregnancy and decrease sharply in the early puerperium. (Adapted from Tyson et al.,[55] with permission.)

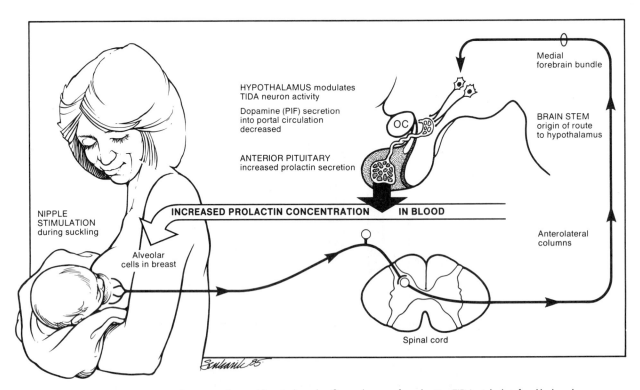

Fig. 7.9 Somatosensory pathways in the suckling-induced reflex release of prolactin. TIDA, tubuloinfundibular dopamine neuron activity; PIF, prolactin-inhibiting factor. (Adapted from Johnson and Everitt,[131] with permission.)

paminergic neurons, which maintain a tonic release of dopamine from the median eminence into the portal vessels flowing into the capillary plexus of the anterior lobe. Dopamine inhibits prolactin release, while suckling removes this inhibitory influence.[36] The effect of suckling is mediated by the dopaminergic neurons in the hypothalamus. Each suckling episode is associated with a rapid rise in plasma prolactin. Prolactin levels peak in 20 to 40 minutes and return to near baseline in about 3 to 4 hours (Fig. 7.10).[55,57,58] Frequent nursing is required to maintain the elevated prolactin levels on which continued milk secretion depends.

Frequent nursing is also necessary to maintain pituitary responsiveness to the nursing stimulus. Studies in animals have indicated that a significant decrease in the suckling-induced rise in plasma prolactin occurs if the nursing interval is prolonged to 16 to 24 hours. After delivery, a delay of 1 to 2 days in the initiation of nursing results in diminished responsiveness of the pituitary. To establish lactation, it is clearly important to put the baby to the breast as early as possible.

The practice still in use in some hospitals to wait 24 to 48 hours before putting the baby to the breast for the first time should be abandoned; it is deleterious, because it diminishes the responsiveness of the pituitary gland to the suckling stimulus to secrete prolactin. This is especially important for mothers who have been delivered by cesarean section and thus have not experienced the surges in prolactin and oxytocin associated with labor. The infant should be put to the breast as soon as possible. Fever after the cesarean section is not a contraindication, and the usual antibiotics given to the mother for infection are not a problem (see Ch. 11).

The proper application of a breast pump also provides adequate stimulus for both oxytocin and prolactin release. A breast pump is useful when a sick infant is hospitalized or a preterm infant is unable to suck.

The suckling-induced increment in plasma prolactin level is quite variable even in the same individual. Like basal prolactin levels, the suckling-induced increment undergoes diurnal variations, the greatest

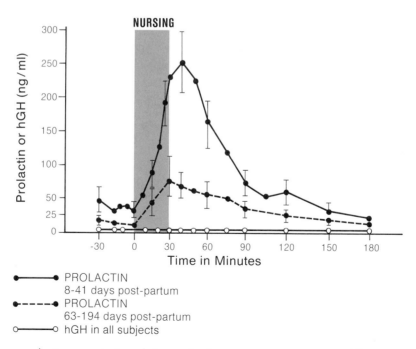

Fig. 7.10 Plasma prolactin concentrations during nursing in postpartum women at two different stages of lactation. Twelve studies were performed on eight women on days 8 to 41 of lactation and six studies on six women on days 63 to 194 of lactation. Plasma growth hormone concentrations are also shown for comparison in all subjects. (Adapted from Noel et al.,[57] with permission.)

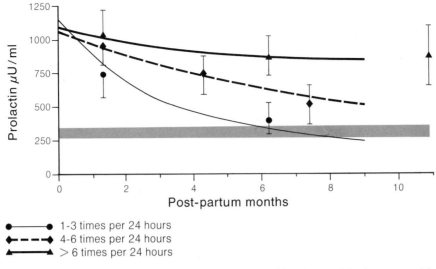

Fig. 7.11 Relationship of mean serum prolactin levels to the duration of lactation and the frequency of suckling (one to three, four to six, and over six times per 24 hours) in groups of African women. The shaded area represents the mean of the prolactin levels for a group of 25 nonlactating women. (From Delvoye et al.,[60] with permission.)

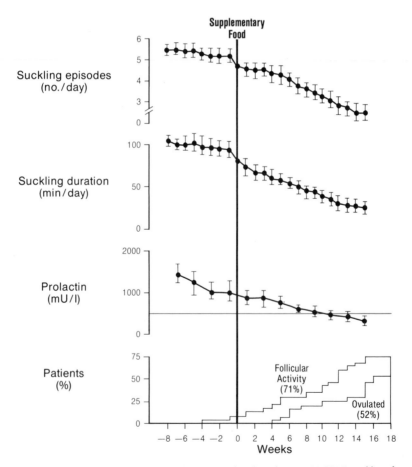

Fig. 7.12 Relationship between introduction of supplementary food and mean (±SEM) suckling frequency, suckling duration, serum prolactin level, and the percentage of women with ovarian activity and ovulation (N = 27). All results were standardized in relation to the time when supplementary feeding was introduced. (From Howie et al.,[61] with permission.)

increment occurring at nighttime and the smallest in the morning.[59] Nighttime feeding should therefore be maintained if problems with insufficient milk occur. The suckling-induced increment in plasma prolactin diminishes with advancing lactation (Fig. 7.10). This change may be due to the decline in nursing frequency that usually takes place in the course of lactation. To maintain elevated plasma prolactin levels for prolonged periods, the mother must nurse at least six times each day.[60,61] In African women, a positive correlation between nursing frequency and the plasma prolactin levels after 8 to 10 months of lactation was observed (Fig. 7.11). Provided that the nursing frequency in American mothers and !Kung mothers was the same, prolactin levels measured in both groups at 10 to 11 A.M. were the same up to 18 months postpartum, and amenorrhea lasted an equally long time.[62] Poor nutrition in lactating mothers is also associated with increased plasma prolactin levels and may contribute to the long periods of lactational amenorrhea observed in the rural areas of many developing countries (Fig. 7.12).

Nicotine diminishes the amount of prolactin released in response to the suckling stimulus.[63] This observation may explain the decreased milk yield in smoking mothers, who, according to several studies, lactate for a shorter time than comparable groups of nonsmoking mothers.

Other Neuroendocrine Responses to Suckling

Suckling elicits a variety of neuroendocrine responses in addition to the classic milk ejection reflex and prolactin release. These include the release of β-endorphin,[64] thyroid-stimulating hormone (TSH),[64] and cholecystokinin.[65] Inhibitory responses also occur, such as suppression of pulsatile luteinizing hormone (LH) release[66] and a selective inhibition of corticotropin-releasing factor (CRF) release in certain stressful situations.[67] In animals the suckling-induced neuroendocrine responses result in behavioral effects that, taken together, promote maternal and feeding behavior; they may have similar, subtle behavioral effects also in lactating women.

Reestablishing Lactation and Augmentation of Milk Yield

Reestablishment of lactation before the breast has undergone complete involution is possible after a period of abstinence from nursing. Frequent nursing or

application of a breast pump for several days is required to establish milk flow. The time needed for reestablishment is usually proportional to the duration of abstinence.

Drugs that stimulate prolactin release, including reserpine, metoclopramide, sulpiride, and thyrotropin-releasing hormone (TRH), have been used to help reestablish lactation. The drugs have also been employed to improve poor lactation, with variable results.[68–71]

Augmentation of poor milk yield is usually best achieved by increasing the nursing frequency, including nighttime nursing, and, in instances of poor sucking activity, by application of a breast pump after each nursing episode to ensure complete emptying of the breasts. Manual expression works as well but is more cumbersome. To relieve stress and anxiety, which inhibit the milk ejection reflex, gentle massage of the neck and shoulders by husband or friend is often helpful.

Involution

Involution of the mammary gland sets in rather abruptly in puerperal women who are not breastfeeding. In lactating women, involution is more gradual as weaning is usually extended over a period of time. The reason for involution is in part hormonal, as prolactin secretion ceases when suckling is terminated. However, mechanical and local factors play an important role in this process, as indicated by the observation that an unsuckled breast undergoes involution, although prolactin secretion is maintained if the other breast is nursed. The flattened alveolar cells cease their secretory activity, and within 24 hours changes in the cellular organelles can be discerned, followed by autophagic activity by lysosomes within the epithelial cells and infiltration of the tissue by leukocytes. The substantial engorgement that follows cessation of nursing also impedes blood flow, further stimulating the necrotic and autophagic changes. The reduction of glandular elements is followed by formation of connective tissue and deposition of adipose tissue, which are completed in about 3 months. After cessation of lactation, the breast usually assumes its prepregnant size, although the glandular tissue does not regress completely,[15] and persistent alteration in the sensitivity of the mammary tissue to hormonal stimulation has been observed.[72] This may be one explanation for why high parity and

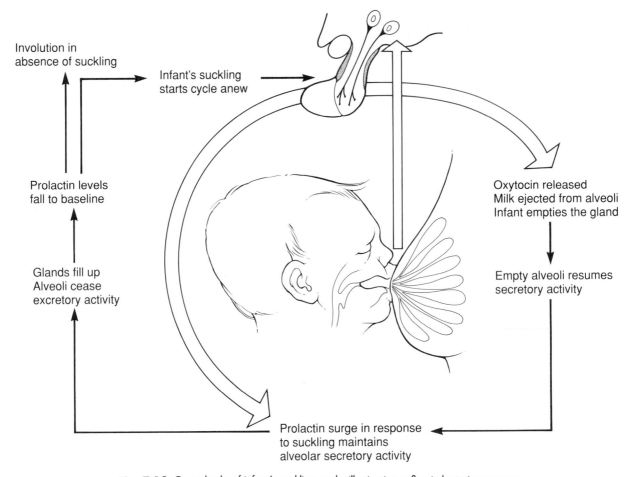

Involution in
absence of suckling

Infant's suckling
starts cycle anew

Prolactin levels
fall to baseline

Glands fill up
Alveoli cease
excretory activity

Oxytocin released
Milk ejected from alveoli
Infant empties the gland

Empty alveoli resumes
secretory activity

Prolactin surge in response
to suckling maintains
alveolar secretory activity

Fig. 7.13 Central role of infant's suckling and milk ejection reflex in lactation success.

birth of the first child at a young age[73] reduce the risk of subsequent cancer of the breast. Lactation and breast-feeding, on the other hand, are not strongly related either positively or negatively to the risk of breast cancer.[74]

Mammogenic and Lactogenic Hormones During Pregnancy and Early Puerperium

A review of the hormonal changes following conception indicates that the levels of all the mammogenic as well as the lactogenic hormones rise during gestation.[75] Signals from the conceptus direct the endocrine changes, leading to mammary gland development, thus assuring the newborn a ready source of nutrition at birth.

At parturition, both mammogenic and lactogenic hormones are near maximal levels. A further rise in plasma prolactin and cortisol levels is associated with the process of labor itself. After parturition and the delivery of the placenta, plasma estrogen and progesterone fall to low levels within a few days, permitting the expression of the lactogenic potential of prolactin, which is strongly suppressed by estrogen and progesterone. Pituitary production of prolactin declines rapidly as a consequence of the abrupt fall in circulating estrogens. Normal nonpregnant levels are reached in 1 to 2 weeks if the mother does not breast-feed.

Because mammary development is almost completed during the second trimester, lactogenesis also

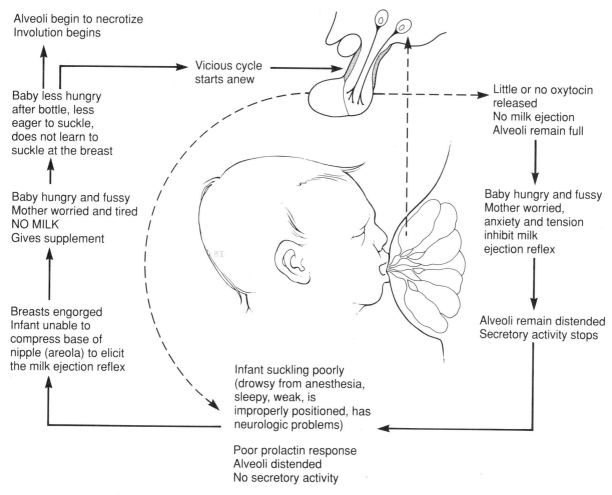

Alveoli begin to necrotize
Involution begins

Vicious cycle
starts anew

Baby less hungry
after bottle, less
eager to suckle,
does not learn to
suckle at the breast

Baby hungry and fussy
Mother worried and tired
NO MILK
Gives supplement

Breasts engorged
Infant unable to
compress base of
nipple (areola) to elicit
the milk ejection reflex

Little or no oxytocin
released
No milk ejection
Alveoli remain full

Baby hungry and fussy
Mother worried,
anxiety and tension
inhibit milk
ejection reflex

Alveoli remain distended
Secretory activity stops

Infant suckling poorly
(drowsy from anesthesia,
sleepy, weak, is
improperly positioned, has
neurologic problems)

Poor prolactin response
Alveoli distended
No secretory activity

Fig. 7.14 Central role of poor suckling and failure to elicit milk ejection reflex in lactation failure. To break the vicious cycle (1) assure mother that she will have enough milk; (2) instruct proper positioning of baby so correct suckling is possible; (3) instruct mother in perioral stimulation of sleepy or lethargic infant; (4) instruct mother to express some milk manually if breast is very engorged so that infant can apply pressure on areola while suckling; (5) instruct mother to nurse frequently, including nighttime (prolactin surge greatest at night) if infant is poor feeder; (6) if all else fails, advise mother to use oxytocin nasal spray at each feeding; (7) if mother suffers fatigue, instruct other members of the family to help with chores.

occurs in mothers who deliver preterm infants. The relative immaturity of the mammary epithelium is reflected in a somewhat different composition of the mother's milk in comparison to milk produced after a term delivery. The composition of preterm milk, discussed in greater detail later, corresponds to the somewhat different requirements for nutrients in preterm infants. Oxytocin has been found to enhance the onset of lactation in mothers delivering preterm.

The Inhibitory Effect of Sex Steroids on Lactogenesis

The mechanism of the inhibitory effect of estrogen on lactogenesis has not yet been clarified. Large doses of estrogen have been found to decrease the amount of prolactin incorporated into the alveolar epithelial cells and to prevent the rise in prolactin receptors that normally occurs in the course of lactation.[76-78]

The inhibitory effect of progesterone is more

clearcut. It inhibits the induction of α-lactalbumin synthesis by prolactin and consequently the synthesis and secretion of milk sugar.[78-81] Administration of prolactin cannot overcome this inhibitory effect. The withdrawal of progesterone is therefore a critical step in lactogenesis. During lactation, progesterone receptors disappear from the mammary gland.[82] It is therefore not surprising that progesterone has no inhibitory effect in established lactation[79] (Figs. 7.13 and 7.14).

ENDOCRINE CONSEQUENCES OF LACTATION

Postpartum Amenorrhea and Return of Ovulation

Postpartum amenorrhea is more prolonged and first ovulation occurs later in lactating women than in those who do not breast-feed. Lactational amenorrhea is one of the principal methods of birth spacing in much of the developing world. Pregnancy rates during lactational amenorrhea vary somewhat in different countries but are always much lower than in nonlactating women and in lactating women in whom menstruation has resumed. The contraceptive protection offered by lactational amenorrhea is comparable to the effectiveness of oral contraceptives or barrier methods.[83]

In nonlactating women ovulation usually occurs 7 to 10 weeks postpartum.[84,85] In lactating women, the anovulatory interval is quite variable and depends on the frequency of nursing episodes each day as well as on the nutritional status of the nursing woman. Those women with very poor nutrition resume ovulatory function much later than do well-nourished mothers. Ovulation precedes the first menstruation in more than one-half of lactating mothers, as judged by monthly endometrial biopsies, vaginal cytology, cervical mucus, and basal body temperature.[84] With advancing lactation, anovulatory bleeding before the first ovulation becomes more prevalent. Plasma progesterone levels measured in a group of lactating women suggested that the first ovulation was followed with an inadequate luteal phase, not considered compatible with fecundity, in about 40 percent of the women.[86] In nonlactating women the first ovulation postpartum was associated with inadequate luteal phase in about 75 percent of the women.[87]

Is it safe for a lactating woman to wait for the first menstruation before beginning contraception? Studies in populations not using any contraception indicate that a significant number of women will become pregnant before the first menstruation, the percentages varying from 1.5 to 13 percent in different countries.[83] Women in the United States have the highest conception rates, 10 to 13 percent.[83] These data indicate that the first ovulation is associated with high fecundity and that it is advisable to begin contraception before resumption of menstruation.

Hormonal Basis for Lactational Amenorrhea

Several factors contribute to lactational amenorrhea: hypothalamic hypofunction, pituitary unresponsiveness, and ovarian refractoriness to gonadotropin stimulation. These changes are related to both gestation and lactation.

In all women, both nursing and nonnursing, the pituitary response to gonadotropin-releasing hormone is suppressed during the early puerperium, returning gradually to normal levels over 6 weeks.[88,89] The positive feedback effect of estrogen on pituitary function is also suppressed. It returns to normal several weeks earlier in nonnursing than in nursing mothers.[90]

Considerable evidence supports the view that high plasma prolactin concentrations are responsible for ovarian hypoactivity in lactating women.[91,92] Estrogen levels remain low, in spite of normal follicle-stimulating hormone (FSH) levels, as long as plasma prolactin levels are elevated over the normal nonpregnant range (Fig. 7.15).[93] At weaning, or when the frequency of nursing falls below a critical value, plasma prolactin levels return to the normal range. Plasma estrogen levels then rise. A preovulatory surge of estrogen usually occurs within 10 to 14 days, followed by an ovulatory surge of LH (Fig. 7.16).[93,94] When postpartum lactation is inhibited by bromocriptine, a dopaminergic drug that selectively inhibits prolactin release, plasma prolactin levels return to baseline values within a few days, sooner than in nonlactating women who have used other methods of lactation suppression (Fig. 7.15).[95] Ovarian responsiveness to FSH is immediately restored in such women, and the first ovulation after delivery occurs within 3 to 4 weeks.

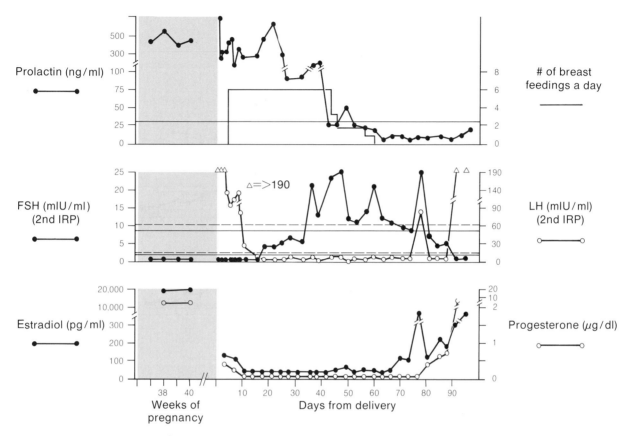

Fig. 7.15 The basal level of prolactin (top) remained raised over the nonpregnant range (indicated by the horizontal line in this and the middle panel) as long as suckling frequency was six per 24 hours but dropped to nonpregnant levels when suckling frequency decreased to two or less. The concentration of FSH returned to normal range within 3 weeks of delivery, while the concentration of LH remained low (middle). Estrogen levels were low (bottom) in spite of normal and even above-normal FSH levels but started to rise when prolactin levels fell to the normal nonpregnant range, and within 3 weeks a surge of estrogen was observed that initiated an ovulatory surge of LH. (From Rolland et al.,[95] with permission.)

Effects of Lactation on Calcium Homeostasis

Low levels of circulating estrogens are characteristic for all lactating women. Concerns have therefore been voiced that lactation may cause osteoporosis, because it also imposes an increased demand for calcium utilization. In the rat, the rate of calcium transfer into the milk exceeds the intestinal capacity to absorb calcium, and extensive demineralization of the skeleton occurs during lactation in this species. In women on a normal vitamin D–replete diet, increased intestinal absorption can meet the demands for calcium transfer into the milk, and little change takes place in the skeleton during pregnancy and lactation.[96–99]

Increased production of 1,25-dihydroxyvitamin D forms a major part of this adjustment. The plasma levels of this metabolite are increased during gestation, but are the same in lactating and nonlactating women six weeks postpartum in spite of about two- to threefold higher intake of vitamin D by the lactating women.[99a] The levels of the inactive metabolite 24,25-dihydroxyvitamin D were lower in lactating women, and urinary excretion of vitamin D and its metabolites is the same. A substantial portion of the maternal vitamin D must therefore be transferred into the milk, and a significant correlation between the vitamin D compounds in maternal plasma and milk has been found.[99b] The parathyroid status of

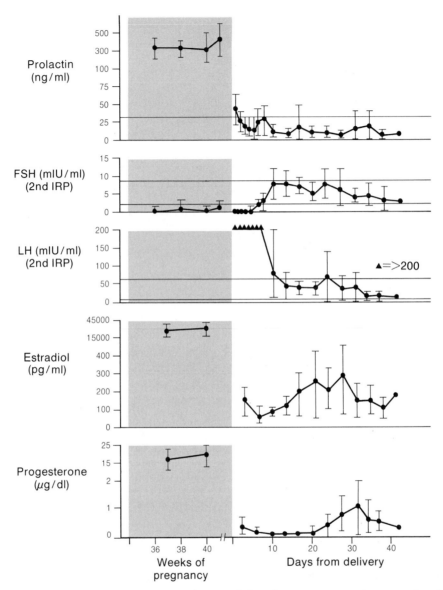

Fig. 7.16 Mean concentrations of prolactin, FSH, LH, estradiol, and progesterone in the puerperium during bromocriptine treatment in nine women. Horizontal lines indicate normal range in menstruating women. During treatment with bromocriptine plasma prolactin dropped immediately to nonpregnant levels, and the concentrations of FSH returned to normal range within 2 weeks. The ovaries responded immediately to the rise in FSH by an increase in estrogen production and subsequent ovulation. The low progesterone levels in these nine women suggest the formation of an inadequate corpus luteum. (From Rolland et al.,[93] with permission.)

lactating women appears to be normal judging from plasma levels of immunoreactive PTH.[99a] The calcitonin status of puerperal women during lactation is still poorly understood; both increased and normal immunoreactive human calcitonin plasma levels have been observed in lactating women whereas in rats a definite increase in calcitonin plasma levels occurs during lactation.[99a] Teenage mothers are at risk for bone demineralization because of their own increased need for calcium and because they often have low dietary intakes of calcium and phosphorus.[100] Women with osteoporosis from pre-existing disease

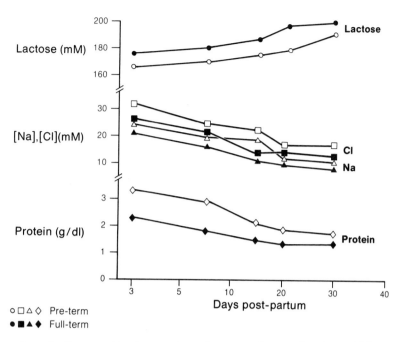

Fig. 7.17 Comparison of milk composition from mothers of preterm infants and mothers of full-term infants in the early puerperium. (Data from Gross et al.,[133] adapted by Neville et al.,[21] with permission.)

may also be at risk of bone mineral loss during lactation.[100a]

THE COMPOSITION OF HUMAN MILK

Colostrum and Mature Milk

During pregnancy a secretion called precolostrum is present in the alveolar lumina. It consists of cellular material and exudates of plasma, with a high concentration of immunoglobulins, lactoferrin, serum albumin, and sodium and chloride ions, but very low levels of lactose.

After birth, this material, colostrum, is secreted at a rate of about 40 ml/day for 3 to 4 days. The sudden increase in alveolar epithelial secretion following parturition results in a rapid increase in lactose, milk proteins, and the total volume of milk. The composition of breast milk therefore gradually changes during the first 1 to 2 weeks until mature milk is secreted. Average values for the major components in colostrum and in mature milk are given in Table 7.1.

The composition of human milk varies at different stages of lactation, at different times of day, during each feed, and even between the breasts. It is therefore difficult to obtain true values for the composition of human milk. (All these variations must be kept in mind in consulting such data as presented in Table 7.2.) The variations in fat content are most marked. Fat concentration rises steadily from the beginning to the end of each feed,[101] and diurnal variations are considerable, with the lowest concentrations around 6 A.M. and the highest around 10 A.M. These differences can be as great as 15 to 30 g/L. The fat content

Table 7.1 The Concentration of the Major Milk Constituents in Colostrum and Mature Milk

Constituent (per dl)	Colostrum	Mature Milk
Total energy (kcal)	54	70
Milk sugar, lactose (g)	5.7	7.1
Fats (g)	2.9	4.5
Proteins (g)	2.3	0.86
Nonprotein nitrogen (g)	—	0.32
Minerals (ash) (mg)	30.8	20.2
Cells (macrophages, neutrophils, lymphocytes)	$7-8 \times 10^6$	$1-2 \times 10^6$

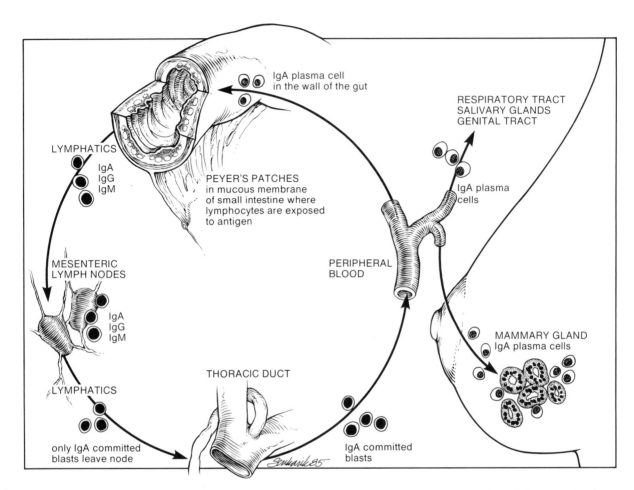

Fig. 7.18 The secretory immune system. Precursor B lymphocytes are exposed to antigens through the specialized epithelium of the Peyer's patches in the lumen of the gut. They are stimulated to divide and migrate into the mesenteric lymph nodes, where they again divide and differentiate into blasts. The IgA-committed lymphoblasts enter the bloodstream via the thoracic duct, where further differentiation takes place in contact with T cells. They "home" to sites of secretory antibody production in the gut, in the respiratory tract, and in the late-pregnancy or lactating mammary gland, where they mature into plasma cells that secrete antibody (IgA). Some of these cells and many macrophages migrate transepithelially into the alveolar lumen. (Adapted from Roux et al.,[116] with permission.)

of human milk increases with advancing lactation, at least up to 84 days postpartum, providing for the increasing caloric requirements of the growing infant. Intake of fat does influence the composition of milk fat, as up to 30 percent of fatty acids in milk can originate in dietary fat.

The stage of lactation influences the protein and carbohydrate contents as well as mineral composition. Initially, protein and salt concentrations are high, but their levels decline 10 to 25 percent during the first week as the secretion of milk is established and then decrease more slowly with advancing lacta-

tion (Fig. 7.17). The influence of dietary protein on the protein content of milk appears to be limited. Intake of protein influences the total amount of milk produced rather than the protein content of milk. The concentration of lactose increases rapidly during the first week and then more slowly, from a mean of 57 to 70 g/L at the end of the first month and to 79 g/L at the end of 6 months.

Preterm Milk

In women who deliver preterm infants, the protein and nonprotein nitrogen concentrations of milk are higher and the lactose concentration lower than in those women who deliver at term. This difference persists for 3 to 5 weeks (Fig. 7.18).[102–104] Because the protein requirement of the preterm infant is higher than that of a term infant, its mother's milk is superior to pooled human milk.[105]

Preterm milk contains higher concentrations of essential long chain fatty acids and polyunsaturated fatty acids than does term milk. The quantities are sufficient to maintain brain growth in preterm infants.[106]

Preterm milk and mature milk contain a high concentration of nonprotein nitrogen, including all essential amino acids. Preterm milk also contains taurine, glycine, leucine, and cysteine, which are considered essential for the preterm infant.

On the other hand, the calcium and phosphorus requirements of the preterm infant, whose relative growth rate is higher than that of the full-term infant, are not always met with human milk. Rickets may develop in small infants despite addition of vitamin D. Supplementation of breast milk with calcium, phosphorus, and protein is therefore recommended for very-low-birth-weight infants. Calcium and phosphorus supplementation is necessary even after the very-low-birth-weight infant is discharged home.[107]

Differences Between Human and Cow's Milk

Although the major constituents are the same in human milk and cow's milk, several significant differences do exist both quantitatively and qualitatively (Table 7.2). In human milk, the caloric content is derived mainly from fats and carbohydrates, up to 95 to 99 percent of which is absorbed in the gut. In cow's milk and formulas, a greater proportion of calories is supplied by proteins that are less easily digested and may cause metabolic and amino acid imbalances. In human milk, 25 to 34 percent of nitrogen is present as nonprotein nitrogen, which provides an immediate source of all essential amino acids, including taurine, a sulfonated amino acid essential for brain development. A large proportion (75 percent) of the proteins in human milk are present as easily digested whey proteins, in contrast to cow's milk, in which casein is the main protein (80 percent). Moreover, the principal whey protein in cow's milk is β-lactoglobulin, a potent allergen. The high casein and butterfat concentrations in cow's milk and many formulas leads to the formation of insoluble curds in the infant's gut.

Table 7.2 Composition of Mature Human Milk and Cow's Milk

Constituent (per dl)	Mature Milk[a] (30 days)	Cow's Milk[b]
Energy (kcal)	70	69
Total solids (g)	12.0	12.7
Lactose (g)	7.3	4.8
Total nitrogen (mg)	171	550
Protein nitrogen (mg)	129	512
Nonprotein nitrogen (mg)	42	32
Total protein (g)	0.9	3.3
Casein (g)	0.4	2.8
Whey protein[c] (g)	0.5	0.19
Lactalbumin (mg)	161	0.6
Lactoferrin (mg)	167	
IgA (mg)	142	
Total fat (g)	4.2	3.7
Unsaturated long-chain fatty acids (g)	2.9	1.0
Calcium (mg)	28	125
Phosphorus (mg)	15	96
Iron (ng)	40	100

[a] Data from Casey and Hambridge.[128]
[b] Data from National Research Council.[129]
[c] Whey protein includes β-lactoglobulin in cow's milk not present in human milk.

The curds bind calcium and inhibit its absorption. The high phosphorous:calcium ratio in cow's milk further decreases calcium absorption.

A much larger proportion of the fatty acids in human milk are unsaturated. Of the unsaturated fats, almost one-third are long-chain polyunsaturated fatty acids, while they make up only one-sixth in cow's milk. Human milk also has a higher cholesterol content, which, together with polyunsaturated fatty acids, is needed for brain development.

In general, the bioavailability of all constituents in human milk is remarkably high and is superior to cow's milk or formulas. Even iron, present in concentrations 20 times lower in human milk than in formulas, is accumulated during the first months of life at the same rate as in formula-fed infants. A smaller volume of breast milk with a smaller caloric content will satisfy the requirements of an infant compared with the larger volume of formula needed.[4] Therefore, formula-fed infants often accumulate more body fat than do breast-fed infants. In addition, the last milk expressed at the end of nursing contains significantly more fat than does early milk.[101] This higher fat concentration may give the infant a sense of satiety, perhaps because fats stimulate the release of cholecystokinin, which in turn acts on the hypothalamic satiety center. Breast-feeding alone can meet the nutritional requirements of the infant for periods from 2 to 15 months, depending on individual variations in milk yield.

Human milk contains significant amounts of epidermal growth factor throughout lactation, whereas cow's milk contains growth factors in the colostral stage only, and cow's milk growth factors are different from those in human milk.[108] Human milk also contains trace elements, vitamins, and enzymes not present in cow's milk.

IMMUNOLOGIC ASPECTS OF BREAST-FEEDING

Immunologic Significance of Colostrum and Milk

The mammary gland forms a part of an immune system that is specifically adapted to provide the immunologically and developmentally immature newborn protection against gastrointestinal and respiratory tract infections.[24,109,110] Experimental and clinical evidence supports a role for immunologic and maturational factors in colostrum that prevent atopic disease as well.[1]

The immunologic significance of colostrum and milk is most obvious in farm animals, the offspring of which invariably succumbs to infection unless fed colostrum and milk. In these animals, the placenta is impermeable to all immunoglobulins during pregnancy. The human infant is less dependent on breast-feeding than are farm animals, because the human placenta does permit transfer of blood-borne antibodies of the IgG class from mother to fetus. Thus the human infant at birth has acquired passive immunity against bacteria and their toxins, reflecting the accumulated experience of the mother. However, the predominant immunoglobulin present in mucosal secretions, secretory IgA, is not transmitted to the fetus in utero. Because the newborn infant is essentially agammaglobulinemic at its mucosal surfaces, the protection provided by the secretory IgA-rich colostrum and milk is of great importance for the establishment of an immune defense against microbial challenges. The mucosal epithelium of the newborn produces

secretory component and is therefore capable of binding both IgA and IgM present in colostrum and milk.[111,112] The secretory IgA forms a protective coating that prevents the passage of infectious microorganisms into the systemic circulation.

Mucosal membranes of newborn infants and preterm infants in particular are permeable to antigens and microorganisms, facilitating access of intestinal antigens, particularly food allergens, into the systemic circulation to evoke a systemic or atopic response. Binding of IgA antibodies to the mucosal surfaces prevents passage of such antigens through the epithelium. Colostrum contains additional factors that facilitate the maturation of the intestinal barrier in newborn infants.[113] Feeding colostrum to preterm infants greatly diminishes infection rates and may protect against necrotizing enterocolitis.[4] The phospholipids in human milk protect the gastric mucosa, as does prostaglandin E_2 (PGE_2) present in human milk. Moreover, human milk contains factors that stimulate the synthesis of PGE_2 in the gastric mucosa.

Immunologically Active Constituents in Human Milk and Colostrum

Human milk contains a number of immunologically active factors, as shown in Table 7.3. They include both soluble antigens and immunocompetent cells, as well as mediators of the immune response.[24–26,109,114] In addition, a host of nonspecific factors are present that singly or together have considerable antibacterial and antiviral activity and promote the growth of beneficial gastrointestinal flora.[110] The bifidus factor, together with the low buffering capacity of human milk, which results in an intestinal pH of 4 to 6, favor the growth of *Lactobacillus bifidus* and suppress the growth of pathogens. The predominant flora of breast-fed infants consists of *L. bifidus*, whereas that of bottle-fed infants consists of *Streptococcus faecalis, Escherichia coli,* and bacteroides.

Studies with farm animals suggest that antibody is the most critical factor in colostrum and milk and that nonspecific factors can only function to augment its specific protective value.[115]

The cells found in the mammary gland and its secretions are not a random collection of maternal leukocytes but represent a selected subpopulation of those cells that migrate from the gut-associated (GALT) and bronchus-associated (BALT) lymphoid

Table 7.3 Immunologically Active Constituents and Resistance Factors in Human Milk and Colostrum

Soluble	Cellular	Other
Immunoglobulins (sIgA, IgA, IgG, IgM, IgE)	Monocytes	Bacterial antigens
Free secretory component	Macrophages	Hepatitis antigen
Immunosecretory mediators (complement, chemotactic factors)	Neutrophils	Rubella virus
Nonspecific factors (lactoferrin, lysozyme, lactoperoxidase, lipids bifidus-factor)	Lymphocytes (B cells, plasma cells, T cells)	Cytomegalovirus
		Other viruses

tissues to other mucosa, where they secrete antibody independent of local antigen contact. They reflect the immunologic response of the mother to pathogens in her environment and, consequently, to that of her newborn infant's (Fig. 7.18).[116]

Most of the cells in milk, approximately 70 to 80 percent, are monocytic phagocytes that differentiate into macrophages during their transepithelial passage. About 15 to 20 percent are neutrophils, and about 10 percent are lymphocytes, including both B cells and T lymphocytes. Highly differentiated inflammatory cells such as polymorphs, basophils, mast cells, atypical mast cells, and eosinophils are largely lacking. The total number of leukocytes in milk is about 1 to 2 million cells/ml during the first days of lactation. Their concentration decreases thereafter, but, because of the increasing volume of milk, their total number remains essentially the same.[19,111] In general, human milk protects against intestinal and respiratory tract pathogens without causing inflammation.

Occasionally, bacteria and viruses (e.g., rubella, cytomegalovirus, hepatitis B, and human immunodeficiency virus [HIV]) are found in the milk of infected subjects; however, neonatal infection with these viruses has not been demonstrated. The breast-fed infant can apparently handle this route of infection even in the case of HIV. Johnson[117] monitored 80 HIV-positive mothers in Haiti and found no instances of viral transmission through breast-feeding.

Maternal Diet and Breast-Feeding

Energy Intake

Today many women are very concerned about diet and weight gain and are afraid that they must "eat for two" while breast-feeding. The recommended energy allowance for lactation, 2,750 kcal/day for a 55 kg

woman (Joint FAO/WHO Group Report, Rome, 1972) may be too high for a sedentary urban population. During pregnancy the maternal organism stores 2 to 4 kg of fat, which is mobilized during lactation, and this must be taken into account when calculating dietary allowances. About 50 percent of the fatty acids in milk originate in tissue stores in well-nourished women; women with little body fat must increase their energy intake correspondingly. A diet consisting on the average of $2{,}350 \pm 250$ kcal/day for a 60 kg woman has been found to provide adequate energy intake while allowing for a gradual reduction in weight to prepregnancy levels.[118,119] A wide variety of personal preferences can be accommodated in a balanced diet. Women on certain extreme vegetarian diets need counseling, however, to avoid the development of deficiency syndromes in their breast-fed infants.

Colic

Maternal diet has long been thought to be associated with the occurrence of infantile colic in breast-fed infants. A double-blind, placebo-controlled trial showed that the elimination of cow's milk from maternal diet had no beneficial effect. However, rates of colic were significantly more frequent on days when the mother ate certain foods (e.g., chocolate, fruits). The rates of colic also increased in proportion to the diversity of foods in the maternal diet, showing that colic cannot be attributed to a single diet component.[120]

Atopic Disease

The possible influence of maternal diet on the incidence of atopic disease has been the focus of considerable attention, but remains poorly understood. Breast-feeding exclusively for the first 6 months provides considerable protection,[1] probably because the intake of foreign allergens is minimized. Allergens from the maternal diet may also gain access to the infant through the mother's milk. In a recent controlled study the presence or absence of two strong allergens, cow's milk and eggs, in maternal diet during the last 3 months of pregnancy and lactation had no significant effect on the development of atopic disease in the infant up to age 18 months.[121] Genetic factors probably have a greater effect than maternal diet during the perinatal period. It seems prudent, however, to avoid allergens known to affect other family members in a family with a strong history of atopic disease.

Breast-Feeding and Diabetes

Diabetic mothers are able to breast-feed and often have reduced insulin requirements during lactation, because the uptake of glucose by the mammary gland is considerable. A group of breast-feeding, insulin-dependent diabetic mothers had at 6 weeks postpartum significantly lower fasting glucose levels (4.6 ± 2.2 mM/L) than did those who had stopped nursing (8.1 ± 2.2 mM/L) or those who bottle-fed (6.7 ± 1.7 mM/L).[122] Diabetic mothers are more prone than are nondiabetic mothers to develop mastitis. They are also more likely to have yeast infections that are transmitted to the infants, and they should be warned and advised about these conditions. Maternal medical complications and contraindications to breast-feeding are discussed in Chapter 22.

CONTRACEPTION DURING LACTATION

Breast-feeding is associated with an extended period of postpartum anovulation, but return of ovulatory function is quite variable in individual women and frequently occurs while they are still nursing. As the first ovulation often occurs before the first menstruation, lactating women who do not wish to become pregnant and who are breast-feeding less than six times daily should be advised to initiate contraception during lactation.[123] Because the introduction of any

supplementary feeding is usually associated with decreased suckling frequency and resumption of ovarian activity, it is recommended that contraception be initiated at this time.[61]

Oral Contraceptives

There is no consensus regarding the safety of contraceptive steroids when given to lactating women.[123,124] Perinatal exposure to estrogens, including those used in most combination pills, may have deleterious effects, short and long term, on the offspring of pregnant or lactating animals. The side effects of diethylstilbestrol on the reproductive organs of female as well as male offspring of mothers given large doses during pregnancy have been clearly documented. Estrogen-containing oral contraceptives may be used because very little steroid appears in the breast milk, but there is at least theoretical concern. Low-dose pills do not appear to inhibit established lactation (see Ch. 22).

Progestational steroids appear to be safer, although their long-term effects are as yet unknown. Progestational steroids are transferred to milk, and measurable quantities have been found in the blood of nursing infants. Concentrations are low and perhaps without physiologic significance, especially with the use of the minipill norgestrel (30 μg/day). Nilsson and Nygren[125] calculated that a fully breast-fed infant would receive approximately 1 μg/month. The low-dose progestins are effective contraceptives in lactating women, who are partially protected by the physiologic effects of lactation. The composition or amount of milk does not appear to be affected in women taking these minipills.[124]

Estrogen-containing contraceptives are more often implicated in suppression of lactation than are progestagen-only preparations. Higher doses of progestational contraceptives have been variously reported to decrease milk yield, have no effect, or increase milk yield or duration of lactation. Few studies have been performed on the effects of steroids on the composition of milk. Several investigations indicate that the total amounts of protein and fat may decrease over a longer period of treatment with various progestagens.[124]

Intrauterine Devices

The use of inert or copper intrauterine devices (IUDs) has no effect on lactation.[123] The influence of progesterone-containing IUDs has not been established. The higher rate of expulsion of IUDs after immediate postpartum insertion is unacceptably high, 20 to 30 percent, with most devices. Delaying the insertion 6 to 8 weeks postpartum dramatically reduces expulsion rates. However, an increased risk of perforation has been reported when an IUD is placed in a lactating woman.[126]

SUPPRESSION OF LACTATION

In the past, women who did not wish to breast-feed, who had a stillborn child, or who suffered from a serious medical complication were given estrogens to suppress lactation. This practice has been discontinued due to concerns about lack of efficacy and potential thromboembolic risk (see Ch. 22).

More recently bromocriptine has been used to suppress lactation. It is a dopaminergic agonist that inhibits the release of prolactin and therefore prevents the secretion of milk.[53] Side effects of this medication include nausea, vomiting, and occasionally hypotension and dizziness. There are no effects on coagulation.[127] Bromocriptine has been reported to be effective in suppressing postpartum lactation, although rebound lactation can occur when the drug is stopped. Most authorities feel that bromocriptine should not be used routinely for lactation suppression, as conservative measures suffice. The absence of suckling stimuli and failure to empty the breast will lead to cessation of lactation in approximately 1 week without the use of medication. However, about 10 percent of women will suffer from painful breast engorgement and milk leakage. Support of the breasts, application of ice packs, and use of analgesics will relieve the condition in 1 to 2 days (see Ch. 22).

REFERENCES

1. Saarinen U, Kajosaari M, Backman A et al: Prolonged breast feeding as a prophylaxis for atopic disease. Lancet 2:163, 1979

2. Appleton JA, McGregor DO: Rapid expulsion of *Trichinella spiralis* in suckling rats. Science 226:70, 1984

3. Crawford MA, Hassam AG, Stevens PA: Essential fatty acid requirements in pregnancy and lactation with special reference to brain development. Prog Lipid Res 20:31, 1981

4. Jelliffe DB, Jelliffe EFP: The uniqueness of human milk. Am J Clin Nutr 24:967, 1977

5. Butte NF, Garza C, O'Brian Smith E, Nichols BL: Human milk intake and growth in exclusively breastfed infants. J Pediatr 104:187, 1984

6. Chandra RK: Long term health consequences of early infant feeding. p. 47. In Atkinson SA, Hanson IA, Chandra RK (eds): Breast Feeding, Nutrition, Infection and Infant Growth in Developed and Emerging Countries. ARTS Biomedical, St. John's, Newfoundland, 1990

7. Bernard-Bonnin A-C, Statchenko S, Girard G: Hospital practices and breast-feeding duration: a meta-analysis of controlled trials. Birth 16:64, 1989

8. Winikoff B, Laukaran VA, Myers D, Stone R: Dynamics of infant feeding: mothers, professionals and the institutional context in a large urban hospital. Pediatrics 77:35, 1986

9. Robinson J, Short R: Changes in breast sensitivity at puberty, during the menstrual cycle, and at parturition. Br Med J 1:1188, 1977

10. Cowie AT, Tindal JS: The Physiology of Lactation. Monographs of the Physiological Society. Edward Arnold, London, 1972

11. Stirling JW, Chandler JA: The fine structure of normal resting terminal ductal lobular unit of the female breast. Virchows Arch Pathol Anat 372:205, 1976

12. Ferguson DJP, Anderson TJ: A morphological study of the changes which occur during pregnancy in the human breast. Virchows Arch Pathol Anat 401:163, 1983

13. Bargmann W, Knoop A: Uber die Morphologie der Milch-Secretion. I. Licht-und Elektronen Mikroskopische Studien an der Milchdruse der Ratte. Z Zellforsch Mikrosk Anat 49:344, 1959

14. Ferguson DJP, Anderson TJ: An ultrastructural study of lactation in the human breast. Anat Embryol 138:349, 1983

15. Helminen HJ, Ericsson JLE: Studies on mammary gland involution. I–III. J Ultrastruct Res 25:193, 214, 228, 1968

16. Tobon H, Salazar H: Ultrastructure of the human mammary gland II. Postpartum lactogenesis. J Clin Endocrinol Metab 40:334, 1975

17. Bargmann W, Fleischhauer K, Knoop A: Uber die

Morphologie der Milchdruse. II. Zugleich eine Kritik am Schema der Sekretions Mechanismus. Z Zellforsch Mikrosk Anat 53:545, 1961

18. Keenan TW, Huang CM, Moore DJ: Lactose synthesis by a Golgi apparatus fraction from rat mammary gland. Nature 228:105, 1970

19. Smith CW, Goldman AS: The cells of human colostrum: in vitro studies of morphology and functions. Pediatr Res 2:103, 1968

20. Smith JJ, Nickerson SC, Keenan TW: Metabolic energy and cytoskeletal requirements for synthesis and secretion by acini for rat mammary glands. Int J Biochem 14:87, 1982

21. Neville MC, Allen JC, Walters C: The mechanisms of milk secretion. In Neville MC, Neifert MR (eds): Lactation: Physiology, Nutrition, and Breast-Feeding. Plenum, New York, 1983

22. Brandtzaeg P: Structure, synthesis and external transfer of mucosa immunoglobulins. Ann Immunol (Paris) 124:C417, 1973

23. Lamm ME: Cellular aspects of immunoglobin A. Adv Immunol 22:223, 1976

24. Hanson LA, Winberg J: Breast milk and defense against infection in the newborn. Arch Dis Child 47:845, 1982

25. Goldman AS, Garza A, Nichols BL, Goldblum RM: Immunologic factors present in human milk during the first year of lactation. J Pediatr 100:563, 1982

26. Ogra SS, Orga PL: Immunological aspects of human colostrum and milk. I. Distribution characteristics and concentrations of immunoglobins. J Pediatr 92:546, 1978

27. Pitelka DR: Cell contacts in the mammary gland. p. 14. In Larson BL, Smith VR (eds): Lactation: A Comprehensive Treatise. Vol. IV. Academic, San Diego, 1978

28. Tobon H, Salazar H: Ultrastructure of the human mammary gland. I. Development of the fetal gland throughout gestation. J Clin Endocrinol Metab 39:443, 1974

29. Raynaud A: Morphogenesis of the mammary gland. p. 3. In Falconer IR (ed): Lactation. University of Pennsylvania Press, Philadelphia, 1971

30. Milligan D, Drife JO, Short RV: Changes in breast volume during normal menstrual cycle and after oral contraceptives. Br Med J 4:494, 1975

31. Dabelow A: Die Milchdruse. p. 277. In Bargmann W (ed): Handbuch der Mikros-kopischen Anatomie des Menschen. Vol. III, Part 3. Springer-Verlag, Berlin, 1957

32. Weisz-Carrington P, Roux ME, Lamm ME: Plasma cells and epithelial immunoglobins in the mouse mammary gland during pregnancy and lactation. J Immunol 199:1036, 1977

33. Linzell JL: Mammary blood flow and methods of identifying and measuring precursors of milk. p. 143. In Larson LB, Smith VR (eds): Lactation: A Comprehensive Treatise. Vol. I. Academic, San Diego, 1974

34. Lyons WR: Hormonal synergism in mammary growth. Proc R Soc Lond [Biol] 149:303, 1958

35. Nandi S: Hormonal control of mammogenesis and lactogenesis in the C3H/He Crgl mouse. Univ Calif Publ Zool 65:4, 1959

36. Neill JD: Prolactin: its secretion and control. p. 469. In Knobil E, Sawyer WH (eds): Handbook of Physiology. Endocrinology. Sect. 7, Vol. 4. American Physiological Society, Washington, DC, 1974

37. Faulkin LJ, DeOme KB: Regulation of growth and spacing of gland elements in the mammary fat pad of the C3H mouse. J Natl Cancer Inst 24:953, 1960

38. Shyamala G, Ferenczy A: Mammary fat pad may be a potential site for initiation of estrogen action in normal mouse mammary glands. Endocrinology 115:1078, 1984

39. Haslam SZ, Gale JJ, Dachler SL: Estrogen receptor activation in normal mammary gland. Endocrinology 114:1163, 1984

40. Topper YJ, Freeman CS: Multiple hormone interactions in the developmental biology of the mammary gland. Physiol Rev 60:1049, 1980

41. Battacharjee M, Vonderhaar BK: Thyroid hormones enhance the synthesis and secretion of lactalbumin by mouse mammary tissue in vitro. Endocrinology. 115:1070, 1984

42. Cross BA, Findlay ALR: Comparative and sensory aspects of milk ejection. p. 245. In Reynolds M, Folley SJ (eds): Lactogenesis: The Initiation of Milk Secretion of Parturition. University of Pennsylvania Press, Philadelphia, 1969

43. Sala NL: The milk ejecting effect induced by oxytocin and vasopressin during human pregnancy. Am J Obstet Gynecol 89:626, 1964

44. Soloff MS, Schroeder BT, Chakraborty J, Pearlmutter AF: Characterization of oxytocin receptors in the uterus and mammary gland. Fed Proc 36:1861, 1977

45. Sala NL, Althabe O: The milk ejecting effect induced by oxytocin during human lactation. Acta Physiol Latino Am 18:88, 1968

46. Wiederman J, Freund M, Stone ML: Oxytocin effect on myoepithelium of the breast throughout pregnancy. J Appl Physiol 19:310, 1964

47. Caldeyro-Barcia R: Milk ejection in women. p. 229. In Reynolds M, Folley SJ (eds): Lactogenesis: The Initia-

tion of Milk Secretion at Parturition. University of Pennsylvania Press, Philadelphia, 1969

48. Fuchs AR, Wagner G: The effect of ethyl alcohol on the release of oxytocin (OT) in rabbits. Acta Endocrinol (Copenh) 44:593, 1963

49. Wagner G, Fuchs AR: Effect of ethanol on uterine activity during suckling in post partum women. Acta Endocrinol (Copenh) 58:133, 1968

50. Dawood MY, Khan-Dawood FS, Wahi RS, Fuchs F: Oxytocin release and plasma anterior pituitary and gonadal hormones in women during lactation. J Clin Endocrinol Metab 52:678, 1981

51. Fuchs AR, Dawood MY, Sumulong L et al: Release of oxytocin and prolactin by suckling in rabbits throughout lactation. Endocrinology 114:462, 1984

52. Johnston AM, Amico JA: A prospective longitudinal study of the release of oxytocin and prolactin in response to infant suckling in long-term lactation. J Clin Endocrinol Metab 622:653, 1986

53. Del Pozo E, Brun del Re R, Varga L, Friesen HG: The inhibition of prolactin section in man by CB-154 (2-Br-alphaergocryptine). J Clin Endocrinol Metab 35:768, 1972

54. Rolland R, Schellekens L: A new approach to the inhibition of puerperal lactation. J Obstet Gynaecol Br Commonw 80:945, 1973

55. Tyson JE, Hwang P, Guyda H, Friesen HG: Studies of prolactin secretion in human pregnancy. Am J Obstet Gynecol 113:14, 1972

56. Selye H, Collip JB, Thomson DL: Nervous and hormonal factors in lactation. Endocrinology 18:237, 1934

57. Noel GL, Such HK, Frantz AG: Prolactin release during nursing and breast stimulation in postpartum and nonpostpartum subjects. J Clin Endocrinol Metab 38:413, 1974

58. Howie PW, McNeilly AS, McArdle T, Smart L: The relationship between suckling-induced prolactin response and lactogenesis. J Clin Endocrinol Metab 50:670, 1980

59. Diaz S, Seron-Ferre M, Cardenas H et al: Circadian variations of basal plasma prolactin: prolactin response to suckling and length of amenorrhea in nursing women. J Clin Endocrinol Metab 68:946, 1989

60. Delvoye P, Demaegd M, Delongne-Desnoeck J: The influence of the frequency of nursing and of previous lactation experience on serum prolactin in lactating mothers. J Biosoc Sci 9:447, 1977

61. Howie PW, McNeilly AS, Houston MJ et al: Effect of supplementary food on suckling patterns and ovarian activity. Br Med J 283:757, 1981

62. Stern JM, Konner M, Herman TN, Reichlin S: Nursing behaviour, prolactin and postpartum amenorrhoea during prolonged lactation in American and !Kung mothers. Clin Endocrinol 25:247, 1986

63. Andersen AN, Lund-Andersen C, Falck Larsen J et al: Suppressed prolactin but normal neurophysin levels in cigarette smoking breast feeding mothers. Clin Endocrinol 17:363, 1982

64. Riskind PN, Millard WJ, Martin JB: Opiate modulation of the anterior pituitary hormone response during suckling in the rat. Endocrinology 114:1232, 1984

65. Uvnas-Moberg K: Release of gastrointestinal peptides in response to vagal activation induced by electrical stimulation, feeding and suckling. J Auton Nerv Syst 9:141, 1983

66. Fox S, Smith M: The suppression of pulsatile luteinizing hormone secretion during lactation in the rat. Endocrinology 115:2045, 1984

67. Lightman S, Young WS III: Lactation inhibits stress-mediated secretion of corticosteroid and oxytocin and hypothalamic accumulation of corticotropin releasing factor and encephalic messenger ribonucleic acids. Endocrinology 124:2358, 1989

68. Kauppila A, Kivinen A, Ylikorkala O: Metoclopramide increases prolactin release and milk secretion in puerperium without stimulating the secretion of TSH or T_3 or T_4. J Clin Endocrinol Metab 52:436, 1981

69. Tyson JE, Perez A, Zanartu J: Human lactational response to oral thyrotropin releasing hormone. J Clin Endocrinol Metab 43:760, 1976

70. Zarate A, Villalobos H, Canales ES et al: The effect of oral administration of thyrotropin releasing hormone on lactation. J Clin Endocrinol Metab 43:301, 1976

71. Ylikorkala O, Kivinen S, Kauppila A: Oral administration of TRH in puerperal women: effects on insufficient lactation, thyroid hormones and prolactin to intravenous TRII. Acta Endocrinol (Copenh) 93:413, 1983

72. Bolander FF Jr: Persistent alterations in hormonal sensitivities of mammary glands from parous mice. Endocrinology 112:1796, 1983

73. MacMahon B, Cole P, Brown JB: Etiology of human breast cancer: a review. J Natl Cancer Inst 50:21, 1974

74. Kvale G, Heuch I: Lactation and cancer risk: is there a relation to breast cancer? J Epidemiol Commun Health 42:30, 1988

75. Fuchs F, Klopper A (eds): Endocrinology of Pregnancy. 3rd Ed. Harper & Row, New York 1983

76. Nolin JM, Bogdanove EM: Effects of estrogen on prolactin (PRL) incorporation by lutein and milk secretory cells and on pituitary PRL secretion in the

postpartum rat: correlations with target cell responsiveness to PRL. Biol Reprod 22:393, 1980

77. Bohnet HG, Gomez F, Friesen HG: Prolactin and estrogen binding sites in the mammary gland of the lactating and nonlactating rat. Endocrinology 101:111, 1977

78. Hayden TJ, Bonney RC, Forsyth IA: Ontogeny and control of prolactin receptors in the mammary gland and liver of virgin, pregnant and lactating rats. J Endocrinol 80:259, 1979

79. Chatterton RT Jr, King WJ, Ward DA, Chien HL: Differential responses of prelactating and lactating mammary gland to similar tissue concentrations of progesterone. Endocrinology 96:861, 1975

80. Kuhn NJ: Progesterone withdrawal as the lactogenic trigger in the rat. J Endocrinol 44:39, 1969

81. Kuhn NJ: Specificity of progesterone inhibition of lactogenesis. J Endocrinol 45:615, 1969

82. Haslam SZ, Shyamala G: Effect of oestradiol on progesterone receptors in normal mammary gland and its relationship with lactation. Biochem J 182:127, 1979

83. Simpson-Herbert M, Huffman S: The contraceptive effect of breast feeding. Stud Fam Plann 12:125, 1981

84. Perez A, Vela P, Masnick GS, Potter RG: First ovulation after childbirth: the effect of breast feeding. Am J Obstet Gynecol 114:1041, 1972

85. Howie PW, McNeilly AS, Houston MJ et al: Fertility after childbirth: ovulation and menstruation in bottle and breast feeding mothers. Clin Endocrinol 17:323, 1982

86. McNeilly AS, Howie PW, Houston MJ: Relationship of feeding patterns, prolactin, and resumption of ovulation postpartum. p. 102. In Zatuchni G, Labbok M, Sciarra J (eds): Research Frontiers in Fertility Regulation. PARFR Series in Fertility Regulation. Vol. 3. Harper & Row, New York, 1981

87. Gray RH, Campbell OM, Zacur HA et al: Postpartum return of ovarian activity in non-breast-feeding women monitored by urinary assays. J Clin Endocrinol Metab 63:645, 1986

88. Tolis G, Guyda H, Pillorger R, Friesen HG: Breast feeding effects on the hypothalamic pituitary gonadal axis. Endocr Res Commun 1:293, 1974

89. LeMaire WJ, Shapiro AG, Rigg ALT, Yang N: Temporary pituitary insensitivity to stimulation by synthetic LRH during the postpartum period. J Clin Endocrinol Metab 38:916, 1974

90. Baird DT, McNeilly AS, Sawers RS, Sharpe RM: Failure of estrogen-induced discharge of leuteinizing hormone in lactating women. J Clin Endocrinol Metab 49:500, 1979

91. Dorrington J, Gore-Langton RE: Prolactin inhibits

oestrogen synthesis in the ovary. Nature 290:600, 1984

92. Wang C, Hsueh AJW, Erickson GF: Prolactin inhibition of estrogen production by cultured rat granulosa cells. Mol Cell Endocrinol 20:135, 1980

93. Rolland R, Lequin RM, Schellekens LA: The role of prolactin in the restoration of ovarian function during the early postpartum period in the human female. Clin Endocrinol 4:15, 1975

94. Weinstein D, Ben-David M, Polishuk WZ: Serum prolactin and the suppression of lactation. Br J Obstet Gynaecol 83:679, 1976

95. Rolland R, DeJong FH, Schellekens LA, Lequin RM: The role of prolactin in the restoration of ovarian function during the early postpartum period in the human: a study during inhibition of lactation by bromergocryptine. Clin Endocrinol 4:23, 1975

96. Lamke B, Brundin JM, Moberg D: Changes in bone mineral content during pregnancy and lactation. Acta Obstet Gynecol Scand 56:217, 1977

97. Lewis P, Rafferty B, Shelley B, Robinson CJ: A suggested physiological role of calcitonin: the protection of the skeleton during pregnancy and lactation. J Endocrinol 49:IX, 1971

98. Lund B, Selnes A: Plasma 1,25-dihydroxyvitamin D levels in pregnancy and lactation. Acta Endocrinol (Copenh) 92:330, 1979

99. Taylor TG, Lewis PE, Balderstone O: Role of calcitonin in protecting the skeleton during pregnancy and lactation. J Endocrinol 66:297, 1975

99a. Hillman L, Sateesha S, Haussler M et al: Control of mineral homeostasis during lactation: interrelationships of 25-hydroxyvitamin D, 24,25-dihydroxyvitamin D, 1,25-dehydroxyvitamin D, parathyroid hormone, calcitonin, prolactin and estradiol. Am J Obstet Gynecol 139:471, 1981

99b. Hollis BW, Pittard WB, Reinhardt TA: Relationships among vitamin D, 25-hydroxyvitamin D, and vitamin D-binding protein concentrations in the plasma and milk of human subjects. J Clin Endocrinol Metab 62:41, 1986

100. Chan GM, Slater P, Ronald N et al: Bone mineral status of lactating mothers of different ages. Am J Obstet Gynecol 144:438, 1982

100a. Hayslip CC, Klein TA, Wray L, Duncan WE: The effects of lactation on bone mineral content in healthy postpartum women. Obstet Gynecol 73(2):588, 1989

101. Hytten FE: Clinical and chemical studies in human lactation. Parts I–III. Br Med J 2:175, 1954

102. Anderson GH, Atkinson SA, Bryan MH: Energy and macronutrient content of human milk during early

lactation from mothers giving birth prematurely and at term. Am J Clin Nutr 34:258, 1981

103. Gross SJ, David RJ, Bauman L et al: Nutritional composition of milk produced by mothers delivering preterm. J Pediatr 96:41, 1980

104. Hohenauer L: Feeding of the mother's expressed breast milk to sick and premature babies: some aspects of practical interest. Eur J Obstet Gynecol Reprod Biol 15:385, 1983

105. Gross SJ: Growth and biochemical response of preterm infants fed human milk or modified infant formula. N Engl J Med 308:237, 1983

106. Clandini MT, Chappell JE, Hein T et al: Human milk as a source of long chain polyunsaturated fatty acids for preterm human infant neural tissues. Nutr Rev 42:247, 1984

107. Abrams SA, Schauler RJ, Garza G: Mineralization in former very-low-birth-weight infants fed either with milk or commercial formula. J Pediatr 112:956, 1988

108. Shing YW, Klagsbrun M: Human and bovine milk contain different sets of growth factors. Endocrinology 115:273, 1984

109. Beer AF, Billingham RE, Head JR: The immunologic significance of the mammary gland. J Invest Dermatol 63:65, 1974

110. Welsh JK, May JT: Anti-infective properties of breast milk. J Pediatr 94:1, 1979

111. Ogra SS, Ogra PL: Characteristics of lymphocyte reactivity and distribution of E-rosette forming cells at different times after the onset of lactation. J Pediatr 92:550, 1978

112. Crago SS, Kalkavy R, Prince SJ, Mesiecky J: Secretory component on epithelial cells is a surface receptor for polymeric immunoglobins. J Exp Med 147:1832, 1978

113. Walker WA: Antigen penetration across the immature gut: effect of immunologic and nutritional factors in colostrum. p. 227. In Ogra P, Dayton DH (eds): Immunology of Breast Milk. Plenum, New York, 1979

114. Goldblum RM, Ahlstedt S, Charlsson B et al: Antibody-forming cells in human colostrum after oral immunization. Nature 257:797, 1975

115. Porter P: Adoptive immunization of the neonate by breast factors. p. 197. In Ogra P, Dayton DH (eds): Immunology of the Breast Milk. Plenum, New York, 1979

116. Roux ME, McWilliams M, Phillips-Quagliata JM: Origin of IgA secreting plasma cells in the mammary gland. J Exp Med 146:1311, 1977

117. Johnson WD: AIDS in Haiti: looking the monster in the eye. Cornell UMC Alumni Q 50:2, 1989

118. Butte NF, Garza C, Stuff JE et al: Effects of maternal diet and body composition on lactational performance. Am J Clin Nutr 39:296, 1984

119. Strode MA, Dewey KG, Lonnerdal B: Effects of short-term caloric restriction on lactational performance of well-nourished women. Acta Pediatr Scand 75:222, 1986

120. Evans RW, Ferguson DW, Allardyce RA, Taylor B: Maternal diet and infantile colic in breast-fed infants. Lancet 1:1340, 1981

121. Lilza G, Dannaeus A, Foucard T, Graff-Lonnevig V: Effect of maternal diet during pregnancy and lactation on the development of atopic disease in infants up to 18 months of age. Clin Exp Al 19:473, 1989

122. Ferris AM, Davidowitz CK, Ingardia CM et al: Lactation outcome in insulin dependent diabetic women. J Am Diet Assoc 88:317, 1988

123. Laukaran VH: Contraceptive choices for lactating women: suggestions for postpartum family planning. Stud Fam Plann 12:156, 1981

124. Hull VJ: The effects of hormonal contraceptives on lactation: current findings, methodological considerations, and future priorities. Stud Fam Plann 12:134, 1981

125. Nilsson S, Nygren K-G: Transfer of contraceptive steroids to human milk. Res Reprod 11:1, 1979

126. Heartwell SF, Schesselman S: Risk of uterine perforation among users of intrauterine devices. Obstet Gynecol 61:31, 1983

127. Nilson P, Meling AB, Abilgaard U: Study of the suppression of lactation and the influence on blood clotting with bromocriptine (CB 154) (Parlodel). Acta Obstet Gynecol Scand 55:39, 1976

128. Casey CE, Hambridge KM: Nutritional aspects of breast-feeding. p. 204. In Neville MC, Neifert MR (eds): Lactation: Physiology, Nutrition, and Breast-Feeding. Plenum, New York, 1983

129. National Research Council: The composition of milks. Bull Natl Res Council: Wash. No. 254, 1953

130. Cowie AT: Lactation. p. 201. In Austin CR, Short RV (eds): Reproduction in Mammals. Book 3. Hormonal Control of Reproduction. 2nd Ed. Cambridge University Press, Cambridge, 1984

131. Johnson M, Everitt B: Essentials of reproduction. p. 321. In Essentials of Reproduction. 2nd Ed. Blackwell Scientific, Oxford, 1984

132. Lincoln DW: Neuroendocrine control of milk ejection. J Reprod Fertil 2:571, 1982

133. Gross ST, David RJ, Bauman L et al: Nutritional composition of milk produced by mothers delivering preterm. J Pediatr 96:641, 1980

SECTION 2
Prenatal Care

Chapter 8

Preconception and Prenatal Care

Timothy R. B. Johnson, Marlene A. Walker, and Jennifer R. Niebyl

The goal of prenatal care is to help the mother maintain her well-being and achieve a healthy outcome for herself and her infant. Education about pregnancy, childbearing, and childrearing is an important part of prenatal care, as are detection and treatment of abnormalities. It has become clear that this process is best realized when begun even prior to pregnancy.

Prenatal care is an excellent example of preventive medicine and is very much a phenomenon of the 20th century. In 1929, the Ministry of Health of Great Britain issued a memorandum on the conduct of prenatal clinics and provided guidelines for their organization that endure to this day.[1] Two recent documents[2,3] addressing the content and efficacy of prenatal care have suggested changes to the prenatal care system, and we believe that during the next decade there will be changes from current practice.

During World War II, when wartime food rationing in England identified expectant and nursing mothers as persons having special dietary requirements, maternal mortality began to fall. In 1942, vitamin tablets were provided for all women in the last 6 months of pregnancy. The decline in maternal mortality was from 3.19 per 1,000 live and stillbirths in 1936 to 0.15 in 1985. The decline in maternal mortality was partly attributed to prenatal care and partly to medical advances in availability of blood transfusions, antibiotics, and management of fluid and electrolyte balance.

MATERNAL MORTALITY

Maternal death is the demise of any woman from any pregnancy-related cause while pregnant or within 42 –6w days of termination of pregnancy, irrespective of the duration and the site of pregnancy. A direct maternal death is an obstetric death resulting from obstetric complications of the pregnancy state, labor, or puerperium; an indirect maternal death is an obstetric death resulting from a disease previously existing or developing during the pregnancy, labor, or the puerperium. It is not directly due to obstetric causes but may be aggravated by the physiologic effects of pregnancy. A nonmaternal death is an obstetric death resulting from accidental or incidental causes unrelated to the pregnancy or its management.

The maternal mortality rate is the number of maternal deaths (direct, indirect, or nonmaternal) per 100,000 women of reproductive age, but, because this denominator is difficult to determine precisely, the National Center for Health Statistics,[4] the World Health Organization, and others define the maternal mortality rate as the number of maternal deaths (indirect and direct) per 100,000 live births. Epidemiologists recognize this as the maternal mortality ratio. The major causes of death in the United States are pulmonary embolism and hypertensive disorders, followed by uterine hemorrhage and sepsis. Furthermore, among 2,475 maternal deaths that occurred in

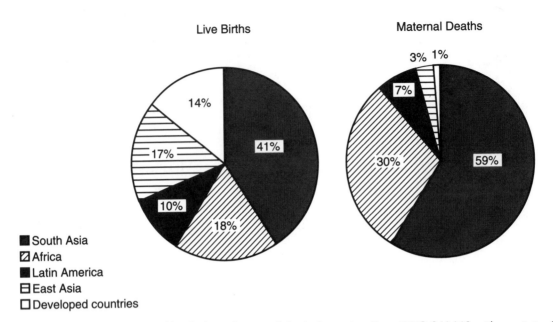

Fig. 8.1 Worldwide distribution of live births and maternal deaths by region. (From WHO 861663, with permission.)

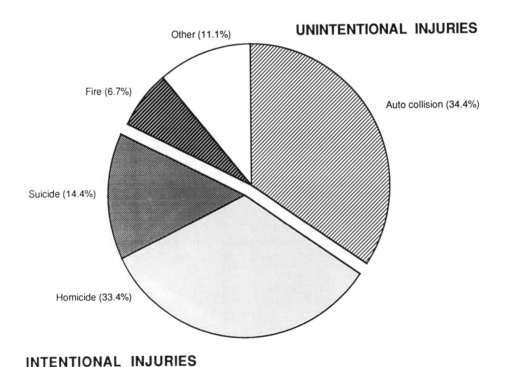

Fig. 8.2 Distribution of deaths due to injury in the United States, 1980–1985 (N = 90). (From MMWR.[36])

the United States from 1974 to 1978, 408 were related to pregnancies with abortive outcomes, and ectopic pregnancy was the most frequent cause of death in this group.

Maternal mortality has been an under-recognized issue worldwide despite an estimated 500,000 maternal deaths per year from pregnancy-related causes.[5] Put in perspective, this is equivalent to six jumbo jet crashes per day with the death of all 250 passengers on board, all of them women in the reproductive years of life. There is also a marked inequity in distribution in that 95 percent of these deaths occur in developing countries (Fig. 8.1). Unfortunately, the United States is undergoing an increase in nonmaternal deaths of pregnant women because of trauma and violence, much of it drug related (Fig. 8.2).

NEONATAL MORTALITY AND MORBIDITY

Historically, in developed countries when decreased maternal mortality was achieved, attention was turned first to fetal mortality and then to fetal morbidity. The stillbirth rate (fetal death rate) is the number of stillborn infants per 1,000 infants born. The neonatal mortality rate is the number of neonatal deaths (deaths in the first 28 days of life) per 1,000 live births. The perinatal mortality combines these two — the number of fetal deaths (stillbirths) plus neonatal deaths per 1,000 total births.

During the past 20 years, new technology has been introduced to assess the fetus antepartum, including electronic fetal monitoring, ultrasound, and amniocentesis, with the fetus emerging as a patient in utero. Prevention of morbidity and of mortality is now the goal. This has made the task of the prenatal clinic more complex, because the two patients can now be given an increasingly sophisticated level of care. At the same time, pregnancy is basically a physiologic process, and the normal pregnant patient may not benefit from this advanced technology. In this situation, the pregnant woman's choices should be respected to best ensure an optimal pregnancy outcome.

Prenatal care is provided at a variety of sites, ranging from the private office to the public health and county hospital clinics, and even to the patient's home. A variety of practitioners are involved, including the public health nurse, nurse practitioner, nurse midwife, physician-in-training, family practitioner, obstetrician, and perinatologist. Each has his or her own interests, experience, and expertise. Prenatal care requires a synthesis of knowledge and experience; in addition, it requires vigilance, compassion, and caring. Obstetricians must optimize their efforts by resourceful use of other professionals and support groups, including nutritionists, childbirth educators, and specialty medical consultants. In fact, most pregnant women are healthy, with normal pregnancies, and they can be followed by an obstetric team including nurses, nurse practitioners, and midwives with an obstetrician available for consultation. The pregnant woman can be followed by midwives who have adequate time to spend on patient education and parenting preparation, while physicians can appropriately concentrate on complicated problems requiring their medical skills. This also provides for improved continuity of care, which is recognized as extremely important for patient satisfaction.

There have been no prospective controlled trials demonstrating efficacy of prenatal care. In retrospective studies, however, patients with increased numbers of visits have improved maternal and fetal outcome. This may be because of self-selection of patients for care who are motivated to take care of themselves in other ways, as women with no prenatal care often come from underprivileged socioeconomic groups.

Efficacy of prenatal care also depends on the quality of care provided by the caretaker. If a blood pressure is recorded as elevated and no therapeutic maneuvers are recommended, this will not change the outcome. Recommendations must be made such as for bed rest to control blood pressure and must be carried out by the patient, whose compliance is essential to alter outcome.

RISK ASSESSMENT

The concept of risk in obstetrics can be examined at many levels. All the problems that arise in pregnancy, whether common complaints or more hazardous diseases, convey some risk to the pregnancy, depending on how they are managed by the patient and her care provider. Risk assessment has received detailed attention in recent years. It has been shown that most women and infants suffering morbidity and mortality come from a small segment of women with high-risk factors; by reassessing risk factors before pregnancy, during pregnancy, and during labor, the ability to identify those at highest risk increases.[6] However, previous preterm birth is the most significant risk factor for preterm delivery, so that risk scoring of primigravidas is of limited value in preventing this condition.[7]

It is important to individualize patient care and to be thorough. The initial visit should include a detailed history and physical and laboratory examinations. The initial history requires that the patient be seen in an office setting. She should not be first seen undressed sitting on an examining table.

PRECONCEPTION EDUCATION

We have reached a level in prenatal care where the optimal time to assess, manage, and treat many pregnancy conditions and complications is before pregnancy occurs.[8,9] The best time to see a woman for prenatal care is when she is considering pregnancy. At that time, much of the risk assessment described later in this chapter can be performed, as well as the basic physical and laboratory evaluations. If there are questions about the history, such as diethylstilbestrol (DES) exposure, family history of fetal anomaly, or previous cesarean delivery, further details can be obtained from family members or from the appropriate medical facility. This is the time to draw a rubella titer and immunize the susceptible patient. Patients need to use contraception for 3 months thereafter (see Ch. 40). It is the time to screen appropriate populations for genetic disease carrier states such as for Tay-Sachs disease or hemoglobinopathies. Resolution of these issues is much easier and less harried without the time limits placed by an advancing pregnancy. Medical conditions such as anemia, urinary tract infection, or hypothyroidism can be fully evaluated and the woman medically treated before pregnancy. If the patient is obese, weight reduction should be completed before pregnancy. Patients in whom risks are very serious should be so counseled, and every attempt should be made to let them make a fully informed decision about pregnancy. Often significant risk factors can be

treated or managed so that risk is reduced during pregnancy.

This concept must not only be a part of obstetric care; prepregnancy counseling must also be emphasized by those who treat women who are at significant risk for pregnancy problems. Women who are followed by other physicians for such problems as diabetes, hypertension, or systemic lupus erythematosus should be seen, evaluated, and counseled prior to pregnancy.

There is evidence that for some conditions such as diabetes mellitus and phenylketonuria medical disease management before conception can positively influence pregnancy outcome. Medical management to normalize the biochemical environment should be discussed with the patient and appropriate management plans outlined before conception (see Ch. 29). Some studies suggest that periconceptional vitamins can reduce the incidence of neural tube defects[10,11] and other anomalies, but the evidence is still conflicting.[12] This is also the time to review drug usage and other practices, such as drinking and smoking (see Ch. 11). Advice can be given about avoiding medications in the first trimester, and general advice can be given concerning diet, exercise, and occupational exposures.

The importance of gestational age dating can be discussed with the patient. Great precision can be achieved with an accurate menstrual calendar predating pregnancy; some women with irregular menses may follow basal body temperatures to document sustained thermogenic rise. Women on oral contraceptives may be advised to stop their pills at least 1 month before attempting pregnancy to help ascertain cycle length.

THE INITIAL PRECONCEPTION OR PRENATAL VISIT

Social and Demographic Risks

Extremes of age are obstetric risk factors. The pregnant teenager has particular nutritional and emotional needs. She is at special risk for sexually transmitted diseases; it has been shown that she benefits particularly from education in areas of childbearing and contraception. The pregnant woman over age 35 years is at increased risk for a chromosomally abnormal child,[13] and she must be so advised. Patients should be asked about family histories of Down syndrome, neural tube defects, hemophilia, hemoglobinopathies, and other birth defects, as well as mental retardation (see Ch. 10). Consultation for genetic counseling and genetic testing, if desired, may be appropriate. The age of the father can be important, as there may be genetic risks to the fetus if the father is older than 55 years.[14] Certain diseases are race-related. Black patients should be screened for sickle cell disease, those of Jewish heritage should be screened for Tay-Sachs disease, and those of Mediterranean descent should be screened for β-thalassemia.

Low socioeconomic status should be identified and attempts to improve nutritional and hygienic measures undertaken. Appropriate referral to federal programs, such as that for women, infants, and children (WIC), and to public health nurses can have real benefits. If a patient has a history of a previous neonatal death or stillbirth, records should be carefully reviewed so that the correct diagnosis is made and recurrence risk appropriately assessed. A history of drug abuse or recent blood transfusion should be elicited. The history of the patient's mother's reproductive record may lead to discovery of DES exposure. The history of medical illnesses should be detailed and records obtained if possible.

Occupational hazards should be identified. If a patient works in a laboratory with chemicals, for example, she should be advised to limit her exposure. Patients whose occupations require heavy physical exercise or excess stress should be informed that they may need to decrease such activity.

Tobacco, alcohol, and recreational drug use can all adversely affect pregnancy and are a critical part of the history. Specific questions concerning smoking, alcohol, and drugs (licit and illicit) should be asked.[15] Regular screening for alcohol and substance use should be carried out using such tools as the T-ACE questionnaire (Table 8.1),[16] and appropriate directed therapy should be made available to those women who screen positive. Women should be urged to stop smoking prior to pregnancy and to drink not at all or minimally once they are pregnant. Drug addiction confers a particularly high risk, and these mothers require specialized care throughout pregnancy (see Ch. 11).

Medical Risk

Family history of diabetes, hypertension, tuberculosis, seizures, hematologic disorders, multiple pregnancies, congenital abnormalities, and reproductive wastage should be elicited. Often a family history of mental retardation, birth defects, or genetic trait is difficult to elicit; these areas should be emphasized at the initial history. A better history may be obtained if patients are asked to fill out a preinterview questionnaire or history form. Any significant maternal cardiovascular, renal, or metabolic disease should be defined. Infectious diseases such as urinary tract disease, syphilis, tuberculosis, or herpes genitalis should be identified. Surgical history with special attention to any abdominal or pelvic operations is noted. A history of previous cesarean birth should include indication, type of uterine incision, and any complications. A copy of the surgical report may be informative. Allergies, particularly drug allergies, should be prominent on the problem list.

Obstetric Risk

Previous obstetric and reproductive history are essential to care in subsequent pregnancy. The gravity and parity should be noted and the outcome for each prior pregnancy recorded in detail. Previous miscarriages not only confer risk and anxiety for another pregnancy loss but also can increase the risk of genetic disease as well as preterm delivery.[17]

Previous preterm delivery is strongly associated with recurrence; it is important to delineate the events surrounding the preterm birth. Did the membranes rupture before labor? Were there painful uterine contractions? Was there bleeding? Were there fetal abnormalities? What was the neonatal outcome? All these questions are vital in determining the etiology and prognosis of the condition, although specific recommendations will vary and the efficacy of routine prevention programs is not clear.[18] DES exposure, incompetent cervix, and uterine anomaly are all conditions that may be known from a previous pregnancy. Previous fetal macrosomia makes glucose screening essential.

It is recommended after all the specific questions to ask the patient a few general questions: What important items have I not asked? What else about you and your pregnancy do I need to know? What problems

Table 8.1   Alcohol Abuse Screening: the T-ACE Questionnaire[a]

T How many drinks does it take to make you feel "high" (can you hold)? (*tolerance;* a positive response consists of two or more drinks)

A Have people *annoyed* you by criticizing your drinking?

C Have you ever felt you ought to *cut down* on your drinking?

E Have you ever had a drink first thing in the morning to steady your nerves or to get rid of a hangover *(eye-opener)*?

Scoring: The tolerance question has substantially more weight (2 points) than the three other questions (1 point each).

[a] These questions were found to be significant identifiers of risk drinking in pregnancy (i.e., alcohol intake potentially sufficient to damage the embryo/fetus).
(From Sokol et al.,[16] with permission.)

Table 8.2   Recommendations for All Women for Prenatal Care

	Preconception or First Visit	Weeks								
		6–8[a]	14–16	24–28	32	36	38	39	40	41
History										
Medical, including genetic	X									
Psychosocial	X									
Update medical and psychosocial		X	X	X	X	X	X	X	X	X
Physical examination										
General	X									
Blood pressure	X	X	X	X	X	X	X	X	X	X
Height	X									
Weight	X	X	X	X	X	X	X	X	X	X
Height and weight profile	X									
Pelvic examination and pelvimetry	X	X								
Breast examination	X	X								
Fundal height			X	X	X	X	X	X	X	X
Fetal position and heart rate			X	X	X	X	X	X	X	X
Cervical examination	X									
Laboratory tests										
Hemoglobin or hematocrit	X	X		X		X				
Rh factor	X									
Pap smear	X									
Diabetic screen				X						
MSAFP			X							
Urine										
Dipstick	X									
Protein	X									
Sugar	X									
Culture		X								
Infections										
Rubella titer	X									
Syphilis test	X									
Gonococcal culture	X	X				X				
Hepatitis B	X									
HIV (offered)	X	X								
Illicit drug screen (offered)	X									
Genetic screen	X									

[a] If preconception care has preceded.

and questions do you have? Leaving time for open-ended questions is the best way to complete the initial visit.

Physical and Laboratory Evaluations

Physical examination should include a general physical examination as well as a pelvic examination. Baseline height and weight as well as prepregnancy weight are recorded. Special attention should be given to the initial vital signs, cardiac examination, and reflexes, because many healthy young women have not had a physical examination immediately before becoming pregnant. Any physical finding that might have an impact on pregnancy (e.g., DES-related changes in the cervix) or that might be affected by pregnancy (e.g., mitral valve prolapse) should be defined. Any factor that might become important later in pregnancy in assessing pathology or disease (e.g., reflexes) should be carefully noted. It is particularly important to perform and record a complete physical examination at this initial visit, because less emphasis will be placed on nonobstetric portions of further examinations as pregnancy progresses in the absence of specific problems or complaints.

The pelvic examination should focus on the uterine size. Before 12 to 14 weeks, size can give a fairly accurate estimate of gestational age. Papanicolaou smear and culture for gonorrhea are done. The cervix should be carefully palpated, and any deviation from normal should be noted. Clinical pelvimetry should be performed and the clinical impression of adequacy noted. The pelvic examination is limited by examiner and patient variation as well as by obesity. If there is any question of difficulty examining the uterus, an ultrasound study is indicated.

Basic laboratory studies are routinely obtained (Table 8.2). Some studies need not be repeated if recent normal values have been obtained, such as at an initial visit following a preconceptional visit or a recent gynecologic examination. Blood studies should include Rh type and screening for irregular antibodies, hemoglobin level, or hematocrit and serologic tests for syphilis and rubella. A urine sample should be obtained and tested for protein and glucose. Screening for asymptomatic bacteriuria has been traditionally done by urine culture, but recent information suggests that screening may be simplified by testing for nitrites and leukocyte esterase.[19]

Tuberculosis screening should also be performed in areas of disease prevalence. Maternal serum α-fetoprotein (MSAFP) screening is offered at 15 to 16 weeks gestation to screen for neural tube defects (see Ch. 10).

The laboratory evaluations outlined above are the minimum standard tests. Specific conditions will require further evaluation. A history of thyroid disease indicates thyroid function testing. Anticonvulsant therapy requires blood level studies to determine adequacy of medication. Identification of problems (e.g., anemia, abnormal glucose level) on screening will mandate further testing.

The American College of Obstetricians and Gynecologists (ACOG) has recently recommended routine screening of all pregnant women for hepatitis B.[20] At minimum, patients at risk for hepatitis should be screened. This includes women of Asian origin, health care workers exposed to blood or blood products, women with previously undiagnosed jaundice or liver disease, parenteral drug abusers, prostitutes, women with tatoos, women with a history of blood transfusion, dialysis or renal transplant patients, women who work or reside in institutions for the retarded, and household contacts of hepatitis B–infected persons. Human immunodeficiency virus (HIV) screening in high-risk populations can also be offered at this time. The recommendations of the Public Health Service Panel[2] for the content of prenatal care are summarized in Table 8.2.

REPEAT PRENATAL VISITS

A plan of visits is outlined to the patient. This has been traditionally every 4 weeks for the first 28 weeks of pregnancy, every 2 to 3 weeks until 36 weeks, and weekly thereafter, if the pregnancy progresses normally.[12,22] A public health service panel recently suggested that this number of visits can be decreased, especially in parous, healthy women,[2] but there are no studies to date evaluating a new regimen of visits. If there are any complications, the visits can be increased appropriately. For example, patients with hypertensive disease may require weekly visits. Fetal heart tones can be documented before week 12 by Doppler devices and generally at week 20 by DeLee-

Hillis stethoscope, and this information can be used for gestational dating.

At regular-interval visits, the patient is weighed, the blood pressure is recorded, and the presence of edema is evaluated. Fundal height is regularly measured with a tape measure, fetal heart tones are recorded, and fetal position is noted. The goal of subsequent pregnancy visits is to assess fetal growth and maternal well-being. In addition, at each prenatal visit, time should be allowed for asking about and discussing any problems and questions the patient may have. Family members should also be encouraged to come to prenatal visits, ask questions, and participate to the degree that the patient wishes.

A pelvic examination is usually only performed on the first visit, after which it is not repeated. In patients at risk of prematurity or in those with a history of DES exposure, however, frequent cervical checks may reveal premature dilatation or effacement.

Further laboratory evaluations are routinely performed at 28 weeks, when the hemoglobin or hematocrit and Rh type and screen for antibodies, as well as the serologic test for syphilis and possibly HIV testing, can be repeated. If the patient is Rh negative and unsensitized, she should receive Rh immunoglobulin prophylaxis at this time. A glucose screening test for diabetes is also appropriately performed at this time (see Ch. 33), and routine fetal movement counting can begin using an organized system (Fig. 8.3).[23] At 36 weeks, a repeat hematocrit, especially in those women with anemia or at risk for peripartum hemorrhage (multipara, repeat cesarean), may be performed. Appropriate cultures for sexually transmitted disease (gonorrhea, herpes) should be obtained as indicated in the third trimester. After 41 weeks from the last menstrual period, the patient should be entered into a screening program for fetal well-being, which may include electronic monitoring tests or ultrasound evaluation (see Ch. 28).

INTERCURRENT PROBLEMS

It is the practice in prenatal care to evaluate the pregnant patient for the development of certain complications. Inherent in these checks is surveillance for intervening problems, an important one being preeclampsia. If a patient shows a tendency to blood pressure elevation at 28 weeks, for example, she should be seen again in a week, not a month. Blood pressure will change physiologically in response to pregnancy, but development of hypertension must be recognized and evaluation and hospitalization appropriately instituted.

Weight gain in pregnancy has been shown to be an important correlate of fetal weight gain and is therefore closely monitored. Too little weight gain should lead to an evaluation of nutritional factors and to an assessment of associated fetal growth. Excess weight gain is one of the first signs of fluid retention, but it may also reflect increased dietary intake or decreased activity. Dependent edema is physiologic in pregnancy, but generalized or facial edema can be a first sign of disease. It is critical here, as in all areas, for the practitioner to understand the normal changes associated with pregnancy in order to accept and explain the normal, but also to manage aggressively any abnormal changes.

Proteinuria is a reflection of urinary tract disease, generally either infection or glomerular dysfunction, possibly caused by preeclampsia. Urinary tract infection should be looked for, and the degree of protein quantitated in a 24-hour urine collection. Glycosuria, while commonly caused by increased glucose filtered through the kidney in pregnancy, warrants evaluation for diabetes, if this is not being checked routinely.

Fetal abnormalities are usually first detected by deviations from the clinical expectation. In some conditions, risk of fetal anomaly will be so high as to prompt some kind of baseline screening or testing (e.g., amniocentesis, ultrasound, fetal echocardiography). At other times, risk only becomes evident during the course of prenatal care. Growth retardation and macrosomia can often be suspected clinically, usually on the basis of an abnormality in fundal growth. Ultrasound can then further define fetal size and weight. For the patient who has a history of these conditions or other predisposing factors, such as hypertension, renal disease, or diabetes, particular vigilance is in order. Excess amniotic fluid is another condition that can be clinically detected, and an etiology for the hydramnios should be sought. In addition to maternal conditions, hydramnios may be caused by fetal disease that can also be defined using ultrasound and that may alter management of the pregnancy.

Detection of a maternal or fetal abnormality will

Fetal Movement Record

HOLLISTER®
maternal/newborn
RECORD SYSTEM

PATIENT IDENTIFICATION

Patient's name _____

_____

_____

G	T	PT	A	L	LMP	mo / day / yr	EDC	mo / day / yr	QUICKENING DATE	mo / day / yr	START DATE	mo / day / yr	NO. OF WEEKS PREGNANT

PATIENT INSTRUCTIONS   ON: mo / day / yr   BY:

BABY'S PHYSICIAN:

IMPORTANT TELEPHONE NUMBERS

DAY/OB CLINIC _____
FETAL ASSESSMENT CENTER _____
NIGHT/LABOR AND DELIVERY: _____

COMMENTS: _____
_____
_____

HOW TO USE THIS RECORD

Counting fetal movements is one way in which you may play an important role in checking the health of your baby. By counting and recording the number of movements made by your baby each day, you create a profile of your baby's activity during the final weeks of your pregnancy.

Instructions for completing this record:

Every day you will note on the record the time you start counting. Beginning at this time, you must keep a count of the number of times your baby kicks or moves until you reach a total of ___ kicks or movements. When you have counted ___ kicks or movements, note on the record the amount of time required for the baby to do this by filling in the square that matches this amount of time. For example, if you started counting Wednesday at 7:30 a.m., and your baby kicked or moved 10 times in 3 hours, fill in the square on the record as shown at the right. There can be a wide variation in the amount babies normally move and also in a woman's perception of those movements. If you experience less than ___ movements after ___ hours counting, simply fill in the actual number of kicks or movements in the shaded column 11.

IMPORTANT

If you experience less than ___ kicks or movements per day for two days in a row, OR if your baby does not kick or move at all for ___ hours in any one day, IMMEDIATELY NOTIFY YOUR DOCTOR OR HOSPITAL LABOR AND DELIVERY STAFF at one of the above listed telephone numbers. This may be an indication that the baby is having a difficult time and needs further testing, but the only way to be certain is to check your baby at the hospital or clinic.

START TIME	M	T	W	T	F
			7:30		

TAKEN TO FEEL MOVEMENTS: 1, 2, 3, 4, 5

FOLD ON THIS LINE

BEGIN HERE

WEEK #	WEEK #	WEEK #	WEEK #	WEEK #	WEEK #
M T W T F S S	M T W T F S S	M T W T F S S	M T W T F S S	M T W T F S S	M T W T F S S

START TIME

HOURS TAKEN TO FEEL MOVEMENTS: 1 2 3 4 5 6 7 8 9 10 11

CONTINUE HERE

WEEK #	WEEK #	WEEK #	WEEK #	WEEK #	WEEK #
M T W T F S S	M T W T F S S	M T W T F S S	M T W T F S S	M T W T F S S	M T W T F S S

START TIME

HOURS TAKEN TO FEEL MOVEMENTS: 1 2 3 4 5 6 7 8 9 10 11

Hollister.

HOLLISTER INCORPORATED, 2000 HOLLISTER DR., LIBERTYVILLE, IL 60048
® TRADEMARK OF HOLLISTER INCORPORATED

5852 108P

Fig. 8.3 Fetal movement record. (Copyright 1988 Hollister Incorporated, Libertyville, IL. Reprinted with permission.)

ACOG ANTEPARTUM RECORD

DATE _____

NAME _____
          LAST   FIRST   MIDDLE

ID # _____ HOSPITAL OF DELIVERY _____

NEWBORNS PHYSICIAN _____   REFERRED BY _____

BIRTHDATE	AGE	RACE	MARITAL STATUS	ADDRESS:		
MO DAY YR		W B O	S M W D SEP			
OCCUPATION ☐ HOMEMAKER ☐ OUTSIDE WORK _____ ☐ STUDENT Type of Work			EDUCATION (LAST GRADE COMPLETED)	ZIP: PHONE: MEDICAID # / INSURANCE		
EMERGENCY CONTACT:				RELATIONSHIP:		PHONE:

TOTAL PREG	FULL TERM	PREMATURE	ABORTIONS INDUCED	ABORTIONS SPONTANEOUS	ECTOPICS	MULTIPLE BIRTHS	LIVING

PAST PREGNANCIES (LAST SIX)

DATE MO / YR	GA WEEKS	LENGTH OF LABOR	BIRTH WEIGHT	TYPE DELIVERY	ANES.	PLACE OF DELIVERY	PERINATAL MORTALITY YES / NO	TREATMENT PRETERM LABOR YES / NO	COMMENTS / COMPLICATIONS

PAST MEDICAL HISTORY

	O Neg + Pos.	DETAIL POSITIVE REMARKS INCLUDE DATE & TREATMENT			
DIABETES			RH SENSITIZED		
HYPERTENSION			TUBERCULOSIS		
HEART DISEASE			ASTHMA		
RHEUMATIC FEVER			ALLERGIES (DRUGS)		
MITRAL VALVE PROLAPSE			GYN SURGERY		
KIDNEY DISEASE / UTI			OPERATIONS / HOSPITALIZATIONS (YEAR & REASON)		
NERVOUS AND MENTAL			ANESTHETIC COMPLICATIONS		
EPILEPSY			HISTORY OF ABNORMAL PAP		
HEPATITIS / LIVER DISEASE			UTERINE ANOMALY		
VARICCSITIES / PHLEBITIS			INFERTILITY		
THYROID DYSFUNCTION			IN UTERO DES EXPOSURE		
MAJOR ACCIDENTS			STREET DRUGS		
HISTORY OF BLOOD TRANSFUSION			OTHER		
USE OF TOBACCO		# CIGS / DAY PRIOR TO PREG _____ # CIGS / DAY NOW _____ AGE ONSET SMOKING _____ YEARS	USE OF ALCOHOL		# DRINKS / WK PRIOR TO PREG _____ # DRINKS / WK NOW _____ AGE ONSET DRINKING _____ YEARS

INFECTION SCREENING	YES	NO			
			PATIENT OR PARTNER HAVE HISTORY OF GENITAL HERPES?		
HIGH RISK AIDS?			RASH OR VIRAL ILLNESS SINCE LAST MENSTRUAL PERIOD?		
HIGH RISK HEPATITIS B?			HISTORY OF STD, GC, CHLAMYDIA, HPV, SYPHILIS?		
LIVE WITH SOMEONE WITH TB OR EXPOSED TO TB?			OTHER?		

Fig. 8.4 ACOG antepartum record. (Copyright 1989 The American College of Obstetricians and Gynecologists, Washington, DC. Reprinted with permission.) (A). (*Figure continues*).

GENETICS SCREENING
INCLUDES PATIENT, BABY'S FATHER, OR ANYONE IN EITHER FAMILY WITH:

	YES	NO		YES	NO
1. PATIENT'S AGE ≥ 35 YEARS?			10. HUNTINGTON CHOREA?		
2. ITALIAN, GREEK, MEDITERRANEAN, OR ORIENTAL BACKGROUND (MCV < 80)?			11. MENTAL RETARDATION?		
3. NEURAL TUBE DEFECT (MENINGOMYELOCELE, OPEN SPINE, OR ANENCEPHALY)?			IF YES, WAS PERSON TESTED FOR FRAGILE X?		
4. DOWN SYNDROME (MONGOLISM)?			12. OTHER INHERITED GENETIC OR CHROMOSOMAL DISORDER?		
5. JEWISH (TAY SACH'S)?			13. PATIENT OR BABY'S FATHER HAD A CHILD WITH BIRTH DEFECT NOT LISTED ABOVE, ≥ 3 FIRST TRIMESTER SPONTANEOUS ABORTIONS, OR A STILLBIRTH?		
6. SICKLE CELL DISEASE OR TRAIT?					
7. HEMOPHILIA?			14. MEDICATIONS OR STREET DRUGS SINCE LAST MENSTRUAL PERIOD?		
8. MUSCULAR DYSTROPHY?			IF YES, AGENT(S)		
9. CYSTIC FIBROSIS?					

COMMENTS _____
_____
_____
_____

PRESENT PREGNANCY

	O Neg + Pos.	DETAIL POSITIVE REMARKS INCLUDE DATE & TYPE RX.			
1. VAGINAL BLEEDING			5. HEADACHE		
2. VAGINAL DISCHARGE / ODOR			6. ABDOMINAL PAIN		
3. VOMITING			7. URINARY COMPLAINTS		
4. CONSTIPATION			8. FEBRILE EPISODE		
			9. OTHER		

COMMENTS _____
_____

_____ **INTERVIEWER'S SIGNATURE** _____

INITIAL PHYSICAL EXAMINATION

DATE _____ / _____ / _____   PRE-PREGNANCY WEIGHT _____   HEIGHT _____   BP _____

1. HEENT	☐ NORMAL	☐ ABNORMAL	12. RECTUM	☐ NORMAL	☐ ABNORMAL	
2. FUNDI	☐ NORMAL	☐ ABNORMAL	13. VULVA	☐ NORMAL	☐ CONDYLOMA	☐ LESIONS
3. TEETH	☐ NORMAL	☐ ABNORMAL	14. VAGINA	☐ NORMAL	☐ INFLAMMATION	☐ DISCHARGE
4. THYROID	☐ NORMAL	☐ ABNORMAL	15. CERVIX	☐ NORMAL	☐ INFLAMMATION	☐ LESIONS
5. BREASTS	☐ NORMAL	☐ ABNORMAL	16. UTERUS	☐ NORMAL	☐ ABNORMAL	☐ FIBROIDS _____ WEEKS
6. LUNGS	☐ NORMAL	☐ ABNORMAL	17. ADNEXA	☐ NORMAL	☐ MASS	
7. HEART	☐ NORMAL	☐ ABNORMAL	18. DIAGONAL CONJUGATE	☐ REACHED	☐ NO	_____ CM
8. ABDOMEN	☐ NORMAL	☐ ABNORMAL	19. SPINES	☐ AVERAGE	☐ PROMINENT	☐ BLUNT
9. EXTREMITIES	☐ NORMAL	☐ ABNORMAL	20. SACRUM	☐ CONCAVE	☐ STRAIGHT	☐ ANTERIOR
10. SKIN	☐ NORMAL	☐ ABNORMAL	21. ARCH	☐ NORMAL	☐ WIDE	☐ NARROW
11. LYMPH NODES	☐ NORMAL	☐ ABNORMAL	22. PELVIC TYPE	GYNECOID	☐ YES	☐ NO

COMMENTS (Number and explain abnormals) _____
_____
_____
_____
_____

_____ **EXAM BY:** _____

Fig. 8.4 _(Continued)_ (B). _(Figure continues.)_

Patient Addressograph

ACOG ANTEPARTUM RECORD

DATE _____

NAME _____
       LAST   FIRST   MIDDLE

ID # _____

PROBLEMS/PLANS (DRUG ALLERGY:)	MEDICATION LIST:	Start date	Stop date
1.	1.		
2.	2.		
3.	3.		
4.	4.		

EDD CONFIRMATION

INITIAL EDD:

LMP ____/____/____ = EDD____/____/____
INITIAL EXAM ____/____/____ = ____ WKS. = EDD____/____/____
ULTRASOUND ____/____/____ = ____ WKS. = EDD____/____/____
INITIAL EDD ____/____/____ INITIALED BY _____

LMP ☐ DEFINITE   MENARCHE_____ (AGE ONSET)
☐ NORMAL AMOUNT/DURATION   MENSES MONTHLY ☐ YES ☐ NO
☐ APPROXIMATE (MONTH KNOWN)   FREQUENCY Q _____ DAYS
☐ UNKNOWN   PRIOR MENSES _____ DATE
                ON BCP'S AT CONCEPTION ☐ NO ☐ YES

HCG – ____/____/____   HCG + ____/____/____

18-20 WEEK EDD UPDATE:

QUICKENING ____/____/____ + 22 WKS. = ____/____/____
FUNDAL HT. AT UMBIL. ____/____/____ + 20 WKS. = ____/____/____
FHT W/FETOSCOPE ____/____/____ + 20 WKS. = ____/____/____
ULTRASOUND ____/____/____ = ____ WKS. = ____/____/____

FINAL EDD ____/____/____ INITIALED BY _____

32-34 WEEK EDD - UTERINE SIZE CONCORDANCE

± 4 OR MORE CMS. SUGGESTS THE NEED FOR ULTRASOUND EVALUATION

VISIT DATE (YEAR_____)													
WEEKS GEST. BEST EST.													
HT FUNDUS (CM.)													
PRESENTATION - VTX, BR, TRANSVERSE													
FHR PRESENT: F=FETOSCOPE O=ABSENT D=DOPTONE													
FETAL MOVEMENT: +=PRESENT D=DECREASED O=ABSENT													
PREMATURITY SIGNS/SYMPTOMS: VAGINAL BLEEDING													
MUCUS SHOW/DISCHARGE													
+ PRESENT CRAMPS/CONTRACTIONS													
O ABSENT DYSURIA													
PELVIC PRESSURE													
CERVIX EXAM (DIL./EFF./STA.)													
BLOOD PRESSURE INITIAL													
REPEAT													
EDEMA + PRESENT O ABSENT													
WEIGHT													
CUMULATIVE WEIGHT GAIN													
URINE: (GLUCOSE/ALBUMIN/KETONES)													
NEXT APPOINTMENT													
PROVIDER													
TEST REMINDERS	8-18 WEEKS CVS/AMNIO/MSAFP			24-28 WEEKS GLUCOSE SCREEN/RhIG									

Fig. 8.4 *(Continued)* (C). *(Figure continues.)*

GUIDELINES: EDUCATION AND LABORATORY

INITIAL LABS	DATE	RESULT	REVIEWED	COMMENTS/ADDITIONAL LAB
BLOOD TYPE	/ /	A B AB O		
RH TYPE	/ /	+ / –		
ANTIBODY SCREEN	/ /	– / +		
HCT/HGB	/ /	_____ % _____ gm/dl		
PAP SMEAR	/ /	NORMAL / ABNORMAL / _____		
RUBELLA	/ /	– / +		
VDRL	/ /	– / +		
GC	/ /	– / +		
URINE CULTURE / SCREEN	/ /	– / +		
HB S AG	/ /	– / +		

8 - 18 WEEK LABS (WHEN INDICATED)	DATE	RESULT		
ULTRASOUND	/ /			
MSAFP	/ /	_____ MOM		
AMNIO/CVS	/ /	– / +		
KARYOTYPE	/ /	46, XX OR 46, XY / OTHER _____		
ALPHA-FETOPROTEIN	/ /	NORMAL _____ ABNORMAL _____		

24 - 28 WEEK LABS (WHEN INDICATED)	DATE	RESULT		
HCT/HGB	/ /	_____ % _____ gm/dl		
DIABETES SCREEN	/ /	1 HR. _____		
GTT (IF SCREEN ABNORMAL)	/ /	____ FBS ____1 HR. ____2 HR. ____3 HR.		
RH ANTIBODY SCREEN	/ /	– / +		
RhIG GIVEN (28 WKS)	/ /	SIGNATURE _____		

32 - 36 WEEK LABS (WHEN INDICATED)	DATE	RESULT		
ULTRASOUND	/ /	– / +		
VDRL	/ /	– / +		
GC	/ /	– / +		
HCT/HGB	/ /	_____ % _____ gm/dl		

OPTIONAL LAB (HIGH RISK GROUPS)	DATE	RESULT		
HIV	/ /			
HGB ELECTROPHORESIS	/ /	AA AS SS AC SC AF		
CHLAMYDIA	/ /	– / +		

PLANS / EDUCATION

	COUNSELED YES NO		COUNSELED YES NO
TOXOPLASMOSIS PRECAUTIONS (CATS/RAW MEAT)_____		TUBAL STERILIZATION_____	
CHILDBIRTH CLASSES_____		VBAC COUNSELING_____	
PHYSICAL ACTIVITY_____		CIRCUMCISION_____	
PREMATURE LABOR SIGNS_____		TRAVEL _____	
NUTRITION COUNSELING_____		**REQUESTS** _____	
METHOD OF ANESTHESIA_____			
BREAST OR BOTTLE FEEDING_____		**OTHER** _____	
NEWBORN CAR SEAT_____			
POSTPARTUM BIRTH CONTROL_____		**TUBAL STERILIZATION** DATE INITIALS	
ENVIRONMENTAL/WORK HAZARDS_____		CONSENT SIGNED ____/____/____ _____	

Fig. 8.4 *(Continued)* (D).

send the clinician down a different and previously unexpected diagnostic and therapeutic path. The practitioner should seek all appropriate consultations so that the warning signs are heeded appropriately.

THE PRENATAL RECORD

As complex as it is, prenatal care should be documented by a prenatal record of good quality (Fig. 8.4). Many of the advances in risk assessment and in regionalization are a direct result of an improvement in this record. Technology allows sophisticated recording, display, and retrieval (often computer based) of prenatal care records, but quality relies on accurate compiling and recording of the information. The record must be complete, yet simple; directive, but flexible; transmittable, legible, and able to display necessary data rapidly. European nations often have one record for uniform care; many U.S. states and regions have adopted records to permit internal consistency, and the ACOG has recently developed the record reproduced here.

The commonly used records accurately reflect the following:

1. Demographic data, obstetric history
2. Medical and family history, including genetic screening
3. Baseline physical examination with emphasis on gynecologic examination
4. Menstrual history, especially last normal menstrual period
5. Information on individual visits
6. Routine laboratory data
7. Problem list
8. Space for special notations and plans

A typical prenatal record covers and records all the appropriate risk factors, documents gestational age and growth, and leaves room for intercurrent problems.

These records must be made available to consultants, and they should be available at the facility where delivery is planned. If transfer is expected, a copy of the prenatal record should accompany the patient.

PRENATAL EDUCATION

Patient education leads to better self-care. As maternal and neonatal outcomes improve, efforts become more sophisticated to improve understanding of, involvement in, and satisfaction with pregnancy and the perinatal period. In this area, more than in any other, the options for paramedical support have expanded. Practitioners and patients have access to a vast array of support persons and groups to assist and advise in the pregnancy and subsequent parenthood. It is the wise practitioner who stays abreast of these advances and integrates them into clinical practice. Patients should be educated about care options and participate in the decision making.

Drugs and Teratogens

At the prepregnancy or first prenatal visit, recommendations for nonpharmacologic remedies for common ailments can be given. They can often be integrated into a discussion of the common aggravations and uncomfortable side effects of pregnancy. Because of widespread use of over-the-counter drugs, the patient should be warned to take only those drugs specifically approved or prescribed to her by her practitioner (see Ch. 11).

Typical patient questions include "May I have my hair dyed?" and "May I paint my room?" If these activities are to be undertaken, exposure to any offensive fumes should be avoided and adequate ventilation is essential.

Radiologic Studies

Dental and radiologic diagnostic procedures should be performed during pregnancy when they are indicated. Dental restorative work especially should be performed to allow optimal maternal nutrition. Elective radiologic studies can safely be delayed until completion of the pregnancy.

Nutrition

One of the earliest purposes of prenatal care was to counsel and ensure that women received adequate nutrition for pregnancy. The health care provider may be influential in correcting inappropriate dietary

Wt gain: ~ 30# → 15# uterine contents - 8# baby   2# ut + 2# AFV
                    → 10# maternal fat/protein   2# placenta
                    → 5# — blood vol 2#
                         — breast 1#
                         — fluid retention 2#

Preconception and Prenatal Care   223

habits. Occasionally, consultation with a registered dietician may be necessary when there is poor compliance or a special medical need such as diabetes mellitus.

Eating wisely means choosing from the four basic food groups daily. Group 1 consists of fruits and vegetables; group 2 of whole-grain or enriched breads and cereals; group 3 of milk and milk products (e.g., cheese); and group 4 of meat, poultry, fish, eggs, nuts, and beans. Four or more daily servings from the first three groups and three or more servings from the fourth make a well-balanced diet. Pregnant women should particularly avoid uncooked meat because of the risk of toxoplasmosis. Pregnant women generally require 15 percent more kilocalories than nonpregnant women, usually 300 to 500 kcal more per day, depending on the patient's weight and activity.

Dietary allowances for most substances increase during pregnancy. According to the 1989 Recommended Daily Allowances only the recommendations for iron, folic acid, and vitamin D double during gestation. The RDA for calcium and phosphorus increase by one-half; the RDA for pyridoxine and thiamine increase by about one-third. The RDAs for protein, zinc, and riboflavin increase by about one-fourth. The recommendation for all other nutrients except vitamin A increase by less than 20 percent (Tables 8.3 and 8.4) and vitamin A not at all as it is thought to be stored adequately. All of these nutrients, with the exception of iron, are supplied by a well-balanced diet. The National Academy of Sciences currently recommends that 30 mg of ferrous iron supplements be given to pregnant women daily, because the iron content of the typical American diet and the iron stores of many women are not sufficient to provide the increased iron required during pregnancy. For those at high nutritional risk, such as some adolescents, women with multiple gestation, heavy cigarette smokers, and drug and alcohol abusers, a vitamin and mineral supplement can be given. Increased iron is needed both for the fetal needs and for the increased maternal blood volume. Thus iron-containing foods should also be encouraged. Iron is found in liver, red meats, eggs, dried beans, leafy green vegetables, whole-grain enriched breads and cereals, and dried fruits. The 30 mg iron supplement is contained in approximately 150 mg of ferrous sulfate, 300 mg of ferrous gluconate, or 100 mg of

ferrous fumarate. Taking iron between meals on an empty stomach will facilitate its absorption.

Because women of higher socioeconomic status have better reproductive performance and fewer low-birth-weight babies than do women of lower socioeconomic status, and because they also consume more protein, it is probably prudent to continue to recommend a generous amount of dietary protein. However, it has not been documented that protein supplementation will improve pregnancy outcome.[24] Acute caloric restriction in a well-nourished population such as occurred during the Dutch famine of 1944 to 1945 caused the average birth weight to drop about 250 g, yet no adverse effects on long-term outcome were observed. These mothers ate a calorie-restricted balanced diet in their second and third trimesters, and placental weight fell proportionally.

Weight Gain

The total weight gain recommended is 25 to 35 lb for normal women. Underweight women may gain up to 40 lb, and overweight women should limit weight gain to 25 lb[24a] (Fig. 8.5). About 2 to 3 lb are from increased fluid volume, 3 to 4 lb from increased blood volume, 1 to 2 lb from breast enlargement, 2 lb from enlargement of the uterus, and 2 lb from amniotic fluid. At term, the infant may weigh approximately 6 to 8 lb and the placenta 1 to 2 lb. A 4- to 6-lb increase in maternal stores of fat and protein are important for lactation. Usually 3 to 6 lb are gained in the first trimester and 0.5 to 1 lb per week in the last two trimesters of pregnancy.

If the patient does not gain 10 lb by midpregnancy, her nutritional status should be carefully evaluated. Inadequate weight gain may be associated with increased risk of a low-birth-weight infant (Fig. 8.6). Inadequate weight gain seems to have its greatest effect in women who are of low or normal weight before pregnancy. Underweight mothers must gain more weight during pregnancy to produce infants of normal weight. Patients should be cautioned against weight loss during pregnancy. Total weight gain in the obese can be modified downward to 15 lb, but less weight gain is associated with lack of expansion of plasma volume and with the risk of intrauterine growth retardation.

When excess weight gain is noted, an assessment for fluid retention is also performed. In the assess-

Table 8.3 1989 Recommended Dietary Allowances

| | Nonpregnant Women | | | | Lactation (Months) | |
	15–18	19–24	25–50	Pregnancy	1–6	7–12
Calories (kcal)						
Protein (g)	44	46	50	60	65	62
Vitamin A (μg RE)	800	800	800	800	1,300	1,200
Vitamin D (μg)	10	5	5	10	10	10
Vitamin E (mg TE)	8	8	8	10	12	11
Vitamin C (mg)	60	60	60	70	95	90
Thiamin (mg)	1.1	1.1	1.1	1.5	1.6	1.6
Riboflavin (mg)	1.3	1.3	1.3	1.6	1.8	1.7
Niacin (mg NE)	15	15	15	17	20	20
Vitamin B_6 (mg)	1.5	1.6	1.6	2.2	2.1	2.1
Folate (μg)	180	180	180	400	280	260
Vitamin B_{12} (μg)	2.0	2.0	2.0	2.2	2.6	2.6
Calcium (mg)	1,200	1,200	800	1,200	1,200	1,200
Phosphorus (mg)	1,200	1,200	800	1,200	1,200	1,200
Magnesium (mg)	300	280	280	320	355	340
Iron (mg)	15	15	15	30	15	15
Zinc (mg)	12	12	12	15	19	16
Iodine (μg)	150	150	150	175	200	200
Selenium μg	50	55	55	65	75	75

(Data from National Academy of Sciences.[35])

ment of edema, some dependent edema in the legs is normal as pregnancy advances because of venous compression by the weight of the uterus. Elevation of the feet and bed rest on the left side will help to correct this problem. Turning the patient from her back to her left side increases venous return from the legs as the pressure on the vena cava is relieved. This maneuver increases the effective circulating blood volume, cardiac output, and thus the blood flow to the kidney. A diuresis will follow, as well as increased blood flow to the uterus.

Limitation of fluids will neither prevent nor correct fluid retention. Salt is not restricted, although patients with hypertension may be advised to decrease salt load.

Rest

During the first trimester, patients are often more tired and should be advised to go to bed earlier or to try to take a nap during the day, if possible. Fatigue often lessens in the second trimester, but, in general, most patients need additional rest during pregnancy.

Activity and Employment

Most patients are able to maintain their normal activity levels in pregnancy. Mothers tolerate pregnancy with considerable physical activity, such as looking after small children, but certainly heavy lifting and excessive physical activity should be avoided. Modification of activity level as the pregnancy progresses is seldom needed, except if the job involves physical danger. Recreational exercises should be encouraged, such as those available in prenatal exercise classes. The patient should be counseled to discontinue activity whenever she experiences discomfort.

Healthy pregnant women may work until their delivery, if the job presents hazards no greater than those encountered in daily life. Strenuous physical exercise, standing for prolonged periods, and work on industrial machines as well as other adverse envi-

Table 8.4 Summary of Recommended Dietary Allowances for Women Aged ≥ 25 – 50 Years, Changes from Nonpregnant to Pregnant, and Food Sources

Nutrient	Nonpregnant	Pregnant	Percent Increase	Dietary Sources
Energy (kcal)	2,200	2,500	+13.6	Proteins, carbohydrates, fats
Protein (g)	50	60	+20	Meats, fish, poultry, dairy
Calcium (mg)	800	1,200	+50	Dairy products
Phosphorus (mg)	800	1,200	+50	Meats
Magnesium (mg)	280	320	+14.3	Seafood, legumes, grains
Iron (mg)	15	30	+100	Meats, eggs, grains
Zinc (mg)	12	15	+25	Meats, seafood, eggs
Iodine (μg)	150	175	+16.7	Iodized salt, seafood
Vitamin A (μg RE)	800	800	0	Dark green, yellow, or orange fruits and vegetables, liver
Vitamin D (IU)	200	400	+100	Fortified dairy products
Thiamin (mg)	1.1	1.5	+36.3	Enriched grains, pork
Riboflavin (mg)	1.3	1.6	+23	Meats, liver, enriched grains
Pyridoxine (mg)	1.6	2.2	+37.5	Meats, liver, enriched grains
Niacin (mg NE)	15	17	+13.3	Meats, nuts, legumes
Vitamin B_{12} (μg)	2.0	2.2	+10	Meats
Folic acid (μg)	180	400	+122	Leafy vegetables, liver
Vitamin C (mg)	60	70	+16.7	Citrus fruits, tomatoes
Selenium (μg)	55	65	+18.2	

(From National Academy of Sciences,[35] with permission.)

ronmental factors may be associated with increased risk of poor pregnancy outcome, and these should be modified as necessary.[25]

Travel

The patient should be advised against prolonged sitting during car travel because of the risk of venous stasis and possible thrombophlebitis. The usual recommendation is a maximum of 6 hr/day driving, with stopping at least every 2 hours for 10 minutes to allow the patient to walk around and increase venous return from the legs. Support stockings are also recommended for prolonged sitting in cars or airplanes.

The patient should be instructed to wear her seatbelt during car travel but to place it under the abdomen as pregnancy advances. It may also be helpful to take pillows along in a car to increase comfort.

If the patient is traveling a significant distance, it might be helpful for her to carry a copy of her medical record with her in case an emergency arises in a strange city. She could also check into the medical facilities in the area or perhaps obtain the name of an obstetrician in the event of a problem.

Immunizations

Because of a theoretical risk to the fetus, pregnant women or women likely to become pregnant should not be given live, attenuated-virus vaccines. Yellow fever and oral polio vaccines may be given to women exposed to maternal infection. Despite theoretical risks, no evidence of congenital rubella syndrome in infants born to mothers inadvertently given rubella vaccine have been reported. Measles, mumps, and rubella viruses are not transmitted by those immunized and can be given to children of pregnant women.

There is no evidence of fetal risk from inactivated virus vaccines, bacterial vaccines, toxoids, or tetanus immunoglobulin, and they should be administered if appropriate.

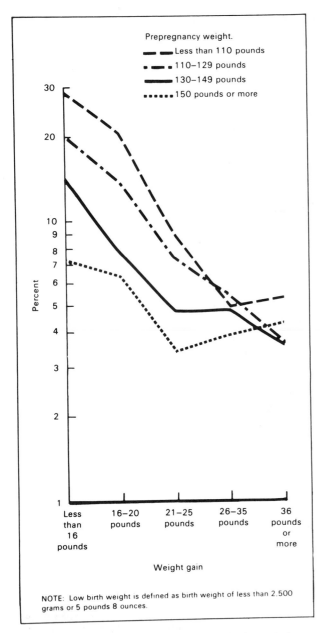

Fig. 8.5 Percent of liveborn infants of low birth weight by maternal weight gain during pregnancy according to mother's prepregnancy weight. 1980. National Natality Survey — United States. (From DHHS Pub. No. [PHS] 86-1922.[37]) Note: Low birth weight is defined as birth weight of less than 2,500 g or 5 pounds 8 ounces.

Nausea and Vomiting in Pregnancy

Nonpharmacologic measures are usually recommended initially to treat nausea and vomiting in early pregnancy. Patients should avoid eating greasy or spicy foods. In addition, frequent small feedings in order to keep some food in the stomach at all times is helpful. A protein snack at night is advised, and the patient is instructed to keep crackers at her bedside so that she can have these before arising in the morning. Drug therapy for nausea in pregnancy is covered in Chapter 11.

Heartburn

Heartburn is a common complaint in pregnancy because of the relaxation of the esophageal sphincter. Overeating contributes to this problem, as do spicy foods. The patient should be advised to save part of her meal for later if she is experiencing postprandial heartburn and also not to eat immediately before lying down. Pillows at bedtime may help. If necessary, antacids may be prescribed. Liquid antacids coat the esophageal lining more effectively than do tablets.

Hemorrhoids

Hemorrhoids are varicose veins of the rectum. Because straining during bowel movements contributes to their aggravation, avoidance of constipation is preventative, and prolonged sitting should also be avoided. Hemorrhoids will often regress after delivery but usually will not disappear completely.

Constipation

Constipation is physiologic during pregnancy with decreased bowel transit time, and the stool may be hardened. Dietary modification with increased bulk such as with fresh fruit and vegetables and plenty of water can usually help this problem significantly. Constipation is aggravated by the addition of iron supplementation; if dietary measures are inadequate, patients may require stool softeners. Additional dietary fibers such as Metamucil (psyllium hydrophilic muciloid) or surface-active agents such as Colace (docusate) are recommended. Laxatives are rarely necessary.

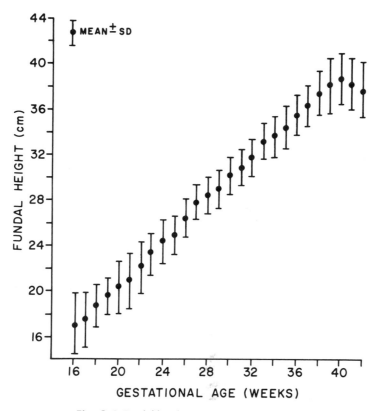

Fig. 8.6 Fundal height versus gestational age.

Urinary Frequency

Often during the first 3 months of pregnancy, the growing uterus places increased pressure on the bladder. Urinary frequency usually will improve as the uterus rises out of the pelvis by the second trimester. However, as the fetus' head engages near the time of delivery, urinary frequency may return as the head presses against the bladder. If the patient experiences pain with urination, it is appropriate to check for infection.

Round Ligament Pain

Frequently, patients will notice sharp groin pains caused by spasm of the round ligaments associated with movement. This is more frequently felt on the right side because of the usual dextrorotation of the uterus. The pain may be helped by application of local heat such as with hot soaks or a heating pad. Patients may awaken at night with this pain after having sud-denly rolled over in their sleep without realizing it. During the daytime, however, modification of activity with gradual rising and sitting down, as well as avoidance of sudden movement, will decrease problems with this type of pain. Analgesics are rarely necessary.

Syncope

Compression of the veins in the legs from the advancing size of the uterus places patients at risk of venous pooling associated with prolonged standing. This may lead to syncope. Measures to avoid this possibility include wearing support stockings and exercising the calves to increase venous return. In later pregnancy, patients may have problems with supine hypotension, a distinct problem when undergoing a medical evaluation such as an ultrasound examination. A left lateral tilt position with wedging below the right hip will help to keep the weight of the pregnancy off the inferior vena cava.

Backache

Backache can be prevented to a large degree by avoidance of excessive weight gain. Exercises to strengthen back muscles can also be helpful. Posture is important, and sensible shoes should be worn, not high heels.

Sexual Activity

No restriction need generally be placed on sexual intercourse. The patient is instructed that pregnancy may cause changes in comfort and sexual desire. Frequently, increased uterine activity is noted after sexual intercourse; it is unclear whether this is due to breast stimulation, female orgasm, or prostaglandins in male ejaculate. In women at risk for preterm labor or with a history of previous pregnancy loss and who note such increased activity, use of a condom or avoidance of sexual activity may be recommended.

Circumcision

Newborn circumcision prevents phimosis and has been shown to decrease the incidence of cancer of the penis. It may result in a decreased incidence of urinary tract infections in children but prospective studies have not confirmed this.[26] Evidence concerning the association of sexually transmitted diseases and circumcision is conflicting. Education in good personal hygiene offers many of the advantages of circumcision without the risks. If circumcision is considered, the benefits and risks should be explained to the parents and informed consent obtained.

Circumcision in the newborn is an elective procedure and should be performed only if the infant is stable and healthy. Local anesthesia may reduce the observed physiologic response to newborn circumcision but has its own inherent risks.

Breast-Feeding

During prenatal visits, the patient should be encouraged to breast-feed her infant. Human milk is the most appropriate nutrient for human infants and also provides significant immunologic protection against infection. Infants who are breast-fed have a lower incidence of infection and require fewer hospitalizations than do infants who are fed formula exclusively.

Other advantages of lactation include economy, convenience, more rapid involution of the uterus, and natural child spacing. The reasons a woman decides to bottle-feed should be explored, as they may be based on a misconception. Encouragement will sometimes convince a hesitant mother who may then be able to nurse successfully.

Working outside the home need not be a contraindication to breast-feeding. Many women who previously would not have considered nursing an option, such as those with careers, are now finding time to breast-feed their infants. Nursing for only a few weeks or months is better than not nursing at all. Women should be aware that alternative ways of breast-feeding can be used to correspond with their work schedules. They can decrease the frequency of lactation to a few times a day in most cases and still continue to nurse. Other women may pump their breasts at work, leaving milk for the child's caretaker during the day and thus providing breast milk to the infant even more frequently. The milk may be collected in containers and if refrigerated is safe to use for 24 hours. For a longer duration, the milk should be frozen. Because freezing and thawing destroys the cellular content, fresh milk is preferred.

There is no need for specific nipple preparation during pregnancy. In one study, women prepared one nipple and not the other with a variety of techniques, including massage and breast creams, and found no difference in the two.[27] Soap and drying agents should not be used on the nipples, which should be washed only with water.

Preparation for Childbirth

The introduction of childbirth education and consumerism has had significant impact on the practice of obstetrics. The success of obstetric practice in preventing disasters has allowed interest to focus on the quality of the child and of the perinatal experience. Studies have shown that prepared childbirth can have a beneficial effect on performance in labor and delivery.[28] The prenatal period should be one in which the patient is exposed to information about pregnancy, normal labor and delivery, anesthesia and analgesia, obstetric complications, and obstetric operations (e.g., episiotomy, cesarean delivery, and forceps or vacuum delivery). The prenatal clinic is an appropriate place to obtain informed consent from the patient for her intrapartum care and management. Certainly, this affords a more dispassionate, quiet, and pain-free environment than the labor and delivery suite.

The education mentioned above is more than can be transmitted by the obstetrician at the initial or the shorter return visits, and patients expect more personal involvement than to be given a book or handout to read. The appropriate place for such education is a series of planned, structured prenatal education classes taught by informed, qualified individuals. These classes can be given in the physician's office, at the hospital, or in free-standing classes. National organizations such as the Childbirth Education Association and the American Society for Psychoprophylaxis in Obstetrics have recognized the need for such instruction and teach prepared childbirth. There are also advantages to office- and hospital-based programs, if the patient volume permits it, because specifics of management and alternatives offered by that practice or hospital can be discussed in these programs. On the other hand, free-standing classes offer the advantage of open-endedness and of presenting many options to the patient, who can then discuss them with her care provider. Many advances in alternative family-centered practice (e.g., allowing fathers in the delivery room and operating room) have come from consumer requests and demands. A pregnant patient often makes a list of what she would like in the peripartum period and to discuss with her practitioner. Thus the care provider can understand her needs and desires, better address these needs and desires if labor and delivery do not proceed normally or as planned, and explain why certain requests are not possible or reasonable.

Signs of Labor

It is important to instruct the patient about certain warning signs that should trigger a call to her care provider or a visit to the hospital. All women should be informed of what to do if contractions become regular, if rupture of membranes is suspected, or if vaginal bleeding occurs. Patients should be given a number to call where assistance is available 24 hours a day.

Prepared Parenthood and Support Groups

As pregnancy progresses, special needs often arise; increasingly, educational support groups are being organized to assist in dealing with such needs. Support groups for families with Down syndrome infants, for mothers of twins, and for women who have had cesarean delivery have all shown that they can meet the special needs of these people. Parenthood is something that all successful obstetric patients face, and, as such, integration of parenting education in prenatal education has merit. Many parents are completely unprepared for the myriad of changes in their lives, and some idea of what to expect is beneficial.

Unsuccessful pregnancies lead to special problems and needs, for which social workers, clergy, and specialized support groups can be invaluable. Miscarriage, stillbirth, and infant death are particularly devastating events, best managed by a team approach with special attention to the needs of the grieving process. Referral to such groups as Compassionate Friends of Miscarriage, Infant Death, and Stillbirth is recommended.

ASSESSMENT OF GESTATIONAL AGE

During the course of the prenatal interview, assessment of gestational age begins with the question, "What was the first day of the last menstrual period?" From that point, the establishment of an estimated date of confinement and confirmation of that date by accumulation of supportive information remains one of the most important tasks of good prenatal care.

Human pregnancy has a duration of 280 days, measuring from the first day of the last menstrual period (LMP) until delivery. The standard deviation is 14 days. It is important to remember that clinicians are measuring menstrual weeks (not conceptional weeks) with an assumption of ovulation and conception based on day 14 of a 28-day cycle. This gives pregnancy the 40-week gestational period in common clinical use. Much confusion exists among patients who try to measure pregnancy in terms of 9 months $(40/4 = 10)$ or who try to measure in conceptional weeks. Another problem exists in women whose menstrual cycles do not follow a 28-day cycle and who therefore do not conceive on day 14 of the menstrual cycle.

It is often helpful to explain to patients and their families that their pregnancy will be described in terms of weeks, rather than months, and that the pregnancy can be broken into three trimesters lasting

1 to 14 weeks, 14 to 28 weeks, and 28 weeks to delivery. The commonly used term "4 months pregnant" has no meaning (one does not know whether this is 16 or 20 weeks), and has no place on a contemporary prenatal record. Every effort should be made to be consistent in usage in order to prevent confusion among patients and among clinicians who may assume care of the pregnancy.

Knowledge of gestational age is critical for obstetric decision making. Generally, in a normal pregnancy, one can extrapolate from gestational age to estimate fetal weight. Throughout pregnancy, these are the two most important determinants of fetal viability and survival. Without accurate knowledge of gestational age, diagnosis of such conditions as postterm pregnancy and intrauterine growth retardation is often impossible. Early detection of multiple gestation is most often made when the size of the uterine fundus is greater than expected for gestation. Appropriate management of preterm labor, previous cesarean section, or a medically complicated pregnancy depends on an accurate estimate of fetal age and size. Within regional perinatal systems, records of gestational age are important for flow of information and patients, and rapid access to consistent and clear data is vital. In such situations, and during prolonged hospitalization, it is sometimes helpful to define gestational age further by using the notation of fractional weeks (27 4/7 weeks). It must be remembered, however, that we are describing a biologic system and that such precision is being used more for ease of communication and organization than for any ability to date the pregnancy with such a degree of accuracy.

Clinical Dating

The most reliable clinical estimator of gestational age is an accurate LMP. Using Naegele's rule, the estimated date of confinement is calculated by subtracting 3 months and adding 1 week from the first day of the LMP. A careful history must be taken from the patient to ensure that the date given is the first day of the period and to determine whether the period was normal, heavy, or light. The date of the previous menstrual period will help to ascertain the length of the cycle. History should also be taken about previous use of oral contraceptives, which might influence ovulation.

Other clinical tools can be used to confirm and support LMP data, and, in cases in which the LMP is inaccurate or unknown, it has been shown that accumulated clinical information from early pregnancy can predict gestational age with an accuracy approaching that of menstrual dating, providing the best obstetric estimate.[29]

The size of the uterus on early pelvic examination, or by direct measurement of the abdomen from the pubic symphysis to the top of the uterine fundus (over the curve), provides useful information. Experienced practitioners can assess the early pregnancy with reproducibility before 12 to 14 weeks. Fundal height measurement in centimeters using the over-the-curve technique approximates the gestational age from 16 to 38 weeks within 3 cm (Fig. 8.6).

The uterus also tends to reach the umbilicus at about 20 weeks, and this too can be assessed when uterine fundal measurements are made.[29] The uterus may be elevated in early pregnancy in a patient with a previous cesarean section, making the fundal height appear abnormally high. Considerable variation in the level of the umbilicus and in the height of patients make this clinical marker variable. Quickening, the first perception of fetal movement by the mother, occurs at predictable times in gestation. In the first pregnancy, quickening is usually noted at about 19 weeks; in subsequent pregnancies, probably because of the experience of the observer, it tends to occur about 2 weeks earlier.[29] It is helpful to ask the woman to mark on a calendar the first time she feels the baby move and to report this date.

Audible fetal heart tones, in addition to being absolute evidence of pregnancy, are another marker of gestational age. Using an unamplified DeLee-Hillis fetoscope, they are generally audible at 19 to 20 weeks.[29] Observer experience, acuity, and the time spent listening can all affect this number, so this guideline may need to be adapted individually.

Use of the electronic Doppler device is widespread and permits detection of the fetal heart by 11 to 12 weeks. Practitioners can set a standard individualized to their own equipment, which can be used as a gestational age marker. If fetal heart tones are not heard at the expected time, an ultrasound is appropriate to look for date and examination discrepancies, polyhydramnios, fetal viability, and twins.

The conversion of a negative urinary pregnancy test to a positive one may be helpful in assessing gestational age, but the sensitivity of the test used must be known in order to interpret the data accurately (see Ch. 3). Home pregnancy tests may be falsely positive, and these tests may be negative if they are performed too early.

Comparison of the various clinical estimators shows that a known date of the LMP to be the most precise predictor. The clinical estimators can be ranked according to decreasing order of accuracy as follows: (1) last menstrual period, (2) the uterus reaching the umbilicus, and (3) fetal heart tone documentation, fundal height measurements, and quickening. Because of inherent biologic variability and differences in examiner acuity, the estimated date of confinement can be predicted with 90 percent certainty only within ±3 weeks by even the best single estimator.[30]

Ultrasound

Ultrasound plays a major role in assessment of size and duration of pregnancy. The National Institutes of Health consensus conference in 1984 concluded that in a low-risk pregnancy followed from the first trimester, routine ultrasound examination was not justified for determining gestational age. However, a long list of indications justify an ultrasound examination.[31] Also, a randomized trial has shown that the risk of a pregnancy being considered overdue was reduced from 8 to 2 percent for patients who received early ultrasound[32] (see Ch. 11). In the future, routine prenatal care may well include use of ultrasound at 16 to 20 weeks for a baseline gestational age measurement and as a screen for fetal abnormalities or multiple gestation.

Ultrasound is an accurate means of estimating gestational age in the first half of pregnancy.[33] The crown–rump length, biparietal diameter, and femur length in the first half of pregnancy correlate closely with age. As pregnancy progresses, however, there is considerable variability in fetal size, and measurement of the fetus is a poor tool for estimation of gestational age in the third trimester (see Ch. 11).

Assessment of Fetal Maturity Before Repeat Cesarean Delivery or Elective Induction of Labor

The ACOG Committee on Obstetrics: Maternal Fetal Medicine[34] states that in a gestation in which 39 weeks have elapsed since the LMP in a patient with normal menstrual cycles and no immediate antecedent use of oral contraceptives, fetal maturity can be assumed if one of the following *clinical criteria* for estimating gestational age are supported by at least one of the following *laboratory determinations:*

Clinical criteria

1. Fetal heart tones have been documented for at least 20 weeks by nonelectronic fetoscope or at least 30 weeks by Doppler
2. Uterine size has been established by pelvic examination prior to 16 weeks of gestation

Laboratory determinations

1. Thirty-six weeks have elapsed since a positive serum or urine human chorionic gonadotropin pregnancy test
2. Ultrasound
   a. Measurement based on the crown–rump length obtained between 6 and 12 weeks of gestation, or
   b. Other ultrasound confirmation of gestational age obtained before 24 weeks of gestation

SUMMARY

Prenatal care is an effective, if incompletely understood and studied, intervention. Preconception care will introduce changes and improve it. Risk assessment (with subsequent elimination or management of risks), health education, advocacy, disease prevention, and appropriate medical management of complications remain the core of the process. Changes in number of visits and improved understanding of the successful components of prenatal care will improve services and efficiency without altering the substance of what has been developed and achieved.

REFERENCES

1. Oakley A: The origins and development of antenatal care. p. 8. In Enkin M, Chalmers I (eds): Effectiveness and Satisfaction in Antenatal Care. Spastics International Medical Publications, Philadelphia, 1982
2. Caring for Our Future: The Content of Prenatal Care. Public Health Service Expert Panel Report. PHS-DHHS, Washington, DC, 1989
3. Chalmers I, Enkin M, Keirse M: Effective care in preg-

nancy and childbirth. Oxford University Press, Oxford, 1989

4. Rochat RW, Koonin LM, Atrach HK, Jewett JF, the Maternal Mortality Collaborative: Maternal mortality in the United States: report from the Maternal Mortality Collaborative. Obstet Gynecol 72:91, 1988

5. Rosenfield A: Maternal mortality in developing countries: an ongoing but neglected "epidemic." JAMA 262:376, 1989

6. Hobel CJ, Hyvarinen MA, Okada DM et al: Prenatal and antepartum high risk screening. 1. Prediction of the high risk neonate. Am J Obstet Gynecol 117:1, 1973

7. Mueller-Heubach E, Guzick DS: Evaluation of risk scoring in a preterm birth prevention study of indigent patients. Obstet Gynecol 160:829, 1989

8. Chamberlain G, Lumley J: Pre-Pregnancy Care: A Manual for Practice. John Wiley, London, 1986

9. Moos MK, Cefalo RC: Preconceptional health promotion: a focus for obstetric care. Am J Perinatol 4:63, 1987

10. Milunsky A, Jick H, Jick S et al: Multi vitamin/folic acid supplementation in early pregnancy reduces the prevalence of neural tube defects. JAMA 262:2847, 1989

11. Mulinare J, Cordero JF, Erickson JD, Berry RJ: Periconceptional use of multivitamins and the occurrence of neural tube defects. JAMA 260:3141, 1988

12. Mills JL, Rhoads GG, Simpson JL et al: The absence of a relation between the periconceptional use of vitamins and neural-tube defects. N Engl J Med 321:430, 1989

13. Hook EB: Rates of chromosome abnormalities at different maternal ages. Obstet Gynecol 58:282, 1981

14. Stene J, Fischer G, Steve E et al: Paternal age effect in Down's syndrome. Am J Hum Genet 40:299, 1977

15. Moore RD, Bone LR, Geller G et al: Prevalence, detection, and treatment of alcoholism in hospitalized patients. JAMA 261:403, 1989

16. Sokol RJ, Martier SS, Ager JW: The T-ACE questions: practical prenatal detection of risk-drinking. Am J Obstet Gynecol 160:863, 1989

17. Creasy RC, Gummer BA, Liggins GC: System for predicting spontaneous preterm birth. Obstet Gynecol 55:692, 1980

18. Main D, Richardson DK, Hadley CB, Gabbe S: Controlled trial of a preterm labor detection program: efficacy and costs. Obstet Gynecol 74:823, 1989

19. Abbasi IA, Hess LW, Johnson TRB Jr et al: Leukocyte esterase activity in the rapid detection of urinary tract and lower genital tract infection in pregnancy. Am J Perinatol 2:311, 1985

20. American College of Obstetricians and Gynecologists: Committee Opinion, Number 78, ACOG, Washington, DC, January 1990

21. American College of Obstetricians and Gynecologists: Standards for Obstetric and Gynecologic Services. 7th Ed. ACOG, Washington, DC, 1989

22. American Academy of Pediatrics/American College of Obstetricians and Gynecologists: Guidelines for Perinatal Care. 2nd Ed. ACOG, Washington, DC, 1988

23. Grant A, Elbourne D, Valentin L, Alexander S: Routine fetal movement counting and risk of antepartum rate death in normally formed singletons. Lancet 2:345, 1989

24. Zlatnik FJ, Burmeister LF: Dietary protein in pregnancy: effect on anthropometric indices of the newborn infant. Am J Obstet Gynecol 146:199, 1983

24a. Food and Nutrition Board, Institute of Medicine, National Academy of Sciences: Nutrition During Pregnancy. p 10. National Academy Press, Washington, DC, 1990

25. Mamelle N, Laumon B, Lazar P: Prematurity and occupational activity during pregnancy. Am J Epidemiol 119:309, 1984

26. American Academy of Pediatrics Task Force on Circumcision. Pediatrics 84:388, 1989

27. Brown MS, Hurloch JT: Preparation of the breast for breast feeding. Nurs Res 24:449, 1975

28. Scott JR, Rose NB: Effect of psychoprophylaxis (Lamaze preparation) on labor and delivery in primiparas. N Engl J Med 294:1205, 1976

29. Andersen HF, Johnson TRB, Flora JD et al: Gestational age assessment. II. Prediction from combined clinical observations. Am J Obstet Gynecol 140:770, 1981

30. Kramer MS, McLean FH, Boyd ME, Usher RH: The validity of gestational age estimation by menstrual dating in term, preterm and postterm gestations. JAMA 260:3306, 1988

31. U.S. Department of Health and Human Services: Ultrasound Imaging In Pregnancy. NIH Publ. No. 84-667. National Institutes of Health, Washington, DC, 1984

32. Saari-Kemppainen A, Karjalainen O, Ylöstalo P, Heinonen OP: Ultrasound screening and perinatal mortality: controlled trial of systematic one-stage screening in pregnancy. Lancet 336:387, 1990

33. Reece EA, Gabrielli S, Degennaro N, Hobbins JC: Dating through pregnancy: a measure of growing up. Obstet Gynecol Surv 44:544, 1989

34. American College of Obstetricians and Gynecologists: Committee Opinion, Number 77, ACOG, Washington, DC, January 1990

35. National Academy of Sciences: Recommended Dietary Allowances. 10th Ed. National Academy Press, Washington, DC, 1989

36. MMWR 37(SS5):26, 1988

37. Taffel S: Maternal Weight Gain and the Outcome of Pregnancy, 1980. No. 21(44). National Center for Health Statistics, Washington, DC, 1986

Chapter 9

Teratology and the Epidemiology of Birth Defects*

Mary Ellen Mortensen, Lowell E. Sever, and Godfrey P. Oakley, Jr.

All pregnant women want to have a normal baby who will develop into a normal, healthy adult. Unfortunately, this wish is not always fulfilled. This chapter considers prenatal environmental influences as a cause of adverse embryologic and fetal maldevelopment. The focus is on structural malformations, but some attention is paid to aberrations in behavior and to other adverse reproductive outcomes. The importance of birth defects as a cause of human mortality, the etiology of birth defects and basic concepts of teratology, epidemiologic methods used to evaluate possible adverse effects of environmental exposures on reproductive outcomes, and data about some specific environmental and occupational exposures are reviewed.

IMPORTANCE OF BIRTH DEFECTS

A country's infant mortality rate is often used as a measure of the health of its children. In general, when the infant mortality rate is high (25 to 150 deaths before age 1 year per 1,000 live births), infectious diseases are a major contributor. When the

rate is less than 25 per 1,000 live births, birth defects, low birth weight, and sudden infant death syndrome (SIDS) become the leading causes, and infectious diseases become relatively unimportant. For example, in the United States in 1986 these three causes of infant mortality accounted for 52 percent of all infant deaths (Table 9.1). Also in 1986, birth defects were the underlying cause of death for 8,005 infants under 1 year of age in the United States. This made birth defects the leading cause of infant mortality, responsible for 20.5 percent of infant deaths. In addition, birth defects were considered to be a contributing cause in another 1,088 deaths.[1]

In developed countries, the public health impact of birth defects can also be shown by calculating "years of potential life lost" because of these conditions. Years of potential life lost is a measure that quantifies the impact of various causes of death on the mortality patterns of the nation. In the United States in 1986, birth defects were the fifth leading cause of years of potential life lost, accounting for 651,523 years, or approximately 5.4 percent of all years of potential life lost that year.[2]

A decrease in infant mortality to no more than 9 infant deaths per 1,000 live births by 1990 was established in 1980 as part of the health objectives for the United States.[3] As part of the *Year 2000 Health Objectives,* a goal of 7 per 1,000 live births is recommended.[4] To reach these goals, deaths caused by birth defects have to be reduced. An important strategy is

233

Table 9.1 Infant Mortality in the United States, 1986

Cause of Death	No. of Deaths	Percent
Birth defects	8,005	20.5
Low birth weight	6,934	17.8
Sudden infant death syndrome	5,337	13.7
Subtotal	20,276	52.0
All other causes	18,681	48.0
Total	38,957	100.0

(Adapted from Centers for Disease Control.[1])

to discover whether there are environmental factors that can cause these adverse reproductive outcomes and reduce exposure to these factors.

Data on morbidity and on the costs of care for infants born with the conditions that are leading causes of infant mortality and potential years of life lost are not readily available. Without a doubt, these conditions have substantial impact on morbidity as well as on the cost of health care and other services (Table 9.2).

EPIDEMIOLOGY OF BIRTH DEFECTS

Epidemiology is concerned with the distribution and determinants (causes) of diseases. A major goal is to identify associations that suggest disease etiology; such knowledge of causal mechanisms can be used to prevent and control disease. In applying epidemiologic methods to examine the causes of birth defects, one is immediately confronted with a challenge: the etiologies of most defects are unknown. Even for defects considered to have polygenic or multifactorial causes, such as cardiac defects, many unanswered questions concerning etiology remain. Table 9.3, based on data from Wilson,[5] shows the distribution of causes of birth defects in humans and the approximate percentages of defects attributable to each.

ETIOLOGY OF BIRTH DEFECTS

Genetic transmission accounts for about 20 percent of birth defects. The number of disorders known to have a genetic basis is increasing, as reference to successive editions of McKusick's catalog of genetic dis-

Table 9.2 Estimated Potential Years of Life Lost Before Age 65 Years — United States, 1987

Cause of Death	Potential Years of Life Lost	Percent of Total	Rank
Unintentional injuries	2,295,710	19.7	1
Cancer	1,821,682	15.1	2
Heart disease	1,534,607	12.7	3
Suicide/homicide	1,342,693	11.1	4
Congenital anomalies	651,523	5.4	5
Prematurity	438,351	3.6	6
Sudden infant death syndrome	313,555	2.6	7
Acquired immunodeficiency syndrome	246,823	2.0	8
Cerebrovascular disease	232,583	1.9	9
Chronic liver diseases and cirrhosis	225,028	1.9	10

Potential years of life lost, up to age 65 years, is the summation from 0 to 65 years of the number of deaths by cause in each age group during 1986 times 75 less age (in years) at death (using a midpoint of 5-year age groups). The Cause of Death categories and rates are from the National Center for Health Statistics.[244]

orders shows.[6,7] The overall percentage of defects attributable to genetic transmission, however, has not changed in any dramatic fashion. Genetic disorders are considered in Chapter 8 and are not discussed further in this chapter.

Chromosomal aberrations, such as aneuploidies, translocations, and deletions, account for about 5 percent of defects. As with the simple genetic disorders, the number of identifiable chromosomally based defects is increasing with advances in cytogenetic methodology. Additional malformation syndromes and cases of mental retardation are probably related to previously unrecognized chromosomal defects. Still, the percentage of all defects that can be attributed to chromosomal causes is small. Chromosomal defects are also discussed in Chapter 8 and are not considered further here.

The general category of environmental causes, in Wilson's categorization,[5] includes both exogenous causes and those related to the maternal environment. Although exogenous factors are mediated by the mother, conditions intrinsic to her can adversely affect intrauterine development. For example, maternal diabetes,[8] maternal phenylketonuria (PKU),[9] and maternal thyroid disease[5] have all been associated with birth defects in the offspring. These fall into Wilson's category of maternal metabolic imbalances, accounting for about 2 percent of the defects.

Although much interest and concern focuses on the exogenous causes of birth defects, in terms of the

recognized causes, such factors are implicated in only about 10 percent of all birth defects. The known environmental causes of human birth defects include acute, high-dose ionizing radiation, maternal infections, drugs, and one chemical pollutant, the organomercurial methylmercury. For this discussion, the term environmental is restricted to those agents or chemical substances that can occur as contaminants in the ambient or occupational environment. The importance of the teratogenic effects of drugs in pregnancy is discussed in Chapter 11, and the teratogenic effects of infections during pregnancy are reviewed in Chapter 40.

TERATOLOGY

Basic Principles

To understand the etiology of birth defects, one must look at what is known about the principles of abnormal development. Although we have noted that only a small percentage of birth defects can be linked to known environmental agents, the search for other similar agents is important. Thus some fundamental aspects of teratology must be considered.

Teratology has been defined as the study of abnormal development; it is directed at understanding the causes and mechanisms of maldevelopment. A teratogen is a substance, organism, or physical agent capable of causing abnormal development. A teratogen can cause abnormalities of structure or function, growth retardation, or death of the organism.

Traditionally, identification and definition of a teratogenic agent were based on its ability to produce structural defects. More recently, the concept of teratogenesis has been expanded to include agents that act during embryonic or fetal development and lead to deviation from normal morphology or function. There is growing interest in exploring the role of prenatal factors in more subtle or difficult-to-ascertain effects, such as growth retardation and developmental and behavioral abnormalities. A major area of current interest is behavioral teratology. Wilson's six general principles of teratology[10] provide a framework for understanding how structural or functional

Table 9.3 Causes of Developmental Defects in Humans

Cause	Percent
Genetic transmission	20
Chromosomal aberrations	5
Environmental causes	
Ionizing radiation	1–2
Infections	1–2
Maternal metabolic imbalances	1–2
Drugs and environmental chemicals	4–6
Interactions/combinations	
Unknown	65–70

(Adapted from Wilson,[5] with permission.)

teratogens may act. These principles are briefly summarized below.

Genotype and Interaction With Environmental Factors

The first of Wilson's principles is that susceptibility to a teratogen depends on the genotype of the conceptus and on the manner in which the genotype interacts with environmental factors. This is perhaps most clearly shown by experiments in which different genetic strains of mice have varied greatly in their susceptibility to teratogens that lead to oral clefts.[11] Some of the variability in responses to human teratogens, such as to phenytoin, relates to genetically-determined differences in activity of the enzyme, epoxide hydrolase.[11a]

Timing of Exposure

The second of Wilson's principles is that susceptibility of the conceptus to teratogenic agents varies with the developmental stage at the time of exposure. This concept of critical stages of development is particularly applicable to alterations in structure. It is during the second to eighth weeks of development after conception—the embryonic period—that most structural defects occur. For such defects, it is believed that there is a critical stage in the developmental process, after which abnormal embryogenesis cannot be initiated. For example, most investigators believe that the neural tube defects (NTDs) anencephaly and spina bifida result from the failure of the neural tube to close. Because this process occurs between 22 and 28 days postconception, any exogenous effect on development must be present at or before this time. Discussions of thalidomide teratogenicity have clearly shown that the effects of the drug differ as a function of the developmental stage at which the pregnant woman took it (Table 9.4).[12] For functional defects, little is known about the existence of critical periods.[13]

Mechanisms

The third of Wilson's principles is that teratogenic agents act in specific ways (mechanisms) on developing cells and tissues in initiating abnormal embryogenesis (pathogenesis). Teratogenic mechanisms are considered separately below.

Table 9.4 Human Malformations Resulting from Maternal Ingestion of Thalidomide

Malformation[a]	Timing of Exposure (Days Since Last Menstrual Period)
Anotia, facial nerve paralysis	35–38
Ear malformations	38–46
Absence of arms	38–45
Phocomelia of arms	39–46
Cardiac malformations	39–45
Duodenal atresia	39–45
Absence of legs	41–44
Phocomelia of legs	41–47

[a] The type of malformation could be related, approximately, to the time when the pregnant woman took the drug. This illustrates the concept of critical or sensitive periods during development. Most of the severe malformations could be attributed to thalidomide ingestion during a critical period between 35 and 50 days after the last menses.
(Data from Lenke and Levy,[9] Wilson,[10] and Fraser.[11])

Manifestations

Wilson's fourth principle is that the final manifestations of abnormal development are death, malformation, growth retardation, and functional disorder. Let us reemphasize that the manifestation may depend on the stage of development at which exposure occurred. Thus a particular teratogen may have one effect if exposure occurs during embryogenesis and another if the exposure was during the fetal period. Embryonic exposure is likely to lead to structural abnormalities or to embryonic death, whereas fetal exposure is likely to lead to functional deficits or growth retardation.

Agent

The fifth of Wilson's principles is that access of adverse environmental influences to developing tissues depends on the nature of the influence (agent). This principle relates to such factors as dosage, maternal metabolism, and placental passage. This is most clearly understood for chemical agents, but the principle also applies to physical agents such as radiation or heat. For an adverse effect to occur, an agent must reach the conceptus, either by being transmitted indirectly through maternal tissues or by directly traversing the maternal body.

Dose Effect

Wilson's sixth and final principle is that manifestations of deviant development increase in degree as dosage increases from the no-effect to the lethal level. This means that the response (e.g., malformation, growth retardation) may be expected to vary according to the dose, duration, or amount of exposure. For most human teratogens, this response is not clearly understood; however, along with the principle of critical stages of development, these concepts are important in supporting causal inferences about human reproductive hazards.

Mechanisms of Teratogenesis

In identifying human teratogens, it is important to consider the mechanisms of teratogenesis, Wilson's third principle. Wilson[10] suggested that the initial changes in developing cells or tissues after teratogenic insult can be categorized into nine mechanisms of teratogenic action. The schema Wilson proposed is that an agent acts via a mechanism that alters normal cellular or biochemical processes. Acting through final common pathways, different alterations can produce similar final defects. The following are suggested mechanisms: gene mutation, chromosomal abnormalities (e.g., breaks and nondisjunction), mitotic interference, altered nucleic acid integrity or function, lack of normal precursors or substrates, altered energy sources, changes in membrane characteristics, osmolar imbalance, and enzyme inhibition. With these mechanisms in mind, it may be easier to understand why such diverse etiologies for spina bifida as maternal hyperthermia and vitamin deficiency have been hypothesized.

In identifying reproductive hazards, relationships among teratogenesis, mutagenesis, and carcinogenesis should be considered.[14] Because these processes may occur through similar mechanisms, this is a logical approach. Hemminki and associates[15] illustrated how various manifestations, classified as teratogenic, mutagenic, or carcinogenic, could result from alterations of DNA. Thus attempts to identify human teratogens should take these potential relationships into account.

CONSIDERATIONS IN IDENTIFYING HUMAN TERATOGENS

Known and Suspected Human Teratogens and Reproductive Toxins

The number of clearly demonstrated human teratogens and reproductive toxins is limited. Table 9.5 lists known and suspected agents in three categories: infectious agents, drugs and chemicals, and physical agents.[16] This chapter focuses on chemicals and physical agents.

The complexity of the issues surrounding, identifying, and regulating teratogens and developmental toxins is illustrated by California's Safe Drinking Water and Toxics Enforcement Act of 1986 ("Proposition 65").[17] Proposition 65 is a law intended to protect California citizens from chemicals that cause cancer, birth defects, or other reproductive effects. A

Table 9.5 Known and Suspected Human Teratogens

Infectious agents	
Cytomegalovirus	T – TOXO
Herpes hominis type II virus	O – varicella
Rubella virus	R – Rubella
Toxoplasma gondii	C – CMV
Treponema pallidum	H – HSV
Varicella virus	S – syphilis

Drugs and chemicals
  Alcohol
  Aminopterin, methylaminopterin (folate antagonists)
  Androgenic hormones
  Busulfan (alkylating agents)
  Coumarin anticoagulants
  Diethylstilbesterol
  Isotretinoin, etretinate, vitamin A excess
  Lead
  Organic mercury compounds
  Phenytoin
  Polybrominated biphenyls (PBBs)
  Polychlorinated biphenyls (PCBs)
  Tetracyclines
  Thalidomide
  Trimethadione
  Valproic acid
Physical agents
  Hyperthermia
  Ionizing radiation

(Adapted from Shepard,[81] with permission.)

key initial step in the process is determining what those chemicals are. To this end, a Governor's Scientific Advisory Panel was established to determine criteria for listing substances "known to cause developmental toxicity." In addition, a group of experts was assembled to review and comment on the criteria. This group published a report that describes their deliberations and suggestions and that illustrates the complexity of the issues involved.[17] This process is an important step in furthering the methods used to identify and regulate human teratogens.

Animal Models for the Study of Human Teratogens

Routine premarket testing of drugs and food additives involves animal testing to determine potential teratogenicity. Established by Food and Drug Administration (FDA) guidelines, the standard protocol includes three phases and requires the use of two animal species,[18] most commonly rats and rabbits. Phase I studies deal with fertility and general reproductive performance: breeding, fertility, nidation, parturition, lactation, and neonatal effects. Phase II, termed teratologic studies, provides information on embryotoxicity and teratogenicity (structural effects). Phase III studies provide information about parturition, lactation, and neonatal effects.

Although important in recognizing potential reproductive toxins and teratogens, animal studies have a number of significant limitations. Extrapolation from animal data may not be relevant to human exposures to an agent because of interspecies differences in metabolism, end-organ response, transport across the placenta, and sensitivity of fetal structures, to name a few. For example, humans and rabbits are both sensitive to the teratogenic effect of thalidomide, but rats are relatively insensitive.[19] There are also problems extrapolating from high, toxic doses to low doses. Most teratologic experiments involve exposure at high doses. Because human exposures typically involve lower doses, effects must then be extrapolated. The assumption often made for such extrapolation is that teratogenic risk is identical at high- and low-dose exposures. This may not be true, so it is not surprising that for many substances teratogenic in animals at high doses, there is little or no evidence of human teratogenicity at low doses.

At present, regulatory agencies are exploring the use of risk assessment methods for developmental toxins. Recently, the Environmental Protection Agency (EPA) published "Guidelines for the Health Assessment of Suspect Developmental Toxicants."[20]

Teratologic testing of drugs and chemicals serves an extremely important public health function. Unfortunately, it does not necessarily prevent exposure of pregnant women to harmful substances. Within the last 5 years, two drugs have been shown to be human teratogens: isotretinoin (Accutane) and valproic acid (Depakene). Although both agents were shown to be teratogenic in animal studies, it was only through human exposure that their teratogenicity in human beings was established. In addition, tens of thousands of chemicals have never been tested for reproductive toxicity or teratogenicity.[14] The limitations of animal testing and the immense number of potentially hazardous substances underscore the need for studies based on human exposure. The remainder of this chapter explores the relevance and application of epidemiologic studies to the identification of teratogens and other reproductive hazards.

CONTRIBUTION OF EPIDEMIOLOGY

Environmental agents are of particular interest and concern, because fetal exposure to these factors is preventable by reducing or eliminating exposure of pregnant women. Of great importance is that the combined forces of epidemiology and teratology are needed to study the effects of environmental exposures on reproductive outcomes.

Although most birth defects probably involve the interaction of genetic and environmental factors, commonly referred to as multifactorial etiology, the relative contributions and specific mechanisms of these genetic and environmental interactions remain unknown. For such defects as NTDs, oral clefts, and congenital heart defects, the genetic contribution is thought to be polygenic — that is, involving the interaction of genes at several loci.[21] It is by applying epidemiologic methods that we attempt to determine the relative contributions of genetic and environmental factors to the etiology of these defects. In addition, epidemiologic methods permit identification of specific agents associated with malformations or other adverse outcomes of pregnancy.[22]

EPIDEMIOLOGIC CONCEPTS

Fundamental to epidemiology is the concept of variation between populations in the frequency of disease occurrence. Epidemiology is based on comparisons. The epidemiologist determines what is occurring at one place compared with another place, what is going on at one time compared with another time, and what is going on with one group of people compared with another group of people. Rates of occurrence are compared; how these rates are determined is of major importance in epidemiology.

Occurrence rates for birth defects are usually expressed in terms of either incidence or prevalence rates at birth. An incidence rate is calculated using cases occurring during a specified period of time and consists of a numerator (the number of new cases of a defect) and a denominator (the population at risk of developing the defect). Incidence rates are expressed in terms of some base population, such as per 1,000 births. An incidence rate gives a measure of the risk of the defect occurring within the population. Many investigators believe it is inappropriate to refer to birth defect rates as incidence rates, because the true population at risk, that is, the number of embryos, is unknown. Thus there is an increasing tendency to refer to the occurrence of birth defects as prevalence at birth.[23] Because the calculation of prevalence requires knowing the number of cases that exist at a point in time, we can define that time point as birth. Thus we determine prevalence at birth because we have information on the number of cases born in a population and on the total number of births.

When we examine the occurrence rates for birth defects, we see that there can be geographic differences in rates.[24] Such differences are found both between countries and between regions within countries. These differences are studied in an effort to identify possible etiologic factors. For example, rates for NTDs increase from west to east in the United States. In 1980, the rates in the western, north central, and south-southeastern regions of the United States were 6.5, 8.2, and 10.7 per 10,000 births, respectively.[25]

Temporal variations in birth defect rates can occur within a population. The interpretation of such variation over time may give insight into etiology. Two kinds of time-related changes are of particular interest: short-term increases, which may be termed epidemics, and long-term secular trends. An example of the former is the epidemic of phocomelia in several European populations during the early 1960s.[24] An example of the latter is the recent decline in NTD rates in several areas of the world.[26] The increase in phocomelia was found to be associated with the introduction of the drug thalidomide. The decline in NTD rates has not been explained and is an example of a trend whose contributing factors need to be identified through epidemiologic study.

EPIDEMIOLOGIC APPROACHES TO THE STUDY OF BIRTH DEFECTS

Epidemiology is the study of the distribution and determinants of disease. Understanding the distribution of disease provides insights into disease determinants. Epidemiology is based on the concept that diseases are not randomly distributed in populations, but rather that groups of individuals with different attributes and exposures differ in terms of their disease risk and frequency. Understanding this uneven distribution can lead to the identification of factors involved in disease etiology.[27] Epidemiologic studies are usually unable to establish causal relationships such as that possible in laboratory animal experiments; however, an association between exposure and an outcome can be very strong and compelling evidence that the outcome results from the exposure.

Epidemiologic studies of birth defects look at associations between exposures and outcomes. Three major issues are involved in this process: (1) the definition and ascertainment of outcomes of interest; (2) the definition, identification, and quantification of exposures or of other risk factors; and (3) the use of epidemiologic and statistical techniques to determine the strength of that association.[27]

Epidemiologic studies of birth defects and other adverse reproductive outcomes present special challenges in terms of definition and ascertainment (identification) of cases and determination of exposure. The definition of what constitutes a case can present major problems in studies of birth defects. Another important problem may be that the completeness of ascertainment varies by source and by defect. For example, one can argue that recent increases in the rates of patent ductus arteriosus (PDA) are due to increases in the incidence of the defect, to better diagnosis, or to increased survival of low-birth-weight infants in whom PDA frequently occurs. Even for defects readily recognizable at birth, such as NTD, differences in sources of case ascertainment can lead to apparent differences in rates of occurrence.[28]

With regard to exposure to exogenous substances, the timing of exposure during the gestational period has a critical role in abnormal development. The ability to define a sensitive period of development and to determine whether exposure occurred during a biologically relevant time window is of critical importance in epidemiologic studies.[23,29] For example, the limb-reduction defects (phocomelia) associated with thalidomide exposure were restricted to days 39 to 47 after the last menses, when limb buds and limbs were forming.[30] Table 9.4 shows some of the malformations of the thalidomide embryopathy in relation to the time after the last menstrual period that exposure occurred.

EPIDEMIOLOGIC STUDY DESIGN

The three general categories of epidemiologic studies are descriptive, analytic, and experimental. The following discussion considers some of the major features of these study designs and relates them to studies of birth defects and other adverse reproductive outcomes.

Descriptive Epidemiology

Case Reports

Most known teratogens and reproductive toxins have been identified through case reports of an unusual number of cases or a constellation of abnormalities. These have come either from astute clinicians who observed something out of the ordinary or from co-workers or others who perceived some abnormal state of health.

For example, the association between maternal rubella and blindness was identified when Gregg[31] diagnosed several cases of an unusual form of congenital cataract temporally related to a rubella epidemic in Australia. On closer questioning, Gregg noted an excess history of rubella among the mothers during their pregnancies.

The thalidomide tragedy was first identified during a discussion of a striking increase in limb malforma-tions when Lenz[32] suggested that these malformations might be related to the use of the drug during pregnancy. Independently, but at about the same time, McBride[33] in Australia noted a high incidence of multiple severe abnormalities in offspring of women who had taken thalidomide during pregnancy. It was through the observations of these two clinicians that the teratogenicity of thalidomide was recognized and the drug was withdrawn from the market.

The above examples can be considered fortuitous in that hazards were not sought out but were observed. They are based on observations by clinicians that something had gone awry. Although the importance of astute observations of abnormal aggregations of cases or patterns of malformations must be recognized, we cannot rely on such methods for identifying health hazards. Furthermore, etiologic speculation based on case reports or case series usually do not lead to a causal agent and are therefore false-positive speculations. Whereas case reports may identify a new teratogen, they can never provide an estimate of the risk of disease after exposure.

Descriptive Studies

Descriptive epidemiologic studies provide information about the distribution and frequency of some outcome of interest. They result in rates of occurrence that can be compared among populations, places, or times. Defining the population at risk is the first step in a descriptive study. The population at risk can be defined geographically (e.g., residents within a state, county, or district) or medically (e.g., patients at a particular hospital). Definition of the population at risk includes the time period under consideration. The population at risk constitutes the *denominator* for calculating rates of occurrence of the outcomes of interest.

The second step in a descriptive study is to determine the *numerator* for calculating rates for comparison. This involves two important concepts: (1) case definition (What defines a case to be counted?) and (2) case ascertainment (How are cases to be identified?). For example, a descriptive study of congenital hypothyroidism must include information about criteria used to diagnose the condition and on how the investigators learned of these cases (ascertainment). From these data, the reader can decide whether all cases during the time of the study, within the population at risk, are likely to have been included.

A recent study of NTDs in Los Angeles County exemplifies the descriptive study.[28] The population at risk was defined as births to Los Angeles County residents occurring in Los Angeles County hospitals during the period 1966 to 1972. Cases were defined as babies for whom birth certificate and/or hospital records recorded the presence of open spina bifida, anencephaly, or encephalocele. Cases were ascertained through the use of multiple sources, including birth, death, and fetal death certificates, hospital newborn records, and records from hospitals to which infants were referred for treatment.

Descriptive studies determine rates; thus they can be compared with one another. However, possible differences in case ascertainment methods must be kept in mind. The Los Angeles County NTD study compared rates based only on vital records ascertainment with rates from other studies in which vital records were used to identify cases. In addition, rates based on all sources of ascertainment were compared with rates from other studies in which multiple sources were used.[28] It would not have been appropriate, however, to have compared rates based on vital records with rates based on multiple sources of ascertainment.

Surveillance Programs

In surveillance programs, an at-risk population is identified and then followed over time to detect outcomes of interest. Cases are included in the program as they occur. These programs provide rates that can be compared and examined at periodic intervals for changes. They are directed at developing baseline data and permitting early recognition of potential problems, and they involve ongoing data collection and analysis.

Birth defect monitoring systems (BDMS) are designed to identify cases occurring in a defined population. The cases are usually ascertained by reviewing vital records or hospital record abstracts or charts. The defined population is a sociopolitical unit, such as a state, but some monitoring programs have been based on discharge data from particular groups of hospitals or births to women residing in a specified metropolitan area.

Two BDMS are operated by the Division of Birth Defects and Developmental Disabilities, Center for Environmental Health and Injury Control, Centers for Disease Control (CDC), Atlanta, Georgia. These two systems—the Birth Defects Monitoring Program (BDMP) and the Metropolitan Atlanta Congenital Defects Program (MACDP)—perform important surveillance functions.[34,35] The two systems follow populations defined differently and differing in sources of case ascertainment. A description and comparison of both systems is available.[35]

Birth Defects Monitoring Program

The BDMP was established by the CDC in 1974 to provide nationwide monitoring of birth defects.[35] The objectives of the BDMP are to act as an early warning system, by providing data on trends of birth defect occurrence and geographic differences in rates, and to serve as a source of cases for epidemiologic studies. The BDMP includes structural and chromosomal disorders, as well as other perinatal problems such as Rh hemolytic disease of the newborn. Cases for the BDMP are ascertained from hospital discharge abstracts submitted by approximately 1,200 hospitals to the Professional Activities Study (PAS) medical audit system of the Commission on Professional and Hospital Activities. Beginning in 1982, approximately 900 hospitals participating in the McDonnell Douglas Health Information System (MDHIS) made such records available to the CDC, and this became an additional data source for BDMP. Though the BDMP data are not from a geographically well-defined population, they are nationwide in scope and represent the largest single source of uniformly collected and coded information on malformed newborns in the United States. Information on slightly fewer than 1 million births per year is reported by the system. The BDMP has been used as a prototype for other surveillance systems, and data from the BDMP are used routinely by state and local health departments.

Metropolitan Atlanta Congenital Defects Program

The MACDP was begun in 1967 as a joint project among the CDC, the Emory University School of Medicine, and the Georgia Mental Health Institute.[36] The MACDP has two primary objectives: (1) to monitor births of infants with malformations to detect changes in incidence or unusual patterns suggestive of environmental influences and (2) to develop a case registry for use in research studies.[35]

Structural, chromosomal, and biochemical abnormalities are included. Any of 158 birth defects identified in infants up to 1 year old whose mothers resided in the five-county Atlanta area at the time of the birth are ascertained through multiple sources. These include hospital and vital records and referral centers such as cytogenetics laboratories and genetic counseling clinics.

Unlike the BDMP, the MACDP involves active case finding and is population based. This means that any infant born and living in metropolitan Atlanta whose birth defect is diagnosed before 1 year of age should be included. The newborn population numbers about 29,000 births per year; cases are identified through multiple sources, not just discharge summaries. In addition, the MACDP, unlike the BDMP, contains linked maternal and infant records.[35]

State-Based Birth Defects Surveillance Systems

In the last 10 years, there has been a dramatic increase in the number of state-based birth defect surveillance systems. As of 1990, about 25 states have birth defects surveillance systems. These programs conduct routine reviews of occurrence rates of specific malformations and attempt to identify increases in rates or clusters of cases. Several of the states are involved in case–control studies using cases from their surveillance program, and others are linking outcome data with environmental databases in an attempt to identify environmental reproductive hazards.[37] A similar approach has been used in other countries as well.[38]

Analytic Epidemiology

Analytic studies are designed to generate or test hypotheses about associations between exposures and outcomes. The detection and quantification of such associations are major epidemiologic concerns. Such associations can be examined at either the group or individual level.

Ecologic Studies

Ecologic studies are important for generating hypotheses about the causes of an outcome such as a birth defect. In such studies, occurrence rates for an outcome are compared between groups thought to differ in terms of some exposure. Studies of this type do not collect information about exposures of individuals. They are most widely used in environmental epidemiology, in which residence in a particular area is often used as an indicator of exposure.

Examples of ecologic studies relevant to reproductive outcome include studies of congenital malformations in communities with vinyl chloride production facilities,[39,40] studies of spontaneous abortions in communities with smelters,[41] and studies of adverse pregnancy outcomes in communities with solvent-contaminated drinking water.[42] Because ecologic studies do not permit the association between exposure and outcome to be tested directly, they often lead to hypotheses that can be tested using other study designs. Ecologic studies can contribute to the development of hypotheses in reproductive epidemiology, but these studies are of limited use.[27] Studies that allow associations between exposure and outcome to be assessed in particular individuals play a much more important role in epidemiologic research.

Cross-Sectional Studies

Cross-sectional studies examine an exposure state and an outcome in groups of individuals at the same time. A sample group is selected, and individuals are categorized as "exposed" or "not exposed" and as "outcome present" or "outcome not present."

Cross-sectional studies test the null hypothesis that exposure and outcome do not occur together in the same individuals more frequently than would be expected by chance. Of interest is an alternate hypothesis of an association between exposure and outcome. Statistical analysis is directed toward determining whether such an association exists and, if so, how strong it is. The same type of statistical reasoning, by different methods, characterizes the analytic study designs considered below.

Case–Control Studies

The case–control study design is the most widely used in reproductive outcome research. In case–control studies, groups of individuals who differ in the presence of some outcome or disease of interest are compared with regard to a history of one or more exposures. The cases are individuals with the outcome under investigation, for example, congenital malformations. The controls are individuals as similar as possible to the cases except that they are without the outcome of interest.

After cases and controls have been identified, the investigator determines whether they differ in terms of the exposure(s) of interest. The hypothesis to be tested is whether individuals who differ in outcome — the cases and controls — differ in exposure as well. How accurately exposure and its timing are determined may vary greatly among studies, but in any study the same methods must be used to identify the exposure of both cases and controls.[27]

The association between outcome and exposure can be tested by using a two-by-two table and the chi-squared test. In addition, the odds ratio, also based on the two-by-two table, can be used to test the strength of the association. The odds ratio in a case–control study gives an estimate of the risk of an outcome, given an exposure. The odds ratio is the probability that a case was exposed divided by the probability that a control was exposed. An odds ratio that exceeds 1 indicates an increased probability of exposure among cases. The higher the odds ratio, the stronger the association between the exposure and the outcome. By calculating the 95 percent confidence interval for the odds ratio — that is, the upper and lower limits within which the true odds ratio is expected to occur 95 percent of the time — the statistical significance of the odds ratio can be determined. If the 95 percent confidence interval does not include an odds ratio of 1, risk is considered statistically significantly elevated.

An important concept in the interpretation of epidemiologic studies is that of *power*. The power of a study, that is, the study's ability to detect a true effect, is often low in reproductive outcome studies. A study's power depends on the size of the study group and on the level of the increased risk. The concept of power becomes important in "negative" studies. Because small numbers are in the sample studied (i.e., few cases), a very large increase in risk must be present to be identified ("statistically significant"). When interpreting the findings of a negative case–control study, one must not overlook the power of the study to detect an association between the particular exposure and the adverse reproductive outcome.[27]

Case–control studies are frequently used in epidemiology for several reasons. In testing etiologic hypotheses, they are applicable to outcomes of infrequent occurrence, and they can be conducted relatively rapidly and inexpensively. One of their disadvantages is that they have a potential for several important types of bias, including bias in recalling exposure, in selecting appropriate controls, and in ascertaining cases. In the case of birth defects studies,

a mother with an abnormal infant is much more likely to think about and remember events in the first trimester of pregnancy that is a control mother with a normal infant; thus recall bias is likely to occur.

Most human studies of potential teratogens have been case–control studies. After suspecting on the basis of case observations that thalidomide was teratogenic, Lenz[43] conducted a case–control study. In ecologic studies of ambient exposure to vinyl chloride, the hypothesis of an association between vinyl chloride exposure and congenital malformations was tested in case–control studies.[40,44,45] The suspected association between valproic acid use and spina bifida was identified through case–control studies.[46]

Cohort Studies = Prospective

Cohort studies use the reverse approach from case–control studies; individuals who differ in exposure history are examined for differences in the occurrence of outcomes of interest. The groups are defined by the presence or absence of exposure to a given factor and then are followed over time and compared for rates of occurrence (i.e., incidence rates) of the outcome of interest.

Cohort studies have three advantages: (1) the cohort is classified by exposure before the outcome is determined, thereby eliminating the exposure recall bias; (2) incidence rates can be calculated among those exposed; and (3) multiple outcomes can be observed simultaneously.

Cohort studies, often called prospective studies, require that groups differing in exposure be followed through time, with outcomes observed. Therefore, these studies tend to be time consuming and expensive. In addition, because occurrence rates for many adverse reproductive outcomes, such as congenital malformations, are low, large samples must be followed for long periods of time. Two main types of cohort studies have been developed: (1) those that identify a cohort and follow it into the future (concurrent cohort study) and (2) those that identify a cohort at some time in the past and follow it to the present (nonconcurrent cohort study).

In both cases, the risks of adverse outcomes are then compared between groups. Cohort studies enable investigators to calculate incidence rates that provide a measure of the risk of an outcome after exposure to an agent of interest. Risk in the exposed group can be compared with the risk in an unexposed group. Most frequently, the ratio of the incidence rate among the exposed to the rate among the unexposed is determined. This ratio, referred to as relative risk, is a measure of how much the presence of exposure increases the risk of the outcome. As with the odds ratio, if the relative risk is greater than unity, an increased risk is associated with exposure. If 95 percent confidence intervals are greater than 1, the increased risk associated with exposure is said to be statistically significant.

A second measure frequently used in epidemiologic studies to relate risk to exposure is *attributable risk* or *population attributable risk*. Attributable risk is equal to the incidence rate among the exposed minus the incidence rate among the unexposed. It estimates the rate of the disease in exposed individuals that can be attributed to the exposure being studied. The attributable risk can also be expressed as the *etiologic fraction*, that is, as the difference between the incidence rates divided by the incidence rate in the exposed population. The etiologic fraction is the proportion of all new cases that are attributable to the exposure of interest.

Only a few large-scale concurrent cohort studies of problems of pregnancy outcome have been conducted. Probably the best known is the Collaborative Perinatal Project, conducted by the National Institute of Neurological and Communicative Disorders and Stroke. In this study, conducted between 1959 and 1966, about 55,000 women and their subsequently born children were studied extensively: the children were examined through age 8 years in a broad spectrum of areas.[47] This study has provided considerable information on the use of drugs in pregnancy, on birth defects, and on many other topics (see Ch. 11).

Numerous studies of reproductive outcome have been conducted by the noncurrent cohort approach. These studies, also known as historical prospective studies, begin by identifying groups who differ in terms of some past exposure and continue by following them to the present and determining outcomes; exposure groups are defined before outcomes are known. A major advantage is that, although the time frame is prospective, investigators do not have to follow the cohort into the future, waiting for events to occur. A disadvantage is that these studies require the ability to determine exposure status retrospectively.

A series of noncurrent cohort studies tested association between smelters and spontaneous abortions.[41] Nordstrom and co-workers[48] compared histories of spontaneous abortions of women who differed in terms of occupational exposure to smelting processes. Later, Beckman and Nordstrom[49] surveyed exposed and unexposed male workers about their wives' histories of spontaneous abortions. In both instances, the findings supported the hypothesis, developed from the ecologic study, of an association between the smelter and spontaneous abortions.

Experimental Epidemiology: Clinical Trials

The most common experimental study design in epidemiology is the clinical trial, in which the efficiency of a prevention or treatment regimen is evaluated. Ideally, in clinical trials, subjects are randomly assigned to different treatment groups. The individuals must be as similar as possible in terms of unknown factors that may affect the response before they are randomly assigned to the treatment groups and receive the different regimens.[50]

The role of vitamin supplements taken during the periconception period in preventing NTD has been evaluated in experimental studies. Smithells and co-workers[51,52] suggested that recurrence risks for NTDs were reduced in women who took the supplements during the period. In their original study, subjects were not randomized into different treatment groups; because of this, their conclusions have been criticized. Some critics have questioned whether the reported differences between the group that took the supplement and the group that did not can be attributed to the vitamins. It should be noted that four observational studies on the potential protective effect of multivitamins were published in 1988 and 1989.[53-56]

Three of these studies show a protective effect,[53,55,56] while the fourth does not.[54] Many investigators feel that the only way the question of whether periconceptional use of multivitamins or folate protects against the development of NTDs can be resolved is through randomized clinical trials such as one currently being conducted by the Medical Research Council in the United Kingdom.[57]

In summary, experimental studies in epidemiology are unique in that they involve intervention as well as observation. In this way, they compare with approaches used in animal studies of teratology and other life sciences and yield results that can be analyzed like other experimental findings. They are limited, however, in what can be ethically tested, namely, treatment or preventive measures, rather than etiologic hypotheses.

OCCUPATIONAL AND ENVIRONMENTAL HAZARDS TO REPRODUCTION

Within the past few years, increased attention has focused on the relationship between adverse reproductive outcomes and exposures to occupational and environmental hazards. Much of the concern about this relationship has grown not out of clearly demonstrated adverse effects, but, rather, out of the possibility of such effects. Numerous books and conferences have addressed the reproductive hazards of chemical and environmental exposures.[58-66]

Among the issues are those that relate to women's rights for equal employment opportunities and the problems of excluding women from some work situations because of potential exposure effects on pregnancy outcomes. Much of the concern has centered on the susceptibility of the embryo and fetus to teratogenic influences; interest has been expanding to embrace a whole gamut of factors in reproductive toxicology.

Adverse Reproductive Outcomes Associated With Occupational and Environmental Exposures

Through a number of mechanisms, occupational or environmental exposures can produce adverse reproductive outcomes.

REPRODUCTIVE OUTCOMES POTENTIALLY ASSOCIATED WITH FETOMATERNAL EXPOSURES

    Altered fertility

    Single-gene defects

    Chromosomal abnormalities

    Spontaneous abortions

    Congenital malformations

(continued)

    Intrauterine growth retardation

    Altered sex ratio

    Perinatal deaths

    Developmental disabilities

    Behavioral disorders

    Malignancies

(From Sever and Hellol,[27] with permission.)

These outcomes include alterations in fertility because of hormonal or gonadal effects and mutations at either the gene or chromosomal level. A variety of adverse outcomes result from direct effects of agents on the products of conception. These range from death at various stages in the life span, to congenital malformations, to developmental disabilities, to cancers recognized in childhood. Another possible outcome is fetal death caused by effects on the intrauterine milieu and the fetomaternal unit. This discussion focuses on three general outcome categories: spontaneous abortions, congenital malformations, and developmental disabilities, such as mental retardation.

Exposure Assessment With Regard to Occupational and Environmental Reproductive Hazards

As a prerequisite to evaluating the reproductive hazards associated with an occupational or environmental agent, one must be able to measure or estimate exposure to potential hazards. A number of investigators have recently addressed the problems associated with this exposure assessment.[14,27,63,66-68]

Considerations concerning occupational exposure can be categorized into three areas: defining and determining exposure, timing of exposure, and problems of mixed exposures.[27] In the first area, which can also be labeled exposure occurrence and measurement,[68] the problems relate to determining what a particular worker is exposed to and then determining the amount of exposure—if such is possible. In many instances, workers may not be aware of the chemical substances to which they are exposed. An important place to begin determining exposure history, however, is to question the worker and to take a job history. When possible, this should be augmented by reviewing the occupational and job history records that the employer maintains. Ideally, the job history will make it possible for the investigator to determine the substances to which the worker was exposed. If so, the exposure records the employer maintains may include data from environmental monitoring.

In studies of reproductive outcome, the timing of exposure is crucial. The critical stages in human development for teratogenesis were discussed earlier in this chapter. Except for exposures associated with mutational events or damage to the reproductive or endocrine systems, exposures must occur within a limited period if they are to produce teratogenic effects. The accuracy with which an employee's exposure can be determined is therefore critical. For example, an agent suspected of causing an NTD could not be implicated as the cause of an infant's neural tube's failing to close if the mother had been exposed to the agent after the fetal neural tube had closed. Many investigators fail to take such matters into account.[23]

Employees can be exposed to a variety of potentially hazardous substances. Because of this, the ability to demonstrate that a specific substance is a reproductive hazard is difficult. Because most occupational exposures are to more than one substance and because it may not be possible to determine the reproductive effects of one agent, occupational groups rather than kinds of exposures are evaluated in many studies. There are studies of laboratory workers[69-71] and of people who work with rubber[72,73] and in which the reproductive performance of workers in particular industries is evaluated.[74,75]

In addition to the problem of mixed occupational exposures, the effects of nonoccupational exposures such as tobacco and alcohol must also be determined. If occupational groups differ in their exposure to these reproductive hazards, it may not be possible to determine whether reproductive effects result from the occupational or the nonoccupational exposure.[14]

In environmental studies, it is particularly difficult to determine exposures. In ecologic studies, measurements or estimates of levels of contaminants in air, soil, or water are used to characterize the exposure of groups of people. In case–control or cohort studies, individual exposures may be determined on the basis of environmental measurements; that is, individual exposures must be estimated on the basis of ambient monitoring, factory releases, or levels of toxic substances in water supplies. This is difficult, as is the determination of timing of such exposures. In the last 5 years interest and research activities have grown in the use of biologic markers of exposure in studies of adverse reproductive outcomes.[76-78]

EXPOSURES THAT MAY LEAD TO ADVERSE REPRODUCTIVE OUTCOMES

We now review what is known about the effects of prenatal exposure to certain occupational and environmental agents. Agents were selected on the bases of the availability of human data and of the authors' impressions of public concern that the agents may cause adverse reproductive effects. Several texts and reviews provide more comprehensive information about the potential teratogenicity and mutagenicity of numerous environmental agents and chemicals.[19,59,60,63-66,79-83]

Known human teratogens number about 30.[81] To date, only two have caused human maldevelopment (cerebral palsy and mental retardation) as a result of environmental contamination: high-dose ionizing radiation and methylmercury. Agents suspected of being teratogens on the basis of animal studies are more numerous, and, when these agents are found to be polluting the environment, there is justifiable concern about potential prenatal exposure and adverse reproductive effects (Table 9.6). The difficulty of demonstrating an association between an environmental hazard and any adverse reproductive outcome must, however, be appreciated.

In a concise review, Heath[84] summarized some of the problems in epidemiologic studies of environmental hazards. Using as examples the childhood leukemia cluster in Woburn, Massachusetts, and the population exposure to waste chemicals at Love Canal, New York, Heath[84] identified three problems: low-dose, nonquantifiable exposures; the long and variable latency between exposure and outcome (disease); and the nonspecific nature of the outcome or disease. As a corollary to the last problem, Heath[84] pointed out that multiple factors probably play a causative role in most outcomes of interest, including birth defects, low birth weight, spontaneous abortion, and cancer. Epidemiologic studies of humans cannot definitely prove that an agent is not a teratogen; they can only show a probability that an agent is

Table 9.6 Occupational and Environmental Agents That May Be Associated With Human Adverse Reproductive Outcomes

Agent	Outcome
Ionizing radiation	
Acute, high dose	Microcephaly, mental retardation, growth retardation
Chronic low dose or before pregnancy	Down syndrome
Methylmercury	Mental retardation, cerebral palsy, deafness, blindness, seizures (abnormal neuronal migration)
Mercury vapor	Cranial defects, ?spontaneous abortion, ?stillbirth
Lead	
High dose	Infertility, spontaneous abortion, growth retardation, psychomotor retardation, seizures, stillbirth
Chronic low dose	Lower IQ, cognitive impairment in speech and language, attention deficit
Lead/arsenic (smelter emissions)	Spontaneous abortion, low birth weight, birth defects
Polychlorinated biphenyls	
High dose	Spontaneous abortion, low birth weight, neuroectodermal dysplasia (skin staining, natal teeth, dysplastic nails, developmental and psychological deficits), abnormal bone calcification
Chronic low dose	Lower birth weight, smaller head circumference, cognitive impairment
Polybrominated biphenyls	
Chronic low dose	?Lower birth weight, ?smaller head circumference, cognitive impairment
Anesthetic Gases	
Chronic low dose	Spontaneous abortion, birth defects
Organic solvents	
Chronic high dose	Developmental impairment, facial dysmorphism, growth retardation (similar to fetal alcohol embryopathy)
Chronic low dose	Spontaneous abortion, CNS malformations, orofacial clefts

or is not a teratogen. An element of uncertainty is always present.

Ionizing Radiation

Acute High Dose

During the 1920s and 1930s, ionizing radiation was used to treat women with pelvic disease; soon afterward, it was identified as the first known environmental human teratogen.[85] Systematic studies of atomic bomb survivors in Japan showed that in utero exposure to high-dose radiation increased the risk of microcephaly and/or mental and growth retardation in the offspring.[86-90] Spontaneous abortions, premature deliveries, and stillbirths may have been increased after exposure to atomic bomb fall-out.[91]

Studies of the Japanese survivors clearly show that distance from the hypocenter—the area directly beneath the detonated bomb—and the gestational age at the time of exposure were directly related to microcephaly and to mental and growth retardation in the infant. In follow-up studies of survivors, the greatest number of children with microcephaly and mental and growth retardation were in the group exposed between 8 and 15 weeks gestation.[90] These findings contrast with those of children exposed in utero during the third trimester and whose mothers were farthest from the hypocenter at the time of exposure. Of 55 children evaluated 20 years later, only 1 was found to be microcephalic and all were of normal intelligence.[87] Although teratogenic effects have been found in several organ systems of animals exposed to acute, high-dose radiation, no structural malformations other than those mentioned above have been reported among humans exposed prenatally.

Using data from animals and outcomes from reported human exposures at various times during pregnancy, Dekaban[92] constructed a timetable for extrapolating acute, high-dose radiation (> 250 rads) to various reproductive outcomes in humans (Table

9.7). Exposure between 2 and 4 weeks gestation (menstrual) is probably embryolethal or else has no demonstrable effect on the offspring. This all-or-nothing response may reflect the embryo's tremendous capacity to recover from sublethal insults. The period between 4 and 11 weeks gestation is the most sensitive in terms of multiple organ effects; it is the time when structural malformations and growth retardation, perhaps because of decreased cell numbers, are most likely to result. From weeks 12 through 16, the central nervous system (CNS) is most sensitive; manifestations at birth are reduced head circumference and mental retardation. The likelihood of these effects occurring decreases after 16 weeks. After 20 weeks, fetal effects are essentially the same as those occurring with postnatal exposure. These are termed radiation sickness, consisting of skin lesions, hair loss, and bone marrow hypoplasia. Although few human data are available to validate the entire timetable, the similarity between animal and known human effects supports Dekaban's proposal.

Dose Threshold

The radiation dose below which no adverse effect occurs is not known. Brent[93] points out that in animal studies the classic findings of growth retardation, structural malformations, and fetal reabsorption cannot be detected at exposures below 25 rad. In a more recent review of embryonic and fetal radiation effects, he contends that the risk of human congenital malformations will not be increased at exposures of 5 rad or less.[83]

Chronic Low Dose

The effects of chronic low-dose radiation on reproduction have not been identified in animals or humans. An increased risk of adverse outcomes was not detected among animals with continuous low-dose exposure (<5 rad) throughout pregnancy.[83]

The relationship between human structural malformations and background radiation has been examined in several epidemiologic studies in different geographic areas. Cosmic radiation was thought to be one factor that contributed to increased rates of anencephalus between 1950 and 1969 in several Canadian cities.[94] Using geologic estimates of natural radioactivity, some investigators have attributed increased malformation rates, including the rate for Down syndrome, to higher radioactivity levels.[95,96] Other studies of the association between estimated cosmic radiation exposure and congenital malformation rates have produced negative results.[97,98] Given that low-dose radiation could be one of a multitude of environmental factors that affect the risk of birth defects, it is not surprising that no consistent relationship is evident.

Mutagenesis

Children exposed in utero to radiation from the atomic bomb were studied over several years for evidence of genetic damage. No evidence was found when six indicators were evaluated: congenital malformations, stillbirth and neonatal death rates, birth weight, sex ratio at birth, anthropomorphic measurements during the first year of life, and mortality in offspring (F1 generation).[85,99,100]

In contrast to the atomic bomb follow-up studies, other investigations have found that mutagenic effects may occur when women are exposed prenatally to diagnostic radiation. These effects include altered sex ratios among the offspring—slightly more females than expected[101]—and abnormal karyotypes in spontaneously aborted fetuses.[102]

Available data provide no conclusive evidence that preconceptional radiographic exposure increases a woman's risk of having an infant with a chromosomal abnormality. Using a retrospective cohort approach, Stevenson and co-workers[103] did not find evidence

Table 9.7   Adverse Pregnancy Outcomes That May Occur Following Maternal High-Dose Ionizing Radiation

Gestational Age At Exposure (Weeks)	Outcome
0–3	Spontaneous abortion or normal
4–11	Microcephaly, mental retardation, microphthalmia, cataracts, growth retardation
12–16	Mental and/or growth retardation
17–19	Same but less severe than at 12–16 weeks
>20	As seen with postnatal exposure: hair loss, skin lesions, bone marrow suppression

(Adapted from Dekaban,[92] with permission.)

that diagnostic radiation before conception increased the risk of Down syndrome. They interviewed women whose radiographic studies were documented in hospital registers. Among women who had borne children, the number of infants with Down syndrome was close to that expected when maternal age was taken into account.

In three case–control studies, mothers of infants with Down syndrome were more likely to report having had fluoroscopy or diagnostic radiographs some time before becoming pregnant.[104-106] The risk of having an infant with a chromosomal abnormality was greatest among women above age 36 years who also reported having had abdominal radiographs.[105] Results of other case–control studies led to the opposite conclusion, that is, that women who have had one or more abdominal radiographs do not have an increased risk of conceiving a child with Down syndrome.[107-109] It may seem confusing that contradictory results follow from similar study designs. The differences among the studies, however, may be greater than the apparent similarities. In addition to differing numbers of study subjects, potentially important differences include whether the radiograph history was validated, how the cases were ascertained, how controls were selected, and whether the controls had normal offspring or infants with nonchromosomal birth defects.

Mutagenic effects in the offspring of irradiated women may be manifested years after the birth of the infant. Compared with nonradiated controls, the estimated risk of leukemia was increased 50 percent for children exposed in utero to radiation during maternal pelvimetry examinations.[110-112] Although this increase seems considerable, it translates into an approximate risk of 1 in 2,000 for exposed versus 1 in 3,000 for unexposed children. As Brent[83] points out, if one were to recommend that pregnancies be terminated whenever exposure from diagnostic radiation occurred because of the increased probability of leukemia in the offspring, 1,999 "exposed pregnancies" would have to be terminated to "prevent" a single case of leukemia.

Ultrasonic Radiation

Widespread use of ultrasound in obstetrics has resulted in concern about possible effects on the fetus. To date, there are no human data that support an increased risk of congenital malformations following in utero exposure.[83,113] Studies in laboratory animals with high-dose ultrasound have shown a variety of fetal effects, including neurologic, developmental, hematologic, genetic, and structural abnormalities.[114,115] Some of these effects may be due to hyperthermia or to tissue destruction resulting from exposure to the continuous and/or high-amplitude ultrasonic radiation used in such studies.[97] By contrast, the diagnostic ultrasound used in medicine is generated in pulses and is low amplitude. No similar or additional risks from the diagnostic use of ultrasound have been documented in humans.[114]

Follow-up studies of human infants exposed to ultrasound in utero have shown no adverse effects. In one large study, exposed and nonexposed infants had similar perinatal outcomes (Apgar scores, gestational age, birth weight, infections) and later neurologic, cognitive, and behavioral function.[113]

Organic Mercury — Methylmercury

Exposure to organic mercury compounds, such as methylmercury or ethylmercury, is not common. In the United States, methylmercury was widely used as a fungicide until the 1960s, when U.S. production was halted because of the compound's toxicity and ability to bioaccumulate. Today in the United States, exposure occurs through the consumption of contaminated fish. Fish may become contaminated when organomercurials are present in water or when bacteria in water convert inorganic mercury to organic mercury, part of a complex environmental mercury cycle.[116]

Methylmercury effects were discovered in 1959 after an epidemic of poisoning in Minamata, Japan, that resulted in fetal neurologic damage with psychomotor retardation, seizures, cerebral palsy, blindness, and deafness.[117] In 1972, similar fetal effects were observed in Iraq after an epidemic of methylmercury poisoning.[118] In both epidemics, breast-fed infants had additional exposure through maternal milk.[117]

Unintentional human exposures have permitted the reproductive effects of methylmercury to be studied more thoroughly than any other environmental pollutant, and these effects have been reviewed extensively.[119-121] The persistence of organic mercury in the body (biologic half-life about 70 days) and its accumulation in hair make it possible to reconstruct prenatal exposure.[122] Methylmercury crosses the placenta easily and accumulates in embryonic and fetal tissues, particularly in brain tissue, at concentrations exceeding those in the mother.[123,124] Methylmercury does not cause obvious structural malformations in humans, so the devastating effects, which may not be obvious at birth, become evident only as abnormal neurologic development proceeds. The developing nervous system of the conceptus and infant is more sensitive to the toxic effects of organic mercury than is that of the adult or older child.[117] For this reason, the infant of an asymptomatic mother can be severely affected.[118,121,125]

Little is known of the human effects of methylmercury at low levels of exposure. Minor neurologic differences, mainly brisker deep tendon reflexes, were found among native Quebec boys exposed in utero compared with boys who had had no such exposure.[126] Low-level methylmercury exposure may, however, be associated with an increased frequency of chromosomal abnormalities[127]; the significance of this finding for adverse health or reproductive effects is unknown.

Nonhuman primates chronically treated with low-dose methylmercury were more likely to experience reproductive failure (nonconception, spontaneous abortion) than were nontreated controls.[128] Prenatal exposure resulted in offspring with impaired visual recognition, consistent with a developmental teratogenic effect.[129-131]

In laboratory animals, methylmercury is embryolethal and causes various structural malformations (exencephaly, limb abnormalities) when high doses are given during critical periods in development.[132] There appears to be no association between similar birth defects and human environmental exposure. Mattison[133] reviewed experimental and human epidemiologic data regarding mercury and other metals, listing the site(s) of action or reproductive outcome studied.

Elemental Mercury (Vapor)

Mercury is an unusual element. At room temperature it is liquid and has a high vapor pressure. Thus vapor concentrations can rapidly rise to toxic concentrations in closed or poorly ventilated areas. The vapor is odorless and colorless, making it virtually nondetectable without special equipment. Mercury vapor is rapidly absorbed through the lungs and, because of its high lipid solubility, easily crosses biologic membranes. Elemental mercury is minimally if at all absorbed from the gastrointestinal tract or through the skin.

Women at risk for exposure work primarily in health-related occupations such as nursing, medicine, dentistry, and dental hygiene. Exposure may occur when dental amalgams are prepared and when thermometers or manometers are broken or mercury is spilled. In recent years, use of encapsulated amalgams has reduced mercury exposure that could occur from dispensing mercury drops and mixing the amalgam materials. Mercury manometers and thermometers are less widely used now, because easy-to-use electronic methods for measuring blood pressure and temperature have been developed. Consequently, mercury exposure in medicine and dentistry in the United States has probably decreased with these developments.

Considering that large numbers of women of childbearing age may have been occupationally exposed to mercury vapor, there is a surprising dearth of animal and human epidemiologic studies of reproductive effects. The only published English language study of the teratogenic effects in animals is in abstract form. In this study, mercury vapor exposure at 0.5 mg/m³ throughout pregnancy resulted in 2 of 115 fetal rats having cranial defects.[134] Exposure during days 10 through 15 of gestation produced increased fetal reabsorption.[133] This vapor concentration is 10 times greater than the occupational limit of 0.05 mg/m³ established by the Occupational Safety and Health Administration[135] and could be expected to cause overt toxicity. Maternal toxicity and illness could also have contributed to the observed fetal effects in the rodent studies.

Animal studies demonstrate the ease with which elemental mercury crosses the placenta. Following mercury vapor exposure, fetal rat blood mercury concentrations were 65 times higher than the corresponding maternal values.[136] The highest mercury concentrations were found in the rat placenta, with average placental to fetal ratios of 2.3.[136] Similar placental accumulation has been confirmed in humans. Placental and fetal membranes from mercury-exposed dental workers contained two to three times more mercury than did tissues taken from unexposed women.[137] The fetal and maternal blood mercury concentrations were similar in both groups, implying that the placental and fetal tissues may act as a barrier at low levels of mercury vapor.[137] At high vapor concentrations that may produce symptoms, mercury readily crosses the human placenta. A 37-week pregnant woman, acutely symptomatic after short-term vapor exposure, gave birth 26 days after the exposure. The normal-appearing infant and mother had blood mercury levels of 3.3 and 3.5 μg/dl, respectively (unexposed levels are usually < 1.0 μg/dl[138]).[139] Unfortunately, long term follow-up of the infant's neurologic and developmental performance was not described.

Occupational studies of chronic mercury vapor exposure have been conducted in male workers. Actual exposure cannot be determined in these studies because of the absence of long-term air mercury monitoring. Using exposure estimates, concentrations as low as 0.026 mg/m³ have been reported to produce intention tremor.[140] Motor and sensory nerve conduction abnormalities and neuropsychologic dysfunction have also been reported in dentists with chronic, presumably low-level mercury vapor exposure.[141,142] To protect the developing conceptus, Koos and Longo[119] recommend that women of childbearing age not be exposed to vapor concentrations exceeding 0.01 mg/m³.

Epidemiologic studies of reproductive effects have been conducted in female dental assistants and dentists. Unfortunately, radiation and anesthetic gases are additional exposures that may confound these studies. Other methodologic problems may include non-verification of the outcome, absence of exposure data, and low survey response rates. As a whole, the limited data provide no conclusive evidence that occupational exposure to mercury vapor is teratogenic or results in other adverse reproductive outcomes. The summary of these studies that follows is intended to emphasize the limited and inadequate data on which this statement is based. The need for more animal and human studies of reproductive effects has been recognized.[143]

In a case–control study of female dentists and dental assistants in Poland, Sikorski and co-workers[144] found an association between increased hair mercury content and self-reports of spontaneous abortion, congenital malformations, and stillbirths. Of note, the rates of these outcomes were not much greater than those expected in the general population, no adjustment was made for maternal age, and there was little difference in mean hair mercury values between the groups. Furthermore, the women were not questioned about fish consumption, a major source of dietary, and thus hair, mercury.[145]

In a large Danish survey of women in several occupations, dental assistants and dentists did not have an increased risk of either self-reported or hospital-recorded spontaneous abortions.[71] In a U.S. survey of female dentists and dental assistants, no association was found between mercury exposure (estimated by the number of dental amalgams prepared per week) and self-reported spontaneous abortion and congenital malformations in the offspring.[146]

Ericson and Kallen[147] used Swedish central birth registry data to study pregnancy outcomes in female dentistry workers during a 5-year period. No measure of actual exposure was available. The low-birth-weight and congenital malformation rates of 4.1 and 4.6 percent, respectively, were similar to overall Swedish rates for these outcomes.[148] Perinatal survival was somewhat better for women in dental occupations than in the general Swedish population.[147]

One explanation offered for the discrepancy between the Polish and Swedish results is that mercury handling and exposure may differ between the two countries.[147] It is also possible that factors other than mercury exposure were responsible for the adverse reproductive outcomes in the Polish workers. For instance, anesthetic gas and ionizing radiation exposures as well as other environmental and nutritional factors may be different. If dental personnel exposures and mercury handling in the United States are similar to those used in Sweden, as one might expect, these results provide some reassurance despite study limitations.

Lead

Since the nineteenth century, exposure to high levels of lead has been known to cause embryotoxicity, growth and mental retardation, increased perinatal mortality, and developmental disability.[148] These adverse reproductive effects were seen when women in occupational settings were exposed to concentrations of lead in air that far exceeded levels allowable today. As a matter of historic interest, unscrupulous vendors sold pills containing lead as an abortifacient at the turn of the century.[149]

Because the nervous system may be more susceptible to the toxic effects during the embryonic and fetal periods than at any other time of life[124] and because maternal and cord blood lead concentrations are directly correlated,[150] lead concentrations in blood should not exceed 25 μg/dl in women of reproductive age.[151] This downward revision from an earlier recommendation of 35 μg/dl represents the lower body burden of lead at which adverse neurobehavioral effects may occur in children.[151,152] In occupational settings, federal standards mandate that women should not work in areas where air lead concentrations can reach 50 μg/cm³, because this may result in blood concentrations above 25 to 30 μg/dl.[153] More recent studies suggest that, in children, subtle but permanent neurologic impairment may occur at an even lower body burden of lead.[154,155] Although controversial, such studies raise the possibility that the occupational standard may inadequately protect the fetus.

Smelter Emissions

Residents of communities near metal smelters may be exposed to increased concentrations of lead as well as to other heavy metals in the air smelter emissions. A series of ecologic studies in Sweden showed an association between residential proximity to a copper smelter and increased rates of spontaneous abortion and low birth weight.[41,156] Neither air nor blood metal concentrations were measured, and risk factors such as socioeconomic status, maternal age, and parity also were not considered in the analysis; thus the association can be questioned. There is good evidence, however, that the duration of maternal occupational lead exposure correlates directly with lead concentrations in cord blood and fetal tissue.[157]

Arsenic

Industrial waste, copper smelter emissions, and some pesticides are sources of environmental pollution with arsenic. Decreased infant birth weight and increased spontaneous abortion rates associated with residential proximity to a copper smelter in Sweden may have resulted from arsenic exposure, because arsenic, lead, and other heavy metals are present in copper smelter emissions.[41,156] Information about exposure to specific metals was not included in those studies. In the same population of smelter workers, occupational arsenic exposure was associated with possibly mutagenic chromosomal aberrations.[158] These workers, however, may have had other potentially mutagenic exposures. Moreover, the estimated degree of arsenic exposure did not correlate well with the frequency of observed chromosomal abnormalities.

In several animal species, arsenic has been shown to be a potent teratogen that produces a spectrum of congenital malformations as well as embryo resorption.[159] Depending on when it is administered, sodium arsenate can cause NTDs, renal dysgenesis, or renal agenesis.[160] Renal effects are thought to be caused by the interference of arsenic with inductive interactions or its destroying cells that form the ureteric bud.[161,162]

The Phenoxy Herbicide 2,4,5-T and Dioxin

2,3,7,8-Tetrachlorodibenzodioxin (TCDD, or dioxin) and other chlorinated dibenzodioxins were produced as contaminants during production of the herbicide 2,4,5-trichlorophenoxyacetic acid (2,4,5-T).[163] This herbicide is no longer marketed in the United States, largely because of concerns about possible teratogenic and fetotoxic effects. Such effects are seen after high doses are administered to animals during critical periods of organogenesis.[164] Data are inadequate to support allegations of adverse reproductive outcomes following human exposure to the dioxin-contaminated herbicide.[165]

Agent Orange, a defoliant used in Vietnam, was a mixture of herbicides, including 2,4,5-T. During the later years of the Vietnam War, public opinion against the ecologic effects of Agent Orange was fueled by reports of birth defects in South Vietnamese babies born to mothers who lived in areas where Agent Orange had been sprayed. The ensuing debate about the potential human teratogenicity of Agent Orange involved numerous federal agencies, and the use of 2,4,5-T containing any chlorodioxin contaminants was cancelled in 1970.[165]

Because 2,4,5-T contained small amounts of TCDD and because long-term human effects were unknown, the U.S. Public Health Service began an immense follow-up of Vietnam veterans. One portion of the study evaluated Vietnam veterans' risks of fathering infants with birth defects. The investigators concluded that "Vietnam veterans who had greater estimated opportunities for Agent Orange exposure did not seem to be at greater risk for fathering babies with all types of defects combined."[166] Vietnam service was, however, associated with a few defects; thus Agent Orange exposure, other Vietnam-related experience, or some unidentified risk factor may have been responsible for the associations.[166] In a subsequent follow-up study, Vietnam and non-Vietnam veterans were interviewed regarding congenital malformations in their offspring. Although Vietnam veterans were more likely to report birth defects in their offspring, hospital records showed similar rates of birth defects for children born to both veteran groups.[167] In contrast, increased CNS, skeletal, and cardiovascular malformations and disease were reported among offspring of Australian Vietnam veterans.[168] This study was less rigorous than its American counterparts, because it was of unconventional case–control design and involved relatively few children whose diagnoses were confirmed by medical record review.

Polychlorinated Biphenyls

Because polychlorinated biphenyls (PCBs) have the properties of thermal stability and heat transfer, they had numerous industrial uses.[169] PCBs are extremely stable and resistant to metabolic or biologic degradation. PCBs have become ubiquitous in the environment because of past dumping or disposal in unregulated landfills and failure to recycle. PCBs are highly lipid soluble, accumulate in fat, and can be found at high concentrations in the breast milk of women despite low concentrations in their blood.[170] Details of PCB biochemistry and toxicology are given elsewhere.[171,172]

Two epidemics of cooking oil contamination are often cited as evidence that high-dose PCBs are hazards to human reproduction. In these epidemics, adults consumed cooking oil tainted with thermally degraded PCBs and developed a disease termed *Yusho* (in Japan) and *Yu-cheng* (in Taiwan). The disease was characterized by chloracne (an acne-form rash), eyelid swelling and discharge, and skin hyperpigmentation.[173] Although PCBs alone are often blamed for these and subsequent health problems, it is clear that heat-degradation products of PCBs (polychlorodibenzofurans [PCDFs] and polychlorinated quarter-

phenyls [PCQs]) contributed significantly to toxicity.[174,175]

High-dose transplacental exposure to the cooking oil resulted in congenital anomalies and low birth weight.[176] Skin and mucosal hyperpigmentation were the most often noted abnormalities.[176] Other anomalies included natal teeth, gingival hyperplasia, exophthalmos, skull calcifications, and delayed bone age.[176]

In 1985, Rogan and co-workers[177] examined 117 children with prenatal and/or breast-milk exposure to the PCB/PCDF/PCQ-contaminated oil. Compared with unexposed children, exposed children demonstrated delayed developmental milestones, psychological deficits, and behavioral abnormalities. Physical abnormalities included shorter stature, lighter weight, and epidermal disorders such as acne, hyperpigmentation, deformed nails, gingival hypertrophy, and tooth chipping.[177] Together these findings suggest a neuroectodermal dysplasia caused by the combined effects of the PCBs and contaminants.[177]

In addition to the teratogenic effects, the contaminated oils led to excessive reproductive losses among exposed women. Increased risks for spontaneous abortion, stillbirth, and infant mortality were documented in the follow-up of a group of Taiwanese women.[178] An unusual phenomenon has been noted with regard to the low birth weight. In follow-up studies, "catch-up" growth occurred in most of the surviving infants, with attainment of normal body weight by 2 years of age.[171,178]

The effects described following cooking oil contamination epidemics should be distinguished from ambient or low-level exposure to PCBs. Low-level PCB maternal exposure can occur throughout life, for example, by consumption of fish from PCB-contaminated waters. Although placental transfer of PCBs occurs,[179] the largest dose is delivered to the nursing infant via breast milk.[170,180] The widespread potential for maternal exposure and PCB transfer to nursing infants has resulted in justifiable concern about reproductive and developmental effects.

Rhesus monkeys fed low levels of PCBs for prolonged periods demonstrate infertility, embryo reabsorption, spontaneous abortion, and intrauterine growth retardation.[181] This species seems to be exquisitely sensitive to PCBs because these effects occur within a range of dietary PCB concentrations considered allowable in certain human foods. In laboratory animals the major effects of chronic low-level exposure are seen in reproduction, immunologic response, and the liver (enzyme induction and tumor development).[182] Induction of liver enzymes, specifically the cytochrome P-450–dependent family of enzymes, has been demonstrated only in humans exposed to high levels of PCBs.[183]

In human epidemiologic studies, maternal PCB exposure via fish consumption is associated with a slight decrease in infant birth weight and head circumference relative to unexposed controls.[184] Neonatal assessment of the same infants provides some evidence that, at low concentrations, PCBs may be behavioral teratogens.[185] At 4 years of age, these infants showed short-term memory impairment that was directly related to the umbilical cord serum PCB concentration.[180]

In an excellent review of behavioral teratology, Fein and associates[186] describe the importance of assessing development as a way to detect subtle behavioral abnormalities. Such behavioral abnormalities may reflect toxicity or permanent impairment caused by prenatal exposure to chemical agents such as PCBs.

Polybrominated Biphenyls

Polybrominated biphenyl (PBB) compounds are structurally similar to PCBs and share characteristics of high lipid solubility and resistance to metabolic or biologic degradation. Fortunately, PBBs are not as widespread environmental contaminants as PCBs because their use has been more limited.

In the United States, PBBs were used as fire-retardants until 1974. In 1973 and 1974, cattle feed distributed in Michigan inadvertently became contaminated with PBBs. Before the contamination was recognized, people in the state thus consumed PBB-tainted meat and poultry. A detailed review of the incident and its health implications is available.[187] In 1977, the health of adult Michigan residents was compared with the health of a similar but unexposed population. The exposed Michigan residents were more likely to have skin, musculoskeletal, and neurologic symptoms, consisting of unusual fatigue and a decreased capacity for intellectual and physical work.[188] Induction of the cytochrome P-450 liver en-

zymes has been demonstrated in highly exposed individuals.[183] Persistent immunologic abnormalities including hypergammaglobulinemia and lymphopenia also have been reported, but the clinical significance of these findings is unknown.[189,190]

Human reproductive effects have not been studied. Fetal mortality in high- versus low-exposure regions of Michigan were not appreciably different after the PBB contamination.[191] As such, the study of fetal mortality is not conclusive because of potential inaccuracies of exposure estimates, the inability to control for confounding variables, and the possibility that mortality may not be the best indicator of PBB reproductive effects.

Transplacental and breast milk PBB exposure to infants was documented in the Michigan incident.[192] An early follow-up study reported that children with higher PBB body burdens scored lower on standardized tests of perceptual-motor, attentional, and verbal abilities.[193] However, later testing of the same children showed that their overall developmental scores were within the normal range.[194] For certain perceptual and perceptual-motor tasks, the scores tended to be inversely related to PBB body burden.[194] Given that PCBs are behaviorial teratogens and that PBBs are structurally and chemically similar to PCBs, one might anticipate similar neurobehavioral effects from prenatal and infant PBB exposure.

Nitrates and Nitrite

Nitrate contamination of drinking water supplies can result from agricultural (fertilizer) run-off, sewerage, or industrial waste. Water-soluble nitrates are readily converted to nitrite ion, an unstable but potent oxidant. In humans, nitrite oxidizes hemoglobin to methemoglobinemia, which has reduced oxygen-carrying capacity. Clinical cyanosis and hypoxemia can result. As early as 1945 published reports described methemoglobinemia in young infants fed milk or formula prepared with nitrate-contaminated water.[195]

The reductase enzyme responsible for restoring hemoglobin to a functional reduced state is deficient during the first months of life, which partially explains the susceptibility of infants to methemoglobinemia.[196] To prevent symptomatic methemoglobinemia in high-risk individuals, the U.S. EPA has established the maximum contaminant level (MCL) in drinking water for nitrate–nitrogen to be 10 mg/L, equivalent to 1 mg/L nitrate–nitrogen.[197] This level is believed to be protective, based on reported cases and on a survey showing that symptomatic infants had consumed water containing much in excess of 10 mg/L of nitrate–nitrogen.[198] The MCL also is protective for pregnant women, who normally have increased methemoglobin concentrations and appear to be susceptible to nitrite-induced methemoglobinemia.[199]

Nitrates and nitrite appear not to be teratogenic in animals.[200,201] Administration of sodium nitrite to pregnant mice stimulated fetal erythropoiesis but did not affect fetal mortality, resorptions, average weight, number of offspring, or incidence of skeletal malformations.[202]

Human epidemiologic studies provide no conclusive evidence that pregnant women who consume low levels of nitrates from drinking water are at increased risk for having a malformed baby. In south Australia an excess of birth defects led to a case–control study examining the relationship between maternal drinking water source (groundwater vs. rainwater) and risk of malformations.[203] The risk of having a malformed infant was increased among women who drank groundwater (relative risk, 2.8; 95 percent confidence interval, 1.6 to 4.4). Risks for NTDs and oral clefts were particularly increased (relative risks, 3.5 and 4.0, respectively). Using estimated nitrate concentration, a dose–response relationship was found with a threefold increased risk at 5 to 15 mg/L nitrates and a fourfold increased risk for greater than 15 mg/L nitrates. Study strengths include case ascertainment and monitoring of water nitrate concentration during the study period. On the other hand, limitations include the assumption that water concentrations were constant during monitoring intervals and that subjects used the same source of drinking water throughout pregnancy. Most notable is the assumption that nitrates rather than some unmeasured drinking water contaminant was responsible. In fact, the seasonal variation in malformation risks suggests that dietary, nutritional, or other environmental factors may have contributed to the increased malformation rates.

A Canadian case–control study found that nitrate exposure from private wells was associated with an increased risk for delivering an infant with a CNS malformation (relative risk, 2.3; 95 percent confidence interval, 0.73 to 7.29).[204] However, the opposite was found with drinking water obtained from other sources: increased nitrate concentration was associated with a decrease in CNS malformations. To assess exposure, the investigators analyzed nitrates in water samples collected at addresses where study subjects lived at the time of delivery. Once again, the study is limited by the lack of information about other possible water contaminants. The contradictory risks associated with drinking water source, independent of nitrate concentration, also suggest that other factors contributed to the observed effects.

Organic Solvents

Large numbers of women are employed in industries that use organic solvents, and women may be exposed through use of household products or drinking water contamination. Not surprisingly, concern has arisen that such exposures may cause any of several adverse reproductive outcomes.

Human health effects of solvent exposure are well known. CNS effects including cortical atrophy, cerebellar degeneration, and loss of intellectual functioning have been documented as a result of chronic, high-dose solvent abuse ("sniffing" or "huffing").[205] Solvent intoxication is an established occupational hazard in such diverse groups as painters and rubber, semiconductor, and dry-cleaning workers. Symptoms may follow inhalation, dermal, or ingestion exposure routes and include headache, nausea, dizziness, and confusion, progressing to CNS depression with loss of consciousness. Chronic exposure to low levels of solvents may lead to neuropsychiatric impairment and to peripheral nerve damage.[206]

Analogous to the health effects described above, maternal solvent abuse by "sniffing" is reported to cause an embryopathy similar to the fetal alcohol syndrome. Hersh and associates[207] described three children with developmental and intellectual impairment, facial dysmorphism, and intrauterine growth retardation whose mothers abused spray paint throughout their pregnancies. Similar dysmorphic features and neurologic impairment have been described in other children born to mothers who chronically abused toluene or unnamed solvents during pregnancy.[208,209]

At lower levels of maternal exposure there is no clear evidence of embryopathic, fetal, or neurobehavioral adverse effects. Epidemiologic studies have examined reproductive outcomes of occupationally as well as environmentally exposed women. Most occupational studies of this subject are case–control designs, with exposure status based on job descriptions and with no actual exposure data (e.g., air concentrations or duration of exposure) available. Multiple solvent exposures are likely, for the most part.[59]

In a series of studies, Holmberg and associates used a compulsory birth defects registry in Finland to examine effects of maternal solvent exposure. In the preliminary reports, the risk of CNS defects was six times more likely and risk of orofacial clefts was 3.5 times more likely with first-trimester maternal exposure.[210-212] Upon reanalysis with additional data 3 years later, the association was no longer statistically significant, and the investigators concluded that still larger numbers of cases with these anomalies were needed for a conclusive study.[213]

Using occupational codes from birth certificates, Olsen[70] reported that mothers who were painters or who worked in a laboratory were no more likely than were unexposed mothers to have children with CNS, gastrointestinal, or limb congenital anomalies. Heidam[71] surveyed Danish women in selected occupations that could result in various chemical exposures. Compared with unexposed women, female painters had a slightly higher risk for spontaneous abortion (odds ratio, 2.9; 95 percent confidence interval, 1 to 8.8). In a study of pregnancy outcomes among women employed at a semiconductor manufacturer, Pastides and associates[214] found an increased risk of spontaneous abortions for women working in the diffusion area (relative risk, 2.18; 95 percent confidence interval, 1.11 to 3.6, compared with nonexposed women). Materials used in the diffusion area include glycol ethers, toxic gases, and various solvents, providing potentially numerous and mixed exposures. Given the small number of pregnancies in exposed and unexposed groups, the investigators consider their results as tentative, pointing out the need for larger prospective studies that include monitoring data to quantify exposure.[214]

To determine if low-level maternal solvent exposure can produce neurobehavioral dysfunction in the offspring, Eskenazi and associates[215] performed developmental evaluations of children with and without prenatal exposure, defined by maternal occupation. Interviews were conducted as long as 4 years after the pregnancy, raising the possibility of maternal recall bias. Developmental and neurobehavioral performance on standardized tests were similar in exposed and unexposed children. Because small differences between groups should have been detectable, the investigators suggested that the exposure levels may have been insufficient to produce an effect. Such findings are reassuring, but, given the known neurobehavioral effects of chronic solvent exposure in adults, additional studies are needed for confirmation. Future studies should evaluate prenatal effects of single or known mixtures of solvents and include more reliable exposure data, if possible.

On numerous occasions, drinking water contamination by organic solvents has resulted from storage tank leaks or hazardous waste leachate. Such contamination is a common "Superfund" issue confronting the U.S. EPA.[216] Affected communities may identify a temporal or geographic clustering of adverse reproductive effects, believing that the contamination has caused the epidemic. To date, there is no published evidence to support such a cause–effect relationship, but at least one study demonstrated an increased risk of spontaneous abortions among women during the time that their drinking water supply was contaminated with trichloroethane and other organic solvents.[42] A hospital-based study was also undertaken in response to community concerns that there were increased numbers of children born with congenital cardiac anomalies to women living in the contaminated area. The increased prevalence of cardiac anomalies was confirmed but was found to be temporally unrelated to the drinking water contamination, making a causal relationship unlikely.[217]

In conclusion, toluene and possibly other organic solvents are probably teratogenic at the high-exposure levels seen with solvent abuse. The risk for the "fetal solvent syndrome" is unknown, and no exposure threshold for effect can be identified at this time. There is no conclusive evidence that low-level exposure increases the risk of congenital malformations or other adverse reproductive outcomes.

In a similar vein, when a pregnant woman asks if it is safe for her to paint the baby's nursery, Scialli[218] wisely advises counseling to minimize exposure without giving the impression that paint is an established developmental toxicant.

Anesthetic Gases

Large numbers of women working in medical and dental professions may be exposed occupationally to anesthetic gases, raising serious concerns about the reproductive hazards of such exposures. There is evidence that chronic first-trimester exposure may increase the risk of spontaneous abortion.[219,220] Despite numerous studies, the question of whether a mother's exposure to anesthetic gas increases the risk of her bearing a congenitally malformed infant is still debated. One argument against a causal relationship is that no pattern of malformations has been found in studies reporting increased birth defect rates following maternal exposure during pregnancy,[221] On the other hand, animal studies have shown that anesthetic gases can be teratogenic at concentrations similar to those experienced by operating room personnel.[222-224] Some investigators have found increased rates of birth defects in infants born to exposed women and have observed a dose-related effect.[219,224,225] In two studies, the rate of congenitally malformed infants was increased among female anesthetists who worked during the first 6 months of pregnancy compared with the rate among female anesthetists who did not work during pregnancy.[226,227] A criteria document prepared by the National Institute for Occupational Safety and Health (NIOSH) contains reviews of animal data and epidemiologic studies published before 1977.[220] More recent reviews are also available.[228,229]

Virtually all epidemiologic studies of exposure to waste anesthetic gas and reproductive outcomes have design problems that affect the interpretation of reported results. Crude estimates of anesthetic gas exposure must be used, because no actual measurements of gas concentrations are available. The specific gases are usually not identified, and exposure to mixtures of anesthetic agents is likely.[220] Many studies have been conducted by survey, with no validation of the responses and often with poor response rates. In such studies selection bias cannot be evaluated, because there is no information about nonresponders. Not validating the reproductive history can lead to misleading results for several reasons. Study subjects may forget or inaccurately recall events that took place years before. Women exposed to an environmental agent are more likely to recall such exposure if they have a spontaneous abortion or a child with a minor malformation, in contrast to women with a normal pregnancy outcome.[230] One last problem pertains to the inherent difficulty of studying spontaneous abortions. To avoid the criticism that reported spontaneous abortions were not validated, investigators in one study considered only patients whose spontaneous abortions required them to be hospitalized.[230] The problem with this approach is that women who have spontaneous abortions do not always require hospitalization, particularly if the abortion occurred during the first trimester or before pregnancy was diagnosed.

Despite problems in study design, epidemiologic evidence supports the view that repeated maternal exposure to waste anesthetic gases during pregnancy should be minimized. Women who work in areas with a potential for repeated anesthetic gas exposure (no gas scavenger system in place) should be aware of the possibility of adverse reproductive effects and decide whether they want to continue to work in the same area during pregnancy or request to be transferred. In settings where anesthetic gases are administered, a gas scavenger system should be used, and particular attention should be given to maintaining that system. A properly functioning gas scavenging system should provide adequate protection from exposure.[220,231] Because there is always uncertainty about completely avoiding exposure to anesthetic gases, however, a woman with a history of pregnancy loss or of having a child with congenital malformations may want to transfer to another work area.[225]

The question of whether pregnant women who undergo general anesthesia are at increased risk for an adverse reproductive outcome is also unresolved. Studies of this question are rare, and the largest is an epidemiologic study that found no increased risk of congenital malformations following surgical general anesthesia in early pregnancy.[232] The present value of this study may be lessened by the fact that data were collected in the 1960s, when anesthetic practices were different and when not all anesthetics currently used were available. There are additional limitations of this or any other study of reproductive risks of general anesthesia during pregnancy: Additional drugs are usually given. The surgical procedure or a complication may be hazardous to the conceptus. Perhaps most important, pregnant women who require surgery are likely to have one or more underlying conditions that may increase the risk of an adverse reproductive outcome, independent of the anesthetic.

THE OBSTETRICIAN'S ROLE IN EVALUATING REPRODUCTIVE RISKS IN AND BEYOND THE WORKPLACE

Limitations of Available Reproductive Toxicity Information

Clinical questions about environmental or occupational exposures causing adverse reproductive outcomes are extremely difficult to answer, and the answers are seldom as helpful as they need to be. The difficulty occurs because the exposure of the patient and fetus is seldom known or measurable. If the exposure is known, there is almost never a study of similar exposure, with a sufficient sample size, that enables a physician to give a reliable estimate of risk or lack thereof.

For all the environmental exposures discussed in this chapter, no threshold is known below which no adverse reproductive outcome can be expected. Except for ionizing radiation and mercury, maximum recommended exposure levels are difficult to quantify.

Most diagnostic radiographs result in exposures of less than 5 rad,[233] and the risk of congenital malformations or developmental delay in the infant probably is negligible at doses below 5 rad.[83] Therefore, under most circumstances, consultation to estimate dosage is not necessary, although it may provide some reassurance to the pregnant patient.

The most readily available data are usually from studies in laboratory animals. Although these data are useful in making judgments about setting standards or marketing an agent, they are seldom helpful in giving accurate risk information to a patient.

Human data usually consist of case reports, which seldom can establish a hazard and never can quantitate the magnitude of the risk. Epidemiologic studies are less often available and frequently have severe limitations in design, execution, analysis, or interpretation. Thus, in most cases, the questions must be answered on the basis of reasoned judgments in the face of inadequate data.

Approach to Occupational Exposure Risk Assessment

The process by which a reasoned judgment can be made follows a logical progression, as summarized in Table 9.8. The steps are described below. Paul and

Table 9.8 Steps in Evaluating Exposures That Can Result in Birth Defects or Other Adverse Reproductive Outcomes

Step/Action	Information Resources
1. Identify the exposure(s)	Material Safety Data Sheet (MSDS); industry (supervisors, industrial hygienists)
2. Characterize extent of exposure(s)	Description of job activities; monitoring data (e.g., air sampling, radiation badge); assessment of exposure routes; biologic sampling (e.g., lead, mercury)
3. Hazard evaluation	Health professionals (occupational/industrial physicians, medical toxicologists, geneticists); regional poison control centers; teratology information services; National Institute for Occupational Safety and Health (NIOSH) criteria documents and technical bulletins; state health departments; on-line databases (National Library of Medicine, Environmental Teratology Information Center, Environmental Mutagen, Carcinogen and Teratogen Department, ReproTox); textbooks and periodicals
4. Risk assessment/judgment	Steps 1 and 2; patient's family, medical, and reproductive history; other relevant exposures (e.g., alcohol, tobacco, drugs-of-abuse), background risk

Himmelstein provide[63] a more detailed description of a similar evaluation process, and a book devoted to this subject will be available soon.[64]

Assessment of potential adverse health effects or toxicity from a chemical exposure begins with correct identification of the agent(s) (Table 9.8). As workers increasingly demanded their right to know the identity and toxicity of chemicals, the U.S. Occupational Safety and Health Administration (OSHA) drafted a regulation and state and local governments have passed so-called "worker right-to-know" laws.[234] One intent of the regulation and laws is to provide workers and physicians with toxicity information about each chemical used in a given workplace. An information sheet, the Material Safety Data Sheet (MSDS), is developed by the chemical manufacturer or distributor, and includes basic identifying and specific toxicity information. Other details of the OSHA regulation and right-to-know laws are reviewed elsewhere.[234,235]

Obstetricians should be aware that copies of MSDSs are available from an employer upon request to any woman who may be occupationally exposed to a hazardous chemical. Supervisors, managers, and industrial hygienists may be able to provide additional identification, particularly when chemicals are mixed or modified through heating or industrial processes.

The next step is to characterize the extent to which the patient is exposed. This can be relatively easy for substances such as lead and other heavy metals quantifiable in blood or urine. The radiation badge properly worn can provide exposure monitoring and should be checked frequently during pregnancy. OSHA has published occupational exposure standards for a large number of chemicals associated with adverse health effects.[135] These chemicals and agents must be monitored in the workplace, and such data may be helpful for exposure assessment.

Most often, however, no biologic or environmental data are available. Instead, the clinician must rely on a detailed description of the patient's job activities, precautions taken to avoid exposure (gloves, respirator, protective clothing, hand washing, and so forth), and any clinical signs or symptoms suggesting excess exposure. All feasible routes of exposure should be considered, including ingestion (common if handwashing is not done before eating), inhalation (especially if hot vapors or odorless gases are produced),

and dermal absorption (increased through irritated skin or prolonged contact with contaminated clothing). Similar considerations apply to nonoccupational exposures as well.

The third step is hazard evaluation. In this context, the physician must determine what is known of the reproductive effects of the chemicals or agents. Because no one can be all-knowing and no single information resource is sufficient for all patient questions, prudence dictates consulting a variety of sources. A partial list is provided in Table 9.8. Physicians specializing in occupational or industrial medicine, medical toxicology, and genetics can be helpful. Such physicians may be affiliated with regional genetics centers or certified regional poison control centers. These centers may be able to recommend other helpful consultants as well. Numerous teratology information services (TISs) provide no-cost physician and patient telephone consultation. These services may vary considerably in how the consultation is provided, whether follow-up is done, nature of the staff qualifications, and the extent of medical supervision. Some TISs also provide a written copy of the consultation to the referring obstetrician. One university-affiliated TIS maintains and updates a reproductive toxicology database (ReproTox) containing summaries of more than 2,000 chemicals and agents.[236] Obstetricians who choose to refer patients to any of these services should be familiar with the kinds of information and follow-up provided.

The U.S. government supports two on line-bibliographic services related to teratology. Requests for either updates or a specific search topic can be sent to the following two agencies:

Environmental Teratology Information Center
Post Office Box 12233
National Institute of Environmental Health Sciences
Maildrop 18-01
Research Triangle Park, NC 27709

Environmental Mutagen, Carcinogen, and Teratogen Information Department
Oak Ridge National Laboratory
Oak Ridge, TN 37830

The National Library of Medicine (NLM) supports

the TOXNET system of toxicology databases. Many university or medical reference librarians and information specialists are trained in searching these databases, which include reproductive as well as general toxicology information. Clinicians can access the NLM databases to perform MEDLINE or TOXNET searches.[237] Individuals can also do their own reproductive toxicology (ReproTox) database searches.[236]

Another federal resource is NIOSH, which publishes recommendations for occupational exposure to a variety of agents or compounds. Each recommendation is supported by a criteria document, providing a comprehensive review of animal and human effects attributable to the specific agent. NIOSH also has a technical information service at its Cincinnati, Ohio, headquarters that may be able to provide in-house reports of investigations as well as NIOSH Technical Bulletins and criteria documents.

The American College of Obstetricians and Gynecologists publishes guidelines for several occupational exposures during pregnancy.[238] These guidelines include information about metals, solvents, and radiation—agents that also may be found as environmental contaminants.

Many state health departments have a division responsible for occupational health issues. Staff may have expertise in industrial hygiene and safety, occupational medicine, and reproductive epidemiology and toxicology. Specific concerns about hazardous occupational exposures or adverse reproductive outcomes related to workplace exposures should be addressed to this division in the health department. In addition, state health departments may be helpful in evaluating associations between environmental exposures and adverse reproductive outcomes.

Numerous off-the-shelf information resources include texts,[19,59,60,64,79,80,164] periodicals, and review articles.[63,81,83,239,243]

The final and most difficult step is formulating an assessment of risk. Chemical identity, extent of exposure, and the reproductive toxicity of the agent must be known. Unfortunately, all these necessary pieces of information are rarely available. If the exposure is known, available information rarely enables a physician to give a reliable estimate of risk. Thus risk assessment is really a process of reasoned judgment. Formulating this judgment requires consideration of many factors, including the best estimate of the nature, extent, duration, and timing of exposure, the patient's medical, reproductive, and genetic history, life-style habits (especially tobacco, alcohol, and drug abuse), and, of course, reproductive toxicity information about the agent. Equally important, the patient should understand that with every pregnancy there is always a background risk for an adverse outcome. Birth defects and other adverse outcomes of pregnancy are relatively common events. Frustrating though it is, the fact remains that it is usual not to know the cause for a given adverse outcome.

After completing this assessment process, the physician will be more familiar with and understand limitations of available information about a particular agent or chemical. The patient's exposure can be considered in the context of other relevant medical information, and this should be explained to the patient in nontechnical language. The physician may be able to recommend ways to decrease or minimize maternal exposure and determine if more close monitoring of the pregnancy is warranted.

CONCLUSION

We know that many chemicals cause birth defects and other adverse reproductive outcomes in animals. A few of these agents are human teratogens or reproductive toxicants. Conceivably, exposure to chemicals could be responsible for a sizable amount of adverse human reproductive outcome, even though the causal role for these chemicals has yet to be shown. Epidemiologic studies may help us to understand what role chemicals play, but we need more accurate assessments of exposure and better identification of the specific reproductive outcomes.

REFERENCES

1. Centers for Disease Control: Contribution of birth defects to infant mortality—United States, 1986. MMWR 38:633, 1989
2. Centers for Disease Control: Changes in premature mortality—United States, 1979–1986. MMWR 37:45, 1988
3. Public Health Service: Pregnancy and infant health. p. 15. In Public Health Service: Promoting Health/Preventing Disease: Objectives for the Nation. U.S. Department of Health and Human Services, Public Health Service, Washington, DC, 1980
4. Public Health Service: Pregnancy and infant health. p. 11-6. In Public Health Service: Promoting Health/

Preventing Disease: Year 2000 Objectives for the Nation (draft). U.S. Department of Health and Human Services, Public Health Service, Washington, DC, 1989

5. Wilson JG: Environmental effects of development—teratology. p. 269. In Assali NS (ed): Pathophysiology of Gestation. Vol 2. Academic Press, San Diego, 1972

6. McKusick VA: Mendelian Inheritance in Man. Johns Hopkins University Press, Baltimore, 1966

7. McKusick VA: Mendelian Inheritance in Man. 9th Ed. Johns Hopkins University Press, Baltimore, 1990

8. Gabbe SG: Congenital malformations in infants of diabetic mothers. Obstet Gynecol Surv 32:125, 1977

9. Lenke RR, Levy HL: Maternal phenylketonuria and hyperphenylalaninemia: an international survey of the outcome of untreated and treated pregnancies. N Engl J Med 303:1202, 1980

10. Wilson JG: Current status of teratology—general principles and mechanisms derived from animal studies. p. 47. In Wilson JG, Fraser FC (eds): Handbook of Teratology. Vol. 1. Plenum Press, New York, 1977

11. Fraser FC: Relation of animal studies to the problem in man. p. 75. In Wilson JG, Fraser FC (eds): Handbook of Teratology. Vol. 1. Plenum Press, New York, 1977

11a. Buehler BA, Delimont D, van Waes M, Finnell RH: Prenatal prediction of risk of the fetal hydantoin syndrome. N Engl J Med 322:1567, 1990

12. Lenz W, Knapp K: Foetal malformations due to thalidomide. Geriatr Med Mthly 7:253, 1962

13. Hook EB: Incidence and prevalence as measures of the frequency of birth defects. Am J Epidemiol 116:743, 1982

14. Sever LE: Reproductive hazards of the workplace. J Occup Med 23:685, 1981

15. Hemminki K, Sorsa M, Vainio H: Genetic risks caused by occupational chemicals. Scand J Work Environ Health 5:307, 1979

16. Shepard TH: Teratogens: an update. Hosp Pract 19:191, 1984

17. Mattison DR, Hanson JW, Kochar DM, Rao KS: Criteria for identifying and listing substances known to cause developmental toxicity under California's Proposition 65. Reprod Toxicol 3:3, 1989

18. Wolkowski-Tyl R: Reproductive and teratogenic effects: no more thalidomides. Am Chem Soc Symp Ser 160:115, 1981

19. Shepard TH (ed): Catalog of Teratogenic Agents. p. 549. The Johns Hopkins University Press, Baltimore, 1986

20. Environmental Protection Agency: Guidelines for the health assessment of suspect developmental toxicants. Fed Register 51:34028, 1986

21. Carter CO: Genetics of common disorders. Br Med Bull 25:52, 1969

22. Sever LE: Epidemiologic approaches to reproductive hazards of the workplace. Birth Defects 18:33, 1982

23. Sever LE: Incidence and prevalence as measures of the frequency of birth defects. Am J Epidemiol 118:608, 1983

24. Leck I: Correlations of malformation frequency with environmental and genetic attributes in man. p. 243. In Wilson JG, Fraser FC (eds): Handbook of Teratology. Vol 3. Plenum Press, New York, 1977

25. Centers for Disease Control: Congenital Malformations Surveillance Report, January–December 1980. Centers for Disease Control, Atlanta, GA, 1982

26. Sever LE, Strassburg MA: Epidemiologic aspects of neural tube defects in the United States: changing concepts and their importance for screening and prenatal diagnostic programs. p. 243. In Mizejewski GJ, Porter IH (eds): Alpha-Fetoprotein and Congenital Disorders. Academic Press, San Diego, 1985

27. Sever LE, Hessol NA: Overall design considerations in male and female occupational reproductive studies. Prog Clin Biol Res 160:15, 1984

28. Sever LE, Sanders M, Monsen R: An epidemiologic study of neural tube defects in Los Angeles County. I. Prevalence at birth based on multiple sources of case ascertainment. Teratology 25:315, 1982

29. Sever LE: Hormonal pregnancy tests and spina bifida. Nature 242:410, 1973

30. Lenz W: Das thalidomid-syndrom. Fortschr Med 81:148, 1963

31. Gregg NM: Congenital cataract following German measles in the mother. Trans Ophthalmol Soc Aust 3:35, 1941

32. Lenz W: Discussion contribution by Dr. W. Lenz, Hamburg, on the lecture by Pfeiffer RA, Kosenow K: On the exogenous origin of malformations of the extremities. Tagung der Rheinisch-Westfalischen Kinderarztevereinigung in Dusseldorf, 1961

33. McBride WG: Thalidomide and congenital abnormalities. Lancet 2:1358, 1961

34. Heath CW Jr, Flynt JW Jr, Oakley GP Jr, Falek A: The role of birth defect surveillance in control of fetal environmental hazards. Postgrad Med J 51:69, 1975

35. Edmonds LD, Layde PM, James LM et al: Congenital malformation surveillance: two American systems. Int J Epidemiol 10:247, 1981

36. Flynt JW Jr, Ebbin AJ, Oakley GP Jr et al: Metropolitan Atlanta congenital defects program. p. 155. In Hook EB, Janerich DT, Porter IH (eds): Monitoring Birth Defects and Environment: The Problem of Surveillance. Academic Press, San Diego, 1971

37. Fan AM, Book SA, Neutra RR, Epstein DM: Selenium

and human health implications in California's San Joaquin Valley. J Toxicol Environ Health 23:539, 1988

38. White FMM, Cohen FG, Sherman G, McCurdy R: Chemicals, birth defects and stillbirths in New Brunswick: associations with agricultural activity. Can Med Assoc J 138:117, 1988

39. Infante PF: Oncogenic and mutagenic risks in communities with polyvinyl chloride production facilities. Ann NY Acad Sci 271:49, 1976

40. Theriault G, Iturra H, Gingras S: Evaluation of the association between birth defects and ambient vinyl chloride. Teratology 27:359, 1983

41. Nordstrom S, Beckman L, Nordenson I: Occupational and environmental risks in and around a smelter in Northern Sweden. III. Frequencies of spontaneous abortion. Hereditas 88:41, 1978

42. Deane M, Swan SH, Harris JA et al: Adverse pregnancy outcomes in relation to water contamination, Santa Clara County, California 1980–1981. Am J Epidemiol 129:894, 1989

43. Lenz W: Thalidomide and congenital abnormalities. Lancet 1:45, 1962

44. Edmonds LD, Falk H, Nissim JE: Congenital malformations and vinyl chloride. Lancet 2:1098, 1975

45. Edmonds LD, Anderson CE, Flynt JW Jr, James LM: Congenital central nervous system malformations and vinyl chloride monomer exposure: a community study. Teratology 17:137, 1978

46. Lammer EJ, Sever LE, Oakley GP: Teratogen update: valproic acid. Teratology 35:465, 1987

47. Sever LE, Olsen AR, Hinds NR et al: NINCDS Collaborative Perinatal Project: A User's Guide to the Project and Data. Vol. I. An Introduction to the History, Scope and Methodology of the Project. Contract NO1-NS-2-2311. National Institute of Neurological and Communicative Disorders and Stroke, Washington, DC, 1983

48. Nordstrom S, Beckman I, Nordenson I: Occupational and environmental risks in and around a smelter in Northern Sweden. V. Spontaneous abortion among female employees and decreased birth weight in their offspring. Hereditas 90:291, 1979

49. Beckman L, Nordstrom S: Occupational and environmental risks in and around a smelter in Northern Sweden. IX. Fetal mortality among wives of smelter workers. Hereditas 97:1, 1982

50. Bracken MB: Design and conduct of randomized clinical trials in perinatal research. p. 397. In Bracken MB (ed): Perinatal Epidemiology. Oxford University Press, New York, 1984

51. Smithells RW, Sheppard S, Schorah CJ et al: Apparent prevention of neural tube defects by periconceptional vitamin supplementation. Arch Dis Child 56:911, 1981

52. Smithells RW, Sheppard S, Schorah CJ et al: Possible prevention of neural-tube defects by periconceptional vitamin supplementation. Lancet 1:339, 1980

53. Mulinare J, Cordero JF, Erickson JD, Berry RJ: Periconceptional use of multivitamins and the occurrence of neural tube defects. JAMA 260:3141, 1988

54. Mills JL, Rhoads GG, Simpson JL et al: The absence of a relation between the periconceptional use of vitamins and neural-tube defects. N Engl J Med 321:430, 1989

55. Milunsky A, Jick H, Jick SS et al: Multivitamin/folic acid supplementation in early pregnancy reduces the prevalence of neural tube defects. JAMA 262:2847, 1989

56. Bower C, Stanley F: Dietary folate as a risk factor for neural tube defects—evidence from a case-control study in Western Australia. Med J Aust 150:613, 1989

57. Wald NJ, Polani PE: Neural-tube defects and vitamins: the need for a randomized clinical trial. Br J Obstet Gynaecol 91:516, 1984

58. Clement Associates: Chemical Hazards to Human Reproduction. Council on Environmental Quality, Washington, DC, 1981

59. Barlow SM, Sullivan FM: Reproductive Hazards of Industrial Chemicals. Academic Press, San Diego, 1982

60. Mattison DR (ed): Reproductive toxicology. Prog Clin Biol Res, Vol. 117, 1983

61. Lockey JE, Lemasters GK, Keye WR Jr (eds): Reproduction: the new frontier in occupational and environmental health research. Prog Clin Biol Res, Vol. 160, 1984

62. Legator MS, Rosenberg M, Zenick H (eds): Environmental Influences on Fertility, Pregnancy and Development. Alan R Liss, New York, 1984

63. Paul M, Himmelstein J: Reproductive hazards in the workplace: what the practitioner needs to know about chemical exposures. Obstet Gynecol 71:921, 1988

64. Paul M (ed): Occupational and Environmental Reproductive Hazards: A Guide for Clinicians. Williams & Wilkins, Baltimore (in preparation)

65. Koren G (ed): Maternal–Fetal Toxicology: A Clinicians' Guide. Marcel Dekker, New York, 1990

66. Hemminki K, Sorsa M, Vainio H (eds): Occupational Hazards and Reproduction. Hemisphere Publishing Corp., Washington, DC, 1985

67. Lemasters GK, Selevan SG: Types of exposure models and advantages and disadvantages of sources of exposure data for use in occupational reproductive studies. Prog Clin Biol Res 160:67, 1984

68. Gordon JE: Assessment of occupational and environmental exposures. p. 450. In Bracken MB (ed): Perinatal Epidemiology. Oxford University Press, New York, 1984

69. Axelsson GA, Lutz C, Rylander R: Exposure to solvents and outcome of pregnancy in university laboratory employees. Br J Ind Med 41:305, 1984

70. Olsen J: Risk of exposure to teratogens amongst laboratory staff and painters. Dan Med Bull 30:24, 1983

71. Heidam LZ: Spontaneous abortions among dental assistants, factory workers, painters, and gardening workers: a follow-up study. J Epidemiol Commun Health 38:149, 1984

72. Monson RR: Occupational Epidemiology. CRC Press, Boca Raton, FL, 1980

73. Lindbohm ML, Hemminki K, Kyyronen P et al: Spontaneous abortions among rubber workers and congenital malformations in their offspring. Scand J Work Environ Health 9:85, 1983

74. Rachootin P, Olsen J: The risk of infertility and delayed conception associated with exposures in the Danish workplace. J Occup Med 25:394, 1983

75. Hemminki K, Kyyronen P, Niemi ML et al: Spontaneous abortions in an industrialized community in Finland. Am J Public Health 73:32, 1983

76. National Research Council Committee on Biological Markers: Biological Markers in Reproductive Toxicology. National Academy Press, Washington, DC, 1989

77. Hattis DB: The promise of molecular epidemiology for quantitative risk assessment. Risk Analysis 6:181, 1986

78. Hulka BS, Wilcosky T: Biological markers in epidemiologic research. Arch Environ Health 43:83, 1988

79. Kirsch-Volders M (ed): Mutagenicity, Carcinogenicity, and Teratogenicity of Industrial Pollutants. Plenum Press, New York, 1984

80. Zielhuis RL, Stijkel A, Verberk MM, van de Poel-Bot M: Health Risks to Female Workers in Occupational Exposure to Chemical Agents. Springer-Verlag, New York, 1984

81. Shepard TH: Human teratogenicity. Adv Pediatr 33:225, 1986

82. Beckman DA, Brent RL: Mechanism of known environmental teratogens: drugs and chemicals. Clin Perinatol 13:649, 1986

83. Brent RL: The effects of embryonic and fetal exposure to x-ray, microwaves, and ultrasound. Clin Perinatol 13:615, 1986

84. Heath CW Jr: Epidemiology of dump exposures. p. 10. In Finberg L (ed): Chemical and Radiation Hazards to Children. Report of the 84th Ross Conference on Pediatric Research. Ross Laboratories, Columbus, OH, 1982

85. Miller RW: Measures of reproductive effects. p. 88. In Finberg L (ed): Chemical and Radiation Hazards to Children. Report of the 84th Ross Conference on Pediatric Research. Ross Laboratories, Columbus, OH, 1982

86. Miller RW: Effects of ionizing radiation from the atomic bomb on Japanese children. Pediatrics 41:257, 1968

87. Wood JW, Johnson KG, Omori Y: In utero exposure to the Hiroshima atomic bomb: an evaluation of head size and mental retardation: twenty years later. Pediatrics 39:385, 1967

88. Wood JW, Johnson KG, Omori Y et al: Mental retardation in children exposed in utero to the atomic bombs in Hiroshima and Nagasaki. Am J Public Health 57:1381, 1967

89. Miller RW: Delayed effects occurring within the first decade after exposure of young individuals to the Hiroshima atomic bomb. Pediatrics 18:1, 1956

90. Yamazaki JN, Schull WH: Perinatal loss and neurological abnormalities among children of the atomic bomb: Nagasaki and Hiroshima revisited, 1949 to 1989. JAMA 264:605, 1990

91. Tabuchi A: Fetal disorders due to ionizing radiation. Hiroshima J Med Sci 13:125, 1964

92. Dekaban AS: Abnormalities in children exposed to x-radiation during various stages of gestation: tentative timetable of radiation injury to the human fetus, part I. J Nucl Med 9:471, 1968

93. Brent RL: Environmental factors: radiation. p. 179. In Brent RL, Harris MI (eds): Fogarty International Series on Preventive Medicine. Vol. 3. DHEW Publ No. 76-853. National Institutes of Health, Bethesda, MD, 1976

94. Archer VE: Anencephalus, drinking water, geomagnetism and cosmic radiation. Am J Epidemiol 109:88, 1979

95. Gentry J, Parkhurst E, Bulin G: An epidemiologic study of congenital malformations in New York state. Am J Public Health 49:497, 1959

96. Kochupiluai N, Verma IC, Grewal MS, Ramalingaswami V: Down's syndrome and related abnormalities in an area of high background radiation in coastal Kenya. Nature 262:60, 1976

97. Brent RL: Radiations and other physical agents. p. 208. In Wilson JG, Fraser FC (eds): Handbook of Teratology. Vol. 1. Plenum Press, New York, 1977

98. Segall A, MacMahon B, Hannigan M: Congenital malformations and background radiation in northern New England. J Chronic Dis 17:915, 1964

99. Wood JW, Keehn RJ, Kawamoto S, Johnson KC: The growth and development of children exposed in utero

to the atomic bombs in Hiroshima and Nagasaki. Am J Public Health 57:1374, 1967

100. Neel JV, Kato H, Schull WJ: Mortality in the children of atomic bomb survivors and controls. Genetics 76:311, 1974

101. Meyer MB, Diamond EL, Merz T: Sex ratio of children born to mothers who had been exposed to x-rays in utero. Johns Hopkins Med J 123:123, 1968

102. Alberman E, Polani PE, Fraser-Roberts JA et al: Parental x-irradiation and chromosome constitution in their spontaneously aborted foetuses. Ann Hum Genet 36:185, 1972

103. Stevenson AC, Mason R, Edwards KD: Maternal diagnostic x-irradiation before conception and the frequency of mongolism in children subsequently born. Lancet 2:1335, 1970

104. Uchida IA, Curtis EJ: A possible association between maternal radiation and mongolism. Lancet 2:848, 1961

105. Uchida IA, Holunga R, Lawler C: Maternal radiation and chromosomal aberrations. Lancet 2:1045, 1968

106. Sigler AT, Lilienfeld AM, Cohen BH, Westlake JE: Radiation exposure in parents of children with mongolism (Down's syndrome). Bull Johns Hopkins Hosp 117:374, 1965

107. Carter CO, Evans KA, Stewart AM: Maternal radiation and Down's syndrome (mongolism). Lancet 2:1042, 1961

108. Marmol JG, Scriggins AL, Vollman RF: Mothers of mongoloid infants in the collaborative project. Am J Obstet Gynecol 104:533, 1969

109. Kinlen LJ, Acheson ED: Diagnostic irradiation, congenital malformations and spontaneous abortion. Br J Radiol 41:648, 1968

110. Stewart A, Kneale GW: Radiation dose effects in relation to obstetric x-rays and childhood cancers. Lancet 1:1185, 1970

111. Stewart A, Webb D, Giles D, Hewitt D: Malignant disease in childhood and diagnostic irradiation in utero. Lancet 2:447, 1956

112. Stewart A, Webb D, Hewitt D: A survey of childhood malignancies. Br Med J 1:1495, 1958

113. Stark CR, Orleans M, Haverkamp AD, Murphy J: Short- and long-term risks after exposure to diagnostic ultrasound in utero. Obstet Gynecol 63:194, 1984

114. Reece EA, Assimakopoulos E, Zheng XZ et al: The safety of obstetric ultrasonography: concern for the fetus. Obstet Gynecol 76:139, 1990

115. Shoji R, Murakami U, Shimizu T: Influence of low-intensity ultrasound irradiation on prenatal development of two inbred mouse strains. Teratology 12:227, 1975

116. World Health Organization: Environmental Health Criteria 1: Mercury. p. 48. WHO, Geneva, 1976

117. Harada M: Minamata disease: a medical report. p. 180. In Smith WE, Smith AM (eds): Minamata. Holt, Rinehart, New York, 1975

118. Bakir F, DamluJi SF, Amin-Zaki M et al: Methylmercury poisoning in Iraq. Science 181:230, 1973

119. Koos BJ, Longo LD: Mercury toxicity in the pregnant woman, fetus, and newborn infant. Am J Obstet Gynecol 126:390, 1976

120. Choi BH: Effects of prenatal methylmercury poisoning upon growth and development of fetal central nervous system. p. 473. In Clarkson TW, Nordberg GF, Sager PR (eds): Reproductive and Developmental Toxicology of Metals. Plenum Press, New York, 1983

121. Marsh DO, Myers GT, Clarkson TW et al: Fetal methylmercury poisoning: clinical and toxicologic data on 29 cases. Ann Neurol 7:348, 1980

122. Clarkson TW: The pharmacology of mercury compounds. Annu Rev Pharmacol 12:375, 1972

123. Tsuchiya H, Mitani K, Kodama K, Nakata T: Placental transfer of heavy metals in normal pregnant Japanese women. Arch Environ Health 39:11, 1984

124. Sandstead HH, Doherty RA, Mahaffey KA: Effects and metabolism of toxic trace metals in the neonatal period. p. 207. In Clarkson TW, Nordberg GF, Sager RP (eds): Reproductive and Developmental Toxicology of Metals. Plenum Press, New York, 1983

125. Pierce PE, Thompson JF, Likosky WH et al: Alkyl mercury poisoning in humans: report of an outbreak. JAMA 220:1439, 1972

126. McKeown-Eyssen G, Ruedy J, Neims A: Methylmercury exposure in northern Quebec. II. Neurologic findings in children. Am J Epidemiol 118:470, 1983

127. Skerfving S, Hansson K, Mangs C et al: Methylmercury-induced chromosome damage in man. Environ Res 7:83, 1974

128. Burbacher TM, Monnett C, Grant KS, Mottet NK: Methylmercury exposure and reproductive dysfunction in the nonhuman primate. Toxicol Appl Pharmacol 75:18, 1984

129. Gunderson VM, Grant KS, Burbacher TM et al: The effect of low-level prenatal methylmercury exposure on visual recognition memory in infant crab-eating macaques. Child Dev 57:1076, 1986

130. Mottet NK, Shaw CM, Burbacher TM: Health risks from increases in methylmercury exposure. Environ Health Perspect 63:133, 1985

131. Gunderson VM, Grant-Webster KS, Burbacher TM, Mottet NK: Visual recognition memory deficits in methylmercury-exposed *Macaca fascicularis* infants. Neurotoxicol Teratol 10:373, 1988

132. Gilani SH: Congenital abnormalities in methylmercury poisoning. Environ Res 9:128, 1975

133. Mattison DR: Female reproductive system. p. 43. In Clarkson TW, Nordberg GW, Sager PR (eds): Reproductive and Developmental Toxicology of Metals. Plenum Press, New York, 1983

134. Steffek AJ, Clayton R, Siew C et al: Effects of elemental mercury vapor exposure on pregnant Sprague-Dawley rats. Teratology 35:59A, 1987

135. American Conference of Governmental Industrial Hygienists: Threshold Limit Values and Biological Exposure Indices for 1988–1989. ACGIH, Cincinnati, 1988

136. Clarkson TW, Magos L, Greenwood MR: The transport of elemental mercury into fetal tissues. Biol Neonate 21:239, 1972

137. Wannag A, Skjaerasen J: Mercury accumulation in placenta and foetal membranes: a study of dental workers and their babies. Environ Physiol Biochem 5:348, 1975

138. Agency for Toxic Substances and Disease Registry: Toxicological Profile for Mercury. p. 65. U.S. Public Health Service, ATSDR, Atlanta, GA, 1989

139. Lein DC, Todoruk DN, Rajani HR et al: Accidental inhalation of mercury vapor: respiratory and toxicologic consequences. Can Med Assoc J 129:591, 1983

140. Fawer RF, DeRibaupierre Y, Juillemin M et al: Measurement of hand tremor induced by industrial exposure to metallic mercury. Br J Ind Med 40:204, 1983

141. Iyer K, Goldgood J, Eberstein A et al: Mercury poisoning in a dentist. Arch Neurol 33:788, 1976

142. Shapiro IM, Sumner AJ, Spitz LK et al: Neurophysiological and neuropsychological function in mercury-exposed dentists. Lancet 1:1147, 1982

143. Agency for Toxic Substances and Disease Registry: Toxicological Profile for Mercury. p. 90. U.S. Public Health Service, ATSDR, Atlanta, GA, 1989

144. Sikorski R, Juszkiewicz T, Paszkowski T, Szprengier-Juszkiewicz T: Women in dental surgeries: reproductive hazards in occupational exposure to metallic mercury. Int Arch Occup Environ Health 59:551, 1987

145. Phelps RW, Clarkson TW, Dershaw TG et al: Interrelationships of blood and hair mercury concentrations in a North American population exposed to methylmercury. Arch Environ Health 35:161, 1980

146. Brodsky JB, Cohen EN, Whitcher C et al: Occupational exposure to mercury in dentistry and pregnancy outcome. J Am Dent Assoc 111:779, 1985

147. Ericson A, Kallen B: Pregnancy outcome in women working as dentists, dental assistants or dental technicians. Int Arch Occup Environ Health 61:329, 1989

148. Rom WN: Effects of lead on the female and reproduction: a review. Mount Sinai J Med 43:542, 1976

149. Hall A: The increasing use of lead as an abortifacient. Br Med J 1:584, 1905

150. Creason JP, Svensgaard DJ, Baumgarner JE et al: Maternal–fetal tissue levels of sixteen trace elements in eight communities. EPA report No. 600:1-78-033. U.S. Environmental Protection Agency, Washington, DC, 1978

151. Centers for Disease Control: Preventing lead poisoning in young children — United States. MMWR 34:66, 1985

152. Needleman HL, Gunnoe C, Leviton A et al: Deficits in psychologic and classroom performance of children with elevated dentine lead levels. N Engl J Med 300:689, 1979

153. Occupational Safety and Health Administration: Occupational exposure to lead. Final standard. Fed Register 43:52952, 1978

154. Needleman HL, Schell A, Bellinger D et al: The long term effects of exposure to low doses of lead in childhood. An 11-year follow-up report. N Engl J Med 322:83, 1990

155. Bellinger D, Leviton A, Waternaux C et al: Longitudinal analyses of prenatal and postnatal lead exposure and early cognitive development. N Engl J Med 316:1037, 1987

156. Nordstrom A, Beckman L, Nordenson I: Occupational and environmental risks in and around a smelter in northern Sweden. I. Variations in birthweight. Hereditas 88:43, 1978

157. Khera AK, Wibberly DC, Dathan JG: Placental and stillbirth tissue lead concentrations in occupationally exposed women. Br J Ind Med 37:394, 1980

158. Nordstrom S, Beckman G, Beckman L, Nordenson I: Occupational and environmental risks in and around a smelter in northern Sweden. II. Chromosomal aberrations in workers exposed to arsenic. Hereditas 88:47, 1978

159. Holmberg RE, Ferm VH: Interrelationships of selenium, cadmium, and arsenic in mammalian teratogenesis. Arch Environ Health 18:873, 1969

160. Ferm VH, Hanlon DP: Metal-induced congenital malformations. p. 383. In Clarkson TW, Nordberg GF, Sager PR (eds): Reproductive and Developmental Toxicity of Metals. Plenum Press, New York, 1983

161. Beaudoin AR: Teratogenicity of sodium arsenate in rats. Teratology 10:153, 1974

162. Burk D, Beaudoin AR: Arsenate-induced renal agenesis in rats. Teratology 16:247, 1977

163. Kimbrough RD: Some fat-soluble stable industrial chemicals. p. 23. In Finberg L (ed): Chemical and Ra-

diation Hazards to Children. Report of the 84th Ross Conference on Pediatric Research. Ross Laboratories, Columbus, OH, 1982

164. Courtney KD, Gaylor DW, Hogan MD et al: Teratogenic evaluation of 2,4,5-T. Science 168:864, 1970

165. Hayes WJ Jr: Pesticides Studied in Man. p. 526. Williams & Wilkins, Baltimore, 1982

166. Erickson JD, Mulinare J, McClain PW et al: Vietnam veterans risks for fathering babies with birth defects. JAMA 252:903, 1984

167. Centers for Disease Control: Centers for Disease Control Vietnam experience study: health status of Vietnam veterans. III. Reproductive outcomes and child health. JAMA 259:2715, 1988

168. Field B, Kerr C: Reproductive behavior and consistent patterns of abnormality in offspring of Vietnam veterans. J Med Genet 25:819, 1988

169. Letz G: The toxicology of PCB's—an overview for clinicians. West J Med 138:534, 1983

170. Schwartz PM, Jacobson SW, Fein G et al: Lake Michigan fish consumption as a source of polychlorinated biphenyls in human cord serum, maternal serum, and milk. Am J Public Health 73:293, 1983

171. Safe S: Polychlorinated biphenyls (PCBs) and polybrominated biphenyls (PBBs): biochemistry, toxicology, and mechanism of action. CRC Crit Rev Toxicol 13:319, 1985

172. Kimbrough RD: Human health effects of polychlorinated biphenyls (PCBs) and polybrominated biphenyls (PBBs). Ann Rev Pharmacol Toxicol 27:87, 1987

173. Kuratsune M, Yoshimura Y, Matsuzaka J, Yamagushi A: Epidemiologic study on yusho, a poisoning caused by ingestion of rice oil contaminated with a commercial brand of polychlorinated biphenyls. Environ Health Perspect 1:119, 1972

174. World Health Organization: Assessment of Health Risks in Infants Associated with Exposure to PCBs and PCDFs in Breast Milk. Report on a WHO Working Group. World Health Organization, Copenhagen, 1988

175. Buser HR: Polychlorinated dibenzofurans (PCDFs) found in yusho oil and used in Japanese PCB. Chemosphere 7:439, 1978

176. Yamashita F, Hayashi M: Fetal PCB syndrome: clinical features, intrauterine growth retardation and possible alteration in calcium metabolism. Environ Health Perspect 59:41, 1985

177. Rogan WJ, Gladen BC, Hung KL et al: Congenital poisoning by polychlorinated biphenyls and their contaminants in Taiwan. Science 241:334, 1988

178. Yen YY, Lan SJ, Ko YC, Chen CJ: Follow-up study of reproductive hazards of multiparous women consuming PCB-contaminated rice oil. Bull Environ Contam Toxicol 43:647, 1989

179. Jacobson JL, Fein GG, Jacobson SW et al: The transfer of polychlorinated biphenyls and polybrominated biphenyls across the human placenta and into maternal milk. Am J Public Health 74:378, 1984

180. Jacobson JL, Jacobson SW, Humphrey HE: Effect of in utero exposure to polychlorinated biphenyls and related contaminants on cognitive functioning in young children. J Pediatr 116:38, 1990

181. Barsotti DA, Marker RJ, Allen JR: Reproductive dysfunction in rhesus monkeys exposed to low levels of polychlorinated biphenyls (Aroclor 1248). Food Cosmet Toxicol 14:99, 1976

182. Kimbrough RD: Laboratory and human studies on polychlorinated biphenyls (PCBs) and related compounds. Environ Health Perspect 59:99, 1985

183. Lambert GH, Kotake AN, Schoeller D: The CO_2 breath tests as monitors of the cytochrome P450 dependent mixed function monooxygenase system. Prog Clin Biol Res 135:119, 1983

184. Fein GG, Jacobson JL, Jacobson SW et al: Prenatal exposure to polychlorinated biphenyls: effects on birth size and gestational age. J Pediatr 105:315, 1984

185. Jacobson JL, Jacobson SW, Fein GG et al: Prenatal exposure to an environmental toxin: a test of the multiple effects model. Dev Psychol 20:523, 1984

186. Fein GG, Schwartz PM, Jacobson SW, Jacobson JL: Environmental toxins and behavioral development. Am Psychologist 38:1118, 1983

187. Fries GF: The PBB episode in Michigan: an overall appraisal. CRC Crit Rev Toxicol 16:105, 1985

188. Anderson HA, Lilis R, Selikoff IJ et al: Unanticipated prevalence of symptoms among dairy farmers in Michigan and Wisconsin. Environ Health Perspect 23:217, 1978

189. Bekesi JG, Roboz JP, Fischbein A, Mason P: Immunotoxicology: environmental contamination by polybrominated biphenyls and immune dysfunction among residents of the state of Michigan. Cancer Detect Prev Suppl 1:29, 1987

190. Roboz J, Greaves J, Bekesi JG: Polybrominated biphenyls in model and environmentally contaminated human blood: protein binding and immunotoxicological studies. Environ Health Perspect 60:107, 1985

191. Humble CG, Speizer FE: Polybrominated biphenyls and fetal mortality in Michigan. Am J Public Health 74:1130, 1984

192. Eyster JT, Humphrey HEB, Kimbrough RD: Partitioning of polybrominated biphenyls (PBBs) in serum, adipose tissue, breast milk, placenta, cord blood, biliary fluid, and feces. Arch Environ Health 38:47, 1983

193. Seagull EAW: Developmental abilities of children exposed to polybrominated biphenyls (PBB). Am J Public Health 73:281, 1983

194. Schwartz EM, Rae WA: Effect of polybrominated biphenyls (PBB) on developmental abilities in young children. Am J Public Health 73:277, 1983

195. Comly HH: Cyanosis in infants caused by nitrates in well water. JAMA 129:112, 1945

196. Ross JD: Deficient activity of DPHN-dependent methemoglobin diaphorase in cord blood erythrocytes. Blood 21:51, 1963

197. U.S. Environmental Protection Agency: National Interim Primary Drinking Water Regulations. p. 5. Publ No. EPA.570/9.76.003. U.S. Environmental Protection Agency, Office of Water Supply, Washington, DC, 1976

198. Walton G: Survey of literature relating to infant methemoglobinemia due to nitrate contaminated water. Am J Public Health 41:986, 1951

199. Skrivan J: Methemoglobin in pregnancy. Acta Univ Carol Med 17:123, 1971

200. Ema M, Kanoh S: Studies on the pharmacological bases of fetal toxicity of drugs: fetal toxicity of potassium nitrate in two generations of rats. Folia Pharmacol Jpn 81:469, 1983

201. Sleight SD, Sinha DP, Uzoukwu M: Effect of sodium nitrite on reproductive performance of pregnant sows. JAVMA 61:819, 1972

202. Globus M, Samuel D: Effect of maternally administered sodium nitrite on hepatic erythropoiesis in fetal CD-1 mice. Teratology 18:367, 1978

203. Dorsch MM, Scragg RKR, McMichael AJ et al: Congenital malformations and maternal drinking water supply in rural South Australia: a case-control study. Am J Epidemiol 119:473, 1984

204. Arbuckle TE, Sherman GJ, Corey PH et al: Water nitrates and CNS birth defects: a population-based case–control study. Arch Environ Health 43:162, 1988

205. King MD: Neurological sequelae of toluene abuse. Hum Toxicol 1:281, 1982

206. Andrews LS, Snyder R: Toxic effects of solvents and vapors. p. 636. In Klaassen CD, Amdur MO, Doull J (eds): Casarett and Doull's Toxicology. The Basic Science of Poisons. 3rd Ed. Macmillan, New York, 1986

207. Hersh JH, Podruch PE, Rogers R, Weisskopf B: Toluene embryopathy. J Pediatr 106:922, 1985

208. Goodwin TM: Toluene abuse and renal tubular acidosis in pregnancy. Obstet Gynecol 71:715, 1988

209. Toutant C, Lippmann S: Fetal solvents syndrome. Lancet 1:1356, 1979

210. Holmberg PC, Nurminen M: Congenital defects of the central nervous system and occupational factors during pregnancy: A case–referent study. Am J Ind Med 1:167, 1980

211. Holmberg PC: Central-nervous-system defects in children born to mothers exposed to organic solvents during pregnancy. Lancet 2:177, 1979

212. Holmberg PC, Hernberg S, Kurppa K et al: Oral clefts and organic solvent exposure during pregnancy. Int Arch Occup Environ Health 50:371, 1982

213. Kurppa K, Holmberg PC, Hernberg S et al: Screening for occupational exposures and congenital malformations. Scand J Work Environ Health 9:89, 1983

214. Pastides H, Calabrese EJ, Hosmer DW, Harris DR: Spontaneous abortion and general illness symptoms among semiconductor manufacturers. J Occup Med 30:543, 1988

215. Eskenazi B, Gaylord L, Bracken MB, Brown D: In utero exposure to organic solvents and human neurodevelopment. Dev Med Child Neurol 30:492, 1988

216. Agency for Toxic Substances and Disease Registry: Toxicological Profile for Trichloroethylene. p. 93. U.S. Public Health Service, ATSDR, Atlanta, GA, 1989

217. Swan SH, Shaw G, Harris JA, Neutra RR: Congenital cardiac anomalies in relation to water contamination, Santa Clara County, California, 1981–1983. Am J Epidemiol 129:885, 1989

218. Scialli AR: Who should paint the nursery? Reprod Toxicol 3:159, 1989

219. Spence AA, Cohen EN, Brown BW et al: Occupational hazards for operating room-based physicians: analysis of data from the United States and the United Kingdom. JAMA 238:955, 1977

220. National Institute for Occupational Safety and Health: Criteria for a Recommended Standard: Occupational Exposure to Waste Anesthetic Gases and Vapors. DHEW Publ No. 77-140. NIOSH, Washington, DC, 1977

221. Spence AA, Knill-Jones RP: Is there a health hazard in anaesthetic practice? Br J Anaesth 50:713, 1978

222. Mazze RE, Wilson AI, Rice SA, Baden JM: Reproduction and fetal development in rats exposed to nitrous oxide. Teratology 30:259, 1984

223. Corbett TH: Cancer and congenital anomalies associated with anesthetics. Ann NY Acad Sci 271:58, 1976

224. Edling C: Anesthetic gases as an occupational hazard —a review. Scand J Work Environ Health 6:85, 1980

225. Vessey MP, Nunn JF: Occupational hazards of anesthesia. Br Med J 281:696, 1980

226. Corbett TH, Cornell RG, Endres JL, Lieding K: Birth

defects among children of nurse-anesthetists. Anesthesiology 41:341, 1974

227. Knill-Jones RP, Moir DD, Rodrigues LV, Spence AA: Anesthetic practice and pregnancy—controlled survey of women anesthetists in the United Kingdom. Lancet 1:1326, 1972

228. Friedman JM: Teratogen update: anesthetic agents. Teratology 37:69,1988

229. Infante PF, Tsongas TA: Anesthetic gases and pregnancy: a review of evidence for an occupational hazard. p. 287. In Hemminki K, Sorsa M, Vainio H (eds): Occupational Hazards and Reproduction. Hemisphere Publishing Corporation, Washington, DC, 1985

230. Axelsson GA, Rylander R: Exposure to anaesthetic gases and spontaneous abortion: response bias in a postal questionnaire study. Int J Epidemiol 11:250, 1982

231. Mattia MA: Anesthesia gases and methylmethacrylate. Am J Nurs 83:73, 1983

232. Heinonen OP, Slone D, Shapiro S: Birth Defects and Drugs in Pregnancy. Publishing Sciences Group, Inc., Littleton, MA, 1977

233. Swartz HM, Reichling BA: Hazards of radiation exposure for pregnant women. JAMA 239:1907, 1978

234. Occupational Safety and Health Administration: Hazard Communication Guidelines for Compliance. Publ No. OSHA 3111. U.S. Department of Labor, OSHA, Washington, DC, 1988

235. Himmelstein JS, Frumkin H: The right to know about toxic exposures: implications for physicians. N Engl J Med 312:687, 1985

236. Reproductive Toxicology Center: ReproTox Database. Reproductive Toxicology Center, Washington, DC

237. U.S. Public Health Service: National Library of Medicine. National Institutes of Health, Bethesda, MD

238. American College of Obstetricians and Gynecologists: Guidelines on Pregnancy and Work. The American College of Obstetricians and Gynecologists, Chicago, 1977

239. Kurzel RB, Cetrulo CL: The effect of environmental pollutants on human reproduction, including birth defects. Environ Sci Technol 15:626, 1981

240. Longo LD: Environmental pollution and pregnancy: risks and uncertainties for the fetus and infant. Am J Obstet Gynecol 137:162, 1980

241. Wilson JG: Teratogenic effects of environmental chemicals. Fed Proc 36:1698, 1977

242. Strobino B, Kline J, Stein ZA: Chemical and physical exposures of parents: effects on human reproduction and offspring. J Early Hum Dev 1:371, 1978

243. Council on Scientific Affairs: Effects of toxic chemicals on the reproductive system. JAMA 253:3431, 1985

244. National Center for Health Statistics: Monthly Vital Statistics Report. Vol. 35, No. 13. National Center for Health Statistics, Washington, DC, 1987

Chapter 10

Genetic Counseling and Prenatal Diagnosis

Joe Leigh Simpson

[handwritten annotation: Major congenital anomaly – 3% causes: chromos .5% single gene 1% multifactorial 1% other .5%]

Approximately 3 percent of liveborn infants have a major congenital anomaly. About one-half of these anomalies are evident at birth; the remainder become evident later in childhood or, less often, during adulthood. Although nongenetic factors may cause malformations, genetic factors are usually responsible. In addition, more than 50 percent of first-trimester spontaneous abortions and at least 5 percent of stillborn infants show chromosomal abnormalities (see Ch. 23). Given such an important role for genetic factors, knowledge of human genetics clearly becomes integral to the practice of modern obstetrics.

This chapter first considers the principles of genetic counseling and genetic screening. Thereafter, disorders amenable to genetic screening and prenatal diagnosis are discussed.

SPECTRUM OF GENETIC DISEASE

Phenotypic variation—normal or abnormal—may be considered in terms of several etiologic categories: (1) chromosomal abnormalities, numerical or structural; (2) single-gene or Mendelian disorders; (3) polygenic and multifactorial disorders, polygenic implying an etiology resulting from cumulative effects of more than one gene and multifactorial implying interaction with environmental factors as well; and (4) teratogenic disorders, caused by exposure to exogenous factors (e.g., drugs) that deleteriously affect an embryo otherwise destined to develop normally. Principles of these mechanisms are reviewed elsewhere.[1]

Chromosomal Abnormalities

From surveys of more than 50,000 liveborn neonates, it has been established that the incidence of chromosomal aberrations is 1:160 (Table 10.1).[2] *[handwritten: liveborns]*

Single-Gene Disorders

In addition to the 0.6 percent of liveborns who are phenotypically abnormal as a result of chromosomal aberrations, about 1 percent exhibit disorders caused by a single-gene mutation. There exist at least 1,864 autosomal dominant, 631 autosomal recessive, and 161 X-linked disorders.[3] Even the most common Mendelian disorders (cystic fibrosis in whites, sickle cell anemia in blacks, β-thalassemia in Greeks and Italians, α-thalassemia in Southeast Asians, Tay-Sachs disease in Ashkenazi Jews) are individually rare. In aggregate, however, Mendelian disorders result in 1 percent of liveborns having a congenital defect.

Polygenic/Multifactorial Disorders

Another 1 percent of neonates are abnormal, but possess a normal chromosomal complement and have not undergone mutation at a *single* genetic locus. It can be deduced that several genes are involved (polygenic/multifactorial inheritance).[1] Included in this

Table 10.1   Chromosomal Abnormalities in Liveborn Infants[a]

Type of Abnormality	Births
Numerical aberrations	
Sex chromosomes	
47,XYY	1/1,000 MB
47,XXY	1/1,000 MB
Other, males	1/1,350 MB
47,X	1/10,000 FB
47,XXX	1/1,000 FB
Other, females	1/2,700 FB
Autosomes	
Trisomies	
13–15 (D group)	1/20,000 LB
16–18 (E group)	1/8,000 LB
21–22 (G group)	1/800 LB
Other	1/50,000 LB
Structural aberrations	
Balanced	
Robertsonian	
t(Dq;Dq)	1/1,500 LB
t(Dq;Gq)	1/5,000 LB
Reciprocal translocations and insertional inversions	1/7,000 LB
Unbalanced	
Robertsonian	1/14,000 LB
Reciprocal translocations and insertional inversions	1/8,000 LB
Inversions	1/50,000 LB
Deletions	1/10,000 LB
Supernumeraries	1/5,000 LB
Other	1/8,000 LB
Total	1/160 LB

[a] Pooled data tabulated by Hook and Hamerton.[2]

[b] Abbreviations: LB, live births; MB, male births; FB, female births.

etiologic category are most common malformations limited to a single organ system. These include hydrocephaly, anencephaly, and spina bifida (neural tube defects), facial clefts (cleft lip and palate), cardiac defects, pyloric stenosis, omphalocele, hip dislocation, uterine fusion defects, and clubfoot (Table 10.2). After the birth of one child with such anomalies, the recurrence risk in subsequent progeny is usually 1 to 5 percent.[1] This frequency is less than would be expected if only a single gene were responsible but greater than that for the general population. The risks of the malformations are also 1 to 5 percent for offspring of affected parents. That recurrence risks are similar for siblings and offspring diminishes the likelihood that environmental causes are the exclusive etiologic factor, because it is unlikely that households in different generations would be exposed to the same teratogen. Further excluding environmental factors as sole etiologic agents are observations that monozygotic twins are much more often concordant (similarly affected) than are dizygotic twins, despite both types of twins sharing a common intrauterine environment.

The above observations are best explained on the basis of polygenic/multifactorial inheritance. Although more than one gene is involved, only a few genes are necessary to produce the number of genotypes necessary to explain recurrence risks of 1 to 5 percent. That is, large numbers of genes and complex mechanisms need not be invoked. Polygenic/multifactorial etiology can thus reasonably be held responsible for most abnormal liveborns who have normal chromosomes and who have no Mendelian mutations.

Table 10.2   Polygenic/Multifactorial Traits[a]

Hydrocephaly (excepting some forms of aqueductal stenosis and Dandy-Walker syndrome)

Neural tube defects (anencephaly, spina bifida, encephalocele)

Cleft lip, with or without cleft palate

Cleft lip, alone

Cardiac anomalies (most types)

Diaphragmatic hernia

Omphalocele

Renal agenesis (unilateral or bilateral)

Ureteral anomalies

Posterior urethral valves

Hypospadias

Müllerian fusion defects

Limb-reduction defects

Talipes equinovarus (clubfoot)

[a] Relatively common traits considered to be inherited in polygenic/multifactorial fashion. For each, normal parents have recurrence risks of 1 to 5 percent after one affected child. After two affected offspring, the risk is higher.

Teratogenic Disorders

About a dozen proved teratogens are known. These are reviewed in Chapter 9.

CLINICAL SPECTRUM OF CHROMOSOMAL ABNORMALITIES

One per 160 liveborn infants has a chromosomal abnormality (Table 10.1). Unlike the case with Mendelian disorders, some generalizations concerning these disorders can be offered. These generalizations may prove helpful to the obstetrician, who may detect such abnormalities during prenatal studies or in the delivery room. In this section the clinical and cytogenetic features characteristic of the common chromosomal abnormalities are reviewed. These and other disorders have been discussed in detail elsewhere, where complete references are provided.[1]

Autosomal Trisomy

Trisomy 21

Trisomy 21 (Down syndrome, mongolism) is the most frequent autosomal chromosomal syndrome, occurring in 1 of every 800 liveborn infants (Table 10.1). The relationship to advanced maternal age is well known. Characteristic craniofacial features include brachycephaly, oblique palpebral fissures, epicanthal folds, broad nasal bridge, a protruding tongue, and small, low-set ears with an overlapping helix and a prominent antihelix (Fig. 10.1). At birth, these infants are usually hypotonic. The mean birth weight in Down syndrome, 2,900 g, is decreased but not as much as in some autosomal syndromes. Other features include irideal Brushfield spots, broad short fingers (brachymesophalangia), clinodactyly (incurving deflections resulting from an abnormality of the middle phalanx), a single flexion crease on the fifth digit, and an unusually wide space between the first two toes. Contrary to widespread opinion, a single palmar crease (Simian line) is not pathognomonic, being present in only 30 percent of individuals with trisomy 21 and in 5 percent of normal individuals. Relatively common internal anomalies include cardiac lesions and duodenal atresia. Cardiac anomalies and increased susceptibility to both respiratory infec-

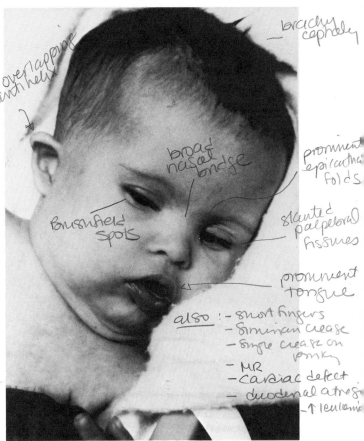

Fig. 10.1 An infant with trisomy 21. (From Simpson and Golbus,[1] with permission.)

tions and leukemia contribute to a reduced life expectancy of approximately 40 years.

Patients with Down syndrome who survive beyond infancy invariably exhibit mental retardation. However, the degree of retardation is generally not as severe as that of many other chromosomal aberrations. Mean IQ is 50 (range, 25 to 70). Although some patients with Down syndrome have been reported with IQs in the 70 to 80 range, 46/47,+21 mosaicism should be suspected in such instances. Females are fertile. Although relatively few trisomic mothers have reproduced, about 30 percent of their offspring are also trisomic. Except possibly for very exceptional cases, affected males are not fertile.

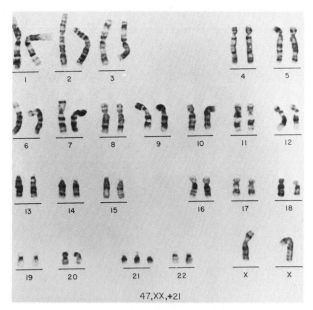

Fig. 10.2 Karyotype of a trisomy 21 cell. Trypsin-Giemsa (GTG) banding. (From Simpson and Golbus,[1] with permission.)

Several different cytogenetic mechanisms may be associated with "clinical Down syndrome," which is actually the result of triplication of a small portion of chromosome 21, namely, band q22. This triplication may be caused either by the presence of an entire additional chromosome 21 or by the addition of only band q22. The latter could be due to a translocation or to other structural rearrangement. Of all cases of Down syndrome, 95 percent have primary trisomy (47 instead of the normal 46 chromosomes) (Fig. 10.2). These cases show the well-known relationship to maternal age. Mosaicism (46/47,+21) cannot be distinguished from those who have the disorder as a result of translocation. Translocations show no definite relationship to parental age and may be either sporadic or familial. The translocation most commonly associated with Down syndrome is that involving chromosomes 14 and 21. With translocation 14/21 Down syndrome, one parent may have the same translocation chromosome, that is, 45,t(14q;21q). For parents with a translocation, the recurrence risk for a child with an unbalanced chromosome com-

plement far exceeds the risk for recurrence of non-disjunction (1 percent). Risks are approximately 10 percent for offspring of female translocation heterozygotes and 2 percent for offspring of male translocation heterozygotes.

Other structural rearrangements resulting in Down syndrome include t(21q;21q), t(21q;22q), and translocations involving chromosome 21 and chromosomes other than a member of group D (chromosomes 13 to 15) or G (chromosomes 21 to 22). In t(21q;21q), no normal gametes can be formed. Thus only trisomic or monosomic zygotes are produced, the latter presumably appearing as preclinical embryonic losses. Parents having the other translocations have a low empiric risk of having offspring with Down syndrome.

Trisomy 13

Trisomy 13 occurs in about 1 per 20,000 live births. Intrauterine and postnatal growth retardation are pronounced, and developmental retardation is severe. Nearly 50 percent of affected children die in the first month, and relatively few survive past 3 years of age. Major characteristic anomalies include holoprosencephaly, eye anomalies (microphthalmia, anophthalmia, or coloboma), cleft lip and palate, polydactyly, and cardiac defects. Other relatively common features include cutaneous scalp defects, hemangiomata on the face or neck, low-set ears with an abnormal helix, and "rocker-bottom" feet (convex soles and protruding heels) (Fig. 10.3).

Trisomy 13 is usually associated with nondisjunctional (primary) trisomy (47,+13). A maternal age effect exists. Translocation is responsible for less than 20 percent of cases, invariably associated with two group D chromosomes (chromosomes 13 to 15) joining at their centromeric regions (Robertsonian translocation). If neither parent has the rearrangement, the risk for subsequent progeny is not increased. If either parent has a balanced 13q;14q translocation, the recurrence risk for an affected offspring is increased but still only about 1 to 2 percent. Homologous 13q;13q parental translocation carries the same dire prognosis as 21q;21q translocation (see above).

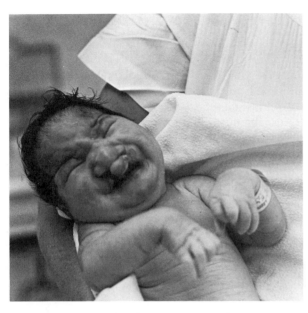

Fig. 10.3 An infant with trisomy 13. (From Simpson and Golbus,[1] with permission.)

Trisomy 18

Trisomy 18 occurs in 1 per 8,000 live births. Trisomy 18 is not infrequently detected among stillborn infants, who interestingly may not be clinically suspected of being trisomic. Among liveborn infants, females are affected more often than males (3:1). Among stillborns and abortuses, however, the sex distribution is more equal.

Facial anomalies characteristic of trisomy 18 include microcephaly, prominent occiput, low-set and pointed "fawnlike" ears, and micrognathia. Skeletal anomalies include overlapping fingers (V over IV, II over III), short sternum, shield chest, narrow pelvis, limited thigh abduction or congenital hip dislocation, "rocker-bottom" feet with protrusion of the calcaneum, and a short dorsiflexed hallu ("hammer toe"). Cardiac and renal anomalies are common.

Birth weight (2,240 g) is below average and fetal movement feeble. The mean survival time for these infants is only a few months. Those surviving show pronounced developmental and growth retardation. Approximately 50 percent develop fetal distress during labor.

Approximately 80 percent of trisomy 18 cases are caused by primary nondisjunction (47,XX,+18 or 47,XY,+18). In such cases, the recurrence risk is about 1 percent.

Other Trisomies

Although trisomies for several other autosomes have been observed in liveborns, such pregnancies more often terminate in abortuses. Trisomies for chromosomes 8, 9, and 14 have been reported. All show mental retardation and various somatic anomalies, but the extent of retardation and the spectrum of anomalies vary. Recurrence risks are assumed to be similar to those for trisomy 21.

Autosomal Deletions or Duplication

Deletions or duplications of portions of autosomes also exist. A single example will suffice for illustrative purposes.

Deletion of a portion of the short arm of chromosome 5(5p) produces the so-called "cri-du-chat" ("cat-cry") syndrome. These babies have a distinctive, monotonic, catlike cry. During infancy, the facies become rounded ("moonlike") because of microcephaly, hypertelorism, a broad nasal bridge, downward slanting of the palpebral fissures, and micrognathia. Ears are low set. As the individual grows older, the facies become elongated, the philtrum shorter, and the cry nonspecific in character. Despite severe mental retardation (mean IQ of 20) and growth retardation, a few patients reach adulthood. Although the size of the deleted segment varies, bands 5p14 and 5p15 are always deficient. The deletion is sporadic in 90 percent of cases, and the recurrence risk is no greater than that for any other couple of comparable parental ages. In 10 percent of these cases, unbalanced translocations or recombinants from inversions are present. In these instances, rearrangements are usually familial.

Many other rare duplication or deficiency syndromes exist. All are characterized by mental retardation and somatic anomalies, but their specific features vary.

Sex Chromosomal Abnormalities

Monosomy X (45,X)

45,X individuals account for approximately 40 percent of gonadal dysgenesis ascertained by gynecologists. The incidence of 45,X in liveborn females is about 1 in 10,000. Because monosomy X accounts for 10 percent of all first-trimester abortions, it can be calculated that more than 99 percent of 45,X conceptuses must end in early pregnancy loss.

Gonadal dysgenesis is usually associated with an abnormal sex chromosomal constitution. Associated complements include not only monosomy X but also structural abnormalities of the X chromosome, such as (1) simple deletion of the short arm, 46,X,del(Xp); (2) simple deletion of the long arm, 46,X,del(Xq); (3) isochromosome for the long arm, 46,X,i(Xq); and (4) ring chromosomes, 46,X,r(X). Mosaicism is frequent, especially with a coexisting 45,X cell line. Both the long arm and short arm of the X chromosome contain determinants necessary for ovarian differentiation and for normal stature. 45,X individuals not only have streak gonads but invariably are short (<150 cm). They usually have various somatic anomalies: renal and cardiac defects, skeletal abnormalities like cubitus valgus and clinodactyly, vertebral anomalies, pigmented nevi, nail hypoplasia, and a low posterior hairline.

Klinefelter Syndrome

Males with two or more X chromosomes have small testes, azoospermia, elevated levels of follicle-stimulating hormone (FSH) and leuteinizing hormone (LH), and decreased testosterone. The most frequent chromosomal complement associated with this phenotype—the Klinefelter syndrome—is 47,XXY. 48,XXXY and 49,XXXXY occur less often.

Mental retardation is uncommon in 47,XXY Klinefelter syndrome but is invariably associated with 48,XXXY and 49,XXXXY. Skeletal, trunk, and craniofacial anomalies occur infrequently in 47,XXY but are common in 48,XXXY and 49,XXXXY. Regardless of the specific chromosomal complement, patients with Klinefelter syndrome all have unquestioned male phenotypes. Although the penis is hypoplastic, hypospadias is uncommon.

Polysomy X in Females (47,XXX; 48,XXXX; 49,XXXXX)

About 1 per 1000 liveborn females has a 47,XXX complement. 47,XXX individuals are seven to eight times more likely to show mental retardation than are individuals in the general population. The absolute risk for mental retardation is 5 to 10 percent, with the IQ usually 60 to 80. Most 47,XXX patients have a normal reproductive system. The theoretical risk of 47,XXX women delivering infants with an abnormal chromosomal complement is 50 percent, given one-half the maternal gametes carrying 24 chromosomes (24,XX). However, the empiric risk is much less. Somatic anomalies may or may not be more frequent in 47,XXX individuals than in 46,XX females. 48,XXXX and 49,XXXXX individuals are invariably retarded and are more likely to have somatic malformations than are 47,XXX individuals.

Polysomy Y in Males (47,XYY and 48,XXYY)

The presence of more than one Y chromosome is also a frequent chromosomal abnormality in liveborn males (1:1000). 47,XYY males are more likely to be tall and display sociopathic behavior than are 46,XY males. The precise prevalence of these features is unknown, however. One estimate is that 1 percent of 47,XYY males will be incarcerated compared with 0.1 percent of 46,XY males. 47,XYY males usually have normal male external genitalia.

GENETIC HISTORY

All obstetrician/gynecologists must attempt to determine whether a couple, or anyone in their families, has a heritable disorder. Obstetric registration forms address this question. Some obstetricians find it helpful to elicit genetic information through the use of questionnaires or check lists that are often constructed in a manner that requires action only to positive responses. Figure 10.4 reproduces the form currently recommended by the American College of Obstetricians and Gynecologists (ACOG).

One should inquire into the health status of first-degree relatives (siblings, parents, offspring), second-degree relatives (nephews, nieces, aunts, uncles, grandparents), and third-degree relatives (first cousins, especially maternal). Adverse reproductive out-

---

Prenatal Genetic Screen*

Name_____ Patient #_____ Date_____

1. Will you be 35 years or older when the baby is due? Yes____No____
2. Have you, the baby's father, or anyone in either of your families ever had any of the following disorders?
   Down syndrome (mongolism) Yes____No____
   Other chromosomal abnormality Yes____No____
   Neural tube defect, i.e., spina bifida (meningomyelocele or open spine), anencephaly Yes____No____
   Hemophilia Yes____No____
   Muscular dystrophy Yes____No____
   Cystic fibrosis Yes____No____
   If yes, indicate the relationship of the affected person to you or to the baby's father:
   _____

3. Do you or the baby's father have a birth defect? Yes____No____
   If yes, who has the defect and what is it? _____
4. In any previous marriages, have you or the baby's father had a child born, dead or alive, with a birth
   defect not listed in question 2 above? Yes____No____
5. Do you or the baby's father have any close relatives with mental retardation? Yes____No____
   If yes, indicate the relationship of the affected person to you or to the baby's father:
   _____

   Indicate the cause, if known: _____
6. Do you, the baby's father, or a close relative in either of your families have a birth defect,
   any familial disorder, or a chromosomal abnormality not listed above? Yes____No____
   If yes, indicate the condition and the relationship of the affected person to you or to the baby's father:
   _____

7. In any previous marriage, have you or the baby's father had a stillborn child or three or
   more first-trimester spontaneous pregnancy losses? Yes____No____
   Have either of you had a chromosomal study? Yes____No____
8. If you or the baby's father are of Jewish ancestry, have either of you been screened for
   Tay-Sachs disease? Yes____No____
   If yes, indicate who and the results: _____
9. If you or the baby's father are black, have either of you been screened for sickle cell trait?
   Yes____No____
   If yes, indicate who and the results: _____
10. If you or the baby's father are of Italian, Greek, or Mediterranean background, have either
    of you been tested for β-thalassemia? Yes____No____
    If yes, indicate who and the results: _____
11. If you or the baby's father are of Philippine or Southeast Asian ancestry, have either of
    you been tested for δ-thalassemia? Yes____No____
    If yes, indicate who and the results: _____
12. Excluding iron and vitamins, have you taken any medications or recreational drugs since becoming
    pregnant or since your last menstrual period? (include nonprescription drugs) Yes____No____
    If yes, give name of medication and time taken during pregnancy: _____

Fig. 10.4 Prenatal genetic screen. Questionnaire for identifying couples having increased risk for offspring with genetic disorders. Any persons replying "YES" to a question should be offered appropriate counseling. If the patient declines further counseling or testing, this should be noted in the chart. Given that genetics is a field in a state of flux, alterations or updates to this form will be required periodically. (From the American College of Obstetricians and Gynecologists,[54] with permission.)

comes such as repetitive spontaneous abortions, still-births, and anomalous liveborn infants should be pursued. Couples having such histories should undergo chromosomal studies to exclude balanced translocations. Genetic counseling may prove sufficiently complex to warrant referral to a clinical geneticist, or it may prove simple enough for the well-informed obstetrician to manage. If a birth defect exists in a second-degree relative (uncle, aunt, grandparent, nephew, niece) or a third-degree relative (first cousin), the risk for that anomaly will usually not prove substantially increased over that in the general population. For example, identification of a second- or third-degree relative with an autosomal recessive trait places the couple at little increased risk for an affected offspring, one exception being if the patient and her husband are consanguineous. However, a maternal first cousin with an X-linked recessive disorder would identify a couple at increased risk for a similar occurrence.

Parental ages should also be recorded. Advanced maternal age (Table 10.3) warrants discussion irrespective of a physician's personal convictions regarding pregnancy termination. Ethnic origin should be recorded to exclude those disorders noted in Table 10.4. Incidentally, the above applies for both gamete donors as well as for couples achieving pregnancy by natural means.

GENETIC COUNSELING

Although genetic counseling may require referral to a clinical geneticist, it is impractical for obstetricians to refer all patients with genetic inquiries. Indeed, obstetricians performing diagnostic procedures such as amniocentesis are obligated to counsel their patients before such a procedure. Salient aspects of the genetic counseling process will therefore be described.

Communication

A first principle of counseling is to employ terms that are readily comprehensible to patients. It is useful to preface remarks with a few sentences recounting the major causes of genetic abnormalities—cytogenetic, single gene, polygenic/multifactorial (can be labeled "complex"), and environmental (teratogens). Writing down unfamiliar words and using tables or diagrams to reinforce important concepts is helpful. Repetition is essential. Allot time for the couple not only to ask questions but also to communicate with one another to formulate their concerns.

Table 10.3 Maternal Age and Chromosomal Abnormalities (Livebirths)[a]

Maternal Age	Risk for Down Syndrome	Total Risk for Chromosome Abnormalities
20	1/1,667	1/526[b]
21	1/1,667	1/526[b]
22	1/1,429	1/500[b]
23	1/1,429	1/500[b]
24	1/1,250	1/476[b]
25	1/1,250	1/476[b]
26	1/1,176	1/476[b]
27	1/1,111	1/455[b]
28	1/1,053	1/435[b]
29	1/1,000	1/417
30	1/952	1/384[b]
31	1/909	1/385[b]
32	1/769	1/322[b]
33	1/625	1/317[b]
34	1/500	1/260
35	1/385	1/204
36	1/294	1/164
37	1/227	1/130
38	1/175	1/103
39	1/137	1/82
40	1/106	1/65
41	1/82	1/51
42	1/64	1/40
43	1/50	1/32
44	1/38	1/25
45	1/30	1/20
46	1/23	1/15
47	1/18	1/12
48	1/14	1/10
49	1/11	1/7

[a] Data of Hook[51] and Hook et al.[52] Because sample size for some intervals is relatively small, confidence limits are sometimes relatively large. Nonetheless, these figures are suitable for genetic counseling.

[b] 47,XXX excluded for ages 20–32 years (data not available).

Table 10.4 Genetic Screening For Various Ethnic Groups

Ethnic Group	Disorder	Screening Test	Definitive Test
Ashkenazi Jews	Tay-Sachs disease	Decreased serum hexosami-dase-A	Chorionic villus sampling (CVS) or amniocentesis for assay of hexosami-dase-A
Blacks	Sickle cell anemia	Presence of sickle cell hemo-globin, confirmatory he-moglobin electrophoresis	CVS or amniocentesis for genotype determination (direct molecular analysis)
Mediterranean people (Greek, Italian in particular)	β-Thalassemia	Mean corpuscular volume (MVC) <80 percent, fol-lowed by hemoglobin electrophoresis	CVS or amniocentesis for genotype determination (direct molecular analysis or RFLP linkage analysis)
Southeast Asians and Chinese (Vietnamese, Laotian, Cambodian, Filipinos)	δ-Thalassemia	MCV <80 percent followed by hemoglobin electrophore-sis (direct molecular stud-ies)	CVS or amniocentesis for genotype determination (direct molecular analysis or RFLP linkage analysis)

Written information (letters or brochures) can serve as a couple's permanent record, allaying misunderstanding and assisting in dealing with relatives. Preprinted forms describing common problems (e.g., advanced maternal age) have the additional advantage of emphasizing that the couple's problem is not unique.

Irrespective of how obvious a diagnosis may seem, confirmation is always obligatory. Accepting a patient's word does not suffice, and neither would accepting a diagnosis made by a physician not highly knowledgeable about the condition. The anomalous individual may need to be examined by the most appropriate authority, and examining first-degree relatives may be required as well if the possibility of an autosomal dominant disorder (e.g., neurofibromatosis) exists. If a definitive diagnosis cannot be made, the physician should not hesitate to say so. Proper counseling requires proper diagnosis.

Nondirective Counseling

In genetic counseling one should provide accurate genetic information yet dictate no particular course of action. Of course, completely nondirective counseling is probably unrealistic. For example, a counselor's unwitting facial expressions may expose his or her unstated opinions. Merely offering antenatal diagnostic services implies approval. Despite the difficulties of being truly objective, one should attempt to provide information and then support the couple's decision.

Psychological Considerations

Psychological defenses underlie all genetic counseling and indeed all communication. If not appreciated, these defenses can impede the entire counseling process. Anxiety is low in couples counseled for advanced maternal age or for an abnormality in a distant relative. As long as the anxiety level remains low, comprehension of information is usually not impaired. However, couples who have experienced a stillborn infant, an anomalous child, or multiple repetitive abortions are more anxious. Their ability to retain information may be hindered.

Couples experiencing abnormal pregnancy outcomes manifest the same grief reactions that occur after the death of a loved one: denial, anger, guilt, bargaining, resolution. One should pay deference to this sequence by not attempting to offer definitive counseling immediately after the birth of an abnormal neonate. Parents must be supported at that time, and the obstetrician should avoid discussing specific recurrence risks for fear of adding to the immediate burden. By 4 to 6 weeks the couple has begun to cope and is more receptive to counseling.

An additional psychological consideration is that of parental guilt. One naturally searches for exogenous factors that might have caused an abnormal outcome. In the process of such a search, guilt may arise. Conversely, a tendency to blame the spouse may arise. Usually guilt or blame is not justified, but occasionally the "blame" is realistic (e.g., in autosomal dominant traits). Fortunately, most couples can be assured that nothing could have prevented a given abnormal pregnancy.

Appreciating the psychological defenses described above helps one to understand the failure of ostensibly intelligent couples to comprehend genetic information.

GENETIC SCREENING

Genetic screening implies routine monitoring for the presence or absence of a given condition in apparently normal individuals. Obstetricians are very familiar with this concept. Screening is now offered routinely for (1) women aged 35 years or older at delivery to detect aneuploidy (e.g., Down syndrome), (2) individuals of certain ethnic groups to identify those heterozygous for a given autosomal recessive disorder, and (3) all pregnant women to detect elevated maternal serum α-fetoprotein to diagnose fetal neural tube defects. In fact, one could theoretically screen for many other genetic disorders. All chromosomal abnormalities could be detected during the prenatal or neonatal period, and almost all disorders of amino acid metabolism are amenable to screening. On the other hand, screening is actually recommended for relatively few disorders, because prerequisites essential for initiating screening programs are not usually met. These prerequisites are discussed.

Capacity to Alter Clinical Management

Although screening to achieve research objectives (such as determining the incidence of a disorder) is sometimes appropriate, widespread testing is ordinarily performed only if an abnormal finding would alter clinical management. Neonates are thus evaluated for those metabolic disorders (e.g., phenylketonuria, hypothyroidism) amenable to dietary or hormonal treatment. However, screening is not attempted for neonates with untreatable disorders. Thus *neonatal* screening is not recommended for chromosomal abnormalities, Tay-Sachs disease, Duchenne muscular dystrophy, and cystic fibrosis. On the other hand, it is reasonable to screen adults to determine whether they are heterozygous for autosomal recessive disorders amenable to prenatal diagnosis. Table 10.4 lists disorders for which screening is currently recommended. The most well-known example in the United States is Tay-Sachs disease, an autosomal recessive disorder for which Ashkenazi Jews are at increased risk (heterozygote frequency 1 per 27). In the United States, Jewish individuals may be uncertain whether they are of Ashkenazic or Sephardic descent; thus obstetricians should screen all Jewish couples and possibly also couples in which only one partner is Jewish. Increasing availability of prenatal diagnostic techniques also renders advisable routine heterozygote detection for β-thalassemia in Italians and Greeks, sickle cell anemia in blacks, and α-thalassemia in Southeast Asians and Filipinos. Mean corpuscular volume (MCV) greater than 80 percent excludes heterozygosity for α- or β-thalassemia. Values less than 80 percent are more likely to reflect iron deficiency anemia than heterozygosity, but additional confirmatory tests are indicated to exclude heterozygosity for the thalassemias.

Population Screening for Cystic Fibrosis

Routine screening is not yet recommended for cystic fibrosis (CF), but some individuals may nonetheless wish to avail themselves of genetic information recently available. About 75 percent of the CF mutations are due to deletion of amino acid 508 (ΔF508), resulting in loss of a phenylalanine residue[4] (Fig. 10.5).

Screening the entire population for the presence or absence of the ΔF508 mutation is worth considering. Indeed, about 50 percent of couples at risk for CF offspring can be identified and thus offered un-

NORMAL

DNA	..*GAA*	*AAT*	*ATC*	*ATC*	*TTT*	*GGT*	*GTT*	*TCC*..
PROTEIN	Glu	Asn	Ile	Ile	Phe	Gly	Val	Ser
POSITION	504	505	506	507	508	509	510	511

CYSTIC FIBROSIS

DNA	..*GAA*	*AAT*	*ATC*	*AT-*	*--T*	*GGT*	*GTT*	*TCC*..
PROTEIN	Glu	Asn	Ile	Ile		Gly	Val	Ser

Fig. 10.5 Schematic drawing illustrating ΔF508 mutation, at least one allele of which is present in 75 percent of cystic fibrosis cases in whites of Northern European ancestry.

equivocal prenatal diagnosis. However, identification of the remaining couples is not possible. Included in this group are matings between two known heterozygotes characterized by one parent having the ΔF508 mutation but the other not having the mutation. This situation is not rare, given that ΔF508 is not found in 25 percent of CF individuals. If one parent has ΔF508 but the other does not, and thus is still of uncertain status with respect to CF heterozygosity, the actual risk of that couple having a CF child is 1 per 400.[4,5] Unfortunately, prenatal diagnosis is not possible except excluding that the fetus inherited the ΔF508 from the known heterozygous parent. Measuring microvillus intestinal enzymes in amniotic fluid is also not helpful, a low value being more likely to connote a false-positive than a true-positive value. Moreover, far lower percentages of at-risk couples are detected in Ashkenazi Jews and in nonwhite populations.[5] In aggregate, these complexities dictate that additional advances, perhaps ability to detect 90 to 95 percent of CF mutations, must be awaited before population screening can be confidently recommended.[6] However, some couples cognizant of these complexities may still elect to be tested.

If a couple has actually had a child with CF, or can identify an affected relative, the discussion above is not germane. Such couples should be screened for the ΔF508 mutation and family studies performed to identify loci informative for linkage analysis if needed

(see below, Detection of Mendelian Disorders by Molecular Techniques).

DIAGNOSTIC PROCEDURES FOR PRENATAL GENETIC DIAGNOSIS

Prenatal genetic diagnosis usually requires obtaining fetal tissue, necessitating an invasive procedure such as amniocentesis or chorionic villus sampling. In this section common techniques and their safety are considered.

Amniocentesis

Technique

Amniocentesis is the aspiration of amniotic fluid, usually performed for genetic purposes at 15 to 16 weeks gestation (menstrual weeks). The procedure has been performed earlier (12 to 14 weeks) in certain centers,[7] but safety at that stage of gestation is not accepted universally.[8] A 22-gauge spinal needle with stylet is usually employed. At 15 to 16 weeks gestation, amniotic fluid volume is sufficient (~200 ml), the uterus is readily accessible to a transabdominal approach, and the interval prior to fetal viability is adequate to permit diagnostic studies. Ultrasound examination is obligatory to determine gestational age, placental position, location of amniotic fluid, and number of fetuses. Ultrasound should be performed concurrently with amniocentesis. Rh-immune globulin should be administered to the Rh-negative, Du-negative, unsensitized patient.

Bloody amniotic fluid is aspirated occasionally; however, this blood is almost always maternal in origin and does not adversely affect amniotic cell growth. By contrast, brown, dark red, or wine-colored amniotic fluid is associated with an increased likelihood of poor pregnancy outcome. The dark color is indicative of intra-amniotic bleeding having occurred earlier in pregnancy, with hemoglobin breakdown products persisting; pregnancy loss eventually occurs in about one-third of such cases. If the abnormally colored fluid shows elevated α-fetoprotein, the outcome is almost always unfavorable (fetal demise or fetal abnormality). Greenish amniotic fluid is the result of meconium staining and is apparently not associated with poor pregnancy outcome.[9]

In multiple gestations, amniocentesis can usually be performed on both or all fetuses.[10,11] Following aspiration of amniotic fluid from the first sac, 2 to 3 ml of indigo carmine, diluted 1:10 in bacteriostatic water, is injected before the needle is withdrawn. A second amniocentesis is then performed, the site determined after visualizing the membranes separating the two sacs. Aspiration of clear fluid confirms that the second (new) sac was entered. Triplets and other multiple gestations can be managed similarly, sequentially injecting dye into successive sacs. Although cross-contamination of cells in multiple gestations appears to be rare, confusion may sometimes arise in interpreting amniotic fluid acetylcholinesterase or α-fetoprotein results.

After amniocentesis, the patient may resume all normal activities. Common sense dictates that strenuous exercise such as jogging or aerobic exercise be deferred for a day or so. The patient should report persistent uterine cramping, vaginal bleeding, leakage of amniotic fluid, or fever; however, physician intervention is almost never required, unless overt abortion occurs.

If only one fetus in a multiple gestation is abnormal, parents will ordinarily have to choose between aborting all fetuses or continuing the pregnancy with one or more normal and one abnormal fetus. Selective termination of a single fetus in the second trimester is possible but cannot be considered standard.[12] The technique is more feasible in the first trimester.[13] In all cases verification that the aborted fetus is truly the abnormal one is crucial.

Safety

Amniocentesis involves potential danger to both mother and fetus, as discussed in detail elsewhere.[11] Actually, maternal risks are quite low; symptomatic amnionitis occurs only rarely (≤ 0.1 percent). Minor maternal complications such as vaginal spotting or amniotic fluid leakage are more frequent but rarely serious.

The frequency of fetal loss following amniocentesis has been addressed by several large studies, most recently a randomized study of 30 to 34-year-old women in Denmark.[14] Even with high-quality concurrent ultrasound and an experienced obstetrician, the procedure-related fetal loss rate should be considered to be about 0.5 percent, possibly higher if the placenta is traversed. Most centers counsel that the risk of abortion secondary to amniocentesis is 0.5 percent or less. At our center, we further state that maternal complications and fetal injuries are "reported but very rare."

Chorionic Villus Sampling

A technique that allows prenatal diagnosis in the first trimester is obviously highly desirable. It would not only permit pregnancy termination early in gestation but also protect patient privacy. Chorionic villus sampling (CVS) is such a technique, available in the United States since 1983 to 1984. Both chorionic villi and amniotic fluid cells offer the same information concerning chromosomal status, enzyme levels, and DNA patterns. The one major exception is that assays requiring amniotic fluid, specifically α-fetoprotein, require amniocentesis.

Technique

CVS can be performed by transcervical, transabdominal, or transvaginal approaches. *Transcervical* CVS is usually performed with a flexible polyethylene catheter that encircles a metal obturator extending just distal to the catheter tip. The outer diameter is usually about 1.5 mm. Introduced transcervically under simultaneous ultrasonographic visualization (Fig. 10.6), the catheter/obturator is directed toward the trophoblastic tissue surrounding the gestational sac. After withdrawal of the obturator, 10 to 25 mg of villi are aspirated through the catheter by negative pressure into a 20- or 30-cc syringe containing tissue culture media. The optimal time for transcervical sampling is 9 to 12 completed gestational weeks.

In *transabdominal* CVS (Fig. 10.7), concurrent ultrasound is used to direct a 19- or 20-gauge spinal needle into the long axis of the placenta. After removal of the stylet, villi are aspirated into a 20-cc syringe containing tissue culture media. Unlike transcervical CVS, transabdominal CVS can be performed

throughout pregnancy. It therefore provides an alternative to chordocentesis (percutaneous umbilical blood sampling) if needed later in pregnancy. If oligohydramnios is present, transabdominal CVS may be the only approach.

A final technique is *transvaginal* CVS, using a spinal needle as in transabdominal CVS. This technique may be preferable for a retroflexed uterus having a posterior placenta. Use of a needle attached to a transvaginal ultrasound probe facilitates the procedure.

Cervical myomas or angulated uteri may preclude transcervical passage of the catheter, although alternative CVS approaches (transabdominal or transvaginal) usually permit sampling in such situations. The transabdominal approach is obviously preferable in the presence of genital herpes, marked cervicitis, or bicornuate uteri. Sampling women sensitized to Rh

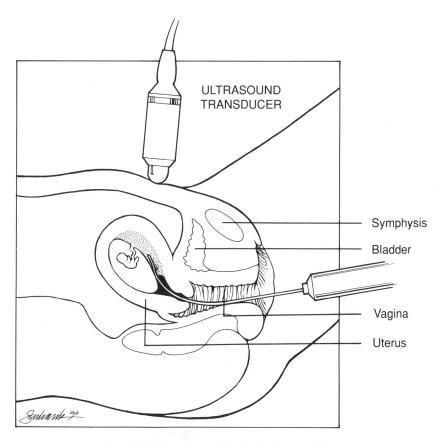

ULTRASOUND TRANSDUCER

Symphysis

Bladder

Vagina

Uterus

Fig. 10.6 Transcervical chorionic villus sampling.

[handwritten margin note: new data re: limb reduction defects ? CVS]

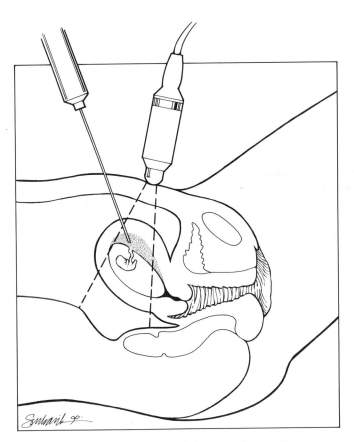

Fig. 10.7 Transabdominal chorionic villus sampling.

should probably be deferred until amniocentesis. Sensitization following CVS is probably no greater than that following amniocentesis, but exacerbating the problem at 10 weeks compared with 16 weeks surely cannot be salutary.

Safety

CVS compares favorably with amniocentesis with respect to safety. A large National Institute of Child Health and Human Development (NICHD) collaborative trial involving seven U.S. centers showed the procedure loss rate of transcervical CVS to be comparable with that of amniocentesis. The absolute excess loss rate for CVS was 0.8 percent, with the 80 percent confidence limit −0.7 to 2.2 percent showing no statistically significant difference. Comparable results were found in a Canadian randomized study.[16] Ear-

lier fears of maternal sepsis have diminished; not a single case was observed among 2,184 women in the NICHD trial. There is also no evidence that birth weight differs among pregnancies having CVS or that other adverse perinatal outcomes (e.g., placental abruption) occur with increased frequency.

The comparative safety of transabdominal and transcervical CVS has also been assessed in a randomized NICHD trial. Transabdominal and transcervical CVS appear equally safe in preliminary analysis.[17]

Preimplantation Prenatal Diagnosis (Embryo Biopsy)

Although CVS offers many advantages when compared with amniocentesis, it still cannot be performed until after organogenesis is nearly complete. There are major disadvantages to this delay.[18] First, earlier diagnosis may be necessary for certain treatment regimens (metabolic, gene insertion). Successful metabolic treatment (dexamethasone) of 21-hydroxylase deficiency detected at CVS is already accepted,[19] but especially propitious circumstances exist for treating this condition, because the genital system is among the last organ systems to differentiate. Second, couples at exceptionally high risk for affected offspring may undergo repeated prenatal diagnosis and termination. An individual with an autosomal dominant disorder transmits a 50 percent risk to any given offspring. The risk is also 50 percent in pseudoautosomal dominant inheritance, a situation in which a homozygote for an autosomal recessive disorder mates a heterozygote for the same disorder. A male with an X-linked recessive trait mated to a heterozygous female has a 50 percent risk for all female offspring. The risk is also very high for some complex chromosomal rearrangements. Third, even couples at lower risks may unfortunately have affected fetuses in successive pregnancies, requiring repeated termination.

For the above reasons, preimplantation diagnosis might be desirable in certain circumstances. Embryos fertilized in vitro or recovered by uterine lavage might be recovered or isolated. In the four-cell mouse embryo, a single cell can be removed safely,[20] and in humans a similar technique has been applied.[21,22] In slightly older embryos, incision of the zona pellucida allows herniation (biopsy) of 10 to 30 cells (trophoectoderm biopsy) (Fig. 10.8). Availability of these few cells is sufficient for diagnosis of molecular defects, given advances in molecular genetics (e.g., polymerized chain reaction) (see Indications for Prenatal Genetic Studies). The safety of human embryonic micromanipulation is not known, but in mice single-cell blastomere biopsy in experienced hands is surprisingly benign.

One can thus envision recovery of embryos by in vitro fertilization or uterine lavage, preimplantation diagnosis, and transfer to the recipient of only genetically normal embryos. Pregnancies requiring metabolic treatment could be identified and treated prior to organogenesis. In the future, genes can surely be inserted to correct the underlying defects. At present, preimplantation genetic diagnosis is not available widely, but its reality can be expected in the foreseeable future.

Analysis of Amniotic Fluid Cells or Chorionic Villi

The obstetrician/gynecologist should be aware of the pitfalls associated with the analysis of chorionic villi or amniotic fluid cells. An obvious problem is that cells may not grow, or growth may be insufficient for proper analysis. Fortunately, culture failures are relatively uncommon. Analysis of maternal rather than fetal cells is another theoretic fear, which fortunately has proved uncommon in experienced hands. In amniocentesis, maternal cell contamination can be minimized by discarding the first few drops of aspirated amniotic fluid. In CVS, examination under a dissecting microscope allows one to distinguish villi from decidua.

Of more pressing concern is the possibility that chromosomal abnormalities in villi or amniotic fluid may fail to reflect fetal status. One reason is that chromosomal aberrations may arise in culture (in vitro). This possibility should be suspected whenever an abnormality is restricted to only one of the several culture flasks or clones from a single amniotic fluid or CVS specimen. In fact, cells containing at least one additional structurally normal chromosome are detected in 1 to 2 percent of amniotic fluid or chorionic villus specimens.[23] If these abnormal cells are limited to a single culture or clone, the phenomenon is termed pseudomosaicism; no clinical significance is attached. True fetal mosaicism, defined as presence of the same abnormality in more than one clone or

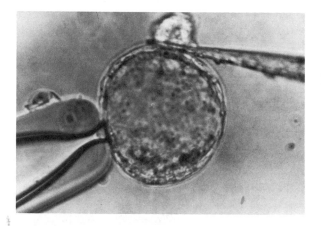

Fig. 10.8 Trophoectoderm biopsy.

culture flask, is rare in amniotic fluid and villi but clinically significant. True mosaicism can be confirmed by studies of the abortus or liveborn in at least 70 to 80 percent of cases[24] and cannot be truly excluded in the remainder.

Chorionic villi divide more rapidly than do amniotic fluid cells. Trophoblasts derived from villi can be accumulated in metaphase within hours of sampling. Analysis of these cells can provide rapid answers. However, discrepancies may arise between short-term trophoblast cultures and long-term cultures initiated from the mesenchymal core of the villi.[25] Discrepancies may further arise between CVS preparations of either type and the embryo. Fortunately, it is possible to recognize and manage these discrepancies, usually by confirmatory amniocentesis and assessment of normal interval growth. In most discrepancies, the fetus proves normal at amniocentesis, having shown normal growth in the interim ("false positive"). In the U.S. collaborative study, which involved 6,033 patients having successful CVS analysis (direct method, long-term culture, or both), there were no incorrect sex predictions.[25] There were also no diagnostic errors involving autosomal trisomies (13, 18, 21), sex chromosomal aneuploidy, or structural aberrations. In none of the 6,033 was a normal cytogenetic diagnosis with CVS followed by birth of an abnormal infant. However, one tetraploidy and two lethal trisomies (16, 22) were diagnosed when the direct method only was used, in no case either cytogenetic follow-up or results with other methods being available. Mosaicism was observed in 0.83 percent of specimens, but confirmed in only one-fourth of the cases. Overall, accuracy is comparable to amniocentesis, although caution is necessary if only the direct method is utilized.

The obstetrician must also realize that the neonatal phenotype cannot always be predicted on the basis of the chromosomal complement in amniotic fluid cells or chorionic villi. If a phenotypically normal parent carries the same balanced translocation as found in the fetus, reassurance usually suffices. On the other hand, if an ostensibly balanced translocation is detected in the fetus but in neither parent (a de novo translocation), the likelihood is 10 percent that the neonate will be phenotypically abnormal.[26] Presumably, the rearrangement is not always truly balanced.

INDICATIONS FOR PRENATAL GENETIC STUDIES

Cytogenetic Disorders

All chromosomal disorders are detectable in utero. It is not appropriate, however, to perform amniocentesis or CVS in every pregnancy, because for many couples the risks of such invasive procedures outweigh diagnostic benefits. Considered below are currently accepted indications.

Advanced Maternal Age

The most common indication for antenatal cytogenetic studies is advanced maternal age. The incidence of trisomy 21 is 1 per 800 liveborn births in the United States, but the frequency increases with age (Table 10.3). Trisomy 21, trisomy 13, trisomy 18, 47,XXX and 47,XXY all increase with advanced age.

It is now standard medical practice in the United States to offer prenatal chromosomal diagnosis to all women who at their expected delivery date will be 35 years or older. The designation of 35 years is largely arbitrary, however, having been chosen at a time when risk figures were available only in 5-year intervals (i.e., 30 to 34 years, 35 to 39 years, 40 to 44 years). Flexibility is thus appropriate when answering inquiries from women younger than age 35 years. Increasing numbers of women aged 33 or 34 years seek prenatal diagnosis.

The risk figures listed in Table 10.3 are applicable only for liveborns. The prevalence of abnormalities at the time when CVS or amniocentesis is performed is somewhat higher.[27,28] For example, the risk for 35-year-old women is about 1 : 270 for Down syndrome at the time of amniocentesis (mid-trimester). That the frequency of chromosomal abnormalities is lower in liveborn infants than in first- or second-trimester fetuses is due to the disproportionate likelihood that fetuses lost spontaneously between the time of prenatal testing (9 to 16 weeks) and term (40 weeks) will have chromosomal abnormalities. Some abnormal fetuses would have died in utero had iatrogenic intervention not occurred in the second trimester. In fact, 5 percent of stillborn infants show chromosomal abnormalities (see Ch. 23).

Observations that low maternal serum α-fetopro-

? not true in studies

AFP sens 25%

Triple screen sens 60%

tein (MSAFP) is associated with increased risk of trisomy are discussed below. A logical corollary might be that normal or slightly elevated MSAFP (e.g., 1.0 to 2.4 multiples of the median [MOM]) decreases the risk of aneuploidy for older women. For this reason, some British workers recommend against amniocentesis in older women (35 to 37 years) having normal or slightly increased MSAFP values. However, most U.S. authorities do not agree because of potential legal hazard.

Previous Child With Chromosomal Abnormality

After the birth of a child, and probably also of an abortus with autosomal trisomy, the likelihood that subsequent progeny will also have autosomal trisomy is increased, even if parental chromosomal complements are normal. The risk is probably not as high as once believed, but parental anxiety still dictates that antenatal chromosomal studies should be discussed for couples having had a trisomy 21 child. A recurrence risk of perhaps 1 percent is appropriate.[29]

Recurrence risk data following the birth of a liveborn infant trisomic for a chromosome other than 21 are limited. A risk of perhaps 1 percent is appropriate for either the same or for a different chromosomal abnormality. Thus antenatal studies should be offered.

Parental Chromosomal Rearrangements

An uncommon but important indication for prenatal cytogenetic studies is the presence of a parental chromosomal abnormality. A balanced translocation is the usual indication, but inversions and other chromosomal abnormalities exist. As discussed above (see Chromosomal Abnormalities), empiric data reveal that theoretic risks for abnormal (unbalanced) offspring are greater than empiric risks. Empiric risks approximate 12 percent for offspring of either male or female heterozygotes having reciprocal translocations.[30] For Robertsonian translocations, risks vary according to the chromosomes involved. For t(14q;21q), risks are 10 percent for offspring of heterozygous mothers and 2 percent for offspring of heterozygous fathers (Fig. 10.9).[30] For other nonhomologous Robertsonian translocations, empiric risks

for liveborns are less than 1 percent. For homologous translocations 21q;21q, all liveborn offspring have trisomy 21. For other homologous Robertsonian translocations (13q;13q or 22q;22q), all pregnancies result in abortions. The other parental chromosomal rearrangement of relevance to prenatal diagnosis is the inversion (see Chromosomal Abnormalities). Counseling is not dissimilar to that offered to individuals having a balanced translocation, although the cytologic mechanism responsible for abnormal offspring differs.

Increased Risk of Aneuploidy Because of Low MSAFP, Low Estriol, and Elevated Human Chorionic Gonadotropin

As discussed in greater detail later in this chapter (see MSAFP Screening), elevated MSAFP can be indicative of an underlying fetal neural tube defect. Low MSAFP is also associated with Down syndrome (Fig. 10.10).[31,32] The diagnosis is made by performing amniocentesis on women who would otherwise not have an invasive diagnostic procedure. Approximately 25 percent of trisomy 21 infants can be detected on the basis of low MSAFP. In evaluating MSAFP, one must take into account maternal weight and gestational age. Overestimating gestational age can be associated with spurious "low" MSAFP values. Most centers now use an algorithm based on age and MSAFP value to calculate a new risk for Down syndrome. If the risk is equal to or greater than that associated with a 35-year-old woman at mid-trimester (i.e., 1/270) counseling for potential amniocentesis is appropriate. In our center we do not inform the patient unless the risk equals this degree. More recently, it has developed that low estriol[33,34] as well as elevated human chorionic gonadotropin (hCG)[35] are similarly associated with aneuploidy, at least with trisomy 21. At present we utilize all three of these hormones to create a new risk figure. By taking into account age (≥ 35 years), MSAFP, estriol, and hCG, approximately 60 percent of trisomy 21 fetuses can be detected.

Prenatal Diagnosis of Mendelian Disorders

Increasing numbers of Mendelian disorders are becoming detectable in utero as new diagnostic techniques become available. Initially only metabolic dis-

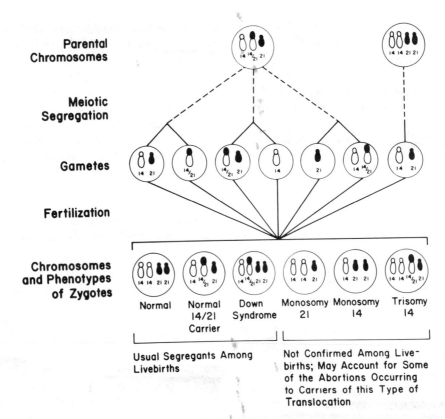

Fig. 10.9 Diagram of possible gametes and progeny of a phenotypically normal individual heterozygous for a Robertsonian translocation between chromosomes 14 and 21. Three of the six possible gametes are incompatible with life. The likelihood that an individual with such a translocation would have a child with Down syndrome is theoretically 33 percent. However, the empirical risk is considerably less. (From Gerbie and Simpson,[50] with permission.)

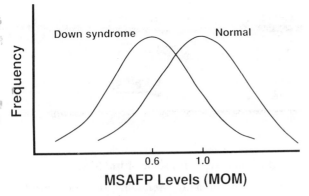

Fig. 10.10 Distributions of MSAFP in the normal population and in a population of women carrying a Down syndrome infant.

orders were detectable, on the basis of enzyme analysis. Antenatal diagnoses of hemoglobinopathies and hemophilia were later accomplished by studying fetal blood, originally obtainable only by fetoscopy. Now, DNA analysis permits many diagnoses using any available nucleated cell (chorionic villi, amniotic fluid cells). The nature of the mutant or absent gene product need not even be known. We can predict confidently that in the foreseeable future all common Mendelian disorders will be detectable. The rapid progress and increasing complexity required to diagnose Mendelian traits dictate close liaison between obstetrician/gynecologist and geneticist.

Inborn Errors of Metabolism

Antenatal diagnosis is possible for approximately 100 inborn errors of metabolism. Most are transmitted in an autosomal recessive fashion, although a few display X-linked recessive or autosomal dominant inheritance. Couples at increased risk will usually be identified because they previously had an affected child. Most metabolic disorders are so rare that it is unreasonable to expect obstetricians who are not geneticists to be fully cognizant of diagnostic possibilities.

Detection of a metabolic error requires that the enzyme be expressed in amniotic fluid cells or in chorionic villi. This requirement is fulfilled by most metabolic disorders, a prominent exception being phenylketonuria (PKU). Fortunately, PKU can be detected by the molecular techniques to be described below. All metabolic disorders detectable in amniotic fluid have proved detectable in chorionic villi. Although cultured cells are usually necessary for diagnosis, occasionally one can arrive at a diagnosis on the basis of a product in amniotic fluid. The most prominent example is 17-α-hydroxyprogesterone, which if elevated indicates adrenal 21-hydroxylase deficiency (congenital adrenal hyperplasia). However, this disorder is best detected by analysis of linked HLA markers in nuclei obtained by CVS.[19]

Genodermatosis and Other Disorders Detectable Solely by Tissue Sampling

If a gene causing a given disorder is not expressed in amniotic fluid or chorionic villi, biochemical analysis of such tissues will provide no information concerning presence or absence of the disorder. However, the gene might still be expressed in other tissues—blood, skin, or liver. Originally obtained through fetoscopically directed biopsy, such tissues have recently been obtained more easily by ultrasound-directed sampling with relatively small (14-gauge) instruments. Procedure-related losses following skin biopsy or other invasive procedures are surely greater than those following CVS or amniocentesis; however, the severity of some disorders justifies tissue sampling if no other diagnostic method is available. In our center we counsel a procedure-related loss of about 2 to 3 percent.[36]

Sampling fetal skin is the only available method for diagnosing dermatologic abnormalities such as epidermolysis bullosa or congenital ichthyosis (harlequin ichthyosis).[36,37] Histologic and electron microscopic analyses of fetal skin are necessary.

Detection of Mendelian Disorders by Molecular Techniques

The advantage of prenatal diagnosis by molecular techniques is that any available nucleated cell can be utilized for diagnosis. All cells contain the same DNA. The gene need not be expressed, unlike the situation when a gene product (enzyme protein) must be analyzed. Through molecular techniques developed within the last decade, Duchenne muscular dystrophy, hemophilia, cystic fibrosis, adult-onset polycystic kidney disease, Huntington's chorea, and other disorders have become detectable.

To appreciate recent clinical advances, the obstetrician/gynecologist must first be aware of the analytic techniques that made possible diagnosis by molecular methods. Pivotal was the discovery of restriction endonucleases. These bacterial enzymes recognize specific sequences five to seven nucleotides in length and cut DNA only at those sequences. Use of restriction enzymes permits DNA to be divided into fragments of reproducible lengths (Figs. 10.11 and 10.12). Analysis of DNA fragments can then proceed. A radioactive or biotinylated gene probe can be used to recognize hybridization (annealing) between complementary single-stranded DNA sequences, one the unknown and one the labeled probe. In challenging unknown DNA (e.g., nuclei derived from villi or amniotic fluid) with a labeled gene probe, the DNA coding for the gene in question will be located from among thousands of other DNA fragments. Diagnoses were initially made on the basis of size differences of the DNA fragments in the region of the gene in question (Fig. 10.12), but sensitive oligonucleotide (allele-specific) probes can now often be used for "dot-blot" DNA analysis (see below).

Integral to facile diagnosis was development of the polymerase chain reaction (PCR) procedure.[38,39] In PCR a target sequence of up to 1 kb can be amplified 10^5- to 10^6-fold (Fig. 10.13). Such amplification utilizes unique DNA primers that flank and are specific for the DNA region in question. The region in question may consist of a portion of a gene containing a

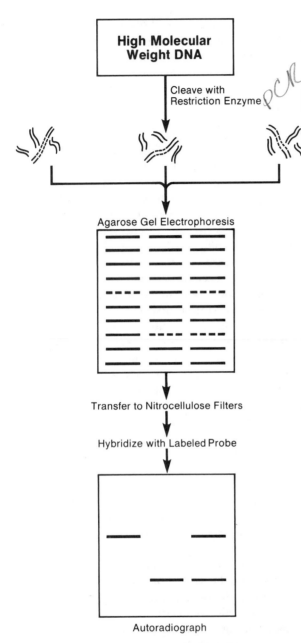

Fig. 10.11 Southern blotting. DNA is cleaved with restriction enzymes and the cleaved DNA separated by size using agarose gel electrophoresis. The gel is then laid on a piece of nitrocellulose, and buffer is allowed to flow through the gel into the nitrocellulose. DNA fragments migrate out of the gel and bind to the filter. A replica of the gel's DNA fragment pattern is thus made on the filter. The filter can then be hybridized to a labeled probe, with DNA fragments hybridizing to the probe identified by the autographic or biotinylated label.

mutation, a polymorphic DNA sequence closely linked to a given locus, or a repetitive DNA sequence characteristic of a given chromosome (the Y long arm). A heat-stable DNA polymerase extracted from *Thermas aquaticus* is also required (Taq polymerase). Incubated in a single tube is the DNA in question, an excess of the four deoxyribonucleoside triphosphates (adenine, thymine, guanine, and cytosine), the unique primers specific for the region being studied, and Taq polymerase. DNA synthesis (amplification) is initiated (cycle 1 in Fig. 10.13). When the temperature is raised, denaturation into single-stranded DNA occurs. Upon cooling, another amplification cycle ensues (cycle 2 in Fig. 10.13). The DNA sequence between primers amplifies in geometric fashion. In 3 to 4 hours 30 to 40 amplifications are achieved.

It is convenient for heuristic purposes to divide Mendelian disorders into those in which molecular basis (i.e., precise nucleotide abnormality) is known and those in which the gene is localized to a given chromosomal region but in which molecular basis is not known.

Diagnosis When the Molecular Basis is Known

Among the known causes of a Mendelian disorder are absence of or point mutation of DNA. If a disorder is known to be characterized by absence of DNA, one can determine whether a probe does or does not recognize (hybridize) the relevant sequence of DNA from an individual of unknown genotype. Failure of hybridization indicates that the individual lacks the DNA sequence in question; thus the disorder must be present. This approach is currently used to diagnose all forms of ∂-thalassemia, 80 percent of Duchenne/Becker muscular dystrophy, about 20 percent of β-thalassemia in the United States, and some forms of hemophilia.

A second approach becomes applicable if the etiology involves a point mutation whose nucleotide sequence is known. In sickle cell anemia, the triplet (codon) designating the sixth amino acid has undergone a mutation from adenine to thymine. As result, codon 6 connotes valine rather than glutamic acid, leading to the abnormal protein (β^S). Fortunately, several restriction enzymes recognize the normal DNA sequence at codons 5, 6, and 7 (Fig. 10.12).

An increasingly useful direct approach involves construction of synthetic probes capable of hybrid-

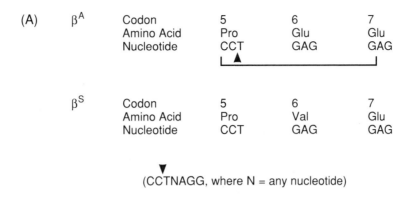

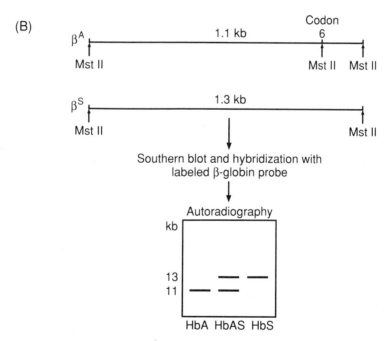

Fig. 10.12 Use of a radioactively labeled gene probe for B-globin for diagnosis of sickle cell anemia. The approach uses the choice of a specific restriction enzyme **(A)** followed by Southern blotting **(B)** to elicit differences in DNA lengths. A mutation of adenine to thymine results in loss of an Mst II restriction recognition site (CCTNAGG, where N = any nucleotide).

izing only to a specific sequence of approximately 15 nucleotides (oligonucleotides). Oligonucleotide probes can be designed to hybridize if and only if the (complementary) DNA of a given individual contains every single nucleotide in its correct sequence. Alter-

ation of even a single nucleotide (e.g., in sickle cell anemia) will result in the oligonucleotide probe failing to hybridize. Sensitivity of oligonucleotide probes can also be enhanced by the use of PCR to amplify the amount of DNA present in the unknown sample.

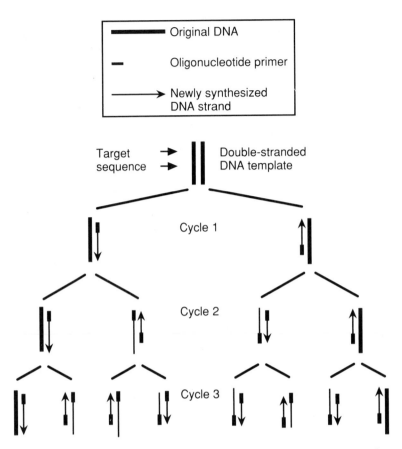

Fig. 10.13 Polymerase chain reaction (PCR). Placing the DNA in question, unique primers and Taq polymerase together results in amplification (cycle 1). When the temperature is raised, denaturation into single-stranded DNA occurs. Upon cooling, a second amplification cycle continues. Continued amplification increases the DNA between primers in logarithmic fashion.

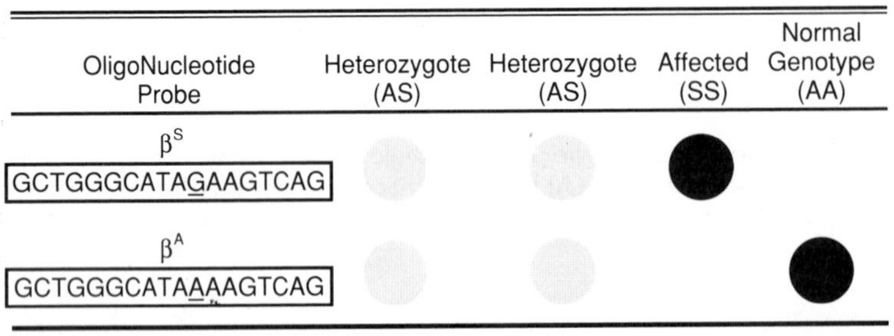

Fig. 10.14 Dot-blot analysis. Oligonucleotides are constructed for sequences unique to normal DNA (β^A) and mutant DNA (β^S) at the sequence responsible for sickle cell anemia. DNA challenged by the oligonucleotide probe will be hybridized if and only if the DNA contains all nucleotides connoted by the probe. Thus, AS individuals will respond to both β^A and β^S probes, whereas AA or SS individuals will respond only to one of the two probes (β^A and β^S, respectively). Homozygous individuals respond with a stronger (darker) signal than do heterozygous individuals. (Modified from Simpson,[53] with permission.)

Diagnoses can thus be made with small amounts of DNA, potentially even single cells. If the allele-specific oligonucleotide hybridizes, it appears as a "dot blot" (Fig. 10.14). Absence of hybridization is signified by absence of the dot. If a given Mendelian disorder is genetically heterogenous (i.e., consisting of several different nucleotide mutations), the various possible mutations can be tested by a panel of oligonucleotide probes (multiplex).

Diagnosis When the Molecular Basis Is Not Known

The molecular approaches described above are applicable only when the precise molecular basis of a disorder is known. Actually, this requirement is fulfilled infrequently. However, prenatal diagnosis may still prove possible on the basis of linkage analysis, taking advantage of the ostensibly innocuous differences in DNA that exist among individuals in the general population.

These clinically insignificant differences in DNA yield differences in DNA fragment lengths after exposure to a given restriction endonuclease. These differences are termed restriction fragment length polymorphisms (RFLPs). The basis of linkage analysis for prenatal diagnosis is that a diagnosis can be made not on the basis of analyzing the mutant gene per se (whose nature may be unknown), but rather on the basis of presence or absence of a nearby marker. Here the marker is a DNA variant capable of being recognized following exposure to a given endonuclease (thus, RFLP).

For illustration of the principle, assume that a given RFLP is known to lie close to or preferably within the mutant gene of interest. One next needs to deduce the relationship of the mutant to the status of the marker. Starting with an individual of known genotype, usually an affected fetus or child, one determines on which parental chromosome a given DNA fragment (RFLP marker) is located (cis–trans relationship). Is the marker located on the chromosome carrying the mutant gene, and is it located on the chromosome carrying the normal gene? Figure 10.15 illustrates a simple example in which the probe hybridizes to a DNA sequence capable of being affected by an RFLP.

There are pitfalls in linkage analysis using RFLP. First, an RFLP may not be informative in a given family. If all family members show identical DNA fragment patterns, that particular RFLP is useless because affected and unaffected individuals cannot be distinguished from each other. If a given RFLP is uninformative, one searches for another RFLP that may be informative. Second, the distance between the mutant gene and the RFLP is crucial, because the likelihood of meiotic recombination is inversely related to this distance. Recall that, during meiosis I, recombination can occur between homologous chromosomes. Genes are linked to one another if, after meiosis I, they remain together more often than expected by chance. Recombination can occur even between closely linked loci; thus prenatal diagnosis based on linkage analysis is less than 100 percent accurate. Using polymorphic markers on both sides of the mutant can minimize but not exclude the likelihood of missing a recombination event.

Despite these caveats, RFLP analysis permits prenatal diagnosis of many disorders not heretofore detectable. Because a potentially limitless number of RFLPs exist, increasing numbers of single gene (Mendelian) disorders can be expected to become detectable. This will especially prove feasible as a more complete map of the human genome is developed. Disorders likely amenable to RFLP analysis that are most likely to be encountered by the obstetrician are Huntington's chorea, PKU, CF, hemophilias A and B, adult-onset polycystic kidney disease, some forms of neurofibromatosis, Duchenne/Becker muscular dystrophy, and β-thalassemia (Table 10.5).

Prenatal Diagnosis and Genetic Screening for Polygenic/Multifactorial Disorders

Failure of neural tube closure during embryogenesis leads to anencephaly, spina bifida (myelomeningocele or meningocele), encephalocele, and other less common midline defects (e.g., lipomeningocele). Anencephaly is not compatible with long-term survival. Spina bifida is compatible with long-term survival, although it is frequently associated with hemiparesis, urinary incontinence, and hydrocephalus.

Anencephaly and spina bifida represent different manifestations of the same pathogenic process. Couples who have had a child with a neural tube defect have an approximate 1 percent risk for any subsequent offspring having spina bifida and a 1 percent risk for subsequent offspring having anencephaly (2

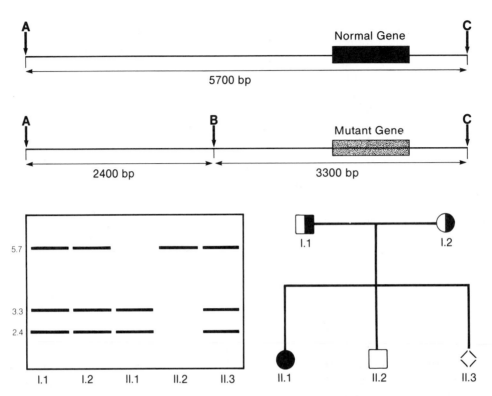

Fig. 10.15 Restriction fragment length polymorphisms (RFLPs), which are invaluable for certain prenatal diagnoses. Suppose a mutant gene is linked to another gene that governs whether or not a restriction site (B) is present. If the repetitive segment is present, DNA is cut by a certain restriction enzyme *(arrow)* to produce 3,300- and 2,400-bp-long fragments. If the segment is not present, the total fragment is 5,700 bp long. The different lengths can function as markers to allow genotypes to be deduced. Suppose two obligate heterozygotes I.1 and I.2 have one affected child (II.1). Suppose further that a probe for the gene hybridizes to the region from A to C. The probe can thus identify three fragments (2,400 and 3,300, 5,700 bp). If the affected child shows only the 2,400- and 3,300-bp fragments, it can be deduced that the mutant allele is in association (i.e., on the same chromosome) with the gene-conferring restriction site B and thus is producing both 2,400- and 3,300-bp fragments. The normal allele must be in association with the allele not conferring restriction B and thus is designated by the 5,700-bp fragment. For simplicity it is assumed that this situation exists in both parents. Genotypes can thus be predicted from DNA analysis of chorionic villi and amniotic fluid cells. Fetus II.3 can be assumed to be heterozygous, because all three fragments (2,400, 3,300, 5,700 bp) are present.

percent for any neural tube defect).[40] This is true irrespective of the type of neural tube defect present in the index case (proband). If a prospective parent has a neural tube defect, the risk is also about 2 percent. Second-degree relatives (nieces, nephews, grandchildren) and third-degree relatives (first cousins) are less likely to be affected. A woman whose sister or brother had a child with a neural tube defect has a 0.5 to 1.0 percent risk for neural tube defect offspring.[40] For reasons that are unclear, risks are slightly lower if the father's sibling had the neural tube defect.

Amniotic Fluid α-Fetoprotein Analysis

Antenatal diagnosis of a neural tube defect can be accomplished by either high-quality ultrasound or assay of amniotic fluid α-fetoprotein (AF-AFP). Through AF-AFP analysis, diagnosis of a neural tube defect is possible in all anencephaly cases and in all except the 5 to 10 percent of spina bifida cases in which skin covers the lesion. Closed lesions are somewhat more common in encephalocele. Ultrasonography by experienced physicians should readily exclude anencephaly, and spina bifida theoretically can be

Table 10.5 Disorders Detectable by DNA Analysis

Direct
  α-Thalassemia
  β-Thalassemia (80 percent worldwide; lower in the United States)
  Duchenne/Becker muscular dystrophy (80 percent)
  Hemophilia A (rare)
  Sickle cell anemia
  Cystic fibrosis (50 percent; 55 to 70 percent in whites of northern European ancestry)
Linkage analysis (restriction fragment length polymorphisms)
  Adrenal 21-hydroxylase deficiency
  β-Thalassemia (20 percent worldwide; higher in United States)
  Cystic fibrosis (50 percent; 30 to 45 percent in whites of northern European ancestry)
  Duchenne muscular dystrophy (20 percent)
  Hemophilia A and B (most forms)
  Neurofibromatosis (some forms)
  Huntington's chorea
  Adult onset polycystic kidney disease

detected by serial views of the vertebral column and third ventricle. Unfortunately, few ultrasonographers state their own sensitivity or specificity for detecting neural tube defects. Until such data are available, AF-AFP analysis should be considered the standard method for detecting neural tube defects.

Amniotic fluid AFP may be spuriously elevated if the amniotic fluid is contaminated with fetal blood. This pitfall can be eliminated if amniotic fluid acetylcholinesterase (AChE) is concurrently assayed. AChE is present in the amniotic fluid of fetuses with open neural tube defects but is absent in normal amniotic fluid. If AChE is absent but fetal hemoglobin is present, the elevated AFP is probably due to fetal blood. Confusion may also arise if amniocentesis is performed earlier than 14 weeks.[41]

Elevated AFP is also associated with certain other polygenic/multifactorial anomalies (e.g., omphalocele, gastroschisis, cystic hygroma) and with certain Mendelian traits (e.g., congenital nephrosis). In these disorders, AChE may or may not be elevated. Ultrasonographic studies should therefore be undertaken to corroborate elevated AF-AFP and to determine the nature of any defect present. On the other hand, failure to detect an anomaly by ultrasound does not necessarily indicate that elevated amniotic fluid AFP was spurious. If amniotic fluid AFP is elevated and AChE is present, I consider the fetus to be abnormal irrespective of ultrasound findings.

MSAFP Screening

Relatively few (5 percent) neural tube defects occur in families who have had previously affected offspring. Thus a method other than a positive family history is needed to identify couples in the general population at risk for a neural tube defect. MSAFP serves this purpose, identifying couples with a negative family history who nonetheless have sufficient risk to justify amniocentesis.

MSAFP is greater than 2.5 MOM in 80 to 90 percent of pregnancies characterized by a fetus with a neural tube defect. Because considerable overlap exists between MSAFP in normal pregnancies and MSAFP in pregnancies characterized by a fetus with a neural tube defect, systematic protocols for evaluating elevated MSAFP values are necessary. In addition to the presence of a neural tube defect, elevated MSAFP occurs for the following reasons: (1) underestimation of gestational age, inasmuch as MSAFP increases as gestation progresses (Fig. 10.16); (2) multiple gestation (60 percent of twins and almost all triplets have MSAFP values that would be elevated if judged on the basis of singleton values); (3) fetal demise, presumably because of fetal blood extravasating into the maternal circulation; (4) Rh disease, cystic hygroma, and other conditions associated with fetal edema; and (5) anomalies other than neural tube defects, again generally characterized by edema or skin defects.

For maximum accuracy of MSAFP screening, the initial assay should be performed at 15 to 18 weeks gestation. Corrections for maternal weight and other factors are necessary, using various algorithms. Obstetricians should expect their referring laboratory to have generated its own normal values and to provide a weight-adjusted MSAFP appropriate for the gestation age. MSAFP should be weight adjusted, for dilutional effects can result in large women having a spuriously low value when MSAFP is actually elevated for women of their weight (Fig. 10.17).

Values of 2.5 MOM or greater in the general population are usually considered elevated. Values above 2.0 MOM are considered elevated in insulin-dependent diabetic women, but in twin gestations MSAFP is

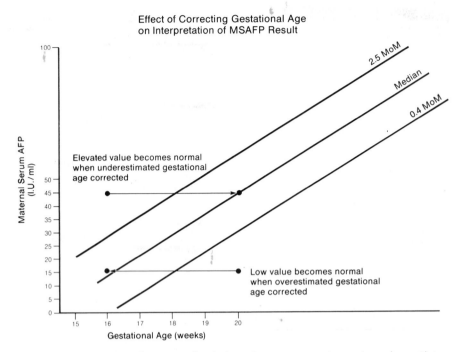

Fig. 10.16 Median maternal serum α-fetoprotein levels throughout gestation. Increasing values with increasing gestational age require accurate dating to interpret low or high MSAFP.

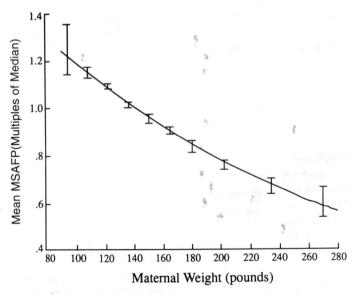

Fig. 10.17 Relationship of MSAFP to maternal weight.

Table 10.6 Likelihood of Having a Fetus With NTD After Various Stages of an MSAFP Screening Program

Time	Risk
Prior to MSAFP	1/1,000
After one elevated MSAFP	1/50
Prior to sonogram	1/30
Prior to amniocentesis	1/15
Amniotic fluid AFP > 5 SD	1/2.2[a]
Acetylcholinesterase present	1/1.1

[a] Approximately equal numbers of neural tube defect (NTD) and other serious abnormalities or fetal demise.

considered abnormal above 4.5 or 5.0 MOM. A second MSAFP sample may or may not be necessary. At our institution, we assay MSAFP again 1 week after the initial sample only if MSAFP is between 2.50 and 2.99 MOM and if gestational age is 18 weeks or less. If not already performed, ultrasound is required to exclude erroneous gestational age, multiple gestations, or fetal demise. Amniocentesis for AFAFP and AChE analyses is then necessary if no explanation for elevated MSAFP is evident at ultrasound.

MSAFP screening identifies 90 percent of anencephaly and 80 to 85 percent of spina bifida, albeit at the cost of 1 to 2 percent of all pregnant women undergoing amniocentesis. Only 1 of approximately 15 women having unexplained elevated serum AFP will prove to have a fetus with a neural tube defect (Table 10.6). If gestational age assessment is determined accurately before MSAFP sampling, the number of women undergoing amniocentesis will be even lower.

Polygenic/Multifactorial Disorders Detectable Only by Ultrasound

Anomalies inherited in polygenic/multifactorial fashion usually carry recurrence risks of 1 to 5 percent for first-degree relatives (siblings, offspring, parent), a risk sufficiently high to justify prenatal diagnosis for many couples. Because the number of genes responsible for these defects is unknown, albeit presumably more than one, diagnosis on the basis of enzyme assays or DNA cannot seriously be proposed at present.

The remaining methods of assessment involve visualization of fetal anatomy, principally by ultrasound. Fetal visualization is also useful for certain Mendelian disorders (e.g., autosomal recessive polycystic kidney disease, X-linked recessive aqueductal stenosis [hydrocephaly], and various skeletal dysplasias).

The typical couple at risk already has had a child with the anomaly in question, thus incurring a 1 to 5 percent risk for another affected child. To alter clinical management, an ultrasound diagnosis should be made by 20 to 24 weeks gestation. This is sufficiently early to weigh the alternative options of termination, fetal surgery, or preterm delivery followed by neonatal surgery. Percutaneous uterine blood sampling and rapid karyotyping[42] or second-trimester transabdominal CVS[43,44] are necessary to exclude chromosomal abnormalities if either of the latter options is pursued. A careful search for other defects is necessary. For hydrocephaly, an isolated anomaly is rare, but for posterior urethral values it is less so.

Antenatal ultrasonography for anomaly detection should be performed only by highly experienced physicians. Physicians scanning obstetric patients only for fetal viability, multiple gestations, and placental location should explicitly inform their patients that anomaly assessment is not being attempted. Casual reassurance of fetal normalcy should be eschewed. It should further be realized that almost no individual has sufficient experience to calculate his or her own specificities or sensitivities.

Future Directions

Few areas of obstetrics and gynecology have shown more rapid advances than prenatal diagnosis. Barely 20 years have passed since the initiation of amniocentesis and prenatal diagnosis, yet diagnosis and genetic screening is now accepted as standard. The next decade will bring further advances, many alluded to previously. Molecular genetic technology can be expected to be available for all common monogenic disorders. Indeed, this would be one of the first benefits of mapping the human genome, a project expected to be finished in 10 to 15 years.[45,46] In addition to greatly expanding the numbers of disorders amenable to prenatal diagnosis, information will be available for genetic screening, identifying more couples at risk prior to the birth of a first affected child. Of note here is the confident expectation that increasing technology will make cost effective screening for a host of disorders in addition to those shown in Table 10.4.

It further seems likely that prenatal genetic diagnosis will move increasingly into the area of fetal treatment as well. We have already alluded to the ability of early diagnosis for metabolic conditions, and worth emphasizing again is the possibility of using preimplantation genetics for gene therapy. Certainly this is an ideal stage at which to insert genes.[18] Of course, the ultimate prenatal diagnosis would involve a noninvasive technique, an area in which a great deal of active work is necessary. There is increasing evidence that fetal cells truly exist in maternal blood,[47,48] based on the presence of Y-specific DNA in the peripheral blood of pregnant women known to be carrying a male fetus. A variety of attempts to isolate fetal cells or fetal DNA are in progress.[49] For example, in our institution we are pursuing the approach of fetal cell sorting followed by in situ hybridization with chromosome-specific probes. Success is not guaranteed and, if achieved, would doubtless first be followed by an invasive diagnostic procedure for confirmation. Nonetheless, the potential exists for noninvasive screening of maternal blood. Perhaps this would be offered to women under age 35 years, with invasive procedures remaining the standard for those having current cytogenetic indications. In any case, obstetricians and gynecologists can expect a host of exciting genetic advances.

REFERENCES

1. Simpson JL, Golbus MS: Genetics in Obstetrics and Gynecology. 2nd Ed. WB Saunders, Philadelphia (in press)
2. Hook EB, Hamerton JL: The frequency of chromosome abnormalities detected in consecutive newborn studies—differences between studies—results by sex and by severity of phenotypic involvement. p. 63. In Hook EB, Porter IH (eds): Population Cytogenetic Studies in Humans. Academic Press, San Diego, CA, 1977
3. McKusick VA: Mendelian Inheritance in Man. 9th Ed. The Johns Hopkins University Press, Baltimore, 1990
4. Riordan JR, Rommens JM, Kerem BS et al: Identification of the cystic fibrosis gene: cloning and characterization of complementary DNA. Science 245:1066, 1989
5. Lemna WK, Feldman GL, Kerem BS et al: Mutation analysis for heterozygote detection and the prenatal diagnosis of cystic fibrosis. N Engl J Med 322:219, 1990
6. Elias S, Annas G, Simpson JL: Carrier screening for cystic fibrosis: implications for obstetrical and gynecological practice. Amer J Obstet Gynecol (in press)
7. Elejalde BR, Elejalde MM, Acuna JM: Prospective study of amniocentesis performed between weeks 9 and 16 gestation: its feasibility, risks, complications and use in prenatal diagnosis. Am J Med Genet 35:188, 1990
8. Verp MS, Simpson JL: Amniocentesis for prenatal genetic diagnosis. p. 305. In Filkins K, Russo J (eds): Human Prenatal Diagnosis. Marcel Dekker, New York, 1990
9. Karp LE, Schiller HS: Meconium staining of amniotic fluid at midtrimester amniocentesis. Obstet Gynecol 50:475, 1977
10. Elias S, Gerbie AB, Simpson JL et al: Genetic amniocentesis in twin gestations. Am J Obstet Gynecol 138:169, 1980
11. Elias S, Simpson JL: Amniocentesis. p. 64. In Milunsky A (ed): Genetic Disorders and the Fetus. 2nd Ed. Plenum Press, New York, 1987
12. Antsaklis A, Politis J, Karagiannopoulos C et al: Selective survival of only the healthy fetus following prenatal diagnosis of thalassemia major in binovular twin gestation. Prenat Diagn 4:289, 1984
13. Evans MI, Fletcher JC, Zador IE et al: Selective first-trimester termination in octuplet and quadruplet pregnancies: clinical and ethical issues. Obstet Gynecol 71:289, 1988
14. Tabor A, Philip J, Madsen M et al: Randomized controlled trial of genetic amniocentesis in 4606 low-risk women. Lancet 1:1287, 1986
15. Rhoads GG, Jackson LG, Schlesselman SE et al: The safety and efficacy of chorionic villus sampling for early prenatal diagnosis of cytogenetic abnormalities. N Engl J Med 320:609, 1989
16. Canadian Collaborative Chorionic Villus Sampling—Amniocentesis Clinical Trial Group: Multicentered randomized clinical trial of chorionic villus sampling and amniocentesis: first report. Lancet 1:1, 1987
17. NICHD Collaborative CVS Study Group: Transcervical and transabdominal CVS are comparably safe procedures for first trimester prenatal diagnosis: preliminary analysis. Am J Hum Genet 47:A278, 1990
18. Simpson JL, Carson SA, Buster JE, Elias S: Future horizons in prenatal genetic diagnosis: preimplantation diagnosis and noninvasive screening. p. 547. In Filkins K, Russo J (eds): Human Prenatal Diagnosis. 2nd Ed. Marcel Dekker, New York, 1990
19. Speiser PW, Laforgia N, Kato K et al: First trimester prenatal treatment and molecular genetic diagnosis of congenital hyperplasia (21-hydroxylase deficiency). J Clin Endocrinol Metab 70:838, 1990
20. Wilton LJ, Trounson AO: Biopsy of preimplantation

mouse embryos: development of micromanipulated embryos and proliferation of single blastomeres in vitro. Biol Reprod 40:145, 1989

21. Handyside AH, Pattinson JK, Renketh RJ et al: Biopsy of human preimplantation embryos and sexing by DNA amplification. Lancet 1:347, 1989

22. Handyside AH, Kontogianni EH, Hardy K et al: Pregnancies from biopsied human preimplantation embryos sexed by Y-specific DNA amplification. Nature 344:768, 1990

23. Simpson JL, Martin AO, Verp MS et al: Hypermodel cells in amniotic fluid cultures: frequency, interpretation, and clinical significance. Am J Obstet Gynecol 143:250, 1982

24. Hsu LYF, Perlis TE: United States survey on chromosome mosaicism and pseudomosaicism in prenatal diagnosis. Prenat Diagn 4:97, 1980

25. Ledbetter DH, Gilbert F, Jackson L et al: Cytogenetic results of chorionic villus sampling: high success rate and diagnostic accuracy in United States Collaborative Study. Am J Obstet Gynecol 162:495, 1990

26. Warburton D: Outcome of cases of de novo structural rearrangements diagnosed at amniocentesis. Prenat Diagn 4:69, 1984

27. Hook EB, Cross PK, Jackson L et al: Maternal age specific rates of 47,+21 and other cytogenetic abnormalities diagnosed in the first trimester of pregnancy of chorionic villus biopsy specimens: comparison with rates expected from observations at amniocentesis. Am J Hum Genet 42:797, 1988

28. Hook EB, Cross PK: Maternal age-specific rates of chromosome abnormalities at chorionic villus study: a revision. Am J Hum Genet 45:474, 1989

29. Stene J, Stene E, Mikkelsen M: Risk for chromosome abnormality at amniocentesis following a child with a non-inherited chromosome aberration. Prenat Diagn 4:81, 1984

30. Boué A, Gallano P: A collaborative study of the segregation of inherited chromosome structural rearrangements in 13,356 prenatal diagnoses. Prenat Diagn 4:45, 1984

31. Merkartz IR, Nitowsky HM, Macri JN et al: An association between low maternal serum alpha fetoprotein and fetal chromosome abnormalities. Am J Obstet Gynecol 148:886, 1984

32. Cuckle HS, Wald NJ, Lindembaum RH: Maternal serum alpha fetoprotein measurement: a screening test for Down syndrome. Lancet 1:926, 1984

33. Canick JA, Knight GJ, Palomaki GE et al: Low second trimester maternal serum unconjugated estriol in pregnancies with Down syndrome. Br J Obstet Gynecol 95:330, 1988

34. Wald NJ, Cuckle HS, Densem JW et al: Maternal serum screening for Down's syndrome in early pregnancy. Br Med J 297:883, 1988

35. Bogart MH, Pandian MR, Jones OW: Abnormal maternal serum chorionic gonadotropin levels in pregnancies with chromosome abnormalities. Prenat Diagn 7:623, 1987

36. Elias S, Easterly N: Prenatal diagnosis of hereditary skin disorders. Clin Obstet Gynecol 4(24):1069, 1981

37. Bakhavev VA, Aivazyan AA, Karetnikova NA et al: Fetal skin biopsy in prenatal diagnosis of some genodermatoses. Prenat Diagn 10:1, 1990

38. Saiki RK, Scharf S, Faloona F et al: Enzymatic amplification of β-globin genomic sequences and restruction site analysis for diagnosis of sickle cell anemia. Science 230:1350, 1985

39. Einstein BI: Current concepts—the polymerase chain reaction: a new method of using molecular genetics for medical diagnosis. N Engl J Med 322:178, 1990

40. Milunsky A: The prenatal diagnosis of neural tube and other congenital defects. p. 453. In Milunsky A: Genetic Disorders and the Fetus. 2nd Ed. Plenum Press, New York, 1987

41. Crandall BF, Hanson FW, Tennant F: Acetylcholinesterase (AChE) electrophoresis and early amniocentesis. Am J Hum Genet 45:A257, 1989

42. Tipton RE, Tharapel AT, Chang HT et al: Rapid chromosome analysis with the use of spontaneously dividing cells derived from umbilical cord blood (fetal and neonatal). Am J Obstet Gynecol 161:1546, 1989

43. Holzgreve W, Miny P, Basarans S et al: Safety of placental biopsy in the second and third trimester. N Engl J Med 317:1159, 1987

44. Shulman LP, Tharapel AT, Meyers CM et al: Direct analysis of cytotrophoblast from second and third trimester placentas: an accurate and very rapid method for detecting fetal chromosome abnormalities. Am J Obstet Gynecol Commun 163:1606, 1990

45. Watson JD: The human genome project: past, present and future. Science 248:44, 1990

46. Cantor CR: Orchestrating the human genome project. Science 248:49, 1990

47. Bianchi DW, Flint AF, Pizzimenti MF et al: Isolation of fetal DNA from nucleated erythrocytes in maternal blood. Proc Natl Acad Sci USA 87:3279, 1990

48. Lo YMD, Patel P, Wainscoat JS et al: Prenatal sex determination by DNA from maternal peripheral blood. Lancet 2:1363, 1989

49. Simpson JL, Elias S: Noninvasive screening for prenatal diagnosis: isolating fetal cells from maternal blood. In Antsaklis AJ (ed) (in press)

50. Gerbie AT, Simpson JL: Antenatal diagnosis of genetic disorders. Postgrad Med 59:129, 1976

51. Hook EB: Rates of chromosomal abnormalities of different maternal ages. Obstet Gynecol 58:282, 1981

52. Hook EB, Cross PK, Schreinemachers DM et al: Chromosomal abnormality rates at amniocentesis and liveborn infants. JAMA 249:2043, 1983

53. Simpson JL: Genetic factors in obstetrics and gynecology. p. 237. In Scott RJ, DiSaia PJ, Hammond CB, Spellacy WN (eds): Danforth's Obstetrics and Gynecology. 6th Ed. JB Lippincott, Philadelphia, 1990

54. American College of Obstetricians and Gynecologists: Antenatal Diagnosis of Genetic Disorders. Technical Bulletin No. 108. ACOG, Washington, DC, 1987

Drugs in Pregnancy and Lactation

Jennifer R. Niebyl

GENERAL TERATOLOGY

Caution with regard to diet and drug ingestion during pregnancy is usually advised. Until recently, the fetus was thought to rest in a privileged site with little exposure to the environment experienced by the mother. The term placental barrier has been in widespread use but is truly a contradiction, as the placenta allows the transfer of many drugs and dietary substances.

Lipid-soluble substances readily cross the placenta, and water-soluble substances pass less well the greater their molecular weight. The degree to which a drug is bound to plasma protein also influences the amount of drug that is free to cross the placenta. Virtually all drugs cross the placenta to some degree, with the exception of large organic ions such as heparin and insulin.

Developmental defects in humans may be from genetic, environmental, or unknown causes. Approximately 25 percent are genetic in origin; drug exposure accounts for only 2 to 3 percent of birth defects. Approximately 65 percent of defects are of unknown etiology but may be from combinations of genetic and environmental factors (see Ch. 9).

The incidence of major malformations in the general population is usually quoted as 2 to 3 percent.[1] A major malformation is defined as either one that is incompatible with survival, such as anencephaly, or one that requires major surgery for correction, such as cleft palate or congenital heart disease. If all minor malformations are also included, such as ear tags or extra digits, the rate may be as high as 7 to 10 percent. The risk of malformation after exposure to a drug must be compared with this background rate.

There is a marked species specificity in drug teratogenesis.[2] For example, thalidomide was not found to be teratogenic in rats and mice but is a potent human teratogen. On the contrary, in certain strains of mice, corticosteroids produce a high percentage of offspring with cleft lip with or without cleft palate, although no studies have shown these drugs to be teratogenic in humans. The Food and Drug Administration (FDA) lists five categories of labeling for drug use in pregnancy:

A. Controlled studies in women fail to demonstrate a risk to the fetus in the first trimester, and the possibility of fetal harm appears remote.
B. Animal studies do not indicate a risk to the fetus; there are no controlled human studies, or animal studies do show an adverse effect on the fetus but well-controlled studies in pregnant women have failed to demonstrate a risk to the fetus.
C. Studies have shown the drug to have animal teratogenic or embryocidal effects, but no controlled studies are available in women or no studies are available in either animals or women.
D. Positive evidence of human fetal risk exists, but benefits in certain situations (e.g., life-threatening situations or serious diseases for which safer

drugs cannot be used or are ineffective) may make use of the drug acceptable despite its risks.

X. Studies in animals or humans have demonstrated fetal abnormalities, or evidence demonstrates fetal risk based on human experience, or both and the risk clearly outweighs any possible benefit.

The classic teratogenic period is from day 31 after the last menstrual period in a 28-day cycle to 71 days from the last period (Fig. 11.1). During this critical period, organs are forming, and teratogens may cause malformations that are usually overt at birth. The timing of exposure is important. Administration of drugs early in the period of organogenesis will affect the organs developing at that time, such as the heart or neural tube. Closer to the end of the classic teratogenic period, the ear and palate are forming and may be affected by a teratogen taken then. Before this period, exposure to a teratogen produces an all-or-none effect. With exposure around conception,

the conceptus usually either does not survive or survives without anomalies.

Because so few cells exist in the early stages, irreparable damage to some may be lethal to the entire organism. If the organism remains viable, however, organ-specific anomalies are not manifested, because either repair or replacement will occur to permit normal development. A similar insult at a later stage may produce organ-specific defects.

Embryology

During the first 3 days after ovulation, development takes place in the fallopian tube. At the time of fertilization, a pronuclear stage exists during which the nuclei from the egg and the sperm retain their integrity within the egg cytoplasm. After the pronuclei fuse, the zygote begins mitotic cell divisions (cleavage). The two-cell stage is reached about 30 hours after fertilization. With continued division, the cells develop into a solid ball of cells (morula), which

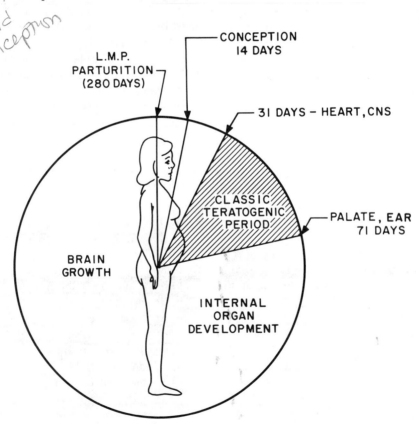

Fig. 11.1 Gestational clock showing the classic teratogenic period. (From Blake and Niebyl,[165] with permission.)

reaches the endometrial cavity about 3 days after fertilization. Thereafter, a fluid-filled cavity forms within the cell mass, at which time the conceptus is called a blastocyst. The number of cells increases from approximately 12 to 32 at the end of the third day to 250 by the sixth day.

Until approximately 3 days after conception, any cell is thought to be totipotential, that is, capable of initiating development of any organ system. For example, separation of cells during this time period can give rise to monozygotic twins, each normal. At the blastocyst stage, cells first begin to differentiate. The blastocyst is located in the uterus, where implantation occurs 6 to 9 days after conception.

One group of cells forms the inner cell mass that will ultimately develop into the fetus. Different tissues will develop from each of the three cell layers. The brain, nerves, and skin will develop from the ectoderm. The lining of the digestive tract, respiratory tract, and part of the bladder as well as the liver and pancreas will develop from the endoderm. Connective tissue, cartilage, muscle, blood vessels, heart, kidneys, and gonads are of mesodermal origin. The group of cells forming the periphery of the blastocyst is termed the trophoblast. The placenta and the fetal membranes will develop from this outer cell layer.

The trophoblast continues to develop, and lacunae form within the previously solid syncytiotrophoblast. The lacunae are the precursors of the intervillous spaces of the placenta, and by 2 weeks after conception maternal blood is found within them. Meanwhile, the cytotrophoblast is forming cell masses that will become chorionic villi.

From the third to the eighth week after conception, the embryonic disc undergoes major developments that lay the foundation for all organ systems. By 4 weeks after conception the fertilized ovum has progressed from one cell to millions of cells. The rudiments of all major systems have differentiated, and the blueprints are set for developmental refinements. The embryo has been transformed into a curved tube approximately 6 mm in length and isolated from the extraembryonic membranes.

At 5 weeks after conception, the embryo begins to assume features of human appearance. The face emerges, with the formation of discernible eyes, nose, and ears. Limbs emerge from protruding buds; digits, cartilage, and muscles develop. The cerebral hemispheres begin to fill the brain area, and the optic stalk becomes apparent. Nerve connections are established between the retina and the brain. The digestive tract rotates from its prior tubular structure, and liver starts to produce blood cells and bile. Two tubes emerge from the pharynx to become bronchi, and the lungs have lobes and bronchioles. The heart is beating at 5 weeks and is almost completely developed by 8 weeks after conception. The diaphragm begins to separate the heart and lungs from the intestines. The kidneys approach their final form at this time. The urogenital and rectal passages separate, and germ cells migrate toward the genital ridges for future transformation into ovaries or testes. Differentiation of internal ducts begins, with persistence of either müllerian or wolffian ducts. Virilization of external genitalia occurs in males. The embryo increases from approximately 6 to 33 mm in length and increases 50 times in weight.

Structurally, the fetus has become straighter, and the tubular neural canal along which the spinal cord develops becomes filled with nerve cells. Ears remain low on the sides of the head. Teeth are forming, and the two bony plates of the palate fuse in the midline. Disruptions during the latter part of the embryonic period lead to various forms of cleft lip and palate. By 10 weeks after the last menstrual period, all major organ systems have become established and integrated.

Management

Development of other organs continues in the second and third trimesters of pregnancy. Some of the anomalies of the uterus from diethylstilbestrol (DES) exposure occurred with exposure as late as 20 weeks, but were not recognized until after puberty. The brain is continuing to develop throughout the pregnancy and the neonatal period. Fetal alcohol syndrome may occur with chronic exposure to alcohol in later stages of pregnancy. Thus the effects of drugs taken in later pregnancy are of concern as well, although they may not be recognized until later in life.

The sensitive serum pregnancy tests can diagnose pregnancy as early as 1 week after conception. However, some urine tests for human chorionic gonadotropin (hCG) such as home pregnancy tests may not be positive until several days after the missed menses.

Thus a patient may not realize she is pregnant until she is already in the critical period.

Patients should be educated about avenues other than the use of drugs to cope with tension, aches and pains, and viral illnesses during pregnancy. Drugs should be used only when necessary. The risk–benefit ratio should justify the use of a particular drug, and the minimum effective dose should be employed. As long-term effects of drug exposure in utero may not be revealed for many years, caution with regard to the use of any drug in pregnancy is warranted.

EFFECTS OF SPECIFIC DRUGS

Estrogens and Progestins

Oral contraceptives and other hormones given in the first trimester of pregnancy have been blamed for a variety of birth defects, but recent studies have not confirmed any teratogenic risk for these drugs. Data from the Collaborative Perinatal Project initially supported the possibility of a risk of cardiac defects after first-trimester exposure to female hormones and oral contraceptives.[3] However, a reevaluation of these data has questioned this risk.[4] Careful review of the records indicated that some patients had taken the medication too early or too late to affect the cardiovascular system. When infants with Down syndrome were excluded, no significant difference in the risk of cardiovascular anomalies remained. Another study of 2,754 infants born to mothers after bleeding in the first trimester suggested no increased risk of first-trimester exposure to progestogens.[5]

In the Collaborative Perinatal Project there was no evidence of teratogenicity of 17α-hydroxyprogesterone caproate (Delalutin) in 162 infants or in 253 infants exposed to progesterone. Johnson et al.[6] studied 43 infants exposed in early pregnancy and found no teratogenic risk. One study, however, presented evidence suggesting that 17α-hydroxyprogesterone caproate may produce hypospadias if given before week 16 of pregnancy.[7] This also has not been confirmed.[5]

It appears that there is little or no risk to oral contraceptives in the first trimester.[8] Because of the medicolegal climate and the conflicting literature, it is wise to do a sensitive pregnancy test before refilling pills in a patient with amenorrhea.

Androgenic Steroids

Androgens may masculinize a developing female fetus. Progestational agents, most often the synthetic testosterone derivatives, may cause clitoromegaly and labial fusion if given before 13 weeks of pregnancy.[9] Danazol has been reported to cause mild clitoral enlargement and labial fusion when given inadvertently at a dosage of 800 mg/day for the first 10 to 12 weeks postconception (Fig. 11.2).[10] The degree of abnormality was correctable by surgery.

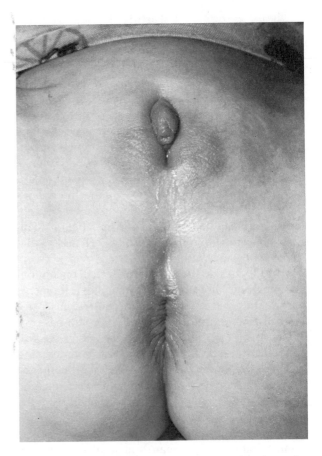

Fig. 11.2 Perineum of a female fetus exposed to danazol in utero. (From Duck and Katayama,[10] with permission.)

Spermicides

Jick et al.[11] initially reported an increased risk of abnormal offspring in mothers who had used spermicides for contraception. In that study, however, women were considered to be users if a prescription for a spermicide had been filled within 600 days of delivery. There was no documentation that the women had ever used the spermicide, certainly not at the critical period for teratogenesis. Also, the medication is available over the counter and could have been used by either group.

Several studies have refuted the association. In the Collaborative Perinatal Project data,[12] 462 women reported spermicide use in the first 4 lunar months, with 438 women also reporting use during the month preceding the last menstrual period. The exposed women had 23 infants with anomalies (5 percent) compared with 4.5 percent in the nonexposed controls, which is not a significant difference.

In the study of Mills et al.,[13] the malformation rate in women using spermicides after their last menstrual period was 4.8 per 1,000 compared with 6.4 per 1,000 in the controls, which is not significantly different. The risks of preterm delivery, a low-birth-weight infant, and spontaneous abortion were no higher in the spermicide-exposed group. Linn et al.[14] studied 12,440 women and found no relationship between contraceptive method and the occurrence of malformations. Clearly, the consensus of the scientific community is that vaginal spermicides are not associated with increased malformations when women use them either just before pregnancy or during pregnancy.[8]

Anticonvulsants

Epileptic women taking anticonvulsants during pregnancy have approximately double the general population risk of malformations.[15] As the general risk is 2 to 3 percent, in epileptic women on anticonvulsants the risk of major malformations is about 5 percent, especially for cleft lip with or without cleft palate and for congenital heart disease. Valproic acid carries approximately a 1 percent risk of neural tube defect (NTD) and possibly other defects; α-fetoprotein screening is appropriate for these patients.[16] Valproic acid appears to cause spina bifida much more often than anencephaly, with a ratio of 5 : 1.[17]

Whenever a drug is claimed to be a teratogen, one can always raise the issues of whether (1) the drug actually is a teratogen and (2) the disease for which the drug was prescribed in some way contributed to the defect. Women with a convulsive disorder, even when they take no anticonvulsant drug, have an increased risk of birth defects; this information has been used to claim that it is the epilepsy rather than the drug that contributes to the birth defect.[18] Of infants born to 305 epileptic women on medication in the Collaborative Perinatal Project, 10.5 percent had a birth defect. Of the offspring of women who had a convulsive disorder and who had not taken phenytoin, 11.3 percent had a malformation. This contrasted with the control group of women who did not have a convulsive disorder and who therefore did not take any antiepileptic drugs, whose total malformation rate was 6.4 percent. The issue is unresolved, as patients who take more drugs during pregnancy usually have more severe convulsive disorders than do those who do not take any anticonvulsants. A combination of more than three drugs or a high daily dose increases the chance of malformations.[19]

Possible causes of malformations in epileptic women on anticonvulsants include the disease itself, a genetic predisposition to epilepsy and malformations, genetic differences in drug metabolism, the specific drugs themselves, and deficiency states induced by drugs such as decreased serum folate. Phenytoin causes decreased absorption of folate and lowering of the serum folate, which has been implicated in birth defects in animals.

Fewer than 10 percent of offspring show fetal hydantoin syndrome,[20] which consists of microcephaly, growth deficiency, developmental delays, mental retardation, and dysmorphic craniofacial features (Fig. 11.3). These features are also found in other syndromes, such as fetal alcohol syndrome, but more common in the fetal hydantoin syndrome is hypoplasia of the nails and distal phalanges (Fig. 11.4). Trimethadione and carbamazepine are also associated with an increased risk of a dysmorphic syndrome.[21]

A genetic metabolic defect in arene oxide detoxification in the infant may increase the risk of a major birth defect.[22] Prenatal diagnosis of epoxide hydrolase deficiency may become available to indicate susceptibility to fetal hydantoin syndrome.[23]

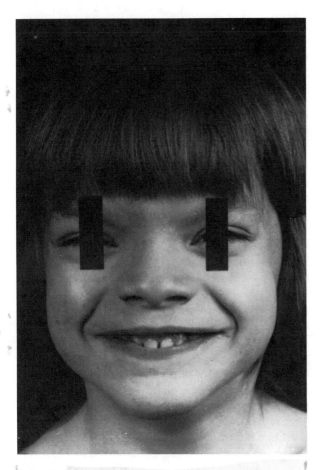

Fig. 11.3 Facial features of the fetal hydantoin syndrome. Note broad, flat nasal bridge, epicanthic folds, mild hypertelorism, and wide mouth with prominent upper lip. (Courtesy of Dr. Thaddeus Kelly, Charlottesville, VA.)

Some women may have taken anticonvulsant drugs for a long period without reevaluation of the need for continuation of the drugs. For patients with idiopathic epilepsy who have been seizure free for 2 years and who have a normal electroencephalogram (EEG), it may be safe to attempt a trial of withdrawal of the drug before pregnancy.[24] Also, if the patient has not been taking her drug regularly, a low blood level may demonstrate her lack of compliance.

If the patient is already pregnant, most authorities agree that the benefits of therapy outweigh the risks of discontinuation of the drug at that point. The blood level of drug should be monitored, monthly if possible, to ensure a therapeutic level but to minimize dosage. As the albumin concentration falls in pregnancy, the total amount of phenytoin measured is decreased because it is highly protein bound. However, the free level, which is the pharmacologically active portion, is unchanged. Neonatologists need to be aware that the patient is on anticonvulsants, because this can affect vitamin K–dependent clotting factors in the newborn; vitamin K supplementation for these mothers has been recommended.[25,26]

Isotretinoin

Isotretinoin (Accutane) is a significant human teratogen. This drug is marketed for treatment of cystic acne and unfortunately has been taken inadvertently by women who were not planning pregnancy.[27] It is labeled as contraindicated in pregnancy (FDA category X), with appropriate warnings that a negative pregnancy test is required before therapy. Of 154 exposed human pregnancies to date, there have been 21 reported cases of birth defects, 12 spontaneous abortions, 95 elective abortions, and 26 normal infants in women who took isotretinoin during early pregnancy.[28] The risk of anomalies in patients studied prospectively is now estimated to be about 25 percent. An additional 25 percent may have mental retardation. The malformed infants have a characteristic pattern of craniofacial, cardiac, thymic, and central nervous system (CNS) anomalies. They include microtia/anotia (small/absent ears) (Fig. 11.5), micrognathia, cleft palate, heart defects, thymic defects, retinal or optic nerve anomalies, and CNS mal-

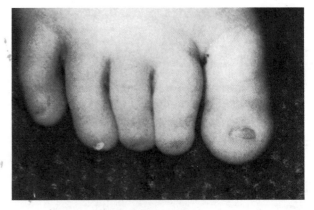

Fig. 11.4 Hypoplasia of toenails and distal phalanges. (From Hanson,[166] with permission.)

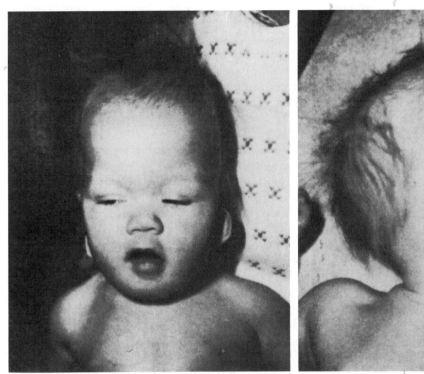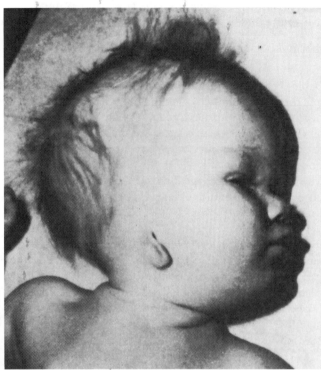

Fig. 11.5 Infant exposed to Accutane in utero. Note high forehead, hypoplastic nasal bridge, and abnormal ears. (From Lot et al.,[167] with permission.)

formations, including hydrocephalus.[28] Microtia is rare as an isolated anomaly yet appears commonly as part of the retinoic acid embryopathy. Cardiovascular defects include great vessel transposition and ventricular septal defects.

Isotretinoin is not stored in tissue, unlike vitamin A, and thus an exposure before pregnancy should not be a risk because the drug would not be detectable in serum 5 days after ingestion.

Topical tretinoin (Retin-A) has not been associated with any teratogenic risk.

Etretinate (Tegison)

Etretinate is marketed for use in psoriasis and may well have a teratogenic risk similar to that of isotretinoin. Case reports of malformations, especially of the CNS,[29] have appeared, but the absolute risk is unknown. Its half-life of several months makes levels cumulative, and the drug carries a warning to avoid pregnancy within 6 months of use.

Vitamin A

There is no evidence that vitamin A itself in normal doses is teratogenic. The levels in prenatal vitamins have not been associated with any documented risk. Eighteen cases of birth defects have been reported after exposure to levels of 25,000 IU of vitamin A or greater during pregnancy,[29] with syndromes similar to those produced by isotretinoin.

Tranquilizers

Conflicting reports of the possible teratogenicity of the various tranquilizers have appeared, including meprobamate (Miltown) and chlordiazepoxide (Librium), but in prospective studies no risk of anomalies has been confirmed.[30,31] In most clinical situations, the risk–benefit ratio does not justify the use of benzodiazepines in pregnancy. A fetal benzodiazepine syndrome has been reported in 7 infants of 36 mothers who regularly took benzodiazepines during pregnancy.[32] Perinatal use of diazepam has been associated with hypotonia, hypothermia, and respiratory depression.

Lithium

According to the International Register of Lithium Babies,[33] 217 infants had been exposed at least during the first trimester of pregnancy, and 25 (11.5 percent) were malformed. Eighteen had cardiovascular anomalies, including six cases of the rare Ebstein's anomaly, which occurs only once in 20,000 in the nonexposed population. Of 60 unaffected infants who were followed to age 5 years, no increased mental or physical abnormalities were noted compared with unexposed siblings.[34]

Lithium is excreted more rapidly in pregnancy; thus serum lithium levels should be monitored. Perinatal effects of lithium have been noted, including hypotonia, lethargy, and poor feeding in the infant. Also, complications similar to those seen in adults taking lithium have been noted in newborns, including goiter, hypothyroidism, and nephrogenic diabetes insipidus. Thus it is usually recommended that drug therapy be changed in pregnant women taking lithium to avoid fetal drug exposure. Alternate drugs such as tricyclic antidepressants should be tried. However, discontinuing lithium is associated with a 70 percent chance of relapse of the affective disorder in 1 year, as opposed to 20 percent in those who continue to take lithium.

Anticoagulants

Warfarin (Coumadin) has been associated with chondrodysplasia punctata, similar to the genetic Conradi-Hünermann syndrome, occurring in about 5 percent of exposed pregnancies. This syndrome includes nasal hypoplasia, bone stippling on radiologic examination, ophthalmologic abnormalities including bilateral optic atrophy, and mental retardation (Fig. 11.6). Even with use only beyond the first trimester, the ophthalmologic abnormalities and mental retardation may occur.[35] Fetal and maternal hemorrhages have also been reported in pregnant women on warfarin, although the incidence can be lowered with careful control of the prothrombin time. The alternative drug heparin does not cross the placenta, because it is a large molecule with a strong negative charge. As it does not have an adverse effect on the fetus when given in pregnancy, heparin should be the drug of choice for patients requiring anticoagulation.

Teaching patients subcutaneous administration of heparin or even administration with an intravenous heparin lock should be no more difficult than teaching patients self-administration of insulin for diabetes.[36] However, some evidence suggests that therapy with 20,000 units/day for more than 20 weeks is associated with bone demineralization;[37] thus the drug should only be used for prolonged periods when clearly necessary.

The risks of heparin during pregnancy may not be justified in patients with only a single episode of thrombosis in the past.[38,39] However, conservative measures should be recommended, such as elastic stockings and avoidance of prolonged sitting or standing.

In patients with cardiac valve prostheses, full anticoagulation is necessary, as low-dose heparin resulted in three valve thromboses (two fatal) of 35 mothers thus treated.[40]

Thyroid and Antithyroid Drugs

Propylthiouracil (PTU) and methimazole (Tapazole) both cross the placenta and cause some degree of fetal goiter. However, the thyroid hormones triiodothyronine (T3) and thyroxine (T4) cross the placenta poorly, so that fetal hypothyroidism produced by antithyroid drugs cannot be corrected satisfactorily by administration of thyroid hormone to the mother. Thus the goal of such therapy during pregnancy is to keep the mother slightly hyperthyroid to minimize fetal drug exposure. As methimazole has been associated with scalp defects in infants,[41] as well as a higher incidence of side effects, PTU is the drug of choice.

Radioactive iodine administered for thyroid ablation or for diagnostic studies is not concentrated by the fetal thyroid until after 12 weeks of pregnancy.[42] Thus, with inadvertent exposures, usually around the time of missed menses, there is no specific risk to the fetal thyroid from ^{131}I or ^{125}I administration.

Cardiovascular Drugs

Digoxin

In 52 exposures, no teratogenicity of digoxin was noted.[43] Blood levels should be monitored in pregnancy to ensure adequate therapeutic levels.

Digoxin-like immunoreactive substances may be mistaken in assays for fetal concentrations of digoxin.

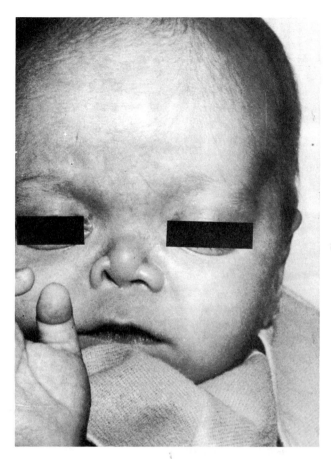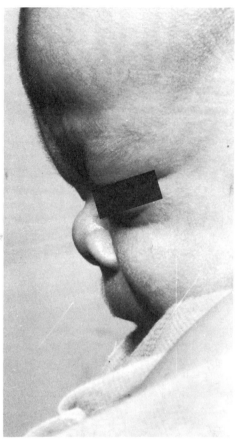

Fig. 11.6 Warfarin embryopathy. Note small nose with hypoplastic bridge. (From Shaul,[168] with permission.)

In one study of fetuses with cardiac anomalies[44] there was no difference in the immunoreactive digoxin levels whether or not the mother had received digoxin. In hydropic fetuses, digoxin may not easily cross the placenta.[45]

Antihypertensive Drugs (see Ch. 30)

α-Methyldopa (Aldomet) has been widely used in pregnancy to treat chronic hypertension. Although postural hypotension may occur, no unusual fetal effects have been noted. Hydralazine (Apresoline) may be used in pregnancy but is usually reserved for treatment of severe preeclampsia.

Propranolol (Inderal) is a β-adrenergic blocking agent in widespread use for a variety of indications. Although theoretically there might be increased uterine contractility in association with the use of this drug, this has not been reported, presumably because the drug is not specific for β_2-receptors in the uterine

wall. No evidence of teratogenicity has been noted to date. One review of 12 cases suggested an increased risk of intrauterine growth retardation (IUGR),[46] but this has not been confirmed in other studies. Bradycardia has been reported in the newborn as a direct effect of a dose of the drug given to the mother within 2 hours of delivery of the infant.[46]

Studies from Scotland suggest improved outcome with the use of atenolol to treat chronic hypertension during pregnancy and do not suggest any of the adverse effects mentioned in isolated case reports in this country.[47]

Antineoplastic Drugs and Immunosuppressants

There is reason to believe that methotrexate, a folic acid antagonist, is a human teratogen, although experience is limited.[48] Infants of two women known to receive methotrexate in the first trimester of pregnancy both had multiple congenital anomalies, including cranial defects and malformed extremities. Eight normal infants were delivered to seven women treated with methotrexate in combination with other agents after the first trimester.

Azothioprine (Imuran) has been used in patients with renal transplants or systemic lupus erythematosus. The frequency of anomalies in 45 women treated in the first trimester was not increased.[48] Two infants had leukopenia, one was small for gestational age, and the others were normal.

Four cases have been reported in which cyclosporine A was used for immunosuppression in renal transplant recipients.[49] Cord blood values of 34 percent and 57 percent of maternal values of cyclosporine A were found at delivery. No adverse effects on the infants were noted.

Antiasthmatics

Theophylline and Aminophylline

Both theophylline and aminophylline are safe to use to treat asthma during pregnancy. No evidence of teratogenic risk was found in 76 exposures in the Collaborative Perinatal Project.[43] Because of increased renal clearance in pregnancy, dosages may need to be increased.

Epinephrine

Minor malformations have been reported with exposure to sympathomimetic amines as a group in 3,082 exposures in the first trimester, usually in commercial preparations used to treat upper respiratory infections.[43]

Terbutaline

Terbutaline (Brethine) has been widely used in the treatment of preterm labor (see Ch. 25). It is more rapid in onset and has a longer duration of action than epinephrine and is preferred for asthma in the pregnant patient. No associated risk of birth defects has been reported. Long-term use has been correlated with an increased risk of glucose intolerance.[50]

Cromolyn Sodium

Cromolyn sodium may be administered in pregnancy, and the systemic absorption is minimal. Teratogenicity has not been reported in humans.

Isoproterenol and Metaproterenol

When isoproterenol (Isuprel) and metaproterenol are given as topical aerosols in the treatment of asthma, the total dose absorbed is usually not significant. With oral or intravenous doses, however, the cardiovascular effects of the agents may result in decreased uterine blood flow and thus they should be used with caution. No teratogenicity has been reported.[43]

Corticosteroids

All the steroids cross the placenta to some degree, but prednisone and prednisolone are inactivated by the placenta. When prednisone or prednisolone are maternally administered, the concentration of active compound in the fetus is less than 10 percent of that in the mother, and therefore they are the drugs of choice for treating medical diseases such as asthma. When corticosteroid effects are desired in the infant such as for lung maturity, β-methasone and dexamethasone are preferred, as these are minimally inactivated by the placenta.

In a study of 145 infants exposed to corticosteroids in the first trimester, no increase in abnormalities was noted.[43] Additional studies of corticosteroid administration during pregnancy have confirmed the lack of teratogenicity in humans.

Iodide

Iodide such as is found in a saturated solution of potassium iodide expectorant (SSKI) crosses the placenta and can produce a very large fetal goiter, which may cause respiratory obstruction in the newborn (Fig. 11.7).[42] Thus, before a patient is advised to take a cough medicine, she should ascertain that it does not contain iodide.

Antiemetics

Remedies suggested to help nausea and vomiting in pregnancy without pharmacologic intervention include taking crackers at the bedside upon first awakening in the morning and before getting out of bed, getting up very slowly, omitting the use of iron tablets, consuming frequent small meals, and eating protein snacks at night. Faced with a self-limited condition occurring at the time of organogenesis, the

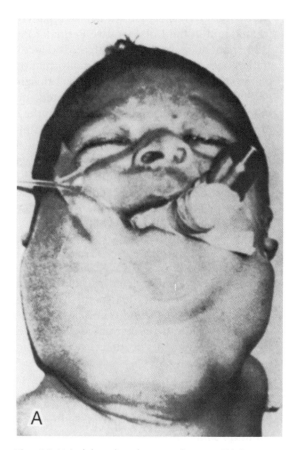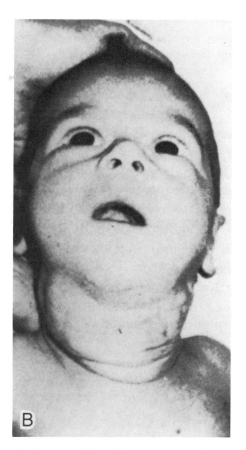

Fig. 11.7 Iodide-induced neonatal goiter. (A) Appearance on the first day of life. (B) Appearance at 2 months of age. (From Senior and Chernoff,[169] with permission.)

clinician is well advised to avoid the use of medications whenever possible and to encourage these supportive measures initially.

Bendectin

Bendectin contained doxylamine 10 mg and pyridoxine (vitamin B_6) 10 mg. It was the drug of choice for nausea and vomiting in pregnancy until the manufacturer stopped producing it in 1983, and it was the only drug the FDA had approved for this indication. Although there is considerable evidence that this agent is not teratogenic, the cost of defense of law suits alleging adverse effects led the company to cease production.

As the incidence of congenital malformations in the general population is 2 to 3 percent, and approximately 10 percent of women take antinauseants in the first trimester of pregnancy, it is not surprising that sporadic cases were reported of infants with malformations who were exposed to Bendectin in early pregnancy. In some case-controlled retrospective studies, teratogenicity was claimed. This was not confirmed, however, in large prospective controlled trials.

Vitamin B_6 is available over the counter and has some efficacy alone. Doxylamine is also available over the counter as Unisom, 25 mg, so that a combination similar to Bendectin can be administered. Doxylamine 25 mg and vitamin B_6 25 mg at bedtime is the usual dose, with one-half of this in the morning and afternoon as necessary.

Although there is no known teratogenicity of the other antiemetics, much less information is available about them.

Meclizine (Bonine)

In one randomized placebo-controlled study, meclizine gave significantly better results than placebo.[51] Prospective clinical studies have provided no evidence that meclizine is teratogenic in humans. In 1,014 patients in the Collaborative Perinatal Project,[43] and an additional 613 patients from the Kaiser Health Plan study,[52] no teratogenic risk was found.

Dimenhydrinate (Dramamine)

No teratogenicity has been noted with dimenhydrinate, but a 29 percent failure rate and a significant incidence of side effects, especially drowsiness, have been reported.[53]

Diphenhydramine (Benadryl)

In 595 patients treated with diphenhydramine in the Collaborative Perinatal Project, no teratogenicity was noted.[43] Drowsiness was a problem.

Trimethobenzamide

Trimethobenzamide (Tigan) is an antinauseant that is not classified as either an antihistamine or a phenothiazine and has been used for nausea and vomiting in pregnancy. The data collected in studies of small numbers of patients are conflicting. In the Kaiser Health Plan study,[52] 193 patients were exposed to trimethobenzamide, and there was a suggestion of excess of congenital anomalies ($p < 0.05$); no concentration of specific anomalies was observed in these children, however, and some of the mothers took other drugs as well. In 340 patients in the Collaborative Perinatal Project,[43] no evidence for association between this drug and malformations was found.

Phenothiazines

Because of the potential for severe side effects, the phenothiazines have not been used routinely in the treatment of mild or moderate nausea and vomiting. Instead, they have been reserved for the treatment of hyperemesis gravidarum. Chlorpromazine has been shown to be effective in hyperemesis gravidarum, and the most important side effect is drowsiness.

Teratogenicity does not appear to be a problem with the phenothiazines when evaluated as a group.

In the Kaiser Health Plan study,[52] 976 patients were treated and in the Collaborative Perinatal Project,[43] 1,309 patients were treated, with no evidence of association between these drugs and malformations. Suspicion of an association between phenothiazines and cardiovascular malformations was noted, however, but was of borderline significance and, in the context of multiple comparisons, was of doubtful import. In one study,[54] chlorpromazine (Thorazine) seemed to be associated with an increased risk of malformations in 141 exposed mothers. In 58 mothers exposed to promethazine (Phenergan) and in 48 mothers exposed to proclorperazine (Compazine), no increased risk of malformations was found.

Emetrol

Emetrol is a phosphorylated carbohydrate solution that acts on the wall of the hyperactive gastrointestinal tract. It reduces smooth muscle contractions in direct proportion to the amount used and is relatively free from toxicity or side effects.

Antihistamines and Decongestants

Patients should be educated that antihistamines and decongestants are only symptomatic therapy for the common cold and have no influence on the course of the disease. Other remedies should be recommended, such as use of a humidifier, rest, and fluids. If medications are necessary, combinations of two drugs should not be used if only one drug is necessary. If the situation is truly an allergy, an antihistamine alone will suffice. If decongestion is necessary, topical nasal sprays will result in a lower dose to the fetus than will systemic medication. In the Collaborative Perinatal Project[43] an increased risk of birth defects was noted with phenylpropanolamine exposure in the first trimester. Although this study has not been repeated, use of over the counter drugs for trivial indications should be discouraged because it is not known if long-term side effects will occur.

Antibiotics and Antiinfective Agents

Because pregnant patients are particularly susceptible to vaginal yeast infections, antibiotics should only be used when clearly indicated. Therapy with antifungal agents may be necessary during or after the course of therapy.

Penicillins

Penicillin derivatives, including penicillin and ampicillin, are apparently safe in pregnancy. In the Collaborative Perinatal Project, 3,546 mothers took penicillin derivatives in the first trimester of pregnancy, with no increased risk of anomalies.[43] There is little experience in pregnancy with the newer penicillins such as piperacillin, mezlocillin, and azlocillin. These drugs, therefore, should be used in pregnancy only when another, better-studied antibiotic is not effective.

Serum levels of the penicillins are lower and their renal clearance is higher throughout pregnancy than in the nonpregnant state.[55] The increase in maternal renal function, because of an increased renal blood flow and glomerular filtration rate, results in a higher renal excretion of drugs such as the penicillins. The expansion of the maternal intravascular volume during the late stages of pregnancy is another factor that affects antibiotic therapy. If the same dose of penicillin or ampicillin is given to both nonpregnant and pregnant women, lower serum levels are attained in the pregnant women because of the distribution of the drug in a larger intravascular volume.

The transplacental passage of penicillin is by simple diffusion. The free circulating portion of the antibiotic crosses the placenta, resulting in a lower maternal serum level of the unbound portion of the drug. Maternal administration of penicillins with high protein binding, e.g., oxacillin, cloxacillin, dicloxacillin, and nafcillin, results in lower fetal tissue and amniotic fluid levels than the administration of poorly bound penicillins, e.g., penicillin G, ampicillin, and methicillin.[56]

The antibiotic is ultimately excreted in the fetal urine and thus into the amniotic fluid. The delay in appearance of different types of penicillins in the amniotic fluid depends primarily on the rate of transplacental diffusion, the amount of protein binding in fetal serum, and the adequacy of fetal enzymatic and renal function. A time delay may occur before effective levels of the antibiotic appear in the amniotic fluid.

Most penicillins are primarily excreted unchanged in the urine, with only small amounts being inactivated in the liver. This is of significance in patients with impaired renal function, a state that requires a reduction in dosage.

Cephalosporins

There is no evidence of teratogenicity of cephalosporins, but the third-generation agents have had limited use during pregnancy. Maternal serum levels of cephalosporins during pregnancy are lower than those in nonpregnant patients receiving equivalent dosages because of a shorter half-life in pregnancy and an increased volume of distribution.[57] They readily cross the placenta to the fetal blood stream and ultimately to the amniotic fluid.

Sulfonamides

Among 1,455 human infants exposed to sulfonamides during the first trimester, no teratogenic effects were noted.[43] The administration of sulfonamides should be avoided in glucose-6-phosphate dehydrogenase–deficient women, because a dose-related toxic reaction can occur, resulting in red cell hemolysis. This is also a theoretical risk to the fetus if the drug is used near the time of delivery, as fetal red cells are normally relatively deficient in glutathione.[58]

Sulfonamides cause no known damage to the fetus in utero, as the fetus can clear free bilirubin through the placenta. However, these drugs might theoretically have deleterious effects if present in the blood of the neonate after birth. The sulfonamides compete with bilirubin for binding sites on albumin, thus raising the levels of free bilirubin in the serum and increasing the risk of hyperbilirubinemia in the neonate.[59] For that reason, it is recommended that an alternate antibiotic be used in the third trimester, if possible. The sulfonamides are easily absorbed orally, and they readily cross the placenta, achieving fetal plasma levels 50 to 90 percent of those attained in the maternal plasma.[60]

Sulfamethoxazole With Trimethoprim (Bactrim, Septra)

Sulfa is often given with trimethoprim to treat urinary tract infections. Controlled trials have failed to show any increased risk of birth defects after first-trimester exposure.[61,62] Although trimethoprim antagonizes folic acid in bacteria, it does not affect the human enzyme system with similar potency.

Sulfasalazine

Because of its relatively poor oral absorption, sulfasalazine is used to treat ulcerative colitis and Crohn's disease. However, it does cross the placenta to the fetal circulation, with fetal concentrations approximately the same as maternal concentrations, although both are low. Neither kernicterus nor severe neonatal jaundice have been reported following maternal use of sulfasalazine even when the drug was given up to the time of delivery.[63]

Nitrofurantoin

Nitrofurantoin is used in the treatment of acute uncomplicated lower urinary tract infections as well as for long-term suppression in patients with chronic bacteriuria. Nitrofurantoin is capable of inducing hemolytic anemia in patients deficient in G6PD and theoretically in infants, whose red blood cells are deficient in glutathione.[58] However, hemolytic anemia in the newborn as a result of in utero exposure to nitrofurantoin has not been published.

No reports linking the use of nitrofurantoin with congenital defects have been located. In the Collaborative Perinatal Project,[43] 590 infants were exposed, 83 in the first trimester, with no increased risk of adverse effects. More recent studies have confirmed these findings.[64,65]

Nitrofurantoin absorption from the gastrointestinal tract varies with the form administered. The macrocrystalline form is absorbed more slowly than the crystalline and is associated with less gastrointestinal intolerance. Because of rapid elimination, the serum half-life is 20 to 60 minutes. Therapeutic serum levels are not achieved, and therefore this drug is not indicated when there is a possibility of bacteremia. Approximately one-third of an oral dose appears in the active form in the urine.

Tetracyclines

The tetracyclines readily cross the placenta and are firmly bound by chelating to calcium in developing bone and tooth structures. This produces brown discoloration of the deciduous teeth, hypoplasia of the enamel, and inhibition of bone growth.[66] The staining of the teeth takes place in the second or third trimester of pregnancy, while bone incorporation can occur earlier. Depression of skeletal growth was particularly common among premature infants treated with tetracycline. Alternate antibiotics are currently recommended during pregnancy.

Hepatotoxicity has been reported in pregnant women treated with tetracyclines in large doses, usually with intravenous administration for pyelonephritis. First-trimester exposure to tetracycline was not found to have any teratogenic risk in 341 women in the Collaborative Perinatal Project[43] or in 174 women in another study.[67]

Aminoglycosides

Streptomycin and kanamycin have been associated with congenital deafness in the offspring of mothers who took these drugs during pregnancy. Ototoxicity was reported with doses as low as 1 g of streptomycin biweekly for 8 weeks during the first trimester.[68] Of 391 mothers who had received 50 mg/kg of kanamycin for prolonged periods during pregnancy, nine children (2.3%) were found to have hearing loss.[69]

Ototoxicity may be increased with simultaneous use of ethacrynic acid.[70] Nephrotoxicity may be increased when used in combination with cephalosporins. Neuromuscular blockade may be potentiated by the combined use of aminoglycosides and curariform drugs and therefore the dosages should be reduced appropriately. Potentiation of magnesium sulfate-induced neuromuscular weakness has also been reported in a neonate exposed to magnesium sulfate and gentamicin.[71]

There is no known teratogenic effect associated with the use of these drugs in the first trimester other than ototoxicity. In 135 infants exposed to streptomycin in the Collaborative Perinatal Project[43] no teratogenic effects were observed. In a group of 1,619 newborns whose mothers were treated for tuberculosis during pregnancy with multiple drugs including streptomycin, the incidence of congenital defects was the same as the healthy control group.[72]

These drugs are poorly absorbed after oral administration and are rapidly excreted by the normal kidney. Because the rate of clearance is related to the glomerular filtration rate, dosage must be reduced in the presence of abnormal renal function. Serum aminoglycoside levels are usually lower in pregnant than in nonpregnant patients receiving equivalent doses because of more rapid elimination.[73,74] Thus it is important to monitor levels to prevent subtherapeutic dosing.

Antituberculosis Drugs

There is no evidence of any teratogenic effect of isoniazid (INH), para-aminosalicylic acid (PAS), rifampin, or ethambutol. In one report, ethionamide was associated with CNS anomalies in 7 of 23 infants exposed to the drug in utero.

Erythromycin

No teratogenic risk of erythromycin has been reported. In 79 patients in the Collaborative Perinatal Project[43] and in 260 in another study,[67] no increased risk of birth defects was noted. Erythromycin estolate has been associated with subclinical reversible hepatotoxicity during pregnancy,[75] and thus other forms are usually recommended.

Erythromycin is not consistently absorbed from the gastrointestinal tract of pregnant women, and the transplacental passage is unpredictable. Both maternal and fetal plasma levels achieved after the administration of the drug in pregnancy are low and vary considerably with fetal plasma concentrations of 5 to 20 percent of those in maternal plasma.[76,77] Thus some authors have recommended that penicillin be administered to every newborn whose mother received erythromycin for the treatment of syphilis.[78] Fetal tissue levels increase after multiple doses.[77] The usual oral dose is 250 to 500 mg every 6 hours, but the higher dose may not be well tolerated in pregnant women who are susceptible to gastrointestinal symptoms.

Clindamycin

No reports linking the use of clindamycin with congenital defects have been found. However, this drug is sufficiently new that it was not included in the Collaborative Perinatal Project.[43]

Clindamycin is nearly completely absorbed after oral administration, and a small percentage is absorbed after topical application. The drug crosses the placenta, achieving maximum cord serum levels of about 50 percent of the maternal serum.[77] It is 90 percent bound to serum protein, and fetal tissue levels increase following multiple dosing.[77] Maternal

serum levels after dosing at various stages of pregnancy are similar to those of nonpregnant patients.[73]

Metronidazole

Studies have failed to show any increase in the incidence of congenital defects among the newborns of mothers treated with metronidazole (Flagyl) during early or late gestation. In one study,[79] 4 of 55 infants treated in early pregnancy had a variety of minor defects; in the Collaborative Perinatal Project,[43] 2 of 31 infants were abnormal, close to the expected incidence. Of 880 additional infants exposed during pregnancy, no difference in any adverse outcome was noted as compared with controls.[80]

Controversy regarding the use of metronidazole during pregnancy was stirred when metronidazole was shown by the Ames test to be mutagenic in bacteria, which correlates with carcinogenicity in animals. However, the doses used were much higher than the doses used clinically, and carcinogenicity in humans has not been confirmed.[81] As some have recommended against its use in pregnancy,[82] metronidazole should only be given for clear-cut indications and its use deferred until after the first trimester if possible.

Lindane

Toxicity in humans after use of topical 1 percent lindane (Kwell) has been observed almost exclusively after misuse and overexposure to the agent. After application of lindane to the skin, however, about 10 percent of the dose used can be recovered in the urine. Although no evidence of specific fetal damage is attributable to lindane, it is a potent neurotoxin and its use during pregnancy should be limited. Pregnant women should be cautioned about shampooing their children's hair, as absorption could easily occur across the skin of the hands of the mother. An alternate drug for lice is usually recommended, such as pyrethrins with piperonyl butoxide (Rid).

Antifungal Agents

Nystatin is poorly absorbed from intact skin and mucous membranes, and topical use has not been associated with teratogenesis.[67]

The imidazoles are absorbed in only small amounts from the vagina.[83] Use of chlotrimazole or miconazole in pregnancy is not known to be associated with congenital malformations. However, in one study a slightly increased risk of first-trimester abortion was noted after use of these drugs, although many associations were examined. These findings were considered not to be definitive evidence of risk.[84] However, use of these drugs should be postponed until after the first trimester if possible for theoretical reasons.

Drugs for Induction of Ovulation

In more than 2,000 exposures, no evidence of teratogenic risk of clomiphene has been noted,[85] and the percentage of spontaneous abortions is close to the expected rate. Although infants are often exposed to bromocriptine in early pregnancy, no teratogenic effects have been observed in more than 1,400 exposed pregnancies.[86,87]

Mild Analgesics

Few pains during pregnancy justify the use of a mild analgesic. Pregnant patients should be encouraged to use nonpharmacologic remedies, such as local heat and rest.

Aspirin

There is no evidence of any teratogenic effect of aspirin in human beings when taken in the first trimester.[43] Aspirin does have significant perinatal effects, however, as it inhibits prostaglandin synthesis. Uterine contractility is decreased, and patients taking aspirin in analgesic doses have delayed onset of labor, longer duration of labor, and an increased risk of going postdates.[88]

Aspirin also causes decreased platelet aggregation, which can cause increased risk of bleeding before as well as at delivery. Platelet dysfunction has been described in newborns within 5 days of ingestion of aspirin by the mother.[89] Aspirin causes permanent inhibition of prostaglandin synthetase in platelets, so that the only way for adequate clotting to occur is for more platelets to be produced.

Prostaglandins are involved in multiple organ systems in the fetus; because aspirin works by inhibiting prostaglandin synthetase, multiple organs may be affected by chronic aspirin use. Of note, prostaglandins mediate the neonatal closure of the ductus arteriosus, and one case has been reported in which taking aspirin close to the time of delivery presumably was related to closure of the ductus arteriosus in utero.[90]

Low-dose aspirin (80 mg/day) may ultimately prove of benefit in prevention of preeclampsia and fetal wastage associated with autoimmune diseases. Wallenburg et al.[91] randomized patients who had positive angiotensin II infusion tests to low-dose aspirin therapy or placebo; the incidence of preeclampsia was reduced in the treated compared with the placebo group (see Ch. 30). Lubbe et al.[92] treated patients with lupus anticoagulant and fetal wastage with prednisone 40–60 mg/day and low-dose aspirin (75 mg/day), with improved fetal outcome (see Ch. 23).

Acetaminophen

Acetaminophen (Tylenol, Datril) has also shown no evidence of teratogenicity. With acetaminophen, inhibition of prostaglandin synthesis is reversible, so that once the drug has cleared, platelet aggregation returns to normal. The bleeding time is not prolonged with acetaminophen, in contrast to aspirin,[93] and the drug is not toxic to the newborn. Thus, if a mild analgesic or antipyretic is indicated, acetaminophen is preferred over aspirin. The absorption and disposition of acetaminophen in normal doses is not altered by pregnancy.[94]

Propoxyphene

Propoxyphene (Darvon) is an acceptable alternative mild analgesic with no known teratogenicity.[43] However, it should not be used for trivial indications, as it has potential for narcotic addiction. Evidence of risk in late pregnancy comes from case reports of infants of mothers who were addicted to propoxyphene and had typical narcotic withdrawal in the neonatal period.[94]

Codeine

In the Collaborative Perinatal Project, no increased relative risk of malformations was observed in 563 codeine users.[43] Codeine can cause addiction and newborn withdrawal symptoms if used to excess perinatally.

Smoking

Smoking has been associated with low birth weight as well as with an increased prematurity rate (see Ch. 23).[96] The spontaneous abortion rate is up to twice that of nonsmokers. Abortions associated with maternal smoking tend to have a higher percentage of normal karyotypes and occur later than those with chromosomal aberrations.[97] An increased perinatal mortality associated with smoking is partly attributable to increased risk of both abruptio placenta and placenta previa as well as premature and prolonged rupture of membranes. Risks of complications and of the associated perinatal loss increase with the number of cigarettes smoked. Discontinuation of smoking during pregnancy can reduce the risk of complications and of perinatal mortality, especially in women at high risk for other reasons. Maternal passive smoking has been associated with a twofold risk of low birth weight at term in one study.[98]

There is also a positive association between smoking and sudden infant death syndrome (SIDS). In these studies, it is not possible to distinguish between apparent effects of maternal smoking during pregnancy and smoking after pregnancy, but both may have a role in increasing the risk.

Alcohol

The fetal alcohol syndrome (FAS) has been reported in the offspring of alcoholic mothers and includes the features of gross physical retardation with onset prenatally and continuing after birth (Fig. 11.8).[99]

In 1980, the Fetal Alcohol Study Group of the Research Society on Alcoholism proposed strict criteria for diagnosis of FAS.[100] These criteria stated that at least one characteristic from each of the following three categories had to be present for a valid diagnosis of the syndrome:

1. Growth retardation before and/or after birth
2. Facial anomalies, including small palpebral fissures; indistinct or absent philtrum; epicanthic folds; flattened nasal bridge; short length of nose; thin upper lip; low set, unparallel ears; and retarded mid-facial development
3. Central nervous system dysfunction, including microcephaly, varying degrees of mental retardation, or other evidence of abnormal neurobehavioral development, such as attention deficit disorder with hyperactivity

None of these features is individually pathognomonic for fetal alcohol exposure. Confirmatory evidence for this diagnosis is a history of heavy maternal drinking during pregnancy.

In the study of Jones et al.,[101] 23 chronically alcoholic women were matched with 46 controls, and the pregnancy outcomes of the two groups were compared. Among the alcoholic mothers, perinatal deaths were about eight times more frequent. Growth

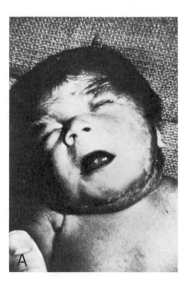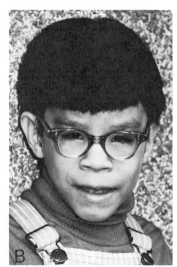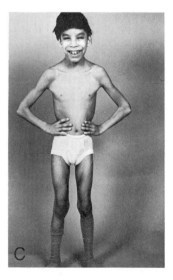

Fig. 11.8 Fetal alcohol syndrome. Patient photographed at (A) birth, (B) 5 years, and (C) 8 years. Note short palpebral fissures, short nose, hypoplastic philtrum, thinned upper lip vermilion, and flattened midface. (From Streissguth,[170] with permission.)

retardation, microcephaly, and an IQ below 80 were considerably more frequent than among the controls. Overall outcome was abnormal in 43 percent of the offspring of the alcoholic mothers compared with 2 percent of the controls.

Ouelette et al.[102] addressed the risks of smaller amounts of alcohol. Nine percent of infants of abstinent or rare drinkers were categorized as having some abnormality. Of infants of moderate drinkers, 14 percent were abnormal, not a significant difference. In heavy drinkers (average daily intake of 3 oz of 100 proof liquor or more), 32 percent of the infants had anomalies. Overall, including anomalies, growth retardation, and abnormal neurologic examination, 71 percent of the children of heavy drinkers were abnormal, which is twice the frequency of abnormality found in the moderate and rarely drinking groups. In this study, an increased frequency of abnormality was not found until 45 ml of ethanol (equivalent to three drinks) daily were exceeded. The study of Mills and Graubard[103] showed that total malformation rates were not significantly higher among offspring of women who had an average of less than one drink per day (77.3 per 1,000) or one to two drinks per day (83.2 per 1,000) than among nondrinkers (78.1 per 1,000). Genitourinary malformations increased with increasing alcohol consumption, however, and thus the possibility remains that for some malformations no safe drinking level exists.

Heavy drinking remains a major risk to the fetus, and reduction even in midpregnancy can benefit the infant. An occasional drink during pregnancy carries no known risk, but no level of drinking is known to be safe.

Sokol et al.[104] has addressed history taking for prenatal detection of risk drinking. Four questions help differentiate patients who drink enough to potentially damage the fetus (Table 11.1). The patient is considered at risk if more than two drinks are required to make her feel "high." The probability of risk drinking increases to 63 percent for those responding positively to all four questions.

Marihuana

No documented teratogenic effect of marihuana used during pregnancy has been noted. In a prospec-

Table 11.1 The T-ACE Questions Found To Identify Women Drinking Sufficiently To Potentially Damage the Fetus.

T	How many drinks does it take to make you feel high (can you hold) *(Tolerance)*?
A	Have people *annoyed* you by criticizing your drinking?
C	Have you felt you ought to *cut down* on your drinking?
E	Have you ever had to drink first thing in the morning to steady your nerves or to get rid of a hangover *(eye-opener)*?

Two points are scored as a positive answer to the tolerance question and one each for the other three. A score of 2 or more correctly identified 69 percent of risk drinkers.
(From Sokol et al,[104] with permission.)

tive study of marihuana use in 35 pregnancies,[105] infants born to users exhibited significantly more meconium staining: 57 percent versus 25 percent in nonusers. However, users tended to come from lower socioeconomic backgrounds than nonusers. Most adverse outcomes of pregnancy were too infrequent to permit reliable comparisons between the groups. Marihuana users had an increased incidence of precipitate labor (<3 hours total); 29 percent compared with 3 percent in the control group.[105]

In another population in which the users and nonusers of marihuana were similar in general health, ethnic background, nutritional habits, and use of tobacco, these differences were not confirmed (19 patients in each group).[106] In the same small group of patients, average use of marihuana six or more times per week during pregnancy was associated with a reduction of 0.8 weeks in the length of gestation, although no reduction in birth weight was noted. One study suggested a mean 73-g decrease in birth weight when urine assays were performed rather than relying on self-reporting.[107]

Cocaine

Cocaine is a CNS stimulant and has local anesthetic and marked vasoconstrictive effects. Cocaine-using women have a higher rate of spontaneous abortion than do controls.[108] Abruptio placenta has been reported to occur immediately after nasal or intravenous administration.[108]

Three studies have suggested an increased risk of

congenital anomalies after first-trimester cocaine use,[109-111] most frequently of the heart and CNS. In the study of Bingol et al.[110] the malformation rate was 10 percent in cocaine users, 4.5 percent in polydrug users, and 2 percent in controls. MacGregor et al.[111] reported a 6 percent anomaly rate compared with 1 percent of controls.

Several studies have also noted increased stillbirths, preterm labor, premature birth, and small for gestational age infants with cocaine use.[107-109,112,113] Dysmorphic features and neurobehavioral abnormalities are also seen.[113]

Aside from causing congenital anomalies in the first trimester, cocaine has been reported to cause fetal disruption[114] presumably because of vascular insufficiency. Bowel infarction has been noted with unusual ileal atresia and bowel perforation. Limb infarction has resulted in missing fingers in a distribution different from the usual congenital limb anomalies. CNS bleeding in utero may result in porencephalic cysts.

Narcotics

Menstrual abnormalities, especially amenorrhea, are common in heroin abusers, although they are not associated with the use of methadone. The goal of methadone maintenance is to bring the patient to a level of approximately 20 to 40 mg/day. The dose should be individualized at a level sufficient to minimize the use of supplemental illicit drugs, because they represent a greater risk to the fetus than do the higher doses of methadone required by some patients. Manipulation of the dose in women maintained on methadone should be avoided in the last trimester because of an association with increased fetal complications and fetal deaths in utero, attributed to fetal withdrawal in utero.[115] As management of narcotic addiction during pregnancy requires a host of social, nutritional, educational, and psychiatric interventions, these patients are best managed in specialized programs.

The infant of the narcotic addict is at increased risk of abortion, prematurity, and IUGR. Withdrawal should be watched for carefully in the neonatal period.

Caffeine

There is no evidence of teratogenic effects of caffeine in humans. The Collaborative Perinatal Project[43] showed no increased incidence of congenital defects in 5,773 women taking caffeine in pregnancy, usually in a fixed-dose analgesic medication. There is conflicting evidence as to whether heavy ingestion of caffeine is associated with increased pregnancy complications. Early studies suggested that ingestion of more than seven to eight cups of coffee per day was associated with low-birth-weight infants, spontaneous abortions, prematurity, and stillbirths.[116,117] However, these studies were not controlled for the use of tobacco and alcohol. In one study controlled for smoking, other drug habits, demographic characteristics, and medical history, no relationship was found between low birth weight or short gestation and heavy coffee consumption.[118] Also, there was no excess of malformations among coffee drinkers. One study suggested an increase in term low-birth-weight infants,[119] less than 2,500 g at greater than 36 weeks, with over 300 mg per day caffeine intake.

Heavy caffeine intake may be a signal of risk in pregnancy, and this history should lead to questioning about other substances that lead to poor pregnancy outcome. Concomitant consumption of caffeine with cigarette smoking may increase the risk of low birth weight.[120] Maternal coffee intake decreases iron absorption and may increase maternal and fetal anemia.[121]

Aspartame (NutraSweet)

Aspartame is metabolized into three products: aspartic acid, methanol, and phenylalanine.[122] Aspartic acid does not readily cross the placenta. The amount of methanol from an aspartame-sweetened beverage is generally less than the content recorded for fruit juices and other natural food sources. Phenylalanine is concentrated on the fetal side of the placenta. Sustained high blood levels of phenylalanine in the fetus associated with maternal phenylketonuria are associated with mental retardation in the infant. With normal ranges of aspartame ingestion, peak phenylalanine levels do not exceed the normal postprandial range, and even with high doses the levels of phenylalanine are still very far below the levels associated with mental retardation. Thus it seems unlikely that use of aspartame in pregnancy would cause any fetal toxicity.

DRUGS IN BREAST MILK

Many drugs can be detected in breast milk at low levels that are not usually of clinical significance to the infant. The rate of transfer into milk depends on the lipid solubility, molecular weight, degree of protein binding, degree of ionization of the drug, and the presence or absence of active secretion. Nonionized molecules of small molecular weight such as ethanol cross easily.[123] If the mother has unusually high blood concentrations such as with increased dosage or decreased renal function, drugs may appear in higher concentrations in the milk. Thus nursing mothers should take the minimum effective dose necessary for therapy.

The amount of drug in breast milk is a variable fraction of the maternal blood level that is proportional to the maternal oral dose. Thus the dose to the infant is usually subtherapeutic, approximately 1 to 2 percent of the maternal dose on the average. This amount is usually so trivial that no adverse effects are noted. In the case of toxic drugs, however, any exposure may be inappropriate. Allergy may also be possible. Long-term effects of even small doses of drugs may yet be discovered. Also, drugs are eliminated more slowly in the infant with immature enzyme systems. As the benefits of breast-feeding are well known, the risk of drug exposure must be weighed against these benefits.

With respect to drug administration in the immediate few days postpartum before lactation is fully established, the infant receives only a small volume of colostrum and thus little drug is excreted via milk at this time. It is helpful to allay fears of patients undergoing cesarean sections that analgesics or other drugs administered at this time will have no known adverse effects on the infant. For drugs requiring daily dosing during lactation, knowledge of pharmacokinetics in breast milk may minimize the dose to the infant. For example, dosing after nursing will decrease the exposure as the blood level will be lowest before the next dose. The American Academy of Pediatrics has reviewed drugs in lactation[124] and categorized the drugs as listed below.

Drugs Commonly Listed as Contraindicated During Breast-Feeding

Cytotoxic Agents

Amethopterin and cyclophosphamide might cause immune suppression in the infant, although data are limited with respect to these and other cytotoxic agents. In general, the potential risks of these drugs would outweigh the benefits of continuing nursing if these were required.

After oral administration to a lactating patient with choriocarcinoma, methotrexate was found in milk in low, but detectable, levels (0.26 μg/100 ml). Most individuals would elect to avoid any exposure to the infant of this drug. However, in environments in which bottle-feeding is rarely practiced and presents practical and cultural difficulties, therapy with this drug would not in itself appear to constitute a contraindication to breast-feeding.[125]

Busulphan has been reported to cause no adverse effect in nursing infants.[126]

Bromocriptine

Bromocriptine is an ergot alkaloid derivative that has an inhibitory effect on lactation and therefore should be avoided. However, in one report a mother taking 5 mg/day for a pituitary tumor was able to nurse her infant.[127]

Ergotamine

Ergotamine in doses used in migraine medications has been reported to be associated with vomiting, diarrhea, and convulsions in the infant and therefore should generally be avoided. However, if a patient requires short-term ergot therapy in the postpartum period for uterine contractility, this is not a contraindication to breast-feeding.

Cimetidine

Cimetidine suppresses gastric acidity and causes CNS stimulation in the infant. As it is concentrated in breast milk, it is usually considered contraindicated during nursing.

Other Drugs

Other drugs generally thought to be contraindicated during breast-feeding include gold salts, which have been associated with rash and inflammation in the kidney and liver, and phenindione, which has been associated with hemorrhage and elevation of the pro-thrombin time in the infant.

Drugs That Require Temporary Cessation of Breast-Feeding

Some drugs dictate only temporary cessation of breast-feeding during administration. These include metronidazole (Flagyl), whose half-life is such that interruption of lactation for 12 to 24 hours after single-dose therapy usually results in negligible exposure to the infant. It is excreted into breast milk with a milk–plasma ratio of about 1.0, and thus, even if the woman continues to nurse, the infant gets a trivial dose.

Radiopharmaceuticals require variable intervals of interruption of nursing to ensure that no radioactivity is detectable in the milk. Intervals generally quoted for gallium 67 are 2 weeks; ^{131}I, 5 days; radioactive sodium, 4 days; and technetium-99, 24 hours. For reassurance, the milk can be counted for radioactivity before nursing is resumed.[128]

Drugs Usually Compatible with Breast-Feeding

Narcotics, Sedatives, and Anticonvulsants

In general, no adverse effects are noted with most of the sedatives, narcotic analgesics, and anticonvulsants. Patients can be reassured that, in normal doses, carbamazepine (Tegretol),[129] phenytoin (Dilantin), magnesium sulfate, codeine, alphaprodine (Nisentil), morphine, and meperidine do not cause any obvious adverse effects in the infants.[130] This is because the dose detectable in the breast milk is approximately 1 to 2 percent of the mother's dose, which is sufficiently low to have no significant pharmacologic activity.

With diazepam, the milk–plasma ratio at peak dose is 0.68, with only small amounts detected in the breast milk.[131] In two patients who took carbamazepine while nursing, the concentrations of the drug in breast milk at 4 and 5 weeks postpartum were similar, about 60 percent of the maternal serum level. No adverse effects were noted in either infant.

In studies in which phenobarbital[132] and phenytoin levels were measured, only small amounts of the drug were detected in the breast milk. Phenobarbital and diazepam are slowly eliminated by the infant, however, and thus accumulation may occur. Women consuming barbiturates or benzodiazepine should observe the infants for sedation. Accumulation does not seem to occur with carbamazepine (Tegretol).[133]

In 10 preeclamptic patients receiving magnesium sulfate 1 g/hr intravenously for 24 hours after delivery, magnesium levels in breast milk were 64 μg/ml compared with 48 μg/ml in controls.[134] Breast milk calcium levels were not affected by magnesium sulfate therapy.

Analgesics

Aspirin is transferred in small amounts into breast milk. Salicylates are usually found in low concentrations, as transport from plasma into milk is not favored because acids exist primarily in the ionized form. The risk is related to high dosages (e.g., 16 300-mg tablets per day in the mother), when the infant may get sufficiently high serum levels to affect platelet aggregation. No harmful effects of acetaminophen have been noted. In one study, 3 mg% was detected in breast milk. In one patient taking propoxyphene (Darvon) in a suicide attempt, the level in the breast milk was one-half that in the serum. A breast-feeding infant could theoretically receive up to 1 mg of propoxyphene a day if the mother were to consume the maximum dose continually.[135] One infant was reported to have poor muscle tone when the mother was taking propoxyphene every 4 hours.

Antihistamines and Phenothiazines

Although the studies are not extensive, no harmful effects have been noted from antihistamines or phenothiazines, and they have not been found to affect milk supply. Decongestants should be avoided in women who are having trouble with milk supply.

Aminophylline

Maximum milk concentrations of aminophylline are achieved between 1 and 3 hours after an oral dose. The nursing infant has been calculated to receive less than 1 percent of the maternal dose with no noted adverse effects. To minimize neonatal drug exposure, however, a nursing mother should try to breast-feed her infant immediately before taking her doses of the drug.[136]

Amphetamines

One report of 103 cases of exposure to amphetamines in breast milk noted no insomnia or stimulation in the infants.[137]

Antihypertensives

After a single 500-mg oral dose of chlorothiazide, no drug was detected in breast milk at a sensitivity of 1 μg/ml.[138] In one mother taking 50 mg of hydrochlorothiazide daily, peak milk levels were about 25 percent of maternal blood levels. The drug was not detectable in the nursing infant's serum, and the infant's electrolytes were normal.[139] Thiazide diuretics may decrease milk production in the first month of lactation.[124]

Propranolol is excreted in the breast milk with milk concentrations after a single 40-mg dose less than 40 percent of peak plasma concentrations. In one patient on continuous dosage of 40 mg four times daily, plasma and breast milk concentrations peaked 3 hours after dosing, and the peak breast milk concentration of 42 ng/ml was 64 percent of the corresponding plasma concentration. After a 30-day regimen of 240 mg/day of propranolol, the predose and 3-hour postdose propranolol concentrations in breast milk were 26 and 64 ng/ml, respectively. Thus an infant ingesting 500 ml/day of milk would ingest a maximum of 21 μg in 24 hours at a maternal dose of 160 mg/day and a maximum of 32 μg in 24 hours at a maternal dose of 240 mg/day. This would represent a dose to the infant of approximately 1 percent of the therapeutic dose. This amount of drug is unlikely to cause any adverse effect.[140–142]

Atenolol is concentrated in breast milk to about three times the plasma level.[143] However, the plasma concentration in the infant after a peak level feeding is less than 10 ng/ml, a level not associated with side effects in the infant. The total infant dose is about 1 percent of the maternal therapeutic dose. As with other drugs, the effect of these small doses is unknown.

Clonidine concentrations in milk are almost twice maternal serum levels.[144] Neurologic and laboratory parameters in the infants were similar to those of untreated mothers.

Anticoagulants

Most mothers requiring anticoagulation can continue to nurse their infants with no problems. Heparin does not cross into milk, and in any case it is not active orally.

At a maternal dose of warfarin (Coumadin) of 5 to 12 mg/day in seven patients with maternal plasma concentrations of 0.5 to 2.6 μg/ml, no warfarin was detected in breast milk or infant plasma at a sensitivity of 0.025 μg/ml. This is probably due to the fact that warfarin is 98 percent protein bound. Thus, 1 L of milk would contain 20 μg of the drug at maximum, an insignificant amount to have an anticoagulant effect.[145] Another report confirms that warfarin appears only in insignificant quantities in breast milk.[146] The oral anticoagulant bishydroxycoumarin (Dicumarol) was given to 125 nursing mothers with no effect on the infants' prothrombin times and no hemorrhages.[147] Thus, with careful monitoring of maternal prothrombin time so that the dosage is minimized and of neonatal prothrombin times to ensure lack of drug accumulation, warfarin may be safely administered to nursing mothers.

This safety does not apply to all oral anticoagulant drugs, however. In one case in which phenindione[148] was being taken by a nursing mother, the infant underwent surgical repair of an inguinal hernia at 5 weeks of age. He developed a large hematoma, and his prothrombin time was found to be elevated.

Corticosteroids

In one patient requiring corticosteroids, breast milk was studied 2 hours after an oral dose of 10 mg of prednisone. The levels in the milk were 0.1 μg/100 ml of prednisolone and 2.67 μg/100 ml of prednisone. Thus an infant taking 1 L of milk would obtain 28.3 μg of the two steroids, an amount not likely to have any deleterious effect.[149]

MacKenzie et al.[150] administered 5 mg of radioactive prednisolone to 7 patients and found 0.14 percent of the sample secreted in the milk in the subsequent 60 hours, a negligible quantity. Thus breast-feeding is not contraindicated in the mother taking corticosteroids. Even at 80 mg/day, the nursing infant would ingest less than 0.1 percent of the dose, less than 10 percent of its endogenous cortisol.[151]

Digoxin

After a maternal dose of 0.25 mg, peak breast milk levels of 0.6 to 1 ng/ml occur, and the milk–plasma ratio at the 4-hour peak is 0.8 to 0.9. This represents a small amount because of significant maternal protein binding. An infant would receive in 24 hours only about 1 percent of the maternal dose,[152] and no adverse effects in nursing infants have been reported.

Antibiotics

Penicillin derivatives are safe in nursing mothers. In the usual therapeutic doses of penicillin or ampicillin, the mother's milk–plasma ratio is only up to 0.2, and no adverse effects are noted in the infants. In susceptible individuals or with prolonged therapy, diarrhea and candidiasis are theoretical concerns.

Dicloxicillin is 98 percent protein bound. If this drug is used to treat breast infections, very little will get into the breast milk and nursing may be continued.

Cephalosporins appear only in trace amounts in milk. In one study after 500 mg IM three times a day of cefazolin, no drug was detected in breast milk.[153] After 2 g of cefazolin IV at the 3-hour peak level, 1.51 μg/ml was detected for a milk–plasma ratio of 0.023. Thus the infant was exposed to only 0.075 percent of the maternal dose.

Infant tooth staining and delayed bone growth because of tetracycline have not been reported after the drug was taken by a breast-feeding mother. This is probably due to the high binding of the drug to calcium and protein, limiting its absorption from the milk. The amount in the milk is about one-half the level in the mother's plasma, and thus the amount of free tetracycline available is too small to be significant.

Sulfonamides only appear in small amounts in breast milk and are not contraindicated during nursing. However, during the first 5 days of life or in premature infants when hyperbilirubinemia may be a problem, the drug is best avoided as it can displace bilirubin from binding sites on albumin. In one study of sulfapyridine, the drug and its metabolites were detected in plasma and milk at levels of 4 to 7 μg/ml, and thus the infant would receive less than 1 percent of the maternal dose. When a mother took sulfasalazine (Azulfidine) 500 mg every 6 hours, the drug was undetectable in all milk samples.

Nitrofurantoin is excreted into breast milk in very low concentrations. In one study the drug could not be detected in 20 samples from mothers receiving 100 mg four times a day.[154]

Erythromycin is excreted into breast milk in small amounts, with milk–plasma ratios of about 0.5. No reports of adverse effects of infants exposed to erythromycin in breast milk have been noted. Clindamycin is excreted into breast milk in low levels, and nursing is usually continued during administration of this drug.

There are no reported adverse effects on the infant of isoniazid administered to nursing mothers, and its use is considered compatible with breast-feeding.[124]

Oral Contraceptives

Estrogen and progestin combined oral contraceptives cause a dose-related suppression of the quantity of milk produced. The use of oral contraceptives containing 50 μg and more of estrogen during lactation has been associated with shortened duration of lactation, decreased milk production, decreased infant weight gain, and decreased composition of nitrogen and protein content of the milk. However, the composition and volume of breast milk may vary considerably even in the absence of birth control pills. Lactation is inhibited to a lesser degree if the pill is started after the immediate postpartum period and with lower doses of estrogen. Although the magnitude of the changes is low, the changes may be of nutritional importance, particularly in malnourished mothers. However, if the patient persists in taking birth control pills while nursing, there is no documented adverse effect of this practice.

An infant consuming 600 ml of breast milk daily

from a mother taking an oral contraceptive that contains 50 μg of the ethinylestradiol receives a daily dosage in the range of 10 ng of the estrogen.[155] The amount of natural estradiol received by infants who consume a similar volume of milk from mothers not taking oral contraceptives is estimated at 3 to 6 ng during anovulatory cycles and at 6 to 12 ng during ovulatory cycles. No consistent long-term adverse effects on children's growth and development have been described. Evidence indicates that D-norgestrel is metabolized rather than accumulated by the infants, and to date no adverse effects have been identified as a result of progestational agents taken by the mother.

Progestin-only contraceptives do not cause alteration of breast milk composition or volume.[156] Thus progestin-only pills would be ideal in the breast-feeding mother.

Alcohol

Alcohol levels in breast milk are similar to those in maternal blood. One report has appeared of intoxication of an infant whose mother ingested 750 mg of port wine in 24 hours.[157] For obvious reasons intoxicated mothers should not breast-feed their babies.

If a moderate social drinker had two cocktails and had a blood alcohol concentration of 50 mg/100 ml, the nursing infant would receive about 82 mg of alcohol, which would produce insignificant blood concentrations.[158] There is no evidence that occasional ingestion of alcohol by a mother is harmful to the infant. However, one study showed that ethanol ingested chronically through breast milk might have a detrimental effect on the motor development, but not the mental development, of the infant.[159]

Lithium

Lithium levels in breast milk are about one-half of the maternal serum levels, but neonatal hypotonia and lethargy have been reported.[160] The benefits of breast-feeding must be weighed against the theoretical risks of the drug.

Propylthiouracil

Propylthiouracil (PTU) is found in breast milk only in small amounts.[161] If the mother takes 200 mg PTU three times a day, the child would receive 149 μg daily, or the equivalent of a 70-kg adult receiving 3 mg/day. Several infants have been studied up to 5 months of age, with no changes found in thyroid parameters, including TSH. Lactating mothers taking PTU can continue to nurse with close supervision of the infant.[161,162] PTU is preferred over methimazole because of its high protein binding (80 percent) and lower breast milk concentrations.[153]

Caffeine

Caffeine has been reported to have no adverse effects in the nursing infant, even after the mother consumes several cups of strong coffee.[163] In one study, the milk level contained 1 percent of the total dose 6 hours after coffee ingestion, which is not enough to affect the infant. If a mother drinks excessive amounts of caffeine and caffeine accumulates in the infant, the infant might show signs of wakefulness. It is therefore recommended that nursing mothers limit their intake to a moderate level.

Smoking

Nicotine can enter the milk but reaches relatively low levels of 0.01 to 0.05 mg/100 ml if 20 cigarettes are smoked per day.[164] Because nicotine is not readily absorbed by the infant's intestinal tract, risks of nicotine are unlikely from breast-feeding. However, the infant may have risks from passive smoking.

CONCLUSIONS

Many medical conditions during pregnancy and lactation are best treated initially with nonpharmacologic remedies. Before a drug is used in pregnancy, the indications should be clear and the risk–benefit ratio justify the drug use. If possible, therapy should be postponed until after the first trimester. In addition, patients should be cautioned about the risks of social drug use such as smoking, alcohol, and cocaine during pregnancy. Most drug therapy does not require cessation of lactation, as the amount excreted into breast milk is sufficiently small to be pharmacologically insignificant.

REFERENCES

1. Wilson JG, Fraser FC (eds): Handbook of Teratology. Plenum Press, New York, 1979
2. Blake DA, Niebyl JR: Requirements and limitations in

reproductive and teratogenic risk assessment. p. 1. In Niebyl JR (ed): Drug Use in Pregnancy. 2nd Ed. Lea & Febiger, Philadelphia, 1988

3. Heinonen OP, Slone D, Monson RR et al: Cardiovascular birth defects and antenatal exposure to female sex hormones. N Engl J Med 296:67, 1977

4. Wiseman RA, Dodds-Smith IC: Cardiovascular birth defects and antenatal exposure to female sex hormones: a reevaluation of some base data. Teratology 30:359, 1984

5. Katz Z, Lancet M, Skornik J et al: Teratogenicity of progestagens given during the first trimester of pregnancy. Obstet Gynecol 65:775, 1985

6. Johnson JWC, Austin KL, Jones GS et al: Efficacy of 17 α-hydroxyprogesterone caproate in the prevention of premature labor. N Engl J Med 293:675, 1975

7. Aarskog D: Maternal progestins as a possible cause of hypospadias. N Engl J Med 300:75, 1979

8. Simpson JL, Phillips OP: Spermicides, hormonal contraception and congenital malformations. Adv Contracept 6:141, 1990

9. Wilkins L: Masculinization of female fetus due to use of orally given progestins. JAMA 172:1028, 1960

10. Duck SC, Katayama KP: Danazol may cause female pseudohermaphroditism. Fertil Steril 35:230, 1981

11. Jick H, Walker AM, Rothman KJ et al: Vaginal spermicides and congenital disorders. JAMA 245:1329, 1981

12. Shapiro S, Slone D, Heinonen OP et al: Birth defects and vaginal spermicides. JAMA 247:2381, 1982

13. Mills JL, Reed GF, Nugent RP et al: Are there adverse effects of periconceptional spermicide use? Fertil Steril 43:442, 1985

14. Linn S, Schoenbaum SC, Monson RR et al: Lack of association between contraceptive usage and congenital malformations in offspring. Am J Obstet Gynecol 147:923, 1983

15. Speidel BD, Meadow SR: Maternal epilepsy and abnormalities of the fetus and newborn. Lancet 2:839, 1972

16. Robert E, Guibaud P: Maternal valproic acid and congenital neural tube defects. Lancet 2:937, 1982

17. Lindhout D, Schmidt D: In utero exposure to valproate and neural tube defect. Lancet 1:1392, 1986

18. Shapiro S, Hartz SC, Siskind V et al: Anticonvulsants and parental epilepsy in the development of birth defects. Lancet 1:272, 1976

19. Nakane Y, Okuma T, Takashashi R et al: Multi-institutional study on the teratogenicity and fetal toxicity of antiepileptic drugs: a report of a collaborative study group in Japan. Epilepsia 21:663, 1980

20. Hanson JW, Smith DW: The fetal hydantoin syndrome. J Pediatr 87:285, 1975

21. Jones KL, Lacro RV, Johnson KA et al: Pattern of malformations in the children of women treated with carbamazepine during pregnancy. N Engl J Med 320:1661, 1989

22. Strickler SM, Miller MA, Andermann E et al: Genetic predisposition to phenytoin-induced birth defects. Lancet 2:746, 1985

23. Buehler BA, Delimont D, VanWaes M et al: Prenatal prediction of risk of the fetal hydantoin syndrome. N Engl J Med 322:1567, 1990

24. Callaghan N, Garrett A, Goggin T: Withdrawal of anticonvulsant drugs in patients free of seizures for two years. N Engl J Med 318:942, 1988

25. Davies VA, Argent AC, Staub H et al: Precursor prothrombin status in patients receiving anticonvulsant drugs. Lancet 1:126, 1985

26. Deblay MF, Vert P, Andre M et al: Transplacental vitamin K prevents haemorrhagic disease of infant of epileptic mother. Lancet 1:1247, 1982

27. Rosa F: Editorial. JAMA 251:3208, 1984

28. Lammer EJ, Chen DT, Hoar RM et al: Retinoic acid embryopathy. N Engl J Med 313:837, 1985

29. Rosa FW, Wilk AL, Kelsey FO: Teratogen update: vitamin A congeners. Teratology 33:355, 1986

30. Rosenberg L, Mitchell AA, Parsella JL et al: Lack of relation of oral clefts to diazepam use during pregnancy. N Engl J Med 309:1282, 1983

31. Czeizel A: Lack of evidence of teratogenicity of benzodiazepine drugs in Hungary. Reprod Toxicol 3:183, 1988

32. Laegreid L, Olegard R, Wahlstrom J et al: Abnormalities in children exposed to benzodiazepines in utero. Lancet 1:108, 1987

33. Linden S, Rich CL: The use of lithium during pregnancy and lactation. J Clin Psychiatry 44:358, 1983

34. Weinstein MR, Goldfield MD: Cardiovascular malformations with lithium use during pregnancy. Am J Psychiatry 132:529, 1975

35. Hill RM, Stern L: Drugs in pregnancy: effects on the fetus and newborn. Drugs 17:182, 1979

36. Goldberg E: Anticoagulants in pregnancy. p. 83. In Niebyl JR (ed): Drug Use in Pregnancy. 2nd Ed. Philadelphia, Lea & Febiger, 1988

37. deSwiet M, Ward PD, Fidler J et al: Prolonged heparin therapy in pregnancy causes bone demineralization. Br J Obstet Gynaecol 90:1129, 1983

38. Tengborn L, Bergqvist D, Matzsch T et al: Recurrent thromboembolism in pregnancy and puerperium: is there a need for thromboprophylaxis? Am J Obstet Gynecol 160:90, 1989

39. Lao TT, deSwiet M, Letsky E et al: Prophylaxis of thromboembolism in pregnancy: an alternative. Br J Obstet Gynaecol 92:202, 1985

40. Iturbe-Alessio I, del Carmen Fonseca M, Mutchinik O et al: Risks of anticoagulant therapy in pregnant women with artificial heart valves. N Engl J Med 315:1390, 1986

41. Mujtaba Q, Burrow GN: Treatment of hyperthyroidism in pregnancy with propylthiouracil and methimazole. Obstet Gynecol 46:282, 1975

42. Burrow GN: Thyroid diseases. p. 229. In Burrow GN, Ferris TF (eds): Medical Complications During Pregnancy. WB Saunders, Philadelphia, 1988

43. Heinonen OP, Slone S, Shapiro S: Birth Defects and Drugs in Pregnancy. Publishing Sciences Group, Littleton, MA, 1977

44. Weiner CP, Landas S, Persoon TJ: Digoxin-like immunoreactive substance in fetuses with and without cardiac pathology. Am J Obstet Gynecol 157:368, 1987

45. Weiner CP, Thompson MIB: Direct treatment of fetal supraventricular tachycardia after failed transplacental therapy. Am J Obstet Gynecol 158:570, 1988

46. Pruyn SC, Phelan JP, Buchanan GC: Long-term propranolol therapy in pregnancy: maternal and fetal outcome. Am J Obstet Gynecol 135:485, 1979

47. Rubin PC, Clark DM, Sumner DJ: Placebo-controlled trial of atenolol in treatment of pregnancy-associated hypertension. Lancet 1:431, 1983

48. Buscema J, Stern JL, Johnson TRB Jr: Antineoplastic drugs in pregnancy. p. 89. In Niebyl JR (ed): Drug Use in Pregnancy. 2nd Ed. Lea & Febiger, Philadelphia, 1988

49. Burrows DA, O'Neil TJ, Sorrells TL: Successful twin pregnancy after renal transplant maintained on cyclosporine A immunosuppression. Obstet Gynecol 72:459, 1988

50. Main EK, Main DM, Gabbe SG: Chronic oral terbutaline therapy is associated with maternal glucose intolerance. Obstet Gynecol 157:644, 1987

51. Diggory PLC, Tomkinson JS: Nausea and vomiting in pregnancy: a trial of meclozine dihydrochloride with and without pyridoxine. Lancet 2:370, 1962

52. Milkovich L, Van den Berg GJ: An evaluation of the teratogenicity of certain antinauseant drugs. Am J Obstet Gynecol 125:244, 1976

53. Cartwright EW: Dramamine in nausea and vomiting of pregnancy. West J Surg Obstet Gynecol 59:216, 1951

54. Rumeau-Rouquette C, Goujard J, Huel G: Possible teratogenic effect of phenothiazines in human beings. Teratology 15:57, 1977

55. Philipson A: Pharmacokinetics of antibiotics in pregnancy and labour. Clin Pharmacokinet 4:297, 1979

56. Kunin CM: Clinical pharmacology of the new penicillins. I. The importance of serum protein binding in determining antimicrobial activity and concentration in serum. Clin Pharmacol Ther 7:166, 1966

57. Dubois M, Delapierre D, Demonty J et al: Transplacental and mammary transfer of cephoxitin. 11th International Congress of Chemotherapy and 19th Interscience Conference on Antimicrobial Agents and Chemotherapy. Boston, MA, 1979

58. Briggs GG, Freeman RK, Yaffe SJ: Drugs in Pregnancy and Lactation. Williams & Wilkins, Baltimore, 1986

59. Nyhan WL: Toxicity of drugs in the neonatal period. J Pediatr 59:1, 1961

60. Monif GFG: Infectious Diseases in Obstetrics and Gynecology. Harper & Row, New York, 1974

61. Ochoa AG: Trimethoprim and sulfamethoxazole in pregnancy. JAMA 217:1244, 1971

62. Brumfitt W, Pursell R: Double-blind trial to compare ampicillin, cephalexin, co-trimoxazole, and trimethoprim in treatment of urinary infection. Br Med J 2:673, 1972

63. Jarnerot G, Into-Malmberg MB, Esbjorner E: Placental transfer of sulphasalazine and sulphapyridine and some of its metabolites. Scand J Gastroenterol 16:693, 1981

64. Hailey FJ, Fort H, Williams JR et al: Foetal safety of nitrofurantoin macrocrystals therapy during pregnancy: a retrospective analysis. J Int Med Res 11:364, 1983

65. Lenke RR, VanDorsten JP, Schifrin BS: Pyelonephritis in pregnancy: a prospective randomized trial to prevent recurrent disease evaluating suppressive therapy with nitrofurantoin and close surveillance. Am J Obstet Gynecol 146:953, 1983

66. Cohlan SQU, Bevelander G, Tiamsic T: Growth inhibition of prematures receiving tetracycline. Am J Dis Child 105:453, 1963

67. Aselton P, Jick H, Mulnsky A et al: First-trimester drug use and congenital disorders. Obstet Gynecol 65:451, 1985

68. Robinson GC, Cambon KG: Hearing loss in infants of tuberculous mothers treated with streptomycin during pregnancy. N Engl J Med 271:949, 1964

69. Nishimura H, Tanimura T: Clinical Aspects of the Teratogenicity of Drugs. Excerpta Medica, Amsterdam, 1976

70. Jones HC: Intrauterine ototoxicity: a case report and review of literature. J Natl Med Assoc 65:201, 1973

71. L'Hommedieu CS, Nicholas D, Armes DA et al: Potentiation of magnesium sulfate-induced neuromuscular weakness by gentamicin, tobramycin, and amikacin. J Pediatr 102:629, 1983

72. Marynowski A, Sianozecka E: Comparison of the incidence of congenital malformations in neonates from healthy mothers and from patients treated because of tuberculosis. Ginekol Pol 43:713, 1972

73. Weinstein AJ, Gibbs RS, Gallagher M: Placental transfer of clindamycin and gentamicin in term pregnancy. Am J Obstet Gynecol 124:688, 1976

74. Zaske DE, Cipolle RJ, Strate RG et al: Rapid gentamicin elimination in obstetric patients. Obstet Gynecol 56:559, 1980

75. McCormack WM, George H, Donner A et al: Hepatotoxicity of erythromycin estolate during pregnancy. Antimicrob Agents Chemother 12:630, 1977

76. Philipson A, Sabath LD, Charles D: Erythromycin and clindamycin absorption and elimination in pregnant women. Clin Pharmacol Ther 19:68, 1976

77. Philipson A, Sabath LD, Charles D: Transplacental passage of erythromycin and clindamycin. N Engl J Med 288:1219, 1973

78. South MA, Short DH, Knox JM: Failure of erythromycin estolate therapy in in utero syphilis. JAMA 190:70, 1964

79. Peterson WF, Stauch JE, Ryder CD: Metronidazole in pregnancy. Am J Obstet Gynecol 94:343, 1966

80. Morgan FK: Metronidazole treatment in pregnancy. Int Congress Symp Ser Roy Soc Med 18:245, 1979

81. Beard CM, Noller KL, O'Fallon WM et al: Lack of evidence for cancer due to use of metronidazole. N Engl J Med 301:519, 1979

82. Finegold SM: Metronidazole. Ann Intern Med 93:585, 1980

83. Tan CG, Good CS, Milne LJR et al: A comparative trial of six day therapy with clotrimazole and nystatin in pregnant patients with vaginal candidiasis. Postgrad Med 50:102, 1974

84. Rosa FW, Baum C, Shaw M: Pregnancy outcomes after first trimester vaginitis drug therapy. Obstet Gynecol 69:751, 1987

85. Asch RH, Greenblatt RB: Update on the safety and efficacy of clomiphene citrate as a therapeutic agent. J Reprod Med 17:175, 1976

86. Riuz-Velasco V, Tolis G: Pregnancy in hyperprolactinemic women. Fertil Steril 41:793, 1984

87. Turkalj I, Braun P, Krupp P: Surveillance of bromocriptine in pregnancy. JAMA 247:1589,1982

88. Collins E, Turner G: Salicylates and pregnancy. Lancet 2:1494, 1973

89. Stuart JJ, Gross SJ, Elrad H et al: Effects of acetylsalicyclic acid ingestion on maternal and neonatal hemostasis. N Engl J Med 307:909, 1982

90. Areilla RA, Thilenius OB, Ranniger K: Congestive heart failure from suspected ductal closure in utero. J Pediatr 75:74, 1969

91. Wallenburg HCS, Dekker GA, Makovitz JW et al: Low-dose aspirin prevents pregnancy-induced hypertension and pre-eclampsia in angiotensin-sensitive primigravidae. Lancet 1:1,1986

92. Lubbe WF, Butler WS, Palmer SJ et al: Lupus anticoagulant in pregnancy. Br J Obstet Gynaecol 91:357, 1984

93. Waltman T, Tricomi V, Tavakoli FM: Effect of aspirin on bleeding time during elective abortion. Obstet Gynecol 48:108, 1976

94. Rayburn W, Shukla U, Stetson P et al: Acetaminophen pharmacokinetics: comparison between pregnant and nonpregnant women. Obstet Gynecol 155:1353, 1986

95. Tyson HK: Neonatal withdrawal symptoms associated with maternal use of propoxyphene hydrochloride (Darvon). J Pediatr 85:684, 1974

96. Berkowitz GS: Smoking and pregnancy. p. 173. In Niebyl JR (ed): Drug Use in Pregnancy. 2nd Ed. Lea & Febiger, Philadelphia, 1988

97. Alberman E, Creasy M, Elliott M et al: Maternal factors associated with fetal chromosomal anomalies in spontaneous abortions. J Obstet Gynecol 83:621, 1976

98. Martin TR, Bracken MB: Association of low birth weight with passive smoke exposure in pregnancy. Am J Epidemiol 124:633, 1986

99. Jones KL, Smith DW, Ulleland CN et al: Patterns of malformation in offspring of chronic alcoholic mothers. Lancet 2:1267, 1973

100. Rosett HL: A clinical perspective of the fetal alcohol syndrome. Alcoholism: Clin Exp Res 4:119, 1980

101. Jones KL, Smith DW, Streissguth AP et al: Outcome of offspring of chronic alcoholic women. Lancet 2:1076, 1974

102. Ouellette EM, Rosett HL, Rosman NP et al: Adverse effects on offspring of maternal alcohol abuse during pregnancy. N Engl J Med 297:528, 1977

103. Mills JL, Graubard BI: Is moderate drinking during pregnancy associated with an increased risk of malformations? Pediatrics 80:309, 1987

104. Sokol RJ, Martier SS, Ager JW: The T-ACE questions: practical prenatal detection of risk-drinking. Am J Obstet Gynecol 160:863,1989

105. Greenland S, Staisch KJ, Brown N et al: The effects of marijuana use during pregnancy: Part 1—a preliminary epidemiologic study. Am J Obstet Gynecol 143:408, 1982

106. Fried PA, Buckingham M, Von Kulmiz P: Marijuana

use during pregnancy and perinatal risk factors. Am J Obstet Gynecol 146:992, 1983

107. Zuckerman B, Frank DA, Hingson R et al: Effects of maternal marijuana and cocaine use on fetal growth. N Engl J Med 320:762, 1989

108. Acker D, Sachs BP, Tracey KJ et al: Abruptio placentae associated with cocaine use. Am J Obstet Gynecol 146:220, 1983

109. Little BB, Snell LM, Klein VR et al: Cocaine abuse during pregnancy: maternal and fetal implications. Obstet Gynecol 73:157, 1989

110. Bingol N, Fuchs M, Diaz V et al: Teratogenicity of cocaine in humans. J Pediatr 110:93, 1987

111. MacGregor SN, Keith LG, Chasnoff IJ et al: Cocaine use during pregnancy: adverse perinatal outcome. Am J Obstet Gynecol 157:686, 1987

112. Keith LG, MacGregor S, Friedell S et al: Substance abuse in pregnant women: recent experience at the Perinatal Center for Chemical Dependence of Northwestern Memorial Hospital. Obstet Gynecol 73:715, 1989

113. Chasnoff IJ, Griffith DR, MacGregor S et al: Temporal patterns of cocaine use in pregnancy. JAMA 261:1741, 1989

114. Chasnoff IJ, Chisum GM, Kaplan WE: Maternal cocaine use and genitourinary tract malformations. Teratology 37:201, 1988

115. Finnegan LP, Wapner RJ: Narcotic addiction in pregnancy. p. 203. In Niebyl JR (ed): Drug Use in Pregnancy. 2nd Ed. Lea & Febiger, Philadelphia, 1988

116. Mau G, Netter P: Kaffee- und alkoholkonsum-risikofaktoren in der schwangerschaft? Geburtsch Frauenheilkd 34:1018, 1974

117. Van den Berg BJ: Epidemiologic observations of prematurity: effects of tobacco, coffee and alcohol. In Reed DM, Stanley FJ (eds): The Epidemiology of Prematurity. Urban and Schwarzenberg, Baltimore, 1977

118. Linn S, Schoenbaum SC, Monson RR et al: No association between coffee consumption and adverse outcomes of pregnancy. N Engl J Med 306:141, 1982

119. Martin TR, Bracken MB: The association between low birth weight and caffeine consumption during pregnancy. Am J Epidemiol 126:813, 1987

120. Beaulac-Baillargeon L, Desrosiers C: Caffeine-cigarette interaction on fetal growth. Am J Obstet Gynecol 157:1236, 1987

121. Munoz LM, Lonnerdal B, Keen CL et al: Coffee consumption as a factor in iron deficiency anemia among pregnant women and their infants in Costa Rica. Am J Clin Nutr 48:645, 1988

122. Sturtevant FM: Use of aspartame in pregnancy. Int J Fertil 30:85, 1985

123. Kesaniema YA: Ethanol and acetaldehyde in the milk and peripheral blood of lactating women after ethanol administration. J Obstet Gynaecol Br Commonw 81:84, 1974

124. American Academy of Pediatrics Committee on Drugs: The transfer of drugs and other chemicals in human breast milk. Pediatrics 72:375, 1983

125. Johns BG, Rutherford CD, Laighton RC et al: Secretion of methotrexate into human milk. Am J Obstet Gynecol 112:978, 1972

126. Bounaneaux Y, Duren J: Busulphan in nursing infants. Ann Soc Belg Med Trop 44:381, 1964

127. Canales ES, Garcia IC, Ruiz JE et al: Bromocriptine as prophylactic therapy in prolactinoma during pregnancy. Fertil Steril 36:524, 1981

128. Berlin CM: The excretion of drugs in human milk. p. 125. In Schwartz RH, Yaffe SJ (eds): Drug and Chemical Risks to the Fetus and Newborn. Alan R Liss, New York, 1980

129. Niebyl JR, Blake DA, Freeman JM et al: Carbamazepine levels in pregnancy and lactation. Obstet Gynecol 53:139, 1979

130. Briggs GG, Freeman RK, Yaffe SJ: Drugs in Pregnancy and Lactation. 2nd Ed. Williams & Wilkins, Baltimore, 1986

131. Cole AP, Hailey DM: Diazepam and active metabolite in breast milk and their transfer to the neonate. Arch Dis Child 50:741, 1975

132. Nau H, Rating D, Hauser I et al: Placental transfer and pharmacokinetics of primidone and its metabolites phenobarbital, PEMA and hydroxyphenobarbital in neonates and infants of epileptic mothers. Eur J Clin Pharmacol 18:31, 1980

133. Pynnonen S, Sillanpaa M: Carbamazepine and mother's milk. Lancet 2:563, 1975

134. Cruikshank DP, Varner MW, Pitkin RM: Breast milk magnesium and calcium concentrations following magnesium sulfate treatment. Am J Obstet Gynecol 143:685, 1982

135. Ananth J: Side effects in the neonate from psychotropic agents excreted through breastfeeding. Am J Psychiatry 135:801, 1978

136. Yurchak AM, Jusko NJ: Theophylline secretion into breast milk. Pediatrics 57:518, 1976

137. Ayd F: Int Drug Ther Newslett 8:33, 1973

138. Weithmann MW, Krees SV: Excretion of chlorothiazide in human breast milk. J Pediatr 81:781, 1972

139. Miller ME, Cohn RD, Burghart PH: Hydrochlorothia-

zide disposition in a mother and her breast-fed infant. J Pediatr 101:789, 1982

140. Bauer JH, Pope B, Zajicek J et al: Propranolol in human plasma and breast milk. Am J Cardiol 43:860, 1979

141. Leviton AA, Marion JC: Propranolol therapy during pregnancy and lactation. Am J Cardiol 32:247, 1973

142. Anderson PO, Salter FJ: Propranolol therapy during pregnancy and lactation. Am J Cardiol 37:325, 1976

143. White WB, Andreoli JW, Wong SH et al: Atenolol in human plasma and breast milk. Obstet Gynecol 63:42S1, 1984

144. Hartikainen-Sorri AL, Heikkinen JE, Koivisto M: Pharmacokinetics of clonidine during pregnancy and nursing. Obstet Gynecol 69:598, 1987

145. Orme ME, Lewis PJ, deSwiet M et al: May mothers given warfarin breastfeed their infants? Br Med J 1:1564, 1977

146. deSwiet M, Lewis PJ: Excretion of anticoagulants in human milk. N Engl J Med 297:1471, 1977

147. Brambel CE, Hunter RE: Effect of Dicumarol on the nursing infant. Am J Obstet Gynecol 59:1153, 1950

148. Eckstein HB, Jack B: Breastfeeding and anticoagulant therapy. Lancet 1:672, 1970

149. Katz FH, Duncan BR: Entry of prednisone into human milk. N Engl J Med 293:1154, 1975

150. MacKenzie SA, Seeley JA, Agnew JE: Secretion of prednisolone into breast milk. Arch Dis Child 50:894, 1975

151. Ost L, Wettrell G, Bjorkhem I et al: Prednisolone excretion in human milk. J Pediatr 106:1008, 1985

152. Loughnan PM: Digoxin excretion in human breast milk. J Pediatr 92:1019, 1978

153. Yoshioka H, Cho K, Takimoto M et al: Transfer of cefazolin into human milk. J Pediatr 94:151, 1979

154. Hosbach RE, Foster RB: Absence of nitrofurantoin from human milk. JAMA 202:1057, 1967

155. Nilsson S, Nygren KG, Johansson EDB: Transfer of estradiol to human milk. Am J Obstet Gynecol 132:653, 1978

156. American Academy of Pediatrics Committee on Drugs: Breast-feeding and contraception. Pediatrics 68:138, 1981

157. Bisdom CJW: Maandschr Kindergeneesk 6:332, 1936

158. Wilson JT, Brown RD, Cherek DR et al: Drug excretion in human breast milk: principles of pharmacokinetics and projected consequences. Clin Pharmacokinet 5:1, 1980

159. Little RE, Anderson KW, Ervin CH et al: Maternal alcohol use during breastfeeding and infant mental and motor development at one year. N Engl J Med 321:425, 1989

160. Sykes PA, Quarrie J, Alexander FW: Lithium carbonate and breast feeding. Br Med J 2:1299, 1976

161. Kampmann JP, Hansen JM, Johansen K et al: Propylthiouracil in human milk. Lancet 1:736, 1980

162. Cooper DS: Antithyroid drugs: to breast-feed or not to breast-feed. Am J Obstet Gynecol 157:234, 1987

163. Illingsworth RS: Abnormal substances excreted in human milk. Practitioner 171:533, 153

164. Vorherr H: Drug excretion in breast milk. Postgrad Med 56:97, 1974

165. Blake DA, Niebyl JR: Requirements and limitations in reproductive and teratogenic risk assessment. p.2. In Niebyl JR (ed): Drug Use in Pregnancy. 2nd Ed. Lea & Febiger, Philadelphia, 1988

166. Hanson JWM: Fetal hydantoin syndrome. Teratology 13:186, 1976

167. Lot IT, Bocian M, Pribam HW, Leitner M: Fetal hydrocephalus and ear anomalies associated with use of isotretinoin. J Pediatr 105:598, 1984

168. Shaul W, Hall JG: Multiple congenital anomalies associated with oral anticoagulants. Am J Obstet Gynecol 127:191, 1977

169. Senior B, Chernoff HL: Iodide goiter in the newborn. Pediatrics 47:510, 1971

170. Streissguth AP: CIBA Foundation Monograph 105. Pitman, London, 1984

Chapter 12

Obstetric Ultrasound: Assessment of Fetal Growth and Anatomy

Frank A. Chervenak and Steven G. Gabbe

Diagnostic ultrasound has emerged as an important tool for antepartum fetal surveillance. This technology has permitted the most accurate assessment of gestational age and has enabled the obstetrician to follow fetal growth serially and to detect fetal growth disorders. In addition, ultrasound has become an essential aid in the safe performance of a variety of diagnostic procedures, including amniocentesis, chorionic villus sampling, and cordocentesis. Finally, the use of real-time ultrasound has permitted the obstetrician to assess fetal well-being through the evaluation of fetal movements, breathing activity, and tone.

BIOPHYSICS OF ULTRASOUND

To use ultrasound most effectively, the obstetrician must understand the basic biophysics of this technique.[1] Sound is a waveform of energy that causes small particles in a medium to oscillate. The frequency of sound refers to the number of peaks or waves that traverse a given point per unit of time and is expressed in Hertz (Hz). Sound with a frequency of one cycle or one peak per second would have a frequency of 1 Hz. Ultrasound applies to high-frequency sound waves exceeding 20,000 Hz. Diagnostic ultrasound instruments operate in a higher range of frequencies, varying from 2 to 10 million Hz, or 2 to 10 megaHertz (MHz).

Ultrasound energy is produced by a transducer containing crystal structures that convert electrical energy to ultrasound waves and the returning echoes to electrical energy. Therefore, each crystal in the transducer acts as both a transmitter and receiver. The power of ultrasound refers to the amount of work being done by the ultrasound field as it interacts with the medium in which the sound waves are propagating and is expressed in terms of watts (W). Most therapeutic equipment operates in the range of 1 to 50 W, while diagnostic and monitoring units use 0.1 to 100 mW. The standard unit used in defining the power of ultrasound equipment is watts per square centimeter (W/cm^2), describing the amount of energy delivered per given surface area. The safety of diagnostic ultrasound is considered below, but one must remember that diagnostic ultrasound equipment generates a sound pulse every 1 millisecond (msec) and that the duration of the pulse is 1 microsecond (μsec). The time the sound pulse is off is 1,000 times greater than the time it is on. Therefore, the duty factor of diagnostic ultrasound, defined as the ratio between the emission of a sound wave and the reception of the sound wave, is $1 : 1,000$ or 0.001. During a 15-minute diagnostic evaluation, the fetus is exposed to only 1 second of ultrasound energy.

PRINCIPLES OF IMAGING

A two-dimensional picture is created when the returning ultrasound echoes are displayed on an oscilloscope screen.[1] The ultrasound signal returning to the transducer is converted to an electrical impulse, and the strength of that electrical impulse is directly proportional to the strength of the returning echo. The density of the medium into which the sound wave has been transmitted and through which it is reflected will determine the strength of the signal. The velocity of the reflected sound wave will be faster and its signal on the oscilloscope brighter after reflection off bone than off tissues that are less dense such as muscle, fat, brain, and water. Air greatly decreases the transmission of sound waves. For this reason, a coupling medium or gel is applied between the surface of the transducer and the skin. A full maternal bladder provides an important window for diagnostic obstetric ultrasound. The bladder displaces gas-filled loops of bowel that would obstruct the propagation of sound, thereby providing a medium that enhances the transmission of the ultrasound waves.

Ultrasound can be used to produce diagnostic images in several ways. In A mode (amplitude modulation), echoes from the reflecting surfaces are displayed as vertical spikes along the baseline of a cathode ray tube. The height of the spike is related to the amplitude of the reflected echo. Although this technique can be used to define the location of some structures, its diagnostic applications are limited. With M mode (motion mode), the reflected echo is displayed as a spot that generates a horizontal line on a moving display. In this way, one can examine the motion of structures against time. This technique has been widely applied in the assessment of cardiac anatomy, including the dimensions of the cardiac chambers, ventricular wall thickness, and valvular motion. B mode (brightness modulation) converts the strength of the returning echoes into signals of varying brightness that are proportional to the amplitude of the returning echo. A storage oscilloscope is used to create a compounded image of the target and in this way produce a two-dimensional picture. Real-time array transducer systems create these images within a fraction of a second. When the image of the fetus is compounded at a rate faster than the flicker fusion rate of the eye, the fetus will appear to be moving in real time. Most often the obstetrician will use a linear array transducer in which a series of crystals are aligned along the transducer. The standard transducer used in these systems is 3.5 MHz. The higher the frequency of the sound, the better the reproduction and resolution, but the shallower the depth of penetration. B-mode sector scanning uses a moving transducer head containing the crystals or a wheel containing multiple transducers that moves through a prescribed sector. Sector scanning facilitates the visualization of structures behind the symphysis pubis. Curvilinear transducers are now available that incorporate the advantages of both the linear array and sector transducers.

Doppler ultrasound differs significantly from the imaging techniques that have been described. In this application of ultrasound, employed in Doppler velocimetry (see Ch. 13) and antepartum and intrapartum fetal heart rate monitoring (see Chs. 13 and 15), the receiver detects shifts in the frequency of the returning sound waves rather than in the amplitude of these reflected echoes. Targets moving toward the receiving transducer produce an increase in the frequency of the echo, while objects moving away decrease the frequency. Doppler ultrasound uses a continuous beam of sound rather than the intermittent transmission that characterizes B-mode ultrasound.

SAFETY OF ULTRASOUND

Concern has been expressed by basic scientists, physicians, and consumers about the safety of diagnostic ultrasound.[2,3] The dissipation of energy from ultrasound can produce heating of the exposed tissues. Ultrasound may also create cavitation or the formation of bubbles and microstreaming, the flow of liquid around these oscillating bubbles. In experimental systems, exposure to high-intensity ultrasound has been associated with alterations in immune response, increases in sister chromatid[4] exchange frequencies, fetal malformations, and growth retardation. However, these effects have *not* been seen with diagnostic ultrasound.

The total ultrasound exposure for a fetus will depend on the number of ultrasound examinations performed, the type of equipment used, and the amount of energy received, which is dependent on the duration of the examination. It has been recommended that the length of each ultrasound study and the type of equipment used be recorded.[3]

The amount of ultrasound energy received by the fetus varies directly with the intensity of the ultrasound signal and is inversely related to the square of its distance from the emitting source. If one is using a 3.5-MHz transducer, which focuses at approximately

8 cm, exposed tissues will receive only 1/64th of the energy originally emitted from the transducer. In considering the intensity of medical ultrasound equipment, one must consider the terms spatial peak (SP) and spatial average (SA).[3] SP is the measurement of the ultrasound beam at its point of maximum intensity, usually on the beam axis. SA refers to the intensity averaged across the beam at its focal point. The ratio of SP to SA intensities ranges from 2 to 4 for unfocused ultrasound fields to as high as 50 at the focal point. Thus far, the safe level of ultrasound intensity has been defined as less than 100 mW/cm^2 for unfocused ultrasound and below 1 W/cm^2 for focused ultrasound.[5] For sequenced linear array transducers, the SP pulse average intensity varies from 0.3 to 69 mW/cm^2.[2,3] The temporal average refers to the intensity of sound averaged from one pulse to the next. Linear array transducers demonstrate a spatial peak temporal average intensity (SPTA) from 0.5 to 12 mW/cm^2. Doppler instruments produce an SPTA of 0.6 to 80 mW/cm^2.

Studies of clinical outcomes of infants exposed to ultrasound have failed to demonstrate any significant effects. Stark et al.[6] reported no decrease in birth weight or impairment of neurologic function. An insignificant increase in dyslexia was observed in infants who had been exposed to ultrasound. Of note, these infants were also more likely to have been low birth weight.

Diagnostic ultrasound has been in use since the late 1950s. Given its known benefits and recognized efficacy for medical diagnosis, including use during human pregnancy, in 1988 the American Institute of Ultrasound in Medicine (AIUM) Bioeffects Committee[5] addressed the clinical safety of such use:

No confirmed biological effects on patients or instrument operators caused by exposure at intensities typical of the present diagnostic ultrasound instruments have ever been reported. Although the possibility exists that such biological effects may be identified in the future, current data indicate that the benefits to patients of the prudent use of diagnostic ultrasound outweigh the risks, if any, that may be present.

In considering the safety of any diagnostic procedure, one must also consider the skill with which the examination has been conducted and the way in which the results are interpreted and utilized. False-positive and false-negative diagnoses appear to be the greatest risk for the patient undergoing an obstetric ultrasound examination. What guidelines should be followed to ensure that an obstetrician is adequately trained in the application of ultrasound? In 1982, the AIUM published guidelines for minimum post-residency training in obstetric and gynecologic ultrasound.[7] These recommendations called for a minimum of 3 months experience in obstetric and gynecologic ultrasound or its equivalent, including 1 month of supervised and documented training in an established ultrasound facility. The training should include basic physics and technique, performance, and interpretation of ultrasound examinations. The guidelines also called for 2 months of practical experience or its equivalent in which at least 200 examinations were performed, followed by continuing education efforts devoted to the expansion of skills in ultrasound diagnosis, including self-assessment examinations when possible.

CLINICAL APPLICATIONS

First Trimester

Ultrasound studies in early pregnancy may not only help to establish gestational age, but also may prove useful in assessing the viability of a gestation in which bleeding has occurred.[8] Documentation of fetal cardiac activity is extremely important. Simpson and his colleagues[9] noted that among 220 women who had a viable pregnancy as evidenced by fetal cardiac activity at 8 weeks gestation, only seven, or 3.2 percent, subsequently experienced a fetal loss. In a study of 466 pregnant patients who presented with a threatened miscarriage, Stabile et al.[8] observed that pregnancy continued in only one-half. However, in those women in whom a live fetus was identified, less than 3 percent subsequently aborted. Using transabdominal ultrasound, Nyberg et al.[10] reported that a living embryo was always detected when the mean gestational sac was greater than 25 mm in average diameter. In addition, a yolk sac was always seen when the mean sac diameter was greater than 20 mm. The absence of these findings suggests the presence of a blighted ovum. Nyberg et al. found that the normal gestational sac grew at a rate of 1.1 mm/day. Therefore, if one finds a gestational sac without an embryo, one may determine the time interval for a follow-up examination by the formula: time interval (in days) = 25 − initial mean sac diameter. When the viability of a pregnancy is in doubt based on ultrasound findings, serial examinations should be undertaken. Ultrasound criteria for a nonviable gestation include a deformed and angular gestational sac, decidual reaction surrounding the sac of less than 2 mm in width, and a sac located low in the uterus.[11]

Transvaginal sonography (TVS) may provide significant advantages, not only for evaluation of the gynecologic patient, but for the assessment of the pregnant patient as well.[12] Most abdominal ultrasound examinations are performed with 3.5- or 5-MHz transducers. With TVS, sound frequencies of up to 7.5 MHz may be utilized.[13] Higher frequencies permit greater resolution of pelvic structures, and, because the probe is closer to the organs of interest, attenuation of sound does not present a problem. Thus TVS may be especially helpful in evaluating an obese patient. As noted above, when performing an abdominal ultrasound examination to assess pelvic

structures, a full bladder is necessary to create an acoustic window. TVS does not require that the bladder be filled prior to a study. Therefore, one need not delay an examination while waiting for bladder filling, and patient discomfort is reduced.

The higher resolution obtained with TVS permits earlier identification of structures in pregnancy (Fig. 12.1). A normal intrauterine pregnancy can be seen approximately 1 week earlier with TVS than with transabdominal ultrasound.[12] By 6 weeks gestation, one can identify a fetal pole and cardiac activity. The normal herniation of the midgut visualized at 8 weeks with TVS should not be confused with an abdominal wall defect (Fig. 12.2). By 12 weeks, the midgut has returned to the abdominal cavity.

TVS may permit earlier identification of pathologic processes such as an ectopic pregnancy (see Ch. 24), blighted ovum, uterine anomaly, or adnexal mass. Timor-Tritsch and Monteagudo[12] noted that, when using TVS, all of the following should be considered evidence of an abnormal pregnancy: a chorionic sac

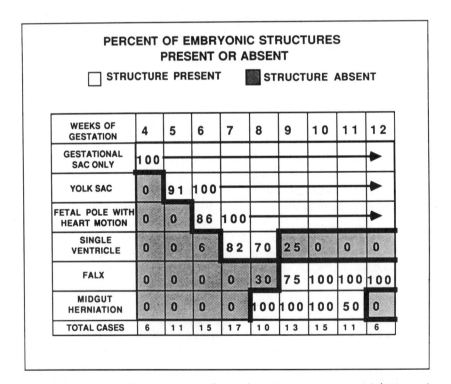

Fig. 12.1 Transvaginal sonography. The percentage of six embryonic structures present (white areas) or absent (gray areas) during the first trimester of pregnancy in patients evaluated with transvaginal sonography. Solid lines separate the weeks of gestation at which a majority of embryos demonstrated a change in sonographic appearance. (From Timor-Tritsch and Monteagudo,[12] with permission.)

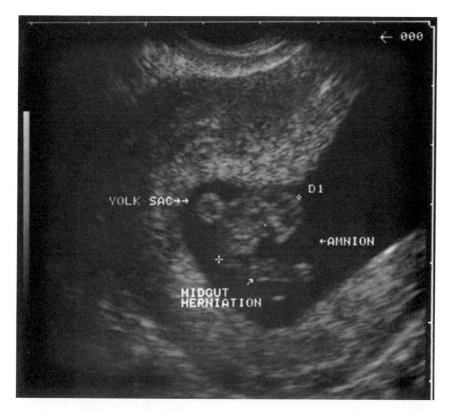

Fig. 12.2 Transvaginal sonography demonstrates a crown–rump length measurement at 8 weeks gestation. The cursors (+) are placed at the top of the fetal head and the fetal rump. Care must be taken to identify the longest fetal diameter but to exclude the lower limbs and yolk sac when making this measurement. Note the midgut herniation, which is normal at this gestational age.

larger than 1 cm (mean diameter) without the presence of a yolk sac, a well-dated pregnancy at 6.5 weeks without fetal cardiac activity, or a pregnancy in which the β-human chorionic gonadotropin (β-hCG) level is 10,800 mIU/ml (IRP) or greater without fetal cardiac activity. They emphasize that one must be certain of the patient's dates before concluding that the absence of an expected finding is consistent with an abnormal pregnancy. In such cases, it is best to repeat the ultrasound study in several days. The ability of TVS to detect major anomalies in the first trimester is also being studied.[14,15] Later in pregnancy, TVS may be employed to assess cervical length in patients at risk for cervical incompetence or preterm delivery and to detect placenta previa.

The early studies of Robinson and Fleming[16] demonstrated that a fetal crown–rump length (Fig. 12.2), a measurement from the top of the fetal head to its rump, could define gestational age between 6 to 10 weeks with an error of about 3 to 5 days (Fig. 12.3). In general, the gestational age of the pregnancy in weeks is equal to 6.5 plus the crown–rump length of the fetus in centimeters. When performing a crown–rump length measurement, care must be taken to avoid confusing the yolk sac with the fetal head. Beyond 12 weeks, the fetus begins to curve and the crown–rump length loses its accuracy. Real-time transabdominal ultrasound will also permit the detection of fetal heart motion by 7 to 8 weeks gestation.

Second Trimester

Assessment of Gestational Age

When performed during the first 18 weeks of gestation, ultrasound permits an extremely accurate assessment of gestational age. The biparietal diameter (BPD) is the measurement most often used for establishing fetal gestational age. Campbell et al.[17] found

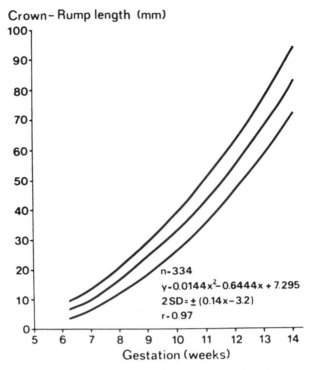

Fig. 12.3 Nomogram showing the correlation between the crown–rump length measurement and gestational age. (From Robinson and Fleming,[16] with permission.)

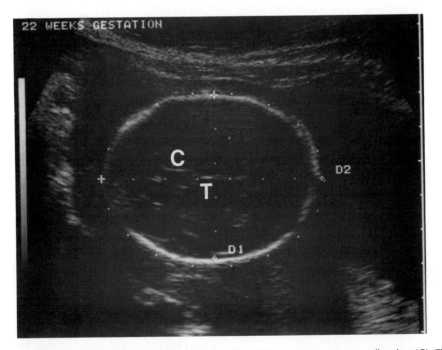

Fig. 12.4 A determination of the BPD at the level of the thalami (T) and cavum septum pellucidum (C). The BPD measurement is made from the outer edge of the skull to the opposite inner edge (D1) and on a line perpendicular to the midline. The occipitofrontal diameter (D2) is also shown. The electronic calipers (dots) have been placed to obtain a measurement of the HC.

the BPD to be the most accurate predictor of the estimated date of confinement (EDC) when performed between 12 and 18 weeks gestation. In their study, the crown–rump length was as predictive of the EDC as was an excellent menstrual history. The transaxial or transverse BPD is best obtained at the level of the thalami and cavum septum pellucidum (Fig. 12.4). The strong midline echo, once thought to be the falx, has now been shown to result from the apposition of the two sides of the brain. The BPD measurement is made from the outer edge of the skull to the inner edge of the opposite side.

From 12 to 28 weeks gestation, the relationship between BPD and gestational age is linear (Fig. 12.5).[18] The error when measuring the BPD using a 3.5-mHz transducer is about 1 to 1.5 mm. This error will be least significant early in gestation when the fetal head is growing rapidly. However, late in gestation, growth of the fetal head slows, and errors of several weeks may be made in estimating gestational age (Table 12.1). In addition, later in gestation the fetal head becomes more elongated in its anteroposterior plane. Such dolichocephaly may be assessed by measuring the cephalic index: the ratio of the BPD divided by the occipital frontal diameter (OFD). This ratio should normally be 0.75 to 0.85. If the ratio falls outside this range, the BPD should not be used to estimate gestational age. Femur length (FL) may be used in such cases. At a given gestational age, a group of fetuses will vary in their BPD. This biologic varia-

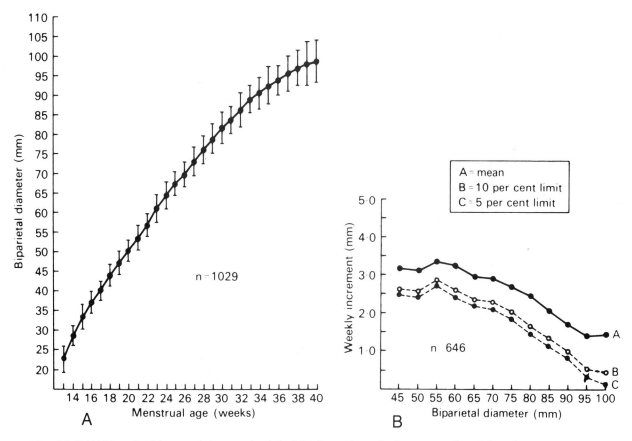

Fig. 12.5 (A) Mean fetal biparietal diameter (mm) ± 2 SD for each week of pregnancy from 13 weeks to term. (B) Mean growth rate of the fetal biparietal diameter. The mean weekly increase in the biparietal diameter is rapid and almost linear from 14 until 30 weeks menstrual age, 3.3 mm/week. The growth slows significantly between 30 and 36 weeks (2.0 mm/week) and then falls rapidly until term, with a mean rate of increase of 1.2 mm/week. (From Campbell,[124] with permission.)

Table 12.1 Ultrasonographic Assessment of Fetal Age

Measurement	Gestational Age (Menstrual Weeks)	Range (Days)
Crown–rump length	5–12	±3
Biparietal diameter	12–20	±8
	20–24	±12
	24–32	±15
	>32	±21
Femur length	12–20	±7
	20–36	±11
	>36	±16

(From Gabbe and Iams,[123] with permission.)

tion is another source of error in estimating gestational age with advancing gestation. Sabbagha and Hughey[19] used serial determinations of BPD in the second and early third trimesters to determine a growth-adjusted sonographic age (GASA). Using this technique, the significance of biologic variation can be reduced by determining the normal growth rate for a given fetus.

Assessment of Fetal Viability

Real-time ultrasound can be used to confirm the presence of fetal death in utero. The absence of fetal cardiac motion as well as the presence of fetal scalp edema and overlapping of the fetal cranial bones confirms a fetal death.

Third Trimester

Evaluation of Fetal Growth

Among the parameters to study when establishing gestational age and evaluating fetal growth are the long bones, especially the femur and humerus, and the abdominal circumference (Fig. 12.6), outer and inner orbital diameters, and transcerebellar diame-

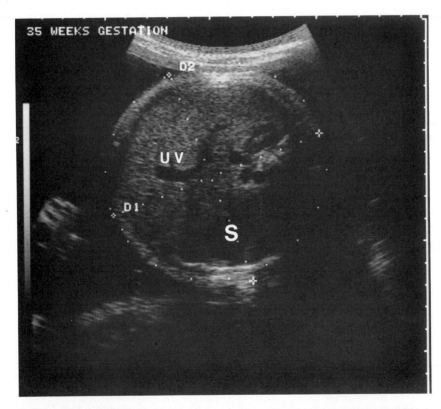

Fig. 12.6 Transverse or axial view of the abdomen demonstrates the fetal stomach (S) and umbilical vein (uv). Note that the abdomen is round and the umbilical vein is well within the substance of the liver. This is the proper level for determination of the fetal AC; electronic calipers (dots) have been placed to make this measurement. The AC may also be calculated using measurements of the anteroposterior (D1) and transverse (D2) abdominal diameters using the following formula: AC = D1 + D2 × 1.57.

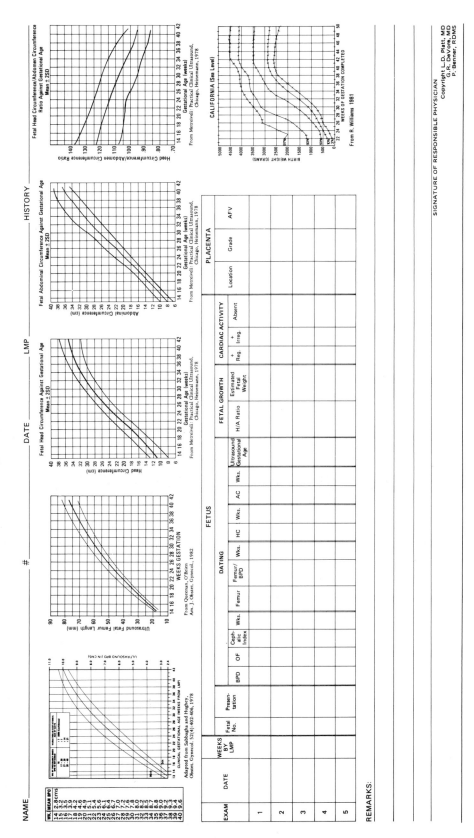

Fig. 12.7 Sequential analysis of ultrasonic fetal growth parameters. (Courtesy of Dr. Lawrence D. Platt, Los Angeles County Women's Hospital, University of Southern California Medical Center, Los Angeles, CA.)

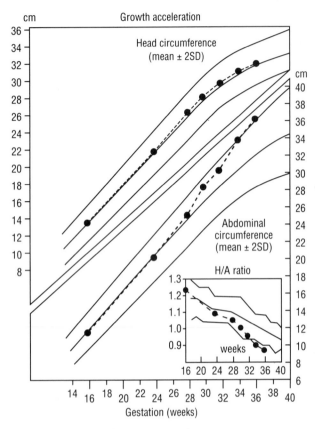

Fig. 12.8 Growth chart in a case of asymmetric macrosomia. While HC growth is preserved, AC growth is accelerated in the third trimester. For this reason, the HC/AC or H/A ratio shown in the lower right corner of the graph is reduced. This growth pattern is characteristic of the accelerated growth of the fetus of the diabetic mother. (From Chudleigh and Pearce,[125] with permission.)

ter. These data are best plotted serially in a graphic format (Fig. 12.7). The uniformity of fetal growth that characterizes early gestation is lost after 20 weeks. Therefore, a single ultrasound study performed late in pregnancy cannot accurately establish gestational age (Table 12.1). Fetal abdominal circumference (AC) or perimeter measured at the level of the umbilical vein has been used not only to assess gestational age but also to detect the presence of intrauterine growth retardation (IUGR) and macrosomia (Fig. 12.8). Composite tables estimating fetal weight have been constructed by several authors and

are usually based on a combination of (1) head size (as measured by BPD or head circumference [HC]), (2) FL, and (3) AC. Tables by Hadlock et al.[20] and Shepard et al.[21] are currently in most common use. Shepard et al. demonstrated that the BPD and fetal AC may be combined to calculate estimates of fetal weight that are likely to be within 10 percent of actual weight.

Abnormal Fetal Growth

Fetal Growth Retardation

This subject is discussed in Chapter 27.

Fetal Macrosomia

Macrosomia has been defined by some investigators as a birth weight in excess of 4,000 to 4,500 g. Other studies, utilizing population-specific growth curves, categorize infants with a birth weight above the 90th percentile as large for gestational age (LGA). Excessive fetal growth resulting in macrosomia has long been recognized as an important cause of perinatal morbidity and mortality, especially in the pregnancy complicated by diabetes mellitus. At delivery, the macrosomic fetus is more likely to suffer shoulder dystocia, traumatic injury, and asphyxia.

Macrosomia in the infant of the diabetic mother (IDM) is characterized by selected organomegaly, with increases in both fat and muscle mass resulting in a disproportionate increase in the size of the abdomen and shoulders. However, brain growth is not altered, and therefore the HC is usually normal. Thus the macrosomia of the IDM is asymmetric. The macrosomic infant of an obese woman without glucose intolerance will demonstrate symmetric macrosomia: excessive growth of *both* the AC and HC.

Antenatal detection of the LGA fetus could allow optimal selection of the route of delivery to reduce the likelihood of birth trauma. Unfortunately, the clinical ability to evaluate fetal size at term remains poor, with only 35 percent of large infants being identified by excessive symphysis–fundal height measurements.[22] Thus diagnostic ultrasound can be a valuable adjunct in the evaluation of suspected macrosomia.

Sonographic estimation of fetal weight has been

employed to detect excessive growth. Using the formula of Shepard et al.,[21] Ott and Doyle[23] determined fetal weight in 595 patients undergoing real-time ultrasound estimation within 72 hours of delivery. Overall, almost 75 percent of LGA infants were detected using an estimated fetal weight (EFW) of more than the 90th percentile as a cut-off for diagnosis. There were a significant number of false positives, as the predictive value of a positive test was only 63.2 percent. An EFW less than the 90th percentile predicted a normally grown fetus in 96 percent of cases. Tamura et al.[24] also applied Shepard's formula in a study of 147 diabetic women during the last 2 weeks of the third trimester and reported a sensitivity of 77 percent in detecting infants with birth weights exceeding the 90th percentile. It must be remembered that formulae for estimation of fetal weight are associated with a 95 percent confidence range of at least 10 to 15 percent. Thus the predicted weight using ultrasonography would have to exceed 4,700 g for all fetuses with weights in excess of 4,000 g to be accurately identified! Miller et al.[25] reported that all formulae for estimating fetal weight, including those of Shepard et al.[21] and Hadlock et al.,[20] significantly underestimated the largest fetuses, those weighing 4,000 to 4,999 g, although the Hadlock et al. formula did show slightly better predictive value.

Measurement of the AC is probably the most reliable sonographic parameter for the detection of macrosomia. Using an AC greater than the 90th percentile obtained within 2 weeks of delivery, Tamura et al.[24] correctly identified 78 percent of LGA fetuses. When both the AC and EFW exceeded the 90th percentile, an LGA infant was correctly diagnosed in 88.8 percent of cases. Bochner et al.[26] used early third-trimester ultrasound measurements of the AC to determine the risk for both macrosomia and birth trauma at term. In a series of 201 women with gestational diabetes mellitus, 36 of 41 cases of macrosomia were identified by the presence of an AC greater than the 90th percentile at 30 to 33 weeks gestation. The false-positive rate was high, with 28 normally grown fetuses having large AC measurements. Of note, the risk for shoulder dystocia was 9.3 percent in the suspected LGA group versus 0.8 percent in the group with a normal AC measurement at 30 to 33 weeks.

Although the HC to AC ratio has been used for the detection of asymmetric IUGR (see Ch. 27), this index has not been well evaluated as a predictor of macrosomia. The HC/AC ratio should be reduced in cases of asymmetric macrosomia, because abdominal size is disproportionately large when compared with head growth (Fig. 12.8). The HC/AC ratio does require an accurate knowledge of gestational age, because the ratio varies throughout pregnancy.

The FL/AC ratio, which is gestational age independent after 21 weeks, has also been employed to detect fetal macrosomia. A low FL/AC ratio should reflect increased AC growth. Using a cut-off of less than 20.5 percent, representing the 10th percentile, Hadlock et al.[27] were able to detect only 63 percent of LGA fetuses. Landon et al.[28] employed a less stringent cut-off of less than 21 percent and could identify only 58 percent of LGA fetuses of diabetic women studied late in the third trimester.

In summary, detection of the macrosomic infant using both clinical *and* ultrasonographic techniques remains challenging. In patients at risk for fetal macrosomia (women who have diabetes mellitus, are obese, or whose pregnancies go beyond 42 weeks), a "growth profile" including ultrasound measurements of estimated fetal weight and HC/AC and FL/AC ratios may identify excessive fetal growth.[29] In patients at low risk for macrosomia, a fundal height measurement 4 cm or greater than expected for gestational age should signal the need for an ultrasound study.

Assessment of Amniotic Fluid Volume

Ultrasound has proved valuable in the evaluation of amniotic fluid volume. Early application of this technology included measurements of the largest vertical pocket of fluid. Oligohydramnios, a reduction in amniotic fluid volume, was diagnosed when the largest pocket of amniotic fluid measured in two perpendicular planes was less than 1 cm. Chamberlain et al.[30] reported this degree of oligohydramnios in 0.85 percent of more than 7,500 patients evaluated. When defined in this way, oligohydramnios was associated with a 40-fold increase in perinatal mortality (187.5/1,000); a 17-fold increase in lethal congenital anomalies such as renal agenesis, polycystic kidney disease, or complete obstruction of the genitourinary system (9.4 percent); and an 8-fold increase in growth retardation (39 percent). Hydramnios or excessive amniotic fluid was diagnosed when the largest pocket of amniotic fluid exceeded 8 cm in two perpendicular planes.[31] In one series of more than 2,500 patients, hydramnios was observed in approximately 2.8 percent. Major fetal malformations were found in 18 percent of these cases. Neural tube defects, obstruction of the fetal gastrointestinal tract, multiple gestations, and fetal hydrops are associated with hydramnios.

Several investigators have questioned the diagnostic accuracy of the largest or maximum vertical pocket concept as an index of overall amniotic fluid volume and perinatal outcome. Bottoms et al.[32] reported that subjective assessment of amniotic fluid volume was as valuable as measurements of the maximum vertical pocket. They did note that suspected fetal growth retardation and suspected post-term gestation were negatively correlated with the maximum vertical pocket, while suspected fetal growth acceleration and increasing birth weight were positively correlated. Hoddick et al.[33] reported poor sensitivity when applying the 1 cm vertical pocket as an index of oligohydramnios for the detection of IUGR.

In an effort to find a more reproducible and quantitative technique to assess amniotic fluid volume, Phelan and colleagues[34,35] developed the amniotic fluid index (AFI).[34,35] The AFI measurement is performed with the patient in the supine or semi-Fowler position. The maternal abdomen is divided into quadrants (Figs. 12.9 and 12.10). The umbilicus is used as one reference point to divide the uterus into upper and lower halves, and the linea nigra is used as the midline to divide the uterus into right and left halves. The ultrasound transducer head is then placed on the maternal abdomen along the longitudinal axis. The transducer head is maintained perpendicular to the floor, and the vertical diameter of the largest amniotic fluid pocket in each quadrant is identified and measured. The total of each of these measurements is summed to obtain the AFI in centimeters. If a fetal extremity or portion of the umbilical cord is observed in the quadrant to be measured, the transducer head is moved slightly to exclude these structures.[36] The technique is extremely reproducible, with intraobserver and interobserver variations averaging 1.0 and 2.0 cm, respectively.[36,37] When the AFI is determined in a patient at 20 weeks gestation or lower, the uterus is divided into halves using the linea nigra, and the largest pocket identified in each half is added to pro-

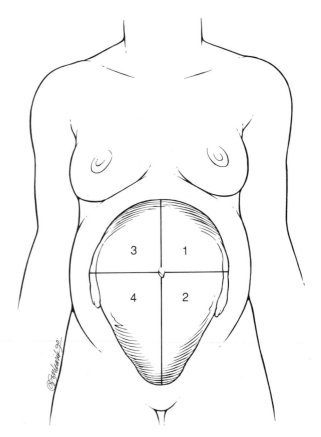

Fig. 12.9 The AFI measurement utilizes ultrasound to assess the depth of fluid pockets in each quadrant of the uterus. Note that the umbilicus divides the uterus into upper and lower halves, and the linea nigra divides the uterus into right and left halves.

duce an AFI. Using this technique, Phelan et al.[34] found that the mean AFI in over 350 pregnancies at 36 to 42 weeks was 12.9 ± 4.6 cm. Patients with an AFI less than 5.0 cm at term were considered to have oligohydramnios, while those with an AFI of 20 cm or greater were considered to have polyhydramnios. When the AFI fell below 5 cm, Rutherford et al.[38] noted that the frequency of nonreactive nonstress tests, fetal heart rate decelerations, meconium staining, cesarean sections for fetal distress, and low Apgar scores increased. Fetal structural anomalies and chromosomal abnormalities are more common in pregnancies with polyhydramnios, as defined by the AFI.[39]

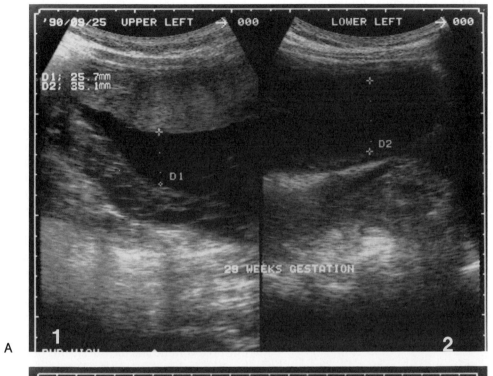

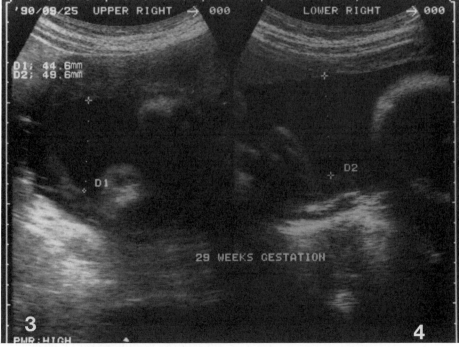

Fig. 12.10 (A & B) Ultrasound determination of the AFI at 29 weeks gestation. The numbers in the corner of each ultrasound section correspond to those in Figure 12.9. The AFI was 15.6 cm, which is normal at this gestational age (see Table 12.1).

Moore and colleagues recently completed several important studies demonstrating the validity of the AFI and establishing normative values for this measurement. In a pregnant sheep model, Moore and Brace[40] first found that the AFI demonstrated a close linear relationship to the actual amount of amniotic fluid and an 88 percent accuracy in quantitating amniotic fluid volume. Moore and Cayle[36] next studied 791 uncomplicated pregnancies prospectively to establish normal values for the AFI (Table 12.2). At term, the mean AFI was 11.5 cm, while the 5th and 95th percentiles were 6.8 cm and 19.6 cm, respectively. These values are similar to those reported by

Phelan et al. Most recently, Moore[41] demonstrated the superiority of the AFI over the maximum vertical pocket in detecting abnormalities of amniotic fluid volume. In that study of 1,178 high-risk patients, oligohydramnios was defined as an AFI less than the 5th percentile for gestational age (7.0 to 9.8 cm), while hydramnios was defined as an AFI greater than the 95th percentile for gestational age (18.5 to 24.9 cm) (Fig. 12.11). The ability of a maximum vertical pocket of 3 cm or less to identify cases with oligohydramnios by AFI was poor, with a sensitivity of only 42 percent and a positive predictive value of 51 percent. Moore noted that 58 percent of cases with oligohydramnios by AFI had normal values when using the largest vertical pocket technique. The detection of polyhydramnios, defined as a maximum vertical pocket of 8.0 cm or greater, was also limited in cases identified to have excessive amniotic fluid by AFI. Values of 3 cm for oligohydramnios and 8 cm for polyhydramnios were developed from the study population of Chamberlain et al.[30] as the 5th and 95th percentiles, respectively.

In summary, while subjective assessment of amniotic fluid volume and measurements of the maximum vertical pocket may be helpful in quantitating amniotic fluid, the AFI appears to have significant advantages. First, this index appears highly reproducible and may therefore be more uniformly utilized by a number of different examiners. Second, the AFI may be applied with greater reliability at each gestational age using the normative values that were developed by Moore and Cayle.[36] Finally, the AFI has greater sensitivity and predictive value in evaluating the pregnancy at risk for oligohydramnios and polyhydramnios.

SONOGRAPHIC EVALUATION OF FETAL ANATOMY

Evaluation of fetal anatomy is an integral part of ultrasound examinations during the second and third trimesters. A basic ultrasound examination should not only document fetal life, fetal number, fetal presentation, gestational age and growth assessment, amniotic fluid volume assessment, and placental localization but should include an evaluation of fetal anatomy as well. The following is meant to represent the *minimal* examination of fetal anatomy that should be part of the basic examination. Sonographic examination of fetal anatomy is often more detailed when it is targeted to look for a certain anomaly.[42–48]

Table 12.2 Amniotic Fluid Index Percentile Values (mm)

| Week | Percentile | | | | | n |
	2.5th	5th	50th	95th	97.5th	
16	73	79	121	185	201	32
17	77	83	127	194	211	26
18	80	87	133	202	220	17
19	83	90	137	207	225	14
20	86	93	141	212	230	25
21	88	95	143	214	233	14
22	89	97	145	216	235	14
23	90	98	146	218	237	14
24	90	98	147	219	238	23
25	89	97	147	221	240	12
26	89	97	147	223	242	11
27	85	95	146	226	245	17
28	86	94	146	228	249	25
29	84	92	145	231	254	12
30	82	90	145	234	258	17
31	79	88	144	238	263	26
32	77	86	144	242	269	25
33	74	83	143	245	274	30
34	72	81	142	248	278	31
35	70	79	140	249	279	27
36	68	77	138	249	279	39
37	66	75	135	244	275	36
38	65	73	132	239	269	27
39	64	72	127	226	255	12
40	63	71	123	214	240	64
41	63	70	116	194	216	162
42	63	69	110	175	192	30

(From Moore and Cayle,[36] with permission.)

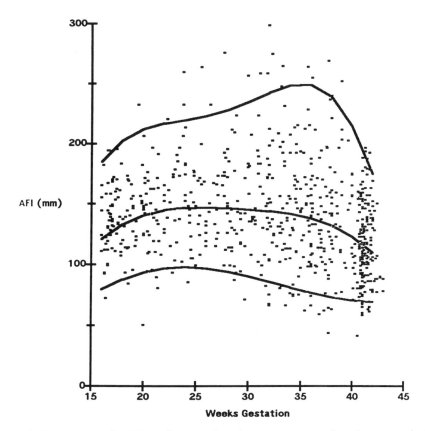

Fig. 12.11 Graph demonstrating the AFI in millimeters plotted against gestational week in a population of normal patients. The upper, middle, and lower lines represent the 95th, 50th, and 5th percentiles, respectively. (From Moore,[41] with permission.)

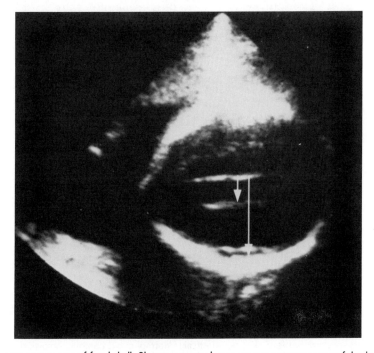

Fig. 12.12 Transverse sonogram of fetal skull. Shorter arrow demonstrates measurement of the lateral ventricle width. Longer arrow represents measurement of the hemispheric width.

The fetal skull should be elliptic, with the cranium ossified and intact. The ventricular system should be evaluated either by assessment of the body of the lateral ventricle (Fig. 12.12) or the atrium (Fig. 12.13). The cerebellum should be visualized (Fig. 12.14). The spine is easier to evaluate in its entirety in the second trimester than in the third. A sagittal sonogram (Fig. 12.15) should be complemented by a series of transverse sonograms (Fig. 12.16) to identify normal anterior and normal posterior ossification elements. An attempt should be made to obtain a four-chambered view of the heart. Ventricles and atria of equal and appropriate sizes and an intact ventricular septum should be observed. (Fig. 12.17). A fetal bladder (Fig. 12.18) and stomach (Fig. 12.19) should be visualized by 14 weeks gestation; kidneys should be identified by 16 weeks (Fig. 12.20). The abdominal wall should be intact (Fig. 12.21). The long bones of at least the lower extremities should be visualized (Figs. 12.22 and 12.23). Although fetal gender may often be identified in the second and third trimesters, this should not be considered an integral part of the examination[42-47] (Figs. 12.24 and 12.25).

ULTRASOUND DIAGNOSIS OF FETAL ANOMALIES

Antenatal ultrasound scanning at 18 to 20 weeks gestation permits the detection of most major fetal structural anomalies. It is important to appreciate, however, that even a thorough ultrasound evaluation during the second trimester will not detect all structural malformations. Such anomalies as hydrocephalus, duodenal atresia, microcephaly, achondroplasia, and polycystic kidneys may not manifest until the third trimester, when the degree of anatomic distortion is sufficient to be sonographically detectable. A useful classification of fetal anomalies is based on the nature of the dysmorphology that permits sonographic detection.

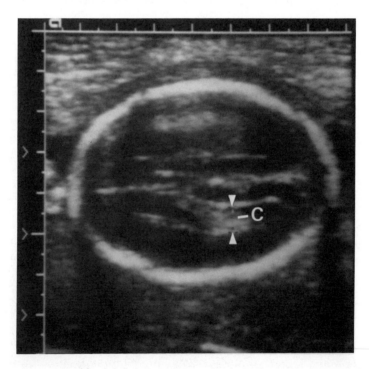

Fig. 12.13 Transverse sonogram of fetal skull demonstrating normal ovoid contour. Arrows define width of the atrium of the lateral ventricle. C, choroid plexus.

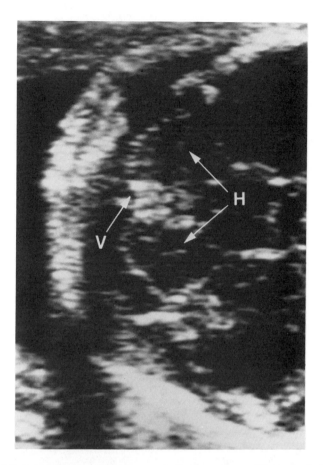

Fig. 12.14 Sonogram demonstrating cerebellar hemispheres (H). V, cerebellar vermis.

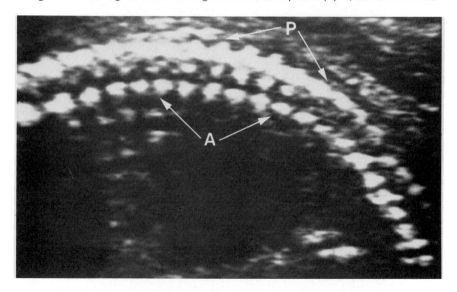

Fig. 12.15 Longitudinal view of the spine demonstrating anterior (A) and posterior (P) ossification elements.

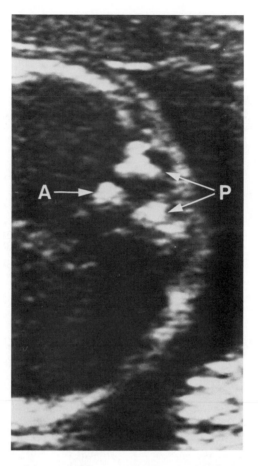

Fig. 12.16 Transverse view of the spine demonstrating anterior (A) and posterior (P) ossification elements.

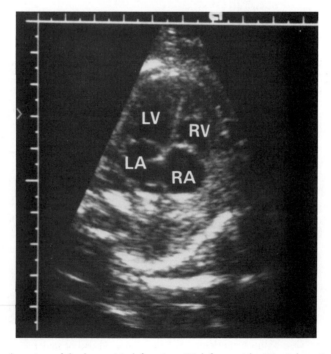

Fig. 12.17 Four-chamber view of the heart. LA, left atrium; LV, left ventricle; RA, right atrium; RV, right ventricle.

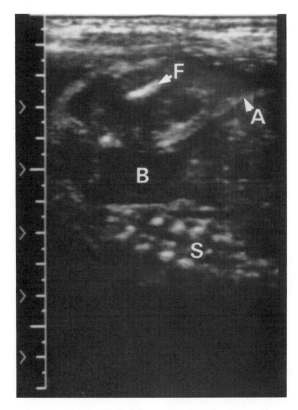

Fig. 12.18 Sonogram demonstrating fetal bladder (B), spine (S), abdominal wall (A), and femur (F).

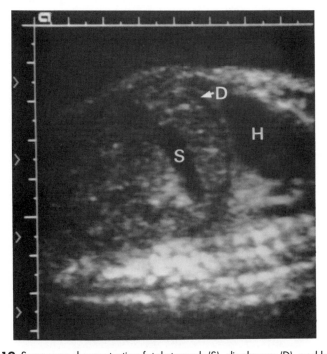

Fig. 12.19 Sonogram demonstrating fetal stomach (S), diaphragm (D), and heart (H).

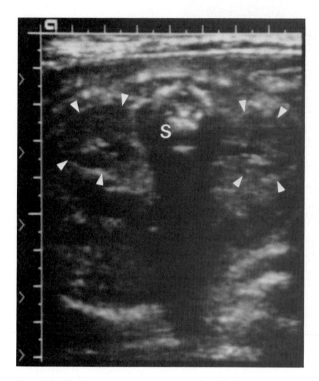

Fig. 12.20 Sonogram demonstrating fetal kidneys outlined by arrows. S, fetal spine.

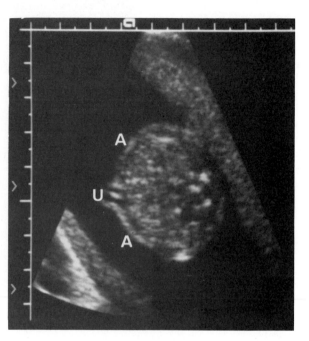

Fig. 12.21 Sonogram demonstrating intact abdominal wall (A) and umbilical cord insertion (U).

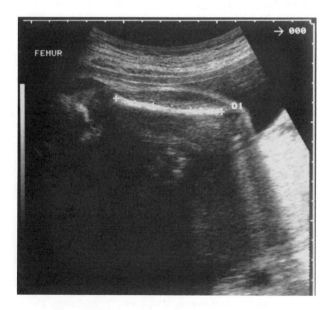

Fig. 12.22 Sonogram demonstrating femur.

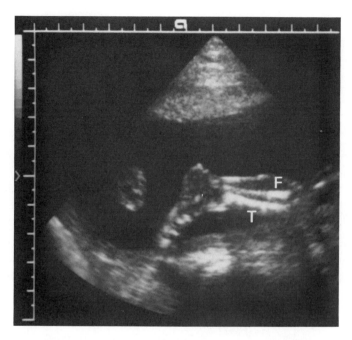

Fig. 12.23 Sonogram demonstrating tibia (T) and fibula (F).

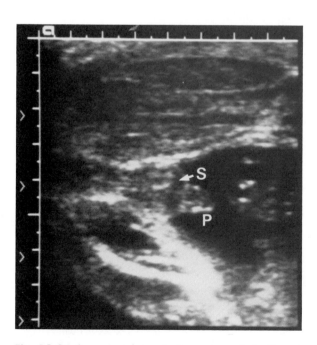

Fig. 12.24 Sonogram demonstrating male genitalia. P, penis; S, scrotum.

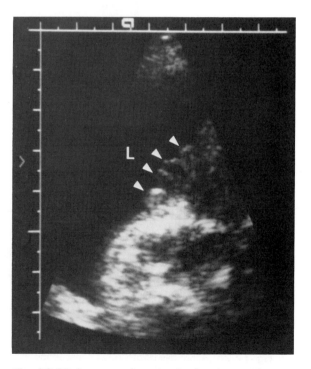

Fig. 12.25 Sonogram demonstrating female genitalia. L, labia.

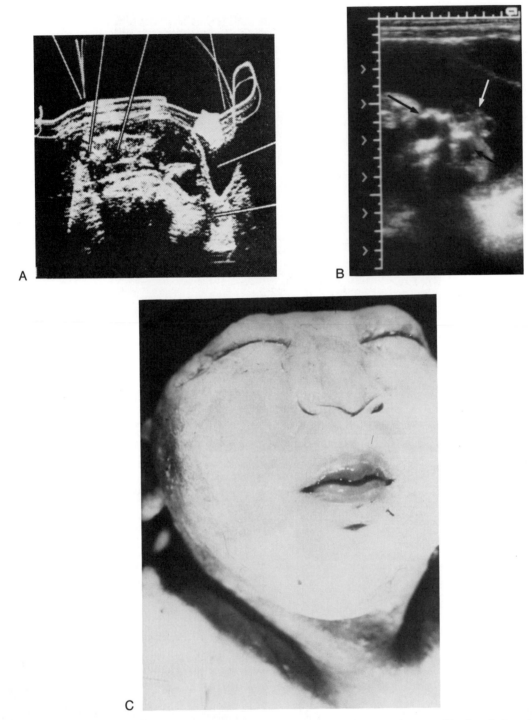

Fig. 12.26 (A) Bistable ultrasound of anencephalic fetus performed in 1971. CP, absence of fetal cephalic pole; FT, fetal trunk; UM, maternal umbilicus; SP, maternal symphysis pubis; B, maternal bladder; CX, internal cervix. (From Campbell et al.,[49] with permission.) (B) Coronal sonogram of fetal head demonstrating anencephaly. Black arrows point to orbits. White arrow points to area cerebrovasculosa. (C) Postmortem photograph of infant with anencephaly.

Absence of a Normally Present Structure

A dramatic example of the absence of a structure normally detected by ultrasound is anencephaly, the absence of calvaria and forebrain. Ultrasound clearly reveals the absence of echogenic skull bones and the presence of a heterogeneous mass of cystic tissue, called the area cerebrovasculosa, which replaces well-defined cerebral structures. In 1972, anencephaly was the first fetal anomaly to be diagnosed with sufficient certainty to support a decision to terminate a pregnancy[49] (Fig. 12.26).

Alobar holoprosencephaly is the absence of midline cerebral structures, resulting from incomplete cleavage of the primitive forebrain. The "midline echo" of the fetal head, normally generated by acoustic interfaces in the area of the interhemispheric fissure, is absent. However, absence of a midline echo is not specific to alobar holoprosencephaly; an additional sonographic sign should be sought to confirm a diagnosis, which may include hypotelorism, nasal anomalies, and facial clefts. The detection of the facial aberration helps to confirm the diagnosis of alobar holoprosencephaly[50] (Fig. 12.27).

The kidneys are normally visualized as bilateral, ovoid, paraspinal masses with echospared renal pelvices. When not visualized, the diagnosis of renal agenesis should be suspected. Severe oligohydramnios and the inability to visualize the bladder support the diagnosis of renal agenesis (Fig. 12.28). Although antenatal diagnosis of renal agenesis is possible, false-positive and false-negative diagnoses occur from inadequate visualization because of the presence of oligohydramnios and simulation of the sonographic appearance of kidneys by the ovoid-shaped adrenal glands.[51]

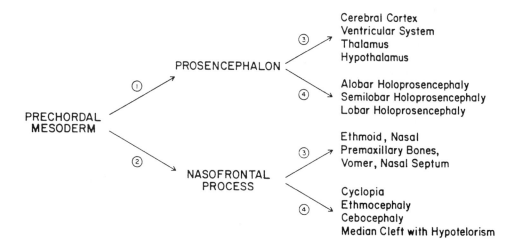

A

① Induces cleavage
② Gives rise to
③ Normal development
④ Abnormal development

Fig. 12.27 (A) Embryology of holoprosencephaly and midline facial defects. *(Figure continues.)*

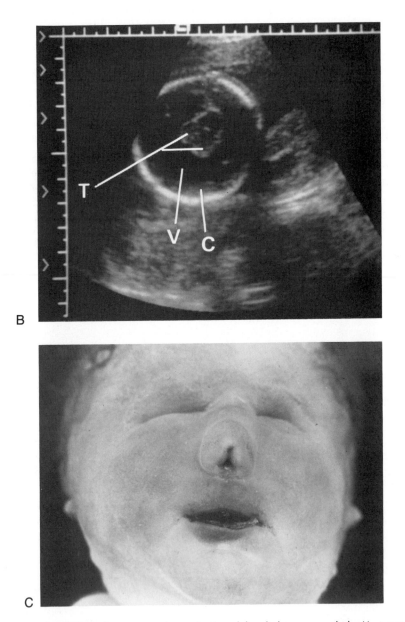

Fig. 12.27 *(Continued).* (B) Cranial sonogram demonstrating alobar holoprosencephaly. V, common ventricle; T, prominent fused thalamus; C, compressed cerebral cortex. (C) Cebocephaly with hypotelorism and normally placed nose with a single nostril. (Figures A and C from Chervenak et al.,[50] with permission.)

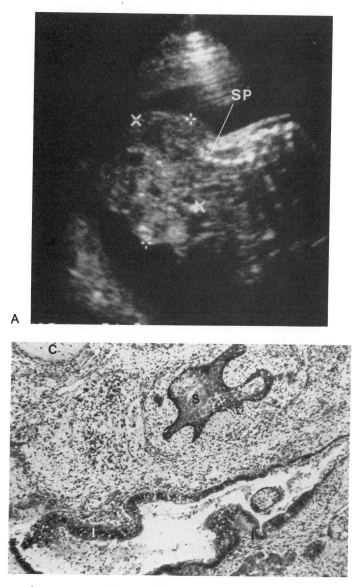

Fig. 12.28 (A) Sonogram of sacrococcygeal teratoma outlined by Xs protruding beneath fetal spine (SP). (B) Histologic section from intracranial teratoma with mature elements of ectodermal, endodermal, and mesodermal origin. S, squamous epithelium; I, intestinal mucosa; C, cartilage. *(Figure continues.)*

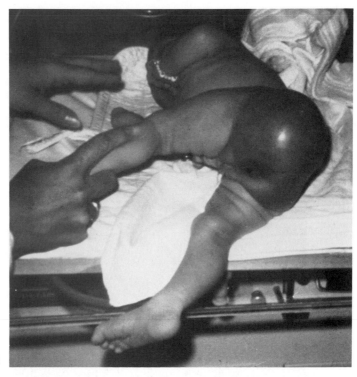

Fig. 12.28 (Continued). (C) Neonate with sacrococcygeal teratoma. (Figures B and C from Chervenak et al.,[52] with permission.)

Presence of an Additional Structure

Masses that distort normal fetal anatomy can be readily identified with ultrasound. Fetal teratomas are the most common neoplasms of the fetus. They are derived from pluripotent cells and are composed of a diversity of tissue foreign to the anatomic site from which they arise. They may be visualized as distortions of fetal contour, often in the sacrococcygeal area or along the fetal midline. The internal sonographic appearance, characterized by irregular cystic and solid areas and occasional calcifications, helps to identify the lesion[52] (Fig. 12.28).

Fetal cystic hygromas are fluid-filled masses of the fetal neck that arise from abnormal lymphatic development. They are generally anechoic, with scattered septations and the presence of a midline septum arising from the nuchal ligament. If the lymphatic disorder causing the hygromas is widespread, it may produce fetal hydrops and intrauterine death[53] (Fig. 12.29).

Fetal hydrops or fetal anasarca may be identified by the distortion of the normal fetal surface by skin edema. Ascites, pleural effusions, and pericardial effusions also may be identified.[54] The etiologies of fetal hydrops are many and varied (Fig. 12.30).

Herniation Through Structural Defects

A common theme in the development of the fetus is the formation of compartments containing vital structures by folding and midline fusion. Incomplete fusion in a variety of locations can lead to defects and herniations of contained structures.[55]

The neural tube and overlying mesoderm begin their closure in the region of the fourth somite, with fusion extending both rostrally and caudally during the fourth week of fetal life.[55] Malformations of the fetal central nervous system account for approximately 40 percent of all anomalies. Incomplete closure at the rostral end of the neural tube produces

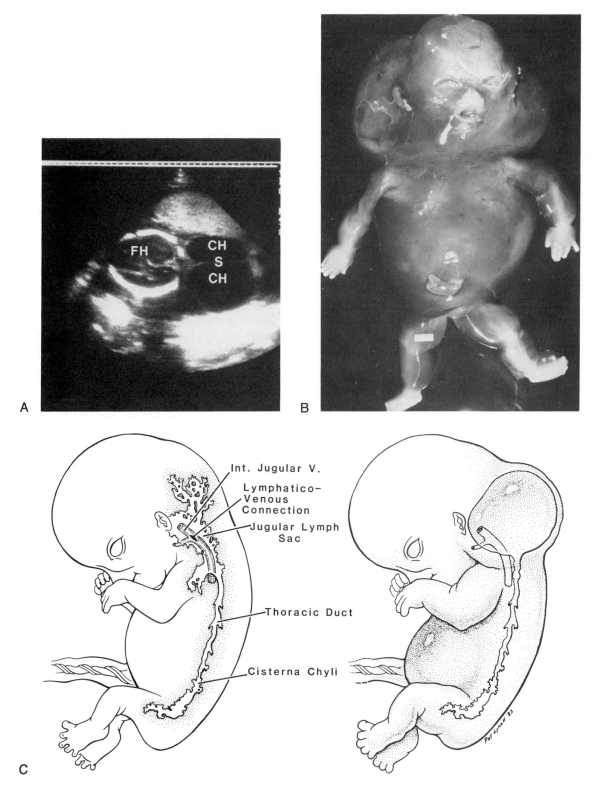

Fig. 12.29 (A) Sonogram demonstrating nuchal cystic hygroma (CH) divided by midline septum (S). FH, fetal head. (B) Postmortem photograph demonstrating fetus with cystic hygroma protruding from posterolateral neck. (From Chervenak et al.,[45] with permission.) (C) Lymphatic system in normal fetus with patent connection between jugular lymph sac and internal jugular vein (left) and fetus with cystic hygroma and hydrops from failed lymphaticovenous connection (right). (From Chervenak et al.,[53] with permission.)

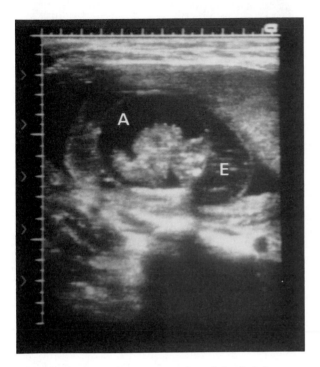

Fig. 12.30 Transverse sonogram through fetal abdomen demonstrating fetal hydrops. E, edema of abdominal wall; A, ascites.

cephaloceles, with herniations of meninges and, frequently, of brain substance through a defect in the cranium[56] (Fig. 12.31). Failed fusion at the caudal end produces spina bifida with protruding meningoceles and meningomyeloceles[57] (Fig. 12.32). Sonographic diagnosis of each of these anomalies depends on the demonstration of a defect in the normal structure of the cranium or spine and of a protruding sac, often containing tissue.

The Arnold-Chiari malformation is an anomaly of the hindbrain that has two components. The first is a variable displacement of a tongue of spinal canal. The second is a similar caudal dislocation of the medulla and fourth ventricle. Most, if not all, cases of spina bifida are complicated by the Arnold-Chiari malformation.[58] Therefore, the Arnold-Chiari malformation can serve as an important marker for spina bifida. Two characteristic sonographic signs (the "lemon" and the "banana") of the Arnold-Chiari malformation have been described. A scalloping of the frontal bones can give a lemon-like configuration, in axial section, to the skull of an affected fetus during the second trimester. The caudal displacement of the cranial contents within a pliable skull is thought to produce this scalloping effect. Similarly, as the cerebellar hemispheres are displaced into the cervical canal, they are flattened rostrocaudally and the cisterna magna is obliterated, thus producing a flattened, centrally curved, banana-like sonographic appearance. In extreme instances, the cerebellar hemispheres may be absent from view during fetal head scanning. These characteristic cranial signs are valuable adjuncts to the sonographer in the search for spina bifida[59] (Fig. 12.33). In a recent prospective study of 1,561 patients, including 130 fetuses with open spina bifida, the lemon and banana sign demonstrated a sensitivity of greater than 95 percent and a positive predictive value of greater than 90 percent before 24 weeks gestation.[60] After 24 weeks, the lemon sign usually disappears, while the banana sign retains its high sensitivity and positive predictive value. In summary, the cranial signs of open spina bifida include a small BPD and HC, lemon sign, banana sign, ventriculomegaly, and obliteration of the cisterna magna.

Omphaloceles result from failure of the intestines to retract from their temporary location in the umbilical cord and the subsequent herniation of other abdominal contents, including both hollow and solid structures contained within a peritoneal sac.[61] Insertion of the umbilical cord into the sac helps to differentiate an omphalocele (Fig. 12.34) from gastroschisis (Fig. 12.35), which has no covering membrane.[61]

The diaphragm forms from four separate structures that fuse to separate the pleural and peritoneal cavities. When a diaphragmatic hernia is present, abdominal contents may be visualized within the chest on transverse sonographic scanning. A disruption in this development of the diaphragm may be seen in the sagittal plane.[62]

Dilatation Behind an Obstruction

When dilatation behind an obstruction occurs, the structural defect itself is rarely seen. Rather, what is observed is the distention of structures behind a defect. Such dilatation is caused by obstruction to the normal flow of cerebrospinal fluid, urine, or swallowed amniotic fluid.

Hydrocephalus is characterized by a relative enlargement of the cerebroventricular system with an

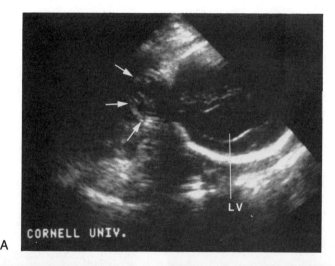

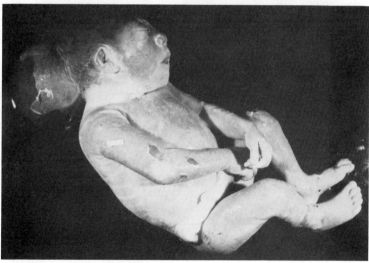

Fig. 12.31 (A) Occipital encephalocele (outlined by arrows). LV, dilated lateral ventricle. (B) Large encephalocele with resultant microcephaly. (From Chervenak et al.,[56] with permission.)

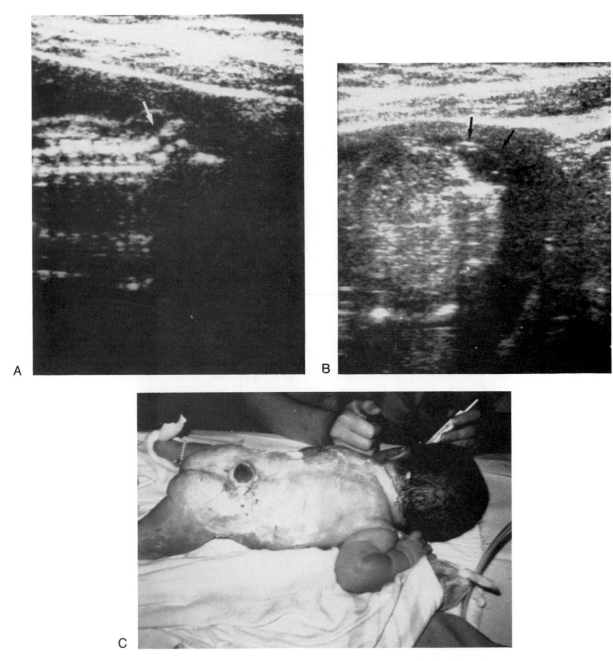

Fig. 12.32 (A) Longitudinal sonogram of fetal spine with arrow pointing to meningomyelocele. (B) Transverse sonogram through fetal spine with arrows pointing to meningomyelocele. (C) Intact lumbosacral meningomyelocele in neonate. (From Chervenak et al.,[45] with permission.)

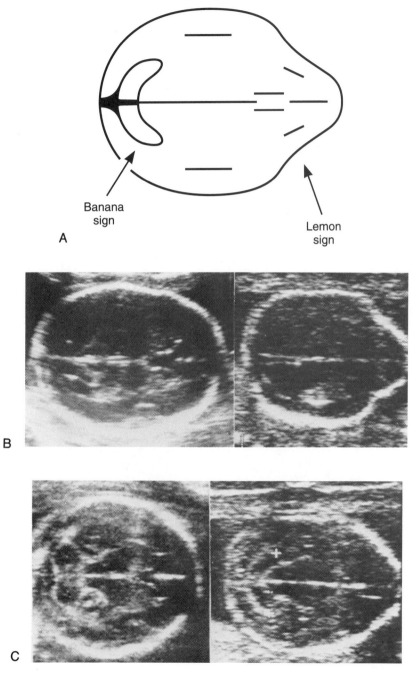

Fig. 12.33 (A) Diagrammatic representation of "banana" and "lemon" signs in fetus with spina bifida. (B) Transverse section of normal fetal head in an 18-week fetus at level of cavum septi pellucidi (left). Transverse section of fetal head at level of cavum septi pellucidi in an 18-week fetus with open spina bifida showing "lemon" sign (right). (C) Suboccipital bregmatic view of fetal head in an 18-week fetus with normal cerebellum and cisterna magna (left). Suboccipital bregmatic view of fetal head in an 18-week fetus with open spina bifida, demonstrating "banana" sign (+). (Figures A–C from Nicolaides et al.,[59] with permission.)

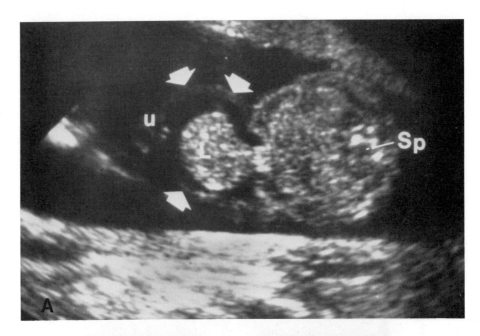

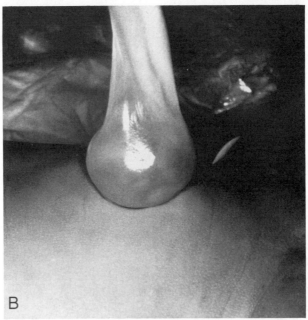

Fig. 12.34 Omphalocele. (A) The surrounding membrane (arrowheads), cord insertion into the apex of the omphalocele (u), liver (L) herniated into the omphalocele sac, and spine (Sp) can be seen. (B) Gross picture of an omphalocele, although smaller than that illustrated in the accompanying ultrasound. Note that the abdominal contents are surrounded by a membrane and protrude into the base of the umbilical cord. (Courtesy of Dr. Harbhajan Chawla, Hahnemann University, Philadelphia, PA.)

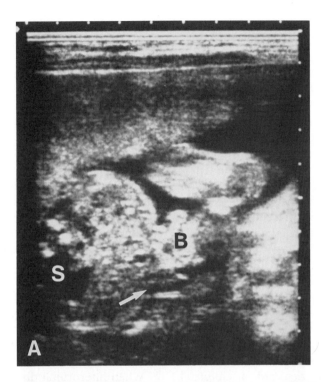

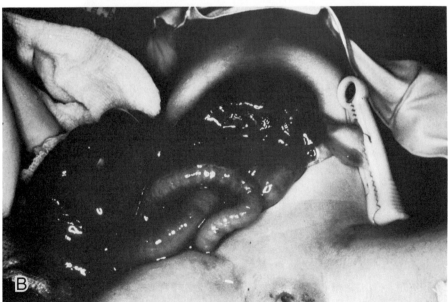

Fig. 12.35 (A) Loops of bowel (B) without a surrounding membrane are characteristic of gastroschisis. The arrow points to the insertion of the umbilical cord. Since the stomach (S) is on the left of the fetus, the site of the bowel herniation is to the right of the umbilical cord. (B) Matted loops of bowel in a neonate with gastroschisis. Note the absence of a surrounding membrane. As in the ultrasound, the abdominal contents are seen to the right of the umbilical cord. (Courtesy of Dr. Harbhajan Chawla, Hahnemann University, Philadelphia, PA.)

accompanying increase of pressure of the cerebrospinal fluid within the fetal head. Hydrocephalus has been successfully diagnosed by a lateral ventricular atrial width greater than 1 cm,[63] an abnormally increased lateral ventricle (LV) to hemispheric width (HW) ratio,[64,65] a dangling choroid plexus,[66] and an asymmetric appearance of the choroid plexus.[67,68] Between 17 to 20 weeks gestation, the LV/HW ratio exceeds 50 percent. This ratio decreases with advancing gestational age, and by term it is normally 33 percent or less.[69] The location of the obstruction may be determined by observing which portions of the ventricular system are enlarged (Fig. 12.36). There is a frequent association of fetal hydrocephalus with other anomalies, especially spina bifida.

Fetal small bowel obstruction may cause dilatation proximal to the area of obstruction. Duodenal atresia has been observed to produce its characteristic "double bubble" sign, consisting of an enlarged duodenum and stomach with narrowing at the pylorus and duodenum (Fig. 12.37). Duodenal atresia is commonly associated with Down syndrome.[70] Obstruction in the lower gastrointestinal tract (e.g., imperforate anus) is generally not detected on antenatal ultrasound unless there is another associated lesion.

Obstructions to urinary flow with proximal dilatation may occur at the ureteropelvic and ureterovesicular junctions. These are commonly unilateral defects, whereas obstruction at the urethra from posterior urethral valves characteristically produces bilateral dilatation of the ureters and renal pelves[71,72] (Fig. 12.38). When a posterior urethral valve produces complete obstruction, renal dysplasia and pulmonary hypoplasia may result.

Abnormal Fetal Biometry

Several fetal anomalies are best diagnosed not by observing alterations in shape or consistency, but by determining abnormalities in size. The science of fetal biometry has generated many nomograms defining normal values for parts of the fetal anatomy at various gestational ages.[73]

Fetal microcephaly is usually the result of an underdeveloped brain. Although commonly associated with cerebral structural malformations, microcephaly may be produced by a brain that is normal in configuration but merely small. The accurate diagnosis of microcephaly has proved challenging because compressive forces within the uterus may distort the shape of the fetal head. The best correlation between microcephaly diagnosed in utero and neonatal microcephaly is made when multiple fetal parameters are measured and suggest an inappropriately small head.[74,75]

A variety of skeletal dysplasias may affect the growth of long bones. Measurement may suggest a particular skeletal dysplasia, depending on which bones are foreshortened. The shape of these bones, their density, the presence of fractures, or the absence of specific bones may aid in differentiating the various bony abnormalities.[76] It may be difficult to determine whether a fetus with long bones that are shorter than expected for gestational age is constitutionally small, is symmetrically growth retarded, or is exhibiting a form of dwarfism. Campbell et al.[77] observed that the fetal femur/foot length ratio is normally 1 at 14 to 40 weeks. Foot growth appears to be spared in cases of skeletal dysplasia. Therefore, a femur/foot length ratio below 0.9 suggests dwarfism. In such cases, other anatomic anomalies should be sought. A normal ratio indicates a normal small or symmetrically growth-retarded fetus.

When interorbital distances are inconsistent with gestational age, hypotelorism or hypertelorism may be suggested. Abnormal distance between the orbits may serve as a clue to several malformation syndromes (e.g., alobar holoprosencephaly and median cleft face syndrome)[78] (Fig. 12.39).

The internal architecture of the kidneys may be difficult to assess in the presence of oligohydramnios. The diagnosis of polycystic kidneys thus is aided by renal measurement. In addition to being echogenic, polycystic kidneys usually are enlarged and display an abnormally increased kidney circumference (KC)/AC ratio.[79,80] The KC/AC ratio normally remains constant at approximately 28 to 30 percent throughout pregnancy.

Absent or Abnormal Fetal Motion

Abnormalities in fetal motion may suggest a malformation that cannot itself be seen. Although the fetus normally can assume contorted positions in utero, the persistence of such an unusual posture over time may suggest an orthopedic or neurologic anomaly such as clubfoot[81] (Fig. 12.40) or arthrogryposis.[82]

The fetal heart is the most conspicuously dynamic part of the fetus. Real-time ultrasound is invaluable in

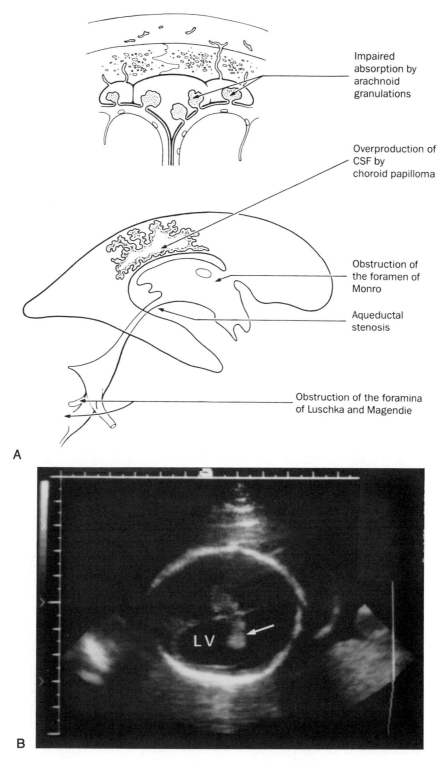

Fig. 12.36 (A) Common sites of obstruction of cerebrospinal fluid flow resulting in ventriculomegaly. (From Chervenak et al.,[45] with permission.) (B) Transverse sonogram of fetal head demonstrating hydrocephalus. LV, dilated lateral ventricle; arrow points to dangling choroid plexus.

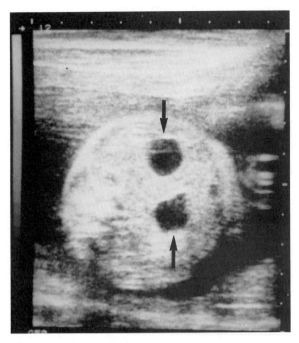

Fig. 12.37 A case of duodenal atresia illustrating the "double bubble" sign. The two hypoechoic areas (arrows) represent the stomach and proximal duodenum.

diagnosing most fetal cardiac anomalies, which comprise approximately 20 to 30 percent of all major anomalies. A four-chamber view of the heart should be obtained in each obstetric ultrasound examination in which fetal anatomy is surveyed, because this view alone may detect 80 to 90 percent of all cardiac malformations. In cases of a suspected fetal arrhythmia, atrial and ventricular rates can be determined.[83–85]

MANAGEMENT OF A PREGNANCY COMPLICATED BY AN ULTRASONICALLY DIAGNOSED FETAL ANOMALY

If a fetal anomaly is diagnosed by obstetric ultrasound, the fetus should be carefully evaluated for other anomalies before management options can be considered. Echocardiography and karyotype determination should usually be part of this evaluation. In a recent series, 23 percent of fetuses referred for echocardiography because of an extracardiac anomaly had congenital heart disease.[86] Approximately one-third of fetuses with structural anomalies have a chromosomal disorder.[87–89] This additional information is invaluable to determine fetal prognosis. For

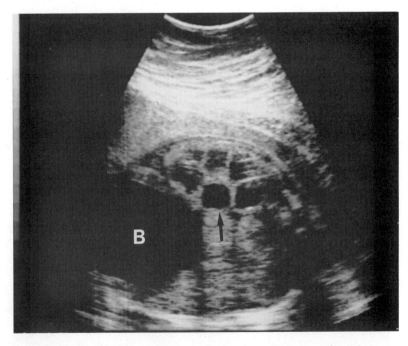

Fig. 12.38 Longitudinal scan at 32 weeks gestation in a fetus with urinary tract outflow obstruction. Note the large bladder (B) and the accompanying hydronephrosis (arrow).

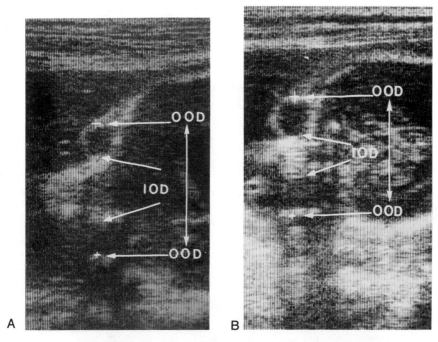

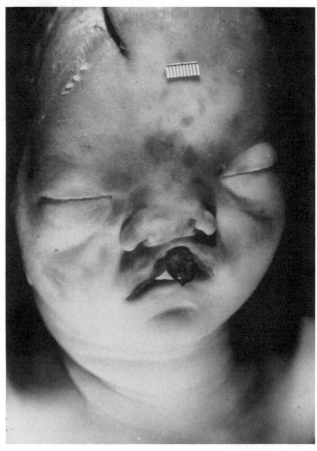

Fig. 12.39 (A) Transverse scan through orbits of fetus affected with median cleft face syndrome demonstrates hypertelorism. Inner orbital distance (IOD) and outer orbital distance (OOD) are increased for gestational age of 31 weeks. (B) Transverse scan through orbits of normal fetus at 37 weeks of gestation demonstrates normal IOD and OOD. (C) Infant with median cleft face syndrome at postmortem examination. Severe hydrocephalus, collapsed cranial bones, flattened nose, and cleft lip with protruding mass are demonstrated. (Figures A–C from Chervenak et al.,[78] with permission.)

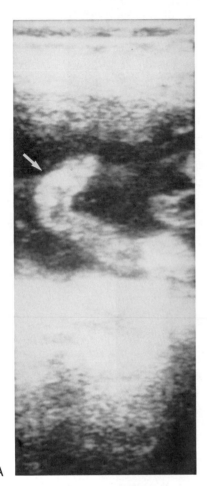
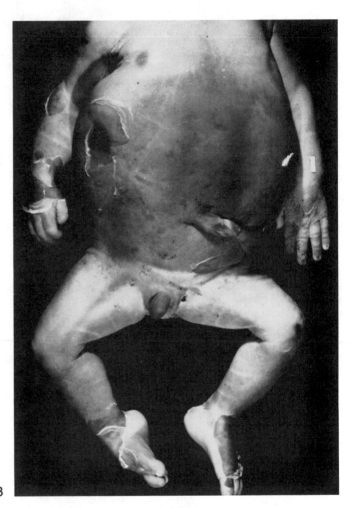

Fig. 12.40 (A) Sonogram demonstrating clubfoot (arrow). (B) Postmortem photograph demonstrating clubfoot.

example, the prognosis for isolated hydrocephalus is substantially better than that for hydrocephalus associated with alobar holoprosencephaly and trisomy 13. Amniocentesis is the most widely utilized technique for determination of fetal karyotype when an ultrasonically diagnosed anomaly is detected, but fetal blood sampling or placental biopsy may be necessary if a rapid result is required.

After the fetal evaluation is completed, the certainties and uncertainties of fetal prognosis should be explained to the pregnant woman. The disclosure requirements of the informed consent process require the physician to present information about the range of available management options: aggressive manage-

ment, termination of pregnancy, nonaggressive management, and cephalocentesis.[90] These disclosure requirements obligate the physician to be objective when presenting this information. That is, the physician is not justified in withholding information about available management options to which he or she might object for reasons of personal conscience.[91]

Aggressive Management

To optimize fetal outcome, there should be an interdisciplinary approach, including specialists in maternal–fetal medicine, neonatology, genetics, pediatric surgery, and pediatric cardiology.[44,92,93] Social work services may provide important support to the family before as well as after birth. Such a team approach is best equipped to address the important questions of where, when, and how the infant should be delivered, as well as the role of invasive fetal therapy.

Most infants with anomalies are best delivered in a referral center with a neonatal intensive care unit experienced in caring for those problems. In such a setting there is immediate access to diagnostic and therapeutic medical and surgical interventions.

Delivery at term is optimal for most fetal anomalies. For some malformations, however, such as hydrocephalus, delivery as soon as fetal lung maturation has occurred may be advisable to expedite corrective neonatal surgery.[94] Rarely, because of the risk of imminent fetal death, an anomaly such as progressive fetal hydrops may necessitate delivery prior to fetal lung maturity.[44]

Most fetuses with anomalies can be delivered vaginally. Cesarean delivery may be necessary to avoid dystocia if certain conditions are present, such as a sacrococcygeal teratoma or conjoined twins. For other anomalies, such as spina bifida, cesarean delivery may be recommended to minimize trauma to fetal tissues.[95]

Rarely, an invasive procedure may be considered during the antenatal period to optimize outcome when there is a sonographically diagnosed anomaly. This approach should only be considered when the natural history of the anomaly diagnosed is dismal and a relatively simple intrauterine correction is possible. The sonographic and karyotypic evaluations described above are especially important before an invasive approach can be considered. The disclosure requirements of the informed consent process necessitate that the experimental nature of invasive fetal therapy at this time and the potential dangers to the fetus and the mother be carefully explained. In addition, it is generally agreed that such an approach after 32 weeks of gestation offers no clear advantage over delivery and neonatal treatment. Given the risk of initiating premature labor and delivery as well as the experimental nature of these procedures, a normal coincident twin is considered to be a contraindication to such an approach.[44,92,96]

The most common form of invasive fetal therapy has been intrauterine shunt placement. The purpose of such a shunt is to drain fluid under high pressure in a fetal organ to the lower pressure of the amniotic fluid. Such a shunt may have a role in the treatment of a complete bladder outlet obstruction that would be expected eventually to result in both renal and pulmonary failure.[96,97] Analysis of fetal urine after bladder aspiration may help to define which fetuses are candidates for this vesicoamniotic shunt.[98] Intrauterine aspiration or shunt placement may also be of value in cases of isolated pleural effusions[99] (Fig. 12.41). In fetal hydrocephalus, however, because current experience does not demonstrate a clear benefit, ventriculoamniotic shunt placement should be avoided.[96,100]

Harrison and his coworkers have pioneered open fetal surgery to manage such conditions as congenital diaphragmatic hernia and complete bladder obstruction. In such cases, hysterotomy and exteriorization of the fetus is performed followed by repair, replacement, and continuation of the pregnancy.[92,101] At this time it is not possible to make a final judgment concerning the place of this fascinating modality in fetal therapy. More clinical experience is needed to clarify both the benefits to the fetus and the risks to the mother.

Termination of Pregnancy

Prior to fetal viability, abortion of any pregnancy is a woman's right as established by *Roe v. Wade.*[102] The option of abortion prior to fetal viability is therefore available to a pregnant woman when *any* fetal anomaly is diagnosed by ultrasound. Ethically, this option is supported by an approach that holds that all of obstetric ethics is essentially a function of the pregnant woman's autonomy[103,104] as well as an approach that holds that autonomous-based obligations to the pregnant woman should be balanced against beneficence-based obligations to her and the fetus that she is carrying.[91]

After fetal viability has been reached, there is limited legal access in the United States to termination of pregnancy because of a fetal anomaly. Ethically, the option of terminating third-trimester pregnancies complicated by fetal anomalies has been defended when there is (1) certainty of diagnosis and (2) either (a) certainty of death as an outcome of the anomaly diagnosed or (b) in some cases of short-term survival, certainty of the absence of cognitive developmental capacity as a result of the anomaly diagnosed. Anen-

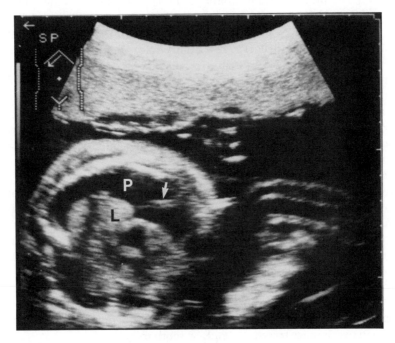

Fig. 12.41 A shunt (arrow) has been placed to drain a pleural effusion (P) in a fetus at 24 weeks gestation. Note the compressed lung (L).

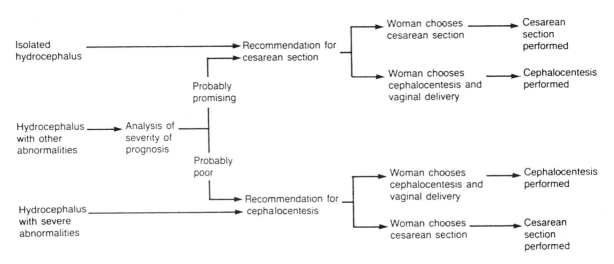

Fig. 12.42 Resolution strategies for conflicts in the intrapartum management of hydrocephalus with macrocephaly. (From Chervenak and McCullough,[107] with permission.)

cephaly is a clear example of a sonographically diagnosed anomaly that meets these criteria.[105]

Nonaggressive Management

The above-mentioned criteria for termination of pregnancy for fetal anomalies during the third trimester are quite restrictive. In addition, even if ethical criteria for third-trimester termination of pregnancy were met, it may not be possible to perform termination in some situations because of legal concerns. Nonaggressive management is the noninclusion of obstetric interventions to benefit the fetus, such as fetal surveillance, tocolysis, cesarean delivery, or delivery in a referral center. Ethically, the option of nonaggressive management for third-trimester pregnancies complicated by fetal anomalies has been defended when there is (1) a very high probability of a correct diagnosis and (2) either (a) a very high probability of death as an outcome of the anomaly diagnosed or (b) a very high probability of severe irreversible deficit of cognitive developmental capacity as a result of the anomaly diagnosed.[106]

Cephalocentesis

When a pregnancy is complicated by fetal hydrocephalus with macrocephaly, there may be a role for cephalocentesis, which is the transabdominal or transvaginal aspiration of cerebrospinal fluid to avoid cesarean delivery. Because the use of cephalocentesis carries a high rate of morbidity and mortality in a fetus shortly before birth, ethical justification is required for its use. This justification can be based on an analysis of beneficence-based and autonomy-based obligations to the pregnant woman and the fetus she is carrying. Such an analysis needs to respect the heterogeneity of fetal hydrocephalus: isolated fetal hydrocephalus, hydrocephalus with severe associated anomalies (such as alobar holoprosencephaly), and hydrocephalus with other associated anomalies (such as an arachnoid cyst)[107] (Fig. 12.42).

WHO SHOULD HAVE AN OBSTETRIC ULTRASOUND EXAMINATION?

The Consensus Development Conference, sponsored by the National Institute of Child Health and Human Development (NICHHD),[3] has supported ultrasound examinations in the following clinical situations:

1. Estimation of gestational age for patients with uncertain clinical dates, or verification of dates for patients who are to undergo scheduled elective repeat cesarean delivery, induction of labor, or other elective termination of pregnancy
2. Evaluation of fetal growth
3. Vaginal bleeding of undetermined etiology in pregnancy
4. Determination of fetal presentation
5. Suspected multiple gestation
6. Adjunct to amniocentesis
7. Significant uterine size/clinical dates discrepancy
8. Pelvic mass
9. Suspected hydatidiform mole
10. Adjunct to cervical cerclage placement
11. Suspected ectopic pregnancy
12. Adjunct to special procedures, such as fetoscopy, intrauterine transfusion, shunt placement, in vitro fertilization, embryo transfer, or chorionic villus sampling
13. Suspected fetal death
14. Suspected uterine abnormality
15. Intrauterine contraceptive device localization
16. Ovarian follicle development surveillance
17. Biophysical evaluation for fetal well-being
18. Observation of intrapartum events
19. Suspected polyhydramnios or oligohydramnios
20. Suspected abruptio placenta
21. Adjunct to external version from breech to vertex presentation
22. Estimation of fetal weight and/or presentation in premature rupture of membranes and/or vertex presentation
23. Abnormal serum α-fetoprotein value
24. Follow-up observation of identified fetal anomaly
25. Follow-up evaluation of placental localization for identified placenta previa
26. History of previous congenital anomaly
27. Serial evaluation of fetal growth in multiple gestation
28. Evaluation of fetal condition in late registrants for prenatal care

The American College of Obstetricians and Gynecologists (ACOG) has concluded that "More studies with large numbers of patients are needed to address the question of the role of routine ultrasound screening."[108] Horger and Tsai[109] surveyed 429 Fellows of the ACOG to determine their pattern of ultrasound use. While 64 percent had ultrasound equipment in their office, only 15 percent scanned every pregnancy. On the other hand, the respondents reported that 70 percent of cases were scanned at least once after 16 weeks gestation. Over 67 percent had detected one or more anomalies, and over 51 percent had missed a malformation. Law suits attributed to ultrasound-related practice activities were reported by 4.7 percent of these obstetricians.

Although the above indications are widely accepted, routine performance of obstetric ultrasound examinations, in the absence of one of the above indications, is widely debated in the United States. Arguments against the routine use of obstetric ultrasound include the failure of randomized clinical trials conclusively to demonstrate a benefit, concerns about unknown bioeffects of ultrasound, potential deleterious effects of false-positive or false-negative sonographic diagnoses, lack of adequately trained personnel to perform the procedures, and cost.[3,110–112] Nevertheless, certain high-risk factors for sonographically detectable fetal anomalies can be identified: family history of congenital anomalies, abnormal maternal serum α-fetoprotein value, maternal diabetes mellitus, medication or radiation exposure, substance abuse, potentially teratogenic maternal infection, and multiple gestation. The presence of such a high-risk factor would be a clear indication for selective ultrasound examination.[113,114]

Routine obstetric ultrasound is performed throughout Europe. Indeed, in Germany the German National Health Insurance Institute has recommended that *two* routine ultrasound examinations be performed on each pregnant woman. Failure to perform these studies would render the obstetrician liable to litigation should complications that could have been detected develop during the pregnancy. The Royal College of Obstetricians and Gynaecologists has concluded that routine obstetric ultrasound examination is justifiable.[2]

Probably the most important advantage of routine ultrasound screening is the detection of unsuspected fetal anomalies. The above-mentioned high-risk factors for fetal anomalies will fail to identify the great majority of congenital abnormalities that occur in pregnancies without established risk factors.[113,114] Routine ultrasound screening has recently been shown to detect fetal anomalies in 1 percent (46/4,353) of pregnant women screened when performed at 18 to 20 weeks.[115] This result is important as it represents the experience in a district general hospital in the United Kingdom, not a referral center. Moreover, most anomalies diagnosed during the third trimester of pregnancy are probably detectable in the second trimester, when management options are not as limited.[116]

In the largest prospective randomized investigation of routine ultrasonography performed in the early second trimester, 9,000 Finnish women were entered in a trial to compare routine ultrasound screening between 16 and 20 weeks with selective screening. Ultrasonography could be performed in the latter group according to usual practice standards. Routine ultrasonography was associated with fewer outpatient clinic visits and antenatal hospitalizations, improved early detection of twins, and detection of patients at risk for placenta previa. There were no differences in the number of labor inductions or mean birth weights in the two groups. Perinatal mortality was significantly lower in the screened than in the control group (4.6/1,000 vs. 9.0/1,000). This reduction by almost one-half was due primarily to early detection of major malformations that led to induced abortion. Additional benefits were the correction of the expected date of delivery by 10 or more days in over 11 percent of the screened group and a decrease in the rate of postmaturity. In contrast to other prospective randomized trials of ultrasound screening, this investigation did not reveal a difference between the two groups in the rate of labor inductions. The investigators concluded that their findings justified routine ultrasound screening of all pregnancies at 16 to 20 weeks for the detection of major congenital anomalies under circumstances in which their elimination by induced abortion is acceptable.[117]

In addition, a routine ultrasound examination permits accurate determination of fetal age.[118] Although this knowledge is not necessary for the success of the majority of pregnancies, it can be helpful later in pregnancy if postmaturity or IUGR is suspected.[119,120] Accurate assessment of gestational age may also be helpful in defining a management plan if *any* obstetric complication, such as premature labor, arises. Early identification of unsuspected multiple gestation or of patients at risk for placenta previa may also result from a routine ultrasound examination.[2] Lastly, an ultrasound examination may provide psychological benefits to the pregnant woman by increasing fetal bonding.[121]

While the debate concerning routine obstetric ultrasound continues, a reasonable strategy for this dilemma is the concept that prenatal informed consent for sonogram (PICS)[122] is a valid indication for obstetric ultrasonography to be added to the 28 above-mentioned indications cited by the Consensus Development Conference. The informed consent process is the means for implementing the clinical strategy of PICS. Shortly after the pregnancy is diagnosed, the woman should be provided with information about the actual and theoretical benefits and harms of a routine ultrasound examination. Thus a routine obstetric ultrasound examination is *offered,* not necessarily recommended. Because the sonographic detection of many fetal anomalies is a proven, not unproven, benefit at this time, withholding this information from pregnant women, and not respecting PICS as a valid justification for obstetric ultrasound, would not appear to be justified.

Lastly, in western Europe there is debate whether routine sonograms should be performed during the first and third, as well as the second, trimesters. A routine first-trimester sonogram may be of value in establishing the integrity of an intrauterine pregnancy as well as detecting some fetal malformations.[12] A routine third-trimester sonogram may be of value to screen for IUGR as well as to detect certain anomalies such as polycystic kidney disease, which would not have been identifiable earlier.[120] Nonetheless, it would appear that, if a *single* routine obstetric ultrasound examination is to be performed, it is best done during the second trimester at about 18 to 20 weeks gestation. This period maximizes the detection of fetal anomalies and still provides that information in time to be useful for management decisions.

REFERENCES

1. Manning F: Ultrasound in perinatal medicine. p. 195. In Creasy RK, Resnik R (eds): Maternal–Fetal Medicine: Principles and Practice. WB Saunders, Philadelphia, 1989
2. Report of the Royal College of Obstetricians and Gynaecologists Working Party on Routine Ultrasound Examination in Pregnancy, December 1984
3. U.S. Department of Health and Human Services: Diagnostic Ultrasound in Pregnancy. NIH Publ. No. 84-667. National Institutes of Health, Washington, DC, 1984
4. Reece EA, Assimakopoulos E, Zheng XZ et al: The safety of obstetric ultrasonography: concern for the fetus. Obstet Gynecol 76:139, 1990
5. American Institute of Ultrasound in Medicine Bioeffects Committee: Bioeffects considerations for the safety of diagnostic ultrasound. J Ultrasound Med 7:1988
6. Stark C, Orleans M, Haverkamp A et al: Short- and long-term risks after exposure to diagnostic ultrasound in utero. Obstet Gynecol 63:194, 1984
7. Guidelines for minimum post-residency training in obstetrical and gynecological ultrasound. In: Official Guidelines and Statements on Obstetrical Ultrasound. American Institute of Ultrasound in Medicine, Bethesda, MD, October 1985
8. Stabile I, Campbell S, Grudzinskas JG: Ultrasonic assessment of complications during first trimester of pregnancy. Lancet 2:1237, 1987
9. Simpson JL, Mills JL, Holmes LB et al: Low fetal loss rates after ultrasound-proved viability in early pregnancy. JAMA 258:2555, 1987
10. Nyberg DA, Mack LA, Laing FC, Patten RM: Distinguishing normal from abnormal gestational sac growth in early pregnancy. J Ultrasound Med 6:23, 1987
11. Nyberg DA, Laing FC, Filly RA: Threatened abortion: sonographic distinction of normal and abnormal gestation sacs. Radiology 158:397, 1986
12. Timor-Tritsch IE, Monteagudo A: Transvaginal ultrasonography: a new frontier. Obstet Gynecol Rep 2:210, 1990
13. Steinkampf MP: Transvaginal sonography. J Reprod Med 33:931, 1988
14. Timor-Tritsch IE, Farine D, Rosen MG: A close look at early embryonic development with the high-frequency transvaginal transducer. Am J Obstet Gynecol 159:676, 1988
15. Cullen MT, Green J, Whetham J et al: Transvaginal ultrasonographic detection of congenital anomalies in the first trimester. Am J Obstet Gynecol 163:466, 1990
16. Robinson H, Fleming J: Critical evaluation of sonar "crown–rump length" measurements. Br J Obstet Gynaecol 82:703, 1975
17. Campbell S, Warsof S, Little D et al: Routine ultrasound screening for the prediction of gestational age. Obstet Gynecol 65:613, 1985

18. Kurtz A, Wapner R, Kurtz R et al: Analysis of biparietal diameter as an accurate indicator of gestational age. J Clin Ultrasound 8:319, 1980

19. Sabbagha R, Hughey M: Standardization of sonar cephalometry and gestational age. Obstet Gynecol 52:402, 1978

20. Hadlock EP, Harrist RB, Carpenter RJ et al: Sonographic estimation of fetal weight. Radiology 150:535, 1984

21. Shepard M, Richard V, Berkowitz R et al: An evaluation of two equations for predicting fetal weight by ultrasound. Am J Obstet Gynecol 142:47, 1982

22. Persson B, Stangenberg M, Lunnell NO et al: Prediction of size of infants at birth by measurement of symphysis fundus height. Br J Obstet Gynaecol 93:206, 1986

23. Ott WJ, Doyle S: Ultrasonic diagnosis of altered fetal growth by use of a normal ultrasound fetal weight curve. Obstet Gynecol 63:201, 1984

24. Tamura RK, Sabbagha RE, Depp R et al: Diabetic macrosomia: accuracy of third trimester ultrasound. Obstet Gynecol 67:828, 1986

25. Miller JM, Korndorffer FA, Gabert HA: Fetal weight estimates in late pregnancy with emphasis on macrosomia. J Clin Ultrasound 14:437, 1986

26. Bochner CJ, Medearis AL, Williams J et al: Early third-trimester ultrasound screening in gestational diabetes to determine the risk of macrosomia and labor dystocia at term. Am J Obstet Gynecol 157:703, 1987

27. Hadlock FP, Harrist RB, Fearneyhough TC et al: Use of femur length/abdominal circumference ratio in detecting the macrosomic fetus. Radiology 154:503, 1985

28. Landon MB, Mintz MC, Gabbe SG: Sonographic evaluation of fetal abdominal growth: predictor of the LGA infant in pregnancies complicated by diabetes mellitus. Am J Obstet Gynecol 160:115, 1989

29. Deter RL, Hadlock FP: Use of ultrasound in the detection of macrosomia: a review. J Clin Ultrasound 13:519, 1985

30. Chamberlain P, Manning F, Morrison I et al: Ultrasound evaluation of amniotic fluid volume. I. The relationship of marginal and decreased amniotic fluid volumes to perinatal outcome. Am J Obstet Gynecol 150:245, 1984

31. Chamberlain P, Manning F, Morrison I et al: Ultrasound evaluation of amniotic fluid volume. II. The relationship of increased amniotic fluid volume to perinatal outcome. Am J Obstet Gynecol 150:250, 1984

32. Bottoms SF, Welch RA, Zador IE et al: Limitations of using maximum vertical pocket and other sonographic evaluations of amniotic fluid volume to predict fetal growth: technical or physiologic? Am J Obstet Gynecol 155:154, 1986

33. Hoddick WK, Callen PW, Filly RA et al: Ultrasonographic determination of qualitative amniotic fluid volume in intrauterine growth retardation: reassessment of the 1 cm rule. Am J Obstet Gynecol 149:758, 1984

34. Phelan JP, Smith CV, Broussard P, Small M: Amniotic fluid volume assessment using the four-quadrant technique in the pregnancy between 36 and 42 weeks' gestation. J Reprod Med 32:540, 1987

35. Phelan JP, Ahn MO, Smith CV et al: Amniotic fluid index measurements during pregnancy. J Reprod Med 32:601, 1987

36. Moore TR, Cayle JE: The amniotic fluid index in normal human pregnancy. Am J Obstet Gynecol 162:1168, 1990

37. Rutherford SE, Smith CV, Phelan JP et al: Four-quadrant assessment of amniotic fluid volume. J Reprod Med 32:587, 1987

38. Rutherford SE, Phelan JP, Smith CV et al: The four-quadrant assessment of amniotic fluid volume: an adjunct to antepartum fetal heart rate testing. Obstet Gynecol 70:353, 1987

39. Carlson DE, Platt LD, Medearis AL et al: Quantifiable polyhydramnios: diagnosis and management. Obstet Gynecol 75:989, 1990

40. Moore TR, Brace RA: Amniotic fluid index (AFI) in the term ovine pregnancy: a predictable relationship between AFI and amniotic fluid volume. In: Proceedings of the 35th Annual Meeting of the Society for Gynecologic Investigation, Baltimore, Maryland, March 1988

41. Moore TR: Superiority of the four-quadrant sum over the single-deepest-pocket technique in ultrasonographic identification of abnormal amniotic fluid volumes. Am J Obstet Gynecol 163:762, 1990

42. Nyberg DA, Mahony BS, Pretorius DH: Diagnostic Ultrasound and Fetal Anomalies: Text and Atlas. Year Book Medical Publishers, Chicago, 1990

43. Romero R, Pilu G, Jeanty P et al: Prenatal Diagnosis of Congenital Anomalies. Appleton & Lange, Norwalk, CT, 1988

44. Seeds JS, Azizkhan RG: Congenital Malformations: Antenatal Diagnosis, Perinatal Management, and Counseling. Aspen Publishers, Rockville, MD, 1990

45. Chervenak FA, Isaacson G, Lorber J: Anomalies of the Fetal Head, Neck and Spine: Ultrasound Diagnosis and Management. WB Saunders, Philadelphia, 1988

46. Vintzileos AM, Campbell WA, Nochimson DJ, Weinbaum PJ: Antenatal evaluation and management of ultrasonically detected fetal anomalies. Obstet Gynecol 69:640, 1987

47. Leopold GR: Antepartum obstetrical ultrasound examination guidelines. J Ultrasound Med 5:241, 1986

48. Filly RA: Level 1, level 2, level 3 obstetric sonography: I'll see your level and raise you one. Radiology 172:312, 1989

49. Campbell S, Johnstone FD, Hold EM et al: Anencephaly: early ultrasonic diagnosis and active management. Lancet 2:1226, 1972

50. Chervenak FA, Isaacson G, Mahoney MJ et al: The obstetric significance of holoprosencephaly. Obstet Gynecol 63:115, 1984

51. Romero R, Cullen M, Grannum P et al: Antenatal diagnosis of renal anomalies with ultrasound. III. Bilateral renal agenesis. Am J Obstet Gynecol 151:38, 1985

52. Chervenak FA, Isaacson G, Touloukian R et al: The diagnosis and management of fetal teratomas. Obstet Gynecol 66:666, 1985

53. Chervenak FA, Isaacson G, Blakemore KJ et al: Fetal cystic hygroma: cause and natural history. N Engl J Med 309:822, 1984

54. Holzgreve W, Curry CJR, Golbus MS: Investigation of nonimmune hydrops fetalis. Am J Obstet Gynecol 150:805, 1984

55. Arey LB: Developmental Anatomy. pp. 245, 465. WB Saunders, Philadelphia, 1974

56. Chervenak FA, Isaacson G, Mahoney MJ et al: The diagnosis and management of fetal cephalocele. Obstet Gynecol 64:86, 1984

57. Hobbins JC, Venus I, Tortora M et al: Stage II ultrasound examination for the diagnosis of fetal abnormalities with an elevated amniotic fluid alpha-fetoprotein concentration. Am J Obstet Gynecol 142:1026, 1982

58. McIntosh R: The incidence of congenital malformations: a study of 5,964 pregnancies. Pediatrics 14:505, 1954

59. Nicolaides KH, Campbell S, Gabbe SG, Guidetti R: Ultrasound screening for spina bifida: cranial and cerebellar signs. Lancet 2:72, 1986

60. Van den Hof MC, Nicolaides KH, Campbell J, Campbell S: Evaluation of the lemon and banana signs in one hundred thirty fetuses with open spina bifida. Am J Obstet Gynecol 162:322, 1990

61. Nakayama DK, Harrison RM, Gross BH et al: Management of the fetus with an abdominal wall defect. J Pediatr Surg 19:408, 1984

62. Marwood RP, Dawson MR, Gross BH et al: Antenatal diagnosis of diaphragmatic hernias. Br J Obstet Gynaecol 88:71, 1981

63. Cardoza JD, Goldstein RB, Filly RA: Exclusion of fetal ventriculomegaly with a single measurement: the width of the lateral ventricular atrium. Radiology 169:711, 1988

64. Chervenak FA, Berkowitz RL, Romero R et al: The diagnosis of fetal hydrocephalus. Am J Obstet Gynecol 147:703, 1983

65. Chervenak FA, Duncan C, Ment LR et al: The outcome of fetal ventriculomegaly. Lancet 2:179, 1984

66. Cardoza JD, Filly RA, Podarsky AE: The dangling choroid plexus: a sonographic observation of value in excluding ventriculomegaly. Am J Radiol 151:767, 1988

67. Benaceraff BR, Birnholz JC: The diagnosis of fetal hydrocephalus prior to 22 weeks. J Clin Ultrasound 15:531, 1987

68. Benaceraff BR: Fetal hydrocephalus: diagnosis and significance. Radiology 169:858, 1988

69. Johnson M, Dunne M, Mack L et al: Evaluation of fetal intracranial anatomy by static and real-time ultrasound. J Clin Ultrasound 8:311, 1980

70. Lees RF, Alford BA, Brenbridge NAG et al: Sonographic appearance of duodenal atresia in utero. AJR 131:701, 1978

71. Hobbins JC, Romero R, Grannum P et al: Antenatal diagnosis of renal anomalies with ultrasound. I. Obstructive uropathy. Am J Obstet Gynecol 148:868, 1984

72. Sanders R, Graham D: Twelve cases of hydronephrosis in utero diagnosed by ultrasonography. J Ultrasound Med 1:341, 1982

73. Deter RL, Harrist RB, Birnholz JC, Hadlock FP: Quantitative Obstetrical Ultrasonography. Churchill Livingstone, New York, 1986

74. Chervenak FA, Jeanty P, Cantraine F et al: The diagnosis of fetal microcephaly. Am J Obstet Gynecol 149:512, 1984

75. Chervenak FA, Rosenberg J, Brigthman RC et al: A prospective study of the accuracy of ultrasound in predicting fetal microcephaly. Obstet Gynecol 69:908, 1987

76. Romero R, Pilu G, Jeanty P et al: Prenatal Diagnosis of Congenital Anomalies. p. 311. Appleton & Lange, Norwalk, CT, 1988

77. Campbell J, Henderson A, Campbell S: The fetal femur/foot length ratio: a new parameter to assess dysplastic limb reduction. Obstet Gynecol 72:181, 1988

78. Chervenak FA, Tortora M, Mayden K et al: Antenatal diagnosis of median cleft face syndrome: sonographic demonstration of cleft lip and hypotelorism. Am J Obstet Gynecol 149:94, 1984

79. Grannum P, Bracken M, Silverman R et al: Assessment of fetal kidney size in normal gestation by comparison of ratio of kidney circumference to abdominal circumference. Am J Obstet Gynecol 136:249, 1980

80. Romero R, Cullen M, Jeanty P et al: The diagnosis of congenital renal anomalies with ultrasound. II. Infan-

tile polycystic kidney disease. Am J Obstet Gynecol 150:259, 1984

81. Chervenak FA, Tortora MN, Hobbins JC: Antenatal sonographic diagnosis of clubfoot. J Ultrasound Med 4:49, 1985

82. Goldberg JD, Chervenak FA, Lipman RA et al: Antenatal sonographic diagnosis of arthrogryposis multiplex congenita. Prenat Diagn 6:45, 1986

83. Allan LD, Crawford DC, Anderson RH et al: Echocardiographic and anatomical correlation in fetal congenital heart disease. Br Heart J 52:542, 1984

84. Copel JA, Pilu G, Green J et al: Fetal echocardiographic screening for congenital heart disease: the importance of the four-chamber view. Am J Obstet Gynecol 157:648, 1987

85. Gertgesell HP (ed): Symposium of fetal echocardiography. J Clin Ultrasound 13:227, 1985

86. Copel JA, Pilu G, Kleinmann CS: Congenital heart disease and extracardiac anomalies: associations and indications for fetal echocardiography. Am J Obstet Gynecol 154:1121, 1986

87. Palmer CG, Miles JH, Howard-Peebles PN et al: Fetal karyotype following ascertainment of fetal anomalies by ultrasound. Prenat Diagn 7:551, 1987

88. Platt LD, DeVore GR, Lopez E et al: Role of amniocentesis in ultrasound-detected fetal malformations. Obstet Gynecol 68:153, 1986

89. Williamson RA, Weiner CP, Patil S et al: Abnormal pregnancy sonogram: selective indication for fetal karyotype. Obstet Gynecol 69:15, 1987

90. Chervenak FA, McCullough LB: An ethically justified, clinically comprehensive management strategy for third-trimester pregnancies complicated by fetal anomalies. Obstet Gynecol 75:311, 1990

91. Chervenak FA, McCullough LB: Does obstetric ethics have any role in the obstetrician's response to the abortion controversy? Am J Obstet Gynecol 163:1425, 1990

92. Harrison M, Golbus M, Filly R: The Unborn Patient. Grune & Stratton, New York, 1984

93. Romero R, Oyarzun E, Sirtori M, Hobbins JC: Detection and management of anatomic congenital anomalies. Obstet Gynecol Clin North Am 15:215, 1988

94. Chervenak FA, Berkowitz RL, Tortora M et al: The management of fetal hydrocephalus. Am J Obstet Gynecol 151:933, 1985

95. Chervenak FA, Duncan D, Ment LR et al: Perinatal management of meningomyelocele. Obstet Gynecol 63:376, 1984

96. Manning FA, Harrison MR, Rodeck C et al: Catheter shunts for fetal hydronephrosis and hydrocephalus: special report. N Engl J Med 315:336, 1986

97. Manning FA, Harman CR, Lange IR et al: Antepartum chronic fetal vesicoamniotic shunts for obstetric uropathy: a report of two cases. Am J Obstet Gynecol 145:819, 1983

98. Anderson RL, Golbus MS: Bladder aspiration. In Chervenak FA, Isaacson G, Campbell S (eds): Textbook of Ultrasound in Obstetrics and Gynecology. Little, Brown, Boston (in press)

99. Rodeck CH, Fisk NM, Fraser DI, Nicolini U: Long-term in utero drainage of fetal hydrothorax. N Engl J Med 319:1135, 1988

100. Clewell WH, Johnson ML, Meier PR et al: A surgical approach to the treatment of fetal hydrocephalus. N Engl J Med 306:1320, 1982

101. Harrison MR, Adzick NS, Longaker MT et al: Successful repair in utero of a fetal diaphragmatic hernia after removal of herniated viscera from the left thorax. N Engl J Med 322:1582, 1990

102. *Roe v. Wade*, 410 U.S. 113, 1973

103. Elias S, Annas GJ: Reproductive Genetics and the Law. Year Book Medical Publishers, Chicago, 1987

104. Annas GJ: Protecting the liberty of pregnant patients. N Engl J Med 316:1213, 1987

105. Chervenak FA, Farley MA, Walters L et al: When is termination of pregnancy during the third trimester morally justifiable? N Engl J Med 310:501, 1984

106. Chervenak FA, McCullough LB: Nonaggressive obstetric management: an option for some fetal anomalies during the third trimester. JAMA 261:3439, 1989

107. Chervenak FA, McCullough LB: Ethical challenges in perinatal medicine: the intrapartum management of pregnancy complicated by fetal hydrocephalus with macrocephaly. Semin Perinatol 11:232, 1987

108. Ultrasound in Pregnancy. ACOG Tech Bull 116, May 1988

109. Horger EO, Tsai CC: Ultrasound and the prenatal diagnosis of congenital anomalies: a medicolegal perspective. Obstet Gynecol 74:617, 1989

110. Thacker SB: Quality of controlled clinical trials. The case of imaging ultrasound in obstetrics: a review. Br J Obstet Gynaecol 92:437, 1985

111. Ewigman B, LeFevre M, Hesser J: A randomized trial of routine prenatal ultrasound. Obstet Gynecol 76:189, 1990

112. Ewigman B, LeFevre M, Bain RP et al: Ethics and routine ultrasonography in pregnancy. Am J Obstet Gynecol 163:256, 1990

113. Kalter H, Warkany J: Congenital malformations: etiologic factors and their role in prevention, part 1. N Engl J Med 308:424, 1983

114. Kalter H, Warkany J: Congenital malformations: etiologic factors and their role in prevention, part 2. N Engl J Med 308:491, 1983

115. Chitty L, Campbell S: Screening with realtime ultra-

sound for fetal anomalies. In Chervenak FA, Isaacson G, Campbell S (eds): Textbook of Ultrasound in Obstetrics and Gynecology. Little, Brown, Boston (in press)

116. Hegge FN, Franklin RW, Watson PT, Calhoun BC: An evaluation of the time of discovery of fetal malformations by an indication-based system for ordering obstetric ultrasound. Obstet Gynecol 74:21, 1989

117. Saari-Kemppainen A, Karjalainen O, Ylostalo P et al: Ultrasound screening and perinatal mortality: controlled trial of systematic one-stage screening in pregnancy. Lancet 2:387, 1990

118. Campbell S, Warsof SL, Little D, Cooper DJ: Routine ultrasound screening for the prediction of gestational age. Obstet Gynecol 65:613, 1985

119. Waldenstrom U, Axelsson O, Nilsson S et al: Effects of routine one-stage ultrasound screening in pregnancy: a randomized controlled trial. Lancet 2:585, 1988

120. Warsof SL, Cooper DJ, Little D, Campbell S: Routine ultrasound screening for antenatal detection of intrauterine growth retardation. Obstet Gynecol 67:33, 1986

121. Cox DN, Wittman BK, Hess M et al: The psychological impact of diagnostic ultrasound. Obstet Gynecol 70:673, 1987

122. Chervenak FA, McCullough LB, Chervenak JL: Prenatal informed consent for sonogram: an indication for obstetric ultrasonography. Am J Obstet Gynecol 161:857, 1989

123. Gabbe SG, Iams JD: Intrauterine growth retardation. p. 169. In Iams JD, Zuspan FP (eds): Manual of Obstetrics and Gynecology. CV Mosby, St. Louis, 1990

124. Campbell S: Fetal growth. p. 288. In Beard RS, Nathanielsz PW (eds): Fetal Physiology in Medicine, The Basis of Perinatology. WB Saunders, Philadelphia, 1976

125. Chudleigh P, Pearce JM: Obstetric Ultrasound. Churchill Livingstone, Edinburgh, 1986

Chapter 13

Antepartum Fetal Evaluation

Steven G. Gabbe

Antenatal care in this century has undergone a sea change. It began as a charitable concern for the indigent, often unmarried mother. As, one by one, the causes of maternal death were eliminated, the focus of care shifted to her unborn baby. Now we are approaching the point where nearly every established pregnancy ends in the birth of a live, surviving baby, and the proper concern of antenatal care is the quality of the product.[1]

Antepartum fetal deaths now account for more than one-half of all perinatal mortality in the United States. As emphasized by Chard and Klopper,[1] the obstetrician must be concerned not only with prevention of this mortality, but also with the detection of fetal compromise and the timely delivery of such infants in an effort to maximize their future potential. This chapter reviews the definition and causes of perinatal mortality, the techniques available for assessing fetal condition, how one may evaluate their diagnostic accuracy, and the clinical application of these techniques to obstetric practice.

THE ETIOLOGY OF PERINATAL MORTALITY

The perinatal mortality rate (PMR) has been defined by the National Center for Health Statistics (NCHS) as the number of late fetal deaths (fetal deaths of 28 weeks or more gestation) plus early neonatal deaths (deaths of infants 0 to 6 days of age) per 1,000 live births plus fetal deaths.[2] A live birth is the complete expulsion or extraction from its mother of a product of conception, irrespective of the duration of the pregnancy, that, after separation, breathes or shows any evidence of life, such as beating of the heart, pulsation of the umbilical cord, or definite movement of voluntary muscles, whether or not the umbilical cord has been cut or the placenta is attached; each product of such a birth is considered liveborn. According to the NCHS, the neonatal mortality rate is defined as the number of neonatal deaths (deaths of infants 0 to 27 days of age) per 1,000 live births; the postneonatal mortality rate, the number of postneonatal deaths (the number of infants 28 to 365 days of age) per 1,000 live births; and the infant mortality rate, the number of infant deaths (deaths of infants under 1 year of age) per 1,000 live births. The definition of PMR provided by the World Health Organization is somewhat different, including the number of fetuses and live births weighing at least 500 g or, when birth weight is unavailable, the corresponding gestational age (22 weeks) or body length (25 cm crown–heel), dying before day 7 of life per 1,000 such fetuses and infants.

Since 1965, the PMR in the United States has fallen steadily by an average of approximately 3 percent per year.[3] The overall PMR reported in 1986 was 13.3/1,000. The total number of fetal deaths recorded has fallen each year from approximately 33,000 in 1980

377

to 29,000 in 1986, and the fetal death rate has declined from 9.2 to 7.7/1,000. While the fetal death rate has fallen 16 percent in the past 6 years, the neonatal mortality rate has declined 21 percent. Of all fetal deaths in the United States, 22 percent now take place between 36 to 40 weeks gestation and approximately 10 percent beyond 41 weeks gestation. While the majority of fetal deaths occur before 32 weeks gestation, Grant and Elbourne[4] have emphasized that in planning a strategy for antepartum fetal monitoring one must examine the risk of fetal death in the population of women who are still pregnant at that point in pregnancy. When this approach is taken, one finds that fetuses at 40 to 41 weeks are at a 3-fold greater risk, and those at 42 or more weeks are at a 12-fold greater risk for intrauterine death than fetuses at 28 to 31 weeks.

The overall pattern of perinatal deaths in the United States appears to have changed considerably during the past 25 years. Data collected between 1959 and 1966 by the Collaborative Perinatal Project reveal that 30 percent of perinatal deaths could be attributed to complications of the cord and placenta.[5] Other major causes of perinatal loss were maternal and fetal infections (17 percent), prematurity (10 percent), congenital anomalies (8 percent), and erythroblastosis fetalis (4 percent). In this series, 21 percent of the deaths were of unknown cause. In 1982, the major cause of early neonatal deaths was attributed to conditions originating in the perinatal period, such as infections, intraventricular hemorrhage, hydrops, meconium aspiration, and maternal complications such as diabetes mellitus and hypertension.[2] Congenital anomalies were the second leading cause of early neonatal death, accounting for 23 percent of such losses, while intrauterine hypoxia and birth asphyxia were responsible for 5 percent. In 1986, congenital anomalies emerged as the leading cause of infant mortality, with approximately 25 percent of deaths attributed to birth defects[6] (Fig. 13.1). Prematurity was the most common cause of mortality among nonmalformed infants. Intrauterine hypoxia and birth asphyxia were responsible for approximately 3 percent of all infant deaths.

Fetal deaths may be divided into those that occur during the antepartum period and those that occur during labor, intrapartum stillbirths. The antepartum death rate in an unmonitored population is approximately 8/1,000. In a recent review, 86 percent of fetal deaths occurred before the onset of labor.[7] Manning et al.[8] point out that antepartum deaths may be divided into four broad categories: (1) chronic asphyxia of diverse origin; (2) congenital malformations; (3) superimposed complications of pregnancy, such as Rh isoimmunization, placental abruption, and fetal infection; and (4) deaths of unexplained cause. If it is to succeed, a program of antenatal surveillance must identify the malformed fetus (see Ch. 12) and recognize those at risk for asphyxia.

Recent data describing the etiology of fetal deaths in the United States are not available. However, Lammer and his colleagues[7] reviewed the causes of 574 fetal deaths in Massachusetts during 1982. For the first time, the fetal mortality rate in that state exceeded the neonatal mortality rate, emphasizing that if further decreases in the PMR are to be achieved, they will need to come from reductions in fetal as well as neonatal mortality. Fetal mortality was higher among women who were black, unmarried, over age 34 years, under age 20 years, of parity 5 or more, and who received no prenatal care or care only in the third trimester. Ten percent of all fetal deaths occurred in multiple gestations, for a fetal mortality rate of 50/1,000, or a rate seven times that of women with singleton pregnancies. More than one-half of all fetal deaths were assigned to either asphyxia or maternal conditions, including hypertension and placental abruption and infarction. Overall, 30 percent of the fetal deaths were assigned to maternal causes, 28 percent to hypoxia, 12 percent to congenital anomalies, and 4 percent to infection. In almost 25 percent, no cause could be identified. Of note, when autopsy data were reviewed, there was disagreement between the fetal death record and autopsy findings in 55 percent of cases.

In summary, based on available data, approximately 30 percent of antepartum fetal deaths may be attributed to asphyxia; 25 percent to maternal complications, especially hypertension, preeclampsia, and placental abruption; 20 percent to congenital malformations; and 5 percent to infection. At least 25 percent of stillbirths will have no obvious etiology.

Can these antepartum fetal deaths be prevented? Grant and Elbourne[4] have noted that "antepartum late fetal death is the component of perinatal mortality that has shown greatest resistance to change over

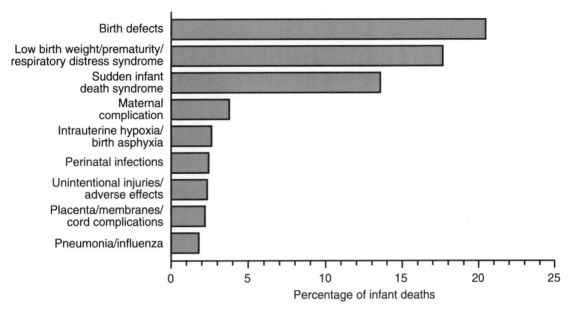

Fig. 13.1 Leading causes of infant mortality—United States, 1986.

recent years. In part, this reflects its relative unpredictability; in part, it reflects the relatively long period of time over which it can occur." Obstetric and pediatric assessors reviewed the circumstances surrounding each case of perinatal death in the Mersey region of England to identify any avoidable factors contributing to the deaths.[9] There were 309 perinatal deaths in this population, consisting of 157 stillbirths and 152 deaths in the first week of life. Of the 309 perinatal deaths, 182 (58.9 percent) were considered to have had avoidable factors. Most avoidable factors were found to be obstetric as compared with pediatric or maternal and social factors. A high proportion (73.8 percent) of normal-birth-weight infants with no fetal abnormalities and no maternal complications had avoidable factors. The failure to respond appropriately to abnormalities during pregnancy and labor, such as abnormal results from the monitoring of fetal growth or intrapartum fetal well-being, significant maternal weight loss, or reported reductions in fetal movement, constituted the largest groups of avoidable obstetric factors. A recent study by Kirkup and Welch[10] confirmed these results in an analysis of avoidable factors contributing to fetal death in nonmalformed infants weighing 2,500 g or more. Pa-

tients at highest risk for fetal death included women of parity 3 or more and those who had no prenatal care before 20 weeks. The Mersey Region Working Party on Perinatal Mortality concluded that, in light of increasing public awareness about obstetric management and, in some instances, an antipathy toward modern procedures, the failure to act on abnormalities discovered during monitoring would assume greater importance.[9] These workers found that in no case was the induction of labor as a result of such monitoring considered an avoidable factor.

A large clinical experience has demonstrated that antepartum fetal assessment can have a significant impact on the frequency and causes of antenatal fetal deaths. Schneider and her colleagues[11] reviewed a decade of experience with antepartum fetal heart rate monitoring from 1974 through 1983. The contraction stress test was used primarily during the first 2 years of the study, followed by the nonstress test. Overall, the perinatal mortality was found to be 22.4/1,000 in the nontested population and 11.8/1,000 in the tested high-risk population, a highly significant difference. The stillbirth rate in the nontested population, 11.1/1,000, was twice that of patients who were followed with antepartum surveillance. When corrected for congenital anomalies, the stillbirth rate in the tested high-risk population was only 2.2/1,000. Of 18 stillbirths within 7 days of testing, the majority were due to congenital anomalies and placental abruption.

In a carefully performed study, Stubblefield and Berek[12] reviewed the causes of perinatal death in term and post-term births at the Boston Hospital for Women. The most frequent cause of death of a term or post-term infant was extrinsic perinatal hypoxia, and the second most common cause was a lethal malformation. Overall, extrinsic perinatal hypoxia accounted for 56.1 percent of the deaths of term infants and 71.4 percent of the deaths of post-term infants. Major malformations were implicated in 26.3 percent of the deaths of term infants. Twenty-nine of the 32 antenatal deaths occurred between 37 and 42 weeks gestation. The investigators concluded that two-thirds of the antenatal deaths were associated with chronic processes such as placental infarction that might have been detected had routine antepartum fetal surveillance been used. In obstetric populations in which high-risk patients are monitored, the majority of stillbirths now occur in what had previously been considered normal pregnancies.[12]

APPLICATION OF ANTEPARTUM FETAL TESTING

Before using antepartum fetal testing, the obstetrician must ask several important questions[13]:

1. Does the test provide information not already known by the patient's clinical status?
2. Can the information be helpful in managing the patient?
3. Should an abnormality be detected, is there a treatment available for the problem?
4. Could an abnormal test result lead to increased risk for the mother and/or her fetus?
5. Will the test ultimately decrease perinatal morbidity and mortality?

Unfortunately, few of the tests commonly employed today in clinical practice have been subjected to prospective and randomized evaluations that can answer these questions.[14] In most cases, the test has been applied and, when good perinatal outcomes were observed, the test has gained further acceptance and has been used more widely. In such cases, one cannot be sure whether it is actually the information provided by the test that has led to the improved outcomes or whether it is the total program of care that has made the difference. When prospective randomized investigations are conducted, large numbers of patients must be studied because many adverse outcomes such as intrauterine death are uncommon even in high-risk populations. While several controlled trials have failed to demonstrate improved outcomes with nonstress testing, the study populations ranged from only 300 to 530 subjects.[15-18]

Table 13.1 lists the information one might predict from an antepartum fetal test. Although one would want to detect intrauterine growth retardation (IUGR) or discover the presence of a significant congenital malformation, the most valuable information provided by antepartum fetal assessment may be that the fetus is well and requires no intervention. In this way, the pregnancy may be safely prolonged and the fetus allowed to gain further maturity. Table 13.2 lists those aspects of obstetric management that might be influenced by antepartum testing. Certainly, one would not want to begin a program of testing unless one were prepared to use the information. For this reason, most testing is initiated at approximately 28 weeks gestation when, if fetal compromise were detected and antenatal delivery were indicated, the fetus would have a good chance for intact survival. Improvements in neonatal care have played a significant role in our application of antepartum fetal testing. Should fetal distress be documented, the neonatal intensive care unit, not the uterus, may be the best place for the fetus.

Table 13.1 Aspects of Fetal Condition That Might Be Predicted by Antepartum Testing

Perinatal death
Intrauterine growth retardation (IUGR)
Fetal distress in labor
Neonatal asphyxia
Postnatal motor and intellectual impairment
Premature delivery
Congenital abnormalities
Need for specific therapy

(Adapted from Chard and Klopper,[1] with permission.)

Table 13.2 Obstetric Management That Might Be Influenced by Antepartum Testing

Preterm delivery
Route of delivery
Bedrest
Observation
Drug therapy
Operative intervention in labor
Neonatal intensive care
Termination of pregnancy for a congenital anomaly

(Adapted from Chard and Klopper,[1] with permission.)

In selecting the population of patients for antepartum fetal evaluation, one would certainly include those pregnancies known to be at high risk of uteroplacental insufficiency (Table 13.3).

The question of routine antepartum fetal surveillance must be carefully examined. Schifrin et al.[19] demonstrated that the results of antepartum fetal testing will more accurately predict fetal outcome than antenatal risk assessment using an established scoring system. Patients judged to be at high risk based on known medical factors but whose fetuses demonstrated normal antepartum fetal evaluation had a lower PMR than did patients considered at low risk whose fetuses had abnormal antepartum testing results. As emphasized by Stubblefield and Berek,[12] routine antepartum fetal evaluation would be necessary to detect most infants dying in utero as the result of hypoxia and asphyxia. It would seem reasonable to consider extending some form of antepartum fetal surveillance to all obstetric patients. As described

below, assessment of fetal activity by the mother may be an ideal technique for this purpose.

STATISTICAL ASSESSMENT OF ANTEPARTUM TESTING

To determine the clinical application of antepartum diagnostic testing, the predictive value of the tests must be considered.[20] This information can most easily be presented in a 2×2 matrix. Table 13.4 presents this matrix using the contraction stress test (CST) and intrauterine fetal death as examples. The sensitivity of the test is the probability that the test will be positive or abnormal when the disease is present. The specificity of the test is the probability that the test result will be negative when the disease is not present. Note that the sensitivity and specificity refer not to the actual number of patients with a positive or abnormal result but to the proportion or probability of these test results. The predictive value of an abnormal test would be that fraction of patients with an abnormal test result who have the abnormal condition, while the predictive value of a normal test would be the fraction of patients with a normal test result who are normal (Table 13.4).

Antepartum fetal tests may be used to screen a large obstetric population to detect fetal disease. In this setting, a test of high sensitivity is preferable, since one would not want to miss patients whose fetuses might be compromised. One would be willing to overdiagnose the problem, that is, to accept some false-positive diagnoses. In further evaluating the patient whose fetus may be at risk and when attempting

Table 13.3 Indications for Antepartum Fetal Monitoring

1. Patients at high risk of uteroplacental insufficiency
   Prolonged pregnancy
   Diabetes mellitus
   Hypertension
   Previous stillbirth
   Suspected IUGR
   Advanced maternal age
2. When other tests suggest fetal compromise
   Suspected IUGR
   Decreased fetal movement
   Rh disease
3. Routine antepartum surveillance

IUGR, intrauterine growth retardation.

Table 13.4 Two-by-Two Matrix of Possible Results for the Contraction Stress Test (CST)

	Perinatal Outcome	
Test Result	Normal (Normal Newborn)	Abnormal (Intrauterine Fetal Death)
Normal (negative CST)	A True negative	B False negative
Abnormal (positive CST)	C False positive	D True positive

Sensitivity = D/(D + B).
Specificity = A/(A + C).
Predictive value of a positive test = D/(C + D).
Predictive value of a negative test = A/(A + B).

to confirm the presence of disease, one would want a test of high specificity. One would not want to intervene unnecessarily and deliver a fetus that was doing well. In this setting, multiple tests may be helpful. When multiple test results are normal, they tend to exclude disease. When all are abnormal, however, they tend to support the diagnosis of fetal disease.

The prevalence of the abnormal condition has great impact on the predictive value of antepartum fetal tests. Table 13.5 presents data for a population of 1,000 patients in whom the prevalence of the disease is 50 percent. The sensitivity of the test being used is 75 percent, and its specificity is 98 percent. These figures are similar to those observed for several antepartum tests now in use. In this setting, an abnormal test result is likely to be associated with a true fetal abnormality. The predictive value of a positive test is 97.4 percent. However, when the prevalence of the disease falls to 2 percent, as it may for intrauterine fetal deaths, even tests with a high sensitivity and specificity are associated with many false predictions (Table 13.6). In this circumstance, an abnormal test is more likely to indicate a false-positive diagnosis ($n = 20$) than it is a true-positive diagnosis ($n = 15$).

In interpreting the results of studies of antepartum testing, obstetricians must consider the application of that test to their own patient populations. If the study has been done in patients at great risk, it is more likely that an abnormal test will be associated with an abnormal fetus. If the obstetrician is practicing in a community with patients who are, in general, at low risk, however, an abnormal test result would more likely be associated with a false-positive diagnosis.

For most antepartum diagnostic tests, a cutoff point used to define an abnormal result must be arbitrarily established.[21] The cutoff point is selected to maximize the separation between the normal and diseased populations (Fig. 13.2). Changing the cutoff will have great impact on the predictive value of the test. For example, suppose that 10 accelerations in 10 minutes were required for a fetus to have a reactive nonstress test (threshold A). The fetus who fulfilled this rigid definition would almost certainly be in good condition. However, many fetuses who failed to achieve 10 accelerations in 10 minutes would also be in good condition but would be judged to be abnormal by this cutoff. In this instance, the test would have many abnormal results. It would be highly sensitive and capture all of the abnormal fetuses, but it would have a low specificity. If the number of accelerations required to pass a nonstress test were lowered to one in 10 minutes, it would decrease the sensitivity of the test (threshold C). That is, one might miss a truly sick fetus. At the same time, however, one would improve the specificity of the test or its ability to predict that percentage of the patients who are normal. Using the criterion of two accelerations of the fetal heart rate in 20 minutes for a reactive nonstress test (threshold B), it is hoped that one will have a test with both high sensitivity and high specificity.

Table 13.6 Two Percent Prevalence

Test Result	Perinatal Outcome	
	Normal	Abnormal
Normal	960 True negative	5 False negative
Abnormal	20 False positive	15 True positive

Sensitivity = 75%.
Specificity = 98%.
Predictive value of a positive test = 42.8% (15/35).
Predictive value of a negative test = 99.4% (960/965).

Table 13.5 Fifty Percent Prevalence

Test Result	Perinatal Outcome	
	Normal	Abnormal
Normal	490 True negative	125 False negative
Abnormal	10 False positive	375 True positive

Sensitivity = 75%.
Specificity = 98%.
Predictive value of a positive test = 97.4% (375/385).
Predictive value of a negative test = 79.6% (490/615).

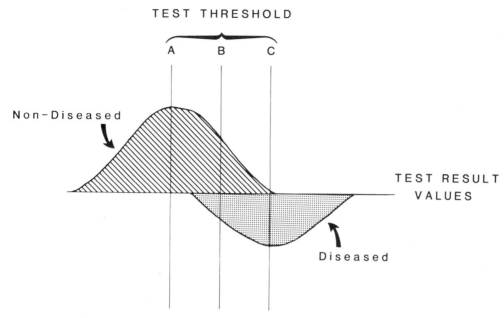

Fig. 13.2 Hypothetical distribution of test results in a normal and diseased population, demonstrating the differences in test sensitivity and specificity with a change in test threshold. Making it more difficult for the fetus to pass the test by raising the test threshold (A) will increase the sensitivity, but decrease the specificity, of the test. On the other hand, making the test easier to pass by decreasing the test threshold (C) will increase the specificity of the test, but decrease the sensitivity. (Adapted from Carpenter and Coustan,[21] with permission.)

BIOCHEMICAL ANALYSES FOR ANTEPARTUM EVALUATION

Biochemical tests, such as urinary and plasma estriols and human placental lactogen, were among the first techniques applied to assess fetal well-being. This approach has been largely abandoned today. These assays were expensive, not always available, and difficult to interpret. Furthermore, they were associated with many false-negative (human placental lactogen) and false-positive (estriol) results.[22]

BIOPHYSICAL TECHNIQUES FOR FETAL EVALUATION

Fetal State

When interpreting tests that monitor fetal biophysical characteristics, one must appreciate that, during the third trimester, the normal fetus may exhibit marked changes in its neurologic state.[22,23] The near-term fetus spends approximately 90 percent of its time in a quiet (state 1F) or active (state 2F) sleep state. Active sleep is associated with rapid eye movements (REM). In fetal lambs, electrocortical activity during REM sleep is characterized by low-voltage, high-frequency waves. The fetus exhibits regular breathing movements and intermittent abrupt movements of its head, limbs, and trunk. The fetal heart rate in active sleep exhibits increased variability and frequent accelerations with movement. During quiet, or non-REM, sleep, the fetal heart rate slows and heart rate variability is reduced. The fetus may make infrequent breathing movements and startled movements. Electrocortical activity recordings at this time reveal high-voltage, low-frequency waves. Near term, periods of quiet sleep may last 20 minutes, and those of active sleep approximately 40 minutes. The mechanisms that control these periods of rest and activity in the fetus are not well established. External factors such as the mother's activity, her ingestion of drugs, and her nutrition may all play a role.

When evaluating fetal condition with the non-stress test or the biophysical profile, one must ask whether a fetus that is not making breathing movements or shows no accelerations of its baseline heart rate is in a quiet sleep state or is neurologically compromised. In such circumstances, prolonging the period of evaluation will usually allow a change in fetal state, and more normal parameters of fetal well-being will appear.

Maternal Assessment of Fetal Activity

Maternal assessment of fetal activity is a simple yet valuable method for monitoring fetal condition. Most patients can understand and follow protocols for counting fetal activity, and this method is obviously inexpensive. Therefore, maternal assessment of fetal activity may be ideal for routine antepartum fetal surveillance.

Studies performed using real-time ultrasonography have demonstrated that during the third trimester the human fetus spends 10 percent of its time making gross body movements and that 30 such movements are made each hour.[24] Periods of active fetal body movement last approximately 40 minutes, while quiet periods last about 20 minutes. Patrick et al.[24] noted that the longest period without fetal movements in a normal fetus was approximately 75 minutes. The mother is able to appreciate about 70 to 80 percent of gross fetal movements. The fetus does make fine body movements such as limb flexion and extension, hand grasping, and sucking, which probably reflect more coordinated central nervous system (CNS) function. However, the mother is generally unable to perceive these fine movements. Fetal movement appears to peak between 9:00 P.M. and 1:00 A.M., a time when maternal glucose levels are falling.[24] In a study in which maternal glucose levels were carefully controlled with an artificial pancreas, Holden et al.[25] found that hypoglycemia was associated with increased fetal movement. Fetal activity does not increase after meals.

Maternal evaluation of fetal activity may reduce fetal deaths caused by asphyxia. Using a sheep model, Natale et al.[26] demonstrated that fetal activity is extremely sensitive to a decrease in fetal oxygenation. A small fall in fetal PO_2 was associated with a cessation of limb movements in the fetal lamb.

Several methods have been used to monitor fetal activity in clinical practice. In general, the presence of fetal movements is a reassuring sign of fetal health. However, the absence of fetal activity requires further assessment before one can conclude that fetal compromise exists. Sadovsky et al.[27] recommended that mothers count fetal activity for 30 to 60 minutes each day, two or three times daily. If the mother has fewer than three movements in an hour, or if she appreciates no movements for 12 hours, which is the movement alarm signal, further evaluation of fetal condition must be made. Rayburn et al.[28] suggested that patients count fetal activity at least 60 minutes each day. Fewer than three movements an hour for 2 consecutive days may be a sign of fetal compromise. Pearson and Weaver[29] advocated the use of the Cardiff Count-to-Ten chart. They found that only 2.5 percent of 1,654 daily movement counts recorded by 61 women who subsequently delivered healthy infants fell below 10 movements per 12 hours. Therefore, they accepted 10 movements as the minimum amount of fetal activity the patient should perceive in a 12-hour period. The patient is asked to start counting the movements in the morning and to record the time of day at which the tenth movement has been perceived. Should the patient not have 10 movements during 12 hours, or should it take longer each day to reach 10 movements, the patient is told to contact her obstetrician. Sadovsky et al.[30] found that, of those techniques currently used in clinical management, the movement alarm signal and the technique of Pearson and Weaver are the most valuable.

Whatever technique is used must be carefully explained to the patient. Draper et al.[31] observed that, while most women are reassured by keeping a fetal activity chart, some do become more anxious. Women who were concerned about monitoring fetal movement complained that they were not given adequate information about variations in fetal activity patterns and maternal perception of movement.

While there will be wide but normal variation in fetal activity and the appreciation of fetal movement by different mothers, with fetal movement counting, the mother and her fetus serve as their own control.[4] Factors that influence maternal assessment of fetal activity include placental location and amniotic fluid volume.[32] If the placenta is anterior, maternal perception of fetal movements may be decreased. Hydramnios will reduce the mother's appreciation of fetal activity. Hydramnios may be associated with a fetal anomaly and should be further evaluated using ultrasonography. Rayburn and Barr[33] reported that 26 percent of fetuses with major malformations show decreased fetal activity as compared with only 4 percent of normal fetuses. Anomalies of the CNS are most commonly associated with decreased activity.

Approximately 80 percent of all mothers will be able to comply with a program of counting fetal activity.[4,34] Maternal factors that influence the evaluation of fetal movement include maternal activity, obesity, and medications. Mothers appear to appreciate fetal movements best when resting in the left lateral recumbent position. Patients should therefore be told to lie down when counting fetal movement, an additional benefit of this approach to fetal evaluation. Obesity decreases maternal appreciation of fetal activity. Maternal medications such as narcotics or barbiturates may depress fetal movement.

Several large clinical studies have demonstrated the efficacy of maternal assessment of fetal activity in preventing unexplained fetal deaths. In a prospective randomized study, Neldam[34] asked one group of 1,562 pregnant patients at 32 weeks gestation to count fetal activity three times each week for 2 hours after their main meals. Fewer than three fetal movements each hour was regarded as a sign of potential fetal compromise and was further evaluated with an ultrasound examination and a nonstress test. In the monitored group of patients, only one stillbirth occurred. Ten stillbirths were noted in a control population of 1,549 women. Overall, 4 percent of patients in the monitored group reported their baby was not moving adequately, a low figure but one similar to that observed in other studies. Of these 60 patients, almost 25 percent were found to have a fetus in distress based on further antepartum testing. Neldam and colleagues attributed the prevention of 14 fetal deaths to the use of maternal assessment of fetal activity.

Rayburn[35] found that in the 5 percent of his patients who reported decreased fetal activity, the incidence of stillbirths was 60 times higher, the risk of fetal distress in labor two to three times higher, the incidence of low Apgar scores at delivery 10 times

greater, and the incidence of severe growth retardation 10 times higher. Rayburn also observed that the normal fetus does *not* decrease activity in the week before delivery.

Using the Cardiff Count-to-Ten chart, Liston et al.[36] noted that 11 of 150 high-risk patients (7.3 percent) reported fewer than 10 movements in a 12-hour period. Two of these patients suffered perinatal deaths, and 33 percent experienced fetal distress in labor. Overall, 60 percent of patients who reported decreased fetal activity did exhibit evidence of fetal compromise. The number of false alarms was quite manageable.

Two recent prospective studies have yielded conflicting results regarding the efficacy of fetal movement counting as a technique for preventing fetal deaths. Grant and his co-workers[37] recruited 68,000 European women who were randomly allocated within 33 pairs of clusters to either routine fetal movement counting using the Cardiff Count-to-Ten method or to standard care. Women counted for an average of almost 3 hours per day, and about 7 percent of the charts showed at least one alarm. Of concern, the rate of compliance for reporting decreased fetal movement was only 46 percent. Furthermore, compliance for charting movements and reporting alarms was lower among women who had a late fetal death. The antepartum death rates for nonmalformed singleton fetuses were equal in both experimental groups. However, in none of the 17 cases in which reduced movements were recognized and the fetus was still alive when the patient arrived at the hospital was an emergency delivery attempted. Why? Grant et al. concluded that intervention was not undertaken because of false reassurance from follow-up testing, especially heart rate monitoring, and because of errors in clinical judgment. One might conclude that this large prospective study failed to demonstrate a reduction in the antepartum fetal death rate as a result of fetal movement counting. However, what it seems to prove most clearly is that patient compliance is an essential part of this program, as is appropriate evaluation of the patient who presents with decreased fetal activity.

In contrast to the study by Grant and his co-workers, an investigation by Moore and Piacquadio[38] demonstrated an impressive reduction in fetal deaths resulting from a formal program of fetal movement counting. Patients used the count-to-ten approach but were told to monitor fetal activity in the evening, a time of increasing fetal movement. Most women observed 10 movements in an average of 21 minutes, and compliance was greater than 90 percent. Patients who did not perceive 10 movements in 2 hours, a level of fetal activity slightly more than five standard deviations below the mean, were told to report immediately for further evaluation. During a 7-month control period, a fetal mortality rate of 8.7/1,000 was observed in 2,519 patients, and 11 of 247 women who came to the hospital with a complaint of decreased fetal movement had already suffered an intrauterine death. During the study period, the fetal death rate fell to 2.1/1,000, and only 1 of 290 patients with decreased fetal movement presented after fetal death had occurred. The number of antepartum tests required to assess patients with decreased fetal activity rose 13 percent during the study period. This investigation has been expanded to include almost 6,000 patients, and a fetal death rate of 3.6/1,000, less than one-half that found in the control period, has been achieved.[39]

In conclusion, there appears to be a clearly established relationship between decreased fetal activity and fetal death. Therefore, it would seem prudent to request that *all* pregnant patients, regardless of their risk status, monitor fetal activity starting at 28 weeks gestation. (Fig. 13.3). The count-to-ten approach developed by Moore seems ideal.

Contraction Stress Test

CST, also known as the oxytocin challenge test, was the first biophysical technique widely applied to antepartum fetal surveillance. In contrast to biochemical assays such as estriol and human placental lactogen, the CST could be performed at any time, and the results were immediately available. It was well known that uterine contractions produced a reduction in blood flow to the intervillous space. Analyses of intrapartum fetal heart rate monitoring had demonstrated that a fetus with inadequate placental respiratory reserve would demonstrate late decelerations in response to hypoxia (see Ch. 15). The CST extended these observations to the antepartum period. The response of the fetus at risk for uteroplacental insufficiency to uterine contractions formed the basis for this test.

Performing the CST

The CST may be conducted in the labor and delivery suite or in an adjacent area, although the likelihood of fetal distress requiring immediate delivery in response to uterine contractions or hyperstimulation is extremely small. The CST should be performed by staff familiar with the principles and technique of such testing. In many institutions, an antenatal diagnostic unit has been developed for this purpose. The patient is placed in the semi-Fowler's position at a 30- to 45-degree angle with a slight left tilt to avoid the supine hypotensive syndrome. The fetal heart rate is recorded using a Doppler ultrasound transducer, while uterine contractions are monitored with the tocodynamometer. Maternal blood pressure is determined every 5 to 10 minutes to detect maternal hypotension.[40] Baseline fetal heart rate and uterine tone are first recorded for a period of approximately 10 to 20 minutes. In some cases adequate uterine activity will occur spontaneously, and additional uterine stimulation will not be necessary. An adequate CST requires uterine contractions of moderate intensity lasting approximately 40 to 60 seconds, with a frequency of three in 10 minutes. These criteria were selected to approximate the stress experienced by the fetus during the first stage of labor. If uterine activity is absent or inadequate, nipple stimulation is used to initiate contractions or intravenous oxytocin is begun. Oxytocin is administered by an infusion pump at 0.5 mU/min. The unfusion rate is doubled every 20 minutes until adequate uterine contractions have been achieved. One does not usually need to exceed 10 mU/min to produce adequate uterine activity. After the CST has been completed, the patient should be observed until uterine activity has returned to its baseline level. With nipple stimulation, the test may take approximately 30 minutes. If oxytocin is needed, 90 minutes may be required to perform the CST.

Contraindications to the test include those patients at high risk for premature labor, such as patients with premature rupture of the membranes, multiple gestation, and cervical incompetence, although the CST

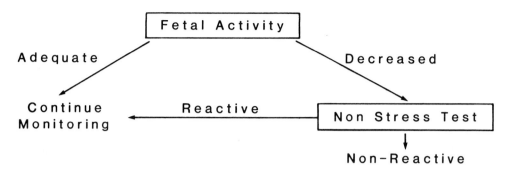

Fig. 13.3 Maternal assessment of fetal activity is a valuable screening test for fetal condition. Should the mother report decreased fetal activity, a nonstress test is performed. In this situation, most nonstress tests will be reactive. However, should a nonreactive nonstress test be observed, further evaluation as outlined in Figure 13.12 is necessary.

has not been associated with an increased incidence of premature labor.[41,42] The CST should also be avoided in conditions in which uterine contractions may be dangerous, such as a previous classical cesarean section or uterine surgery and placenta previa.

Interpreting the CST

The interpretation of the CST has varied from study to study. However, most investigators have utilized the definitions proposed by Freeman,[43] as presented in Table 13.7. In an attempt to decrease the frequency of suspicious tests that would require further evaluation, Martin and Schifrin[44] used the "10-min-

ute window" concept. A positive test would be any 10-minute segment of the tracing that includes three contractions, all showing late decelerations. A negative test is one in which no positive window is seen and there is at least one negative window, three uterine contractions in 10 minutes with no late decelerations (Figs. 13.4 and 13.5). The CST would be read as negative and not suspicious if an occasional late deceleration were seen but a negative window was also present. Schifrin has advocated that the term equivocal rather than suspicious be used for a CST with an occasional late deceleration but no negative window. Equivocal implies that one is unable to make a deter-

Table 13.7 Interpretation of the Contraction Stress Test

Interpretation	Description	Incidence (%)
Negative	No late decelerations appearing anywhere on the tracing with adequate uterine contractions (3 in 10 minutes)	80
Positive	Late decelerations that are consistent and persistent, present with the majority (>50 percent) of contractions without excessive uterine activity; if persistent late decelerations seen before the frequency of contractions are adequate, test interpreted as positive	3–5
Suspicious	Inconsistent late decelerations	5
Hyperstimulation	Uterine contractions closer than every 2 minutes or lasting >90 seconds, or five uterine contractions in 10 minutes; if no late decelerations seen, test interpreted as negative	5
Unsatisfactory	Quality of the tracing inadequate for interpretation or adequate uterine activity cannot be achieved	5

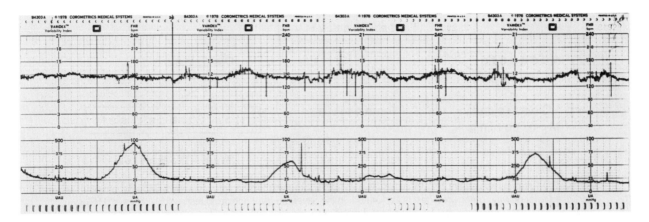

Fig. 13.4 A reactive and negative contraction stress test. With this result, the contraction stress test would ordinarily be repeated in 1 week.

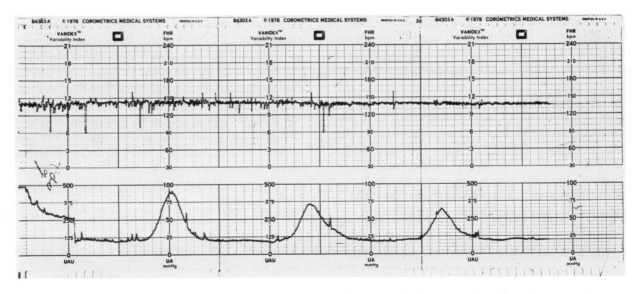

Fig. 13.5 A nonreactive and negative contraction stress test. After this result, the test would ordinarily be repeated in 24 hours.

mination of fetal condition based on the available information. A CST with both a positive and a negative window would be interpreted as positive.

Variable decelerations that occur during the CST may indicate the presence of oligohydramnios. In such cases, ultrasonography should be performed to assess amniotic fluid volume.

A negative CST has been consistently associated with good fetal outcome. A negative result therefore permits the obstetrician to prolong a high-risk preg-

nancy safely. In a series of 679 pregnancies complicated by a prolonged gestation, Freeman et al.[45] reported no perinatal deaths when the CST was used as the primary method of surveillance. Of 337 women with a previous intrauterine fetal death, none had a stillbirth during a pregnancy in which they were followed with CSTs.[46] Similarly, Gabbe et al.[47] noted no fetal deaths within 1 week of a negative CST in 198 pregnancies complicated by insulin-dependent diabetes. Other studies have shown the incidence of perinatal death within 1 week of a negative CST to be less than 1/1,000.[48-50] Many of these deaths, however, can be attributed to cord accidents, malformations, placental abruption, and acute deterioration of glucose control in patients with diabetes mellitus. Thus the CST, like most methods of antepartum fetal surveillance, cannot prevent acute fetal compromise. If the CST is negative, a repeat study is usually scheduled in 1 week. While testing patients with a weekly CST is practical, it is also arbitrary. Changes in the patient's clinical condition may warrant more frequent studies.

A positive CST has been associated with an increased incidence of intrauterine death, late decelerations in labor, low 5-minute Apgar scores, IUGR, and meconium-stained amniotic fluid (Fig. 13.6).[50] In a prospective and blind study, Ray et al.[51] observed three fetal deaths in 15 patients with positive CSTs. The incidence of low Apgar scores in this group was

53 percent. Overall, the likelihood of perinatal death after a positive CST has ranged from 7 to 15 percent. On the other hand, there has been a significant incidence of false-positive CSTs that, depending on the end point used, will average approximately 30 percent.[40] The positive CST is more likely to be associated with fetal compromise if the baseline heart rate lacks accelerations or "reactivity" and if the latency period between the onset of the uterine contraction and the onset of the late deceleration is less than 45 seconds.[52,53]

There is no doubt that the high incidence of false-positive CST results is one of the greatest limitations of this test, as such results could lead to unnecessary premature intervention. False-positive CSTs may be due to misinterpretation of the tracing; supine hypotension, which decreases uterine perfusion; uterine hyperstimulation, which is not appreciated using the tocodynamometer; or an improvement in fetal condi-

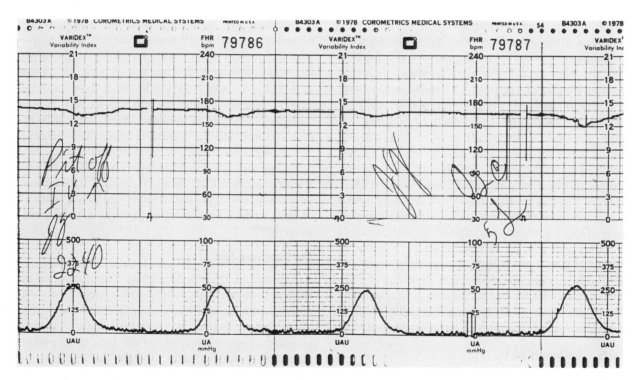

Fig. 13.6 A nonreactive and positive contraction stress test. At 40 weeks gestation, this patient reported no fetal activity for 18 hours. A nonstress test was nonreactive, and the contraction stress test was positive. Induction of labor was begun. Rupture of membranes yielded meconium-stained amniotic fluid. Soon thereafter, the patient underwent delivery by cesarean section for fetal distress. The infant weighed 7 lb and had Apgar scores of 2 at 1 minute and 8 at 5 minutes. (Courtesy of Dr. Dennis R. Johnson, York Hospital, York, PA.)

tion after the CST has been performed. The high false-positive rate also indicates that a patient with a positive CST need not necessarily be delivered by elective cesarean section. If a trial of labor is to be undertaken after a positive CST, the cervix should be favorable for induction so that direct fetal heart rate monitoring and careful assessment of uterine contractility with an intrauterine pressure catheter can be performed. False-positive results are not increased when the CST is used early in the third trimester.[54] A negative or positive CST obtained between 28 and 33 weeks gestation appears to have the same diagnostic significance as it would later in gestation.

A suspicious or equivocal CST should be repeated in 24 hours. Most of these tests will become negative. Bruce et al.[55] did observe that 5 of 67 patients (7.5 percent) with an initially suspicious CST exhibited positive tests on further evaluation. In 36 patients the CST became negative, whereas in 26 patients it remained suspicious. Like the suspicious CST, a test that is unsatisfactory or shows hyperstimulation should be repeated in 24 hours.

Several investigators have now performed follow-up studies of children who demonstrated a positive CST. Scanlon et al.[56] found that infants delivered within 24 hours of a positive CST showed poor state organization and reflexive performance. By contrast, Crane and co-workers[57] evaluated 12 children 5.5 months to 4.75 years after a positive CST and observed that most had grossly normal neurologic and psychologic development. Beischer et al.[58] assessed 45 children ranging in age from 2 months to 8 years, 9 months whose antenatal heart rate tests exhibited "critical fetal reserve," fetal heart rate baseline variability of less than 5 beats per minute (bpm), absence of accelerations, and late decelerations in response to Braxton Hicks contractions. In only four cases was significant neurologic impairment detected. An important determinant in the long-term outcome for these children would be the early recognition of fetal distress and the prevention of intrapartum asphyxia.

Nipple Stimulation in the CST

At the present time, most centers utilize nipple stimulation to produce the uterine contractions needed for the CST. With nipple stimulation, the CST can generally be completed in less time, and an intravenous infusion is not required. Therefore, this approach would appear to be an ideal first step in performing a CST.

Several methods have been used to induce adequate uterine activity.[59,60] The patient may first apply a warm moist towel to each breast for 5 minutes. If uterine activity is not adequate, the patient is asked to massage one nipple for 10 minutes. Using this protocol, Oki et al.[59] achieved adequate uterine contractions in 30 minutes or less in 87.5 percent of 657 patients tested. The incidence of negative tests (72 percent) and positive tests (2 percent) was not different from that seen with the oxytocin-induced CST. Huddleston et al.[61] reported great success using intermittent nipple stimulation. The patient gently strokes the nipple of one breast with the palmar surface of her fingers through her clothes for 2 minutes and then stops for 5 minutes. This cycle is repeated only as necessary to achieve adequate uterine activity. In a series of 193 patients and 345 CSTs, 97 percent of the tests required only three cycles of stimulation. The average time for a CST performed in this way was 45 minutes, and 67.5 percent of the patients completed their tests in 40 minutes or less. The nipple stimulation CST was negative in 80.3 percent of patients and positive in 2.6 percent of patients. All the patient's in the series of Huddleston et al. were able to achieve adequate uterine contractions with nipple stimulation, and none required an oxytocin infusion. Intermittent rather than continuous nipple stimulation is important in avoiding hyperstimulation. Defined as contractions lasting more than 90 seconds or five or more contractions in 10 minutes, hyperstimulation has been reported in approximately 2 percent of tests when intermittent nipple stimulation is employed.[62,63]

The Nonstress Test

As Hammacher[64] noted in 1969, "the fetus can be regarded as safe especially if reflex movements are accompanied by an obvious increase in the amplitude of oscillations in the basal fetal heart rate." This observation that accelerations of the fetal heart rate in response to fetal activity, uterine contractions, or stimulation reflect fetal well-being has formed the basis for the nonstress test (NST), the most widely applied technique for antepartum fetal evaluation.

In late gestation, the healthy fetus exhibits an average of 34 accelerations above the baseline fetal heart rate each hour.[65] These accelerations, which average 20 to 25 bpm in amplitude and approximately 40 seconds in duration, require intact neurologic coupling between the fetal CNS and the fetal heart.[65] Fetal hypoxia will disrupt this pathway. At term, fetal accelerations are associated with fetal movement more than 85 percent of the time, and more than 90 percent of gross movements are accompanied by accelerations. Fetal heart rate accelerations may be absent during periods of quiet fetal sleep. Studies by Patrick et al.[65] demonstrated that the longest time between successive accelerations in the healthy term fetus is approximately 40 minutes. However, the fetus may fail to exhibit heart rate accelerations for up to 80 minutes and still be normal.

While an absence of fetal heart rate accelerations is most often due to a quiet fetal sleep state, CNS depressants such as narcotics and phenobarbital, as well as the β-blocker propranolol can reduce heart rate reactivity.[66,67] Chronic smoking is known to decrease fetal oxygenation through an increase in fetal carboxyhemoglobin and a decrease in uterine blood flow. In these patients, fetal heart rate accelerations are also decreased.[68]

Performing the NST

The NST is usually performed in an outpatient setting. In most cases, only 10 to 15 minutes are required to complete the test. It has virtually no contraindications, and few equivocal test results are observed. The patient may be seated in a reclining chair, with care being taken to ensure that she is tilted to the left to avoid the supine hypotensive syndrome.[69] The patient's blood pressure should be recorded before the test is begun and then repeated at 5- to 10-minute intervals. Fetal heart rate is recorded using the Doppler ultrasound transducer, and the tocodynamometer is applied to detect uterine contractions or fetal movement. Fetal activity may be recorded by the patient using an event marker or noted by the staff performing the test. The most widely applied definition of a reactive test requires that at least two accelerations of the fetal heart rate of 15 bpm amplitude and 15 seconds duration be observed in 20 minutes of monitoring (Fig. 13.7).[69] Because almost all accelerations are accompanied by fetal movement, fetal movement need not be recorded with the accelerations for the test to be con-

sidered reactive. However, fetal movements do provide another index of fetal well-being.

If the criteria for reactivity are not met, the test is considered nonreactive (Fig. 13.8). The most common cause for a nonreactive test will be a period of fetal inactivity or quiet sleep. Therefore, the test may be extended for an additional 20 minutes with the expectation that fetal state will change and reactivity will appear. Keegan et al.[70] noted that approximately 80 percent of tests that were nonreactive in the morning became reactive when repeated later the same day. In an effort to change fetal state, some clinicians have manually stimulated the fetus or attempted to increase fetal glucose levels by giving the mother orange juice. There is no evidence that such efforts will increase fetal activity.[71,72] If the test has been extended for 40 minutes and reactivity has not been seen, a CST or biophysical profile should be performed. Of those fetuses that exhibit a nonreactive NST, approximately 25 percent will have a positive CST on further evaluation.[69,73,74] Reactivity that occurs during preparations for the CST has proved to be a reliable index of fetal well-being.

Overall, on initial testing, 85 percent of NSTs will be reactive and 15 percent will be nonreactive (Fig. 13.9).[69] Fewer than 1 percent of NSTs will prove unsatisfactory because of inadequately recorded fetal heart rate data. On rare occasions, a sinusoidal heart rate pattern may be observed as described in Chapter 15. This undulating heart rate pattern with virtually absent variability has been associated with Rh isoimmunization, fetal anemia, and fetal asphyxia. In one of the earlier reports on the use of NST, Rochard et al.[75] described a sinusoidal pattern in 20 of 50 pregnancies complicated by Rh isoimmunization. One-half of these pregnancies ended in a perinatal death, and 40 percent of the surviving infants required prolonged hospitalization. Only 10 percent of the babies with a sinusoidal pattern had an uncomplicated course.

The NST is most predictive when normal or reactive. Overall, a reactive NST has been associated with a perinatal mortality of approximately 5/1,000.[69,76] At least one-half of the deaths of babies dying within 1 week of a reactive test may be attributed to placental abruption or cord accidents. The perinatal mortality rate associated with a nonreactive NST, 30 to 40/1,000, is significantly higher, for this group includes

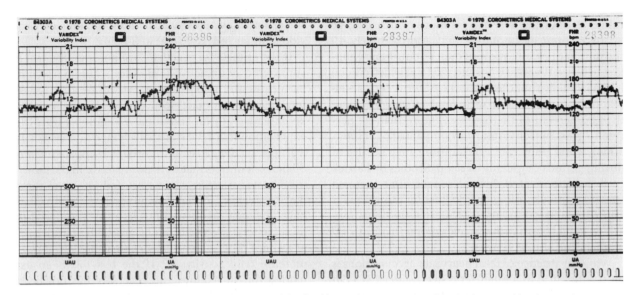

Fig. 13.7 A reactive nonstress test. Accelerations of the fetal heart that are greater than 15 bpm and last longer than 15 seconds can be identified. When the patient appreciates a fetal movement, she presses an event marker on the monitor, creating the arrows on the lower portion of the tracing.

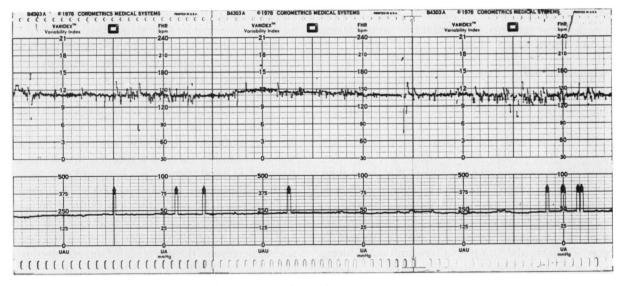

Fig. 13.8 A nonreactive nonstress test. No accelerations of the fetal heart rate are observed. The patient has perceived fetal activity as indicated by the arrows in the lower portion of the tracing.

those fetuses who are truly asphyxiated.[69,76] On the other hand, when considering perinatal asphyxia and death as end points, a nonreactive NST has a considerable false-positive rate. Most fetuses exhibiting a nonreactive NST will not be compromised but will simply fail to exhibit heart rate reactivity during the

40-minute period of testing. Malformed fetuses also exhibit a significantly higher incidence of nonreactive NSTs.[77] Overall, the false-positive rate associated with the nonreactive NST is approximately 75 to 90 percent.[69]

The likelihood of a nonreactive test is substantially

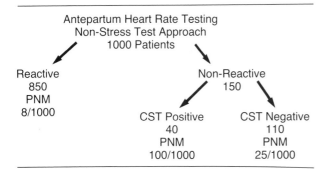

Antepartum Heart Rate Testing
Non-Stress Test Approach
1000 Patients

Reactive
850
PNM
8/1000

Non-Reactive
150

CST Positive
40
PNM
100/1000

CST Negative
110
PNM
25/1000

Fig. 13.9 Results of nonstress testing in 1,000 high-risk patients. In general, 85 percent of the nonstress tests will be reactive and 15 percent nonreactive. Of those patients with a nonreactive nonstress test, approximately 25 percent will have a positive contraction stress test on further evaluation. The highest perinatal mortality (PNM) will be observed in patients with a nonreactive nonstress test and positive contraction stress test. Patients with a nonreactive nonstress test and negative contraction stress test will have a perinatal mortality rate higher than that found in patients whose nonstress test is initially reactive. (Perinatal mortality rates based on data from Evertson et al.[74].)

increased early in the third trimester.[78] Between 24 and 28 weeks gestation, approximately 50 percent of NSTs are nonreactive.[79] Both Lavin et al.[80] and Druzin et al.[81] have reported that 15 percent of NSTs remain nonreactive between 28 and 32 weeks. After 32 weeks, the incidence of reactive and nonreactive tests is comparable to that seen at term. Aladjem et al.[82] emphasized that before 27 weeks gestation the normal fetal heart rate response to fetal movement may in fact be a bradycardia. Nevertheless, when accelerations of the baseline heart rate are seen during monitoring in the late second and early third trimesters, the NST has been associated with fetal well-being.

Several investigators have extended the NST in an attempt to separate the fetus in a period of prolonged quiet sleep from those who are hypoxemic and/or asphyxiated.[83–85] In three studies, approximately 3 percent of fetuses tested remained nonreactive after 80 to 90 minutes of evaluation. Brown and Patrick[83] noted that all NSTs that were to become reactive did so by 80 minutes or remained nonreactive for up to 120 minutes. Two stillbirths and one neonatal death occurred in seven cases with prolonged absence of reactivity. The mean arterial cord pH at delivery in this group was 6.95! In 27 pregnancies in which the fetus failed to exhibit accelerations during 80 min-

utes of monitoring, Leveno et al.[84] reported 11 perinatal deaths. In that study, IUGR was documented in 74 percent of cases, oligohydramnios in 81 percent, fetal acidosis in 41 percent, meconium staining of the amniotic fluid in 30 percent, and placental infarction in 93 percent. Therefore, if the NST is extended and a persistent absence of reactivity is observed, the fetus is likely to be severely compromised.

Vibroacoustic stimulation may be utilized to change fetal state from quiet to active sleep and shorten the length of the NST (Fig. 13.10). Most studies have employed an electronic artificial larynx (EAL), which generates sound pressure levels measured at 1 m in air of 82 dB, with a frequency of 80 Hz and a harmonic of 20 to 9,000 Hz.[86] Whether it is the acoustic or vibratory component of this stimulus that alters fetal state is unclear. Gagnon et al.[87] reported that a low-frequency vibratory stimulus applied at term changed fetal state within 3 minutes and was associated with an immediate and sustained increase in long-term fetal heart rate variability, heart rate accelerations, and gross fetal body movements. Stimulation with an EAL may produce a significant increase in the mean duration of heart rate accelerations, the mean amplitude of accelerations, and the total time spent in accelerations.[88] Kuhlman and Depp[89] reported that the auditory brain stem response in the fetus is functional at 26 to 28 weeks gestation. Therefore, vibroacoustic stimulation may be helpful after 26 weeks. Druzin noted that the incidence of reactive NSTs after stimulation with an EAL was significantly increased after 26 weeks gestation.[89a] Using an EAL, the incidence of nonreactive NSTs was reduced from 12.6 to 6.1 percent in a retrospective study and from 14 to 9 percent in a prospective investigation.[90,91] A reactive NST after vibroacoustic stimulation appears to be as reliable an index of fetal well-being as spontaneous reactivity. However, those fetuses that remain nonreactive even after vibroacoustic stimulation may be at increased risk for poor perinatal outcome.[89] In a study conducted by Trudinger and Boylan,[92] intrapartum fetal distress, growth retardation, and low Apgar scores were increased in fetuses that were nonreactive after acoustic stimulation. In most medical centers that use vibroacoustic stimulation, the baseline fetal heart rate is first observed for 5 minutes.[86] If the pattern is nonreactive, a stimulus of 3 seconds or less is applied near the fetal head. If the NST remains nonreactive,

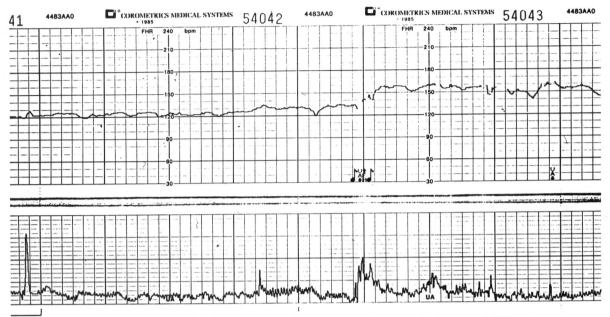

Fig. 13.10 Reactive nonstress test after vibroacoustic stimulation. The stimulus was applied in panel 54042 at the point marked by the musical notes. A sustained fetal heart rate acceleration was produced.

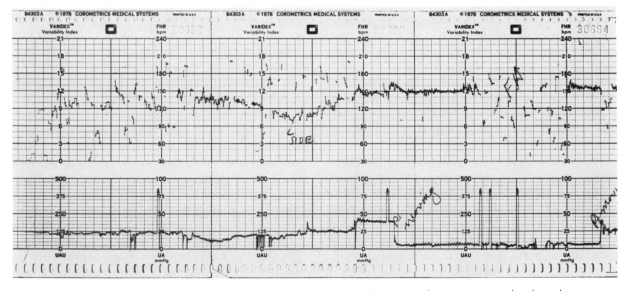

Fig. 13.11 A nonstress test in this primigravid patient of 43 weeks gestation reveals a spontaneous bradycardia (panel 30692). The fetal heart rate has fallen from a baseline of 150 to 100 bpm. Upon induction of labor, the patient required a cesarean section for fetal distress associated with severe variable decelerations. The amniotic fluid was decreased in amount and was meconium stained.

the stimulus is repeated at 1-minute intervals up to three times. If there continues to be no response to vibroacoustic stimulation, further evaluation should be carried out with a CST or biophysical profile.

Could the sound generated by an EAL damage the fetal ear? Using intrauterine microphones, Smith and his colleagues[93] documented baseline intrauterine sound levels of up to 88 dB during labor. Transabdominal stimulation with an EAL increased these levels minimally, up to 91 to 111 dB. In a follow-up study of 20 neonates exposed in utero to vibroacoustic stimulation, no abnormalities in auditory acuity were reported.[94] Therefore, it is unlikely that the short acoustic pulses generated by the EAL present a risk to the fetus. In summary, vibroacoustic stimulation may be helpful in shortening the time required to perform an NST and may be especially useful in medical centers where large numbers of NSTs are done.

Significant fetal heart rate bradycardias have been observed in 1 to 2 percent of all NSTs.[95–100] Druzin et al.[95] defined such bradycardias as a fetal heart rate of 90 bpm or a fall in the fetal heart rate of 40 bpm below the baseline for 1 minute or longer (Fig. 13.11). This definition has been most widely applied. In a review of 121 cases, bradycardia was associated with increased perinatal morbidity and mortality, particularly antepartum fetal death, cord compression, IUGR, and fetal malformations.[100] At least one-half of the NSTs associated with such bradycardias will be nonreactive. The incidence of low 5-minute Apgar scores is significantly higher in this group. If a bradycardia is observed, an ultrasound examination should be performed to assess amniotic fluid volume and to detect the presence of anomalies such as renal agenesis. When expectant management has been followed, such bradycardias have been associated with a perinatal mortality rate of 25 percent. Several reports have therefore recommended that delivery be undertaken if the fetus is mature. When the fetus is premature, one might elect to administer corticosteroids to accelerate fetal lung maturation before delivery. Continuous fetal heart rate monitoring is necessary if expectant management is followed.

In most cases, mild variable decelerations are not associated with poor perinatal outcome. Meis et al.[101] reported that variable decelerations of 20 bpm or more below the baseline heart rate but lasting less than 10 seconds were noted in 50.7 percent of pa-

tients having an NST. While these decelerations were more often associated with a nuchal cord, they were not predictive of fetal distress, IUGR, or more severe variable decelerations during labor. Phelan[86] has added, however, that when mild variable decelerations are observed, even if the NST is reactive, an ultrasound examination should be done to detect oligohydramnios. A low amniotic fluid index and mild variable decelerations increase the likelihood of a cord accident.

In selected high-risk pregnancies, the false-negative rate associated with a weekly NST may be unacceptably high.[102,103] Boehm et al.[104] reported a reduction in the fetal death rate in their high-risk population from 6.1 to 1.9/1,000 when the frequency of the NST was increased from once to twice weekly. Barrett et al.[102] emphasized that in pregnancies complicated by IUGR and diabetes mellitus, twice-weekly testing should be utilized. In reviewing the literature, they noted that the fetal death rate within 1 week after a nonreactive NST was significantly increased in both diabetes mellitus (14/1,000) and IUGR (20/1,000). Miyazaki and Miyazaki[105] reported an 8 percent false-negative rate in 125 prolonged gestations evaluated with the NST. In the prolonged pregnancy and IUGR, oligohydramnios may occur, leading to cord compression and fetal demise. Real-time ultrasonography to assess amniotic fluid volume has clearly proved important in such cases. Barss and co-workers[106] reviewed the incidence of stillbirths within 1 week of a reactive test in patients with a prolonged gestation. For the general high-risk population, a false-negative rate of 2.7/1,000 was reported. Although the incidence in pregnancies complicated by a prolonged gestation was not higher (2.8/1,000), Barss and colleagues noted that even this low rate can be considered excessively high in view of the fact that these fetuses are otherwise normal and mature. In summary, it appears that the frequency of the NST should be increased to twice weekly in pregnancies complicated by diabetes mellitus, prolonged gestation, and IUGR.[104]

Which antepartum heart rate test is best? The NST has proved to be an ideal screening test and remains the primary method for antepartum fetal evaluation at most medical centers. It can be quickly performed in an outpatient setting and is easily interpreted. In contrast, the CST is usually performed near the labor and delivery suite, may require an intravenous infusion of oxytocin, and may be more difficult to interpret. In initial studies, a reactive NST appeared to be as predictive of good outcome as a negative CST. Nevertheless, as more data have been gathered, it appears that the ability of the CST to stress the fetus and to evaluate its response to intermittent interruptions in intervillous blood flow provides an earlier warning of fetal compromise. Murata et al.[107] found that, in the dying fetal rhesus monkey, the fetal pH at which late decelerations appear is significantly higher (7.32) than the pH at which fetal heart rate accelerations disappear (7.22). In a large collaborative project in which 1,542 patients were evaluated primarily with the NST and 4,626 with the CST, Freeman et al.[108] observed that the corrected perinatal mortality associated with a reactive NST, 3.2/1,000, was significantly higher than that observed with a negative CST, 1.4/1,000. While both fetal death rates are extremely low for a high-risk population, that associated with the CST is clearly better.

The healthy fetus should exhibit a reactive baseline heart rate with no late decelerations when a CST is performed. However, as the fetus deteriorates, one will first observe late decelerations and, finally, the most ominous fetal heart rate pattern, the nonreactive NST and positive CST (Fig. 13.6).[48,53,109] When a nonreactive NST is followed by a positive CST, the incidence of perinatal mortality has been approximately 10 percent, fetal distress has occurred in most laboring patients, and IUGR has been reported in 25 percent of cases. The unusual combination of a reactive NST and a positive CST has been associated with a higher incidence of IUGR and late decelerations in labor than that seen with a negative CST.[110] Freeman et al.[108] proposed that patients with a positive CST but a reactive NST be delivered if the lecithin/sphingomyelin (L/S) ratio is mature. If the L/S ratio is immature, the patient may be followed with daily NSTs as long as they remain reactive. A biophysical profile might be helpful in this situation. Although some investigators have found no increase in perinatal deaths in patients demonstrating a nonreactive NST followed by a negative CST,[49] other workers have found this combination to be associated with a perinatal mortality of 25 to 50/1,000 (Fig. 13.9).[111,112] Conse-

quently, repeating the NST in 24 hours appears the prudent course in such cases (Fig. 13.12).

Fetal Biophysical Profile

The use of real-time ultrasonography to assess antepartum fetal condition has enabled the obstetrician to perform an in utero physical examination and to evaluate dynamic functions reflecting the integrity of the fetal CNS.[113] As emphasized by Manning et al.,[114] "fetal biophysical scoring rests on the principle that the more complete the examination of the fetus, its activities, and its environment, the more accurate may be the differentiation of fetal health from disease states."

Fetal breathing movements were the first biophysical parameter to be assessed using real-time ultrasonography. It is thought the fetus exercises its breathing muscles in utero in preparation for postdelivery respiratory function. With real-time ultrasonography, fetal breathing movement (FBM) is evidenced by a downward movement of the diaphragm and abdominal contents and by an inward collapsing of the chest. Fetal breathing movements become regular at 20 to 21 weeks and are controlled by centers on the ventral surface of the fourth ventricle of the fetus.[115] They are observed approximately 30 percent of the time, are seen more often during REM sleep, and, when present, demonstrate intact neurologic control. While the absence of FBM may reflect fetal asphyxia, this finding can also indicate that the fetus is in a period of quiet sleep.[22,23]

Several factors other than fetal state and hypoxia can influence the presence of FBM. As maternal glucose levels rise, FBMs become more frequent, and, during periods of maternal hypoglycemia, FBMs decrease. Maternal smoking will also reduce FBMs, probably as a result of fetal hypoxemia.[116] Narcotics that depress the fetal CNS will also decrease FBM.

Platt and colleagues[117] were among the first to examine the ability of FBM to predict perinatal outcome. Using real-time ultrasonography, they judged FBM to be present if at least one episode of FBM of at least 60 seconds duration was observed within any 30-minute period of observation. Of 136 fetuses studied, 116 (85 percent) exhibited FBM. The incidence of fetal distress was significantly higher in fetuses

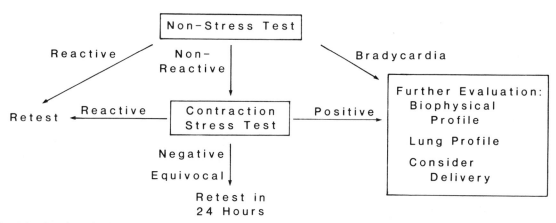

Fig. 13.12 A branched testing scheme using the nonstress test, contraction stress test, and biophysical profile. Delivery is considered when the nonstress test is nonreactive and the contraction stress test is positive. Delivery is also considered when a bradycardia is observed during the nonstress test. The fetal biophysical profile may be used to decrease the incidence of unnecessary premature intervention.

without FBM, 60 percent (12/20), as was the incidence of low Apgar scores at 5 minutes, 50 percent (10/20). The comparable figures for fetuses demonstrating FBM were 3 percent (4/116) for fetal distress and 4 percent (5/116) for low Apgar scores.

Further research demonstrated that the evaluation of FBM could be used to distinguish the truly positive CST from a false-positive CST. Those fetuses that displayed FBM but had a positive CST were unlikely to exhibit fetal distress in labor. However, when a fetus failed to show FBM and demonstrated late decelerations during the CST, the likelihood of fetal compromise was great. A pattern emerged from these studies that as long as one antepartum biophysical test was normal the likelihood that the fetus would have a normal outcome was high.[118,119] As the number of abnormal tests increased, however, the likelihood that fetal asphyxia was present increased as well.

Using these principles, Manning et al.[120] developed the concept of the fetal biophysical profile score. These workers elected to combine the NST with four parameters that could be assessed using real-time ultrasonography: FBMs, fetal movement, fetal tone, and amniotic fluid volume. FBMs, fetal movement, and fetal tone are mediated by complex neurologic pathways and should reflect the function of the fetal CNS at the time of the examination. On the other hand, amniotic fluid volume should provide informa-

tion about the presence of chronic fetal asphyxia. One additional parameter, placental grading, has been added by some investigators.[115,121]

Vintzileos et al.[115] stressed that those fetal biophysical activities that are present earliest in fetal development are the last to disappear with fetal asphyxia. The fetal tone center in the cortex begins to function at 7.5 to 8.5 weeks. Fetal tone would therefore be the last fetal parameter to deteriorate with worsening asphyxia. The fetal movement center in the cortex nuclei is functional at 9 weeks and would be more sensitive than fetal tone. As noted above, FBMs become regular at 20 to 21 weeks. Finally, fetal heart rate control, residing within the posterior hypothalamus and medulla, becomes functional at the end of the second trimester and early in the third trimester. An alteration in fetal heart rate would theoretically be the earliest sign of fetal asphyxia.

A fetal biophysical profile score was developed that is similar to the Apgar score used to assess the condition of the newborn.[120] The presence of a normal parameter, such as a reactive NST, was awarded 2 points, while the absence of that parameter was scored as zero. The highest score a fetus can receive is 10, while the lowest score is zero. The biophysical profile may be used as early as 26 to 28 weeks gestation. Twice weekly testing is recommended in pregnancies complicated by IUGR, diabetes mellitus, prolonged gestation, and hypertension with proteinuria. The criteria most recently proposed by Manning and the clinical actions recommended in response to these scores are presented in Tables 13.8 and 13.9. Regardless of a low score on the biophysical profile, Manning has emphasized that vaginal delivery is attempted if other obstetric factors are favorable.

In a prospective blinded study of 216 high-risk patients, Manning and colleagues[120] found no perinatal deaths when all five variables described above were normal, but a perinatal mortality rate of 60 percent in fetuses with a score of zero. Fetal deaths were increased 14-fold with the absence of fetal movement, and the perinatal mortality rate was increased 18-fold if FBMs were absent. Any single test was associated with a significant false-positive rate ranging from 50 to 79 percent. However, combining abnormal variables significantly decreased the false-positive rate to as low as 20 percent. The false-negative rate, that is, the incidence of babies who were compromised but who had normal testing was quite low, ranging from a perinatal mortality rate of 6.9/1,000 for infants with normal amniotic fluid volume to 12.8/1,000 for fetuses demonstrating a reactive NST. These investigators found that in most cases the biophysical profile and the NST could be completed within a relatively short time, each requiring approximately 10 minutes.

Manning et al.[122] have recently presented their experience with 26,780 high-risk pregnancies followed with the biophysical profile. It should be noted that since 1984 a routine NST was not performed if all of the ultrasound parameters were found to be normal for a score of 8.[123] An NST was performed when one ultrasound finding was abnormal. The corrected PMR in this series was 1.9/1,000, with less than one fetal death per 1,000 patients within 1 week of a normal profile. Of all patients tested, almost 97 percent had a score of 8, which means that only 3 percent required further evaluation for scores of 6 or less. In a study of 525 patients with scores of 6 or less, poor perinatal outcome was most often associated with either a nonreactive NST and absent fetal tone or a nonreactive NST and absent FBM.[124] A significant inverse linear relationship was observed between the last biophysical profile score and both perinatal morbidity and mortality (Figs. 13.13, 13.14).[122] The false-positive rate, depending on the end point used, ranges from 75 percent for a score of 6 to less than 20 percent for a score of 0. The ultrasound examination performed for the biophysical profile has the added

Table 13.8 Technique of Biophysical Profile Scoring

Biophysical Variable	Normal (Score = 2)	Abnormal (Score = 0)
Fetal breathing movements	At least one episode of >30 seconds duration in 30 minutes observation	Absent or no episode of ≥30 seconds duration in 30 minutes
Gross body movement	At least three discrete body/limb movements in 30 minutes (episodes of active continuous movement considered a single movement)	Up to two episodes of body/limb movements in 30 minutes
Fetal tone	At least one episode of active extension with return to flexion of fetal limb(s) or trunk; opening and closing of hand considered normal tone	Either slow extension with return to partial flexion or movement of limb in full extension or absent fetal movement
Reactive fetal heart rate	At least two episodes of acceleration of ≥15 bpm and 15 seconds duration associated with fetal movement in 30 minutes	Fewer than two accelerations or acceleration <15 bpm in 30 minutes
Qualitative amniotic fluid volume	At least one pocket of amniotic fluid measuring 2 cm in two perpendicular planes	Either no amniotic fluid pockets or a pocket <2 cm in two perpendicular planes

(Adapted from Manning et al.,[215] with permission.)

Table 13.9 Management Based on Biophysical Profile

Score	Interpretation	Management
10	Normal infant; low risk of chronic asphyxia	Repeat testing at weekly intervals; repeat twice weekly in diabetic patients and patients at ≥42 weeks gestation
8	Normal infant; low risk of chronic asphyxia	Repeat testing at weekly intervals; repeat testing twice weekly in diabetics and patients at ≥42 weeks gestation; oligohydramnios is an indication for delivery
6	Suspect chronic asphyxia	If ≥36 weeks gestation and conditions are favorable, deliver; if at <36 weeks and L/S <2.0, repeat test in 4–6 hours; deliver if oligohydramnios is present
4	Suspect chronic asphyxia	If ≥32 weeks gestation, deliver; if <32 weeks, repeat score
0–2	Strongly suspect chronic asphyxia	Extend testing time to 120 minutes; if persistent score ≥4, deliver, regardless of gestational age

(Adapted from Manning et al.,[122,215] with permission.)

advantage of detecting previously unrecognized major fetal anomalies.

The biophysical profile correlates well with fetal acid–base status. Vintzileos et al.[125] studied 124 patients undergoing cesarean section *before* the onset of labor. Deliveries were undertaken for severe preeclampsia, elective repeat cesarean section, growth retardation, breech presentation, placenta previa, and fetal macrosomia. Acidosis was defined as an umbilical cord arterial pH less than 7.20. The earliest manifestations of fetal acidosis were a nonreactive NST and loss of FBMs. With scores of 8 or more, the mean arterial pH was 7.28, and only 2 of 102 fetuses were acidotic. For 13 fetuses with scores of 5 to 7, the mean pH was 7.19, and 69 percent were acidotic. Nine fetuses with scores of 4 or less had a mean pH of 6.99, and all were acidotic.

Is an NST needed if all ultrasound parameters of the biophysical profile are normal? Prospective and blinded studies by Platt et al.[126] and Manning et al.[127] using both the biophysical profile and the NST have demonstrated that each of these tests is a valuable predictor of normal outcome. As emphasized by Eden et al.,[128] however, the NST will allow the detection of fetal heart rate decelerations. In the presence of reduced amniotic fluid, these decelerations may be associated with a cord accident. Eden et al.[128] re-

ported that when spontaneous fetal heart rate decelerations lasting at least 30 seconds with a decrease of at least 15 bpm are seen in the presence of normal amniotic fluid, there is an increased likelihood of late decelerations in labor and cesarean section for fetal distress.

Several additional drawbacks of the biophysical profile should be considered. Unlike the NST and the CST, unless the biophysical profile is videotaped, it cannot be reviewed. If the fetus is in a quiet sleep state, the biophysical profile can require a long period of observation. Studies have not been done to assess the effects of fetal stimulation with an EAL, for example, on the predictive value of this test. Finally, the present scoring system does not consider the impact of hydramnios. In a pregnancy complicated by diabetes mellitus, the presence of excessive amniotic fluid is of great concern.

DOPPLER VELOCIMETRY

For decades, obstetricians have attempted to measure blood flow in the fetal and uteroplacental circulations. The techniques applied have usually been invasive or have required the use of radioactive tracers.

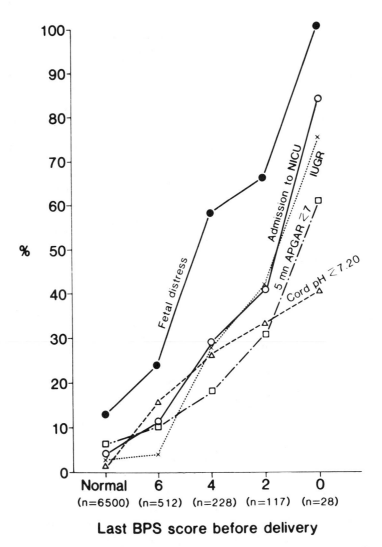

Fig. 13.13 The relationship between five indices of perinatal morbidity and last biophysical profile score before delivery. A significant inverse linear correlation is observed for each variable. (From Manning et al.,[122] with permission.)

Most recently, the principle of Doppler ultrasound has been utilized to measure blood flow in the uterine and fetal vessels.

The Doppler effect is the key principle upon which flow studies are based.[129] We have all noted that the frequency of sound produced by an ambulance siren changes as the ambulance approaches us and then passes. The pitch of the siren becomes higher as the ambulance comes closer and lower after it has passed. Similarly, a moving column of red blood cells will scatter and reflect a beam of ultrasound with a fre-

quency shift proportional to the velocity of the blood flow. In other words, the frequency of the reflected sound is proportional to the speed of the moving red blood cells. Determining blood flow velocity will provide an indirect assessment of changes in blood flow. Calculation of flow velocity is derived from the equation

$$f_d = 2\, f_o \frac{V\cos\theta}{c}$$

where f_d is the change in ultrasound frequency or

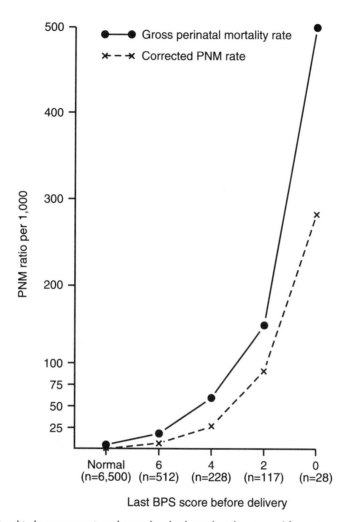

Fig. 13.14 The relationship between perinatal mortality, both total and corrected for major anomalies, and the last biophysical profile score before delivery. A highly significant inverse and exponential relationship is observed. (From Manning et al.,[122] with permission.)

Doppler shift, f_o is the transmitted frequency of the incident ultrasound, V is the velocity of the reflector or red blood cells, θ is the angle between the beam and the direction of movement of the reflector or red blood cells, and c is the velocity of sound in the medium (Fig. 13.15). The speed of sound in tissues is 1,540 m/sec. The number 2 in the equation accounts for the time spent from the transmission of the sound signal at its origin to its return. The value for cosine θ

approaches 1 as θ approaches 0. Volume flow may be calculated by multiplying the mean velocity times the cross-sectional area of the vessel as measured by ultrasound. The velocity of sound in tissues is constant, and the frequency of the incident ultrasound is fixed by the transducer. Therefore, if the angle between the blood vessel studied and the ultrasound beam remains constant, the Doppler shift frequency, f_d, will be directly proportional to the flow velocity, V.

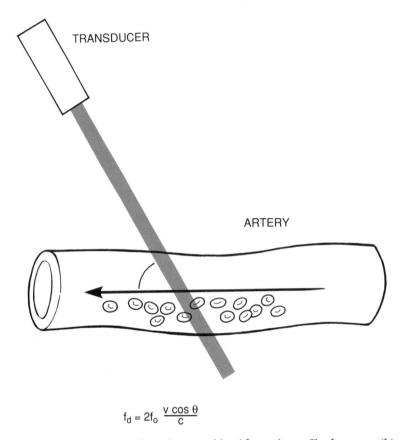

$$f_d = 2f_o \frac{v \cos \theta}{c}$$

Fig. 13.15 Application of the Doppler principle to determine blood flow velocity. The frequency (f_o) of the ultrasound beam directed at a moving column of red blood cells with velocity V will be increased to f_d in proportion to V and the cosine of the angle of intersection of the vessel by the beam (theta).

The frequency of ultrasound used in Doppler velocimetry studies is 3 to 5 MHz. Velocities are measured in meters per second.

Duplex systems to assess blood flow combine real-time imaging with pulsed wave Doppler. The vessel to be insonated can be identified, and the ultrasound beam generated from a single piezo electric crystal is placed across that vessel using range gating. Duplex systems have been applied to study blood flow in the fetal aorta and cerebral circulation.

Technical and practical problems must be considered when utilizing a duplex Doppler system.[129] Theta, the angle of the beam to the vessel insonated, should ideally be kept below 30 degrees and should not exceed 55 degrees. As this angle increases, large errors may be made in estimating flow velocity. One must accurately measure the diameter of the vessel studied to calculate its cross-sectional area. Because the radius is squared to calculate the area of the blood vessel, a small error in this measurement can produce a major error in estimating volume flow. The beam must be placed uniformly across the vessel so that the flow of all red blood cells is in the same direction and with the same velocity. The high pass or thump filter used to remove low frequency signals generated from the vessel wall also eliminates low flow velocities and may lead to an overestimation of mean blood flow velocity. If the thump filter is set too high, low frequency end-diastolic velocities may be eliminated. Because blood flow is usually expressed in milliliters per kilogram per minute, one must also accurately estimate the fetal weight. Finally, duplex Doppler systems are quite expensive.

For the above reasons, continuous-wave Doppler systems have been more widely applied.[129,130] These units, which are considerably less expensive, use both an emitting crystal and a receiving crystal at frequencies of 2 to 10 MHz. They also employ considerably less power (<25 mW/cm²) than the pulsed Doppler systems (100 to 1,000 mW/cm²). Continuous wave systems do not allow one to image the vessel to be insonated. Rather, one must depend on the identification of characteristic waveforms produced by maternal and fetal vessels.

Continuous-wave Doppler systems generate flow velocity waveforms that reflect the distribution and intensities of the Doppler frequency shifts over time.[129,130] As long as the angle of insonation and the transmitted frequency of the ultrasound beam are constant, these frequency shifts are directly proportional to changes in flow velocity within the vessel. The upswing of the frequency shift reflects stroke volume or cardiac contractility, while the downswing reflects vessel compliance and indicates peripheral resistance.

A variety of angle-independent indices have been developed to quantify the flow velocity waveforms produced.[130] It must be emphasized that these indices do not measure blood flow itself. Most commonly used is the peak systolic (S)/diastolic (D) ratio, the S/D ratio, also known as the A/B ratio (Figs. 13.16, and 13.17). The greater the diastolic flow, the lower the ratio. As peripheral resistance increases, diastolic flow falls, and the S/D ratio increases. The pulsatility index is calculated as the systolic value minus diastolic value divided by the mean of the velocity waveform profile (S − D/mean). An additional ratio, the resistance index, or Pourcelot ratio, is expressed as S − D/S. The latter two ratios are useful when the diastolic flow is absent or reversed.

As noted above, vessels within the maternal circulation and fetoplacental unit produce characteristic waveforms.[131] In addition, waveforms generated from maternal vessels can obviously be distinguished from waveforms in the fetal circulation by the slower heart rate. During the first trimester, the uterine ar-

tery normally demonstrates high pulsatility, as demonstrated by systolic flow followed by reduced diastolic flow (Fig. 13.18).[131] This pattern results from high downstream resistance in the uterine vessels, which causes reflection of the incident pressure pulse and dampens the diastolic portion of that pulse. A diastolic notch can also be identified early in gestation. By the end of the second trimester, flow velocity waveforms in the normal uterine artery demonstrate a systolic peak associated with a large diastolic component, indicating decreased resistance in the placental bed (Fig. 13.19).[131,132] Increased resistance in the placental bed has been associated with IUGR and is reflected by a reduction in end-diastolic flow.

The normal umbilical artery demonstrates a peak in systole with a large amount of end-diastolic flow, reflecting decreased placental resistance (Figs. 13.16, and 13.17).[130] There is a progressive reduction in pulsatility and an increase in diastolic flow throughout gestation. Abnormal umbilical artery flow shows decreased end-diastolic flow or, in extreme situations, absent or reversed end-diastolic flow (Figs. 13.20, and 13.21).[130,133]

When evaluating flow velocity waveforms, it is important that at least three to five waveforms be obtained at different angles of insonation. The fetus should be in a quiet state. Fetal breathing movements shorten the cardiac cycle, increasing end-diastolic frequencies and decreasing the S/D ratio. When studying the umbilical artery, it is important to demonstrate flow in the umbilical vein in the opposite direction to verify that the umbilical artery has been insonated. Umbilical vein velocities can be seen as a continuous band across the lower portion of the umbilical artery flow waveform.

The criteria for normal flow velocity waveforms in both maternal and fetal circulations have been reported by many investigators.[131,134,135] Umbilical artery waveforms are characterized by a progressive decline in S/D ratio from early pregnancy until term. This change reflects growth of small muscular arteries in the tertiary stem villi of the placenta. By 30 weeks gestation, the S/D ratio in the umbilical artery should be below 3 (Fig. 13.22).[134] In the uterine artery, increased diastolic flow is noted at 14 to 20 weeks, reflecting trophoblastic invasion of the spiral arterioles. Thereafter, there is minimal decline in the S/D ratio. The uterine artery S/D ratio should fall

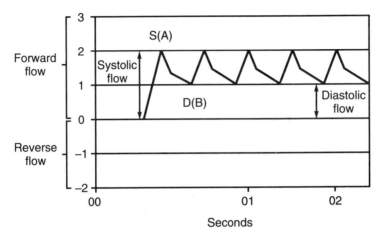

Fig. 13.16 Diagram of a normal umbilical artery flow velocity waveform. Note the forward flow during both systole and diastole, the latter indicating low resistance in the placental bed. (Adapted from Warsof and Levy,[130] with permission.)

below 2.6 by 26 weeks gestation.[131] Furthermore, the diastolic notch seen early in gestation should disappear. Abnormal uterine artery waveforms in the second trimester may herald the subsequent development of preeclampsia (Fig. 13.23).

The broadest application of Doppler flow has been in the study of the pregnancy at risk for or demonstrating IUGR. This subject is discussed in detail in Chapter 27. In summary, an elevation in the S/D ratio in the umbilical artery may precede the onset of growth retardation. When IUGR has been identified, an abnormal umbilical S/D ratio may be more predic-

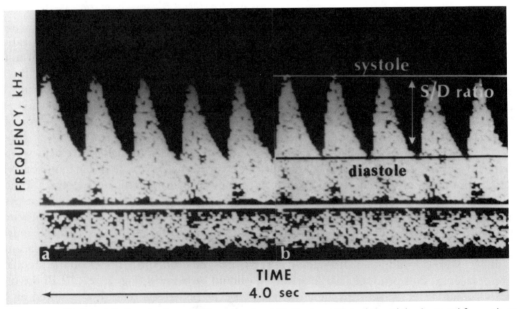

Fig. 13.17 Doppler flow velocity waveforms of the normal umbilical artery. Note that umbilical arterial flow velocities are recorded above the baseline, while nonpulsatile umbilical vein flow in the opposite direction is found below the baseline (a). Measurement of the systolic/diastolic or S/D ratio is also illustrated (b). (From Bruner et al.,[217] with permission.)

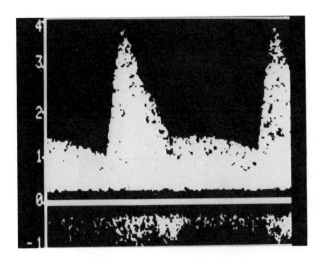

Fig. 13.18 Flow velocity waveform of the uterine artery early in the second trimester. Note the high pulsatility as demonstrated by systolic flow followed by reduced diastolic flow. While this pattern is normal at this time in gestation, during the third trimester, this finding would represent an abnormal uterine artery flow velocity waveform.

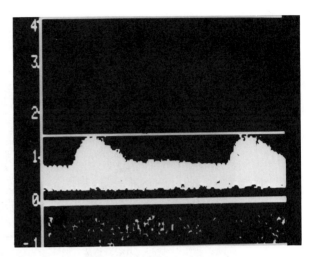

Fig. 13.19 Flow velocity waveform in the normal uterine artery during the third trimester. Note the systolic peak associated with a large diastolic component, indicating decreased resistance in the placental bed.

tive of neonatal morbidity than the NST.[136] The absence of end-diastolic flow in the pregnancy complicated by growth retardation has been associated with intrapartum fetal distress and an increased perinatal mortality rate.[130,133]

How accurate do changes in umbilical artery flow velocity waveform indices reflect alterations in fetal blood flow? Using a sheep model, Trudinger et al.[137] embolized the umbilical placental circulation with microspheres each day for 9 days in late gestation. The umbilical artery S/D ratio rose at 4 days, reflecting increased vascular resistance in the placental bed. Umbilical blood flow did not fall significantly until the end of the study period. Morrow and Ritchie,[138] using a similar experimental model, reported a progressive increase in the S/D ratio leading to absent and then reversed diastolic flow. These changes produced by embolization of the umbilical artery are similar to those seen in the human fetus with IUGR. Increasing the fetal hematocrit and blood viscosity by 100 percent had little effect on the S/D ratio. These investigators also observed that hypoxia did not alter the S/D ratio and concluded that abnormalities in the umbilical artery flow velocity waveform reflect placental pathology and not asphyxial changes. Copel et

al.[139] made similar observations using a sheep model in which umbilical blood flow and S/D ratio were measured shortly after embolization. In that study, normal umbilical artery S/D ratios were found even in the presence of fetal acidosis. It appears then that while the umbilical artery S/D ratio can provide an approximation of umbilical artery flow, it best reflects changes in placental vascular resistance. How the fetus has responded to this placental abnormality and whether it is hypoxemic cannot be judged by flow velocity waveform indices.

How do Doppler studies compare with other techniques for antepartum fetal surveillance? Devoe and his colleagues[140] evaluated 1,000 consecutive high-risk pregnancies using the NST, a measurement of amniotic fluid volume, and umbilical artery velocimetry. The PMR associated with this approach was 2.1/1,000. Using perinatal mortality, fetal distress, low 5-minute Apgar score, and neonatal acidosis as end points, each method had a specificity over 90 percent. Sensitivities ranged from 69 percent for the NST to 21 percent for the S/D ratio. The positive predictive value for any abnormal test was 54 percent but increased to 100 percent when *all* of the tests were abnormal. The best predictive values for Doppler studies were found in pregnancies complicated by

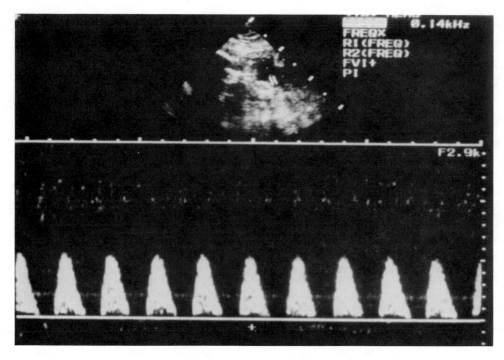

Fig. 13.20 Absent end-diastolic flow in the umbilical artery in a pregnancy complicated by severe IUGR. Note the systolic peak without evidence of diastolic flow. The real-time ultrasound image that allows visualization of the vessel to be studied, in this case the umbilical artery, can be seen in the upper portion of the figure.

hypertension and IUGR. Overall, however, the NST was found to be the best single test.

In conclusion, while Doppler velocimetry has provided important information about physiologic changes in the uteroplacental and fetal circulations, further clinical investigation must be performed to determine if this technology provides more accurate information than current techniques for antepartum fetal surveillance.

THE ASSESSMENT OF FETAL PULMONARY MATURATION

This section reviews those techniques that enable the obstetrician to predict accurately the risks of respiratory distress syndrome (RDS) for the infant requiring premature delivery and that help to avoid the unnecessary tragedy of iatrogenic prematurity. RDS is caused by a deficiency of pulmonary surfactant, an antiatelectasis factor that is able to maintain a low stable surface tension at the air–water interface within alveoli. Surfactant decreases the pressure

needed to distend the lung and prevents alveolar collapse (see Ch. 21). The type II alveolar cell is the major site of surfactant synthesis. Surfactant is packaged in lamellar bodies, discharged into the alveoli, and carried into the amniotic cavity with pulmonary fluid.

Phospholipids account for more than 80 percent of the surface active material within the lung, and more than 50 percent of this phospholipid is dipalmitoyl lecithin. The latter is a derivative of glycerol phosphate and contains two fatty acids as well as the nitrogenous base choline. Other phospholipids contained in the surfactant complex include phosphatidylglycerol (PG), phosphatidylinositol (PI), phosphatidylserine (PS), phosphatidylethanolamine (PE), sphingomyelin (S), and lysolecithin. PG is the second most abundant lipid in surfactant and significantly improves its properties.

An accurate assessment of gestational age and fetal maturity is essential before an elective induction of labor or cesarean section or before the delivery of a patient whose fetus may not have matured normally,

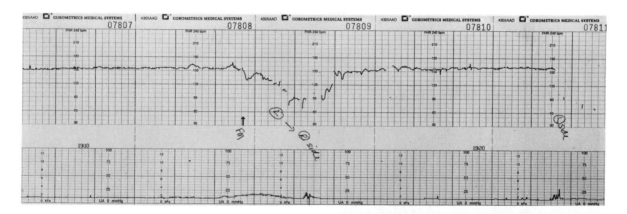

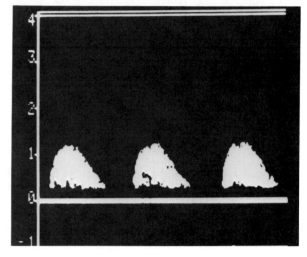

Fig. 13.21 The patient, a 27-year-old, primigravid, class C diabetic, was hospitalized for preeclampsia at 32 weeks gestation. Her nonstress test was nonreactive. The fetal biophysical profile at this time was 6. The following day, the patient's nonstress test remained nonreactive and revealed spontaneous fetal heart rate decelerations with uterine contractions (A). The biophysical profile score at this time was 2. Prior to delivery by primary cesarean section, a Doppler flow study was performed which revealed absent end diastolic flow (B). A normally grown, 1,650-g, female infant was delivered with Apgar scores of 8 at 1 minute and 8 at 5 minutes. The umbilical arterial pH was 7.23, with a base excess of −1.6. The placenta was small and calcified. The baby required oxygen by hood for 24 hours but had no significant morbidity.

such as a growth-retarded fetus or the fetus of a poorly controlled diabetic mother. Many of the techniques used in clinical practice in the past not only failed to predict gestational age but also provided little information about fetal pulmonary maturation.[141]

Prior to the now common practice of using ultrasound to establish gestational age and amniotic fluid studies to assess fetal pulmonary maturation, iatrogenic prematurity was an important clinical problem. In 1975, Goldenberg and Nelson[142] concluded that untimely or unwarranted intervention was responsible for 15 percent of their cases of RDS. In a similar study, Hack et al.[143] observed that 12 percent of all infants with RDS in their neonatal intensive care unit were born after elective deliveries. None of these infants had had documentation of pulmonary maturation before delivery. In 1977, Maisels et al.[144] reported their experience with 18 cases of RDS in neonates born after elective intervention. The L/S ratio was used in only one case and ultrasound dating in three.

Several changes in clinical practice appear to have decreased the incidence of RDS caused by iatrogenic prematurity. Patients who have had a previous low transverse cesarean section are now being encouraged to attempt a vaginal birth. In such cases, because the onset of spontaneous labor is awaited, documentation of fetal pulmonary maturation prior to elective intervention is not required. Berkowitz et al.[145] noted a marked reduction in cases of iatrogenic RDS at their institution. Between 1970 and 1973, elective delivery without adequate documentation of fetal maturity occurred in 11 of 63 pregnancies (11.1 percent) resulting in RDS. In contrast, from 1980 to 1983, only 1 of 71 pregnancies (1.4 percent) delivered electively

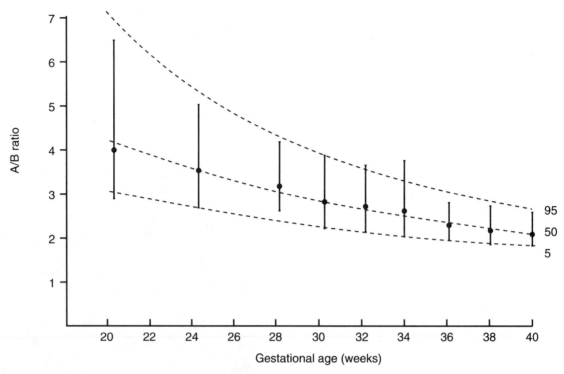

Fig. 13.22 Normal reference values for the S/D or A/B ratio in the umbilical artery throughout gestation. The 95th, 50th, and 5th percentiles are shown at each gestational age. Note that the ratio falls below 3 after 30 weeks gestation. (From Thompson et al.[134] with permission.)

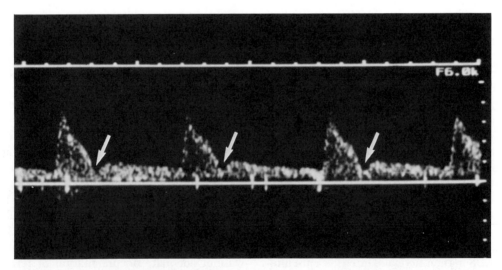

Fig. 13.23 The patient, a 30-year-old primigravida at 30 weeks gestation, had an ultrasound performed for lagging uterine growth. Estimated fetal weight was 910 g, and the amniotic fluid volume was reduced. A Doppler flow study demonstrated notching of the uterine artery. Within 12 hours, the patient developed hypertension with a blood pressure of 180/110 mmHg, proteinuria, hyperreflexia, and a headache. She was delivered by primary cesarean section of a 975-g infant who did well in the nursery.

resulted in RDS. Berkowitz et al. concluded that this decline in iatrogenic RDS presumably reflects increased availability of ultrasound and fetal lung maturity studies and advances in the application and interpretation of these diagnostic procedures.

ASSESSMENT OF FETAL PULMONARY MATURITY

Available methods for evaluating fetal pulmonary maturity may be divided into four categories: (1) quantitation of pulmonary surfactant, such as the L/S ratio; (2) measurement of surfactant function, including the shake test; (3) evaluation of amniotic fluid turbidity; and (4) association with placental grade and cephalometry using ultrasonography.

Quantitation of Pulmonary Surfactant

The L/S Ratio

The L/S ratio, developed by Gluck and associates,[146,147] has proved to be the most valuable assay for the assessment of fetal pulmonary maturity. The amniotic fluid concentration of lecithin increases markedly at approximately 35 weeks gestation, while sphingomyelin levels remain stable or decrease. Rather than determine the concentration of lecithin that could be altered by variations in amniotic fluid volume, Gluck and co-workers used sphingomyelin as an internal standard and compared the amount of lecithin with that of sphingomyelin. Amniotic fluid sphingomyelin exceeds lecithin until 31 to 32 weeks, when the L/S ratio reaches 1. Lecithin then rises rapidly, and an L/S ratio of 2.0 is observed at approximately 35 weeks. Wide variation in the L/S ratio at each gestational age has been noted. Nevertheless, a ratio of 2.0 or greater has repeatedly been associated with pulmonary maturity. In more than 2,100 cases, a mature L/S ratio predicted the absence of RDS in 98 percent of neonates.[148] With a ratio of 1.5 to 1.9, approximately 50 percent of infants will develop RDS. Below 1.5, the risk of subsequent RDS increases to 73 percent. Thus the L/S ratio, like most indices of fetal pulmonary maturation, rarely errs when predicting fetal pulmonary maturity, but is frequently incorrect when predicting subsequent RDS.[149] Many neonates with an immature L/S ratio will not develop RDS.

Several important variables must be considered in interpreting the predictive accuracy of the L/S ratio.

A prolonged interval between the determination of an immature L/S ratio and delivery will necessarily increase the number of falsely immature results. If not processed immediately, the amniotic fluid sample should be frozen at -20 degrees C.[150] At room temperature, phospholipases will destroy amniotic fluid phospholipids and decrease the ratio. The L/S ratio can also be altered by varying the centrifugal force employed in the initial centrifugation. Excessively low speeds of centrifugation may yield false high L/S values, while high speeds increase the false-negative results. Cherayil et al.[151] concluded that $3,000 \times g$ for 10 minutes provides maximum precision. It is probably best to discard amniotic fluid samples heavily contaminated by blood or meconium, because the effects of these compounds on the determination of the L/S ratio are quite unpredictable.[152,153] Blood has been reported to both increase and decrease the ratio, while meconium can produce falsely mature results. The presence of PG in a blood- or meconium-stained amniotic fluid sample or a specimen collected from the vaginal pool remains a reliable indicator of pulmonary maturity.[154] PG is not normally found in blood, and meconium generally does not interfere with the identification of PG.[155,156] While Gluck proposed that the cold acetone precipitation step provides a semiquantitative concentration of the most surface-active dipalmitoyl lecithin, some investigators have questioned its value.[157] When the L/S ratio reaches 2.0, approximately 45 to 50 percent of amniotic fluid lecithin is precipitable.[146] Gluck et al.[146] employed reflectance densitometry to determine the final L/S ratio. However, planimetric techniques that measure the area of the spots are comparable up to ratios of 3.0. It is essential that obstetricians know the analytic technique used in their laboratories. If the method has been modified, the critical L/S ratio of 2.0 may not apply.

Many perinatal processes alter the final interpretation of the L/S ratio. Surfactant deficiency, immaturity, and intrapartum complications are the prime factors in determining the pathogenesis of RDS.[158] Birth asphyxia may lead to RDS in many infants despite an L/S ratio greater than 2.0. In earlier studies, infants with severe Rh disease and infants of diabetic mothers were reported to have developed RDS during the neonatal period with mature L/S ratios; more recent data indicate that the L/S ratio is reliable in both high-risk conditions.[159,160] Kjos and her colleagues[160] found no cases of RDS caused by surfactant deficiency in a study of 54 pregestational and 472 gestational diabetics.

In subsequent studies, Gluck and associates emphasized that full assessment of fetal pulmonary maturity, the lung profile, requires determination of the L/S ratio, percent precipitable lecithin, and the acidic phospholipids PI and PG.[147,161] The latter are separated by two-dimensional thin-layer chromatography. A rapid L/S ratio may be performed in approximately 1 hour. Determinations of the L/S ratio and lung profile require approximately 5 ml amniotic fluid and take 2.5 to 3 hours to complete. PI appears at 26 to 30 weeks gestation, increases in parallel with the rise in L/S ratio at 35 to 36 weeks, and then decreases. PG, which does not appear until 35 weeks gestation and increases rapidly between 37 to 40 weeks, is a marker of completed pulmonary maturation. Most infants who lack PG but who have a mature L/S ratio fail to develop RDS. However, PG may provide further insurance against the onset of RDS despite asphyxia. Using the total lung profile can significantly reduce the number of falsely immature L/S ratios, as some infants with L/S ratios below 2.0 do demonstrate PG.[162] This combination has been noted in cases of accelerated pulmonary maturation observed in severe pregnancy-induced hypertension and prolonged premature rupture of the membranes.[163,164] Pulmonary maturation is also accelerated in twin gestations, with a mature L/S ratio being reached at 31 to 32 weeks gestation.[165] Regardless of birth weight, sex, or zygosity, L/S ratios have been found to be concordant in twin pregnancies. PG can be produced by some bacteria such as *Gardnerella vaginalis, Listeria,* and *Escherichia coli,* and false-positive results for PG have been reported in amniotic fluid specimens collected from the vagina.[166]

Slide Agglutination Test for PG

A rapid immunologic semiquantitative agglutination test (Amniostat-FLM) can be used to determine the presence of PG.[166-170] The sensitivity of this assay has recently been increased, and it can now detect PG at a concentration greater than 0.5 µg/ml of amniotic fluid.[170] The test takes 20 to 30 minutes to perform and requires only 1.5 ml amniotic fluid. Besides being highly sensitive, several studies have found a positive Amniostat-FLM to correlate well with the presence of PG by thin-layer chromatography and the absence of subsequent RDS. In a recent study evaluating samples from the vaginal pool and those obtained by amniocentesis, the overall concordance for the Amniostat-FLM and thin-layer chromatography results was 89 percent.[170] No cases of RDS were observed when the Amniostat-FLM assay demonstrated PG. This technique can be applied to samples contaminated by blood and meconium.

Microviscosimeter

The relative lipid content of amniotic fluid may be evaluated by fluorescence depolarization analysis.[171-174] The lipid-soluble dye 1,6-diphenyl-1,3,5-hexatriene is incubated for 30 minutes with the amniotic fluid specimen, and the amount of dye absorbed into the phospholipid membrane structures within the fluid is determined by measuring the fluorescence of polarized light with the microviscosimeter (Felma, Elscint). The fluorescence polarization or P value falls as the L/S ratio rises. Few falsely mature results have been reported with P values ranging from less than 0.310 to 0.336. In a study of 105 pregnancies complicated by diabetes, Simon et al.[175] found the L/S ratio and fluorescence polarization to have equal predictive values. Specimens contaminated with blood cannot be used for this analysis. One disadvantage of this technique is the high cost of the microviscosimeter. The test is technically easier and faster than the L/S ratio, but, because of the financial considerations mentioned above, is not widely used in this country.

An improved fluorescence polarization assay has recently been developed that utilizes the TDx Analyzer, an automated fluorescence polarimeter that is used for therapeutic drug monitoring.[175a,b,c] This technique does require a different fluorescent probe. In this system, polarization values above 0.260 are associated with a low risk of RDS.[175d] Because the TDx Analyzer is widely available, this procedure may become a helpful, rapid screening test for fetal pulmonary maturation.

Disaturated Phosphatidylcholine

Disaturated phosphatidylcholine (DSPC) is the major component of fetal pulmonary surfactant. The concentration of DSPC in amniotic fluid can be measured by a technique that separates it from unsaturated lecithin using osmium tetroxide. Torday et al.[176] showed a DSPC concentration of 500 µg/dl amniotic fluid to be consistent with fetal lung maturity and a small risk of subsequent RDS. Although this test may be more sensitive and specific than the L/S ratio, it is also somewhat more complicated to perform. The results could be altered by oligohydramnios or polyhydramnios.

Measurement of Surfactant Function

Shake Test

In 1972, Clements and colleagues[177] described the shake test, an assay of surfactant function that evaluates the ability of pulmonary surfactant to generate a stable foam in the presence of ethanol. Ethanol, a nonfoaming competitive surfactant, eliminates the contributions of protein, bile salts, and salts of free fatty acids to the formation of a stable foam. At an ethanol concentration of 47.5 percent, stable bubbles that form after shaking are due to amniotic fluid lecithin. The concentration of ethanol used in the assay is critical, and the technique must be followed carefully. This test should therefore be performed in a laboratory setting by experienced personnel. It is not a bedside procedure. A positive test result—a complete ring of bubbles at the meniscus with a 1 : 2 dilution of amniotic fluid—is rarely associated with neonatal RDS. False predictions of maturity are more frequent in complicated pregnancies.[178] At least 75 percent of negative shake tests may be falsely immature. Contamination with blood or meconium may produce falsely mature results.[148,179,180] The shake test may also be altered by changes in amniotic fluid volume. The shake test must be regarded as a screening procedure that yields useful information if mature.

Foam Stability Index

The test is based on the manual foam stability index (FSI), a variation of the shake test designed by Sher et al.[181] The kit currently available contains test wells with a predispensed volume of ethanol. The addition of 0.5 ml amniotic fluid to each test well in the kit produces final ethanol volumes of 44 to 50 percent. A control well contains sufficient surfactant in 50 percent ethanol to produce an example of the stable foam end point. The amniotic fluid/ethanol mixture is first shaken, and the FSI value is read as the highest value well in which a ring of stable foam persists.[182]

This test appears to be a reliable predictor of fetal lung maturity.[183-185] Subsequent RDS is very unlikely with an FSI value of 47 or more. The methodology is simple, and the test can be performed at any time of day by persons who have had only minimal instruction. The assay appears to be both extremely sensitive, with a high proportion of immature results being associated with RDS, and moderately specific, with a high proportion of mature results predicting the absence of RDS. Contamination of the amniotic fluid specimen by blood or meconium invalidates the FSI results. It could be used as a screening test when the L/S ratio is not available.

Tap Test

This recently developed test provides a rapid semiquantitative measurement of surfactant function.[186] The test is performed by mixing 1 ml of amniotic fluid with 1 drop of 6N hydrochloric acid and then adding approximately 1.5 ml of diethyl ether. A 6 × 150 mm test tube is briskly tapped three or four times, creating an estimated 200 to 300 bubbles in the ether or top layer. In amniotic fluid from the mature fetus, the bubbles quickly rise from the bottom layer of amniotic fluid to the surface and break down, while in amniotic fluid from an immature fetus the bubbles are stable or break down slowly. Note that these end points are opposite those used in the shake test. The cutoff for maturity has been set at five bubbles. If no more than five bubbles persist in the ether layer, the test is considered mature. The test is read at 2, 5, and 10 minutes. Fluid obtained from either amniocentesis or a freely flowing vaginal pool may be used. Amniotic fluid contaminated by blood, meconium, or vaginal mucus should be centrifuged before the assay is performed.

Socol[186] evaluated the tap test in 332 patients who delivered within 72 hours of amniotic fluid analysis. The predictive value for mature tests was greater than 95 percent, while the predictive value for immature tests ranged from 40 to 60 percent. These results were comparable with those obtained with phospholipid profiles. Fluid contaminated by blood or meconium or obtained from the vaginal pool did not demonstrate an increased incidence of falsely mature tests. While further studies are needed, the tap test may prove to be valuable as a screening test, particularly if a phospholipid profile is not available.

Evaluation of Amniotic Fluid Turbidity

Visual Inspection

During the first and second trimesters, amniotic fluid is yellow and clear. It becomes colorless in the third trimester. By 33 to 34 weeks gestation, cloudiness and flocculation are noted, and, as term approaches, vernix appears. Amniotic fluid with obvious vernix will usually have a mature L/S ratio.[187]

Optical Density

Sbarra and co-workers[188,189] assessed the relationship between the optical density (O.D.) of fresh amniotic fluid at 650 nm and the L/S ratio. This method is thought to evaluate the turbidity changes in amniotic fluid that are dependent on the total amniotic fluid phospholipid concentration. Although a wavelength of 400 nm was originally used, interference by pigments from meconium, bilirubin, and hemolyzed blood led to a choice of 650 nm. An O.D. of 0.15 or greater at this wavelength correlates extremely well with a mature L/S ratio and the absence of RDS.[190,191] Falsely immature results were observed in 6 to 8 percent of Sbarra's patients but have exceeded 30 percent in other studies.[192] Hydramnios may decrease amniotic fluid turbidity and could contribute to these findings. Because the test requires only a spectrophotometer and can be performed rapidly, the O.D.$_{650}$ is a valuable screening test. The test must be performed on a clear amniotic fluid specimen, as contamination with blood or meconium invalidates the results.

Placental Grading and Cephalometry

With the exception of amniotic fluid specimens obtained from the vaginal pool, the evaluation of fetal pulmonary maturation requires that a sample of amniotic fluid be obtained by amniocentesis. In the past, third-trimester amniocentesis was associated with significant fetal and maternal risks.[193] Fetal complications have included bleeding from laceration of the placenta or umbilical cord, fetomaternal bleeding, premature labor and premature rupture of the membranes, placental abruption, and traumatic injury. Maternal complications, though rare, have included hemorrhage, in some cases from perforation of the uterine vessels, abdominal wall hematomas, Rh isoimmunization, and infection.

Ultrasound guidance for third-trimester amniocentesis has significantly decreased the risks of the procedure. In a review of seven studies that included 4,115 third-trimester amniocenteses, the frequency of complications was 3 percent for rupture of the membranes within 24 hours, 7 percent for a bloody tap, 4.4 percent for failed amniocentesis, 3.3 percent

for labor within 24 hours, 1 percent for fetal trauma, and 0.05 percent for fetal death.[194]

Golde and Platt[195] stressed that a bloody tap warrants careful observation. At term, the fetal blood volume is relatively small, and fetal bleeding may have disastrous consequences. These investigators recommend that when a bloody tap occurs, the patient be monitored continuously with electronic fetal heart rate monitoring until an Apt test or Kleihauer-Betke test confirms that the blood is of maternal origin and that the fetus has demonstrated no evidence of distress. Should fetal distress occur, delivery is performed by cesarean section. When fetal blood is recovered, the fetus is delivered if its pulmonary status is mature even if it has not exhibited fetal distress. For those fetuses with pulmonary immaturity, Golde and Platt recommend treatment with corticosteroids and delivery thereafter.

In an effort to avoid the traumatic complications of amniocentesis, several investigators have examined the correlation between placental morphology on ultrasonography and fetal pulmonary maturation. In 1979, Grannum et al.[196] described four stages of placental maturation based on the appearance of the basal and chorionic plates of the placenta and the placental substance (Table 13.10 and Fig. 13.24). With progression from the least mature placenta, grade 0, to the most mature placenta, grade 3, one observes increasing deposition of calcium within the placental septa. The fallout areas seen in the grade 3 placenta are thought to represent holes in the center of the cotyledon corresponding to the flow of blood from the maternal spiral arterioles. Grannum et al. noted an excellent correlation between the presence of a grade 3 placenta and a mature L/S ratio. This parallel maturation between the fetal lung and placenta has been confirmed by several examiners. Harman et al.[197] reported that 93 percent of grade 3 placentas were associated with a mature L/S ratio and 75 percent with the presence of PG. Kazzi et al.[198] attempted to refine this classification by describing as mature only those placentas that are entirely grade 3. Placentas that have a grade 3 appearance in one portion but that are less mature in other areas are judged intermediate. In this series, no fetus with a mature or entirely grade 3 placenta developed RDS. Unfortunately, at term only approximately 18 percent of patients will demonstrate a grade 3 placenta. Furthermore, the observation of a grade 3 placenta in preg-

Table 13.10 Summary of Placental Grading[a]

Section of Placenta	Placental Grade			
	0	1	2	3
Chorionic plate	Straight and well defined	Subtle undulations	Indentations extending into placenta but not to basal layer	Indentations communicating with basal layer
Placental substance	Homogeneous	Few scattered EGAs	Linear echogenic densities (commalike densities)	Circular densities with echo-spared areas in center; large, irregular densities casting acoustic shadows
Basal layer	No densities	No densities	Linear arrangement of small EGAs (basal stippling)	Large and somewhat confluent basal EGAs; can create acoustic shadows

[a] EGAs, echogenic areas.
(From Grannum et al.,[196] with permission.)

nancies complicated by maternal hypertension, diabetes mellitus, IUGR, and Rh isoimmunization cannot reliably be associated with a mature L/S ratio.[199-202] In summary, it appears that the presence of a grade 3 placenta in an uncomplicated pregnancy at term strongly suggests fetal pulmonary maturation.[203]

Other investigators have assessed the correlation between the biparietal diameter (BPD) and fetal pulmonary maturation.[204-207] Gross et al.[204] reported that in 294 pregnancies the presence of a BPD of 9.0 cm or more was associated with a gestational age of at least 38 weeks in 97 percent of cases, with the presence of PG in 87 percent of patients, and with the absence of RDS in all infants. These workers estimated that more than one-third of all amniocenteses in their series could have been eliminated using the predictive value of the BPD. Several investigators have now confirmed that a BPD of at least 9.2 cm will reliably predict the absence of RDS in uncomplicated pregnancies. This approach should not be used in patients with diabetes mellitus.

In summary, ultrasound parameters that correlate with fetal pulmonary maturation may be helpful when the risk of amniocentesis is increased, as with an anterior placenta. However, as emphasized by Hadlock et al.,[208] the most appropriate use of ultrasound in predicting fetal lung maturity is early documentation of gestational age so that elective delivery later in pregnancy can be safely undertaken.

Determination of Fetal Pulmonary Maturation in Clinical Practice

A large number of techniques are now available to assess fetal pulmonary maturation (Tables 13.11 and 13.12). Several rapid screening tests, including the microviscosimeter, FSI, O.D._{650}, and Amniostat-FLM appear to be highly reliable in the mature state. In an uncomplicated pregnancy, when a screening test such as the FSI demonstrates fetal pulmonary maturation, one can safely proceed with delivery. This approach is also extremely cost effective.[209,210] However, if the screening test is immature, the L/S ratio and lung profile should be used. Similarly, in complicated pregnancies, such as those with diabetes mellitus, IUGR, and Rh isoimmunization, the L/S ratio and lung profile should be determined to assess fetal pulmonary maturation. As noted above, in an uncomplicated pregnancy at term, when an amniocentesis would be difficult because of placental or fetal location, placental grade and fetal BPD may be

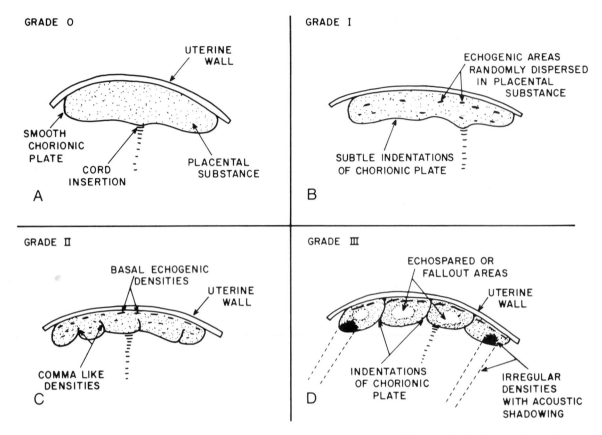

Fig. 13.24 The four stages of placental maturation based on the appearance of the basal and chorionic plate of the placenta and the placental substance. (From Grannum et al.,[197] with permission.)

used as an indirect measure of fetal pulmonary maturity.

PUTTING IT ALL TOGETHER

How can one most efficiently use all the techniques available for antepartum fetal surveillance? Obstetricians should take a "diagnosis-specific" approach to testing. That is, they must consider the pathophysiology of the disease process that will be evaluated and then select the best method or methods of testing for that problem. For example, in the pregnancy complicated by significant Rh isoimmunization, one might want to use serial evaluations of fetal hemoglobin, as well as perform frequent assessments of the fetus with ultrasound to detect evidence of hydrops. In a pregnancy complicated by diabetes mellitus, careful moni-toring of maternal glucose levels should accompany antepartum heart rate testing. By contrast, in a pregnancy complicated by suspected growth retardation, one would want to make serial evaluations of amniotic fluid volume with ultrasound to detect oligohydramnios.

In a prolonged pregnancy, one would use a parallel testing scheme. In this situation, the obstetrician is not concerned with fetal maturity but rather with fetal well-being. Several tests are performed at the same time, such as antepartum fetal heart rate testing and the biophysical profile. It is acceptable in this high-risk situation to intervene when a single test is abnormal. One is willing to accept a false-positive test result to avoid the intrauterine death of a mature and otherwise healthy fetus.

On the other hand, in most other high-risk pregnancies, such as those complicated by diabetes melli-

Table 13.11 Assessment of Fetal Lung Maturity

Test	Principle	Mature Level
L/S ratio	Quantity of surfactant lecithin compared with sphingomyelin	≥ 2.0 (method dependent)
Lung profile	Includes determination of L/S ratio, percentage precipitable lecithin, PG, and PI	L/S ratio ≥ 2.0; $>50\%$ acetone precipitable lecithin, 15–20% PI, 2–10% PG
Amniostat-FLM[a]	Immunologic test with agglutination in presence of PG	Test positive with PG ≥ 0.5 μg/ml amniotic fluid
Disaturated phosphatidylcholine (DSPC)	Direct measure of primary phospholipid in surfactant	≥ 500 μg/dl
Microviscosimeter[a]	Fluorescence depolarization used to determine phospholipid membrane content	$p < 0.310 - 0.336$
Shake test[a]	Generation of stable foam by pulmonary surfactant in presence of ethanol	Complete ring of bubbles 15 minutes after shaking at 1 : 2 diluation
Lumadex-FSI[a]	Modification of manual foam stability index; stable foam in presence of increasing concentration of ethanol	≥ 47
Optical density[a]	Evaluates turbidity changes dependent on total phospholipid concentration	At 650 nm, ≥ 0.15

[a] Denotes screening test.
(Adapted from Gabbe,[216] with permission.)

Table 13.12 Assessment of Fetal Lung Maturity

Test	Advantages	Disadvantages
L/S ratio	Few falsely mature values; not altered by changes in amniotic fluid volume	Many falsely immature values, long turn around time, special laboratory equipment required
Lung profile	Reduces falsely immature L/S ratios; PG not altered by blood, meconium	Requires more time and equipment than L/S ratio
Amniostat-FLM[a]	Rapid, few falsely mature tests; can be used with contaminated specimens	Many falsely immature results
Disaturated phosphatidylcholine (DSPC)	Few falsely mature tests; may reduce falsely immature tests	May be altered by changes in amniotic fluid volume
Microviscosimeter[a]	Few falsely mature tests; fast, easily performed	Requires expensive equipment
Shake test[a]	Few falsely mature tests; fast, easily performed	Concentration of reagents critical; many falsely immature results
Lumadex-FSI[a]	Few falsely mature tests; fast, easily performed	Concentration of reagents critical; some falsely immature results
Optical density at 650 nm[a]	Few falsely mature tests; fast, easily performed	Many falsely immature results; need clear amniotic fluid

[a] Denotes screening test.
(Adapted from Gabbe,[216] with permission.)

tus or hypertension, it is preferable to allow the fetus to remain in utero as long as possible. In these situations, a branched testing scheme is used. To decrease the likelihood of unnecessary premature intervention, the obstetrician uses a series of tests and, under most circumstances, would only deliver a premature infant when all parameters suggest fetal compromise. In this situation, one must consider the likelihood of neonatal RDS as predicted by the lung profile and review these risks with colleagues in neonatology.

Maternal assessment of fetal activity would appear to be an ideal first-line screening test for both high-

risk and low-risk patients. The use of this approach may decrease the number of unexpected intrauterine deaths in so-called normal pregnancies. Although a negative CST has been associated with fewer intrauterine deaths than a reactive NST, the NST appears to have significant advantages in screening high-risk patients. It can be easily and rapidly performed in an outpatient setting. The nipple stimulation CST provides an excellent alternative for those who favor primary use of the CST, particularly in the prolonged pregnancy and in those cases complicated by diabetes mellitus and IUGR. Most clinicians, however, use the

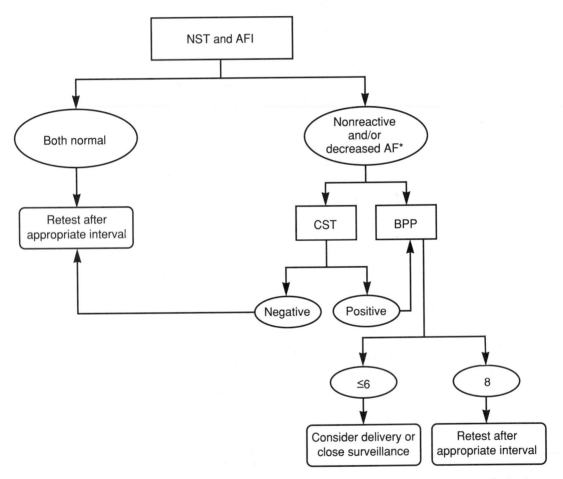

Fig. 13.25 Flow chart for antepartum fetal surveillance in which the nonstress test (NST) and amniotic fluid index (AFI) are used as the primary methods for fetal evaluation. A nonreactive NST and/or decreased amniotic fluid (AF) are further evaluated using either the contraction stress test (CST) or the biophysical profile (BPP). Further details regarding the use of the biophysical profile are provided in Table 13.9. *If the fetus is mature and amniotic fluid volume is reduced, delivery should be considered before further testing is undertaken. (Adapted from Finberg et al.,[113] with permission.)

biophysical profile or CST to assess fetal condition further in patients exhibiting a persistently nonreactive NST. This sequential approach may be particularly valuable in avoiding unnecessary premature intervention.

Figure 13.25 presents a practical testing scheme that has been utilized successfully by several medical centers.[86,113,211,212] The NST, an indicator of present fetal condition, is combined with an amniotic fluid index (AFI) (see Ch. 12), a marker of long-term status. Vibroacoustic stimulation may be used to shorten the time required to achieve a reactive NST. While most patients are evaluated weekly, patients with diabetes mellitus, IUGR, or a prolonged gestation are tested twice weekly. If the NST is nonreactive or if the AFI is abnormal, either a CST or a biophysical profile may be performed. Note that in the mature fetus with decreased amniotic fluid, delivery should be considered. Using this approach, Clark et al.[211] reported no unexpected antepartum fetal deaths in a series of 2,628 high-risk pregnancies. Vibroacoustic stimulation shortened the mean testing time to 10 minutes. Only 2 percent of all NSTs were nonreactive. However, 17 percent of these were followed by a positive CST or a biophysical profile score of 4 or less. Clark et al. have extended their experience with this technique to include an additional 3,005 tests. One fetus died 2 days after a reactive NST because of a cord accident. Therefore, only one fetal death has been observed in almost 9,000 tests after a reactive NST and a normal AFI! In a series of 6,543 fetuses, Vintzileos et al.[213] also reported no fetal deaths caused by hypoxia within 1 week of a reactive NST and an ultrasound study demonstrating normal amniotic fluid.

Finally, tests of any kind can only do so much. As emphasized by Wilson and Schifrin[214]:

. . . improvement does not lie with tests alone. It is axiomatic that informed and interested personnel must translate test results into meaningful clinical activity and communicate thoroughly with the patient.

REFERENCES

1. Chard T, Klopper A: Introduction in Placental Function Tests. Springer-Verlag, New York, 1982
2. Friede A, Rochat R: Maternal mortality and perinatal mortality: definitions, data, and epidemiology. p. 35. In Sachs B (ed): Clinical Obstetrics. PSG, Littleton, MA, 1985
3. Vital Statistics of the United States, Vol. II—Mortality, 1986. U.S. Department of Health and Human Services, Public Health Service, Washington, DC, 1988
4. Grant A, Elbourne D: Fetal movement counting to assess fetal well-being. p. 440. In Chalmers I, Enkin M, Keirse MJNC (eds): Effective Care in Pregnancy and Childbirth. Oxford University Press, New York, 1989
5. Naeye RL: Causes of perinatal mortality in the United States Collaborative Perinatal Project. JAMA 238: 228, 1977
6. CDC: Contribution of birth defects to infant mortality—United States, 1986. MMWR 38:633, 1989
7. Lammer EJ, Brown LE, Anderka MT, Guyer B: Classification and analysis of fetal deaths in Massachusetts. JAMA 261:1757, 1989
8. Manning FA, Lange IR, Morrison I, Harman CR: Determination of fetal health: methods for antepartum and intrapartum fetal assessment. p. 6. In Leventhal J (ed): Current Problems in Obstetrics and Gynecology. Year Book Medical Publishers, Chicago, 1983
9. Mersey Region Working Party on Perinatal Mortality: perinatal health. Lancet 1:491, 1982
10. Kirkup B, Welch G: "Normal but dead": perinatal mortality in non-malformed babies of birthweight 2–5 kg and over in the Northern Region in 1983. Br J Obstet Gynaecol 97:381, 1990
11. Schneider EP, Hutson JM, Petrie RH: An assessment of the first decade's experience with antepartum fetal heart rate testing. Am J Perinatol 5:134, 1988
12. Stubblefield P, Berek J: Perinatal mortality in term and post-term births. Obstet Gynecol 56:676, 1980
13. Duenhoelter J, Whalley P, MacDonald P: An analysis of the utility of plasma immunoreactive estrogen measurements in determining delivery time of gravidas with a fetus considered at high risk. Am J Obstet Gynecol 125:889, 1976
14. Mohide P, Keirse MJNC: Biophysical assessment of fetal well-being. p. 477. In Chalmers I, Enkin M, Keirse MJNC (eds): Effective Care in Pregnancy and Childbirth. Oxford University Press, New York, 1989
15. Flynn AM, Kelly J, Mansfield H et al: A randomized controlled trial of non-stress antepartum cardiotocography. Br J Obstet Gynaecol 89:427, 1982
16. Brown VA, Sawers RS, Parsons RJ et al: The value of antenatal cardiotocography in the management of high-risk pregnancy: a randomized controlled trial. Br J Obstet Gynaecol 89:716, 1982
17. Lumley J, Lester A, Anderson I et al: A randomized

trial of weekly cardiotocography in high-risk obstetric patients. Br J Obstet Gynaecol 90:1018, 1983

18. Kidd LC, Patel NB, Smith R: Non-stress antenatal cardiotocography—a prospective randomized clinical trial. Br J Obstet Gynaecol 92:1156–1159, 1985

19. Schifrin B, Foye G, Amato J et al: Routine fetal heart rate monitoring in the antepartum period. Obstet Gynecol 54:21, 1979

20. Stempel L: Eenie, meenie, minie, mo . . . what do the data really show? Obstet Gynecol 144:745, 1982

21. Carpenter M, Coustan D: Criteria for screening tests for gestational diabetes. Am J Obstet Gynecol 144:768, 1982

22. Manning FA: Assessment of fetal condition and risk: analysis of single and combined biophysical variable monitoring. Semin Perinatol 9:168, 1985

23. Van Geijn HP, Griffin RL, Caron FJM et al: Heart rate and behavioral states in the near term fetus, abstracted. Tenth Conference on Fetal Breathing Movements and Other Fetal Measurements. Malmo, Sweden, 1983:55

24. Patrick J, Campbell K, Carmichael L et al: Patterns of gross fetal body movements over 24-hour observation intervals during the last 10 weeks of pregnancy. Am J Obstet Gynecol 142:363, 1982

25. Holden K, Jovanovic L, Druzin M, Peterson C: Increased fetal activity with low maternal blood glucose levels in pregnancies complicated by diabetes. Am J Perinatol 1:161, 1984

26. Natale R, Clewlow F, Dawes G: Measurement of fetal forelimb movements in the lamb in utero. Am J Obstet Gynecol 140:545, 1981

27. Sadovsky E, Yaffe H, Polishuk W: Fetal movement monitoring in normal and pathologic pregnancy. Int J Gynaecol Obstet 12:75, 1974

28. Rayburn W, Zuspan F, Motley M, Donaldson M: An alternative to antepartum fetal heart rate testing. Am J Obstet Gynecol 138:223, 1980

29. Pearson J, Weaver J: Fetal activity and fetal well being: an evaluation. Br Med J 1:1305, 1976

30. Sadovsky E, Ohel G, Havazeleth H et al: The definition and the significance of decreased fetal movements. Acta Obstet Gynecol Scand 62:409, 1983

31. Draper J, Field S, Thomas H: Women's views on keeping fetal movement charts. Br J Obstet Gynaecol 93:334, 1986

32. Sorokin Y, Dierker L: Fetal movement. Clin Obstet Gynecol 25:719, 1982

33. Rayburn W, Barr M: Activity patterns in malformed fetuses. Am J Obstet Gynecol 142:1045, 1982

34. Neldam S: Fetal movements as an indicator of fetal well being. Lancet 1:1222, 1980

35. Rayburn W: Antepartum fetal assessment. Clin Perinatol 9:231, 1982

36. Liston R, Cohen A, Mennuti M, Gabbe S: Antepartum fetal evaluation by maternal perception of fetal movement. Obstet Gynecol 60:424, 1982

37. Grant A, Valentin L, Elbourne D, Alexander S: Routine formal fetal movement counting and risk of antepartum late death in normally formed singletons. Lancet 2:345, 1989

38. Moore TR, Piacquadio K: A prospective evaluation of fetal movement screening to reduce the incidence of antepartum fetal death. Am J Obstet Gynecol 160:1075, 1989

39. Moore TR, Piacquadio K: Study results vary in count-to-10 method of fetal movement screening. Am J Obstet Gynecol 163:264, 1990

40. Collea J, Holls W: The contraction stress test. Clin Obstet Gynecol 25:707, 1982

41. Antepartum Fetal Surveillance. ACOG Tech Bull 107:1 1987

42. Braly P, Freeman R, Garite T et al: Incidence of premature delivery following the oxytocin challenge test. Am J Obstet Gynecol 141:5, 1981

43. Freeman R: The use of the oxytocin challenge test for antepartum clinical evaluation of uteroplacental respiratory function. Am J Obstet Gynecol 121:481, 1975

44. Martin C, Schifrin B: Prenatal fetal monitoring. p. 155. In Aladjem S, Brown A (eds): Perinatal Intensive Care. C.V. Mosby, St. Louis, MO, 1977

45. Freeman R, Garite T, Modanlou H et al: Postdate pregnancy: utilization of contraction stress testing for primary fetal surveillance. Am J Obstet Gynecol 140:128:1981

46. Freeman RK, Dorchester W, Anderson G, Garite TJ: The significance of a previous stillbirth. Am J Obstet Gynecol 151:7, 1985

47. Gabbe SG, Mestman JH, Freeman RK et al: Management and outcome of diabetes mellitus, classes B–R. Am J Obstet Gynecol 129:723, 1977

48. Evertson L, Gauthier R, Collea J: Fetal demise following negative contraction stress tests. Obstet Gynecol 51:671, 1978

49. Grundy H, Freeman RK, Lederman S, Dorchester W: Nonreactive contraction stress test: clinical significance. Obstet Gynecol 64:337, 1984

50. Freeman R, Anderson G, Dorchester W: A prospective multiinstitutional study of antepartum fetal heart rate monitoring. I. Risk of perinatal mortality and morbidity according to antepartum fetal heart rate test results. Am J Obstet Gynecol 143:771, 1982

51. Ray M, Freeman R, Pine S et al: Clinical experience with the oxytocin challenge test. Am J Obstet Gynecol 114:1, 1972

52. Bissonnette J, Johnson K, Toomey C: The role of a trial of labor with a positive contraction stress test. Am J Obstet Gynecol 135:292, 1979

53. Braly P, Freeman R: The significance of fetal heart rate reactivity with a positive oxytocin challenge test. Obstet Gynecol 50:689, 1977

54. Gabbe S, Freeman R, Goebelsmann U: Evaluation of the contraction stress test before 33 weeks' gestation. Obstet Gynecol 52:649, 1978

55. Bruce S, Petrie R, Yeh S-Y: The suspicious contraction stress test. Obstet Gynecol 51:415, 1978

56. Scanlon J, Suzuki K, Shea E, Tronick E: A prospective study of the oxytocin challenge test and newborn neurobehavioral outcome. Obstet Gynecol 54:6, 1979

57. Crane J, Anderson B, Marshall R, Harvey P: Subsequent physical and mental development in infants with positive contraction stress tests. J Reprod Med 26:113, 1981

58. Beischer N, Drew J, Ashton P et al: Quality of survival of infants with critical fetal reserve detected by antenatal cardiotocography. Am J Obstet Gynecol 146:662, 1983

59. Oki EY, Keegan KA, Freeman RK, Dorchester W: The breast-stimulated contraction stress test. J Reprod Med 32:919, 1987

60. Keegan KA, Helm DA, Porto M et al: A prospective evaluation of nipple stimulation techniques for contraction stress testing. Am J Obstet Gynecol 157:121, 1987

61. Huddleston J, Sutliff G, Robinson D: Contraction stress test by intermittent nipple stimulation. Obstet Gynecol 63:669, 1984

62. Curtis P, Evens S, Resnick J et al: Patterns of uterine contractions and prolonged uterine activity using three methods of breast stimulation for contraction stress tests. Obstet Gynecol 73:631, 1989

63. Devoe LD, Morrison J, Martin J et al: A prospective comparative study of the extended nonstress test and the nipple stimulation contraction stress test. Am J Obstet Gynecol 157:531, 1987

64. Hammacher K: The clinical significance of cardiotocography. p. 80. In Huntingford P, Huter K, Saling E (eds): Perinatal Medicine, 1st European Congress, Berlin. Academic, New York, 1969

65. Patrick J, Carmichael L, Chess L, Staples C: Accelerations of the human fetal heart rate at 38 to 40 weeks' gestational age. Am J Obstet Gynecol 148:35, 1984

66. Margulis E, Binder D, Cohen A: The effect of propranolol on the nonstress test. Am J Obstet Gynecol 148:340, 1984

67. Keegan K, Paul R, Broussard P et al: Antepartum fetal heart rate testing. III. The effect of phenobarbital on the nonstress test. Am J Obstet Gynecol 133:579, 1979

68. Phelan J: Diminished fetal reactivity with smoking. Am J Obstet Gynecol 136:230, 1980

69. Lavery J: Nonstress fetal heart rate testing. Clin Obstet Gynecol 25:689, 1982

70. Keegan K, Paul R, Broussard P et al: Antepartum fetal heart rate testing. V. The nonstress test—an outpatient approach. Am J Obstet Gynecol 136:81, 1980

71. Druzin M, Gratacos J, Paul R et al: Antepartum fetal heart rate testing. XII. The effect of manual manipulation of the fetus on the nonstress test. Am J Obstet Gynecol 151:61, 1985

72. Eglinton G, Paul R, Broussard P et al: Antepartum fetal heart rate testing. XI. Stimulation with orange juice. Am J Obstet Gynecol 150:97, 1984

73. Keegan K, Paul R: Antepartum fetal heart rate testing. IV. The nonstress test as a primary approach. Am J Obstet Gynecol 136:75, 1980

74. Evertson L, Gauthier R, Schifrin B et al: Antepartum fetal heart rate testing. I. Evolution of the nonstress test. Am J Obstet Gynecol 133:29, 1979

75. Rochard F, Schifrin B, Goupil F et al: Nonstressed fetal heart rate monitoring in the antepartum period. Am J Obstet Gynecol 126:699, 1976

76. Phelan J: The nonstress test: a review of 3,000 tests. Am J Obstet Gynecol 139:7, 1981

77. Phillips W, Towell M: Abnormal fetal heart rate associated with congenital abnormalities. Br J Obstet Gynaecol 87:270, 1980

78. Natale R, Nasello C, Turliuk R: The relationship between movements and accelerations in fetal heart rate at twenty-four to thirty-two weeks' gestation. Am J Obstet Gynecol 148:591, 1984

79. Bishop E: Fetal acceleration test. Am J Obstet Gynecol 141:905, 1981

80. Lavin J, Miodovnik M, Barden T: Relationship of nonstress test reactivity and gestational age. Obstet Gynecol 63:338, 1984

81. Druzin ML, Fox A, Kogut E et al: The relationship of the nonstress test to gestational age. Am J Obstet Gynecol 153:386, 1985

82. Aladjem S, Vuolo K, Pazos R et al: Antepartum fetal testing: evaluation and redefinition of criteria for clinical interpretation. Semin Perinatol 5:145, 1981

83. Brown R, Patrick J: The nonstress test: how long is enough? Am J Obstet Gynecol 141:646, 1981

84. Leveno K, Williams M, DePalma R et al: Perinatal outcome in the absence of antepartum fetal heart rate acceleration. Obstet Gynecol 61:347, 1983

85. Devoe L, McKenzie J, Searle N et al: Clinical sequelae of the extended nonstress test. Am J Obstet Gynecol 151:1074, 1985

86. Phelan JP: Antepartum fetal assessment—newer techniques. Semin Perinatol 12:57, 1988

87. Gagnon R, Foreman J, Hunse C et al: Effects of low-frequency vibration on human term fetuses. Am J Obstet Gynecol 161:1479, 1989

88. Gagnon R, Hunse C, Foreman J: Human fetal behavioral states after vibratory stimulation. Am J Obstet Gynecol 161:1470, 1989

89. Kuhlman KA, Depp R: Acoustic stimulation testing. Obstet Gynecol Clin North Am 15:303, 1988

89a. Druzin ML, Edersheim TG, Hutson JH et al: The effect of vibroacoustic stimulation on the nonstress test at gestational ages of thirty-two weeks or less. Am J Obstet Gynecol 161:1476, 1989

90. Smith CV, Phelan JP, Paul RH et al: Fetal acoustic stimulation testing: a retrospective experience with the fetal acoustic stimulation test. Am J Obstet Gynecol 153:567, 1985

91. Smith CV, Phelan JP, Platt LD et al: Fetal acoustic stimulation testing. II. A randomized clinical comparison with the nonstress test. Am J Obstet Gynecol 155:131, 1986

92. Trudinger BJ, Boylan P: Antepartum fetal heart rate monitoring: value of sound stimulation. Obstet Gynecol 55:265, 1980

93. Smith CV, Satt B, Phelan JP et al: Intrauterine sound levels: intrapartum assessment with an intrauterine microphone. Am J Perinatol 7:312, 1990

94. Ohel G, Horowitz E, Linder N et al: Neonatal auditory acuity following in utero vibratory acoustic stimulation. Am J Obstet Gynecol 157:440, 1987

95. Druzin M, Gratacos J, Keegan K et al: Antepartum fetal heart rate testing. VII. The significance of fetal bradycardia. Am J Obstet Gynecol 139:194, 1981

96. Phelan J, Lewis P: Fetal heart rate decelerations during a nonstress test. Obstet Gynecol 57:228, 1981

97. Pazos R, Vuolo K, Aladjem S et al: Association of spontaneous fetal heart rate decelerations during antepartum nonstress testing and intrauterine growth retardation. Am J Obstet Gynecol 144:574, 1982

98. Dashow E, Read J: Significant fetal bradycardia during antepartum heart rate testing. Am J Obstet Gynecol 148:187, 1984

99. Bourgeois F, Thiagarajah S, Harbert G: The significance of fetal heart rate decelerations during nonstress testing. Am J Obstet Gynecol 150:215, 1984

100. Druzin ML: Fetal bradycardia during antepartum testing: further observations. J Reprod Med 34:47, 1989

101. Meis P, Ureda J, Swain M et al: Variable decelerations during non-stress tests (NST): a sign of fetal compromise? Society of Perinatal Obstetricians, Fourth Annual Meeting, San Antonio, TX, 1984

102. Barrett J, Salyer S, Boehm F: The nonstress test: an evaluation of 1,000 patients. Am J Obstet Gynecol 141:153, 1981

103. Miller JM Jr, Horger EO III: Antepartum heart rate testing in diabetic pregnancy. J Reprod Med 30:515, 1985

104. Boehm FH, Salyer S, Shah DM et al: Improved outcome of twice weekly nonstress testing. Obstet Gynecol 67:566, 1986

105. Miyazaki F, Miyazaki B: False reactive nonstress tests in postterm pregnancies. Am J Obstet Gynecol 140:269, 1981

106. Barss V, Frigoletto F, Diamond F: Stillbirth after nonstress testing. Obstet Gynecol 65:541, 1985

107. Murata Y, Martin C, Ikenoue T et al: Fetal heart rate accelerations and late decelerations during the course of intrauterine death in chronically catheterized rhesus monkeys. Am J Obstet Gynecol 144:218, 1982

108. Freeman R, Anderson G, Dorchester W: A prospective multiinstitutional study of antepartum fetal heart rate monitoring. II. Contraction stress test versus nonstress test for primary surveillance. Am J Obstet Gynecol 143:778, 1982

109. Slomka C, Phelan J: Pregnancy outcome in the patient with a nonreactive nonstress test and a positive contraction stress test. Am J Obstet Gynecol 139:11, 1981

110. Devoe L: Clinical features of the reactive positive contraction stress test. Obstet Gynecol 63:523, 1984

111. Druzin M, Gratacos J, Paul R: Antepartum fetal heart rate testing. VI. Predictive reliability of "normal" tests in the prevention of antepartum death. Am J Obstet Gynecol 137:746, 1980

112. Kadar N: Perinatal mortality related to nonstress and contraction stress tests. Am J Obstet Gynecol 142:931, 1982

113. Finberg HJ, Kurtz AB, Johnson RL et al: The biophysical profile: a literature review and reassessment of its usefulness in the evaluation of fetal well-being. J Ultrasound Med 9:583, 1990

114. Manning FA, Morrison I, Lange IR et al: Fetal assessment based on fetal biophysical profile scoring: experience in 12,620 referred high-risk pregnancies. Am J Obstet Gynecol 151:343, 1985

115. Vintzileos A, Campbell W, Ingardia C, Nochimson D: The fetal biophysical profile and its predictive value. Obstet Gynecol 62:271, 1983

116. Gennser G, Marsal K, Brantmark B: Maternal smoking and fetal breathing movements. Am J Obstet Gynecol 123:861, 1975

117. Platt L, Manning F, Lemay M, Sipos L: Human fetal breathing: relationship to fetal condition. Am J Obstet Gynecol 132:514, 1978

118. Manning F, Platt L, Sipos L, Keegan K: Fetal breath-

ing movements and the nonstress test in high-risk pregnancies. Am J Obstet Gynecol 135:511, 1979

119. Schifrin B, Guntes V, Gergely R et al: The role of real-time scanning in antenatal fetal surveillance. Am J Obstet Gynecol 140:525, 1981

120. Manning F, Platt L, Sipos L: Antepartum fetal evaluation: development of a fetal biophysical profile. Am J Obstet Gynecol 136:787, 1980

121. Vintzileos AM, Campbell WA, Feinstein SJ et al: The fetal biophysical profile in pregnancies with grade III placentas. Am J Perinatol 4:90, 1987

122. Manning FA, Harman CR, Morrison I et al: Fetal assessment based on fetal biophysical profile scoring. Am J Obstet Gynecol 162:703, 1990

123. Manning FA, Morrison I, Lange IR et al: Fetal biophysical profile scoring: selective use of the nonstress test. Am J Obstet Gynecol 156:709, 1987

124. Manning FA, Morrison I, Harman CR et al: The abnormal fetal biophysical profile score. V. Predictive accuracy according to score composition. Am J Obstet Gynecol 162:918, 1990

125. Vintzileos AM, Gaffney SE, Salinger LM et al: The relationship between fetal biophysical profile and cord pH in patients undergoing cesarean section before the onset of labor. Obstet Gynecol 70:196, 1987

126. Platt L, Eglinton G, Sipos L et al: Further experience with the fetal biophysical profile. Obstet Gynecol 61:480, 1983

127. Manning F, Lange I, Morrison I et al: Fetal biophysical profile score and the nonstress test: a comparative trial. Obstet Gynecol 64:326, 1984

128. Eden RD, Seifert LS, Kodack LD et al: A modified biophysical profile for antenatal fetal surveillance. Obstet Gynecol 71:365, 1988

129. Burns PN: Doppler flow estimations in the fetal and maternal circulations: principles, techniques and some limitations. p. 43. In Maulik D, McNellis D (eds): Reproductive and Perinatal Medicine VIII: Doppler Ultrasound Measurement of Maternal–Fetal Hemodynamics. Perinatology Press, Ithaca, NY, 1987.

130. Warsof SL, Levy DL: Doppler blood flow and fetal growth retardation. p. 158. In Gross TL, Sokol RJ (eds): Intrauterine Growth Retardation, A Practical Approach. Year Book Medical Publishers, Chicago, 1989

131. Fleischer A, Schulman H, Farmakides G et al: Uterine artery Doppler velocimetry in pregnant women with hypertension. Am J Obstet Gynecol 154:806, 1986

132. Ducey J, Schulman H, Farmakides G et al: A classification of hypertension in pregnancy based on Doppler velocimetry. Am J Obstet Gynecol 157:680, 1987

133. Reed KL, Anderson CF, Shenker L: Changes in intra-

cardiac Doppler blood flow velocities in fetuses with absent umbilical artery diastolic flow. Am J Obstet Gynecol 157:774, 1987

134. Thompson RS, Trudinger BJ, Cook CM et al: Umbilical artery velocity waveforms: normal reference values for A/B ratio and Pourcelot ratio. Br J Obstet Gynaecol 95:589, 1988

135. Hendricks SK, Sorensen TK, Wang KY et al: Doppler umbilical artery waveform indices—normal values from fourteen to forty-two weeks. Am J Obstet Gynecol 161:761, 1989

136. Trudinger BJ, Cook CM, Jones L et al: A comparison of fetal heart rate monitoring and umbilical artery waveforms in the recognition of fetal compromise. Br J Obstet Gynaecol 93:171, 1986

137. Trudinger BJ, Stevens D, Connelly A et al: Umbilical artery flow velocity waveforms and placental resistance: the effects of embolization of the umbilical circulation. Am J Obstet Gynecol 157:1443, 1987

138. Morrow R, Ritchie K: Doppler ultrasound fetal velocimetry and its role in obstetrics. Clin Perinatol 16:771, 1989

139. Copel JA, Schlafer D, Wentworth R et al: Does the umbilical artery systolic/diastolic ratio reflect flow or acidosis? Am J Obstet Gynecol 163:751, 1990

140. Devoe LD, Gardner P, Dear C et al: The diagnostic values of concurrent nonstress testing, amniotic fluid measurement, and Doppler velocimetry in screening a general high-risk population. Am J Obstet Gynecol 163:1040, 1990

141. Strassner H, Nochimson D: Determination of fetal maturity. Clin Perinatol 9:297, 1982

142. Goldenberg R, Nelson K: Iatrogenic respiratory distress syndrome. Am J Obstet Gynecol 123:617, 1975

143. Hack M, Fanaroff A, Klaus M et al: Neonatal respiratory distress following elective delivery: a preventable disease? Am J Obstet Gynecol 126:43, 1976

144. Maisels M, Rees R, Marks K et al: Elective delivery of the "term" fetus—an obstetrical hazard. JAMA 238:2036, 1977

145. Berkowitz GS, Chang K, Chervenak FA et al: Decreasing frequency of iatrogenic neonatal respiratory distress syndrome. Am J Perinatol 3:205, 1986

146. Gluck L, Kulovich M, Borer R et al: The interpretation and significance of the lecithin/sphingomyelin ratio in amniotic fluid. Am J Obstet Gynecol 120:142, 1974

147. Kulovich M, Hallman M, Gluck L: The lung profile. Am J Obstet Gynecol 135:57, 1979

148. Harvey D, Parkinson C, Campbell S: Risk of respiratory distress syndrome. Lancet 1:42, 1975

149. Creasy G, Simon N: Sensitivity and specificity of the L/S ratio in relation to gestational age. Am J Perinatol 1:302, 1984

150. Blumenfeld T: Clinical laboratory tests for fetal lung maturity. Pathol Ann 10:21, 1975

151. Cherayil G, Wilkinson E, Borkowf H: Amniotic fluid lecithin/sphingomyelin ratio changes related to centrifugal force. Obstet Gynecol 50:682, 1977

152. Buhi W, Spellacy W: Effects of blood or meconium on the determination of the amniotic fluid lecithin/sphingomyelin ratio. Am J Obstet Gynecol 121:321, 1975

153. Tabsh K, Brinkman C, Bashore R: Effect of meconium contamination on amniotic fluid lecithin:sphingomyelin ratio. Obstet Gynecol 58:605, 1981

154. Stedman C, Crawford S, Staten E et al: Management of preterm premature rupture of membranes: assessing amniotic fluid in the vagina for phosphatidylglycerol. Am J Obstet Gynecol 140:34, 1981

155. Strassner H, Golde S, Mosley G et al: Effect of blood in amniotic fluid on the detection of phosphatidylglycerol. Am J Obstet Gynecol 138:697, 1980

156. Hill L, Ellefson R: Variable interference of meconium in the determination of phosphatidylglycerol. Am J Obstet Gynecol 147:339, 1983

157. Hobson DW, Spillman T, Cotton DB: Effect of acetone precipitation on the clinical prediction of respiratory distress syndrome when utilizing amniotic fluid lecithin/sphingomyelin ratios. Am J Obstet Gynecol 154:1023, 1986

158. Thibeault D, Hobel C: The interrelationship of the foam stability test, immaturity, and intrapartum complications in the respiratory distress syndrome. Am J Obstet Gynecol 118:56, 1974

159. Horenstein J, Golde SH, Platt LD: Lung profiles in the isoimmunized pregnancy. Am J Obstet Gynecol 153:443, 1985

160. Kjos SL, Walther FJ, Montoro M et al: Prevalence and etiology of respiratory distress in infants of diabetic mothers: predictive value of fetal lung maturation tests. Am J Obstet Gynecol 163:898, 1990

161. Kulovich M, Gluck L: The lung profile. II. Complicated pregnancy. Am J Obstet Gynecol 135:64, 1979

162. Hallman M, Teramo K: Measurement of the lecithin/sphingomyelin ratio and phosphatidylglycerol in amniotic fluid: an accurate method for the assessment of fetal lung maturity. Br J Obstet Gynaecol 88:806, 1981

163. Obladen M, Merritt T, Gluck L: Acceleration of pulmonary surfactant maturation in stressed pregnancies: a study of neonatal lung effluent. Am J Obstet Gynecol 135:1079, 1979

164. Yambao T, Clark D, Smith C, Aubry R: Amniotic fluid phosphatidylglycerol in stressed pregnancies. Am J Obstet Gynecol 141:191, 1981

165. Leveno K, Quirk J, Whalley P et al: Fetal lung maturation in twin gestation. Am J Obstet Gynecol 148:405, 1984

166. Schumacher RE, Parisi VM, Steady HM et al: Bacteria causing false positive test for phosphatidylglycerol in amniotic fluid. Am J Obstet Gynecol 151:1067, 1985

167. Halvorsen PR, Gross TL: Laboratory and clinical evaluation of a rapid slide agglutination test for phosphatidylglycerol. Am J Obstet Gynecol 151:1061, 1985

168. Benoit J, Merrill S, Rundell C et al: Amniostat-FLM: an initial clinical trial with both vaginal pool and amniocentesis samples. Am J Obstet Gynecol 154:65, 1986

169. Saad SA, Fadel HE, Fahmy K et al: The reliability and clinical use of a rapid phosphatidylglycerol assay in normal and diabetic pregnancies. Am J Obstet Gynecol 157:1516, 1987

170. Towers CV, Garite TJ: Evaluation of the new Amniostat-FLM test for the detection of phosphatidylglycerol in contaminated fluids. Am J Obstet Gynecol 160:298, 1989

171. Golde S, Vogt J, Gabbe S, Cabal L: Evaluation of the Felma microviscosimeter in predicting fetal lung maturity. Obstet Gynecol 54:639, 1979

172. Golde S, Mosley G: A blind comparison study of the lung phospholipid profile, fluorescence microviscosimetry, and the lecithin/sphingomyelin ratio. Am J Obstet Gynecol 136:222, 1980

173. Simon N, Williams G, Fairbrother P et al: Prediction of fetal lung maturity by amniotic fluid fluorescence polarization, L:S ratio, and phosphatidylglycerol. Obstet Gynecol 57:295, 1981

174. Barkai G, Mashiach S, Lanzer D et al: Determination of fetal lung maturity from amniotic microviscosity in high-risk pregnancy. Obstet Gynecol 59:615, 1982

175. Simon NV, Levisky JS, Lenko PM: The prediction of fetal lung maturity by amniotic fluid fluorescence polarization in diabetic pregnancy. Am J Perinatol 4:171, 1987

175a. Tait JF, Franklin RW, Simpson JB, Ashwood ER: Improved fluorescence polarization assay for use in evaluating fetal lung maturity. I. Development of the assay procedure. Clin Chem 32:248, 1986

175b. Foerder CA, Tait JF, Franklin RW, Ashwood ER: Improved fluorescence polarization assay for use in evaluating fetal lung maturity. II. Analytical evaluation and comparison with the lecithin/sphingomyelin ratio. Clin Chem 32:255, 1986

175c. Ashwood ER, Tait JF, Foerder CA et al: Improved fluorescence polarization assay for use in evaluating fetal lung maturity. III. Retrospective clinical evaluation and comparison with the lecithin/sphingomyelin ratio. Clin Chem 32:260, 1986

175d. Tait JF, Foerder CA, Ashwood ER et al: Prospective clinical evaluation of an improved fluorescence polarization assay for predicting fetal lung maturity. Clin Chem 33:554, 1987

176. Torday J, Carson L, Lawson E: Saturated phosphatidylcholine in amniotic fluid and prediction of the respiratory-distress syndrome. N Engl J Med 301:1013, 1979

177. Clements JA, Platzker A, Tierney D et al: Assessment of the risk of the respiratory-distress syndrome by a rapid test for surfactant in amniotic fluid. N Engl J Med 286:1081, 1972

178. Morrison J, Whybrew W, Bucovaz E: The L/S ratio and shake test in normal and abnormal pregnancies. Obstet Gynecol 52:410, 1978

179. Sproule W, Greene M, Whitfield C: Amniotic fluid bubble stability test as screening procedure for predicting the risk of neonatal respiratory distress. Am J Obstet Gynecol 119:653, 1974

180. Wagstaff T, Bromham D: A comparison between the lecithin–sphingomyelin ratio and the "shake test" for the estimation of surfactant in amniotic fluid. Br J Obstet Gynaecol 80:412, 1973

181. Sher G, Statland B, Freer D, Hisley J: Performance of the amniotic fluid foam stability–50 percent test: a bedside procedure for the prenatal detection of hyaline membrane disease. Am J Obstet Gynecol 134:705, 1979

182. Sher G, Statland B: Assessment of fetal pulmonary maturity by the Lumadex Foam Stability Index Test. Obstet Gynecol 61:444, 1983

183. Golde S, Stabler M, Mosley G: A prospective comparison of the Lumadex-FSI, A650, Foam Stability Test, and Lung Profile. Society of Perinatal Obstetricians, Third Annual Meeting, San Antonio, 1983

184. Lipshitz J, Whybrew W, Anderson G: Comparison of the Lumadex-foam stability test, lecithin: sphingomyelin ratio, and simple shake test for fetal lung maturity. Obstet Gynecol 63:349, 1984

185. Lockitch G, Wittmann BK, Snow BE et al: Prediction of fetal lung maturity by use of the Lumadex-FSI test. Clin Chem 32:361, 1986

186. Socol ML: The tap test: confirmation of a simple, rapid, inexpensive, and reliable indicator of fetal pulmonary maturity. Am J Obstet Gynecol 162:218, 1990

187. Hastwell G: Amniotic fluid: visual assessment of fetal maturity. Lancet 1:349, 1975

188. Sbarra A, Selvaraj R, Cetrulo C et al: Positive correlation of optical density at 650 nm with lecithin/sphin-

gomyelin ratios in amniotic fluid. Am J Obstet Gynecol 130:788, 1978

189. Cetrulo C, Sbarro S, Selvaraj R et al: Amniotic fluid optical density and neonatal respiratory outcome. Obstet Gynecol 55:262, 1980

190. Turner R, Read J: Practical use and efficiency of amniotic fluid OD 650 as a predictor of fetal pulmonary maturity. Obstet Gynecol 61:551, 1983

191. Khouzami V, Beck J, Sullivant H et al: Amniotic fluid absorbance at 650 nm: its relationship to the lecithin/sphingomyelin ratio and neonatal pulmonary sufficiency. Am J Obstet Gynecol 147:552, 1983

192. Plauche W, Faro S, Wycheck J: Amniotic fluid optical density: relationship to L/S ratio, phospholipid content, and desquamation of fetal cells. Obstet Gynecol 58:309, 1981

193. Galle P, Meis P: Complications of amniocentesis: a review. J Reprod Med 27:149, 1982

194. Newton ER, Cetrulo CL, Kosa DJ: Biparietal diameter as a predictor of fetal lung maturity. J Reprod Med 28:480, 1983

195. Golde S, Platt L: The use of ultrasound in the diagnosis of fetal lung maturity. Clin Obstet Gynecol 27:391, 1984

196. Grannum P, Berkowitz R, Hobbins J: The ultrasonic changes in the maturing placenta and their relation to fetal pulmonic maturity. Am J Obstet Gynecol 133:915, 1979

197. Harman C, Manning F, Stearns E et al: The correlation of ultrasonic placental grading and fetal pulmonary maturation in five hundred sixty-three pregnancies. Am J Obstet Gynecol 143:941, 1982

198. Kazzi G, Gross T, Sokol R et al: Noninvasive prediction of hyaline membrane disease: an optimized classification of sonographic placental maturation. Am J Obstet Gynecol 152:213, 1985

199. Spirt B, Gordon L: The placenta as an indicator of fetal maturity: fact and fancy. Semin Ultrasound 5:290, 1984

200. Tabsh K: Correlation of real-time ultrasonic placental grading with amniotic fluid lecithin/sphingomyelin ratio. Am J Obstet Gynecol 145:504, 1983

201. Kazzi G, Gross T, Rosen M et al: The relationship of placental grade, fetal lung maturity, and neonatal outcome in normal and complicated pregnancies. Am J Obstet Gynecol 148:54, 1984

202. Gast MJ, Ott W: Failure of ultrasonic placental grading to predict severe respiratory distress in a neonate. Am J Obstet Gynecol 146:464, 1983

203. Shah YG, Graham D: Relationship of placental grade to fetal pulmonary maturity and respiratory distress syndrome. Am J Perinatol 3:53, 1986

204. Gross T, Sokol R, Kazzi G et al: When is an amniocentesis for fetal maturity unnecessary in nondiabetic pregnancies at risk? Am J Obstet Gynecol 149:311, 1984

205. Golde S, Petrucha R, Meade K et al: Fetal lung maturity: the adjunctive use of ultrasound. Am J Obstet Gynecol 142:445, 1982

206. Golde SH, Tahilramaney MP, Platt LD: Use of ultrasound to predict fetal lung maturity in 247 consecutive elective cesarean deliveries. J Reprod Med 29:9, 1984

207. Slocum WA, Martin JN Jr, Martin RW et al: Third-trimester biparietal diameter as a predictor of fetal lung maturity. Am J Perinatol 4:266, 1987

208. Hadlock FP, Irvin JF, Roecker E et al: Ultrasound prediction of fetal lung maturity. Radiology 155:469, 1985

209. Garite TJ, Freeman RK, Nageotte MP: Fetal maturity cascade: a rapid and cost-effective method for fetal lung maturity testing. Obstet Gynecol 67:619, 1986

210. Herbert WNP, Chapman JF: Clinical and economic considerations associated with testing for fetal lung maturity. Am J Obstet Gynecol 155:820, 1986

211. Clark SL, Sabey P, Jolley K: Nonstress testing with acoustic stimulation and amniotic fluid volume assessment: 5,973 tests without unexpected fetal death. Am J Obstet Gynecol 160:694, 1989

212. Mills MS, James DK, Slade S: Two-tier approach to biophysical assessment of the fetus. Am J Obstet Gynecol 163:12, 1990

213. Vintzileos AM, Campbell WA, Nochimson DJ et al: The use and misuse of the fetal biophysical profile. Am J Obstet Gynecol 156:527, 1987

214. Wilson R, Schifrin B: Is any pregnancy low risk? Obstet Gynecol 55:653, 1980

215. Manning F, Baskett T, Morrison I, Lange I: Fetal biophysical profile scoring: a prospective study in 1,184 high-risk patients. Am J Obstet Gynecol 140:289, 1981

216. Gabbe S: Recent advances in the assessment of fetal maturity. J Reprod Med 23:277, 1979

217. Bruner JP, Gabbe SG, Levy DW et al: Doppler ultrasonography of the umbilical cord in normal pregnancy. J Perinatol (in press)

SECTION 3
Intrapartum Care

Chapter 14

Labor and Delivery

William F. O'Brien and Robert C. Cefalo

MANAGEMENT OF LABOR AND DELIVERY

Definitions

Labor can be defined as progressive dilatation of the uterine cervix in association with repetitive uterine contractions. This definition serves to exclude instances in which cervical dilatation occurs without uterine contractions such as an incompetent cervix. Also excluded are uterine contractions that occur without true progressive dilatation, as is common in the latter stage of pregnancy. Labor can be either spontaneous or induced, either term or preterm. The physiology of labor is reviewed in Chapter 6.

Normal Mechanisms of Labor

Stages and Phases of Labor

Normal labor is a continuous process, but for reasons of study it has been divided into three stages, with the first stage further subdivided into three phases. The first stage of labor is the interval between the onset of labor and full cervical dilatation. The second stage of labor is the interval between full cervical dilatation and the delivery of the infant. The third stage of labor encompasses the period between the delivery of the infant and the delivery of the placenta.

The first stage of labor has been subdivided by Friedman[1] in his classic studies in 1967 on the course of labor. Analyzing the progress of spontaneous labor by graphically plotting cervical dilatation against time, he described three phases. A latent phase of variable duration was defined as the period between the onset of labor and the point at which a change in the slope of cervical dilatation is noted. A phase of maximal dilatation was defined as that period of labor when the rate of cervical dilatation was maximal. This phase usually began at 2 to 3 cm dilatation. A short deceleration phase followed the acceleration phase and was terminated at full cervical dilatation. It should be noted that not all investigators have accepted the validity of a separate deceleration phase. A descent phase was described that usually coincides with the second stage of labor. Investigators examining various ethnic groups have demonstrated that, fortunately, the parameters of progression in labor do not differ among these populations.[2] A listing of the average and fifth centile limits of progression in labor is given in Table 14.1.

The Mechanisms of Labor

The most usual presentation of the fetus to the birth canal is the vertex presentation wherein the occiput of the fetus is the lowermost part with regard to the longitudinal axis of the mother. This presentation occurs in approximately 95 percent of all term labors. The mechanisms of labor, also known as the cardinal mechanisms, refer to the changes in the position of the fetal head during passage through the birth canal.

427

Table 14.1 Progression of Spontaneous Labor

Parameter	Mean or Median	5th Centile
Nulliparas		
Total duration	10.1 hr	25.8 hr
Stages		
First	9.7 hr	24.7 hr
Second	33.0 min	117.5 min
Third	5.0 min	30.0 min
Latent phase (duration)	6.4 hr	20.6 hr
Maximal dilatation (rate)	3.0 cm/hr	1.2 cm/hr
Descent (rate)	3.3 cm/hr	1.0 cm/hr
Multiparas		
Total duration	8.2 hr	19.5 hr
Stages		
First	8.0 hr	18.8 hr
Second	8.5 min	46.5 min
Third	5.0 min	30.0 min
Latent phase (duration)	4.8 hr	13.6 hr
Maximal dilatation (rate)	5.7 cm/hr	1.5 cm/hr
Descent (rate)	6.6 cm/hr	2.1 cm/hr

Data from Friedman.[63]

Because of the asymmetry of the shape of both the fetal head and the maternal bony pelvis, such rotations are required for the average-sized fetus to accomplish passage through the birth canal. These rotations of the fetal head are accomplished by the propulsive force of uterine activity occurring during labor. The cardinal movements of labor are usually described as (1) engagement, (2) descent, (3) flexion, (4) internal rotation, (5) extension, (6) external rotation, and (7) expulsion. As noted above, a division into distinct movements occurring at separate times is artificial. Obviously, descent occurs throughout the passage through the birth canal, as does flexion of the fetal head.

Engagement

In the normal flexed position, the largest transverse diameter of the fetal head is the biparietal diameter (Fig. 14.1). Engagement is the descent of the biparietal diameter of the fetal head to a level below the plane of the pelvic inlet. When this has occurred, the head is said to be engaged. Clinically, engagement is usually measured by palpation of the presenting part of the occiput. If the lowest portion of the occiput is

at or below the level of the maternal ischial spines, station 0, engagement has usually taken place. This is because the average distance between the plane of the pelvic inlet and the ischial spines is approximately 5 cm, while the distance between the biparietal plane

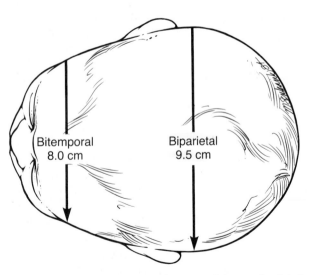

Bitemporal
8.0 cm

Biparietal
9.5 cm

Fig. 14.1 Average transverse diameters of the term fetal skull.

and the lowermost part of the occiput averages 3 to 4 cm. Engagement is considered an important clinical parameter, as it demonstrates that, at least at the level of the pelvic inlet, the maternal bony pelvis is sufficiently large to allow the descent of the fetal head. It should be noted that, although engagement is classically listed as one of the cardinal movements of labor, engagement often occurs before the onset of true labor, especially in nulliparas.

Descent

Because the obvious purpose of labor is the expulsion of the fetus through the birth canal, descent is the most important component of labor. Descent of the fetus is not continuous, however; it usually occurs in a discontinuous fashion, with the greatest rate of descent in the deceleration phase of the first stage of labor and during the second stage of labor.

Flexion

Flexion of the fetal head is a passive motion whereby the presenting diameters of the fetal head to the maternal pelvis are optimized (Fig. 14.2). Although flexion of the fetal head onto the chest is present, to some degree, in most fetuses before labor, complete flexion with the placement of the fetal chin on the thorax usually occurs only during the course of labor.

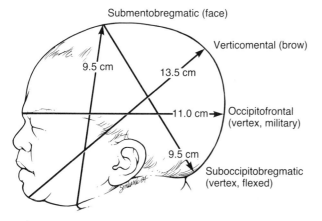

Fig. 14.2 Possible presenting diameters of the average term fetal skull.

Internal Rotation

During internal rotation, the fetal occiput gradually rotates from its original position (usually transverse with regard to the birth canal) toward the symphysis pubis or, less commonly, toward the hollow of the sacrum. As in flexion, this rotation is passive with regard to the fetus and again facilitates the presentation of the smallest possible diameters of the fetal head to the birth canal. As the musculature of the pelvic floor, including the coccygeus and ileococcygeus muscles, form a V-shaped hammock diverging anteriorly, the occiput of the fetus (the widest portion of the presenting part) rotates toward the symphysis pubis, allowing the widest portion of the fetus to transverse the birth canal at its area of greatest dimension.

Extension

Extension occurs after the fetus has descended to the level of the maternal vulva. This descent brings the base of the occiput into contact with the inferior margin of the symphysis pubis. At this point the birth canal curves upward. The fetal head is delivered by extension from the flexed to the extended position, rotating around the symphysis pubis. The forces responsible for this motion are the downward force exerted on the fetus by the uterine contractions associated with the upward forces exerted by the muscles of the pelvic floor. In combination, these forces form a diagonal vector resulting in extension of the fetal head.

External Rotation

After delivery of the head, the forces exerted on the head by the maternal bony pelvis and its musculature are relieved. At this point, the unopposed forces of the fetal musculature assume precedence and the fetus resumes its normal "face-forward" position, with the occiput and spine lying in the same plane.

Expulsion

After external rotation of the fetal head, further descent brings the anterior shoulder to the level of the symphysis pubis. The shoulder is delivered in much the same manner as the head, with rotation of the anterior shoulder under the symphysis pubis. After the shoulders, the rest of the body is usually quickly delivered.

Management of Normal Labor and Delivery

Initial Assessment

As in all patient care encounters, initial management of labor should include an appropriate history, physical examination, and necessary laboratory testing. At 36 weeks gestation (or earlier if premature labor is likely), the patient's prenatal record should be available to personnel in the labor area. When the patient is admitted, prenatal data should be reviewed, with pertinent information transferred to the labor record. Besides updating the history in the prenatal chart, significant new data that have accrued since the last antepartum visit should be obtained. Of special attention are the time of onset of contractions, status of the fetal membranes, the presence or absence of vaginal bleeding, a notation of fetal activity, history of allergies, time and content of last ingestion of food or fluids, and use of any medications. An admitting physical examination should include the patient's vital signs, notation of fetal position and presentation, reporting of the fetal heart rate as well as frequency, duration, and quality of uterine contractions. If no contraindications to pelvic examination exist, the degree of cervical dilatation, effacement, status of the membranes, and type and station of the presenting part should be noted.

Risk Status Assignment

Based on information from the prenatal record as well as on information gleaned from the initial assessment of the patient, an assignment of her risk status should be made. Identification of the high-risk patient is critical in the proper management of labor and delivery. Approximately 20 percent of pregnant women who can be identified antenatally as high risk account for 55 percent of poor pregnancy outcomes. In addition, 5 to 10 percent of pregnant women are identified as high risk only during the course of labor, and these patients result in 20 to 25 percent of poor pregnancy outcomes. It is important to realize, however, that approximately 20 percent of perinatal morbidity and mortality arise from a group of patients who are assessed to be at low risk. Therefore, all

women require adequate surveillance throughout labor and delivery.

Standard Procedures

Over the course of the last decade, significant changes in the policies of institutions and physicians regarding once routinely recommended procedures such as shaving of perineal hair, enemas, showers, intravenous catheters, and positioning during labor and delivery have occurred. Modern management methods include the involvement of the patient and her family in these decisions, which are based on informed and prudent guidelines formulated by the health care team. Upon admission patients who have had no prenatal care should undergo a complete history and physical examination, blood count, blood typing, Rh determination, and urine testing. Those patients who have had antepartum care require only a urine sample to be tested for the presence of protein and glucose, a determination of hematocrit, blood count, and submission to the laboratory of a specimen of blood to be available in the event of subsequent need for cross-matching.

Management of Labor in Patients Without Identifiable Risks

After the patient has been admitted, she should be introduced to the members of the health care team who will be responsible for her care. An assessment of the quality of the uterine contractions as well as cervical examinations at appropriate intervals should be performed to detect evidence of any abnormality of the labor. Vaginal examinations should be kept to the minimum required for the evaluation of the labor pattern. Cleansing of the perineum with an antiseptic and the use of a sterile lubricant may decrease potential contamination. The fetal heart rate should be recorded at least every 30 minutes during the first stage of labor. The heart rate should be auscultated immediately after uterine contractions. During the second stage of labor, the fetal heart rate should be auscultated at least every 15 minutes, and preferably after each uterine contraction. Because inhalation anesthesia may be needed for cesarean birth or for management of complications of the third stage of labor, oral intake should be limited to small sips of water, ice chips, or hard candies. Aspiration pneumonitis, a major cause of anesthetic-associated maternal mortality, is related to the acidity of gastric contents. The use of a clear antacid such as 0.3 M sodium citrate during the course of labor has been recommended by many authors.

Preparation for delivery should be started with consideration given to the patient's parity, the progression of labor, presentation of the fetus, and complications of the labor. For patients without identifiable risks, delivery may be conducted either in birthing rooms or in traditional delivery areas. Although the lithotomy position is generally used for vaginal delivery in the United States, many patients and physicians prefer the lateral or Sims position, or the partial sitting position. During delivery, maternal blood pressure and pulse should be evaluated and recorded every 10 minutes.

Management of Labor in High-Risk Patients

Continuous electronic fetal monitoring is recommended for patients identified as high risk. Internal uterine pressure monitoring provides important information regarding the quality and quantity of contractions. Abnormal findings by electronic fetal monitoring should be described and interpreted by qualified obstetric personnel. An assessment of fetal scalp capillary pH can be performed in situations of potential fetal distress and may clarify suspicious or confusing fetal heart rate patterns. In patients at high risk, if no specific problems have been identified during the course of labor, management should proceed in a manner similar to that recommended for low-risk patients.

ASSISTED SPONTANEOUS DELIVERY

The goals of assisted spontaneous delivery are the reduction of maternal trauma, prevention of fetal injury, and initial support of the newborn.

Episiotomy

An episiotomy is an incision into the perineal body made before delivery to enlarge the area of the outlet and thereby facilitate delivery. Although there is general agreement that episiotomy is indicated in cases of arrested or protracted descent or accompanying forceps or vacuum delivery, the role of prophylactic epis-

iotomy is widely debated. Cited advantages include the substitution of a straight surgical incision for ragged spontaneous lacerations, reduction in the duration of the second stage, and reduction of trauma to the pelvic floor musculature. Although elective episiotomy has been advocated principally as a method to reduce the likelihood of subsequent pelvic relaxation,[3] this association has never been proved.[4]

Disadvantages of episiotomy include increased blood loss, especially if the incision is made too early, and possibly an increase in trauma over that which would have occurred spontaneously. Although a mediolateral episiotomy may serve to reduce the likelihood of third-degree lacerations, this procedure is considerably more painful than a median episiotomy and is performed less frequently than in the past. In view of the lack of objective evidence on the value of prophylactic episiotomy and the often emotional nature of the issue, the decision to perform an episiotomy is best left to the individual physician and to the patient.

In the absence of complicating factors such as rectal or perineal lesions, a medial episiotomy is preferred. The incision should be performed when the fetal head has distended the vulva to 2 to 3 cm unless earlier delivery is indicated. Care should be taken to displace the perineum from the fetal head. The size of the incision will depend on the length of the perineum but is generally one-half the length of the perineum.

Although an episiotomy may be performed with a scalpel, incisions are usually made with a straight Mayo scissors. The incision should be placed vertically into the midline of the perineal body and be of sufficient size to increase the area of the introitus without compromise of the anal sphincter.

Mediolateral episiotomies are less likely to be associated with damage to the anal sphincter or the rectal mucosa. This advantage is usually offset by greater difficulty in repair, increased blood loss, and a more painful postpartum course.

Although proper repair of rectal damage caused by extension of a median episiotomy rarely results in long-term morbidity, abnormalities in this area such as inflammatory bowel disease or prior surgery may indicate mediolateral episiotomy as the procedure of choice. Mediolateral episiotomy is performed by incision at a 45-degree angle from the inferior portion of the hymenal ring. The length of the incision is less critical than with median episiotomy, but longer incisions require more lengthy repair. The side to which the episiotomy is performed is usually dictated by the dominant hand of the obstetrician, as a right-sided episiotomy is more easily performed by a right-handed individual. For both median and mediolateral episiotomies, the incision should be extended vertically up the vaginal mucosa for a distance of approximately 2 to 3 cm.

Delivery of the Head

In the vertex presentation, the fetal head is delivered by extension. The goal of assisted delivery of the head is the prevention of rapid delivery. If extension does not occur with ease, assistance in the form of a modified Ritgen's maneuver may be provided. The hand, protected by a sterile towel, is placed on the perineum and the fetal chin palpated. The chin is then gently pressed upward, effecting extension of the fetal head.

After expulsion of the head, external rotation is allowed. If the cord is palpable around the neck, it should be looped over the head; if not reducible, it should be doubly clamped and cut. Mucus should be aspirated from the fetal mouth, oropharynx, and nares. Although usually performed with a bulb syringe, in the presence of meconium, thorough aspiration with a DeLee suction catheter reduces the risk of meconium aspiration syndrome.

Delivery of the Shoulders and Body

Once the fetal airway has been cleared, the physician places his or her hands along the parietal bones of the fetus, and the mother is asked to bear down gently. The fetus is directed posteriorly until the anterior shoulder has passed beneath the symphysis.

After delivery of the anterior shoulder, the mother should be asked to pant. The fetus is slowly directed anteriorly until the posterior shoulder passes the perineum.

After delivery of the shoulders, the fetus should be grasped with the palm of one hand above the shoulders and with the other hand along the spine. The infant should be cradled as delivery is completed either spontaneously or with a gentle maternal push. Once delivered, the infant should be held securely and wiped dry with a sterile towel, and any mucus remaining in the airway is suctioned.

Cord Clamping

After delivery, there is a net transfer of blood from the placenta to the infant. Spasm of the umbilical artery occurs within approximately 1 minute of birth. However, the remaining communication between the neonate and placenta, the umbilical vein, permits passage of blood for up to 3 minutes after birth. The pressure gradient for the flow in the umbilical vein depends on intrauterine pressure and neonatal venous pressure. Because these pressures are usually fairly low during the immediate postdelivery period, gravitational effects are important. The physician can therefore influence the degree of postnatal placental transfusion both by the interval between delivery and cord clamping and by altering the height at which the infant is held after delivery. In most instances, the volume of this transfusion is not important, and the timing of the cord clamping is dictated by convenience. Because intentional manipulation of the volume of transfusion can result in either relative hypervolemia or hypovolemia of the neonate, such procedures should be reserved for unusual situations.[5]

PELVIMETRY AND LABOR

Pelvic Shapes, Planes, and Diameters

It is intuitively obvious that successful vaginal delivery is dependent on the relative size of the fetus and the maternal pelvis. Not surprisingly, therefore, a great deal of information has accumulated about the size and shape of the female pelvis. Measurements of great precision have been made directly in cadavers and using radiographic techniques in large numbers of women. In general, these measurements have divided the pelvis into a series of planes that must be traversed by the fetus during passage through the birth canal. It should be kept in mind, however, that these planes describe the bony limits of the pelvis, and consideration of the influence of the soft tissues of the birth canal has been rare.

The bony pelvis is a bowl-shaped structure open at the anterior inferior margin. It is bounded anteriorly

Table 14.2 Pelvic Types and Characteristics

Type	Shape	Posterior Sagittal Diameter	Prognosis
Gynecoid	Round	Average	Good
Anthropoid	Long, oval	Long	Good
Android	Heart shaped	Short	Poor
Platypelloid	Flat, oval	Short	Poor

by the pubic portion of the innominate bones, which are joined in the midline at the symphysis pubis. The lateral margins are the innominate bones, which are joined by synchondroses to the sacrum that, along with the coccyx, forms the posterior margin. The true pelvis lies below the linea terminalis, which demarcates the line of fusion between the iliac and ischial portion of the innominate bones.

The most commonly measured planes are the pelvic inlet and the midplane. The pelvic inlet (obstetric conjugate) is bounded anteriorly by the posterior border of the symphysis pubis, posteriorly by the sacral promontory, and laterally by the linea terminalis. As the shape of this plane varies considerably, the measurement of its transverse diameter is conventionally made at the widest point. The mid-pelvic plane is bounded laterally by the inferior margins of the ischial spines, anteriorly by the lower margin of the symphysis pubis, and posteriorly by the sacrum (usually S4 or S5).

Pelves have been classified into four basic types based on the shape of the inlet. This classification, based on the radiographic studies of Caldwell et al.,[6] separates those with favorable characteristics (gynecoid, anthropoid) from those with less efficient utilization of space within the pelvis (android, platypelloid). The differing types are usually described according to their shapes, as demonstrated in Table 14.2. The distinguishing feature between favorable and unfavorable types is the amount of space posterior to the greatest transverse diameter. This space is most easily characterized by the posterior sagittal diameter extending from the sacral promontory to the greatest transverse diameter. Unfortunately, this simple characterization of pelvic types does not com-

pletely characterize the pelvis, because in reality many women fall into intermediate classes and distinctions become arbitrary.

Clinical Pelvimetry

Although many external measurements of the female pelvis have been advocated as predictive of pelvic size, only a few such measurements enjoy current usage. The most commonly used is the diagonal conjugate. This important measurement is the distance from the inferior border of the symphysis pubis to the sacral promontory. It is an easily obtainable index of the obstetric conjugate and therefore the anteroposterior diameter of the pelvic inlet.

The measurement is made by positioning the tip of the middle finger at the sacral promontory and noting the point on the hand that contacts the symphysis pubis. The diagonal conjugate is generally 1.5 to 2.0 cm longer than the obstetric conjugate.

The second clinical measurement still in use is the bi-ischial diameter. With the patient in the lithotomy position, the ischial tuberosities are palpated and the distance between them measured. A value of greater than 8 cm is considered adequate. A small measurement may imply a generally small pelvis or convergence of the pelvic side walls.

Other characteristics of the pelvis may be noted on digital examination but only described qualitatively (small, average, large). These include the angulation of the pubic rami beneath the pubic arch, the apparent size of the ischial spines, the size of the sacrospinous notch, and the degree of curvature of the sacrum and coccyx. Although the qualitative nature of these measurements detracts from their general utility, they may supply significant information about the overall shape of the pelvis.

Radiographic Pelvimetry

Although pelvic measurement has been accepted for centuries as an adjunct for the management of labor, precision in pelvic measurements was not achieved prior to the advent of radiographic pelvimetry. Initial enthusiasm for the use of this technique, however, was later tempered by an increasing appreciation of the potential hazards of radiation to the fetus. Although used much less frequently today, radiographic pelvimetry still plays an important role in the

Table 14.3 Average and Critical Limit Values for Pelvic Measurements by Radiographic Pelvimetry

Diameter	Average Value	Critical Limit
Inlet		
AP (cm)	12.5	10.0
T (cm)	13.0	12.0
Total (cm)	25.5	22.0
Area (cm²)	145.0	123.0
Midplane		
AP (cm)	11.5	10.0
T (cm)	10.5	9.5
Total (cm)	22.0	20.0
Area (cm²)	125.0	106.0

management of some patients, especially those with breech presentation.

Systems of radiographic pelvimetry rely primarily on anteroposterior (AP) and transverse (T) views of the pelvis. These systems compensate for magnification by inclusion of a metallic ruler to which measurements are compared or by calculation of film object distances.

The systems developed by Thoms and by Colcher and Sussman depend on comparisons between the diameters measured to tables of average and critical limits. The most commonly used measurements are the AP and T diameters and their totals at the pelvic inlet and at the pelvic midplane. Commonly used values for these measurements are listed in Table 14.3. It should be noted that the critical limits cited imply that a high likelihood of cephalopelvic disproportion may exist.

A popular modification of this technique is a calculation of areas as popularized by Mengert.[7] He demonstrated that below a critical limit (85 percent of the mean value) labor was associated with a high rate of cesarean birth or with difficult deliveries.

A major disadvantage of these systems is the lack of information on fetal size. This deficiency is addressed by the technique originally described by Ball.[8] In this system, corrected values for the diameters of the planes are used to calculate spheres to which the calculated volume of the fetal cranium is compared. The criteria for disproportion rely on the deficit between the calculated capacities of the pelvic planes and the volume of the fetal cranium.

Risks of X-Ray Pelvimetry

The primary concern governing the use of x-ray pelvimetry is exposure of the fetus to ionizing radiation. This concern has been based on several retrospective studies that have demonstrated a higher incidence of childhood malignancy in infants exposed to x-ray in utero.[9,10] Although these studies suffer from serious methodologic flaws with respect to scientific proof and a number of reports have failed to detect such an association, they are supported by firm theoretical considerations, and it is prudent to consider antenatal pelvimetry potentially carcinogenic for the fetus.

Allowing for this potential hazard, the risks and benefits of the procedure must be carefully weighed. The likelihood of childhood malignancy based on these retrospective studies is approximately 1 cancer per 5,000 infants exposed. This risk is quite small in comparison to the hazard of perinatal mortality associated with cephalopelvic disproportion. Data from the Collaborative Perinatal Study document a perinatal death rate of 17.9 per 1,000 in the presence of maternal dystocia.[11] This potentially favorable risk-benefit ratio, however, must be considered in light of the real benefits derived. In most recent reports, the results of x-ray pelvimetry were not used to guide clinical management, and the fetus therefore gained little benefit from the study. Clearly, a potentially hazardous procedure with results that are not likely to influence management has little place in sound medical practice. On the other hand, x-ray pelvimetry may be helpful in labors complicated by breech presentations. Most authorities agree that the hazards of breech presentation are sufficient to warrant radiographic pelvimetry for cases in which vaginal delivery is contemplated.[12] Perinatal mortality for vaginal breech delivery in the presence of abnormal pelvimetry findings ranges from 2.2 to 8.5 percent.[13] Recognizing these hazards as well as the potential limitations of x-ray pelvimetry, most modern authors have recommended that women with pelvic diameters of less than average size are best managed by cesarean birth.[14,15] Although these stringent criteria serve to exclude approximately one-half the candidates for vaginal delivery, they have achieved acceptable levels of perinatal morbidity in this hazardous setting.

Obstetric Palpation — Leopold's Maneuvers

Although abdominal palpation of the gravid uterus for the diagnosis of fetal lie and presentation dates back to antiquity, a codified method of examination was first described by Leopold and Sporlin in 1894. Palpation is divided into four separate maneuvers that can identify fetal landmarks and reveal fetomaternal relationships. Although abdominal examination has several limitations (small fetus, obese mother, polyhydramnios, multiple gestation), and ascertainment of fetal position and station are less precise than vaginal examination, the procedure is safe and well tolerated and may add valuable information to the management of labor.

Leopold's maneuvers consist of a series of four palpations of the uterus. Over the years the numerical sequence has varied, but the objectives remain the same. Basically, Leopold's maneuvers answer four questions:

1. *What is at the fundus?* With the patient lying supine and her knees comfortably flexed, the examiner stands at her side facing her head. The examiner's hands (which are warm, it is hoped) are placed at the fundus of the uterus. Palpation with the tips of the fingers ascertains the presence or absence of a fetal pole (vertical versus transverse lie) and the nature of the fetal pole. The fetal breech is larger, less well defined, and less ballottable than the cranium.
2. *Where are the spine and small parts?* After examination of the fundus, the lateral walls of the uterus are examined. In vertical lies, the sides will be usually occupied by the fetal back and small parts (extremities). The location of the fetal spine is determined by the characteristic properties of the spine, a long, firm, linear structure. The small parts are characterized by their different contours and occasionally by rapid movement. The fingers of one hand are used for palpation, while the other hand fixes the fetus.
3. *What is presenting in the pelvis?* The examiner now turns toward the feet of the patient. The fingertips are placed laterally above the symphysis and

brought toward the midline. When the fetus is encountered, the characteristics of the fetal pole are noted. In addition, the degree of descent of the fetal pole beneath the symphysis is noted as an indication of the station of the presenting part.
4. *Where is the cephalic prominence?* In cephalic presentations, a point of the fetal head may be noted as a protuberance that arrests the hand outlining the fetus. As the hands are moved along the lateral walls of the fetus toward the pelvis, either the occiput or the chin will be encountered, if the head is not deep within the pelvis. If the head is neither flexed nor extended, the chin (located on the same side as the small parts) will be prominent. In deflexed attitudes (face presentation), the occiput will be encountered below the fetal spine. If the head is well flexed, neither structure will be prominent.

For most patients, the information gleaned from Leopold's maneuvers will be sufficient for the diagnosis of position and station. Rather than being considered an alternative, abdominal palpation should be viewed as a valuable adjunct to vaginal examination.

DISORDERS OF LABOR

Abnormal Patterns

Abnormal patterns of labor are defined by deviation from the norms for the phases of labor as defined earlier in this chapter. For all phases except the latent phase, the abnormality may be either protraction or arrest (an arrested latent phase implies that labor has not truly begun). Because these disorders differ considerably in implication and management, they will be discussed separately.

Prolonged Latent Phase

The latent phase of labor is defined as the period of time starting with the onset of regular uterine contractions and terminated by the onset of the active phase. Based on the criteria listed in Table 14.1, this phase is considered prolonged if it exceeds approximately 20 hours in nulliparas or 14 hours in multiparas. Although the duration of this phase of labor apparently has little direct implication on perinatal mortality, prolongation can certainly be taxing to the mother and her attendants. In many women, cervical effacement during the latent phase, especially in the nulliparas entering labor prior to significant effacement, presents a problem.

The basis for management of a prolonged latent phase consists of recognition of possible etiologies and individualized treatment.[16] Although less frequently encountered today than when Friedman originally studied this group, oversedation must be considered. Most patients will simply be those who have entered labor without substantial cervical effacement. For these women the process that normally occurs over weeks must be compressed into hours.

Unless there is a maternal or fetal indication for expeditious delivery, most authorities agree that the management of choice consists of therapeutic rest. This allows the patient a respite from the physical and emotional rigors of labor and can aid in the distinction between true and false labor. Because this therapeutic rest is generally induced with a rather large dose of morphine (15 to 20 mg), it is essential that an evaluation of the myometrial contraction pattern and cervical examination be made to exclude those patients entering into the active phase.

After several hours of rest (usually sleep), approximately 85 percent of patients thus treated will progress to the active phase. Approximately 10 percent will cease to have contractions, and the diagnosis of false labor may be made. For the approximately 5 percent of patients in whom therapeutic rest fails and in patients for whom expeditious delivery is indicated, oxytocin infusion may be used.

Two other methods of management must be condemned. Amniotomy holds little benefit for the patient with prolonged latent phase and may serve only to increase the risk of intrauterine infection or cord prolapse. Finally, cesarean birth for this indication alone benefits neither the fetus nor the mother.

Disorders of the Active Phase

Cervicographic and Manometric Analysis of Labor

The major classification of abnormalities of the active phase of labor is based on the cervicographic analysis of labor. According to this classification, abnormalities are defined by their departure from the normal pattern of cervical dilatation.[17] In addition to this system, a number of investigators have proposed a classification based on the electromechanical state of the uterus.[18,19] Inefficient uterine activity is divided into hypertonic and hypotonic dysfunction. Hypotonic dysfunction reflects an insufficient generation of action potentials from the myometrial pacemaker, inadequate propagation of the signal throughout the myometrium, or lack of mechanical response to the signal. Hypertonic dysfunction includes a group of disorders associated with contractions that are generated in the lower pole of the uterus or in multiple sites. In either circumstance, the contraction pattern fails to result in cervical effacement and dilatation.

In the clinical setting, the distinction between hypotonic and hypertonic dysfunction is made on the basis of clinical and manometric criteria. Hypotonic dysfunction occurs in both nulliparas and multiparas and may be seen at any point during labor. It is often an indication of relative cephalopelvic disproportion, malposition, or maternal fatigue. Uterine contractions are infrequent, of low amplitude, and are accompanied by low or normal baseline pressures. Maternal discomfort is minimal. Hypertonic dysfunction is primarily a condition of nulliparas and is usually associated with early labor. Frequent contractions of low amplitude are often associated with an elevated baseline pressure. Maternal discomfort is significant and backache frequent. In addition to hypertonic and hypotonic dysfunction, cervicographic abnormalities of labor may be eutonic in which manometric parameters of uterine activity are normal.

Primary Dysfunctional Labor

Primary dysfunctional labor is defined as active-phase dilatation that occurs at a rate less than the fifth centile. This value is 1.2 cm/hr in nulliparas and 1.5 cm/hr in multiparas (Fig. 14.3). An example of this disorder is shown in Figure 14.4.

What is considered optimal management of primary dysfunctional labor is a major distinction between the American and British schools of labor management. The American approach is based on the studies of Friedman and Sachtleben[20] in which amniotomy, oxytocin, and sedation had little effect, while physiologic support and further observation seemed to provide the best course. The British approach, exemplified by the reports from the National

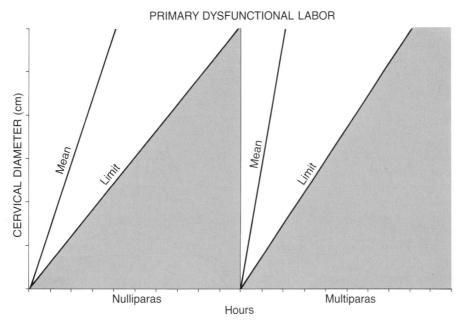

PRIMARY DYSFUNCTIONAL LABOR

CERVICAL DIAMETER (cm)

Mean Limit

Nulliparas

Mean Limit

Multiparas

Hours

Fig. 14.3 Mean and lower limit for rate of cervical dilatation in nulliparas and multiparas. Rates below the 5th centile signify primary dysfunctional labor.

Maternity Hospital in Dublin, includes prompt amniotomy and oxytocin infusion.[21] Despite these major differences in approach, several important similarities exist. Both groups acknowledge the importance of recognition of primary dysfunctional labor as a frequent predecessor of secondary arrest of labor and as a risk factor for perinatal mortality. Gravidas exhibiting this disorder require careful maternal and fetal surveillance. In addition, both groups agree that primary dysfunctional labor alone is not an indication for cesarean birth.

Secondary Arrest of Cervical Dilatation and Combined Disorders of Active Phase

Secondary arrest was defined by Friedman and Sachtleben[22] as cessation of a previously normal dilatation for a period of 2 hours (Fig. 14.4). It should be noted that this definition is somewhat artificial, and arrests of 1 hour have been associated with an increase in second-stage abnormalities and fetal morbidity.

A combined disorder of active-phase dilatation is defined as arrest of dilatation occurring when the patient has previously exhibited primary dysfunctional labor (Fig. 14.4). In Friedman's series, this group of patients had a less favorable outcome with regard to vaginal delivery than did patients with secondary arrest alone.

Although less controversial than primary dysfunctional labor, management of arrest in the active phase varies considerably. As noted earlier, radiographic pelvimetry is advocated by some but is generally considered to be of little value in the treatment of this disorder. Ambulation has been reported to be beneficial, but the number of patients managed by this method has been quite limited.[23] Although a "trial of labor" is advocated universally, a uniform definition of such a trial is lacking.

While realizing these difficulties, a generally accepted management approach would consist of a careful examination followed by amniotomy and initiation of intrauterine monitoring if indicated. The examination should include an assessment for signs of fetal distress, maternal fatigue, or excessive fetal size. A detailed vaginal examination should be performed to verify cervical dilatation, fetal station, presentation, and position. Clinical pelvimetry should be performed with notation of overall pelvic capacity and pelvic type. Unusual causes of dystocia such as uterine leiomyomata, ovarian tumors, vaginal cysts or

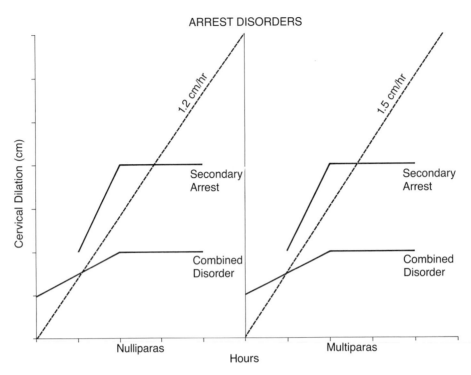

Fig. 14.4 Active phase-arrest disorders. Combined disorder implies an arrest in a gravida previously exhibiting primary dysfunctional labor.

septa, as well as fetal malformations should be considered.

If the uterine activity is noted to be optimal, then further stimulation of the myometrium by oxytocin infusion should be undertaken only with extreme caution, if at all. If, however, hypotonic uterine dysfunction exists and no other cause of arrest has been noted, oxytocin infusion may be used with a high degree of success and safety.

The optimum duration of this "trial of labor" is poorly defined. Fortunately, the large majority of patients (70 to 80 percent in Friedman's series) respond successfully and resume progression of cervical dilatation. Although precise information is difficult to obtain, most authorities cite continued arrest over 2 to 4 hours as an indication for cesarean birth. It must be noted, however, that even in the group in which progress is noted there is an increased frequency of second-stage abnormalities and operative deliveries.

Abnormalities of the Second Stage

The second stage of labor is the interval between full cervical dilatation and delivery of the infant. Abnormalities of the second stage may be either protraction or arrest of descent. Arrest of descent, sometimes referred to as failure of descent, occurs rarely in normal presentations.

Protraction of descent has been defined as descent occurring at less than 1 cm/hr in nulliparas and 2 cm/hr in multiparas.[24] This definition, however, suffers from two major flaws. First, the accuracy and precision of estimation of fetal station is considerably less than the estimation of cervical dilatation. Second, the location of the presenting part within the birth canal is noted in terms of station. Because the length of the birth canal varies considerably and is generally between 11 and 15 cm, estimation of change in station, descent in centimeters per hour, is difficult.

These problems notwithstanding, it is clear that gravidas may exhibit protracted descent with etiologies similar to those seen for primary dysfunctional labor. The potential fetal risk inherent in a prolonged second stage has been known for some time. Studies from the early 1950s documented increasing infant mortality correlating with the length of the second stage.[25] Reviews of electronic fetal heart rate tracings obtained during this phase have documented a high incidence of variable decelerations and prolonged decelerations.[26] The gradual fall in fetal scalp capillary pH that occurs throughout labor is accelerated during the second stage.[27]

Until recently, these factors led to a policy of intervention whenever the second stage exceeded 2 hours in length. Subsequent experience, however, has demonstrated that when electronic fetal monitoring is employed, operative intervention may be avoided provided that descent is progressive.[28]

Arrest of descent, on the other hand, is more accurately diagnosed (at least when both examinations are conducted by a single examiner) and is more urgent. As in arrest of dilatation, this disorder requires prompt reevaluation of uterine contractility, maternal and fetal well-being, and cephalopelvic relationships. Obvious problems such as hypotonic dysfunction, overdistended bladder, strong perineal resistance, conduction anesthesia, or ineffectual bearing down should be treated appropriately with a high expectation of success. In the absence of such factors, however, very careful judgment is required. Estimation of fetopelvic relationships, including station, caput formation, molding, palpation of the fetal head above the symphysis, and malrotation is mandatory. For patients in whom low forceps delivery is possible, this is the procedure of choice. When a low forceps delivery is not possible, the choice among mid-forceps delivery, vacuum extraction, oxytocin infusion, or cesarean birth is extremely difficult and controversial. In view of the emotional problems in making such decisions, consultation is often helpful.

STIMULATION OF UTERINE ACTIVITY

Measurements of Uterine Activity

Parameters of uterine activity usually measured during labor include the frequency, duration, and intensity of contractions. In addition, with the use of direct pressure monitors, baseline tone may be determined. Three major techniques for the measurement of uterine contractions are commonly employed. The oldest of these is palpation, performed by resting a hand on the uterine fundus. The examiner notes the frequency, apparent duration, and relative intensity of contractions (subjectively rated as +1 to +3). The major advantages of palpation include simplicity and the direct contact between patient and examiner.

Disadvantages include the inability to measure intensity or duration of contractions accurately, lack of information concerning baseline tone, difficulty of measurement in the obese patient, and inability to correlate fetal heart rate patterns with uterine contractions.

External tocodynamometry measures the change in shape of the abdominal wall as a function of uterine contractions. Although sharing most of the disadvantages of palpation, this method does permit graphic display of uterine activity in relationship to fetal heart rate patterns.

The most precise method of determination of uterine activity is the direct method. Direct measurements require the insertion of a fluid-filled catheter directly into the uterine cavity, usually through the cervix after rupture of the membranes.

The quantification of uterine activity has received a considerable amount of attention since the pioneering studies of Caldeyro-Barcia and Posiero during the 1950s.[18] These studies demonstrated that cervical dilatation can be considered as an exponential function of uterine work (uterine pressure time).[29] The most commonly used units of uterine activity are the Montevideo Unit (average intensity frequency/10 min) and the Uterine Activity Unit (1 mmHg/min).[30]

Clinically all measurements of uterine activity demonstrate marked interpatient and intrapatient variation. Although some definitions of active management include augmentation of all patients with suboptimal uterine activity, current policies in the United States indicate that intervention is not required unless an abnormality in the progression of labor is documented. When such an abnormality is noted and uterine activity is not optimal (i.e., contractions of less than 50 mmHg every 3 minutes or below 250 Montevideo Units),[31] administration of an oxytocic agent is recommended.

Oxytocic Agents

Oxytocin is a peptide hormone that is stored and released from the posterior pituitary gland. It consists of eight amino acids, six of which it shares with the neuropeptide vasopressin. Oxytocin was first successfully purified in 1951 and was identified and synthetically prepared in 1953. Only intravenous solutions of oxytocin are approved for induction and augmentation of labor. Commercial solutions contain 10 IU/ml oxytocin (1 mg of synthetic oxytocin is equivalent to 450 IU). Oxytocin infusions have as their most important mechanism of action the stimulation of myometrial contractions. This action is dependent on the degree or responsiveness of the myometrium. Sensitivity of the uterus to oxytocin varies with the hormonal milieu in gestation and increases between weeks 20 and 40 of pregnancy. Stimulation of myometrial activity appears to depend on an increase in the permeability of myometrial cells to sodium ions. Very high infusion rates of oxytocin have been associated with hypertension, and bolus injections may cause hypotension. However, when administered intravenously as dilute solutions at recommended rates, few cardiovascular side effects are noted.

Oxytocin in the form of crude pituitary extracts has been used in clinical obstetrics since the early 1900s. Because of the extreme variability in myometrial stimulation associated with these crude extracts, early enthusiasm was tempered by disastrous results from uterine hyperactivity with fetal compromise and maternal damage. With standardization of synthetic preparations and an understanding of the importance of strict control of the infusion rate, oxytocin infusion has become an accepted and effective form of therapy.

The recommended rate of administration of oxytocin is usually that which stimulates normal labor. This rate may vary from 0.5 mIU/min to greater than 30 mIU/min, although some authorities recommend a maximal rate of 20 mIU/min.[32,33] Even at low infusion rates, however, contractions associated with oxytocin do not truly mimic spontaneous uterine contractions, as the rate of rise in intrauterine pressure appears to be greater than that seen in spontaneous labor.[34] Recent studies have demonstrated that, when used in patients demonstrating a protraction disorder, oxytocin infusion rates greater than 6 mIU/min are rarely required.[35] Approximately 30 to 40 minutes are needed for the full effect of an increase in dosage to be evident in the contraction pattern.

Despite the frequent use of oxytocin in clinical obstetrics, considerable debate still exists as to its proper utilization. Some authorities recommend the use of oxytocin only following radiographic pelvimetry or when uterine contractions are infrequent, of low amplitude, or both. Other investigators recommend oxytocin infusion whenever a protraction disorder of labor has been documented, despite apparently adequate uterine contractility. Regardless of these variations, it is clear that the use of an oxytocin infusion is associated with a high rate of success. Overall, approximately 80 percent of patients with documented disorders of labor respond to oxytocin infusion with subsequent progression of labor and vaginal delivery.[22]

Prostaglandins

Prostaglandins are a group of 20-carbon compounds derived from unsaturated fatty acids that possess high degrees of biologic activity. In the human, the major precursor for prostaglandins is arachidonic acid. Prostaglandin synthesis depends on the release of arachidonic acid from triglyceride esters and subsequent conversion by a group of enzymes collectively known as prostaglandin synthetases.

Although a large number of prostaglandins and prostaglandin-like substances exist, most obstetric interest has centered on prostaglandin F_2 (PGF_2) and prostaglandin E_2 (PGE_2). Both prostaglandins are potent stimulators of myometrial activity.

Myometrial contractility in response to prostaglandins, unlike that with oxytocin, is not greatly dependent on the duration of pregnancy. This activity has led to the widespread use of prostaglandins in midtrimester abortion and following intrauterine death.

The effects of prostaglandins have been compared with those of oxytocin in the term patient regarding both induction and augmentation of labor. These studies have generally failed to demonstrate a superiority of prostaglandins in terms of efficacy.[36] It is unlikely that prostaglandins will replace oxytocin for these indications.

ACTIVE MANAGEMENT OF LABOR

The increasing incidence of cesarean births noted in the United States during the 1970s has prompted an examination of the standard of methods used for labor management. Considerable interest has been directed toward the disparity in the incidences of cesarean birth in the United States and Ireland. O'Driscoll et al.[37] have maintained that the low rate of cesarean birth at the National Maternity Hospital in Dublin is due to a philosophy of labor management known as active management. The basic principles of active management include

1. Strict criteria for admission to the labor suite
2. Early amniotomy
3. Hourly cervical examinations
4. Oxytocin administration for dilatation rates less than 1 cm/hr
5. High (by American standards) concentrations of oxytocin in patients requiring augmentation
6. Expected durations of less than 12 hours for the first stage of labor and 2 hours for the second stage

Adherence to these principles at the National Maternity Hospital in Dublin has been associated with a primary cesarean birth rate of 5 to 6 percent. Direct comparison of cesarean birth rates between countries is difficult, however. As demonstrated by Levens et al.,[38] the rate of cesarean births depends on a number of demographic factors, including age and race, in addition to the method of management. Also of concern is the difficulty in ensuring that infrequent events, such as fetal injury, are comparable with differing methods of management. Although there have been reports that adoption of the principles of active management at hospitals in North America has resulted in a decrease in the rate of cesarean births,[39] the studies have not been prospectively controlled and the problem of relative fetal safety of active management remains.

FORCEPS DELIVERY AND VACUUM EXTRACTION

Types and Specialized Functions

Although obstetric forceps vary greatly in design, all types consist of two separate portions that are inserted into the vagina sequentially. Each blade is moved into the correct position, opposing the fetal head prior to the joining (locking) of the blades.

Each half consists of the blade proper (which is applied to the fetal head), a shank, and a handle. The halves are joined by a lock usually located at the junction of the shanks and the handles. The overall architecture of a forceps is determined by two curves, the cephalic curve, which allows for the area of the fetal head, and the pelvic curve, compensating for the curvature of the birth canal.

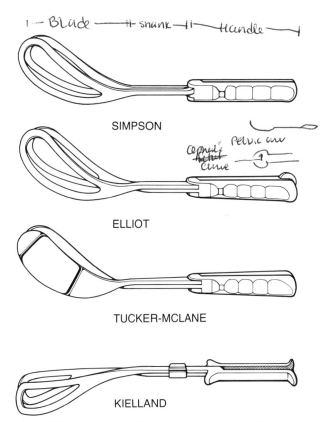

Fig. 14.5 Lateral view of some obstetric forceps. The pelvic curve, a prominent feature of classic instruments, is lacking in the Kielland forceps.

The blades may be either solid or fenestrated, and most forceps designs are available in either type. The most commonly used forceps types use either the "English" lock, in which the articulation is fixed, or the "sliding" lock, which permits movement between the forceps halves along the longitudinal axis of the shanks. The shanks may be either separated or overlapping. Instruments are illustrated in Figures 14.5 and 14.6.

Forceps may be divided into major groups according to their intended use. Most instruments fall into the "classic" category. These forceps have a fixed lock and a pelvic curve yielding a concave longitudinal axis. Three commonly used instruments are the Simpson forceps (fenestrated blade, separated shanks), the Elliot forceps (fenestrated blade, overlapping shanks), and the Tucker-McLean forceps (solid blade, overlapping shanks). The forceps in this

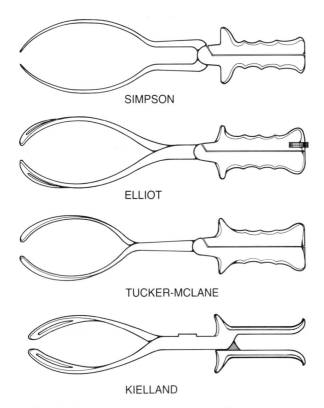

SIMPSON

ELLIOT

TUCKER-MCLANE

KIELLAND

Fig. 14.6 Anteroposterior view of some forceps. Note the difference between the separated shanks of the Simpson forceps and the overlapping shanks of the Elliot forceps.

category are primarily intended for use when the fetal head does not require rotation prior to delivery.

The second major category includes the "specialized" forceps. These instruments have been designed to facilitate delivery in cases requiring rotation of the fetal head (Kielland, Barton) or for breech delivery (Piper). The Kielland forceps differ from classic instruments in that the pelvic curve has been modified such that the blades lie below rather than above the plane of the shanks. This modification facilitates rotation of the forceps about a point rather than around a circle as is required with the classic instruments. Second, these forceps use a sliding lock, enabling the user to adjust for asynclitism of the fetal head.

The Barton forceps have decreased in popularity over the past 20 years. Designed for use in a platypelloid pelvis, these forceps allow traction with the fetal head in a transverse position until the introitus has been reached. The Piper forceps have blades below the plane of elongated shanks. These modifications are designed to facilitate application to the aftercoming head in breech delivery.

Classification of Forceps Delivery

Forceps deliveries are classified according to the station of the fetal head at the time of application. Although all systems of classification use station as the primary criterion, the number of divisions included vary. The Committee on Obstetrics: Maternal and Fetal Medicine of the American College of Obstetricians and Gynecologists, has recently offered the following classification:[40]

1. *Outlet forceps*—Application of forceps when the scalp is visible at the introitus without separating the labia, the fetal skull has reached the pelvic floor, the fetal head is at or on the perineum, and the angle between the anteroposterior line and the sagittal suture does not exceed 45 degrees
2. *Low forceps*—Application when the leading point of the skull is at station +2 or more, subclassified as to whether the angle between the sagittal suture and anteroposterior line exceeds 45 degrees
3. *Mid-forceps*—Application of forceps when the head is engaged but the presenting part is above station +2

Older classifications include forceps to the unengaged head, in which the fetal head is floating and ballottable above the brim of the true pelvis, and low-mid-forceps, in which the fetal biparietal diameter is at or below the level of the ischial spines, with the presenting part within a fingerbreadth of the perineum between contractions.

Indications and Contraindications

Few areas in obstetrics have been surrounded with as much controversy as the use of obstetric forceps. Since the introduction of forceps delivery, the potential for causing fetal damage has been clearly recognized. With the development of cesarean birth as an accepted method of management, the use of high forceps delivery for the living fetus has been universally abandoned. Low forceps delivery, once considered optimal management in the United States,[3] is now often considered meddlesome and unnecessary and has decreased considerably in popularity.

The major controversy, however, surrounds mid-forceps delivery. As a group, infants delivered by this method demonstrate an increased incidence of perinatal mortality, perinatal morbidity, and long-term neurologic defects.[41,42] Opponents of the continued use of this technique argue that these data suggest that mid-forceps delivery should be abandoned in a manner similar to high forceps.[43,44]

Proponents of the continued usage of mid-forceps believe that the great majority of infants with poor outcome after mid-forceps delivery result from deliveries that are considered difficult.[45] Because current terminology does not permit distinction among the varying degrees of fetal hazard involved with the procedure, all mid-forceps deliveries have been condemned. Studies in which mid-forceps have been associated with poor outcome, moreover, are retrospective in nature and subject to the problems of multiple confounding variables that may have significantly biased the outcome.[46] The Committee on Obstetrics: Maternal and Fetal Medicine of the American College of Obstetricians and Gynecologists has suggested that outlet forceps may be used to shorten the second stage of labor when it is in the best interests of the mother or fetus. More difficult forceps delivery (low forceps or mid-forceps) may be considered when the second stage is prolonged, for fetal distress, or for maternal indications such as cardiac disease or exhaustion. Although it is unlikely that this controversy will be resolved in the near future, all authorities agree that mid-forceps deliveries should be reserved for competent operators following careful consideration of the potential fetal risks.

Prerequisites for Forceps Delivery

All forceps deliveries require that several criteria be met before the application of the forceps:

1. The membranes must be ruptured.
2. The cervix must be fully dilated.
3. The operator must be fully acquainted with the use of the instrument.
4. The position and station of the fetal head must be known with certainty.
5. Adequate maternal anesthesia for proper application of the forceps must be present.

6. The maternal pelvis must be adequate in size for atraumatic delivery.
7. The characteristics of the maternal pelvis must be appropriate for the type of delivery being considered.
8. The fetal head must be engaged.

Mid-forceps deliveries require that strong consideration be given to alternative approaches such as administration of oxytocin, cesarean birth, or simply expectant management. Cases in which instrument rotation is considered may prove amenable to digital or manual rotation. Specifically hazardous are mid-forceps deliveries in which the fetus is less than 2,500 g or greater than 4,500 g, or when there has been an abnormality in the progression of labor.[47]

Technique of Application and Delivery

Before attempting forceps application, the patient should be properly prepared and positioned. The patient should be placed in the lithotomy position and cleansed and draped in the usual manner. The bladder, if full, should be emptied by catheterization. Adequate anesthesia is mandatory for both maternal and fetal safety. Although little anesthesia may be required for easily performed outlet forceps, low-forceps and mid-forceps procedures require properly administered and monitored conduction of general anesthesia.

A thorough examination of the fetal position and characteristics of the maternal pelvis is mandatory. Exact knowledge of fetal position, station, and degree of asynclitism is essential to proper application. If the maternal pelvis appears to be inadequate in size or to possess unfavorable characteristics for the proposed procedure (e.g., rotation in an android or platypelloid pelvis), the procedure should be reconsidered.

Before application of the forceps, the operator should perform a "phantom application" by positioning the forceps in front of the perineum in the correct position of the final application. This "phantom application" aids in the evaluation of proper placement.

Outlet Forceps

Because by definition an outlet forceps delivery always requires the sagittal suture of the fetal skull to be within 45 degrees of directly anteroposterior, correction for fetal position prior to application is usually not required. In the occiput anterior (OA) position, following separation of the blades of the forceps, the left blade is held by the right hand of the operator. The handle is held loosely in the left hand so that the position of the forceps is essentially vertical. The blade is then introduced directly posteriorly and guided in an arc by the right (intravaginal) hand along the left side of the maternal pelvis to the correct position along the left parietal bone of the fetus. The hand of the operator is then removed from the vagina, allowing the blade of the forceps to remain in place. The remaining half of the forceps is then inserted in a similar manner, except that the right blade is held in the left hand and guided to the right parietal bone of the fetus.

Following the application, the handles are brought together and locked. Before the initiation of traction, it is mandatory that the application be checked for correct positioning.

Checking the Application

Safe use of obstetric forceps requires proper application to the fetus. Proper application involves a true cephalic placement (biparietal, bimalar). The application of compressive or tractive forces to any other area of the fetal skull may result in serious cranial or neurologic damage. Proper application must be determined by assessing the position of the forceps in relation to three landmarks on the fetal skull. The first check determines the position of the plane of the shanks with regard to the posterior fontanelle. The median angle of the fontanelle should be located halfway between the blades of the forceps and approximately 1 to 1.5 cm above the plane of the shanks. The second check requires that the sagittal suture be perpendicular to the plane of the shanks throughout its length. The third check is to ensure that the blades of the forceps are sufficiently applied to the parietal bones. Only 1 to 1.5 cm of the blades should be palpable beyond the fetal skull (if the blades are fenestrated, no more than a fingertip should be able to be inserted). If all criteria for proper application are not met, readjustment must be made before attempts at traction or rotation. An illustration of proper application is given in Figure 14.7.

Low Forceps and Mid-Forceps

Application of the forceps for low forceps and mid-forceps deliveries when the fetal head is directly OA or occiput posterior (OP) is identical to that for outlet forceps. In cases where fetal position is rotated more than slightly (ROA, LOA, ROP, LOP), attempts at manual or digital rotation should be made prior to instrument rotation. If this fails, following a phantom application the forceps should be applied such that the posterior blade is inserted first. For the LOA and ROP positions this is the left blade; for ROA and LOP this is the right blade. The blades are inserted according to the same principles as for low forceps, remembering that the proper location of the shanks is dictated by the position of the fetal skull, not the axis of the maternal pelvis. Thus, after application, the shanks of the forceps will point toward either the left (LOA, ROP) or right (ROA, LOP) shoulder of the operator. In cases in which the right blade is the posterior blade, the shanks of the forceps must be rotated around each other (left under right) for locking to take place. After application, the three checks of proper application are made and, if necessary, the blades are adjusted.

If the fetal head is not flexed, flexion is accomplished before rotation. Because forceps of the classic type include a prominent pelvic curve, rotation of the handles of the forceps must be about an arc. This rotation is carried out until the sagittal suture rests in the direct anteroposterior position. After rotation, the position of the forceps should be rechecked before traction.

Occiput Transverse Positions

Forceps delivery from the occiput transverse position is best accomplished with the use of specialized forceps. These instruments (Keilland, Barton) require considerable skill and experience, and their use has decreased greatly in recent years. The design and use of these instruments differs greatly from the classic forceps.

In the gynecoid or anthropoid pelvis, the Kielland forceps permit the rotational axis of the forceps to be in line with the plane of the fetus. Thus the rotation can be accomplished without the need for a large sweeping motion of the handles of the forceps during rotation. Two main methods of application of the Kielland forceps have come into popular usage. The "classical" or "inversion" method entails the application of the anterior blade of the forceps beneath the symphysis pubis, with the cephalic curve of the blade following the curve of the undersurface of the symphysis pubis. The application is carried on until the forceps have been applied in apposition to the ante-

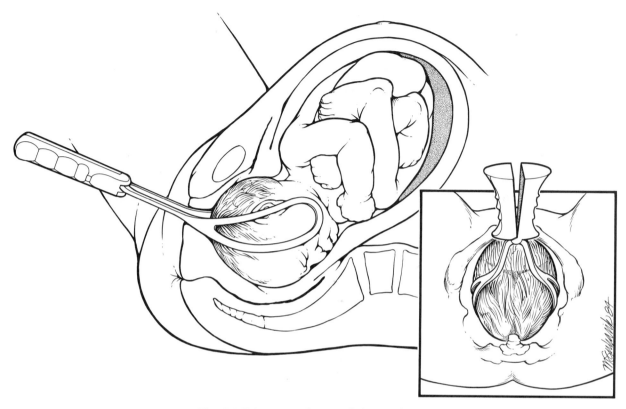

Fig. 14.7 Proper application of obstetric forceps.

rior surface of the fetal head. This blade is rotated at 180 degrees so that the cephalic curve of the blade corresponds with the cephalic curve of the fetus. The second blade is then applied directly to the posterior parietal region of the fetus.

The "wandering" application of the anterior blade is made in a manner similar to that of a classic forceps, with insertion posteriorly and rotation about either the frontal or the occipital region of the fetus to lie eventually in apposition to the anterior ear of the fetus. The second or posterior blade is then applied as in the classic application. After application and checks of proper positioning, the head is flexed and rotation is accomplished so that the head comes into the occiput anterior position. At this point, delivery is accomplished by traction either with the Kielland forceps or by reapplication of a classic type of forceps. If the Kielland forceps are used for traction, care must be taken to protect the posterior wall of the vagina. If the handles are raised as the head is delivered, lacerations of the posterior vaginal wall may result.

The Barton forceps are used when there is a transverse arrest of the fetus within a pelvis of the platypel-

loid type. The anterior blade is hinged and is applied in a wandering maneuver similar to that described for the Kielland forceps. The posterior blade, which has a sharp cephalic curve, is applied directly. After a check for proper application, traction is applied without rotation using a traction handle. Rotation to the occiput anterior position is not accomplished until the fetus is at the outlet.

Traction

After the application of forceps, delivery is accomplished according to the principle of axis traction; force is applied in a plane perpendicular to the plane of the pelvis at which the fetal head lies. The pelvis is curved in a reversed J shape, and it is in this direction that the series of force vectors should be applied. When the fetal head lies at the mid-pelvis, traction is directed posteriorly; at the pelvic floor, horizontally; and before expulsion, anteriorly.

To produce traction according to these changing vectors, axis traction may be accomplished either manually or via axis-traction attachments. Manual traction is applied via the Saxtorph-Pajot maneuver.

The vector is generated by force applied downward or upward on the shanks with one hand while the other hand pulls outward on the handles. Although this method is adequate for delivery from low stations, axis traction is best accomplished via the use of attachments that guide the operator continuously throughout the proper path of traction. The most commonly used axis-traction attachment is fastened at the finger guards of the classic instruments.

The Use of Vacuum Extraction

First popularized by Malmstrom[48] during the mid-1950s, the use of vacuum extraction–assisted delivery has become widespread in Europe. The classic instrument consists of a disc-shaped cup through which a vacuum of up to 0.8 kg/cc^2 is applied to the fetal scalp. This suction induces a caput succedaneum (chignon) within the cup to which tractional force is applied during uterine contractions. Although a number of studies have compared vacuum extraction with forceps deliveries, no definitive comparison has been made, and the choice of instrument appears to remain one of operator preference.

The indications and contraindications to vacuum extraction are essentially the same as those for forceps delivery. An advantage of vacuum extraction, however, is that delivery may be accomplished with minimal maternal analgesia.

Currently available instruments include metal cups in three sizes (40, 50, and 60 mm) and Silastic cups, which are cone shaped. Manually or electrically operated vacuum sources are available, but the latter are preferred.

The cup should be applied to the fetal head away from the fontanelles, with care being taken that no maternal tissue is entrapped within the cup. After application, a vacuum is established at 0.2 kg/cc^2 as the cup is held in place. The vacuum is raised every 2 minutes by intervals of 0.2 kg/cc^2 until a final vacuum of 0.7 to 0.8 kg/cc^2 is reached. These slow increments in vacuum are necessary for the proper development of the chignon.

Once a proper vacuum has been reached, traction may begin. One hand is used for traction, while the other maintains the fetal head in flexion and confirms that the cup has remained in place. Traction is applied in conjunction with uterine contractions only.

The vacuum should not be maintained for longer than 30 minutes.

THE THIRD STAGE OF LABOR

The interval between delivery of the infant and delivery of the placenta with attached umbilical cord and fetal membranes lasts less than 10 minutes in most women and occurs within 15 minutes in approximately 95 percent of all deliveries. Separation of the placenta is a consequence of continued uterine contractions following expulsion of the fetus. These contractions reduce the area of the uterine placental bed with subsequent disruption of the placental attachment along a plane in the spongiosa layer of the decidua vera. Continued powerful and prolonged contractions serve to control blood loss from the spiral arteries through compression and transport the placenta from the fundus into the lower uterine segment.

Because placental separation relies solely on uterine contractions, interference with this process by techniques such as fundal compression or traction on the umbilical cord can increase the incidence of complications such as hemorrhage or uterine inversion. During this interval, proper management requires only gentle palpation of the uterine fundus for uterine contractions and observation for excessive blood loss.

Although most authorities agree that the use of oxytocic agents is valuable in the reduction of blood loss during the third stage, the timing of administration varies between institutions. On the basis of controlled trials, dilute intravenous oxytocin appears to be superior to intravenous or intramuscular ergometrine.[49] Timing of administration, however, is controversial. Administration immediately following delivery may reduce total blood loss but can hamper management in cases involving an undiagnosed second twin or placenta accreta. In the United States, administration after delivery of the placenta appears to be the most common practice. During the interval between delivery of the infant and separation of the placenta, the physician should conduct a careful and thorough examination of the cervix, vagina, and perineum unless his or her assistance is required with neonatal resuscitation. The uterine fundus should be examined transabdominally to ensure that it is firm and that the uterine size is appropriate.

In the absence of anesthesia, intravaginal exploration for obstetric trauma can be quite uncomfortable, and the mother should be notified in advance of the procedures to be performed. Three or four fingers of one hand placed against the posterior vaginal wall and depressed will provide excellent visualization of the vagina and cervix in most cases. Using a sponge forceps, the obstetrician should grasp the anterior lip of the cervix and visualize the entire rim of the cervix either simultaneously or sequentially. If a laceration is seen, its length and position should be noted for subsequent repair.

After cervical inspection, a surgical sponge should be rolled and placed in the forceps. The instrument is then placed in the vagina and the sponge used to elevate the vaginal apex. This will permit complete visualization of both vaginal side walls for evidence of lacerations or hematoma formation.

Perineal inspection involves examination of the anteroposterior fourchette, the vaginal vestibule, hymenal ring, perineal body, external rectal sphincter, and the rectal mucosa. Examination of the rectal sphincter and mucosa is especially important, as failure to recognize injuries to these structures can result in serious morbidity.

Separation of the placenta is usually rapidly followed by its passage into the lower uterine segment. This event can usually be detected by the occurrence of the classic signs of placental detachment. These include (1) a gush of blood from the vagina, (2) descent of the umbilical cord, (3) a change in shape of the uterine fundus from discoid to globular, and (4) an increase in the height of the fundus as the lower uterine segment is distended by the placenta. After separation, the placenta, cord, and membranes should be delivered by maternal expulsive efforts along with gentle traction on the umbilical cord. Excessive traction will only serve to increase the likelihood of tearing of the membranes.

After passage of the placenta through the vulva, membranes that are still adhered to the decidua are usually separated simply by the weight of the placenta. If this does not occur, gentle traction on the membranes with a ring forceps may be required.

After delivery, the placenta, cord, and membranes should be examined. The cord should be inspected for length, presence of knots, and number of vessels. The placenta and membranes should be examined for signs of tearing or missing pieces. A vessel coursing along the membranes should arouse suspicion of an accessory lobe. The need for manual intrauterine exploration is controversial. Although some authorities believe that manual exploration is indicated in all deliveries,[50] in the absence of adequate anesthesia this may be quite difficult and uncomfortable to the patient. Intrauterine exploration is required when there is suspicion of retained tissue or when there is excessive uterine bleeding.[51]

INDUCTION OF LABOR

Induction of labor is the initiation of uterine contractions before the spontaneous onset of labor by medical and/or surgical means for the purpose of delivery. It may be categorized as elective or indicated. Before the decision to induce labor, the physician should document the type of induction and that the patient had been informed and accepts the indications, the methods, and potential complications, including the possibility of delivery by cesarean section.

Indicated Induction

In general, induction of labor may be indicated when the benefit of delivery to the mother and/or fetus outweighs the potential problem if the pregnancy continues. There may be maternal or fetal indications. These conditions may arise if the maternal medical or surgical condition worsens under expectant therapy or if there is evidence of impaired intrauterine existence. If obstetric data confirm that the pregnancy is at term or if fetal pulmonary maturity has been documented, the decision to induce labor is not difficult. At times, however, the benefit of a premature delivery of a fetus from a hostile intrauterine environment may outweigh the potential problems associated with prematurity.

Before induction, a thorough evaluation of the patient is indicated. This process as well as the indications for the induction should be documented on the chart. The pediatricians should be notified of the induction so that they can make specific plans of management for the neonate.

The maternal pelvis should be assessed as to its

Table 14.4 Bishop Prelabor Scoring System

Factor	Score			
	0	1	2	3
Dilatation (cm)	Closed	1–2	3–4	≥5
Effacement (%)	0–30	40–50	60–70	≥80
Station	−3	−2	−1.0	+1, +2
Consistency	Firm	Medium	Soft	
Position of cervix	Posterior	Mid-position	Anterior	

adequacy for vaginal delivery. This assessment may be performed by clinical rather than radiographic pelvimetry. The fetal presentation should be vertex, and the fetus should not be macrosomic. In 1964 Bishop[52] evaluated multiparous patients for elective induction of labor and developed a score for different variables found from the vaginal examination. This scoring system suggested by Bishop has provided valid parameters for evaluating all patients prior to the induction of labor.[53,54] Table 14.4 represents a modification of Bishop's method for predicting the ease of inductibility in which a score of 0, 1, 2, or 3 is given for dilatation, effacement, consistency, and position of the cervix and for station of the vertex. A total score of 9 or above indicates that induction of labor should be successful. Ideally, the best results are obtained when prelabor contractions have contributed to the formation of the lower uterine segment; the cervix is soft in consistency, 50 percent effaced, 2 cm or more dilated, and anterior in position; and the vertex is engaged in the pelvis. If spontaneous prelabor has not occurred and the cervix is not favorable, it may take 10 to 12 hours of good uterine contractility to "ripen" the cervix. It should be recognized that the induction process attempts to accomplish in hours what may take several days of spontaneous prelabor.

Indications

The following are accepted, but not all-inclusive, maternal or fetal indications for induction of labor: preeclampsia, eclampsia, premature rupture of membranes, chorioamnionitis, abruptio placenta, fetal death, suspected fetal distress as evidenced by biophysical indicators, prolonged gestation, diabetes mellitus, chronic hypertension, renal disease, or isoimmunization.

Contraindications

In general, any contraindication to spontaneous labor and delivery per vagina should be a contraindication to induced labor. Contraindications may include, but are not limited to, the following: previous uterine incision secondary to metroplasty, extensive myomectomy, or cesarean section; cephalopelvic disproportion resulting from abnormalities of pelvic bones or malpresentation of fetus (e.g., shoulder, complete or footling breech); invasive cervical carcinoma; central or total placenta previa; or an active or culture-proven genital herpes infection. Grand multiparity and uterine overdistention secondary to multiple gestation or hydramnios are relative contraindications.

Methodology

Surgical

Stripping of Membranes

Digitally separating the chorioamniotic membrane from the wall of the cervix and lower uterine segment appears to release prostaglandins produced locally from the membranes and adjacent decidua.[55,56] Prostaglandins may be involved in stimulating myometrial contractions and the onset of labor. In addition, the method may excite an autonomic neural reflex and/or cause the release of maternal oxytocin from the posterior pituitary that may initiate labor.[57] For stripping or sweeping of the membranes to be successful, the vertex should be well applied to the cervix. Risks of this technique include the potential for introducing uterine infection, bleeding from an unsuspected placenta previa, and accidental rupture of the membranes. Because the effects of membrane stripping are not predictable and the efficacy of this method has not been proved, it should not be used alone or as a routine practice for induction.

Amniotomy

In patients with a high Bishop score, artificial rupture of the membranes has been reported to be 88 percent successful in inducing labor.[58] The technique of amniotomy involves perforation of the chorioamniotic membranes, which are palpable through the cervix and digitally retracting the membranes over the vertex. In addition to retracting the membranes, the amniotic fluid should be released without dislodging the vertex. The amount and character of the fluid should be noted and documented.

Advantages of amniotomy are (1) high success rate, (2) observation of the amniotic fluid for blood or meconium, (3) ready access for an intrauterine pressure catheter, a direct fetal scalp electrode, and fetal scalp blood sampling. Risks include (1) umbilical cord prolapse, (2) adverse change in fetal position, (3) prolonged rupture of membranes and increased risk of ascending uterine and/or fetal infection, (4) fetal injury, and (5) rupture of vasa previa and subsequent fetal hemorrhage. With due caution and attention, many of the risks can be avoided. Amniotomy has been associated with greater frequency of disalignment of fetal cranial bones.[59] The significance of these findings on fetal outcome is yet to be determined.

Before amniotomy, the vertex should be well applied to the cervix and engaged in the pelvis to prevent prolapse of the umbilical cord. Amniotomy may be performed with a toothed clamp (Allis) or a plastic hook (Amnihook, Hollister, Chicago). Vaginal examination is first performed to evaluate the cervix and station of the vertex. One or two fingers of the examining hand are introduced into the cervix, and the membranes are swept away from the cervix. The membranes are then ruptured by passing the instrument through the cervical canal across the examining hand usually aside the examining finger or in the groove formed between two examining fingers. Whether an Amnihook or Allis clamp is chosen, it is gently applied to the membranes and turned, either hooking and/or scratching the membranes. The opening in the membranes is widened and the membranes retracted over the vertex by blunt dissection with the examining finger. The time of the amniotomy and the presence of meconium or blood in the fluid must be documented in the chart. Bleeding may occur and if persistent should be investigated for a maternal or fetal source. The application of a fetal scalp electrode or introduction of an intrauterine pressure catheter should be completed prior to removing the examining fingers.

After amniotomy, a thorough cervical examination should attempt to uncover prolapse of the cord. The fetal heart rate should be carefully monitored electronically or by auscultation for evidence of fetal distress. The fetal heart rate may increase transiently postamniotomy. However, decelerations or bradycardia of the fetal heart rate are rare without overt or occult umbilical cord prolapse.

Stripping of the membranes and/or amniotomy may initiate labor through the release of arachidonic acid and the subsequent formation of prostaglandins. Maternal plasma levels of 13,14-dihydro-15-keto-prostaglandin F have increased markedly within a short time after amniotomy.[53] If the vertex is well engaged and the leaking of the fluid minimal, ambulation may further facilitate the onset of labor. If uterine contractions do not ensue after 2 to 4 hours, then intravenous oxytocin should be initiated.

Medical: Oxytocin

In 1948 Theobald et al.[60] initiated the use of oxytocin given by intravenous drip for the induction of labor. Synthetic oxytocin is available as a solution for intravenous or intramuscular use and as a nasal spray. In the United States, only the intravenous solution has been approved by the Food and Drug Administration for medically indicated induction of labor when fetal viability is expected. Oxytocin will stimulate myometrial contractions. However, variability in patient sensitivity and response to oxytocin is the rule rather than the exception. The safest method and the most predictable results are obtained with a properly regulated continuous intravenous infusion of a dilute solution.

During the first stage of spontaneous labor, endogenous oxytocin from the posterior pituitary is released in spurts: initially at low levels and with increasing levels during the second stage.[61] With continuous intravenous oxytocin infusion, plasma oxytocin concentration increases during the first 20 minutes. After 20 minutes, the concentration of plasma oxytocin does not change significantly. The amount of oxytocin being metabolized by placental oxytocinase appears to be equal to the amount infused. The mean plasma oxytocin half-life is 3 to 4 minutes, with a range of 2 to 7 minutes. A rapid fall in plasma levels occurs after the intravenous infusion is discontinued.

A primary intravenous line of an electrolyte-containing solution with a large-bore catheter or needle is started and administered at a rate sufficient to keep the vein open. A stock solution containing 10 USP units (1 ml) of synthetic oxytocin is added to 500 ml of 5 percent dextrose in water. One ml of 1/1,000 heparin is also added to the stock solution. A large syringe (usually 60 ml) is filled from the diluted oxytocin stock solution, and the syringe is placed in a controlled infusion pump. The prepared solution from the syringe is next connected or piggybacked into the primary line through a sidearm near the intravenous insertion site in the patient's arm. The 500-ml standard stock solution containing the oxytocin should never be connected directly to the patient.

The rate of administration is usually recommended as that which produces contractions every 2 to 3 minutes, lasting 60 to 90 seconds with 50 to 60 mmHg intrauterine pressure and a resting uterine tone of 10 to 15 mmHg if intrauterine pressure monitoring is used. Dosage may vary from 0.5 to 30 to 40 mU/min of oxytocin. Induction is started with 0.5 mU/min, and the rate is doubled every 15 to 20 minutes until uterine activity that stimulates normal labor in both quality and quantity of contractions is obtained. It is unusual for a patient to require more than 20 to 40 mU/min of oxytocin to achieve myometrial contractions that mimic spontaneous labor and to achieve satisfactory changes in cervical dilatation. As labor

progresses, the frequency and intensity of contractions may increase. The infusion rate of oxytocin can then be reduced to prevent hyperstimulation.

Control of the intravenous dose is best achieved by using a constant infusion pump. If a pump is not available, the dosage of oxytocin may be regulated by a manually controlled infusion of a dilute solution of 10 USP units in 1,000 ml or 5 percent dextrose/normal saline infusion. Monitoring of uterine contractions and fetal heart rate is recommended throughout the induction and is best accomplished with continuous electronic monitoring. Constant surveillance of uterine activity is recommended to avoid uterine hyperstimulation. Electronic fetal heart rate monitoring may facilitate the detection of fetal distress by documenting fetal heart rate decelerations in response to uterine contractions.

A thorough knowledge of the pharmacologic and physiologic actions of oxytocin and appropriate techniques for monitoring the mother and fetus are mandatory for all personnel administering oxytocin. They must be qualified to identify complications and be able to take immediate action when problems arise. A written protocol for oxytocin administration that has been approved by the appropriate hospital staff should be available on the labor and delivery floor.

COMPLICATIONS

Hypercontractility

The most frequently encountered complication of intravenously administered oxytocin is uterine hyperstimulation. Hyperstimulation refers to excessive frequency of contractions (polysystole) and/or increased uterine tone (hypertonus), which may produce fetal distress, abruptio placenta, or uterine rupture. The use of electronic monitoring has increased the early detection of these potentially lethal maternal and/or fetal complications.

Oxytocin-induced uterine activity appears to be more frequently associated with uterine hypertonus and hyperactivity than spontaneous labor.[62] If the uterus is overstimulated, placental gas exchange may be jeopardized, leading to fetal acidosis or hypoxemia. Because intravenous oxytocin has a short half-life, one can expect uterine relaxation with improved intervillous blood flow and gas exchange to follow soon after the infusion has been discontinued. In the presence of hyperstimulation, the patient should also be turned to her side and oxygen administered.

Water Intoxication

Oxytocin is related structurally and functionally to vasopressin. As such, it shares the effects of vasopressin, or antidiuretic hormone (ADH). The use of regulatory infusion pumps and electrolyte-containing solutions can help to prevent water intoxication, which can lead to hyponatremia, confusion, convulsions, coma, congestive heart failure, and death. The ADH effect is rarely seen when the dosage of oxytocin remains below 20 mU/min. Fluid overload and hyponatremia may be prevented by strict intake and output recordings, use of balanced salt infusions, and avoiding prolonged administration of an oxytocin infusion of 20 to 40 mU/min.

Hypertension

A constant intravenous infusion of dilute oxytocin not exceeding 20 mU/min usually has no effect on blood pressure. However, in the presence of preeclampsia or with an infusion rate of 20 to 40 mU/min, slight elevation of blood pressure can occur.

Uterine Rupture

Uterine rupture may occur with the use of oxytocin. This obstetric disaster is more common in grand multiparous patients, in women who have undergone prior uterine surgery, with fetal malpresentations, and with a markedly overdistended uterus. These conditions are recommended contraindications to the use of oxytocin. After uterine rupture, contractions may cease even if the oxytocin infusion is continued.

Amniotic Fluid Embolism

Amniotic fluid embolism has been seen in patients undergoing oxytocin-induced labor, especially if the indication for the induction is fetal demise and the membranes are artificially ruptured.

Elective Induction

In a strict sense, elective induction of labor may be defined as a termination of pregnancy without an indication. In a broader sense, elective induction of labor refers to the initiation of labor when control over the timing of labor may be beneficial, such as in patients who live a great distance from the hospital and/or have a history of rapid labors. Elective induction of labor should not be attempted for the convenience of the patient or physician. Two major problems associated with elective induction are iatrogenic prematurity and increased cesarean delivery because of failed induction. In the event of a bad outcome that developed as a result of an elective induction of labor, the burden of proof must demonstrate that the risk of allowing the pregnancy to continue exceeded that of the induction. Prerequisites for the technique of elective induction include all that has been outlined above for an indicated induction. It must be noted that in 1978 the Food and Drug Administration ruled that injectable oxytocin not be used for elective induction of labor.

To avoid iatrogenic prematurity, a detailed assessment of fetal maturity as outlined in Chapter 8 must be made.

Combined Medical – Surgical Methods

A combination of the above methods is frequently employed for the induction of labor. A constant infusion of dilute intravenous oxytocin and artificial rupture of the membranes after the initiation of labor appears to be a successful technique. Other clinicians prefer to rupture the membranes first, and, if labor has not ensued in several hours, they then begin intravenous oxytocin administration.

The Future

Investigations have focused on the use of the synthetic PGE_2 and PGF_2 to ripen the cervix before amniotomy or oxytocin induction. These prostaglandin preparations are not used to induce labor in a viable pregnancy at term. Such compounds as ergot derivatives, quinine, sparteine sulfate, subcutaneous or intramuscular oxytocin, or nasal oxytocin spray are mentioned only for historical interest and should not be used for the induction of labor.

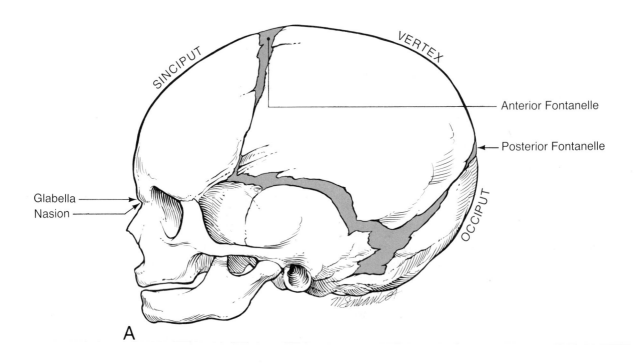

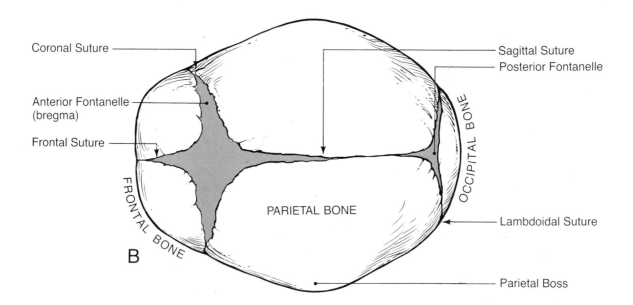

Fig. 14.8 Landmarks on the fetal skull for determination of fetal position.

GLOSSARY

Asynclitism: When the biparietal diameter of the fetal head is parallel to the planes of the pelvis, the head is in synclitism. The sagittal suture is midway between the front and back of the pelvis. When either the anterior or posterior parietal bone precedes the sagittal suture, asynclitism is present.

Attitude: The relationship of the fetal parts to each other. This usually refers to the position of the head with regard to the trunk.

Dilatation: Also referred to as dilation. The degree of patency, expressed in centimeters of diameter, of the internal os of the cervix.

Denominator: A reference point on the fetus used to determine position. These points include landmarks in the fetal skull (Fig. 14.8), the fetal chin, the sacrum, and the acromion.

Effacement: A process that occurs in the latter part of pregnancy and labor by which the cervix is drawn intra-abdominally by the uterine corpus. This process is demonstrable by a shortening and thinning of the remaining intravaginal portion of the cervix. Effacement is expressed as the percentage by which the length of the cervix has been reduced and ranges from 0 percent (no reduction in length) to 100 percent (no cervix palpable below the fetal presenting part).

Engagement: Engagement occurs when the largest transverse diameter of the presenting part has descended past the plane of the pelvic inlet. Engagement is diagnosed clinically when the leading bony portion of the fetal head is at or below the level of the ischial spines (station 0 or more).[40]

Labor: Repetitive uterine contractions associated with progressive cervical dilatation. Labor may be spontaneous or induced, term or preterm.

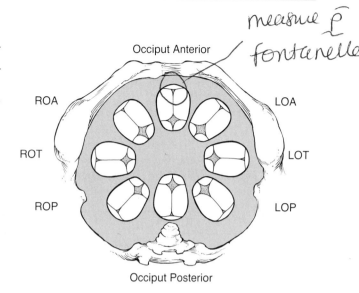

measure p̄ fontanelle

Fig. 14.9 Possible positions for a fetus with a vertex presentation.

Lie: Relationship between the long axis of the fetus and that of the mother.

Position: Relationship between the denominator of the fetus (occiput in cephalic presentations) and the vertical (anterior, posterior) and horizontal (right, left) planes of the birth canal. Examples for cephalic and face presentations are shown in Figures 14.9 and 14.10.

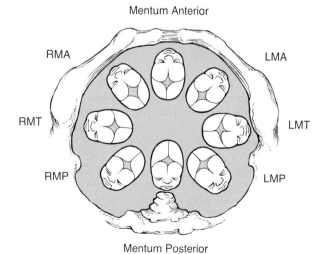

Fig. 14.10 Possible positions for a fetus with a face presentation.

Presentation: The fetal part that lies closest to the pelvic inlet. The three main presentations are cephalic (vertex), breech, and shoulder.

Station: The degree of descent of the presenting part of the fetus through the birth canal. The estimated distance, in centimeters, between the leading bony portion of the fetal head and the level of the maternal ischial spines.[40] The level of the ischial spines is station 0. The stations below the spines are designated +1 for 1 cm below the spines to +5, which is the perineum. Similarly, the level of the inlet is 5 cm above the spines and is designated station −5.

REFERENCES

1. Friedman EA: Labor: Clinical Evaluation and Management. Appleton-Century-Crofts, E. Norwalk, CT 1967
2. Duignan NM, Studd JWW, Hughes AO: Characteristics of normal labour in different racial groups. Br J Obstet Gynaecol 82:593, 1975
3. DeLee JB: The prophylactic forceps operation. Am J Obstet Gynecol 1:34, 1920
4. Goodlin RC: On protection of the maternal perineum during birth. Obstet Gynecol 62:393, 1983
5. Yao AC, Lind J: Placental transfusion. Am J Dis Child 127:128, 1974
6. Caldwell WE, Moloy HC, D'Esposo DA: Studies on pelvic arrests. Am J Obstet Gynecol 36:928, 1938
7. Mengert WF: Estimation of pelvic capacity. JAMA 138:169, 1948
8. Friedman EA: The therapeutic dilemma of arrested labor. Contemp Obstet Gynecol 11:34, 1978
9. Diamond EL, Schnierler H, Lillienfeld AM: The ratio of intrauterine radiation to subsequent mortality and development of leukemia in children: a prospective study. Am J Epidemiol 97:283, 1973
10. Harvey EB, Boice JD, Honeyman M, Flannery JT: Prenatal x-ray exposure and childhood cancer in twins. N Engl J Med 312:541, 1985
11. Niswander K, Gordon M, Berendes H et al: The Women and Their Pregnancies: the Collaborative Perinatal Study of the National Institute of Neurological Disease and Stroke. Washington DC, U.S. Department of Health Education and Welfare, 1972
12. O'Brien WF, Cefalo RC: Evaluation of x-ray pelvimetry and abnormal labor. Clin Obstet Gynecol 25:157, 1982
13. Benson WL, Boyce DC, Vaughn DL: Breech delivery in the primigravida. Obstet Gynecol 40:417, 1972
14. Joyce DN, Giva-Osagie F, Stevenson GW: Role of pelvimetry in active management of labour. Br Med J 4:405, 1975
15. Collea JV, Chen C, Quilligan EJ: The randomized management of frank breech presentation: a study of 208 cases. Am J Obstet Gynecol 137:235, 1980
16. Friedman EA, Sachtleben MR: Dysfunctional labor. I. Prolonged latent phase in the nullipara. Obstet Gynecol 17:135, 1961
17. Friedman EA: The functional divisions of labor. Am J Obstet Gynecol 109:274, 1971
18. Caldeyro-Barcia R, Posiero JJ: Physiology of uterine contractions. Clin Obstet Gynecol 3:386, 1960
19. Jeffcoate TN, Baker K, Martin RB: Inefficient uterine action. Surg Gynecol Obstet 95:257, 1952
20. Friedman EA, Sachtleben MR: Dysfunctional labor. II. Protracted active phase dilatation in the nullipara. Obstet Gynecol 17:566, 1961
21. O'Driscoll K, Meagher P: Active Management of Labor. WB Saunders, London, 1980
22. Friedman EA, Sachtleben MR: Dysfunctional labor. III. Secondary arrest of dilatation in the nullipara. Obstet Gynecol 19:576, 1962
23. Read JA, Miller FC, Paul RH: Randomized trial of ambulation versus oxytocin for labor enhancement: a preliminary report. Am J Obstet Gynecol 139:699, 1981
24. Friedman EA, Satchtleben MR: Station of the fetal presenting part. V. Protracted descent patterns. Obstet Gynecol 36:558, 1970
25. Hellman LM, Prystowski H: The duration of the second stage of labor. Am J Obstet Gynecol 63:1223, 1952
26. Gaziano EP, Freeman DW, Bendel RP: FHR variability and other heart rate observations during second stage labor. Obstet Gynecol 56:42, 1980
27. Jacobson L, Rooth G: Interpretative aspects on the acid base composition and its variation in fetal scalp blood and maternal blood during labour. J Obstet Gynaecol Br Commonw 78:971, 1971
28. Cohen W: Influence of the duration of the second stage of labor on perinatal outcome and puerperal morbidity. Obstet Gynecol 49:266, 1977
29. Harbert GM: Uterine contractions. Clin Obstet Gynecol 25:177, 1980
30. Huey JR, Miller FC: The evaluation of uterine activity: a comparative analysis. Am J Obstet Gynecol 135:2, 1979

31. Miller FC: Uterine activity, labor management, and perinatal outcome. Semin Perinatal 2:181, 1978
32. Turnbull AC, Anderson ABM: Induction of labour. J Obstet Gynaecol Br Commonw 5:32, 1968
33. Toaff ME, Herzoni J, Toaff R: Induction of labour by pharmacological and physiological doses of intravenous oxytocin. Br J Obstet Gynaecol 85:101, 1978
34. Seitchick J, Chatkoff ML: Intrauterine pressure waveform characteristics in hypocontractile labor before and after oxytocin administration. Am J Obstet Gynecol 123:426, 1975
35. Seitchick J, Castillo M: Oxytocin augmentation of dysfunctional labor. I. Clinical data. Am J Obstet Gynecol 144:899, 1982
36. Simons CL: Prostaglandins and labor problems and benefits. Contemp Obstet Gynecol 12:91, 1978
37. O'Driscoll K, Foley M, MacDonald D: Active management of labor as an alternative to cesarean section for dystocia. Obstet Gynecol 63:485, 1984
38. Levens K, Cunningham C, Pritchard J: Cesarean section: an answer to the house of Horne. Am J Obstet Gynecol 153:838, 1985
39. Akoury HA, Brodie G, Caddick R et al: Active management of labor and operative delivery in nulliparous women. Am J Obstet Gynecol 158:255, 1988
40. ACOG Committee Opinion, Obstetric Forceps. Number 71. The American College of Obstetricians and Gynecologists, Washington D.C. 1989.
41. Friedman EA, Niswander KR, Sachtleben MR, Naftaly N: Dysfunctional labor. X. Immediate results to the infant. Obstet Gynecol 106:776, 1969
42. Friedman EA, Sachtleben MR, Bresky PA: Dysfunctional labor. XII. Long-term effects on the infant. Am J Obstet Gynecol 127:779, 1977
43. Bowes WA, Bowes C: Current role of the midforceps operation. Clin Obstet Gynecol 23:549, 1980
44. Chez RA: Midforceps delivery: is it an anachronism? Contemp Obstet Gynecol 15:82, 1980
45. Dudley AG, Markham SM, McNil O: Elective versus indicated midforceps delivery: a comparative study. Obstet Gynecol 37:19, 1971
46. Richardson DA, Evans MI, Cibils LA: Midforceps delivery: a critical review. Am J Obstet Gynecol 145:621, 1983
47. Hughey MJ, McElin TW, Lussky R: Midforceps operations in perspective. I. Midforceps rotation operations. J Reprod Med 20:253, 1978
48. Malmstrom T: Vacuum extractor: an obstetrical instrument. Acta Obstet Gynecol Scand 33:1, 1954
49. Sorbe B: Active pharmacologic management of the third stage of labor. Obstet Gynecol 52:694, 1978
50. Thierstein ST, Jahn HC, Lange K: Routine third-stage exploration of the uterus. Obstet Gynecol 10:269, 1957
51. Blanchette H: Elective manual exploration of the uterus after delivery: a study and review. J Reprod Med 19:13, 1977
52. Bishop EH: Pelvic scoring for elective induction. Obstet Gynecol 24:260, 1964
53. Friedman EA, Niswander KR, Bayonet-Rivera NP, Sachtleben MR: Relation of pre-labor evaluation to inductibility and the course of labor. Obstet Gynecol 29:539, 1966
54. Friedman EA, Niswander KR, Bayonet-Rivera NP, Sachtleben MR: Prelabor status evaluation. II. Weighted score. Obstet Gynecol 29:539, 1967
55. Liggins GC: Initiation of parturition. Br Med Bull 35:145, 1979
56. Seilers SM, Hodgson HT, Mitchell MD et al: Release of prostaglandins after amniotomy is not mediated by oxytocin. Br J Obstet Gynaecol 87:43, 1980
57. Chard T: The physiology of labor and its initiation. In Chard T, Richards M (eds): Benefits and Hazards of the New Obstetrics. JB Lippincott, Philadelphia, 1977
58. Booth JH, Kurdizak VB: Elective induction of labor: a controlled study. Can Med Assoc J 103:245, 1970
59. Baumgarten K: Advantages and disadvantages of low amniotomy. J Perinatal Med 4:2, 1976
60. Theobald GW, Graham A, Campbell J et al: The use of posterior pituitary extract in physiological amounts in obstetrics. Br Med J 2:123, 1948
61. Dawood YM: Oxytocin: new data may help establish the ideal dose. Contemp Obstet/Gynecol 13:181, 1979
62. Seitchek J, Castillo M: Oxytocin augmentation of dysfunctional labor. I. Clinical data. Am J Obstet Gynecol 144:899, 1982
63. Friedman EA: Labor: Clinical Evaluation and Management. Appleton-Century-Crofts, East Norwalk, CT, 1978, p. 49

Chapter 15

Intrapartum Fetal Evaluation

Roy H. Petrie

There is little argument that the changes relating to intrapartum fetal evaluation that were introduced during the past two to three decades have significantly altered obstetrics itself and the concepts relating to obstetrics more than any other recent factor. Within the decade 1960 to 1970, reasonably sophisticated fetal surveillance systems, including intermittent fetal blood acid–base determinations and continuous electronic fetal heart rate monitoring, were introduced with the expectation that stillbirths and neonatal neurologic injury caused by intrapartum hypoxemia could be significantly reduced or eliminated.

Indeed some centers with knowledgeable and dedicated personnel have realized some or all of these expectations. However, in prospective, randomized studies, the incidence of neurologic damage and perinatal death associated with the use of electronic fetal heart rate monitoring is not significantly lower than that documented with older methods of fetal surveillance, including intermittent fetal heart rate auscultation by stethoscope or Doppler and the presence of meconium-stained amniotic fluid. Consequently, the use of the newer techniques for intrapartum fetal evaluation has been downplayed by some individuals and groups who offer recommendations for patient management in these areas.

Although it has been demonstrated that electronic fetal heart rate monitoring is associated with an increased incidence of delivery by cesarean section

without demonstrable improvement in perinatal outcome, there has been little interest in reverting to the more traditional fetal monitoring techniques, especially in those patients judged to be at high risk. The reasons for this reluctance to revert to the older and simpler fetal surveillance techniques are multiple, but chief among them include (1) the undisputed reliability and assurance (>98 percent) that a good fetal/neonatal outcome is associated with normal continuous fetal heart rate data and/or acid–base combination, which safely allows continuation of labor; (2) the unacceptably great expense involved in providing the one-on-one nursing that is almost mandatory to perform intermittent fetal heart rate auscultation; and (3) the knowledge that, although nonreassuring continuous fetal heart rate data may not be uniformly associated with poor perinatal outcome, it does provide a warning of potential problems and a gauge of fetal response to actions undertaken to improve fetal condition.

HISTORICAL PROSPECTIVE

Although breakthroughs in the early 1900s, including the introduction of clean milk supplies, helped to improve neonatal outcome, it was not until the 1940s and 1950s that serious attention was directed to the high rates of neonatal morbidity and fetal mortality. It had been known for some time that many fetuses died in utero before the onset of labor. A significant number of fetuses entered labor alive but were still-born at delivery. That labor was a risk factor for neonatal morbidity and fetal mortality was well accepted. Abnormalities in placentation, infection, trauma, dystocia, fetopelvic disproportion, and asphyxia were all recognized as risk factors that could compromise fetal condition.

Despite their appreciation of these dangers, before the mid-1900s obstetricians could do little to change the poor perinatal outcomes. Few diagnostic techniques were available for antepartum evaluation of fetal well-being. Even if fetal jeopardy had been recognized, except at full dilatation and with reasonable descent into the pelvis, it was impossible to expedite delivery without the expectation of marked maternal morbidity and mortality. With the introduction of antibiotics, blood grouping and typing, and safe pharmacologic agents to stimulate uterine contractions, coupled with the recognition of normal and abnormal patterns of labor, it became feasible to terminate a gestation or labor safely using oxytocin stimulation, early forceps delivery, or cesarean section. Once pregnancy and labor could be interrupted safely, information about the antepartum and intrapartum conditions of the fetus became a vital necessity if an improvement in perinatal outcome was to be accomplished.

The early investigative efforts of such researchers as Barcroft,[1] Barron,[2] Apgar,[3] Freda,[4] and James and co-workers[5] described fetal physiology during labor in response to the stresses of the labor process. Their observations included the potential for reduction of blood flow from mother to placenta and from the placenta to the fetus. The mechanism for fetal damage and death in such cases was identified as an insufficient supply of oxygen to the fetus secondary to a reduction in blood flow from the mother to the intervillous space or from the placenta to the fetus. Inadequate fetal oxygenation decreases or eliminates the supply of adenosine triphosphate (ATP) derived from the Krebs cycle and mandates that ATP be obtained from the Embden-Meyerhoff pathway. This pathway not only yields significantly less ATP but also creates lactic acid as a byproduct. As lactate accumulates, it causes fetal brain cells to swell and finally to rupture. With sufficient brain cell necrosis, fetal damage or death can occur.

If one could determine when there was a significant potential for the reduction of blood flow from the mother to the placenta, or from the placenta to the fetus, and if it was safe to remove the fetus from the uterus prior to the normal termination of labor, a remedial aspect of labor as a risk factor could be identified and treated. By the mid-1960s to early 1970s, an understanding of fetal respiratory physiology was developed that provided a basis for diagnostic techniques that could be used to detect fetal compromise. Saling,[6] Hammacher et al.,[7] Hon and Quilligan,[8] Caldeyro-Barcia et al.,[9] and others developed technologies during the 1950s and early 1960s that allowed the clinician, for the first time, to monitor fetal status during labor. By the late 1960s and early 1970s, equipment for intrapartum fetal evaluation had become commercially available.

One last change was needed before significant improvement in fetal outcome could be attempted. This change was related to the philosophy of management for mother and fetus. Through the mid- to late 1960s, the obstetrician was primarily concerned with the well-being of the mother at the termination of the reproductive process. Little if any attention was paid to the fetus. The guiding philosophy was that, if the perinatal outcome was unsatisfactory, the mother and father could try again. With a better understanding of basic fetal physiology and an appreciation that clinical management could change fetal condition, attention shifted from the mother to her fetus. Although one can never ignore or forget the potential for maternal morbidity or mortality, it became apparent that improved perinatal outcomes required deliveries with less hypoxia, less anesthesia and analgesia, and less trauma. Therefore, an increasing number of cesarean sections were performed to reduce the potential for fetal damage or death from asphyxia. During the past decade and a half, the cesarean section rate has risen from 3 to 4 percent to a rate of 15 to 25 percent. Obviously, not all these operative deliveries are performed for fetal distress. But the clinical lesson has been learned that with improved effort relating to diagnosis and management, fetal morbidity and mortality, especially that related to asphyxia, could be reduced. Accordingly, many institutions have, over the past decade and a half, shown dramatic reductions in perinatal mortality from 30 in 1,000 to 6 to 8 in 1,000. Many believe that a considerable portion of this improvement has been due to skilled intrapartum fetal surveillance.

METHODOLOGIES FOR INTRAPARTUM FETAL EVALUATION

In an effort to determine which fetus is likely to experience a reduction in oxygenation and to develop fetal distress during labor, obstetricians looked at a number of potential indicators of fetal jeopardy. The presence of meconium in the amniotic fluid, fetal movement, fetal acid–base balance, fetal heart rate, and fetal respiration have been evaluated as indicators of fetal condition.

Before the routine clinical use of fetal heart rate and acid–base monitoring during labor, Fenton and Steer[10] reviewed the steps by which fetal heart rate and meconium have come to be regarded as indicators of fetal stress during labor. These investigators found that fetal heart rate was probably first described by Marsac in 1650 and subsequently by Mayor in 1815 and by Kergaradec in 1822. In 1843, Kennedy reported with considerable detail the changes in the fetal heart rate noted during pregnancy and labor, as did Bodson, who described signs of fetal distress in which there was "excessive frequency, great irregularity, or marked slowing of the fetal heart rate." In 1903, von Winckel indicated that a fetal heart rate above 160 or below 100 bpm should be regarded as evidence of distress. However, Lund found no evidence of asphyxia in nearly 60 cases with a heart rate above 160 bpm. By contrast, Fitzgerald and McFarlane noted that more than 60 percent of babies with a heart rate above 160 bpm were born in only fair, poor, or depressed condition. The same investigators observed that when the rate was below 120 bpm almost 60 percent of the babies were compromised. Subsequently, obstetricians of the present generation have noted increased perinatal mortality and morbidity with a fetal heart rate greater than 160 to 180 bpm or below 100 to 120 bpm.

In patients with meconium, particularly thick meconium, the incidence of fetal and neonatal morbidity is increased when compared with gestations without meconium. Fenton and Steer[10] noted that the passage of meconium during labor was first described as an indicator of fetal distress by Schwartz in 1858. In reviewing the literature, these workers found that a perinatal mortality of approximately 8 percent was reported when meconium was present alone. Subsequently Steer reported a mortality of 4.5 percent. However, McCall and Fulsher as well as Berger observed patients without changes in fetal heart rate but with meconium who had no apparent fetal distress and were in good condition at birth.

Fenton and Steer[10] then investigated the combination of an abnormal fetal heart rate and meconium. Holman and co-workers noted that this combination was associated with a mortality of 7.2 percent. If the fetal heart rate was irregular but not slow, and meconium was found, the mortality increased to 35 percent. A slow fetal heart rate and meconium was reported to have a mortality of 18.4 percent by Walker. Resnick subsequently described a group of infants whose delivery was expedited by forceps or cesarean section. In this series, a normal fetal heart rate with lightly stained meconium was associated with a perinatal mortality rate of 3 percent. When the heart rate was abnormal and the amniotic fluid was thickly stained with meconium, the mortality rose to 32 percent. To determine the significance of these two indicators of fetal distress, Fenton and Steer looked at almost 8,000 deliveries over a 2-year interval. Fetal distress was present in 9.9 percent of these cases. These investigators found that the combination of thick meconium and a fetal heart rate under 100 bpm was associated with a perinatal mortality of 22.2 percent. They also noted that meconium alone, or the slowing of the heart rate alone, was not a sufficient indicator of fetal distress to warrant intervention. In 1962, these workers found that fetal survival was directly correlated with the interval between discovery of the signs of fetal distress and delivery. They concluded that 30 minutes was a critical interval.

In a paper written after the institution of routine clinical utilization of both continuous fetal heart rate and intermittent acid–base evaluation, Miller et al.[11] substantiated the earlier findings of Fenton and Steer.[10] They noted that the incidence of Apgar scores below 7 at 5 minutes was 3.5 times higher when meconium was present. In agreement with Fenton and Steer, Miller et al. confirmed that meconium alone was a relatively poor indicator of fetal and neonatal jeopardy unless an abnormal fetal heart rate or other risk factor was present. For example, Miller and Read[12] observed that the presence of meconium in a prolonged pregnancy was associated with a normal but significantly lower fetal capillary pH level than was a prolonged pregnancy without meconium.

During the late 1940s and 1950s, a number of investigators made attempts to correlate fetal condition with fetal heart rate.[13,14] Could an insult to the fetus be associated with an aberration in the fetal heart rate? It was soon appreciated that fetal heart rate counted over a period of time and expressed as a mean (e.g., 150 bpm averaged over 4 to 5 minutes) was an inadequate measurement. A number of investigators[15,16] demonstrated that the use of a stethoscope is also inadequate for the evaluation of stress and the heart rate reaction to stress. Seasoned clinicians, using stethoscopically derived fetal heart rate data, were wrong at least one-third of the time in their evaluation of heart rate information.

To understand the effects of physiologic stress and the responses of the fetal heart rate, the clinician needed a continuous record of heart rate. Accordingly, investigators began to plot by hand fetal heart rate in a beat-by-beat manner. Subsequently, an electronic system, the current fetal heart rate monitor, was developed to do this function automatically. One of a number of systems is used to detect each fetal heart beat, calculate its rate instantaneously, and plot it on graph paper. The fetal heart rate tracing may then be compared with continuously recorded uterine activity data.

In 1961, Saling[6] introduced the first direct assessment for fetal well-being during labor. Relying on the biochemical principles by which a decrease in fetal oxygenation would diminish the production of ATP by the Krebs cycle and cause the Embden-Meyerhoff pathway to be utilized, Saling proposed that the production of H^+ ion in the form of lactate would cause the pH of the fetus to drop. Reviewing the biochemical responses during hypoxia, Saling chose to look at fetal pH rather than the PO_2 level for two reasons: (1) the level of PO_2 fluctuated quite rapidly during labor and the drift in readings of the PO_2 electrode did not permit precise monitoring and (2) pH values provided a good overall representative evaluation of fetal acid–base balance. A number of investigators around the world have substantiated Saling's original work and advocated the use of pH and base deficit

measurements to differentiate between chronic and acute fetal distress.[17–19]

Fetal capillary blood samples may provide other important information. In pregnancies complicated by Rh isoimmunization, capillary blood can be utilized to determine the fetal hematocrit and bilirubin levels. It is possible to cross-match fetal blood with a 40 to 80 microliter sample in anticipation of an immediate neonatal transfusion after delivery. The fetal platelet count can be measured in pregnancies complicated by idiopathic thrombocytopenic purpura. Glucose determinations have been made on fetal capillary blood obtained from the fetus of a diabetic mother during labor.

A number of investigators, including Rayburn[20] and Sadovsky and Yaffe,[21] have reported the value of counting fetal movement during the antepartum period as an indicator of fetal well-being. During labor, fetal movement cannot be perceived by many mothers. Nevertheless, when fetal movement is appreciated during labor, it can be a reassuring finding.

Researchers[22,23] have attempted to relate fetal breathing movements during the antepartum period or during the course of labor to fetal well-being. Unfortunately, the technology for continuous surveillance of fetal breathing has not become available. Furthermore, during the intrapartum period, a rather marked reduction in fetal breathing episodes is normal and can be expected.

INTERMITTENT FETAL HEART RATE MONITORING

Low-Risk Patients

When using a stethoscope or fetoscope or a portable Doppler device, the fetal heart rate is generally monitored and recorded during a contraction and for 30 seconds following the contraction. The standard practice is to record fetal heart rate every 30 minutes following a contraction during the active phase of the first stage of labor and at least every 15 minutes in the second stage of labor. Although these temporal recommendations are made, there are no data that support the validity of these intervals.

In early latent phase labor, many obstetricians prefer to have the patients ambulate until they have advanced into latent phase labor rather than discharge them until labor progresses. Intermittent fetal heart rate monitoring during ambulation is frequently performed at intervals of 45 to 60 minutes or until contractions become regular at 3 to 4 minute intervals.

High-Risk Patients

In the high-risk group, the fetal heart rate is intermittently obtained and recorded every 15 minutes during the first stage of labor and every 5 minutes during the second stage of labor. The heart rate is preferably obtained during and 30 seconds following a uterine contraction.

Using auscultation, abnormalities related to basal rate, variability, and perhaps postcontraction[21] slowing may be identified. When these changes are noted, additional fetal surveillance is warranted. Frequently continuous internal fetal heart rate monitoring with appropriate fetal blood acid – base determination are used to clarify an abnormality of the ausculated fetal heart rate.

CONTINUOUS FETAL HEART RATE MONITORING

To evaluate the effects of intrapartum stress on the fetus, it is necessary to determine the fetal heart rate on a beat-to-beat basis. With each beat of the fetal heart, a new calculation of rate is made based on what the fetal heart rate would be if all temporal intervals between beats were (1) the same as that between the last two heart beats and (2) uniform during 1 minute. Ideally, there should be no averaging of heart rate over a given interval or a given number of beats. The data collected should also be displayed continuously. This type of calculation is impossible to achieve with a stethoscope, because the heart rate auscultated by the human ear must be averaged over a given number of beats in seconds or minutes, and this averaging destroys the physiologic detail.

To record the fetal heart rate continuously and instantaneously, a signal must be obtained each time the heart beats, and some mechanical or electronic device must measure the interval between two successive heart beats, calculate the fetal heart rate, and plot each successive rate that is calculated. Such determinations of the fetal heart rate have been made using the Doppler ultrasonographic technique, phonocardiographic monitors with a microphone, and fetal electrocardiographic (ECG) signals collected either

from the maternal abdomen with multiple electrodes or from a single electrode attached to the fetus. In clinical practice, the utilization of an ultrasound transducer on the maternal abdominal wall or an electrode attached to the fetal scalp has become the standard technique for collecting fetal heart rate data. With the scalp electrode, the R wave of the fetal QRS complex initiates counting by the cardiotachometer of the monitor. The cardiotachometer determines the time between each R wave (the R – R interval), and a rate in beats per minute is generated. For example, an R – R interval difference of 500 msec or 0.5 second would produce an instantaneous rate of 120 bpm.

To evaluate uterine contractions or uterine activity, two methods have been developed. A tocodynamometer may be placed on the maternal abdomen overlying the gravid uterus and secured with a belt encircling the midsection of the body. The tocodynamometer detects alterations in the curvature of the abdomen resulting from changes in the configuration of the contracting uterus. Because no direct measurements are obtained, this system will not provide quantitative data on the strength or amplitude of contractions. However, the tocodynamometer will accurately record the frequency of contractions and show with reasonable accuracy the duration of the contractions. The second system for collecting information about uterine contractility requires the insertion of a small catheter filled with sterile water into the chorioamniotic sac after rupture of the membranes. The fluid-filled catheter is attached to a strain gauge and placed at a level that corresponds to the midpoint of the vertical axis of the uterus. Accurate pressure readings can then be obtained that indicate the onset, strength or amplitude, and duration of uterine contractions.

External Monitoring

In some cases, it may be clinically undesirable or impossible to rupture the membranes. Similarly, the obstetrician may not wish to place a fetal electrode or intrauterine pressure catheter. In these situations, the external form of fetal monitoring utilizing a tocodynamometer and ultrasound transducer can usually be applied (Fig. 15.1). An ultrasound transducer is affixed to the maternal abdomen at a position overlying the fetal heart so that sound waves can be trans-

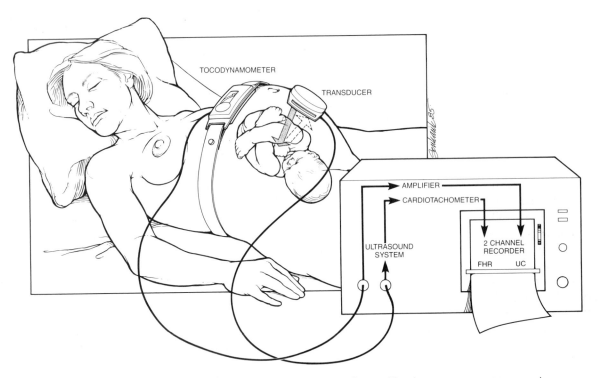

Fig. 15.1 Instrumentation for external monitoring. Contractions are detected by the pressure-sensitive tocodynamometer, amplified, and then recorded. Fetal heart rate is monitored using the Doppler ultrasound transducer, which both emits and receives the reflected ultrasound signal that is then counted and recorded.

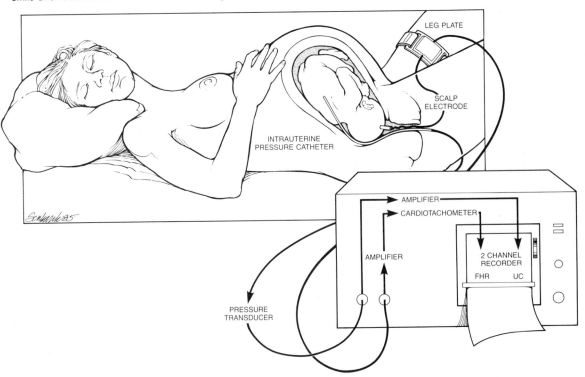

Fig. 15.2 Techniques used for direct monitoring of fetal heart rate and uterine contractions. Uterine contractions are assessed with an intrauterine pressure catheter connected to a pressure transducer. This signal is then amplified and recorded. The fetal electrocardiogram is obtained by direct application of the scalp electrode, which is then attached to a leg plate on the mother's thigh. The signal is transmitted to the monitor, where it is amplified, counted by the cardiotachometer, and then recorded.

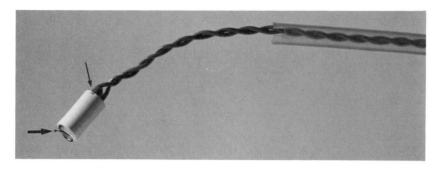

Fig. 15.3 Fetal spiral electrode used for direct monitoring of the fetal heart rate. The thick arrow points to the stainless steel spiral; the thin arrow designates the reference electrode.

mitted toward the fetal heart valves. As the valves move, the reflected sound waves return to the transducer, permitting an accurate assessment of fetal heart rate activity.

The mitral and aortic valves generally provide four events during each systole: mitral opening, mitral closure, aortic opening, and aortic closure. With four different signals, the electronic counting device of the fetal monitor, the cardiotachometer, will, at random, pick one of these four signals to count. This process introduces a certain amount of "false" heart rate variability into the calculation of fetal heart rate when one considers that the first event may be used for one beat, the last event for the next beat, one of the two intermediate events for subsequent beats, and so forth. Systems have been developed that use a directional depth-range Doppler system, permitting continuous monitoring of only one of these signals. While this method can provide a more accurate index of heart rate variability, it is too expensive for routine clinical monitoring. As the fetus moves in utero, the ultrasound transducer must be adjusted to maintain a good signal. This may be especially true in the obese patient. Similarly, the external tocodynamometer transducer may need adjustment in position or in tension to obtain a good recording of uterine contractions. There are few complications or side effects of external monitoring, although difficulty may be encountered in interpreting heart rate and uterine activity data if the recording is of poor quality.

Internal Monitoring

Internal monitoring requires the spontaneous or artificial rupture of the chorioamnion (Fig. 15.2). Usually, the cervix needs to be dilated 1 to 2 cm before the uterine pressure catheter can be inserted and the fetal electrode attached. The electrode is placed during a vaginal examination. With the examiner's finger inserted through the cervical os against the fetal scalp, a cartilaginous plate is first identified. The obstetrician must be certain the electrode will not be placed over the fetal face or fontanel. An electrode introducer is next inserted along the finger to come to rest against the fetal vertex. Turning the top part of the introducer two and one-half to three times will cause the spiral electrode to become attached to the fetal scalp. The introducer is removed, and the ends of the wires from the electrode are connected to a maternal leg plate that contains a ground lead and is attached to the fetal monitor. The fetal electrode is composed of two parts (Fig. 15.3). The spiral electrode itself is attached to the fetus and the circuit closed when a second electrode, or reference, comes in contact with electrolyte-containing secretions in the maternal vagina. It is also possible for the maternal ECG signal to be conducted through a dead fetus to the fetal electrode and be amplified and counted by the fetal monitor's cardiotachometer. The use of real-time ultrasonography to evaluate fetal cardiac valvular action can resolve this question quickly and perhaps avoid an unnecessary operative delivery. The scalp electrode allows the patient more freedom of movement than does the ultrasound transducer, because fetal movement will not alter the quality of the signal. During placement of the internal monitoring apparatus, the patient should remain in a lateral position to avoid hypotension secondary to vena caval compression.

After the electrode has been attached, a catheter for the determination of uterine activity is inserted.

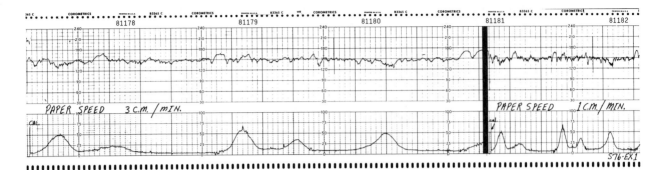

Fig. 15.4 Internal fetal heart rate data gathered at the standard recording speed of 3 cm/min for the first portion. The same data are being recorded at a speed of 1 cm/min in the last segment. Normal long-term and short-term variabilities are present. Note that the uterine activity channel has been calibrated so that the intrauterine pressure readings can be measured correctly.

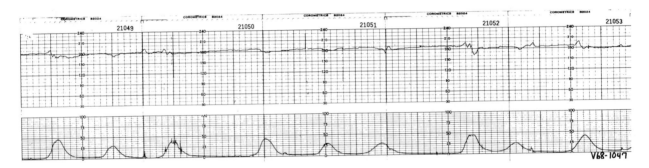

Fig. 15.5 Internal monitoring. A baseline tachycardia is noted at a rate of 180 to 190 bpm. Uterine activity is occurring every 2 to 3 minutes, with an intensity of 30 to 45 mmHg and a normal resting tone of 5 mmHg.

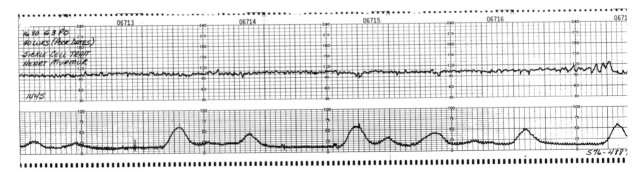

Fig. 15.6 Internal heart rate monitoring and an external tocodynamometer are being utilized. A fetal heart rate bradycardia at 100 to 110 bpm with good variability over the 20-minute interval is displayed. The small undulating aspects of the uterine pressure recording represent maternal respiration.

The soft plastic intrauterine catheter is filled with sterile water to avoid corrosion of the pressure strain gauge, which may occur with dextrose and water or saline. The catheter should be filled with fluid before it is introduced to avoid the possibility of an air embolus. The soft, fluid-filled catheter is inserted through a stiffer plastic guide. The guide is moved along the examiner's finger, which has been positioned just inside the cervix between the fetal presenting part and the cervix. To prevent perforation of the uterus, the guide must be passed no further than the examiner's fingers. The intrauterine pressure catheter is then manually pushed through the guide until it is halfway up the uterine cavity, a distance of approximately 18 inches from the tip of the catheter to the labia minora. (Most commercial manufacturers now place a marker at the 18-inch level.) The catheter is next attached to the strain gauge. Utilizing a three-way stopcock, the catheter is flushed to remove any vernix or air, and the strain gauge is calibrated. As with the fetal electrode, the use of an intrauterine pressure catheter allows the patient considerably more mobility. With a sufficiently long electrode lead, the patient may be able to walk about or sit down. Prefilled intrauterine catheters are now available. These catheters are easily calibrated, but are considerably more expensive.

By convention, instantaneously calculated fetal heart rate and uterine activity are recorded on graph paper driven at a uniform speed. The paper speed is usually 3 cm/min, although 1 cm/min may be employed to save paper. The vertical scaling is 30 to 240 bpm over 7 cm and 0 to 100 mmHg (torr) over 4 cm. Thick vertical lines are placed at 1-minute intervals (Fig. 15.4). After delivery, the heart rate tracing should be clearly labeled with the date, the patient's name, her identification number, and important clinical information. The tracing may be microfilmed and should be kept as a permanent part of the patient's medical record.

Potential complications resulting from the placement and use of the fetal electrode and intrauterine pressure catheter include cord prolapse, endometritis, infection of the fetal scalp at the site of electrode attachment, uterine rupture when introducing the catheter, and disruption of placental implantation. These complications are very uncommon (see discussion later in this chapter).

PHYSIOLOGIC CONTROL OF FETAL HEART RATE (see Ch. 4)

Baseline Heart Rate

Over a number of years, it has been noted that the mean human fetal heart rate varies between 120 and 160 bpm; however, rates of 90 to 180 are not uncommon or necessarily abnormal. Persistent periods (≥ 10 minutes) of heart rate above 160 bpm are classified as a baseline tachycardia. Periods (≥ 10 minutes) of fetal heart rate below 120 bpm are known as fetal bradycardia. Persistent intervals of tachycardia or bradycardia are more likely to be associated with hypoxia than is a normal heart rate (Figs. 15.5 and

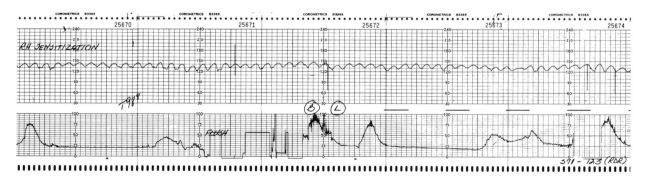

Fig. 15.7 With internal monitoring, the sinusoidal heart rate pattern with its undulating characteristics is demonstrated. Note that the intrauterine pressure catheter is flushed, and the patient's position is changed from the back (B) to the left (L) side.

15.6). Fetal tachycardia has also been identified in cases complicated by maternal fever, fetal infection, maternal thyrotoxicosis, fetal anemia, and fetal tachyrhythmias. If the patient has received β-sympathomimetic drugs or parasympatholytic agents such as atropine, fetal tachycardia may also be observed. Fetal bradycardia can be seen in patients treated with β-blockers such as propranolol and in the fetus with congenital heart block. Women with systemic lupus erythematosus may produce an antibody that crosses the placenta and damages the conduction system of the fetal heart, thereby causing congenital heart block.

Although it occurs infrequently, a sinusoidal heart rate may have great clinical importance. This baseline heart rate is usually within a normal range of 120 to 160 bpm. However, it has a somewhat smooth, undulating pattern of uniform long-term variability with an amplitude of 5 to 20 bpm that resembles a sine wave. There is an absence of short-term variability. The sinusoidal heart rate (Fig. 15.7) has often been associated with fetal anemia, as in Rh isoimmunization. The physiologic mechanism for this pattern is unknown. Some investigators believe that it represents aberrant neurologic control of the heart rate that may result from anemia or hypoxia. Sinusoidal-like heart rate patterns can be seen following the administration of some narcotic analgesics and related agents. Whenever a persistent sinusoidal baseline heart rate pattern is noted, it is advisable to collect fetal scalp capillary blood for an acid–base determination.

Heart Rate Variability

Perhaps the most reliable indicator of fetal well-being available to the obstetrician is the finding of normal beat-to-beat heart rate variability (Fig. 15.8). Fetal heart rate variability can only be appreciated when it is continuously and instantaneously calculated and recorded on a beat-by-beat basis. Heart rate variability represents the interplay between the cardioinhibitory and cardioaccelerator centers in the fetal brain stem. It is unusual for a heart rate under normal nervous system control to be steady at any one consistent rate. Rather, there is considerable variation or short-term variability on a beat-to-beat basis, usually ranging from 3 to 8 bpm around an imaginary average heart rate. Fluctuation or long-term variability

occurs as well, usually having a cyclicity of three to five cycles per minute (cpm)[24] (Fig. 15.8). The presence of normal fetal heart rate variability is one of the best indicators of intact integration between the central nervous system and heart of the fetus. While the loss of heart rate variability may suggest fetal hypoxia, other factors may be responsible, including a fetal sleep state, drugs that depress the central nervous system (CNS), a fetal tachycardia of more than 180 bpm, and anomalies of the heart and CNS.[25] A fetus of 28 weeks or more gestational age should demonstrate normal variability. When evaluating beat-to-beat variability, the external or ultrasonographic system cannot be utilized as a precise indicator of variability with one exception. When a flat heart rate is observed with ultrasound techniques, close correlation between the external and internal system can be anticipated (Figs. 15.9 and 15.10). The external system, when working properly, can permit adequate evaluation of long-term or 3 to 5 bpm variability.

The clinical significance of short-term variability or beat-to-beat variability has been assessed for a number of years. To date, no clinically significant difference between long-term and short-term variability is uniformly apparent or clinically significant. Wherever there is good beat-to-beat variability present on a heart rate tracing without other indicators of loss of fetal well-being, the likelihood of delivering a significantly jeopardized fetus is exceedingly low. Even when other parameters suggest fetal distress, the presence of good beat-to-beat variability is generally a reassuring finding.[26]

Exaggerated or increased fetal heart rate variability (> 25 bpm) may be representative of a shifting P_{O_2} and P_{CO_2} relationship mediated by the barochemoreceptors. Without the presence of repetitive decelerations, there is generally no significant change in fetal oxygenation or fetal status (Fig. 15.11).[27] The presence of increased fetal heart rate variability that is followed by loss of beat-to-beat variability can be ominous.

Fetal Arrhythmias

As long as the fetal QRS wave is clear and regular, the fetal heart rate will be instantaneously counted and expressed in beats per minute for each fetal heart rate. However, occasional electrical and/or mechanical interference from external and/or internal

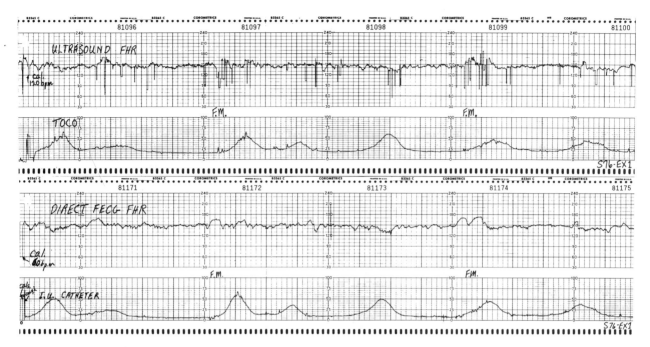

Fig. 15.8 The use of external monitoring with ultrasound and a tocodynamometer (top), with the same data being recorded using an internal system with a fetal electrode and an intrauterine pressure catheter (bottom). Note that the characteristics of the heart rate channel are similar but with considerable noise or increased variability (top), reflecting the recording characteristics of the ultrasound system. Nevertheless, long-term variability with its cyclicity can still be appreciated. The tocodynamometer is positioned to approximate the calibrated intrauterine pressure reading. However, by turning the calibration knob on the tocodynamometer, one can position uterine activity information anywhere on the vertical scale for uterine activity.

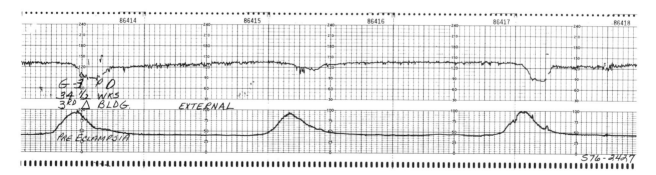

Fig. 15.9 A case complicated by third-trimester bleeding in which external heart rate and uterine activity data are collected. Note the presence of persistent late decelerations with only three contractions in 20 minutes as well as the apparent loss of variability of the fetal heart rate. The rise in baseline tone on the uterine activity channel cannot be evaluated with the external system.

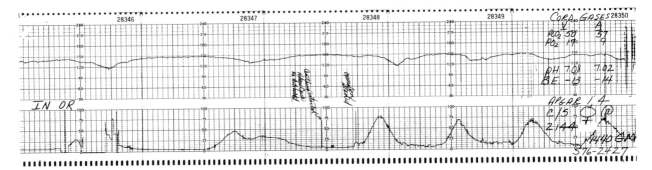

Fig. 15.10 The same patient described in Figure 15.9 following a double set-up examination that ruled out a placenta previa and allowed placement of an internal monitoring system. Note that the flat heart rate demonstrated in Figure 15.9 is indeed found when internal monitoring is used. After delivery by cesarean section, the attending staff have listed all pertinent data, including Apgar scores, weight, sex, cord pH, and respiratory gases for cord vein and artery.

sources may be introduced, and the clarity and reliability of the fetal heart rate tracing can be lost. Such interference has often been referred to as "noise" or artifact. Interference caused by mechanical sources usually creates a pattern of artifact that is random. In evaluating this problem, one should confirm that all electrical connections are secure. The obstetrician should be certain that the scalp electrode is firmly fastened and that the wires to the leg plate have not loosened. When one suspects the presence of a fetal heart rate arrhythmia, the ECG signal on the oscilloscope should be inspected. To evaluate a fetal ar-

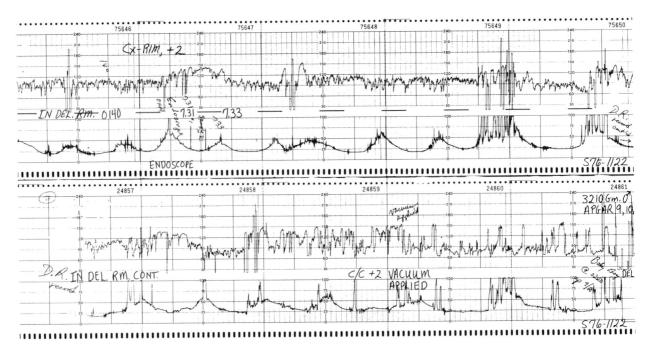

Fig. 15.11 Exaggerated variability with a baseline bradycardia of 90 to 110 bpm. Note accelerations. Concern about this tracing led to evaluation of the fetal scalp pH, which was found to be normal (7.31, 7.33). When the baseline fell further, it was elected to deliver the infant using the vacuum extractor (panel 24859). The 3,210-g male had Apgar scores of 9 and 10, consistent with accelerations, exaggerated variability, and the fetal capillary pH values.

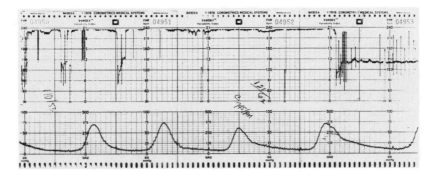

Fig. 15.12 The patient, a 26-year-old, gravida 6, para 3, aborta 2, entered spontaneous labor at 37 weeks gestation. Monitoring with a scalp electrode and an external tocodynamometer demonstrates a fetal supraventricular tachycardia approaching 240 bpm in panels 04950 through 04952. In panel 04953, the fetal heart returns to a normal baseline rate of 140 bpm. The patient was delivered vaginally of a 3,300-g male infant with Apgar scores of 9 and 9. The infant required digitalization for a persistent tachycardia during the neonatal period. The conversion of the heart rate from the supraventricular tachycardia to a normal rate at the end of this tracing may have been due to vagal stimulation secondary to pressure on the fetal head. Antenatal treatment of the fetus with a supraventricular tachycardia has included maternal therapy with propranolol, verapamil, and digitalis. Fewer than 10 percent of fetuses with a supraventricular tachycardia will demonstrate a cardiac malformation. (From Bergmans et al,[77] with permission.)

rhythmia optimally, one should obtain a continuous tracing from an ECG monitor attached directly to the fetal heart rate monitor. In this way, the obstetrician can evaluate the presence of the P, QRS, and T waves of the fetal signal.

While many fetal cardiac arrhythmias are transient and of little clinical significance, some have been associated with fetal compromise (Fig. 15.12). Fetal supraventricular tachycardia may lead to heart failure and hydrops. The fetus with complete heart block will usually demonstrate a rate of 50 to 70 bpm. Approximately 40 percent of these infants will have congenital heart disease, particularly a ventricular septal defect. Fetal heart failure and hydrops have also been associated with congenital heart block.

Periodic Changes

Important periodic changes in fetal heart rate have been observed in association with uterine contractions. Transient slowing of the fetal heart rate with uterine contractions is known as a deceleration, while a transient increase is known as an acceleration. The four patterns of clinical significance are accelerations and early, variable, and late decelerations. Only two mechanisms alter fetal heart rate: (1) a reflex response secondary to the nervous control of the heart by direct nervous innervation or by humoral control of the autonomic nervous system and (2) transient

slowing of the heart when fetal myocardial hypoxia is present.

Early Deceleration

With an early deceleration, the fetal heart rate demonstrates a slowing or deceleration as a contraction begins, reaching its lowest point just as the acme of the contraction is reached and returning to baseline levels just as the contraction is finished. The heart rate never falls below 100 bpm (Fig. 15.13). This deceleration is known as an early deceleration because it starts early in the contraction phase. The early deceleration is felt to be due to pressure on the fetal head as it moves down the birth canal, and the mechanism is one of reflex slowing mediated by the vagus nerve with release of acetylcholine at the sinoatrial node commensurate with the pressure applied to the fetal vertex. Accordingly, this pattern can be blocked by the use of a vagolytic drug such as atropine. These early decelerative changes are innocuous and can be observed throughout labor without alteration in fetal condition, acid–base status, or neonatal or long-term outcome.

Variable Deceleration

The variable deceleration is a reflex-mediated change in fetal heart rate, again mediated by the vagus nerve, but generally caused by umbilical cord compression

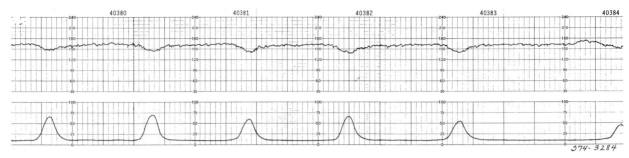

Fig. 15.13 Internal monitoring demonstrates a baseline heart rate of approximately 160 bpm, minimal to moderate short-term variability, and persistent early decelerations with each contraction.

that may occur as a result of the cord being around the baby's neck, under the baby's arm, or between some part of the fetus and the uterine wall (Fig. 15.14). This pattern is often seen in association with oligohydramnios. As the umbilical cord is compressed, fetal peripheral resistance increases. Fetal PO_2 falls and PCO_2 rises. Baroreceptors and chemoreceptors fire, causing a swift and somewhat erratic release of acetylcholine at the sinoatrial node with a sharp angular drop in heart rate, usually to a range below 100 bpm. The variable deceleration may begin before the onset of a contraction, with the onset of a contraction, or following the onset of a contraction. This change in fetal heart rate can be blocked to some degree by the administration of atropine but is not affected by the administration of oxygen or improvement in fetal PO_2. The variable deceleration is the most common periodic pattern noted during labor

and generally can be corrected by changing maternal position to alleviate cord compression.

If the fetal heart rate does not fall below 80 bpm and the duration of the deceleration is short, cord compression is usually of minimal clinical significance. However, with moderate and severe variable decelerations (Table 15.1), a significant reduction in umbilical blood flow may occur. Carbon dioxide accumulates in the fetal compartment, causing a transient respiratory acidosis. If the decelerations are severe and repetitive, hypoxia and metabolic acidosis may result. Fetal myocardial hypoxemia may then produce a delayed recovery to baseline. If this occurs, great care must be taken to eliminate this stress; otherwise, the fetus may require early delivery. When the fetal heart rate falls below 60 bpm, loss of nodal control of the heart resulting in momentary "cardiac arrest" may occur. In summary, repetitive variable

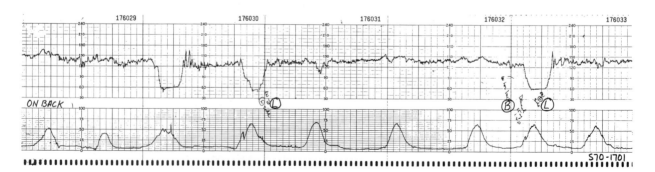

Fig. 15.14 Internal monitoring reveals uterine contractions every 2 to 3 minutes of 50 to 60 mmHg intensity and a baseline of 5 to 10 mmHg. Variable decelerations occur intermittently, providing adequate intervals between contractions for CO_2 and O_2 exchange and fetal recovery.

Table 15.1 Principles of Grading Variable and Late Decelerations

Criteria of Grading	Mild	Moderate	Severe
Variable deceleration; level to which FHR drops and duration of deceleration	<30-sec duration, irrespective of level >80 bpm, irrespective of duration	<70 bpm, >30–<60 sec 70–80 bpm, >60 sec	<70 bpm, >60 sec
Late deceleration; amplitude of drop in FHR	70–80 bpm, <60 sec <15 bpm	15–45 bpm	>45 bpm

bpm, beats per minute; FHR, fetal heart rate.
(From Kubli et al,[33] with permission.)

decelerations represent reflex vagally mediated heart rate changes; however, repetitive moderate and severe variable decelerations over a prolonged interval may result in a direct myocardial hypoxic depression of heart rate.

Late Deceleration

A transient but repetitive deceleration of the fetal heart rate noted to occur late in the contraction phase, well after the contraction is under way, is known as a late deceleration (Figs. 15.15 and 15.16). It reaches its lowest point after the acme of the contraction has been achieved and then returns to the baseline rate after the contraction is over. Initially, late decelerations represent a reflex vagally mediated response and are associated with normal heart rate variability. Recent investigations have demonstrated that late decelerations result from fetal hypoxia, triggering a chemoreceptor response and transient fetal hypertension stimulating fetal baroreceptors. Late decelerations indicate uteroplacental insufficiency and decreased intervillous exchange between mother and fetus with intermittent fetal hypoxia. As the uterine contraction peaks, limiting intervillous blood flow, fetal oxygenation is impaired. Poorly oxygenated blood ultimately reaches the fetus—hence the late timing of the deceleration. Late decelerations may occur with placental abruption (Fig. 15.17B), excessive uterine activity of either a spontaneous or pharmacologically induced nature, and maternal hypotension, anemia, or ketoacidosis. Even if mild late decelerations of only 5 to 10 bpm are noted but are found to be repetitive, there is a reasonable potential for fetal hypoxia and acidosis (see Fig. 15.16).

How long the fetus can tolerate such intermittent hypoxia without injury is unknown. Steps should therefore be taken to reverse this pattern by improving fetal oxygenation. If the mother is hypotensive, normal blood pressure should be restored. If excessive uterine activity is present, oxytocin should be discontinued and administration of a tocolytic agent considered. If late decelerations persist and the fetus becomes acidemic, direct myocardial depression will result. Such cases may be characterized by late decelerations with absent heart rate variability. In the dying fetus, late decelerations give way to a marked bradycardia.

Occasionally two fetal heart rate patterns may be seen together. This combination has been called a mixed pattern (Fig. 15.18). In managing such cases, clinical decisions should be based on the worst component of the mixed pattern. Whatever the origin of the fetal hypoxia with late deceleration, it must be corrected, or the infant must be delivered to avoid damage.

Accelerations

Transient increases in fetal heart rate associated with uterine contractions or fetal movement are known as accelerations and are usually indicators of a fetus that is adequately oxygenated (Fig. 15.17). In some cases, accelerations result from partial cord occlusion. With cord compression, the umbilical vein may be compressed, producing fetal hypotension and a baroreceptor-mediated increase in heart rate. Acid–base determinations during accelerations almost uniformly demonstrate a normal fetal pH.

Summary

A healthy fetus is characterized by a normal heart rate and by the absence of significant repetitive heart rate decelerations. The presence of fetal heart rate accel-

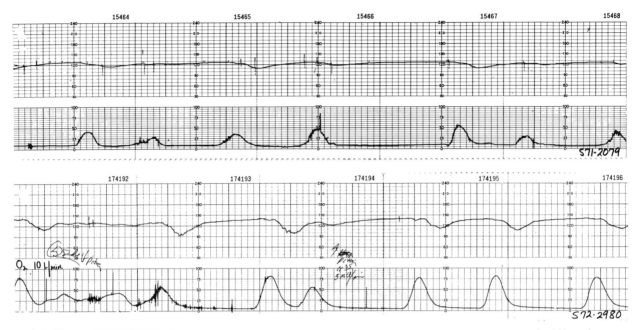

Fig. 15.15 (Top) Internal monitoring shows complete loss of beat-to-beat variability with the presence of mild late decelerations. (Bottom) More marked late decelerations are noted, again with loss of variability. In panel 174192, oxygen is administered, the patient is turned to her left side, and the oxytocin infusion is decreased.

erations and normal heart rate variability strengthens the diagnosis of fetal well-being. A potentially compromised fetus is characterized by the presence of significant repetitive decelerations and/or by an abnormal baseline fetal heart rate. The absence of fetal heart rate accelerations and the loss of fetal heart rate variability tend to support the diagnosis of fetal stress or distress. The presence of repetitive decelerations, repetitive moderate to severe variable decelerations, a sinusoidal pattern, and a baseline tachycardia, particularly when associated with diminished fetal heart rate variability, all indicate the need to obtain further

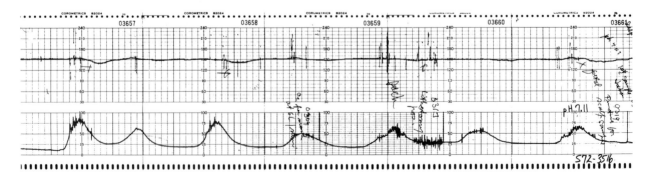

Fig. 15.16 With internal monitoring, very mild late decelerations are noted with loss of beat-to-beat variability. However, note the fetal capillary pH value of 7.11, indicative of a rather marked acidosis. As expected, a fetal heart rate acceleration is not seen with scalp puncture.

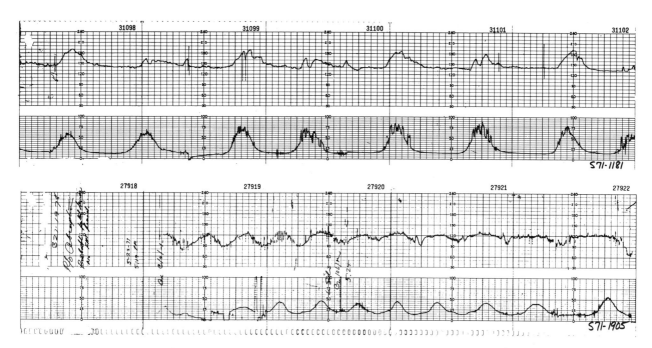

Fig. 15.17 (Top) Internal monitoring is used, and accelerations are noted with each contraction. (Bottom) It is difficult to judge the baseline heart rate, making it difficult to determine whether there are persistent repetitive accelerations or persistent repetitive late decelerations. This differential may be critical; if the baseline heart rate cannot be established, a measurement of fetal capillary pH or base deficit can be most helpful.

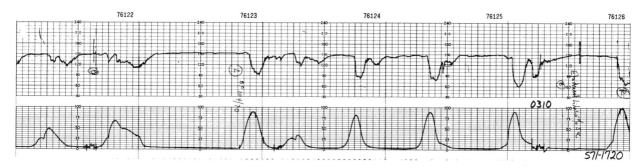

Fig. 15.18 Using internal monitoring, a mixed variable–late pattern is noted. Generally the periodic pattern begins as a variable deceleration with a slow return to baseline, indicative of a late deceleration. The potential fetal compromise associated with the fetal heart rate pattern should be judged by the worst component of the pattern, the late deceleration.

Table 15.2.   Relationship of Fetal Heart Rate Pattern, Fetal Acid–Base, 5-Minute Apgar Score, and Umbilical Acid–Base

Pattern	Fetal Scalp Blood pH	5-Min Apgar Scores ≥ 7 (%)	Umbilical pH ≥ 7.25 (%)
Normal tracing	7.33 ± 0.01	92	91
Accelerations	7.34 ± 0.01	91	97
Early decelerations	7.33 ± 0.01	92	93
Variable decelerations	7.30 ± 0.01	78	77
Late decelerations	7.29 ± 0.01	63	66

(Data from Tejani et al[78] and Tejani N et al.[79])

information about fetal status. This usually involves the collection of fetal scalp capillary blood for the determination of fetal acid–base balance.

FETAL ACID–BASE EVALUATION

Blood Collection for Respiratory Gases

In the early 1960s, Saling,[6,28] a German obstetrician, introduced an innovative technique for obtaining accurate data about fetal well-being. This new method was based on the acquisition of fetal blood for the determination of acid–base status. For the first time, the obstetrician could assess fetal pH and oxygenation during labor. Over the next 15 years, fetal blood sampling became an integral aspect of intrapartum surveillance in many institutions.

Over the three decades since fetal surveillance by acid–base determinations of capillary blood was introduced, a number of studies have been performed

that have verified the validity of this form of monitoring. The supporting data have come from animal models in which central blood values have been correlated with capillary scalp pH,[26] studies comparing cord acid–base[27–29] data with capillary values, and studies relating both cord and fetal capillary acid–base determinations to neonatal performance and outcome.[30,31] Since the introduction of fetal heart rate monitoring, a number of investigators have demonstrated the linear correlation between the severity of heart rate patterns and the degree of acidosis present (Tables 15.2 and 15.3).[32–34]

During labor, fetal acidosis may result from impaired fetomaternal exchange. A transient fall in fetal pH may be due to acute umbilical cord compression, which leads to the rapid accumulation of carbon dioxide and a respiratory acidosis. Of greater concern is inadequate fetal oxygenation because of impaired oxygen–carbon dioxide exchange in the intervillous space. When there is inadequate fetal

Table 15.3   Relationship Between Qualitative Periodic Fetal Heart Rate Changes and Mean Fetal pH

Pattern	Kubli[33]	Beard (1971)[80]	Tejani (1975)[78]
Normal tracing	7.30 ± 0.04	7.34 ± 0.06	7.33 ± 0.01
Accelerations		7.34 ± 0.03	7.34 ± 0.01
Early decelerations	7.30 ± 0.04	7.33 ± 0.05	7.33 ± 0.01
Variable decelerations (all)		7.31 ± 0.05	7.30 ± 0.01
Moderate	7.26 ± 0.04		
Severe	7.15 ± 0.07		
Late decelerations (all)		7.28	7.29 ± 0.01
Moderate	7.21 ± 0.05		
Severe	7.12 ± 0.07		

oxygenation for energy production and the aerobic processes for generating ATP fail, the anaerobic (Embden-Meyerhoff) pathway of energy production is used. Lactic acidosis is generated, and fetal pH falls. Accordingly, if sufficient hypoxia and acidosis develop, brain damage or death from asphyxia may result. The collection of fetal blood for pH and respiratory gas evaluation, when performed at the appropriate time, may alert the obstetrician to impending fetal jeopardy and permit correction of the underlying problem or delivery by whatever route is safest for mother and fetus.

A number of investigators[6,25] have found that a pH value of 7.25 or greater is normal for the fetus during labor. The pH range of 7.20 to 7.24 has been referred to by some investigators as a preacidotic range. Many investigators believe a fetal capillary pH value of 7.19 or less indicates potential fetal acidosis and, if substantiated on two collections 5 to 10 minutes apart, represents sufficient acidosis to warrant termination of labor. A number of investigators have demonstrated that it is uncommon to find significant damage until a pH range of less than 7.10 is noted, and this value may be as low as 7.00. Normal umbilical blood and fetal capillary pH and respiratory gas values are given in Tables 15.4 and 15.5. The fetal capillary scalp pH value will normally decline in early labor from approximately 7.30 to 7.25 at delivery. In clinical practice, a trend of serial pH determinations correlated with the clinical setting is probably of greater importance than the absolute value of one or two pH determinations (Fig. 15.19). It should be remembered that heart rate variability provides an important commentary on the severity of ominous periodic patterns. The fetus with normal heart rate variability and late decelerations will have a significantly higher scalp pH than will the fetus with decreased variability and late decelerations.

Table 15.4 Normal Umbilical Cord Blood-Gas Values

	Vein	Artery
pH	7.34 ± 0.15	7.28 ± 0.15
Po_2	30 ± 15	15 ± 10
Pco_2	35 ± 8	45 ± 15
Base deficit	5 ± 4	7 ± 4

Table 15.5 Fetal Capillary Blood Respiratory Gas Values

Normal	Respiratory Acidosis	Metabolic Acidosis
pH 7.25–7.40	Decreased	Decreased
Po_2 18–22	Usually stable	Decreased
Pco_2 40–50	Increased	Usually stable
Base deficit 0–11	Usually stable	Increased

Maternal acidosis may occasionally cause fetal acidosis secondary to equilibration of H^+ ions across the placenta. When maternal acidosis is associated with fetal acidosis, the comparison of maternal and fetal base deficit can be used to distinguish the truly hypoxic fetus. A freely flowing maternal venous blood sample can be used for these analyses. Fetal pH is usually about 0.1 pH unit below the maternal value. When maternal acidosis is observed, every effort should be made to determine the etiology (e.g., sepsis, ketoacidosis, or dehydration) and appropriate correction undertaken. Maternal respiratory alkalosis associated with hyperventilation has been reported to elevate fetal pH falsely.

The base deficit (excess) is an indication of fetal buffer reserves available to neutralize H^+ ions or fixed acids. The base deficit can be clinically useful as an indicator of impending loss of fetal well-being when pH values are satisfactory, but the fetal heart rate pattern is cause for concern. The longer the fetus is exposed to recurrent stress, the more likely its acid–base status will suddenly deteriorate. With recurrent stress, stable pH values, and a rising base deficit, the temporal interval before deterioration of fetal condition becomes progressively shorter. When base deficit values are compared with pH values and fetal heart rate patterns, there is a more reliable association of base deficit and the severity of the fetal heart rate patterns. Accordingly, the judicious clinical use of base deficit as an indicator of fetal well-being, especially with confusing fetal heart rate data, should be encouraged, especially now that newer equipment can perform this evaluation more easily (Table 15.6).

To collect fetal blood, the chorioamnion must be ruptured and the cervix must be sufficiently dilated, approximately 2 to 2.5 cm, to provide exposure to the

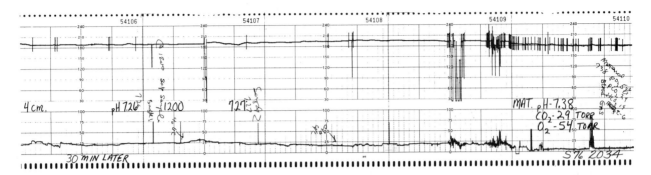

Fig. 15.19 This pregnancy has been complicated by viral pneumonia. Meconium is present, and there is a baseline fetal tachycardia (190 bpm) with loss of variability. For this reason, baseline fetal acid–base determinations were obtained and were found to be normal (7.26, 7.27). Maternal pH and respiratory gas values confirm her pulmonary problems.

fetal scalp. The presenting part must be sufficiently low in the pelvis to remain reasonably immobile. When the fetus is presenting as a breech, fetal blood can be obtained from the buttocks. After appropriate cleansing of the vulvar area, and after the application of sterile drapes, a conical vaginal endoscope is passed through the vagina and cervix so that the small end of the endoscope comes to rest against the fetal scalp at a site not overlying a suture line or fontanel. Amniotic fluid, blood, mucous, and meconium are removed by the use of sponges on a long holder. Once the scalp is cleaned, a small amount of silicone is spread over the exposed area. The layer of silicone has two purposes: it smoothes the fetal hair for easier visualization of the scalp, and it provides a smooth surface on which a globule of fetal capillary blood can form. Using a 2×2 mm microscalpel set in a plastic guard, the fetal scalp is punctured. To aid in the collection of blood, this puncture should be performed just as the beginning of a contraction so that scalp blood flow is facilitated. A long glass heparinized cap-

illary tube is then introduced into the endoscope and, using gravity, the fetal blood is collected into the capillary tube. The tube holds approximately 250 μl of blood when full. Newer instruments require only 25 to 40 μl of fetal blood for determination of pH and respiratory gases. A pH value alone may be determined with as little as 20 μl of blood.

Fetal blood sampling can be performed with the mother's hips elevated or in the conventional dorsal lithotomy position. It can also be performed with the mother in the lateral Sims position on a flat bed. After the fetal blood sample has been collected, pressure should be applied to the puncture site by a sponge on a long holder. Pressure is continued through the completion of two contractions and the puncture site then observed through a third contraction. If there is no bleeding from the puncture site, the endoscope can be removed. However, if bleeding continues, additional pressure may be required. Rarely, pressure alone will not provide adequate hemostasis, and a metal clip may be applied across the puncture site. Cases have been reported in which an emergency cesarean section was required because of continued fetal hemorrhage. Such fetuses often have an unrecognized genetic or pharmacologically induced bleeding disorder.[35,36] Sampling an area of fetal scalp that has been traumatized may give a falsely low pH. Caput formation should not alter the pH.

Unless the fetal blood sample will be processed immediately, one end of the capillary tube should be stopped with sealing clay, and a small metal rod or

Table 15.6 Base Deficit (Excess)[a] in Fetal Capillary Blood

Base (mEq/L)	Indication
0–9	Normal
9–11	Borderline
>11	Potential metabolic acidosis

[a] Base deficit and base excess have the same numerical value; however, a positive value is used for base deficit and a negative value for base excess, i.e., a base deficit of 6 is the same as a base excess of −6.

"flea" introduced into the other end of the capillary tube. Using a magnet, the fetal blood sample should then be mixed with the heparin by moving the metal rod from one end of the tube to the other. The second end of the capillary tube should be sealed with clay and the tube placed on ice until the pH and/or acid–base determinations can be performed. Ideally, the equipment for these determinations should be present in a laboratory near the obstetric suite. Labor floor personnel can become familiar with the equipment and perform these analyses should a technician be unavailable.

Until the introduction of continuous fetal heart rate monitoring during the early 1970s, fetal scalp sampling alone was used to monitor fetal well-being in known high-risk situations, including diabetes mellitus and hypertension. Because of the intermittent nature of this technique, many fetal blood samples were needed to assess fetal condition. With the introduction of continuous fetal heart rate monitoring, fetal acid–base surveillance in labor has assumed two roles as part of the overall fetal surveillance system. First, in those high-risk situations in which chronic fetal distress may be present at the onset of labor, such as intrauterine growth retardation (IUGR) or a prolonged pregnancy, many obstetricians feel more comfortable obtaining baseline pH and/or respiratory gas determinations in early labor to determine fetal status at that point and as a subsequent comparative marker. Second, because most obstetricians are comfortable with the diagnostic accuracy of normal fetal heart rate data, they use intermittent acid–base determinations only when the heart rate patterns are unclear or confusing.

Fetal Stimulation, Accelerations, and pH/Buffer Evaluation

Clark et al.[37] investigated the utilization of evoked fetal heart rate accelerations during scalp stimulation at the collection of fetal capillary blood. These investigators found that during the scalp blood sampling process, when the scalp was stimulated and an acceleration of 15 bpm lasting 15 seconds occurred, the fetal pH value was almost always 7.22 or greater. Unfortunately the reverse does not hold true, and several normal fetuses did not accelerate with scalp stimulation.

A number of investigators have used vibro-acoustic fetal stimulation to evoke a fetal heart rate accelera-

tion. An artificial larynx, generating 82 dB of mixed noise and vibration, is placed on the maternal abdomen approximately one-third the distance from the symphysis pubis to the xiphoid process. A stimulation interval of 2 to 5 seconds is used. This may evoke a fetal heart rate acceleration. Such fetal heart rate accelerations have been associated with a fetus that is in good condition physiologically. Polzin et al.[38] have demonstrated, using continuous internal fetal heart rate monitoring, that a 5-second vibro-acoustic stimulation to the fetus resulting in either a 10-bpm acceleration lasting 10 seconds or a 15-bpm acceleration lasting 15 seconds will correlate with a mean pH value of 7.29 ± 0.07. Unfortunately, some healthy fetuses will not respond with an acceleration to this stimulation. Studies relating vibro-acoustically stimulated fetal heart rate accelerations to base deficit (excess) appear promising.

Umbilical blood gas values are often used to relate intrapartum fetal heart rate data to acid–base status and neonatal condition at birth.[32] These data help to establish the state of fetal oxygenation at birth.[39,40] A doubly clamped, 10 to 30 cm segment of umbilical cord is obtained and, using two preheparinized 1 to 2 ml syringes, samples of blood are collected from the umbilical artery and vein. These samples are then analyzed for respiratory gases (see Tables 15.2 to 15.4). Some investigators now advocate obtaining cord blood gas measurements after all deliveries.[40] These data will confirm normal acid–base status in 98 percent of vigorous newborns and nearly 80 percent of infants judged to be depressed at birth. Cord blood gas studies may be most helpful when a delivery is performed for fetal distress, when the condition of the newborn differs from that which would have been expected on the basis of the course of labor or fetal heart rate tracing, and when one delivers an infant at greater risk for subsequent neurologic handicap, such as IUGR, prolonged pregnancy, or preterm birth.

FETAL THERAPY

Amnioinfusion

In 1983, Miyazaki and Taylor[41] first described the use of amnioinfusion with saline to relieve variable or prolonged decelerations. Saline warmed to 37 degrees C is infused through an internal pressure catheter attached to a three-way stopcock. This catheter is separate from that used to monitor uterine activity. Nageotte et al.[42] subsequently demonstrated several clinical uses for this technique and added data regarding its safety and reliability. Amnioinfusion could be used to prevent fetal distress when persistent unremitting variable decelerations were a problem. Most often this technique has been of value in labor complicated by premature rupture of the membranes, IUGR, and post-dates gestation.

Sadovsky et al.[43] have evaluated the benefits of amnioinfusion in labors complicated by meconium in an effort to reduce the concentration of meconium bathing the fetus. In this setting, amnioinfusion significantly decreased the thickness of meconium, the likelihood of significant meconium below the vocal cords, and the incidence of neonatal acidemia.

Several different protocols for amnioinfusion have been developed. Usually 500 to 1,000 ml of saline is administered initially, followed by a continuous infusion of 150 to 200 ml per hour as long as the decelerative pattern persists. Once the pattern has been ameliorated, a maintenance infusion of 10 to 20 ml per minute is continued. Until recently, it was recommended that the saline be warmed to body temperature. The use of saline at room temperature has been demonstrated to be as safe and effective.[44]

Tocolysis

The primary stress that the fetus must tolerate during labor is the contraction itself. When uterine activity of any origin or type exceeds the fetus' tolerance for reduced oxygenation, fetal stress and possible fetal distress follow. Generally the manifestation of excessive uterine activity includes hypoxic or reflex fetal heart rate decelerations, loss of variability, or baseline changes. Often when such situations arise it is reasonable to attempt to reduce uterine activity to a level that the fetus is able to tolerate rather than to deliver the fetus operatively at a time when the pH may be low and the PCO_2 elevated. This technique of intrauterine resuscitation has been popular in many parts of the world for a number of years[45] and has recently become more widely applied in the United States.[46] One or two parenteral injections of tocolytic agents such as 0.5 mg of subcutaneous terbutaline or 4 to 6 g of intravenous magnesium sulfate have been used for this purpose. Although the response of the worrisome fetal heart rate pattern to this therapy may be used to judge fetal status, it is often advisable to assess fetal acid–base status, particularly a base deficit, following resolution to confirm a physiologically normal fetus. Using tocolysis in this manner, a significant number of deliveries by cesarean section can be eliminated, particularly when this approach is utilized late in the first stage or early in the second stage of labor. When it has been decided to proceed to delivery by cesarean section for fetal distress, a single injection of a tocolytic agent will frequently reduce uterine activity, thereby allowing some recovery before delivery occurs.

Management of Fetal Stress and Distress

In an effort to reduce morbidity and mortality secondary to intrapartum hypoxia, it seems reasonable to use and integrate all available fetal data-collecting systems. Accordingly, because continuous fetal heart rate monitoring provides the only currently available system for instantaneous continuous data collection from the fetus and particularly because its diagnostic accuracy for confirming fetal well-being is no less than 98 percent, it is logical to use this as the primary system. Because fetal heart rate monitoring is less able to identify the fetus that is truly in distress, it also appears reasonable to add intermittent fetal capillary blood collection for acid–base values to supplement fetal heart rate monitoring. Using both systems, the diagnostic accuracy for *fetal compromise* approaches that for the diagnosis of well-being using fetal heart rate only. In the ideal setting, the obstetrician should be intimately familiar with both techniques. A protocol for intrapartum monitoring with fetal heart rate evaluation supplemented by acid–base determinations is given below. Although not completely ideal, and in some instances overtly conservative, it is well within the capability of most obstetric units. When followed, this protocol has the potential to reduce the number of fetuses born in an asphyxiated or damaged condition.

General Principles

1. All high-risk patients should be monitored internally as soon as it is clinically feasible. If an external technique is used and there is flattening

of the baseline, an internal electrode should be used to assess true heart rate variability.

2. For a mixed fetal heart rate pattern, the patient should be managed according to the most ominous pattern.

3. In the presence of maternal fever, a satisfactory fetal scalp capillary blood determination should not be relied on solely as an indication of fetal well-being. Sepsis may cause fetal compromise despite a normal pH.

4. When a fetal blood sample is obtained, a simultaneous sample of free-flowing maternal venous blood should be obtained for acid–base determination and comparison with fetal pH.

5. When meconium is present or the gestation is thought to be prolonged, and especially if both are present, a fetal scalp capillary blood sample should be obtained as soon as it is clinically feasible for baseline acid–base determinations.

6. If there is an abnormal fetal heart rate pattern, such as a confusing pattern, late or severe variable decelerations, a baseline tachycardia, or loss of variability that is not drug induced, a fetal scalp capillary blood sample should be obtained at that time for a baseline acid–base determination or as soon as it is clinically feasible (Fig. 15.19). If fetal scalp sampling cannot be performed, a fetal stimulation test should be done to assess acid–base status.

Management of Fetal Heart Rate Patterns

Early Deceleration

In the vast majority of patients, the maximal deceleration does not fall below 100 bpm. This pattern is usually associated with uncomplicated labor and delivery, and thus no management correction is in order. If the maximal deceleration falls below 100 bpm and is repetitive, a vaginal examination should be performed to check for a prolapsed cord. The fetal heart rate pattern may be observed with subsequent contractions and managed expectantly as a cord-variable pattern described below with the use of fetal scalp capillary acid–base determinations.

Late Deceleration

With repetitive late decelerations, the following steps should be initiated:

1. If oxytocin is in use, discontinue it. When the pattern has been corrected, and after appropriate reevaluation, oxytocin may be restarted.

2. Start oxygen at 5 to 6 L/min with a tight-fitting face mask.

3. Check maternal blood pressure; if the mother is hypotensive, correct the hypotension as follows:
   a. Change the maternal position (e.g., back to left lateral to right lateral, leg elevation).
   b. Increase the rate of administration of electrolyte-containing intravenous fluids maximally.
   c. If the hypotension is thought to be secondary to regional anesthesia, consult with an obstetric anesthesiologist regarding the possible use of a vasopressive agent (e.g., ephedrine 15 mg IV).

4. Assess fetal acid–base status with a fetal stimulation test or collection of fetal blood. Obtain a free-flowing maternal venous blood sample if fetal capillary blood sample acid–base determination is utilized. Fetal scalp capillary blood may be collected from maternal positions other than the dorsolithotomy position.

After acid–base status has been determined, if the above measures do not correct the pattern of decelerations, the obstetrician should prepare for delivery by the method that is quickest and safest for both mother and fetus (i.e., alert the operating room, shave the abdomen, and so forth):

1. If the late deceleration pattern persists and fetal acid–base status is satisfactory (pH > 7.24) or if an acceptable fetal heart rate acceleration is obtained, if delivery is not too far off, and if it is decided to allow labor to continue, confirmation of satisfactory fetal acid–base status must be determined at 20-minute intervals as long as late decelerations are observed. If such repetitive sampling cannot be done, delivery of the fetus is in order (Figs. 15.20 and 15.21). A base deficit will often help determine whether the fetus is at significant risk for metabolic acidosis.

2. If the fetal capillary blood pH is in the pathologic range (< 7.20) and the maternal venous blood pH is normal, fetal capillary pH should be repeated immediately.
   a. If the second fetal pH is in the normal range,

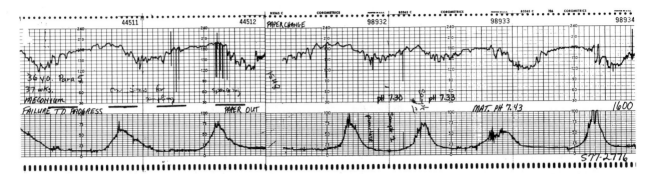

Fig. 15.20 Baseline tachycardia with persistent late decelerations is noted using internal monitoring. Good variability is present, and uterine activity is not excessive. The differentiation between stress and distress is made in this case by obtaining a fetal capillary pH (panel 98932), which is in the normal range, at 7.30 and 7.33. A free-flowing maternal venous pH is 7.43. If there is concern about buffer reserve, a fetal base deficit could add additional information, especially if one anticipates imminent delivery.

sampling is repeated in 20 minutes to ensure a satisfactory value.

b. If the second fetal sample is in the prepathologic range (7.20 to 7.24), the sample is repeated in 15 to 20 minutes.

c. If the second fetal sample is also in the pathologic range (<7.20), the patient is delivered by the method that is quickest and safest for both the mother and the fetus. Of note, the use of a tocolytic agent such as intravenous ritodrine or terbutaline to arrest labor and allow recovery of the fetus before delivery is being used in many centers.

3. If the maternal venous sample has an abnormal pH, maternal acidosis with a pH <7.35, and is associated with a low fetal pH value, steps must be taken to improve the mother's condition. The difference in fetal and maternal base deficit may also be checked. If vaginal delivery does not appear imminent, cesarean section may be required.

Variable Deceleration

When variable decelerations are mild and not repetitive, the pattern is usually associated with good fetal outcome. However, variable decelerations may worsen as labor progresses. If they become repetitive, fall below 90 bpm at their nadir, and last longer than 60 seconds, fetal condition can deteriorate. This type of pattern is usually seen during the late first and the second stages of labor.

Should the variable deceleration begin as or progress to an ominous variable deceleration pattern, the following steps should be initiated:

1. If oxytocin is in use, discontinue it. When the pattern has been corrected, and after appropriate reevaluation, oxytocin may be restarted.

2. Unless clinically contraindicated (e.g., suspected placenta previa), a vaginal examination should be performed immediately to check for a prolapsed cord and to determine the progress of labor.

3. Maternal hypotension should be identified and corrected.

4. Maternal position should be changed: left lateral, right lateral, Trendelenburg, reverse Trendelenburg, knee–chest, or supine.

5. Oxygen is started at 5 to 6 L/min with a tight-fitting face mask.

6. If uterine activity is excessive, the use of intravenous tocolysis with terbutaline or magnesium sulfate may be considered, especially if delivery is not thought to be too far distant.

If these management measures do not correct the pattern, and if the variable decelerations worsen, reaching a nadir of less than 90 bpm with progressive lengthening to 60 seconds and longer:

1. The obstetrician should prepare for delivery by the method that is quickest and safest for both

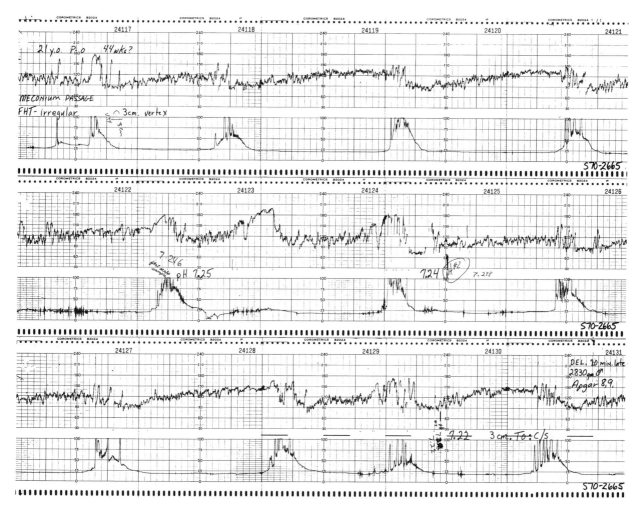

Fig. 15.21 (Top) A tracing of this possibly prolonged gestation (44 weeks?) complicated by meconium passage revealing accelerations with contractions (panel 24117) but late decelerations after each contraction. The baseline heart rate shows exaggerated variability. (Middle) For these reasons, fetal capillary pH values were obtained (panels 24122 and 24125) and were found to be 7.25 and 7.24. (Bottom) Because of borderline or preacidotic values, the pH was repeated 20 minutes later and is now 7.22 (panel 24129). Because the patient had made no progress during 1 hour of labor and had meconium with a probable prolonged pregnancy, a cesarean section was performed before further deterioration of fetal condition occurred. Apgar scores at delivery were 8 and 9.

mother and fetus (i.e., alert the operating room, shave the abdomen, and so forth).

2. Access fetal acid–base status by a stimulation test or by analysis of fetal capillary blood. A free-flowing maternal venous blood sample may be obtained and fetal scalp capillary blood taken for acid–base determination. Care should be exercised to obtain the fetal capillary blood sample

after the deceleration has returned to the baseline and just before the next contraction. There is rapid diffusion of CO_2 across the placenta. With the alleviation of cord compression, wide variations in fetal pH values may occur, depending on the timing of scalp sampling. Great care must therefore be taken in interpreting the values. Because the initial respiratory acidosis of variable

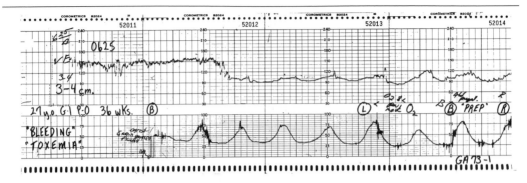

Fig. 15.22 Internal monitoring is used for this nullipara at 36 weeks with pregnancy-induced hypertension and bleeding. Internal monitoring demonstrates good heart rate variability. The intrauterine pressure catheter, following appropriate calibration (panel 52011), demonstrates an elevated resting tone (30 mmHg) and frequent contractions, suggesting placental abruption. Note that the heart rate falls in panel 52012, and the patient is taken to the operating room for a cesarean section, where a "total abruption" was found.

decelerations may shortly progress to a metabolic acidosis unless cord compression is corrected, pH, PCO_2, and a base deficit represent useful fetal blood determinations in the management of these cases. The base deficit should not be allowed to exceed 10 or 11 with a pH of <7.2 unless delivery is imminent.

3. Immediate delivery can be delayed if a safe vaginal delivery is expected within 20 to 30 minutes unless the fetal heart rate pattern or the acid–base status of the fetus worsens acutely.

Prolonged Sudden Deceleration

Occasionally, an unexpected and often unexplained prolonged deceleration may occur. The fetal heart rate will drop below 80 bpm, and the deceleration can last several minutes. Such sudden prolonged decelerations may be related to

1. Uterine hyperactivity, usually oxytocin related (Fig. 15.22)
2. Fetal manipulation (e.g., vaginal examination, blood sampling) (Fig. 15.23)

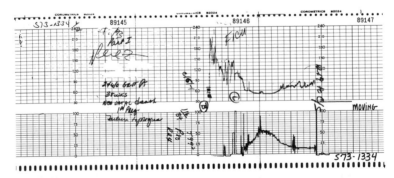

Fig. 15.23 In preparation for oxytocin augmentation of labor for failure to progress, an internal pressure catheter was placed and an electrode attached to the fetal scalp. Note that with the attachment of the fetal electrode the fetal heart rate suddenly decelerates to approximately 50 bpm, with a slow and irregular return. Some fetuses are very sensitive to manipulation of the scalp and can have a sudden prolonged deceleration mediated by the vagus nerve. This patient was taken to the operating room and observed. The fetal heart rate returned to a normal level in a few minutes, and subsequently the patient was vaginally delivered of a healthy baby.

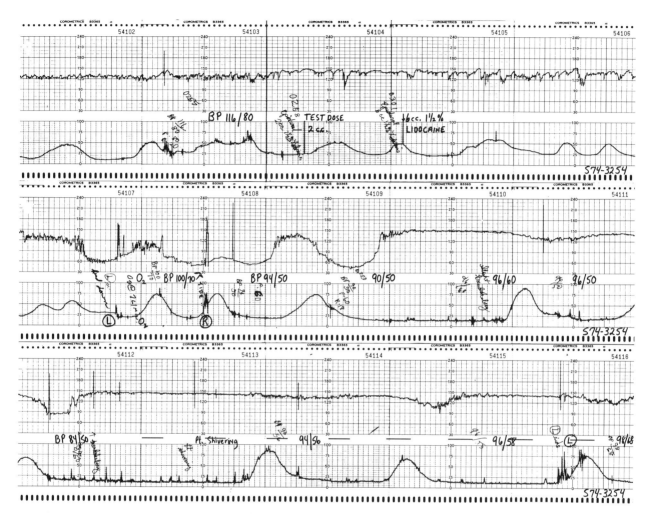

Fig. 15.24 (Top) Normal fetal heart rate and uterine activity data with an internal monitoring system. The blood pressure is normal, and a test dose of a local anesthetic agent is used in preparation for epidural anesthesia. Approximately 3.5 minutes after the test dose, additional local anesthetic is administered. (Middle) Heart rate decelerations are noted (panels 54107 to 54109), along with a fall in maternal blood pressure. These decelerations appear to be of both reflex and hypoxic etiologies. Heart rate variability is reduced in panel 54110 and remains so throughout the remainder of the tracing. (Bottom) Late decelerations are seen in panels 54111 to 54116. Similar heart rate changes may be noted after administration of a paracervical block.

3. Conduction anesthesia with hypotension (Fig. 15.24)
4. Supine hypotension
5. Maternal respiratory arrest (convulsions, high spinal anesthesia, intravenous narcotics) (Fig. 15.25)

If the deceleration has no remedial cause, careful observation of the fetal heart rate after recovery should be maintained. If the deceleration should occur a second or third time, corrective measures need to be instituted and preparation for immediate delivery undertaken. If at all possible, delivery should be accomplished 10 to 15 minutes into the recovery period to allow the fetus to benefit from intrauterine resuscitation.

Should a prolonged sudden deceleration occur, the following steps should be instituted:

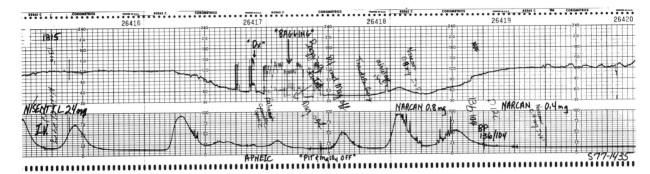

Fig. 15.25 Before this recording, the patient had received the narcotic analgesic Nisentil. An additional dose of 24 mg was given intravenously at the onset of this tracing, followed by a marked fall in fetal heart rate in panel 26417. The patient had suffered a respiratory arrest because of the Nisentil, and the change in fetal heart rate can be attributed to hypoxia. The mother was intubated and "bagged" to reestablish respiration. The narcotic antagonist Narcan was administered, and, with the establishment of normal maternal respiration, the fetal heart rate returned to a normal level.

1. Consider the causes of prolonged decelerations and attempt to correct them, including tocolytic therapy for excessive uterine activity.
2. Change maternal position until an effective position is found.
3. Perform a vaginal examination, unless uncontraindicated, to check for cord prolapse and the progress of labor.
4. Institute oxygen at 5 to 6 L/min with a tight-fitting face mask.
5. Increase the infusion of intravenous fluids.

If these measures do not resolve the problem and vaginal delivery is not imminent after 5 minutes of a fetal heart rate at 60 bpm, delivery by cesarean section is indicated. If these steps do alleviate the deceleration, assessment of fetal acid–base status by a fetal stimulation test or by fetal and maternal acid–base determinations should be obtained 5 to 15 minutes after the fetal heart rate has recovered. If the fetal pH is 7.25 or less, a second sample should be obtained within 15 minutes or until the pH is 7.25 or greater.

Sinusoidal Fetal Heart Rate Pattern

If a sinusoidal pattern occurs and is unrelated to the administration of narcotics, a fetal scalp blood sample for acid–base determination should be obtained. A fetal hematocrit may also be performed to detect the presence of fetal anemia. If abnormal values are found, immediate delivery should be considered. The neonatal staff should also be informed of the fetal blood values so that they can prepare for immediate newborn resuscitation and/or transfusion.

RISK VERSUS BENEFIT OF INTRAPARTUM EVALUATION

Without question, the outstanding value of fetal heart rate monitoring during the intrapartum period is the reasonably sensitive ability of this technique to confirm fetal well-being and to permit labor to continue without unnecessary intervention. Unfortunately, this method of surveillance is less able to identify accurately if the fetus is clearly in distress. Accordingly, in utilizing fetal heart rate monitoring alone, a large number of fetuses that are in good condition and that show no clinical evidence of morbidity may be delivered by "emergency" measures.

Most of the criticism of fetal heart rate monitoring has been aroused by this deficiency. Banta and Thacker[47] reviewed the world literature and could find no statistical evidence that fetal heart rate surveillance reduced perinatal morbidity or mortality. In contrast, a number of small studies have shown fetal heart rate monitoring to be of clinical value.[48,49] Critics, both old and new, have pointed out that fetal heart rate monitoring should not have been introduced without an adequate prospective, randomized, double-blind trial.

A few large prospective investigations have recently failed to demonstrate that continuous fetal heart rate monitoring is associated with an improved perinatal outcome. The study conducted by MacDonald and his colleagues[51,52] in Dublin included more than 13,000 patients. This investigation demonstrated a twofold increase in the incidence of neonatal asphyxial convulsions and persistently abnormal neurologic examinations in the offspring of patients followed with intermittent auscultation as compared with continuous electronic fetal heart rate monitoring. Four years later, however, evaluation of 9 children in the electronic fetal heart rate monitoring group and 21 in the intermittent auscultation group who survived after neonatal seizures showed that three children in each group had cerebral palsy.[53] Cerebral palsy was also identified in a fourth child in the electronic fetal heart rate monitoring group who had a transiently abnormal neurologic examination during the neonatal period. An additional eight children in the electronic fetal heart rate monitoring group and seven in the intermittent auscultation group who had not had abnormal neurologic signs in the neonatal period were found to have cerebral palsy. In total, 16, or almost 80 percent, of the 22 cases of cerebral palsy had not shown clinical evidence suggestive of intrapartum asphyxia. The incidence of cerebral palsy was nearly identical in both groups, 1.8 : 1,000 for electronic fetal heart rate monitoring and 1.5 : 1,000 for intermittent auscultation. The authors concluded that, compared with intermittent auscultation, electronic fetal heart rate monitoring had little, if any, protective effect against cerebral palsy. Overall, it appears that no more than 20 percent of cases of cerebral palsy are associated with intrapartum events.[54]

Recent studies have also failed to demonstrate improved outcomes in preterm infants followed with continuous heart rate monitoring as compared with periodic auscultation. Luthy et al.[55] observed no significant differences for low 5-minute Apgar scores, intrapartum acidosis, intracranial hemorrhage, or frequency of cesarean section in a randomized trial of preterm singleton pregnancies with fetal weights of 750 to 1,750 g. At 18 months of age, 93 children in the electronic fetal heart rate monitoring group were not found to differ from the 96 premature infants in the intermittent auscultation group in mean mental development scores and psychomotor development.[56] In the electronic fetal heart rate monitoring group, the risk of cerebral palsy increased with the duration of abnormal fetal heart rate patterns, reaching 67 percent when the abnormal pattern lasted 91 minutes or more. Of note, 13 of the children found to have cerebral palsy did not manifest an abnormal heart rate pattern on electronic fetal heart rate monitoring or intermittent auscultation during labor. The authors conclude that, when compared with a structured protocol of intermittent auscultation, electronic fetal heart rate monitoring did not improve neurologic outcome for children born prematurely.

Over the past decade and a half, marked improvements in perinatal morbidity and mortality have been reported around the world coincident with the utilization of fetal heart rate and acid–base surveillance techniques.[57,58] While no direct cause and effect can be demonstrated, such data certainly support the use of continuous fetal heart rate monitoring. It is the opinion of the American College of Obstetricians and Gynecologists, as reported in its technical bulletins,[59,60] that continuous fetal heart rate monitoring with acid–base support and appropriate intermittent monitoring by auscultation or Doppler ultrasound are of equal value for the monitoring of the fetus. Some investigators have emphasized that, on a statistical basis, there is little advantage to continuous fetal heart rate monitoring for the normal fetus. Few clinicians will deny that occasional cord accidents and other unforeseen problems may arise that cannot be detected by standard auscultatory techniques. It must also be emphasized that in most studies comparing electronic monitoring to auscultation, auscultation has been carried out by a single nurse at the bedside. Such staffing is not possible in most institutions.[61]

Acid–base determinations can decrease the number of false-positive diagnoses of fetal distress.[59,60] Although Beard and associates[31] demonstrated a good correlation between acid–base values and Apgar score at delivery, many investigators remained concerned about false-negative diagnoses and about the reliability of acid–base data in the presence of fetal heart rate patterns indicative of potential fetal jeopardy. If the fetal heart rate tracing showed late decelerations but the scalp pH was normal, is it wise to wait until fetal acidosis can be documented before undertaking delivery? Bowe et al.[30] found that 10.4

percent of fetuses with good acid–base values had Apgar scores below 7 at delivery (Table 15.7). They reported the 1-minute Apgar scores, which reflect fetal status at birth and the type of resuscitative efforts that will be necessary. Hutson et al.[62] reevaluated this false-normal group of patients using the 5-minute Apgar score and found that by 5 minutes only 1.7 percent of fetuses with good scalp pH values had a low Apgar score, a risk most clinicians find acceptable (Table 15.8).

In recent years, the obstetrician has by the courts and the judicial system been held to increasingly higher standards for perinatal outcome. The delivery of a damaged infant in the absence of a clearly documented chart with accurate data relating to labor, fetal condition, management plan, and delivery process has unfortunately been related to medical negligence. Not surprisingly, the obstetrician now is always aware of the continuous scrutiny of the judicial system and its review process. In dealing with high-risk situations and in response to the medicolegal climate, the obstetrician may resort more frequently to cesarean section (Figs. 15.26 to 15.29).[58]

Unfortunately, as described above, the use of continuous fetal heart rate monitoring has not demonstrated a significant decrease in certain poor outcomes such as cerebral palsy.[63–67] In some cases, particularly those with a confusing heart rate tracing, the use of additional fetal surveillance in the form of acid–base data may allow a more logical approach to the problem.

For every new technique certain risks or potential problems must be addressed and integrated into the day-to-day utilization of the method. For the external fetal monitoring systems, the most likely risk is the potential to misinterpret heart rate or uterine activity tracings because of inadequate or confusing data. The circuitry of many external heart rate monitors

Table 15.7 One-Minute Apgar Score (355 Patients)

Fetal pH	Apgar Score	
	1 – 6	7 – 10
≥ 7.20	10.4% (false normal)	64.4%
≤ 7.19	17.6%	7.6% (false abnormal)

(From Hutson et al,[62] with permission.)

Table 15.8 Five-Minute Apgar Score (355 Patients)

Fetal pH	Apgar Score	
	1 – 6	7 – 10
≥ 7.20	1.7% (false normal)	—
≤ 7.19	—	—

(From Hutson et al,[62] with permission.)

dictates that once the fetal heart rate exceeds 180 bpm or falls below 90 bpm, the machine will either halve or double the rate. Errors in interpretation (Fig. 15.29) can easily be made if this electronic editing is not understood. When this occurs, one needs mentally to place that section of displaced heart rate information in its proper position.

Internal fetal heart rate monitoring involves breaking the skin or scalp to attach the electrode. In rare cases, a small pustule may form at the electrode site. The incidence of this infectious problem has been reported to be between 1 in 500 and 1 in 2,000 cases.[68] These lesions can generally be treated by drainage and topical antibiotics.

Many clinicians believe that an internal pressure catheter will increase the risk of chorioamnionitis and postpartum endomyometritis. Most studies have failed to confirm this suspicion. There is no doubt, however, that the longer an intrauterine catheter and electrode are in situ before a cesarean section is performed, the greater the likelihood of postpartum febrile morbidity.[69,70]

Occasionally, when inserting the intrauterine pressure catheter, the stiff plastic guide may penetrate the myometrium. Accordingly, the obstetrician must guard against this complication and avoid extending the guide beyond his or her finger. It is exceedingly uncommon for the soft plastic intrauterine pressure catheter to penetrate the myometrium.

Collecting fetal scalp blood requires a 2 mm incision into the scalp that penetrates to the level of the cartilaginous plate. Occasionally, excess bleeding may be noted, but pressure usually controls this problem. In approximately 20,000 patients, significant fetal bleeding was encountered in only two or three cases. As with the scalp electrode, a pustule or local infection may be noted at the incision site. The incidence of this complication has been reported to

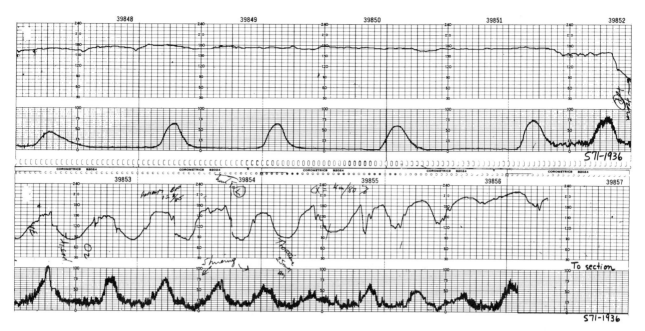

Fig. 15.26 (Top) Unexplained baseline fetal tachycardia. Heart rate variability is poor. The patient suffered a shaking chill (panel 39852), as reflected in the ''jitteriness'' of the uterine activity tracing. (Bottom) With the chill, and presumably with increased maternal oxygen consumption, severe late decelerations occurred. A baseline fetal scalp pH performed earlier may have been helpful in the management of this case.

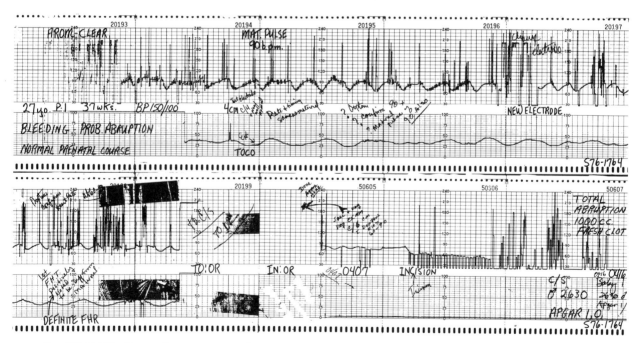

Fig. 15.27 (Top) Internal monitoring reveals a heart rate that is indistinguishable from the maternal heart rate. A new electrode is applied (panel 20196), and (Bottom) the heart rate remains unchanged. Today, the immediate use of real-time ultrasound to look at fetal cardiac motion would help differentiate a true fetal heart rate bradycardia from a maternal heart rate that is being transmitted through a dead fetus. The use of ultrasound in these situations has been invaluable. At cesarean section in this case, a total abruption was found.

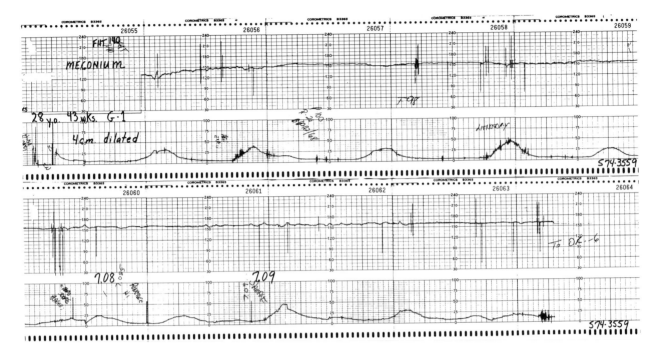

Fig. 15.28 (Top) Essentially normal fetal heart rate and uterine activity are noted in this nullipara at 43 weeks with meconium. No periodic patterns are noted, but minimal heart rate variability is seen. (Bottom) Because of the fetal metabolic acidosis that may occur in this setting, a baseline fetal capillary pH was obtained on two occasions (panels 26060 and 26061). The values were 7.08 and 7.09. Thereafter, this patient was quickly delivered by cesarean section. In this case, fetal capillary scalp sampling clearly benefited the fetus.

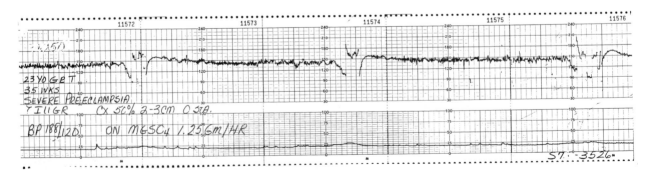

Fig. 15.29 External tracing containing three variable decelerations. At the bottom of each deceleration, data are missing, and it appears that the heart rate has jumped to the 160 to 170 bpm range. In reality, this monitor is doubling the true heart at the bottom of the deceleration. To interpret this tracing, one needs to move the data mentally back down to the bottom of the deceleration, their proper place. With an external fetal heart rate monitor, the reverse can happen when the heart rate is at 180 bpm or higher. The monitor may halve the rate to 90 bpm.

be 1 in 1,000 cases.[71] Again, most perinatologists believe that the value of these data in clinical management offsets the potential for neonatal morbidity.

Overall, the benefits of the internal monitoring system when compared with external monitoring outweigh the potential risks by providing significant additional data, including precise quantitation of both long-term and short-term variability, continuous fetal heart rate data (even when the fetus and/or mother are moving), and accurate uterine activity data with quantitation of frequency, duration, and amplitude of contractions.

Some patients believe that both forms of fetal surveillance are too technical and restrictive and that they interfere with the birth process. They find this unnatural and therefore unneeded.[72-76] Generally, when an appropriate explanation is given to these patients, they realize that the benefits of the added information achieved far outweigh any perceived liability.[76] An occasional patient simply refuses any form of fetal surveillance. When appropriate explanations have been given and the patient still declines the process, it is generally advisable to have two independent observers document in the chart that the patient refuses "usual and customary forms of intrapartum fetal surveillance" in order to establish the facts that (1) the surveillance was offered, (2) the reasons for its use were explained, and (3) the complications that can arise from not using these forms of monitoring were known to the patient and were fully understood at the time of refusal.

REFERENCES

1. Barcroft J: Researches on Pre-Natal Life. Charles C Thomas, Springfield, IL, 1947
2. Barron DH: The exchange of the respiratory gases in the placenta. Neonatal Stud 1:3, 1952
3. Apgar V: A proposal for a new method of evaluation of the newborn infant. Curr Res Anesth Analg 32:260, 1953
4. Freda V: Hemolytic disease. Clin Obstet Gynecol 16:72, 1973
5. James LS, Weisbrot IM, Prince CE et al: The acid–base status of human infants in relation to birth asphyxia and the onset of respiration. J Pediatr 52:379, 1958
6. Saling E: Neues Vorgehen zur Untersuchung des Kindes unter der Gebrut. Arch Gynakol 197:108, 1961
7. Hammacher K, Huter KA, Bokelmann J et al: Foetal heart frequency and perinatal condition of foetus and newborn. Gynaecologia (Basel) 166:348, 1968
8. Hon EH, Quilligan EJ: The classification of fetal heart rate. II. A revised working classification. Conn Med 31:779, 1967
9. Caldeyro-Barcia R, Casacuberta C, Busros R et al: Correlation of intrapartum changes in fetal heart rate with fetal blood oxygen and acid–base balance. p. 205. In Adamsons K (ed): Diagnosis and Treatment of Fetal Disorders. Springer-Verlag, New York, 1968
10. Fenton AN, Steer CM: Fetal distress. Am J Obstet Gynecol 83:354, 1962
11. Miller FC, Sacks DA, Yeh S-Y: Significance of meconium during labor. Am J Obstet Gynecol 130:473, 1978
12. Miller FC, Read JA: Intrapartum assessment of the postdate fetus. Am J Obstet Gynecol 141:516, 1981
13. Dawes GS, Handler JJ, Mott JC: Some cardiovascular responses in foetal, newborn and adult rabbits. J Physiol (Lond) 139:123, 1957
14. Assali NS, Holm L, Parker H: Regional blood flow and vascular resistance in response to oxytocin in the pregnant sheep and dog. J Appl Physiol 16:1087, 1961
15. Hon EH: The electronic evaluation of the fetal heart rate. Am J Obstet Gynecol 75:1215, 1958
16. Miller FC, Pearse KE, Paul RH: Fetal heart rate pattern recognition by the method of auscultation. Obstet Gynecol 64:332, 1984
17. Wood C, Lumbley J, Renou P: A clinical assessment of foetal diagnostic methods. J Obstet Br Commonw 74:823, 1967
18. Beard RW: Fetal blood sampling. Br J Hosp Med 3:523, 1970
19. Hon EH, Khazin AF: Biochemical studies of the fetus. II. Fetal pH and Apgar scores. Obstet Gynecol 33:237, 1969
20. Rayburn WF: Clinical significance of maternal perceptible fetal motion. Am J Obstet Gynecol 138:210, 1980
21. Sadovsky E, Yaffe H: Daily fetal movement recording and fetal prognosis. Obstet Gynecol 41:6, 1973
22. Patrick J, Campbell LK, Carmichael L et al: Patterns of human fetal breathing during the last 10 weeks of pregnancy. Obstet Gynecol 56:24, 1980
23. Patrick J, Challis J: Measurement of human fetal breathing movements in healthy pregnancies using a real-time scanner. Semin Perinatol 4:275, 1980
24. Martin CB: Physiology and clinical use of fetal heart rate variability. Clin Perinatol 9:339, 1982
25. Zalar RW Jr, Quilligan EJ: The influence of scalp sampling on the cesarean section rate for fetal distress. Am J Obstet Gynecol 123:206, 1975
26. Paul RH, Suidan AK, Yeh SY et al: Clinical fetal moni-

toring. VII. The evaluation and significance of intrapartum baseline fetal heart rate variability. Am J Obstet Gynecol 123:206, 1975

27. Hutson JM, Mueller-Heubach E: Diagnosis and management of intrapartum reflex fetal heart rate changes. Clin Perinatol 9:325, 1982

28. Saling E: Technik der endoskopischen microblutentnahme am feten. Geburtshilfe Frauenheilkd 24:464, 1964

29. Adamsons K, Beard RW, Cosmi EV et al: The validity of capillary blood in the assessment of the acid–base state of the fetus. p. 175. In Adamsons K (ed): Diagnosis and Treatment of Fetal Disorders. Springer-Verlag, New York, 1968

30. Bowe ET, Beard RT, Finster M et al: Reliability of fetal blood sampling. Am J Obstet Gynecol 107:279, 1970

31. Beard RW, Morris ED, Clayton SG: pH of fetal capillary blood as an indication of the condition of the fetus. J Obstet Gynecol Br Commonw 74:812, 1967

32. Wilble JL, Petrie RH, Koons A et al: The clinical use of umbilical cord acid–base determinations in perinatal surveillance and management. Clin Perinatol 9:387, 1982

33. Kubli FW, Hon EH, Khazin AF et al: Observations on heart rate and pH in the human fetus during labor. Am J Obstet Gynecol 104:1190, 1969

34. Low JA, Cox MJ, Karchmar EJ et al: The prediction of intrapartum fetal metabolic acidosis by fetal heart rate monitoring. Am J Obstet Gynecol 139:299, 1981

35. Mountain KR, Hirsh J, Gallus AS: Neonatal coagulation defect due to anticonvulsant drug treatment in pregnancy. Lancet 1:265, 1970

36. Webb MT, Petrie RH, Pippenger CE: Fetal circulatory collapse during induction of labor in pregnant patient with epilepsy. Am J Obstet Gynecol 130:727, 1978

37. Clark SL, Gimovsky ML, Miller FC: Fetal heart rate response to scalp blood sampling. Am J Obstet Gynecol 144:706, 1982

38. Polzin GB, Blakemore KJ, Petrie RH, Amon E: Fetal vibro-acoustic stimulation: magnitude and duration of fetal heart rate accelerations as a marker of fetal health. Obstet Gynecol 72(4):621, 1988

39. Gilstrap LC, Leveno KJ, Burris J et al: Diagnosis of birth asphyxia on the basis of fetal pH, Apgar score, and newborn cerebral dysfunction. Am J Obstet Gynecol 161(3):825, 1989

40. Thorp JA, Sampson JE, Parisi VM, Creasy RK: Routine umbilical cord blood gas determinations? Am J Obstet Gynecol 161(3):600, 1989

41. Miyazaki FS, Taylor NA: Saline amnioinfusion for relief of variable or prolonged decelerations. Am J Obstet Gynecol 146:670, 1983

42. Nageotte MP, Freeman RK, Garite TJ, Dorchester W: Prophylactic intrapartum amnioinfusion in patients with preterm premature rupture of membranes. Am J Obstet Gynecol 153:557, 1985

43. Sadovsky Y, Amon E, Bade M, Petrie RH: Prophylactic amnioinfusion during labor complicated by meconium: a preliminary report. Am J Obstet Gynecol 161(3):613, 1989

44. Nageotte MP, Bertucci L, Towers CV et al: Prophylactic amnioinfusion or thick meconium: a prospective study. Society of Perinatal Obstetricians, Tenth Annual Meeting, Houston, Texas, 1990

45. Caldeyro-Barcia R, Magaña JM, Castillo JB et al: A new approach to the treatment of acute intrapartum fetal distress. Perinatal Factors Affecting Human Development. Proceedings of the Special Session held during the Eighth Meeting of the PAHO Advisory Committee on Medical Research, June 10, 1969

46. Reece EA, Chervenak FA, Romero R, Hobbins JC: Magnesium sulfate in the management of acute intrapartum fetal distress. Am J Obstet Gynecol 148(1):104, 1984

47. Banta HD, Thacker S: Assessing the costs and benefits of electronic fetal monitoring. Obstet Gynecol Surv 34:627, 1979

48. Kelso IM, Parsons RJ, Lawrence GF et al: An assessment of continuous fetal heart rate monitoring in labor: a randomized trial. Am J Obstet Gynecol 131:526, 1978

49. Renou P, Chang A, Anderson I et al: Controlled trial of fetal intensive care. Am J Obstet Gynecol 113:573, 1972

50. Leveno KJ, Cunningham FG, Nelson S et al: A prospective comparison of selective and universal electronic fetal heart rate monitoring in 34,995 pregnancies. N Engl J Med 315:615, 1986

51. MacDonald D, Grant A, Sheridan-Pereira M et al: The Dublin randomized controlled trial of intrapartum fetal heart rate monitoring. Am J Obstet Gynecol 152:524, 1985

52. Boylan P, MacDonald D, Grant A et al: The Dublin fetal monitoring trial. Society of Perinatal Obstetricians, Fourth Annual Meeting, San Antonio, Texas, 1984

53. Grant A, O'Brien N, Joy M-T et al: Cerebral palsy among children born during the Dublin randomised trial of intrapartum monitoring. Lancet II:1233, 1989

54. Editorial: Cerebral palsy, intrapartum care, and a shot in the foot. Lancet II:1251, 1989

55. Luthy DA, Shy KK, vanBelle G et al: A randomized trial of electronic fetal monitoring in preterm labor. Obstet Gynecol 69:687, 1987

56. Shy KK, Luthy DA, Bennett FC et al: Effects of elec-

tronic fetal heart rate monitoring, as compared with periodic auscultation, on the neurologic development of premature infants. N Engl J Med 322:588, 1990

57. Shamsi HH, Petrie RH, Steer CM: Changing obstetrical practices and amelioration of the perinatal outcome in a university hospital. Am J Obstet Gynecol 133:855, 1979

58. Rosen MG: Consensus report by the Task Force on Cesarean Childbirth. NIH, Hyattsville, MD. U.S. Department of Health and Human Services, Public Health Service, National Institutes of Health, NIH Publ. #82-2067, 1981

59. American College of Obstetricians and Gynecologists: Assessment of Fetal and Newborn Acid–Base Status. Technical bulletin No. 127. ACOG, Washington, DC 1989

60. American College of Obstetricians and Gynecologists: Intrapartum Fetal Heart Rate Monitoring. Technical bulletin No. 132. ACOG, Washington, DC, 1989

61. Freeman R: Intrapartum fetal monitoring—a disappointing story. N Engl J Med 322:624, 1990

62. Hutson JM, Bowe ET, Petrie RH: The reliability of fetal acid–base determinations for prediction of normal Apgar scores: a reappraisal using the 5 minute score, abstracted. Soc Perinatal Obstet 99, 1982

63. Newell SJ, Green SH: Diagnostic classification of the aetiology of mental retardation in children. Br Med J 294:163, 1987

64. Sims ME, Turkel SB, Halterman G, Paul RH: Brain injury and intrauterine death. Am J Obstet Gynecol 151(6):721, 1985

65. Jenkins HM: Thirty years of electronic intrapartum fetal heart rate monitoring: discussion paper. J R Soc Med 82:210, 1989

66. Prentice A, Lind T: Fetal heart rate monitoring during labour—too frequent intervention, too little benefit? Lancet II:1375, 1987

67. Brown NA: Congenital "brain damage." Reprod Toxicol 6:1, 1987 Page 1.

68. Ledger WJ: Complications associated with invasive monitoring. Semin Perinatol 2:187, 1978

69. Gassner CB, Ledger WJ: The relationship of hospital-acquired maternal infection to invasive intrapartum monitoring techniques. Obstet Gynecol 126:33, 1976

70. Gibbs RS, Listwa HM, Read JA: The effect of internal fetal monitoring on maternal infection following cesarean section. Obstet Gynecol 48:653, 1976

71. Bowe ET: Fetal blood sampling. Bull Sloane Hosp Women 13:11, 1967

72. Starkman M: Psychological responses to the use of the monitor during labor. Psychosom Med 38:269, 1976

73. Shields D: Maternal reactions to fetal monitoring. Am J Nurs 3:2110, 1978

74. Jackson JE, Vaughan M, Black P et al: Psychological aspects of fetal monitoring: maternal reaction to the position of the monitor and staff behavior. J Psychosom Obstet Gynecol 2:97, 1983

75. Dulock HL, Herron M: Women's response to fetal monitoring. J Obstet Gynecol Neonatal Nursing 5:68s, 1976

76. Molfese V, Sunshine P, Bennett A: Reactions of women to intrapartum fetal monitoring. Obstet Gynecol 59:706, 1982

77. Bergmans MG, Jonker GJ, Kock CLV: Fetal supraventricular tachycardia: review of the literature. Obstet Gynecol Surv 40:61, 1985

78. Tejani N, Mann N, Bhakthavathsalan A, Weiss R: Correlation of fetal heart rate–uterine contraction patterns with fetal scalp blood pH. Obstet Gynecol 46:392, 1975

79. Tejani N, Mann L, Bhakthavathsalan A: Correlation of fetal heart rate patterns and fetal pH with neonatal outcome. Obstet Gynecol 48:460, 1976

80. Beard RW, Filshie GM, Knight CA et al: The significance of the changes in the continuous fetal heart rate in the first stage of labor. J Obstet Gynaecol Brit Commonw 78:865, 1971

Chapter 16

Obstetric Anesthesia

David H. Chestnut and Charles P. Gibbs

The word *anesthesia* encompasses all techniques used by anesthesiologists: general anesthesia, regional anesthesia, local anesthesia, and analgesia. Traditionally, general anesthesia includes four stages during which not only sensation but also consciousness and motor and reflex activities are gradually lost. During stage I, termed analgesia, memory and sensitivity to pain fade, yet consciousness and protective reflexes such as swallowing and laryngeal closure persist. Inhalation analgesia may be used for vaginal delivery, commonly in combination with local infiltration or pudendal block. Alone, this degree of anesthesia is not sufficient for even minor surgical incisions, including episiotomy. Stage II, the excitement stage, borders consciousness and unconsciousness. The patient may be agitated and uncooperative. Protective laryngeal reflexes may be either hyperactive or obtunded. Anesthesiologists avoid the second stage by keeping the patient in stage I or by rapidly inducing stage III with the aid of fast-acting barbiturates and muscle relaxants. The patient must also pass through this stage on awakening. Induction of and emergence from general anesthesia are usually the most dangerous times for the patient, because marked cardiovascular, respiratory, and laryngeal reflex changes occur.

Stage III, which is used for most surgical procedures, has four planes. As anesthesia deepens, it progressively depresses the central nervous, cardiovascu-

lar, and respiratory systems. Laryngeal reflexes nearly disappear; thus vomiting or regurgitation render the patient particularly susceptible to aspiration unless her airway is protected by an endotracheal tube. Stage IV terminates in death.

Anesthesiologists can produce all stages of general anesthesia. With the proper dose, concentration, and combination of agents, a specific anesthetic technique is matched to the requirements of a given procedure. The requirements for general anesthesia for cesarean section differ considerably from those for craniotomy, cholecystectomy, or exploratory laparotomy for a ruptured ectopic pregnancy, yet all these patients will be rendered unconscious, immobile, and pain free.

Balanced general anesthesia is the type of general anesthesia employed for obstetrics; it usually refers to various combinations of barbiturates, inhalation agents, opioids, and muscle relaxants as opposed to high concentrations of potent inhalation agents alone. General anesthesia is used in obstetrics mainly for cesarean section and rarely is required for vaginal delivery.

Regional analgesia/anesthesia uses local anesthetics to provide sensory as well as various degrees of motor blockade over a specific region of the body. In obstetrics, regional techniques include major blocks, such as spinal and lumbar or caudal epidural, as well as minor blocks, such as paracervical, pudendal, and

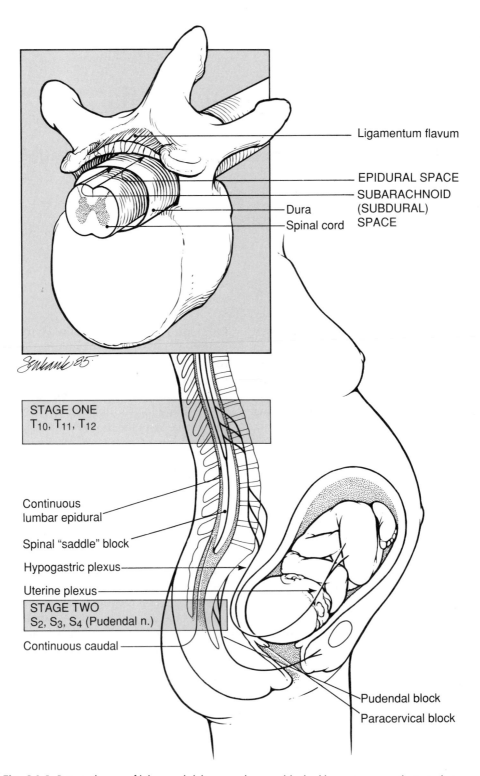

Ligamentum flavum

EPIDURAL SPACE

SUBARACHNOID (SUBDURAL) SPACE

Dura

Spinal cord

STAGE ONE
T_{10}, T_{11}, T_{12}

Continuous lumbar epidural

Spinal "saddle" block

Hypogastric plexus

Uterine plexus

STAGE TWO
S_2, S_3, S_4 (Pudendal n.)

Continuous caudal

Pudendal block

Paracervical block

Fig. 16.1 Pain pathways of labor and delivery and nerves blocked by various anesthetic techniques.

local infiltration (Fig. 16.1). In some cases, the anesthesiologist may combine a local anesthetic and opioid for epidural or spinal administration.

PAIN PATHWAYS

Pain during the first stage of labor results primarily from cervical dilatation and secondarily from uterine contractions themselves. Painful sensations travel from the uterus via visceral afferent (sympathetic) nerves that enter the spinal cord through the posterior segments of thoracic spinal nerves 10, 11, and 12 (Fig. 16.1). Pain during the second stage of labor results primarily from distention of the pelvic floor, vagina, and perineum by the presenting part of the fetus. (Some physicians contend that uterine contractions themselves may also contribute to pain during the second stage.) The sensory fibers of sacral nerves 2, 3, and 4 (i.e., the pudendal nerve) transmit painful impulses from the perineum to the spinal cord (Fig. 16.1).

PERSONNEL

An anesthesiologist is a physician who has completed 4 years of postgraduate residency training in anesthesia. A nurse anesthetist is a registered nurse (with variable background and training) who has completed an 18-month training program sponsored by the American Association of Nurse Anesthetists. Most states require that nurse anesthetists be supervised or directed by a physician. Ideally, an anesthesiologist assumes this role, which results in an efficient anesthesiologist/anesthetist team. Such an anesthesiologist/anesthetist team provides anesthesia for 62.3 percent of operations in the United States. Anesthesiologists working independently provide anesthesia for 23.3 percent of operations. Nurse anesthetists, independent of anesthesiologists, provide anesthesia for 7.6 percent of operations, usually in smaller hospitals.[1] In this situation, the operating surgeon or obstetrician will, or must, assume the role of supervisor. When anesthetic-related untoward events occur, the nonanesthesiologist supervising a nurse anesthetist often will be ultimately responsible for the treatment and outcome of those events. The American Society of Anesthesiologists and the American College of Obstetricians and Gynecologists recently issued the Joint Statement on the Optimal Goals for Anesthesia Care in Obstetrics.[2] That statement recommends that there be a qualified anesthesiologist responsible for all anesthetics in every hospital providing obstetric care. The statement notes: "The administration of general or regional anesthesia requires numerous medical judgements and technical skills. Nurse anesthetists are not trained as physicians and cannot be expected to make medical decisions. Obstetricians seldom have sufficient training or experience in anesthesia to allow them to properly supervise nurse anesthetists."[2]

PAIN AND STRESS

When considering obstetric anesthesia, reasonable questions include the following: How painful is labor? How stressful is labor? What are the effects of pain and stress? What role does anesthesia play? Melzack and colleagues[3] provided perhaps the most sophisticated, enlightened, and in-depth study of labor pain. Using the McGill Pain Questionnaire, which measures intensity and quality of pain, these investigators quantified and described the reaction of 87 nulliparous and 54 parous patients to labor pain. When pain-rating index scores were assigned to each parturient's description of labor pain and compared with those of other patients suffering different kinds of pain, 59 percent of nulliparous and 43 percent of parous patients described their labor pain in terms more severe than did those suffering back and cancer pain. More than 50 percent of the obstetric patients described their pain as sharp, cramping, and intense; more than 33 percent as aching, throbbing, stabbing, shooting, heavy, and exhaustive; and 25 percent of nulliparous patients and 9 percent of parous patients as horrible or excruciating. In contrast, only 24 percent of parous patients and 9 percent of nulliparous patients described the pain as relatively minor. Although those with childbirth training reported less pain than those without such training, the differences were small. Eighty-one percent of trained patients requested epidural anesthesia compared with 82 percent of those without training. The most substantial predictors of pain intensity proved to be socioeconomic status and prior menstrual difficulties.

How does the body respond to the pain and stress of labor? Does the response affect mother, fetus, or

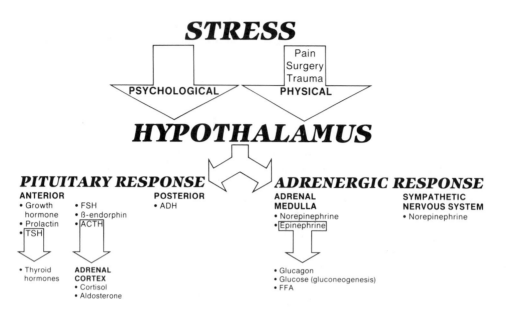

Fig. 16.2 The stress response.

both? Most investigators have described and quantified the body's response to stress in terms of the release of certain hormones, namely, adrenocorticotropic hormone (ACTH), cortisol, catecholamines, and β-endorphins (Fig. 16.2).

What kind of response does labor invoke? The following have been reported: prolonged increases of plasma cortisol levels in early labor,[4] increases of both ACTH and cortisol during labor and immediately postpartum,[5] and increases in epinephrine, norepinephrine, and β-endorphins throughout labor.[6-9] These are the same responses described during other types of pain,[10] surgical stress,[11] and even hypoxia.[12,13] Thus many of the hormones associated with stress are elevated during labor.

What are the effects of these hormones on pregnancy? Elevated epinephrine levels are found in patients with anxiety and prolonged labor, which is not surprising, considering the well-known uterine relaxant effects of β-adrenergic agents.[14] Animal studies indicate that both epinephrine and norepinephrine can decrease uterine blood flow and cause fetal asphyxia.[15-17] Furthermore, these alterations may occur without clinical signs, because uteroplacental blood flow can change in the absence of heart rate and blood pressure change.[16] Maternal psychological

stress can detrimentally affect the fetal cardiovascular system and acid–base status as demonstrated in baboons and monkeys.[18-20] In pregnant sheep, catecholamines increase and uterine blood flow decreases after both painful and nonpainful stimuli (Fig. 16.3). In humans, sudden noise and flashing lights predictably increase maternal heart rate. Not so predictably, fetal heart rate responds similarly within 45 seconds.[21] Fear produces similar effects.[21]

If one accepts that anxiety, pain, and labor are forms of stress and that stress may be harmful, can anesthesia, by alleviating pain, minimize the effects of that stress? Epidural anesthesia has prevented increases in both cortisol and 11-hydroxycorticosteroid levels during labor,[22,23] but systemically administered opioids did not.[24] Epidural anesthesia also attenuates elevations of epinephrine,[6] norepinephrine,[7] and β-endorphin levels.[25] Presumably, regional anesthesia blocks afferent stimuli to the hypothalamus and thus inhibits the body's response to stress.[26] Some of the responses to the stress of labor and the effects of epidural anesthesia on these responses are presented in Figure 16.4.

What of the fetus? There is convincing evidence that anesthesia, sedation, or both effectively decrease asphyxia-inducing effects of psychologically induced

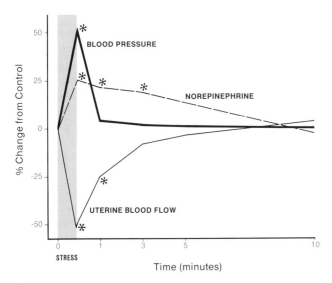

* Significantly different
  from control, P<0.05

Fig. 16.3 Effects of electrically induced stress (30 to 60 seconds) on maternal mean arterial blood pressure, plasma norepinephrine levels, and uterine blood flow. (Modified from Shnider et al.,[229] with permission.)

stress in monkey and baboon fetuses.[19,20,27] Furthermore, acid–base status of human infants whose mothers receive epidural anesthesia during the first stage of labor is less altered than when mothers do not receive regional anesthesia. During the second stage of labor, the salutary effects of anesthesia may be limited to the mother.[28,29]

To summarize, labor and delivery can be stressful to both mother and fetus. Anesthesia, particularly regional anesthesia, can reduce and sometimes prevent the harmful effects of that stress.

ANESTHESIA FOR LABOR

Psychoprophylaxis

Psychoprophylaxis is a nonpharmacologic method of minimizing the perception of painful uterine contractions. Relaxation, concentration on breathing, gentle massage (effleurage), and husband participation contribute to its effectiveness. One of the method's most valuable contributions is that it is often taught in prepared childbirth classes where patients learn about the physiology of pregnancy and the normal processes of labor and delivery. In many instances, husband and wife may even visit the hospi-

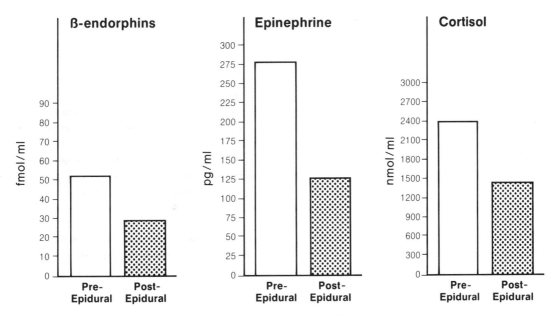

Fig. 16.4 Effects of epidural analgesia on the response to stress.

tal and the labor and delivery suites before labor. Thus the fear of the unknown is largely mitigated.

Although psychoprophylactic techniques may discourage the use of drugs, not all patients are alike and not all will be satisfied with psychoprophylaxis.[30] The greatest disadvantage is the potential for believing the use of drug-induced pain relief is a sign of failure and will harm the child. Those who believe that accepting analgesia is a sign of failure do not understand that some labors are longer than others or more painful than others and that some patients have lower pain thresholds than others. Furthermore, there are times when anesthesia will be *required* for vaginal or cesarean delivery. In these instances, both mother and fetus should benefit from all that modern medicine can provide. Anyone who doubts that modern anesthetic techniques can be applied to the pregnant patient without harm to her or to her unborn child need only reflect that approximately 25 percent of all births in the United States today are cesarean births. All these patients receive anesthesia, yet few believe that such anesthesia results in harm to the fetus, and no one would suggest that these patients avoid anesthesia. If a mother is led to believe that she is a failure by "giving in" to anesthesia, which may have been indicated for forceps delivery or cesarean section, and her infant has a deficit resulting from an unrelated etiology, both she and her husband could believe that the anesthesia caused the problem and live the rest of their lives bearing a tragic and unnecessary sense of guilt.

Systemic Opioid Analgesia

Opioids (also known as narcotics) are drugs possessing morphine-like pharmacologic actions.[31] Morphine and codeine are natural alkaloids derived from opium, which is obtained from unripe seed capsules of the poppy plant. Opioids such as hydromorphone and heroin are semisynthetic compounds made by a simple alteration of the morphine molecule. Meperidine, alphaprodine, and fentanyl are synthetic compounds resembling morphine.[32] All opioids provide pain relief and a sense of euphoria, hence their use in obstetrics. However, opioids also produce respiratory depression, the degree of which is usually comparable for equipotent analgesic doses. Also, all opioids freely cross the placental barrier to the newborn.[33-35] Therefore, the risk associated with opioids for obstet-

rics is obvious—all can produce respiratory depression in both mother and newborn.[36-39] Nevertheless, when used properly, they can be safe and effective.

In the past, because large doses of the long-acting opioids (e.g., morphine) were given intramuscularly throughout labor, depressant effects on the infant were observed.[40,41] Currently, morphine is rarely used for pain relief during labor. Instead, smaller doses of other opioids are used and are administered via the more predictable intravenous route. Therefore, recent reports detail little neonatal depression.[42-45] In addition, anesthesiologists recently have begun to give opioids (with or without local anesthetics) via the epidural or subarachnoid (i.e., spinal) space. Opioids may then bind to opioid receptors in the spinal cord and thereby produce segmental analgesia.

The immediate treatment for respiratory depression caused by opioids is ventilation. Infants depressed by opioids may be sleepy and may not breathe adequately. Initially they typically are not hypoxic, hypercarbic, or acidotic; however, if they are not ventilated, hypoxia, hypercarbia, and acidosis will result. Hypoxia and acidosis (not opioids *per se*) may cause neonatal injury. If properly cared for, infants with opioid-induced depression will suffer no ill effects. Proper care includes ventilation, oxygenation, gentle stimulation, and the judicious use of the opioid antagonist naloxone. Positive-pressure ventilation is the single most effective measure and can be provided via face mask or intubation. Without ventilation, other measures are fruitless.

Naloxone, 0.1 mg/kg, should be given intravenously if possible, but it can be given intramuscularly or subcutaneously. This dose (i.e., 0.1 mg/kg) is higher than that previously recommended and should ensure an increased likelihood of effectiveness.[46] It may be repeated in 3 to 5 minutes if there is no immediate response. If there is no response after two or three doses, the depression is most likely not due to opioid effect.[46] Nursery personnel should be advised when naloxone has been given because it has a short duration of action, and therefore repeat administration may be necessary in the nursery. Naloxone should not be used prophylactically. Specifically, it should not be given to the mother just before delivery. Pain relief afforded the mother by the opioid will be antagonized. Furthermore, because of the unpredictability of placental transfer, it is difficult to estimate how much naloxone would get to the infant. Indeed, naloxone may not be necessary at all. It should not be given routinely to all opioid-exposed newborns.[46] Finally, naloxone should not be given to infants of opioid-dependent mothers, because this may precipitate withdrawal in the physically dependent newborn infant.[46] Naloxone is a useful drug that should be available whenever opioids are used. However, it is an adjunct to ventilation, not a substitute for it.

Opioids also may produce neurobehavioral changes in the newborn, and these changes may persist for as long as 2 to 4 days.[47-49] Although some have indicated that the effects may persist and be influential in later life, such has not been proved true.[50] In fact, the significance of neurobehavioral changes in general is open to question. It is doubtful that any decisions regarding choice of agent should be made on the basis of neurobehavioral tests.

An important and significant disadvantage of opioid analgesia is the prolonged effect of these agents on gastric emptying. Labor itself prolongs gastric emptying. When opioids are used, the effect is compounded, and, if general anesthesia becomes necessary, the risk of aspiration is increased.[51]

Morphine

Morphine is now primarily used to provide sedation and rest during the early prodromal stages of labor. With intramuscular administration, the onset of analgesia occurs in 10 to 20 minutes and lasts for approximately 2.5 to 4 hours. With intravenous administration, the onset of analgesia is less than 3 to 5 minutes and lasts approximately 1.5 to 2 hours.[32] Occasionally, bradycardia will follow an injection of morphine. Also, α-blockade may occur and result in orthostatic hypotension. One of the more frequent and bothersome side effects of morphine is nausea and vomiting. Urinary retention is also common. As with most opioids, a small amount of morphine is eliminated in the urine unchanged. The remainder is gradually detoxified by the liver.

Meperidine

Meperidine is perhaps the most commonly used opioid intrapartum; 100 mg is roughly equianalgesic to 10 mg morphine, but purportedly it has a less de-

pressive effect on respiration.[37] Usually, 25 mg is administered intravenously, or 50 to 75 mg is given intramuscularly. Shnider and Moya[36] showed that both timing and dosage influence neonatal depression. When administered within 1 hour of delivery, little depression of Apgar scores or time to sustained respiration occurs. With a 50-mg intramuscular dose, the greatest depression occurs during the second hour; when 75 to 100 mg is administered, the depression extends through the second and third hours. Notably, when secobarbital, 100 mg, is added, depression extends even further to the fourth hour after administration.[36] The peculiar metabolism of meperidine may partially explain the lack of depression in the first hour. Part of meperidine is metabolized to an active metabolite, normeperidine. Thus, although the increase and decrease of meperidine concentrations take place immediately in both mother and fetus, the increase of the active metabolite normeperidine is slow and thereby exerts its effect on the newborn during the second hour after administration.[34,52] Furthermore, Kuhnert and colleagues[53,54] observed that multiple doses of meperidine result in greater accumulation of both meperidine and normeperidine in fetal tissues.

Intramuscularly the analgesic action of meperidine begins in approximately 10 to 20 minutes and persists for 2 to 3 hours. Lazebnik and colleagues[55] recently noted that plasma concentrations of meperidine are higher after deltoid injection than after gluteus muscle injection. They suggested that the deltoid muscle might be the preferred intramuscular site during labor. Intravenously, the onset of analgesia begins almost immediately and lasts approximately 1.5 to 2 hours. Side effects are similar to those of morphine except that tachycardia occasionally results rather than bradycardia. As with morphine, nausea and vomiting are frequent, and there is considerable delay in gastric emptying. Slightly less urinary retention occurs with meperidine than with morphine.[32]

Alphaprodine

Alphaprodine is a short-acting drug that is given in an intramuscular or subcutaneous dose of 20 to 40 mg or in an intravenous dose of 10 to 20 mg. Its onset of action is similar to that of meperidine; however, the duration of action with the intravenous route is briefer (i.e., approximately 45 minutes).[32] But alphaprodine may produce more respiratory depression than expected.[56] Formerly a popular opioid in many obstetric units, alphaprodine is currently not commercially available in the United States.

Butorphanol

Butorphanol is one of the new synthetic agonist–antagonist opioid analgesic drugs. One to 2 mg is administered intravenously and compares favorably with 40 to 80 mg of meperidine.[42,43,57] Nausea and vomiting appear to occur less with butorphanol than with other opioids.[42,43] The major advantage is a ceiling effect for respiratory depression; that is, respiratory depression from multiple doses appears to plateau.[58,59] The major side effects are somnolence and dizziness.

Nalbuphine

Nalbuphine is another synthetic agonist–antagonist opioid. Its analgesic potency is similar to that of morphine when compared on a milligram per milligram basis. As with butorphanol, a purported advantage of nalbuphine is its ceiling effect for respiratory depression.[60] It may cause less maternal nausea and vomiting than meperidine, but it tends to produce more maternal sedation and dizziness.[61]

Patient-Controlled Opioid Analgesia

In some centers opioids are administered by patient-controlled intravenous infusion. The infusion pump is programmed to give a predetermined dose of drug upon patient demand. The physician may program the pump to include a lock-out interval (that is, there is a minimum interval between doses of drug). Thus the physician may limit the total dose administered per hour. Advantages of this method include the fact that some patients appreciate the sense of autonomy, as well as the fact that one avoids lengthy delays between doses. There are conflicting data as to whether this practice results in a decreased or increased total dose of opioid during labor.[62–64]

Sedatives

Sedatives do not possess analgesic qualities and are most often used early in labor to relieve anxiety or to augment the analgesic qualities and reduce the nausea associated with opioids. All sedatives and hypnotics cross the placental barrier freely. Perhaps the most

important aspect of these drugs is that they, unlike the opioids, have no known antagonists. Those most frequently used are barbiturates, phenothiazines, and benzodiazepines.

Barbiturates

Because barbiturates and other sedatives are not analgesic, patients may be less able to cope with pain than if they had received no pharmacologic assistance at all; that is, normal coping mechanisms may be blunted.[65,66] Although barbiturates can depress both cardiovascular and respiratory functions in mother and newborn, low doses have little effect. The combination of barbiturate (100 mg secobarbital) with opioid (50 to 100 mg meperidine) increases the degree of newborn depression.[36] In addition, effects that do occur may persist for a prolonged time. For example, attention span can be depressed for as long as 2 to 4 days.[67] Thus these drugs should rarely be used during labor.

Phenothiazines

Promethazine is perhaps the most widely used phenothiazine. However, propiomazine, promazine, and hydroxyzine are also common. When given in small doses in combination with an opioid, these drugs do not seem to produce additional neonatal depression.[68–70] However, like the barbiturates, these agents rapidly cross the placenta and, in large doses, can depress the fetus for a significant period. Also like the barbiturates, they have no known antagonist.

Benzodiazepines

Diazepam was the first widely used benzodiazepine. A major disadvantage of diazepam is that it disrupts temperature regulation in newborns, which renders them less able to maintain body temperature.[71] The drug may persist in the fetal circulation for as long as 1 week.[72] As with many drugs, beat-to-beat variability of the fetal heart rate is reduced markedly even with a single intravenous dose (i.e., 5 to 10 mg).[73] However, these doses have little effect on acid–base or clinical status of the newborn.[74] Sodium benzoate, a buffer in the injectable form of diazepam, competes with bilirubin binding to albumin. Thus unbound bilirubin is increased and could be a threat to infants susceptible to kernicterus.[75]

Recently midazolam was introduced into clinical

practice. Unlike diazepam, midazolam is water soluble, and it is shorter acting than diazepam.[76] There are conflicting data regarding its effects on the fetus/ neonate.[77,78]

A disadvantage of all the benzodiazepines is their tendency to cause maternal amnesia. This can be a significant disadvantage if the drug is given near the time of delivery.[79]

Scopolamine

An anticholinergic sedative that also has amnesic effects, scopolamine has no analgesic effects and often results in bizarre behavior and total amnesia of the event. It is doubtful that scopolamine has any place in modern obstetrics.

Lumbar Epidural Analgesia/Anesthesia

Epidural blockade is a major regional anesthetic technique in which local anesthetic is injected into the epidural space. Epidural blockade may be used to provide *analgesia* during labor, or surgical *anesthesia* for vaginal delivery or cesarean section. A large-bore needle (16-, 17-, or 18-gauge) is used to locate the epidural space. Next, a catheter is inserted through the needle, and the needle is removed over the catheter. Local anesthetic is injected through the catheter, which remains taped in place to the mother's back to enable subsequent injections throughout labor (Figs. 16.1 and 16.5). Thus it is often called continuous epidural analgesia. A test dose of local anesthetic is given first to check for the possibility that the catheter was unintentionally placed in the subarachnoid (spinal) space or in a blood vessel. Single-dose techniques are occasionally used for vaginal delivery or for cesarean section when the duration of pain is expected to be brief. For the single-dose technique, the catheter is omitted.

Two forms of epidural anesthesia are used for labor: lumbar and caudal. The catheter is placed via a lumbar interspace in the former and via the sacral hiatus in the latter (Fig. 16.1). More local anesthetic is necessary for the caudal technique, because the local anesthetic must fill the entire sacral canal before filling the epidural space up to T10; 15 to 20 ml of local anesthetic is required. In contrast, for the lumbar technique, 8 to 10 ml (and often less) suffices, because the local anesthetic is injected much closer to its site of action.

For the caudal approach, because the local anesthetic is injected at the sacral area, sacral nerves 2, 3, and 4 are always affected. Because these nerves innervate the pelvic floor, the muscles of the pelvic floor will become insensitive and relaxed throughout labor. Moreover, the patient's legs will be affected and occasionally will be rendered immobile, depending on the strength of the local anesthetic. Pressure exerted on the pelvic floor by the descending vertex plays a major role in ensuring proper rotation of the fetal head to the occiput anterior position, and resistance may not be adequate to rotate the head when muscles of the pelvic floor are relaxed. Thus an increase in occiput transverse or occiput posterior positions may result with the caudal technique. Also, because the patient's perception of pressure on the perineum by the presenting part is a stimulus for her to increase voluntary effort, blocking or minimizing this perception may prolong the second stage. For these reasons, the caudal approach is less favorable.

Most anesthesiologists now prefer the lumbar approach and use a technique described as segmental epidural anesthesia (Fig. 16.6). Because nerves that carry painful impulses during the first stage of labor are small sympathetic nerves and because they are easily blocked, only the smallest amount and the weakest effective concentration of local anesthetic is injected via the L2-3, L3-4, or L4-5 interspace. Thus both sensation and motor function of the perineum and lower extremities remain mostly intact. The patient can move about and perceive the impact of the presenting part on the perineum. If perineal anesthesia is needed for delivery, a larger concentration and dose of local anesthetic can be administered at that time through the catheter (Fig. 16.6). Alternatively, for perineal anesthesia, the obstetrician can perform a pudendal block or local infiltration of the perineum.

The segmental epidural technique, when performed properly, is effective and safe for both mother and fetus. In most instances, total or near-total pain relief is accomplished without resorting to depressant and sometimes disorienting drugs. The mother remains awake, alert, and aware of her surroundings. She can communicate with her husband, her physician, and the nursing personnel. She will remember and appreciate her entire labor and delivery. Finally, because anesthesia can be extended

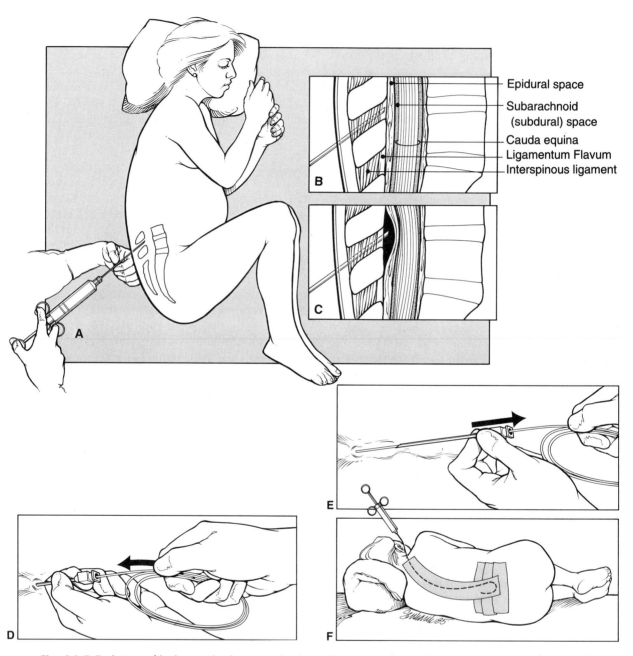

Fig. 16.5 Technique of lumbar epidural puncture by the midline approach. (A) This side view shows left hand held against patient's back, with thumb and index finger grasping hub. Attempts to inject solution while point of needle is in the interspinous ligament meet resistance. (B) Point of needle is in the ligamentum flavum, which offers marked resistance and makes it almost impossible to inject solution. (C) Entrance of the needle's point into epidural space is discerned by sudden lack of resistance to injection of saline. Force of injected solution pushes dura-arachnoid away from point of needle. (D) Catheter is introduced through needle. Note that hub of needle is pulled caudad toward the patient, increasing the angle between the shaft of the needle and the epidural space. Also note technique of holding the tubing: it is wound around the right hand. (E) Needle is withdrawn over tubing and held steady with the right hand. (F) Catheter is immobilized with adhesive tape. Note the large loop made by the catheter to decrease risk of kinking at the point where the tube exits from the skin. (From Bonica,[32] with permission.)

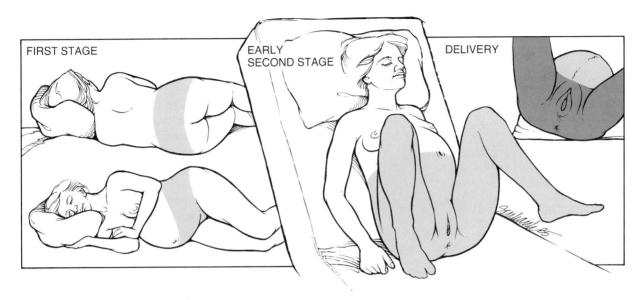

Fig. 16.6 Segmented epidural analgesia for labor and delivery. A single catheter is introduced into the epidural space and advanced so that its tip is at L2. Initially, small volumes of low concentrations of local anesthetic are used to produce segmental analgesia. For the second stage, the analgesia is extended to the sacral segments by injecting a larger amount of the same concentration of local anesthetic, with the patient in the semirecumbent position. After internal rotation, a higher concentration of local anesthetic is injected to produce motor block of the sacral segments and thus achieve perineal relaxation and anesthesia. The wedge under the right buttock causes the uterus to displace to the left. (From Bonica,[230] with permission.)

to the perineum at the time of delivery, the obstetrician can accomplish whatever kind of delivery is necessary, spontaneous or instrumental, with or without an episiotomy.

Even though the advantages would seem to make epidural anesthesia the ideal anesthetic technique, and many believe it to be so, there are disadvantages. These include hypotension, local anesthetic toxicity, allergic reaction, high or total spinal, neurologic injury, spinal headache, and, in some cases, adverse effects on progress of labor. For the most part, these represent side effects and complications. (Contraindications are discussed in the section on anesthesia for cesarean section.)

Hypotension

Hypotension is defined variably, but most often it is defined as a systolic blood pressure less than 100 mmHg or a 20 percent decrease from control values. It occurs after approximately 10 percent of epidural blocks given during labor, but the incidence has been reported to be as low as 1.4 percent in some large series.[80-84] Hypotension occurs primarily as a result of sympathetic blockade. Local anesthetics block not only pain fibers but sympathetic fibers as well, which normally maintain blood vessel tone. When these fibers are blocked, vasodilatation results and blood pools in the lower extremities, decreasing the return of blood to the right side of the heart. Cardiac output then decreases, and hypotension results. Hypotension threatens the fetus by decreasing uterine blood flow and threatens the mother by decreasing cerebral blood flow. When hypotension is recognized promptly and treated effectively, very little, if any, untoward effects accrue to either (Table 16.1).[85-87] However, in the acutely or chronically compromised fetus, hypotension can result in further compromise if not treated immediately.[88]

Treatment of hypotension begins with prophylaxis, which demands an intravenous catheter and an infusion of 500 to 1,000 ml Ringer's lactate or normal saline solution. The infusion fills the expanded vascular space caused by vasodilatation. Glucose is easily transported across the placenta; therefore, dextrose-

Table 16.1 Epidural Analgesia: Hypotension Vs. No Hypotension[a]

	Hypotension[b] (N = 5)	No Hypotension (N = 20)
Umbilical artery		
pH	7.269	7.311
BE (mEq/L)	−1.4	−1.3
Po$_2$ (mmHg)	23.6	23.2
SaO$_2$ (%)	48.2	50.2
Umbilical vein		
pH	7.344	7.366
BE (mEq/L)	−1.8	−1.5
Po$_2$ (mmHg)	41.0	33.7
SvO$_2$ (%)	84.6	72.0

[a] Values are means; they indicate that properly treated hypotension need not result in a compromised fetus.

[b] Hypotension was severe enough to be treated with the vasopressor ephedrine.

(Modified from James et al.,[167] with permission.)

containing solutions are avoided for this purpose because they can cause neonatal hypoglycemia.[89] Left uterine displacement must be maintained during the block because compression of the inferior vena cava and aorta may decrease cardiac output and/or uteroplacental perfusion. Proper treatment depends on immediate diagnosis. To diagnose hypotension the person administering the anesthesia must be present and attentive, which means not being involved in anything else that cannot be abandoned. Once diagnosed, hypotension is corrected by increasing the rate of intravenous fluid infusion and exaggerating left uterine displacement. If these simple measures do not suffice, a vasopressor is indicated, and the vasopressor of choice is ephedrine, given in 5- to 10-mg doses. Ephedrine is a mixed α- and β-agonist, and it is less likely to compromise uteroplacental perfusion than the pure α-agonists.[90] α-Adrenergic agents such as methoxamine or phenylephrine are avoided in most cases (Fig. 16.7).

Local Anesthetic Toxicity

The incidence of systemic local anesthetic toxicity (high blood concentrations of local anesthetic) after lumbar epidural analgesia is less than 0.5 percent.[91] Most often, toxicity occurs when the anesthetic is injected into a vessel rather than into the epidural space or when too much is administered even though injected properly. Occasionally, the dosage can be miscalculated: 1 ml of 1 percent lidocaine contains 10 mg of lidocaine, not 1 mg. All local anesthetics have maximal recommended doses that should not be exceeded. For example, the maximum recommended dose of lidocaine is 4 mg/kg when used without epinephrine and 7 mg/kg when used with epinephrine. (Epinephrine delays and decreases the uptake of local anesthetic into the bloodstream.) Package inserts for all local anesthetics contain dose information (Table 16.2).

Local anesthetic reactions have two components, central nervous system (CNS) and cardiovascular.

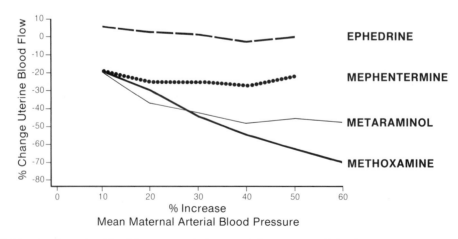

Fig. 16.7 Changes in uterine blood flow at equal elevations of mean arterial blood pressure after vasopressor administration (pregnant ewes). (From Ralston et al.,[90] with permission.)

Table 16.2 Maximal Recommended Doses of Common Local Anesthetics

Local Anesthetic	Without Epinephrine		With Epinephrine[a]	
	mg/kg	Dose (mg/70 kg)	mg/kg	Total (mg/70 kg)
Bupivacaine	2.5	175	3.0	225
Chloroprocaine	11.0	800	14.0	1,000
Etidocaine	4.0	300	5.5	400
Lidocaine	4.0	300	7.0	500
Mepivacaine	5.0	400	—	—
Tetracaine	1.5	100	—	—

[a] All epinephrine concentrations 1 : 200,000.

Usually, the CNS component precedes the cardiovascular component. Prodromal symptoms of the CNS reaction include excitation, bizarre behavior, ringing in the ears, and disorientation. These symptoms may culminate in convulsions, which are usually brief. After the convulsions, depression follows and manifests predominantly by the postictal state. The cardiovascular component of the local anesthetic reaction usually begins with hypertension and tachycardia but is soon followed by hypotension, arrhythmias, and in some instances cardiac arrest. Thus the cardiovascular component also has excitant and depressant characteristics. Usually the CNS and cardiovascular components are widely separated, because it takes a significantly higher blood concentration of local anesthetic to cause the cardiovascular symptoms than it does the CNS symptoms. Thus one frequently sees the CNS component without the more serious cardiovascular component. Bupivacaine may represent an exception to this principle.[92,93] There are reports of several patients who experienced serious arrhythmias and marked cardiovascular depression after administration of 0.75 percent bupivacaine, and most physicians now believe that there is minimal distinction between the two types of reactions to bupivacaine. Moreover, resuscitation of these patients was difficult or impossible, probably because of the drug's prolonged blocking effect on sodium channels.[94] Indeed there now is laboratory evidence that bupivacaine is more cardiotoxic than equianalgesic doses of other amide local anesthetics[94] and that pregnancy may enhance that cardiotoxicity.[95] Several manufacturers of bupivacaine have recommended that the 0.75 percent concentration not be used in obstetric patients and that the drug be contraindicated for paracervical block.[96] Of course, it is possible to give the same total dose of bupivacaine by giving a larger volume of 0.5 percent bupivacaine. In other words, use of a more dilute concentration of drug does not guarantee safety. Thus it is important that the physician give bupivacaine, or any other local anesthetic, by slow, incremental injection.[97]

The bupivacaine controversy has resulted in greater emphasis on the administration of a safe and effective test dose (to exclude unintentional intravenous or subarachnoid injection of local anesthetic) before injection of a therapeutic dose of local anesthetic. Many anesthesiologists give a test dose that includes 15 μg of epinephrine.[98,99] An increase in heart rate of at least 25 to 30 bpm would signal intravascular injection. Others have questioned whether an epinephrine-containing test dose is the best choice in obstetric patients.[100]

Treatment of a local anesthetic reaction depends on recognizing the signs and symptoms as they occur. Again, to recognize the signs and symptoms, one must be present. If possible, once prodromal symptoms arise, the injection of local anesthetic should be stopped. However, if convulsions have already occurred, treatment is aimed at maintaining proper oxygenation and preventing the patient from harming herself. Convulsions use considerable amounts of oxygen, which results in hypoxia and acidosis (Table 16.3).[101] Adequate oxygenation is essential for both mother and fetus, because a hypoxic mother results in a hypoxic and acidotic fetus. Should the convulsions continue for more than a brief period, small intravenous doses of thiopental (25 to 50 mg) or diazepam (5 to 10 mg) are useful. In obstetrics, because of the adverse effects of diazepam on the neonate, thiopental would be the agent of choice. Occasionally succinylcholine is used for paralysis to prevent the muscular activity associated with the convulsions and to facilitate ventilation and perhaps intubation. Before using thiopental, diazepam, or succinylcholine, consideration must be given to the depressant effects that these agents will add to the depressant phase of the local anesthetic reaction. Therefore, appropriate equipment and personnel must be available to maintain oxygenation, a patent airway, and cardiovascular

Table 16.3 Blood-Gas Determinations During and After Local Anesthetic-Induced Convulsions

Convulsion	Time	Oxygen (L/min)	Blood-Gas Values				
			pH	Pco₂ (mmHg)	Po₂ (mmHg)	HCO₃ (mEq/L)	Base Excess (mEq/L)
Patient 1							
1st	9:50:00	10[a]	—	—	—	—	—
2nd	9:50:30		7.27	48	48	21.5	−4
3rd	9:51:00		—	—	—	—	—
4th	9:53:00		7.09	59	33	17.1	−10
Cessation	9:54:00		—	—	—	—	—
	9:55:30		7.01	71	210	17.2	−11
	10:22:00	6[b]	7.25	48	99	20.5	−5
		Room air	7.56	25	106	22.5	0
Patient 2							
1st	9:47:00	10[a]	—	—	—	—	—
2nd	9:47:30		6.99	76	87	17.4	−10.2
3rd	9:48:00		—	—	—	—	—
Cessation	9:50:00		—	—	—	—	—
	10:02:00		7.16	54	140	18.5	−6.9

[a] Bag and mask with oral Guedel airway and artificial respiration.
[b] Nasal prongs.
(Modified from Moore et al.,[101] with permission.)

support. Resuscitation of the pregnant patient is essentially the same as that of the nonpregnant patient except that left uterine displacement should be maintained. Usually this means that the uterus will have to be lifted off the inferior vena cava manually for resuscitation with the patient supine.

Allergy to Local Anesthetics

There are two classes of local anesthetics: amides and esters. A true allergic reaction to an amide-type local anesthetic (e.g., lidocaine, bupivacaine, mepivacaine, etidocaine) is extremely rare. Allergic reactions to the esters (2-chloroprocaine, procaine, tetracaine) are also rare but occur more often. Generally, when a patient says she is "allergic" to local anesthetics, she is referring to what is perhaps a normal reaction to the epinephrine that is occasionally added to local anesthetics, particularly by dentists. Epinephrine can cause increased heart rate, pounding in the ears, and nausea, symptoms that may be interpreted as an allergy. It is therefore important to document any history of allergy. Was there a rash? Hives? Difficulty breathing? If so, which local anesthetic was used? If a specific local anesthetic can be identified, choosing one from the other class should be safe.

High Spinal or "Total Spinal" Anesthesia

This complication occurs when the level of anesthesia rises dangerously high, resulting in paralysis of the respiratory muscles, including the diaphragm. The incidence of total spinal anesthesia after epidural anesthesia is less than 0.03 percent and after spinal anesthesia is 0.1 percent.[91] Total spinal anesthesia can result from a miscalculated dose of drug, unintentional subarachnoid injection during an epidural block, or improper positioning of a patient after spinal block with hyperbaric local anesthetic solutions. Motor nerves to the diaphragm, the major respiratory muscle, emanate from C3 to C5; therefore, the anesthetic must be at this level before phrenic nerve paralysis results. Moreover, the phrenic nerve is a large motor nerve, which requires considerable local anesthetic for complete block. Because the accessory muscles of respiration are paralyzed earlier, their paralysis may result in apprehension and anxiety. The patient usually can breathe adequately as long as the diaphragm is not paralyzed. However, treatment must be individualized, and dyspnea, real or imagined, should always be considered an effect of paralysis until proved otherwise. In addition to respiratory symptoms, cardiovascular components, including hypotension and even cardiovascular collapse, may occur.

Treatment of total spinal anesthesia includes rapidly assessing the true level of anesthesia. Therefore, to determine the precise level of anesthesia, persons who perform major regional anesthesia should be thoroughly familiar with dermatome charts (Fig. 16.8). Furthermore, these persons should also recognize what a certain sensory level of anesthesia means in regard to innervation of other organs or systems. For example, a T4 sensory level may represent total sympathetic nervous system blockade. Numbness and weakness of the fingers and hands indicates that the level of anesthesia has reached the cervical level (C6 to C8), which is dangerously close to the innervation of the diaphragm. If the diaphragm is not paralyzed, the patient is breathing adequately, and cardiovascular stability is maintained, oxygen, a simple explanation, and assurance that things will eventually be better may suffice. If the patient continues to be anxious or if the level of anesthesia seems to be involving the diaphragm, then assisted ventilation is indicated. Occasionally, this can be accomplished with a bag and face mask without rendering the patient unconscious. Most often, however, endotracheal intubation will be necessary. If so, induction of general anesthesia will facilitate the process. Cardiovascular support is provided as necessary. If the person administering regional anesthesia is well acquainted with the signs and symptoms of high spinal anesthesia and its treatment,

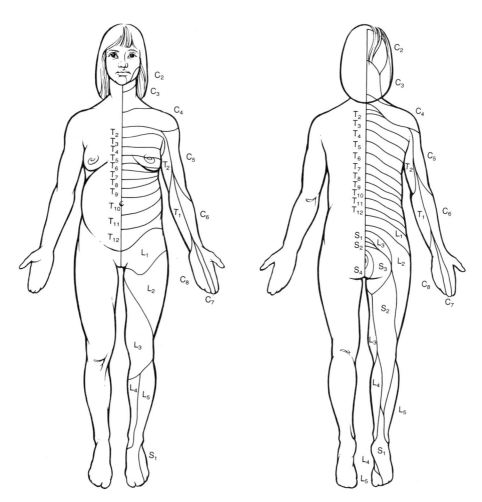

Fig. 16.8 Dermatome chart. (Adapted from Haymaker and Woodhall,[231] with permission.)

serious sequelae should be extremely rare. The onset is easy to diagnose, and the treatment is relatively simple. However, the same admonition applies as with hypotension and local anesthetic toxicity: early symptoms cannot be diagnosed if the person administering the block is not present and attentive.

Paralysis and Nerve Injury

Paralysis after either epidural or spinal anesthesia is extremely rare; even minor injuries such as footdrop and segmental loss of sensation are rare. All forms of nerve injury occur in less than 1 in 10,000 applications of regional anesthesia.[102] More serious injuries are even less frequent. Today, commercially prepared drugs, ampules, and disposable needles make infection and caustic injury nearly unheard of. Several years ago there were several cases of neurologic deficit after use of 2-chloroprocaine, primarily after unintentional subarachnoid (i.e., spinal) injection of large volumes of the drug.[103-105] These cases prompted performance of several laboratory studies to evaluate any potential neurotoxicity of 2-chloroprocaine. The earlier formulation of 2-chloroprocaine contained the antioxidant 0.2 percent sodium bisulfite. Currently the consensus is that 2-chloroprocaine itself is not neurotoxic, but that the low pH of the local anesthetic solution and the inclusion of the sodium bisulfite together may produce neurodysfunction.[106] The current formulation of 2-chloroprocaine does not contain sodium bisulfite. Curiously, there have been recent reports of transient back pain after epidural use of the new formulation of 2-chloroprocaine in nonpregnant patients.[107,108]

When nerve damage follows regional analgesia during obstetric or surgical procedures, the anesthetic technique must be suspect. Nerve damage can result from other causes, however. For example, incorrectly positioned stirrups may cause nerve injury after both gynecologic and obstetric procedures.[109-111] Also, nerve damage can be secondary to a difficult forceps application.[109-111] During abdominal procedures, overzealous or prolonged application of pressure with retractors on sensitive nerve tissues may result in injury.[109-111] Fortunately, most neurologic deficits after labor and delivery are minor and transient.[112] Nonetheless, one should consider consultation with a neurologist or neurosurgeon. One of the more dramatic and correctable forms of

nerve damage follows compression of the spinal cord by a hematoma that has formed during the administration of spinal or epidural anesthesia, presumably from accidental puncture of an epidural vessel. If the condition is diagnosed early, usually with the aid of a neurologist or neurosurgeon, the hematoma can be removed by laminectomy and the problem resolved without permanent damage. Fortunately, this is a very rare complication. Nonetheless, spinal and epidural blocks are contraindicated if clotting is abnormal. Any prolonged motor or sensory deficit after regional anesthesia should be investigated immediately and thoroughly.

Spinal Headache

Spinal headache may follow uncomplicated spinal anesthesia. This complication can also occur when, during the process of administering an epidural block, the dura is punctured and spinal fluid leaks out (i.e., "wet tap"). The incidence of this complication varies between 1 and 3 percent, and its occurrence depends on the experience of the person performing the epidural.[80] Once a "wet tap" occurs, a spinal headache results in perhaps 50 percent of patients. (The incidence is much less following spinal anesthesia, because smaller needles are used.) Characteristically, the headache is more severe in the upright position and is relieved by the prone position. The headache is thought to be caused by loss of cerebral spinal fluid, which allows the brain to settle and thus meninges and vessels to stretch. Hydration, abdominal binders, and the prone position have all been advocated as prophylactic measures. However, most anesthesiologists now agree that, other than hydration, these actions are of little value.[113] In some hands, epidural saline injected through the catheter has proven to be an effective prophylactic measure.[114]

Treatment of the headache, once it has occurred, may be initiated with oral analgesics and continued hydration. If these simple measures do not prove immediately effective, an epidural blood patch is placed. Approximately 15 ml of the patient's own blood are placed aseptically into the epidural space; the blood coagulates over the hole in the dura and prevents further leakage.[115] Patients can be released within 1 to 2 hours.[116] Patients should be instructed to avoid coughing or straining at stool for the first several days after performance of the blood patch; a stool softener is recommended. The epidural blood patch has been found to be remarkably effective and nearly complication free.[117-119] There remains controversy whether one should perform a prophylactic blood patch before the onset of spinal headache.[120-123]

Because epidural anesthesia is associated with these side effects and complications, those who administer it must be thoroughly familiar not only with the technical aspects of its administration but also with the signs and symptoms of complications and their treatment. Specifically, the American Society of Anesthesiologists and the American College of Obstetricians and Gynecologists stated: "Persons administering or supervising obstetric anesthesia should be qualified to manage the infrequent but occasionally life-threatening complications of major regional anesthesia such as respiratory and cardiovascular failure, toxic local anesthetic convulsions, or vomiting and aspiration. Mastering and retaining the skills and knowledge necessary to manage these complications require adequate training and frequent application."[2]

Effects on Labor and Method of Delivery

One of the more controversial aspects of regional anesthesia for obstetrics is the question of whether these techniques influence the length and pattern of labor, the incidence of malposition, and the use of forceps. The perspectives of the anesthesiologist and the obstetrician differ when trying to answer these questions. The anesthesiologist is concerned primarily with relieving pain and sees regional anesthesia as the ideal method because it depresses neither mother nor fetus, provides exceptional pain relief, and even optimal operating conditions for the obstetrician. The obstetrician, although concerned with pain relief, is also concerned with the progress of labor and the method of delivery.

Reports on the effects of epidural anesthesia on labor are numerous and conflicting. How does one interpret these conflicting data?

Study Design

Most published studies of the effect of epidural anesthesia on progress of labor are retrospective and, if prospective, are nonrandomized. Studies that compare patients who received epidural anesthesia versus those who did not are typically biased in favor of the nonepidural group of patients. Specifically, patients who have rapid, uncomplicated labor are less likely to ask for, and even if they ask for are less likely actually to receive, epidural anesthesia. In other words, the epidural group will include more patients with dysfunctional, difficult, and complicated labors. In fact, it is possible that the very reason why some, but not all, parturients request and receive epidural anesthesia may relate to a greater likelihood of abnormal labor. On the other hand, it is also problematic when one attempts to evaluate the influence of epidural anesthesia on labor by use of historical controls. For example, if one compares the incidence of mid-forceps delivery after the introduction of epidural anesthesia to a hospital (e.g., in 1989) versus the incidence of mid-forceps delivery before the use of epidural anesthesia in that hospital (e.g., in 1979), one might note no change in the incidence of mid-forceps delivery and therefore conclude that the introduction of epidural anesthesia did not affect the incidence of mid-forceps delivery. The problem with that approach is that other changes in obstetric practice may have occurred during that 10-year interval. For example, some obstetricians are less willing to perform difficult mid-forceps delivery today than they were a decade ago. Therefore, it would be inappropriate to conclude that epidural anesthesia did not influence the incidence of mid-forceps delivery in that hospital.

Variation in Epidural Technique

A second difficulty with interpretation of existing studies is that epidural anesthesia is not a generic procedure. Unfortunately, many obstetricians, and even some anesthesiologists, consider epidural anesthesia during labor as a generic procedure. For example, one does not make a blanket conclusion that all oral contraceptives increase the risk of vascular complications in young women. Today we know that complications associated with oral contraceptives are dose related and also may even vary with the choice of the estrogen and progestin component. Similarly, the influence of epidural anesthesia on the progress of labor may vary according to the choice and dose of the local anesthetic administered. In general, anesthesiologists today use more dilute solutions of local anesthetic for epidural anesthesia than were used a decade ago. There is greater attention to titrating the dose of the local anesthetic to the specific needs of the patient. For example, Naulty and colleagues[124] made an abrupt change in their epidural anesthetic technique in June 1987. Specifically, they had been providing epidural anesthesia during labor with either 1.5 percent lidocaine or 0.25 to 0.5 percent bupivacaine, but they changed their technique to include 0.125 to 0.25 percent bupivacaine with fentanyl. They then compared the results during the 9 months before the change versus those during the 9 months after the change. They noted a significant decrease in the percentage of patients admitted for labor who eventually underwent cesarean section. Specifically, during the 9 months before the change, 19.6 percent of patients in labor underwent cesarean section, whereas after the change 15.1 percent required cesarean section. Furthermore, there was a significant decrease in the percentage of patients who received epidural anesthesia and who subsequently underwent cesarean section. Finally, the incidence of forceps deliveries decreased from 17.3 percent before the change to 6.3 percent after the change.

Another potential source of variation in management and outcome is the timing of administration of epidural anesthesia. Although controversial, many physicians believe that institution of anesthesia during the latent phase of the first stage of labor is more likely to delay the progress of labor. Friedman[125] stated:

Spinal anesthesia given prior to the onset of the phase of dilatation in the first stage of labor will impede progress of the latent phase, and forestall the normal progressive changes of late labor. It would seem that spinal block given after the latent phase has ended, in a patient whose labor is otherwise normal, and to a level which does not exceed that necessary for uterine pain relief (tenth thoracic) should not influence labor. The general impression of *caudal* or *epidural* anesthesia as it affects labor is that of negligible influence unless misused.

The Committee on Obstetrics: Maternal and Fetal Medicine of the American College of Obstetricians and Gynecologists issued a statement about dystocia. Regarding the latent phase of labor, they stated: "The latent phase may be prolonged by excessive medication and inappropriate timing of conduction anesthesia." Regarding the active phase, they stated: "The normal active phase tends to be resistant to the inhibitory effects of the usual amounts of analgesia. At times, further sedation or epidural anesthesia, hydration, or ambulation may be advantageous." Furthermore, the Committee stated: "A hypertonic pattern may be observed in the active phase. Prolongation of a hypertonic pattern may result in maternal exhaustion, marked pain, and decreased uteroplacental blood flow. The combination of sedation, epidural anesthesia and oxytocin infusion may prove effective."[126]

The problem with delaying institution of epidural anesthesia until the onset of the active phase of labor is that it is often difficult to make that diagnosis prospectively. Furthermore, it is also inappropriate to delay institution of epidural anesthesia until the patient has reached an arbitrary cervical dilatation. For example, approximately 50 percent of patients will enter the active phase of labor by 4 cm cervical dilatation, but a minority will not enter active labor until more than 5 cm cervical dilatation.[127] If one delays institution of epidural anesthesia until the patient reaches an arbitrary dilatation (e.g., 5 cm cervical dilatation), one will subject some patients to unnecessary periods of severe pain. On the other hand, earlier institution of epidural anesthesia may slow labor in some patients. This is problematic in situations when the obstetrician is reluctant to augment labor with oxytocin.

Management of the Second Stage

A third problem with interpretation of studies of epidural anesthesia and progress of labor relates to the indication for performance of instrumental delivery. In general, an obstetrician is more likely to perform elective forceps delivery in a comfortable patient with effective epidural anesthesia than in an uncomfortable patient with no anesthesia. Furthermore, heretofore some obstetricians have arbitrarily terminated the second stage at 2 hours in nulliparous patients and at 1 hour in parous patients. There is evidence that effective epidural analgesia may slightly prolong the second stage of labor.[128,129] But a delay in the second stage is not necessarily harmful to infant or to mother, provided there is normal electronic fetal heart rate monitoring and adequate maternal hydration and analgesia.[128,130-132] Indeed, the American College of Obstetricians and Gynecologists recently defined a prolonged second stage as more than 3 hours in nulliparous patients *with* regional anesthesia as compared with more than 2 hours in nulliparous patients *without* regional anesthesia.[133]

Prospective Studies of Epidural Anesthesia and Progress of Labor

Unfortunately, there are few prospective, randomized studies of the effect of epidural anesthesia on the progress of labor. The fact that epidural anesthesia provides analgesia superior to other techniques causes physicians to be reluctant to randomize patients to a nonepidural group. Robinson and colleagues[134] randomized 386 parturients to receive either epidural anesthesia or systemic analgesia (i.e., meperidine with inhalation analgesia) during labor. They noted that "epidural block was more effective than systemic analgesia in the relief of pain and discomfort in all stages of labour." They also noted that there was a significant increase in the incidence of instrumental delivery in the epidural group. Unfortunately, the randomization occurred before final consent was obtained. Patients were free to withdraw from the study after they learned their group assignment, and many did. Only 93 of the original patients completed the study. One can suspect that more patients with a long, difficult labor dropped out of the systemic analgesia group. This suspicion is confirmed when one notes that there was a threefold increase in the incidence of induction of labor in the epidural group. Furthermore, patients in the epidural group received 0.5 percent bupivacaine, a concentration higher than that used by most anesthesiologists today. Finally, the authors did not report the incidence of cesarean section in either group.

Recently, Philipsen and Jensen[135] reported the only other published study in which patients were randomized to receive either epidural anesthesia or opioid during the first stage of labor. Patients in the epidural group received 0.375 percent bupivacaine, although the authors noted that they attempted to produce a segmental block from T10 to L1. They also stated: "In an attempt to retain the bearing-down reflex and to allow the mother to take active part in the second stage of labour, the analgesic effect was allowed to wear off at the beginning of the second stage and a top-up dose was not given if the cervix was dilated beyond 8 cm." There was no significant difference between groups in the method of delivery.

Thirty-three of 57 (58 percent) women in the epidural group versus 34 of 54 (63 percent) women in the meperidine group had spontaneous delivery. Fourteen of 57 (25 percent) women in the epidural group versus 14 of 54 (26 percent) women in the meperidine group underwent instrumental vaginal delivery.

There are several studies in which nulliparous patients already receiving epidural anesthesia were randomized with respect to management of epidural anesthesia during the second stage.[128,136–138] Phillips and Thomas[136] reported no increase in duration of the second stage, and a nonsignificant decrease in the incidence of instrumental delivery, in 28 nulliparous women who received additional epidural bupivacaine (i.e., 0.25 percent) at complete cervical dilatation compared with 28 women who received no additional bupivacaine. However, this study was randomized but nonblinded, and it is unclear as to how the two groups actually differed, as there was no significant difference between groups in total dosage of bupivacaine or in mean number of doses of bupivacaine (i.e., four doses per patient in each group).

Chestnut and colleagues[137] performed a study in which nulliparous patients already receiving a continuous epidural infusion of 0.75 percent lidocaine were randomized to receive either additional 0.75 percent lidocaine or saline placebo after 8 cm cervical dilatation. The epidural infusion of lidocaine or saline placebo was continued in all patients until delivery. Maintenance of the epidural infusion of 0.75 percent lidocaine until delivery did not prolong the second stage or increase the frequency of instrumental delivery, but it also did not reliably provide second-stage analgesia or perineal anesthesia. Specifically, women who continued to receive epidural lidocaine until delivery did not clearly perceive that they had better analgesia than did women who received saline placebo.

Subsequently, Chestnut and colleagues[128] performed a study in which nulliparous women already receiving a continuous epidural infusion of 0.125 percent bupivacaine were randomized to receive either additional 0.125 percent bupivacaine or saline placebo beyond 8 cm cervical dilatation. Patients continued to receive the epidural infusion of bupivacaine or saline placebo until delivery. Maintenance of the epidural infusion of bupivacaine until delivery resulted in a second-stage analgesia that was clearly superior to that provided by replacement of the bupivacaine with placebo. Infusion of bupivacaine until delivery prolonged the second stage of labor approximately 30 minutes, and it also increased the incidence of instrumental delivery. However, maintenance of epidural bupivacaine analgesia did *not* result in an increased incidence of abnormal position of the vertex, and it did *not* result in a more frequent performance of cesarean section. Furthermore, there were nonsignificant tendencies toward better neonatal condition in the bupivacaine group as evaluated by umbilical cord blood acid–base status and Apgar scores.

Recommendations

What can be concluded from these studies of epidural anesthesia and the progress of labor? *First,* it is probably preferable to avoid institution of epidural anesthesia during early, latent-phase labor in most patients. In general, epidural anesthesia should not be instituted until the obstetrician is satisfied that the labor is active, that is, until the patient is having regular contractions and the cervix is dilating progressively. But it is difficult to assign a specific cervical dilatation as indicating the time to administer epidural anesthesia; for some it will be 3 to 4 cm and for others, 4 to 6 cm. Psychoprophylactic techniques are probably most effective during the latent phase of labor and will allow many patients to forego supplemental analgesia during that period. However, physicians should recognize that some patients experience severe pain during latent-phase labor. This is especially true if the patient is receiving intravenous oxytocin. It is best to individualize decisions regarding timing of epidural anesthesia. Thus, in some patients, early institution of epidural anesthesia may be appropriate.

Second, it is preferable to use dilute solutions of local anesthetic rather than more concentrated solutions. For example, 0.25 percent bupivacaine will provide satisfactory analgesia in most patients, and it is rarely necessary to give a more concentrated solution of bupivacaine for analgesia during labor.

Third, the obstetrician should recognize that a brief period of decreased uterine activity often follows the institution of epidural anesthesia. In some patients, there is a brief period of decreased uterine activity followed by reestablishment of the contraction pattern and resumption of normal labor (Fig. 16.9).[139] In some patients, epidural anesthesia may accelerate labor, perhaps by decreasing maternal concentrations of catecholamines. At least one study has documented a favorable influence of epidural anesthesia in patients with discoordinate uterine contractions and prolonged labor.[140] But, in other patients, analgesia may seem to slow or to stop labor for more than a brief period. In such patients, the obstetrician should be willing to augment labor by giving oxytocin intravenously.

Fourth, there remains disagreement regarding whether it is advisable to add epinephrine to the therapeutic dose of local anesthetic. Some anesthesiologists add epinephrine to local anesthetic solutions to

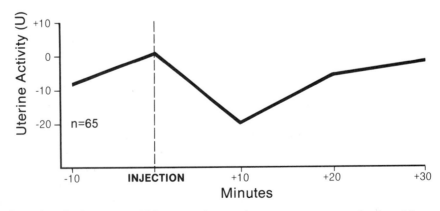

Fig. 16.9 Effect of epidural injections of lidocaine with epinephrine on uterine activity levels in 65 cases. (From Lowensohn et al.,[139] with permission.)

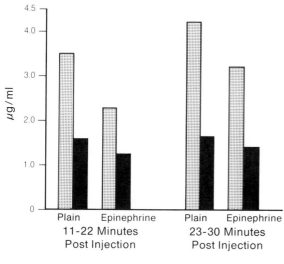

Fig. 16.10 Histogram of mean maternal and cord plasma concentrations of lidocaine, 20 ml 2 percent solution with or without the addition of 1 : 250,000 epinephrine, in patients who were delivered 11 to 22 minutes or 23 to 30 minutes after administration of lidocaine by the lumbar epidural route. (From Thomas et al.,[232] with permission.)

produce vasoconstriction in the area where the local anesthetic is injected. In this way, the blood absorbs smaller amounts of anesthetic over a longer time period. Thus there is a decreased concentration of local anesthetic in the maternal blood, and less local anesthetic crosses the placenta to the fetus (Fig. 16.10). Also, the addition of epinephrine may result in a more solid block, especially if one is administering lidocaine. On the other hand, some studies have demonstrated that the addition of epinephrine to local anesthetic solution is more likely to decrease uterine activity than administration of local anesthetic without epinephrine. In one study, plain lidocaine decreased uterine activity briefly in 16 patients but increased it in 14 patients. In contrast, lidocaine with epinephrine (1:200,000) decreased uterine activity in 39 patients and increased it in only 12. Furthermore, mean uterine activity (Montevideo Units) decreased much more when epinephrine was used (Fig. 16.11).[84] Another study reported similar results in uterine activity but no significant effect of epinephrine on the length and progression of labor.[141] Recently other studies have also suggested that the addition of epinephrine to local anesthetic does not

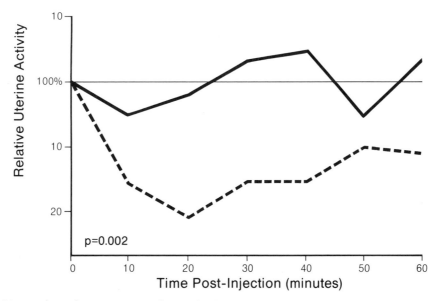

Fig. 16.11 Mean values of uterine activity after epidural administration of lidocaine (solid line) or lidocaine with epinephrine (dotted line). (From Matadial and Cibils,[84] with permission.)

prolong the duration of labor.[142-145] This is especially likely to be true if a very dilute concentration of epinephrine is administered.[142-145]

Fifth, should epidural anesthesia be continued or discontinued during the second stage of labor? We believe that it is inappropriate to withhold analgesia *routinely* during the second stage. Johnson et al.[146] concluded: "Voluntary effort is decreased in some patients in the second stage of labor with spinal and peridural analgesia. Since this is not a consistent finding, and some patients actually exhibited increased capability for bearing down after the anesthesia, it must be an individual reaction without the actual loss of ability." It is important to understand that epidural anesthesia during labor is not a generic procedure. For example, in one study[137] maintenance of the infusion of local anesthetic until delivery did not prolong the second stage or increase the incidence of instrumental delivery, but it also did not reliably provide second-stage analgesia. In a similar study[128] performed at the same institution, infusion of a different local anesthetic until delivery provided excellent second stage analgesia, but it prolonged the second stage and increased the incidence of instrumental delivery. In the first study,[137] the block during the second stage was clearly inadequate in most patients, while in the second study[128] the block was probably excessive in some patients. Clearly, a dense epidural block may decrease the ability of some patients to push effectively. On the other hand, other patients will push more effectively in the presence of analgesia. In clinical practice, it seems best to individualize patient management. If the block is too dense and the patient cannot push effectively, then there should be diminution of the level and/or intensity of analgesia. In other patients, the block should be maintained or strengthened. The optimal approach is to provide a reasonable level of analgesia consistent with the parturient's ability to push effectively. Of course, it is also important that patients be actively coached in pushing.

Sixth, one should avoid arbitrary termination of the second stage. As noted earlier, the American College of Obstetricians and Gynecologists recently redefined the "normal" limits of the duration of the second stage in patients with and without regional anesthesia.[133] Indeed, in some patients with effective epidural analgesia, it may be appropriate to allow a second stage of more than 3 hours, provided that there is continued progress in descent of the vertex.

Seventh, it is important to recognize that risk to mother and infant of instrumental delivery performed under the ideal conditions provided by spinal or epidural anesthesia may differ from the risk of instrumental delivery performed without adequate anesthesia. Indeed, regional anesthesia may well allow for more complete cooperation by the patient, a more accurate application of the forceps, and a more gently controlled birth.

There remain several unresolved questions with regard to optimal management of epidural anesthesia during labor. *First,* does *continuous infusion* of local anesthetic affect labor differently than intermittent epidural bolus injection? Recently the continuous epidural infusion technique has become popular. Purported advantages of continuous epidural infusion during labor include (1) a more stable level of analgesia, (2) reduced risk of hypotension, (3) reduced risk of systemic toxicity, (4) reduced risk of total spinal block, and (5) convenience for the anesthesiologist.[147] An infusion pump delivers a dilute solution of local anesthetic by continuous positive pressure. A potential disadvantage of continuous epidural infusion is that it tends to discourage individualization of the dose of local anesthetic in an individual patient. Thus there is a tendency to give more local anesthetic than one would give if one were using the intermittent epidural bolus injection technique. For example, there have been at least five controlled comparisons of the continuous epidural infusion of bupivacaine versus intermittent epidural bolus injection of bupivacaine.[148-152] In each study, patients in the continuous infusion group received more bupivacaine than did patients in the intermittent bolus group. It is unclear whether the increased dose of bupivacaine is clinically significant and represents a disadvantage. Furthermore, it is unclear whether the continuous epidural infusion technique has more or less effect on the progress of labor and method of delivery than does the intermittent epidural bolus injection technique.

Second, is it advantageous to add opioid to the solution of local anesthetic and thereby reduce the total dose of local anesthetic and the extent of maternal motor block? Chestnut and colleagues[153] observed that the continuous epidural infusion of 0.0625 percent bupivacaine – 0.0002 percent fentanyl produced first-stage analgesia similar to that provided by the infusion of 0.125 percent bupivacaine alone. Women who received bupivacaine – fentanyl experienced less intense motor block, but they did *not* have a shorter second stage or a lower incidence of instrumental delivery than did women who received bupivacaine alone. A legitimate criticism of that study is that the epidural infusion was discontinued at full cervical dilatation in both groups. Had the infusion been continued until delivery, it is possible that there would have been a difference between groups in the method of delivery. This question deserves further investigation.

Third, should there be more frequent use of oxytocin during the second stage of labor? Goodfellow and colleagues[154] noted a significant increase in maternal blood concentrations of oxytocin between the onset of full cervical dilatation and crowning of the fetal head in patients *without* epidural anesthesia, but they did not observe a similar increase in patients *with* epidural anesthesia. Similarly, Bates and colleagues[155] observed significantly less uterine activity during the second stage in patients *with* epidural anesthesia compared with patients *without* epidural anesthesia. Both groups of investigators recommended increased utilization of oxytocin during the second stage in order to increase the chance of spontaneous vaginal delivery.

Fourth, is there a role for delayed pushing during the second stage? Maresh and colleagues[130] reported a study of 76 nulliparous patients with epidural anesthesia who were randomly assigned to early pushing or late pushing in the second stage. There was a significant increase in the duration of the second stage but a nonsignificant decrease in the frequency of instrumental delivery in the late-pushing group. The increased second-stage duration was not associated with an increase in fetal heart rate abnormalities or a decrease in Apgar scores or umbilical cord blood pH. It is possible that patients become exhausted when asked to push too early during the second stage. Indeed, it may be preferable to allow the force of uterine contractions to deliver the vertex to a station at which maternal pushing might be effective.

Paracervical Block

Paracervical block anesthesia, a simple, effective procedure when performed properly, is used most commonly by obstetricians. Usually, 5 to 6 ml of a low concentration of local anesthetic without epinephrine (e.g., 1 percent lidocaine or 1 or 2 percent 2-chloroprocaine) is injected into the mucosa of the cervix at either 4 and 8 or 3 and 9 o'clock; an Iowa trumpet prevents deep penetration of the needle (Fig. 16.12). The duration of anesthesia depends on the local anesthetic used. Several manufacturers of bupivacaine have recommended that bupivacaine, the longest acting local anesthetic, be contraindicated for obstetric paracervical block (see discussion of local anesthetic toxicity, above). In the past, paracervical block enjoyed considerable favor, particularly when anesthesiologists were not available to provide major regional

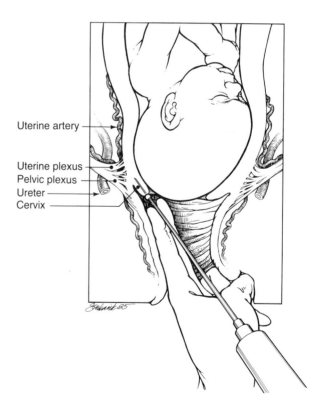

Fig. 16.12 Technique of paracervical block. Schematic coronal section (enlarged) of lower portion of cervix and upper portion of vagina shows relation of needle to paracervical region. (Modified from Bonica,[32] with permission.)

Uterine artery
Uterine plexus
Pelvic plexus
Ureter
Cervix

techniques. Disadvantages of the technique are that the block can only be applied during the first stage of labor and that it must be reapplied frequently during the course of a long labor. Furthermore, it has the widely recognized, *major* disadvantage of fetal bradycardia, which occurs in 2 to 70 percent of applications. It occurs within 2 to 10 minutes and lasts from 3 to 30 minutes. Although usually benign, it can be associated with fetal acidosis and occasionally with fetal death.[156–158]

There is no consensus regarding the mechanism of postparacervical block bradycardia. The theories include (1) high blood concentrations of local anesthetic in the fetus, (2) uterine artery vasoconstriction, and (3) postparacervical block increase in uterine activity. A high blood concentration is feasible, because the local anesthetic is injected close to the uterine artery. The anesthetic would traverse the wall of the uterine artery, pass directly to the fetus, and thus result in a high blood concentration and subsequent bradycardia.[156] Clinical support for this theory is that infants who suffer bradycardia frequently have higher anesthetic blood concentrations than do their mothers.[156] Alternatively, the bradycardia may result from uterine artery vasoconstriction secondary to a direct effect of the local anesthetic on the uterine artery.[159,160] This effect has been demonstrated in vitro on human uterine arteries[159] (Fig. 16.13) and is supported by uterine blood flow studies in animals.[160]

The fetal electrocardiogram (ECG) pattern during one of these episodes after paracervical block suggests hypoxia, a finding that supports the uterine artery vasoconstriction theory.[161] Although high concentrations of local anesthetic are required to produce vasoconstriction during the administration of a paracervical block, high concentrations are deposited close to the uterine artery (Fig. 16.12). It is unlikely that such levels are obtained with other forms of regional anesthesia. The third theory is based on the possibility that local anesthetic injected directly into the uterine musculature increases uterine tone.

Some have suggested that manipulation of the fetal head, the uterus, or the uterine vasculature during institution of the block might produce reflex bradycardia. It is possible that no one theory is adequate to explain all cases of postparacervical block bradycardia. Regardless of etiology, the severity and duration of the bradycardia correlate with the incidence of fetal acidosis and subsequent neonatal depression. Freeman and colleagues[161] reported a significant fall in pH and a rise in base deficit only in those fetuses with bradycardia persisting more than 10 minutes. Paracervical block should be used cautiously at all times and should not be used at all in mothers with fetuses in either acute or chronic distress.

To conclude this section on anesthesia for labor, Table 16.4 shows the frequency with which the various forms of anesthesia are used. The data are

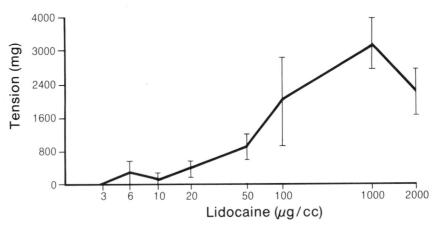

mean ±SEM, n=9

Fig. 16.13 Dose–response curve of the pregnant human uterine artery to lidocaine hydrochloride (mean ± SEM; N = 9). (From Gibbs and Noel,[159] with permission.)

Table 16.4 Anesthetic Procedures Used for Labor in 1981 According to Delivery Service

Delivery Service (births/year)	No Anesthesia (%)	Narcotics Barbiturates Tranquilizers (%)	Paracervical Block (%)	Epidural Block (%)
<500	45	37	6	9
500–1,499	33	53	5	13
>1,500	27	52	5	22
All hospitals	32	49	5	16

(From Gibbs et al.,[162] with permission.)

from a joint American Society of Anesthesiologists/ American College of Obstetricians and Gynecologists survey of 1,200 hospitals in the United States.[162]

ANESTHESIA FOR VAGINAL DELIVERY

Pain relief for vaginal delivery can be achieved in a number of ways. Some patients will require no anesthesia. For those who do, the goal is to match the patient's wishes with the requirements of the delivery without subjecting either mother or fetus to unnecessary risk.

Local Anesthesia

In the form of perineal infiltration, local anesthesia is widely used and very safe. Spontaneous vaginal deliveries, episiotomies, and perhaps use of outlet forceps can be accomplished with this simple technique. Local anesthetic toxicity may occur if large amounts of local anesthetic are used or in the unlikely event that an intravascular injection occurs. Usually, 5 to 15 ml of 1 percent lidocaine suffices. Philipson and colleagues[163] demonstrated the rapid and significant transfer of lidocaine to the fetus after perineal infiltration. In 5 of 15 infants, the concentration of lidocaine at delivery was greater in the umbilical vein than in the mother (Table 16.5).[163]

Pudendal Block

Pudendal block is a minor regional block that also is widely used, reasonably effective, and very safe. The obstetrician, using an Iowa trumpet and a 20-gauge needle, injects 5 to 10 ml of local anesthetic just below the ischial spine. Because the hemorrhoidal nerve

may be aberrant in 50 percent of patients,[164] some physicians prefer to inject a portion of the local anesthetic somewhat posterior to the spine (Fig. 16.14). For those inexperienced at identifying the ischial spine, the bony prominence at the inner canthus of one's eye provides a reasonable facsimile of a small and somewhat sharp ischial spine. Although a transperineal approach to the ischial spine is possible, most prefer the transvaginal approach. One percent lidocaine or mepivacaine or 2 percent 2-chloroprocaine is used.

The technique is satisfactory for all spontaneous vaginal deliveries and episiotomies and for some outlet or low forceps deliveries, but may not be sufficient for deliveries requiring additional manipulation. For example, a difficult breech delivery or a delivery necessitating more than outlet forceps may require more pain relief, relaxation, and cooperation than pudendal block can ensure. Likewise, a pudendal block may not provide enough anesthesia for the successful and controlled release of shoulder dystocia. In these instances, as in any others that require significant manipulation, more extensive anesthesia will be required. Ideally, such requirements should be anticipated before the event.

More than with perineal infiltration, the potential for local anesthetic toxicity exists with pudendal block because of the proximity of large vessels close to the site of injection (Fig. 16.14). Therefore, aspiration before injection is particularly important. Furthermore, the potential for large amounts of local

Table 16.5 Lidocaine Concentrations at Delivery in Maternal Plasma and Umbilical Cord Vein After Perineal Infiltration

Sample (N = 15)	Concentration (ng/ml)	
	Mean ± SD	Range
Maternal plasma		
Peak concentration	648 ± 666	60–2,400
At delivery	548 ± 468	33–1,474
Umbilical cord vein	420 ± 406	45–1,380
Fetal:maternal ratio[a]	1.32 ± 1.46	0.05–4.66

[a] Ratio of level in cord vein to level in maternal vein at delivery (mean of individual ratios, not ratio of means).

(From Philipson et al.,[163] with permission.)

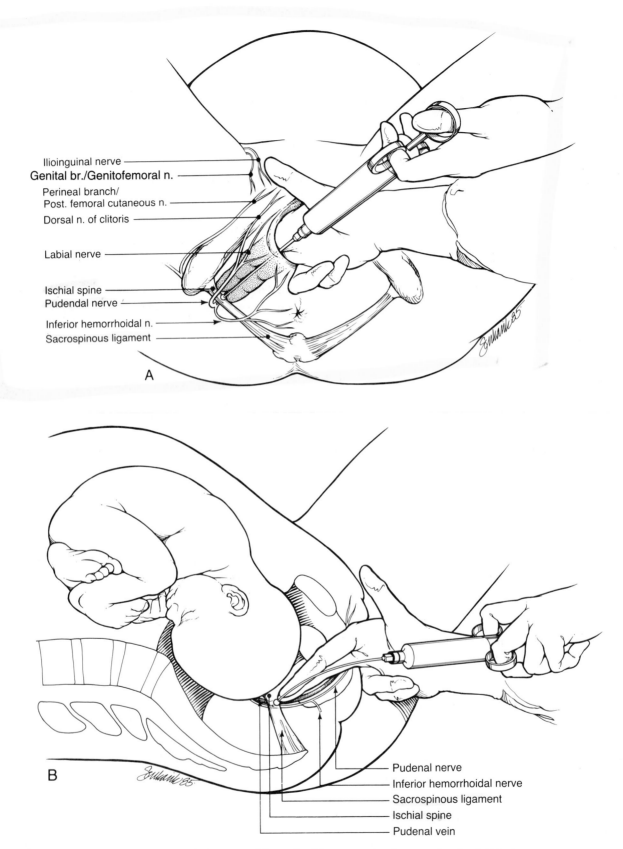

Fig. 16.14 (A, B) Anatomy of the pudendal nerve and techniques of pudendal block.

anesthetic to be used increases when perineal and labial infiltration are required in addition to the pudendal block. In these instances, it is important to monitor closely the amount of local anesthetic given (see discussion of local anesthetic toxicity, above).

Inhalation or Intravenous Analgesia

An anesthesiologist or nurse anesthetist administers inhalation or intravenous analgesia (stage I anesthesia), which provides varying degrees of pain relief and amnesia but maintains protective laryngeal and cough reflexes. Most often the obstetrician will add local infiltration or a pudendal block. The anesthesiologist will frequently question the patient to determine the level of anesthesia and to ensure that deeper planes of anesthesia are avoided. Such precautions are important because, if the patient becomes unconscious and passes beyond stage I, all the hazards associated with general anesthesia are possible, including inadequate airway, hypoxia, and aspiration. Because continual assessment of the patient's state of consciousness is required and is sometimes difficult, only anesthesiologists or nurse anesthetists should administer inhalation analgesia. Furthermore, this technique requires the use of the increasingly complicated anesthesia machine, misuse of which can prove disastrous. Most frequently, the anesthesiologist uses 40 or at most 50 percent nitrous oxide or, for intravenous analgesia, ketamine, 0.25 mg/kg. (This latter agent may be particularly effective for the patient who cannot or will not tolerate an anesthetic face mask.) Less commonly, the anesthesiologist may administer a subanesthetic concentration of a potent halogenated agent (e.g., halothane, enflurane, isoflurane) for a brief period.

Inhalation or intravenous analgesia alone will not be sufficient for performing episiotomies or repairing perineal lacerations. Therefore, these techniques usually require supplemental pudendal block or perineal infiltration. The combined effects of both techniques are additive and satisfactory for spontaneous vaginal deliveries, most outlet forceps deliveries, and even some manipulative deliveries. Inhalation or intravenous analgesia renders some patients amnesic of the event, a characteristic that is often undesirable.

Spinal (Subarachnoid) Block

A saddle block is a spinal block in which the level of anesthesia is limited to little more than the perineum, that is, the saddle area; thus true saddle blocks are rarely used. Spinal anesthesia is reasonably easy to perform and usually provides total pain relief in the blocked area. Therefore, spontaneous deliveries, forceps deliveries, and episiotomies can be accomplished easily. Likewise, complicated deliveries that require extensive manipulation can be effected in a controlled and pain-free manner. Although the ability to push may be compromised somewhat, the advantage of having a cooperative patient who is receptive to suggestion and able to cooperate because she is pain free may outweigh the disadvantage of moderately diminished strength.

Usually spinal anesthesia is achieved by injecting 4 mg hyperbaric tetracaine or 20 to 35 mg hyperbaric lidocaine into the subarachnoid space through a 22-, 25-, or 26-gauge spinal needle. (It is preferable to use the smallest possible needle, because the smaller the needle, the less the risk of spinal headache.) Because the solution is hyperbaric relative to cerebral spinal fluid, the most important determinant of anesthesia level is gravity. The level is most easily controlled by varying the position of the patient. For example, the head-down position causes the level to rise. Other factors may also contribute to the level of anesthesia: amount of drug, volume injected, speed of injection, and height of the patient. Less controllable factors include the Valsalva maneuver, coughing, and straining, any of which will cause the level to rise. If one injects the local anesthetic during a contraction, a higher than expected level of anesthesia may occur. Thus it is best not to inject the local anesthetic during a uterine contraction. Finally, left uterine displacement is maintained by a wedge or by some other effective device placed under the right hip.

Because spinal anesthesia is sometimes administered by persons other than anesthesiologists and is technically easy to perform, the single most important fact to understand is that it is a major regional block; it is not a procedure to be taken lightly. All hazards associated with major blocks are possible, including hypotension and "total spinal" (see the discussion of lumbar epidural anesthesia for labor, above). Although these complications can occur, they should not result in disaster if diagnosed early and treated appropriately. The person who administers spinal anesthesia must never leave the patient unattended without ensuring that another competent individual will assume responsibility for monitoring the blood pressure and level of anesthesia. Usually, the level of the spinal block will be complete and fixed within 5 to 10 minutes. However, sometimes the level continues to creep upward for 20 minutes or longer.

Single-Dose Caudal and Lumbar Epidural Anesthesia

Single-dose epidural anesthesia techniques are used much less frequently than in the past. The relative difficulty and the large amounts of local anesthetic required are significant disadvantages for the caudal technique. Usually, when these techniques are used they are instituted during labor as continuous techniques and maintained for the delivery. They then provide the same advantages as spinal anesthesia.

General Anesthesia

General anesthesia is rarely indicated for vaginal delivery. Whether given for a brief or a prolonged period of time, general anesthesia engenders considerable risk and should therefore not be used without strong indication. An unanticipated difficult breech, shoulder dystocia, or internal version and extraction of a second twin represent rare indications for general anesthesia. Also, general anesthesia may rarely be indicated for difficult forceps delivery in a patient in whom major regional anesthesia is contraindicated. When general anesthesia is indicated, the technique specific for cesarean section is used, including administration by experienced and competent personnel, rapid sequence induction, and endotracheal intubation (see the discussion on anesthesia for cesarean section, below). For breech delivery or delivery of a second twin, one may administer a high concentration of a potent halogenated agent (e.g., halothane, enflurane, isoflurane) to effect uterine and perhaps cervical relaxation. Equipotent doses of any of these three agents will provide equivalent uterine relaxation.[165]

Table 16.6 lists the frequencies with which the various forms of anesthesia are used for vaginal delivery.

ANESTHESIA FOR CESAREAN SECTION

The patient can be either asleep or awake during cesarean section. For those who wish to be awake, either spinal anesthesia or lumbar epidural anesthesia are used most commonly. In the United States, general anesthesia is used for 41 percent of cesarean births, and spinal and epidural anesthesias are used for 34 and 21 percent, respectively (Table 16.7).[162] Local anesthesia for cesarean section is possible but only rarely used.[166]

Either general anesthesia or regional anesthesia should be safe for the infant; studies have reported Apgar scores and blood gas values as essentially the same for infants of mothers choosing either technique (Table 16.8).[167-169] In recent years some authors suggested that Apgar scores and acid–base analysis evaluated brain stem activity, but not the higher centers. Therefore, neurobehavioral testing for the newborn was developed.[170] The testing involves eliciting and observing the quality of the infant's responses to certain stimuli in the early postpartum hours; a trained person can accomplish the testing in approximately 15 minutes. Results indicate that infants of mothers who receive regional anesthesia achieve somewhat higher scores than those whose mothers receive general anesthesia, and infants do somewhat better when ketamine is the induction agent for general anesthesia than when thiopental is

Table 16.6 Anesthetic Procedures Used for Vaginal Delivery in 1981 According to Delivery Service

Delivery Service (births/year)	No Anesthesia (%)	Local or Pudendal Block (%)	Inhalational Analgesia (%)	Preexisting Epidural Block (%)	Spinal Block (%)	General Anesthesia (%)
<500	27	59	4	7	5	2
500–1,499	13	68	7	11	7	3
>1,500	11	54	5	20	11	3
All hospitals	15	59	6	14	9	3

(From Gibbs et al.,[162] with permission.)

Table 16.7 Anesthetic Procedures Used for Cesarean Section in 1981 According to Delivery Service

Delivery Service (births/year)	Lumbar Epidural Block (%)	Spinal Block (%)	General Anesthesia (%)
<500	12	37	46
500–1,499	16	35	45
>1,500	29	33	35
All hospitals	21	34	41

(From Gibbs et al.,[162] with permission.)

used.[171] Moreover, regarding the choice of local anesthetic for regional anesthesia, infants were originally thought to do better after 2-chloroprocaine and bupivacaine than after lidocaine and mepivacaine.[170,172] Recently, however, lidocaine has been "exonerated" and is associated with neurobehavioral scores equal to those when mothers have received 2-chloroprocaine or bupivacaine.[81] When the Food and Drug Administration (FDA) appointed a committee to study neurobehavioral changes in newborns after anesthesia, the committee concluded that, although anesthetic agents can alter neurobehavioral performance, there was no evidence that they affect later development.[50] Therefore, neurobehavioral considerations do not weigh heavily in the choice of anesthesia or anesthetic agent; the choice can be based on the preferences of the mother, the obstetrician, and the anesthesiologist as well as on the demands of the particular clinical situation.

General Anesthesia

Advantages of general anesthesia for cesarean section
  Many patients prefer not to be awake during a major operation.
  General anesthesia provides total pain relief.
  Operating conditions are optimal.

Disadvantages of general anesthesia for cesarean section
  Many patients wish to experience the birth consciously.
  There is a slight risk of fetal depression.
  Intubation causes hypertension and tachycardia, which may be particularly dangerous in severely preeclamptic patients.
  Intubation can be difficult or impossible.
  Aspiration of stomach contents is possible.

Two complications, failure to intubate and aspiration, continue to be major causes of maternal mortality.[173-176] Because these two disadvantages of general anesthesia are of considerable and significant threat to the mother, many anesthesiologists now prefer regional anesthesia over general anesthesia. To understand how these complications arise, the obstetrician should be aware of the sequence of events during general anesthesia. Furthermore, there may be times when the obstetrician must participate in difficult decisions concerning anesthetic management. Those decisions may affect the lives and well-being of both mother and infant.

Premedication

Premedication, an otherwise routine part of general anesthesia that usually employs sedative or opioid agents, is omitted because these agents cross the placenta and can depress the fetus. Sedation should be unnecessary if the procedure is explained well.

Table 16.8 Elective Cesarean Section — Blood-Gas and Apgar Scores

	General Anesthesia[a] (N = 20)	Epidural Anesthesia[a] (N = 15)	Spinal Anesthesia[b] (N = 15)
Umbilical vein			
pH	7.38	7.359	7.34
Po_2 (mmHg)	35	36	37
Pco_2 (mmHg)	38	42	48
Apgar <6			
1	1	0	0
5	0	0	0
Umbilical artery			
pH	7.32	7.28	7.28
Po_2 (mmHg)	22	18	18
Pco_2 (mmHg)	47	55	63
BE (mEq/L)	−1.80	−1.60	−1.40

[a] Data from James et al.[167]
[b] Data from Datta and Brown.[88]

Antacids

As soon as it is known that the patient requires cesarean section, be it with regional or general anesthesia, 30 ml of a clear, nonparticulate antacid, such as 0.3 M sodium citrate,[177] Bicitra,[178] or Alka Seltzer, 2 tablets in 30 ml water,[179] is administered to decrease gastric acidity in order to ameliorate the consequences of aspiration, should it occur. The chalky white particulate antacids are avoided because they can produce lung damage (Fig. 16.15).[180]

Left Uterine Displacement

As during labor, the uterus may compress the inferior vena cava and the aorta during cesarean delivery; aortocaval compression is detrimental to both mother and fetus. The duration of anesthesia makes little difference when left uterine displacement is practiced; however, when patients remain supine, Apgar scores decrease as time of anesthesia increases.[181]

Regarding this latter point (i.e., anesthesia time or

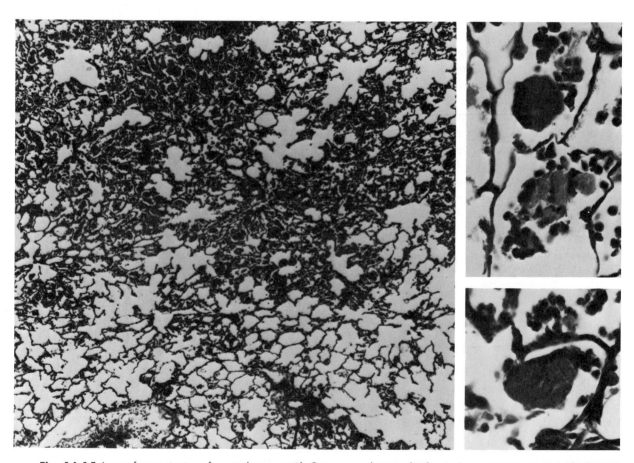

Fig. 16.15 Lung after aspiration of particulate antacid. Compare with normal saline in Figure 16.16. Note marked extensive inflammatory reaction. The alveoli are filled with polymorphonuclear leukocytes and macrophages in approximately equal numbers. Insets at right show large and small intra-alveolar particles surrounded by inflammatory cells (48 hours). Later, the reaction changed to an intra-alveolar cellular collection of clusters of large macrophages with abundant granular cytoplasm, in some of which were small amphophilic particles similar to those seen in the insets. No fibrosis or other inflammatory reaction was seen (28 days). (From Gibbs et al.,[180] with permission.)

induction-to-delivery time), more recent data indicate that the induction-to-delivery time is not the crucial time. Rather, it is the uterine incision-to-delivery interval that is predictive of neonatal status.[182] A uterine-incision interval of less than 90 seconds is optimal, whereas an incision-to-delivery interval of 90 to 180 seconds is less satisfactory; after 180 seconds, the incidence of newborn depression is significantly increased. Therefore, it seems that uterine manipulation and difficulty of the delivery are significant factors for the fetus during cesarean section.

Preoxygenation

Because patients become unconscious and paralyzed, it is best to wash all nitrogen from the lungs and to replace it with oxygen. This is especially important in pregnant patients, because functional residual capacity is decreased and pregnant patients become hypoxemic more quickly than nonpregnant patients during periods of apnea.[183] Therefore, *before* starting induction, 100 percent oxygen is administered via face mask for 2 to 3 minutes. In situations of dire emergency, four vital capacity breaths of 100 percent oxygen via a tight circle system will provide similar benefit.[184] Thus, should untoward events occur, the patient can tolerate them for a longer period without becoming hypoxic. This simple, safe, effective maneuver should not be neglected.

Induction

The anesthesiologist rapidly administers thiopental, a short-acting barbiturate, or ketamine to render the patient unconscious. An appropriate dose of either agent has little, if any, effect on the fetus.[185,186]

Muscle Relaxant

Immediately after administration of thiopental or ketamine, the anesthesiologist gives a muscle relaxant to facilitate intubation. Succinylcholine, a rapid-onset, short-acting muscle relaxant, remains the agent of choice in most patients.

Cricoid Pressure

In rapid-sequence induction, as the thiopental or ketamine begins to take effect and the patient approaches unconsciousness, an assistant applies pressure to the cricoid cartilage, which is just below the thyroid cartilage, and does not release the pressure until an endotracheal tube is placed, its position verified, and the cuff on the tube inflated.[187,188] Pressure on the cricoid closes off the esophagus and is extremely important in preventing aspiration should regurgitation or vomiting occur. It is a simple, safe, effective maneuver that should not be omitted.

Intubation

Usually intubation proceeds smoothly. However, in approximately 5 percent of patients, it will be difficult or delayed. In some (e.g., approximately 0.3 to 0.5 percent of patients) it will be impossible. When the delay is prolonged or the intubation impossible, the situation becomes a crisis in which the critical factor is to deliver oxygen to the now unconscious and paralyzed patient. Also, because it is during this induction sequence (i.e., before the airway is secured with an endotracheal tube) that the patient is most at risk from aspiration, any delay increases the risk.[174] It is therefore particularly important during a difficult intubation that the person applying cricoid pressure not release that pressure until told to do so by the anesthesiologist.

Proper Tube Placement

Before the operation begins, the anesthesiologist must ensure that the endotracheal tube is properly positioned within the trachea. End-tidal CO_2 analysis is the preferred method of confirming that the tube is within the trachea.[189] Of course, the anesthesiologist will also confirm that breath sounds are bilateral and equal. If the endotracheal tube is not in the trachea (and therefore is likely in the esophagus), the tube must be removed immediately and the entire situation reassessed. In some instances, the attempt will be repeated. Otherwise, the anesthesiologist will allow the patient to awaken (wherein lies the virtue of the short-acting drugs thiopental and succinylcholine), and another course of action will be chosen. Until the patient completely awakens, ventilation with bag and face mask and continuous application of cricoid pressure may be necessary. Once the patient is awake and breathing spontaneously, the anesthesiologist must choose between awake intubation or regional anesthesia. In most cases, if the endotracheal tube is incorrectly placed, the operation should not proceed until the airway is secure, because the patient cannot be allowed to awaken after the abdomen is opened. If the operation proceeds and ventilation cannot be accomplished, hypoxia, hypercarbia, and cardiac arrest can result; the fetus also will suffer.

When cesarean section is not urgent, the decision to delay the operation and to allow the mother to awaken is easy. However, if the operation is being done because of fetal distress, allowing the mother to awaken may further jeopardize the fetus. It is helpful if one continues fetal heart rate monitoring before and even during induction of anesthesia. (In most situations of fetal distress, one can leave the fetal scalp electrode in place until delivery. At that time the circulating nurse can reach under the drapes and disconnect the scalp lead.) Fetal heart rate monitoring may guide anesthetic and obstetric management in situations of failed intubation. Rarely, in situations of dire fetal distress, the anesthesiologist and obstetrician may jointly decide to proceed with cesarean section while the anesthesiologist provides oxygenation, ventilation, and anesthesia by face mask ventilation with cricoid pressure. In these emergency situations, it may be necessary to have additional trained personnel to provide assistance. After delivery, the obstetrician should obtain temporary hemostasis and then halt surgery while the anesthesiologist secures the airway by fiberoptic or blind nasal intubation.

The obstetrician and anesthesiologist should address these issues before they become emergent. Such instances should be the subject of combined obstetric/anesthesia conferences during which the concerns of all can be presented and discussed. The anesthesiologist performing a rapid-sequence induction is in a position comparable to the obstetrician confronted with the vaginal delivery of a breech presentation: the anesthesiologist has an unconscious and paralyzed mother whose airway is not yet established, and the obstetrician must deliver the largest part of the baby last. In both instances, one acts before the outcome is certain. In both instances, considerable clinical skill and judgment must be exercised.

Nitrous Oxide and Oxygen

Once the endotracheal tube is in place, a 50:50 mixture of nitrous oxide and oxygen is added to provide analgesia. Such a mixture is safe for both mother and fetus.[190]

Potent Inhalation Agent

Usually, in addition to the nitrous oxide, an analgesic quantity (low concentration) of a potent inhalation agent (e.g., halothane, enflurane, isoflurane) will be added to provide amnesia and additional analgesia. These agents, in low concentrations, are not harmful to mother or fetus. Also, uterine relaxation does not occur, and bleeding is not excessive.[191,192] If one does not add a potent inhalation agent, there will be an unacceptably high incidence of maternal awareness and recall. Even with the use of one of these agents, maternal awareness and recall occasionally occur. Therefore, it is important that all operating room personnel use discretion in conversation and conduct themselves as if the patient were awake.

Postdelivery

Usually the concentration of nitrous oxide can be increased after delivery. In addition, either the potent inhalation agent is continued or an opioid is added to supplement the nitrous oxide and oxygen.

Oxytocin Administration

Ten to 30 units/L is infused intravenously. Bolus injections are avoided, because they can cause hypotension and tachycardia.[193]

Extubation

Because the patient can aspirate while awakening as well as during induction, extubation is not done until the patient is awake and can respond appropriately to commands. Coughing and bucking do not necessarily indicate that the patient is awake, merely that she is in the second stage, the excitement stage, of anesthesia. It is during this period of anesthesia that laryngospasm is most likely to occur should any foreign body, including the endotracheal tube or bits of stomach contents, stimulate the larynx. The patient must therefore be awake and conscious, not merely active, before extubation.

Recovery

The most important requirement of the recovery room is the presence of personnel trained appropriately and assigned no other duties than those required for the recovery process. The recovery room must contain adequate facilities and should provide care comparable to that provided patients who have received general or regional anesthesia for other surgical procedures.[2,194-196]

Aspiration

Aspiration is a serious and often fatal complication of general anesthesia and therefore deserves specific attention. In most instances it can be prevented. When it cannot, the consequences depend in part on the volume and nature of the aspirate. The conventional wisdom is that patients are at risk when their stomach contents are greater than 25 ml and when the pH of those contents is less than 2.5.[197] There are several reasons why the pregnant patient is particularly at risk. The enlarged uterus increases intra-abdominal pressure and thus intragastric pressure.[198] The gastroesophageal sphincter is distorted by the enlarged uterus, making it less competent, possibly explaining the high incidence of heartburn that occurs during pregnancy.[199,200] Concentrations of progesterone are increased during pregnancy. Progesterone is a smooth muscle relaxant, and thereby it delays gastric emptying and relaxes the gastroesophageal sphincter. Gastrin, the hormone that increases both acidity and volume of gastric contents, is increased during pregnancy,[201] and motilin, a hormone that speeds gastric emptying, is decreased during pregnancy.[202] Labor itself delays gastric emptying,[203] as do opioids.[204] Many patients undergo cesarean section after a prolonged labor, during which they may have received several doses of opioids.[51]

Not all cases of aspiration are the same. The severities of lung damage, morbidity, and mortality vary

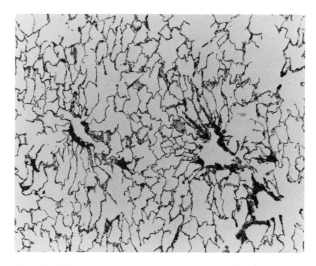

Fig. 16.16 Lung after aspiration of normal saline. Essentially normal lung histology. (From Gibbs and Modell,[233] with permission.)

and depend on the type of material aspirated. Less acid (pH greater than 2.5) liquid significantly decreases PaO_2 physiologically but has very little histologic effect. Liquids with a pH of less than 2.5 decrease PaO_2 further and cause a burn in the lungs that results in hemorrhage, exudate, and edema histologically. The type of aspiration that produces the most severe physiologic and histologic alterations is partially digested food. PaO_2 decreases more than with any other type of aspiration, and lung damage is considerably more destructive[205] (see Table 16.9 and Figs. 16.15 to 16.19).

The variability of the effects is important to the obstetrician and the anesthesiologist. Because the necessity of a cesarean section cannot always be predicted, oral intake of anything but small sips of water or ice chips should be prohibited during labor. Eating food during labor is unnecessary and dangerous and should not be encouraged or allowed. Acid liquid can be neutralized safely and effectively with clear antacids or an H_2-receptor antagonist.[177-179,206,207] Partially digested food, however, causes significant hypoxia and lung damage even at a pH level as high as 5.9.[205] Therefore, the most important and critical preventive measure by the obstetrician is the advice not to eat before coming to the hospital, which should be accompanied by a thorough explanation of the necessity for such advice.

Table 16.9 Arterial Blood-Gas Tensions and pH of Dogs 30 Minutes After Aspiration of 2 cc/kg of Various Materials

Aspirate		Response		
Composition	pH	PaO_2 (mmHg)	$PaCO_2$ (mmHg)	pH
Saline	5.9	61	34	7.37
HCl	1.8	41	45	7.29
Food particles	5.9	34	51	7.19
Food particles	1.8	23	56	7.13

(From Gibbs and Modell,[233] with permission.)

Regional Anesthesia

ADVANTAGES OF REGIONAL ANESTHESIA

The patient is awake and can participate in the birth of her child.

There is little risk of drug depression or aspiration and no intubation difficulties.

Newborns generally have good neurobehavioral scores.

The mother can be given 100 percent oxygen.

The father is more likely to be allowed in the operating room.

DISADVANTAGES OF REGIONAL ANESTHESIA

Many patients prefer not to be awake.

An inadequate block may result.

Hypotension, perhaps the most common complication of regional anesthesia, occurs during 25 to 75 percent of spinal or epidural procedures.[208-214]

Total spinal anesthesia may occur.

Local anesthetic toxicity may occur.

Although extremely rare, permanent neurologic sequelae may occur.

There are several contraindications.

Hemorrhage is a firm contraindication to regional anesthesia. The blood volume of a hemorrhaging patient is too low for the vascular tree. One compensatory mechanism is vasoconstriction, which reduces the size of the vasculature, making it more commensurate with the blood volume. Major regional anesthesia produces sympathetic blockade, which not only hampers the compensatory mechanism but also dilates the vasculature and makes the discrepancy between volume and vasculature even greater.

Other contraindications to regional anesthesia include infection at the site, coagulopathy, patient refusal, and perhaps some varieties of heart disease. For example, most obstetricians and anesthesiologists have considered epidural anesthesia to be the anesthetic technique of choice for patients with mitral

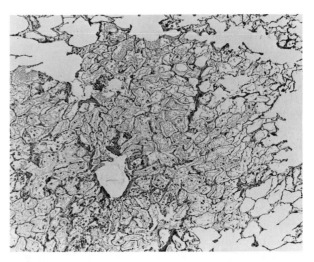

Fig. 16.17 Lung after aspiration of liquid acid. Note hemorrhage (red blood cells) and edema. Lung architecture has remained intact. (From Gibbs and Modell,[233] with permission.)

valvular disease, but have considered regional anesthesia to be contraindicated in other patients with aortic stenosis, pulmonary hypertension, and/or a right-to-left shunt. The latter group of patients cannot tolerate a decrease in systemic vascular resistance and/or a decrease in venous return of blood to the right side of the heart.[215] Recently there have been several reports of successful administration of epidural anesthesia to patients with aortic stenosis[216] and Eisenmenger syndrome.[217] However, it must be remembered that these reports represent small numbers of cases. Because regional anesthesia results in widespread sympathetic blockade, the pathophysiology of these forms of heart disease would most often dictate that regional anesthesia be provided. If one chooses to give regional anesthesia to such patients, it is clear that single-dose spinal or epidural anesthesia is inappropriate. Rather, there should be slow, careful induction of epidural anesthesia performed by an anesthesiologist with experience in the use of epidural anesthesia in high-risk obstetric patients. Intrathecal or epidural *opioid* analgesia does not decrease systemic vascular resistance and cause hypotension and has emerged as an attractive choice of analgesia *during labor.*[218-220]

Fetal distress as a contraindication to regional anesthesia is relative to the type and the degree of fetal distress. If the fetal distress is severe and acute, most often one should not take the additional time neces-

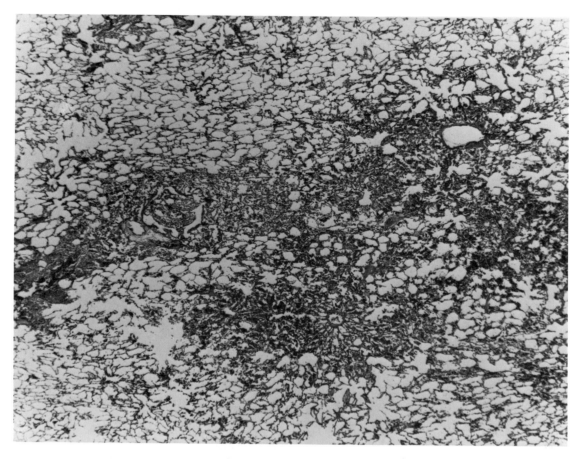

Fig. 16.18 Lung after aspiration of nonacid food particles at pH 5.9. Note inflammatory response around bronchioles and in lung tissues. Edema and hemorrhage exudates are visible. Most of the reaction surrounds the bronchioles. On higher magnification, food particles can be seen as well as polymorphonuclear leukocytes and macrophages. Lung architecture has remained intact. (From Gibbs and Modell,[233] with permission.)

sary to perform a regional technique. Also, if hypotension occurs, the risk to the already compromised fetus is increased. Lesser degrees of fetal distress may well be compatible with regional anesthesia.[221,222] For example, if an epidural catheter has been placed earlier, a partial level of anesthesia already exists, and there is hemodynamic stability, extension of epidural anesthesia may be appropriate for cesarean section. The anesthesiologist may give additional local anesthetic while the urethral catheter is inserted and the abdomen is prepared and draped. Often there will be satisfactory anesthesia when the surgeon is ready to make the skin incision. If not, the ongoing fetal heart rate pattern will dictate whether a delay is acceptable. When partial but inadequate epidural anesthesia results, one may consider supplemental local infiltra-

tion of local anesthetic. Because the anesthesiologist may have already given a large dose of local anesthetic, the obstetrician should consult with the anesthesiologist to determine the proper choice and concentration of local anesthetic in order to avoid local anesthetic toxicity. (For example, if the anesthesiologist has given lidocaine epidurally, and the patient has an area of inadequate anesthesia, the obstetrician might infiltrate the skin with 1 percent 2-chloroprocaine.)

An improved fetal heart rate tracing may allow one to wait for satisfactory extension of epidural anesthesia, or it may allow the anesthesiologist to perform epidural or spinal anesthesia de novo. Again, this illustrates the usefulness of continuing fetal heart rate monitoring before and during induction of anesthe-

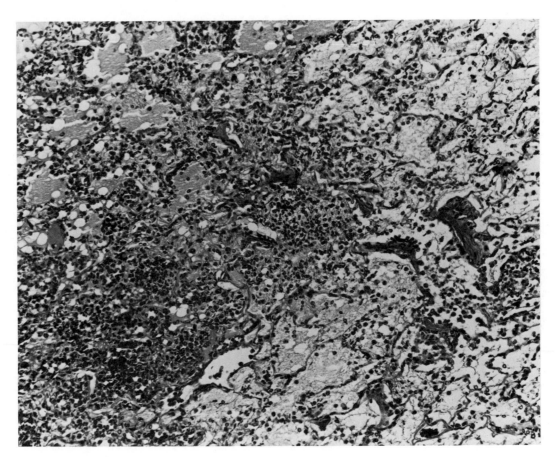

Fig. 16.19 Lung after aspiration of acid food particles at pH 1.8. Hemorrhage exudate and edema are more extensive. Also actual breakdown of alveolar walls and lung architecture has occurred. (From Gibbs and Modell,[233] with permission.)

sia. In the absence of satisfactory epidural anesthesia and in the presence of ongoing acute fetal distress, rapid sequence induction of general anesthesia is usually indicated for cesarean section. However, one should not indiscriminantly perform rapid sequence induction of general anesthesia. A history and/or suspicion of difficult intubation should prompt performance of either awake intubation or regional anesthesia, despite the presence of fetal distress. One should not endanger the mother in an effort to deliver a distressed fetus.

Finally, in healthy patients, the choice between epidural and spinal anesthesia will primarily rest with the anesthesiologist. Most consider spinal block to be easier and quicker to perform, and most believe that the resulting anesthesia will be more solid and complete. On the other hand, hypotension is probably more

frequent and the potential for spinal headache greater depending on the size of the needle used. Perhaps the most significant advantage of spinal anesthesia is that it requires considerably less local anesthetic, and therefore the potential for local anesthetic toxicity is less. Either technique is satisfactory, however, and should provide safe, effective anesthesia for mother, newborn, *and* obstetrician.

Local Anesthesia

The obstetrician can use local anesthesia to perform a cesarean section but must be thoroughly familiar with the recommended maximal dosages of the anesthetic used because large amounts of it may be necessary (Table 16.2). The obstetrician should give a dilute solution of local anesthetic (e.g., 0.5 percent lidocaine or 1.0 percent 2-chloroprocaine) to allow for administration of a sufficiently large volume. (It may be necessary to dilute a stock solution of 1 percent lidocaine or 2 percent 2-chloroprocaine to provide the recommended dilute solution.) The patient must be familiar with the procedure and willing to cooperate. When the technique is used successfully, the operation must be done skillfully and with minimal tissue trauma. Such requirements are often difficult to meet during an emergency cesarean section, particularly one for severe fetal distress or massive hemorrhage. When a major operation proceeds with local anesthesia, the initial stages of the operation may be accomplished easily, but later the need may arise to progress more rapidly or to use maneuvers that require more tugging and pulling than anticipated. For example, the fetal head may be impacted in the pelvis, or a uterine vein may be lacerated. In these situations the obstetrician must proceed with extreme haste, and a patient under local anesthesia may not be able to tolerate the manipulation. With an anesthesiologist in attendance, general anesthesia can be instituted immediately and the situation resolved. Therefore, the obstetrician must seriously consider all consequences before beginning an emergency cesarean section without an anesthesiologist in attendance.

Occasionally local anesthesia is elected in the patient for whom a regional block is technically impossible or contraindicated (e.g., after back injury or surgery) so that the patient can be awake for the delivery of the infant. In these cases, after delivery of the infant general anesthesia is usually initiated, if necessary, for completion of the operation.

PLACENTAL TRANSFER

FACTORS INFLUENCING PLACENTAL TRANSFER FROM MOTHER TO FETUS

Drug

    Molecular weight

    Lipid solubility

    Ionization, pH of blood

    Spatial configuration

continued

Maternal

    Uptake into bloodstream

    Distribution via circulation

    Uterine blood flow

        Amount

        Distribution (myometrium versus placenta)

Placental

    Circulation: intermittent spurting arterioles

    Lipoid membrane: Fick's law of simple diffusion

Fetal

    Circulation: ductus venosus, foramen ovale, ductus arteriosus

---

Essentially, all anesthetic agents except muscle relaxants cross the placenta.[223–226] Actually, even very large nonclinical doses of muscle relaxants will cross. That muscle relaxants do not generally cross the placental barrier is one of the major factors that enables anesthesiologists to utilize general anesthesia for cesarean section without causing fetal paralysis.

Placental transfer of any agent begins with uptake of the agent into the bloodstream of the mother and thus distribution to all internal organs, one of which is the uterus. The distribution of uterine blood flow determines the final common pathway to the uterus and placenta. Eighty percent of uterine blood flow goes to the area of the placenta, while 20 percent goes to the myometrium and thus never comes into contact with either placenta or fetus.[227] The intermittent spurting character of the maternal spiral arterioles also prevents a portion of the drug in blood distributed to the uterus from reaching the placental circulation and fetus. Because not all these spiral arterioles are functioning at the same time, some of the anesthetic bypasses the area of exchange and remains in the maternal circulation.

Once in the fetal circulation, a part of the drug will travel directly to the liver, where some will be "soaked up," some will be metabolized, and some will eventually reach the inferior vena cava. The other part will be shunted directly across the ductus venosus into the inferior vena cava. That portion of drug reaching the inferior vena cava will proceed to the right atrium, where some will enter the right ventricle, and hence to the pulmonary artery, where all but 10 percent will be shunted directly across the ductus arteriosus to the lower part of the systemic circulation, bypassing the cerebral circulation. The remainder of the drug that reaches the right atrium will be shunted across the foramen ovale into the left atrium, left ventricle, and out the aorta into the upper part of the fetal circulation, which includes the brain, where the greatest effect ocurs. Thus, even with this very brief description of the fetal circulation, it is easy to see how the mother can be affected by a certain concentration of drug without the fetus being affected.

Because the placenta has the properties of a lipid membrane, most drugs and all anesthetic agents cross by a mechanism called simple diffusion. The physico-chemical factors governing transfer across a lipid membrane by simple diffusion is described by Fick's law[223]:

$$Q/T = [K\,A(C_m - C_f)]/X$$

where Q/T is the rate of diffusion, K is the diffusion constant of the drug, A is the available area, C_m is the maternal blood concentration, C_f is the fetal blood concentration, and X is the thickness of the membrane. Thus the amount of drug that crosses the placenta increases as concentrations in the maternal circulation and total area of the membrane increase and decreases as the thickness of the membrane increases. The effective surface area of the human placenta is approximately 11 m², and its thickness is approximately 3.5 μm. The diffusion constant, K, accounts for the properties of the drug itself, including molecular weight, spatial configuration, degree of ionization, lipid solubility, and protein binding. For example, bupivacaine is highly protein bound, a characteristic that some believe explains why fetal blood concentrations of it are so much lower than with other local anesthetics. On the other hand, bupivacaine is also highly lipid soluble, and the more lipid soluble a drug is, the more freely it passes through a lipid membrane. Furthermore, once in the fetal system, lipid solubility enables the drug to be taken up by fetal tissues rapidly, which again contributes to the lower blood concentration of the agent.

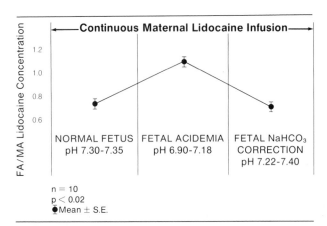

Fig. 16.20 Fetal–maternal arterial (FA/MA) lidocaine ratios were significantly higher ($p < 0.02$) during fetal acidemia than during control or where pH was corrected with bicarbonate. $N = 10$; mean $\pm$ SE. (From Biehl et al,[228] with permission.)

The degree of ionization of a drug is also important. Most drugs exist in both an ionized and nonionized state. It is the nonionized state that freely crosses lipid membranes. Drugs such as muscle relaxants are highly ionized; thus very little crosses to the fetus. The degree of ionization is influenced by the pH of the medium. For example, local anesthetics are more ionized at lower pH values. Such factors become clinically relevant in obstetrics, because occasionally the pH of the mother's blood will be 7.4, while that of the fetus will be 7.0 or less. In this instance, the nonionized portion of the drug in the maternal circulation crosses to the fetus, becomes ionized, and thus remains in the fetus (Fig. 16.20).[228]

SUMMARY

Obstetric anesthesia has much to offer the obstetric patient. However, as in many other areas of medicine, anesthesia can be dangerous when used inappropriately. To make best use of the available techniques, cooperation and continued communication must exist between all parties: obstetrician, anesthesiologist, and patient.

REFERENCES

1. Orkin FW: The Geographical Distribution of Anesthesia Care Providers in the United States. Committee on Manpower, American Society of Anesthesiologists, Park Ridge, IL, 1983

2. Joint Statement on the Optimal Goals for Anesthesia Care in Obstetrics. American Society of Anesthesiologists/American College of Obstetricians and Gynecologists, Washington, DC 1988

3. Melzack R, Taenzer P, Feldman P, Kinch RA: Labour is still painful after prepared childbirth training. Can Assoc Med J 125:357, 1981

4. Burns JK: Relation between blood levels of cortisol and duration of human labour. J Physiol (Lond) 254:12P, 1976

5. Tuimala RJ, Kauppila JI, Haapalahti J: Response of pituitary–adrenal axis on partial stress. Obstet Gynecol 46:275, 1975

6. Lederman RP, McCann DS, Work B Jr: Endogenous plasma epinephrine and norepinephrine in last-trimester pregnancy and labor. Am J Obstet Gynecol 129:5, 1977

7. Falconer AD, Powles AB: Plasma noradrenaline levels during labour: influence of elective lumbar epidural blockade. Anaesthesia 37:416, 1982

8. Goland RS, Wardlaw SI, Stark RI, Frantz AG: Human plasma beta-endorphin during pregnancy, labor, and delivery. J Clin Endocrinol Metab 52:74, 1981

9. Fletcher JE, Thomas TA, Hill RG: Beta-endorphin and parturition. Lancet 1:310, 1980

10. Rossier J, French ED, Rivier C et al: Foot-shock induced β-endorphin levels in blood but not brain. Nature 270:618, 1977

11. Dubois M, Pickar D, Cohen MR et al: Surgical stress in humans is accompanied by an increase in plasma beta-endorphin immunoreactivity. Life Sci 29:1249, 1981

12. Wardlaw SL, Stark RI, Bazi L, Frantz AG: Plasma beta-endorphin and beta-lipotropin in human fetus at delivery: correlation with arterial pH and Po_2. J Clin Endocrinol Metab 49:888, 1979

13. Yanagida H, Corssen G: Respiratory distress and beta-endorphin–like immunoreactivity in humans. Anesthesiology 55:515, 1981

14. Lederman RP, Lederman E, Work BA Jr, McCann DS: The relationship of maternal anxiety, plasma catecholamines, and plasma cortisol to progress in labor. Am J Obstet Gynecol 132:495, 1978

15. Adamsons K, Mueller-Heubach E, Myers RE: Production of fetal asphyxia in the rhesus monkey by administration of catecholamines to the mother. Am J Obstet Gynecol 109:248, 1971

16. Rosenfeld CR, Barton MD, Meschia G: Effects of epinephrine on distribution of blood flow in the pregnant ewe. Am J Obstet Gynecol 124:156, 1976

17. Roman-Ponce H, Thatcher WW, Caton D et al: Effects of thermal stress and epinephrine on uterine blood flow in ewes. J Anim Sci 46:167, 1978

18. Myers RE: Maternal psychological stress and fetal asphyxia: a study in the monkey. Am J Obstet Gynecol 122:47, 1975

19. Morishima HO, Yeh M-N, James LS: Reduced uterine blood flow and fetal hypoxemia with acute maternal stress: experimental observation in the pregnant baboon. Am J Obstet Gynecol 134:270, 1979

20. Morishima HO, Pedersen H, Finster M: The influence of maternal psychological stress on the fetus. Am J Obstet Gynecol 131:286, 1978

21. Copher DE, Huber CP: Heart rate response of the human fetus to induced maternal hypoxia. Am J Obstet Gynecol 98:320, 1967

22. Maltau JM, Eielsen OV, Stokke KT: Effect of the stress during labor on the concentration of cortisol and estriol in maternal plasma. Am J Obstet Gynecol 134:681, 1979

23. Buchan PC, Milne MK, Browning MCK: The effect of continuous epidural blockade on plasma 11-hydroxycorticosteroid concentrations in labour. J Obstet Gynaecol Br Commonw 80:974, 1973

24. Thorton CA, Carrie LES, Sayers I et al: A comparison of the effect of extradural and parenteral analgesia on maternal plasma cortisol concentrations during labour and the puerperium. Br J Obstet Gynaecol 83:631, 1976

25. Abboud TK, Sarkis F, Hung TT et al: Effects of epidural anesthesia during labor on maternal plasma beta-endorphin levels. Anesthesiology 59:1, 1983

26. Abboud TK, Artal R, Henriksen EH et al: Effects of spinal anesthesia on maternal circulating catecholamines. Am J Obstet Gynecol 142:252, 1982

27. Myers R, Myers SE: Use of sedative, analgesic, and anesthetic drugs during labor and delivery: bane or boon? Am J Obstet Gynecol 133:83, 1979

28. Pearson JF, Davies P: The effect of continuous lumbar epidural analgesia upon fetal acid–base status during the first stage of labour. J Obstet Gynaecol Br Commonw 81:971, 1974

29. Pearson JF, Davies P: The effect of continuous lumbar epidural analgesia upon fetal acid–base status during the second stage of labour. J Obstet Gynaecol Br Commonw 81:975, 1974

30. Beazley JM, Leaver EP, Morewood JHM, Bircumshaw J: Relief of pain in labour. Lancet 1:1033, 1967

31. Jaffee JH, Martin WR: Narcotic analgesics and antagonists. p. 245. In Goodman LS, Gilman A (eds): The Pharmacological Basis of Therapeutics. 5th Ed. Macmillan, New York, 1975

32. Bonica JJ: Principles and Practice of Obstetric Analgesia and Anesthesia. p. 234. FA Davis, Philadelphia, 1967

33. Shute E, Davis ME: The effect on the infant of morphine administered in labor. Surg Gynecol Obstet 57:727, 1933

34. Kuhnert BR, Kuhnert PM, Tu AL, Lin DCK: Meperidine and normeperidine levels following meperidine administration during labor. II. Fetus and neonate. Am J Obstet Gynecol 133:909, 1979

35. Pittman KA, Smyth RD, Losada M et al: Human perinatal distribution of butorphanol. Am J Obstet Gynecol 138:797, 1980

36. Shnider S, Moya F: Effects of meperidine on the newborn infant. Am J Obstet Gynecol 89:1009, 1964

37. Way WL, Costley EC, Way EL: Respiratory sensitivity of the newborn infant to meperidine and morphine. Clin Pharmacol Ther 6:454, 1965

38. Gillam JS, Hunter GW, Darner CB, Thompson GR: Meperidine hydrochloride and alphaprodine hydrochloride as obstetric analgesic agents. Am J Obstet Gynecol 75:1105, 1958

39. Powell PO Jr, Savage JE: Nisentil in obstetrics. Obstet Gynecol 2:658, 1953

40. Gordon DWS, Pinker GD: Increased pethidine dosage in obstetrics associated with the use of nalorphine. J Obstet Gynaecol Br Commonw 65:606, 1958

41. Walker PA: Drugs used in labour: an obstetrician's view. Br J Anaesth 45(suppl):787, 1973

42. Hodgkinson R, Huff RW, Hayashi RH, Husain FJ: Double-blind comparison of maternal analgesia and neonatal neurobehaviour following intravenous butorphanol and meperidine. J Int Med Res 7:224, 1979

43. Quilligan EJ, Keegan KA, Donahue MJ: Double-blind comparison of intravenously injected butorphanol and meperidine in parturients. Int J Gynaecol Obstet 18:363, 1980

44. Miller FC, Mueller E, McCart D: Maternal and fetal response to alphaprodine during labor: a preliminary study. J Reprod Med 27:439, 1982

45. Rayburn WF, Smith CV, Parriott JE, Woods RE: Randomized comparison of meperidine and fentanyl during labor. Obstet Gynecol 74:604, 1989

46. Committee on Obstetrics: Maternal and Fetal Medicine: Naloxone Use in Newborns. American College of Obstetricians and Gynecologists, Washington, DC, 1989

47. Brackbill Y, Kane J, Manniello RL, Abramson D: Obstetric premedication and infant outcome. Am J Obstet Gynecol 118:377, 1974

48. Stechler G: Newborn attention as affected by medication during labor. Science 144:315, 1964

49. Corke BC: Neurobehavioural responses of the newborn: the effect of different forms of maternal analgesia. Anaesthesia 32:539, 1977

50. Kolata GB: Scientists attack report that obstetrical medications endanger children. Science 204:391, 1979

51. Nimmo WS, Wilson J, Prescott LF: Narcotic analgesics and delayed gastric emptying during labour. Lancet 1:890, 1975

52. Kuhnert BR, Kuhnert PM, Tu AL et al: Meperidine and normeperidine levels following meperdine administration during labor. I. Mother. Am J Obstet Gynecol 133:904, 1979

53. Kuhnert BR, Philipson EH, Kuhnert PM, Syracuse CD: Disposition of meperidine and normeperidine following multiple doses during labor. I. Mother. Am J Obstet Gynecol 151:406, 1985

54. Kuhnert BR, Kuhnert PM, Philipson EH, Syracuse CD: Disposition of meperidine and normeperidine following multiple doses during labor. II. Fetus and neonate. Am J Obstet Gynecol 151:410, 1985

55. Lazebnik N, Kuhnert BR, Carr PC et al: Intravenous, deltoid, or gluteus administration of meperidine during labor? Am J Obstet Gynecol 160:1184, 1989

56. Forrest WH Jr, Bellville JW: Respiratory effects of alphaprodine in man. Obstet Gynecol 31:61, 1968

57. Maduska AL, Hajghassemali M: A double-blind comparison of butorphanol and meperidine in labour: maternal pain relief and effect on the newborn. Can Anaesth Soc J 25:398, 1978

58. Nagashima H, Karamanian A, Malovany R et al: Respiratory and circulatory effects of intravenous butorphanol and morphine. Clin Pharmacol Ther 19:738, 1976

59. Kallos T, Caruso FS: Respiratory effects of butorphanol and pethidine. Anaesthesia 34:633, 1979

60. Romagnoli A, Keats AS: Ceiling effect for respiratory depression by nalbuphine. Clin Pharmacol Ther 27:478, 1980

61. Wilson CM, McClean E, Moore J, Dundee JW: A double-blind comparison of intramuscular pethidine and nalbuphine in labour. Anaesthesia 41:1207, 1986

62. Robinson JO, Rosen M, Evans JM et al: Self-administered intravenous and intramuscular pethidine. Anesthesia 35:763, 1980

63. Podlas J, Breland BD: Patient-controlled analgesia with nalbuphine during labor. Obstet Gynecol 70:202, 1987

64. Rayburn W, Leuschen MP, Earl R et al: Intravenous meperidine during labor: a randomized comparison between nursing — and patient-controlled administration. Obstet Gynecol 74:702, 1989

65. Clutton-Brach JC: Some pain threshold studies with particular reference to thiopentone. Anaesthesia 15:71, 1960

66. Dundee JW: Alterations in response to somatic pain associated with anaesthesia. II. The effect of thiopentone and pentobarbitone. Br J Anaesth 32:407, 1960

67. Irving FC: Advantages and disadvantages of the barbiturates in obstetrics. RI Med J 28:493, 1945

68. Powe CE, Kiem IM, Fromhagen C, Cavanagh D: Propiomazine hydrochloride in obstetrical analgesia: a controlled study of 520 patients. JAMA 181:290, 1962

69. Benson C, Benson RC: Hydroxyzine–meperidine analgesia and neonatal response. Am J Obstet Gynecol 84:37, 1962

70. Zsigmond EK, Patterson RL: Double-blind evaluation of hydroxyzine hydrochloride in obstetric anesthesia. Anesth Analg 46:275, 1967

71. Owen JR, Irani SF, Blair AW: Effect of diazepam administered to mothers during labour on temperature regulation of neonate. Arch Dis Child 47:107, 1972

72. Cree JE, Meyer J, Hailey DM: Diazepam in labour: its metabolism and effect on the clinical condition and thermogenesis of the newborn. Br Med J 4:251, 1973

73. Hahn E: An Atlas of Fetal Heart Rate Patterns. Hardy Press, New Haven, CT, 1968

74. Yeh SY, Paul RH, Cordero L, Hon EH: A study of diazepam during labor. Obstet Gynecol 43:363, 1974

75. Schiff D, Chan G, Stern L: Fixed drug combinations and the displacement of bilirubin from albumin. Pediatrics 48:139, 1971

76. Wilson CM, Dundee JW, Moore J et al: A comparison of the early pharmacokinetics of midazolam in pregnant and nonpregnant women. Anaesthesia 42:1057, 1987

77. Ravlo O, Carl P, Crawford ME et al: A randomized comparison between midazolam and thiopental for elective cesarean section anesthesia. II. Neonates. Anesth Analg 68:234, 1989

78. Bland BAR, Lawes EG, Duncan PW et al: Comparison of midazolam and thiopental for rapid sequence anesthetic induction for elective cesarean section. Anesth Analg 66:1165, 1987

79. Camann W, Cohen MB, Ostheimer GW: Is midazolam desirable for sedation in parturients? Anesthesiology 65:441, 1986

80. Crawford JS: The second thousand epidural blocks in an obstetric hospital practice. Br J Anaesth 44:1277, 1972

81. Abboud TK, Khoo SS, Miller F et al: Maternal, fetal, and neonatal responses after epidural anesthesia with bupivacaine, 2-chloroprocaine, or lidocaine. Anesth Analg 61:638, 1982

82. Jouppila R, Jouppila P, Karinen JM, Hollmen A: Segmental epidural analgesia in labour: related to the progress of labour, fetal malposition and instrumental delivery. Acta Obstet Gynaecol Scand 58:135, 1979

83. Kandel PF, Spoerel WE, Kinch RAH: Continuous epidural analgesia for labour and delivery: review of 1000 cases. Can Med Assoc J 95:947, 1966

84. Matadial L, Cibils LA: The effect of epidural anesthesia on uterine activity and blood pressure. Am J Obstet Gynecol 125:846, 1976

85. Datta S, Kitzmiller JL, Naulty JS et al: Acid–base status of diabetic mothers and their infants following spinal anesthesia for cesarean section. Anesth Analg 61:662, 1982

86. James FM, Greiss FC Jr, Kemp RA: An evaluation of vasopressor therapy for maternal hypotension during spinal anesthesia. Anesthesiology 33:25, 1970

87. Brizgys RV, Dailey PA, Shnider SM et al: The incidence and neonatal effects of maternal hypotension during epidural anesthesia for cesarean section. Anesthesiology 67:782, 1987

88. Datta S, Brown WU: Acid–base status in diabetic mothers and their infants following general or spinal anesthesia for cesarean section. Anesthesiology 47:272, 1977

89. Kenepp NB, Shelley WC, Kumar S et al: Effects on newborn of hydration with glucose in patients undergoing caesarean section with regional anesthesia. Lancet 1:645, 1980

90. Ralston DH, Shnider SM, deLorimier AA: Effects of equipotent ephedrine, mataraminol, mephentermine, and methoxamine on uterine blood flow in the pregnant ewe. Anesthesiology 40:354, 1974

91. Ralston DH, Shnider SM: The fetal and neonatal effects of regional anesthesia in obstetrics. Anesthesiology 48:34, 1978

92. Albright GA: Cardiac arrest following regional anesthesia with etidocaine or bupivacaine. Anesthesiology 51:285, 1979

93. deJong RH, Gamble CA, Bonin JD: Bupivacaine-induced cardiac arrhythmias and plasma cation concentrations in normokalemic cats. Regional Anesth 8:104, 1983

94. Clarkson CW, Hondeghem LM: Mechanism for bupivacaine depression of cardiac conduction: fast block of sodium channels during the action potential with slow recovery from block during diastole. Anesthesiology 62:396, 1985

95. Morishima HO, Pedersen H, Finster M et al: Bupivacaine toxicity in pregnant and nonpregnant ewes. Anesthesiology 63:134, 1985

96. Abbott Laboratories: Letter to doctors: urgent new recommendations about bupivacaine. Astra Pharma-

ceutical Products, Inc., Breon Laboratories, Westboro, MA, 1984

97. Writer WDR, Davies JM, Strunin L: Trial by media: the bupivacaine story. Can Anaesth Soc J 31:1, 1984

98. Moore DC, Batra MS: The components of an effective test dose prior to epidural block. Anesthesiology 55:693, 1981

99. Abraham RA, Harris AP, Maxwell LG, Kaplow S: The efficacy of 1.5 percent lidocaine with 7.5 percent dextrose and epinephrine as an epidural test dose for obstetrics. Anesthesiology 64:116, 1986

100. Leighton BL, Norris MC, Sosis M et al: Limitations of epinephrine as a marker of intravascular injection in laboring women. Anesthesiology 66:688, 1987

101. Moore DC, Crawford RD, Scurlock JE: Severe hypoxia and acidosis following local anesthetic-induced convulsions. Anesthesiology 53:259, 1980

102. Dripps RD, Eckenhoff JE, Vandam LD: Long-term follow-up of patients who received 10,098 spinal anesthetics: failure to discover major neurological sequelae. JAMA 156:1486, 1954

103. Ravindran RS, Bond VK, Tasch MD et al: Prolonged neural blockade following regional analgesia with 2-chloroprocaine. Anesth Analg 59:447, 1980

104. Reisner LS, Hochman BN, Plumer MH: Persistent neurologic deficit and adhesive arachnoiditis following intrathecal 2-chloroprocaine injection. Anesth Analg 59:452, 1980

105. Moore DC, Spierdijk J, Van Kleef JD et al: Chloroprocaine neurotoxicity: four additional cases. Anesth Analg 61:155, 1982

106. Gissen AJ, Datta S, Lambert D: The chloroprocaine controversy. II. Is chloroprocaine neurotoxic? Regional Anesth 9:135, 1984

107. Fibuch EE, Opper SE: Back pain following epidurally administered Nesacaine-MPF. Anesth Analg 69:113, 1989

108. Levy L, Randel GI, Pandit SK: Does chloroprocaine (Nesacaine MPF) for epidural anesthesia increase the incidence of backache? Anesthesiology 71:476, 1989

109. Cole JT: Maternal obstetric paralysis. Am J Obstet Gynecol 52:374, 1946

110. Goldstein PJ: The lithotomy position. p. 142. In Martin JT (ed): Positioning in Anesthesia and Surgery. WB Saunders, Philadelphia, 1978

111. Deppe G, Hercule J, Gleicher N: Sciatic nerve injury complicating surgical removal of retroperitoneal tumor. Acta Obstet Gynaecol Scand 63:369, 1984

112. Ong BY, Cohen MM, Esmail A et al: Paresthesias and motor dysfunction after labor and delivery. Anesth Analg 66:18, 1987

113. Carbaat PAT, van Crevel H: Lumbar puncture headache: controlled study on the preventive effect of 24 hours' bed rest. Lancet 2:1133, 1981

114. Craft JB, Epstein BS, Coakley CS: Prophylaxis of dural-puncture headache with epidural saline. Anesth Analg 52:228, 1973

115. Szeinfeld M, Ihmeidan IH, Moser MM et al: Epidural blood patch: evaluation of the volume and spread of blood injected into the epidural space. Anesthesiology 64:820, 1986

116. Ravindran RS: Epidural autologous blood patch on an outpatient basis. Anesth Analg 63:962, 1984

117. DiGiovanni AJ, Galbert MW, Wahle WM: Epidural injection of autologous blood for postlumbar-puncture headache. II. Additional clinical experiences and laboratory investigation. Anesth Analg 51:226, 1972

118. Abouleish E, de la Vega S, Blendinger I, Tio TO: Long-term follow-up of epidural blood patch. Anesth Analg 54:459, 1975

119. Abouleish E, Wadhwa RK, de la Vega S et al: Regional analgesia following epidural blood patch. Anesth Analg 54:634, 1975

120. Loeser EA, Hill GE, Bennett GM, Sederberg JH: Time vs. success rate for epidural blood patch. Anesthesiology 49:147, 1978

121. Quaynor H, Corbey M: Extradural blood patch—why delay? Br J Anaesth 57:538, 1985

122. Berrettini WH, Simmons-Alling S, Nurnberger JI: Epidural blood patch does not prevent headache after lumbar puncture. Lancet 1:856, 1987

123. Cheek TG, Banner R, Sauter J, Gutsche BB: Prophylactic extradural blood patch is effective. Br J Anaesth 61:340, 1988

124. Naulty JS, Smith R, Ross R: The effect of changes in labor analgesic practice on labor outcome, abstracted. Anesthesiology 69:A660, 1988

125. Friedman EA: Effects of drugs on uterine contractility. Anesthesiology 26:409, 1965

126. Committee on Obstetrics: Maternal and Fetal Medicine: Dystocia: Etiology, Diagnosis, and Management Guidelines. American College of Obstetricians and Gynecologists, Washington, DC, 1983

127. Peisner DB, Rosen MG: Transition from latent to active labor. Obstet Gynecol 68:448, 1986

128. Chestnut DH, Vandewalker GE, Owen CL et al: The influence of continuous epidural bupivacaine analgesia on the second stage of labor and method of delivery in nulliparous women. Anesthesiology 66:774, 1987

129. Kilpatrick SJ, Laros RK: Characteristics of normal labor. Obstet Gynecol 74:85, 1989

130. Maresh M, Choong KH, Beard RW: Delayed pushing with lumbar epidural analgesia in labour. Br J Obstet Gynaecol 90:623, 1983

131. Cohen WR: Influence of the duration of second stage labor on perinatal outcome and puerperal morbidity. Obstet Gynecol 49:266, 1977

132. Pearson JF: The effect of continuous lumbar epidural analgesia on maternal acid–base balance and arterial lactate concentration during the second stage of labour. J Obstet Gynaecol Br Commonw 80:225, 1973

133. Committee on Obstetrics: Maternal and Fetal Medicine: Obstetric Forceps. American College of Obstetricians and Gynecologists, Washington, DC, 1988

134. Robinson JO, Rosen M, Evans JM et al: Maternal opinion about analgesia for labor. Anaesthesia 35:1173, 1980

135. Philipsen T, Jensen NH: Epidural block or parenteral pethidine as analgesic in labour: a randomized study concerning progress in labour and instrumental deliveries. Eur J Obstet Gynecol Reprod Biol 30:27, 1989

136. Phillips KC, Thomas TA: Second stage of labour with or without extradural analgesia. Anaesthesia 38:972, 1983

137. Chestnut DH, Bates JN, Choi WW: Continuous infusion epidural analgesia with lidocaine: efficacy and influence during the second stage of labor. Obstet Gynecol 69:323, 1987

138. Johnsrud ML, Dale PO, Lovland B: Benefits of continuous infusion epidural analgesia throughout vaginal delivery. Acta Obstet Gynecol Scand 67:355, 1988

139. Lowensohn RI, Paul RH, Fales S et al: Intrapartum epidural anesthesia: an evaluation of effects on uterine activity. Obstet Gynecol 44:388, 1974

140. Maltau JM, Andersen HT: Epidural anaesthesia as an alternative to caesarean section in the treatment of prolonged, exhaustive labour. Acta Anaesthesiol Scand 19:349, 1975

141. Craft JB, Epstein BS, Coakley CS: Effect of lidocaine with epinephrine versus lidocaine (plain) on induced labor. Anesth Analg 51:243, 1972

142. Abboud TK, David S, Nagappala S et al: Maternal, fetal, and neonatal effects of lidocaine with and without epinephrine for epidural anesthesia in obstetrics. Anesth Analg 63:973, 1984

143. Abboud TK, Sheik-ol-Eslam A, Yanagi T et al: Safety and efficacy of epinephrine added to bupivacaine for lumbar epidural analgesia in obstetrics. Anesth Analg 64:585, 1985

144. Abboud TK, DerSarkissian L, Terrasi J et al: Comparative maternal, fetal, and neonatal effects of chloroprocaine with and without epinephrine for epidural anesthesia in obstetrics. Anesth Analg 66:71, 1987

145. Eisenach JC, Grice SC, Dewan DM: Epinephrine enhances analgesia produced by epidural bupivacaine during labor. Anesth Analg 66:447, 1987

146. Johnson WL, Winter WW, Eng M et al: Effect of pudendal, spinal, and peridural block anesthesia on the second stage of labor. Am J Obstet Gynecol 113:166, 1972

147. Morrison DH, Smedstad KG: Continuous infusion epidurals for obstetric analgesia. Can Anaesth Soc J 32:101, 1985

148. Nadeau S, Elliott RD: Continuous bupivacaine infusion during labour: effects on analgesia and delivery, abstracted. Can Anaesth Soc J 32:S70, 1985

149. Bogod DG, Rosen M, Rees GAD: Extradural infusion of 0.125 percent bupivacaine at 10 ml h^{-1} to women during labour. Br J Anaesth 59:325, 1987

150. Gaylard DG, Wilson IH, Balmer HGR: An epidural infusion technique for labor. Anaesthesia 42:1098, 1987

151. Hicks JA, Jenkins JG, Newton MC et al: Continuous epidural infusion of 0.075 percent bupivacaine for pain relief in labour: a comparison with intermittent top-ups of 0.5 percent bupivacaine. Anaesthesia 43:289, 1988

152. Smedstad KG, Morrison DH: A comparative study of continuous and intermittent epidural analgesia for labour and delivery. Can J Anaesth 35:234, 1988

153. Chestnut DH, Owen CL, Bates JN et al: Continuous infusion epidural analgesia during labor: a randomized, double-blind comparison of 0.0625 percent bupivacaine/0.0002 percent fentanyl versus 0.125 percent bupivacaine. Anesthesiology 68:754, 1988

154. Goodfellow CF, Hull MGR, Swaab DF et al: Oxytocin deficiency at delivery with epidural analgesia. Br J Obstet Gynaecol 90:214, 1983

155. Bates RG, Helm CW, Duncan A, Edmonds DK: Uterine activity in the second stage of labour and the effect of epidural analgesia. Br J Obstet Gynaecol 92:1246, 1985

156. Shnider SM, Asling JH, Holl JW, Margolis AJ: Paracervical block anesthesia in obstetrics. I. Fetal complications and neonatal morbidity. Am J Obstet Gynecol 107:619, 1970

157. Tafeen CH, Freedman HL, Harris H: Combination continuous paracervical and continued pudendal nerve block anesthesia in labor. Am J Obstet Gynecol 100:55, 1968

158. Teramo K, Widholm O: Studies of the effects of anesthetics on foetus. I. The effect of paracervical block with mepivacaine upon fetal-base values. Acta Obstet Gynaecol Scand 46(suppl 2):1, 1967

159. Gibbs CP, Noel SC: Response of arterial segments from gravid human uterus to multiple concentrations of lignocaine. Br J Anaesth 45:409, 1977

160. Greiss FC Jr, Still JG, Anderson SG: Effects of local

anesthetic agents on the uterine vasculatures and myometrium. Am J Obstet Gynecol 124:889, 1976

161. Freeman RK, Gutierrez NA, Ray ML et al: Fetal cardiac response to paracervical block anesthesia. Part I. Am J Obstet Gynecol 113:583, 1972

162. Gibbs CP, Krischer J, Peckham BM et al: Obstetric anesthesia: a national survey. Anesthesiology 65:288, 1986

163. Philipson EH, Kuhnert BR, Syracuse CD: Maternal, fetal, and neonatal lidocaine levels following local perineal infiltration. Am J Obstet Gynecol 149:403, 1984

164. Klink EW: Perineal nerve block: an anatomic and clinical study in the female. Obstet Gynecol 1:137, 1953

165. Munson ES, Embro WJ: Enflurane, isoflurane and halothane and isolated human uterine muscle. Anesthesiology 46:11, 1977

166. Ranney B, Stanage WF: Advantages of local anesthesia for cesarean section. Obstet Gynecol 45:163, 1975

167. James FM III, Crawford JS, Hopkinson R et al: A comparison of general anesthesia and lumbar epidural analgesia for elective cesarean section. Anesth Analg 56:228, 1977

168. Magno R, Kjellmer I, Karlsson K: Anaesthesia for cesarean section. III. Effects of epidural analgesia on the respiratory adaptation of the newborn in elective caesarean section. Acta Anaesthesiol Scand 20:73, 1976

169. Datta S, Alper MH: Anesthesia for cesarean section. Anesthesiology 53:142, 1980

170. Scanlon JW, Brown WU Jr, Weiss JB, Alper MH: Neurobehavioral responses of newborn infants after maternal epidural anesthesia. Anesthesiology 40:121, 1974

171. Hodgkinson R, Bhatt M, Kim SS et al: Neonatal neurobehavioral tests following cesarean section under general and spinal anesthesia. Am J Obstet Gynecol 132:670, 1978

172. McGuinness GA, Merkow AJ, Kennedy RL, Erenberg A: Epidural anesthesia with bupivacaine for cesarean section: neonatal blood levels and neurobehavioral responses. Anesthesiology 49:270, 1978

173. Marx GF, Finster M: Difficulty in endotracheal intubation associated with obstetric anesthesia. Anesthesiology 51:364, 1979

174. Gibbs CP, Rolbin SH, Norman P: Cause and prevention of maternal aspiration. Anesthesiology 61:111, 1984

175. Turnbull AC, Tindall VR, Robson G et al: Report on Confidential Enquiries Into Maternal Deaths in England and Wales 1979–1981. Her Majesty's Stationery Office, London, 1986

176. Morgan M: Anaesthetic contribution to maternal mortality. Br J Anaesth 59:842, 1987

177. Gibbs CP, Spohr L, Schmidt D: The effectiveness of sodium citrate as an antacid. Anesthesiology 57:44, 1982

178. Gibbs CP, Banner TC: Effectiveness of Bicitra as a preoperative antacid. Anesthesiology 61:97, 1984

179. Chen CT, Toung TJ, Cameron JL: Alka-Seltzer® for prophylactic use in prevention of acid aspiration pneumonia. Anesthesiology 57:A103, 1982

180. Gibbs CP, Schwartz DJ, Wynne JW et al: Antacid pulmonary aspiration in the dog. Anesthesiology 51:380, 1979

181. Crawford JA, Burton M, Davies P: Time and lateral tilt at caesarean section. Br J Anaesth 44:477, 1972

182. Datta S, Ostheimer GW, Weiss JB et al: Neonatal effect of prolonged anesthetic induction for cesarean section. Obstet Gynecol 58:331, 1981

183. Archer GW, Marx GF: Arterial oxygen tension during apnoea in parturient women. Br J Anaesth 46:358, 1974

184. Norris MC, Dewan DM: Preoxygenation for cesarean section: a comparison of two techniques. Anesthesiology 62:827, 1985

185. Kosaka Y, Takahashi T, Mark LC: Intravenous thiobarbiturate anesthesia for cesarean section. Anesthesiology 31:489, 1969

186. Peltz B, Sinclair DM: Induction agents for cesarean section: a comparison of thiopental and ketamine. Anaesthesia 28:37, 1973

187. Sellick BA: Cricoid pressure to control regurgitation of stomach contents during induction of anesthesia. Lancet 2:404, 1961

188. Sellick BA: Rupture of the oesophagus following cricoid pressure? Anaesthesia 37:213, 1982

189. American Society of Anesthesiologists: Standards for Basic Intra-Operative Monitoring. American Society of Anesthesiologists, Park Ridge, IL, 1986

190. Marx GF, Joshi CW, Orkin LR: Placental transmission of nitrous oxide. Anesthesiology 32:429, 1970

191. Moir DD: Anaesthesia for caesarean section: an evaluation of a method using low concentrations of halothane and 50 percent of oxygen. Br J Anaesth 42:136, 1970

192. Warren TM, Datta S, Ostheimer GW et al: Comparison of the maternal and neonatal effects of halothane, enflurane, and isoflurane for cesarean delivery. Anesth Analg 62:516, 1983

193. Andersen TW, DePadua CB, Stenger V, Prystowsky H: Cardiovascular effects of rapid intravenous injection of synthetic oxytocin during elective cesarean section. Clin Pharmacol Ther 6:345, 1965

194. Orkin LR, Shapiro G: Admission assessment and general monitoring. Int Anesthesiol Clin 21:3, 1983

195. Aldrete JA, Kroulik D: A postanesthetic recovery score. Anesth Analg 49:924, 1970

196. Fisher TL: Responsibility for care in recovery rooms. Can Med Assoc J 102:78, 1970

197. Roberts RB, Shirley MA: Reducing the risk of acid aspiration during cesarean section. Anesth Analg 53:859, 1974

198. Spence AA, Moir DD, Finlay WEI: Observations on intragastric pressure. Anaesthesia 22:249, 1967

199. Greenan J: The cardio-oesophageal junction. Br J Anaesth 33:432, 1961

200. Williams MH: Variable significance of heartburn. Am J Obstet Gynecol 42:814, 1941

201. Attia RR, Ebeid AM, Fischer JE, Goudsouzian NG: Maternal fetal and placental gastrin concentrations. Anaesthesia 37:18, 1982

202. Christofides ND, Ghatei MA, Bloom SR et al: Decreased plasma motilin concentrations in pregnancy. Br Med J 285:1453, 1982

203. Davison JS, Davison MC, Hay DM: Gastric emptying time in late pregnancy and labour. J Obstet Gynaecol Br Commonw 77:37, 1970

204. Holdsworth JD: Relationship between stomach contents and analgesia in labour. Br J Anaesth 50:1145, 1978

205. Schwartz DJ, Wynne JW, Gibbs CP et al: The pulmonary consequences of aspiration of gastric contents at pH values greater than 2.5. Am Rev Respir Dis 121:119, 1980

206. Eyler SW, Cullen BF, Murphy ME, Welch WD: Antacid aspiration in rabbits: a comparison of Mylanta and Bicitra. Anesth Analg 61:288, 1982

207. Hodgkinson R, Glassenberg R, Joyce TH et al: Comparison of cimetidine (Tagamet®) with antacid for safety and effectiveness in reducing gastric acidity before elective cesarean section. Anesthesiology 59:86, 1983

208. James FM III, Dewan DM, Floyd HM et al: Chloroprocaine vs. bupivacaine for lumbar epidural analgesia for elective cesarean section. Anesthesiology 52:488, 1980

209. Caritis SN, Abouleish E, Edelstone DI, Mueller-Heubach E: Fetal acid–base state following spinal or epidural anesthesia for cesarean section. Obstet Gynecol 56:610, 1980

210. Belfrage P, Irestedt L, Raabe N, Arner S: General anaesthesia or lumbar epidural block for caesarean section? Effects on the foetal heart rate. Acta Anaesthesiol Scand 21:67, 1977

211. Corke BC, Datta S, Ostheimer GW et al: Spinal anaesthesia for caesarean section: the influence of hypotension on neonatal outcome. Anaesthesia 37:658, 1982

212. Downing JW, Houlton PC, Barclay A: Extradural analgesia for caesarean section: a comparison with general anaesthesia. Br J Anaesth 51:367, 1979

213. Fox GS, Smith JB, Namba Y, Johnson RC: Anesthesia for cesarean section: further studies. Am J Obstet Gynecol 133:15, 1979

214. Gibbs CP, Werba JV, Banner TE et al: Epidural anesthesia: leg-wrapping prevents hypotension. Anesthesiology 59:A405, 1983

215. Mangano DT: Anesthesia for the pregnant cardiac patient. p. 345. In SM Shnider, G Levinson (eds): Anesthesia for Obstetrics. 2nd Ed. Williams & Wilkins, Baltimore, 1987

216. Easterling TR, Chadwick HS, Otto CM, Benedetti TJ: Aortic stenosis in pregnancy. Obstet Gynecol 72:113, 1988

217. Spinnato JA, Kraynack BJ, Cooper MW: Eisenmenger's syndrome in pregnancy: epidural anesthesia for elective cesarean section. N Engl J Med 304:1215, 1981

218. Ahmad S, Hawes D, Dooley S et al: Intrathecal morphine in a parturient with a single ventricle. Anesthesiology 54:515, 1981

219. Abboud TK, Raya J, Noveihed R, Daniel J: Intrathecal morphine for relief of labor pain in a parturient with severe pulmonary hypertension. Anesthesiology 59:477, 1983

220. Pollack KL, Chestnut DH, Wenstrom KD: Anesthetic management of a parturient with Eisenmenger's syndrome. Anesth Analg 70:212, 1990

221. Marx GF, Luykx WM, Cohen S: Fetal–neonatal status following caesarean section for fetal distress. Br J Anaesth 56:1009, 1984

222. Chestnut DH: Fetal distress. p. 385. In James FM, Dewan DM, Wheeler AS (eds): Obstetric Anesthesia: The Complicated Patient. 2nd Ed. FA Davis, Philadelphia, 1988

223. Moya F, Thorndike V: Passage of drugs across the placenta. Am J Obstet Gynecol 84:1778, 1962

224. Dilts PV: Placental transfer. Clin Obstet Gynecol 24:555, 1981

225. Ralston DH: Perinatal pharmacology. p. 50. In Shnider SM, Levinson G (eds): Anesthesia for Obstetrics. 2nd Ed. Williams & Wilkins, Baltimore, 1987

226. Alper MH: What drugs cross the placenta and what happens to them in the fetus? p. 1. In Hershey SG (ed): Refresher Courses in Anesthesiology. Vol. 4. American Society of Anesthesiologists, Park Ridge, IL, 1976

227. Makowski EL, Meschia G, Droegemueller W, Battaglia

FC: Distribution of uterine blood flow in the pregnant sheep. Am J Obstet Gynecol 101:409, 1968

228. Biehl D, Shnider SM, Levinson G, Callender K: Placental transfer of lidocaine: effects of fetal acidosis. Anesthesiology 48:409, 1978

229. Shnider SM, Wright RG, Levinson G et al: Uterine blood flow and plasma norepinephrine changes during maternal stress in the pregnant ewe. Anesthesiology 50:526, 1979

230. Bonica JJ: Obstetric Analgesia and Anesthesia. World Federation of Societies of Anesthesiologists, Amsterdam, 1980

231. Haymaker L, Woodhall B: Peripheral Nerve Injuries. WB Saunders, Philadelphia, 1945

232. Thomas J, Climmie CR, Long G, Nighjoy LE: The influence of adrenaline on the maternal plasma levels and placental transfer of lignocaine following lumbar epidural administration. Br J Anaesth 41:1031, 1969

233. Gibbs CP, Modell JH: Management of aspiration pneumonitis. p. 1293. In Miller RD (ed): Anesthesia. 3rd Ed. Vol. 2. Churchill Livingstone, New York, 1990

Chapter 17

Malpresentations

John W. Seeds

Near term or during labor, the fetus normally assumes a longitudinal lie and presents the cephalic pole at the maternal pelvis, and the fetal vertex is flexed on the neck (Fig. 17.1). In approximately 5 percent of cases, however, deviation occurs from this normal lie, presentation, or flexion attitude, and such deviation constitutes a fetal malpresentation. Malpresentation is associated with danger to both the mother and the fetus and historically has led to a variety of operative maneuvers intended to facilitate delivery. Historically, interventions have included destructive operations leading predictably to fetal death. Later, manual or instrumental attempts to convert the malpresentation to a more favorable one were developed. Internal podalic version followed by a complete breech extraction was advocated as a clinical solution to many malpresentations. However, such manipulative attempts to achieve vaginal delivery are associated with unacceptably high fetal or maternal morbidity or mortality. Thus their use is now discouraged. More recently, cesarean delivery has become the recommended alternative to manipulative vaginal techniques when normal progress toward delivery is not observed.

This chapter examines each of the various malpresentations, those features of a pregnancy considered responsible for the abnormality, and the mechanics of labor and vaginal delivery unique to each situation. Those characteristics of specific fetal malpresenta-

tions are reviewed that suggest that no intervention is needed in contrast to the clinical findings that might justify expedient abdominal delivery.

Generally, factors associated with malpresentation result in (1) diminished vertical polarity of the uterine cavity, (2) increased or decreased fetal mobility, or (3) fetal presenting part blocked from entering the maternal pelvis (Table 17.1). The association of great parity with malpresentation is presumably related to laxity of maternal abdominal muscular support and therefore loss of the normal vertical uterine polarity. Placentation either high in the fundus or low in the pelvis (Fig. 17.2) is another factor that diminishes the likelihood of a fetus comfortably assuming a longitudinal axis. Both prematurity and hydramnios permit increased fetal mobility; hence increased probability of a noncephalic presentation in labor. By contrast, such conditions as autosomal trisomies and myotonic dystrophy result in decreased fetal muscle tone and strength and decreased fetal mobility and are associated with an increased incidence of malpresentation. Furthermore, preterm birth involves a fetus disproportionately small for the maternal pelvis. In these cases, pelvic engagement and descent can occur despite extreme deflexion attitudes. Because deflection attitudes require the passage of a bulkier fetal profile, they are seen less frequently with a larger fetus. Finally, the cephalopelvic disproportion seen with severe fetal hydrocephalus or with a contracted

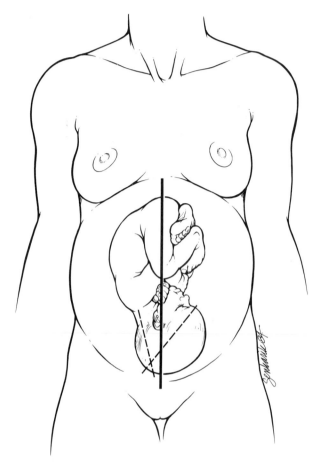

Fig. 17.1 Frontal view of a fetus occupying a longitudinal lie (dark vertical line), with the fetal vertex properly flexed on the neck.

Table 17.1 Etiologic Factors in Malpresentation

Maternal	Fetal
Great parity	Prematurity
Pelvic tumors	Multiple gestation
Pelvic contracture	Hydramnios
Uterine malformation	Macrosomia
	Hydrocephaly
	Trisomies
	Anencephaly
	Myotonic dystrophy
	Placenta previa

pelvis is frequently implicated as an etiology of malpresentation because engagement of the fetal head is prevented.

ABNORMAL AXIAL LIE

The fetal "lie" indicates the alignment of the fetal spine with that of the mother. The normal fetal lie is longitudinal and by itself does not necessarily indicate whether the cephalic pole or the breech is presenting. If the fetal spine or long axis crosses that of the mother, the fetus may be said to occupy a transverse or oblique lie (Fig. 17.3), resulting in a shoulder or

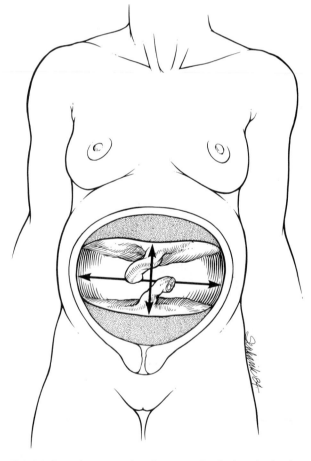

Fig. 17.2 Implantation of a placenta either high in the fundus or across the lower segment of the uterus would alter the normal vertical capacity of the uterine cavity, as illustrated here, and increase the probability of malpresentation.

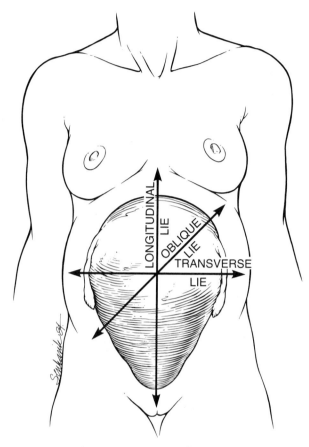

Fig. 17.3 These vectors demonstrate the three major possible axes that a fetus may occupy. A fetal lie does not necessarily indicate whether the vertex or the breech is closest to the cervix.

arm presentation (Fig. 17.4). The presentation is termed unstable if the fetal membranes are intact and there is great fetal mobility.[1,2]

Abnormal fetal lie is diagnosed on average in approximately 1 in 300 instances, or 0.33 percent.[1,3–9] Prematurity is a factor, with abnormal lie reported to occur in approximately 2 percent of pregnancies at 32 weeks, or six times the rate reported to occur at term.[10] Persistence of a transverse, oblique, or unstable lie beyond 35 or 38 weeks is of major clinical significance, requiring a systematic clinical approach. Unexpected spontaneous rupture of membranes without a fetal part filling the pelvic inlet carries a high risk of cord prolapse, fetal distress, and maternal morbidity and mortality if neglected. In such cases,

Hourihane[11] in 1968 and Edwards and Nicholson[7] in 1969 recommended elective hospitalization to permit observation and early recognition of cord prolapse. Phalen et al.[12] reported a series of 29 patients with transverse lie diagnosed at or beyond 37 weeks gestation and managed expectantly. Eighty-three percent (24 of 29) spontaneously converted to breech (9 of 24) or vertex (15 of 24) before labor; however, the overall cesarean delivery rate was 45 percent, and there were two cases of cord prolapse, one uterine rupture, and one neonatal death. These authors conclude that external version is indicated if transverse lie persists to 39 weeks. If an attempted version is unsuccessful, elective cesarean should be considered.[12]

Great parity, prematurity, pelvic contracture, and abnormal placentation are the most commonly reported clinical settings associated with abnormal lie.[3,6–10] Although Cockburn and Drake[4] reported no etiology in 30 to 79 percent of their cases, other investigators have frequently observed one of the four conditions cited above.[1,9,13] Any factor that destroys the normal vertical polarity of the uterine cavity encourages an abnormal lie.[4,11]

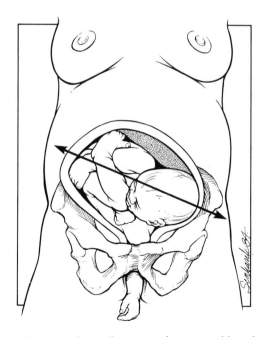

Fig. 17.4 Frontal view illustrating a fetus in an oblique lie with a shoulder or arm presenting.

Diagnosis may be accomplished by inspection, palpation, or vaginal examination, but successful prenatal detection has been observed in as few as 41 percent of cases before labor.[4] A fetal loss rate of 9.2 percent[4] has been reported with early diagnosis, whereas a mortality of 27.5 percent has been seen when the diagnosis was delayed.[4] It is therefore clear that careful attention to the antenatal diagnosis of abnormal lie can be vital to achieve the best fetal outcome.

Reported perinatal mortality for unstable or transverse lie (corrected for lethal malformations or extreme prematurity) varies from 3.9 percent[11] to 24 percent,[2] with maternal mortality reported to be as high as 10 percent. Maternal deaths are usually related to infection after premature rupture of membranes, hemorrhage secondary to abnormal placentation, complications of operative intervention for cephalopelvic disproportion, or traumatic delivery.[8,10] Fetal loss is primarily associated with neglect, prolapsed cord, or traumatic delivery.[10] Cord prolapse occurs 20 times as often with abnormal axial lie as it does with a vertex presentation. The risk of fetal death varies with the type of obstetric intervention. Fetal mortality of 0 to 10 percent has been reported for cesarean birth compared with 25 to 90 percent when internal podalic version and breech extraction is performed.[4,5,8–10,14] A mortality of only 6 percent is reported for external version and vertex vaginal delivery.[9,10]

There is a consensus that the normally grown infant at term cannot undergo a safe delivery from an axial malposition.[1,5,8,15] A transverse/oblique or unstable lie after 35 to 38 weeks should thus lead to consideration of placenta previa or contracted pelvis.[11] Ultrasound would not only identify placental location but also allow prenatal diagnosis of many of the fetal malformations associated with an abnormal lie. Admission to the hospital in anticipation of labor or spontaneous rupture of membranes has been recommended to permit immediate examination for cord prolapse.[3] If admission is not feasible, careful instructions to the patient regarding prompt presentation to the hospital in the event of spontaneous rupture of membranes or the onset of labor must be provided.[8]

Some clinicians believe that external version is contraindicated because it is often unsuccessful[4,15] and may carry a higher fetal loss rate than cesarean delivery.[4,9,10] However, if placenta previa and cephalopelvic disproportion can be reasonably excluded and if the fetal heart rate can be monitored throughout the procedure, a judicious attempt at external version is a reasonable alternative to expectant management or primary cesarean delivery.[5,8] Intact membranes and the absence of active labor are recommended prerequisites, although external version may be possible in early labor or even with ruptured membranes if the fetus is sufficiently mobile and cord prolapse can be excluded.[4] In the series reported by Edwards and Nicholson,[7] which included 254 patients at 38 to 39 weeks gestation, fetal lie polarized spontaneously in 20 percent of cases, while another 20 percent ruptured membranes or entered spontaneous labor before scheduled admission at 39 weeks. In the 60 percent of cases remaining after exclusion of cephalopelvic disproportion and placenta previa, oxytocin induction with fetal monitoring was begun. After contractions were established, external version was attempted; if successful, amniotomy was performed with a fetal pole over or in the pelvic inlet. Eighty-six of 96 cases thus managed were delivered vaginally, with fetal distress occurring in only four cases.[7] There were no fetal losses. Prophylactic induction would be feasible only with a cervix sufficiently dilated to permit artificial rupture of membranes. Visualization with real-time ultrasound can facilitate the version, providing the operator continuous feedback on fetal position. Prior consultation with an anesthesiologist is recommended to permit prompt cesarean delivery in the event of fetal distress or cord prolapse, both of which are possible complications.

If external version is impractical, unsuccessful, or unavailable, if spontaneous rupture of the membranes has occurred, or if active labor has begun with an abnormal lie, cesarean section is the treatment of choice.[2,4,15] There remains no place for internal podalic version and breech extraction in the management of transverse/oblique lie or unstable presentation in singleton pregnancies because of an unacceptably high rate of fetal and maternal complications.[3]

A persistently abnormal axial lie, particularly if accompanied by ruptured membranes, might also alter the actual technique of cesarean section. Although a low transverse cervical incision has many surgical advantages, up to 25 percent of transverse incisions require vertical extension in the case of an abnormal lie to allow access to a vertex trapped in the muscular fundus.[4,15] Furthermore, the lower uterine segment is often poorly developed. Therefore, in cases of transverse or oblique lie with ruptured membranes and a poorly developed lower segment, a low vertical incision is more prudent. After the peritoneal cavity has been entered, extrauterine version at the time of cesarean section has been described. In 1979, Pelosi et al.[15] reported that such an approach resulted in easier surgical delivery and more often permitted the use of a low transverse incision. However, in many cases with ruptured membranes, oligohydramnios, and a poorly developed lower uterine segment, even intraoperative version would not be easily accomplished.

DEFLECTION ATTITUDES

The normal "attitude" of the fetal vertex during labor is one of full flexion on the neck, with the fetal chin tucked against the upper chest. Deflection attitudes involve various degrees of deflection or even extension of the fetal head on the spine (Fig. 17.5). Spontaneous conversion to a more normal flexed attitude or further extension of an intermediate deflection to a fully extended position will commonly occur as labor progresses. Although safe vaginal delivery is possible in most cases, experience indicates that cesarean section is the only appropriate alternative to spontaneous vaginal delivery when dysfunctional labor is associated with a deflection attitude.

Face Presentation

A face presentation is characterized by a longitudinal lie and full extension of the fetal head on the spine, with the occiput against the upper back (Fig. 17.6).[13] The fetal chin is used as the point of designation. For

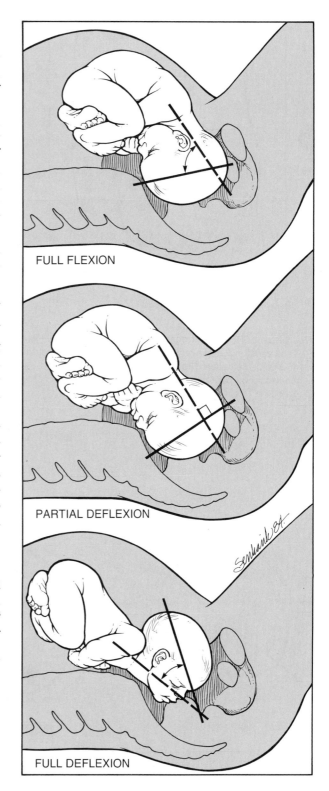

FULL FLEXION

PARTIAL DEFLEXION

FULL DEFLEXION

Fig. 17.5 (Top view) Normal attitude with the fetal occipitofrontal plane describing an acute angle with the axis of the cervical spine. (Middle view) Intermediate deflexion attitude with the occipitofrontal plane of the fetal skull describing a right angle with the axis of the fetal cervical spine. (Bottom view) Full deflexion attitude or face presentation, where the occipitofrontal plane is hyperextended on the axis of the cervical spine.

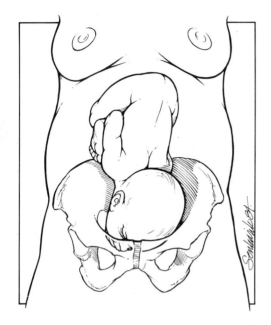

Fig. 17.6 Frontal view of a fetus entering the pelvic inlet with the fetal vertex fully deflexed on the cervical spine demonstrating a face presentation. The fetal occiput (cephalic prominence) would be palpable on the same side of the maternal uterus as the fetal back.

example, a fetus presenting by the face whose chin is in the right posterior quadrant of the maternal pelvis would be called a right mentum posterior (RMP) (Fig. 17.7). The reported incidence of face presentation ranges from 0.14 to 0.54 percent,[9,16-21] averaging about 0.2 percent, or 1 in 500 live births overall. Reported perinatal mortality, corrected for nonviable malformations and extreme prematurity, varies from 0.6 percent[22] to 5 percent,[23] averaging approximately 2 to 3 percent.

All clinical factors known to increase the general rate of malpresentation (Table 17.1) have been implicated in face presentation, but in addition, Browne and Carney[13] reported that as many as 60 percent of infants with a face presentation were malformed. Anencephaly, for instance, is seen in approximately one-third of cases of face presentation.[6,24,25] Frequently observed maternal factors include a contracted pelvis or cephalopelvic disproportion in 10 to 40 percent of cases.[1,13,17,20] In addition, high parity and prematurity are repeatedly associated with face presentation.[6,9,16,17,19,26] In a review of face presentation, Duff[18] found that one of these etiologic factors was identified in up to 90 percent of face presentations.

Early diagnosis is important for proper management. Diagnosis can be suspected anytime abdominal palpation finds the cephalic prominence on the same side of the maternal abdomen as the fetal back (Fig. 17.8); however, face presentation is more often dis-

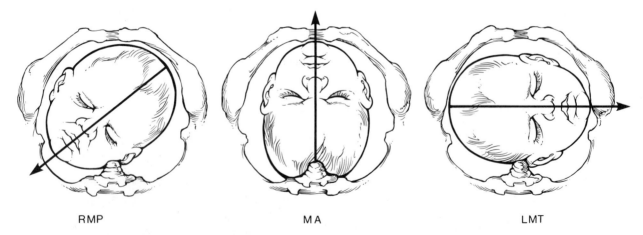

RMP   M A   LMT

Fig. 17.7 Three pelvic views of the fetus demonstrating the various positions the fetus might occupy in a face presentation. The point of designation is the fetal chin or mentum. (A) Right mentum posterior (RMP). (B) Mentum anterior (MA). (C) Left mentum transverse (LMT).

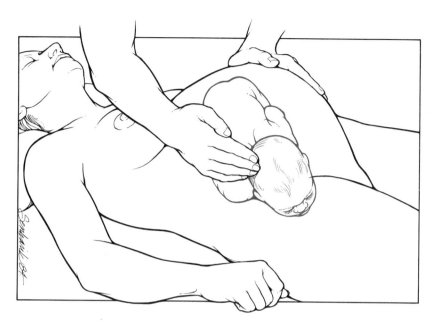

Fig. 17.8 Palpation of the maternal abdomen in the case of a full-deflexion attitude or face presentation should reveal the cephalic prominence on the same side of the maternal abdomen as the fetal back.

covered by vaginal examination and confirmed by radiography or ultrasound. In practice, fewer than 1 in 20 infants with a face presentation is diagnosed abdominally.[22] In fact, only one-half of these infants are diagnosed by any means to be face presentation prior to the second stage of labor,[20,22,25,27] and one-half of the remaining cases are undiagnosed until delivery.[20,23] Early detection can be important, however, as perinatal mortality appears to be substantially increased with delayed diagnosis.[17]

Mechanism of Labor

Knowledge of the early mechanism of labor for the face presentation is incomplete. Many infants with a face presentation probably begin labor in the less extended brow position. With descent into the pelvis, the forces of labor press the fetus against maternal soft tissues; full extension of the spine results. The labor of a face presentation must include engagement, descent, internal rotation generally to a mentum anterior position, and delivery by flexion under the symphysis (Fig. 17.9). However, flexion of the occiput may not always occur. Borrell and Fernstrom[28] have proposed that delivery in the full ex-

tended attitude is more common than was previously thought.

The prognosis for labor with a face presentation depends on the orientation of the fetal chin. At diagnosis, 60 to 80 percent of infants with face presentation are mentum anterior,[6,20,22,29] 10 to 12 percent are mentum transverse,[6,22,29] and 20 to 25 percent are mentum posterior.[6,20,22,29] Almost all infants presenting mentum anterior will achieve spontaneous or easily assisted vaginal delivery in the absence of cephalopelvic disproportion (CPD).[6,22,30,31] Furthermore, most mentum transverse infants will rotate to the mentum anterior position and deliver vaginally.[6,16] Even 25 to 33 percent of mentum posterior infants will rotate and deliver vaginally in the mentum anterior position.[6,16,20] In reviewing 51 cases of persistent face presentation, Schwartz et al.[29] found that the mean birth weight of those infants in mentum posterior who did rotate and deliver vaginally was 3,425 g compared with 3,792 g for those infants who did not rotate and deliver vaginally. Persistence of mentum posterior with an infant of normal size, however, increases the probability of functional disproportion and makes safe vaginal delivery probably impossible.

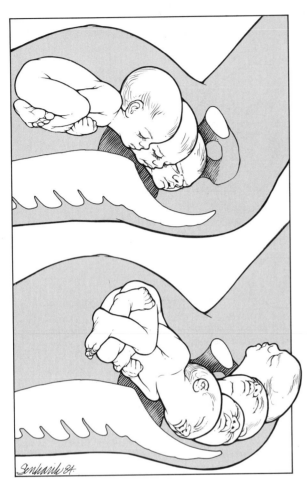

Fig. 17.9 Descent and delivery of a fetus in a face presentation. The fetus may engage and descend in a mentum anterior position or engage in a mentum posterior as illustrated here, internally rotating for delivery from the mentum anterior position.

There is little evidence, though, that a properly monitored trial of labor in the case of an infant of average size or smaller is unsafe.

Overall, 70 to 80 percent[6,20,22,23] of infants with face presentations can be delivered vaginally, either spontaneously or by low forceps. However, 12 to 30 percent require cesarean section. Manual attempts to convert the face to a flexed attitude or to rotate a posterior position to a more favorable mentum anterior are rarely successful and increase both maternal and fetal risks.[1,16,22,25,32] Internal podalic version with breech extraction as a remedy for face presentation is contraindicated. Campbell[22] reported fetal losses of

up to 60 percent with such maneuvers. Maternal deaths from uterine rupture and trauma after version extraction have also been documented. Spontaneous delivery or cesarean section are therefore the preferred routes of delivery for maternal safety as well.[1,16,22,25]

Prolonged labor is a common and ominous feature of face presentation[6,9,26] and has itself been associated with an increased number of intrapartum deaths.[17] Therefore, prompt attention to an arrested labor pattern is essential. The choice between augmentation of a dysfunctional labor or primary cesarean delivery rests on assessment of uterine activity, pelvic adequacy, and fetal condition. Fetal distress is common. Salzmann et al.[25] observed a 10-fold increase in fetal distress with face presentation. Several other investigators have also found that abnormal fetal heart rate patterns occur more often with face presentation.[16,18] Continuous intrapartum electronic fetal monitoring of a fetus with this malposition is therefore mandatory. Extreme care must be exercised in the placement of an electrode, as ocular and cosmetic damage might result from this device. If external Doppler heart rate monitoring is inadequate and an internal electrode is necessary, placement of the electrode on the fetal chin is preferred over any part of the upper face.

Potential neonatal sequelae of face presentation make prenatal pediatric consultation important. Laryngeal and tracheal edema resulting simply from the presence of the birth process might require immediate nasotracheal intubation.[33] Nuchal teratomas or simple goiter, fetal anomalies that might have caused the malpresentation, require expert neonatal care.

In summary, successful management of a face presentation includes early diagnosis, use of electronic fetal heart rate monitoring, and delivery by cesarean section in cases of maternal or fetal distress or arrest of descent or dilatation.[1,9,16,18,20] Delivery by cesarean section has been recommended for all term-sized infants with mentum posterior. If fetal heart rate patterns are reassuring and steady progress is observed, however, rotation may occur, permitting safe vaginal delivery.[6,10,16]

Radiographic pelvimetry might be useful for the intrapartum management of the face presentation, because both CPD and fetal anomalies are common. However, in the presence of progressive descent and dilatation, its value is uncertain.[6] No clear contraindication has been found to oxytocin augmentation of hypotonic secondary arrest of labor provided CPD can be ruled out and the fetus monitored carefully.[18,23] However, these prerequisites for safe augmentation of dysfunctional labor with a face presentation may be difficult to satisfy.

Although cesarean section has been reported in up to 60 percent of cases of face presentation,[18,27] safe vaginal delivery can be expected in most cases of face presentation. Cesarean section is more often required for delivery of the primagravida with a term infant in the mentum posterior position. Nevertheless, in any case with a face presentation making steady progress toward delivery, surgical intervention is cautiously reserved.[9] When progress is arrested despite adequate labor or if fetal distress is identified, delivery by cesarean section is preferred to all other possible interventions.

BROW PRESENTATION

An infant with a brow presentation occupies a longitudinal axis, with a partially deflexed cephalic attitude, midway between full flexion and full extension (Fig. 17.10).[1,13] The frontal bones become the point of designation. If the anterior fontanel is on the mother's left side, with the sagittal suture in the transverse pelvic axis, the fetus would be in a left frontum transverse position (Fig. 17.11). The reported incidence of brow presentation varies widely between 1 : 670[34] and 1 : 3,433,[35] averaging approximately 1 in 1,500 deliveries.[36] Brow presentation will be detected more often in early labor before flexion occurs to a normal attitude. Less frequently, further extension results in a face presentation.

Perinatal mortality corrected for lethal anomalies and very low birth weight varies from 1.28 to 8 percent.[37] In reviewing 88,988 deliveries, Ingolfsson[38] found that corrected perinatal mortality rates for fetuses presenting by the brow depended on the mode of delivery. Ingolfsson observed that the highest rate of loss, 16 percent, was associated with manipulative vaginal birth.[38]

Causative factors for brow presentation encompass most of those listed in Table 17.1 and are similar to those clinical circumstances associated with face presentation. Cephalopelvic disproportion, prematur-

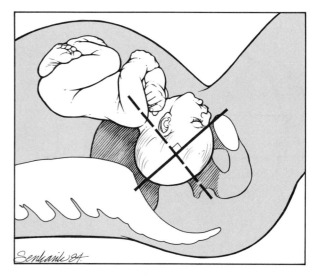

Fig. 17.10 This fetus demonstrates an intermediate deflexion attitude known as a brow presentation. The occipitofrontal plane of the fetal cranium describes a right angle with the axis of the cervical spine. This fetus is in a frontum anterior position.

ity, and great parity are often emphasized and have been implicated in more than 60 percent of cases of persistent brow presentation.[1,6,35,39,40] In general, factors that delay or prevent engagement are associated with a persistent brow presentation.

Detection of a brow presentation by abdominal palpation may be possible but is unusual in practice. More often, a brow is detected on vaginal examination. As in the case of a face presentation, late diagnosis is more likely. Fewer than 50 percent of brow presentations are detected before the second stage of labor, with most of the remainder undiagnosed until delivery.[34,38-40] Frontum anterior is reportedly the most common position at diagnosis, occurring about twice as often as either transverse or posterior positions. Although the initial position at diagnosis may be of only limited prognostic value, Skalley and Kramer[49] reported the cesarean section rate to be higher with frontum transverse or frontum posterior.

A persistent brow presentation requires that the largest (mento-occipital) diameter of the fetal head engage in the pelvic inlet and negotiate the midplane and the outlet.[41] This process is possible only with a large pelvis or a small infant or both. However, the majority of brow presentations convert spontaneously by flexion or further extension to either a vertex

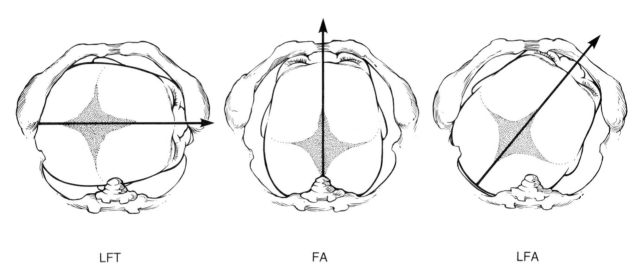

LFT   FA   LFA

Fig. 17.11 The frontal area of the fetus in a brow presentation is the point of designation when describing fetal position. (A) Fetus in the left frontum transverse position. (B) Frontum anterior position. (C) Left frontum anterior position.

or a face presentation and would then be managed accordingly.[34,35] The earlier the diagnosis is made the more likely conversion will occur spontaneously. Fewer than one-half of infants with persistent brow presentations are reported to undergo spontaneous delivery, but in most cases a trial of labor is not contraindicated.[6,37]

Prolonged labors have been observed in 33 to 50 percent of brow presentations,[6,20,26,35,39,40] and secondary arrest is not uncommon.[34] Conversion of the brow to a more favorable position with forceps is contraindicated,[34,35,39] as are attempts at manual conversion, although Abell[36] reported some success. One unexpected cause of persistent brow presentation may be an open fetal mouth pressed against the vaginal wall, bracing the head and preventing both flexion and extension[28,35] (Fig. 17.12). Borrell and Fernstrom[28] observed this to be a major cause of persistent brow and reported success manually elevating the head and closing the mouth. Such a maneuver could also lead to cord prolapse or fetal trauma, however, and therefore should only be undertaken with great caution.

In most cases of brow presentation, as with face presentation, minimal manipulation yields the best results,[1,35,42] assuming of course no fetal distress occurs. Ingolfsson[38] concluded, however, that expectancy is justified only with a large pelvis, a small infant,

and adequate progress. If a brow presentation persists with a large baby, successful delivery is unlikely, and cesarean section might be most prudent.[20,26] However, because spontaneous flexion or extension can occur unpredictably, intervention by cesarean section before arrest of spontaneous progress would seem premature.

Vaginal delivery of an uncompromised term-sized infant as a brow presentation is unlikely. Some clinicians have reported radiographic pelvimetry to be useful in discriminating those cases more likely to deliver vaginally from those unlikely to do so. Cruikshank and White[6] noted that 91 percent of cases with adequate pelvic dimensions converted spontaneously to a vertex or face presentation and delivered vaginally, while only 20 percent showing some form of pelvic contraction did so. It must be recalled, however, that CPD is itself a common etiologic factor in brow presentation. Therefore, pelvimetry in cases of brow presentation would be expected to identify a large number of cases with diminished pelvic dimensions. On the other hand, 20 percent of patients with contracted pelvic measurements as seen on x-ray film had a successful vaginal delivery. In summary, there is no good evidence that a carefully monitored trial of labor in the case of a brow presentation is detrimental to either mother or fetus.

When arrest of progress occurs as a result of inade-

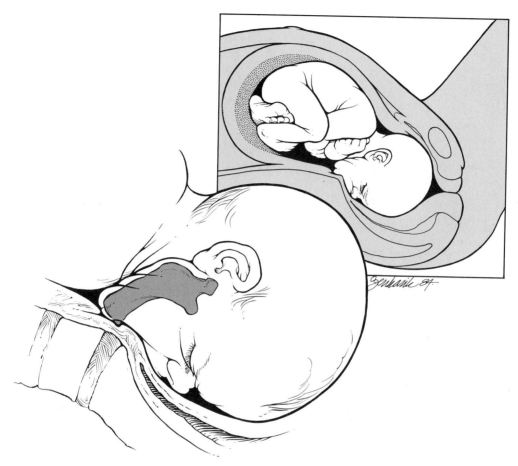

Fig. 17.12 Illustration of the possibility that an open fetal mouth in contact with the vaginal wall may prevent a fetus from converting an intermediate deflexion attitude by either flexion or further extension and therefore result in a persistent brow.

quate uterine contractions, oxytocin augmentation of labor can be considered if continuous fetal monitoring is available. Resumption or initiation of labor should, however, result in prompt and clear progress toward vaginal delivery. If such progress does not occur, cesarean section is preferable to prolonged augmentation.

COMPOUND PRESENTATION

Whenever an extremity is found prolapsing beside the presenting part, it is termed a compound presentation[43] (Fig. 17.13). The reported incidence ranges from 1 in 377 to 1 in 1,213 deliveries.[6,43–45] The com-

bination of an upper extremity and the vertex is most common.[6,43–46]

This diagnosis should be suspected with an arrest of labor in the active phase or failure to engage during active labor.[45] The diagnosis is made by vaginal examination, which will reveal an irregular mobile tissue mass adjacent to the presenting part. Diagnosis late in labor is common, and as many as 50 percent of persistent compound presentations are not diagnosed until the second stage.[43] This delay may not be detrimental, because it is probable that only these persistent cases will require any significant attention.

Although maternal age, race, parity, and pelvic size have all been implicated in the etiology of compound

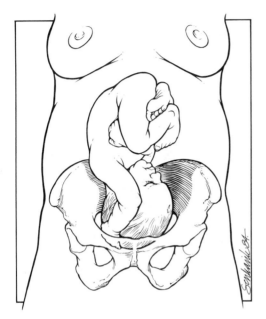

Fig. 17.13 Frontal view of a fetus occupying a longitudinal lie and demonstrating a compound presentation of a vertex and a hand.

presentation,[44,45] prematurity is the most consistently associated clinical finding.[6,43] It is primarily the very small fetus that is at great risk of persistent compound presentation. In late pregnancy, external cephalic version of a fetus in breech position may increase the risk of a compound presentation; in such cases the combination is more often that of a lower extremity and the vertex.[47]

Perinatal mortality with compound presentation is consistently elevated, with an overall rate of 93 per 1,000 reported by Cruikshank and White[6] in 1973. Higher losses of 17 and 19 percent have been reported when the foot prolapses.[44] As with other malpresentations, fetal risk can be directly related to the method of management. A fetal mortality rate of 4.8 percent has been noted if no intervention is required. This figure increases to 14.4 percent with intervention other than a cesarean section. A 30 percent fetal mortality rate has been observed with internal podalic version and breech extraction.[44] There is probably some selection bias in these figures, because it is likely that only the more difficult cases became candidates for manipulative intervention. Nevertheless, when

intervention is necessary, cesarean section appears to be the only safe choice.

Fetal risk in the case of compound presentation is specifically associated with birth trauma and cord prolapse. Cord prolapse occurs in 11 to 20 percent of cases[6,44,45] and is the most frequent single complication of this malpresentation.[43] It probably occurs because the extremity splints the presenting part and provides an irregular fetal aggregate that incompletely fills the pelvic inlet. In addition to the hypoxic risk of cord prolapse, common fetal morbidity includes neurologic and musculoskeletal damage to the involved extremity.

Despite these risks, labor is not necessarily contraindicated with a compound presentation. However, the prolapsed extremity should not be manipulated.[43-45,48,49] As the presenting part descends, the accompanying extremity usually retracts. The prognosis, however, is variable. Cruikshank and White[6] found that 75 percent of vertex/upper extremity combinations will deliver spontaneously, whereas Weissberg and Weingold[49] reported that spontaneous vaginal delivery of a foot/vertex combination is less likely. Occult or undetected cord prolapse is possible, and therefore continuous electronic fetal heart rate monitoring is indicated.

The primary indications for surgical intervention are cord prolapse and failure to progress.[6] Cesarean section is the only appropriate clinical intervention,[43] as both version extraction and attempts at repositioning the prolapsed extremity are associated with unacceptably high fetal and maternal morbidity and mortality and are to be avoided.[44,45] Breen and Wiesmeien[43] found that 2 percent of patients with compound presentation required abdominal delivery, whereas Weissberg and O'Leary[45] reported cesarean section to be necessary in 25 percent of cases. Protraction of the second stage of labor has been noted to occur more frequently with persistent compound presentation, and dysfunctional labor patterns are said to be common.[43] Again, as in other malpresentations, spontaneous resolution occurs more often and surgical intervention is therefore less frequently necessary in those cases diagnosed early in labor. Persistent compound presentation is more likely with a small infant, as is the prognosis for successful vaginal delivery. Persistent compound presentation with a term-sized infant has a poor prognosis

Table 17.2 Breech Categories

	Overall Proportion of Breeches (%)	Risk of Cord Prolapse (%)	Proportion With Prematurity (%)
Frank breech	48–73[31,47,50,52,73]	0.5[71]	38[50]
Complete	4.6–11.5[31,50,52,73]	4–6[71]	12[50]
Footling[a]	12–38[31,50,52]	15–18[71]	50[50]

[a] Increased with very low birth weight.

for safe vaginal delivery, and cesarean delivery is usually necessary for an atraumatic result.

BREECH PRESENTATION

The infant presenting as a breech occupies a longitudinal axis with the cephalic pole in the uterine fundus.[1] This presentation occurs in 3 to 4 percent of labors overall, although it is reported in 7 percent of pregnancies at 32 weeks[1,50] and in 25 percent of pregnancies of less than 28 weeks duration.[50] The three types of breech are noted in Table 17.2. The infant in the frank breech position is flexed at the hips with extended knees. The complete breech is flexed at both joints, and the footling breech has one or both hips extended (Fig. 17.14).

The diagnosis of breech presentation may be made by abdominal palpation or vaginal examination and confirmed by ultrasound or x-ray film.[1] Prematurity, fetal malformations, and polar placentation are commonly observed causative factors. There is a history of previous breech presentation in 20 percent of cases.[1] High rates of breech presentation are noted in certain genetic disorders, including trisomies 13, 18, and 21, Potter syndrome, and myotonic dystrophy.[51] Thus conditions that alter fetal muscular tonus and mobility also increase the frequency of breech birth.

Mechanisms and Conduct of Labor

The two most important elements for the safe conduct of vaginal breech delivery are continuous electronic fetal monitoring and a policy of noninterference until spontaneous delivery of the breech to the umbilicus has occurred. Early in the course of labor, appropriate preparations should be made for immediate cesarean section should that be necessary. Anesthesia should be available, the operating room readied, and appropriate informed consent obtained. Two obstetricians should be in attendance as well as a pediatric team. The instrument table should be prepared in the customary manner, with the addition of Piper forceps and extra towels. There is no contrain-

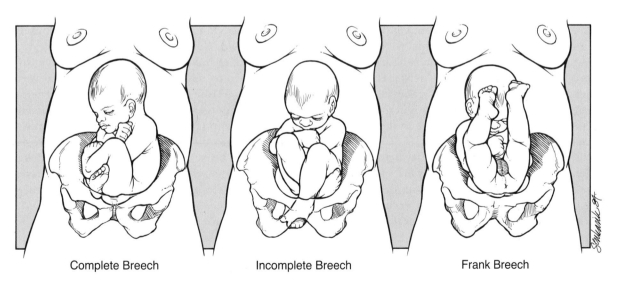

Complete Breech   Incomplete Breech   Frank Breech

Fig. 17.14 Three possible breech presentations. The complete breech demonstrates flexion of the hips and flexion of the knees. The incomplete breech demonstrates intermediate deflexion of one hip and knee. The frank breech shows flexion of the hips and extension of both knees.

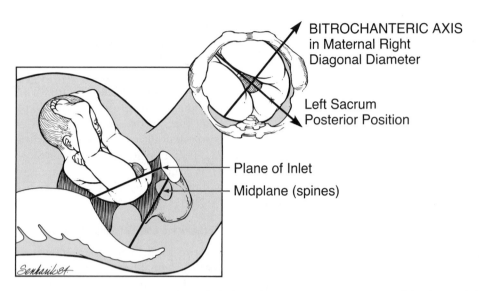

Fig. 17.15 Breech of a fetus entering the pelvis with the bitrochanteric axis occupying one of the diagonal diameters of the pelvis, while the sacrum lies in the opposite diagonal diameter.

dication to cautious conduction analgesia once labor is well established.

The infant presenting in the frank breech position usually enters the pelvic inlet in one of the diagonal pelvic diameters (Fig. 17.15). Engagement has occurred when the bitrochanteric diameter of the fetus has passed the plane of the inlet, although by vaginal examination the presenting part might only be palpated at −1 or −2 station relative to the maternal ischial spines. As the breech descends and encounters the levator ani muscle sling, internal rotation usually occurs to bring the bitrochanteric diameter into anteroposterior (AP) axis of the pelvis. The point of designation in a breech labor is the fetal sacrum. When the bitrochanteric diameter is in the AP axis of the pelvis, the fetal sacrum will lie in the transverse pelvic diameter (Fig. 17.16).

With further descent, the breech will present at the outlet and begin to emerge, usually in a sacrum transverse or slightly oblique orientation, depending on the shape of the pelvis. Crowning occurs when the bitrochanteric diameter passes under the pubic rami. A generous episiotomy should be cut, most often in the midline, just as crowning occurs. As the infant emerges, rotation begins, usually toward a sacrum anterior position. This direction of rotation may reflect the greater capacity of the hollow of the posterior pelvis to accept the fetal small parts. It is impor-

tant to emphasize that operator intervention is not yet indicated or helpful other than to cut the episiotomy and encourage maternal expulsive efforts.

Premature or overly aggressive assistance may adversely affect the breech birth in two ways. First, cervical dilatation must be maximized and complete dilatation sustained for sufficient duration to retard retraction of the cervix and entrapment of the aftercoming head. Rushing the delivery of the trunk might significantly diminish the effectiveness of this process. Second, the safe descent and delivery of the breech infant must be the result of expulsive forces from above to maintain flexion of the fetal vertex. Any traction from below in an effort to speed delivery would encourage deflexion of the vertex and result in the presentation of the large occipitofrontal fetal cranial profile to the pelvic inlet (Fig. 17.17). Such an event could be catastrophic. The safe breech delivery of an average-sized infant therefore depends predominantly on maternal expulsive forces, not on traction from below.

As the frank breech emerges further, the fetal thighs should be pressed firmly against the fetal abdomen, often splinting and protecting the umbilicus and cord. As the umbilicus appears over the maternal perineum, the operator may decompose the breech by aligning his or her fingers medial to one thigh, then the other, and pressing laterally (Fig. 17.18). This

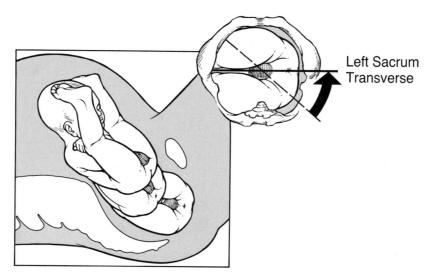

Fig. 17.16 With descent of the breech, the bitrochanteric axis generally rotates toward the anteroposterior pelvic dimension, while the sacrum moves to the transverse axis.

results in external rotation of the thigh at the hip, flexion at the knee, and usually delivery of one and then the other leg. The fetal trunk should then be wrapped with a towel for secure handling. With only support of the fetal trunk, further descent is seen in response to expulsive forces from the mother.

When the scapulae appear at the outlet, the operator may slip his or her fingers over the fetal shoulder from the fetal back (Fig. 17.19), follow the humerus, and, again with a lateral movement, rotate first one and then the other arm across the chest and out over the posterior vagina. Gentle rotation of the fetal

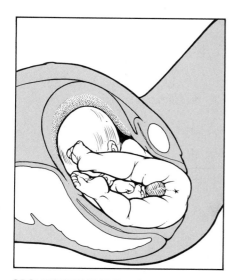

SPONTANEOUS EXPULSION

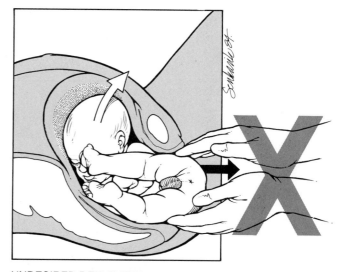

UNDESIRED DEFLEXION

Fig. 17.17 (A) Fetus emerging from the vaginal outlet spontaneously, while the uterine contraction maintains flexion of the fetal head. (B) Inappropriate aggressive traction on the fetal breech might result in undesired extension of the fetal head or even entrapment of one fetal arm behind the head (nuchal arm).

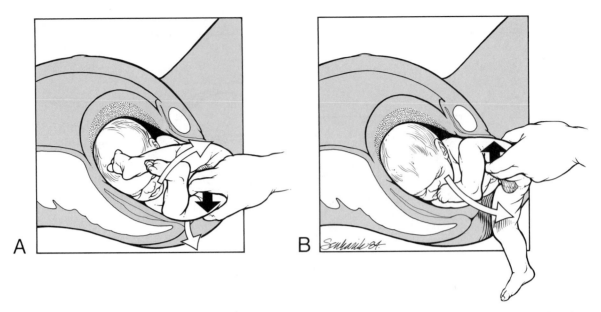

Fig. 17.18 After the spontaneous expulsion of the breech (A), lateral rotation of the thighs on the hips should result in easy delivery of the legs (B).

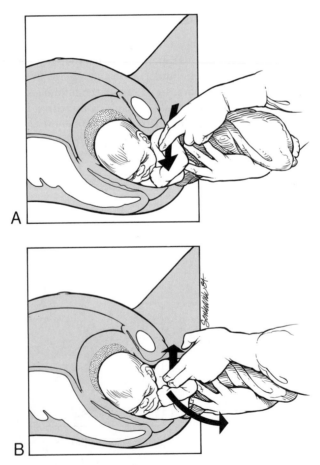

Fig. 17.19 After delivery of the legs, the operator in (A) medially rotates the infant's left arm across the chest for (B) delivery of the left arm.

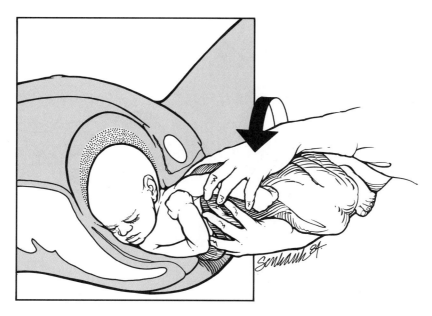

Fig. 17.20 After delivery of the anterior arm, the fetus may be rotated counterclockwise, facilitating delivery of the right arm.

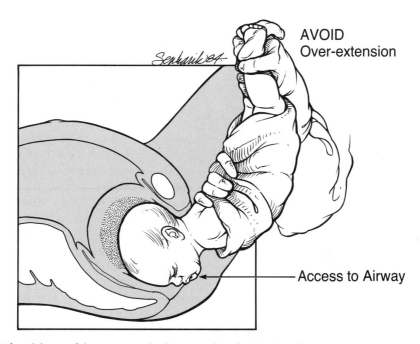

Fig. 17.21 After delivery of the arms, gentle elevation of the fetal trunk will permit access to the fetal airway. Excessive elevation of the fetal trunk may lead to fetal cervical injury and is unnecessary.

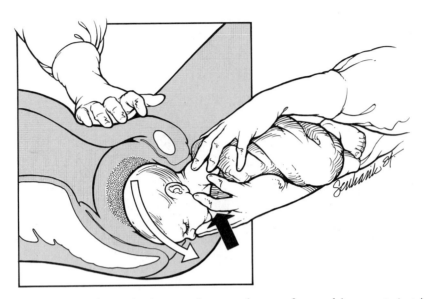

Fig. 17.22 The heavy arrow indicates the direction of pressure from two fingers of the operator's right hand on the fetal maxilla. This maneuver assists in maintaining appropriate flexion of the fetal vertex, as does moderate suprapubic pressure from an assistant along with optimal maternal expulsive forces.

trunk counterclockwise for the delivery of the right arm and clockwise for the left arm will assist in their rotation and delivery (Fig. 17.20). Overzealous traction on the fetus might result in entrapment of an arm between the fetal occiput and the symphysis, a nuchal arm. This condition is to be avoided, as it makes safe delivery much more difficult. The chin and the face of the infant will now appear at the outlet, and its airway may be cleared and suctioned (Fig. 17.21).

With maternal expulsive efforts alone, spontaneous controlled delivery of the head will often occur. If it does not, two alternatives are available. First, in an attempt to maximize flexion of the fetal vertex, the operator may place two fingers on the fetal maxillary ridge (not the fetal mandible) and with pressure and gentle downward traction assist the delivery (Fig. 17.22). Although maxillary pressure will maximize cephalic flexion, the main force effecting delivery remains the mother. Alternatively, an assistant supports and elevates the fetus as the operator kneels and applies Piper forceps directly to the fetal vertex (Fig. 17.23). It is important that the assistant elevate the fetal trunk no more than necessary, as hyperextension of the fetal neck is a dangerous possibility.

Close examination of Piper forceps will demonstrate that the pelvic curvature characteristic of other

forceps has been eliminated. This modification allows direct application to the fetal head, because the elevated fetal trunk would prevent the normal application of traditional forceps from below. The forceps are inserted into the vagina from beneath the fetus. The right blade should be inserted with the right hand along the right maternal sidewall and placed against the left fetal parietal bone. The left blade should then be inserted by the left hand along the left maternal sidewall and placed against the right fetal parietal bone. Forceps application controls the fetal head and prevents extension of the head on the neck. Gentle downward traction on the forceps with the fetal trunk supported on or near the forcep shanks will result in controlled delivery of the vertex (Fig. 17.24). Routine use of Piper forceps to the aftercoming head may be advisable both to ensure control of the delivery and to maintain optimal operator proficiency in anticipation of future deliveries when the use of this instrument might be absolutely necessary.

Any arrest of spontaneous progress in labor necessitates cesarean section. Any evidence of fetal compromise or sustained cord compression based on continuous electronic fetal monitoring should also result in prompt cesarean section. Vaginal interventions directed at facilitating delivery of the breech compli-

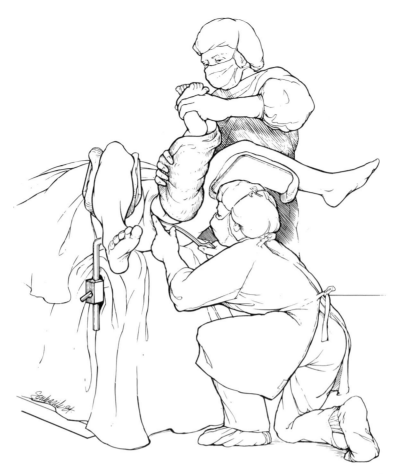

Fig. 17.23 While an assistant supports the fetal trunk, the operator on one knee applies Piper forceps to the fetal vertex directly.

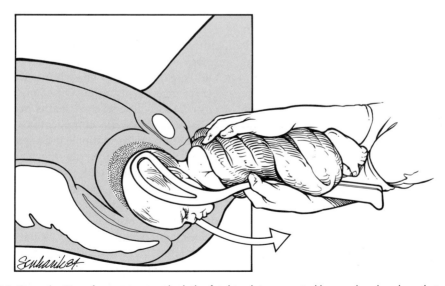

Fig. 17.24 Once the Piper forceps are applied, the fetal trunk is supported by one hand and gentle traction on the forceps, as illustrated by the arrow, in the direction of the pelvic axis results in a controlled delivery.

cated by an arrest of spontaneous progress are discouraged, because fetal and maternal morbidity and mortality are both greatly increased.

The mechanisms of descent and delivery of the footling and the complete breech are not unlike those of the frank breech described above, except one or both legs might already be delivered and thus not require decomposition. The risk of cord prolapse or entanglement is greater, hence the increased possibility of emergency cesarean section. Furthermore, the footling and complete breech are not as effective a dilator of the cervix as either the vertex or the larger aggregate profile of the thighs and buttocks of the frank breech, which might increase the risk of entrapment of the aftercoming head. As a result of these considerations, primary cesarean section has been advocated for these breech presentations.

Management of Breech Second Twin

Approximately one-third of all twin gestations present as vertex/breech (i.e., first twin vertex, second twin breech).[53] The appropriate management of these pregnancies is unclear, with some investigators advocating cesarean delivery and others recommending vaginal delivery.[53-56] Blickstein et al.[53] compared the obstetric outcome of 39 cases of vertex/breech twins to the outcomes of 48 vertex/vertex twins. Although the breech second twin had a higher incidence of low birth weight and a longer hospital stay, these authors found no basis for elective cesarean in this situation. Laros and Dattel[54] studied 206 twin pairs and likewise found no clear advantage to arbitrary cesarean delivery because of specific presentation.

The management alternatives in the case of the vertex/breech twin pregnancy in labor include cesarean delivery, vaginal delivery of the first twin and attempted external version of the second, or breech, extraction. Gocke et al.[55] studied the outcome of management of 136 pairs of vertex/nonvertex twins weighing over 1,500 g and concluded that breech extraction of the second twin appeared to be a safe alternative to cesarean delivery.[55] Vaginal delivery followed by external version can be a viable alternative. Ultrasound in the delivery room with direct visualization of the fetus during the attempt can facilitate an otherwise difficult procedure. Often there is a transient decrease in uterine activity after the delivery of the first baby, and this brief period of relaxation can be taken advantage of.

Internal podalic version/extraction of the second twin can also benefit from ultrasound guidance. The goal of the operator is to insert his or her hand into the uterus, identify and grasp both fetal feet with membranes intact, and apply traction to bring the feet into the pelvis and out the introitus, leaving membranes intact until both feet are at the introitus.[56] Maternal expulsive efforts should remain the major force in leading to descent of the fetus. Membranes are ruptured, and the delivery is managed as any footling breech delivery would be managed. The operator can often have difficulty identifying the feet, however, and ultrasound available in the delivery room can facilitate the identification of the fetal feet.

In the case of a breech extraction, and perhaps more often with a breech extraction in the case of the smaller baby, the fetal head can become caught in the cervix. It can be useful in such a case to insert the operator's entire hand into the uterus to cup the fetal head, withdrawing the hand with the fetal head in it.[57] This splinting technique has also been promoted for the safe extraction of the breech at the time of cesarean delivery.[57]

Breech-Perinatal Mortality and Method of Delivery

The reported overall perinatal mortality associated with breech presentation varies from 9 to 25 percent.[1,52,58] The perinatal mortality rate is three to five times that of the nonbreech infant at term,[59-61] and some authors have shown mortalities to be increased and Apgar scores lower with breech presentation at every stage of gestation. Other observers have suggested that these excess deaths are largely due to lethal anomalies and complications of prematurity, adding that malformations and prematurity are both found more frequently among breech infants. Excluding anomalies and extreme prematurity, the corrected perinatal mortality is calculated by some investigators to be near zero regardless of the method of delivery for normal breech infants over 2,500 g.[62]

Despite consideration by some authors of the "corrected" perinatal mortality of breech infants, the infant presenting by the breech has been reported to be at higher risk before, during, and after labor than the comparable infant presenting as a vertex.[1,63-65] At least a portion of the recent and striking increase in the rate of cesarean sections is a response to this reported higher risk in the case of the breech infant.[66-69] In 1980, Collea[50] observed that 29 percent of primary cesarean operations performed at his institution during a 12-month period were performed on infants in the breech presentation. The National Institutes of Health Consensus Report in 1981 found that 12 percent of cesarean section deliveries in 1978 were performed for breech presentation and that this indication contributed 10 to 15 percent to the overall rise in the rate of cesarean births.[65] Although measurably greater risks face the breech infant,[70] the method of delivery alone may or may not contribute to those risks.[71,72] There are many who believe that abandonment of vaginal delivery for the breech has occurred prematurely.[73,74]

The major dangers facing the breech infant are summarized in Table 17.3. While prematurity and birth defects account for a large fraction of the fetal losses associated with breech presentation, there remains an excess of birth trauma and the supposition that vaginal birth may be responsible for some preventable fetal deaths or morbidity. Given the increased likelihood of malformations and extreme prematurity, settlement of the issue of which is the safest method for delivery of the breech requires comparisons of infants comparable in all characteristics except mode of delivery. Indeed, in some series, improved perinatal survival has been reported for breeches born by cesarean section,[58,61,62,70,75] and

Table 17.3 Incidence of Complications Seen With Breech Presentation

Complication	Incidence
Intrapartum fetal death	Increased 16-fold[1]
Intrapartum asphyxia	Increased 3.8-fold[1,70,80]
Cord prolapse	Increased 5-20-fold[1,50,58,71]
Birth trauma	Increased 13-fold[50]
Arrest of aftercoming head	8.8 percent[50]
Spinal cord injuries with deflexion	21 percent[30,95]
Major anomalies	6-18 percent[1,58,88]
Prematurity	16-33 percent[31,52,64,67,72,80,81]
Hyperextension of head	5 percent[94]

there is evidence that the method of delivery may impact on the quality of survival as well. In 1979, Westgren et al.[76] found functional neurologic defects by 2 years of age in 24 percent of breech infants born vaginally, but only in 2.5 percent of those breech infants of similar weights and gestational ages born by cesarean delivery. However, in comparing 175 breech infants having a 94 percent cesarean delivery rate with 595 historical controls having a 22 percent rate of abdominal delivery, Green et al.[69] found no significant differences in outcome. Faber-Nijholt et al.[77] reviewed neurologic outcome in 348 infants born in breech position. Examinations were performed on 239 children from 3 to 10 years of age. No statistically significant differences were notable between breech infants delivered vaginally and properly matched vertex controls. These authors concluded that breech outcome relates to degree of prematurity, impact of pregnancy complications, and presence of malformations as well as birth trauma or asphyxia. The benefit of arbitrary cesarean section in the case of breech presentation therefore remains uncertain.

Type of Breech and Risk

The various categories of breech presentation clearly demonstrate dissimilar risks. Therefore, management plans might vary in these situations.[78,79] The premature breech, the breech with a hyperextended head, and the footling breech are subcategories that have been shown repeatedly to have extraordinarily high rates of fetal loss and complicated vaginal deliveries. Incomplete dilatation and cephalic entrapment may be more frequent. In general, for these three breech presentations, cesarean section appears to optimize fetal outcome and is therefore recommended.

Low birth weight (less than 2,500 g) is a confounding factor in approximately one-third of all breech presentations.[31,52,64,67,72,80,81] While the benefit of cesarean section to the perinatal rate of the 1,500- to 2,500-g breech infant has remained controversial,[11,35,58,80, 82-87] improved survival when abdominal delivery is employed has often been found in the 1,000- to 1,500-g weight group.[64,84] Traumatic morbidity is reported decreased in both groups by cesarean section, including a lower rate of both intra- and periventricular hemorrhage in the low-birth-weight infant delivered by cesarean.[87] Although some advocate a trial of labor in the frank breech infant weighing over 1,500 g, others recommend such a course only when the infant exceeds 2,000 g.[35,67,72,88] It is relevant that there are proportionately fewer frank breech presentations in the low-birth-weight group.[31,64] In fact, most infants weighing less than 1,500 g and presenting as a breech have been found to be footling breeches.[88] Although most deaths in the very-low-birth-weight breech group are due to prematurity or lethal anomalies,[80,83,88,89] cesarean section has been shown by some to decrease corrected perinatal mortality in this weight group compared with that in similar-sized vertex presentations.[64,90] Other authors suggest that improved survival in these studies is incorrectly attributed to cesarean delivery and instead relates to improved neonatal care of the premature infant when compared with the outcomes of historical controls.[91] When vaginal delivery of the preterm breech is chosen or is unavoidable, however, conduction anesthesia and the use of forceps for delivery of the aftercoming head appears to decrease fetal morbidity and mortality.[80,92,93]

A second high-risk category is the breech presentation with a deflexed head. Hyperextension of the fetal head has been consistently associated with a high (21 percent) risk of spinal cord injury if the breech is delivered vaginally.[30,94,95] In such cases, it is important to differentiate simple deflexion of the head from clear hyperextension.[96] Ballas et al.[96] have shown that simple deflexion carries no excess risk. The issue of simple deflexion of the fetal vertex as opposed to hyperextension is similar to the relationships between the occipitofrontal cranial plane and the axis of the fetal cervical spine illustrated in Figure 17.5. Often, as labor progresses, spontaneous flexion will occur in response to fundal forces.

Finally, the footling breech, not uncommon at term and even more common in the preterm breech, carries a prohibitively high (16 to 19 percent) risk of cord prolapse during labor. Furthermore, in many cases cord prolapse may become manifest only late in labor, after a commitment to vaginal delivery has been made.[64,83] Cord prolapse necessitates prompt delivery by cesarean section. To decrease cord compression, the presenting part should be elevated with the examining hand until the cesarean section has started. In addition, the footling breech is a poor

cervical dilator, and cephalic entrapment may be more frequent.

Controversy continues surrounding the method of delivery for the frank or complete breech, as the cesarean section rate for breech presentation increases to 70 to 90 percent without a continued or proportional drop in perinatal mortality.[66–68] Maternal mortality is clearly higher with cesarean section delivery, ranging from 0.2 to 0.43 percent.[71,78] Maternal morbidity is also measurably higher with abdominal delivery. Some institutions report a 50 percent incidence of postoperative maternal morbidity compared with as little as 5 percent with vaginal delivery.[71] In an attempt to balance both maternal and fetal risks, several management plans have been designed to select appropriate candidates for a trial of labor.

In 1965, Zatuchni and Andros[81] retrospectively analyzed 182 breech births. Of those reviewed, 25 infants had poor outcomes. These workers concluded that scoring six clinical variables at the time of admission (Table 17.4) identified those patients destined to manifest serious problems in labor and allowed prompt and appropriate intervention. While there might be inherent doubts about conclusions drawn from a small retrospective database using a system wherein the parturient herself could increase the score by presenting later in labor, at least three subsequent prospective studies applied the Zatuchni-

Table 17.4 Zatuchni-Andros System

| Factor | Points Scored on Presentation in Labor | | |
	0	1	2
Parity	Gravida 1	Multipara	—
Gestational age (weeks)	39	38	37
Estimated weight (lb)	8	7–8	7
Previous breech	None	One	2 or more
Dilatation (cm)	2	3	≥4
Station	≥−3 or more	−2	≤−1

(From Zatuchni and Andros,[81] with permission.)

Andros system and found it to be both sensitive and accurate.[97-99] A Zatuchni-Andros score of less than 4 in these studies accurately predicted poor outcomes in patients with infants presenting as a breech. Furthermore, in applying the scoring system, only 21 to 27 percent of patients failed to qualify for a trial of labor.[97,98]

Because most reports dealing with the risks of breech presentation and method of delivery have been retrospective, serious doubts exist about the validity of such recommendations as much of the data were gathered prior to the modern era of neonatal care and to the common use of continuous electronic fetal monitoring. In an extremely important study, Collea et al.[71,100] selected singleton term frank breech infants with an estimated fetal weight of between 2,500 and 3,800 g in mothers with adequate radiographic pelvimetry and prospectively randomized the cases into two groups. The first group underwent immediate cesarean section, whereas the second group was given a trial of labor. Intrapartum monitoring was used in all patients. The majority, or 82.6 percent, of those patients allowed to labor delivered vaginally without a perinatal loss.[100] There were no maternal deaths, although 36 percent of patients experienced some postpartum morbidity.[71] In a similar study, O'Leary[101] allowed those frank breeches estimated to be between 2,500 and 3,500 g in women with a large pelvis to labor vaginally. He used radiographic pelvimetry, ultrasound, and the Zatuchni-Andros score and paid close attention to the labor curve in selecting candidates for cesarean section. The results were similar to those described by Collea et al.[100] Neither group of investigators found that oxytocin induction of labor was contraindicated if all other criteria were satisfied.[100,101] However, both concluded that augmentation of secondary arrest was not appropriate. Nulliparity or multiparity were not found to be accurate prognostic indicators.[31,102] In a similar study, Gimovsky et al.[103] randomized 105 nonfrank term breech infants and found that 44 percent achieved a safe vaginal delivery. There were no differences in neonatal outcome. Most cesarean sections were performed for arrested progress. Using similar criteria, Flanagan et al.[104] more recently found that a trial of labor in the selected term frank breech resulted in vaginal delivery in 73 percent of

cases, with no increase in maternal or neonatal morbidity or mortality rates. They estimated that with the application of external version to a known breech population and a trial of labor for selected frank breech infants, the cesarean rate for these pregnancies could be safely cut in half.[104]

In conclusion, there does seem to be a place for vaginal delivery of the uncomplicated term frank breech of average size through a normal pelvis if there is normal progress in labor and heart rate monitoring is reassuring.[101] The apparent safety of a trial of labor in selected cases, however, is not without dispute.[105] Furthermore, using properly sensitive monitoring techniques, many nonfrank breech infants might be safely delivered vaginally.[103] If one were to calculate from the known incidences of prematurity, nonfrank breech presentation, poor Zatuchni-Andros score, contracted pelvis, fetal distress, and hyperextended attitude, it could be estimated that only 25 to 28 percent of patients would meet the necessary criteria for a trial of labor.[106] But the factors are not simply additive, and many will coexist. Thus it is more likely that 50 percent would qualify for a trial of labor.[107]

Table 17.5 summarizes those factors that impact on

Table 17.5 Management of the Breech

A trial of labor appears safe if
   Estimated fetal weight $\geq 2,500$ g and $\leq 3,800$ g[1,100]
   Frank breech presentation[100,101]
   Adequate x-ray pelvimetry[1,71,100]
   Flexed fetal head[1]
   Availability of continuous electronic fetal
      monitoring[71,100,101]
   Zatuchni-Andros score ≥ 4[81,99,101]
   Capability for rapid cesarean birth[1]
   Absence of maternal or fetal distress[101]
   Good labor progress[71,100]
   Availability of experienced attendants
A cesarean delivery is considered prudent with
   Fetal weight ≥ 800 g and $\leq 1,500$ g[11,80,88]
   Footling breech presentation[1,71,100]
   One or more contracted pelvic diameters[71,100,101]
   Hyperextension of fetal head[95]
   Zatuchni-Andros score < 4[81,99,101]
   Absence of expertise in vaginal delivery
   Evidence of fetal distress[1,71,100]
   Secondary arrest of progress[71,100]

the decision to deliver a breech vaginally or by cesarean section. The obvious implication of the dramatically decreased experience in training programs with vaginal breech deliveries is that the danger to the infant will rise with the absence of appropriate training. Therefore, obstetric inexperience itself will constitute an indication for cesarean section. Such a circumstance appears unavoidable. Certainly, in no case should a woman with an infant presenting as a breech be allowed to labor unless (1) anesthesia coverage is immediately available, (2) a cesarean section can be undertaken promptly, (3) continuous fetal monitoring is used, and (4) the delivery is attended by a pediatrician and two obstetricians experienced with vaginal breech birth. The ultimate decision belongs to the patient. The decision is made with the advice of her obstetrician. The apparent conflict of interest involves the increase in maternal risk associated with cesarean delivery versus the possibly increased risk of neonatal morbidity or perinatal mortality associated by some investigators with vaginal delivery of the breech.

External Version

External cephalic version, the third alternative to vaginal delivery or cesarean section for the breech infant, is espoused as vigorously by some investigators as it is discouraged by others.[52,59,107–110] Many have found that consistent application of this technique significantly reduces the incidence of breech presentation in labor and is associated with few complications such as cord compression or placental separation.[108–110] Reported success of external version varies from 60 to 75 percent, with a similar percentage of these remaining vertex to labor.[111–115] Ylikorkala and Hartikainen-Sorri[110] found that while many infants in breech presentation before 34 weeks will convert spontaneously to a cephalic presentation, few will do so afterward. A careful, gentle, repetitive external version technique applied weekly after 34 weeks was successful in converting over two-thirds of cases, reducing their breech presentation rate by 50 percent.[110] In a randomized trial of external cephalic version in low-risk pregnancies between 37 and 39 weeks, Van Dorsten and colleagues[107] were successful in 68 percent of 25 cases in the version group. Four of the 23 controls converted to a vertex presentation spontaneously before labor. All those in whom external version was successful presented in labor as vertex.[107] Gentle constant pressure applied in a relaxed patient with constant fetal heart rate surveillance are elements of the method stressed by all investigators.[52,59,107] Methodology varies, although the "forward roll" technique enjoys wider support than the "back flip" (Fig. 17.25).[107]

Tocolysis and ultrasound during the procedure may also be helpful, but reports of benefit from tocolysis are conflicting. Most studies are not randomized trials.[114] Robertson et al.[112] in a randomized trial including 58 patients at 37 to 41 weeks gestation with breech presentation, found no benefit from β-mimetic tocolysis. The success rate was 66.7 percent with tocolysis and 67.8 percent without tocolysis.[112] Factors associated with failure of version included obesity, deep pelvic engagement of the breech, oligohydramnios, and posterior positioning of the fetal back.[113] Fetomaternal transfusion has been reported to occur in up to 6 percent of patients undergoing external version.[116] Rh-negative unsensitized women should, therefore, receive Rh immune globulin.

SHOULDER DYSTOCIA

Shoulder dystocia is diagnosed when, after the delivery of the fetal head, further progress toward expulsion of the infant is prevented by impaction of the fetal shoulders within the maternal pelvis. This requires specific efforts to relieve the obstruction and allow delivery (Fig. 17.26).

Although it happens infrequently, the clinician does not soon forget a difficult case of shoulder dystocia. Generally occurring at the end of a difficult labor, the fetal head may be delivered spontaneously or by forceps, but the neck is retracted. Often, the fetal head appears to be drawn back with the chin against the maternal thigh or thighs. It may be difficult to suction the infant's mouth because of its close approximation to the perineum. As maternal expulsive efforts are more vigorously encouraged, the fetal head becomes plethoric, and the danger to the infant becomes apparent if delivery cannot be promptly accomplished.

Shoulder dystocia has been reported in 0.15 to 1.7 percent of all vaginal deliveries.[117–120] Although some observers have reported an apparent increase in the incidence in recent years,[117] others have disputed

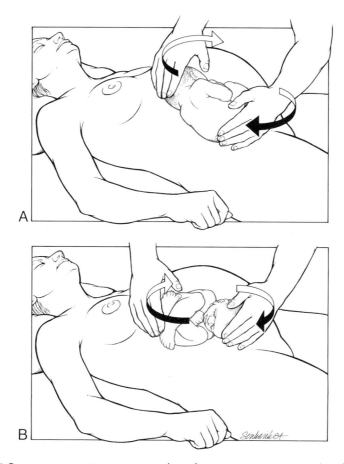

Fig. 17.25 (A & B) Operator attempting to convert a breech to a vertex presentation by effecting a forward roll movement in the fetus. The use of ultrasound simultaneously facilitates this maneuver. Tocolysis is controversial.

such a trend,[121] believing instead that the data only reflect increased reporting.

All investigators have documented increased perinatal morbidity and mortality with shoulder dystocia.[117] Mortality varies from 21 to 290 in 1,000 when shoulder girdle impaction occurs, and neonatal morbidity has been reported to be immediately obvious in 20 percent of infants.[119] In reviewing 131 macrosomic infants, Boyd et al.[121] found that one-half of all cases of brachial palsy occurring in macrosomic infants accompanied the diagnosis of shoulder dystocia. Severe asphyxia was observed in 143 of 1,000 births with shoulder dystocia compared with 14 of 1,000 overall.[121] Fetal morbidity is not always immediately apparent. McCall[122] found 28 percent of infants born with shoulder dystocia to demonstrate some

neuropsychiatric dysfunction at 5- to 10-year follow-up. Fewer than one-half of these children had immediate morbidity.

Although shoulder dystocia has traditionally been strongly associated with macrosomia, up to one-half of cases of shoulder dystocia occur in neonates under 4,000 g.[123,124] However, Acker et al.[124] found that the relative probability of shoulder dystocia in the 7 percent of infants over 4,000 g was 11 times greater than the average, and in the 2 percent of infants over 4,500 g it was 22 times greater. With macrosomia or continued fetal growth beyond term, the trunk and particularly the chest grow larger relative to the head. The chest circumference exceeds the head circumference in 80 percent of cases.[123] The arms also contribute to the greater dimensions of the upper body. Within a

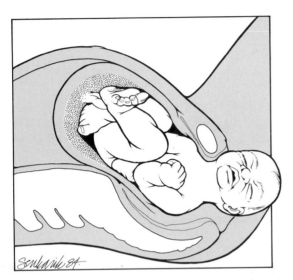

Fig. 17.26 After delivery of the head of this fetus, the right shoulder has become impacted behind the pubic symphysis. Heroic and desperate traction on the head is dangerous and will not be helpful.

barely adequate pelvis, such bulk might easily block fetal rotation from a disadvantageous AP to the more desirable oblique diameter. Macrosomia has the strongest correlation with shoulder dystocia of any clinical feature. Other clinical factors associated with shoulder dystocia appear to be related to macrosomia as well and include maternal obesity,[121,125] previous birth of an infant weighing more than 4,000 g,[121,123,125] diabetes,[125,126] prolonged gestation,[121,125] prolonged second stage,[125] prolonged deceleration phase (8 to 10 cm),[117] and instrumental midpelvic delivery.[126] Increased maternal age and excess maternal weight gain have been found to increase the risk of macrosomia and shoulder dystocia by some but not all investigators.[121,125,126]

Because excess fetal size is strongly associated with shoulder dystocia, it is relevant to review that subject briefly. Macrosomia has been variously defined as a birth weight of more than 4,000 g or more than 4,500.[119,121,127–129] A male predominance is routinely observed, and the condition is associated with the clinical features described above. The two most common complications seen with macrosomia are postpartum hemorrhage and shoulder dystocia.[125] Golditch and Kirkman[128] observed shoulder dystocia in 3

percent of deliveries of infants weighing between 4,100 and 4,500 g and in 8.2 percent of those over 4,500 g. Benedetti and Gabbe[119] reported that fetal injury occurred in 47 percent of infants weighing more than 4,000 g who were delivered from the midpelvis and had shoulder dystocia.

Clinical efforts to detect macrosomia prenatally could be helpful in anticipating problems with delivering the shoulders at delivery. Such efforts, however, have had imperfect results. Parks and Ziel[125] found that, of 110 macrosomic infants, the diagnosis was made prenatally in only 20 percent. The clinical estimate of birth weight was more than 3 lb in error in 6 percent.

Ultrasonic techniques promoted for the detection of macrosomia include the estimation of fetal weight using a variety of fetal dimensions and the comparison of chest to head circumference.[117,123] There is a growing trend to consider cesarean delivery of any infant with an estimated weight over 4,500 g, or any infant of a diabetic mother with an estimated weight over 4,000 g.[124,126] Any consideration of elective abdominal delivery based on estimated fetal weight, however, must consider the technical error of the method. If 90 percent confidence is desired that the actual fetal weight is at least 4,000 g, the ultrasonic estimate in the case of most current methods must exceed 4,600 g. This is because the ultrasonic estimation of fetal weight carries an error of at least plus or minus 10 percent (one standard deviation). Furthermore, the fetal vertex is often too deeply engaged in the pelvis to allow accurate measurement of head circumference. Estimated fetal weight should be only one of several factors considered in the management of the laboring patient. In the case of a diabetic, obese patient with an estimated fetal weight over 4,500 g and making poor progress in labor, cesarean section may be the most prudent course of action. However, in most other cases, the risks of cesarean to the mother, the accuracy of prediction of macrosomia, and the alternative of a carefully monitored trial of labor should be discussed. Gross et al.[130] carefully reviewed the clinical characteristics of 394 mothers delivering infants over 4,000 g and concluded that, although birth weight, prolonged deceleration phase, and length of second stage were all individually predictive, no prospective model adequately discrimi-

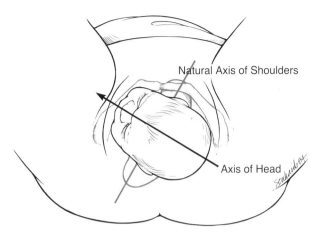

Fig. 17.27 After delivery of the vertex, this fetal head has reassumed a natural relationship to the shoulders, which are in the opposite oblique diameter of the maternal pelvis.

nated the infant destined to sustain trauma from shoulder dystocia from the infant not destined to sustain trauma.[130]

Normally, after the delivery of the head, external rotation (restitution) occurs, returning the head to its natural perpendicular relationship to the shoulder girdle. The fetal saggital suture is usually oblique to the AP diameter of the outlet, and the shoulders occupy the opposite oblique pelvic diameter (Fig. 17.27). As the shoulders descend in response to maternal pushing, the anterior shoulder emerges from its oblique axis under one of the pubic rami. If, however, the anterior shoulder descends in the AP diameter of the outlet and the fetus is relatively large for the outlet, impaction behind the symphysis can occur, and further descent is blocked.[120,131] Shoulder dystocia also occurs with an extremely rapid delivery of the head, as can occur with vacuum extraction or forceps. It could also result from overzealous external rotation of the fetal vertex by the operator.

The first consideration of treatment is anticipation and preparation. Anticipation involves primarily the prenatal suspicion of macrosomia by clinical and ultrasonic methods. One must be aware of the clinical features that have been cited that place a pregnancy at high risk for macrosomia and therefore for shoulder dystocia.

Such deliveries are best managed in a delivery room. Deliveries in bed increase the difficulty of reducing a shoulder dystocia, because the bedding precludes fullest use of the posterior pelvis and outlet. Many investigators also suggest that blood be prepared, because postpartum hemorrhage is more likely. Strong consideration for cesarean section is recommended when a prolonged second stage occurs in association with macrosomia.

Once a vaginal delivery has begun, the obstetrician must resist the temptation to rotate the head to a transverse axis. Maternal expulsive efforts should be used rather than traction. Gentle manual pressure on the fetal head inferiorly and posteriorly will push the posterior shoulder into the hollow of the sacrum, increasing the room for the anterior shoulder to pass under the pubis (Fig. 17.28). If such efforts do not result in delivery, shoulder dystocia is diagnosed.

A deliberate, planned sequence of efforts should then be initiated. One must not pull desperately on the fetal head. Fundal expulsive efforts, including maternal pushing and fundal pressure, should be temporarily stopped. Aggressive fundal pressure often worsens the impaction. In many cases, only moderate suprapubic pressure is necessary to disimpact the anterior shoulder and allow for delivery (Fig. 17.29). If this is not effective, the operator's hand may be

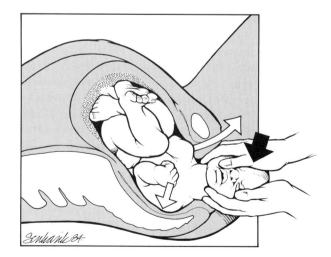

Fig. 17.28 Gentle pressure on the fetal vertex in a dorsal direction will move the posterior fetal shoulder deeper into the maternal pelvic hollow, usually resulting in easy delivery of the anterior shoulder.

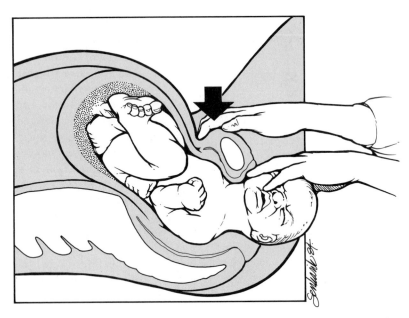

Fig. 17.29 Moderate suprapubic pressure is often the only additional maneuver necessary to disimpact the anterior fetal shoulder.

passed behind the occiput into the vagina, and the anterior shoulder may be pushed forward to the oblique where, with maternal efforts and gentle posterior pressure, delivery should occur (Fig. 17.30).[117,118] Alternatively, the posterior shoulder may be pushed forward, through a 180 degree arc, and passed under the pubic ramus as in turning a screw. As the posterior shoulder rotates anteriorly, it will often deliver.[123,132,133]

Many authorities have advocated delivery of the posterior arm and shoulder should these methods fail. The operator's hand is passed into the vagina, following the posterior arm of the fetus to the elbow. The arm is flexed and swept out over the chest and the perineum (Fig. 17.31). In some cases, delivery will now occur without further manipulation. In others, rotation of the trunk bringing the freed posterior arm anteriorly is necessary.[117,118,123,132]

Deliberate fracture of the clavicle is possible and will significantly facilitate delivery by diminishing the rigidity and size of the shoulder girdle. It is best if the pressure is exerted in a direction away from the lung to avoid puncture. Sharp instrumental transsection of the clavicle is not recommended, as lung puncture is common with such a technique, and infection of the

bone through the open wound is a serious complication.

Gonik et al.[134] described an interesting maternal manipulation consisting of hyperflexion of maternal legs on the maternal abdomen that results in flattening of the lumbar spine and ventral rotation of the maternal pelvis and symphysis (Fig. 17.32). This maneuver may increase the useful size of the posterior outlet, resulting in easier disimpaction of the anterior shoulder. More recently, these authors showed that this technique (McRoberts maneuver) significantly reduces shoulder extraction forces, brachial plexus stretching, and the likelihood of clavicular fracture.[135]

Two techniques rarely used in the United States for the management of shoulder dystocia include vaginal replacement of the fetal head with cesarean delivery (Zavanelli maneuver) and subcutaneous symphysiotomy. Sanberg[136] recently reviewed 15 published cases of the Zavanelli maneuver, with remarkable results. Seven of eight infants managed with this technique and delivered by cesarean after replacement of the fetal head for intractable shoulder dystocia had a good outcome. One infant was stillborn.[136] Subcutaneous symphysiotomy has been practiced in remote

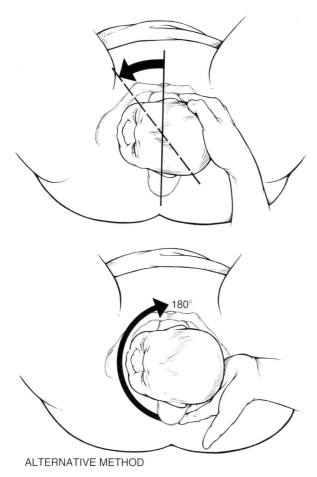

ALTERNATIVE METHOD

Fig. 17.30 Delivery may be facilitated by counterclockwise rotation of the anterior shoulder to the more favorable oblique pelvic diameter as illustrated here, or alternatively clockwise rotation of the posterior shoulder. During these maneuvers, expulsive efforts should be stopped.

areas of the world for many years as an expedient alternative to cesarean delivery with very good results.[137] However, neither of these techniques is widely or often used in obstetric practice in this country. The attempted implementation of either method by the inexperienced practitioner before the trial of more conventional remedies carries grave risk to the child, the mother, and the clinician.

In summary, many cases of shoulder dystocia are predictable, to a degree, and most will respond to any

or all of the methods outlined above. Which specific method is used is probably not as critical as the practice of a careful, methodical approach to the problem and the avoidance of desperate, potentially traumatic traction. There may not be any complication of labor and delivery, where forethought is more important to success than shoulder dystocia.

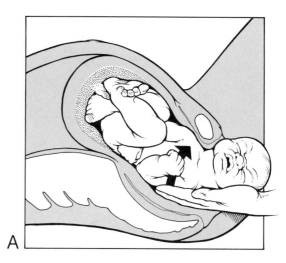

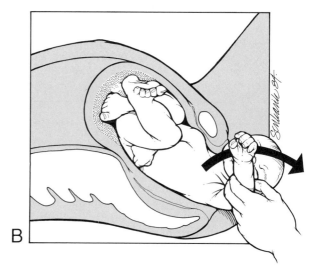

Fig. 17.31 If less invasive maneuvers fail to produce disimpaction, delivery should be facilitated by manipulative delivery of the posterior arm by inserting a hand into the posterior vagina (A) and ventrally rotating the arm at the shoulder with delivery over the perineum (B).

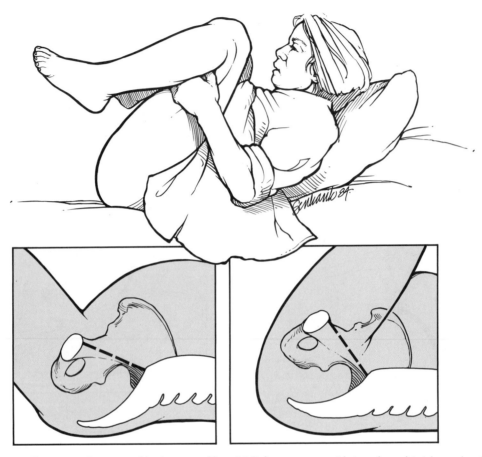

Fig. 17.32 Sharp ventral rotation of both maternal hips (McRoberts maneuver) brings the pelvic inlet and outlet into a more vertical alignment, facilitating delivery of the fetal shoulders.

REFERENCES

1. Pritchard JA, MacDonald PC: Williams Obstetrics. 16th Ed. Appleton-Century-Crofts, New York, 1980
2. Yates MJ: Transverse foetal lie in labour. J Obstet Gynaecol Br Commonw 71:245, 1964
3. MacGregor WG: Aetiology and treatment of the oblique, transverse and unstable lie of the foetus with particular reference to antenatal care. J Obstet Gynaecol Br Commonw 71:237, 1964
4. Cockburn KG, Drake RF: Transverse and oblique lie of the foetus. Aust NZ J Obstet Gynaecol 8:211, 1968
5. Sandhu SK: Transverse lie. J Indian Med Assoc 68:205, 1977
6. Cruikshank DP, White CA: Obstetric malpresentations—twenty years' experience. Am J Obstet Gynecol 116:1097, 1973
7. Edwards RI, Nicholson HO: The management of the unstable lie in late pregnancy. J Obstet Gynaecol Br Commonw 76:713, 1969
8. Flowers CE: Shoulder presentation. Am J Obstet Gynecol 96:145, 1966
9. Johnson CE: Abnormal fetal presentations. Lancet 84:317, 1964
10. Johnson CE: Transverse presentation of fetus. JAMA 187:642, 1964
11. Hourihane MJ: Etiology and management of oblique lie. Obstet Gynecol 32:512, 1968
12. Phalen JP, Boucher M, Mueller E et al: The nonlaboring transverse lie. J Reprod Med 31:184, 1986
13. Browne ADH, Carney D: Management of malpresentations in obstetrics. Br Med J 5393:1295, 1964
14. Cackins LA, Pearce EWJ: Transverse presentation. Obstet Gynecol 9:123, 1957

15. Pelosi MA, Apuzzio J, Fricchione D et al: The intra-abdominal version technique for delivery of transverse lie by low segment cesarean section. Am J Obstet Gynecol 136:1009, 1979
16. Benedetti TJ, Lowensohn RI, Truscott AM: Face presentation at term. Obstet Gynecol 55:199, 1980
17. Copeland GN, Nicks FI, Christakos AC: Face and brow presentations. NC Med J 29:507, 1968
18. Duff P: Diagnosis and management of face presentation. Obstet Gynecol 57:105, 1981
19. Groenig DC: Face presentation. Obstet Gynecol 2:495, 1953
20. Magid R, Gillespie CF: Face and brow presentation. Obstet Gynecol 9:450, 1957
21. Prevedourakis CN: Face presentation. Am J Obstet Gynecol 94:1092, 1966
22. Campbell JM: Face presentation. Aust NZ Obstet Gynaecol 5:231, 1965
23. Dede JA, Friedman EA: Face presentation. Am J Obstet Gynecol 87:515, 1963
24. Gomez HE, Dennen EH: Face presentation. Obstet Gynecol 8:103, 1956
25. Salzmann B, Soled M, Gilmour T: Face presentation. Obstet Gynecol 16:106, 1960
26. Mostar S, Akactin E, Babuna C: Deflexion attitudes. Obstet Gynecol 28:49, 1966
27. Cucco UP: Face presentation. Am J Obstet Gynecol 94:1085, 1966
28. Borrell U, Fernstrom I: The mechanism of labor. Radiol Clin North Am 5:73, 1966
29. Schwartz A, Dgani R, Lancet M et al: Face presentation. Aust NZ Obstet Gynaecol 26:172, 1986
30. Abroms IF, Bresnan MJ, Zuckerman JE et al: Cervical cord injuries secondary to hypertension of the head in breech presentations. Obstet Gynecol 41:369, 1973
31. Adams CM: Review of breech presentation. SD J Med 32:15, 1979
32. Gold S: The conduct and management of face presentations. J Int Coll Surg 43:253, 1965
33. Lansford A, Arias D, Smith BE: Respiratory obstruction associated with face presentation. Am J Dis Child 116:318, 1968
34. Meltzer RM, Sachtleban MR, Friedman EA: Brow presentation. Am J Obstet Gynecol 100:255, 1968
35. Kovacs SG: Brow presentation. Med J Aust 2:820, 1970
36. Abell DA: Brow presentation. S Afr Med J 47:1315, 1973
37. Levy DL: Persistent brow presentation—a new approach to management. South Med J 69:191, 1976
38. Ingolfsson A: Brow presentations. Acta Obstet Gynecol Scand 48:486, 1969
39. Bednoff SL, Thomas BE: Brow presentation. NY J Med 67:803, 1967
40. Skalley TW, Kramer TF: Brow presentation. Obstet Gynecol 15:616, 1960
41. Moore EJT, Dennen EH: Management of persistent brow presentation. Obstet Gynecol 6:186, 1955
42. Jennings PN: Brow presentation with vaginal delivery. Aust NZ J Obstet Gynaecol 8:219, 1968
43. Breen JL, Wiesmeien E: Compound presentation—a survey of 131 patients. Obstet Gynecol 32:419, 1968
44. Goplerud J, Eastman NJ: Compound presentation. Obstet Gynecol 1:59, 1953
45. Weissberg SM, O'Leary JA: Compound presentation of the fetus. Obstet Gynecol 41:60, 1973
46. Dignam WJ: Difficulties in delivery, including shoulder dystocia and malpresentations of the fetus. Clin Obstet Gynecol 19:577, 1976
47. Ang LT: Compound presentation following external version. Aust NZ J Obstet Gynaecol 19:213, 1978
48. Douglas HGK, Savage PE: An unusual case of compound presentation. J Obstet Gynaecol Br Commonw 77:1036, 1970
49. Weissberg SM, Weingold AB: Compound presentation of the fetus. NY J Med 67:936, 1967
50. Collea JV: Current management of breech presentation. Clin Obstet Gynecol 23:525, 1980
51. Braun FHT, Jones KL, Smith DW: Breech presentations as an indicator of fetal abnormality. J Pediatr 86:419, 1975
52. Fall O, Nilsson BA: External cephalic version in breech presentation under tocolysis. Obstet Gynecol 53:712, 1979
53. Blickstein I, Schwartz-Shoham Z, Lancet M: Vaginal delivery of the second twin in breech presentation. Obstet Gynecol 69:774, 1987
54. Laros RK, Dattel BJ: Management of twin pregnancy: the vaginal route is still safe. Am J Obstet Gynecol 158:1330, 1988
55. Gocke SE, Nageotte MP, Garite T et al: Management of the nonvertex second twin: primary cesarean section, external version, or primary breech extraction. Am J Obstet Gynecol 161:111, 1989
56. Rabinovici J, Reichman B, Serr DM et al: Internal podalic version with unruptured membranes for the second twin in transverse lie. Obstet Gynecol 71:428, 1988
57. Druzin ML: Atraumatic delivery in cases of malpresentation of the very low birth weight fetus at cesarean section: the splint technique. Am J Obstet Gynecol 154:941, 1986
58. Kubli F: Risk of vaginal breech delivery. Contrib Gynecol Obstet 3:80, 1977

59. Hibbard LT, Schumann WR: Prophylactic external cephalic version in an obstetric practice. Am J Obstet Gynecol 116:511, 1973

60. Kauppila O, Gronroos M, Aro P et al: Management of low birth weight breech delivery—should cesarean section be routine? Obstet Gynecol 57:289, 1981

61. Rovinsky JJ, Miller JA, Kaplan S: Management of breech presentation at term. Am J Obstet Gynecol 115:497, 1973

62. Lyons ER, Papsin FR: Cesarean section in the management of breech presentation. Am J Obstet Gynecol 130:558, 1978

63. de la Fuente P, Escalante JM, Hernandez-Garcia JM: Perinatal mortality in breech presentations. Contrib Gynecol Obstet 3:108, 1977

64. Goldenberg RL, Nelson KG: The premature breech. Am J Obstet Gynecol 127:240, 1977

65. NIH consensus development statement on cesarean childbirth. Obstet Gynecol 57:537, 1981

66. Mansani FE, Cerutti M: The risk in breech delivery. Contrib Gynecol Obstet 3:86, 1977

67. Seitchik J: Discussion of "breech delivery—evaluation of the method of delivery on perinatal results and maternal morbidity" by Bowes et al. Am J Obstet Gynecol 135:970, 1979

68. Wolter DF: Patterns of management with breech presentation. Am J Obstet Gynecol 125:733, 1976

69. Green JE, McLean F, Smith LP et al: Has an increased cesarean section rate for term breech delivery reduced the incidence of birth asphyxia, trauma, and death? Am J Obstet Gynecol 142:643, 1982

70. Brenner WE, Bruce RD, Hendricks CH: The characteristics and perils of breech presentation. Am J Obstet Gynecol 118:700, 1974

71. Collea JV, Rabin SC, Weghorst GR et al: The randomized management of term frank breech presentation—vaginal delivery versus cesarean section. Am J Obstet Gynecol 131:186, 1978

72. DeCrespigny LJC, Pepperell RJ: Perinatal mortality and morbidity in breech presentation. Obstet Gynecol 53:141, 1979

73. Graves WK: Breech delivery in twenty years of practice. Am J Obstet Gynecol 137:229, 1980

74. Niswander KR: Discussion of "the randomized management of term frank breech presentation—vaginal delivery versus cesarean section" by Collea et al. Am J Obstet Gynecol 131:193, 1978

75. Spanio P, Elia F, DeBonis F et al: Fetal-neonatal mortality and morbidity in cesarean deliveries. Contrib Gynecol Obstet 3:130, 1977

76. Westgren M, Ingemarsson I, Svenningsen NW: Long-term follow-up of preterm infants in breech presentation delivered by cesarean section. Dan Med Bull 26:141, 1979

77. Faber-Nijholt R, Huisjes JH, Touwen CL et al: Neurological follow-up of 281 children born in breech presentation—a controlled study. Br Med J 286:9, 1983

78. Bowes WA, Taylor ES, O'Brien M et al: Breech delivery—evaluation of the method of delivery on perinatal results and maternal morbidity. Am J Obstet Gynecol 135:965, 1979

79. Lewis BV, Sene Viratne HR: Vaginal breech delivery or cesarean section. Am J Obstet Gynecol 134:615, 1979

80. Cruikshank DP, Pitkin RM: Delivery of the premature breech. Obstet Gynecol 50:367, 1977

81. Zatuchni GI, Andros GJ: Prognostic index for vaginal delivery in breech presentation at term. Am J Obstet Gynecol 93:237, 1965

82. Cruikshank DP: Premature breech [letter to the editor]. Am J Obstet Gynecol 130:500, 1978

83. Woods JR: Effects of low birth weight breech delivery on neonatal mortality. Obstet Gynecol 53:735, 1979

84. Ulstein M: Breech delivery. Ann Chir Gynaecol Fenn 69:70, 1980

85. Weissman A, Blazer S, Zimmer EZ et al: Low birth-weight breech infant: short term and long term outcome by method of delivery. Am J Perinatol 5:289, 1988

86. Anderson G, Strong C: The premature breech: caesarean section or trial of labour? J Med Ethics 14:18, 1988

87. Tejani N, Verma U, Shiffman R et al: Effect of route of delivery on periventricular/intraventricular hemorrhage in the low-birth-weight fetus with a breech presentation. J Reprod Med 32:911, 1987

88. Karp LE, Doney JR, McCarthy T et al: The premature breech—trial of labor or cesarean section? Obstet Gynecol 53:88, 1979

89. Mann LI, Gallant JM: Modern management of the breech delivery. Am J Obstet Gynecol 134:611, 1979

90. Dvenhoelter JH, Wells CE, Reisch JS et al: A paired controlled study of vaginal and abdominal delivery of the low birth weight breech fetus. Obstet Gynecol 54:310, 1979

91. Cox C, Kendall AC, Hommers M: Changed prognosis of breech-presenting low birthweight infants. Br J Obstet Gynaecol 89:881, 1982

92. Milner RDG: Neonatal mortality of breech deliveries with and without forceps to the aftercoming head. Br J Obstet Gynaecol 82:783, 1975

93. Milner RDG: Neonatal mortality of breech deliveries

with and without forceps to the aftercoming head. Contrib Gynecol Obstet 3:113, 1977

94. Caterini H, Langer A, Sama JC et al: Fetal risk in hyperextension of the fetal head in breech presentation. Am J Obstet Gynecol 123:632, 1975

95. Daw E: Hyperextension of the head in breech presentation. Am J Obstet Gynecol 119:564, 1974

96. Ballas S, Toaff R, Jaffa AJ: Deflexion of the fetal head in breech presentation. Obstet Gynecol 52:653, 1978

97. Bird CC, McElin TW: A six year prospective study of term breech deliveries utilizing the Zatuchni-Andros prognostic scoring index. Am J Obstet Gynecol 121:551, 1975

98. Mark C, Roberts PHR: Breech scoring index. Am J Obstet Gynecol 101:572, 1968

99. Zatuchni GI, Andros GJ: Prognostic index for vaginal delivery in breech presentation at term. Am J Obstet Gynecol 98:854, 1967

100. Collea JV, Chein C, Quilligan EJ: The randomized management of term frank breech presentation—a study of 208 cases. Am J Obstet Gynecol 137:235, 1980

101. O'Leary JA: Vaginal delivery of the term breech. Obstet Gynecol 53:341, 1979

102. Selvaggi L, Chieppa M, Loizzi P et al: Intrapartum mortality among breech deliveries. Contrib Gynecol Obstet 3:99, 1977

103. Gimovsky ML, Wallace RL, Schifrin BS et al: Randomized management of the non-frank breech presentation at term—a preliminary report. Am J Obstet Gynecol 146:34, 1983

104. Flanagan TA, Mulchahey KM, Korenbrot CC et al: Management of term breech presentation. Am J Obstet Gynecol 156:1492, 1987

105. Bingham P, Lilford RJ: Management of the selected term breech presentation: assessment of the risks of selected vaginal delivery versus cesarean section for all cases. Obstet Gynecol 69:965, 1987

106. Quilligan EJ: Response to discussion of "the randomized management of term frank breech presentation—a study of 208 cases" by Collea et al. Am J Obstet Gynecol 137:242, 1980

107. Van Dorsten JP, Schifrin BS, Wallace RL: Randomized control trial of external cephalic version with tocolysis in late pregnancy. Am J Obstet Gynecol 141:417, 1981

108. Hanley BJ: Editorial—fallacy of external version. Obstet Gynecol 4:124, 1954

109. Thornhill PE: Changes in fetal polarity near term spontaneous and external version. Am J Obstet Gynecol 93:306, 1965

110. Ylikorkala O, Hartikainen-Sorri A: Value of external version in fetal malpresentation in combination with use of ultrasound. Acta Obstet Gynecol Scand 56:63, 1977

111. Stine LE, Phalen JP, Wallace R et al: Update on external cephalic version performed at term. Obstet Gynecol 65:642, 1985

112. Robertson AW, Kopelman JN, Read JA et al: External cephalic version at term: is a tocolytic necessary? Obstet Gynecol 70:896, 1987

113. Fortunato SJ, Mercer LJ, Guzick DS: External cephalic version with tocolysis: factors associated with success. Obstet Gynecol 72:59, 1988

114. Marchick R: Antepartum external cephalic version with tocolysis: a study of term singleton breech presentations. Am J Obstet Gynecol 158:1339, 1988

115. Scaling ST: External cephalic version without tocolysis. Am J Obstet Gynecol 158:1424, 1988

116. Marcus RG, Crewe-Brown H, Krawitz S et al: Fetomaternal haemorrhage following successful and unsuccessful attempts at external cephalic version. Br J Obstet Gynaecol 82:578, 1975

117. Hopwood HG: Shoulder dystocia—fifteen years' experience in a community hospital. Am J Obstet Gynecol 144:162, 1982

118. Pritchard JA, MacDonald PC: Williams Obstetrics. 16th Ed. Appleton-Century-Crofts, New York, 1980

119. Benedetti TJ, Gabbe SG: Shoulder dystocia—a complication of fetal macrosomia and prolonged second stage of labor with midpelvic delivery. Obstet Gynecol 52:526, 1978

120. Swartz DP: Shoulder girdle dystocia in vertex delivery—clinical study and review. Obstet Gynecol 15:194, 1960

121. Boyd ME, Usher RH, McLean FH: Fetal macrosomia—prediction, risks, and proposed management. Obstet Gynecol 61:715, 1983

122. McCall JO: Shoulder dystocia—a study of aftereffects. Am J Obstet Gynecol 83:1486, 1962

123. Seigworth GR: Shoulder dystocia—review of 5 years' experience. Obstet Gynecol 28:764, 1966

124. Acker DB, Sachs BP, Friedman EA: Risk factors for shoulder dystocia. Obstet Gynecol 66:762, 1985

125. Parks DG, Ziel HK: Macrosomia—a proposed indication for primary cesarean section. Obstet Gynecol 52:407, 1978

126. Acker DB, Gregory KD, Sachs BP et al: Risk factors for Erb-Duchene palsy. Obstet Gynecol 71:389, 1988

127. Modanlou HD, Dorchester WL, Thorosian A et al: Macrosomia—maternal, fetal, and neonatal implications. Obstet Gynecol 55:420, 1980

128. Golditch IM, Kirkman K: The large fetus—

management and outcome. Obstet Gynecol 52:26, 1978

129. Modanlou HD, Komatsu G, Dorchester W et al: Large-for-gestational-age neonates: anthropometric reasons for shoulder dystocia. Obstet Gynecol 60:417, 1982

130. Gross TL, Sokol RJ, Williams T et al: Shoulder dystocia: a fetal-physician risk. Am J Obstet Gynecol 156:1408, 1987

131. Hibbard LT: Shoulder dystocia. Obstet Gynecol 34:424, 1969

132. Barnum CG: Dystocia due to the shoulders. Am J Obstet Gynecol 50:459, 1949

133. Gross SJ, Shime J, Farine D: Shoulder dystocia: pre-dictors and outcome. Am J Obstet Gynecol 156:334, 1987

134. Gonik B, Stringer CA, Held B: An alternate maneuver for management of shoulder dystocia. Am J Obstet Gynecol 145:882, 1983

135. Gonik B, Allen R, Sorab J: Objective evaluation of the shoulder dystocia phenomenon: effect of maternal pelvic orientation on force reduction. Obstet Gynecol 74:44, 1989

136. Sandberg EC: The Zavanelli maneuver extended: pro-gression of a revolutionary concept. Am J Obstet Gynecol 158:1347, 1988

137. Hartfield VJ: Symphysiotomy for shoulder dystocia [letter]. Am J Obstet Gynecol 155:228, 1986

Chapter 18

Obstetric Hemorrhage

Thomas J. Benedetti

ASSESSMENT AND TREATMENT OF BLOOD LOSS

It is critical that the obstetrician be able to estimate rapidly the blood volume deficit in the pregnant patient. Although some have proposed that the pregnant woman fails to show the usual signs and symptoms of blood loss, there is little scientific evidence to support this hypothesis. The confusion may have arisen from an incomplete understanding of the physiologic responses to volume loss and lack of appreciation of normal volume expansion of pregnancy. The normal pregnant patient frequently loses 500 ml of blood at the time of vaginal delivery and 1,000 ml at the time of cesarean section. Appreciably more blood can be lost without clinical evidence of a volume deficit as a result of the 40 percent expansion in blood volume that occurs by 30 weeks of pregnancy.

To understand why the pregnant patient does not exhibit early signs of volume loss, it is important to understand the normal physiologic responses to hemorrhage. When 1,000 ml is rapidly removed from the circulatory blood volume, vasoconstriction occurs in both the arterial and venous compartments to preserve essential body organ flow. In addition, if the volume loss has occurred more than 4 hours earlier, significant fluid shifts from the interstitial space into the intravascular space will partially correct the volume deficit. This movement of fluid, termed transcapillary refill, can replace as much as 30 percent of lost volume. In more chronic bleeding states, the final blood volume deficit can amount to as little as 70 percent of the actual blood lost.

CLASSIFICATION OF HEMORRHAGE

A standard classification for volume loss secondary to hemorrhage is illustrated in Table 18.1. Hemorrhage can be classified as one of four classes, depending on the volume lost. The determination of the class of hemorrhage reflects the volume deficit, which may not be the same as the volume loss. Because the average 60-kg pregnant woman has a blood volume of 6,000 ml at 30 weeks, an unreplaced volume loss of less than 900 ml falls into class 1. Such patients rarely exhibit signs or symptoms of volume deficit.

A blood loss of 1,200 to 1,500 ml is characterized as a class 2 hemorrhage. These individuals will begin to show expected physical signs, the first being a rise in pulse rate and/or possibly a rise in respiratory rate. Tachypnea is a nonspecific response to volume loss and, although a relatively early sign of mild volume deficit, is frequently overlooked. A doubling of the respiratory rate may be observed in this circumstance. If the patient appears to be breathing rapidly, the minute ventilation is usually twice its normal value. This finding should not be interpreted as an encouraging sign, but rather one of impending problems.

Table 18.1 Classification of Hemorrhage in the Pregnant Patient[a]

Hemorrhage Class	Acute Blood Loss[b]	Percentage Lost
1	900	15
2	1,200–1,500	20–25
3	1,800–2,100	30–35
4	2,400	40

[a] Total blood volume = 6,000 ml.

[b] In the usual clinical setting, very few episodes of volume loss occur without some infusion of intravenous fluids, usually crystalloid-containing solutions such as Ringer's lactated solution, or normal saline. Therefore, the amount of blood loss preceding physical signs and symptoms will usually exceed the values listed.

(Adapted from Baker,[57] with permission.)

Patients with class 2 hemorrhage will frequently have orthostatic blood pressure changes and may have decreased perfusion of the extremities. However, this amount of blood loss will not usually result in the classic cold, clammy extremities. Rather, a more subtle test is needed to document this phenomenon. One can simply squeeze the hypothenar area of the hand for 1 to 2 seconds and then release the pressure. A patient with normal volume status will have an initial blanching of the skin, followed within 1 to 2 seconds by a return to the normal pink coloration. A patient who has a volume deficit of 15 to 25 percent will have delayed refilling of the blanched area of the hand.

Narrowing of the pulse pressure is another sign of class 2 hemorrhage. A thorough understanding of blood pressure readings is necessary to interpret subtle volume changes in the pregnant patient. The blood pressure may be viewed as having three components: diastolic pressure, pulse pressure, and systolic pressure. The diastolic pressure reflects the amount of systemic vasoconstriction present, the pulse pressure indicates stroke volume, and the systolic pressure denotes the interrelationship between the level of vasoconstriction and the stroke volume. While pulse pressure is a good clinical approach to the assessment of stroke volume in a given patient, it is not a reliable method of monitoring stroke volume in larger groups of patients because of individual variations in the many factors that can alter stroke volume (age, aortic stiffness). However, monitoring this pa-

rameter in a given patient will provide earlier signs of hypovolemia and reduced blood flow than either systolic or diastolic pressure used individually.

When a patient loses blood, compensatory mechanisms are activated that help ensure perfusion to vital body organs (brain, heart). The initial response, vasoconstriction, diverts blood away from nonvital body organs (skin, muscle, kidney). Blood loss results in sympathoadrenal stimulation, which causes a rise in diastolic pressure. Because the systolic pressure is usually maintained with small volume deficits (15 to 25 percent), the first blood pressure response seen with volume loss is narrowing of the pulse pressure (120/70 mmHg to 120/90 mmHg). That is, pulse pressure changes from 50 mmHg to 30 mmHg. When pulse pressure drops to 30 mmHg or less, the patient should be carefully evaluated for other signs of volume loss.

Class 3 hemorrhage is defined as blood loss sufficient to cause overt hypotension. In the pregnant patient, this usually requires a blood loss of 1,800 to 2,100 ml. These patients exhibit marked tachycardia (120 to 60 bpm) and may have cold, clammy skin and tachypnea (respiratory rate of 30 to 50 per minute).

In class 4 patients, the volume deficit exceeds 40 percent. These patients are in profound shock and frequently have no discernible blood pressure. They may have absent pulses in their extremities and are oliguric or anuric. If volume therapy is not quickly begun, circulatory collapse and cardiac arrest will soon result.

The hematocrit is another clinical method frequently used to estimate blood loss. After acute blood loss, the hematocrit will not change significantly for at least 4 hours, and complete compensation requires 48 hours. Infusion of intravenous fluids can alter this relationship, resulting in earlier lowering of measured hematocrit. When significant hemorrhage is thought to have occurred, a hematocrit should always be obtained. If this result shows a significant fall from a previous baseline value, a large amount of blood has been lost. Measures should immediately be taken to evaluate the source of the loss and whether the hemorrhage is ongoing but unrecognized.

Cesarean section is a frequent cause of excessive blood loss. It must be remembered that narcotics, which are frequently used for pain relief in the immediate postoperative period, can significantly reduce the ability of the sympathetic nervous system to effect vasoconstriction of the arterial and venous compartments. If these medications are given to a hypovolemic patient, serious hypotension can result. Signs and symptoms of hypovolemia should always be sought before the postoperative patient is given narcotic analgesics on the first postpartum day.

URINE OUTPUT — "THE WINDOW OF BODY PERFUSION"

In hypovolemic patients, urine output must be carefully monitored. In many cases, the urine output will fall before other signs of impaired perfusion are manifest. By contrast, adequate urine volume in patients who have not received diuretics strongly suggests that perfusion to vital body organs is adequate.

There is reasonable correlation between renal blood flow and urine output. If the urine output is low, renal blood flow is often low as well. When there is a rapid decrease in renal blood flow, there is usually a reduction in urine output. In such cases, renal blood flow tends to shift from the outer renal cortex to the juxtamedullary portion of the renal cortex. Glomerular filtration rate (GFR) is further reduced, but absorption of water and sodium is increased because there are fewer glomeruli and longer loops of Henle in this region. Urine will become more concentrated and will have a lower concentration of sodium and a higher osmolarity. With a gradual fall in renal blood flow, the urine sodium and osmolarity will often be affected before any significant fall in urine output. A urine sodium concentration of less than 10 to 20 mEq/L or a urine–serum osmolar ratio of greater than 2 usually indicates reduced renal perfusion.

BLOOD LOSS IN SEVERE PREECLAMPSIA

Major blood loss in a patient with severe preeclampsia may present a confusing picture. One must be aware of the altered hemodynamic status of these patients to appreciate the extent of the volume loss and to ensure appropriate fluid replacement. In severe preeclampsia, the blood volume has frequently failed to expand and is similar to that of a nonpregnant person. These patients will not have the protective effect of the usual volume expansion of pregnancy and will show signs of blood loss earlier. In these cases, however, blood pressure can be a misleading indicator of volume. A blood pressure appropriate for a previously normotensive patient could indicate serious volume depletion in the preeclamptic woman. It is especially important to record serial pressures. If the blood pressure shows a significant drop during the immediate postoperative or postpartum period, a volume deficit should be suspected because hypertension usually persists for days to weeks in patients with severe preeclampsia.

When significant hemorrhage occurs in the woman with hypertension, it may be important to supplement the crystalloid fluid resuscitation with colloidal fluids pending the availability of the best colloid, whole blood. Albumin (5 percent) should be given in the ratio of 500 ml of albumin for every 4 L of crystalloid. This form of therapy will help to compensate for the low albumin and total protein concentrations present in the patient with severe preeclampsia. It is not uncommon for these women to have total protein levels less than 5.0 g/dl, with an albumin concentration below 2.5 g/dl. If crystalloid fluids alone are given, massive fluid accumulation in the already overexpanded extravascular space can occur and may result in cerebral edema as well as pulmonary edema.[1]

TREATMENT

Patients showing signs of class 2 or greater volume loss should receive crystalloid intravenous fluids pending the arrival of blood and blood products. The infusion rate should be rapid, between 1,000 and 2,000 ml in 30 to 45 minutes, or faster if the patient is obviously hypotensive. This infusion may serve as a therapeutic trial to help determine the amount of blood lost. If the physical signs and symptoms return to normal and remain stable after this challenge, no further therapy may be needed. If blood loss has been severe and the patient continues to bleed, however, this favorable response may be only transient. In this situation, typed and cross-matched blood should be given. The initial administration of a balanced salt solution will reduce the amount of whole blood needed to restore an adequate blood volume.[2]

BLOOD AND BLOOD PRODUCTS

The use of whole blood has been discouraged by blood banking centers around the United States. In obstetrics, the main indication for whole blood rather than component therapy is massive blood loss requiring more than a 2,000-ml replacement (see Table 18.2).

An anticoagulant (cpda-1) is used to preserve whole blood. This compound contains c, a calcium chelating agent; p, phosphate, to maintain ATP levels; d, dextrose, food for red blood cells (RBCs) and for preservation of 2,3-diphosphoglyceric acid (DPG) levels; and a, adenine, to preserve adenosine triphosphate (ATP) levels. Maintenance of ATP is essential to preserve the RBC sodium pump and cell shape, both of which affect cell survival. A byproduct of the normal glycolytic pathway in the RBC, 2,3-DPG causes a shift to the right of the oxyhemoglobin dissociation curve. This shift permits more oxygen to be dissociated from the hemoglobin molecule and released into the tis-

sues. Despite these alterations, the useful life of a unit of whole blood is only 21 days.

The storage of whole blood has significant effects on its cellular elements as well as coagulation factors. After 24 hours, white blood cells (WBCs) and platelets are either absent or nonfunctional. After 7 days, levels of Factors V and VIII have fallen 50 percent or more. There remains a large amount of plasma protein in stored blood, however, for which reason it remains the agent of choice for transfusion in the face of major hemorrhage.

MASSIVE BLOOD TRANSFUSION

Massive transfusion is an ill-defined term but can generally be thought of as the replacement of a patient's entire blood volume in 24 hours.[3] In a pregnant patient, this is usually 10 or more units of blood. Massive transfusion is a medical emergency that often requires the ultimate in surgical and medical skills. Administrative skills are also essential, because usually a

Table 18.2 Blood Replacement

Product	Cost/Unit[a]	Contents	Volume (cc)	Effect
Whole blood	$57	RBC (2,3-DPG) WBC (not functional after 24 hours) Coagulation factors (50 percent V, VIII after 7 days) Plasma proteins	500	Increase volume (ml/ml) Increase hematocrit 3 percent/unit
Packed red cells	$57	RBC, same as whole blood WBC, less than whole blood Plasma proteins—few	240	Same RBC as whole blood Less risk febrile or WBC transfusion reaction Increase hematocrit 3 percent/unit
Platelets	$28	55×10^6 platelets/unit Few WBC	50	Increase platelet count 5,000–10,000 μl/unit Give six packs minimum
Fresh frozen plasma	$25	Clotting factors V, VIII, fibrinogen	250	Only source of factors V, XI, XII Increase fibrinogen 10 mg percent/unit
Cryoprecipitate	$13	Factor VIII 25 percent fibrinogen von Willebrand's factor	40	Increase fibrinogen 10 mg percent/unit
Albumin 5 percent	$25	Albumin	500	
Albumin 25 percent	$25	Albumin	50	

Abbreviations: RBC, red blood cells; WBC, white blood cells.
[a] Data from Puget Sound Blood Center (1990).

number of physicians from various medical specialties are involved in the care of such a patient. Events may be occurring so rapidly and clinical circumstances changing from hour to hour that clear lines of communication between the various physicians must be maintained. During an acute hemorrhage requiring prolonged surgical management, such as a placenta accreta with bladder involvement, it is optimal to have one member of the obstetric team whose job is to coordinate blood replacement and to monitor laboratory results, which are the basis for choosing which components to replace. Communication between the surgeon and the anesthesiologist regarding volume and coagulation status is essential and may be compromised because each physician is heavily involved in his or her own work.

The essentials of management of the patient requiring massive transfusion are maintenance of circulation, blood volume, oxygen carrying capacity, hemostasis, colloid osmotic pressure, and biochemical balance. As soon as it is apparent that more than 2 units of blood will be required, preparations should be made to have a significant quantity of whole blood available if possible. After 4 units of packed red cells are given, it is preferable to use whole blood because plasma will provide both the coagulation factors and proteins needed to maintain hemostasis and colloid osmotic pressure. If whole blood is not available, earlier laboratory testing for coagulation deficiencies should be performed because more component therapy will probably be required. As soon as it becomes apparent that massive transfusion therapy will be required, baseline coagulation tests should be ordered and the laboratory notified that more tests will be coming on a periodic basis. These tests should include complete blood count (CBC), platelet count, fibrinogen, prothrombin time (PT), and partial thromboplastin time (PTT). The laboratory must be alerted regarding the life-threatening nature of the problem, and it must give these tests top priority. A turnaround time of 15 minutes should be the goal.

Previous algorithms for massive transfusion advised transfusion with platelets and fresh frozen plasma after a certain number of units of blood had been used. However, with modern laboratory testing, the overuse of these products can be limited. In general, microvascular oozing will be apparent at platelet counts below $50,000/\mu l$. This drop usually requires the replacement of 1.5 blood volumes. However, counts may drop to this level or below in the face of a consumptive process (e.g., disseminated intravascular coagulation [DIC]) prior to the loss of 15 units of blood (see DIC, below). In addition, platelet function itself may be impaired in patients undergoing massive transfusion. If there is continued surgical evidence of microvascular bleeding in the face of laboratory tests near the critical levels, more replacement should be given.

If whole blood is available, there will often be no need for the transfusion of fresh frozen plasma, because many of the coagulation factors are present in stored blood. However, if packed cells are used, frequent monitoring of the PT should be performed. When the PT is prolonged by greater than 5 seconds, fresh frozen plasma should be used. In the face of DIC there will also be prolongation of the PTT and a fall in fibrinogen. In this case, cryoprecipitate should also be used as a source of Factor VIII and fibrinogen.

Metabolic derangements are frequently mentioned when massive transfusion is discussed. However, traditional formulas for using alkalating agents or calcium supplements are probably unnecessary. Hypocalcemia is a theoretical problem, but clinical syndromes from this problem are infrequently described and the possible complications of prophylactic calcium infusion may be more harmful than hypocalcemia. Hypocalcemia can be clinically important is if it is combined with hyperkalemia and hypothermia. This triad can lead to cardiac arrhythmias, and, if the blood cannot be warmed above four degrees centigrade before transfusion, close attention should be paid to the electrocardiogram. If arrhythmias are noted, supplemental calcium should be considered.

Acid–base problems can arise in the event of massive transfusion. However, citrate toxicity is rarely a problem, because the healthy liver can metabolize citrate in 1 unit of blood in 5 minutes. Unless transfusion rates exceed 1 unit per 5 minutes or the liver is previously diseased, citrate toxicity should not be a problem. Although stored blood has an acid pH, acidosis is uncommon because the metabolism of citrate produces alkalosis. Prolonged acidosis is more often the result of hypoperfusion and shock than is blood replacement. Blood gas measurement should guide the therapy with bicarbonate in this instance.

Packed Red Blood Cells

Packed red blood cells (PRBCs) are the most effective and efficient way to provide increased oxygen carrying capacity to the anemic patient. Unless a patient has suffered massive blood loss, PRBCs and crystalloid will satisfy most clinical needs. Because this product has small amounts of WBCs and isohemagglutinins (anti-A and anti-B), its use reduces the incidence of nonhemolytic transfusion reactions compared with that of 1 unit of whole blood. However, care should be taken to administer PRBCs with normal saline rather than Ringer's lactated or dextrose solutions, which can cause the blood to clot or the red cells to lyse.

Platelets

One unit of platelets is derived from 1 unit of whole blood and has a shelf life of 72 hours. Transfusion of 1 unit of platelets can be expected to raise the platelet count between 5,000 and 10,000/μl. A single unit of platelets should never be given, the smallest single dose of clinical value being 4 to 6 units. Platelets should be administered rapidly, over 10 minutes, with repeat laboratory evaluation performed 2 hours after infusion. For the obstetric patient, it is important that the platelets be ABO and Rh specific, because the platelet concentrate usually contains some RBCs that can potentially sensitize an Rh-negative woman. It must also be remembered that six packs of platelets have a volume effect if multiple doses are used. Each unit of platelets carries the transfusion risk of 1 unit of blood.

Platelet administration is frequently considered in patients with DIC, massive hemorrhage, severe preeclampsia, and idiopathic thrombocytopenia (ITP). In each of these conditions, the absolute levels at which a platelet transfusion is indicated may vary depending on the time course of the thrombocytopenia (more chronic forms will result in less hemostatic defects than acute loss), the need to perform a surgical procedure, the etiology of the inciting event producing thrombocytopenia, and the level of blood pressure elevation and the bleeding time. In general, platelet counts below 50,000/μl or bleeding times

longer than 15 minutes will require transfusion prior to or during surgery.

Cryoprecipitate

Prepared by warming fresh frozen plasma and collecting the precipitate, cryoprecipitate contains significant amounts of Factor VIII fibrinogen and von Willebrand's factor. Cryoprecipitate is used primarily in patients with von Willebrand's disease and in patients with a normal blood volume who require factor replacement. Except for Factor VIII, the same coagulation factors are available in this product as in fresh frozen plasma, but in only 15 percent of the volume. As with platelets, cryoprecipitate should be ABO and Rh specific. One unit of cryoprecipitate will raise the serum fibrinogen 10 mg/dl. This preparation should be used when significant hypofibrinogenemia must be treated.

Fresh Frozen Plasma

Fresh frozen plasma contains all the coagulation factors present in cryoprecipitate, including appreciably higher levels of Factor VIII. Fresh frozen plasma should be administered when both volume replacement and coagulation factors are needed. The main clinical indication for this therapy will be the massively hemorrhaging patient. If bleeding continues after the transfusion of 4 to 5 units of blood, a coagulation screen should be checked to see whether the replacement of clotting factors and platelets is indicated. If coagulation parameters, PT, and PTT are abnormal, 1 unit of fresh frozen plasma should be administered for every 4 units of transfused blood.

Transfusion Risks

PRBCs, fresh frozen plasma, cryoprecipitate, and platelets have the same risk of transmitting infectious diseases as 1 unit of whole blood. Table 18.3 lists the common risks of blood transfusion when blood is procured from volunteer donors. Blood obtained from paid sources can be expected to have higher rates of many of the complications listed in Table 18.3.

Autologous Transfusion

Primarily as the result of fear of acquiring the human immunodeficiency virus (HIV) from blood transfusion, patients have in recent years begun to inquire

Table 18.3 Risks of Blood Transfusion

Complication	Incidence of Complication	Incidence of Death
Human immunodeficiency virus	1/250,000	1/500,000
Hepatitis B	1/100,000	1/2,000,000
Non-A, non-B hepatitis	1/50	Not known
Hemolytic transfusion reaction	—	1/600,000
Nonhemolytic transfusion reaction	1/100	1/10,000,000

(Adapted from Hewitt and Machin,[3] with permission.)

about the feasibility of autologous blood transfusion if they should require transfusion during childbirth. Autologous transfusion can be accomplished in two ways. In the most common approach, blood is collected from the patient and stored during the weeks before delivery. This presents some logistic problems for the pregnant patient, because 3 weeks is the longest time that the blood can be stored and most patients' hematocrit level will only allow the donation of 1 unit of blood. Only 100 patients donating 139 units of blood have been studied to date with regard to fetal effects of this procedure.[4-7] Single cases of fetal bradycardia with recovery and requiring emergency cesarean section have been reported. Maternal hypotension associated with transfusion has also been reported. It is still probably premature to conclude that this procedure is safe for the fetus. More studies of short- and long-term results will be needed to evaluate completely antenatal autologous blood donation.

A second type of autologous donation can occur at the time of excessive blood loss. Intraoperative autotransfusion has been reported in obstetric patients at the time of ruptured ectopic pregnancy and recently after delayed cesarean hysterectomy. This technique has some limitations in the obstetric setting. Heavy bacterial contamination is a contraindication, and the use during cesarean section should also be avoided because of the possibility of amniotic fluid, fetal debris, and bacterial contamination. However, in the case of cesarean hysterectomy with massive bleeding or delayed reoperation because of continued bleeding, this technique can be considered.[8]

The chance of acquiring HIV from a unit of donated and screened blood is on the order of 1 in 1 million. Furthermore, when blood transfusion is clinically indicated, there is usually the need for more blood than the patient is able to donate unless the

blood is frozen, which dramatically increases the cost of the procedure. The pregnant patient inquiring about this practice should be carefully counseled that the chance of needing a blood transfusion is about 1 in 80 overall or higher if she has placenta previa or requires emergency cesarean section.[9,10] That fact, coupled with the low risk of acquiring HIV from a donated unit of blood, makes the a priori risk of contracting AIDS as a result of transfusion during childbirth on the order of 1 in 25 to 50 million.

ANTEPARTUM HEMORRHAGE

Abruptio Placenta

The premature separation of the normally implanted placenta from its attachment to the uterus is called abruptio placenta or placental abruption. This event occurs with a frequency of approximately 1 in 120 births, but accounts for nearly 15 percent of perinatal mortality. Diagnosis of placental abruption is certain when inspection of the placenta shows an adherent retroplacental clot with depression or disruption of the underlying placental tissue; however, this may not always be found if the abruption is of recent onset. Clinical findings indicating placental abruption include the triad of external or occult uterine bleeding, uterine hypertonus and/or hyperactivity, and fetal distress and/or fetal death. Placental abruption can be broadly classified into three grades that correlate with clinical and laboratory findings.

Grade 1: Slight vaginal bleeding and some uterine irritability are usually present. Maternal blood pressure is unaffected, and the maternal fibrinogen level is normal. The fetal heart rate pattern is normal.

Grade 2: External uterine bleeding is mild to moderate. The uterus is irritable, and tetanic contractions may be present. Maternal blood pressure is maintained, but the pulse rate may be elevated, and postural blood volume deficits may be present. The fibrinogen level is usually reduced to 150 to 250 mg percent. The fetal heart rate often shows signs of fetal distress.

Grade 3: Bleeding is moderate to severe but may be concealed. The uterus is tetanic and painful. Maternal hypotension is frequently present, and fetal death has occurred. Fibrinogen levels are often reduced to less than 150 mg percent; other coagulation abnormalities (thrombocytopenia, factor depletion) are present.

Incidence

The reported incidence of placental abruption varies from 1 in 86 to 1 in 206 births.[11] This variability reflects differing criteria for diagnosis as well as the increased recognition in recent years of milder forms of the disorder. Grade 1 placental abruption is found in about 40 percent, grade 2 in about 45 percent, and grade 3 in 15 percent of clinically recognized cases of placental abruption.[11,12] Eighty percent of all cases will occur before the onset of labor.[13]

Etiology

The primary etiology of placental abruption is unknown, but several reports have identified statistically significant correlations with common obstetric complications. Studies have suggested an increased incidence of abruption[14,15] in patients with advanced parity or age, maternal smoking, poor nutrition, cocaine use, and chorioamnionitis.[16,17] However, some of these data may have been subject to selection bias, as only populations of low socioeconomic status were evaluated. The U.S. Perinatal Collaborative project performed during the years 1959 to 1966 found no relationship between age or parity and abruption.[18] A recent population-based study in Washington state also failed to show a relationship between placental abruption and either maternal age or parity.[19]

Maternal hypertension (> 140/90 mmHg) seems to be the most consistently identified factor predispos-

ing to placental abruption.[20] This relationship is true for all grades of placental abruption but is most strongly associated with grade 3 abruption, in which 40 to 50 percent of cases are found to have hypertensive disease of pregnancy.[18,20] Intrapartum hypertension significantly increases the risk of abruption, but one study failed to show a relationship between the antenatal detection of hypertension and placental abruption.

External maternal trauma is an uncommon but important cause of placental abruption. One to 2 percent of grade 3 abruptions have been attributed to maternal trauma.[20,21] Despite this reportedly low incidence, the present-day utilization of high-speed automobile transportation without adequate passenger restraints and the increasing recognition of physical abuse of the mother make it incumbent on the obstetrician to consider placental abruption when a history of trauma is elicited. Unfortunately, the physical evidence of trauma may be minimal and still be associated with placental abruption that can progress from grade 1 to 3 within 24 hours. Figure 18.1 illustrates fetal heart rate tracings 8 hours apart in a patient who was involved in an automobile accident.

Rapid decompression of the overdistended uterus is an uncommon cause of placental abruption. The two clinical situations in which this can occur are patients with multiple gestations and those with polyhydramnios. The true incidence of placental abruption in twins and other multiple gestations is difficult to ascertain. Abruption usually occurs after the delivery of the first fetus. Delivery of the second twin usually follows soon after, before a retroplacental clot has time to form. Rapid decompression of the uterus should be avoided in a patient with polyhydramnios. Amniotic fluid should be slowly released by amniocentesis before the induction of labor or once spontaneous labor has been established.

In the past, folic acid deficiency, a short umbilical cord, and the supine hypotensive syndrome had been suggested as etiologies for placental abruption. Further evidence has shown, however, that these factors are unlikely causes of placental abruption.

There is a significant recurrence rate for placental abruption. This figure has been reported to vary from 5 to 17 percent.[13,15,20] If a patient has suffered an abruption in two pregnancies, the chance for recurrence is 25 percent. Unfortunately, no published data

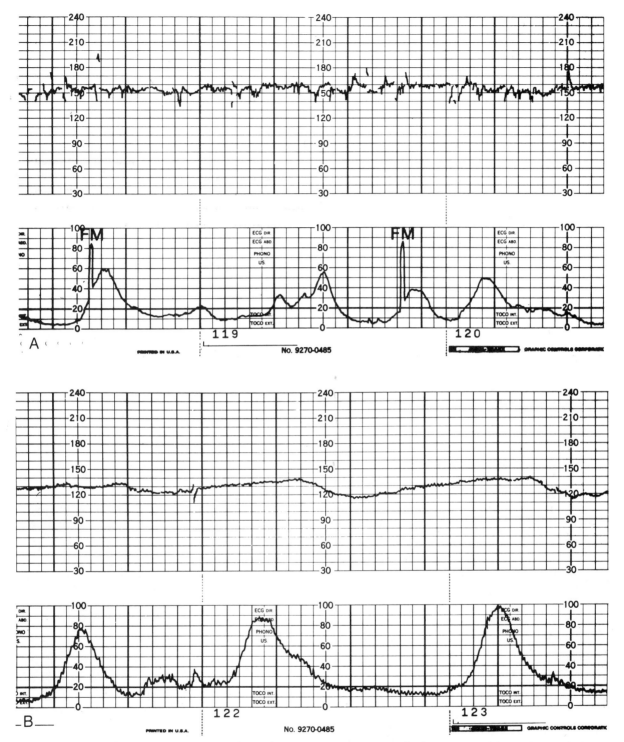

Fig. 18.1 (A) A fetal heart rate tracing at 37 weeks gestation in a patient involved in an automobile accident in which the maternal abdomen struck the steering wheel. Fetal movements were present, and no periodic changes were observed. Uterine contractions were occurring every 2 to 3 minutes. (B) Eight hours later, repetitive late decelerations are now present. An asphyxiated fetus was delivered, and evidence of grade 3 placental abruption was found at the time of delivery.

are available to document a prospective plan of management that will reduce this unacceptably high risk.

Diagnosis and Management

Vaginal bleeding in the third trimester of pregnancy is the hallmark of placental abruption and should always prompt an investigation to determine its etiology. After appropriate physical and laboratory examination of the mother and fetus, ultrasound evaluation of the uterus, placenta, and fetus has become the standard of care (Fig. 18.2). The other common and potentially life-threatening cause of third-trimester bleeding, placenta previa, should be recognized in nearly all cases in which it is present. If ultrasound examination fails to show a placenta previa and if other local causes of vaginal bleeding (including cervical or vaginal trauma, labor, or malignancy) have been ruled out, placental abruption becomes a more likely diagnosis.

In the initial studies evaluating ultrasound, less than 2 percent of cases were definitively identifiable with ultrasound. Recent advances in ultrasound imaging and interpretation have most likely improved this rate.

Ultrasound can identify three predominant locations for placental abruption. These are subchorionic or marginal (between the placenta and the myometrium), retroplacental (between the placenta and the myometrium), and preplacental (between the placenta and the amniotic fluid). Hematomas identified by ultrasound during the early phases of vaginal bleeding and pain are most likely to be hyperechoic or isoechoic compared with the placenta. As the hematoma resolves, it will become hypoechoic within 1 week and sonolucent within 2 weeks.[22] Because of the changing character of the hematoma, misinterpretation of a hematoma as uterine myoma, succinturiate placental lobe, chorioangioma, or molar pregnancy has been reported.

The location and extent of the placental abruption identified on ultrasound has definite clinical significance. Retroplacental hematomas carry a worse prognosis for fetal survival than does subchorionic hemorrhage. The size of the hemorrhage is also predictive of fetal survival. Large retroplacental hemorrhages (>60 ml, >50 percent) are associated with a 50 percent or greater fetal mortality, whereas a similar-sized subchorionic hemorrhage is associated with a 10 percent mortality.[23]

Gestational age at the time of presentation is an

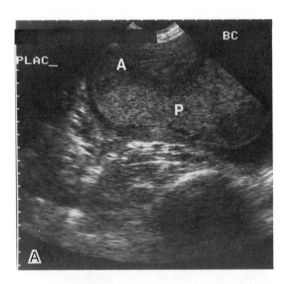
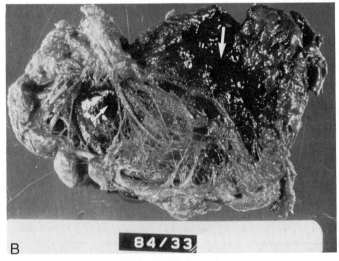

Fig. 18.2 (A) Ultrasound study at 18 weeks gestation demonstrating a hypoechoic area (A) representing retroplacental bleeding and an enlarged placenta (P). This patient had chronic hypertension. She presented with intermittent dark red vaginal bleeding and abdominal pain, a picture consistent with a chronic abruption. (B) At delivery, the placenta revealed a large clot (small arrow) and fresh hemorrhage (large arrow). The fibrous bands bridging the clot are also consistent with chronic abruption.

important prognostic factor. Of patients presenting at less than 20 weeks, 82 percent can be expected to have a term delivery despite evidence of placental separation. If the presentation occurs after 20 weeks gestation, only 27 percent will deliver at term.

Nearly 80 percent of patients who eventually prove to have a placental abruption will present with vaginal bleeding. The remaining 20 percent of patients fail to exhibit external signs of bleeding. These patients have a concealed abruption and are commonly diagnosed as premature labor. Such cases must be watched very carefully. On some occasions, the abruption may progress despite successful tocolysis, and fetal death may result. Other classic signs of placental abruption include increased uterine tenderness and tone. These findings are uncommon (17 percent) unless the abruption is grade 2 or 3.[12]

Once the diagnosis of placental abruption has been entertained, precautions should be taken to deal with the possible life-threatening consequences for both mother and fetus. At least 4 units of blood should be available for maternal transfusions. A large-bore (16-g) intravenous line must be secured and the infusion of a crystalloid solution begun. Blood should be drawn for hemoglobin and hematocrit determinations and coagulation studies (fibrinogen, platelet count, fibrin degradation products, PT, PTT). A red-topped tube should also be obtained and used to perform a clot test. This test, a "poor man's" fibrinogen assay, will often give critical information before the laboratory can document a coagulation defect. If a clot does not form within 6 minutes or forms and lyses within 30 minutes, a coagulation defect is probably present and the fibrinogen level is less than 150 mg percent. Because fetal distress will develop in as many as 60 percent of patients who present with a live fetus, continuous fetal monitoring should be used to record fetal heart rate and document uterine activity.

In the patient with a term fetus in whom the diagnosis of grade 1 abruption is made, close observation for signs of fetal or maternal compromise is essential. If the fetus is known to be mature, controlled delivery should be accomplished by induction of labor while the mother and fetus are in stable condition.

The occurrence of a grade 1 placental abruption with a preterm fetus presents greater challenge. Often, a vicious circle is established in which a small placental abruption stimulates uterine irritability, further separating the placenta until fetal compromise becomes evident. In carefully selected cases, it may be possible to inhibit uterine contractions so long as there are no signs of acute fetal distress and no ultrasonographic evidence of intrauterine growth retardation (IUGR). Magnesium sulfate has far less adverse cardiovascular side effects than do β-sympathomimetic agents and would seem to be a good choice in this circumstance. A comparison of tocolytic therapy versus observation alone has never been evaluated in a clinical trial. Any attempt to arrest preterm labor in known or suspected abruption should be weighed against the likelihood for survival and morbidity if the infant were delivered.

In most cases of placental abruption, delivery will be the treatment of choice. During labor, careful attention must be paid to several maternal and fetal parameters. Because 60 percent of fetuses may exhibit signs of intrapartum fetal distress, continuous fetal heart rate monitoring is essential. In a similar manner, continuous monitoring of maternal volume status is important. An indwelling Foley catheter will permit accurate assessment of maternal urine output. Serial maternal hematocrit determinations should be made regularly at intervals of 2 to 3 hours. The goal of therapy should be to maintain a maternal urine output of 1 ml/min and a hematocrit of at least 30 percent. An updated flow sheet at the bedside permits the clinician to follow maternal vital signs, urine output, laboratory values, and critical clotting parameters.

Placental abruption frequently stimulates the clotting cascade, resulting in DIC. Intravascular fibrinogen is converted to fibrin by activation of the extrinsic clotting cascade. In the usual clinical setting, platelets and clotting Factors V and VIII are also depleted. Serial measurements of plasma fibrinogen provides valuable information regarding the coagulation status of the patient and will help to estimate the volume of blood loss that has occurred.

The normal maternal fibrinogen concentration in the third trimester is 450 mg percent. In grade 1 abruptions, there is often no alteration in this value and no evidence of DIC. However, when the fibrinogen value drops below 300 mg percent, significant coagulation abnormalities are usually present. Nearly all these women will require blood transfusion to maintain a normal circulating volume. If the presenting fibrinogen level is less than 150 mg percent, most patients will have already lost 2,000 ml of blood. The signs and symptoms of such blood loss may not be obvious because, as noted earlier, the normal hypervolemia of pregnancy protects the mother from a volume loss that a nonpregnant individual could not tolerate. In the case of grade 3 placental abruption, the mean blood loss is 2,500 ml or more.[24] In patients with grade 2 and grade 3 abruption, rapid crystalloid infusion of at least 1,000 ml pending the availability of whole blood should be done. Two to 3 ml of crystalloid should be given for each 1 ml of blood lost to maintain euvolemia.

If urine output fails to reach 30 ml/hr despite adequate volume replacement, then consideration should be given to inserting a central venous pressure (CVP) catheter to determine the adequacy of intravascular volume. This catheter is best inserted through a site in the arm rather than the neck or subclavian area because of the severe coagulopathy that is often present. The absolute level of CVP is less important than the response of the CVP to volume infusion, as long as the CVP is less than 7 cmH$_2$O in response to the preceding 250-ml aliquot. If this response has been achieved but the urine output is still inadequate, consideration should be given to replacing the CVP catheter with a pulmonary artery catheter. This circumstance is uncommon unless there is intrinsic heart disease or severe preeclampsia or if the patient has already suffered critical renal ischemia and is in acute renal failure.

Placental abruption is a clinical circumstance in which whole blood transfusion is indicated. Many blood banking facilities are now advocating component therapy for most clinical situations, especially elective surgery. In the patient with placental abruption, whole blood is preferred, because it supplies the needed volume that packed cells do not provide, and, depending on the length of storage, it may contain clotting factors, especially fibrinogen. The use of whole blood replacement often abrogates the need for additional factor replacement.

Considerable controversy remains regarding the appropriate method of delivery in patients with placental abruption. Concern exists for the fetal outcome in such cases. A number of patients present with a live fetus, only to have that fetus die undelivered while awaiting vaginal delivery.[11,14] Retrospective re-

views show a trend for increased fetal survival in patients who have undergone delivery by cesarean section once the maternal condition has been stabilized. However, none of these reports surveyed a period in which intrapartum fetal monitoring was routine. A recent study using electronic fetal monitoring demonstrated that excellent fetal survival can be expected if cesarean section is reserved for cases with fetal distress or for traditional obstetric indications.[12]

The management of mothers with severe coagulopathy and/or fetal demise is also controversial. Restoration of a normal blood volume is the sine qua non of treatment in these patients. Once adequate volume status has been achieved, attention can be given to effecting delivery. Some clinicians believe that if placental abruption has progressed to fetal death and severe coagulopathy, delivery by cesarean section will result in the quickest resolution of maternal problems. However, this is usually an unwise choice, because operating on such a patient in the presence of a coagulopathy can be hazardous. Fibrinogen levels lower than 125 mg percent lead to generalized bleeding from all surgical incisions. Even in the face of a severe coagulopathy, induction to delivery times of up to 18 hours may result in no greater complication rate than a shorter but arbitrary time limit as long as maternal volume status is maintained with whole blood.[13]

When cesarean delivery is necessary, extravasation of blood into the uterine muscle producing red to purple discoloration of the serosal surface will be found in 8 percent of patients. This finding, known as a couvelaire uterus, has been feared to result in a high incidence of uterine hemorrhage secondary to atony. However, atony is the exception rather than the rule, and most patients with a couvelaire uterus demonstrate an appropriate response to the infusion of oxytocin. Hysterectomy should be reserved for cases of atony and hemorrhage unresponsive to conventional uterotonics.

Placenta Previa

Placenta previa is defined as the implantation of the placenta over the cervical os. There are three recognized variations of placenta previa: total, partial, and marginal (Fig. 18.3). In total placenta previa, the cervical os is completely covered by the placenta. This type presents the most serious maternal risk, as it is

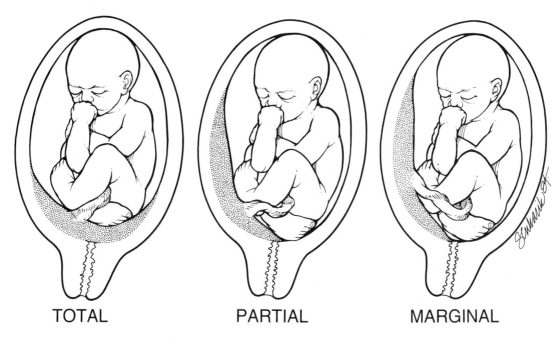

TOTAL   PARTIAL   MARGINAL

Fig. 18.3 Three variations of placenta previa.

associated with greater blood loss than either marginal or partial placenta previa. The frequency of total placenta previa has been reported to be as low as 20 percent[25] or as high as 43 percent.[26] Partial placenta previa is defined as the partial occlusion of the cervical os by the placenta and occurs in 31 percent of diagnosed cases. A marginal placenta previa is characterized by the encroachment of the placenta to the margin of the cervical os. It does not cover the os. Differentiation of the latter two degrees of placenta previa is dependent on the dilatation of the cervix and the method of diagnosis (ultrasound or direct examination).

A leading cause of third-trimester hemorrhage, placenta previa presents classically as painless bleeding. Bleeding is thought to occur in association with the development of the lower uterine segment in the third trimester. Placental attachment is disrupted as this area gradually thins in preparation for the onset of labor. When this occurs, bleeding results from the implantation site, as the uterus is unable to contract adequately to stop the flow of blood from the open vessels.

The incidence of placenta previa is stated to be 1 in 250 live births.[26] However, this figure may be influenced by the makeup of the population from which the data were derived. The most important factor in the development of placenta previa is previous cesarean section. The risk for placenta previa occurring in the pregnancy following a cesarean section is 1 percent.[25,26] Placenta previa should be suspected in all patients presenting with bleeding after 24 weeks gestation. Seventy percent of patients who are eventually shown to have placenta previa will present with painless vaginal bleeding. Twenty percent will have evidence of uterine activity accompanying vaginal bleeding; the remaining patients will have the diagnosis made incidentally at time of cesarean section or at ultrasound examination performed for another indication.

Patients with third-trimester bleeding should be treated in a manner similar to that outlined in the section on abruptio placenta (e.g., maternal stabilization, blood studies, fetal monitoring). Once fetal and maternal status have been stabilized, ultrasound evaluation should be performed to establish the diagnosis (Fig. 18.4). Gestational age at the time of the ultrasound examination greatly influences the incidence of placenta previa. At 17 weeks gestation, evidence of placental tissue covering the cervical os will be found

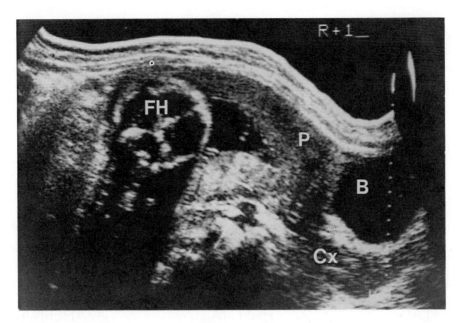

Fig. 18.4 This ultrasound examination at 34 weeks gestation in a patient with painless vaginal bleeding revealed a placenta previa (P) covering the cervical os (Cx). The maternal bladder (B) and fetal head (FH) are also shown.

in 5 to 6 percent of all patients.[26] However, more than 90 percent of these will resolve by term.[27] This phenomenon has been termed "placental migration." It is unlikely the placenta actually separates and reattaches throughout the second and third trimesters. The changes in architecture secondary to differential growth of the lower uterine segment during the second and third trimesters probably account for this observation.

Once the diagnosis of placenta previa is made, management decisions depend on the gestational age, amount of bleeding, fetal condition, and presentation. In the patient who is unequivocally at 37 weeks gestation with evidence of uterine activity or with persistent bleeding, a double setup examination should be performed. The double setup should be done in an operating room, with full preparation made to be able to perform an emergency cesarean section should excessive vaginal bleeding follow the examination. Some have questioned the need to confirm the ultrasound diagnosis of placenta previa by physical examination. With a central placenta previa or history of prior cesarean section, abdominal delivery is prob-

ably the delivery method of choice. However, vaginal delivery in patients with marginal placenta previa who present in labor has occurred in my experience in each of the two academic institutions in which I have practiced. In addition, vaginal delivery in the presence of marginal or partial placenta previa can safely occur, because the fetal head descends past the placenta and tamponades the bleeding edge.

In performing a double setup examination, the patient should be prepped and draped for cesarean section. The anesthesiologist should be present and the operating room team ready. The patient should first undergo a careful speculum examination, which may reveal placental tissue in the cervical os. If the diagnosis of placenta previa cannot be made with a speculum examination, the obstetrician should next examine the vaginal fornices. Fullness in the fornices suggests the presence of the placenta extending down toward the cervix. Finally, examining fingers should be carefully introduced into the cervical os to detect the placenta.

In the patient who is remote from term (24 to 36 weeks gestation), expectant management is the treatment of choice. The essence of this approach is maintenance of the fetus in a healthy intrauterine environment without jeopardizing maternal condition. Maternal blood loss should be replaced to maintain the maternal hematocrit between 30 and 35 percent. This RBC volume will provide a margin of safety in the event of a large hemorrhage. Even an initial blood loss in excess of 500 ml can be expectantly managed with adequate volume replacement.

Although maternal hemorrhage is the greatest concern, the obstetrician must remember that fetal blood can also be lost during the process of placental separation. Rh immunoglobulin should be given to all at-risk patients with third-trimester bleeding who are Rh negative and unsensitized. A Kleihauer-Betke preparation of maternal blood should also be done in all Rh-negative women. This test will detect the occasional patient with a fetomaternal hemorrhage of greater than 30 ml. Thirty-five percent of infants whose mothers require antepartum transfusion will themselves be anemic and require transfusion when delivered.[26] K-B= >1%

Twenty percent of patients with placenta previa will show evidence of uterine contractions. Because a vaginal examination to document cervical dilatation is absolutely contraindicated, it is difficult to make a firm diagnosis of preterm labor. Although no controlled studies are available to show the efficacy of tocolytic therapy in such cases, some studies document that it can be safely attempted.[26] The choice of agents in this situation can be critical. If β-mimetics are used in the presence of maternal hypovolemia, serious maternal hypotension can result (Fig. 18.5). In addition, the use of β-mimetics will produce maternal tachycardia, making the evaluation of maternal volume status more difficult. For these reasons, magnesium sulfate has become the agent of choice for the treatment of patients in preterm labor with placenta previa at the University of Washington. Infusion of a 6-g loading dose followed by 3 g/hr or more is often necessary to control uterine irritability because of the increased maternal GFR. Once the patient has been stabilized on magnesium sulfate, the use of oral β-mimetics is an appropriate choice provided that euvolemia has been achieved. Newer treatments, such as continuous subcutaneous β-mimetic infusion, also offer promise in controlling uterine activity in this group of patients. Patients may occasionally require

more than 1 week of continuous intravenous tocolytic therapy. Such treatment is considered justified, because, before 33 weeks gestation, each day that the fetus remains in utero reduces its stay in the neonatal intensive care nursery by 2 days.[28] The use of antenatal corticosteroids to accelerate fetal pulmonary maturity is effective in some patients.[29,30] However, the U.S. National Collaborative Study failed to find a significant benefit in many groups of patients who were previously thought to be candidates for such treatment.[31] Meta-analysis of all studies on steroids to accelerate fetal pulmonary maturity does show an effect in reducing respiratory distress syndrome and mortality. Given a high incidence of respiratory distress syndrome in the infants of mothers requiring delivery after failed expectant management (24 to 41 percent),[26,32] the use of antenatal steroids in patients presenting between 26 to 32 weeks should be considered. However, there are no data on safety or efficacy of repeated weekly doses of steroids administered during a prolonged maternal hospital course.

If the mother responds to conservative management, she should be treated with bed rest, preferably in the hospital setting. Blood should always be available for maternal transfusion in the event of sudden hemorrhage. Although this is a costly treatment, recent studies suggest that, when total expenses for both mother and baby are calculated, this strategy is more cost effective than rest at home.[32] An additional reason for continued hospitalization is the observation that one-half of all patients requiring early delivery because of failed expectant management do so because of excessive bleeding with or without uterine contractions. Approximately 25 to 30 percent of patients can be expected to complete 36 weeks gestation without labor or repetitive bleeding forcing earlier delivery. In these patients, amniocentesis should be performed and, if the analysis of amniotic fluid documents pulmonary maturity, cesarean section planned.

When encountering a patient with placenta previa, the possibility of a placenta accreta or one of its variations, placenta percreta or placenta increta, should be considered (Fig. 18.6).[33] In this condition, the placenta forms an abnormally firm attachment to the uterine wall. There is absence of the decidua basalis and incomplete development of the fibrinoid layer. The placenta can be attached directly to the myome-

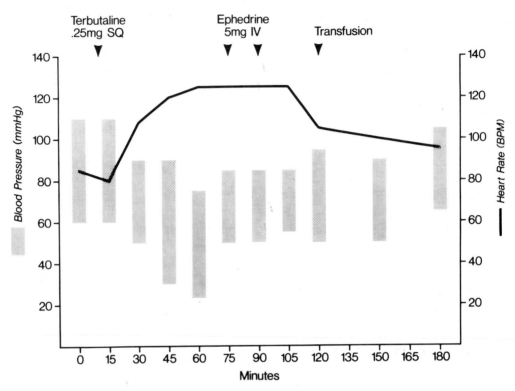

Fig. 18.5 Blood pressure and heart rate response to terbutaline administration in a bleeding patient with placenta previa. Hypotension, which developed acutely, is somewhat resistant to ephedrine and crystalloid administration.

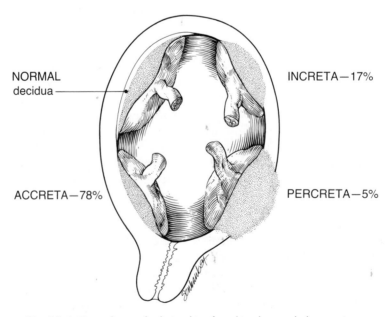

Fig. 18.6 Uteroplacental relationships found in abnormal placentation.

trium (accreta), invade the myometrium (increta), or penetrate the myometrium (percreta). Prior cesarean section or other uterine surgery are the factors most often associated with this problem. In patients without prior uterine surgery who have placenta previa, the incidence of placenta accreta will be 4 percent. In patients with previous cesarean delivery who have placenta previa, the incidence of placenta accreta is between 16 and 25 percent. Most of the patients with placenta accreta in this instance will require cesarean hysterectomy.[26,34,35] However, in cases in which uterine preservation is highly desired and no bladder invasion has occurred, bleeding has been successfully controlled by packing of the lower uterine segment with subsequent removal of the pack through the vagina within 24 hours.[36]

Complete placenta accreta encountered after vaginal delivery may permit other treatment options. Bleeding may be minimal unless the placenta has partially separated. If no cleavage plane is identified and a placenta accreta is suspected, one should first make preparations for the possibility of major postpartum blood loss. At least 4 units of blood should be on hand and an anesthesiologist present in the delivery room. The patient should be in a suite in which a laparotomy can be performed, and surgical instruments for hysterectomy should be sterilized and ready. Whenever possible, the obstetrician should discuss the likely diagnosis with the patient and review possible treatment options.

Three therapeutic plans may be considered. If uterine preservation is not important, or if maternal blood loss is excessive, hysterectomy offers the best chance for survival and will minimize morbidity.[37] If uterine preservation is important, an effort can be made to remove as much of the placenta as possible and then treat the patient with oxytocics and antibiotics. This option is probably most useful when there is significant bleeding from a partially separated placenta with only a focal accreta. For the patient who wishes to maximize her chances for uterine preservation and who is not actively bleeding, the placenta may be left in situ. The umbilical cord should be ligated and cut as close to its base as possible. The patient should then be treated with antibiotics. This approach has been successful when bleeding has not necessitated more aggressive surgical procedures.[38]

Third-Trimester Fetal Bleeding

A rare but important cause of third-trimester bleeding is that associated with rupture of a fetal vessel. This event is often the result of a velamentous insertion of the umbilical cord and occurs in 0.1 to 1.8 percent of pregnancies. In this instance, the cord inserts at a distance from the placenta, and its vessels must traverse between the chorion and amnion without the protection of Wharton's jelly. When the fetal vessel ruptures, often acute vaginal bleeding is associated with an abrupt change in the fetal heart rate. The fetal heart rate pattern often shows an initial fetal tachycardia followed by bradycardia with intermittent accelerations. Short-term variability is frequently maintained.

[VASA PREVIA]

One must have a high index of suspicion to make the correct diagnosis. In most instances, one must make the diagnosis rapidly and institute definitive therapy, delivery, to optimize fetal outcome. The fetal mortality in this condition has been reported to be greater than 50 percent.[39,40] Figure 18.7 illustrates the fetal heart rate tracing of a successfully treated case of spontaneous rupture of a velamentous insertion of the fetal vessel.

On occasion, examining the blood passed vaginally by the Apt test will reveal its fetal origin. The Apt test is performed by first mixing one part of bloody vaginal fluid with 5 to 10 parts tap water. This mixture is then centrifuged for 2 minutes. The supernatant must be pink to proceed with the test. One then mixes 5 parts of the supernatant with 1 part of 1 percent (0.25 N) sodium hydroxide. This mixture is again centrifuged for 2 minutes. A pink color indicates the presence of fetal blood; a yellow-brown color indicates maternal blood. The basis of the test is that adult oxyhemoglobin is less resistant to alkali than is fetal oxyhemoglobin. During the reaction with sodium hydroxide, adult oxyhemoglobin is converted to alkaline globin hematin.[34]

POSTPARTUM HEMORRHAGE

Acute blood loss is the most common cause of hypotension in obstetrics. Hemorrhage usually occurs immediately preceding or after the delivery of the placenta. At term, approximately 600 ml/min of blood flows through the placental site. Excessive blood loss

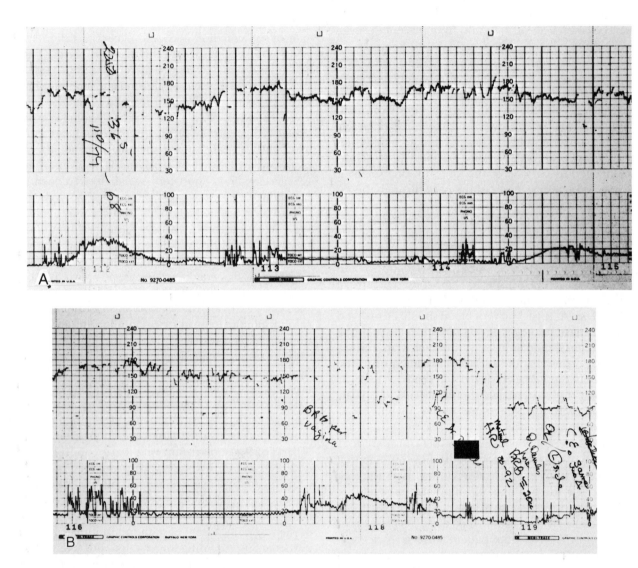

Fig. 18.7 Fetal heart rate tracing after rupture of a velamentous insertion of the cord. (A) Normal fetal heart rate tracing in early labor at term showing accelerations but no other changes. (B) Just before panel 118, bright red vaginal bleeding is noted. Shortly thereafter, the fetal heart rate is noted to be 80 to 90 bpm. *(Figure continues.)*

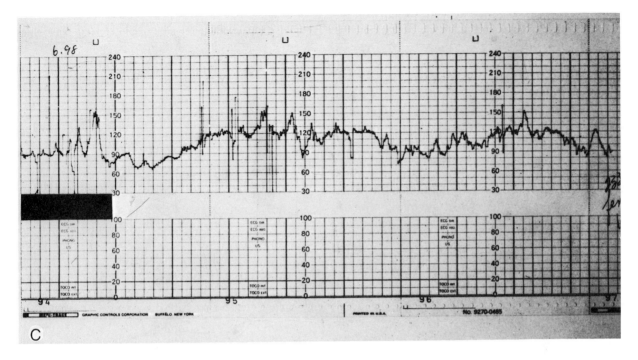

C

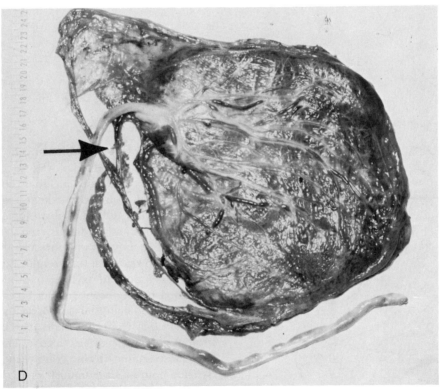

D

Fig. 18.7 *(Continued)* (C) In the delivery room, the fetal heart rate tracing shows the characteristic bradycardia–tachycardia heart rate response as the fetus attempts to compensate for acute blood loss. An emergency cesarean section was performed, and an anemic fetus was delivered. After rapid volume infusion and resuscitation, the infant survived and is developing normally. (D) Examination of the placenta showed a velamentous insertion of the umbilical cord and a lacerated fetal vessel as a result of spontaneous rupture of the membranes. In this case, the unprotected fetal vessels passed over the cervical os, a vasa previa.

most commonly results when the uterus fails to contract after the delivery of its contents. Effective hemostasis after separation of the placenta is dependent on contraction of the myometrium to compress severed vessels. Failure of the uterus to contract can usually be attributed to myometrial dysfunction and retained placental fragments. Factors predisposing to myometrial dysfunction include overdistention of the uterus as in multiple pregnancy and hydramnios, oxytocin-stimulated labor, general anesthesia with halothane, and amnionitis.

Upon encountering postpartum hemorrhage, manual digital exploration of the uterus should be quickly accomplished to rule out the possibility of retained placental fragments (Fig. 18.8). If retained tissue is not detected, manual massage of the uterus should be

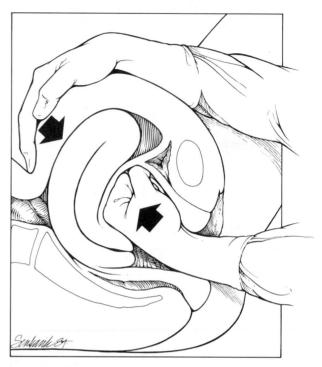

Fig. 18.9 Manual compression and massage of the uterus to control bleeding from uterine atony.

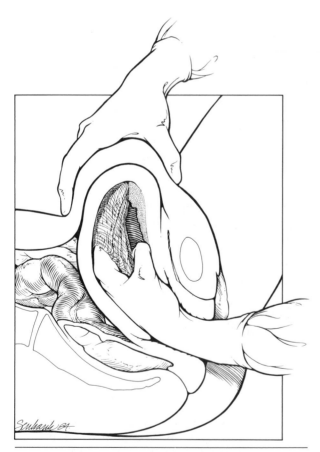

Fig. 18.8 Digital exploration of the uterus and removal of retained membranes. A sponge has been wrapped around the examiner's fingers.

started (Fig. 18.9). Simultaneously, pharmacologic methods should be employed to control uterine bleeding. Initial therapy includes the administration of a dilute solution of oxytocin, usually 10 to 20 units of oxytocin in 1,000 ml of physiologic saline solution. The solution can be administered in rates as high as 500 ml in 10 minutes without cardiovascular complications. However, an intravenous bolus injection of as little as 5 units of oxytocin may be associated with maternal hypotension, further stressing an already compromised maternal cardiovascular system. When oxytocin fails to produce adequate uterine contraction, ergonovine may be effective. This ergot alkaloid will cause tetanic uterine contractions that may persist for hours after administration. This medication should be given intramuscularly whenever possible in a dose of 0.2 mg. Intravenous usage has been associated with transient, but severe hypertension. This reaction is more likely to occur in women with pre-existing hypertension, a relative contraindication to oxytocin use.

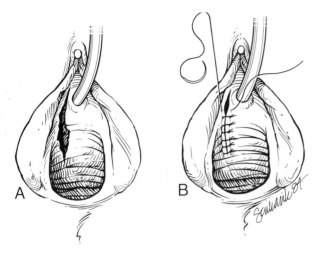

Fig. 18.10 Repair of an anterior periurethral laceration. Either running or interrupted sutures can be used. An indwelling catheter is placed before the repair is made.

As an alternative to ergonovine, prostaglandin $F_{2\alpha}$ has been used successfully to treat postpartum uterine atony. Initial studies were performed with the naturally occurring compound, which required direct intrauterine injection. The total dose used was 1 to 2 mg diluted in 10 to 20 ml of saline.[41] Recently, clinical trials of the synthetic 15-methyl-$F_{2\alpha}$ prostaglandin produced promising results.[42] Many clinicians now believe this prostaglandin should be used if oxytocin has failed to arrest hemorrhage from uterine atony. This compound should be given in 0.25-mg doses in the deltoid muscle every 1 to 2 hours. As many as five doses may be administered without adverse effect. Experience at the University of Washington supports these observations, as the routine availability of this agent in the delivery unit has arrested a number of otherwise uncontrollable hemorrhages.

When pharmacologic methods fail to control hemorrhage from atony, surgical measures should be undertaken to arrest the bleeding before it becomes life-threatening. However, before a laparotomy, a careful inspection of the vagina and cervix should be

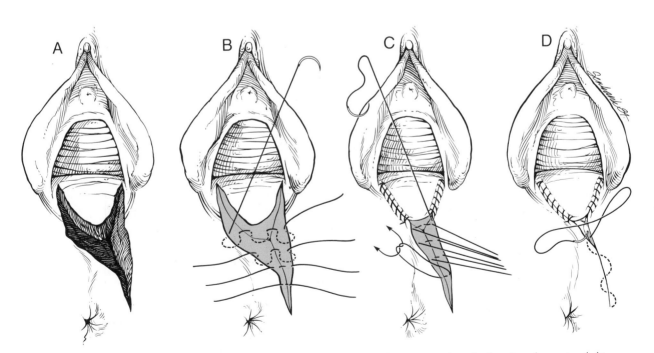

Fig. 18.11 Repair of a second-degree laceration. A first-degree laceration involves the fourchet, the perineal skin, and the vaginal mucous membrane. A second-degree laceration also includes the muscles of the perineal body. The rectal sphincter remains intact.

made to confirm that the uterus is the source of the bleeding.

If the uterus is found to be contracted appropriately and no placental fragments are retained within the uterus, a laceration of maternal soft tissues is the likely cause of continued vaginal bleeding. Careful inspection of the cervix and vagina will often indicate the source of the bleeding. Figures 18.10 through 18.13 respectively illustrate second-, third-, and fourth-degree lacerations of the perineum and techniques for their repair. Adequate exposure for the repair of such lacerations is critical, and, if needed, assistance should be summoned to aid in retraction.

In cervical laceration, it is important to secure the base of the laceration that is often a major source of bleeding. However, this area is frequently the most difficult to suture. Valuable time can be lost trying to expose the angle of such a laceration. A helpful technique to use in these cases, especially when help is limited or slow in responding, is to start to suture the laceration at its proximal end, using the suture for traction to expose the more distal portion of the cer-

vix until the apex is in view (Fig. 18.14). This technique has the added advantage of arresting significant bleeding from the edges of laceration.

Ligation of the ascending branch of the uterine arteries should be attempted as a first step if hemorrhage is unresponsive to oxytocin or prostaglandin (Fig. 18.15).[43] Next, the hypogastric artery should be exposed and suture ligated or occluded with hemostatic clips. If this slows but does not stop the bleeding, temporary occlusion of the ovarian vessels bilaterally may be attempted. This can be accomplished with digital pressure or with rubber-sleeved clamps. It may be an especially useful technique if the patient is of low parity and future childbearing is of great importance. Successful pregnancy has been reported after all major pelvic vessels were ligated to arrest postpartum hemorrhage.[44] If childbearing has been completed or if the patient develops hypovolemia not easily corrected with transfusion, rapid hysterectomy should be performed (see Ch. 20). If the patient's blood loss temporarily exceeds the capacity for replacement, the aorta should be manually compressed

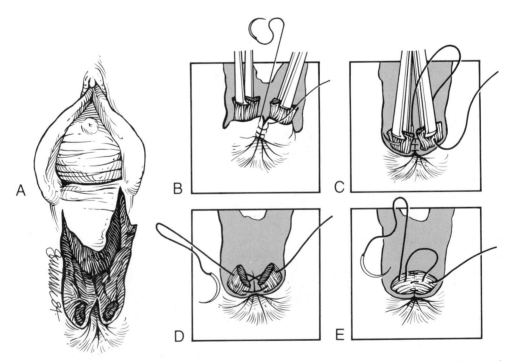

Fig. 18.12 Repair of the sphincter after a third-degree laceration. A third-degree laceration extends not only through the skin, mucous membrane, and perineal body, but includes the anal sphincter. Interrupted figure of eight sutures should be placed in the capsule of the sphincter muscle.

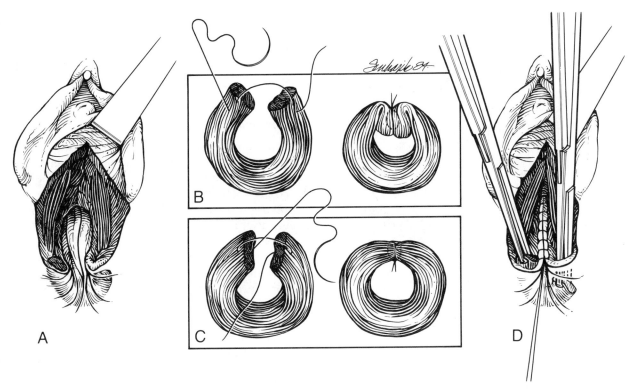

Fig. 18.13 Repair of a fourth-degree laceration. This laceration extends through the rectal mucosa. (A) The extent of this laceration is shown, with a segment of the rectum exposed. (B) Approximation of the rectal submucosa. This is the most commonly recommended method for repair. (C) Alternative method of approximating the rectal mucosa in which the knots are actually buried inside the rectal lumen. (D) After closure of the rectal submucosa, an additional layer of running sutures may be placed. The rectal sphincter is then repaired.

with the heel of the surgeon's hand. This maneuver effectively removes the lower one-third of the body from the circulation. It will often allow added minutes for volume infusion and for surgical assistance to be readied before definitive surgical therapy.

Pelvic Hematoma

Blood loss leading to cardiovascular instability is not always visible. In some instances traumatic laceration of blood vessels may lead to the formation of a pelvic hematoma. Pelvic hematomas may be divided into three main types: vulvar, vaginal, and retroperitoneal.

Vulvar Hematoma

This type of hematoma results from laceration of vessels in the superficial fascia of either the anterior or posterior pelvic triangle. The usual physical signs are

subacute volume loss and vulvar pain. The blood loss in this case is limited by Colles' fascia and the urogenital diaphragm. In the posterior area, the limitations are the anal fascia. Because of these fascial boundaries, the mass will extend to the skin, and a visible hematoma will result (Figs. 18.16 and 18.17).

Treatment in these cases requires the volume support outlined previously. Surgical management calls for wide linear incision of the mass through the skin and evacuation of blood and clots. As this condition is often the result of bleeding from small vessels, the lacerated vessel will not usually be identified. Once the clot has been evacuated, the dead space can be closed with sutures. The area should then be compressed by a large sterile dressing and pressure applied. Efforts to pack the cavity are usually futile, only serving to create further bleeding. An indwelling catheter should be placed in the bladder at the start of

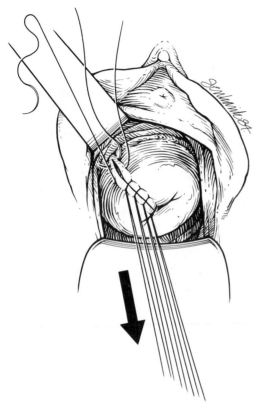

Fig. 18.14 Repair of a cervical laceration, which begins at the proximal part of the laceration, using traction on the previous sutures to aid in exposing the distal portion of the defect.

the surgical evacuation and left in place for 24 to 36 hours. Compression can be removed after 12 hours.

Vaginal Hematoma

Vaginal hematomas can result from trauma to maternal soft tissues during delivery. These hematomas are frequently associated with a forceps delivery but may occur spontaneously; they are less common than vulvar hematomas. In a vaginal hematoma, blood accumulates in the plane above the level of the pelvic diaphragm (Fig. 18.18). It is unusual for large amounts of blood to collect in this space. The most frequent complaint in such cases is severe rectal pressure. Examination will reveal a large mass protruding into the vagina.

Vaginal hematomas should be treated by incision of the vagina and evacuation. As with vulvar hematomas,

it is uncommon to find a single bleeding vessel as the source of bleeding. The incision need not be closed, as the edges of the vagina will fall back together after the clot has been removed. A vaginal pack should be inserted to tamponade the raw edges. The pack is then removed in 12 to 18 hours.

Retroperitoneal Hematoma

Retroperitoneal hematomas are the least common of the pelvic hematomas, but are the most dangerous to the mother. Symptoms from a retroperitoneal hematoma may not be impressive until the sudden onset of hypotension or shock. A retroperitoneal hematoma occurs after laceration of one of the vessels originating from the hypogastric artery (Fig. 18.19). Such lacerations may result from inadequate hemostasis of the uterine arteries at the time of cesarean section or after rupture of a low transverse cesarean section scar during a trial of labor. In these patients, blood may dissect up to the renal vasculature.

Treatment of this life-threatening condition involves surgical exploration and ligation of the hypogastric vessels on both the lacerated side and the contralateral side if unilateral ligation does not arrest the bleeding. On occasion, it may be possible to open the hematomas and identify the bleeding vessel.

Umbrella Pack

Use of an umbrella pack to control bleeding after hysterectomy is a valuable technique in desperate situations (Fig. 18.20). This technique may be needed after cesarean hysterectomy complicated by persistent bleeding from the vaginal cuff. Such hemorrhage may be encountered after massive blood loss secondary to the washout of platelets or as a result of DIC. In either instance, it may be impossible to control the generalized oozing from the vaginal cuff except with pressure. The umbrella pack will often permit one to tamponade the bleeding surfaces until coagulation factors and platelets can be given and, in addition, enables the surgeon to close the abdomen without the fear of continued blood loss.

The pack itself should be a bag or sack of nonadhesive material. A small garbage bag serves the purpose very well. The bag can be inserted through the vagina or at laparotomy. When abdominal placement is possible, the bag should be filled with 2-inch gauze packing through the vagina to ensure an orderly packing

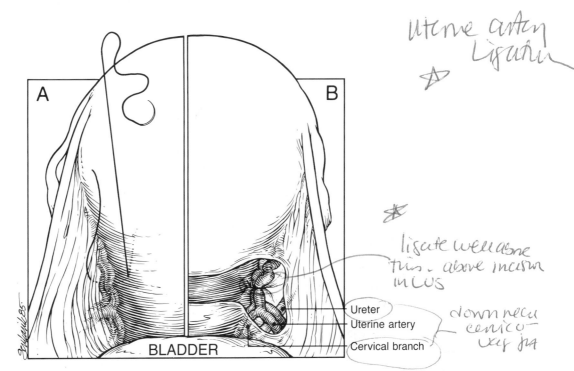

Fig. 18.15 Ligation of the uterine artery. This anterior view of the uterus demonstrates the placement of a suture around the ascending branch of the uterine artery and vein as described by O'Leary and O'Leary.[43] Note that 2 to 3 cm of myometrium medial to the vessels has been included in the ligature. The vessels are not divided.

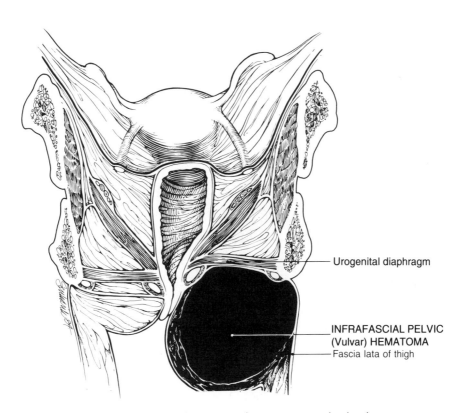

Fig. 18.16 Vulvar hematoma, showing anatomic landmarks.

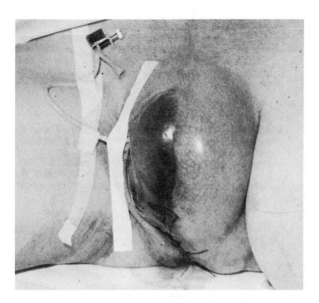

Fig. 18.17 Photograph of vulvar hematoma before evacuation.

that will facilitate removal at a future time. The bag should be filled with enough gauze to occlude the open vaginal cuff completely and present enough resistance to prevent expulsion when a weight is attached to the end of the pack.

Once the pack is in true pelvis and the gauze has been inserted, a 1,000-ml intravenous bag should be tied to the umbrella pack and traction applied. Traction should be maintained for 24 hours. After 24 hours, the traction may be relieved, but the bag should be left in place for an additional 12 hours. After 36 hours, the gauze packing should be removed by pulling on the tail that has been left protruding through the vagina. After the gauze has been evacuated, the bag should be removed.

Two major complications of this procedure include infection and urinary obstruction. The latter can be obviated by the use of an indwelling Foley catheter. The danger of infection is an ever-present one but is usually of secondary importance in the acute events

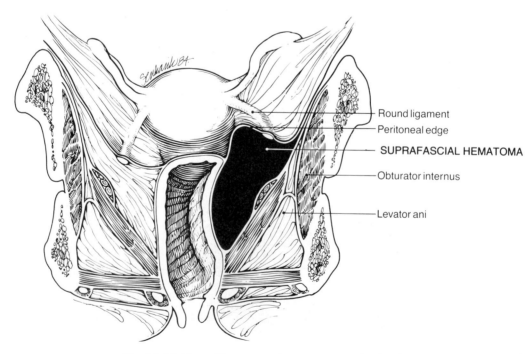

Fig. 18.18 Vaginal hematoma showing anatomic landmarks.

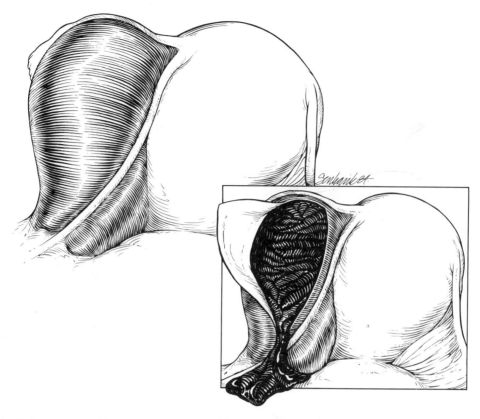

Fig. 18.19 Retroperitoneal hematoma as a result of laceration of one of the branches of the hypogastric artery. Evacuation of the hematoma is illustrated in the accompanying panel.

surrounding such massive bleeding. Prophylactic antibiotics should be used.

Inversion of the Uterus

Occasionally the third stage of labor is complicated by partial delivery of the placenta followed by rapid onset of shock in the mother. These events characterize uterine inversion. Hypotension usually results before significant blood loss has occurred. The inexperienced obstetrician may mistake an inversion of the uterus for a partially separated placenta or aborted myoma.

Uterine inversion is an uncommon but life-threatening event. Since 1970, the reported incidence has been 1 in 2,000 deliveries.[45] Inversion of the uterus is termed incomplete if the corpus does not pass through the cervix, complete if the corpus passes through the cervix, and prolapsed if the corpus ex-

tends through the vaginal introitus. Uterine inversion usually occurs in association with a fundally inserted placenta. Although earlier studies implicated the use of excessive cord traction and the Crede maneuver as causes of uterine inversion, recent studies have failed to document this association.[45]

Treatment of uterine inversion should include fluid therapy for the mother and restoration of the uterus to its normal position. The latter, best accomplished using the technique illustrated in Figure 18.21, should be attempted immediately upon recognition of the inversion. Separation of the placenta before replacement of the uterus will only increase maternal blood loss.[46] If possible, the uterus should be replaced without removing the placenta. Initial efforts to replace the uterus should be made without the use of uterine-relaxing agents. If initial efforts fail, the use of either β-mimetic agents or magnesium sulfate should be tried. The choice of these agents

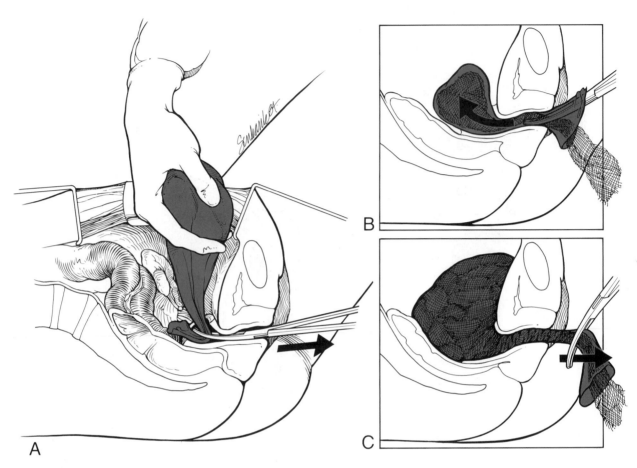

Fig. 18.20 Abdominal placement of an umbrella pack to control hemorrhage from the vaginal cuff. (A) Vaginal route for insertion of gauze packing. The pack is pulled downward over the vaginal cuff (B) and is secured (C).

depends on the maternal vital signs. In the case of severe maternal hypotension, magnesium sulfate is probably the best choice. These agents have been reported to be safe and associated with 85 to 90 percent success rate in patients failing initial replacement without pharmacologic therapy. In 10 to 15 percent of remaining cases, general anesthesia should be employed.[47]

Subacute inversion of the uterus occurs when the corpus has protruded through the cervix and the cervix and lower uterine segment have subsequently contracted, thereby trapping the corpus. In this instance, general anesthesia is necessary for restoration of the uterus to its proper anatomic position.

Occasionally, it is impossible to reposition the subacutely inverted uterus vaginally; laparotomy is then

necessary. Figure 18.22 shows the surgical technique used to correct this problem. Initially, a combination of vaginal pressure and traction from above on the round ligaments should be attempted. However, this maneuver may not always be successful, and one may have to resort to a vertical incision on the posterior aspect of the lower uterine segment to replace the uterus.

Once the uterine inversion has been corrected, the anesthetic agents used for uterine relaxation should be discontinued and oxytoxic agents given to produce uterine contraction. If oxytocin fails to contract the uterus, prostaglandin $F_{2\alpha}$ should be used. The same dosage and intervals used in arresting postpartum hemorrhage with uterine atony are appropriate in this circumstance.

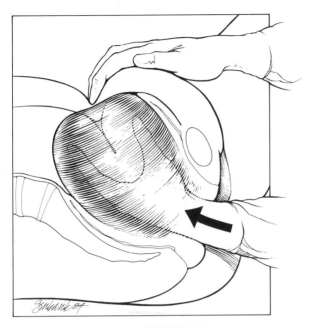

Fig. 18.21 Manual replacement of an inverted uterus.

Coagulation Disorders

Continued bleeding in the third stage of labor that is unresponsive to usual treatment should cause the clinician to consider uncommon but serious maternal coagulation disorders.

Von Willebrand's Disease

Von Willebrand's disease (VWD) is a hemorrhagic disorder that affects both men and women. This coagulopathy is inherited in an autosomal dominant pattern and is characterized by the following laboratory abnormalities: prolonged bleeding time, decreased Factor VIII activity, decreased Factor VIII–related antigen, and decreased von Willebrand factor. The latter is a plasma factor that is essential for proper platelet function and aggregation.

VWD, an autosomal dominant disorder, is quite variable in its clinical course, severity, and laboratory abnormalities, even in the same patient. It is therefore possible for a patient with this disorder to go undetected throughout pregnancy until bleeding problems develop postpartum. The usual increase in Factor VIII coagulant activity associated with pregnancy can also mask VWD. Only those patients with

very low levels (<5 percent) before gestation fail to exhibit this rise.

When VWD is diagnosed before parturition, Factor VIII activity should be monitored serially, with cryoprecipitate transfusion given to keep the Factor VIII activity near term at 40 percent. If Factor VIII levels are inadequate, the patient should be given one bag of cryoprecipitate per 10-kg body weight 24 hours before the planned induction of labor or cesarean section. This infusion will immediately restore the Factor VIII activity level, but it will take 24 hours for the associated platelet defect to be corrected. If one suspects this disorder in a patient with unexplained postpartum hemorrhage, coagulation studies should be ordered and a hematologist consulted. However, since time is often limited, it would be prudent to notify the blood bank that cryoprecipitate may be needed emergently. In this situation, at least 6 units of cryoprecipitate are required, to be given every 12 hours for the next 3 to 5 days.[48]

Amniotic Fluid Embolism

Amniotic fluid embolism (AFE) is a rare but frequently fatal obstetric emergency clinically recognized in approximately 1 of 30,000 deliveries. The mortality rate for mothers suffering from AFE is 50 percent.[49] The definitive diagnosis of AFE can be made by the demonstration of fetal squames and lanugo in the pulmonary vascular space. The clinical presentation of the syndrome is reflected by five signs that usually occur in the following sequence: (1) respiratory distress, (2) cyanosis, (3) cardiovascular collapse, (4) hemorrhage, and (5) coma. In one-half of patients surviving the initial cardiovascular crisis, a life-threatening bleeding diathesis will develop.

The cardiorespiratory effects of acute intravascular injection of amniotic fluid have been studied in pregnant ewes.[50] The initial response to the intravascular injection of amniotic fluid was hypotension. A 40 percent decrease in mean arterial pressure was followed by a 100 percent increase in mean pulmonary artery pressure. Little change occurred in the left atrial pressure or the pulmonary artery wedge pressure. A 40 percent fall in cardiac output was associated with the rapid rise in pulmonary artery pressure. These changes resulted in a two- to threefold increase in pulmonary vascular resistance and a two- to threefold decrease in systemic vascular resistance.

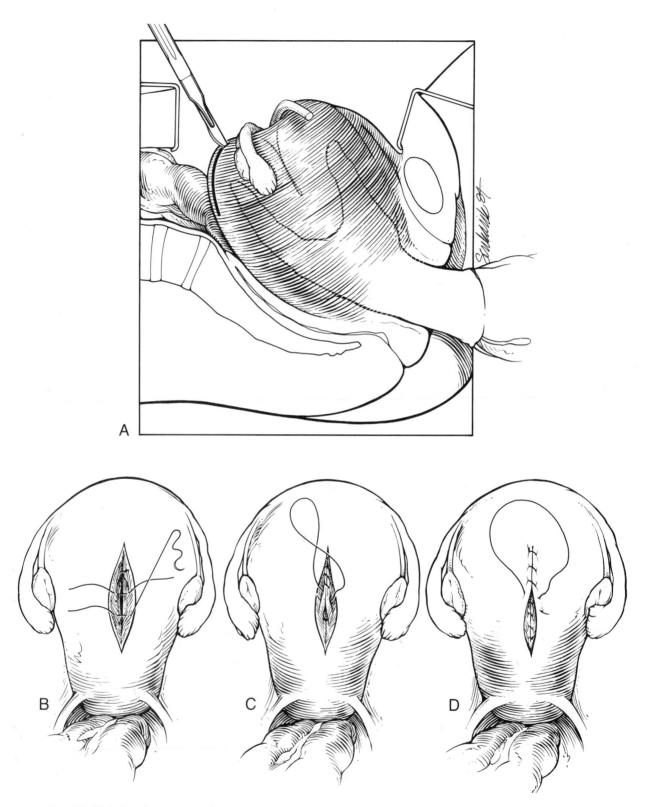

Fig. 18.22 Surgical restoration of an inverted uterus. Note the incision on the posterior aspect of the uterus and subsequent repair.

In contrast to these findings in sheep, intravascular injection of amniotic fluid in rhesus monkeys failed to produce cardiovascular changes similar to the syndrome observed in humans.[51]

Only scanty information is available on which to base the treatment of the initial syndrome. Early airway control usually necessitating endotracheal intubation has been stressed in the few patients surviving the full-blown syndrome.[52,53] Once maximal ventilation and oxygenation has been achieved, attention should be paid to restoration of cardiovascular equilibrium. Central monitoring of fluid therapy with a pulmonary artery catheter is essential. This catheter also provides a mechanism for definitive diagnosis. Pulmonary arterial blood may be aspirated and stained for the presence of fetal squames, lanugo hair, and mucin. The treatment of shock in the early phase of the syndrome unaccompanied by massive blood loss has not been well studied. Recent data suggest that the hypotension results from myocardial failure and that efforts should be used to provide myocardial support. These include inotropic agents as well as volume therapy.[54] Other investigators have observed reduced systemic vascular resistance and have used vasopressor therapy such as ephedrine or levarterenol with success.[53] If the patient survives the initial cardiorespiratory collapse, there is a 40 to 50 percent risk of the development of a coagulopathy within 1 to 2 hours. Disseminated intravascular coagulation results in the depletion of fibrinogen, platelets, and coagulation factors, especially Factors V, VIII, and XIII. The fibrinolytic system is activated as well.[55] Supportive coagulation and volume therapy (whole blood and fresh frozen plasma) have also been shown to improve survival.[52,53]

I have had personal experience with three cases of amniotic fluid embolism. All were managed with supportive therapy without the use of heparin or fibrinolytic inhibitors. Two patients survived, and one died of irreversible hypotension and pulmonary failure before the development of the coagulopathy.

DIC

DIC results from the loss of local control of the body's clotting mechanisms. Normally, there are four essential elements in the maintenance of local control of the hemostatic system: vascular integrity, platelet function, the coagulation system, and clot lysis.[56] The body must maintain vascular integrity for the survival of the organism. To minimize blood loss, any break in this system initiates the entire hemostatic cascade.

Platelets play an essential role in initiating and localizing clot formation. Platelets circulate until they encounter a break in vascular integrity. They then adhere to the damaged endothelium and release adenosine diphosphate, recruiting additional platelets to form an adhesive mass of platelets. Once the platelet plug extends past the site of damaged endothelium, platelets interact with the normal vessel wall and produce prostacyclin. This substance inhibits further platelet aggregation and localizes the platelet plug to the site of injury.

Platelets also localize the formation of fibrin by the coagulation cascade. Coagulation factors circulate in an inactive form. Aggregated platelets and injured tissue provide a phospholipid surface on which the coagulation factors can act. Once the factors are activated, fibrin is produced. The action of the coagulation cascade is limited to a localized area by a decrease in the amount of activated factors. These factors are reduced by (1) the reticuloendothelial system, (2) dilution by rapid blood flow, and (3) neutralization by a circulating protein (antithrombin 3).

Once a clot has formed, the reestablishment of normal circulation depends on the orderly removal of the clot. Clot lysis is usually a localized process that must proceed in a timely fashion because rapid lysis would lead to rebleeding. Clot lysis is limited in two ways. First, because both depend on Factor XII, the coagulation cascade and lytic processes are triggered simultaneously. Second, activated plasminogen or plasmin is inactivated by antiplasmin, which circulates in concentrations 10 times that of plasminogen. The orderly progression of clot lysis is facilitated by the incorporation of plasminogen directly into the clot, protecting it from rapid neutralization by antiplasmin. Activation of plasminogen within the clot can then proceed at a local level.

During DIC, the body is forming and lysing fibrin clots throughout the circulation rather than in the localized physiologic process as usually happens at all times. Therefore, the loss of localization of the clotting process is the main defect in DIC. The lytic process may be activated as well but occurs only in response to the activation of the clotting system.

In obstetrics, DIC causing hemorrhage may involve any of the four mechanisms involved in the localization process. However, it is uncommon for DIC to be initiated by a failure of vascular integrity. Similarly, a platelet abnormality leading to diffuse platelet aggregation is an unlikely cause of hemorrhage in obstetrics. However, activation of the coagulation cascade by the presence of large amounts of tissue phospholipids is a common stimulus for DIC in obstetrics. Such conditions include abruptio placenta, retained dead fetus, and amniotic fluid embolism. These tissue phospholipids contribute to the utilization of large amounts of clotting factors and lead to a consumption coagulopathy. Once this widespread coagulation has taken place, the lytic process is called into action. The degradation of large amounts of fibrin produces fibrin split products, or fibrin degradation products. These factors have their own physiologic activity and, when present in large amounts, contribute to bleeding by inhibiting fibrin cross-linking and producing platelet dysfunction.

The platelet count and fibrinogen level are the most clinically useful indications in evaluating the patient with DIC. They may be measured on a 1- to 2-hour basis to provide an accurate reflection of the activity of the coagulation process. PT and PTT are usually abnormal during DIC but are less helpful in evaluating the ongoing severity of the disorder. Because platelets and fibrinogen have a half-life of 4 to 5 days, they are not immediately replaced by the body's own mechanisms and will give an accurate reflection of ongoing consumption as well as the effectiveness of factor replacement.

The sine qua non of successful management of DIC is treatment of the initiating event. Once the cause has been located and treated, the process should resolve. However, depleted factors must be restored to permit orderly repair of injured tissues. Successful therapy involves the replacement of essential factors faster than the body is consuming them. These factors are platelets, coagulation factors derived from fresh frozen plasma or cryoprecipitate, and fibrinogen supplied by cryoprecipitate or fresh frozen plasma. Monitoring replacement therapy should be initiated 20 minutes after the intravenous administration of these products. The obstetrician should attempt to achieve a platelet count of more than $100,000/\mu l$ and a fibrinogen level of more than 150 mg/dl. In obstetric conditions complicated by hemorrhage, heparin has no use and will only cause the bleeding to worsen.

REFERENCES

1. Benedetti TJ, Quilligan EJ: Cerebral edema in severe pregnancy induced hypertension. Am J Obstet Gynecol 137:860, 1979
2. Shires GT: Management of hypovolemic shock. Bull NY Acad Med 55:139, 1979
3. Hewitt PE, Machin SJ: Massive blood transfusion. Br Med J 300:107, 1990
4. Davis R: Banked autologous blood for caesarean section. Anaesth Intens Care 7:358, 1979
5. Druzin ML, Wolf CF, Edersheim TG et al: Donation of blood by the pregnant patient for autologous transfusion. Am J Obstet Gynecol 159:1023, 1988
6. Herbert WN, Owen GH, Collins ML: Autologous blood storage in obstetrics. Obstet Gynecol 72:166, 1988
7. Kruskall MS, Leonard S, Klapholz H: Autologous blood donation during pregnancy: analysis of safety and blood uses. Obstet Gynecol 70:938, 1987
8. Grimes DA: A simplified device for intraoperative autotransfusion. Obstet Gynecol 72:947, 1988
9. Chestnut DH, Dewan DM, Redick LF et al: Anesthetic management for obstetric hysterectomy: a multiinstitutional study. Anesthesiology 70:607, 1989
10. Celayeta MA: Comment: tocolysis in placenta previa. Drug Intell Clin Pharmacol 28:828, 1988
11. Knab D: Abruptio placentae. Obstet Gynecol 52:625, 1978
12. Hurd W, Miodovnik M, Hertzberg V, Lavin J: Selective management of abruptio placentae: a prospective study. Obstet Gynecol 61:467, 1983
13. Pritchard J: Obstetric hemorrhage. p. 485. In Pritchard J, MacDonald P (eds): Williams Obstetrics. Appleton-Century-Crofts, New York, 1980
14. Paterson ML: The aetiology and outcome of abruptio placentae. Acta Obstet Gynecol Scand 58:31, 1979
15. Hibbard B, Jeffcoate T: Abruptio placentae. Obstet Gynecol 27:155, 1966
16. Townsend RR, Laing FC, Jeffrey RB: Placental abruption associated with cocaine abuse. Am J Roentgenol 150:1339, 1988
17. Darby MJ, Caritis SN, Shen-Schwarz S: Placental

abruption in the preterm gestation: an association with chorioamnionitis. Obstet Gynecol 74:88, 1989

18. Naeye R, Harkness WL, Utts J: Abruptio placentae and perinatal death: a prospective study. Am J Obstet Gynecol 128:740, 1977

19. Krohn M, Voight L, McKnight B et al: Correlates of placental abruption in birth certificate data. Br J Obstet Gynaecol 94:333, 1987

20. Pritchard J: The genesis of severe placental abruption. Am J Obstet Gynecol 208:22, 1970

21. Douglas RG, Stromme WE: Operative Obstetrics. Appleton-Century-Crofts, New York, 1976

22. Nyberg DA, Cyr DR, Mack LA, Wilson DA, Shuman WP: Sonographic spectrum of placental abruption. Am J Roentgenol 148:161, 1987

23. Nyberg DA, Mack LA, Benedetti TJ et al: Placental abruption and placental hemorrhage: correlation of sonographic findings with fetal outcome. Radiology 358:357, 1987

24. Pritchard J, Brekken A: Clinical and laboratory studies on severe abruptio placentae. Am J Obstet Gynecol 97:681, 1967

25. Brenner W, Edelman D, Hendricks C: Characteristics of patients with placenta previa and results of "expectant management." Am J Obstet Gynecol 132:180, 1978

26. Cotton D, Ead J, Paul R, Quilligan EJ: The conservative aggressive management of placenta previa. Am J Obstet Gynecol 17:687, 1980

27. Rizos N, Doran T, Miskin M et al: Natural history of placenta previa ascertained by diagnostic ultrasound. Am J Obstet Gynecol 133:287, 1979

28. Perkins R: Discussion of paper. Am J Obstet Gynecol 149:323, 1984

29. Liggins GC, Howie RN: A controlled trial of antepartum glucocorticoid treatment of RDS. Pediatrics 50:515, 1972

30. Ballard RB, Ballard PL, Goanberg P, Sinderman S: Prenatal administration of betamethasone for prevention of respiratory distress syndrome. J Pediatr 94:97, 1979

31. Collaborative Group on Antenatal Steroid Therapy: Effect of antenatal dexamethasone administration on the prevention of respiratory distress syndrome. Am J Obstet Gynecol 141:276, 1981

32. d'Angelo L, Irwin L: Conservative management of placenta previa: a cost benefit analysis. Am J Obstet Gynecol 149:320, 1984

33. Breen J, Neubecker R, Gregori C, Franklin J: Placenta accreta, increta and percreta. Obstet Gynecol 49:43, 1977

34. Read J, Cotton D, Miller F: Placenta accreta: changing clinical aspects and outcome. Obstet Gynecol 56:31, 1980

35. Nielsen TF, Hagberg H, Ljungblad U: Placenta previa and antepartum hemorrhage after previous cesarean section. Gynecol Obstet Invest 27:88, 1989

36. Druzin ML: Packing of lower uterine segment for control of postcesarean bleeding in instances of placenta previa. Surg Gynecol Obstet 169:543, 1980

37. Fox HG: Placenta accreta. Obstet Gynecol Surv 27:475, 1972

38. Gemmell AA: Unusual case of adherent placenta treated in unorthodox manner. J Obstet Gynecol 49:43, 1947

39. Torrey EW: Vasa previa. Am J Obstet Gynecol 63:146, 1952

40. Sirivongs B: Vasa previa report of 3 cases. J Med Assoc Thai 57:261, 1974

41. Takagi S, Yuoshida T, Togo Y et al: The effects of intramyometrial injection of prostaglandin $F_{2\alpha}$ on severe postpartum hemorrhage. Prostaglandins 12:565, 1980

42. Hayashi R, Castillo M, Noah M: Management of severe postpartum hemorrhage due to uterine atony using an analog of prostaglandin $F_{2\alpha}$. Obstet Gynecol 58:426, 1981

43. O'Leary JL, O'Leary JA: Uterine artery ligation in control of intractable postpartum hemorrhage. Am J Obstet Gynecol 94:920, 1966

44. Mengert WE, Burchell RC, Blumstein R, Daskal J: Pregnancy after bilateral ligation of internal iliac and ovarian arteries. Obstet Gynecol 34:664, 1969

45. Watson P, Desch N, Bowes W: Management of acute and subacute puerperal inversion of the uterus. Obstet Gynecol 55:12, 1980

46. Kitchin JD, Thiagaraja MMBS, May HV, Thornton WJ: Puerperal inversion of the uterus. Am J Obstet Gynecol 123:51, 1975

47. Brar HS, Greenspoon JS, Platt LD, Paul RH: Acute puerperal uterine inversion: new approaches to management. J Reprod Med 34:173, 1989

48. Walker EH, Dormandy KM: The management of pregnancy in von Willebrand's disease. J Obstet Gynaecol Br Commonw 75:459, 1968

49. Courtney LD: Amniotic fluid embolism. Obstet Gynecol Surv 29:169, 1974

50. Reis RC, Pierce WA, Behrendt DM: Hemodynamic effects of amniotic fluid embolism. Surg Gynecol Obstet 129:45, 1969

51. Stolte L, vanKessel H, Seelen H et al: Failure to produce the syndrome of amniotic fluid embolism by infusion of amniotic fluid and meconium into monkeys. Am J Obstet Gynecol 98:694, 1967

52. Resnik R, Swartz WH, Plummer MH et al: Amniotic fluid embolism with survival. Obstet Gynecol 47:295, 1976

53. Schaef RH, Campo TD, Civetta JM: Hemodynamic alterations and rapid diagnosis in a case of amniotic fluid. Anesthesiology 45:155, 1977

54. Clark S, Montz FJ, Phelan JP: Hemodynamic alterations associated with amniotic fluid embolism: a reappraisal. Am J Obstet Gynecol 151:617, 1985

55. Ratnoff OD, Vosburgh GH: Observations on the clotting defect in amniotic fluid embolism. N Engl J Med 247:970, 1952

56. Fischbach DP, Fogdall RP: Coagulation: The Essentials. Williams & Wilkins, Baltimore, 1981

57. Baker RN: Hemorrhage in obstetrics. Obstet Gynecol Annu 6:295, 1977

Chapter 19

Critical Care Obstetrics

William C. Mabie

INTRODUCTION

In the past decade, several large obstetric services in the United States have established intensive care units (ICUs). Although only about 1 percent of obstetric patients require intensive care, these units offer several benefits: (1) intensive observation and organization allows for prevention or early recognition and treatment of complications; (2) familiarity with invasive hemodynamic monitoring permits personnel to exert prompt rational treatment of hemodynamically unstable patients; (3) continuity of care is improved before and after delivery; and (4) residents and fellows learn a great deal about intensive care and about the management of rare medical complications of pregnancy.[1]

This chapter is divided into two sections: basic principles and clinical management. In the first, indications, insertion technique, and physiologic principles involved in using the Swan-Ganz catheter in obstetrics are considered. In the second, pregnancy-specific diseases and medical complications of pregnancy that often require intensive care are discussed.

BASIC PRINCIPLES OF CRITICAL CARE

Indications for Invasive Hemodynamic Monitoring

The mainstay of intensive obstetric care is pulmonary artery catheterization, common indications for which are listed in Table 19.1. Many of the indications occur in patients with severe preeclampsia or eclampsia. The Swan-Ganz catheter is useful in differentiating cardiogenic from noncardiogenic forms of pulmonary edema. It may also be used to guide diuretic therapy and manipulations of cardiac output such as preload and afterload reduction or inotropic therapy (Table 19.2). In patients with oliguria, the catheter may be used to assess volume status. In preeclampsia it has been shown that central venous pressure is not adequate for assessing volume status.[2,3] The change in wedge pressure in response to a fluid challenge is the most important guide to intravascular volume. While invasive hemodynamic monitoring is not necessary for acute resuscitation from hemorrhagic shock, it is useful in the subsequent 24 to 72 hours to guide fluid therapy in complex cases in which it is not clear if internal bleeding is continuing or if oliguria, pulmonary edema, liver dysfunction, or severe coagulopathy are present. In septic shock, invasive monitoring allows manipulation of cardiovascular parameters with fluid and inotropic therapy as well as assessment of response to therapy through such parameters as oxygen delivery and consumption. In the adult respiratory distress syndrome, the catheter is used to exclude cardiogenic pulmonary edema and to guide supportive therapy with mechanical ventilation, positive end-expiratory pressure, intravenous fluids, diuretics, and inotropic agents. New York Heart Association Class 3 and 4 cardiac patients require invasive monitoring for fluid, drug therapy, and anesthesia management during labor and delivery. The final in-

Table 19.1 Indications for Pulmonary Artery
Catheterization in Obstetrics

Pulmonary edema
Oliguria
Massive hemorrhage
Septic shock
Adult respiratory distress syndrome
Class 3 and 4 cardiac disease
Respiratory distress of unknown cause

dication includes patients in whom the contribution of cardiac or pulmonary disease to respiratory distress is unclear by clinical examination. The pulmonary artery catheter can help to differentiate heart failure from pneumonia, pulmonary emboli, adult respiratory distress syndrome, and chronic pulmonary disorders.

Risks Versus Benefits in Catheter Insertion

Complications associated with invasive hemodynamic monitoring include pneumothorax, ventricular arrhythmias, air embolism, pulmonary infarction, pulmonary artery rupture, sepsis, local vascular thrombosis, intracardiac knotting, and valvular damage.[4] The Swan-Ganz catheter was introduced into clinical practice in 1970.[5] Complications have decreased over the years at least partially because of better physician and nurse awareness. The incidence of pneumothorax has decreased from 1 to 6 percent in the early literature to less than 0.1 percent. Pulmonary infarction has been reduced from 7.2 percent in 1974 to 0 to 1.3 percent as reported in recent studies. Pulmonary artery rupture has fallen from 0.1 to 0.2 percent to almost zero. Local vascular thrombosis has decreased with heparin-bonded catheters, and septicemia has fallen from 2 to 0.5 percent. Yet all complications have not been eliminated.[6]

Interpretive error may also be considered a complication. It may result from improper calibration, air or blood in the lines, use of a digital readout instead of hard copy printout, and failure to measure wedge pressure at end expiration when pleural pressure is zero.[6]

The continuous generation of data can be mesmerizing. The obstetrician may spend excessive time calibrating, debugging, and collecting data, yet ignore such equally important aspects as the fetal heart rate tracing or the progress of labor.

The main benefit of pulmonary artery catheterization is its ability to provide information that clinical examination alone cannot supply.[6] The technique is more accurate than clinical assessment in determining the cause of shock or assessing the etiology of pulmonary edema. Two studies have shown that prediction of cardiac output and wedge pressure based on history, physical examination, and chest x-ray are about 75 percent accurate in coronary care unit patients[7,8]; however, three studies have shown that wedge pressure and cardiac output may be accurately predicted by clinical criteria only about one-half of the time in a more heterogeneous group of general ICU patients. Furthermore, information from invasive monitoring made a difference in treatment with fluids, diuretics, vasopressors, or vasodilators about 50 percent of the time.[9–11]

Does use of the Swan-Ganz catheter improve outcome? This question has not been answered rigorously for obstetric patients. There is some evidence for improved outcome in patients with acute myocar-

Table 19.2 Definitions of Hemodynamic Terms

Wedge pressure: A measure of left ventricular preload. The pulmonary artery wedge pressure is obtained with a balloon-tipped catheter advanced into a branch of a pulmonary artery until the vessel is occluded, forming a free communication through the pulmonary capillaries and veins to the left atrium. A true wedge position is in a lung zone where both pulmonary artery and pulmonary venous pressures exceed alveolar pressure.

Preload: Initial stretch of the myocardial fiber at end diastole. Clinically the right and left ventricular end-diastolic pressures are assessed by the central venous pressure and wedge pressure, respectively.

Afterload: Wall tension of the ventricle during ejection. Best reflected by systolic blood pressure.

Contractility: The force of myocardial contraction when preload and afterload are held constant.

dial infarction and low cardiac output.[12] There is also evidence of improved outcome in critically ill postoperative patients managed with invasive monitoring targeted to specific hemodynamic end points (e.g., wedge pressure, cardiac index, and oxygen delivery).[13] It is important to recognize that the Swan-Ganz catheter is only a monitoring device that can improve patient care and outcome only if the data generated are accurately interpreted and treatment exists for the condition present.[6]

Inserting the Swan-Ganz Catheter

Technique for Cannulating the Internal Jugular Vein

A pulmonary artery catheter can be inserted in several sites—internal jugular, external jugular, subclavian, basilic, and femoral veins. The right internal jugular is most commonly used because it provides a straight path to the right side of the heart and it has the lowest complication rate (Fig. 19.1). The internal jugular vein emerges from the base of the skull to enter the carotid sheath, which also contains the carotid artery and vagus nerve. Initially the internal jugular vein is posterior and lateral to the carotid artery. However, in the lower portion of the neck it lies lateral and slightly anterior to the carotid artery. The lower portion of the internal jugular vein lies within the triangle formed by the sternal and clavicular heads of the sternocleidomastoid muscle and the clavicle. It is within this triangle that the internal jugular vein is best cannulated (Fig. 19.2).

If the patient is obese or muscular with a short neck, place a small pillow or rolled towel under the shoulders to extend the neck. Have the patient turn her head 60 degrees to the contralateral side. The right internal jugular vein is usually easier to cannulate, and one avoids the risk of injuring the thoracic duct on the left. The patient is asked to raise her head so that the sternal and clavicular heads of the sternocleidomastoid muscle can be palpated. The carotid artery is palpated; the vein lies lateral to it. The patient is then placed in Trendelenburg position to distend the veins and to prevent air embolism. Several commercial trays containing the necessary equipment are available for central venous cannulation using the Seldinger technique (i.e., over a guidewire)

(Fig. 19.3). The procedure is performed under continuous electrocardiographic (ECG) monitoring.

After the skin is prepped and a sterile drape is applied to the area, the junction of the two heads of the sternocleidomastoid muscle at the apex of the triangle is infiltrated with 1 percent lidocaine. A 1.5-inch, 22-gauge needle with a 10-cc syringe may be used to locate the internal jugular vein. When the vein is found and the needle is withdrawn, the tract must be kept in the mind's eye. A large bore (18-gauge needle) can next be used to follow this path for cannulation of the internal jugular vein. I prefer a slightly different technique in which the vein is cannulated directly using a Teflon catheter over a steel needle that is used for routine intravenous therapy (18-gauge Cathlon). The needle enters at the apex of the triangle at about 30 degrees from the horizontal plane and is pointed along the medial border of the clavicular head of the sternocleidomastoid muscle toward the ipsilateral nipple. The needle is advanced with constant suction until a return of blood is obtained. Occasionally both sides of the vein will be traversed; however, withdrawing the needle slowly and maintaining suction will result in a return of blood. The flexible cannula is then advanced off the needle and is left in place in the vein. The most common problems are failing to locate the vein and puncturing the carotid artery. Usually the latter will be recognizable by pulsatile blood flow. However, pressure monitoring is occasionally required to determine if the catheter is in the carotid artery. If the carotid has been inadvertently cannulated, the needle can be removed and direct pressure applied for 5 minutes. Another attempt may be made on the right or it may be necessary to go to the left side to insert the catheter.

The J wire (guidewire) is then inserted through the Teflon plastic catheter. This is an important step. If the J wire is introduced easily and moves back and forth freely, one feels confident in placing the vessel dilator and introducer over the J wire. If, on the other hand, one encounters resistance and the patient complains of pain, it is necessary to remove the J wire and aspirate from the catheter to make sure that its position still lies within the vein. Once the J wire is in place, a scalpel blade (No. 11) is used to enlarge the

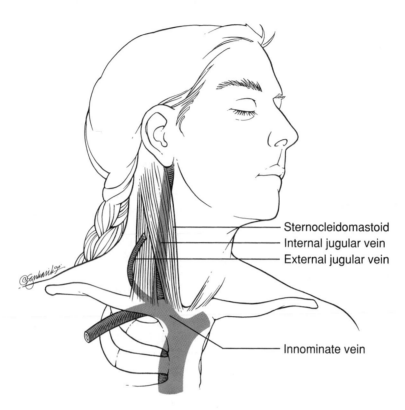

Fig. 19.1 Anatomic relationship of the internal jugular vein and the sternocleidomastoid muscle. The carotid artery lies just medial to the internal jugular vein.

incision. The vessel dilator and introducer are then slipped as one over the guidewire, using firm pressure and a twisting motion, which is particularly important as the catheter passes between the ribs and into the chest. The vessel dilator and guidewire are then withdrawn. Blood should flow freely into the introducer sidearm. Air is removed from the system, and an intravenous infusion is started.

Inserting the Pulmonary Artery Catheter

The catheter is removed from its sterile packaging. The balloon is checked by inflating with 1.5 cc of air and then deflated passively. The distal port is connected to the transducer that will be used for pulmonary artery pressure monitoring and is flushed with heparinized saline. The same is repeated for the proximal infusion port and the central venous pressure port. If disposable transducers are used, it is important to check their calibration and to ensure

that all transducers are zeroed to the midchest level. The integrity of the thermostatic wire is then checked by connecting the Swan-Ganz catheter to the cardiac output computer. The computer should register room temperature. The sterility sheath is then placed over the catheter. The tip of the catheter is moved up and down and the oscilloscope checked for pressure variation. The catheter is placed into the introducer, with the curvature of the catheter directed to the patient's left side. After the catheter has been advanced to about 15 cm, the balloon is inflated with 1.5 cc of air. The ECG and pressure tracing are observed continuously as the catheter is advanced into the right ventricle. The right ventricle is recognized by its low diastolic pressure (0 to 5 mmHg). Once in the right ventricle, the catheter is moved quickly into the pulmonary artery. The pulmonary artery is recognized because its diastolic pressure is higher than that of the ventricle. The catheter is then passed out to the

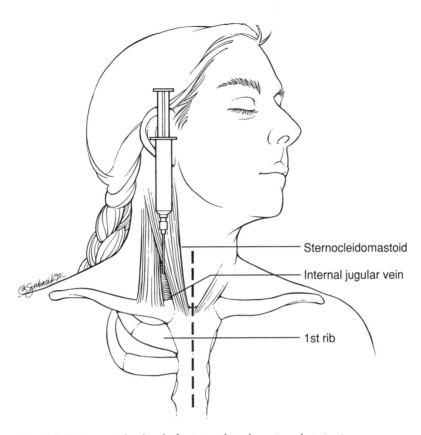

Fig. 19.2 Anatomic landmarks for internal jugular vein catheterization.

Sternocleidomastoid

Internal jugular vein

1st rib

wedge position, which is usually at approximately the 40-cm mark on the catheter. The wedge tracing is a damped tracing that has a, c, and v waves similar to the right atrium (see below). The wedge pressure is usually slightly lower than the pulmonary artery diastolic pressure. When the balloon is emptied passively, the pulmonary artery tracing should reappear. The introducer is then sewn into place. Antibiotic ointment and an occlusive dressing are applied.

If frequent premature ventricular contractions or ventricular tachycardia develop when the Swan-Ganz catheter passes into the right ventricle, the balloon should be deflated and the catheter withdrawn immediately. If the pulmonary artery is not encountered after 30 cm of catheter has been inserted, the catheter is probably coiling in the ventricle. A chest x-ray should be obtained after the procedure to confirm proper placement of the catheter and to rule out pneumothorax. The strip chart recording of the pas-

sage through the heart is then examined, and the right atrial, right ventricular, pulmonary artery, and wedge pressures are obtained at end expiration.

Hemodynamic Waveforms

The right atrial pressure tracing (Fig. 19.4A) consists of three distinct waves—a, c, and v. The a wave is a small wave caused by atrial systole. The declining pressure that immediately follows the a wave is called the x descent. The c wave may or may not appear as a distinct wave. It reflects the increase in right atrial pressure produced by closure of the tricuspid valve. The negative wave following the c wave is called the x^1 descent. The v wave is caused by right atrial filling and concomitant right ventricular systole, which causes the leaflets of the closed tricuspid valve to bulge back into the right atrium. The y descent immediately follows the v wave. The pressure changes produced by the a, c, and v waves are usually within 3 to 4 mmHg of

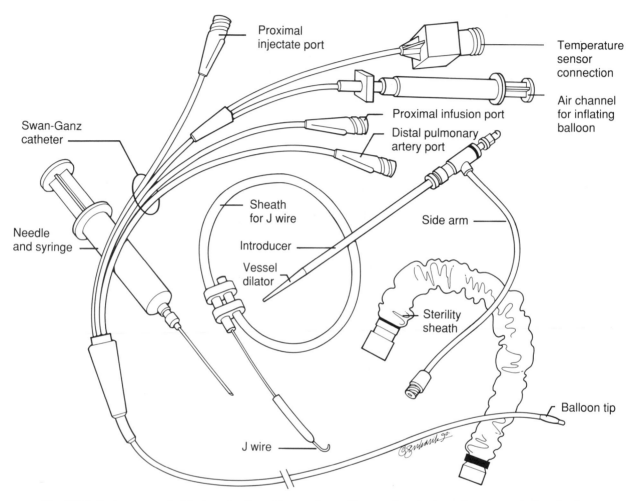

Fig. 19.3 Equipment needed for inserting Swan-Ganz catheter. The use of each piece of equipment is described in detail in the text.

each other so that the mean pressure is taken. The normal resting mean right atrial pressure is 2 to 6 mmHg. Elevated right atrial pressures may occur in the following conditions: right ventricular failure, tricuspid stenosis and regurgitation, cardiac tamponade, constrictive pericarditis, pulmonary hypertension, chronic left ventricular failure, and volume overload.

The phases of systole and diastole in the right ventricular pressure tracing can be divided into seven events. Systolic events include (1) isovolumetric contraction, (2) rapid ejection, and (3) reduced ejection.

Diastolic events include (4) isovolumetric relaxation, (5) early diastole, (6) atrial systole, and (7) end diastole (Fig. 19.4B).

The pulmonary artery pressure tracing is shown in Figure 19.4C. There is a sharp rise in pressure, followed by a decline in pressure as the volume decreases. When the right ventricular pressure falls below the level of the pulmonary artery pressure, the pulmonary valve snaps shut. This sudden closure of the valve leaflets causes the dicrotic notch in the pulmonary artery pressure tracing. Normal pulmonary artery systolic pressure is 20 to 30 mmHg. Normal

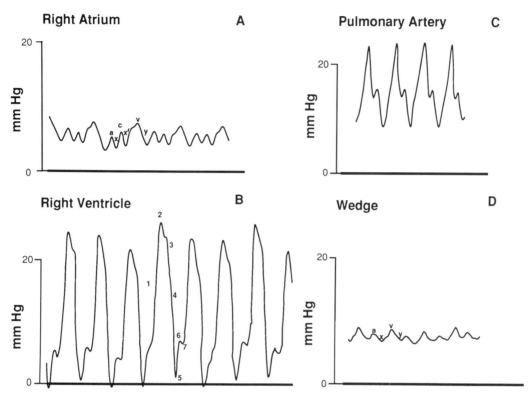

Fig. 19.4 (A–D) Pulmonary artery catheter placement. Waveforms and normal pressures. (Adapted from Daily and Schroeder,[101] with permission.)

end-diastolic pressure is 8 to 12 mmHg. Elevated pulmonary artery pressures are seen in pulmonary disease, primary pulmonary hypertension, mitral stenosis or regurgitation, left ventricular failure, and intracardiac left-to-right shunts. Hypoxia increases pulmonary vascular resistance and pulmonary artery pressure.

When a small branch of the pulmonary artery is occluded by inflation of the balloon on the Swan-Ganz catheter, the pressure tracing reflects left atrial pressure. The waveform looks similar to the right atrial pressure tracing described above (Fig. 19.4A). The a wave of the wedge pressure is produced by left atrial contraction followed by the x descent (Fig. 19.4D). The c wave is produced by closure of the mitral valve, but is usually not seen. The v wave is produced by filling of the left atrium and bulging back of the mitral valve during ventricular systole. The decline following the v wave is called the y de-

scent. The normal resting mean wedge pressure is 6 to 12 mmHg. Elevated wedge pressure is seen in left ventricular failure, mitral stenosis or regurgitation, cardiac tamponade, constrictive pericarditis, and volume overload.[14]

Determining the Hemodynamic Profile

Cardiac output is measured by the thermodilution cardiac output computer using five (10-cc) injections of iced saline. Highest and lowest values are discarded with the mean of the three remaining values recorded. The following measured hemodynamic variables are then used to calculate the rest of the hemodynamic profile: heart rate, blood pressure, pulmonary artery pressure, pulmonary capillary wedge pressure, central venous pressure, cardiac output, and patient height and weight. The derived variables include cardiac index, stroke volume and index, systemic vascular resistance and index, pulmonary vascu-

Table 19.3 Derived Hemodynamic Parameters

Parameter	Abbreviation	Formula	Units
Pulse pressure	PP	$BP_{syst} - BP_{diast}$	mmHg
Mean arterial pressure	MAP	$BP_{diast} + 1/3\ PP$	mmHg
Cardiac index	CI	$\dfrac{CO}{BSA}$	$L \cdot min^{-1} \cdot m^2$
Stroke volume	SV	$\dfrac{CO \times 1{,}000}{HR}$	ml
Stroke index	SI	$\dfrac{SV}{BSA}$	ml/beat/m^2
Systemic vascular resistance	SVR	$\dfrac{MAP - CVP}{CO} \times 80$	dynes $\cdot$ sec $\cdot$ cm^{-5}
Systemic vascular resistance index	SVRI	$SVR \times BSA$	dynes $\cdot$ sec $\cdot$ cm^{-5} $\cdot$ m^2
Pulmonary vascular resistance	PVR	$\dfrac{\overline{PAP} - PCWP}{CO} \times 80$	dynes $\cdot$ sec $\cdot$ cm^{-5}
Pulmonary vascular resistance index	PVRI	$PVR \times BSA$	dynes $\cdot$ sec $\cdot$ cm^{-5} $\cdot$ m^2
Left ventricular stroke work	LVSW	$SV \times MAP \times 0.136$	g/m
Left ventricular stroke work index	LVSWI	$\dfrac{LVSW}{BSA}$	g/m/m^2
Right ventricular stroke work	RVSW	$SV \times \overline{PAP} \times 0.136$	g/m
Right ventricular stroke work index	RVSWI	$\dfrac{RVSW}{BSA}$	g/m/m^2

BP_{syst}, systolic blood pressure; BP_{diast}, diastolic blood pressure; CO, cardiac output; HR, heart rate; BSA, body surface area; $\overline{PAP}$, mean pulmonary artery pressure; PCWP, pulmonary capillary wedge pressure.

lar resistance and index, and left and right ventricular stroke work and indices (Table 19.3 provides formulae).[15]

Oxygen Transport

Arterial oxygen content is the sum of the oxygen bound to hemoglobin and that dissolved in plasma as described by the equation

$$CaO_2 = (Hgb \times 1.36 \times SaO_2) + (PaO_2 \times 0.003)$$

where 1.36 is the ml of oxygen bound to 1 g of hemoglobin (Hgb), SaO_2 is the arterial oxygen saturation, and 0.003 is the solubility coefficient of oxygen in human plasma. If $SaO_2 = 1.0$ or 100 percent saturated, Hgb = 15 g/dl, and $PaO_2 = 100$ mmHg, then

$$CaO_2 = (15 \times 1.36 \times 1.0) + (100 \times 0.003)$$
$$= 20 + 0.3$$
$$= 20\ ml/dl$$

The amount of oxygen dissolved in the plasma usually does not make a significant contribution to CaO_2.

Mixed venous blood gives an estimate of the balance between oxygen supply and demand. For example, in low cardiac output states with a high rate of peripheral oxygen extraction, mixed venous oxygen tension ($P\overline{v}O_2$) will be low. Normal $P\overline{v}O_2$ ranges from 35 to 45 mmHg, and mixed venous oxygen saturation ($S\overline{v}O_2$) ranges from 0.68 to 0.76. Mixed venous oxygen content is measured on blood drawn from the pulmonary artery rather than from the superior vena cava or the right atrium. This is necessary because inferior vena cava blood has a higher oxygen saturation than superior vena cava blood and because drainage of coronary sinus blood into the right atrium contaminates the chamber with markedly desaturated blood because of the high myocardial oxygen extraction rate. After blood from the three sources passes through the right ventricle, it is thoroughly mixed.[15] A true mixed venous sample can thus be obtained. Mixed venous oxygen content is calculated as follows:

$$C\overline{v}O_2 = (Hgb \times 1.36 \times S\overline{v}O_2) + (P\overline{v}O_2 \times 0.003)$$

If $Hgb = 15$ g, $S\overline{v}O_2 = 0.75$, and $P\overline{v}O_2 = 40$ mmHg, then

$$\begin{aligned}C\overline{v}O_2 &= (15 \times 1.36 \times 0.75) + (40 \times 0.003)\\ &= 15 + 0.12\\ &= 15 \text{ ml/dl}\end{aligned}$$

The arteriovenous oxygen content difference is described by the equation

$$A - \overline{V}O_2 = CaO_2 - C\overline{v}O_2$$

Substituting the above calculations,

$$A - \overline{V}O_2 = 20 - 15 = 5 \text{ ml } O_2/\text{dl}$$

The normal range of the arteriovenous oxygen content difference is 3.5 to 5.0 ml/dl.

Oxygen delivery ($\dot{D}O_2$) is the product of CaO_2 and cardiac output (CO) as expressed by the equation

$$\dot{D}O_2 = CO \times CaO_2 \times 10$$

If cardiac output equals 5 L/min, then

$$\dot{D}O_2 = 5 \times 20 \times 10 = 1{,}000 \text{ ml/min}$$

Oxygen delivery is normally about 1,000 ml/min. Oxygen consumption ($\dot{V}O_2$) is the amount of oxygen that diffuses into the tissues and is expressed by the equation

$$\begin{aligned}\dot{V}O_2 &= CO \times (CaO_2 - C\overline{v}O_2) \times 10\\ &= 5 \times 5 \times 10 = 250 \text{ ml/min}\end{aligned}$$

Oxygen consumption is normally about 250 ml/min.[16]

Cardiopulmonary Profile

In aggregate, the hemodynamic and oxygen transport parameters described above provide invaluable information for the management of clinical problems. The data shown in Table 19.4 were derived from a single patient with severe preeclampsia near term. Among the measured variables, one notes borderline tachycardia, elevated blood pressure, and normal pulmonary artery pressure, wedge pressure, central venous pressure, and cardiac output. Arterial

and mixed venous blood gases are also normal, as are all of the derived variables. Because blood pressure = cardiac output × systemic vascular resistance, the hypertension seems to result from a systemic vascular resistance that is inappropriately high for the level of cardiac output.

Oxyhemoglobin Dissociation Curve

Some familiarity with the oxyhemoglobin dissociation curve is necessary to understand oxygen transport and the influence of shifts in the curve. Acidosis, increased red cell 2,3-diphosphoglycerate (DPG), and fever shift the curve to the right, thus reducing the hemoglobin affinity for oxygen and increasing oxygen unloading in the tissues. Alkalosis, reduced red cell 2,3-DPG, and hypothermia cause the curve to shift to the left, with the opposite effects on tissue oxygenation. As shown in Figure 19.5, hemoglobin is 50 percent saturated (P_{50}) at a PaO_2 of 27 mmHg. A PaO_2 of 60 mmHg correlates with an oxygen saturation of about 90 percent. Therefore, little is gained in oxygen saturation by increasing PaO_2 much higher than 60 mmHg. On the other hand, below a PaO_2 of 60 mmHg, small changes in PaO_2 result in large changes in oxygen saturation. A PaO_2 less than 20 mmHg is incompatible with life.[16]

Hemodynamic Support

Cardiac output is determined by four factors: preload, afterload, rate, and contractility. According to the Frank-Starling principle, the force of striated muscle contraction varies directly with the initial muscle length. The relationship between myocardial fiber length and fiber shortening can be graphically described by the curve in Figure 19.6. Fiber length can best be equated with preload or filling volume of the ventricle. To allow clinical estimation of preload the pressure correlate of the filling volume is used (i.e., right or left ventricular end-diastolic pressure). Varying compliance will alter the pressure–volume relationship. For example, a poorly compliant left ventricle resulting from myocardial hypertrophy or ischemia requires higher intracavitary pressure to achieve a specific end-diastolic volume or fiber stretch.[17]

Afterload is defined as the wall tension of the ventricle during ejection. This is best reflected by the

Table 19.4   Cardiopulmonary Profile in Severe Preeclampsia

Measured Variable	Patient Value	Normal Values for Pregnancy
Heart rate (HR)	93	60–100 bpm
Blood pressure (BP)	180/105 (130)	70–100 mmHg
Pulmonary artery pressure (PAP)	23/9 (14)	10–20 mmHg
Pulmonary capillary wedge pressure (PCWP)	7	6–12 mmHg
Central venous pressure (CVP)	3	1–7 mmHg
Cardiac output (CO)	7.29	5.0–7.5 L/min
Height	149	NA cm
Weight	67.3	NA kg
Inhaled oxygen fraction (FIO_2)	0.21	0.21
Hemoglobin	10.6	11.0–13.5 g/dl
Arterial pH (pHa)	7.35	7.36–7.45
Arterial partial pressure of oxygen (PaO_2)	94	80–100 mmHg
Arterial partial pressure of carbon dioxide ($PaCO_2$)	31	28–32 mmHg
Arterial oxygen saturation (SaO_2)	0.97	0.95
Mixed venous oxygen tension ($P\bar{v}O_2$)	44	35–45 mmHg
Mixed venous oxygen saturation ($S\bar{v}O_2$)	0.74	0.68–0.76
Body surface area (BSA)	1.71	NA m²
Cardiac index (CI)	4.26	$3.0–4.6 \text{ L} \cdot \text{min}^{-1} \cdot \text{m}^2$
Stroke volume (SV)	78.4	60–90 ml/beat
Stroke index (SI)	45.8	35–53 ml/beat/m²
Systemic vascular resistance (SVR)	1,393	$800–1,500 \text{ dynes} \cdot \text{sec} \cdot \text{cm}^{-5}$
Systemic vascular resistance index (SVRI)	2,382	$1,360–2,550 \text{ dynes} \cdot \text{sec} \cdot \text{cm}^{-5} \cdot \text{m}^2$
Pulmonary vascular resistance (PVR)	77	$50–150 \text{ dynes} \cdot \text{sec} \cdot \text{cm}^{-5}$
Pulmonary vascular resistance index (PVRI)	132	$85–255 \text{ dynes} \cdot \text{sec} \cdot \text{cm}^{-5} \cdot \text{m}^2$
Left ventricular stroke work index (LVSWI)	81.1	42–54 g/m/m²
Arterial oxygen content (CaO_2)	14.3	20 ml/dl
Mixed venous oxygen content ($C\bar{v}O_2$)	10.8	15 ml/dl
A-V oxygen content difference ($C[a - \bar{v}]O_2$)	3.46	3.5–5.0 ml/dl
Oxygen delivery ($\dot{D}O_2$)	1040	1,000 ml/dl
Oxygen consumption ($\dot{V}O_2$)	252	250 ml/dl

systolic blood pressure. In the absence of aortic or pulmonary stenosis, vascular resistance in the appropriate bed—systemic or pulmonary—will determine the afterload for that side of the heart. The effect of afterload on ventricular output is shown in Figure 19.7.[17]

Heart rate has a marked effect on cardiac output (i.e., cardiac output = heart rate × stroke volume). Increases in heart rate are accomplished at the expense of diastolic filling time, systolic emptying time being rate independent. Marked increases in heart rate may lead to circulatory depression when they cause myocardial ischemia or when reduced diastolic filling or loss of atrial "kick" prevent adequate ventricular preload. As a general rule, heart rates exceeding (220 − age)/min reduce cardiac output and myocardial perfusion.[18]

Contractility is defined as the force of ventricular contraction when preload and afterload are held constant. An increase in contractility is associated with an increase in stroke volume despite no change in preload. Factors that affect contractility include sympathetic impulses, catecholamines, acid–base and electrolyte disturbances, ischemia, loss of myocardium, hypoxia, and drugs or toxins. A third heart sound, distant heart sounds, and a narrow pulse pressure suggest impaired contractility. Radionuclide ventriculograms and two-dimensional (2D) echocardiography allow determination of ventricular size and contractile state. Effects of altered myocardial contractility on cardiac output at a given preload are shown in Figure 19.8.[17,18]

Figure 19.9 shows Starling curves that summarize the effects of increases and decreases of preload, af-

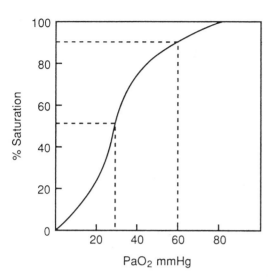

Fig. 19.5 The oxyhemoglobin dissociation curve of normal blood. Hemoglobin is 50 percent saturated at a PaO$_2$ of 27 mmHg. A PaO$_2$ of 60 mmHg correlates with an oxygen saturation of about 90 percent.

terload, and contractility on ventricular function. The agents used to treat hemodynamic instability are grouped in Table 19.5. The therapeutic rationale for supporting the cardiovascular system based on the Frank-Starling relationship is illustrated in Figure 19.10.

The primary adjustment to improve low cardiac output is to optimize preload using volume administration. Because of the lack of correlation between measurements on the right and left sides of the heart in patients with significant cardiopulmonary disease, pulmonary capillary wedge pressure is monitored to optimize left ventricular preload and to avoid pulmonary edema. If blood pressure and cardiac output do not respond to fluids (e.g., a pulmonary capillary wedge pressure of approximately 15 mmHg), then a positive inotropic agent may be needed to increase myocardial contractility. Dopamine is the drug of choice in most situations. It is utilized because its activity is modified at different doses. At 2 to 3 μg/kg/min, renal and splanchnic vasodilatation occur. Positive inotropy occurs up to 10 μg/kg/min. Vasoconstriction predominates over 10 μg/kg/min. These dose ranges reflect a predominance of action only.

There is a great deal of overlap and individuality of response. The usual therapeutic range for dopamine in clinical practice is 1 to 10 μg/kg/min. When the requirement exceeds this, a more potent vasopressor such as norepinephrine is added, and the dopamine is decreased to renotonic doses in the hope that renal blood flow will be preserved.

Afterload may be manipulated with vasodilators in cardiac failure or in low cardiac output states secondary to severe hypertension. Vasodilators have varying effects on arterial and venous resistances. Nitroglycerin, which is predominantly a venodilator, may cause a greater reduction in preload than in afterload. Nitroprusside, an equal arterial and venular vasodilator, may be preferred; however, marked decreases in systemic vascular resistance result in hypotension, poor perfusion, and myocardial ischemia. The use of a vasodilator requires careful observation of the adequacy of intravascular volume and the net effect on cardiac output.[17]

CLINICAL MANAGEMENT

Preeclampsia

The etiology, pathophysiology, and management of preeclampsia are discussed in Chapter 30. Although the indications for invasive hemodynamic monitoring in preeclampsia have not been firmly established, Swan-Ganz monitoring has been recommended for the management of pulmonary edema, oliguria, refractory hypertension, and epidural anesthesia and as a guide to volume expansion in efforts to prolong pregnancy in early-onset severe preeclampsia.[19,20] These indications are rather broad. The great majority of preeclamptic women can be managed with clinical acumen. Invasive hemodynamic monitoring is needed most in complex cases with multiple organ dysfunction or preexisting cardiac disease or in obese patients with pulmonary edema in whom clinical examination is compromised. Thus the main value of invasive monitoring in preeclampsia is as a research tool to study the pathophysiology of the disease, to define hemodynamic subsets of patients, and to evaluate the hemodynamic effects of drugs, anesthesia, and other interventions.

The cardiovascular hemodynamics of normal human pregnancy have been investigated over the

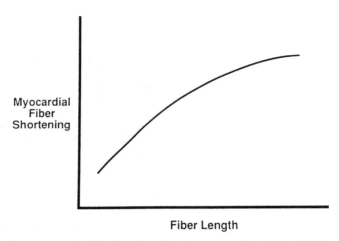

Fig. 19.6 Starling curve relating myocardial fiber length to fiber shortening. (From Rosenthal,[17] with permission.)

years with many techniques for measuring cardiac output, including the Fick principle,[21-24] dye dilution,[25-27] thermodilution,[20,28-30] radioiodinated human serum albumin,[31] echocardiography (M-mode, 2D, and Doppler),[32-37] and transthoracic electrical impedance.[38-40] While there is now some consensus on the hemodynamics of normal pregnancy, the data are conflicting.[41] Nearly every author reports different results. There is even more disagreement when one examines serial longitudinal studies of cardiac output in pregnancy and post partum and the effects of position change, exercise, labor, delivery,

and anesthesia. The same lack of agreement is found in studies of preeclampsia. In addition to the above sources of variability, the lack of agreement among hemodynamic studies in preeclamptic patients has been attributed to differences in the definition of preeclampsia, variable severity and duration of disease, underlying cardiac or renal disease, small numbers of patients in each series, technique for measuring cardiac output, and therapeutic interventions before study entry. In addition, the dynamic minute-to-minute fluctuation of the cardiovascular system makes it difficult to standardize conditions under

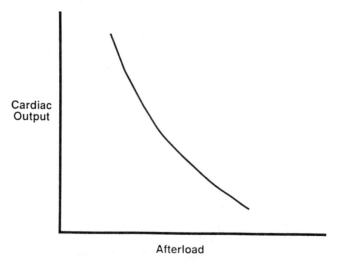

Fig. 19.7 Relationship of afterload to cardiac output at a constant preload. (From Rosenthal,[17] with permission.)

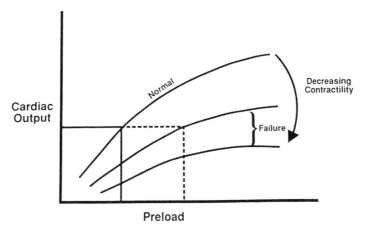

Fig. 19.8 Cardiac function curves demonstrating downward displacement secondary to decreased contractility and failure. Dotted line represents increased preload demands in failure. (From Rosenthal,[17] with permission.)

which observations are made and limits the value of a single point on a continuum.

Hemodynamics of Normal Pregnancy

Table 19.6 summarizes several of the invasive hemodynamic studies in normal pregnancy. These data represent patients in the third trimester lying in the lateral recumbent position. As previously noted, the mean values for each parameter are quite variable, and there is a broad range (e.g., Ueland et al.[26] found a mean cardiac output of 6.7 L/min, ranging from 3.7 to 8.4 L/min). Three of the more important recent studies done with the Swan-Ganz catheter are those by Groenendijk et al.,[29] Wallenburg,[20] and Clark et al.[30] Groenendijk et al. and Wallenburg reported cardiac index, while Clark et al. reported cardiac output. Using 1.7 m² for the mean body surface area to convert cardiac index to cardiac output results in a mean output of 7.6 L/min and 6.8 L/min, respectively, for the two Dutch studies compared with 6.2 ± 1.0 L/min in the study by Clark et al. Corresponding systemic vascular resistances are slightly

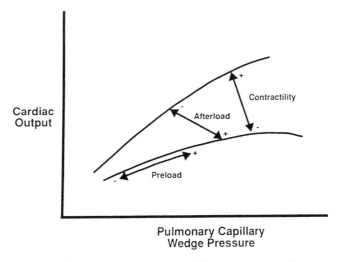

Fig. 19.9 Alteration in Starling curve of ventricular function caused by increases and decreases in preload, afterload, and contractility. (From Rosenthal,[17] with permission.)

Table 19.5 Hemodynamic Therapy

Decreased preload	Decreased afterload	Contractility
Crystalloid	Volume	Dopamine
Colloid	Inotropic support	Dobutamine
Blood	Vasopressors	Epinephrine
	Norepinephrine	Calcium[a]
	Phenylephrine	Digitalis[b]
	Metaraminol	
Increased preload	Increased afterload	
Diuretics	Arterial dilators	
Furosemide	Hydralazine	
Ethacrynic acid	Diazoxide	
Mannitol	Mixed arteriovenous dilators	
Venodilators	Nitroprusside	
Furosemide	Trimethaphan	
Nitroglycerin	Venous dilators	
Morphine	Nitroglycerin	

[a] May produce marked increase in systemic vascular resistance.

[b] Of questionable value and safety for acute management.

(Adapted from Rosenthal,[17] with permission.)

lower in the Dutch studies, although wedge pressures and central venous pressures agree among the three investigations. After synthesizing the hemodynamic data reported in Table 19.6, I propose a normal range for hemodynamic parameters in the third trimester of pregnancy (Table 19.7).

Hemodynamics of Preeclampsia

The cardiovascular hemodynamics of preeclampsia are uncertain, having been reported to range from a low output–high resistance state to a high output–low resistance state. In an insightful analysis, Hankins et al.[42] categorized studies by therapy prior to insertion of the Swan-Ganz catheter. They felt that much of the variation in the reported data was related to prior treatment (e.g., intravenous fluids, magnesium sulfate, and hydralazine). This categorization of studies has been expanded in Table 19.8.

Actually, prior treatment is only one factor in determining hemodynamics. Before therapy, Cotton et al.[43] found wedge pressure, cardiac output, and systemic vascular resistance to be within the normal range. The findings of Nisell et al.[44] on cardiac output and systemic vascular resistance agreed with those of Cotton et al. On the other hand, Groenendijk et al.,[29] Wallenburg,[20] and Belfort et al.[45,46] found low wedge pressure, normal to low cardiac index, and elevated

systemic vascular resistance. In the fluid restriction group,[47-52] all but Hankins et al.[48] found a normal wedge pressure, and all authors found a normal to slightly elevated cardiac output and systemic vascular resistance. With volume expansion, wedge pressure was normal to high in studies by Rafferty and Berkowitz[53] and by Phelan and Yurth[54] but low in the study by Rolbin et al.[55] Cardiac output was elevated in all three studies, and systemic vascular resistance was normal. In the final group in which prior fluid administration and drug therapy were unclear, results were similar to those with the fluid restriction group, with normal wedge pressure and normal to slightly elevated cardiac output and systemic vascular resistance.[28,56-59]

Phelan and Yurth[54] were the first to propose that a spectrum of hemodynamic changes characterized preeclampsia. The two extremes of the spectrum are represented by the data of Wallenburg[20] and Mabie et al.[50]

Wallenburg's data support the traditional view of preeclampsia—that of a volume-contracted, vasospastic state. He found a low wedge pressure, low cardiac output, and high systemic vascular resistance in 44 untreated nulliparous preeclamptic patients. In 22 patients who had received various therapies and had been referred to his center, a wide range of hemo-

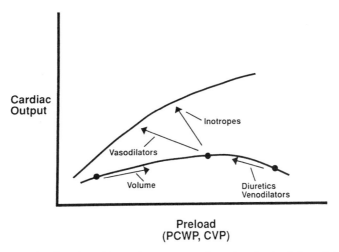

Fig. 19.10 Treatment approaches for altered hemodynamic states based on Starling's law of the heart. PCWP, pulmonary capillary wedge pressure; CVP, central venous pressure. (From Rosenthal,[17] with permission.)

dynamics was found. He concluded that the untreated patient was significantly volume depleted and that the wide spectrum of hemodynamic findings present in the treated group resulted from prior therapy and from other variables such as labor, multiparity, and preexisting hypertension. Thus the disparity in cardiac outputs, peripheral resistances, and wedge pressures among various studies was not due to the hemodynamic variability of preeclampsia but rather to differences in patient selection and therapeutic intervention prior to invasive monitoring.

Mabie et al.[50] studied the hemodynamics of 49 subjects with severe preeclampsia at a large referral center. Despite a heterogeneous population of referred and nonreferred patients, pretreated and nonpretreated individuals, a generally consistent profile emerged. Preeclampsia was in general a high cardiac output state associated with an inappropriately high peripheral resistance. Although the systemic vascular resistance was within the normal range, it was still inappropriately high for the elevated cardiac output. The failure of the circulation to dilate in the setting of increasing cardiac output appeared to be a characteristic feature of preeclampsia. The normal wedge pressure and central venous pressures found in their study suggested central redistribution of intravascular volume if the generally accepted reports of decreased plasma volume in preeclampsia are correct.

They postulated splanchnic venoconstriction as the mechanism for this volume shift. Mabie et al. also noted that while the hemodynamic profile is variable in preeclampsia, it is variable in virtually every other type of experimental and naturally occurring hypertension. They pointed out that Wallenburg had minimized the variable hemodynamic presentation of his untreated group in that 15 percent or more had wedge pressures greater than 8 mmHg, indicating normal central blood volume.

Although there is a wide range of hemodynamic findings, comparing the mean cardiac output and systemic vascular resistance from studies in Table 19.6 to those in Table 19.7 may be instructive. Mean cardiac output is 6.0 L/min and mean systemic vascular resistance is 1,171 dynes · sec · cm^{-5} in the normotensive, third-trimester patient. In severe preeclampsia, mean cardiac output is 8.0 L/min and mean systemic vascular resistance is 1,418 dynes · sec · cm^{-5}. Thus cardiac output and systemic vascular resistance both tend to be higher in preeclampsia.

In summary, it is too early to draw firm conclusions about the central hemodynamics of preeclampsia. However, there are several points that most authors agree on: (1) preeclampsia includes a spectrum of hemodynamic findings with variable wedge pressures, cardiac outputs, and systemic vascular resistances; (2) pulmonary vascular resistance is unaf-

Table 19.6 Invasive Hemodynamic Findings During the Third Trimester of Normal Pregnancy

Author (Year)	Method of Determination	No. of Patients	MAP (mmHg)	HR (bpm)	SV (ml)	CO (L/min)	SVR (dynes · sec · cm⁻⁵)	CI (L · min⁻¹ · m²)	SVRI (dynes · sec · cm⁻⁵ · m²)	PCWP (mmHg)	CVP (mmHg)
Hamilton[21] (1949)	Fick					4.6					
Werko[22] (1954)	Fick	11	99	83	71	6.5					
Bader et al.[23] (1955)	Fick	11	90	96	58	5.5	1,244	3.4		5	
Walters et al.[25] (1966)	Dye dilution	15		78	79	6.2					
Kerr[24] (1968)	Fick	5	86	84	76	6.3	1,119				
Smith[31] (1970)	RIHSA	10	79			4.5					
Ueland et al.[26] (1972)	Dye dilution	13		86	79	6.7	1,056				
Lim and Walters[27] (1979)	Dye dilution	23	86	80	93	7.8	1,540				
Lees[28] (1979)	Thermodilution	14	85	84		5.9	1,145				
Groenendijk et al.[29] (1984)	Thermodilution	4	95	84			886	4.5		9	
Wallenburg[20] (1988)	Thermodilution	7	83	80				4.0	1,629	6	4
Clark et al.[30] (1989)	Thermodilution	10	90	83		6.2	1,210			8	4

MAP, mean arterial pressure; HR, heart rate; SV, stroke volume; CO, cardiac output; SVR, systemic vascular resistance; CI, cardiac index; SVRI, systemic vascular resistance index; PCWP, pulmonary capillary wedge pressure; CVP, central venous pressure.

fected; and (3) systemic vascular resistance is elevated. If not above the normal range for pregnancy, systemic vascular resistance is at least inappropriately high for the level of cardiac output.

Effects of Volume Expansion in Preeclampsia

Because many studies have shown either contracted plasma volume in preeclampsia[60,61] or low wedge pressures,[20,29,45,46] volume expansion has been advocated in the treatment of severe preeclampsia. A few studies of malignant hypertension in the nonpregnant patient have also advocated volume expansion to prevent circulatory collapse precipitated by vasodilator therapy.[62] Advocates of volume expansion have shown that it causes no rise or fall in blood pressure, yet it does cause an increase in cardiac output and a fall in systemic vascular resistance. They suggest that volume expansion prevents precipitous falls in blood pressure during vasodilator

therapy; thus uteroplacental circulation is not compromised.[63–66]

Kirshon et al.[67] managed 15 primigravid patients with severe preeclampsia using the following protocol:

1. Colloid osmotic pressure was optimized to 17 mmHg with infusions of 25 percent albumin.
2. Pulmonary capillary wedge pressure was optimized to 10 to 15 mmHg with 5 percent albumin infusion.
3. Mean arterial pressure was reduced by 20 percent or to a mean of 106 mmHg with intravenous nitroglycerin, nitroprusside, or hydralazine.

The results were compared with those from a control group undergoing Swan-Ganz catheterization but not having volume expansion. The only benefit derived from volume expansion was an absence of acute

Table 19.7 Normal Hemodynamic Parameters for the Third Trimester of Pregnancy

Heart rate	60–100 bpm
Mean arterial pressure	70–100 mmHg
Pulmonary capillary wedge pressure	6–12 mmHg
Central venous pressure	1–7 mmHg
Cardiac output	5.0–7.5 L/min
Cardiac index	3.0–4.6 L · min^{-1} · m^2
Stroke volume	60–90 ml
Systemic vascular resistance	800–1,500 dynes · sec · cm^{-5}
Systemic vascular resistance index	1,360–2,550 dynes · sec · cm^{-5} · m^2
Pulmonary vascular resistance	50–150 dynes · sec · cm^{-5}
Pulmonary vascular resistance index	85–255 dynes · sec · cm^{-5} · m^2

fetal distress after initiation of antihypertensive therapy. Six of 15 patients (40%) still developed fetal distress in labor, suggesting that volume expansion does not affect the overall incidence of fetal distress. No pulmonary edema occurred, but nearly all patients required furosemide postpartum to control wedge pressures.

There are other arguments against volume expansion. The effects of volume loading are transient. If colloid is used, it may "leak" into the alveoli, while crystalloid decreases oncotic pressure, which is already depressed in preeclampsia. In 8 of 10 preeclamptic patients described by Benedetti et al.,[68] colloid had been given prior to the onset of pulmonary edema. Postpartum mobilization of extravascular fluid further predisposes the preeclamptic patient to pulmonary edema.[48] While volume overload may be avoided with central hemodynamic monitoring, such monitoring is not without risk.[4] Moreover, numerous studies indicate that monitoring central venous pressure alone is not adequate in severe pre-

eclampsia.[2,3] Furthermore, volume expansion seems to be counterproductive in that it makes patients more refractory to vasodilators, necessitating higher doses. On the contrary, in the treatment of hypertensive emergencies in the nonpregnant patient, a loop diuretic is advised for its synergistic effect with other antihypertensive agents.[69] Finally, part of the hemodynamic instability characteristic of severe preeclampsia is caused by baroreflex dysfunction. Wasserstrum et al.[52] looked at Δ heart rate/Δ blood pressure and Δ cardiac index/Δ blood pressure in response to hydralazine-induced decreases in blood pressure. A high baseline blood pressure was associated with a dramatic reduction in baroreflex sensitivity and control of blood pressure. Baroreflex dysfunction has been described in many other forms of hypertension as well. In summary, it is not yet clear whether or in what circumstances volume expansion is indicated in preeclampsia.[70]

Pulmonary Edema in Preeclampsia

Pulmonary edema in preeclampsia may be divided into cardiogenic (wedge pressure > 18 mmHg) and noncardiogenic (wedge pressure < 18 mmHg) forms, as summarized in Table 19.9. Cardiogenic pulmonary edema may result from systolic dysfunction or impaired myocardial contractility (e.g., peripartum cardiomyopathy). It may also result from diastolic dysfunction or impaired myocardial relaxation. Patients with left ventricular hypertrophy caused by chronic hypertension develop diastolic dysfunction, which precedes the development of systolic dysfunction by several years. These patients, who have thick walls and stiff ventricles, require high filling pressures and are thus predisposed to develop hydrostatic pulmonary edema if they retain excess sodium and water during late pregnancy or receive an iatrogenic fluid overload. Combined systolic and diastolic dysfunction usually occurs in elderly multiparas with long-standing, severe hypertension.[71,72]

Noncardiogenic pulmonary edema results either from a pulmonary capillary leak or from narrowing of the colloid osmotic pressure (COP)–wedge pressure gradient.[73] Plasma proteins such as albumin, globulins, and fibrinogen exert osmotic pressure to hold water in the vasculature, counteracting hydrostatic pressure, which pushes water out of the vasculature. Interstitial COP and interstitial hydrostatic pressure

Table 19.8 Invasive Hemodynamic Findings in Severe Preeclampsia and Eclampsia

Author	No. of Patients	PCWP (mmHg)	CVP (mmHg)	CO (L/min)	CI (L · min⁻¹ · m²)	SVR (dynes · sec · cm⁻⁵)	SVRI (dynes · sec · cm⁻⁵ · m²)
No therapy							
Cotton et al.[43]	5	12.0	6.0	7.6	4.8	1,350	2,256
Nisell et al.[44]	21			7.6		1,160	
Groenendijk et al.[29]	10	3.3		5.3	2.8	1,943	
Wallenburg [20]	44	4.0	1.0		3.0		2,970
Belfort et al.[45]	10	5.0	2.0		3.0	2,392	
Belfort et al.[46]	6	6.0	6.0		3.2	1,965	
Magnesium, hydralazine, fluid restriction							
Benedetti et al.[47]	10	6.0	3.0	7.4	4.7	1,322	
Hankins et al.[48]	8	3.9	1.0	6.7	4.3	1,357	
Cotton et al.[49]	45	10.0	4.0	7.5	4.1	1,496	2,726
Mabie et al.[50]	41	8.3	4.8	8.4	4.4	1,226	2,293
Wasserstrum et al.[51]	8	7.9	3.4		3.7		3,066
Wasserstrum et al.[52]	7	11.0	4.0		4.2		
Magnesium, hydralazine, volume expansion							
Rafferty and Berkowitz[53]	3	7.0		11.0	6.2	917	
Phelan and Yurth[54]	10	16.4	9.7	9.3	5.4	1,042	
Rolbin et al.[55]	4	5.2		9.7	5.2	1,040	
Unclear about previous treatment							
Graham and Goldstein[56]	10			8.8			
Newsome et al.[57]	11				5.0	1,078	
Lees[28]	14			5.8		1,590	
Cotton et al.[58]	6	9.0	2.0		3.5		3,330
Clark et al.[59]	9	9.2	4.1	8.5	4.2	1,388	

PWCP, pulmonary capillary wedge pressure; CVP, central venous pressure; CO, cardiac output; CI, cardiac index; SVR, systemic vascular resistance; SVRI, systemic vascular resistance index. All studies were performed using the Swan-Ganz thermodilution technique except in the study by Nisell et al., who used dye dilution.

have similar antagonistic effects on the other side of the membrane.

Normal intravascular COP in the nonpregnant state is 25.4 ± 2.3 mmHg, whereas normal wedge pressure (a measure of pulmonary vascular hydrostatic pressure) is 6 to 12 mmHg.[74] Therefore, the normal COP–wedge gradient is about 12 mmHg. A COP–wedge gradient of 4 or less has been associated with an increased risk of pulmonary edema.[75] The normal COP in pregnancy at term is 22.4 ± 0.5 mmHg. With delivery accompanied by blood loss and crystalloid replacement, COP decreases to 15.4 ± 2.1 mmHg.[76,77] With preeclampsia, COP has been reported to fall from 17.9 ± 0.7 to 13.7 ± 0.5 mmHg postpartum.[78] This narrowing of the COP–wedge gradient reflects predisposition to pulmonary edema.

Pulmonary edema associated with preeclampsia–eclampsia usually occurs postpartum.[68,79] Serum al-

bumin decreases because of renal losses, impaired liver synthesis, and blood loss with crystalloid replacement. Wedge pressure increases because of delayed mobilization of extravascular fluid. Beginning 24 to 72 hours postpartum, edema fluid is mobilized and returned to the intravascular space faster than the diseased kidneys can excrete it. Iatrogenic fluid overload may also contribute to raising the wedge pressure; however, elevations in filling pressure may not be significant enough to account for pulmonary edema without simultaneous lowering of the intravascular COP.

Oliguria in Preeclampsia

Oliguria has been variously defined—for example, urine output less than 30 ml/hr × 3 hours,[59] less than 30 ml/hr × 2 hours,[80] less than 0.5 ml/kg/hr × 2 hours,[81] and less than 500 ml/24 hours.[82] The patho-

Table 19.9 Causes of Pulmonary Edema in Preeclampsia

Cardiogenic	Noncardiogenic
Systolic dysfunction	Increased capillary permeability
Diastolic dysfunction	Narrowed COP–wedge gradient
Combined	Decreased COP
	Delayed mobilization of extravascular fluid
	Iatrogenic fluid overload

COP, colloid osmotic pressure.

genesis of oliguria in severe preeclampsia is not well defined, and appropriate management remains unsettled.

Clark et al.[59] studied nine patients with severe preeclampsia and oliguria (<30 ml/hr × 3 hours) using the Swan-Ganz catheter. Eight patients were in labor and one was postpartum. Three hemodynamic subsets were defined. In category 1, five patients had low wedge pressures, normal cardiac indices, and elevated systemic vascular resistances. Their oliguria improved with volume expansion. In category 2, three patients had normal to high wedge pressures and cardiac indices and normal systemic vascular resistances. These patients responded to fluid and/or afterload reduction with hydralazine. They were felt to have renal arterial spasm as the cause of their oliguria. In category 3, a single patient had high wedge pressure, low cardiac index, and high systemic vascular resistance. She responded to hydralazine and volume restriction. Clark et al. advocated placement of a pulmonary artery catheter to guide management of oliguric patients with severe preeclampsia.

Lee et al.[80] compared urinary diagnostic indices to wedge pressure in seven oliguric, preeclamptic patients. Although urine sodium was high in six patients, indicating intrinsic renal disease, most of the other parameters indicated prerenal disease (e.g., urine osmolality, urine/plasma urea nitrogen, urine/plasma creatinine, renal failure index, and fractional excretion of sodium). Swan-Ganz readings showed predominantly normal wedge pressures (mean 8.7 mmHg, range 4 to 14), indicating euvolemia. Lee et al. concluded that oliguria is a poor index of volume status in preeclamptic women and that urinary diagnostic indices may be misleading if used to guide fluid management in these patients.

Kirshon et al.[81] studied the hemodynamic and renal function effects of low-dose dopamine (1 to 5 μg/kg/min) in six antepartum, oliguric patients with severe preeclampsia. Cardiac output increased from 6.8 ± 1.8 to 8.0 ± 2.3 L/min. Blood pressure, central venous pressure, and wedge pressure did not change significantly from baseline. Urine output increased from a mean of 21 ± 10 to 43 ± 23 ml/hr. The fractional excretion of sodium, negative free water clearance, and osmolal clearance increased during dopamine therapy. The best response in urine flow was seen in patients with the highest wedge pressures. No adverse maternal or fetal effects were noted.

Barton et al.[82] randomized 31 patients into nifedipine (10 mg) or placebo groups, treated every 4 hours beginning immediately after delivery and continuing for 48 hours. Nifedipine did not have a marked effect on blood pressure, because the patients were not very hypertensive; however, the investigators observed almost a doubling of urine output (3,934 vs. 2,057 ml) during the first 24 hours after delivery in the nifedipine-treated group. The mechanism of the beneficial effect on urine flow is unknown, but it may have been related to increased renal blood flow or to a natriuretic effect of nifedipine on the proximal convoluted tubule.

One of the first considerations in the oliguric patient is simply to be certain that the Foley catheter is not displaced from the urethra or malfunctioning. It may be helpful to irrigate the catheter with sterile saline and to note whether full return of the irrigant is obtained. Further evaluation of the oliguric patient requires many factors to be considered: antepartum versus postpartum oliguria, history, physical examination, postural changes in blood pressure, blood loss, intake and output, medications, hematocrit, blood urea nitrogen, creatinine, and electrolytes. Urinary diagnostic indices are noninvasive and inexpensive tests, but they must be interpreted with caution in preeclampsia. Prerenal findings suggesting the need for volume expansion include urine sodium less than 20 meq/L, urine osmolality more than 500 mOsm/kg, urine/plasma urea nitrogen more than 8, urine/plasma creatinine more than 40, renal failure index less than 1, and fractional excretion of sodium less than 1.

In treating the oliguric patient, a fluid challenge may be given. For example, 500 ml of normal saline may be administered intravenously over 30 minutes on two occasions. At least 1 hour should be allowed to observe a response in urine output. A trial of furosemide may be given if the patient is thought to be euvolemic or volume overloaded. Dopamine or nifedipine may be tried. Finally, a Swan-Ganz catheter may be placed to categorize the central hemodynamics and to guide therapy.

Cardiac Disease

A more complete discussion of cardiac disease is found elsewhere in this volume (see Ch. 31). However, the role of invasive monitoring in certain cardiac lesions will be considered here. Most New York Heart Association class 3 and 4 patients should have invasive hemodynamic monitoring during labor and delivery. In some patients with complex congenital heart disease, placement of a pulmonary artery catheter is not recommended, because the anatomic defect makes it difficult to determine where the catheter is located.

Mitral Stenosis

In the pregnant patient, mitral stenosis is the principal lesion resulting from rheumatic heart disease. Patients with mitral stenosis may have a reasonable cardiac output, albeit relatively fixed. They cannot increase their cardiac output in response to a greater oxygen demand. Normal pregnancy results in increased blood volume, heart rate, and stroke volume. Thus the pregnant patient with mitral stenosis has a shorter time to get a larger amount of blood across a stenotic valve, resulting in increased left atrial pressure. Because there are no valves in the pulmonary circuit, increased right-sided pressures and eventually right ventricular failure occur. The patient with mitral stenosis is thus closer to being in pulmonary edema when she is pregnant than when she is not pregnant.

Clark et al. used invasive hemodynamic monitoring to study 10 pregnant patients with mitral stenosis. A major finding was that postpartum autotransfusion of blood from the contracting uterus resulted in a 10 ± 6 mmHg increase in wedge pressure. This increase in blood volume was thought to explain the occurrence of pulmonary edema in the early postpartum period in patients with mitral stenosis. Clark et al.[83] suggested the following protocol for management using a pulmonary artery catheter: (1) keep the heart rate less than 90 beats/min with a β-blocker (e.g., propranolol or esmolol) to allow sufficient diastolic filling time; (2) maintain wedge pressure during labor at 12 to 14 mmHg with furosemide or fluid restriction in anticipation of a postpartum increase in wedge pressure of 10 mmHg; and (3) use epidural anesthesia to relieve pain and anxiety, thus reducing oxygen demand.

Hypertrophic Obstructive Cardiomyopathy

Resulting from asymmetric hypertrophy of the interventricular septum, hypertrophic obstructive cardiomyopathy may be of varying severity. These patients have four cardiac problems: (1) diastolic dysfunction, (2) sudden death caused by ventricular arrhythmias, (3) obstruction to left ventricular outflow produced by systolic anterior motion of the mitral valve, and (4) mitral regurgitation. During labor, patients should be kept "wet" and "slow." Sufficient fluid should be given so that there is no obstruction to left ventricular outflow, and heart rate should be controlled with a β-blocker if necessary to allow sufficient diastolic filling time.[84]

Eisenmenger Syndrome

Eisenmenger syndrome usually results from an unrecognized ventricular septal defect or from a patent ductus arteriosus. Because of their long-standing left-to-right shunt, these patients develop medial hypertrophy of the pulmonary vasculature and pulmonary hypertension. After many years, pulmonary artery pressures equal or exceed systemic pressures; thus shunt reversal occurs. Ideally, these women should not undertake a pregnancy, because the maternal mortality rate is 25 to 50 percent.[85] During pregnancy, systemic vascular resistance falls because of the vasodilatory effects of estrogen, progesterone, prolactin, prostaglandins, and the arteriovenous shunt in the placenta. Pulmonary vascular resistance remains high and fixed. As pregnancy progresses, these patients will shunt more and more blood right-to-left, thus bypassing their lungs. In labor, they require adequate preload and must be well hydrated before epidural anesthesia is given.[86] A Swan-Ganz catheter is useful to guide management during labor and delivery; however, it is technically difficult to insert a pulmonary artery catheter in patients with severe pulmonary hypertension and to maintain it in position, because it often migrates back into the right ventricle. A distressing feature of Eisenmenger syndrome is sudden death approximately 5 days postpartum. The cause is unknown, but is possibly related to pulmonary embolism or to arrhythmia. Hypoxia creates a vicious cycle of pulmonary vasoconstriction resulting in increased right-to-left shunting, which in turn results in more hypoxia.

Dilated Cardiomyopathy

Patients with poor systolic function are at risk for congestive heart failure in the peripartum period. These patients are usually diagnosed by history, physical examination, chest x-ray, and echocardiography. Invasive hemodynamic monitoring guides fluid management, inotropic therapy, and afterload reduction and prepares patients for the vicissitudes of labor (e.g., hemorrhage, epidural hypotension, or cesarean section). Other problems include thromboemboli and both atrial and ventricular arrhythmias.[87]

Tocolytic-Induced Pulmonary Edema

Some patients given tocolytics for preterm labor develop pulmonary edema. Early reports suggested the incidence to be as high as 5 percent.[88] With widespread knowledge of this complication, the incidence is now less than 1 percent. Pulmonary edema has occurred with ritodrine, terbutaline, isoxsuprine, and other β-agonists, as well as with magnesium sulfate. It has occurred both antepartum and postpartum. The mechanism of tocolytic-induced pulmonary edema is unknown. One of the problems in evaluating the cause is that patients often have a complex clinical course with many interrelating occurrences such as multiple drug administration, blood loss, blood transfusion, anesthesia, vaginal delivery, or cesarean section.[89] Perhaps the best explanation for pulmonary edema in this setting is that β-mimetics increase antidiuretic hormone release.[90] Urine output falls, and the hematocrit is diluted down.[91] Indeed, in many of the early cases abruptio placenta or occult bleeding was suspected when, during the evaluation of dyspnea, these patients were found to have had a 5 to 10 point fall in hematocrit. Iatrogenic fluid overload may also have contributed. Nevertheless, invasive he-

modynamic monitoring has usually revealed normal wedge pressure, suggesting noncardiogenic pulmonary edema. A significant percentage of patients with tocolytic-induced pulmonary edema do not have a fall in hematocrit. Corticosteroids given to accelerate fetal lung maturity have been blamed, but the mineralocorticoid effect is probably minimal, thus playing no significant role in the development of pulmonary edema. Other proposed mechanisms include myocardial ischemia, endotoxin released from occult chorioamnionitis, high-output cardiac failure, idiosyncratic drug reaction, unrecognized heart disease, reduced intravascular COP, and hypokalemia. Pulmonary edema rarely occurs before 24 hours of parenteral therapy and is rare with oral therapy. Predisposing factors include multiple gestation, anemia, low maternal weight, and aggressive fluid-loading. A strategy for prevention includes

1. Attention to contraindications to tocolytic therapy
2. Careful intake and output, with total fluid administration limited to 2,500 ml/day
3. Recognition of predisposing factors
4. Limitation of parenteral therapy to 24 hours

Patients with tocolytic-induced pulmonary edema usually respond to discontinuation of the drug and administration of oxygen, morphine, and furosemide. Acute respiratory failure requiring mechanical ventilation may still be seen, however. The duration of pulmonary edema is quite variable, ranging from a few hours to 3 to 4 days.[89]

Septic Shock

Clinical criteria for the diagnosis of septic shock include hypotension, temperature disturbance (either high or low), and an identifiable source of infection. With the decline in criminal abortions, septic shock is now rare in obstetrics. The condition is still seen in patients with pyelonephritis, urinary tract instrumentation, chorioamnionitis, ruptured appendix, necrotizing fasciitis, toxic shock syndrome, and sepsis from venous or arterial lines. The predominate organisms are gram negative, although gram-positive organisms and fungi may also cause septic shock. At least one-third of patients with a clinical diagnosis of septic shock have negative blood cultures. Predisposing factors include pregnancy, diabetes mellitus, cirrhosis, leukemia, carcinoma, cancer chemotherapy, steroid therapy, and other immunosuppressive therapy.[92]

Pathophysiologic mechanisms involve bacterial products (endotoxin) reacting with cell membranes and activating the coagulation and complement systems. Prostaglandins, thromboxanes, platelet-activating factor, bradykinin, myocardial depressant factor, and cachectin or tumor necrosis factor are generated. Catecholamines, glucocorticoids, histamine, serotonin, and central nervous system opioids are also released. Cell death is the result of direct or indirect effects of these substances and tissue anoxia. The latter is partially due to maldistribution of tissue blood flow and reduction of effective blood volume.

Complications of septic shock include coagulation defects, adult respiratory distress syndrome (ARDS), renal failure, cardiac failure, liver dysfunction, gastrointestinal injury, reticuloendothelial suppression, and cerebral dysfunction.

The most important aspect of management is to control the primary cause. Surgery should not be postponed to stabilize the patient. Her condition will only deteriorate until the septic focus is removed or drained. Intravascular volume should be optimized. The superiority of colloid over crystalloid therapy has not been established, and cost concerns favor the latter. Cultures should be obtained and antibiotics started. β-Adrenergic agonists such as dopamine, dobutamine, and isoproterenol may be needed if hypotension does not respond to fluids. Corticosteroids are no longer recommended in septic shock.[93,94] Naloxone, lidocaine, indomethacin, and prostaglandins have improved survival in animal models of endotoxin shock; however, studies in humans either have not been performed or are inadequately designed to allow accurate interpretation.[92]

Adult Respiratory Distress Syndrome

ARDS is characterized by diffuse infiltrates, marked intrapulmonary shunting, and decreased lung compliance. Neonatal respiratory distress syndrome is caused by surfactant deficiency and a compliant chest wall. By contrast, in ARDS surfactant deficiency is a secondary change, with the chest wall not compliant. The main problem in ARDS is noncardiogenic pulmonary edema resulting from increased permeability of the alveolar–capillary membrane. Stimulated polymorphonuclear (PMN) leukocytes appear to be major offenders, adhering to endothelial surfaces and releasing toxic oxygen species and mediators of inflammation (e.g., leukotrienes, thromboxanes, and prostaglandins). The initial capillary leak produces interstitial edema followed by alveolar edema, atelectasis, interstitial inflammation, and pulmonary fibrosis. Other intermediary agents in addition to PMN leukocytes must be involved in the pathogenesis of ARDS, because granulocytopenic patients with acute leukemia also develop the syndrome.

The lung can respond in only a limited number of ways to injury. Therefore, the causes of ARDS are many: bacterial, viral, fungal, and pneumocystis infections; aspiration; inhalation of toxins or irritants; drug overdose; head trauma; pancreatitis; fat embolism; amniotic fluid embolism; sepsis; systemic lupus erythematosus; Goodpasture syndrome; and cardiopulmonary bypass. The main causes of ARDS in the obstetric population are gram-negative sepsis, particularly with pyelonephritis; varicella or influenza pneumonia; aspiration pneumonia; and amniotic fluid embolism.

Management of ARDS involves treating the underlying cause, maintaining oxygenation with mechanical ventilation and positive end-expiratory pressure, normalizing acid–base derangements, and limiting the accumulation of extravascular lung water. Positive end-expiratory pressure reduces shunting and improves matching of ventilation and perfusion, which allows the use of lower inhaled oxygen fractions. Noncardiogenic pulmonary edema is treated with loop diuretics and fluid restriction to maintain the wedge pressure as low as is compatible with satisfactory oxygen delivery and urine output. Death is most commonly caused by sepsis and multiple organ failure rather than by ARDS itself.[95] In survivors with previously normal lung function, the long-term prognosis is remarkably good. Pulmonary function tests and arterial blood gases return to normal 4 to 6 months after respiratory failure. In some patients, severe fibrotic residua make complete resolution unlikely.[96]

Diabetic Ketoacidosis

Diabetic ketoacidosis (DKA) is due to a relative or absolute insulin deficiency and to an excess of insulin counterregulatory hormones. Although the type I insulin-dependent diabetic is more likely to develop

DKA, type II noninsulin-dependent diabetics may also develop DKA with sufficient provocation. Investigation of the cause reveals medical illness, usually infection, in 50 percent of the patients. The omission of insulin accounts for an additional 20 percent, and in 30 percent of cases no precipitating cause can be identified.

Symptoms include polyuria, polydipsia, vomiting, vague abdominal pain, hyperventilation, stupor, and coma. Laboratory diagnosis is based on hyperglycemia, ketonemia, and a serum pH less than 7.35. In practice, a urinalysis showing $4+$ glucose and large ketones is all that is required for the diagnosis of DKA. Other laboratory features may include an anion gap [$Na - (Cl + HCO_3) > 12$ meq/L], hyponatremia, hyperkalemia, elevated serum urea nitrogen and creatinine, and elevated serum amylase unrelated to pancreatitis.

Some aspects of DKA are different in pregnancy. Patients may have significant DKA with only a modest degree of hyperglycemia. An example of this would be a patient with pH 7.01, Pco_2-7 mmHg, Po_2-132 mmHg, and blood sugar 180 mg/dl. The cause of DKA with modest hyperglycemia is not well understood, but may result from the fetus constantly removing glucose, from the expanded blood volume of pregnancy, or from rapid clearance of glucose in the urine because of increased glomerular filtration rate. In some cases, glucose administration will be required as substrate for the insulin needed to clear ketonemia. Sodium bicarbonate therapy is normally withheld in the nonpregnant patient until the pH is less than 7.10 or 7.00 because of concern about rapid alkalinization shifting the oxyhemoglobin dissociation curve to the left and metabolic alkalosis occurring as ketones are metabolized to bicarbonate. In pregnancy, bicarbonate should be given for a pH less than 7.20 because of the risk of intrauterine fetal demise. Decreased fetal heart rate variability and late decelerations may occur during DKA. This will usually resolve with correction of the maternal metabolic disturbance. Cesarean section for fetal distress will usually not be required. β-Mimetic drugs and steroids given for preterm labor may worsen glucose control in the diabetic. Magnesium sulfate or nifedipine may be a better tocolytic agent in the diabetic. Treatment of DKA is otherwise the same as for nonpregnant adults.

During the history and physical examination, special attention should be paid to patency of the airway; mental status; cardiovascular, pulmonary, and renal status; source of infection; and state of hydration. Immediate biochemical evaluation should include blood and urine glucose and ketones by Chemstrip and Ketostix, respectively. Plasma glucose, blood gases and pH, electrolytes, blood urea nitrogen, chest x-ray, ECG, and cultures may be obtained. One liter of normal saline may be given in the first hour, followed by 0.5 N saline at a rate depending on the state of hydration. Usually 3 to 5 L of crystalloid will be needed in the first 24 hours. Seven units of regular insulin may be given intravenously and 7 units intramuscularly, followed by a constant infusion of 7 to 10 units per hour. Plasma glucose should be determined hourly and electrolytes and blood gases every 4 hours as needed. All laboratory data, intake and output, and medications should be recorded in an organized fashion. If glucose does not fall 10 percent in the first hour, the rate of insulin infusion may be doubled. The biologic effect of insulin is only 10 to 20 percent of normal during DKA. When plasma glucose reaches 250 mg/dl, 5 percent dextrose in water should be added to the regimen. Intravenous glucose and insulin are continued until the urine is cleared of ketones. Unless the serum potassium is more than 5.5 meq/L or if renal insufficiency is present, potassium replacement (20 to 40 meq/L) should begin with the initial insulin therapy. Sodium bicarbonate (44 or 88 meq in 1 L of 0.5 N saline) may be given until the arterial pH is more than 7.20. Phosphate supplementation is unnecessary. As soon as the patient can eat, she may be restarted on subcutaneous NPH insulin twice daily, with regular insulin before each meal based on a sliding scale. Making the transition from intravenous to subcutaneous insulin is often the trickiest part of managing DKA.[97]

Thyroid Storm

The diagnosis of thyroid storm is based on three clinical criteria: (1) exaggerated manifestations of hyperthyroidism, (2) rectal temperature greater than 101 degrees F, and (3) central nervous system changes. Alterations in mental state vary from confusion to psychosis to coma. Other common findings include tachycardia out of proportion to fever, arrhythmias, cardiac failure, diarrhea, abdominal pain, vomiting, jaundice, and dehydration.[98]

Interestingly, serum thyroxine (T4) and triiodothyronine (T3) levels may be no higher during thyroid storm than they were weeks earlier. Thyroid storm seems to involve loss of refractoriness to the effects of thyroid hormone. There have been reports of thyroid storm with normal serum T3 levels, presumably illness interfering with normal peripheral conversion of T4 to T3.[99] Thyrotoxic crisis associated with pregnancy usually occurs in the early postpartum period. Other precipitating causes include infection, trauma, surgery, myocardial infarction, diabetic ketoacidosis, and cessation of antithyroid drugs.

Treatment of thyroid storm involves the following general measures: (1) replace fluids, glucose, and electrolytes; (2) lower temperature with acetaminophen or a cooling blanket; (3) treat precipitating factors (e.g., infection or trauma); and (4) treat cardiac failure with oxygen and diuretics. Treatment of cardiac failure may involve β-blocker therapy, in which case invasive monitoring may be indicated to balance the reduction in heart rate against the negative inotropic effect. Heart failure because of thyrotoxicosis in pregnancy is normally seen in patients with longstanding hyperthyroidism and poor control. Left ventricular ejection fraction is increased at rest in the hyperthyroid state, but there is a significant decrease in ejection fraction during exercise. This cardiomyopathy is reversible with treatment of the underlying thyrotoxicosis.

Specific measures for treating thyroid storm include antithyroid drugs, glucocorticoids, iodides, and propranolol. Propylthiouracil 600 to 1,000 mg administered orally or via nasogastric tube followed by 300 to 600 mg/day prevents further hormone production and blocks peripheral conversion of T4 to T3. Methimazole 60 to 100 mg orally followed by 30 to 60 mg daily may be substituted for propylthiouracil, although the former has caused scalp defects in the fetus and does not block peripheral conversion of T4 to T3. Iodides given at least 1 hour after the initial dose of propylthiouracil block thyroid hormone release. The 1-hour delay is to allow propylthiouracil to block hormone synthesis and to avoid buildup of thyroid hormone stores in the gland. Iodides may be given as Lugol's solution 30 drops orally daily in divided doses, sodium iodide 500 mg intravenously every 8 to 12 hours, or as radiographic contrast drugs

ipodate or iopanoic acid 1 g orally daily. Hydrocortisone 300 mg intravenously in divided doses daily or equivalent amounts of oral prednisone or dexamethasone may be administered to cover the patient for relative adrenal insufficiency and to inhibit peripheral conversion of T4 to T3. Propranolol decreases the peripheral effects of thyroid hormone and also blocks the peripheral conversion of T4 to T3. It may be given orally 40 to 80 mg every 4 to 6 hours or intravenously 1 mg every 10 minutes up to five doses.

After initial clinical improvement, iodides and glucocorticoids may be discontinued, and antithyroid drugs can be continued until the patient becomes euthyroid. Ablative therapy with radioactive iodine or surgery is indicated in nearly all patients after an episode of thyroid storm. In pregnancy, ablative therapy should be postponed until after delivery.[100]

REFERENCES

1. Mabie WC, Sibai BM: Treatment in an obstetric intensive care unit. Am J Obstet Gynecol 162:1, 1990
2. Benedetti TJ, Cotton DB, Read JC, Miller FC: Hemodynamic observations in severe preeclampsia with a flow-directed pulmonary artery catheter. Am J Obstet Gynecol 136:467, 1980
3. Cotton DB, Gonik B, Dorman KF, Harrist R: Cardiovascular alterations in severe pregnancy-induced hypertension: relationship of central venous pressure to pulmonary capillary wedge pressure. Am J Obstet Gynecol 151:962, 1985
4. Robin ED: The cult of the Swan-Ganz catheter. Ann Intern Med 103:445, 1985
5. Swan HJ, Ganz W, Forrester J et al: Catheterization of the heart in man with the use of a flow-directed balloon-tipped catheter. N Engl J Med 283:447, 1970
6. Mathay MA, Chatterjee K: Bedside catheterization of the pulmonary artery: risks compared with benefits. Ann Intern Med 109:826, 1988
7. Forrester JC, Diamond G, Swan HJ: Correlative classification of clinical and hemodynamic function after acute myocardial infarction. Am J Cardiol 39:137, 1977
8. Bayliss J, Norell M, Ryan A et al: Bedside hemodynamic monitoring: experience in a general hospital. Br Med J (Clin Res) 287:187, 1983
9. Connors AF Jr, McCaffree DR, Gray BA: Evaluation of right heart catheterization in the critically ill patient without acute myocardial infarction. N Engl J Med 308:263, 1983
10. Eisenberg PR, Jaffe AS, Schuster DP: Clinical evalua-

tion compared to pulmonary artery catheterization in the hemodynamic assessment of critically ill patients. Crit Care Med 12:549, 1984

11. Fein AM, Goldberg SK, Wahlenstein MD et al: Is pulmonary artery catheterization necessary for the diagnosis of pulmonary edema? Am Rev Respir Dis 129:1006, 1984

12. Gore JM, Goldberg RJ, Spodick DH et al: A community-wide assessment of the use of pulmonary artery catheters in patients with acute myocardial infarction. Chest 92:721, 1987

13. Shoemaker WC, Appel PL, Bland R et al: Clinical trial of an algorithm prediction in acute circulatory failure. Crit Care Med 10:390, 1982

14. Daily EK, Schroeder JS: Techniques in Bedside Hemodynamic Monitoring. CV Mosby, St. Louis, 1989

15. Sprung CL, Rackow EC, Civetta JM: Direct measurements and derived calculations using the pulmonary artery catheter. p. 105. In Sprung CL (ed): The Pulmonary Artery Catheter. University Park Press, Baltimore, 1983

16. Snyder JV: Oxygen transport: the model and reality. p. 3. In Snyder JV, Pinsky MR (eds): Oxygen Transport in the Critically Ill. Year Book Medical Publishers, Chicago, 1987

17. Rosenthal MH: Intrapartum intensive care management of the cardiac patient. Clin Obstet Gynecol 24:789, 1981

18. Marini JJ, Wheeler AP: Critical Care Medicine—The Essentials. Williams & Wilkins, Baltimore, 1989

19. Clark SL, Cotton DB: Clinical indications for pulmonary artery catheterization in the patient with severe preeclampsia. Am J Obstet Gynecol 158:453, 1988

20. Wallenburg HCS: Hemodynamics in hypertensive pregnancy. p. 73. In Rubin PC (ed): Hypertension in Pregnancy. 1st Ed. Elsevier Publishers, Amsterdam, 1988

21. Hamilton HFH: The cardiac output in normal pregnancy as determined by the Cournand right heart catheterization technique. J Obstet Gynaecol Br Emp 56:548, 1949

22. Werko L: Pregnancy and heart disease. Acta Obstet Gynecol Scand 33:162, 1954

23. Bader RA, Bader ME, Rose DJ, Braunwald E: Hemodynamics of rest and exercise in normal pregnancy as studied by cardiac catheterization. J Clin Invest 34:1524, 1955

24. Kerr MG: Cardiovascular dynamics in pregnancy and labor. Br Med Bull 24:19, 1968

25. Walters WAW, MacGregor WG, Hills M: Cardiac output at rest during pregnancy and the puerperium. Clin Sci 30:1, 1966

26. Ueland K, Akamatsu TJ, Eng M et al: Maternal cardio-

vascular dynamics VI. Cesarean section under epidural anesthesia without epinephrine. Am J Obstet Gynecol 114:775, 1972

27. Lim YL, Walters WAW: Hemodynamics of mild hypertension in pregnancy. Br J Obstet Gynaecol 86:198, 1979

28. Lees MM: Central circulatory responses in normotensive and hypertensive pregnancy. Postgrad Med J 55:311, 1979

29. Groenendijk R, Trimbos JBMJ, Wallenburg HCS: Hemodynamic measurements in preeclampsia: preliminary observations. Am J Obstet Gynecol 150:232, 1984

30. Clark SL, Cotton DB, Lee W et al: Central hemodynamic assessment of normal term pregnancy. Am J Obstet Gynecol 161:1439, 1989

31. Smith RW: Cardiovascular alterations in toxemia. Am J Obstet Gynecol 107:979, 1970

32. Easterling TR, Watts DH, Schmucker BC, Benedetti TJ: Measurement of cardiac output during pregnancy: validation of Doppler technique and clinical observations in preeclampsia. Obstet Gynecol 69:845, 1987

33. Katz R, Karliner JS, Resnik R: Effect of a natural volume overload state (pregnancy) on left ventricular performance in normal human subjects. Circulation 58:434, 1978

34. Lee W, Rokey R, Cotton DB: Noninvasive maternal stroke volume and cardiac output determinations by pulsed Doppler echocardiography. Am J Obstet Gynecol 158:505, 1988

35. Mashini IS, Albazzaz SJ, Fadel HE et al: Serial noninvasive evaluation of cardiovascular hemodynamics during pregnancy. Am J Obstet Gynecol 156:1208, 1987

36. Robson SC, Hunter S, Moore M, Dunlop W: Hemodynamic changes during the puerperium: a Doppler and M-mode echocardiographic study. Br J Obstet Gynaecol 94:1028, 1987

37. Rubler S, Damani P, Pinto ER: Cardiac size and performance during pregnancy estimated by echocardiography. Am J Cardiol 40:534, 1977

38. Masaki DI, Greenspoon JS, Ouzounian JG: Measurement of cardiac output in pregnancy by thoracic electrical bioimpedance and thermodilution. Am J Obstet Gynecol 161:680, 1989

39. Milsom I, Forssman L, Sivertsson R, Dottori O: Measurement of cardiac stroke volume by impedance cardiography in the last trimester of pregnancy. Acta Obstet Gynecol Scand 62:473, 1983

40. Easterling TR, Benedetti TJ, Carlson KL, Watts DH: Measurement of cardiac output in pregnancy by thermodilution and impedance techniques. Br J Obstet Gynaecol 96:67, 1989

41. Elkayam U, Gleicher N: Hemodynamics and cardiac function during normal pregnancy and the puerperium. p. 5. In Elkayam N, Gleicher N (eds): Cardiac Problems in Pregnancy. 2nd Ed. Alan R. Liss, New York, 1990

42. Hankins GDV, Cunningham FG, Pritchard JA: Cardiopulmonary consequences of hypertension during pregnancy and puerperium. Suppl 8, p. 1. In Pritchard JA, MacDonald PC, Gant NF (eds): Williams Obstetrics. 17th Ed. Appleton-Century-Crofts Publishers, East Norwalk, CT, 1986

43. Cotton DB, Gonik B, Dorman K: Cardiovascular alterations in severe pregnancy-induced hypertension: acute effects of magnesium sulfate. Am J Obstet Gynecol 148:162, 1984

44. Nisell H, Lunell NO, Linde B: Maternal hemodynamics and impaired fetal growth in pregnancy-induced hypertension. Obstet Gynecol 71:163, 1988

45. Belfort MA, Uys P, Dommisse J, Davey DA: Hemodynamic changes in gestational proteinuric hypertension: the effects of rapid volume expansion and vasodilator therapy. Br J Obstet Gynaecol 96:634, 1989

46. Belfort MA, Anthony J, Buccimazza A, Davey DA: Hemodynamic changes associated with intravenous infusion of the calcium antagonist verapamil in the treatment of severe gestational proteinuric hypertension. Obstet Gynecol 75:970, 1990

47. Benedetti TJ, Cotton DB, Read JC, Miller FC: Hemodynamic observations in severe preeclampsia with a flow-directed pulmonary artery catheter. Am J Obstet Gynecol 136:465, 1980

48. Hankins GDV, Wendel GD, Cunningham FG, Leveno KJ: Longitudinal evaluation of hemodynamic changes in eclampsia. Am J Obstet Gynecol 150:506, 1984

49. Cotton DB, Lee W, Huhta JC, Dorman KF: Hemodynamic profile of severe pregnancy-induced hypertension. Am J Obstet Gynecol 158:523, 1988

50. Mabie WC, Ratts TE, Sibai BM: The central hemodynamics of severe preeclampsia. Am J Obstet Gynecol 161:1443, 1989

51. Wasserstrum N, Kirshon B, Willis R et al: Quantitative hemodynamic effects of acute volume expansion in severe preeclampsia. Obstet Gynecol 73:546, 1989

52. Wasserstrum N, Kirshon B, Rossavik IK et al: Implications of sino-aortic baroreceptor reflex dysfunction in severe preeclampsia. Obstet Gynecol 74:34, 1989

53. Rafferty TD, Berkowitz RL: Hemodynamics in patients with severe toxemia during labor and delivery. Am J Obstet Gynecol 138:263, 1980

54. Phelan JP, Yurth DA: Severe preeclampsia. 1. Peripartum hemodynamic observations. Am J Obstet Gynecol 144;17, 1982

55. Rolbin SH, Cole AFD, Hew EM: Hemodynamic monitoring in the management of severe preeclampsia and eclampsia. Can Anesth Soc J 28:363, 1981

56. Graham C, Goldstein A: Epidural anesthesia and cardiac output in severe preeclamptics. Anaesthesia 35:709, 1980

57. Newsome LR, Bramwell RS, Curling PE: Severe preeclampsia: hemodynamic effects of epidural anesthesia. Anesth Analg 65:31, 1986

58. Cotton DB, Longmire S, Jones MM et al: Cardiovascular alterations in severe pregnancy-induced hypertension: effects of intravenous nitroglycerin coupled with blood volume expansion. Am J Obstet Gynecol 154:1053, 1986

59. Clark SL, Greenspoon JS, Adahl D, Phelan JP: Severe preeclampsia with persistent oliguria: management of hemodynamic subsets. Am J Obstet Gynecol 154:490, 1986

60. Chesley LC: Hypertensive Disorders in Pregnancy. 1st Ed. p. 203. Appleton-Century-Crofts, East Norwalk, CT, 1978

61. Hays PM, Cruikshank DP, Dunn LJ: Plasma volume determination in normal and preeclamptic pregnancies. Am J Obstet Gynecol 151:958, 1985

62. Cohn JD: Paroxysmal hypertension and hypovolemia. N Engl J Med 275:643, 1966

63. Goodlin RC, Cotton DB, Haesslein H: Severe edema-proteinuria-hypertension gestosis. Am J Obstet Gynecol 132:595, 1978

64. Gallery EDM, Delprado W, Gyory AZ: Antihypertensive effect of plasma volume expansion in pregnancy-associated hypertension. Aust NZ J Med 11:20, 1981

65. Sehgal NN, Hitt JR: Plasma volume expansion in the treatment of preeclampsia. Am J Obstet Gynecol 138:165, 1980

66. Wasserstrum N, Cotton DB: Hemodynamic monitoring in severe pregnancy-induced hypertension. Clin Perinatol 13:781, 1986

67. Kirshon B, Moise KJ, Cotton DB et al: Role of volume expansion in severe preeclampsia. Surg Gynecol Obstet 167:367, 1988

68. Benedetti TJ, Kates R, Williams V: Hemodynamic observations in severe preeclampsia complicated by pulmonary edema. Am J Obstet Gynecol 152:330, 1985

69. Ferguson RK, Vlasses PA: Hypertensive emergencies and urgencies. JAMA 255:1607, 1986

70. Duncan SLB: Does volume expansion in preeclampsia help or hinder? Br J Obstet Gynaecol 96:631, 1989

71. Harizi RC, Bianco JA, Alpert JS: Diastolic function of the heart in clinical cardiology. Arch Intern Med 148:99, 1988

72. Mabie WC, Ratts TE, Ramanathan KB, Sibai BM: Cir-

culatory congestion in obese hypertensive women: a subset of pulmonary edema in pregnancy. Obstet Gynecol 72:553, 1988

73. Ingram R, Braunwald E: Pulmonary edema: cardiogenic and noncardiogenic. p. 544. In Braunwald E (ed): Heart Disease. 3rd Ed. WB Saunders, Philadelphia, 1988

74. Moise KJ, Cotton DB: The use of colloid osmotic pressure in pregnancy. Clin Perinatol 13:827, 1986

75. Rackow EC, Fein IA, Leppo J: Colloid osmotic pressure as a prognostic indication of pulmonary edema and mortality in the critically ill. Chest 72:709, 1977

76. Gonik B, Cotton DB, Spillman T et al: Peripartum colloid osmotic pressure changes: effects of controlled fluid management. Am J Obstet Gynecol 151:812, 1985

77. Cotton DB, Gonik B, Spillman T, Dorman KF: Intrapartum to postpartum changes in colloid osmotic pressure. Am J Obstet Gynecol 149:174, 1984

78. Benedetti TJ, Carlson RW: Studies of colloid osmotic pressure in pregnancy-induced hypertension. Am J Obstet Gynecol 135:308, 1979

79. Sibai BM, Mabie BC, Harvey CJ, Gonzalez AP: Pulmonary edema in severe preeclampsia-eclampsia: analysis of thirty-seven consecutive cases. Am J Obstet Gynecol 156:1174, 1987

80. Lee W, Gonik B, Cotton DB: Urinary diagnostic indices in preeclampsia-associated oliguria: correlation with invasive hemodynamic monitoring. Am J Obstet Gynecol 156:100, 1987

81. Kirshon B, Lee W, Mauer MB, Cotton DB: Effects of low-dose dopamine therapy in the oliguric patient with preeclampsia. Am J Obstet Gynecol 159:604, 1988

82. Barton JR, Hiett AK, Conover WB: The use of nifedipine during the postpartum period in patients with severe preeclampsia. Am J Obstet Gynecol 162:788, 1990

83. Clark SL, Phelan JP, Greenspoon J et al: Labor and delivery in the presence of mitral stenosis: central hemodynamic observations. Am J Obstet Gynecol 152:984, 1985

84. Oakley GDG, McGarry K, Limb DG et al: Management of pregnancy in patients with hypertrophic cardiomyopathy. Br Med J 1:1749, 1979

85. Gleicher D, Midwall J, Hockberger D et al: Eisenmenger's syndrome in pregnancy. Obstet Gynecol Surv 34:721, 1979

86. Spinnato JA, Kraynack BJ, Cooper MW: Eisenmenger's syndrome in pregnancy: epidural anesthesia for elective cesarean section. N Engl J Med 304:1215, 1981

87. O'Connell JB, Costanzo-Nordin MR, Subramanian R et al: Peripartum cardiomyopathy: clinical, hemodynamic, histologic, and prognostic characteristics. J Am Coll Cardiol 8:52, 1986

88. Katz M, Robertson PA, Creasy RK: Cardiovascular complications associated with terbutaline treatment for preterm labor. Am J Obstet Gynecol 139:605, 1981

89. Mabie WC, Pernoll ML, Witty JB et al: Pulmonary edema induced by betamimetic drugs. S Med J 76:1354, 1983

90. Schrier RW, Lieberman R, Ufferman RC et al: Mechanism of antidiuretic effect of beta adrenergic stimulation. J Clin Invest 51:97, 1972

91. Kleinman G, Nuwayhid B, Rudelstorfer R et al: Circulatory and renal effects of β-adrenergic receptor stimulation in pregnant sheep. Am J Obstet Gynecol 149:865, 1984

92. Root RK, Jacobs R: Septicemia and septic shock. p. 502. In Wilson JD, Braunwald E, Isselbacher KJ et al (eds): Harrison's Principles of Internal Medicine. 12th Ed. McGraw-Hill, New York, 1991

93. Bone RC, Fisher CJ Jr, Clemmer TP et al: A controlled clinical trial of high-dose methylprednisolone in the treatment of severe sepsis and septic shock. N Engl J Med 317:653, 1987

94. Hinshaw L, Peduzzi P, Young E et al: Effects of high-dose glucocorticoid therapy in patients with clinical signs of systemic sepsis: the Veterans Administration Systemic Sepsis Cooperative Study Group. N Engl J Med 317:659, 1987

95. Raffin TA: ARDS: mechanisms and management. Hosp Pract 22(11):65, 1987

96. Montgomery AB, Stager MA, Carrico CJ et al: Causes of mortality in patients with the adult respiratory distress syndrome 132:485, 1985

97. Kitabchi AE: Low-dose insulin therapy in diabetic ketoacidosis: fact or fiction? Diabetes Metab Rev 5:337, 1989

98. Singer PA, Mestman JH: Thyroid storm need not be lethal. Contemp OB/GYN 22:135, 1983

99. Ahmad N, Cohen MP: Thyroid storm with normal serum triiodothyronine level during diabetic ketoacidosis. JAMA 245:2516, 1981

100. Mestman JH: Severe hyperthyroidism in pregnancy. p. 262. In Clark SL, Phelan JB, Cotton DB (eds): Critical Care Obstetrics. Medical Economics Books, Oradell, NJ, 1987

101. Daily EK, Schroeder JP: Hemodynamic Waveforms: Exercises in Identification and Analysis. CV Mosby, St. Louis, 1983

Chapter 20

Cesarean Delivery and Other Surgical Procedures*

Richard Depp

INTRODUCTION

Cesarean birth has become the most common hospital-based operative procedure in the United States, accounting for more than 25 percent of all live births.[1] The increase has been attributed to the liberalization of indications for "fetal distress" and breech presentations, as well as elective repeat cesarean sections.[2] In many medical centers the overall rate would be significantly higher if there had not been a change in attitude facilitating acceptance of vaginal birth after cesarean section.[3]

Despite its dramatic impact on society, little attention has been focused on the cumulative consequences of this major surgical procedure with its implications not only for the current pregnancy but also for future reproduction. We know that the cesarean delivery–associated maternal mortality rate is approximately 20 per 100,000 births in the United States.[4] Taken as an isolated end point, it is obviously an infrequent complication. However, there are no reliable data regarding the cumulative long-term morbidity associated with cesarean birth. Cesarean delivery has many possible untoward consequences: an

---

* Both author and editors recognize the tautology of the term cesarean section. Both words connote incision. Therefore, cesarean birth or cesarean delivery would be preferable. However, almost universal usage of the term cesarean section dictates that confusion might ensue if other designations were substituted in this text.

increased risk for postpartum infectious morbidity, despite antibiotic prophylaxis; an increased risk of significant blood loss and need for transfusion with the associated problems of blood and blood product replacement; and an increased risk of anesthetic accidents. Surgical techniques and procedural complications are discussed in this chapter; indications for cesarean section are also presented, and the controversies surrounding a trial of labor and vaginal birth after cesarean section (VBAC) are discussed.

In this chapter, "cesarean section" or "cesarean delivery" is used to describe the delivery of a fetus through a surgical incision of the anterior uterine wall. This definition does not include nonsurgical expulsion of the embryo/fetus from the uterine cavity or tubes following uterine rupture or ectopic pregnancy.

HISTORY OF CESAREAN SECTION

The origin of the term "cesarean section" is likely the product of two separate reports in 1581 and 1598, the former making reference to "Cesarean" and the second to "Sections." However, the origin of the term "cesarean" is somewhat more uncertain. The hypothesis that Julius Caesar was the product of a cesarean birth is unlikely to be true in view of the probability of fatality associated with the procedure in ancient times and the observation that his mother corresponded with him during his campaigns in Europe many years later. The term may have as its origin the Latin verb *cadere,* to cut; the children of such births were referred to as *caesones.* It is also possible that the term stems from the Roman law known as *Lex Regis,* which mandated postmortem operative delivery so that the mother and child could be buried separately; the specific law is referred to historically as *Lex Cesare.*[5]

Although cesarean delivery with the expectation of possible survival of the mother and fetus was proposed in the late 1700s and was first performed in the early 1800s, the procedure was not popularized until the late 1920s. The fear of infection was pervasive in early times. As a consequence, early physicians employed a number of techniques to modify that risk. Eduardo Porro performed the first successful cesarean hysterectomy on a living woman in 1876.[6] The Porro procedure combined subtotal cesarean hysterectomy with marsupialization of the cervical stump.[7] Shortly thereafter, Max Sänger in Leipzig published his work explaining the principles and technique of cesarean section, including aseptic preparation, with special emphasis on a two-step uterine closure using silver wire and silk and careful attention to hemostasis.[8,9] Sänger felt that the employment of this approach would obviate the growing tendency for cesarean hysterectomy because of fear of hemorrhage and infection. It is interesting to note that Sänger attributed much of the early development of suture material to American frontier surgeons, including Frank Polin of Springfield, Kentucky, who in 1852 had reported the use of silver wire sutures in surviving patients who had undergone cesarean delivery.[10] The introduction of suture material, which enabled the surgeon to control bleeding, was of monumental importance in the evolution of the procedure. Nevertheless, death from peritonitis remained a major threat.

Approximately 30 years later, extraperitoneal cesarean delivery was first described by Frank[11] (1907) and subsequently modified by Latzko[12] (1909) and Waters (1940). Subsequently, Krönig (1912) realized that extraperitoneal cesarean birth not only minimized the effects of peritonitis but also allowed access to the lower uterine segment through a vertical midline incision, which could then be covered with peritoneum, an approach that led to the modern-day low vertical procedure.[13] Later, Beck[14] (1919) and DeLee[15] (1922) modified the Krönig approach and introduced it in the United States. Finally, Kerr[16] (1926) developed the low transverse incision, which is most commonly employed throughout the world today.

The Changing Rate of Cesarean Birth

The change in the overall cesarean section rate is dramatically demonstrated by data from the Chicago Lying-In Hospital, which had a fivefold increase in the cesarean section rate from 0.6 percent in 1910 to 3 percent in 1928.[17] By 1963, an overall incidence of approximately 5 percent was considered optimal.[18] Indications for cesarean section have continued to become significantly more liberal. In 1970, the overall cesarean birth rate for the United States had risen to 15.2 percent and that for Canada to 13.9 percent.[19] Cesarean delivery rates have increased even more in the past 20 years. Recent data summarizing the change from 1965 to 1985 indicate an increase in the overall cesarean birth rate from 4.5 to 23 percent.[20] As we enter the last decade of the twentieth century, cesarean rates in some institutions approximate 30 percent. Some physicians have employed cesarean delivery as an answer to all potential problems; an extreme was reached in 1985, when the following was asked: "If an informed patient opts for prophylactic cesarean section at term, can it be denied?"[21]

There are many reasons for the increase in the cesarean section rate, and they are complexly interrelated. Early liberalization of the indications for cesarean section rose out of the increased availability of effective antibiotics, safer blood banking, and a greater tendency for obstetrics to be practiced in facilities delivering large numbers of patients. Even socioeconomic factors have played a role. The widespread availability of contraceptive and sterilization techniques has resulted in smaller family size and greater emphasis on the importance of "quality survival" for the newborn, not simply survival.

Continuous electronic fetal heart rate (FHR) monitoring use has become widespread even in low-risk patients. The apparent effect is an increase in the cesarean section rate for so-called "fetal distress."

Women are delaying childbirth. Nulliparous patients constitute an increased proportion of laboring women, thereby increasing the likelihood of dystocia and other medical complications such as preeclampsia that further increase the likelihood of cesarean delivery. It is well known that cesarean delivery rate increases with advancing age. In the United States between 1980 and 1985, the number of births in patients at least 30 years of age increased from 20 to 25 percent of all deliveries.[22] Finally, repeat cesarean sections have risen as a product of the increasing rate of primary cesarean births.

Dystocia as an indication has been liberalized, and forcep deliveries fell into relative disfavor in some medical centers. For the interval 1972 to 1980, Placek et al.[23] reported a decline in forceps delivery from 37 to 18 percent, which parallels the increase in the cesarean delivery rate from 7 to 17 percent.[23] Vaginal breech deliveries have been abandoned by many clinicians in favor of delivery by cesarean section. Most breech presentations are now delivered by cesarean section with rates in some medical centers as high as 79[22] and 92[24] percent.

Medicolegal pressures have also impacted on the liberalization of indications. Concern regarding potential malpractice action for failure to intervene at an alleged "standard" time increased dramatically in the 1980s, particularly among physicians in traditional private practice. Statistics to support this concept indicate that private nulliparous patients are more likely than clinic patients to undergo cesarean delivery if dystocia or malpresentation or so-called "fetal distress" is diagnosed.[25] The practice of obstetrics has become more defensive. Many obstetricians have concluded that a physician is unlikely to be sued for an unnecessary cesarean delivery. On the other hand, the obstetrician may be criticized in hindsight for failure to perform an earlier cesarean delivery that "may have" resulted in better outcome.

As the indications for primary cesarean section were expanded, it is not surprising that "prior cesarean delivery" became an ever-increasing indication for cesarean birth. By 1964, nearly one-half of all cesarean deliveries at The New York Hospital were based on the indication of prior cesarean birth.[18] Similar data were reported from California in 1970, where repeat cesarean sections accounted for 35 to 50 percent of all cesarean deliveries.[26]

Cesarean Section and Perinatal Mortality

That cesarean birth offers major improvements in outcome has, with few exceptions, yet to be proven. Although it is easy to hypothesize that the increase in cesarean deliveries over the past two decades has impacted favorably on perinatal outcome, few data exist to support this conclusion. There was also hope that birth-related newborn morbidity, including cerebral palsy, could be dramatically reduced by liberalizing the indications for cesarean section. Unfortunately, there are no data to suggest a decline in the incidence of cerebral palsy despite 15 years of major perinatal advances. Perinatal mortality and morbidity for the most part remain predominantly a function of gestational age, abnormal fetal growth, and congenital anomalies. It is more likely that continued improvement in perinatal outcome is the product of widespread changes in perinatal care.[27] Furthermore, the perinatal outcome is more likely to be related to indication for delivery than the route of delivery.

There has been a heated international debate regarding the relative benefits of cesarean birth. O'Driscoll and Foley[28] have compared improvements in perinatal outcome at the National Maternity Hospital in Dublin, Ireland, where cesarean delivery rates have remained stable at less than 5 percent between 1965 to 1980, with improvements in the United States, where rates have increased from slightly less than 5 percent in 1965 to more than 15 percent in 1980. Because the perinatal mortality rate at the National Maternity Hospital has progressively fallen from 42.1 to 16.8 per 1,000 births, despite a low cesarean delivery rate, one is forced to consider that although cesarean delivery, per se, is a contributor to better perinatal outcome, it is likely to be less important than the overall improvement in obstetrical care. It may be as Leveno et al.[29] suggest, that the truth lies somewhere in between. Moreover, the data of O'Driscoll and Foley[28] are limited by their emphasis on mortality rather than morbidity. Perinatal outcome as reflected by intrapartum fetal deaths and neonatal seizures was significantly decreased at Parkland Hospital, Dallas, in association with a low cesarean delivery rate of 10.1 percent. While such comparative data are of interest, it is likely that the populations in Dublin and Dallas are quite different.

There are no well-documented prospective trials demonstrating benefit to the fetus or to the mother that would justify the extent of the increase in the cesarean section rate. Despite an awareness that there is a potential problem, we may have entered a cycle that will be difficult to reverse. Many physicians recently trained in obstetrics have had inadequate exposure to operative vaginal procedures and consequently later often opt for a procedure with which they are familiar, cesarean delivery. Furthermore, our specialty is increasingly dominated by the emergence of the subspecialty of maternal–fetal medicine. The traditional obstetrician "teacher" with many years of clinical hands-on experience has been replaced by the young subspecialist who may have greater in-depth scientific knowledge, particularly related to high-risk obstetric problems and invasive procedures, but who often lacks experience or interest in operative vaginal procedures. The questions now are, how do we conduct the necessary clinical trial of vaginal delivery versus cesarean section, and, if operative vaginal delivery is proven safe, who will train physicians to perform these procedures?

There is an obvious need to evaluate the current cesarean birth rates. Respected clinicians vary greatly in their acceptance of procedures such as mid-forceps or vaginal delivery of the breech, whether a singleton or one of a multiple gestation. This author continues to believe that labor can be managed more scientifically, that VBAC is a rational approach in many centers, that at least 50 percent of breeches can safely be delivered vaginally, and that selective vaginal breech delivery is possible, even for the very-low-birth-weight (VLBW) fetus (weighing less than 1,500 g). In the years 1985 to 1987, my primary cesarean section rate was approximately 16 percent in a referral "high-risk" practice, a number in accord with a theoretically ideal rate of 15 to 16 percent.[30]

INDICATIONS FOR CESAREAN DELIVERY

Indications for cesarean delivery can be categorized (Table 20.1) in several ways. Some strictly benefit the fetus, whereas others are largely done for maternal indications such as to avoid maternal hemorrhage, reduce the potential spread of malignancy, avoid the repeated need for additional procedures such as abdominal cerclage in future pregnancies, and prevent

uterine rupture. Some indications will benefit *both* mother and fetus. Some indications are well accepted even though selectively applied on a subjective basis. Placenta previa or conjoined twins are universally accepted as indications for cesarean birth. On the other hand, several indications such as a breech presentation or a VLBW fetus are controversial. It is not feasible to discuss all indications for cesarean delivery in this chapter.

Fetal Indications

Fetal indications for cesarean birth are in large part designed to minimize long-term consequences of intrapartum asphyxia and/or delivery-related trauma. Accepted indications often employed selectively include the following: "significant" nonremediable, nonreassuring FHR patterns, commonly associated with progressive loss of variability; various categories of breech presentation at risk for head entrapment and/or cord prolapse; the VLBW fetus; and major fetal congenital anomalies such as hydrocephalus, gastroschisis or omphalocele, in which a planned, controlled delivery may be desirable.

Approximately 1 to 3 percent of all laboring patients undergo a cesarean delivery for a nonremediable and nonreassuring FHR pattern (see Ch. 14). Many clinicians will designate this indication as fetal distress. The cesarean section rate and the precise criteria for fetal distress vary considerably from hospital to hospital and among individual practitioners. In large part, that variation reflects the subjective nature of the interpretation of continuous FHR. In 1978, Haddad and Lundy[31] estimated that approximately 50 percent of cesarean births performed for such nonreassuring FHR patterns in their hospital were not justified on independent peer review.

Maternal–Fetal Indications

Placental abnormalities such as placenta previa or placental abruption in which hemorrhage poses a significant risk to both mother and fetus, as well as labor "dystocia," including absolute cephalopelvic disproportion when the latter can be diagnosed, are indica-

Table 20.1   Commonly Reported Indications for Cesarean Delivery

Indications	Selective	Subjective	Controversial[a]	Universally Accepted[b]
Fetal				
Non reassuring FHR	✓	✓		✓
Breech, frank	✓		✓	
Breech, non-frank	✓		✓	
Breech, preterm	✓		✓	
Very low birth weight (<1,500 g)	✓		✓	
Herpes simplex virus	✓			
Immune thrombocytopenic purpura	✓			
Congenital anomalies, major	✓		✓	
Maternal–fetal				
Cephalopelvic disproportion (relative)	✓	✓		✓
Failure to progress	✓	✓		✓
Placental abruption	✓	✓		✓
Placenta previa				✓
Absolute pelvic disproportion		✓		✓
Maternal				
Obstructive benign and malignant tumors	✓	✓		✓
Large vulvar condyloma	✓	✓		
Cervical cerclage (abdominal)	✓			
Prior vaginal colporrhaphy	✓			
Conjoined twins				✓

[a] Controversy regarding need for universal application.

[b] Universally accepted if selective/subjective criteria present.

tions offering a potential benefit to both mother and fetus. In their extreme, each can pose maternal risks of hemorrhage, uterine rupture and infection, and fetal risks of asphyxia.

Dystocia is a term used to describe indications for cesarean birth following an "abnormal labor." The clinician will often attribute these procedures to either "cephalopelvic disproportion" (CPD) or "failure to progress" (FTP). Cephalopelvic disproportion is a relative term; cesarean births most often involve a normal-sized infant.[32]

Maternal Indications

There are only a few indications for cesarean delivery that are solely maternal. They include mechanical obstructions of the vagina from large vulvovaginal condylomata, advanced lower genital tract malignancy, and placement of a permanent abdominal cerclage with a desire for future pregnancies.

INFORMED CONSENT

The patient and her partner should participate in the decision-making process leading to cesarean delivery. There is considerable variation in both the style and substance of obtaining informed consent for cesarean birth. Although there is certainly merit to nondirected counseling, it should be somewhat obvious that it is difficult to transmit a minimum of 8 years of training and a number of years of clinical experience into a 5- to 10-minute discussion for informed consent, particularly when stress and emotions are high. The provision of informed consent involves walking a fine line; it is part of the so-called "art" of medicine. Much of the information provided will depend on whether the procedure is scheduled or unplanned. A key feature in the process is physician–patient rapport and associated patient trust of the managing physician. Current practice patterns often dictate that the patient receive care from several members of a large group practice, in which case rapport is not always optimal. Some patients want a detailed explanation, while others desire whatever the doctor advises. Sadly, much of what is discussed is often not understood or forgotten when stress is high. Provision of too much information may overwhelm the patient. On the other hand, provision of inadequate or unbalanced information may result in a decision that the patient later regrets.

When time is not an issue, the patient should be informed about the standard risks of any operative procedure, namely, infection and hemorrhage, as well as major complications associated with anesthesia. Injury at the time of cesarean delivery to a nearby organ, including bladder and ureters, is a rare complication that is not ordinarily discussed. Should vaginal delivery be an acceptable alternative, the patient may benefit from knowledge regarding the relative risks and benefits of that approach.

In the case of primary cesarean delivery for conditions such as breech presentation, much of the focus of the discussion generally relates to the potential and theoretical fetal advantages of cesarean birth, often with little mention of the severalfold increase in maternal morbidity and mortality associated with a cesarean section and its complications.

The patient should not be asked, "Do you want to do everything possible for your baby?" There are as yet few data to suggest that a cesarean birth, except in the presence of selective indications, has a beneficial effect with regard to survival and long-term outcome. Should cesarean section be considered for a VLBW fetus, it may be advantageous to review the anticipated weight and gestational age specific rate of intact survival by either route and the higher risk of respiratory distress with an elective cesarean birth.

Contingencies may also be important. Should the physician anticipate a repeat cesarean section in a patient with a current diagnosis of anterior placenta previa, informed consent may include some discussion regarding the potential need for hysterectomy for placenta accreta, as well as the potential need for transfusion and its associated risks (see Ch. 18). When an elective cesarean section likely to require blood replacement is anticipated, autologous transfusion should be discussed.

SURGICAL PRINCIPLES AND OPERATIVE PROCEDURE

Skin Preparation

The preparation of the patient's skin in the operating room ordinarily includes mechanical removal of obvious foreign material, cleansing of skin folds and umbilicus, and application of a bactericidal solution. Despite years of clinical research, there are few prospective randomized studies to demonstrate benefit of any of the various skin cleansing preparations, or even hand washing agents, over another. In general, much of what the physician does is based on long-standing surgical principles. Some perspective into this aspect of surgical practice is provided by Masterson,[33] who has indicated that "a surgeon probably would have a lower wound infection rate if he/she did not wash the patient's skin before surgery, than if he/she shaved the patient's operative site the night before surgery." The same author has also indicated that "preoperative skin preparation, whether it is the patient's or the surgeon's, should be a brief event. Successful wound healing is determined more by what is done in the wound than what is done on the wound."

An abdominal incision interrupts the body's first line of defense against infection. The primary objective of skin preparation for cesarean delivery is to reduce the risk of wound infection by decreasing the bacteria flora of the patient's abdominal wall along the anticipated incision site. Bacteria such as *Staphylococcus aureus*, which may be normal inhabitants of the hair follicle, may be reduced in the process, but are not totally eliminated. Fortunately "transient" flora are easier to remove from the skin than are the "resident" flora that are attached to the skin by adhesion or adsorption and require friction for removal.

Under ordinary circumstances, the number of flora in any one area is relatively stable. The relative risk of infection with skin incisions varies, to some extent, according to the site of the incision; the availability of moisture, which promotes bacterial colonization; and the presence of lipid secretion by sebaceous glands. The indigenous "resident" flora of the skin are mainly diphtheroids and gram-positive rods, including aerobic *Corynebacterium* and anaerobic *Propionibacterium.* Gram-negative organisms can proliferate in moist areas such as under a panniculus or air-tight dressing.[34] The aerobic corynebacteria diphtheroids are the most common organisms in areas of moist skin. The diphtheroids seldom cause clinical infection and are actually important in the ecology of skin by suppressing *Staphylococcus epidermidis* and *S. aureus.*

In contrast to the normal resident skin flora whose numbers are normally stable, "transient" flora are deposited on the skin and in the incision/wound from the environment and, as a consequence, vary greatly in type and number. Other factors that determine whether a wound infection will occur include host resistance, virulence of the organisms deposited on the skin/incisional wound, presence and amount of tissue destruction, size and reactivity of the suture material, and vascularity of the incision site. In the case of cesarean delivery, leakage of cervical and vaginal secretions into the pelvis and transmittal to the skin incision site is also a contributing factor.

The questions to be addressed in the selection of a preoperative skin preparation should include the following. Is the preparation safe relative to skin allergic reactions? Is it fast acting? Does it have broad antibacterial properties that will decrease the number of microorganisms on the intact skin?[35] In practical terms, when agents are compared, there is little if any difference between most preparations.[36] Both 0.5 to 4.0 percent chlorhexidene and 4 percent povidone-iodine have been studied. Most institutions employ a povidone-iodine solution, which has some theoretical benefit over 4 percent chlorhexidene in 4 percent isopropyl alcohol[37] despite the known risk of skin reactions with povidone-iodine.[38]

Overall, the rate of wound infection is approximately 6 to 8 percent whether the skin preparation is sprayed or mechanically scrubbed. It is likely that simple application by painting or spraying is as effective, if not more effective, than the traditional approach of long-term mechanical scrubbing.[36,39] There are also data that suggest that a rapid alcohol preparation followed by application of iodine-impregnated sterile drapes may safely reduce skin preparation time to 1 to 2 minutes.[40]

Preparation of the vagina prior to cesarean section is seldom an issue with the exception of instances in which a cesarean hysterectomy is planned. Preparation of the vagina is intended to reduce postoperative infection. However, if the clinician decides to use prophylactic antibiotics, it is doubtful that there is any additional benefit to be gained from preoperative preparation of the vagina with an antiseptic preparation. Should a cesarean hysterectomy be planned, simple irrigation of the vagina with a saline solution will dilute the concentration of bacteria in the vagina and may provide additional benefit.

Hair Removal

A major, but unheralded change in preoperative obstetric management of peri-incisional hair has occurred in the last decade. In general, the only reasons to remove hair from the intended operative site is to eliminate hair that will mechanically interfere with the surgeon's approximation of the wound edges and with adhesion and removal of postoperative dressings.[41] Hair is sterile.[42] Removal of hair with a razor may increase wound infection rates by creating breaks in the skin for bacterial entry.[43] Should shaving be required, it is best done in the operating room. Alexander et al.[43] have shown that clipping the hair the morning of surgery results in a significantly lower infection rate than does clipping the hair the evening prior to surgery or shaving at any time.

Suture Selection

Sutures are synthetic or nonsynthetic. The latter are derived from gut, cotton, or silk. Sutures can be further divided into absorbable and nonabsorbable types (Table 20.2). In turn, synthetic suture types are braided or monofilament. The braided absorbable sutures are either coated (Vicryl or Dexon Plus) or noncoated (Dexon S).

The ideal suture offers knot security, minimal tissue inflammatory reaction, and tensile strength compatible with the inherent healing properties of the tissue to be reapproximated. It is also desirable that the suture be flexible, pliable and easy to handle, resistant to infection, and reabsorbed at a predictable rate. The selection of the suture material to be used should also be based on how rapidly the particular tissue heals. For instance, chromic cat gut is often appropriate for visceral organs like the bladder, peritoneum, and vagina, surfaces that generally heal

Table 20.2 Categories of Commonly Employed Suture Material

	Absorbable	Nonabsorbable
Nonsynthetic	Plain gut Chromic gut	Silk Cotton
Synthetic	Polyglycolic acid (Dexon) Polygalactin 910 Polydioxanone (PDS) Polyglyconate (Maxon)	Polypropylene monofilament (Surgilene, Prolene) Braided (Dacron, Mersilene)

quickly, particularly in pregnancy. As a consequence, these organs require suture material that maintains tensile strength for a relatively short time.[44] In contrast, skin and fascia heal more slowly; thus the suture selected should provide more long-term tensile strength. For example, fascia regains only 25 percent of its original strength after 20 days of healing; wounds will thus readily dehisce if the fascial layer is not closed properly. Nonabsorbable synthetic sutures such as polypropylene (Prolene) and polybutester (Novafil) are strong and dependable and are frequently used to repair fascia and for mass closure. Monofilament nylons, Maxon, and PDS are also useful.[45]

The *United States Pharmacopeia* (USP) categorizes suture materials as nonabsorbable if tensile strength is maintained for more than 60 days. Knot security is maintained for several weeks longer with synthetic absorbable sutures than with chromic cat gut. When using the synthetic sutures, it is recommended that the clinician add two more knots with longer tails to ensure knot security because these sutures may slip when knots are not properly tied. Unfortunately, many of the newer synthetic absorbable sutures do not handle as well as the natural ones. As a result, manufacturers have introduced coated synthetic sutures (Dexon Plus, coated Vicryl) that have less memory and lie more easily.

Each suture type has definite advantages and disadvantages. Should the clinician desire to maintain tensile strength in fascial and subcuticular tissue over longer intervals (e.g., patients who have diabetes, are infected, or on corticosteroid therapy), the newer synthetic monofilament absorbable sutures such as polyglyconate (Maxon) and polydioxanone (PDS)

may be preferable because they support the tissues in the wound adequately for more than 6 weeks.

Nonabsorbable monofilament sutures such as Prolene and Novafil may be the suture of choice for closing the patient at risk of infection because they do not allow bacteria to invade and colonize the interstices of the braided polyfilament sutures. This feature is particularly important in infected abdominal wall fascia, where tensile strength is crucial and chronic inflammation least desirable.

Synthetic sutures offer the benefits of decreased tissue reactivity, prolonged and predictable strength, and low coefficients of friction. Monofilament synthetic sutures elicit somewhat less tissue reaction than their braided counterparts: both are less reactive than their nonsynthetic absorbable and nonabsorbable counterparts. The larger the gauge of the suture, the greater the likelihood of adhesion formation.[46]

ABDOMINAL INCISIONS

Selection of Incision Type

The surgeon may choose either a vertical or transverse skin incision (Fig. 20.1) when performing a cesarean delivery. The actual incision chosen is in large part based on the surgeon's past experience and on consumer pressures favoring a low transverse incision.[47,48] The midline vertical, transverse Maylard, and transverse Pfannenstiel incisions are the three most commonly employed incision types. Transverse Cherney and paramedian vertical incisions are seldom used.

There has been a significant increase recently in the use of transverse incisions as opposed to the traditional low vertical incision. Preferably the obstetrician is comfortable with several types of incision and is prepared to make a selective decision for each patient's need. The choice should be based on the relative simplicity and speed of the various incisions, the desired exposure, the estimated fetal weight, the anticipated cosmetic results, and the risk factors for infection or dehiscence. In general, vertical incisions allow more rapid access to the lower uterine segment, have less blood loss, provide greater feasibility for incisional extension around the umbilicus, and allow easier examination of the upper abdomen. In pregnancy, speed of entry through a midline vertical incision is facilitated by the common occurrence of diastasis of the rectus muscles.

Although transverse incisions are somewhat more time consuming, the difference in time of entry between the two incision types may be only 30 to 60 seconds in the hands of an experienced clinician. Transverse incisions are preferred cosmetically, are generally less painful, have been associated with a lower risk of subsequent herniation, and yet provide equal, if not better, visualization of the pelvis. Some argue that there is a lower incidence of postoperative pulmonary complications when a transverse incision is used, particularly in patients with preexisting pulmonary problems such as obstructive lung disease.[49] Whether a transverse incision is less subject to dehiscence and herniation[50,51] remains controversial.

A number of surgical principles are relevant regardless of the incision selected. The surgeon and surgical assistant should apply traction at right angles to the intended incision site in a symmetric manner so that the incision is developed in a uniform vertical plane through its length and depth. The "Allis" test may be used to determine if the abdominal incision will be large enough. An Allis clamp is 15 cm long and, if it fits easily between retractors placed at the ends of the incision, little difficulty will be encountered in delivering the fetus.[52] There is no reason to disturb the fat from the adjacent fascia unless there is difficulty in exposing the fascial edges. Such efforts will simply increase the risk of postoperative seromas and develop unnecessary dead space.

The Pfannenstiel and Maylard incisions are the most commonly employed transverse incisions for cesarean delivery. The Maylard incision is quicker, pro-

vides better lateral pelvic and midabdominal visualization, requires less dissection and elevation of the anterior abdominal wall during entry and tissue retraction, and makes a repeat procedure somewhat easier than does the Pfannenstiel.

The Maylard incision (Fig. 20.1) differs from the Pfannenstiel incision in that it involves transverse incision of both the anterior rectus sheath and the rectus muscles bilaterally using either knife or cautery.[53] In the nonobese patient, the skin incision is ordinarily at least 3 to 4 cm above the symphysis. Should there be a large panniculus, the incision may be made considerably higher to avoid placement of the incision on the under surface of the panniculus. The superficial inferior epigastric vessels, which can be observed in the lateral extremes of the incision, may be individually ligated. Incision of the rectus

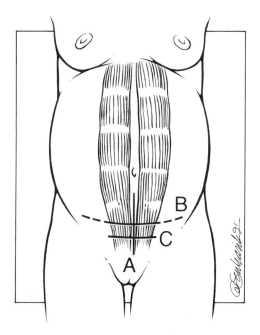

Fig. 20.1 The obstetrician most commonly uses one of three abdominal incisions: (A) midline, (B) Maylard, and (C) Pfannenstiel. Hatched lines indicate possible extension. (Modified from Baker and Shingleton,[194] with permission.)

muscles is accomplished by placing two fingers or clamps beneath each rectus muscle and lifting the muscles in such a way as to allow surgical incision with either a knife or cutting cautery between the fingers or clamps. In most cesarean procedures, pelvic exposure is sufficient if only the medial two-thirds of the rectus muscles are incised. This avoids the necessity to separate surgically the deep inferior epigastric vessels, as may be necessary in more extensive gynecologic cases. Nonetheless, the surgeon should palpate for these vessels. Should extension of the incision be necessary, these vessels should be isolated and ligated to avoid hematoma formation. Those favoring a Cherney modification believe it is preferable to partial transsection of the rectus muscles, a technique required with the Maylard incision.[54] After separation of the rectus muscles, the transversalis fascia and peritoneum are then incised transversely, as opposed to the Pfannenstiel incision in which they are incised vertically.

The Pfannenstiel incision (Fig. 20.1) is a curvilinear incision. The incision is generally made at a point approximately 3 to 4 cm above the symphysis pubis at the level of pubic hair line. The determination of its lateral extension should, to some extent, be a function of the estimated fetal size. Symmetry of the incision can be facilitated by traction of the skin in a cephalad direction during incision that, when released, will result in a curvilinear incision. The incision is generally extended to the lateral border of the rectus muscles.

The inferior and superior margin of the fascial incision is elevated to facilitate blunt dissection of the fascial sheath from the underlying rectus muscles. Individual perforating blood vessels between muscle and fascia will require ligation or coagulation to achieve adequate hemostasis. Sharp separation of the muscles from the median raphe, which is facilitated by upward traction on the anterior rectus sheath, is extended superiorly to the level of the umbilicus. Once the rectus muscles are adequately exposed, they are retracted laterally to reveal the underlying transversalis fascia and peritoneum, which is entered via a midline vertical incision in a manner similar to that of a low vertical abdominal incision.

Surgeons vary as to the technique used for incising the peritoneum. Some prefer initial entry by scalpel with subsequent inferior and superior extension with scissors. Others use the scalpel for the entirety of the incision because it is theoretically less traumatic. Once the surgeon becomes familiar with this technique, it allows somewhat faster entry than do scissors. Nonetheless, either technique is appropriate. The site of initial peritoneal entry chosen should be at least half-way toward the umbilicus so as to avoid bladder injury, particularly in patients undergoing repeat cesarean section; the peritoneum should be "tented" between two hemostats or pickups and palpated to ascertain that there is no adherent bowel, omentum, or even bladder. The peritoneal cavity may be entered using a scalpel or scissors. Should the planned peritoneal incision be in a vertical direction, the peritoneal incision is first extended superiorly for greater exposure and then inferiorly to a point just above the superior pole of the bladder.

Special Considerations

Skin Incision in the Obese Patient

The obese patient is at significant additional risk for wound complications. Reported wound complication rates are 4 and 29 percent in nonobese versus obese patients respectively.[55] Should the patient be massively obese, it is best to use an incision that does not involve the underside of the panniculus, an area that is more heavily colonized with bacteria and is difficult to prepare surgically, to keep dry, and to inspect in the postoperative period. The surgeon may choose either a vertical midline incision, which is developed periumbilically both above and below the umbilicus, or, alternatively, a transverse incision closer to the umbilicus. In either case, the objective is to enter the abdomen directly over the lower uterine segment. The actual selection of the site of incision, whether it be vertical or transverse, can be made by retracting the panniculus in a caudad direction so as to place the incision directly overlying the uterine segment.

In closing the fascia of an obese patient, placement of the sutures in the fascia should be at least 1.5 cm from the cut margin. Should there be major risk factors other than obesity, the clinician may consider use of (1) Smead-Jones monofilament polypropylene internal retention sutures or (2) interrupted or figure-of-eight sutures using either polyglycolic acid or other delayed absorption sutures like monofilament polyglyconate or polydioxanone.

It is also acceptable to use a running continuous large-gauge monofilament polypropylene suture in closing the fascial incision. This technique offers the theoretical advantages of distributing tension equally over the continuity of the incision line and increasing the speed of wound closure, thus minimizing the risk of foreign material within the wound. Sutures should not be locked, a technique that reduces vascularization and potentially slows wound healing. Indeed, Shepherd et al.[56] encountered no wound dehiscences employing a mass closure technique in over 200 high-risk gynecology patients. If this approach is employed, sutures should be placed at least 1.5 to 2 cm lateral to the cut margin of the fascia, with successive bites approximately 1.5 cm apart along the longitudinal axis of the incision. A large needle is used in closure. Some advocate placement of a clip on the short end of the suture to avoid knot disruption. If the wound is not entirely dry, closed drainage (anterior to the fascia) exited through separate stab wounds may be employed for 24 to 72 hours until wound drainage is less than 20 cc in 24 hours. Subcutaneous sutures may be used and the skin closed with suture staples, left in place for 10 to 14 days. Some surgeons employ prophylactic postoperative nasal gastric suction, placed during surgery, for the first 24 hours to avoid distention.

Placenta Accreta

Although the incidence of placenta accreta has been reported to be approximately 1 in 2,500 deliveries, the incidence increases to approximately 4 percent in patients with a placenta previa.[57] This association is particularly marked in the patient with a previous cesarean section. Under such circumstances the incidence of placenta accreta may approach 25 percent.[58] For this reason the physician contemplating a cesarean section for placenta previa, particularly a repeat cesarean section, should be prepared for the possibility of total abdominal hysterectomy.

Uterine Incisions

The most commonly employed uterine incisions (Table 20.3 and Fig. 20.2) are the low transverse incision originally advocated by Kerr[16] and the low vertical incision, originally proposed by Krönig.[13] A low transverse (Kerr incision) is employed in more than 90 percent of all cesarean births. The transverse inci-

Table 20.3 Surgical Considerations in Selection of Uterine Incision

Low Segment Incisions	Transverse	Vertical
Technical ease of		
Extension of incision	−	+
Bladder dissection	+	−
Uterine closure	+	−
Reperitonealization	+	−
Benefits vs. risks		
Uterine rupture (subsequent)	+	−
Lateral extension into uterine vessels	−	+
Extension inferiorly	+	−
Intraoperative bleeding	+	−
Subsequent adhesions	+	−

+, advantage to incision.

sion has the following advantages over a vertical incision: less risk of entry into the upper uterine segment, greater ease of entry, less bladder dissection, less operative blood loss, less repair and easier reperitonealization, and less likelihood of adhesion formation to bowel or omentum should it not be possible to apply the bladder flap above the top of the incision line. Importantly, in subsequent pregnancies the obstetrician can feel more comfortable offering a VBAC because there is less likelihood of uterine rupture.[59]

In contrast, a vertical incision (classic or low vertical) may be advantageous when the patient has not been in labor and the lower uterus is poorly developed or if the fetus is not in a cephalic presentation. Should a transverse incision be performed under such circumstances, there is a greater likelihood of lateral extension of the incision into the vessels of the broad ligament. However, individualization is reasonable. For instance, I generally prefer a vertical incision for a transverse lie. However, a low transverse incision is certainly feasible when the lower uterine segment is well developed, as may be the case when the patient presents in active labor with advanced cervical dilatation.

The classic uterine incision involves the upper active uterine segment. Its primary advantage is the rapidity of entry into the uterus. Furthermore, some physicians believe that the incision is useful in the presence of an anterior placenta previa, reducing the potential for maternal and fetal hemorrhage.[60] De-

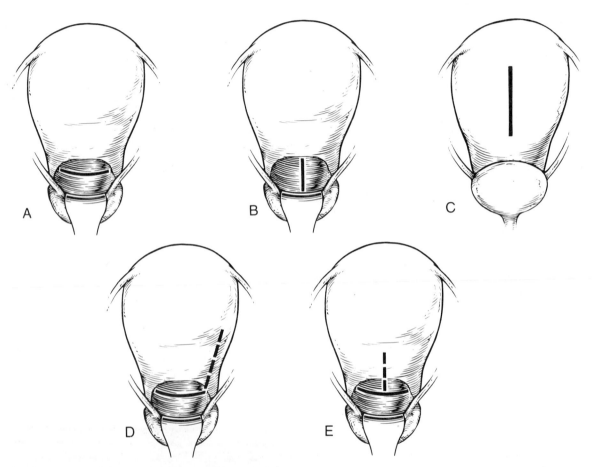

Fig. 20.2 Uterine incisions for cesarean delivery. (A) Low transverse incision. The bladder is retracted downward, and the incision is made in the lower uterine segment, curving gently upward. If the lower segment is poorly developed, the incision can also curve sharply upward at each end to avoid extending into the ascending branches of the uterine arteries. (B) Low vertical incision. The incision is made vertically in the lower uterine segment after reflecting the bladder, avoiding extension into the bladder below. If more room is needed, the incision can be extended upward into the upper uterine segment. (C) Classic incision. The incision is entirely within the upper uterine segment and can be at the level shown or in the fundus. (D) J incision. If more room is needed when an initial transverse incision has been made, either end of the incision can be extended upward into the upper uterine segment and parallel to the ascending branch of the uterine artery. (E) T incision. More room can be obtained in a transverse incision by an upward midline extension into the upper uterine segment.

spite these advantages, the incision is seldom performed except when it is not possible to expose the lower uterine segment or when a hysterectomy is planned. Complications encountered after a classic incision include subsequent adhesions and greater risk of uterine rupture with later pregnancies.[61] Patients who have had a prior classic incision should

consider an appropriately timed elective repeat cesarean birth because of the risk of uterine rupture even before labor has started.

The theoretical advantages of the low vertical (Krönig) incision over the classic incision are similar to those of the low transverse incision. However, unlike the classic incision, there may occasionally be a caudad (inferior) extension of incision into the cervix and vagina or even into the bladder. Although the low vertical (Krönig) incision is theoretically limited to the lower uterine segment, in reality it often involves the upper segment.

PERFORMING THE CESAREAN SECTION

Development of Bladder Flap

After entry into the lower abdomen, the obstetrician should palpate the uterus to determine the degree and direction of uterine rotation. Some obstetricians insert moistened laparotomy pads into each lateral peritoneal gutter prior to making the uterine incision to absorb amniotic fluid and blood escaping from the incision. This approach may have particular advantage when there is a strong suspicion of amnionitis. In most instances the uterus is dextrorotated such that the left round ligament may be visualized more anteriorly and closer to the midline than is the right. The uterovesical peritoneum (serosa) is grasped in the midline and incised with Metzenbaum scissors. The scissors are then inserted between the peritoneum and underlying myometrium. A retroperitoneal space is developed bluntly with the scissors, tenting the peritoneum bilaterally to the lateral margins of the lower uterine segment. The peritoneal reflection is then incised bilaterally in an upward direction and the bladder separated from the underlying lower uterine segment with blunt dissection. The lower portion of the vesicouterine fold is then grasped with forceps and the bladder lifted anteriorly, allowing blunt separation from the lower uterine segment. In some patients undergoing repeat cesarean birth, it may be necessary to dissect sharply the filmy adhesions connecting the lower uterine incision to the posterior aspect of the bladder. Once the dissection is complete in the midline, the fingers may be carefully swept laterally in each direction to free the bladder more completely. After the bladder flap is adequately developed, a universal retractor or bladder blade is used to retract the bladder anteriorly and inferiorly to facilitate exposure of the intended incision site.

Low Transverse Cesarean Incision

The uterine incision (Fig. 20.2A) is begun 1 to 2 cm above the site of the original upper margin of the bladder. A small incision is first made with a scalpel in the lower uterine segment through the myometrium to the fetal membranes. Continuous suction should be available to facilitate visualization of the operative field and to evacuate amniotic fluid should the incision perforate through the fetal membranes. Care should be taken to avoid laceration of the fetus, which is an occasional complication, especially when the lower uterine segment is thin or when expeditious delivery of the fetus is required. After suctioning, the incision may be extended laterally to the margin of the lower uterine segment by either (1) using bandage scissors, taking care to avoid fetal fingers and toes; or (2) spreading the incision with each index finger, particularly if the lower uterine segment is thin. It is important to curve the incision upward (cephalad) so as to maximize incisional length and avoid extension into the uterine vessels. Splitting the uterine incision using the index fingers will result in more rapid entry; however, there is greater likelihood for unpredictable extension with this method, particularly if the lower segment is not fully effaced. Inspection of the lateral margin of the low transverse incision is facilitated by lateral retraction.

Should the placenta be located in the anterior lower uterine segment, entry can be accomplished by one of three methods. First, the clinician can simply dissect through the placenta; this carries the risk of short-term fetal hemorrhage. Second, the placenta can be separated from the lower uterine segment, facilitating lateral exposure of the fetus. Finally, a classic uterine incision can be employed.

Once the fetus is visualized, the retractors are removed and the fetal head elevated through the uterine incision with the operator's fingers or forceps. Moderate transabdominal fundal pressure is useful in facilitating expulsion.

Low Vertical Incision

Should the fetus present as a breech or transverse lie, particularly back down, there is often advantage to a low vertical (Figs. 20.2B and 20.3) uterine incision, particularly if the lower uterine segment is not well developed. The bladder is displaced downward to expose the lower uterine segment more inferiorly so that the low vertical incision will be less likely to extend into the upper segment. Once the lower uterine incision is exposed, an incision is made at the lowest margin of the incision and extended cephalad with either bandage scissors or knife. On occasion it may

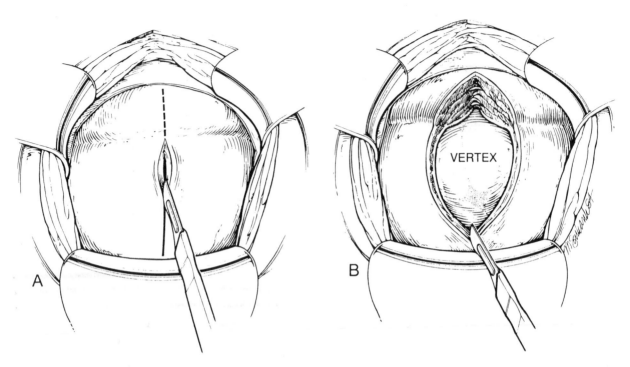

Fig. 20.3 Low vertical incision. (A) Ideally, a vertical incision is contained entirely in the lower uterine segment. (B) Extension into the upper uterine segment, either inadvertently or by choice, is common.

be necessary to extend the incision into the upper active uterine segment. Should such an extension be required, it should be noted in the operative report. The patient should also be advised of this occurrence and its relative importance in future pregnancies. She will have a higher risk of uterine rupture should a subsequent VBAC be attempted.

Although cesarean incisions are traditionally categorized into low vertical and classic types, the performance of a true low vertical incision that does not enter the upper contractile portion of the uterus is actually uncommon. Although the clinical implication is that the low vertical incision poses less risk in a subsequent VBAC, the risk of rupture is nonetheless probably greater than that of a true low transverse incision.

Classic Cesarean Incision

The initial incision (Fig. 20.2C) is made with a scalpel 1 to 2 cm above the bladder reflection. Once the fetus or membranes are visualized the incision is extended

cephalad with bandage scissors, the size of the incision varying with the estimated size of the fetus.

Delivery of the Fetus

Upon completion of the uterine incision, retractors are removed and a hand is inserted into the uterine cavity to elevate the fetal head through the uterine incision. Initial efforts to deliver the presenting part through the uterine incision will indicate the adequacy of the uterine incision. Should the head be deeply wedged within the pelvis, it can be dislodged by an assistant applying upward pressure through the vagina. The head may also be delivered with short-handled Simpson forceps. Once delivery of the fetal head is completed the nose and oropharynx are suctioned with a bulb syringe. If meconium is present, suction should be accomplished with continuous wall suction. When suctioning is complete, expulsion of the remainder of the newborn is facilitated by moderate uterine fundal pressure. The cord is then doubly clamped and cut, and the infant is transferred to the resuscitation team.

Should evaluation of umbilical cord gases be desired, the umbilical cord is first clamped close to the placenta so as to maintain filling of the umbilical arteries and vein and second clamped close to the newborn and then doubly clamped in each location so as to isolate a 10 to 15 cm segment of cord for blood sampling. Umbilical cord gas data may be desirable in high-risk circumstances, such as fetal growth retardation, preterm birth, breech presentations, amnionitis, the presence of thick meconium, or cesarean delivery for nonreassuring FHR findings.

Operative Techniques for the Preterm Fetus

The uterine incision to be used for the delivery of the preterm fetus is best selected after entry into the maternal abdomen. At least 50 percent of cases will require a low vertical or classic incision for indications such as malpresentation or a poorly developed lower uterine segment. Among 174 VLBW cesarean births at Los Angeles County Women's Hospital, a low transverse incision was performed in 31 percent of cases, a low vertical incision in 47 percent, and a classic uterine incision in 22 percent.[62] Using ultrasound, Morrison[63] prospectively evaluated the width of the lower uterine segment in the absence of labor and found its transverse dimension to be 0.5, 1.0, and 4.0 cm at 20, 28, and 34 weeks, respectively. Thus without significant labor, the lower uterine segment will probably not be sufficiently developed to provide an adequate transverse dimension for removal of the fetus. The complications of performing a low transverse incision in the absence of adequate development of the lower uterine segment include difficult removal of the fetus, lateral extension of the incision into the broad ligament and uterine vessels, and downward extension of the incision into the cervix and the vagina. It is noteworthy that intraoperative complications including injury to the bladder, broad ligament laceration, and uterine artery laceration are more common at preterm than term cesarean birth. The complication rate is independent of incision type.[64]

Cesarean Delivery of the Breech Presentation

Should an elective cesarean section be planned, it is desirable, prior to performing the procedure, to confirm that the breech has not converted spontaneously to a vertex or to a more unfavorable transverse lie. The lie of the fetus can be verified by palpation prior

to making the uterine incision. In the case of a transverse lie, the vertex or the buttocks of the breech can often be guided into a position underlying the planned site of the uterine incision. Should the lower uterine segment be well developed, a transverse or vertical uterine incision can be used. However, a vertical incision is often preferable should the cervix be long and closed, the lower uterine segment poorly developed, or if the breech has converted to a backdown transverse lie.

The head of a preterm breech infant may be trapped if the incision is not made large enough.[62] Although cesarean section is often elected to minimize fetal trauma, the actual delivery mechanism via the cesarean incision is very similar to that of the vaginal route. The surgeon should thus anticipate and conduct the delivery process in such a way as to minimize both compression of fetal organs and hyperextension of the fetal neck. The mechanism for delivery of the breech is discussed elsewhere (see Ch. 17). However, should there be evidence of head entrapment, the first action should be to extend the abdominal incision and to enlarge the uterine incision. Occasionally it may be necessary to incise perpendicular to a transverse incision (T-Shaped incision) or to extend the transverse incision upward parallel to the uterine artery (J incision) (Fig. 20.2D,E). Both the T and J incisions are more subject to uterine rupture with subsequent pregnancies.

Repair of the Uterine Incision

Once the newborn is delivered, the incision is inspected for bleeding sites that can be clamped with either Ring forceps or Allis clamps until the incision is sutured. Oxytocin administration on the delivery of the fetus is particularly important following classic cesarean section to facilitate uterine contraction and to reduce blood loss. The placenta can be delivered immediately, either with gentle traction on the umbilical cord or manually if there is no major bleeding about the uterine incision. The placenta should be inspected for possible missing cotyledons.

Closure of the uterine incision is aided by manual delivery of the uterus through the abdominal incision.[65] Delivery of the uterine fundus through the abdominal incision facilitates uterine massage and observation of uterine tone, as well as routine examination of the adnexa and tubal ligation. Its primary disadvantages are peritoneal discomfort and possible nausea and vomiting in patients under inadequate regional anesthesia. The uterine fundus may then be covered with a moistened laparotomy pad and the uterine incision inspected for obvious bleeding points, which are controlled with clamps until suture closure can be accomplished. The uterine cavity is then inspected and wiped clean with a dry laparotomy sponge to remove fetal membranes and placental fragments. If the patient has not been in labor, it may be advantageous to dilate the cervix gently to facilitate later lochial drainage. The dilating instrument should then be discarded from the operating field. Control of uterine bleeding is facilitated by massaging the uterus and administering 20 units of oxytocin in 1 L of a dilute intravenous crystalloid solution.

Midline placement of a ring forceps or Allis clamp may be used to elevate the lower portion of the low transverse uterine incision, facilitating visualization of the field and approximating the incision. If bleeding is encountered along the margins of the incision, a ring forcep or Allis clamp should be placed at the site of bleeding; routine placement of more than the one midline clamp in the absence of bleeding simply clutters the field. The perimeter of the uterine incision is then inspected to locate bleeding vessels and to localize the true margins of the uterine incision. Allis clamps can be placed at the angles of the incision to control bleeding and to identify the end of the incision. If the incisional margin is not inspected in this way, on occasion the posterior wall of the lower uterine segment may balloon anteriorly and be confused with the lower margin of the transverse incision. Failure to recognize this problem can result in complete closure of the uterine cavity (i.e., superior edge of incision to posterior uterine wall).

Reapproximation of the low transverse uterine incision is generally performed in two layers (Fig. 20.4) using zero or double zero chromic suture or similar absorbable synthetic suture such as Vicryl, the second layer inverting the first. The initial suture should be placed lateral to the angle of a transverse incision or inferior to the lower margin of a vertical incision. Subsequent stitches may be run in a continuous locking manner to the opposite end of the incision. The sutures may be placed through the entire myometrium. Although some have stressed the importance of avoiding incorporation of decidua in the suture for

concern of later development of endometriosis in the scar, this is a remote possibility.[66] Although many routinely use a continuous locking suture, there is questionable advantage to routine suture-locking along the entire margin, except at sites of obvious oozing. Locking sutures increase the likelihood of tissue ischemia and can limit potential wound healing. This remains a controversial issue. When the low transverse uterine segment is particularly thin, it is possible to reapproximate the uterine margins with a single suture layer. Once the first layer is complete, a second continuous layer (Lembert or Cushing) of chromic or similar suture is placed to invert the first layer. The inversion of a transverse incision may be accomplished with either a vertical or horizontal stitch, the latter requiring more frequent placement of the needle upon the needle holder. Once reapproximation is completed, the incision should once again be inspected for bleeding points, which should be individually ligated, coagulated, or controlled with figure-of-eight sutures.

Closure of a classic cesarean incision (Fig. 20.5) ordinarily is very similar. Should the uterine wall be unusually thick, it may be necessary to use a third layer. Repair of the incision can be done in several ways. A common method is to employ continuous 0 or 1 chromic cat gut suture in layers, the first layer approximating the inner one-half of the uterine wall thickness in a continuous locking manner. A second and occasionally a third layer of continuous locking suture is then used to approximate the uterine musculature. It may be desirable to bury the knot (at the superior end of the incision) of the outer suture line. This can be done by initiating suture entry within the incision, exiting laterally, then reentering from the lateral margin of the opposing side, and exiting medially, followed by knot placement. It is also desirable to invert the visceral peritoneum (serosa) in an attempt to reduce the likelihood of later adhesions of bowel or omentum to the incision line above the bladder flap. Again, the operative record should state the type of uterine incision, and the patient should be informed about the incision and its impact on care in subsequent pregnancies, including the advisability against a future attempt at a VBAC.[61]

Once the surgeon is satisfied that the uterine incision is reapproximated satisfactorily and all lacerations and extensions have been exposed and appro-

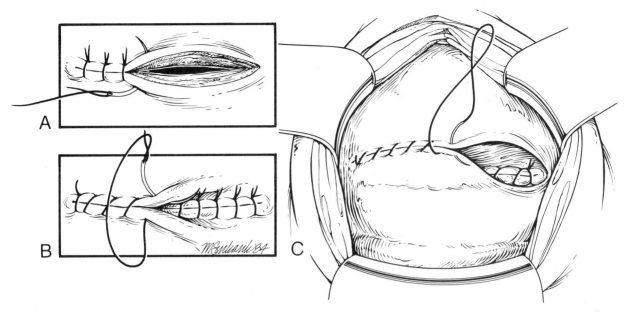

Fig. 20.4 Closure of low transverse incision. (A) The first layer can either be interrupted or continuous. A continuous locking suture is less desirable, despite its reputed hemostatic abilities, because it may interfere with incision vasculature and, hence, with healing and scar formation. (B) A second inverted layer created by using a continuous Lembert's or Cushing's stitch is customary but is really needed only when apposition is unsatisfactory after application of the first layer. Inclusion of too much tissue produces a bulky mass that may delay involution and interfere with healing. (C) The bladder peritoneum is reattached to the uterine peritoneum with fine suture.

priately repaired, the cephalad (superior) and caudad (inferior) folds of the vesicouterine peritoneum may be reapproximated with a running double or triple zero chromic or similar reabsorbable suture. Alternatively, some clinicians no longer reapproximate the peritoneum over the low transverse incision. Although much of an exposed classic incision can be covered with the reapproximated bladder flap, on occasion it may be advantageous to imbricate any exposed edges of the incision to cover raw surfaces and thus reduce the likelihood of later adhesion formation. Before closing the abdomen, the uterus, fallopian tubes, and ovaries should be examined for unsuspected pathology. Should surgical sterilization or ovarian cystectomy be required, this is accomplished before replacing the uterus into the abdominal cavity.

Abdominal Closure

If used, laparotomy pads are removed and, where indicated, the abdominal contents, lateral gutters, and cul-de-sac inspected and suctioned. The operating team should confirm that the needle and sponge counts are correct. There is no need to reapproximate the peritoneum or rectus muscles. However, if the obstetrician routinely closes the anterior peritoneum, this is generally accomplished with a 2-0 chromic cat gut or similar synthetic suture. The transversalis muscle is included in the lower half of the vertical peritoneal incision closure.

The rectus fascia is then closed with either interrupted or continuous (nonlocking) sutures. Suture choice is important in wound healing. If the suture is absorbed too rapidly, tensile strength is reduced, thus increasing the likelihood of wound breakdown. Chromic suture should be avoided when possible. Selection of a suture for its duration of strength is particularly important in patients at risk for wound dehiscence. Unlike their chromic counterparts, synthetic braided sutures maintain tensile strength throughout fascial healing. They are predictably broken down by hydrolysis. In contrast, gut suture has less tensile strength and is degraded less pre-

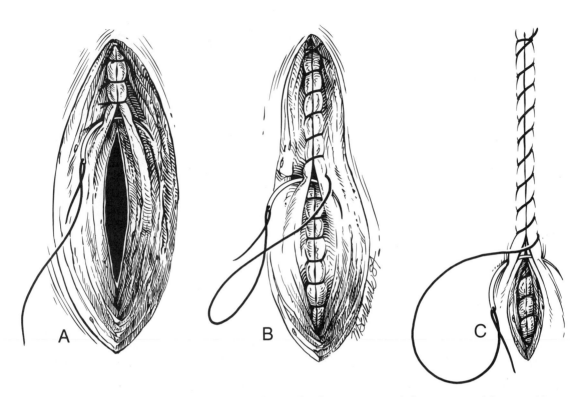

Fig. 20.5 Repair of a classic incision. Three-layer closure of a classic incision, including inversion of the serosal layer to discourage adhesion formation. The knot at the superior end of the incision of the second layer can be buried by medial to lateral placement of the suture from within the depth of the incision and subsequent lateral to medial reentry on the opposing side with resultant knot placement within the incision.

dictably. Local infection may also result in more rapid loss of strength. If the surgeon is dealing with a patient at risk for wound breakdown, such as patients on chronic corticosteroid therapy, delayed absorbable material such as PDS or polyglyconate (Maxon) or permanent material such as nylon or polypropylene (Prolene) may have merit.

Once an appropriate suture is chosen, care should be taken in selecting the site of suture placement for fascial closure. In most instances of wound dehiscence, the suture remains intact but has cut through the tissue in which it has been placed. One study indicates that this problem is responsible for up to 88 percent of disrupted wounds.[67] Large bites using larger gauge suture material are less likely to transect tissue than are small bites with narrow-gauge suture material. Suture entry and exit sites should be well beyond the 1-cm inner zone of collagenolysis at the margin of the wound. Should sutures be placed

within this inner zone, there is greater tendency for them to pull through, leading to dehiscence and possible evisceration. Sutures should be placed at approximately 1-cm intervals.

It is acceptable to use a running suture in closing the fascia in patients with a clean incision. Fagniez et al.[68] were not able to demonstrate a difference in dehiscence rates in a randomized prospective trial of 3,135 patients employing a running versus interrupted polyglycolic acid suture in midline incisions. Approximation of fascia should allow maintenance of adequate blood flow; unnecessarily tight sutures will cause hypoxia and potentially interfere with predictable wound healing.[69,70] Should a patient be at high risk for wound dehiscence, it is preferable that the fascia not be closed with continuous suturing, particularly on a vertical incision. If the patient is at high risk for abdominal distention and wound breakdown, a mass or Smead-Jones (Fig. 20.6) closure is

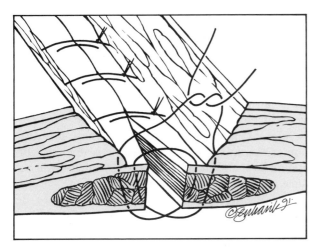

Fig. 20.6 Modification of far-near, near-far Smead-Jones suture. Suture passes deeply through lateral side of anterior rectus fascia and adjacent fat, crosses the midline of the incision to pick up the medial edge of the rectus fascia, then catches the near side of the opposite rectus sheath, and, finally, returns to the far margin of the opposite rectus sheath and subcutaneous fat. (Modified from ACOG,[195] with permission.)

preferable. This closure is mechanically more sound and allows for a 30 percent increase in abdominal girth.

It is generally not necessary to reapproximate the subcutaneous tissue unless the patient is markedly obese, in which case subcutaneous closure will facilitate skin closure. Nor, as noted above, is it necessary to close the peritoneum. No difference in rates of dehiscence was noted between patients who underwent peritoneal closure and those who did not in one large randomized trial.[71] Skin may be closed with staples or a subcuticular stitch. Steristrip adhesive tape (3M Surgical Products, St. Paul, MN) can be used to reduce tension on subcuticular sutures. If staples are used, they should be replaced with Steristrips four days after surgery to decrease scarring.

Intraoperative Complications

The patient undergoing cesarean delivery is at risk for many of the same intra- and postoperative complications as is the patient having a vaginal delivery. Management problems more commonly associated with cesarean delivery, as well as conditions such as uterine

atony and placenta accreta, which are also discussed in Chapter 18, are reviewed in this section.

Although injury to bladder, bowel, or ureters is uncommon, many competent obstetricians, despite careful surgical technique, will encounter complications. When they occur, the primary responsibilities are to identify the injury and its extent, to repair the common complications, and to obtain consultation should injuries be extensive or more complex.

Uterine Lacerations

Lacerations of the lower uterine incision are particularly common when a low transverse incision is used in the presence of a macrosomic fetus or a noncephalic presentation. Fortunately, these lacerations are usually easily sutured as long as they only extend laterally to the margin of the myometrium or inferiorly into the vagina. Care must be taken to avoid ligation of the ureters. In most circumstances, the lateral apex of the extension can be identified and the suture placed just lateral to that point. Should there be extension into the broad ligament in proximity to the ureters, it may be necessary to open the broad ligament and identify the ureters before suture placement. Rarely, there may be an advantage to retrograde placement of a No. 8 French ureteral catheter into the ureters. This can be accomplished transurethrally or by performing a vertical incision in the dome of the bladder to visualize the ureteral orifices. The bladder can then be repaired with an initial continuous 2-0 chromic suture followed by a second imbricating layer of 2-0 suture.

Bladder Injuries

Injury to the bladder is an infrequent, but recognized complication of cesarean delivery. Bladder injury may also occur at the time of uterine rupture, particularly in patients with a prior cesarean delivery. While rates as high as 10 to 14 percent have been reported,[72] the incidence has decreased somewhat in women attempting VBAC.[73,74] Nonetheless, the possibility of bladder injury should be considered in patients undergoing cesarean section following a failed VBAC. Cystotomy as a complication of cesarean hysterectomy has been noted to occur in approximately 4 to 5 percent of procedures.[75,76] In most cases the injury occurs at the bladder base and can, to some extent, be prevented by mobilizing the bladder from the lower uterine segment and upper vagina prior to making the uterine incision. Recently more widespread use of the transverse abdominal incision has increased the likelihood of bladder dome injury upon entering the abdomen. Although the risk of bladder injury can be minimized by preoperative catheterization of the bladder and careful entry into the peritoneal cavity, it is not always possible to avoid injury to the base of the bladder during a repeat cesarean section. When the bladder is more adherent than usual, sharp dissection of the "webbing" between the bladder base and the lower uterine segment and vagina, as opposed to blunt dissection with a sponge stick or gauze-covered finger, will reduce, but not eliminate, the incidence of unplanned cystotomy.

Should a bladder laceration be encountered, the bladder may be repaired with a two-layer closure with 2-0 or 3-0 chromic. Surgeons may differ significantly in their surgical approach to repair. Controversies focus on the use of continuous versus interrupted sutures, on whether it is important to avoid including the mucosa in the suture line, and on the duration of catheter drainage. The issues are probably of little significance when the cystotomy is in the dome of the bladder. However, a cystotomy in the bladder base is more likely to present problems, because the bladder base is thinner and receives less blood flow. There is also a possibility of laceration into the trigone and injury to the ureteral orifices. Should the trigone be lacerated, there may be an advantage to inserting a ureteral catheter under direct visualization. After the bladder has been repaired, a catheter can be left in place for 7 to 10 days.[74,77]

Ureteral Injury

Although one does not frequently think of ureteral injury during cesarean delivery, this complication has been reported in up to 1 in 1,000 cesarean deliveries.[74] Ureteral injury is also increased with cesarean hysterectomy, with rates of 0.2 to 0.5 percent being documented.[75,76] In most instances, injury occurs during efforts to control bleeding arising from lateral extension of the uterine incision; unfortunately, the injury often goes unrecognized intraoperatively. Should lateral extension of an incision occur in the anatomic region of the ureter, opening the anterior leaf of the broad ligament while controlling blood loss with direct pressure will often facilitate more accurate suture placement, which will diminish the potential for ureteral injury.

Gastrointestinal Tract Injury

Injuries to the bowel are also rare, but nonetheless are reported to occur once in approximately 1,300 cesarean sections.[62] Prior abdominal surgery and pelvic/abdominal infection leading to adhesion formation are common risk factors. Sharp scalpel incision limited to a site of transparent peritoneum will reduce inadvertent bowel or bladder injury.

Should adhesions require lysis to gain access to the lower uterine segment, they should be sharply dissected with scissors tips pointed away from the bowel. Small defects in bowel serosa can be closed simply with interrupted silk sutures on an atraumatic needle. Full-thickness lacerations should be repaired in a double-layer closure, employing a transverse closure of a longitudinal laceration, to minimize the possibility of narrowing the bowel lumen.[78] The mucosa can be closed with running or interrupted 3-0 or 4-0 chromic sutures. The muscular and serosal layers are then closed with a similar-sized interrupted silk suture. In the event that there are multiple full-thickness small bowel injuries or the colon or sigmoid is entered, consultation with a gynecologic oncologist or general surgeon is appropriate. The small bowel may require resection and reanastomosis. Primary closure of small colon lacerations ($<$ 1 cm) is indicated using a double-layer closure as described above.[79] More extensive injury associated with fecal contamination may require a temporary colostomy. In either case, antibiotic therapy, with clindamycin or gentamicin, should be provided to cover gram-negative bacteria.

Uterine Atony

Initial efforts to control uterine atony include uterine massage and medical therapy with (1) intravenous oxytocin, 20 to 40 units/L; (2) methergotamine 0.2 mg or ergonovine administered intramuscularly; or (3) 15 methylprostaglandin $F_{2\alpha}$ (Hemabate), which can be administered either intramuscularly or directly into the myometrium. Should the initial dose of prostaglandin be insufficient, successive dosages of 250 μg, up to a total dose of 1.0 to 1.5 mg can be used. Should medical treatment fail, the surgeon must decide between ligation of the uterine arteries (see Fig.

18.15), hypogastric artery ligation, and hysterectomy. Uterine or hypogastric artery ligation may be the desirable approach should the patient be stable cardiovascularly and desirous of future pregnancy. Hypogastric artery ligation can be accomplished by ligation of the ascending branch, which can usually be found at the inferior and lateral extreme of the low transverse incision ascending retroperitoneally within the broad ligament (Fig. 20.7). Unfortunately, even hypogastric artery ligation is actually successful in less than one-half of the cases.[80]

Should uterine or hypogastric artery ligation also fail to control the hemorrhage and the decision is made to proceed to hysterectomy, the surgeon should anticipate an average blood loss of approximately 1,500 to 2,000 cc. If the patient is cardiovascularly unstable or if there is technical difficulty, in certain cases it may be desirable to perform a supracervical hysterectomy.

Placenta Accreta

Placenta accreta is the second most common indication for hysterectomy (obstetric hemorrhage being the first).[81,82] Approximately 25 percent of patients having a cesarean section for placenta previa in the presence of a prior uterine incision subsequently require cesarean hysterectomy for placenta accreta. The risk of placenta accreta appears to increase with the number of prior incisions. This obstetric complication may be increasing in frequency[58] because of the increasing incidence of previous cesarean sections.

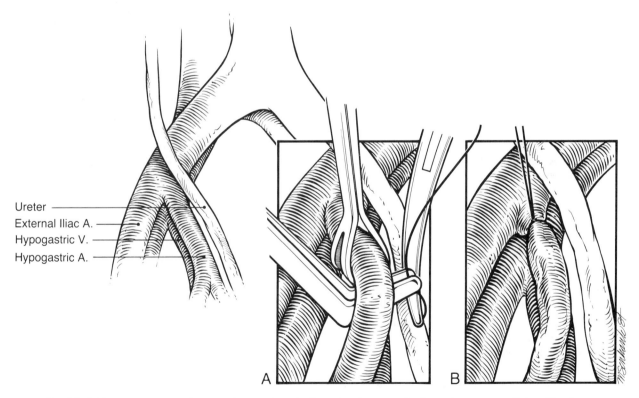

Ureter
External Iliac A.
Hypogastric V.
Hypogastric A.

A   B

Fig. 20.7 Hypogastric artery ligation. Approach to the hypogastric artery via the peritoneum, parallel and just lateral to the ovarian vessels, exposing the interior surface of the posterior layer of the broad ligament. The ureter will be found attached to the medial leaf of the broad ligament. The bifurcation of the common iliac artery into its external and internal (hypogastric) branches is exposed by blunt dissection of the loose overlying areolar tissues. Identification of these structures is essential. (A,B) To avoid traumatizing the underlying hypogastric vein, the hypogastric artery is elevated by means of a Babcock clamp before passing an angled clamp to catch a free tie. (Adapted from Breen et al.,[196] with permission.)

If the accreta is focal and the patient desires future pregnancies, it may be possible to excise the site of trophoblastic invasion, over-sewing bleeding areas with several figure-of-eight sutures. If that is not possible, hysterectomy should be initiated. A complete hysterectomy will usually be required because a placenta accreta commonly involves the lower uterine segment, and, in such cases, a supracervical hysterectomy will not be effective in controlling the bleeding.

Drainage of the Abdominal Incision

The purpose of the drain is to remove the bacterial growth media that can act as a site of infection and reduce potential spaces within the wound. There are few indications for prophylactic drainage, because cesarean delivery is a relatively "short" procedure and operative time and tissue devitalization are ordinarily not an issue. Prophylactic drainage is most commonly employed in situations in which there is an expectation of fluid accumulation in association with likely contamination of the wound, particularly in obese patients.[83] Therapeutic drainage is seldom, if ever, indicated with cesarean delivery or cesarean hysterectomy unless there is a coincidental abscess. Should an abscess be encountered, a continuous suction drain should be inserted via a separate stab wound at a site away from the incision.[84] In some instances in which there is a suspicion of heavy contamination, particularly in morbidly obese patients, it may be better to plan secondary wound closure, as opposed to drainage.

Extraperitoneal Cesarean Delivery

Extraperitoneal cesarean section (Fig. 20.8) is mentioned largely for historical purposes. In the era prior to antibiotics, extraperitoneal cesarean delivery was an alternative to cesarean hysterectomy as a means to reduce the risk of infection in patients with chorioamnionitis; Frank[11] and Latzko[12] were prominent early proponents. The operation differs from the more commonly employed modern procedures in that an effort is made to avoid penetrating the peritoneum. The uterus is approached through the space of Retzius, exposing one lateral aspect of the lower uterus and bladder. The bladder is then dissected from its lateral approximation to the anterior surface of the lower uterus and retracted so as to expose the lower uterine segment. Although this procedure is seldom done today, there remain advocates for its use.[85] One prospective study comparing three groups (extraperitoneal cesarean delivery without antibiotic prophylaxis versus extraperitoneal cesarean delivery with antibiotic prophylaxis versus transperitoneal cesarean section with antibiotic prophylaxis) found that extraperitoneal cesarean delivery was not as effective as systemic prophylactic antibiotics in the prevention of postoperative endomyometritis.[86]

POSTMORTEM CESAREAN SECTION

Postmortem cesarean section originated with the Catholic Church, which mandated its performance to accomplish baptism. In 1747, the King of Sicily condemned a physician to death for not performing a postmortem cesarean section.[87] Obstetric texts continued to discuss the possibility of postmortem cesarean section, despite rather dismal success and considerable debate among noted clinicians. If a postmortem cesarean delivery is anticipated, successful perinatal outcome will depend on preexisting fetal status and on the knowledge that death can be reliably anticipated in the near future. There are a number of determinants that favorably affect outcome. They include (1) a gestational age compatible with fetal survival, (2) delivery within 10 minutes of cessation of maternal circulation, (3) prompt availability of appropriately trained staff and equipment, and (4) access to personnel capable of neonatal resuscitation. Unfortunately, in many instances it is not possible to provide one or more of the above, and for this reason, outcome is often poor.

Katz et al.[88] described 269 cases of postmortem cesarean births between 1879 and 1986 in the English literature. Only 188 infants survived. In recent history, normal survival following postmortem cesarean section has been primarily limited to instances in which the baby was delivered within 5 minutes after maternal death. The likelihood of a normal outcome decreased to approximately 10 to 15 percent in the 6- to 15-minute interval and to less than 15 percent at 16 or more minutes after death. The current consen-

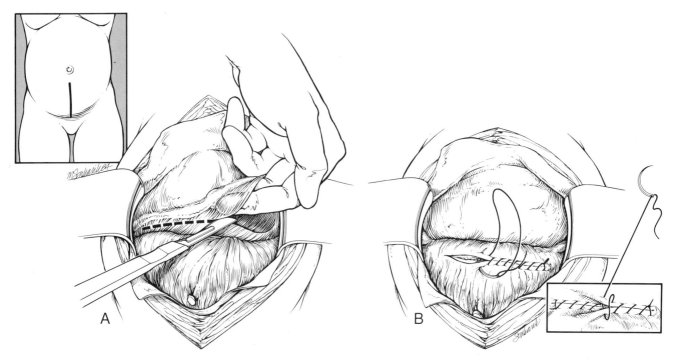

Fig. 20.8 Waters extraperitoneal section. (A) One step in the Waters operation is illustrated. The transversalis fascia has been opened and the vesical peritoneum separated from the muscularis of the bladder dome by sharp dissection. At this point, the uterovesical fold of bladder peritoneum is isolated and is being cut free to expose the lower uterine segment. (B) A successful dissection has left the lower uterine segment widely exposed without having entered the peritoneal cavity. The remainder of the operation is similar to a low transverse cesarean section, except that it will not be necessary to close either a bladder flap or the peritoneum.

sus is that postmortem cesarean birth may be performed at any time that a viable fetus or the potential for one exists, even without the consent of a family member.[88] Thus the current recommendation is that, if clinically possible, a postmortem section should be begun within 4 to 5 minutes after initiation of cardiopulmonary resuscitation for cardiac arrest. Delivery will also diminish uterine compression of the inferior vena cava in the supine position. For this reason, delivery of the fetus may actually increase the effectiveness of cardiopulmonary resuscitation.

There are limited data with which to assess the ability of modern life-support equipment to maintain the mother for an extended period. A recent case report described a mother supported for 10 weeks to gain time for fetal maturation.[89]

PREOPERATIVE AND INTRAOPERATIVE FLUID GUIDELINES

Extracellular (interstitial and intravascular) water constitutes approximately one-third of total body water and 20 percent of total body weight. Ordinary daily physiologic fluid needs approximate 2,000 to 2,500 ml. In the pregnant patient, daily physiologic fluid losses are estimated to be 1,000 ml in excess of urinary output and include urinary output (800 to 1,500 ml), insensible loss (800 ml) from both skin and lungs, and stool loss (200 ml). Insensible loss in the laboring patient can be considerably greater.

Because insensible fluid loss increases significantly in the laboring patient, the woman about to undergo a cesarean section for CPD may be quite dehydrated. She may have had little fluid intake since the onset of labor and have increased fluid loss due to the physical exertion and rapid breathing movements associated with labor. The bleeding patient or the patient about to receive epidural anesthesia is particularly sensitive to the effects of dehydration.

There will be little problem with dehydration if intravenous fluid intake has been maintained at 100 to 125 ml per hour. Should this not be the case, fluid losses can be estimated based on the average hourly need (100 to 125 ml) times the cumulative number of hours since the time of last fluid intake. Adjustments, which may vary from center to center, should be made for ice chips and other fluid intake. An additional intravenous fluid load is required prior to the administration of epidural anesthesia.

Intravenous Fluids Commonly Used:

1. Sodium chloride (0.9 percent isotonic saline) is an isotonic solution containing 310 mOsm. This solution is commonly used to expand plasma volume as well as to correct mild degrees of hyponatremia.
2. Lactated Ringer's solution is also an isotonic solution, containing multiple electrolytes in a concentration similar to that found in human plasma. This solution is also used to expand plasma volume and may be preferable to isotonic saline during the first 24 postoperative hours.
3. Sodium chloride 0.45 percent is a hypotonic (half normal) solution that is useful in the provision of postoperative fluid needs after the first 24 hours, when volume expansion is no longer needed.

Fluid and Electrolyte Replacement

Should the patient be only mildly hypovolemic in the first 24 hours, normal isotonic saline or Ringer's lactate solution in 5 percent dextrose are preferable to more hypotonic solutions because there is greater retention of fluids in the intravascular space providing volume expansion. In contrast, infusion of a 5 percent dextrose in water solution will result in distri-

bution of fluid evenly throughout all water spaces, two-thirds being in the intracellular space. Should hypovolemia be more significant, particularly in association with low intravascular colloid osmotic pressure, administration of an albumin-containing solution may minimize the effects of loss of fluids into the interstitial space. Under such circumstances, it may on occasion be advisable to employ a central venous pressure line or a Swan-Ganz catheter.

Special Considerations for Preoperative Fluids

Some patients such as those with vomiting, diarrhea, or fever may require additional fluids. The presence of a fever may increase the need for intravenous fluid replacement, generally on the order of 15 percent above basal levels for every degree centigrade above normal body temperature.[90]

Intraoperative Fluids

Fluid needs during surgery are generally determined by the anesthesiologist or nurse anesthetist and are largely directed to the replacement of blood loss, insensible losses, and urinary output. In general, isotonic solutions are used to maintain adequate circulating blood volume. Actual blood or plasma replacement is rarely needed during cesarean section.

Intraoperative fluid requirements, apart from blood replacement, range from 500 to 1,000 ml per hour, up to a maximum of 3 L in a 4-hour interval under ordinary surgical conditions. Such replacement is associated with a low incidence of renal failure and pulmonary edema in instances in which there has been obstetric hemorrhage.[91]

POSTOPERATIVE COMPLICATIONS

Maternal Morbidity and Mortality

The reported incidence of maternal morbidity and mortality following cesarean delivery varies greatly from series to series, but is consistently severalfold higher than that following vaginal delivery. The increase in part is a result of the complications that required the cesarean delivery and in part is a result of the risk associated with any surgical procedure. Nonetheless, even when morbidity and mortality arising from the indication leading to cesarean delivery have been excluded, maternal morbidity remains severalfold higher for cesarean section than for vaginal delivery.[92] It is important to remember that data describing morbidity for a primary cesarean section do not include the consideration of long-term consequences such as the need for repeat cesarean births.

In a review of approximately 400,000 cesarean births performed between 1965 and 1978, maternal death occurred in 1 in 1,635 procedures.[4] In that series, approximately one-half of the deaths were attributable to the procedure. In another series, Sachs et al.[93] reviewed 121,000 cesarean births performed in Massachusetts from 1976 to 1984; seven (5.8 per 100,000) of 27 total deaths (22 per 100,000) arose as a result of the procedure itself. Lower rates have been described, the most remarkable being in the Boston Hospital for Women study that reported no maternal mortality in 10,231 cesarean deliveries.[94]

Major sources of morbidity and associated mortality relate to complications of maternal sepsis, anesthesia, and thromboembolic disease and its complications. Each has been discussed in Chapters 16 and 40. Much has been done in recent years to reduce the impact of anesthesia-related mortality largely through increased availability of qualified anesthesia personnel and the implementation of rigid protocols, including routine use of antacids prior to cesarean delivery, as well as routine protocols for intubation. Other common causes of morbidity arising from cesarean delivery include hemorrhage and injury to the urinary tract.[95,96]

Endomyometritis

Postpartum infection is the most frequent complication arising from cesarean delivery. Should prophylactic antibiotics not be used, the incidence of postcesarean endomyometritis varies from as low as 5 to 10 percent to as high as 70 to 85 percent, with a mean of 35 to 40 percent in most series.[97,98] The rate is largely dependent on socioeconomic status and whether the cesarean delivery is a primary procedure. The lowest incidence occurs in middle- and upper-income women undergoing a scheduled cesarean delivery; the highest occurs in the young indigent patient undergoing primary cesarean delivery after an extended labor and prolonged membrane rupture. Age and socioeconomic status may influence the incidence of infection because they reflect general health and host

immunocompetence. The other major risk factors include length of labor, duration of membrane rupture, and number of vaginal examinations. These factors exert their effects by influencing the size of the bacterial inoculum. Other weaker risk factors include length of surgery, preoperative hematocrit, intraoperative blood loss, duration of internal fetal monitoring, experience of the surgeon, and type of anesthesia.

Prior to the advent of modern broad-spectrum antibiotics with activity against both anaerobic and aerobic gram-negative bacilli, the incidence of severe complications arising from endomyometritis was as high as 4 to 5 percent.[99,100] When blood cultures were obtained, the frequency of associated bacteremia was approximately 10 percent.[97,99] Prophylactic antibiotics at the time of cesarean delivery reduce the postoperative infection rate to approximately 5 percent.[99,100] With the advent of modern antibiotics the incidence of life-threatening complications, including pelvic abscess, septic shock and septic pelvic thrombophlebitis, is now less than 2 percent.

Microbiology

Endomyometritis is a polymicrobial infection that is almost always caused by bacteria arising from the lower genital tract. There are four major groups of principal pathogens: aerobic streptococci, anaerobic gram-positive cocci, and aerobic and anaerobic gram-negative bacilli.[97] In some cases *Mycoplasma hominis* and *Chlamydia* can cause intrauterine infection.[101] Microorganisms most frequently recovered from patients with bacteremia include *E. coli*, group B streptococci, *Bacteroides* species, anaerobic gram-positive cocci, and *Gardnerella vaginalis*. *M. hominis* has also been isolated.[102,103]

Clinical Diagnosis

Endomyometritis is commonly suspected following cesarean delivery when the patient demonstrates a temperature of at least 100.4°F, associated in many instances with tachycardia, lower abdominal pain, uterine and, in some cases, adnexal tenderness above that ordinarily experienced with a cesarean incision, and lower abdominal peritoneal irritation. These systems and signs usually develop 24 to 48 hours following cesarean delivery. The onset may be relatively earlier with group B streptococci. In most instances, the diagnosis is made by exclusion after considering the differential diagnosis of breast infection, urinary tract infection, and atelectasis if the procedure was performed under general anesthesia.

Laboratory Evaluation

In most instances, the initial work-up is limited to clinical history and physical examination plus evaluation of the differential white cell blood count, hematocrit, and urinalysis to rule out urinary tract infection. Should the clinical impression be endomyometritis, many physicians will not obtain cultures. Although blood cultures can be drawn for aerobic and anaerobic organisms, it is quite difficult to attain a reliable culture specifically from the endometrial cavity. Use of a double-lumen catheter (Meditech, Watertown, MA) that contains a small biopsy brush[104] decreases the likelihood of contamination by normal endocervical canal and upper vaginal bacterial flora. In some circumstances, pelvic ultrasound or a computed tomographic scan of the pelvis, and on occasion of the abdomen, may be of value should an abscess or ovarian vein thrombosis be suspected.

Therapy

Once the diagnosis of endomyometritis is established, antibiotic therapy can be initiated with one of the following regimens: clindamycin plus an aminoglycoside; an extended-spectrum cephalosporin (Moxalactam, Cefotetan, Cefoxitin, or Cefotaxime); an extended-spectrum penicillin, or a metronidazole-penicillin-aminoglycoside combination. Should the patient be seriously ill, the combination of clindamycin plus gentamicin is preferable. If the patient received cephalosporin prophylaxis, treatment with a penicillin may be a better choice because enterococci may be one of the predominant organisms. Parenteral antibiotic therapy should generally be continued for at least 24 hours following the return to a normal temperature and resolution of symptoms. Subsequent to this point, Duff[105] believes that therapy may be discontinued. Oral antibiotic therapy is not required.

Most patients will respond rather promptly by 72 hours. If there has not been a reasonable response to antibiotics, the differential diagnosis should include resistant microorganisms, mastitis, infected retained products of conception, a wound infection or pelvic abscess, and septic pelvic thrombophlebitis. Even appendicitis should occasionally be considered, particularly if the discomfort is unilateral. Collagen vascular disease, drug fever, and factitious fever are other potential considerations.[97] On occasion, the infection may spread outside the uterine cavity, leading to parametritis and, rarely, to septic pelvic thrombophlebitis and peritonitis.

Should a wound infection be identified, it should be incised and drained; however, it is not necessary to change antibiotics. If the clinical impression is bacterial resistance, antibiotic therapy should be modified. In the absence of a wound infection, the principal microorganisms likely to be resistant to initial treatment are the aerobic gram-negative bacilli, enterococci, and *Bacteroides* species. Penicillin should be added to the treatment regimen to provide coverage against enterococci if the patient is receiving clindamycin plus an aminoglycoside. If the patient is receiving single-agent therapy, one can change treatment to clindamycin plus penicillin and an aminoglycoside *or* simply add an aminoglycoside to improve coverage of aerobic gram-negative bacilli. When improved coverage of anaerobes is desired, clindamycin or metronidazole should be used.

Wound Complications

Risk Factors for Poor Wound Healing and Wound Infection

Identifiable medical risk factors that increase the likelihood of poor wound healing include diabetes mellitus and malnutrition. Surgical risk factors to be considered are the duration of surgery, the use of drains, the suture material chosen, and the closure technique employed. Postoperative factors include asthma, pulmonary complications and associated coughing, and vomiting.[106,107] In rare cases, other risk factors such as ascites, long-term corticosteroid therapy, anemia, or prior irradiation may exist.

Wound infection rates following cesarean delivery vary according to patient population from 2.5 to 16.1 percent.[106] Determinants include local wound conditions and patient host resistance. Infection rates will vary according to whether the cesarean delivery is performed as an elective repeat procedure with intact membranes or follows labor, particularly with ruptured membranes. Risk factors for wound infection interact in a complex manner, making it difficult to determine the independent contribution of any one factor.

Many studies demonstrate a substantial increase in wound infections with increasing duration of membrane rupture, long labors, and more frequent vaginal examinations.[108-111] Amnionitis and possibly meconium passage are additional risk factors. Up to 75 percent of amniotic fluid cultures done at the time of primary cesarean delivery are positive, with an average of 3.5 organisms, 44 percent being highly virulent bacteria.[112] Flora isolated from amniotic fluid and wound infections exist in a synergistic system of aerobes and anaerobes similar to the situation with endometritis. *S. aureus, E. coli, Proteus mirabilis, Bacteroides* species, and *group B streptococci* are common isolates; clostridial species are infrequent.[113] Even in the absence of ruptured membranes, patients in preterm labor with unrecognized chorioamnionitis may have pathogens consistent with bowel flora.[114]

Methods to Reduce Wound Infection

Some determinants of wound infection (diabetes mellitus, amnionitis, obesity, and alcoholism) are to a large degree beyond the control of the obstetrician. However, the obstetrician who knows the potential risk factors does have the option to employ a number of measures selectively to minimize the risk of wound infection and wound breakdown. These measures include (1) clipping hair in the incision site (as opposed to shaving pubic and abdominal hair), if the abdomen is prepared the night prior to surgery; (2) preoperative skin preparation, including careful cleansing of the umbilicus and abdomen prior to surgery; (3) sterile technique; (4) wound hemostasis; (5) selective use of prophylactic antibiotics; (6) avoidance of unnecessary suture material, particularly in the patient at risk for a wound infection or breakdown; (7) closed-system drainage if the patient is obese or the wound is "wet" in the absence of an obvious bleeder as opposed to open Penrose drains; (8) skin closure with suture rather than a skin stapler; and (9) delayed wound closure if the wound is grossly contaminated by bowel contents.

Although it is difficult to determine the magnitude of preventable wound infections, Emmons et al.[115] suggest that the approximately 25 percent of wound infections that are associated with *S. aureus* represent a potentially preventable condition that presumably arises from exogenous sources. Sixty (5.4 percent) consecutive wound infections were studied among 1,104 women undergoing cesarean delivery. Wound infections caused by cervical–vaginal flora were associated with prolonged labor, particularly with greater duration of FHR monitoring; with more frequent vaginal examinations; and with organisms isolated from the endometrium at cesarean section. In contrast, women with wound infections caused by *S. aureus* had neither prolonged labor nor *S. aureus* isolated at cesarean delivery.[115]

When closing the wound, a balance must be maintained between adequate hemostasis and significant tissue devitalization. Excessive use of electrocautery may result in unnecessary tissue damage and reduced host resistance. Seroma or hematoma formation reduces tissue oxygen tension and phagocyte penetration. Tissues should be carefully reapproximated without major tension. Unnecessarily tight placement of sutures may interfere with adequate tissue oxygenation, which is essential to bacterial phagocytosis.[116]

Morbid obesity is a risk factor for wound infection, regardless of the degree of contamination and length of the procedure.[117] Adipose tissue is relatively fragile and tends to heal relatively poorly. As a result, careful handling of the subcutaneous tissue is important. However, there is uncertainty as to the best surgical approach. Gallup[51] recommends a midline incision, a superficial closed suction drain, a nonabsorbable monofilament fascial closure with a Smead-Jones technique, and avoidance of subcutaneous suture. Others favor a transverse incision.[118] The recommendation to avoid subcutaneous suture is based on the observation that the suture material acts as an additional foreign body in a wound that is already predisposed to infection.

Management of Wound Infection

If fever develops in the postoperative period, careful inspection of the wound will often lead to early diagnosis and treatment. Diagnosis of a wound infection is relatively obvious in the febrile patient if the wound is inflamed and indurated, or if drainage of purulent material is observed on palpation. Should an infection be found, the involved area must be opened to allow drainage and debrided to clean the wound margins. A Gram stain and culture for anaerobic and aerobic organisms should be obtained and systemic antibiotics employed to cover the anticipated organisms within the wound. Culturing tissue debris from the wound improves the isolation of anaerobic organisms. Once the infection is controlled, the surgeon must then decide between the inconvenience for the patient associated with healing by secondary intention versus the risk of recurrent infection should secondary closure be elected.

Fascial Dehiscence

Dehiscence of a wound through the fascia is infrequent, occurring in approximately 5 percent of wound infections.[111] Dehiscence is suggested by the presence of a large amount of discharge from the wound. If loops of small bowel protrude through the incision, the small bowel should be immediately covered with wet sterile dressings and emergency closure performed in the operating room. The wound should be opened and inspected in the operating room under sterile conditions. If a dehiscence is confirmed, the wound should be cleansed, debrided and closed with either Smead-Jones or retention sutures (Fig. 20.6).

Sonography as Potential Diagnostic Aid

Resistance to antibiotic therapy may be an indication for sonography or other imaging techniques (Figs. 20.9 to 20.11) to rule out retained uterine products, as well as seromas, hematomas, or abscesses in the abdominal wall, pelvis, or occasionally the uterine incision. While sonography offers immediate evaluation of the pelvis in the patient resistant to therapy, computed tomography (CT) may be preferable in some cases because it allows complete assessment of the entire peritoneal cavity and may identify fresh hemorrhage within a fluid collection as well as ovarian vein thrombosis. Sonography with a 5- or 7-mHz short-focus transducer also allows detailed examination of the abdominal wall for seromas, hematomas, and abscesses. The sonogram may be normal in the presence of a wound infection. Abscesses commonly present as complex, predominantly cystic masses, occasionally containing fluid levels. A complete examination of the abdomen including the subphrenic space may on occasion reveal a subphrenic abscess; however, these are often difficult to visualize, particularly if there are multiple small abscesses. Scanning the patient in different positions may facilitate more

adequate visualization of the subphrenic space. Care should be taken not to mistake the accumulation of subdiaphragmatic fluid for a pleural effusion in the patient with severe preeclampsia. On occasion, a subcapsular liver hematoma may be observed. Sonography may occasionally be difficult in the presence of bowel distention, particularly with the usual placement of the abdominal incision. However, sonography permits the evaluation of peristalsis at the site of a fluid-filled structure (bowel) and, where indicated, may facilitate sonographically guided percutaneous aspiration of a suspected abscess.[119]

By the first postpartum day, the uterus will be at or below the level of the umbilicus. On ultrasound, the uterine wall thickness will vary from 3 to 6.5 cm, being slightly thicker in multiparous patients as compared with primiparas.[120] The uterine wall ordinarily appears homogenous with an occasional subtle irregularity.[121] The endometrial cavity often presents as a slit whose anterior/posterior diameter varies from 0.5 to 1.3 cm.[120] The uterine incision may present a variable sonographic appearance following cesarean section.[122] Strong echoes may arise from the suture material. It is not unusual to see small seromas and hematomas of the uterine incision under the bladder flap. Should a significant fluid collection be observed around the uterine incision in a febrile patient, an abscess should be considered (Fig. 20.9).

When a postpartum abdominal ultrasound examination is performed, the patient should have a full bladder. This will facilitate displacement of the normal anteflexed puerperal uterus posteriorly, positioning the endometrial cavity at right angles to the sound waves and improving visualization.[123] In addition, bladder filling will frequently push any gas-filled loops of bowel out of the pelvis, thus facilitating visualization of the cul-de-sac, adnexa, and uterus. Transvaginal scanning may be helpful if the abdomen is distended, the incision site interferes with adequate abdominal imaging, or the patient is unable to tolerate the pressure of abdominal scanning.

Sonographic findings suggesting endometritis may include a dilated fluid- or gas-filled uterine cavity and fluid in the cul-de-sac. Sonographic evidence of an empty uterus will eliminate the possibility of retained products. However, an abnormal scan may represent either the normal retention of blood or retained products of conception.[124] Abscesses may present

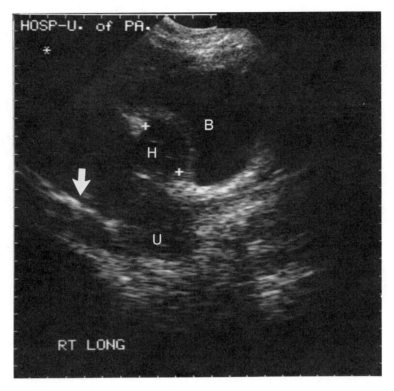

Fig. 20.9 Ultrasound of infected bladder flap hematoma marked by cursors (+). The patient presented approximately 1 week after cesarean delivery with fever. She responded to antibiotics. Note that the full bladder (B) enhances visualization of the hematoma (H). The arrow designates the endometrial cavity of the uterus (U).

with characteristic fluid and gas collections, shaggy walls, and internal echoes in association with cul-de-sac fluid accumulations indicating peritonitis. If gas is detected on sonogram, gas-forming organisms such as *E. coli* or *Clostridium perfringens* may be present. CT may be used to diagnose ovarian vein thrombophlebitis.[125]

Urinary Complications

Urinary tract infections are second to endomyometritis as a cause of postcesarean febrile morbidity. The reported incidence varies from as low as 2 percent to as high as 16 percent.[126] In one study, approximately 7 percent of postoperative clean-catch urine specimens had at least 10^5 bacteria per milliliter in culture. One percent of patients had both bacteriuria and endomyometritis.[127] Urethral catheterization contributes to 80 percent of nosocomial urinary tract infections in hospitalized patients, particularly when indwelling catheters are used. The incidence is increased with longer duration of catheter use, in diabetic patients and in patients who are critically ill.[128] Attention to detail in terms of proper preparation and insertion of the catheter and use of a closed drainage system have decreased this risk.

Gastrointestinal Complications

Most patients undergoing cesarean section have little if any gastrointestinal problems postoperatively. However, anesthesia and narcotics employed to treat postoperative pain may contribute to bowel dysfunction. As a result, an occasional patient may have postoperative nausea or mild transient abdominal distention in the first 24 hours.

Ileus should be suspected if prolonged nausea or vomiting together with signs such as abdominal distention, absence of bowel sounds, and failure to pass flatus are persistent. Distended loops of bowel with or without air fluid levels on x-ray will provide confirmatory evidence. In most instances simply withholding

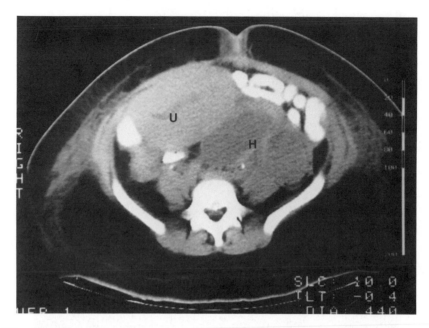

Fig. 20.10 CT scan of pelvis 6 days after a cesarean section showing left-sided broad ligament hematoma (H). The uterus (U) is displaced to the right. The patient responded to antibiotics. (Courtesy of Dr. Michael Blumenfeld, Department of Obstetrics and Gynecology, Ohio State University, Columbus, OH.)

oral intake, adequate fluid replacement, and observations is sufficient. If the ileus is persistent, nasogastric suction may be required.

Actual mechanical bowel obstruction may initially present as an ileus, but is commonly associated with peristaltic rushes and high-pitched bowel sounds in conjunction with symptoms of nausea, vomiting, and abdominal distension. Once again, some patients will respond to conservative management, including restriction of oral intake, placement of a nasogastric tube, or possibly even a long tube. The key to success is maintenance of not only fluids and electrolytes but also of hematocrit and serum protein. Should conservative therapy fail, surgical consultation and possible exploration may be required.

Thromboembolic Disorders

The risk of thrombosis increases during pregnancy because of both higher levels of coagulation factors and diminished fibrinolysis. These changes peak near term and immediately after delivery. Deep venous thrombophlebitis (DVT) of the lower extremities occurs in approximately 0.24 percent of all deliveries.[129,130] The risk of DVT after cesarean delivery is approximately three to five times greater than after vaginal delivery.[131] Compounding risk factors include obesity, inability to ambulate, advanced maternal age, and higher parity. Should the DVT go untreated, approximately 15 to 25 percent of patients will develop pulmonary emboli and 15 percent will sustain a fatal pulmonary embolus (PE). However, if recognized early and treated appropriately, the risks of PE and death are reduced to 4.5 and 0.7 percent, respectively.[130,132]

Classic symptoms for DVT include unilateral leg pain, tenderness and swelling. A 2-cm difference in leg circumference between the affected and normal limb is generally required for diagnosis. Other clinical signs include edema, a palpable cord, and a change in limb color. A positive Homan's sign (calf pain on passive dorsiflexion of the foot) or a positive Lowenberg test (pain distal to the site of rapid inflation of a blood pressure cuff to 100 mmHg) suggests DVT.

Unfortunately, the first sign of DVT may be the occurrence of a PE, which may present with symp-

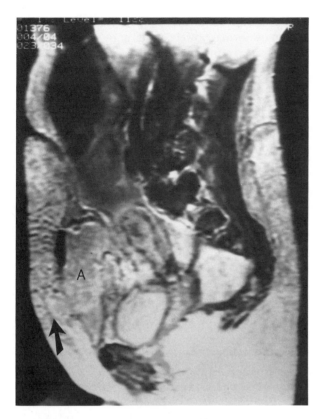

Fig. 20.11 MRI scan of abdominal wall abscess. This patient presented 1 week after a cesarean section with fever and an abdominal mass. The differential diagnosis included an intraperitoneal infection with extension or a wound abscess. This MRI shows a wound abscess (A) above fascia that extended to the abdominal wall (arrow). The abscess responded to drainage and antibiotics.

is sensitive in approximately 95 percent of proximal thromboses, but is not as effective as Doppler for pelvic vessel thrombosis and will generally identify most cases, especially above the calves. Should Doppler and IPG be inconclusive, ascending venography, the most accurate of the three tests, should be performed. IPG can be used as a first-line test postpartum in the non-lactating mother. Should PE be suspected, a baseline arterial blood gas, chest x-ray, and electrocardiogram, as well as prothrombin time and partial thromboplastin time, should be obtained. Oxygen therapy should also be administered. Once the diagnosis has been established, heparin therapy should be started (see Ch. 31).

Septic Pelvic Thrombophlebitis

Approximately 0.5 to 2 percent of patients with endomyometritis or wound infection will develop septic pelvic thrombophlebitis,[135] a more common complication of cesarean section than of vaginal delivery. In large part, this is a result of the higher rate of endomyometritis in patients undergoing cesarean delivery. Largely a diagnosis of exclusion, septic pelvic thrombophlebitis occurs most commonly on the right side and may be suspected should there be fever and unilateral pain. Although tenderness about the incision site may make detection difficult, occasionally one will be able to palpate a tender, rope-like abdominal mass extending laterally and cephalad from the uterus. Sonographic examination of the lower abdomen and pelvis or computed tomography may be of assistance in the diagnosis (see Fig. 40.21).

POSTOPERATIVE MANAGEMENT

Postoperative Analgesia

Analgesia should be provided in a dose and frequency that will neither obtund nor cause respiratory depression and yet allow the patient (1) to avoid the consequences of extremes in analgesic blood levels resulting in unnecessary pain and (2) to cooperate with normal postoperative management. The patient receiving inadequate analgesia may, in an effort to protect her wound, maintain a shallow breathing pattern without deep breaths and, hence, develop atelectasis.[136]

toms of tachypnea (90 percent), dyspnea (80 percent), pleuritic chest pain with or without splinting (> 70 percent), apprehension (approximately 60 percent), tachycardia (40 percent), and cough (> 50 percent).[133,134] Other findings include atelectatic rales, a friction rub, accentuated second heart sound, or a gallop. Patient evaluation is complicated in the post-cesarean section patient, since splinting from incisional pain and tachypnea are not unusual findings. Doppler studies have a sensitivity of 90 percent for popliteal, femoral, or iliac thromboses, but only 50 percent for calf involvement because of abundant collateral vessels. Impedance plethysmography (IPG)

Commonly employed analgesics include meperidine (50–75 mg) or morphine (10 mg, depending on maternal size) administered intravenously or intramuscularly every 3 to 4 hours. Intrathecal or epidural narcotic administration employed with agents such as morphine can also be used for postoperative anesthesia, which may last as long as 30 hours following delivery, providing an advantage to a patient who has undergone a regional block.[137]

Ambulation

Early ambulation is important in reinstitution of inflation of the most dependent alveoli and the prevention of pulmonary complications, particularly in the patient who has had general anesthesia. Early ambulation also promotes the return of normal urinary and bowel activity. Under most circumstances, the uncomplicated patient can be allowed to sit up within 8 to 12 hours following cesarean section, even after epidural anesthesia.

The patient generally can ambulate within the first day after surgery. By the second day she can shower without fear of injury to the incision. Depending on complications and availability of care at home, hospital discharge may occur by the third to fifth postpartum day. The mother's activities at home for the first week should be limited to personal care and to care of the newborn. By the third to fourth week, the patient can generally resume most activities at home.

Oral Intake

Active bowel sounds are commonly not observed until the second postoperative day. Nonetheless, in most instances the patient will easily tolerate oral fluids the day after surgery. Only rarely, when the patient has been septic or there has been extensive intra-abdominal manipulation, will there be a need to withhold oral fluids, even though the patient may have diminished bowel sounds and not pass gas. Most clinicians feel comfortable in providing clear liquids and ice chips with only a small amount of liquid as soon as nausea subsides to relieve complaints of a dry mouth. The progression of the diet also varies according to clinician. Some advance the patient rapidly to a regular diet, whereas others institute a progression to a full liquid diet by 48 hours, awaiting the return of normal bowel sounds and passage of flatus to indicate return of colonic function. Few wait beyond the third postoperative day to institute a regular diet.

Bladder Management

The urinary catheter is ordinarily removed within 12 to 24 hours following surgery unless there have been intraoperative complications.

Postoperative Wound Care

The incision is generally covered for the first day with a light dressing, until the wound is sealed. The dressing is removed after the first postoperative day.

Laboratory Studies

Blood loss arising from an uncomplicated cesarean delivery is approximately 1,000 ml.[138] As a consequence, the postoperative hematocrit may be expected to change by approximately 2 to 3 percent during the initial 2 days following surgery, independent of hydration status.

Postoperative Fluids

The normal postpartum period is generally characterized by mobilization of the physiologic accumulation of fluid during pregnancy. As a consequence, large volumes of intravenous fluids are seldom required after cesarean delivery. In the low-risk patient. fluid replacement needs during a 24-hour interval are generally only 1,000 ml above urinary output. Three liters of a salt-containing solution will thus generally suffice during the first 24 hours unless urinary output falls below 30 ml per hour. Under certain circumstances there may be increased requirements for fluids: following prolonged labor, febrile illness, vomiting, diarrhea, or even prior use of diuretics or salt restriction. Additional needs may be required in more complex patients. Potassium is ordinarily not needed during the first 24 hours in uncomplicated patients because of intracellular potassium release from cell destruction. After the first 24 hours, intravenous fluid replacement with 5 percent dextrose in 0.45 percent sodium chloride is commonly employed, unless volume expansion is an issue. If it is anticipated that the patient will require prolonged intravenous fluids, potassium may be administered as 60 to 80 mEq/day. Should the patient be oliguric, potassium is generally not given until the patient has normal urinary output.

REDUCING THE CURRENT CESAREAN SECTION RATE

A concerted effort should be made to reduce the current cesarean section rate. Cesarean births increase health-care costs and pose considerable additional risk for maternal morbidity with only marginal proven fetal benefits. Although it is likely that a proportion of the increase in cesarean delivery is justified, it is also likely that the primary rate can be decreased in a selective manner for certain indications. If physicians are truly to impact on repeat cesarean deliveries, they must make an effort to limit primary cesarean sections. In 1980 the National Institutes of Health sponsored a Consensus Development Conference to consider the issue of cesarean delivery in the United States.[19] That conference recommended that efforts be made to diminish the impact of elective repeat cesarean delivery and the diagnosis of "dystocia" because these two indications had contributed a major proportion of the recent cesarean section cases. Bottoms et al.[139] have concluded that cesarean delivery for dystocia and repeat cesarean deliveries should be points of primary review. If primary indications are more tightly controlled, the number of candidates for repeat cesarean section will be reduced accordingly. Management alternatives that may reduce the cesarean section rate include VBAC, a more rational approach to the management of dystocia, better markers of intrapartum fetal condition, external version of the breech or transverse lie, and selective vaginal delivery of the breech presentation.

Indirect Indicators of Room for Improvement

Blumenthal et al.[140] noted a significant difference between the incidence of dystocia in public versus private patients and concluded that the difference was probably the result of differences in indications employed in the two groups. The issue is a complex one. The etiology of differences in cesarean birth rates is as yet unresolved and probably multifactorial. While it has been suggested that physician convenience may be operative in the decision process to perform cesarean sections in private patients, Phillips et al.[141] were unable to demonstrate the predictable distribution of nonscheduled cesarean births that would support this hypothesis.

Indications Susceptible to Reduction

Repeat cesarean sections currently constitute 30 to 40 percent of cesarean births. The cesarean section rate rose 44 percent between 1978 and 1984, and 47 percent of the rise was due to the performance of elective repeat cesarean deliveries.[2] Fortunately, the VBAC concept is gaining more widespread acceptance. Recently the American College of Obstetricians and Gynecologists (ACOG) released guidelines indicating that women with one prior transverse cesarean section should be counseled to undergo a trial of labor. That recommendation acknowledged that neither oxytocin for induction or augmentation nor epidural anesthesia are contraindicated.

There is also likely to be significant room for improvement in the current cesarean delivery rate for CPD. The lower cesarean section rate in the Dublin series is largely attributable to a lower rate for dystocia. O'Driscoll et al.[142] conclude that much of their success in maintaining a low cesarean section rate is attributable to aggressive utilization of oxytocin in nulliparous patients as well as greater use of VBAC and liberal criteria for vaginal breech deliveries. There is also likely to be significant room for improvement in the current rate of cesarean births for the breech presentation and nonreassuring FHR patterns during labor. Although vaginal delivery can be justified in up to 50 percent of term breech presentations, cesarean births for breech constitute only 10 to 15 percent of all cesarean deliveries, and thus a 50 percent reduction is not likely to have a major impact on the overall cesarean section rate.

VAGINAL BIRTH AFTER CESAREAN SECTION

In the United States, approximately 10 percent of women who deliver will have had a prior cesarean delivery. Anderson and Lomas concluded that elective repeat cesarean delivery was responsible for two-thirds of the increase in cesarean deliveries in their community between 1979 and 1982 and suggested that a reduction in the cesarean birth rate can be achieved only by addressing the self-perpetuating contribution of the indication of previous cesarean birth.[143] Few changes within the specialty of obstetrics and gynecology offer greater potential impact to more women than that of VBAC.

The previously held concept of "once a cesarean, always a cesarean" is no longer mandated. Should a trial of labor be offered to this group, more than 50 percent of patients will achieve a successful vaginal delivery, thus offering the hope of vaginal delivery to an additional 5 percent of all gravidas. The potential financial impact of a successful national VBAC program is approximately one-half billion dollars savings, if one assumes a repeat cesarean section rate of only 6 percent and 3.4 million births.[144]

Despite early reports in the 1960s that the concept of VBAC was both feasible and safe,[145] the American obstetrician had been reluctant to accept this major modification in health care delivery. As late as 1987, more than 90 percent of women with prior cesarean deliveries had a repeat cesarean delivery.[2] Much of the initial failure to accept VBAC may have been the result of 1985 guidelines established by the ACOG that included requirements not considered to be feasible in many community hospitals across the United States.[146] However, acceptance is becoming more widespread as reports documenting the safety and efficacy of VBAC continue to be published. In response, the guidelines published by ACOG in 1988 are more liberal.[147]

Maternal and Fetal Mortality

Overall, VBAC success rates have increased significantly as clinicians have become more confident with this approach. Successful vaginal delivery was achieved in 67 percent of 3,214 cases between 1950 and 1980.[144,148] A recent summary of 6,258 women who attempted VBAC indicated that 5,356 (86 percent) were successful with no maternal mortality, thus comparing favorably with an expected mortality of at least 1 death per 1,000 cesarean sections. In that series there were five fetal deaths and one uterine dehiscence of a prior vertical incision.[144] Furthermore, the fetal risk for patients considering VBAC is no higher than that of patients delivering by elective repeat cesarean section, ranging from 2 to 3 per-

cent.[149] Even the increased use of oxytocin during VBAC has not increased the risk of morbidity or mortality.[1,3,150,150a]

Uterine Dehiscence/Rupture Following VBAC

Dehiscence has a distinctly different clinical connotation than "uterine rupture," which occasionally arises as a complication of prolonged oxytocin use in multiparous patients or following obstetric manipulations such as internal version or extraction.[151,152] Uterine incisional dehiscence is commonly used to describe the occult rupture that is occasionally observed in patients with a prior low transverse incision. A useful operational definition of dehiscence is a uterine scar separation that does not penetrate the uterine serosa, does not produce hemorrhage, and does not cause a major clinical problem.[3]

Using the above definition, patients with previous cesarean section who attempt VBAC are at no higher risk, antepartum or early intrapartum, for dehiscence than are those having an elective repeat cesarean section.[3] Indeed, dehiscence of a previous uterine incisional scar has remained constant (1 per 150 laboring patients) over the past 50 years despite changing practice patterns.[152] A 1961 report[145] is instructive relative to the risk for uterine dehiscence/rupture associated with VBAC. In that series of 130 patients, 65 percent were able to achieve a successful vaginal delivery, despite approximately one-third of the patients having had prior classic cesareans. The type of incision was unknown in another 11 percent, but the scars were "classical in type."[145] In a more recent series involving over 2,600 patients, dehiscence was noted in only 1.5 percent of 1,465 patients having a successful VBAC versus 5.1 percent of 331 patients undergoing cesarean delivery for failed VBAC. These numbers are not significantly different from the dehiscence rates in control patients who did not plan a trial of labor.[3]

The advent of the low cervical segment incision together with better control of postcesarean infections has decreased the risk of uterine incision dehiscence during subsequent pregnancies. Significantly higher rates for dehiscence were reported in an early series after prior cesarean for placenta previa, abruptio placenta, or fetal distress than in patients having a prior cesarean section for CPD.[61,153] Although the basis for this difference is not certain, it may be that

[handwritten marginalia: Most were prior to admission / Classical incision > LSCS & slave rate of dehiscence but risk fetal death ↑]

cesarean delivery for FTP occurred after thinning of the lower uterine segment, decreasing the likelihood of incisional extension into the upper segment. Cesarean section for other indications may occur prior to thinning, thus increasing the risk of an upper segment incision and subsequent dehiscence. Alternatively, the origin of uterine scar dehiscence may be a function of the healing process of the primary uterine incision. Although the risk of dehiscence for VBAC is low, there are factors that do increase the risk. Further data are required.

Maternal mortality and intrapartum fetal death as a result of dehiscence of a low transverse uterine incision are uncommon, particularly when the fetus is monitored continuously. The data with regard to fetal death in association with dehiscence of a vertical incision is less reassuring. In one review of published American studies involving 5,400 patients prior to 1980, there were no maternal deaths from uterine rupture, even those involving classic uterine scars.[159] There were 30 uterine ruptures (0.55 percent) arising from prior classic cesarean sections. Although no maternal deaths were encountered, fetal deaths were observed in 17 (56.7 percent) cases in which there was dehiscence of a fundal incision. In contrast, lower uterine segment dehiscence occurred in 25 instances (0.46 percent) with no maternal deaths and only 3 (12 percent) fetal losses. Most fetal deaths arising from uterine dehiscence occurred either prior to admission or prior to the advent of widespread employment of continuous electronic FHR monitoring.

Resolving Controversies

Many theoretical concerns have been resolved as clinicians have gained increased experience and confidence regarding the relative safety of VBAC. In most cases there are benefit versus risk considerations that have impacted favorably on the willingness to consider alterations in practice patterns that would not have been possible even 10 years ago.

Oxytocin and VBAC

The decision to use oxytocin in a VBAC is significant because of a hypothesized increase in the risk of uterine rupture/dehiscence. However, this hypothesis has not been confirmed. Use of oxytocin and the duration of its administration have not had a major impact on the rate of uterine dehiscence.[59,150a]

In a summary of several series in which oxytocin was used,[155] 35 percent (1,111) of 3,211 VBAC patients received oxytocin. One hundred twenty-three (11 percent) patients received oxytocin for induction. Use of oxytocin is associated with a two- to threefold increased probability of repeat cesarean delivery. When VBAC failure rates of patients receiving oxytocin are compared with those not receiving oxytocin, failure is significantly higher in the oxytocin group (32 percent vs. 14 percent), presumably reflecting selection bias toward those receiving oxytocin. If there is an early response to oxytocin, one can expect a greater probability of success. In contrast, if a patient fails to progress within approximately 2 hours, cesarean section becomes considerably more likely.[156] Failure to achieve vaginal delivery in the oxytocin group is thus primarily a function of CPD. In those cases requiring cesarean delivery, 78 percent were attributable to CPD in the oxytocin group versus only 60 percent in the patients receiving no oxytocin.[155]

Surprisingly, when oxytocin is used, success rates for vaginal delivery were similar for the induction (60 percent) and augmentation (68 percent) groups. The relative safety of oxytocin use appears to be substantiated by a low rate of uterine dehiscences/ruptures. Dehiscence was observed in only 43 (3.9 percent) cases.[155] One series has actually reported that the overall dehiscence rate was similar in the oxytocin (4.7 percent) and the nonoxytocin (5.3 percent) groups.[3] Similar safety has been observed using prostaglandin gel for cervical ripening.[157]

Estimated Fetal Weight and Oxytocin

An estimated fetal weight above 4,000 g increases the likelihood of labor dystocia, particularly when the estimate exceeds 4,500 g. When attempting VBAC, the use of oxytocin and a birth weight of at least 4,000 g is associated with a significantly lower probability of success.[158] Although there is no contraindication to a VBAC for a fetus estimated to weigh 4,000–4,500 g, success is likely to be diminished.

Epidural Anesthesia in VBAC

Despite the theoretical concern that anesthesia may mask the signs and symptoms of otherwise painful dehiscence/rupture, recent experience seems to indicate otherwise.[159,160] In balance, the theoretical risk is small when compared with the benefit of pain relief. Epidural anesthesia also offers quick access to safe anesthesia should cesarean section be required. On the basis of information to date, there appears to be little reason to withhold epidural anesthesia. In fact, it may be the reassurance that the patient will have adequate pain relief during labor that encourages her to consider VBAC.

It is important to emphasize that uterine dehiscence is usually followed by a good outcome for both mother and fetus. Flamm et al.[161] could only identify one case in which a uterine incisional scar separation resulted in fetal death in a *monitored* patient. Flamm[144] later reported that 30 percent of 1,692 women attempting VBAC in institutions in which VBAC was widely practiced were given epidural anesthesia with no maternal or fetal deaths. Although two instances of uterine rupture were observed, both fetuses survived because of detection of nonreassuring FHR patterns. In one instance, the patient actually experienced pain despite the epidural.

Regional anesthesia does not appear to obscure the symptoms associated with uterine rupture. Carlson et al.[162] reported two cases with uterine scar rupture in which the patients were aware of uterine pain and tenderness despite epidural anesthesia. This confirmed an earlier report by Crawford.[163] A review of six VBAC cases complicated by uterine rupture indicated that epidural anesthesia did not mask the signs and symptoms of uterine separation at the site of a previous low transverse incision.[164] In most instances a significant alteration in FHR pattern, or occasionally an alteration in uterine contraction pattern, is the presenting sign. The alteration in uterine contraction pattern may appear as increased frequency and intensity of contractions if monitored externally. If monitored with an internal pressure catheter, a loss of intrauterine pressure may be observed. Moreover, even in the unanesthetized patient, uterine or scar tenderness, a sign of uterine rupture, occurs in only 25 percent of patients.[165]

A more legitimate, though controversial, concern is that epidural anesthesia, particularly when used with epinephrine, may increase the need for cesarean delivery or mid-forceps delivery by reducing uterine activity.[166,167] This would reduce the incentive for effective maternal pushing in the second stage of labor and limit spontaneous rotation of the fetal head nor-

mally anticipated with descent of the vertex into the maternal pelvis.[168,169] However, if this occurs, the epidural can be discontinued during the second stage of labor.

Multiple Gestation and Abnormal Fetal Lie

Clinical acceptance of VBAC in patients with multiple gestations or breech presentations remains highly controversial. However, no data contraindicate a VBAC trial in a frank breech presentation if the obstetrician is comfortable with selective vaginal breech delivery. Multiple gestation theoretically increases the risk for uterine rupture/dehiscence because it is associated with increased distention of the uterus. While there are no data demonstrating an increased risk in this setting, more information regarding VBAC in multiple gestation is required before this can be universally recommended.

Prior Cesarean Indications as a Prognostic Indicator

One of the first questions to arise in considering a VBAC is the likelihood for a vaginal birth. Some patients will desire current data regarding success rates according to the indication for the prior cesarean birth. The prognosis will depend in large part on whether the prior indication is "recurring" or "nonrecurring." VBAC success is increased by a history of a prior vaginal delivery (85 percent),[150,156] absence of prior CPD, absolute fetal weight less than 4,000 g, smaller relative fetal weight (50 versus 84 percent) than the index pregnancy,[156] and response to oxytocin stimulation within 2 hours.[156] When oxytocin is required, absence of a prior CPD predicts VBAC success.[150] Even though the success rate is reduced in patients whose prior cesarean section was for CPD, more than 60 percent of these patients will still achieve a vaginal delivery.

VBAC success according to indication for prior cesarean section has been summarized (Table 20.4) in a recent review.[170] For ease of analysis, it is convenient to divide prior indications into "recurring" and "nonrecurring" categories. If a patient has a history of a prior cesarean delivery for a nonrecurring condition, breech presentation, fetal distress, and conditions such as placenta previa, abruption, or maternal hemorrhage, the likelihood of a successful trial of labor is quite high, approximating the success rate for

Table 20.4 VBAC Success in Patients With Recurring Causes (in series with at least 50 cases for that indication) and Nonrecurring Causes (in series with at least 30 cases for that indication)

Prior Indication	No. of Patients	Success No. (%)
Recurring causes		
CPD/FTP	1,794	1,233 (69)
Prolonged Labor	154	107 (70)
Nonrecurring causes		
Breech presentation	791	681 (86)
Fetal distress	374	307 (82)
Abruptio previa	88	72 (82)

(Adapted from Eglinton,[170] with permission.)

the so-called low-risk nulliparous patient particularly if the patient has had a prior vaginal delivery.[149]

Cephalopelvic Disproportion/Failure to Progress

Inherent clinical biases would suggest that patients with a previous cesarean delivery for FTP or CPD would likely be unsuccessful. Rather, the data suggest that most women who had a prior cesarean for "failure to progress" or "relative cephalopelvic disproportion" deserve a trial of labor in a subsequent pregnancy. The most pessimistic estimate indicates a probability of success of approximately 50 percent following a prior cesarean for CPD. One study was particularly instructive,[171] as both pregnancies were managed by the same protocol. In the initial pregnancy, all patients received oxytocin augmentation prior to a diagnosis of FTP in labor. Despite the seeming importance of a well-managed prior labor trial, the success rates for the subsequent VBAC was 69 percent.

Prior Vaginal Delivery

Although all patients have a relatively high rate for a successful VBAC attempt, the success rate is predictably higher for patients with a prior vaginal delivery. The success rates for VBAC are increased to over 80 percent in women who have had a prior vaginal birth.[145,172] While Paul et al.[149] were unable to demonstrate a significant impact of prior vaginal birth, the overall success rate in their series was over 80 percent. It may be that the impact of vaginal birth prior

to cesarean section exerts its effect only in patient populations in which VBAC trials were less aggressive.

Multiple Prior Cesarean Sections

Current ACOG guidelines do not specify a maximum number of prior cesarean births as a criteria for VBAC. Several studies suggest that a VBAC is safe in a patient with two or more prior cesareans and can be managed in a similar manner to that of patients with only one incision, with few complications.[3,145,149,173-175] Not all agree with this recommendation, however.[176] Experience with patients with three or more incisions is especially limited and at this time deserves more extensive study.

Suggested Guidelines for VBAC

In 1985, the ACOG Committee on Obstetrics recommended that a physician capable of performing a cesarean delivery be "immediately available" during a trial of labor. The suggested response time for an urgent cesarean birth was 30 minutes.[177] As a consequence, there was initially some concern regarding compliance with this recommendation. In a small series, Porreco and Meier[178] evaluated the likelihood for an urgent cesarean birth, employing the 30-minute rule, in patients with and without a prior cesarean section. The requirement for a delivery within 30 minutes was similar, namely, 1.2 percent (two cases) in patients with no prior cesarean section and 1.4 percent in those with a previous low transverse incision. The indication for the repeat procedure was not urgent in most patients. Most patients had failed to progress in the first or second stage. The two patients with a prior low transverse incision who required an urgent cesarean birth were found to have an intact scar at the time of surgery.[178] The Canadian Consensus Conference[179] on cesarean childbirth came to a similar conclusion, noting the probability of urgent cesarean delivery to be 2.7 percent among 11,819 births. In that study, accumulated from four prospective studies, symptomatic dehiscence occurred in only 0.22 percent of births. The Canadian panel suggested guidelines similar to those recommended by the ACOG.

More recently, the ACOG has published guidelines recommending VBAC in women with one prior low transverse cesarean delivery. A trial of labor is also considered reasonable with two prior cesarean deliveries. Oxytocin and epidural anesthesia may be used. A prior classic cesarean delivery is a contraindication to a VBAC trial. At the present time, additional data are required before a definitive statement can be made regarding the advisability of VBAC in patients with twin gestations, breech presentations, a fetus estimated to weigh at least 4,000 g, or a prior low vertical incision. Minimum requirements commonly include availability of anesthesia and nursing personnel, the establishment of a large bore intravenous line, access to 24-hour blood banking, continuous electronic FHR monitoring, and selective intrauterine pressure monitoring.[147]

Informed Consent for VBAC

The need for specific consent from a patient attempting VBAC seems somewhat superfluous if one accepts that the inherent risks of a VBAC are no greater than those of an attempted vaginal delivery in other patients. Because likelihood of a successful VBAC is only minimally dependent on the indication for the prior cesarean delivery, the physician should present the chances of success in a positive sense. Obviously written consent can be obtained; however, an equally reasonable approach would be to indicate in the patient's prenatal record that the patient has been informed that labor following a prior cesarean delivery is an acceptable alternative to routine repeat cesarean delivery with only minor attendant risks that are unlikely to be significantly greater than those of a repeat cesarean section.

Fetal Monitoring, Oxytocin, and Anesthesia

Management of the patient undergoing a VBAC is similar to that of patients undergoing vaginal delivery.[177] Continuous electronic FHR monitoring with at least external tocodynamometry should be employed, and a physician capable of performing a cesarean delivery should be "immediately available" in case a cesarean section is required. It appears reasonable to use oxytocin and epidural anesthesia as long as contraindications do not exist. The liberalization of indications for oxytocin use has also increased to include even those patients with two or more prior cesarean births.[3] The indications for oxytocin use are the same as those for patients without a history of a prior cesarean section. Oxytocin should be used in general accordance with guidelines stated in the ACOG Technical Bulletin No. 119.[180,181]

Detection of Uterine Dehiscence/Rupture

Fortunately, it appears that the clinician can be alerted to the possibility of uterine dehiscence or rupture in most instances on the basis of nonreassuring FHR patterns. Some have recommended the routine use of intrauterine pressure catheters. However, this is probably not necessary and does not guarantee a uterine rupture will be detected. I have observed one case of uterine rupture in which there was no change in the intrauterine pressure curves.

Routine uterine exploration following a successful VBAC trial is a controversial issue. Advocates of routine exploration argue that failure to identify a defect does not allow for rational consideration of risk and benefits should a subsequent VBAC trial be considered. It is their belief that should exploration detect a significant defect that is connected with the peritoneal cavity, particularly when associated with excessive bleeding, laparotomy should be performed to either repair the defect or perform a hysterectomy. On the other hand, those who do not recommend routine exploration argue that the examination is often difficult. Furthermore, repair is generally unnecessary if a small defect is discovered that does not open into the peritoneum and is not associated with symptomatic bleeding. These patients can be followed expectantly with careful observation of vital signs and serial hematocrit determinations. In the presence of active bleeding, a laparotomy must be performed.

The decision to attempt a VBAC is also often clouded by other clinical factors such as the need for a postpartum tubal ligation. However, even the patient intending to have a postpartum tubal ligation may wish to consider a VBAC trial. In one study, 13 percent of successful VBAC patients had a postpartum tubal ligation with only minor prolongation of their hospital stay.[182]

CESAREAN HYSTERECTOMY

Indications

Cesarean hysterectomy is usually an emergency procedure. The incidence of emergency hysterectomy following cesarean section is less than 1 percent if one considers only cases that cannot be treated conservatively. In a typical series, emergency indications requiring hysterectomy included atony (43 percent), placenta accreta (30 percent), uterine rupture (13 percent), extension (unplanned) of a low transverse incision (10 percent), and leiomyoma preventing uterine closure and hemostasis.[81]

Extension of a uterine incision into the uterine vessels is an uncommon indication for hysterectomy. However, it may pose a therapeutic dilemma. Although hemorrhage may be quite significant, consideration should be given to the alternative of hypogastric or uterine artery ligation, as opposed to hysterectomy, depending on the patient's parity and desires for future pregnancy. Ligation of the anterior division of one or both hypogastric or internal iliac arteries may decrease the arterial pulse pressure up to 85 percent distal to the point of the ligation, thus allowing clot formation.[183] Alternatively, it is possible to ligate the uterine arteries.[184] However, before ligating the uterine vessels, it may be advisable to identify by either palpation or direct visualization the ureter, which may be in close proximity.[73]

Nonemergency or Planned Cesarean Hysterectomy

The incidence of planned cesarean hysterectomy has fallen in recent years. Desire for permanent sterilization and elimination of long-term risks for later uterine pathology had been felt in the past to be acceptable indications, but the risks of ureteral injury and hemorrhage requiring transfusion usually outweigh the benefits. Indications for a planned cesarean hysterectomy include coexisting uterine pathology such as large symptomatic myomata, or carcinoma in situ. Because diagnosis of carcinoma in situ of the cervix can be confirmed during pregnancy by colposcopy, vaginal delivery is a preferred alternative once invasive disease is excluded. However, in some instances the patient may be noncompliant, and cesarean hysterectomy may then be considered.[185] An occasional case may be performed for microinvasive disease. Rarely, invasive cancer of the cervix may be treated with a primary cesarean delivery followed by radical hysterectomy with pelvic lymphadenectomy.[186,187] Elective cesarean hysterectomy as a means to achieve sterilization is generally felt to carry excessive risks, because of the unquestioned increase in operative morbidity.

Technique for Total Hysterectomy

The operative technique employs the general principles for abdominal hysterectomy in the nongravid state. Although the uterine vessels are considerably larger than in the nonpregnant state, tissue planes are more easily developed. Polyglycolic acid or chromic catgut suture (0- or 1-gauge) may be used throughout the procedure. In initiating the surgical procedure, the surgeon should direct attention to adequate development of the bladder flap, use of overlapping sutures for successive vascular pedicles, selective as opposed to mass placement of clamps and sutures to control bleeders, inspection of the bladder for an inadvertent cystotomy, localization of the ureter should a lateral laceration be the indication for the procedure, and avoidance of excessive removal of vaginal length, particularly when the cervix is completely effaced.

It is advisable to mobilize the bladder extensively in the midline approximately to a point 2 cm below the cervical vaginal junction and to some extent laterally. This will result in displacement of the bladder and ureters caudad or inferiorly. Separation of the bladder from the underlying lower segment can be accomplished in most instances with gentle blunt dissection. On occasion, however, the bladder flap may be adherent, requiring sharp dissection.

After delivery of the fetus, the placenta need not be removed unless noted to be separating spontaneously. It is often desirable to proceed directly to insertion of a self-retaining retractor to facilitate exposure. The uterine fundus is then delivered through the incision, and constant traction is maintained on the uterus to maximize pedicle exposure, facilitate development of tissue planes, and stretch the uterine veins, thereby narrowing their lumen and reducing venous blood loss. If a vertical uterine incision has been made, it is often convenient for the assistant to hook an index finger in the upper extreme of the uterine incision to manipulate the fundus and to expose the operative site. If the placenta is still in place, it can be removed, if bleeding of the uterine incision is excessive. Further bleeding can be controlled by a variety of techniques including use of oxytocin, ligation of individual bleeders, or even closure of the uterine incision. In many instances, however, it is possible to complete the isolation of the uterine pedicles in a time period that approximates that required to close the uterine incision.

Once the bladder separation is completed, the round ligaments (Fig. 20.12) are then clamped using Haney or Kocher clamps, cut, and ligated with transfixing sutures. The previously made vesicouterine peritoneum (serosa) incision is then extended laterally and superiorly across the anterior leaf of the broad ligament through the point of the previously incised round ligaments. It is seldom necessary to remove the ovaries.

Placement of the utero-ovarian clamps is facilitated by perforation of the avascular portion of the posterior leaf of the broad ligament adjacent to the uterus just inferior to the fallopian tube, utero-ovarian ligaments, and ovarian vessels. The ovaries should be inspected, and, if found to be normal, the utero-ovarian ligament and tube are then ligated by means of a free tie with the intent to provide enough room to insert two clamps, either atraumatic (e.g., Masterston) or crushing (e.g., Haney), between the previously placed utero-ovarian free tie and the uterus. The resultant pedicle is then doubly clamped close to the uterus, incised, and ligated with a transfixing suture (Fig. 20.12B). An attempt should be made to avoid placement of the clamps or ligature across ovarian tissue, which may result in immediate or delayed bleeding. Some surgeons will quickly ligate the opposing uterine pedicle so as to remove the second clamp from the operative field, while avoiding back-bleeding.

There is considerable variation regarding subsequent technique. Variation involves the use of two versus three clamps for each pedicle, use of single versus double ligation of vascular pedicles, the relative desirability for skeletonization of vessels in the broad ligament, and the relative need for an additional step to separate and individually ligate the uterosacral ligaments. Many surgeons incise the avas-

cular portion of the broad ligaments and skeletonize the uterine vessels, particularly the large uterine veins. The ascending uterine vessels adjacent to the uterus near their origin are then identified and doubly clamped, incised, and ligated, either singularly or doubly. The surgeon should attempt to place the clamp tip at right angles to the ascending uterine vessels and close to the uterine margin. Placement of the clamps on this vascular pedicle is quite easy should the cervix be long and uneffaced. However, if the lower segment is well developed, soft, and without distinct margins, palpation of the lateral margin of the lower uterine segment (between thumb and forefinger straddling the intended broad ligament pedicle) will facilitate closer approximation of the clamp tip to the uterine margin, reducing the likelihood of back-bleeding. A variation of the two-clamp technique is presented in Figure 20.13. Prior to placement of the clamps on the uterine vessel, it is often useful to confirm that the bladder is displaced, and, should ureteral location be an issue, the ureter can be palpated between the forefinger and thumb. Once the ascending vessels are ligated, pedicles containing descending branches of the uterine vessels and cardinal and uterosacral ligaments are clamped (doubly or singularly) with either Haney-type curved clamps or Ochsner-type straight clamps, attempting to place the clamps as close to the cervix as possible. Placement of the Haney or Kocher straight clamps should be done in such a way as to slide off the lateral substance of the cervix so that the clamp tip is inferior to the margin of the cardinal ligament after reconfirming that the bladder reflection is retracted away from the intended site of clamp placement. The resultant wedge-shaped pedicle is then incised and sutured. Inclusion of the adjacent more superior uterine pedicle in the tie may reduce bleeding between the two pedicles. Should the lower uterine segment be well developed, it may be necessary to develop more than one pedicle for each cardinal ligament. Successive additional pedicles are clamped, incised, and suture ligated until the surgeon is confident that the cardinal ligaments and uterosacral ligaments have been separated and the level of the lateral vaginal fornix is reached (Fig. 20.14). Although some surgeons individually identify and ligate the uterosacral ligaments, many incorporate the uterosacral ligaments in the lower cardinal pedicle.

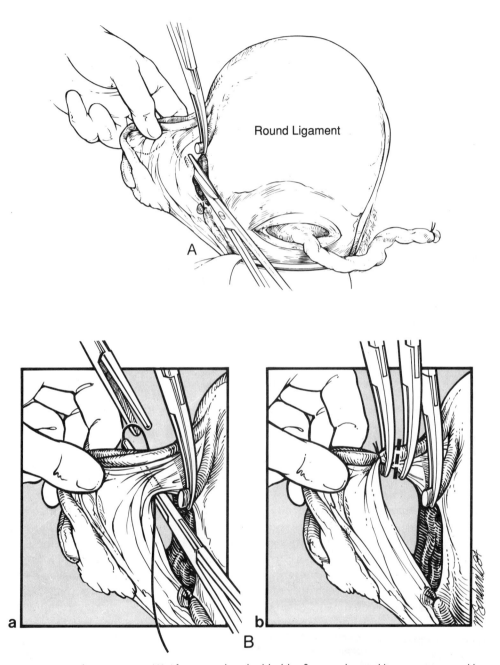

Fig. 20.12 Cesarean hysterectomy. (A) After extending the bladder flap, each round ligament is cut and ligated. The posterior leaf of the broad ligament can be opened for a short distance, taking care to incise only the surface layer. The avascular space beneath the utero-ovarian ligament may be opened by blunt finger dissection to isolate the adnexal pedicle. (B) (a) A free tie is passed through the avascular space and firmly tied. The advantage of this tie is to secure the vessels within the pedicle before it is cut. (b) The adnexal pedicle is doubly clamped and cut. In addition, a transfixing suture will then be placed around the pedicle.

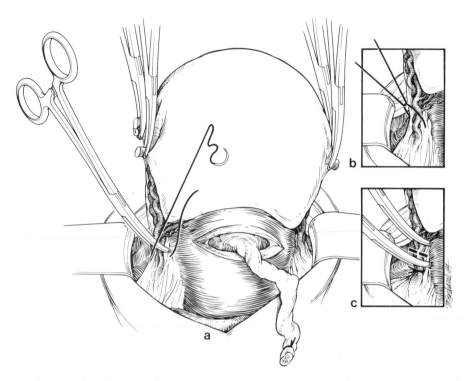

Fig. 20.13 (A) The ascending branches of the uterine artery are clamped, cut, and a suture is placed just below the tip of the hemostat and immediately next to the uterine wall. (B) After removing the hemostat, the suture is tied, thus securing the vessels before they are cut. (C) The pedicle is regrasped just above the tie and then doubly ligated.

Separation of the cervix from its vaginal attachments can be quite difficult should the lower uterine segment be well effaced. One should be careful to avoid both incomplete removal of the cervix and excessive removal of the upper vagina. In some instances it is possible to palpate and milk superiorly the lower margin of the cervix by palpating the approximate site with thumb and forefinger placed anteriorly and posteriorly about the cervicovaginal junction. Should identification of the cervicovaginal junction not be possible by external palpation, the surgeon may insert the index finger either through the cervical canal or through a vertical incision in the anterior lower uterine segment into the upper vagina to locate the cervical vaginal margin (Fig. 20.15) Should the latter method be employed to locate the lower margin of the cervix, once the cervix is freed from the vagina, the circulating nurse should re-glove the surgeon. After the margin is identified, a curved Haney clamp can then be placed on each angle of the vagina and the

tissue incised entering the vaginal vault. The cervix can be circumcised from its vaginal attachments and inspected to ensure that it has been completely excised. The two angles of the resultant vaginal cuff are identified and clamped (Fig. 20.16). The vaginal angle containing the vaginal artery can then be secured by a variety of techniques. Some incorporate the vaginal angle to the cardinal and uterosacral ligaments via a lock loop suture (Fig. 20.17). The vaginal cuff may be closed, using interrupted or continuous sutures. Many surgeons close the vaginal cuff, particularly if the pelvis is dry and there are no major additional risks for cuff infection. Should the surgeon elect to close the vagina, closure can be achieved in either one or two layers (Fig. 20.18). Alternatively, the cuff can be left open by running a locking circumferential suture about the cuff margins to minimize vaginal cuff bleeding and facilitate drainage; some prefer figure-of-eight sutures.

Upon completion of the procedure, the cul-de-sac

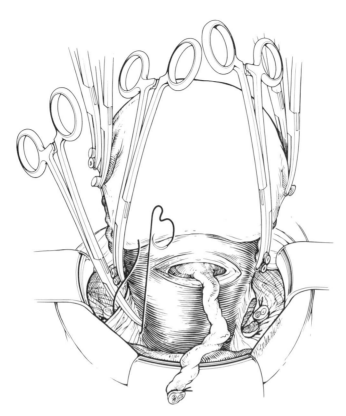

Fig. 20.14 The cardinal ligaments are clamped at their point of insertion, cut, and singly ligated. Because these structures are hypertrophied, several bites may be necessary. Some physicians clamp, cut, and ligate the uterosacral ligaments separately.

and peritoneal gutters are suctioned of blood and accumulated debris and all previous pedicles examined for bleeding points. Bleeding sites should be individually controlled by picking up as little tissue as possible to avoid ligation or kinking of the ureters. Once the surgeon is assured that hemostasis is adequate and that there have been no lacerations of the bladder, the pelvis may be irrigated. The pelvic floor can then be reperitonealized using a continuous suture. Recently some surgeons have discontinued the process of reperitonealizing the pelvic floor and simply allow the sigmoid and bladder to fall into place over the vaginal cuff. This approach may also minimize the admittedly small chance of suturing the ureter during reperitonealization. The surgeon may avoid attachment of the ovarian pedicles to the angle of the vagina by suturing the ovarian pedicle to the ipsilateral round ligament.

Should the surgeon decide to reperitonealize (Fig. 20.19), closure can be initiated by inverting the pedicle of the ligated fallopian tube and ovarian ligament retroperitoneally, avoiding fixation of the ovary in the cul-de-sac. A continuous suture reapproximates the medial and lateral leaves of the broad ligament, burying the round ligament stump and approximating the anterior vesicouterine peritoneum over the vaginal vault to the cul-de-sac peritoneum on the posterior margin of the vagina. The procedure is then conducted in reverse order on the opposing side.

Subtotal Hysterectomy

The obstetrician should usually plan to perform a total hysterectomy. However, in some circumstances a subtotal hysterectomy may be desirable because it is simpler, particularly should the pathology be confined to the upper uterine segment and the surgeon

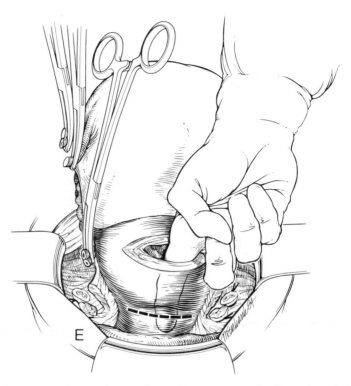

Fig. 20.15 Because the cervix is elongated, it may be useful to insert an index finger through the cervical canal to demarcate the vaginal incision and to ensure complete removal of the cervix and avoid unnecessary removal of vaginal length.

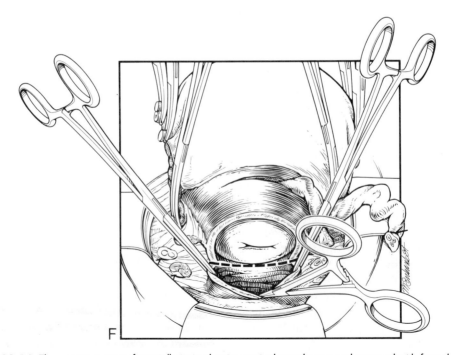

Fig. 20.16 The vagina is circumferentially incised at its cervical attachment and grasped with four clamps.

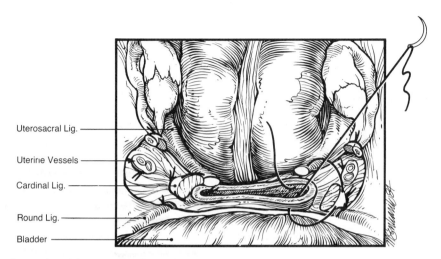

Fig. 20.17 The angles of the vaginal cuff are closed with sutures to include the cardinal and uterosacral ligaments, thus providing fascial support to the vaginal vault. A simple loop suture is commonly used at this location to reduce the likelihood of breakage during the stage of postoperative edema.

Uterosacral Lig.

Uterine Vessels

Cardinal Lig.

Round Lig.

Bladder

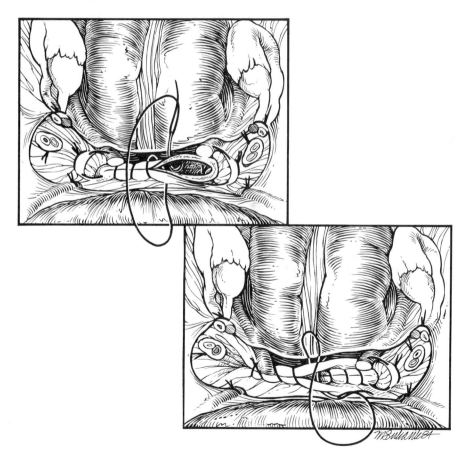

Fig. 20.18 There are a number of methods of closing the vaginal cuff. Illustrated is a two-layer closure. The first layer closes the vagina, and the second layer closes the endopelvic fascia. Many operators prefer to leave the cuff "open" by employing one continuous suture that circles the cuff, approximating the cut edge to its surrounding fascia.

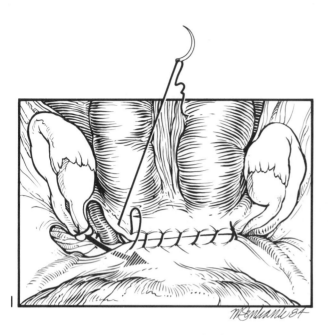

Fig. 20.19 The bladder flap is closed with a continuous suture that inverts the pedicles of the round ligaments and adnexae. Note that these structures have not been attached to the vaginal cuff.

judge that removal of the cervix will significantly prolong the duration of surgery in a patient who is cardiovascularly unstable.

Once the ascending uterine artery and vein are doubly clamped and the pedicles cut and ligated as in a total hysterectomy, the cervix is amputated at the level of the pedicles. In amputating the cervix it may be useful to cone the amputation downward toward the canal (Fig. 20.20A). The resultant cervical stump can be closed with several interrupted sutures. Some surgeons doubly suture ligate the ascending uterine vessels by the angles of the cervix (Fig. 20.20B) to minimize the risk of angle bleeding. Additional bleeding points are ligated and reperitonealization performed in a fashion similar to that required for total hysterectomy.

Complications

The major complications of cesarean hysterectomy are increased blood loss and occasional injury to either bladder or ureters.[188] Complications following cesarean hysterectomy, although similar to those following nonobstetric total abdominal hysterectomy,

occur with greater frequency. Total hysterectomy may add 30 to 60 minutes to operating and anesthesia time and is almost always associated with additional blood loss of at least 500 ml. Operating time will vary depending on whether the procedure is emergent or elective, the surgeon's experience, the degree of development of the lower uterine segment, coincidental pelvic pathology such as leiomyomata, obesity, and the presence of ureteral or bladder laceration. Cystotomy as a complication of cesarean hysterectomy has been noted to occur in approximately 4 to 5 percent of procedures.[75,76] The incidence of ureteral injury during cesarean delivery has been reported to be as high as 1 in 1,000 cesarean deliveries.[74] Ureteral injury is increased even further with cesarean hysterectomy, with rates of 0.2 to 0.5 percent being observed.[75,76] Ureteral injury may occur when excessive tissue is picked up in an attempt to control bleeding or when suture placement follows accidental laceration of a large vessel at the base of the broad ligament. Laceration of the bladder may occur coincident with uterine rupture or during an attempt to develop the bladder flap, particularly in the patient with prior cesarean deliveries. On occasion it will be necessary to remove the adnexae in order to achieve hemostasis.

Postoperative hematoma formation in either the broad ligaments or vaginal cuff is relatively uncommon. Such hematomas may become secondarily infected, producing a cuff abscess. Alternatively, there is the possibility of delayed arterial hemorrhage from the angle of the vaginal cuff.

ELECTIVE MYOMECTOMY AND APPENDECTOMY

The propriety of performing an elective myomectomy or appendectomy during a cesarean section is a matter of dispute. The majority opinion is that, with the possible exception of a subserosal myoma on a thin pedicle, myomectomy is contraindicated because achieving hemostasis may be difficult. Others assert that hemostasis will be excellent because of the action of the contracting uterus. A better argument for abstention is the knowledge that most myomas will involute to an insignificant size during the puerperium. Although the risk of elective appendectomy is quite low, there are no figures to prove that the benefits to

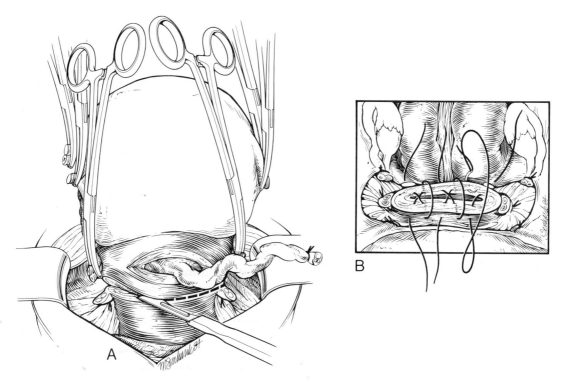

Fig. 20.20 Subtotal hysterectomy. (A) The cervix is incised just below the level of the ligated pedicles of the uterine arteries, amputating the uterine corpus from its cervical stump. (B) The cervical stump may be closed with several interrupted figure-of-eight sutures; reperitonealization is then accomplished as in a total hysterectomy.

be gained are greater than the possible surgical complications.

COINCIDENTAL OVARIAN NEOPLASMS AT CESAREAN DELIVERY

Should an ovarian neoplasm be discovered at the time of cesarean delivery, the surgeon should first rule out the possibility of a theca lutein cyst or the rare luteoma of pregnancy. Other ovarian neoplasms should be excised, sparing the ovary whenever possible.

POSTPARTUM STERILIZATION

Tubal ligation in the postpartum period offers several major advantages. The patient is often only subjected to one anesthesia (epidural) for the labor and delivery and the ligation process. Should that not be possible, there is still the benefit of only abbreviated hospital-

ization at a time when maternal responsibilities are less than will be the case just weeks later. Furthermore, additional preoperative work-up is not necessary for a second procedure. Increased tissue vascularity and edema pose a theoretical risk of more difficult hemostasis, and possibly contribute to the somewhat higher failure rate compared with interval procedures.

A variety of methods of sterilization are available either at the time of cesarean delivery or during the postpartum period. The tubes can be occluded by banding, clipping, resection, or fulguration. In selecting a method for tubal sterilization, consideration should be given to two factors: effectiveness relative to later sterility and reversibility, should the patient later desire reversal. A rational decision for tubal occlusion may later be proven wrong by different circumstances, particularly should sterilization be performed at a young age. Patients are also more likely to regret sterilization procedures performed in associa-

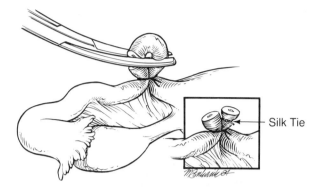

Fig. 20.21 Pomeroy sterilization. A knuckle of tube is ligated with absorbable suture, and a small segment is being excised. Note that the ligation is performed at a site that will favor reanastomosis, should that become desirable. Some surgeons place an extra tie of nonabsorbable suture around the proximal stump as added protection against recanalization.

tion with the stress of pregnancy than considered interval procedures.

From the point of view of later reversibility, the use of clips is probably the best method of sterilization, because clips produce the least damage. Occlusion within the tubal isthmus is desirable should later reanastomosis be attempted, because an isthmic–isthmic reapproximation is most likely to succeed. Salpingectomy, cornual resection, extensive fulguration, and fimbriectomy limit the choices for those patients who later seek restoration of fertility. The timing of the operation relative to the time of birth has little impact. In some instances when there is some concern regarding potential newborn outcome, the procedure may be best postponed.

Postoperative complications are infrequent. Hemorrhage is the most commonly encountered problem. Although patient discomfort associated with the procedure may increase the length of hospitalization by 1 day or more, significant discomfort is seldom encountered after 1 or 2 weeks.

Techniques

Incision

In the early puerperium the tubes are easily isolated through a small abdominal incision, since the uterus is enlarged and the abdominal wall is lax. A small, periumbilical incision offers the most cosmetic result

and least postpartum discomfort. However, a small 3- to 4-cm midline vertical or transverse incision at the level of the fundus is often used. The only disadvantage to such a small incision is one of limited exposure that may increase the risk of inadvertent ligation of a round ligament rather than a tube. If the operation is delayed, or if the patient has had previous adnexal surgery and adhesions are anticipated, a transverse or midline vertical incision may be desirable.

Pomeroy Technique

The Pomeroy technique is the most popular means of postpartum sterilization (Fig. 20.21) because of its simplicity and effectiveness. As originally described, a small knuckle of each tube is picked up approximately 1 inch from its cornual insertion and ligated with a single loop of absorbable suture (plain catgut). A small section of the isolated tubal segment is then resected and submitted to the pathologist to document that the tubal lumina have been interrupted. Presumably the remaining segments of tube will separate when the suture is absorbed, leaving a gap between the proximal and distal ends. A modification wherein the proximal ends of each resected tube are also ligated with a nonabsorbable suture is employed by some in an attempt to reduce the likelihood of recanalization of the proximal tubal lumen. The modified operation has a failure rate of approximately 1 in 500.

Uchida Technique

Some clinicians advocate the Uchida technique because of its low failure rate and the theoretically reduced risk of associated disturbance of ovarian blood supply. This technique is more complicated than the Pomeroy technique and requires the surgeon to separate the muscular portion of the tube from its serosal cover, which is then cut and ligated. The proximal segment is then buried in the leaves of the broad ligament, leaving the distal segment exteriorized (Fig. 20.22).

Irving Technique

Although the Irving operation is slightly more complicated than other techniques, it may have the lowest failure rate. After transecting and ligating the cut ends of the tubes, a tunnel is created by blunt dissection into the adjacent uterine wall at the insertion of

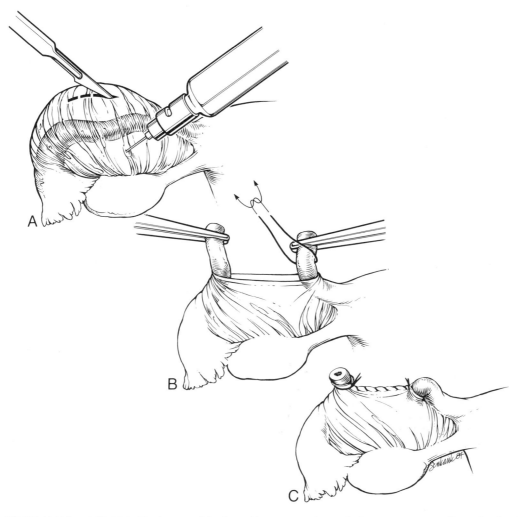

Fig. 20.22 Uchida sterilization. The leaves of the broad ligament and peritubal peritoneum are infiltrated with saline so that the tube can be easily isolated from these structures, divided, and ligated. The broad ligament is then closed, burying the proximal stump between the leaves and including the distal stump in the line of closure.

the round ligament, a less vascular area. The proximal segment of each tube is carried into the depth of the tunnel by means of a traction suture and transfixed there by an interrupted suture (Fig. 20.23). The cut end of each distal segment is then buried between the leaves of the broad ligament or may be left exposed in the modified Irving procedure.

Kroener Fimbriectomy

Excision of the distal portion of each tube (Fig. 20.24) and ligation of the cut ends of the tube with nonabsorbable suture (silk) is a highly effective procedure.

However, because tubal fimbriae have been excised, reversal of this procedure is not likely.

Other Techniques

Simple ligation of the tubes is not acceptable because of a failure rate approximating 20 percent. The Madliner technique involves ligation of previously crushed tubal loops, and the Aldridge technique results in surgical placement of the free end of each tube in the leaves of the broad ligament. Both techniques are less effective than the methods described

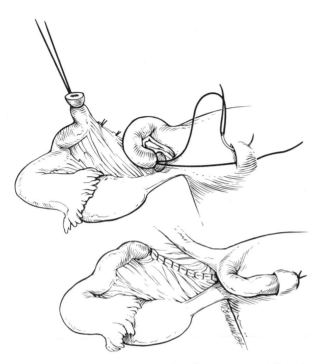

Fig. 20.23 Irving sterilization. The tube is transected 3 to 4 cm from its insertion, and a short tunnel is created by means of a sharp-nosed hemostat in either the anterior or posterior uterine wall. The cut end of the tube can then be buried in the tunnel and, if necessary, further secured by an interrupted suture at the opening of the tunnel. The distal cut end is buried between the leaves of the broad ligament.

above. On the other hand, no method of tubal sterilization is completely effective.[189]

Counseling for Tubal Ligation

Patient counseling may include a discussion of the risk of failure, alternative methods of contraception including male sterilization, and procedural complications. Some clinicians include a review of the variety of tubal techniques available, as well as the possibility of adverse long-term effects on ovarian function and sexual interest. A sufficient interval should be allowed following the provision of consent to satisfy the legal requirements of various jurisdictions and, of equal importance, to permit the patient and her family to reconsider their decision. Despite attempts to provide detailed information, a number of patients will later desire reversal of the procedure. Because reversal is not always possible, tubal steriliza-

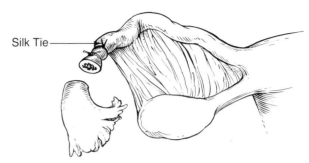

Fig. 20.24 Kroener sterilization. After transecting the distal tube and its fimbria, the proximal tube is religated with a non-absorbable suture to protect against recanalization.

tion should only be recommended as a permanent procedure.

ACUTE ABDOMEN IN PREGNANCY

Appendicitis

Appendicitis is the most common acute surgical condition of pregnancy, with an incidence of 1 in 2,000 births. It is encountered with relatively the same frequency in every trimester as well as the puerperium. The diagnosis is reputed to be more difficult and likely to be delayed because the clinical picture tends to be masked by the symptoms and physical changes of pregnancy.[190] Some of the factors confusing the diagnosis are the nausea, vomiting, and abdominal discomfort of early pregnancy, upward displacement of the appendix by the expanding uterus (Fig. 20.25), laxity of the abdominal wall, round ligament spasm, physiologic leukocytosis, and elevated sedimentation rate.

Diagnosis

Despite these confusing factors, the signs and symptoms of appendicitis in pregnancy are similar to those in the nonpregnant patient. The initial visceral pain is typically gradual in onset, often colicky (denoting an element of obstruction), and usually referred to the epigastrium or periumbilical area. During the first trimester, the pain localizes in the right lower quadrant as the overlying parietal peritoneum becomes

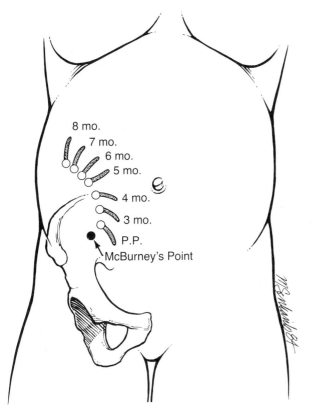

8 mo.
7 mo.
6 mo.
5 mo.
4 mo.
3 mo.
P.P.
McBurney's Point

Fig. 20.25 Locations of the appendix in pregnancy. As modified from Bauer et al.,[191] the approximate location of the appendix during succeeding months of pregnancy is diagrammed. In planning an operation, it is better to make the abdominal incision over the point of maximum tenderness unless there is a great disparity between that point and the theoretical location of the appendix. (Modified from Bauer et al.,[191] with permission.)

involved. Past the fourth month, the appendix has been displaced upward and laterally. At 6 months, the point of maximal thickness is above the iliac crest, and, at 8 months, it rises to the level of the right costal margin.[191] Usually, anorexia accompanied by nausea and vomiting begin 1 to 2 hours after the onset of pain. Right lateral rectal tenderness is commonly found and about one-half of the patients will have abdominal muscle spasm or guarding. Moving the uterus tends to intensify pain in the appendiceal area. By placing the patient on her left side, the clinician can sometimes differentiate pain of uterine origin. If the uterus is the source of the pain, abdominal wall tenderness will diminish as the uterus falls away from the examining fingers.

The patient's temperature can be normal but is usually moderately elevated, up to 101°F. Because of the physiologic leukocytosis of pregnancy, significant alterations of the white blood count depend on finding either a rising count over a period of observation or an increasing left shift. A urinalysis is usually negative unless the inflamed appendix is retroperionteal and lying in close proximity to the right ureter. Roentgenographic studies are rarely helpful. A culdocentesis may demonstrate inflammatory fluid, both before or after rupture.

If the appendix ruptures, either peritonitis follows or the uterus forms the median wall of a localized abscess. In either case, abortion or labor is the usual consequence. As the uterus is emptied, a walled off abscess tends to rupture, producing generalized peritonitis. For these reasons, early diagnosis and operation on all suspicious cases is particularly important. Diagnostic laparoscopy in doubtful cases encountered during early pregnancy may help to avoid an unnecessary laparotomy.

The differential diagnosis includes pyelonephritis, round ligament pain, a placental accident, torsion of an ovarian cyst, degenerating myomata, pancreatitis, and cholecystitis. Appendicitis can also be confused with early labor and postpartum endomyometritis.

Management

A transverse muscle-splitting incision over the point of maximum tenderness is usually adequate and can easily be extended if necessary. If the appendix is unruptured, the incision is closed without drainage. Neither antibiotics nor tocolytic agents are necessary, and abortion or premature labor are unlikely.

When the appendix is ruptured, the patient should receive multiple antibiotic therapy, including an agent effective against anaerobic organisms. Suction drainage through a flank incision will be needed for an abscess or generalized peritonitis. Cul-de-sac drainage is contraindicated, and a cesarean section should be avoided unless a compelling obstetric indication exists. The incision should be separately drained, or the skin should be left open for secondary

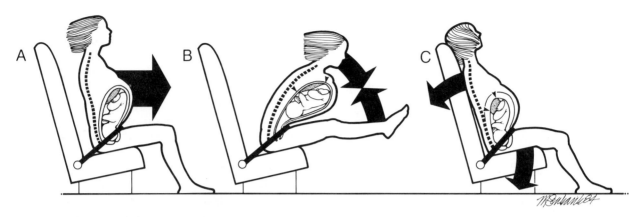

Fig. 20.26 Seatbelt injury. The mechanisms by which placental separation might be produced by a waist-type seatbelt are illustrated. (A) The force of a collision propels the body forward. (B) Acute flexion of the trunk results in elongation of the uterus, including elongation of the site of placental attachment. (C) As the trunk recoils, the placental site is shortened and the posterior wall of the uterus collides with the vertebral column. (Redrawn from Lees and Singer,[197] with permission.)

closure. The value of tocolytic agents to prevent preterm labor in this setting has not been proved.

Acute Cholecystitis

Cholecystitis is more common in pregnancy, presumably because of extrinsic pressure interfering with the circulation and drainage of the gallbladder. The incidence is approximately 1 in 4,000 pregnancies, and attacks are more often associated with increasing age, increasing gravidity, and a history of previous attacks. Preexisting gallstones are rarely a cause of cholecystitis in pregnancy because the ability of the gallbladder to contract is inhibited by high levels of progesterone.

The clinical picture is no different from that in the nonpregnant patient. An attack usually begins with biliary colic, nausea, and vomiting. If the common duct is obstructed by a stone, the pain persists and often radiates to the subscapular area. There is right subcostal tenderness along with fever (i.e., 101 degrees F) and increasing leukocytosis. An ultrasonic study is useful to detect the presence of stones or dilatation of the common duct.[192] If stones are present and Murphy's sign is positive, a diagnosis of cholecystitis is virtually assured.

In most cases, medical therapy suffices. An appropriate antibiotic such as a cephalosporin is combined with intravenous fluids, nasogastric suction, antispasmodics, and analgesics with the expectation of recovery in 48 hours or less. If common duct obstruction or

pancreatitis develops, a cholecystectomy or cholecystotomy will be necessary and should not be delayed. Abortion or cesarean section is not indicated. However, there is considerable risk of premature labor following the operative procedure.

Intestinal Obstruction

Mechanical bowel obstruction, a rare complication of pregnancy, usually involves small bowel, is most commonly due to an adhesive band or hernia, and is more likely to be encountered in the second half of pregnancy. Although the clinical picture is variable, typical symptoms include colicky midabdominal pain that increases in severity and may become diffuse and constant as the bowel distends. In the early stages, bouts of pain are accompanied by reflex vomiting. Later, fecal vomiting may occur. There is usually generalized distention without signs of peritoneal irritation. Dehydration and electrolyte imbalance may intervene. If peristaltic rushes are present, a presumptive diagnosis can be made. Repeated roentgenographic studies are indicated despite the theoretical risks of radiation exposure to the fetus. Significant findings include gaseous distention, intraluminal fluid levels, a stepladder arrangement of small bowel loops, and a paucity of large bowel gas. Initial treatment includes an attempt to decompress the small intestine with a long tube plus hydration and correction of any electrolyte imbalance. If after 6 to 8

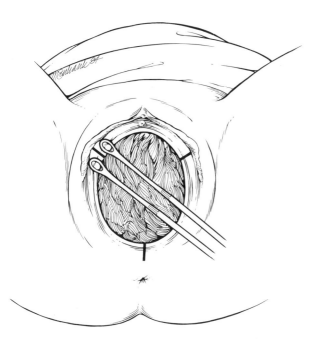

Fig. 20.27 Duhrssen's incision. The location and length of Duhrssen's incisions may be delineated by grasping the cervical rim with two pairs of sponge forceps at the intended point of incision. Either two or three incisions will be sufficient, and repair with interrupted absorbable sutures usually results in satisfactory healing.

hours the patient's response is unsatisfactory, an operation should be done before bowel necrosis and perforation are established. The uterus rarely interferes with the operation and should not be disturbed. If labor follows, a well-repaired abdominal incision will remain intact. The value of postoperative tocolytic agents is speculative.

Trauma

Uterine injury as a result of external trauma is highly unlikely in early pregnancy. However, in later pregnancy, the uterus becomes an abdominal organ. The fetus is well protected by its amniotic fluid cushion, but placental separation can occur as a result of a direct blow or hypovolemic shock. The distortion of the uterus produced by the sudden compression of a waist-type seat belt can also produce placental separation (Fig. 20.26). Uterine rupture is a less likely consequence of a direct blow or seatbelt compression. Another possibility is a penetrating wound from a knife or bullet.

In the management of traumatic injuries, it is essential to institute supportive care promptly to minimize damage to the fetus. Uterine rupture as well as some cases of placental separation will require a celiotomy. Gunshot wounds must also be explored. In the event of a stab wound, an operation can sometimes be avoided if a fistulogram demonstrates that the parietal peritoneum has not been penetrated.

MISCELLANEOUS PROCEDURES (Duhrssen's incisions)

In rare circumstances it may be necessary to incise the cervix as a means to expedite vaginal delivery. Entrapment of the aftercoming head in breech deliveries often following a rapidly progressive labor with expulsion of the fetal body through a partially dilated cervix is probably the most common example. This indication is most likely to involve a preterm breech because of the disproportion between the large fetal head and relatively small body. In such cases, Duhrssen's incisions of the cervix may be attempted.[193] Two or three radial incisions are made in the cervix at the 2, 6, and 10 o'clock positions (Fig. 20.27). To avoid major hemorrhage, the procedure should seldom if ever be done unless the cervix is at least 7 cm dilated and completely effaced. The incision is facilitated by placement of right angle retractors in the vagina with direct visualization of the remaining cervix which is then incised with either bandage or Mayo scissors. Following the delivery, the cervical incisions are repaired in the same fashion as a cervical laceration (see Fig. 18.14).

REFERENCES

1. Rutkow I: Obstetric and gynecologic operations in the United States. 1979 to 1984. Obstet Gynecol 67:755, 1986
2. Shiono PA, McNellis D, Rhoads GS: Reasons for the rising cesarean delivery rates 1978–1984. Obstet Gynecol 69:696, 1987
3. Phelan JP, Clark SL, Diaz F et al: Vaginal birth after cesarean. Am J Obstet Gynecol 157:1510, 1987
4. Petitti DB: Maternal mortality and morbidity in cesarean section. Clin Obstet Gynecol 28:763, 1985
5. Horley JMG: Cesarean section. Clin Obstet Gynecol 7:529, 1980
6. Harris RP: The results of the first fifty cases of cesar-

ean ovarohysterectomy 1869–1880. Am J Med Sci 80:129, 1880

7. Porro E: Della Amputazione Utero-ovarica. Milan, 1876

8. Sanger M: My work in reference to the cesarean operation. Am J Obstet Dis Women Child 20:593, 1887

9. Sanger M: Speaking before the German Gynecology Association 1885. Am J Obstet Dis Women Child 19:883, 1886

10. Eastman NJ: The role of Frontier America in the development of cesarean section. Am J Obstet Gynecol 24:919, 1932

11. Frank F: Suprasymphysial delivery and its relation to other operations in the presence of contracted pelvis. Arch Gynaekol 81:46, 1907

12. Latzko W: Ueber den extraperitonealen Kaiserschnitt. Zentralbl Gynaekol 33:275, 1909

13. Krönig B: Transperitonealer Cervikaler Kaiser-Schnitt. p. 879. In Doderlein A, Krönig B (eds): Operative Gynakologie. 1912

14. Beck AC: Observations on a series of cesarean sections done at the Long Island College Hospital during the past six years. Am J Obstet Gynecol 79:197, 1919

15. DeLee JB, Cornell EL: Low cervical cesarean section (laparotrachelotomy). JAMA 79:109, 1922

16. Kerr JMM: The technique of cesarean section with special reference to the lower uterine segment incision. Am J Obstet Gynecol 12:729, 1926

17. DeLee JB: Principles and Practice of Obstetrics. 6th Ed. WB Saunders, Philadelphia, 1933

18. Douglas RG, Birnbaum SJ, MacDonald FA: Pregnancy and labor following cesarean section. Am J Obstet Gynecol 86:961, 1963

19. Cesarean Childbirth: Report of a Consensus Development Conference Sponsored by the National Institute of Child Health and Human Development. DHHS Pub. No. 82-2067. Government Printing Office, Washington, DC, 1981

20. Notzon FC, Placek PJ, Taffel SM: Comparisons of national cesarean-section rates. N Engl J Med 316:386, 1987

21. Feldman GB, Freiman JA: Prophylactic cesarean section at term? N Engl J Med 312:1264, 1985

22. Taffel SM, Placek PJ, Liss T: Trends in the United States cesarean section rate for the 1980–1985 rise. Am J Public Health 77:955, 1987

23. Placek PJ, Taffel SM, Keppel KG: Maternal and Infant Characteristics Associated With Cesarean Section Delivery. DHHS Publ. No. (PHS) 84-1232. National Center for Health Statistics, Hyattsville, MD, 1983

24. Green JE, McLean F, Smith LP et al. Has an increased cesarean section rate for term breech delivery reduced the incidence of birth asphyxia, trauma and death? Am J Obstet Gynecol 142:643, 1982

25. Haynes de Regt RH, Minkoff HL, Feldman J, Schwarz RH: Relation of private or clinic care to the cesarean birth rate. N Engl J Med 315:619, 1986

26. Hibbard LT: Changing trends in cesarean section. Am J Obstet Gynecol 125:798, 1976

27. Williams RL, Harvesiv WE: Cesarean section, fetal monitoring, and perinatal mortality. Am J Public Health 69:874, 1979

28. O'Driscoll K, Foley M: Correlation of decrease in perinatal mortality and increase in cesarean section rate. Obstet Gynecol 61:1, 1983

29. Leveno KJ, Cunningham FG, Pritchard JA: Cesarean section: an answer to the House of Horne. Am J Obstet Gynecol 153:838, 1985

30. Mann LI, Gallant J: Modern indications for cesarean section. Am J Obstet Gynecol 135:437, 1979

31. Haddad H, Lundy LE: Changing indications for cesarean section: a 38 year experience at a community hospital. Obstet Gynecol 51:133, 1978

32. NIH Consensus Development Task Force Statement on Cesarean Childbirth. Am J Obstet Gynecol 139:902, 1981

33. Masterson BJ: Skin preparation. Clin Obstet Gynecol 31:736, 1988

34. Larson E: Handwashing and skin physiologic and bacteriologic aspects. Infect Control 6:14, 1985

35. The tentative final monograph for over-the-counter topical antimicrobial products. Fed Reg 43:1210, 1978

36. Ritter MS, French MLV, Eitzen HE, Gioe TJ: The antimicrobial effectiveness of operative-site preparative agents. J Bone Joint Surg 62:826, 1980

37. Dineen P: Hand-washing degerming: a comparison of povidone-iodine and chlorhexidine. Clin Pharmacol Ther 23:63, 1978

38. Steere AC, Mallison GF: Handwashing practices for the prevention of nosocomial infections. Ann Intern Med 83:683, 1975

39. Brown TR, Ehrlich CE, Stehman FB et al: A clinical evaluation of chlorhexidine gluconate spray as compared with iodophor scrub for preoperative skin preparation. Surg Gynecol Obstet 158:363, 1984

40. Alexander JW, Aerni S, Plettner JP: Development of a safe and effective one-minute preoperative skin preparation. Arch Surg 120:1357, 1985

41. Garner JS: CDC guidelines for the prevention and

control of nosocomial infections: guideline for prevention of surgical wound infections, 1985. Am J Infect Control 14:71, 1986

42. Price PB: The bacteriology of normal skin: a new quantitative test applied to a study of the bacterial flora and the disinfectant action of mechanical cleansing. J Infect Dis 63:301, 1938

43. Alexander JW, Fischer JE, Boyajian M et al: The influence of hair-removal methods on wound infections. Arch Surg 118:347, 1983

44. Kenady DE: Management of abdominal wounds. Surg Clin No Am 64:803, 1984

45. Bucknall TE: Abdominal wound closure: choice of suture. J R Soc Med 74:580, 1981

46. Holtz C: Adhesion induction by suture of varying tissue reactivity and caliber. Int J Fertil 27:134, 1982

47. Ellis H, Coleridge-Smith PD, Joyce AD: Abdominal incisions — vertical or transverse? Postgrad Med J 60:407, 1984

48. Greenall MJ, Evans M, Pollack AV: Mid-line or transverse laparotomy? A random controlled clinical trial. Br J Surg 67:188, 1980

49. Becquemin J-P, Piquet J, Becquemin M-H et al: Pulmonary function after transverse or midline incision in patients with obstructive pulmonary disease. Int Care Med 11:247, 1985

50. Mowat J, Bonnar J: Abdominal wound dehiscence after cesarean section. Br Med J 2:256, 1971

51. Gallup DG: Modification of celiotomy techniques to decrease morbidity in the obese gynecologic patient. Am J Obstet Gynecol 150:171, 1984

52. Finan MA, Mastrogiannis DS, Spellacy WN: The "Allis" test for easy cesarean delivery. Am J Obstet Gynecol 164:772, 1991

53. Maylard AE: Direction of abdominal incisions. Br Med J 2:895, 1907

54. Cherney LS: A modified transverse incision for low abdominal operations. Surg Gynecol Obstet 72:92, 1941

55. Pitkin RM: Abdominal hysterectomy in obese women. Surg Gynecol Obstet 142:532, 1976

56. Shepherd JH, Cavanagh D, Riggs D et al: Abdominal wound closures using a non-absorbable single layer technique. Obstet Gynecol 61:248, 1983

57. Read JA, Cotton DB, Miller FC: Placenta accreta: changing clinical aspects and outcome. Obstet Gynecol 56:31, 1980

58. Clark SL, Koonings PP, Phelan JP: Placenta previa-accreta and previous cesarean section. Obstet Gynecol 66:89, 1985

59. Tahilramaney MP, Boucher M, Eglinton GS et al: Previous cesarean section and trial of labor: factors related to uterine dehiscence. J Reprod Med 29:17, 1984

60. Pritchard JA, McDonald PC, Gant NF (eds): Williams Obstetrics. 17th Ed. Appleton-Century-Crofts, Norwalk, CT, 1985

61. Pedowitz P, Schwartz RM: The true incidence of silent rupture of cesarean section scars: a prospective analysis of 403 cases. Am J Obstet Gynecol 74:1701, 1957

62. Janovic R: Incision of the pregnant uterus and delivery of low birthweight infants. Am J Obstet Gynecol 152:971, 1985

63. Morrison J: The development of the lower uterine segment. Aust NZ J Med 12:182, 1972

64. Nielson TF, Hokegard KH: Cesarean section and intraoperative surgical complications. Acta Obstet Gynaecol Scand 63:103, 1984

65. Hershey DW, Quilligan EJ: Extraabdominal uterine exteriorization at cesarean section. Obstet Gynecol 52:189, 1978

66. Chatterjee SK: Scar endometriosis: a clinicopathologic study of 17 cases. Obstet Gynecol 56:81, 1980

67. Sanz LE: Choosing the right wound closure technique. Contemp Ob/Gyn 21:142, 1983

68. Fagniez PL, Hay JM, Lacaine F et al: Abdominal midline incision closure. Arch Surg 120:1351, 1985

69. Sanders RJ, Diclementi D, Ireland K: Principles of abdominal wound closure. II. Prevention of wound dehiscence. Arch Surg 112:1184, 1977

70. Stone IK, vonFraunhofer JA, Masterson BJ: The biomechanical effects of tight suture closure upon fascia. Surg Gynecol Obstet 163:448, 1986

71. Elkins TE, Stovall TG, Warren J: Histological evaluation of peritoneal injury and repair: implications for adhesion formation. Obstet Gynecol 70:225, 1987

72. Raghaviah NV, Devi AI: Bladder injury associated with rupture of the uterus. Obstet Gynecol 46:573, 1975

73. Eglinton GS, Phelan JP, Yeh S-Y et al: Outcome of a trial of labor after prior cesarean delivery. J Reprod Med 29:3, 1984

74. Eisenkop SM, Richman R, Platt LD et al: Urinary tract injury during cesarean section. Obstet Gynecol 60:591, 1982

75. Michal A, Begneaud WP, Hawes TP Jr: Pitfalls and complications of cesarean section hysterectomy. Clin Obstet Gynecol 12:660, 1969

76. Barclay DL: Cesarean hysterectomy: a thirty year experience. Obstet Gynecol 35:120, 1970

77. Everett HS, Mattingly RF: Urinary tract injuries resulting from pelvic surgery. Am J Obstet Gynecol 71:502, 1956

78. Shires GT: Trauma. p. 199. In Schwartz SI (ed): Principles of Surgery. McGraw-Hill, New York, 1984

79. Carey LC, Catalano PW: The intestinal tract in relation to gynecology. p. 449. In Mattingly RF, Thompson JD (eds): TeLinde's Operative Gynecology. 6th ed. JB Lippincott, Philadelphia, 1985

80. Clark SL, Phelan JP, Yeh SY et al: Hypogastric artery ligation for the control of obstetric hemorrhage. Obstet Gynecol 66:353, 1985

81. Clark SL, Yeh S-Y, Phelan JP et al: Emergency hysterectomy for the control of obstetric hemorrhage. Obstet Gynecol 64:376, 1984

82. Hayashi RH, Castillo MS, Noah ML: Management of severe postpartum hemorrhage due to uterine atony using an analogue of prostaglandin F_2. Obstet Gynecol 58:426, 1981

83. Shaffer D, Benotti PN, Bothe A Jr et al: Subcutaneous drainage in gastric bypass surgery. Infect Surg 5:716, 1986

84. Cruse PJE, Foord R: A five-year prospective study of 23,649 surgical wounds. Arch Surg 107:206, 1973

85. Perkins RP: Extraperitoneal section: a viable alternative. Contemp Ob/Gyn 9:55, 1977

86. Wallace RL, Eglinton GS, Yonekura ML et al: Extraperitoneal cesarean section: a surgical form of infection prophylaxis? Am J Obstet Gynecol 148:172, 1984

87. Duer EL: Postmortem delivery. Am J Obstet Gynecol 12:1, 1879

88. Katz VL, Dotters DJ, Droegemueller W: Perimortem cesarean delivery. Obstet Gynecol 68:571, 1986

89. Field DR, Gates EA, Creasy R et al: Maternal brain death during pregnancy: medical and ethical issues. JAMA 260:816, 1988

90. Metheny NM. Fluid Balance. 1st Ed. JB Lippincott, Philadelphia, 1984

91. Shires GT, Canizaro PC: Fluid and electrolyte management of the surgical patient. p. 45. In Schwartz S (ed): Principles of Surgery. McGraw-Hill, New York, 1984

92. Rubin GL, Peterson HB, Rochat RW et al: Maternal death after cesarean section in Georgia. Am J Obstet Gynecol 139:681, 1981

93. Sachs BP, Yeh J, Acker D, Driscoll S et al: Cesarean section – related maternal mortality in Massachusetts, 1954–1985. Obstet Gynecol 71:385, 1988

94. Frigoletto FD, Phillipe M, Davies IJ et al: Avoiding iatrogenic prematurity with elective repeat cesarean section without the use of routine amniocentesis. Am J Obstet Gynecol 137:521, 1980

95. Baskett TF, McMillen RM: Cesarean section: trends and morbidity. Can Med Assoc J 125:723, 1981

96. Danforth DN: Cesarean section. JAMA 253:811, 1985

97. Duff P: Pathophysiology and management of postcesarean endomyometritis. Obstet Gynecol 67:269, 1986

98. Vorherr H: Puerperal genitourinary infection. In Sciarra J (ed): Gynecology and Obstetrics. Vol 2, Chapter 91, p. 1. Harper & Row, Philadelphia, 1982

99. Schwartz WH, Grolle K: The use of prophylactic antibiotics in cesarean section: a review of the literature. J Reprod Med 26:595, 1981

100. Cartwright PS, Pittaway DE, Jones HE et al: The use of prophylactic antibiotics in obstetrics and gynecology: a review. Obstet Gynecol Surv 39:537, 1984

101. Hoyme UB, Kiviat N, Eschenbach DA: Microbiology and treatment of late postpartum endometritis. Obstet Gynecol 68:226, 1986

102. Bryan CS, Reynolds KL, More EE: Bacteremia in obstetrics and gynecology. Obstet Gynecol 64:155, 1984

103. Reimer LG, Reller LB: *Gardnerella vaginalis* bacteremia: a review of thirty cases. Obstet Gynecol 64:155, 1984

104. Duff P, Gibbs RS, Blanco JD et al: Endometrial culture techniques in puerperal patients. Obstet Gynecol 61:217, 1983

105. Duff P: Diagnosis and management of post cesarean endomyometritis. p. 403. In Phelan JP, Clark SL (eds): Cesarean Delivery. Elsevier, New York, 1988

106. Mead PB: Managing infected abdominal wounds. Contemp Ob/Gyn 14:69, 1979

107. Wallace D, Hernandez W, Schlaerth JB et al: Prevention of abdominal wound disruption utilizing the Smead-Jones closure technique. Obstet Gynecol 56:26, 1980

108. Hawrylyshyn PA, Bernstein P, Papsin FR: Risk factors associated with infection following cesarean section. Am J Obstet Gynecol 139:294, 1981

109. Green SL, Sarubbi FA: Risk factors associated with postcesarean section febrile morbidity. Obstet Gynecol 49:686, 1977

110. Nielson TF, Hokegard KH: Postoperative cesarean section morbidity: a prospective study. Am J Obstet Gynecol 146:911, 1983

111. Gibbs RS, Blanco JD, St Clair PJ: A case–control study of wound abscess after cesarean delivery. Obstet Gynecol 62:498, 1983

112. Gall SA Jr, Gall SA: Diagnosis and management of postcesarean wound infections. p. 388. In Phelan JP,

Clark SL (eds): Cesarean Delivery. Elsevier, New York, 1988

113. Sweet RL, Yonekura ML, Hill G et al: Appropriate use of antibiotics in serious obstetric and gynecologic infections. Am J Obstet Gynecol 136:719, 1983

114. Gall SA: Infections in the female genital tract. Comp Ther 9:34, 1983

115. Emmons SL, Krohn M, Jackson M, Eschenbach DA: Development of wound infections among women undergoing cesarean section. Obstet Gynecol 72:559, 1988

116. Kuhn HH, Ullman U, Kuhn FW: New aspects on the pathophysiology of wound infection and wound healing — the problem of lowered oxygen pressure in the tissue. Infection 13:52, 1985

117. Polk HC: Operating room acquired infection: a review of pathogenesis. Am Surg 45:349, 1979

118. Krebs HB, Helmkamp BF: Transverse periumbilical incision in the massively obese patient. Obstet Gynecol 63:241, 1984

119. Gerzof SG, Robbins AH, Johnson WC et al: Percutaneous catheter drainage of abdominal abscesses: a five year experience. N Engl J Med 305:653, 1981

120. Lee CY, Madrazo BL, Drukker GH: Ultrasonic evaluation of the postpartum uterus in the management of postpartum bleeding. Obstet Gynecol 58:227, 1981

121. Gross BH, Callen PW: Ultrasound of the uterus. p. 227. In Callen PW (ed): Ultrasonography in Obstetrics and Gynecology. Philadelphia, WB Saunders, 1982

122. Burger NF, Dararas B, Boes EGM: An echographic evaluation during the early puerperium of the uterine wound after cesarean section. J Clin Ultrasound 10:271, 1982

123. Lavery J, Gadwood KA: Postpartum sonography. p. 509. In Sanders RC, Jones E (eds): Ultrasonography in Obstetrics and Gynecology. 4th ed. Appleton-Century-Crofts Medical, Norwalk, CT, 1991

124. Malvern J, Campbell S, May P: Ultrasonic scanning of the puerperal uterus following secondary postpartum haemorrhage. Br J Obstet Gynecol 80:320, 1973

125. Shaffer PB, Johnson JC, Bryan D et al: Diagnosis of ovarian vein thrombophlebitis by computed tomography. J Comput Assist Tomogr 5:436, 1981

126. Farrell SJ, Andersen HF, Work BA Jr: Cesarean section: indications and postoperative morbidity. Obstet Gynecol 56:696, 1980

127. Rehu M, Nilsson CG: Risk factors for febrile morbidity associated with cesarean section. Obstet Gynecol 56:269, 1980

128. Fowler JE Jr, Marshall V: Nosocomial catheter-associated urinary tract infection. Infect Surg 2:43, 1983

129. Bonnar J: Venous thromboembolism and pregnancy. Clin Obstet Gynecol 8:455, 1981

130. Villasanta U: Thromboembolic disease in pregnancy. Am J Obstet Gynecol 93:142, 1965

131. Stead RB: Regulation of hemostasis. p. 27. In Goldhaber AZ (ed): Pulmonary Embolism and Deep Venous Thrombosis. WB Saunders, Philadelphia, 1985

132. Hirsh J, Cade JF, Gallus AS: Anticoagulants in pregnancy: a review of indications and complications. Am Heart J 83:301, 1972

133. Laros RK, Alger LS: Thromboembolism and pregnancy. Clin Obstet Gynecol 22:871, 1979

134. Rosenow ED III, Osmundson PJ, Brown ML: Pulmonary embolism. Mayo Clin Proc 56:161, 1981

135. Duff P, Gibbs RS: Pelvic vein thrombophlebitis: diagnostic dilemma and therapeutic challenge. Obstet Gynecol Surv 38:365, 1983

136. Bartlette RH, Brennan ML, Gazzaniga AB et al: Studies on the pathogenesis and prevention of postoperative pulmonary complications. Surg Gynecol Obstet 137:925, 1973

137. Rosen MA, Hughes SC, Shnider SM: Epidural morphine for the relief of postoperative pain after cesarean delivery. Anesth Analg 62:666, 1983

138. Metcalfe J, Ueland K: Maternal cardiovascular adjustments to pregnancy. Prog Cardiovasc Dis 16:363, 1974

139. Bottoms SF, Rosen MG, Sokol RJ: The increase in the cesarean birth. N Engl J Med 302:559, 1980

140. Blumenthal NJ, Harris RS, O'Connor MC et al: Changing cesarean section rates experience at a Sydney obstetric teaching hospital. Aust NZ J Obstet Gynaecol 24:246, 1984

141. Phillips RN, Thornton J, Gleicher N: Physician bias in cesarean sections. JAMA 248:1082, 1982

142. O'Driscoll K, Foley M, MacDonald D: Active management of labor as an alternative to cesarean section for dystocia. Obstet Gynecol 63:485, 1984

143. Anderson GM, Lomas J: Determinants of the increasing cesarean birth rate. N Engl J Med 311:887, 1984

144. Flamm BL: Vaginal birth after cesarean section: controversies old and new. Clin Obstet Gynecol 28:735, 1985

145. Riva H, Teich J: Vaginal delivery after cesarean section. Am J Obstet Gynecol 81:501, 1961

146. ACOG Newsletter: vaginal birth after cesarean. Focus New Guidelines 29, 1985

147. ACOG: Guidelines for vaginal delivery after a previous cesarean birth. Committee on Maternal and Fetal Medicine. ACOG, Washington, DC, 1988

148. Lavin JP, Stephens RJ, Miodovnik M et al: Vaginal delivery in patients with a prior cesarean section. Obstet Gynecol 59:135, 1982

149. Paul RH, Phelan JP, Yeh S: Trial of labor in the patient with a prior cesarean birth. Am J Obstet Gynecol 151:297, 1985

150. Horenstein JP, Phelan JP: Previous cesarean section: the risks and benefits of oxytocin usage in a trial of labor. Am J Obstet Gynecol 151:564, 1985

150a. Rosen MG, Dickinson JC, Westhoff CL: Vaginal birth after cesarean: A meta-analysis of morbidity and mortality. Obstet Gynecol 77:465, 1991

151. Plauche WC, Von Almen W, Mueller R: Catastrophic uterine rupture. Obstet Gynecol 64:792, 1984

152. Eden RD, Parker RT, Gall SA: Rupture of the pregnant uterus: a 53 year review. Obstet Gynecol 68:671, 1986

153. Salzmann B: Rupture of the low-segment cesarean section scars. Obstet Gynecol 23:460, 1964

154. O'Sullivan M, Fumia F, Holsinger K et al: Vaginal delivery after cesarean section. Clin Perinatol 8:131, 1981

155. Horenstein J, Phelan JP: Vaginal birth after cesarean: the role of oxytocin. p. 484. In Phelan JP, Clark SL (eds): Cesarean Delivery. Elsevier, New York, 1988

156. Silver RK, Gibbs RS: Prediction of vaginal delivery in patients with a previous cesarean section who require oxytocin. Am J Obstet Gynecol 156:57, 1987

157. Mackenzie IZ, Bradley S, Embrey MP: Vaginal prostaglandins and labor induction for patients previously delivered by cesarean section. Br J Obstet Gynecol 91:7, 1984

158. Phelan JP, Eglinton GS, Horenstein JM et al: Previous cesarean birth: trial of labor in women with macrosomic infants. J Reprod Med 29:36, 1984

159. Brundenell M, Chakravarti S: Uterine rupture in labour. Br Med J 2:122, 1975

160. O'Driscoll K: An obstetrician's view of pain. Br J Anaesth 47:1053, 1975

161. Flamm BL, Dunnett C, Fischermann E et al: Vaginal delivery following cesarean section: use of oxytocin augmentation and epidural anesthesia with internal tocodynamic and internal fetal monitoring. Am J Obstet Gynecol 148:759, 1984

162. Carlson C, Lybell-Lindahl G, Ingemarsson I: Extradural block in patients who have previously undergone cesarean section. Br J Anaesth 52:827, 1980

163. Crawford JS: The epidural sieve and MBC (minimal blocking concentration): a hypothesis. Anaesthesia 31:1278, 1976

164. Uppington J: Epidural analgesia and previous cesarean section. Anaesthesia 38:336, 1983

165. Golan A, Sandbank O, Rubin A: Rupture of the pregnant uterus. Obstet Gynecol 56:349, 1980

166. Lowensohn RI, Paul RH, Fales S et al: Intrapartum epidural anesthesia: an evaluation of effects on uterine activity. Obstet Gynecol 44:388, 1974

167. Akamatsu TJ, Bonica JJ: Spinal and extradural analgesia-anesthesia for parturition. Clin Obstet Gynecol 17:183, 1974

168. Kaminski HM, Stafl A, Aiman J: The effect of epidural analgesia on the frequency of instrumental obstetric delivery. Obstet Gynecol 69:770, 1987

169. Chestnut DH, Owen CL, Bates JN et al: Continuous infusion epidural analgesia during labor: a randomized, double-blind comparison of 0.625% bupivacaine/0.0002% fentanyl vs 0.125% bupivacaine. Anesthesiology 68:754, 1988

170. Eglinton GS: Effect of previous indications for cesarean on subsequent outcome. p. 476. In Phelan JP, Clark SL (eds): Cesarean Delivery. Elsevier, New York, 1988

171. Seitchik J, Rao VRR: Cesarean delivery in nulliparous women for failed oxytocin-augmented labor: route of delivery in subsequent pregnancy. Am J Obstet Gynecol 143:393, 1982

172. Clark CL, Eglinton GS, Beall M et al: Effect of indication for previous cesarean section on subsequent delivery outcome in patients undergoing a trial of labor. J Reprod Med 29:33, 1984

173. Saldana LR, Schulman H, Reuss L: Management of pregnancy after cesarean section. Am J Obstet Gynecol 135:555, 1979

174. Martin JN, Harris BA, Huddleston JF et al: Vaginal delivery following previous cesarean birth. Am J Obstet Gynecol 146:255, 1983

175. Porreco RP, Meier RP: Trial of labor in patients with multiple previous cesarean sections. J Reprod Med 28:770, 1983

176. Cesarean sections and cesarean hysterectomy. p. 445. In Cunningham FG, Macdonald PC, Gant NF (eds): Williams Obstetrics. Appleton & Lange, Norwalk, CT, 1989

177. ACOG: Practice perspective: guidelines for vaginal delivery after previous cesarean birth. Newsletter. ACOG, Washington, DC, 1985

178. Porreco RP, Meier RP: Repeat cesarean — most unnecessary. Contemp Obstet Gynecol 21:55, 1984

179. Hannah W: Final statement of the panel from the National Consensus Conference on Aspects of Cesarean Birth, Hamilton, Ontario, Canada, 1986

180. ACOG: Induction and augmentation of labor. Tech Bull No. 49, 1978

181. ACOG: Induction and augmentation of labor. Tech Bull No. 119, 1987

182. Meier P, Porreco R: Trial of labor following cesarean section: a two year experience. Am J Obstet Gynecol 144:671, 1982

183. Burchell CR: Physiology of internal iliac artery ligation. J Obstet Gynecol Br Commonw 75:642, 1968

184. Clark SL, Phelan JP: Surgical control of obstetric hemorrhage. Contemp Ob/Gyn 24:70, 1984

185. Barclay DL, Clark SL, Plauche WC: Cesarean hysterectomy: update tape. Am Coll Obstet Gynecol 11, 1986

186. Sall S, Rini S, Pineda A: Surgical management of invasive carcinoma of the cervix in pregnancy. Obstet Gynecol 118:1, 1974

187. Thompson JD, Caputo TA, Franklin EW III et al: The surgical management of invasive cancer of the cervix in pregnancy. Am J Obstet Gynecol 121:853, 1975

188. Plauche WC, Gruich FG, Bourgeois MO: Hysterectomy at the time of cesarean section: analysis of 108 cases. Obstet Gynecol 58:459, 1981

189. Shepard MK: Female contraceptive sterilization. Obstet Gynecol Surv 29:739, 1974

190. Gomez A, Wood M: Acute appendicitis in pregnancy. Am J Surg 137:180, 1979

191. Bauer JL, Reis RA, Arens RA: Appendicitis in pregnancy with changes in position and areas of normal appendix in pregnancy. JAMA 98:1359, 1932

192. Stauffer RA, Adams A, Wygal J et al: Gallbladder disease in pregnancy. Am J Obstet Gynecol 144:661, 1982

193. Duhrssen A: On the value of deep cervical incisions and episiotomy in obstetrics. Arch Gynaekol 37:27, 1890

194. Baker, Shingleton: Clin Obstet Gynecol 31:701, 1988

195. ACOG: Prolog. p. 187. In Gynecologic Oncology and Surgery. ACOG: Washington, DC, 1991

196. Breen J, Cregori CA, Kindzierski JA: Hemorrhage in gynecologic surgery. p. 438. In Complications in Obstetric and Gynecologic Surgery. Harper & Row, Hagerstown, MD, 1981

197. Lees DH, Singer A: Gynecological Surgery. Vol 6. Wolfe, 1983

SECTION 4
Postpartum Care

Chapter 21

The Neonate

Adam A. Rosenberg

The first 4 weeks of an infant's life, the neonatal period, are marked by the highest mortality rate in all of childhood. The greatest risk occurs during the first several days after birth. Critical to an infant's survival during this period is its ability to adapt successfully to extrauterine life. During the early hours after birth, the newborn must assume responsibility for thermoregulation, metabolic homeostasis, and respiratory gas exchange, as well as undergo the conversion from fetal to postnatal circulatory pathways. This chapter reviews the physiology of a successful transition as well as the implications of circumstances that disrupt this process. Implicit in these considerations is the understanding that the newborn reflects the sum total of its genetic and environmental past as well as any minor or major insults to which it was subjected during gestation and parturition. The period of neonatal adaptation then is most meaningfully viewed as a continuum with fetal life.

CARDIOPULMONARY TRANSITION

Pulmonary Development

Lung development and maturation require a carefully regulated interaction of anatomic, physiologic, and biochemical processes. The outcome of these events provides an organ with adequate surface area, sufficient vascularization, and the metabolic capability to sustain oxygenation and ventilation during the

neonatal period. Four stages of morphologic lung development have been identified in the human fetus[1,2]:

1. Embryonic period—conception to 5 weeks
2. Pseudoglandular period—5th to 16th weeks
3. Canalicular period—16th to 24th weeks
4. Terminal sac period—24th week to term

The lung arises as a ventral diverticulum from the foregut during the fourth week of gestation. During the ensuing weeks, branching of the diverticulum occurs, leading to a tree of narrow tubules with thick epithelial walls composed of columnar-type cells. By 16 weeks, the conducting portion of the tracheobronchial tree up to and including terminal bronchioles has been established. The vasculature derived from the pulmonary circulation develops concurrently with the conducting airways, and by 16 weeks all preacinar blood vessels are formed.[3] The canalicular stage is characterized by differentiation of the airways, with widening of the lumina and thinning of the epithelium. In addition, primitive respiratory bronchioles begin to form, marking the start of the gas-exchanging portion of the lung. Vascular proliferation continues, along with a relative decrease in mesenchyme, bringing the vessels closer to the airway epithelium. The terminal sac stage is marked by the development of the gas-exchanging portion of the tracheobronchial tree (acinus) composed of respiratory bronchioles, alveolar ducts, terminal saccules, and finally alveoli. During this stage, the pulmonary vessels continue to proliferate with the airways and surround the developing air sacs.[3] Postnatal lung growth is characterized by generation of alveoli. At birth, there are approximately 20 million airspaces and by 8 years of age, 300 million.[4]

In early gestation, respiratory epithelial cells are simple and columnar in type. A slow transition from columnar epithelium to the lining of a fully developed alveolus starts during the fifth month.[5] By the time of birth, the epithelial lining of the gas-exchanging surface is thin and continuous with two alveolar cell types (types I and II). Type I cells contain few subcellular organelles, while type II cells contain abundant mitochondria, endoplasmic reticulum, Golgi apparatus, and osmiophilic lamellar bodies now known to contain surfactant (Fig. 21.1). Buckingham and Avery[6] first suggested that these inclusions could be the source of a material that lowered surface tension at the alveolar–air surface. Klaus et al.[7] and Orzalesi et al.[8] subsequently provided support for this suggestion. The first group correlated the presence of os-

miophilic inclusions with surface activity in lung extracts of dog, cat, rat, mouse, rabbit, and human subjects while also demonstrating that surface tension was not reduced by extracts from toad and pigeon lungs, which did not contain inclusions. In the second set of studies, electron microscopic examination revealed osmiophilic lamellar bodies at 120 days gestation in fetal lambs (term, 145 days). The appearance of normal surface activity of lung extracts follows this by only a few days. The number of cells with inclusions as well as the number of inclusions increased toward term. Similar observations have been made in developing human lung.[9] Conclusive evidence that the type II cell synthesizes, stores, and releases surface-active phospholipids has come from studies with mixed cell cultures from lungs.[10]

Because of the development of high surface forces along the respiratory epithelium when breathing begins, the availability of surfactants in terminal airspaces is critical for postnatal lung function. Just as surface tension acts to reduce the size of a bubble in water, so too it acts to reduce lung size, promoting atelectasis. This is described by the LaPlace relationship, which states that the pressure P within a sphere is directly proportional to surface tension T and inversely proportional to the radius of curvature r (Fig. 21.2).

In 1929, von Neergaard[11] was the first to evaluate the importance of surface forces in pulmonary physiology. He determined the pressure–volume characteristics of liquid- and air-filled lungs and observed that transpulmonary pressures were two to three times as great when lungs were distended with air. The only difference in the two situations was the presence of an air–liquid interface in the air-filled lung. He concluded that a considerable portion of elastic recoil in the lung was due to surface forces. Mead et al.[12] later described similar pressure–volume characteristics of saline- and air-filled dog lungs over a full volume range. Their focus centered on an explanation for hysteresis, that is, separation of inflation and deflation curves (Fig. 21.3) in air-filled lungs. Transpulmonary pressure at a given volume was greater during inflation than for a similar volume during deflation. This phenomenon was attributed to the effect of surface forces.

Subsequent to the observations of Mead et al., Clements[13] demonstrated the property of lung ex-

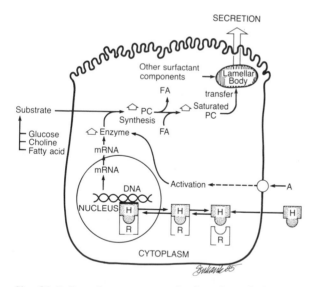

Fig. 21.1 Type II pneumocyte with a hypothetical scheme for the synthesis and release of surfactant to the alveolar lining layer. A, activator; H, hormone (e.g., corticosteroid); R, receptor; FA, fatty acid; DNA, deoxyribonucleic acid; mRNA, messenger ribonucleic acid coding for synthesis of specific enzymes; PC, phosphatidylcholine. (Adapted from Ballard,[319] with permission.)

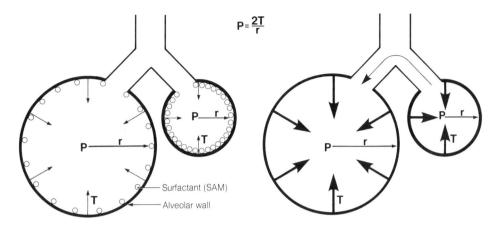

$$P = \frac{2T}{r}$$

Surfactant (SAM)
Alveolar wall

Fig. 21.2 LaPlace's law. The pressure, P, within a sphere is directly proportional to surface tension, T, and inversely proportional to the radius of curvature, r. In the normal lung, as alveolar size decreases, surface tension is reduced because of the presence of surfactant. This serves to decrease the collapsing pressure that needs to be opposed and maintains equal pressures in the small and large interconnected alveoli. (Adapted from Netter,[320] with permission.)

tracts to lower surface tension as surface area was decreased. These studies were carried out with a surface balance, a device in which the material to be investigated is added to a surface and alternately compressed and expanded with measurement of tension. Figure 21.4 shows that the surface tension of water is independent of the area of the surface and has a value

of 70 dyn/cm. If detergent is added to the water, surface tension falls but remains independent of surface area. However, lung extract generates a curve relating surface area to tension. This curve has two important features. One is that the smaller the area, the lower the surface tension. If this behavior is extrapolated to the lung, smaller alveoli will have a lower surface tension than larger alveoli. This will serve to prevent smaller alveoli from inflating larger ones (Fig. 21.2) as well as to avoid the collapse of

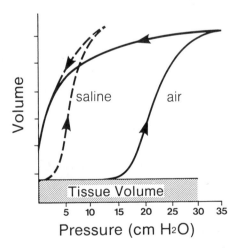

Fig. 21.3 Air and saline pressure volume curves of excised dog lungs. (Adapted from Avery and Said,[321] with permission.)

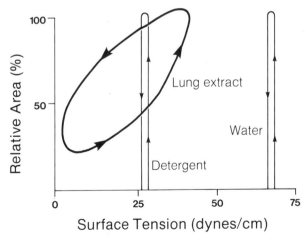

Fig. 21.4 Plots of surface tension and area obtained with a surface balance. (Adapted from Clements,[13] with permission.)

alveoli as their radii decreases on exhalation. Second, the curve demonstrates the same hysteresis that is seen in the pressure–volume curve of the lung. For a given surface area, surface tension is greater during expansion than in compression, corresponding to the circumstance in the lung in which higher pressures are required to achieve a given volume during inflation than deflation. Application of the physiologic data explains several critical functions of surfactant in the neonatal lung: (1) low alveolar surface tension at low lung volumes reduces the work of expanding the lung during inspiration, (2) alveolar stability is maintained over a wide range of local volumes, and (3) alveoli are kept dry by decreasing inward-acting forces that would tend to pull in water from pulmonary capillaries.

Regardless of the total duration of pregnancy in a number of mammalian species examined, the presence of surfactant or evidence of increased phosphatidylcholine (PC) production is demonstrable at 85 to 90 percent of term.[14,15] Tissue stores of surfactant are considerable at term (Fig. 21.5).[16,17] Surfactant is released from storage pools into fetal lung fluid at a basal rate during late gestation. Secretion is stimulated by labor and the initiation of air breathing.[16] Potential mediators of surfactant secretion include mechanical distention of the lung and β-agonists. Ekelund et al.[18] have pointed out that β-agonists could be beneficial to the fetus by causing increased surfactant release. However, prolonged fetal exposure could result in depletion of stores, with resulting surfactant deficiency.

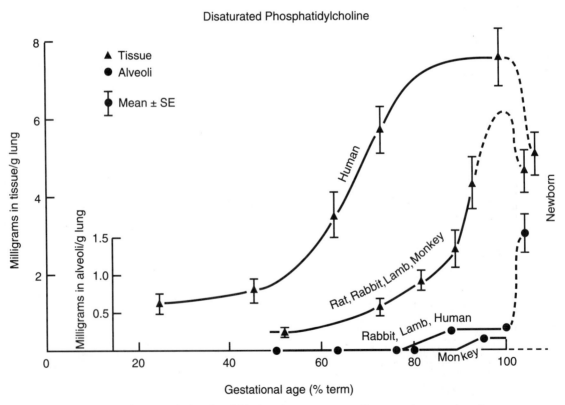

Fig. 21.5 Accumulation of saturated phosphatidylcholine during gestation. Gestational age is plotted as percentage of term. (Adapted from Clements and Tooley,[17] with permission.)

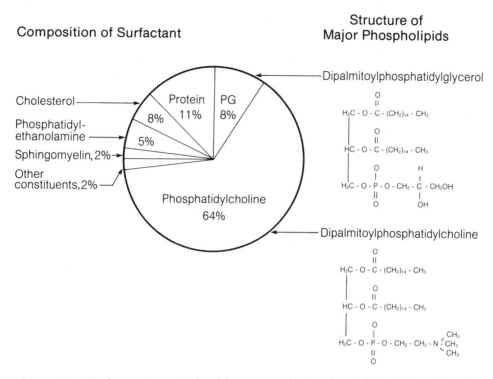

Fig. 21.6 Composition of surface active material and the structure of major phospholipids. (Adapted from Perelman et al.,[322] with permission.)

The composition of pulmonary surfactant is depicted in Figure 21.6. The predominance of PC is evident. PC molecules obtained from tissues other than lung have a saturated fatty acid at the 1-carbon position and an unsaturated inhabitant at the 2-carbon position. In surfactant, PC has saturated fatty acids (usually palmitic acid) at both positions. This degree of saturation appears to be critical for its surface-tension-lowering ability.[19] Phosphatidylglycerol (PG) is another constituent of surfactant, the precise role of which is incompletely defined but appears to relate to pulmonary maturity. Much has been learned in recent years about the protein content of surfactant. Three species of nonserum surfactant-associated proteins have been identified.[20] These proteins are thought to play important roles in the structural organization, function, and metabolism of surfactant. Surfactant protein A is the most abundant and serves to increase the rate of surface film formation. Proteins B and C are hydrophobic and play a role in rapid spreading of surfactant and in decreasing surface tension at the air–liquid interface.

A number of hormones contribute to the regulation of pulmonary phospholipid metabolism. The importance of glucocorticoids has been demonstrated in a number of species. In 1969, Liggins[21] found dexamethasone injected into fetal lambs to lead to premature delivery. He also noted that the lungs of vaginally delivered lambs were partially aerated, suggesting advanced lung maturation. DeLemos et al.[22] confirmed this possibility by injecting fetal lambs with hydrocortisone and demonstrating accelerated lung maturation. Accelerated appearance of surfactant as well as increased numbers of lamellar bodies were observed in a fetal rabbit model after steroid injection,[23,24] while administration of steroid to the amniotic cavity of a baboon was found to cause an increase in the lecithin/sphingomyelin ratio and functional maturity of the lung.[25] β-Adrenergics and thyroid hormone appear to act synergistically with steroids to accelerate pulmonary maturation.[20] Thus there appears to be multihormonal input, but only glucocorticoids have been shown to increase production of all the known lipid and protein components of surfac-

Table 21.1 Clinical Trials of Glucocorticoids in Human Pregnancy

Study[a]	Patient No. Total (Drug/Control)	Time From First Dose	Percent Respiratory Distress Syndrome (RDS) (Drug/Control)	Comments
Liggins and Howie[26]	219 (122/97) 168 (93/75)	All patients >24 hr	9.0/25.8[b] 4.3/24.0[b]	1. Maximum effect at 26 to 32 weeks gestation 2. Lower mortality in the treated group 3. Increased fetal death in treated pregnancies with preeclampsia
Block et al.[27]	110 (57/53) 65 (36/29)	All patients >24 hr	8.7/22.6[b] 11.1/20.7	1. Overall mortality—no difference; <32 weeks gestation—lower mortality in the treated group
Papageorgiou et al.[28]	61 (29/32)	>24 hr	20.7/59.4[b]	1. Lower mortality in the treated group 2. RDS, when present, less severe in the treated group 3. Increased incidence of hypoglycemia in treated babies
Taeusch et al.[29]	115 (50/65) 95 (30/65)	All patients >48 hr	14.0/22.0 7.0/22.0[b]	1. Overall mortality—no difference; less mortality from RDS in treated group 2. RDS, when present, less severe in the treated group 3. Increased maternal infection in the treated group
Doran et al.[30]	137 (75/62)	All patients >48 hr	5.0/17.0[b]	1. Maximum effect at 29 to 32 weeks gestation 2. Lower mortality in the treated group 3. RDS, when present, less severe in the treated group
Collaborative[31]	720 (361/359) 295 (151/144)	All patients >24 hr; <7 days	12.7/18.1[b] 9.3/20.1	1. Maximum effect at 30 to 34 weeks gestation; singleton females 2. No difference in mortality 3. Shorter hospitalization for treated infants[32] 4. No short-term or long-term[33] side effects

[a] All prospective studies.

[b] Significant to at least $p < 0.05$.

tant. Although the exact mechanism of action of steroids is still not entirely clear, there is considerable evidence from human trials that maternal administration of steroids can decrease the incidence and severity of hyaline membrane disease (Table 21.1).

The First Breaths

A critical step in the transition from intrauterine to extrauterine life is the conversion of the lung from a dormant fluid-filled organ to one capable of gas exchange. This requires aeration of the lungs, establishment of an adequate pulmonary circulation, ventilation of the aerated parenchyma, and diffusion of oxygen and carbon dioxide through the alveolar–capillary membranes. This process has its roots in utero as fetal breathing.

Fetal Breathing

Fetal breathing has been documented in a variety of animal species, but the majority of experiments have taken place in fetal sheep.[34,35] The onset of breathing in the fetal sheep has been noted as early as 40 days of gestation. By days 90 through 115, breathing is almost continuous, with rare apneic pauses of less than 2 minutes duration. However, from day 115 to term, breathing is episodic, with long apneic periods interspersed among periods of respiratory activity. The predominant respiratory pattern is one of rapid, irregular movements varying in amplitude at a rate of 60 to 120 per minute. This pattern is associated with rapid eye movement (REM) sleep. A much less frequently observed activity is characterized by isolated, slow gasps (1 to 4 per minute) unassociated with any particular stage of sleep. Human fetal breathing is quite similar to that observed in fetal sheep.[36] Respiratory activity is initially detectable at 11 weeks. The most prevalent pattern is rapid, small-amplitude movements (60 to 90 per minute) present 60 to 80 percent of the time. Less commonly, irregular low-amplitude movements interspersed with slower larger-amplitude movements are seen.

Numerous investigations of the mechanisms that control fetal breathing have been performed in the last 25 years in the hope that an understanding of these controls would provide an answer to the question of what initiates the change from episodic breathing in utero to regular, continuous postnatal respiration. The following statements summarize data from a variety of sources.[35,37–41]

1. Normal fetal breathing movements do not appear to be regulated by central or peripheral chemoreceptors over the usual physiologic range of gas tensions seen in the fetus.
2. In response to a decrease in oxygen tension, the fetus interrupts or slows respiratory activity.
3. Hypercarbia generally acts to increase fetal respiration, but less so than postnatally.
4. Respiratory activity seems to be regulated by factors operative during REM sleep, a condition in which respiratory drive is heavily modified by cortical activity.

The role of fetal breathing in the continuum from fetal to neonatal life is still not completely understood. It seems probable that fetal respiratory activity is essential to the development of chest wall muscles (including diaphragm)[34] and serves as a regulator of lung fluid volume and thus lung growth.[35]

Control of Neonatal Respiration

A variety of stimuli present at the time of birth could have a role in initiating postnatal respiration (Table 21.2). James et al.[42] in 1958 noted that varying degrees of asphyxia occurred with all forms of delivery. This asphyxia, if not too prolonged, was thought to act through chemoreceptors to initiate breathing in the infant. Six years later, Harned et al.[39] observed that breathing begins so promptly after birth that a reflex must be involved. With a series of experiments performed in fetal sheep, Harned and colleagues examined factors responsible for the initiation of post-

Table 21.2 Potential Sensory Inputs to the Respiratory Center

Input	Example
General	
Proprioceptive	Position, gravity
Tactile	Pain, handling
Auditory	Noise
Visual	Light
Thermal	Cold
Reflexes	
Nonchemical	Pulmonary stretch, baroceptors
Chemical	Peripheral and central chemoreceptors responding to blood gas changes

(Modified from Nelson,[324] with permission.)

natal respiration.[39,40,43] Umbilical cord occlusion, associated with marked carotid chemoreceptor activation, provided the most reliable stimulus for sustained respiratory activity. This response was blocked by division of the carotid sinus nerves. These data indicate a crucial role for carotid body input to the medullary respiratory center in initiating respiration. Activation of the carotid bodies after cord occlusion is likely due to the collective effects of a falling P_{O_2}, a rising P_{CO_2}, and decreased blood flow to the region. This drop in carotid blood flow provides an explanation for the postnatal increase in sensitivity of the carotid chemoreceptors to changes in blood gas tensions.[41] More recently, it was shown that prostaglandins may also be involved in the transition from periodic fetal to continuous postnatal respiration.[44,45] Changes in temperature have also been shown to have a role in the initiation of respiration, with cold stimulating increased respiratory activity.[46] The role of the other factors listed in Table 21.2 is less well documented.[47]

With the establishment of sustained respiratory activity, the maintenance of this regular effort becomes of chief importance. The peripheral chemoreceptors so instrumental in the initiation of respiration do not appear to be essential to continued rhythmic breathing.[48] At this point, the response of central chemoreceptors in the medulla is more critical.[48,49] Reflex activity from the lungs and chest play a role as well in the breathing pattern of the newborn infant.[50] There is also considerable excitatory input from nonrespiratory sources, on which rhythmic respiratory activity may depend.[51] Neonatal responses to hypoxia and hypercarbia appear to be species dependent. Although these responses are mature in the neonatal lamb,[52] the human neonate does not possess fully developed sensitivity to changes in either P_{O_2} or P_{CO_2}. The characteristic response to hypoxia is a brief hyperpnea followed by ventilatory depression,[53] while the response to hypercarbia increases with advancing gestational or postnatal age.[54]

Mechanics of the First Breath

With its first breaths, the neonate must overcome several forces resisting lung expansion: (1) viscosity of fetal lung fluid, (2) resistance provided by lung tissue itself, and (3) the forces of surface tension at the air–liquid interface.[55] Viscosity of fetal lung fluid is a major factor as the neonate attempts to displace fluid present in the large airways. As the passage of air moves toward small airways and alveoli, surface tension becomes more important. Resistance to expansion by the lung tissue itself is less significant.

The physiology of the first breaths was first elegantly studied by Karlberg and colleagues[56,57] and more recently reexamined by Milner and Vyas.[58] The process begins as the infant passes through the birth canal. The intrathoracic pressure caused by vaginal squeeze is up to 200 cmH$_2$O.[58,59] With delivery of the head, approximately 5 to 28 ml of tracheal fluid is expressed. Subsequent delivery of the thorax causes an elastic recoil of the chest. With this recoil, up to 30 ml of air could enter the airways.[59] The term newborn possesses a functional residual capacity (FRC) of about 100 ml (1 dl), so this passive entry of air would aid the infant significantly in initial lung expansion. That amount of air would be enough to fill much of the large airway tree, overcoming the forces of viscosity of fetal lung fluid. However, Milner and Vyas[58] were unable to confirm this passive entry of air into the tracheobronchial tree. In their studies, during escape of the baby from the birth canal, no more than 2 ml of air entered the lungs before the onset of active respiratory efforts. In the interval between delivery and the first diaphragmatic inspiration, other factors have also been proposed that might aid the neonate with its first breath. Bosma and Lind[60] demonstrated distention and contraction of the pharynx during this interval. This "frog breathing" could serve to force small amounts of air into the airways. Furthermore, it has been proposed that if some amount of pulmonary capillary flow has been established, "capillary erection" could serve to expand the walls of crumpled air sacs.[61] Under normal circumstances, the contribution of both these mechanisms is probably minimal.

The initial breath is characteristically a short inspiration followed by a more prolonged expiration (Fig. 21.7).[56-58] Considerable negative intrathoracic pressure during inspiration is provided by diaphragmatic contraction. Karlberg and colleagues[56,57] found it necessary to achieve an opening pressure of 20 to 40 cmH$_2$O before a change in lung volume was seen in 5 of 11 babies examined. However, Milner and Vyas[58] were unable to confirm this. Air entered the lungs as soon as intrathoracic pressure began to fall.

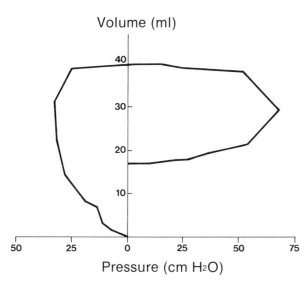

Volume (ml)

Pressure (cm H₂O)

Fig. 21.7 Pressure volume loop of the first breath. Air enters the lung as soon as intrathoracic pressure falls and expiratory pressure greatly exceeds inspiratory pressure. (Modified from Milner and Vyas,[58] with permission.)

The volume of this first breath varies between 30 and 67 ml and correlates with intrathoracic pressure. The expiratory phase is quite prolonged as the infant's expiration is opposed by intermittent closure at the pharyngolaryngeal level[60] with the generation of large positive intrathoracic pressure. This serves to aid both in maintenance of an FRC and with fluid removal from the air sacs. The residual volume after this first breath ranges between 4 and 30 ml, averaging 16 to 20 ml. There are really no major systematic differences among the first three breaths, demonstrating similar pressure patterns of decreasing magnitude. The FRC rapidly increases with the first several breaths and then more gradually. By 30 minutes of age, most infants attain a normal FRC with uniform lung expansion.[62] The presence of functional surfactant is instrumental in the accumulation of an FRC.[16]

Normal expansion and aeration of the neonatal lung is also dependent on removal of fetal lung liquid. Factors involved in this process are (1) the thoracic squeeze during delivery, (2) a marked increase in pulmonary lymph flow, and (3) removal via the pulmonary circulation.[63,64] The importance of the thoracic squeeze has recently been questioned. Removal of pulmonary fluid was thought to begin after birth,[65]

but Mescher et al.[66] demonstrated, in a fetal lamb model, that fluid flow from the trachea decreased during the 48 hours prior to birth. Bland et al.[67] were subsequently able to demonstrate that lung lymph becomes more dilute during labor. Finally, Bland and colleagues[68] found no difference in lung water between a group of rabbits delivered vaginally and a group delivered by cesarean section after experiencing labor. A group delivered by cesarean section without labor had increased lung water. Cumulatively, these studies tend to support the greater importance of labor as a stimulus to increase fluid removal rather than the thoracic squeeze. This is further supported by studies in human infants.[58] Although inspiratory pressures and volume changes were similar to those seen in vaginally delivered infants, babies born by elective cesarean section were less likely to establish an FRC with the initial breath. By contrast, babies born by emergency cesarean section after labor behaved more like vaginally delivered infants. The inability to form an FRC in elective operative deliveries might be attributable to more fluid in the lungs during the first 6 hours of life.[64] The mechanism responsible for the reduction in fetal lung liquid prior to birth is unknown. However, this adaptive process may be the result of late gestation fetal hormone changes. In particular, catecholamines have been implicated.[64] Thus β-adrenergics given to inhibit preterm labor may benefit the fetus by reducing lung water content prior to birth.

Postnatally, within 15 and 30 minutes of birth, there is a marked increase in pulmonary lymph flow.[63] In the term infant about 11 percent of lung fluid is removed via this route and the remainder through the pulmonary circulation. Removal of liquid from the lungs then continues for several hours after birth.

Circulatory Transition

The circulation in the fetus (Fig. 21.8) has been studied in a variety of species using several techniques (see Ch. 4). These studies have been the subject of a number of excellent reviews.[69–73]

Umbilical venous blood, returning from the placenta, has a P_{O_2} of about 30 to 35 mmHg. About 40 to 60 percent of this blood, depending on circumstances, passes through the liver (mainly to the middle and left lobes). This blood will ultimately enter the inferior vena cava (IVC) through the hepatic veins.

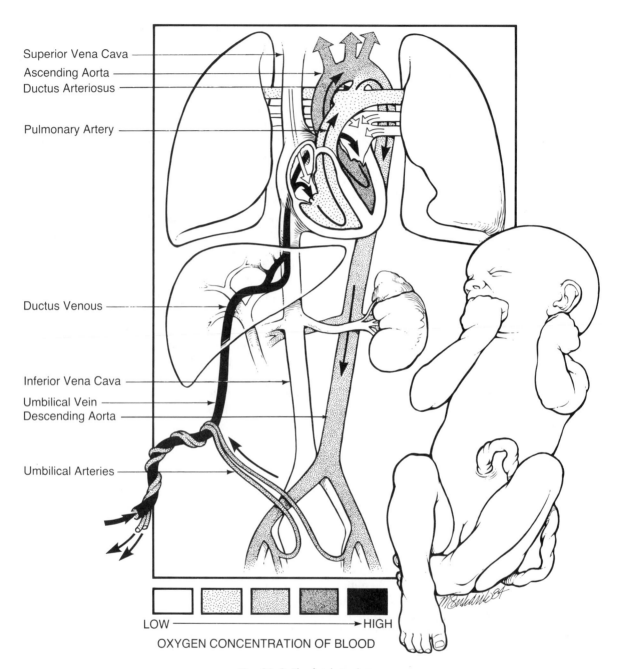

Superior Vena Cava

Ascending Aorta

Ductus Arteriosus

Pulmonary Artery

Ductus Venous

Inferior Vena Cava

Umbilical Vein

Descending Aorta

Umbilical Arteries

LOW → HIGH

OXYGEN CONCENTRATION OF BLOOD

Fig. 21.8 The fetal circulation.

The remainder bypasses the hepatic circulation via the ductus venosus, which empties directly into the IVC. As it enters the heart, most of the IVC blood is deflected by the crista dividens through the foramen ovale to the left atrium. The remainder of left atrial blood is the small amount of venous return from the pulmonary circulation. Almost all the return from the superior vena cava (SVC) and the coronary sinus passes through the tricuspid valve to the right ventricle, with only 2 to 3 percent crossing the foramen ovale. In the near-term fetus, the combined ventricular output is about 450 ml/kg/min.[74] Two-thirds of the cardiac output is from the right ventricle, and one-third is from the left ventricle. The blood in the left ventricle has a Po_2 of 25 to 28 mmHg and is distributed to the coronary circulation, brain, head, and upper extremities, with the remainder (10 percent of combined output) passing into the descending aorta. The major portion of the right ventricular output (60 percent of combined output) is carried by the ductus arteriosus to the descending aorta, with only 7 percent of combined output going to the lungs. Thus 70 percent of combined output passes through the descending aorta, with a Po_2 of 20 to 23 mmHg to supply the abdominal viscera and lower extremities. Fifty percent of combined output will go through the umbilical arteries to the placenta. This arrangement provides blood of a higher Po_2 to the critical coronary and cerebral circulations and serves to divert venous blood to where oxygenation occurs.

The diversion of right ventricular output away from the lungs through the ductus arteriosus is due to the very high pulmonary vascular resistance (PVR) in the fetus. This high pulmonary pressure results from chronic exposure to a low Po_2, causing vasoconstriction and an increase in the medial muscle layer in pulmonary arteries.[71,75] Gaseous expansion of the lungs at birth is associated with a dramatic decline in PVR and an increase in pulmonary blood flow. The factors involved in the decline of PVR include ventilation alone, a decrease in Pco_2, and, most importantly, an increase in Po_2.[71,76] With the increase in pulmonary flow, left atrial return increases with a rise in left atrial pressure (Table 21.3). The foramen ovale is a flap valve, and, when left atrial pressure increases over that on the right side, the opening is functionally closed. It is still possible to demonstrate patency with insignificant right to left shunts in the first 12 hours of life in a human neonate, but in a 7- to 12-day newborn such a shunt is rarely seen, although anatomic closure is not complete for a longer time.[70]

With occlusion of the umbilical cord, the large runoff of blood to the placenta is interrupted, causing an increase in systemic pressure.[76] This, coupled with the decrease in right-sided pressures, serves to reverse the shunt through the ductus arteriosus to a predominantly left to right shunt. By 15 hours of age, shunting in either direction is physiologically insignificant.[77]

Table 21.3 Pressures in the Perinatal Circulation

	Fetal (mmHg)	Neonatal (mmHg)
Right atrium	4	5
Right ventricle	65/10	40/5
Pulmonary artery	65/40	40/25
Left atrium	3	7
Left ventricle	60/7	70/10
Aorta	60/40	70/45

(Modified from Nelson,[324] with permission.)

Although functionally closed by 4 days of age,[78] the ductus is not irreversibly and anatomically occluded for 1 month. The role of an increased oxygen environment in ductal closure is well established.[79] Recently, prostaglandin metabolism has been shown to play an important role in ductal patency in utero and in closure after birth.[80] The ductus venosus is functionally occluded shortly after the umbilical circulation is interrupted.[69]

Shortly after birth in the neonatal lamb, resting cardiac output is about 400 ml/kg/min.[81] This represents an increase in left ventricular output from about 150 (fetal) to 400 (postnatal) ml/kg/min, while right ventricular output increases from 300 (fetal) to 400 (postnatal) ml/kg/min. The most dramatic increase in individual organ blood flow is that to the lungs (30 to 400 ml/kg/min). Myocardial, renal, and gastrointestinal blood flows also increase, while adrenal, cerebral, and carcass flows decrease.[74,82] Possible factors operative in these circulatory changes include catecholamines, the renin–angiotension system, plasma arginine vasopressin, thyroid hormone, and prostaglandins.[74]

ABNORMALITIES OF CARDIOPULMONARY TRANSITION

Birth Asphyxia

Even normal infants may experience some asphyxia during the birth process. A variety of circumstances can exaggerate the degree of asphyxia, resulting in a depressed infant, including (1) acute interruption of umbilical blood flow, as occurs during cord compression; (2) premature placental separation; (3) maternal hypotension or hypoxia; (4) any of the above superimposed on chronic uteroplacental insufficiency; and (5) failure to execute a proper resuscitation.[83] Other contributing factors include anesthetics and analgesics used in the mother, mode and difficulty of delivery, maternal health, and prematurity.

Fortunately, some characteristics of the newborn provide protection from these insults. It has been recognized for many years that fetal and newborn animals in a variety of species are able to tolerate a significant degree of asphyxia. The resistance to asphyxia can be correlated with the animal's maturity, with species less mature at birth exhibiting the greatest reserve. This reserve can be related to the glycogen content of tissues, especially in the heart.[84,85] A second protective feature is the circulatory response to asphyxia, with a redistribution of cardiac output in an effort to maintain flow and oxygen delivery to the coronary and cerebral circulations.[86]

The neonatal response to asphyxia follows a predictable pattern demonstrable in a number of species. Dawes[47] investigated the responses of the newborn rhesus monkey (Fig. 21.9). After delivery, the umbilical cord was tied and the monkey's head was placed in a plastic bag. Within about 30 seconds, a short series of respiratory efforts began. These were interrupted by a convulsion or a series of clonic movements accompanied by an abrupt fall in heart rate. The animal then lay inert with no muscle tone. Skin color became progressively cyanotic and then blotchy because of vasoconstriction in an effort to maintain systemic blood pressure. This initial period of apnea lasted about 30 to 60 seconds. The monkey then began to gasp at a rate of three to six per minute. The gasping lasted for about 8 minutes, becoming weaker terminally. The time from onset of asphyxia to last gasp could be related to postnatal age and maturity at birth; the more immature the animal, the longer the time. Secondary or terminal apnea followed and, if resuscitation was not quickly initiated, death ensued. As the animal progressed through the phase of gasping and then on to terminal apnea, heart rate and blood pressure continued to fall, indicating hypoxic depression of myocardial function. As the heart failed, blood flow to critical organs decreased, resulting in organ injury. In the asphyxiated newborn, arterial oxygen saturation drops to approximately 10 percent in 2 minutes, PaCO₂ increases at a rate of 10 mmHg per minute, and pH drops by 0.1 unit per

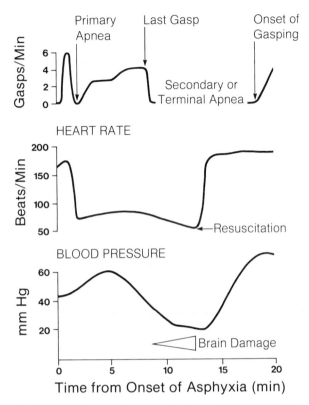

Fig. 21.9 Schematic depiction of changes in rhesus monkeys during asphyxia and on resuscitation by positive pressure ventilation. (Adapted from Dawes,[47] with permission.)

minute.[87,88] Associated with anaerobic glycolysis, there is an increase in lactate, while serum potassium increases because of failure of the ATP-dependent Na,K pump.

The response to resuscitation has also been described in great detail and is qualitatively similar in all species, including humans.[47,89,90] During the first period of apnea, almost any physical or chemical stimulus will cause the animal to breathe. If gasping has already ceased, the first sign of recovery with initiation of positive pressure ventilation is an increase in heart rate. The blood pressure then rises, rapidly if the last gasp has only just passed, but more slowly if the duration of asphyxia has been longer. The skin then becomes pink, and gasping ensues. Rhythmic spontaneous respiratory efforts become established after a further interval. For each 1 minute past the last gasp, 2 minutes of positive-pressure breathing is required before gasping begins and 4 minutes to reach rhythmic breathing.[88] Not until some time later do the spinal and corneal reflexes return. Muscle tone gradually improves over the course of several hours.

Delivery Room Management of the Newborn

A number of situations during pregnancy, labor, and delivery place the infant at increased risk for asphyxia: (1) maternal diseases, such as diabetes and hypertension, third-trimester bleeding, and prolonged rupture of membranes; (2) fetal conditions, such as prematurity, multiple births, growth retardation, fetal anomalies, and rhesus isoimmunization; and (3) conditions related to labor and delivery, including fetal distress, meconium staining, breech presentation, and administration of anesthetics and analgesics.

When an asphyxiated infant is expected, a resuscitation team should be in the delivery room. The team should have at least two persons, one to manage the airway and one to monitor heart rate and provide whatever assistance is needed. The necessary equipment for an adequate resuscitation is listed in Table 21.4. The equipment should be checked regularly and should be in a continuous state of readiness.

Steps in the resuscitation process[91] are as follows (Fig. 21.10):

1. Dry the infant well and place the baby under the radiant heat source.
2. Gently suction the oropharynx and nose.
3. Assess the infant's condition (Table 21.5). The best criteria to assess are the infant's respiratory effort (apneic, gasping, regular) and heart rate (> or <100). A depressed heart rate indicative of hypoxic myocardial depression is the single most reliable indicator of the need for resuscitation.[90,92]
4. Generally, infants with heart rates over 100 bpm will require no further intervention. Infants with heart rates less than 100 bpm with apnea or irregular respiratory efforts should be vigorously stimulated by rubbing the baby's back with a towel while blowing oxygen over the face.
5. If the baby fails to respond to 15 to 20 seconds of stimulation, proceed to bag and face mask ventilation, using a soft mask that seals well around the mouth and nose. For the initial inflations, pres-

sures of 30 to 40 cmH$_2$O may be necessary to overcome surface active forces in the lungs. A 1- to 2-second inspiratory time may be helpful as well.[93] In the premature infant even higher pressures (40 to 60 cmH$_2$O) may be needed. Adequacy of ventilation is assessed by observing expansion of the infant's chest with bagging and a gradual improvement in color, perfusion, and heart rate. After the first few breaths, attempts should be made to lower the peak pressure. Rate of bagging should not exceed 40 bpm.

6. Most neonates can be effectively resuscitated with a bag and face mask. However, if there is not a

Table 21.4 Equipment for Neonatal Resuscitation

Clinical Needs	Equipment
Thermoregulation	Radiant heat source with platform, mattress covered with warm sterile blankets, servo control heating, temperature probe
Airway management	*Suction:* bulb suction, DeLee suction apparatus, wall vacuum suction with sterile catheters
	Ventilation: manual infant resuscitation bag connected to pressure manometer capable of delivering 100 percent oxygen, appropriate masks for term and preterm infants
	Intubation: neonatal laryngoscope with #0 and #1 blades; endotracheal tubes —2.5, 3.0, and 3.5 mm OD with calgiswab stylet
Gastric decompression	Nasogastric tubes—5.0 and 8.0 Fr
Administration of drugs/volume	Sterile umbilical catheterization tray, umbilical catheters (3.5 and 5.0 Fr), volume expanders (Ringer's lactate, Plasmanate), drug box with appropriate neonatal vials and dilutions (Table 21.7), sterile syringes and needles
Transport	Warmed transport isolette with oxygen source and manual resuscitator

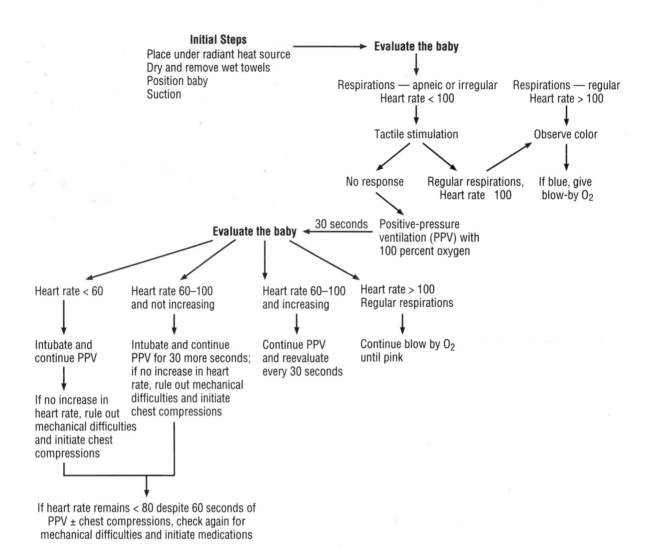

Fig. 21.10 Delivery room management of the newborn. HR, heart rate; PPV, positive-pressure ventilation.

Table 21.5 The Apgar Scoring System

Sign	0	1	2
Heart rate	Absent	<100/min	>100/min
Respiratory effort	Apneic	Weak, irregular, gasping	Regular
Reflex irritability[a]	No response	Some response	Facial grimace, sneeze, cough
Muscle tone	Flaccid	Some reflexion	Good flexion of arms and legs
Color	Blue, pale	Body pink, hands and feet blue	Pink

[a] Elicited by suctioning the oropharynx and nose.

(Modified from Apgar,[92] with permission.)

favorable response in 30 to 40 seconds, one must proceed to intubation:

a. The head should be stable, with the nose in the sniffing position (pointing straight upward).

b. Insert the laryngoscope blade, and sweep the tongue to the left.

c. Advance the blade to the base of the tongue, and identify the epiglottis.

d. Pick up the endotracheal tube with the right hand.

e. Slide the laryngoscope anterior to the epiglottis, and gently lift along the angle of the handle of the laryngoscope.

f. Identify the vocal cords.

g. Insert the tube in the right side of the mouth, and visualize the tube passing through the vocal cords.

h. Ventilate as described above.

i. Failure to respond to intubation and ventilation can result from (i) mechanical difficulties (Table 21.6), (ii) profound asphyxia with myocardial depression, and (iii) inadequate circulating blood volume.

j. The mechanical causes listed in Table 21.6 should be quickly ruled out. Check to be sure the endotracheal tube passes through the vocal cords. Occlusion of the tube should be suspected when there is resistance to bagging and no chest wall movement. If the endotracheal

Table 21.6 Mechanical Causes of Failed Resuscitation

Category	Examples
Equipment failure	Malfunctioning bag, oxygen not connected or running
Endotracheal tube malposition	Esophagus, right mainstem bronchus
Occluded endotracheal tube	
Insufficient inflation pressure to expand lungs	
Space-occupying lesions in the thorax	Pneumothorax, pleural effusions, diaphragmatic hernia
Pulmonary hypoplasia	Extreme prematurity, oligohydramnios

Table 21.7 Neonatal Drug Doses

Drug	Dose	How Supplied
Epinephrine	0.1 ml/kg	1 : 10,000 dilution
Sodium bicarbonate[a]	1–2 mEq/kg	0.5 mEq/ml
Volume[b]	10 ml/kg	Plasmanate, whole blood, 5 percent albumin, Ringer's lactate
Naloxone (Narcan)[c]	0.1 mg/kg	0.4 mg/ml

[a] For correction of metabolic acidosis only after adequate ventilation has been achieved; give slowly over several minutes.

[b] Infuse slowly over several minutes.

[c] After proceeding with proper airway management and other resuscitative techniques.

tube is in place, not occluded, and equipment functioning, a trial of bagging with higher pressures is indicated. The other causes listed in Table 21.6 are rare compared with equipment failure or tube problems. A pneumothorax is characterized by asymmetric breath sounds not corrected by repositioning the tube above the carina. Pleural effusions usually occur with fetal hydrops, while a diaphragmatic hernia should be ruled out in the setting of asymmetric breath sounds and a scaphoid abdomen. Pulmonary hypoplasia should be considered if the pregnancy has been complicated by oligohydramnios. *It is very unusual for a neonatal resuscitation to require either cardiac massage or drugs.* Almost all newborns respond to ventilation with 100 percent oxygen.

k. If mechanical causes are ruled out, external cardiac massage should be performed for persistent heart rate at less than 100 bpm. Compression of 1 to 1.5 cm should be performed at a rate of 120 bpm. There is no need to pause for ventilation while doing cardiac massage.

l. If drugs are needed (Table 21.7), the drug of choice is 0.1 ml/kg of 1 : 10,000 epinephrine through the endotracheal tube or an umbilical venous line. Sodium bicarbonate 1 to 2 mEq/kg of the neonatal dilution can be used for a *documented* metabolic acidosis. If volume loss is suspected (e.g., documented blood loss with clinical evidence of hypovolemia), 10 ml/kg of a volume expander (5 percent albumin, plasmanate) should be administered through an umbilical venous line.

The appropriateness of continued resuscitative efforts should always be reevaluated in an infant who fails to respond to all of the above efforts. Today resuscitative efforts are made even in "apparent stillbirths," that is, infants whose 1 minute Apgar scores are 0 to 1. However, efforts should not be sustained in the face of little or no improvement over a reasonable period of time (i.e., 10 to 15 minutes).

A few special circumstances merit discussion at this point. Infants in whom respiratory depression secondary to narcotic administration is suspected may be given naloxone (Narcan). However, this should not be done until the airway has been managed and the infant resuscitated in the usual fashion. A second special group consists of infants in whom respiratory problems are anticipated. This includes all infants less than 32 weeks old, infants of diabetic mothers, and infants with erythroblastosis fetalis. These infants are all at increased risk for neonatal asphyxia secondary to inadequate ventilation in the delivery room. Intubation should be undertaken much more quickly in these infants, with less time taken attempting stimulation and bag and face mask ventilation.

Finally, there is the issue of meconium-stained amniotic fluid. Meconium aspiration syndrome (MAS) is a form of aspiration pneumonia that occurs most often in term or post-term infants who have passed meconium in utero (8 to 16 percent of all deliveries[94,95]). Death rates as high as 28 percent have been reported[96] despite improvements in ventilator management. Therefore, efforts have turned toward prevention of aspiration. Gregory et al.[94] and Ting and Brady[97] showed that routine tracheal suctioning of all infants delivered through meconium-stained amniotic fluid can significantly decrease the incidence of MAS and result in a less severe clinical picture if the disease is present.

This work was extended by Carson et al.,[95] who instituted a trial of oro- and nasopharyngeal suctioning as soon as an infant's head was delivered on to the perineum and before delivery of the shoulders. Suc-

tion was performed by the obstetrician using a DeLee suction catheter before the initiation of respiration. The delivery was then completed and the infant taken to the pediatrician for direct laryngoscopy. If meconium was noted at or below the vocal cords, tracheal suction was performed. Two results were evident from this study. First, incidence of meconium aspiration was dramatically reduced by this procedure. Second, the presence of meconium at or below the vocal cords after the obstetrician had suctioned was unusual. This finding is in marked contrast to the 56 percent incidence of meconium in the trachea reported by Gregory et al.[94] in the absence of obstetric suctioning on the perineum. Finally, Linder et al.[98] demonstrated increased morbidity with tracheal suctioning of vigorous neonates delivered from meconium-stained amniotic fluid compared with a group in which tracheal suctioning was not performed. On the basis of these data, a reasonable approach to these infants has been developed.

1. The obstetrician carefully suctions the oro- and nasopharynx after delivery of the head with a DeLee suction apparatus.
2. The delivery is then completed and the baby given to the resuscitator.
3. If the baby is active and breathing and requires no resuscitation, the airway need not be inspected to avoid the risk of causing a vagal bradycardia.
4. Any infant in need of resuscitation *must* have the airway checked before instituting positive-pressure ventilation.

Sequelae of Birth Asphyxia

The incidence of birth asphyxia varies between 1 and 5 percent, depending on criteria utilized in making the diagnosis.[99,100] As would be expected, the incidence increases in infants of lower gestational age. In a study involving more than 38,000 deliveries, MacDonald et al.[99] reported an incidence of 0.4 percent in infants greater than 38 weeks and 62.3 percent in those less than 27 weeks. The acute sequelae that need to be managed in the neonatal period are listed in Table 21.8. It is evident that widespread organ injury occurs. If the infant survives, the major long-term concern is permanent central nervous system

Table 21.8   The Acute Sequelae of Asphyxia

System	Manifestations
Central nervous system	Cerebral edema, seizures, and hemorrhage
Cardiac	Papillary muscle necrosis—transient tricuspid insufficiency, cardiogenic shock
Pulmonary	Aspiration syndromes (meconium, clear fluid), acquired surfactant deficiency, persistent pulmonary hypertension
Renal	Acute tubular necrosis
Adrenal	Hemorrhage with adrenal insufficiency
Hepatic	Enzyme elevations, liver failure
Gastrointestinal	Necrotizing enterocolitis
Metabolic	Hypoglycemia, hypocalcemia
Hematologic	Clotting disturbances

(CNS) damage. The problem is identifying criteria that can provide information about the risk of future problems for a given infant. Apgar scores have been the most frequently analyzed variable. Low 1- and 5-minute scores do correlate with an increased risk for mortality and morbidity.[101,102] However, most infants with low scores, even at as late as 10 minutes of age, are normal at follow-up examination. Persistently low Apgar scores at 15 to 20 minutes of age are increasingly predictive of poor CNS outcome.[102] Brown and colleagues[100] used a more sophisticated set of criteria, including specific antepartum disorders, fetal distress, abnormal Apgar scores (<3 at 1 minute and 5 at 5 minutes), need for mechanical ventilation, abnormal acid–base states, and severe postpartum respiratory distress in making the diagnosis of asphyxia. Of 760 infants who satisfied criteria for asphyxia, 94 who demonstrated neurologic symptomatology, including feeding difficulties, apneic and cyanotic spells, apathy, seizures, and high-pitched cry, were selected for careful neurologic evaluation. These infants were followed to 21 months of age, with 20 deaths and 24 infants found with significant handicap.

This experience has been corroborated by Robertson and Finer,[103] who have shown that long-term outcome can be correlated most closely with the severity of the neonatal neurologic syndrome. It is also important to keep in mind that the circulatory response to hypoxia is to redistribute blood flow to provide adequate oxygen delivery to critical organs (e.g., brain, heart) at the expense of other organs. Thus it is hard to imagine an insult severe enough to damage the brain without evidence of other dysfunction. This concept has been examined by Perlman and Tack,[104] who demonstrated a clinical relationship between renal injury and neurologic outcome in asphyxiated infants.

The long-term neurologic sequelae of intrapartum asphyxia are cerebral palsy with or without associated cognitive deficits and epilepsy.[105,106] Although cerebral palsy can be related to intrapartum events, the large majority of cases are of unknown cause.[106,107] Furthermore, cognitive deficits and epilepsy, unless associated with cerebral palsy, cannot be related to asphyxia or to other intrapartum events.[105,106] To attribute cerebral palsy to peripartum asphyxia, there must be an absence of other demonstratable causes, substantial or prolonged intrapartum asphyxia (fetal heart rate abnormalities, fetal acidosis), and clinical evidence during the first days of life of neurologic dysfunction in the infant.[105,108]

NEONATAL NEUROLOGY

Intraventricular Hemorrhage

Although related most closely to degree of prematurity, periventricular hemorrhage (PVH) and intraventricular hemorrhage (IVH) should also be considered within the context of sequelae of asphyxia. The incidence of this complication is 25 to 35 percent in infants weighing less than 2,000 g or at 34 weeks gestation.[109] In those infants under 28 weeks gestation, the incidence is considerably higher.

Bleeding originates in the subependymal germinal matrix located ventrolateral to the lateral ventricles. This cellular region is a source of developing glial cells. The vascularity of this region is characterized by an immature capillary structure that is poorly supported by surrounding matrix.[109] A proposed pathogenesis derived from a review of available information recently summarized by Volpe[109] is presented in Figure 21.11. The critical predisposing event is likely an ischemia–reperfusion injury to the capillaries in

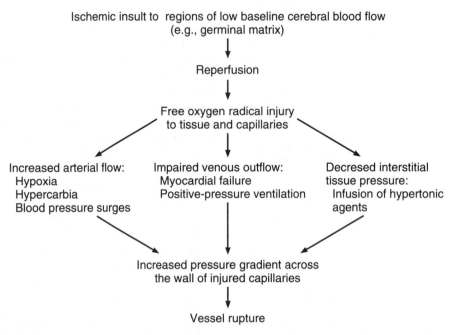

Fig. 21.11 Pathogenesis of periventricular/intraventricular hemorrhage in the preterm infant.

the germinal matrix. Physiologic data from beagle puppies have shown the germinal matrix is a low blood flow region prone to ischemia.[110] Furthermore, IVH is most reliably produced in these puppies by a sequence of hemorrhagic hypotension followed by hypertension.[111] The amount of bleeding is then influenced by a variety of factors that affect the pressure gradient across the injured capillary wall. Other extrinsic factors, including thrombocytopenia[112] and coagulation abnormalities,[113] have been implicated as well. Bleeding can extend into the ventricular cavity. This pathogenic scheme also applies to intraparenchymal bleeding (venous infarction in a region rendered ischemic) and periventricular leukomalacia (PVL; ischemia in a watershed region of arterial supply).

Clinically, there are three recognizable syndromes of PVH–IVH.[114] The first is the classic presentation of a major hemorrhage and is called the catastrophic syndrome—a rapid neurologic deterioration consisting of deep stupor or coma, apnea, seizures, nonreactive pupils, and flaccid quadriparesis. Along

with this occurs systemic hypotension, falling hematocrit, a bulging anterior fontanel, and metabolic acidosis. A second clinical syndrome is a more subtle saltatory deterioration evolving over hours to days. This syndrome is seen more with smaller hemorrhages or in infants experiencing a series of small bleeds. Finally, routine computed tomography (CT) scanning and ultrasound have pointed out the fact that the most common presentation is silent. These infants do not have a recognized clinical event; rather, the bleed is identified on "routine" scan. Up to 50 percent of bleeds occur at less than 24 hours of age, and virtually all occur by day 4 of life.[115]

A number of grading systems are available to evaluate severity of bleeds shown on CT scan[116] or ultrasound[117] (Table 21.9). Outcome has been related to severity of the initial hemorrhage.

The outcome of infants with PVH–IVH must be considered from the standpoint of short- and long-term effects. In the short term, mortality does not occur related to small (grades I and II) bleeds. Larger bleeds have a mortality rate of 10 to 20 percent. Post-

Table 21.9 Classification of Intraventricular Hemorrhage

Grade	Definition
I	Subependymal hemorrhage
II	Intraventricular hemorrhage without ventricular dilatation
III	Intraventricular hemorrhage with ventricular dilatation
IV	Intraventricular hemorrhage with associated parenchymal hemorrhage

(From Papile et al.,[116] with permission.)

hemorrhagic ventriculomegaly develops within 2 weeks of the bleeding and is related to the amount of intraventricular blood.[109] This complication is uncommon in grade I and II bleeds, but occurs in virtually all bleeds with a large amount of intraventricular blood. Long-term neurologic outcome is dependent on several factors, but in largest part is determined by the extent of parenchymal injury.[117] Important predictors of motor and cognitive deficits are the amount of intraparenchymal blood[118] and the presence of extensive PVL.[119] Only an approximate relationship exists between neurologic outcome and amount of intraventricular blood.[120] Other poor prognostic features are progressive posthemorrhagic ventriculomegaly[121] and cerebral atrophy.[122]

An encouraging note is that outcome has improved in recent years because of a decrease in both incidence and severity of bleeds.[123] This improvement is likely related to better obstetric and neonatal care during the initial hours of life, better fluid management, and better control of ventilator support. The result is an amelioration of several of the factors important to the genesis of PVH–IVH (Fig. 21.11).

As with many neonatal disorders, the goal of management of PVH–IVH is prevention. Some success has been achieved through improved perinatal and neonatal management (see above). In addition, several pharmacologic agents have been used postnatally in an effort to alter the pathogenesis of PVH–IVH. Vitamin E (by ameliorating oxygen free-radical damage) and ethamsylate (by stabilizing the immature capillary) have shown the most promise, reducing both the incidence and severity of hemorrhages.[124,125] Because PVH–IVH likely has a perinatal onset, administration of agents antenatally is an exciting approach

to this disorder. Antenatal phenobarbital (mechanism unknown) and vitamin K (improves coagulation deficiencies) have shown some promise.[126–128]

Seizures

Newborns rarely have well-organized tonic–clonic seizures caused by incomplete cortical organization and a preponderance of inhibitory synapses. Volpe[129] has classified newborn seizures into four essential types. The first is the subtle seizure characterized by ocular phenomena, oral-buccal-lingual movements, peculiar limb movements (e.g., bicycling movements), autonomic alterations, and apnea. Clonic seizures are characterized by rhythmic (one to three jerks per second) movements that can be focal or multifocal. The third seizure type is focal or generalized tonic seizures marked by extensor posturing. The fourth sei-

Table 21.10 Differential Diagnosis of Neonatal Seizures

Diagnosis	Comments
Hypoxic-ischemic encephalopathy	Most common etiology (60 percent), onset first 24 hours
Intracranial hemorrhage	≤15 percent of cases; PVH/IVH, subdural or subarachnoid bleeds
Infection	12 percent of cases
Hypoglycemia	SGA, IDM
Hypocalcemia, hypomagnesemia	Low-birth-weight infant, IDM
Hyponatremia	Rare, seen with syndrome of inappropriate secretion of antidiuretic hormone (SIADH)
Disorders of amino and organic acid metabolism, hyperammonemia	Associated acidosis, altered level of consciousness
Pyridoxine dependency	Seizures refractory to routine therapy; cessation of seizures after administration of pyridoxine
Developmental defects	Other anomalies, chromosomal syndromes
Drug withdrawal	10 percent of cases

PVH/IVH, periventricular/intraventricular hemorrhage; SGA, small for gestational age; IDM, infant of diabetic mother.

zure type is myoclonic activity that is distinguished from clonic seizures by the more rapid speed of the myoclonic jerk and the predilection for flexor muscle groups. The differential diagnosis of neonatal seizures is presented in Table 21.10.[130] The most frequent cause of neonatal seizures is hypoxic ischemic encephalopathy, with the second leading cause being intracranial hemorrhage. The prognosis for neonatal seizures is dependent on the cause. Difficult to control seizure activity caused by hypoxic ischemic encephalopathy and hypoglycemic seizures in particular have a high incidence of long-term sequelae.

BIRTH INJURIES

Birth injuries are those sustained during labor and delivery. Many are avoidable with improved obstetric care, as indicated by a decrease in their incidence as a cause for perinatal mortality from 1953[131] to 1970.[132] However, birth injuries remain the eighth most common cause of neonatal death.[132] The overall incidence of birth injury (excluding cephalohematomas) is 7 per 1,000 live births.[133] Factors predisposing to birth injury include macrosomia, cephalopelvic disproportion, shoulder dystocia, prolonged or difficult labor, precipitous delivery, abnormal presentations (including breech), and use of forceps (especially mid-forceps). Injuries range from minor (requiring no therapy) to life threatening (Table 21.11).

Soft tissue injuries are most common. Most are related to dystocia and to the use of forceps. Accidental lacerations of the scalp, buttocks, and thighs may be inflicted with the scalpel during cesarean section. Cumulatively, these injuries are of a minor nature and respond well to therapy. Hyperbilirubinemia, particularly in the premature, is the major neonatal complication related to soft tissue damage.

A cephalohematoma occurs in 0.2 to 2.5 percent of live births.[134] It is caused by rupture of blood vessels that traverse from the skull to the periosteum. The bleeding is subperiosteal and therefore limited by suture lines, with the most common site of bleeding being over the parietal bones. Associations include prolonged or difficult labor and mechanical trauma from forceps. Linear skull fractures beneath the hematoma have been reported in 5.4 percent of cases,[134] but are of no major consequence except in the unlikely event that a leptomeningeal cyst devel-

ops. Most cephalohematomas are reabsorbed in 2 weeks to 3 months. Depressed skull fractures are also seen in neonates, but most do not require surgical elevations.

Intracranial hemorrhages related to trauma include subdural and subarachnoid bleeds.[135] With improvements in obstetric care, subdural hemorrhages fortunately are now rare. Three major varieties of subdural bleeds have been described: (1) tentorial laceration with rupture of the straight sinus, vein of Galen, or lateral sinus; (2) falx laceration, with rupture of the inferior sagittal sinus; and (3) rupture of the superficial cerebral veins.[135] The clinical symptomatology is related to the location of bleeding. With tentorial laceration, bleeding is infratentorial, causing brain stem signs and a rapid progression to death. Falx tears will cause bilateral cerebral signs until blood extends infratentorially to the brain stem. Subdural hemorrhage over the cerebral convexities can cause several clinical states, ranging from an asymptomatic newborn to one with seizures and focal neurologic findings. Infants with lacerations of the tentorium and falx have a poor outlook. By contrast, the prognosis for subdural hemorrhage is much better,

Table 21.11 Birth Injuries

Classification	Example
Soft tissue injuries[a]	Lacerations, abrasions, bruising, fat necrosis
Skull injuries	Cephalohematoma,[a] fractures
Intracranial hemorrhage	Subdural, subarachnoid
Nerve injuries	Facial n.,[a] brachial plexus,[a] phrenic n., recurrent laryngeal n. (vocal cord paralysis), Horner's syndrome
Fractures	Clavicle,[a] facial bones, humerus, femur
Dislocations	
Eye injuries	Subconjunctival and retinal hemorrhages[a]
Torticollis[b]	
Spinal cord injuries	
Visceral rupture	Liver, spleen
Scalp laceration[a]	Fetal scalp electrode, pH
Scalp abscess[a]	Fetal scalp electrode, pH

[a] More common occurrences.

[b] Secondary to hemorrhage into the sternocleidomastoid muscle.

with more than one-half the survivors being normal. Primary subarachnoid hemorrhage is the most common variety of neonatal intracranial hemorrhage.[135] Clinically, these infants are often asymptomatic, although they may present with a characteristic seizure pattern. The seizures begin on day 2 of life, and the infants are "well" between convulsions. In general, the prognosis for subarachnoid bleeds is good.

Trauma to peripheral nerves produces another major group of birth injuries. In one study,[136] the incidence of nerve injuries and fractures had actually increased in the last 20 years, a fact the investigators attributed to increased use of mid-forceps associated with epidural anesthesia. Brachial plexus injuries are caused by stretching of the cervical roots during delivery. Upper arm palsy (Erb-Duchenne), the most common brachial plexus injury, is caused by injury to the fifth and sixth cervical nerves, whereas lower arm paralysis (Klumpke) results from damage to the eighth cervical and first thoracic nerves. Damage to all four nerve roots produces paralysis of the entire arm. Outcome for these injuries is variable, with about 15 percent of infants left with significant residua.[137] Facial palsy is another fairly common injury caused either by pressure from the sacral promontory as the infant passes through the birth canal or by forceps. Most of these palsies resolve, although in some infants paralysis is persistent.[138]

Another fairly common group of injuries, bony fractures, results from traumatic delivery. The majority of these fractures involve the clavicle and result from shoulder dystocia or breech extractions that require vigorous manipulations. Clinically many of these fractures are asymptomatic, and symptoms when present are mild. Prognosis for clavicular as well as limb fractures is uniformly good.

Spinal cord injuries are a relatively infrequent but often severe form of birth injury. Accurate incidence is difficult to assess, because symptomatology mimics other neonatal diseases and autopsies often do not include a careful examination of the spine. The type of lesion varies from localized hemorrhage in the anterior cornua to complete destruction of the cord at one or more levels.[138] Excessive longitudinal traction is thought to be the most important cause of neonatal spinal injury,[139] with hyperextension of the head in a footling breech particularly dangerous.[138] Clinical syndromes include death or stillbirth caused by high cervical or brain stem lesions, long-term survival of infants with paralysis from birth, and minimal neurologic symptoms or spasticity.[140]

RESPIRATORY DISTRESS

The establishment of respiratory function at birth is dependent on expansion and maintenance of air sacs, clearance of lung fluid, and provision of adequate pulmonary perfusion. In many premature and other high-risk infants, developmental deficiencies or unfavorable perinatal events hamper a smooth respiratory transition. Furthermore, a neonate has a limited number of ways to respond symptomatically to a variety of pathophysiologic insults. The presentation of respiratory distress is among the most common symptom complexes seen in the newborn, and may be secondary to both noncardiopulmonary and cardiopulmonary etiologies (Table 21.12). The major clinical symptom in these infants is an elevation of the respiratory rate to greater than 60 breaths per minute with or without cyanosis, nasal flaring, intercostal and sternal retractions, and expiratory grunting. The retractions are the result of the neonate's respiratory efforts to expand a lung with poor compliance utilizing a very compliant chest wall. The expiratory grunt is caused by closure of the glottis during expiration in an effort to increase expiratory pressure and help to maintain FRC. The evaluation of such an infant requires utilization of history, physical examination, and laboratory data to arrive at a diagnosis. It is important to consider causes other than those related to the heart and lungs, because one's natural tendency is to focus immediately on the more common cardiopulmonary etiologies.

Cardiovascular causes of respiratory distress in the neonatal period can be divided into two major groups—those with structural heart disease and those with persistent right to left shunting through fetal pathways and a structurally normal heart. A cardiac defect, some of which may resolve without intervention, is present in approximately 1 percent of live births.[141] Infants presenting in the first week of life with symptoms include those with cyanosis and those with signs of congestive heart failure. In one series, these two groups made up 85 percent of the patients seen.[142] Examples of cyanotic heart disease include transposition of the great vessels, tricuspid atresia, certain types of truncus arteriosus, total anomalous pulmonary venous return, and right-sided outflow

Table 21.12 Respiratory Distress in the Newborn

Noncardiopulmonary	Cardiovascular	Pulmonary
Hypo- or hyperthermia	Left-sided outflow obstruction	Upper airway obstruction
Hypoglycemia	Hypoplastic left heart	Choanal atresia
Metabolic acidosis	Aortic stenosis	Vocal cord paralysis
Drug intoxications; withdrawal	Coarctation of the aorta	Meconium aspiration
Central nervous system insult	Cyanotic lesions	Clear fluid aspiration
Asphyxia	Transposition of the great vessels	Transient tachypnea
Hemorrhage	Total anomalous pulmonary	Pneumonia
Neuromuscular disease	venous return	Pulmonary hypoplasia
Werdnig-Hoffman disease	Tricuspid atresia	Primary
Myopathies	Right-sided outflow obstruction	Secondary
Phrenic nerve injury		Hyaline membrane disease
Skeletal abnormalities		Pneumothorax
Asphyxiating thoracic dystrophy		Pleural effusions
		Mass lesions
		Lobar emphysema
		Cystic adenomatoid malformation

obstruction, including tetralogy of Fallot and pulmonary stenosis or atresia. Although cyanosis is the central feature in these disorders, tachypnea will develop in many infants because of increased pulmonary blood flow or secondary to metabolic acidosis from hypoxia. Infants with congestive heart failure generally have some form of left-sided outflow obstruction. Left to right shunt lesions such as ventricular septal defect do not present with increased pulmonary blood flow and consequent congestive heart failure until pulmonary vascular resistance is low enough to permit a significant shunt (usually 3 to 4 weeks of age at sea level). Infants with left-sided outflow obstruction generally do well the first day or so until the source of systemic flow, the ductus arteriosus, closes. With ductal closure, dyspnea, tachypnea, and tachycardia develop, followed by rapid progression to congestive heart failure and metabolic acidosis. On examination, these infants all have pulse abnormalities. With hypoplastic left heart syndrome and critical aortic stenosis, pulses are profoundly diminished in all extremities, while infants with coarctation of the aorta and interrupted aortic arch will have differential pulses when the arms and legs are compared.

The syndrome of persistent pulmonary hypertension (PPH), also known as persistence of the fetal circulation (PFC), occurs when the normal postnatal decrease in pulmonary vascular resistance does not occur. High pulmonary artery pressures, typical of in utero existence, persist, maintaining right to left shunting across the patent ductus arteriosus and foramen ovale. Most infants with PPH are full term or postmature and have experienced perinatal asphyxia. Other clinical associations include hypothermia, MAS, hyaline membrane disease, polycythemia, neonatal sepsis, chronic intrauterine hypoxia, pulmonary hypoplasia, and premature closure of the ductus arteriosus in utero.[143,144]

On the basis of developmental considerations, these infants can be separated into three groups[144]: (1) acute vasoconstriction caused by perinatal hypoxia, (2) prenatal increase in pulmonary vascular smooth muscle development, and (3) decreased cross-sectional area of the pulmonary vascular bed caused by inadequate vessel number. In the first group of infants, failure of PO_2 to increase at birth results in persistently elevated pulmonary pressures. Several lines of evidence support the second etiology of PPH. Information from human autopsies[145] and animal studies[146] supports the concept that chronic intrauterine hypoxia can cause increased pulmonary arterial and arteriolar muscularization. Rises in pulmonary arterial pressure during fetal life, independent of hypoxia, have also been shown to increase pulmonary vascular smooth muscle development. Levin et al.[147] demonstrated increased medial musculature in animals either by increasing systemic blood pressure or by constricting the ductus arteriosus. Both manipulations lead to increases in pulmonary artery pressure. The third group includes infants who have suffered abnormal development of lung vessels resulting in a decrease in the total cross-sectional area of the pulmonary vascular bed. This may occur when there is a primary abnormality in lung growth (e.g., congenital hypoplasia) or from impaired growth secondary to extrinsic compression (e.g., diaphragmatic hernia[148]). Clinically, the syndrome is characterized by cyanosis, often unresponsive to increases in FIO_2, respiratory distress, an onset at less than 24 hours, evidence of right ventricular overload, systemic hypotension, acidosis, and no evidence of structural heart disease.

Infants with PPH make up the majority of patients who are treated in some centers with extracorporeal membrane oxygenation (ECMO).[149] When conventional medical therapy fails, infants are placed on bypass with blood exiting the baby from the right atrium and returning to the aortic arch after passing through a membrane oxygenator. Over several days pulmonary hypertension resolves, and the infants are weaned from ECMO back to conventional ventilator therapy. This treatment can save infants who otherwise would have died with conventional therapy, but it has major side effects that must be considered prior to utilization.

Of the causes of respiratory distress related to the airways and pulmonary parenchyma listed in Table 21.12, the major concerns in a term infant include transient tachypnea, aspiration syndromes, and congenital pneumonia. The syndrome of transient tachypnea (wet lung or type II respiratory distress syndrome) presents as respiratory distress in nonasphyxiated term infants or slightly preterm infants. The clinical features include various combinations of cyanosis, grunting, flaring, retracting, and tachypnea during the first hours after birth. The chest x-ray is the key to the diagnosis, with prominent perihilar streaking and fluid in the interlobar fissures (Fig. 21.12). The symptoms generally subside in 12 to 24 hours, although they can persist longer. The preferred explanation for the clinical features is delayed reabsorption of fetal lung fluid.[150] Transient tachypnea is seen more commonly in infants delivered by elective cesarean section, presumably secondary to the importance of labor and possibly passage through

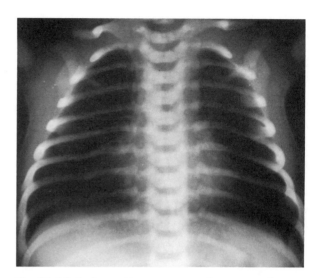

Fig. 21.12 Radiographic appearance of transient tachypnea of the newborn.

the vaginal canal on removal of lung liquid (see Mechanics of the First Breath).

At delivery, the neonate may aspirate clear amniotic fluid or fluid mixed with blood. Whether infants can aspirate a sufficient volume of clear fluid to cause symptoms is controversial. However, there are a group of infants whose clinical course is more prolonged (4 to 7 days) and severe than that of infants with transient tachypnea. These infants have a radiologic picture similar to transient tachypnea often associated with more marked hyperexpansion. Occasionally, the infiltrates are quite impressive, with evidence of far more fluid than is seen with transient tachypnea.

MAS occurs in full-term or postmature infants. The perinatal course is often marked by fetal distress and low Apgar scores. These infants exhibit tachypnea, retractions, cyanosis, overdistended and barrel-shaped chest, and coarse breath sounds. Chest x-ray reveals coarse, irregular pulmonary densities with areas of diminished aeration or consolidation (Fig. 21.13). There is a high incidence of air leaks, and many of the infants exhibit persistent pulmonary hypertension.[151] The pathophysiology of the pulmonary problems relate to airway obstruction, resulting in air trapping (partial) and atelectasis (complete), as well as a chemical pneumonitis. The approach to this disease now centers on prevention.

The lungs represent the most common site for es-

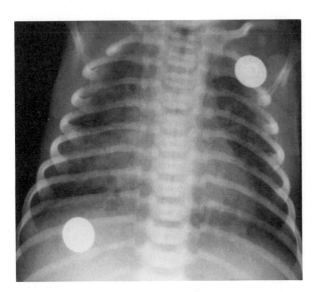

Fig. 21.13 Radiographic appearance of meconium aspiration syndrome.

tablishment of infection in the neonate. Both bacterial and viral infections can be acquired before, during, or after birth. The most common route of infection, particularly for bacteria, is ascending from the genital tract before or during labor. Thus prolonged rupture of the membranes in excess of 24 hours is a major predisposing factor.[152] Major pathogens include group B β-hemolytic streptococcus, gram-negative enterics, and *Listeria monocytogenes*.[153] Infants with congenital pneumonia present with symptomatology from very early in life, including tachypnea, retractions, grunting, nasal flaring, and cyanosis. The chest x-ray pattern is often indistinguishable from other neonate causes of respiratory distress, particularly hyaline membrane disease (HMD).[154]

Despite improved understanding and recent advances, HMD remains the most common etiology for respiratory distress in the neonatal period. Although unusual at greater than 37 weeks gestation, the incidence increases from 5 percent at 35 to 36 weeks to 65 percent in infants of 29 to 30 weeks delivered vaginally and with higher rates in infants delivered abdominally.[155] It was the initial reports of Avery and Mead[156] demonstrating a high surface tension in extracts of lungs from infants dying of respiratory distress syndrome that led to the present understanding of the role of surfactant in the pathogenesis of HMD.

The deficiency of surfactant in the premature infant increases alveolar surface tension and, according to LaPlace's law (Fig. 21.2) increases the pressure necessary to maintain patent alveoli. The end result is poor lung compliance and progressive atelectasis. The infant must expend a great deal of effort to breathe, and respiratory failure ensues. The result of respiratory failure is a combined metabolic and respiratory acidosis, further impairing surfactant production,[157,158] and hypoxia causing pulmonary arteriolar vasoconstriction with a right to left shunt across the ductus arteriosus and foramen ovale.[159] Hypoxemia and hypoperfusion result in alveolar epithelial damage, with increased capillary permeability and leakage of plasma into alveolar spaces. The materials in plasma and cellular debris combine to form the characteristic hyaline membrane seen pathologically.[160] The recovery phase is characterized by regeneration of alveolar cells, including type II cells, with an increase in surfactant activity.

Clinically, neonates with HMD demonstrate tachypnea, nasal flaring, subcostal and intercostal retractions, cyanosis, and expiratory grunting. As the infant begins to tire with progressive disease, apneic episodes occur. If some intervention is not undertaken at this point, death ensues. The radiologic appearance of the lungs is what would be expected in an extensive atelectatic process. The infiltrate is diffuse, with a ground-glass appearance. Major airways are air filled and contrast with the atelectatic alveoli, creating the appearance of air bronchograms while the diaphragms are elevated because of profound hypoexpansion (Fig. 21.14).

Acute complications of HMD include infection, air leaks, and persistent patency of the ductus arteriosus. Increased rates of infection are related to prematurity as well as breaks in the superficial barriers of protection by endotracheal tubes and indwelling lines. Air leaks are caused by the intrapleural pressure developed by the neonate attempting to expand noncompliant lungs as well as pressure generated by ventilator therapy. Persistent patency of the ductus arteriosus in these infants is primarily a developmental phenomenon. The incidence of a clinically important patent ductus arteriosus (PDA) in term infants at sea level is 0.4 percent, whereas in infants less than 1,750 g it is 15.3 percent.[161] The problem is also more common in infants with HMD compared with controls of similar gestational age.[161] PDA tends to be

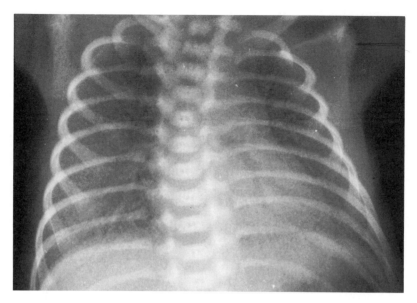

Fig. 21.14 Radiographic appearance of hyaline membrane disease.

most troublesome in very small infants (less than 1,200 g), often requiring medical or surgical ligation, whereas in larger infants spontaneous closure is more frequent. Medical closure is accomplished utilizing the prostaglandin synthetase inhibitor indomethacin.[162] The clinical signs of PDA include a murmur (usually systolic only), bounding pulses, hyperactive precordium, tachypnea, and tachycardia. Many infants will also demonstrate increased pulmonary vascularity and increasing heart size on chest x-ray.[161] Clinical symptomatology generally becomes apparent as the infant's HMD is resolving, with associated decrease in pulmonary vascular resistance allowing left to right shunting through the PDA. It has been suggested, however, that the PDA may play an important role in the early course of respiratory distress in the very-low-birth-weight infant.[163]

Of perhaps more concern than acute complications are the long-term sequelae suffered by infants with HMD. The major long-term consequences are chronic lung disease requiring prolonged ventilator and oxygen therapy and significant neurologic impairment. In 1967, Northway et al.[164] first described the syndrome of bronchopulmonary dysplasia in infants surviving severe HMD requiring mechanical ventilation. Clinically the condition is now defined by the following criteria[165]: (1) a respiratory disorder that begins with acute lung injury during the first 2

weeks of life, (2) 28 or more days of postnatal age, and (3) significant clinical, radiologic, and blood gas tension abnormalities. Using these criteria, the incidence is now estimated at about 50 percent in preterm infants requiring mechanical ventilation.[165-166] The severity is variable, ranging from very mild pulmonary dysfunction to severe disease with high in-hospital mortality, frequent readmissions for respiratory exacerbations after nursery discharge, and a higher incidence of neurodevelopmental sequelae compared with very-low-birth-weight controls.[166,167] These problems are more apparent in infancy as general health, pulmonary function, and developmental delays tend to improve after the first 2 to 3 years of life.[167,168] Factors involved in the etiology of chronic lung disease are gestational age, elevated inspired oxygen concentration, positive-pressure ventilation, and severity of underlying disease.

One of the exciting areas in neonatology is the development of surfactant replacement therapy for the management of hyaline membrane disease. Modified natural surfactant, which is extracted by alveolar lavage or from lung tissue (usually bovine) and then modified by selective addition and/or removal of components, and true artificial surfactant, which is a mixture of synthetic compounds that may or may not be components of natural surfactant, have been extensively studied[169-180] (Table 21.13). In most stud-

Table 21.13 Controlled Clinical Trials of Surfactant Administration

Study	Preparation	Patients (Treated/Control)	Study Type	Percent Neonatal Mortality	Percent Chronic Lung Disease Among Survivors	Comments
Morley et al.[169]	Artificial (dry); DPPC, 70 percent; PG, 30 percent	55 (22/33)	Prevention	Control, 24; treated, 0	Not studied	1. Surfactant group with decreased respiratory support[a] 0 to 6 hours 2. No difference in air leaks[b] between groups
Halliday et al.[170]	Artificial (liquid); DPPC	100 (49/51)	Prevention	Control, 12; treated, 12	Control, 16; treated, 19	1. No difference in incidence and severity of RDS between groups 2. No difference in air leaks between groups
Hallman et al.[171]	Natural (human–liquid)	45 (22/23)	Rescue	Control, 26; treated, 14	Control, 47; treated, 16	1. Lower respiratory support first 3 days in the surfactant group 2. Fewer air leaks in the surfactant group
Kwong et al.[172]	Natural (calf–liquid); DPPC, 80 percent; protein, 1 percent	27 (14/13)	Prevention	Control, 15; treated, 7	Control, 82; treated, 46	1. Less severe RDS; less respiratory support the first 48 hours in the surfactant group 2. No difference in air leaks between groups
Enhorning et al.[173]	Natural (calf–liquid); DPPC, 80 percent; protein, 1 percent	72 (39/33)	Prevention	Control, 18; treated, 3	Control, 81; treated, 58	1. Less respiratory support the first 48 hours in the surfactant group 2. Fewer air leaks in the surfactant group
Merritt et al.[174]	Natural (human–liquid)	69 (31/29)	Prevention	Control, 52; treated, 16	Control, 64; treated, 19	1. Less respiratory support over the first week in the surfactant group 2. Fewer air leaks with surfactant

Study	Type of surfactant	No. (M/F)	Rescue/Prevention		Results
Gitlin et al.[175]	Natural (cow–liquid)	41 (18/23)	Rescue	Control, 26; treated, 17	Control, 41; treated, 27	1. Less respiratory support over the first 72 hours in the surfactant group 2. Fewer air leaks in the surfactant group
Raju et al.[176]	Natural (bovine–liquid); DPPC, 74 percent; protein, 1 percent	30 (17/13)	Rescue	Control, 46; treated, 12	Control, 57; treated, 60	1. Lower respiratory support during first 72 hours in the surfactant group 2. PDA more frequent in surfactant group 3. Fewer air leaks in surfactant group
Ten Centre Study Group[177]	Artificial (liquid)	308 (159/149)	Prevention	Control, 27; treated, 14	Not studied	1. Less serious RDS over the first 10 days with surfactant 2. No difference in air leaks
Collaborative European Multicenter Study Group[178]	Natural (porcine–liquid); DPPC, 70 percent; protein, 1.5 percent	146 (77/69)	Rescue	Control, 51; treated, 31	Control, 53; treated, 23	1. Lower respiratory support first 24 hours in the surfactant group 2. Fewer air leaks in the surfactant group
Kendig et al.[179]	Natural (calf–liquid)	65 (34/31)	Prevention	Control, 26; treated, 24	Control, 48; treated, 46	1. Less respiratory support first 72 hours with surfactant 2. Fewer air leaks with surfactant
Horbar et al.[180]	Natural (cow–liquid)	159 (78/81)	Rescue	Control, 17; treated, 17	Control, 54; treated, 54	1. Less respiratory support first 72 hours with surfactant 2. Fewer air leaks with surfactant

[a] Respiratory support defined as ventilator rate, pressure, and/or inspired concentration of oxygen.

[b] Air leak defined as pneumothorax or pulmonary interstitial emphysema.

Abbreviations: DPPC, dipalmityl phosphatidylcholine; PG, phosphatidyl glycerol; RDS, respiratory distress syndrome (hyaline membrane disease); PDA, patent ductus arteriosus.

723

ies, these agents (administered intratracheally) have shown efficacy in decreasing the severity of acute HMD and the frequency of air leak complications. Efficacy has been demonstrated when used in the delivery room or when used as a rescue treatment for established HMD. Although each individual study has not shown a decrease in mortality or the incidence of chronic lung disease, together the studies do suggest a decrease in both mortality and pulmonary morbidity.

NEONATAL THERMAL REGULATION

Physiology

The human newborn is a homeotherm possessing the ability to maintain a stable core body temperature over a range of environmental temperatures.[181,182] The range of environmental temperatures over which the neonate can operate is narrower than that of an adult due to the infant's inability to dissipate heat effectively in warm environments and, more critically, to maintain temperature in response to cold. For example, in the nude human adult, the lower limit of the control range is 0 degrees C, while in the full term infant it is approximately 23 degrees C.[181,183]

Heat Production

Heat is produced at the rate of approximately 4.8 cal/liter oxygen consumed.[182] For core temperature to remain stable, heat production must equal heat loss. In the adult, heat production in response to cold can come from voluntary muscle activity, involuntary muscle activity (shivering), and nonshivering chemical thermogenesis. While some increase in activity and shivering have been observed,[183,184] nonshivering thermogenesis is the most important means of increased heat production in the cold-stressed newborn. Nonshivering thermogenesis can be defined as an increase in total heat production without detectable (visible or electrical) muscle activity.[185] From both animal[186] and human observations,[187] it has been inferred that the site of this increased heat production is brown fat. Brown fat is more abundant in newborns than adults, accounting for 2 to 6 percent of total body weight.[181] It is located between the scapulae; around the muscles and blood vessels of the neck, axillae, and mediastinum; between the esopha-

gus and trachea; and around the kidneys and adrenal glands. Brown fat differs both morphologically and metabolically from white fat. The cells contain more mitochondria and fat vacuoles and have a richer blood and sympathetic nerve supply. Its metabolism is stimulated by norepinephrine released through sympathetic innervation causing triglyceride hydrolysis.[186,188]

Both term and preterm neonates are able to increase oxygen consumption and thus heat production in response to cold stress.[183,184,188,190] In full-term infants the metabolic rise caused by cooling averages 110 percent during the first few hours after birth at an environmental temperature of 23 degrees C and increases to 170 percent at the end of the first week of life. In prematures, the metabolic rise after cooling to 23 degrees C averages 42 percent on day 1 and increases to 90 percent during the first week. These values reach those of full-term infants before the premature has attained its expected birth date. In general, the response in the premature is much more variable than that seen in the term newborn.

Heat Loss

Heat loss to the environment is dependent on both an internal temperature gradient (from within the body to the surface) and an external gradient (from the surface to the environment). The infant can change the internal gradient by altering vasomotor tone and, to a lesser extent, by postural changes that decrease the amount of exposed surface area. The external gradient is dependent on purely physical variables. Heat transfer from the surface to the environment involves four routes: (1) radiation, (2) convection, (3) conduction, and (4) evaporation. Radiant heat loss, heat transfer from a warmer to a cooler object that is not in contact, is dependent on the temperature gradient between the objects. Heat loss by convection to the surrounding gaseous environment is dependent on air speed and temperature. Conduction or heat loss to a contacting cooler object is minimal in most circumstances. Heat loss by evaporation describes cooling secondary to water loss at the rate of 0.6 cal/g water evaporated and is affected by relative humidity, air speed, exposed surface area, and skin permeability. In infants in excessively warm environments, under overhead radiant heat sources, or in very immature infants with thin, permeable skin, evaporative

Table 21.14 Neonatal Response to Thermal Stress

Stressor	Response	Term	Preterm
Cold	Vasoconstriction	++	++
	↓ Exposed surface area (posture change)	+/−	+/−
	↑ Oxygen consumption	++	+
	↑ Motor activity; shivering	+	−
Heat	Vasodilation	++	++
	Sweating	+	−

++, maximum response; +, intermediate; +/−, may have a role; −, no response.

losses increase considerably. In the average 2-kg infant under basal conditions, 40 percent of heat loss occurs by radiation, 33 percent by convection, 24 percent by evaporation, and 3 percent by conduction.[191]

Compared with an adult, the newborn is compromised in its ability to conserve as well as dissipate heat. Conservation of heat is impaired because of a large surface area to body weight ratio and less tissue insulation because of less subcutaneous fat.[192] Brück[183] estimated heat loss per unit body weight in the newborn to be about four times that of an adult. With a cold stress, heat is conserved chiefly by vasoconstriction in both mature and immature neonates. When the environment is too warm, heat loss is augmented by vasodilation of skin vessels and an increase in evaporative heat loss by sweating. Sweating is present in term infants when rectal temperatures rise above 37.2 degrees C.[183,193] With sweating, evaporative heat losses can increase two- to fourfold in term babies, but this is not enough to prevent a rise in core temperature. Babies born prematurely are even further compromised. Table 21.14 summarizes the neonate's efforts to maintain a stable core temperature in the face of cold or heat stress.

Neutral Thermal Environment

Although most available information confirms that the human neonate is a homeotherm, the range of temperatures over which core body temperature remains stable is narrower than in an adult and decreases with decreasing gestational age. It is therefore advantageous to maintain an infant in a neutral thermal environment (Fig. 21.15). A neutral thermal environment makes minimal demands on the neonate's energy reserves, core body temperature being regulated by changes in skin blood flow and posture. Body temperature remains normal, while oxygen consumption and heat production are minimal and match heat loss.[194] With a drop in environmental temperature out of the thermoneutral range, the infant will increase oxygen consumption and thus heat production to keep up with heat losses and maintain a stable core temperature. Core temperature will be maintained until heat loss exceeds the infant's ability to increase heat production further. Adamsons et al.[184] demonstrated that this increase in oxygen consumption is related linearly to both environmental temperature and the gradient between the infant's surface temperature and environmental temperature. When the infant is placed in an environment warmer than neutral thermal zone, hyperthermia rapidly occurs because of the neonate's inability to dissipate heat, and an increase in oxygen consumption that ensues as the infant's body temperature rises.

The neutral thermal environment for a given infant depends on size, gestational age, and postnatal age.[190] Increased size provides increased insulation, hence less heat loss. Increases in age result in increased heat production per unit area. Oxygen consumption in the term and preterm infant is approximately 4.6 ml/kg/min in the first hours of life.[183,190,194] In the term newborn, a rapid rise in oxygen consumption occurs initially, with a continued slower increase over the first 2 weeks of life. In the term low-birth-weight infant, the increase is initially slower, but eventually oxygen consumption exceeds that observed in the term normally grown infant. In the preterm newborn, oxygen consumption rises more slowly over the first several weeks than in the term infant. The optimal thermal environment for naked babies and cot-nursed (dressed and bundled) babies has been defined (Fig. 21.16).[194,195] It is important to note that the environmental temperatures shown in Figure 21.16 are operative temperatures for an infant in an incubator. The operative temperature can differ from the measured environmental temperature because of changes in relative humidity and temperature of the incubator walls. Incubator wall temperature will vary as a function of room temperature. In general, maintaining the abdominal skin temperature at 36.5 degrees C minimizes oxygen consumption.[197]

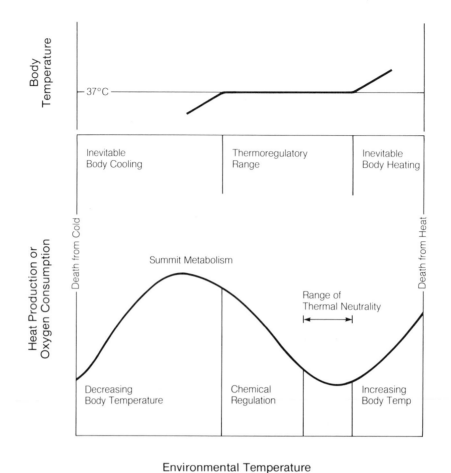

Fig. 21.15 Effect of environmental temperature on oxygen consumption and body temperature. (Adapted from Klaus et al.,[181] with permission.)

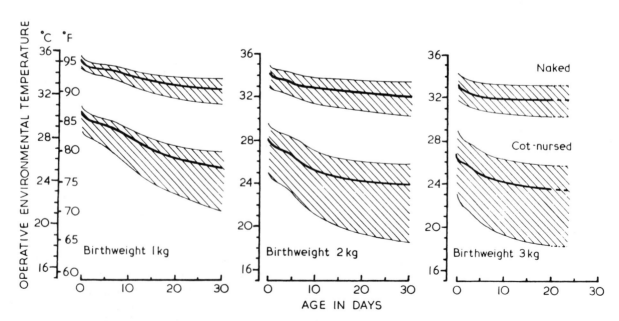

Fig. 21.16 Range of environmental temperatures to maintain naked or cot-nursed 1-kg, 2-kg, and 3-kg infants in a neutral thermal environment. (From Hey,[191] with permission.)

Clinical Applications

Delivery Room

In utero, fetal thermoregulation is the responsibility of the placenta and is dependent on maternal core temperature, with fetal temperature 0.5 degrees C higher than maternal temperature.[185] At birth, the infant's core temperature drops rapidly from 37.8 degrees C because of evaporation from its wet body and radiant and convective losses to the cold air and walls of the room. Heat loss can occur at a rate of 0.2 cal/kg/min in the term infant and at a greater rate in prematures and sick or unstable infants.[185] Even with an increase in oxygen consumption to the maximum capability of the newborn (15 ml/kg/min), the infant can produce only 0.075 cal/kg/min and will rapidly lose heat. Measures taken to reduce heat loss after birth depend on the clinical situation. For the well term infant, drying the skin and wrapping the baby with warm blankets is sufficient. Wet infants exposed to room air lose nearly five times more heat than do those who are dried and warmed.[198] When it is necessary to leave an infant exposed for close observation or resuscitation, the infant should be dried and placed under a radiant heat source.[198,199] Room temperature can be elevated as an added precaution for the low-birth-weight infant.

The thermal environment can alter the recovery from the acidosis of birth asphyxia during the first 2 hours of life.[200] Babies in a cool environment showed a rise in metabolic rate, a slower recovery from acidosis, and hyperventilation. On transfer from the delivery room to the nursery, attention to minimizing heat loss must continue. For the well, normally grown infant, continued insulation with blankets will suffice. However, transfer of an unstable full-sized neonate or any low-birth-weight infant should be carried out in a transport isolette.

Nursery

Babies are cared for in the newborn nursery wrapped in blankets in bassinets (cot nursed), in isolettes, or under a radiant heat source. Healthy full-term infants (weighing > 2.5 kg) need only be clothed and placed in a bassinet under a blanket. A nursery temperature of 25 degrees C should be adequate (Fig. 21.16). Infants weighing 2 to 2.5 kg who are either slightly premature or growth retarded should be allowed 12

to 24 hours to stabilize in an isolette and then advanced to a bassinet.

Lower-birth-weight babies (< 2 kg) will require care in either isolettes or under radiant heat sources. Adequate thermal protection of the low-birth-weight infant is essential. Several groups have demonstrated decreased mortality in low-birth-weight infants kept in warmer environments.[201-203] This is especially important for the very-low-birth-weight infant (< 1.5 kg), who often does not behave like a mature homeotherm.[204] These neonates can react to a small change in environmental temperature with a change in body temperature rather than a change in oxygen consumption. Silverman et al.[201] were able to demonstrate a threefold increase in survival for infants weighing less than 1 kg kept in incubators at 31.7 degrees C as compared with those kept in incubators at 28.9 degrees C. In the premature, warmer environments have also been shown to hasten growth.[205]

The isolette, which heats by convection, is the most commonly used heating device for the low-birth-weight nude infant. The major source of heat loss while in a neutral thermal environment is radiant to the walls of the isolette. The magnitude of this loss is predictable if room temperature is known. These losses can be minimized using the newer double-walled isolettes in which the inner wall temperature is very close to the air temperature within the isolette.

In the very-low-birth-weight infant (< 1.5 kg), evaporative losses must also be considered. Wu and Hodgeman[206] demonstrated a rate of insensible water loss of 37 ml/kg/day for infants less than 1.5 kg versus a loss of 18 ml/kg/day for infants greater than 1.5 kg cared for in an isolette with abdominal skin temperature kept at 36.5 degrees C and relative humidity at 35 percent. These losses can be minimized by increasing the relative humidity in the isolette. An isolette permits adequate observation of the infant and is suitable for caring for most sick low-birth-weight or full-sized infants. Once clinical status has been stabilized the child can be dressed, which will afford increased thermal stability.

Radiant heaters can also be used to ensure thermal stability of both low-birth-weight and full-sized infants. Radiant warmers are used most effectively for short-term warming during initial resuscitation and stabilization as well as for performing procedures. They provide easy access to the infant while assuring thermal stability. The main heat losses are by convection, which can be quite significant because of variable air speed in a room, and by evaporation.

Factors Affecting Thermoregulation

Several factors are known to affect the newborn's ability to maintain a stable core body temperature. The ability to increase oxygen consumption with a cold stress is impaired if the infant is hypoxic. Oliver and Karlberg[207] found breathing 15 percent oxygen to interfere with an infant's ability to increase oxygen consumption in response to cold stress; Scopes and Ahmed[208] showed the metabolic response to be impaired at a PaO_2 value of 45 to 55 mmHg and abolished at a PaO_2 value of 30 mmHg in a group of babies suffering from HMD. Conversely, it is critical in a baby who has impaired gas exchange because of HMD to maintain a neutral thermal environment and avoid increasing oxygen demand. In the newborn, narcotics or diazepam used during labor affect postnatal temperature regulation,[209,210] as do anesthetics that are cutaneous vasodilators.[185]

Neonatal Cold Injury

Neonatal cold injury is a consequence of excessive cold exposure most commonly seen in both term and preterm infants born unexpectedly outside the hospital. Clinical features include poor feeding, lethargy, coolness of skin, bright red color, edema, and occasionally sclerema (hardening of the skin associated with reddening and edema), slow and shallow respiratory effort, and bradycardia.[211] Metabolic derangements include metabolic acidosis, hypoglycemia, hyperkalemia, and elevated blood urea nitrogen. The infant should be warmed slowly in an isolette set at an operative temperature of 2 degrees C higher than the infant's core body temperature.

NEONATAL NUTRITION AND GASTROENTEROLOGY

At birth, the newborn infant must assume various functions performed during fetal life by the placenta. Cardiopulmonary transition and thermoregulation have already been discussed. The final critical task for the newborn is the assimilation of calories, water, and electrolytes.

Nutritional Requirements

The required caloric, water, and electrolyte intake of the newborn is dependent on its body stores and normal rate of expenditure. Body composition varies considerably with gestational age.[212,213] The average 1-kg neonate is 85 percent water, 10 percent protein, and 3 percent fat as compared with 74 percent water, 12 percent protein, and 11 percent fat at term. Carbohydrate stores in the term infant are eight times higher. Rates of expenditure differ as well. Although basal metabolic rate is lower in premature than in term infants, the premature infant frequently has increased metabolic demand secondary to cold stress, respiratory work, and so on. The small-for-gestational-age (SGA) infant provides another special consideration, possessing a higher basal metabolic rate per kilogram than a normally grown infant.[214]

Water and Electrolyte

Maintenance water requirements are dependent on oxygen consumption and rate of generation of renal solute. Other pertinent factors, especially for the premature infant, include variation in insensible water losses[215] and low renal concentrating ability.[206] An individual infant's water requirement can be determined by measuring urine and stool losses and estimating insensible losses through skin and mucosa. It is normal during the first 3 to 4 postnatal days for an infant to experience a weight loss of up to 10 percent as the physiologic contraction of extracellular body fluid takes place. Maintenance electrolyte requirements are 2 to 3 mEq/kg/day for sodium, chloride, and bicarbonate and 1 to 2 mEq/kg/day for potassium. During periods of rapid growth, requirements will be higher.

Calories

Caloric needs are primarily dependent on oxygen consumption. The character of the feeding also affects caloric needs by altering specific dynamic action and fecal losses. The average caloric requirement for a normal full-term infant through the first year of life is estimated to be about 100 to 110 kcal/kg/day.[216] The needs of the low-birth-weight infant are more variable, but for most 120 kcal/kg/day is adequate (Table 21.15). Standard infant formulas and breast milk provide approximately 20 kcal/ounce. There-

Table 21.15 Caloric Requirements of the Well Premature Infant

Factor	kcal/kg/day
Resting expenditure	50
Intermittent activity	15
Occasional cold stress	10
Specific dynamic action[a]	8
Fecal losses	12
Growth allowance	25
Total	120

[a] The metabolic increase caused strictly by the ingestion of food.

(From Sinclair et al.,[213] with permission.)

fore, volumes of 150 to 180 ml/kg/day will provide the necessary caloric intake of 100 to 120 kcal/kg/day for the average term or preterm infant. However, some sick premature infants have excessive caloric demands and are also limited by their ability to tolerate larger fluid volume. In these cases, more concentrated preparations (24 to 30 kcal/ounce), including those formulas designed specifically for the premature, can be utilized.

Protein

Both the quantity and quality of protein intake are important for adequate growth, particularly for the premature infant. Suggested intakes range from 2.0 to 4.0 g/kg/day (3.0 to 3.5 g/kg/day for the premature).[217,218] The "gold standard" for amino acid content is that which provides a plasma aminogram as close as possible to that seen with human milk.[218] Infants who receive inappropriately high protein intakes or an unbalanced amino acid intake are at risk of developing hyperammonemia, azotemia, metabolic acidosis acutely, and a lower IQ long term.[219–221] Inadequate protein intake results in growth failure.

Fat and Carbohydrate

Normal full-term infants fail to absorb 10 to 15 percent of ingested fat, while the low-birth-weight infant malabsorbs considerably more.[222] Important factors relating to fat absorption are the nature of the fat ingested as well as pancreatic and hepatic function. Human milk fat and certain mixtures of vegetable fat are better tolerated than butter fat. Medium-chain triglycerides are generally well tolerated by both term

and premature infants. Fat should provide 30 to 54 percent total calories, with 3 percent of total calories in the form of linoleic acid.[216]

Intestinal disaccharidases develop early in fetal life, with lactase reaching mature levels at term.[223] Both term and preterm infants can digest lactose, the major sugar in human milk and standard infant formulas, although there is some evidence that digestion may not be fully efficient the first several days of life.[224] Carbohydrate represents 40 to 50 percent of total calories in most formulas as well as human milk. These levels are more than adequate to maintain normal blood glucose levels and prevent ketosis.

Vitamins and Minerals

Published requirements are available for all major minerals and vitamins for term and preterm infants.[217,225,226] Information on trace minerals[217,225,226] is available as well.

Infant Feeding

For the well term or slightly preterm infant, institution of oral feeds within the first 4 hours of life is reasonable practice. For infants who are SGA or large for gestational age (LGA), feeds within the first hour or two of life may be indicated to avoid hypoglycemia. Premature infants (<34 weeks gestation) who are unable to nipple feed present a more complex set of circumstances. In addition to an inability to suck and swallow efficiently, such infants face a number of problems: (1) relatively high caloric demand; (2) small stomach capacity; (3) incompetent esophageal–cardiac sphincter, leading to gastroesophageal reflux; (4) poor gag reflex, creating a tendency for aspiration; and (5) decreased digestive capability (especially for fat). These infants can initially be supported adequately with parenteral nutrition followed by institution of nasogastric tube feedings when their cardiopulmonary status is stable.

Although a wide range of infant formulas satisfy the nutritional needs of most neonates, breast milk remains the standard on which formulas are based. The distribution of calories in human milk is 7 percent protein, 55 percent fat, and 38 percent carbohydrate.[222] The whey:casein ratio is 60:40, allowing ease of protein digestion, while fat digestion is augmented by the presence of a breast milk lipase. In addition to easy digestibility, the amino acid makeup is well suited for the newborn. Despite the low levels of several vitamins and minerals, bioavailability is high. Besides the nutritional features, other advantages of breast-feeding include (1) the presence of a variety of host resistance factors, including secretory IgA and several cellular components thought to decrease the incidence of upper respiratory and gastrointestinal infections in infancy[227]; (2) the suggestion that breast-feeding may decrease the frequency of eczema or other allergic reactions and improve the prognosis of childhood asthma[228]; (3) promotion of maternal–infant bonding; and (4) lower cost as compared with bottle-feeding.

The major area of controversy regarding breast milk has been its use for the small premature infant. Concern has centered around the amount of protein, calcium, phosphorus, and sodium present in human milk.[229] Recent reports have pointed out that protein concentration in the breast milk of a mother delivering a preterm infant is higher than that in a mother giving birth at term and is adequate to permit satisfactory growth.[230,231] Of continued concern have been reports of rickets in very small premature infants fed solely breast milk.[232] The levels of calcium and phosphorus are too low, and these elements should be supplemented in the small premature.[231]

Under certain circumstances, breast-feeding might be deleterious. For example, phenylketonuria (PKU), a condition requiring special nutritional products, precludes breast feeding. The presence of environmental pollutants has been documented in breast milk, but to date no serious side effects have been reported. Most drugs do not contraindicate breast-feeding, but there are a few exceptions.[233] These include cytotoxic agents and some antithyroid medications. Radiopharmaceuticals necessitate temporary cessation of breast-feeding. Transmission of some viral infections via breast milk is a concern as well. Mothers who are hepatitis surface antigen B positive should not breast-feed; insufficient data are available regarding cytomegalovirus and herpes. Finally, there is the insufficient milk syndrome and breast-feeding failure. Monographs that deal with this as well as other more minor breast-feeding problems are available for mother and physician.[234,235] The obstetrician and pediatrician should serve as a source of knowledge and, most importantly, support.

Neonatal Hypoglycemia

Glucose is a major fetal fuel transported by facilitated diffusion across the placenta.[236] After birth, before an appropriate supply of exogenous calories is provided, the newborn must maintain blood glucose through endogenous sources. This homeostasis is dependent on an adequate supply of gluconeogenic substrates (amino acids, lactate, glycerol), functionally intact hepatic glycogenolytic and gluconeogenic enzyme systems, and a normal endocrine system integrating and modulating these processes. Hepatic glycogen stores are almost entirely depleted within the first several hours after birth. Fat stores are then used for energy, while glucose levels are maintained by hepatic gluconeogenesis.[237]

In utero, fetal blood glucose concentration is 20 to 30 percent lower than maternal levels. In the healthy unstressed neonate, glucose falls over the first 1 to 2 hours after birth, stabilizes at a minimum of about 40 mg/dl, and then rises to 45 to 60 mg/dl.[238] Hypoglycemia can be defined as blood glucose levels less than 40 mg/dl.[239] Infants at risk for hypoglycemia are those with (1) inadequate stores of fuel, (2) hyperinsulinemia, (3) inborn errors of metabolism, and (4) endocrinopathies.[237]

Infants without adequate stores of fuel include premature and SGA infants. The highest incidence of hypoglycemia (67 percent) occurs in infants who are premature and growth retarded.[240] All these infants fail to benefit from third-trimester increments in fat and glycogen stores. Their plight is exacerbated by a brain size and surface area disproportionately greater than the size of the liver and immaturity of the pathways on which mobilization of fuels depend. Demand will also be increased by cold stress, work of breathing, and anoxia. Onset of hypoglycemia in these infants is usually within the first 4 to 6 hours of life.

The classic hyperinsulinemic neonate is the infant of a diabetic mother.[241] The pathophysiology in these infants is elevated maternal and thus fetal glucose levels, causing fetal pancreatic β-cell hyperplasia and hyperinsulinemia. This causes increased hepatic glucose uptake and glycogen synthesis, accelerated lipogenesis, and augmented protein synthesis. Pathologic correlates include hypertrophy of the myocardium, hepatomegaly, and a generalized increase in body fat.

Thus many of these infants are LGA, although mothers with diabetic vascular disease often give birth to SGA infants. The hyperinsulinemic state leads to early hypoglycemia after interruption of the maternal glucose supply, often at less than 1 hour of age. These infants are also physiologically immature for dates, resulting in increased incidence of HMD for a given gestational age.[242] Other clinical problems experienced by these babies include transient tachypnea, polycythemia, asymmetric septal hypertrophy of the heart, renal vein thrombosis, hypocalcemia, hyperbilirubinemia, birth trauma, and increased incidence of congenital anomalies. There is now evidence that the rate of congenital malformations can be altered by maintaining excellent control of maternal diabetes early in pregnancy.[243] Other less common hyperinsulinemic states include erythroblastosis fetalis, Beckwith syndrome, and primary islet cell disorders (nesidioblastosis). Inborn errors of metabolism (e.g., glycogen storage disease) and endocrinopathies of the counterregulatory hormones (e.g., hypopituitarism) are other rare causes of neonatal hypoglycemia.

Symptoms of hypoglycemia include jitteriness, seizures, cyanosis, respiratory distress, apathy, hypotonia, and eye rolling.[244] However, many infants, particularly prematures, are asymptomatic. Because of the risk of subsequent brain injury,[245,246] hypoglycemia, when present, should be aggressively treated. However, the single best treatment is prevention by identifying infants at risk, including prematures, SGA, LGA, and any stressed infant. These newborns should have blood glucose screened with glucose oxidase impregnated strips. All values less than or equal to 40 mg/dl should be confirmed with a laboratory or rapid glucose analyzer measurement of whole blood glucose.[247] Treatment is provided by early institution of feeds or an intravenous glucose infusion at a rate of 6 mg/kg/min.

Congenital Gastrointestinal Surgical Conditions

There are several congenital surgical conditions of the gastrointestinal tract that interfere with a normal transition. Many of these conditions can be diagnosed with antenatal ultrasound, allowing transfer of the mother to a perinatal center for delivery.

Gastrointestinal Tract Obstruction

Tracheoesophageal fistula and esophageal atresia is characterized by a blind esophageal pouch and a fistulous connection between either the proximal or distal esophagus and the airway.[248] Eighty-five percent of infants with this condition have the fistula between the distal esophagus and the airway. Polyhydramnios is common because of the high level of gastrointestinal obstruction. Infants present in the first hours of life with copious secretions, choking, cyanosis, and respiratory distress. Diagnosis can be confirmed with chest x-ray after careful placement of a nasogastric tube to the point where resistance is met. The tube will be seen in the blind pouch. If a tracheoesophageal fistula is present to the distal esophagus, gas will be present in the abdomen.

Infants with high intestinal obstruction present early in life with either bilious or nonbilious vomiting. In duodenal atresia, vomitus will not contain bile, while malrotation with midgut volvulus and high jejunal atresia are characterized by bilious vomiting. Malrotation and midgut volvulus involve torsion of the intestine around the superior mesenteric artery, causing occlusion of the vascular supply of most of the small intestine. If not treated promptly, the infant can lose most of the small bowel to ischemic injury. Therefore, *bilious vomiting* in the neonate demands immediate attention and evaluation. Diagnosis of high intestinal obstruction can be confirmed with x-rays. Duodenal atresia is characterized by a double bubble sign (stomach and dilated duodenum). Diagnosis of midgut volvulus can be confirmed with a contrast enema, looking for malposition of the cecum and/or an upper gastrointestinal tract series, looking for contrast not to pass the ligament of Treitz.

Low intestinal obstruction presents with increasing intolerance of feeds (spitting progressing to vomiting), abdominal distention, and decreased or absent stool. Differential diagnosis of lower intestinal obstruction includes imperforate anus, Hirschsprung's disease, meconium plug syndrome, small left colon, colonic and ileal atresia, and meconium ileus. Plain x-ray film of the abdomen will show gaseous distention, with air through a considerable portion of the bowel and air fluid levels. Diagnosis of meconium ileus, meconium plug, and small left colon syndrome can be made by appearance on contrast enema. Rectal biopsy looking for absence of ganglion cells will confirm the diagnosis of Hirschsprung's disease.

Abdominal Wall Defects

Omphalocoeles[249] are formed by incomplete closure of the anterior abdominal wall after return of the midgut. The size of the defect is variable, but usually the omphalocoele sac contains some intestine, stomach, liver, and spleen. The abdominal cavity is small and underdeveloped. The umbilical cord can be seen to insert onto the center of the omphalocoele sac. There is a high incidence of associated anomalies, including cardiac, other gastrointestinal anomalies, and chromosomal syndromes (trisomy 13). Delivery room treatment involves covering the defect with sterile warm saline to prevent fluid loss and nasogastric tube decompression.

Gastroschisis[249] is a defect in the anterior abdominal wall *lateral* to the umbilicus with no covering sac, with the herniated viscera usually limited to intestine. Furthermore, the intestine has been exposed to amniotic fluid and has a thickened, beefy red appearance. The herniation is thought to occur as a rupture through an ischemic portion of the abdominal wall. Other than intestinal atresia, associated anomalies are uncommon. Acute therapy is as described for omphalocoele.

Diaphragmatic Hernia

Diaphragmatic hernia is a congenital malformation that consists of herniation of abdominal organs into the hemithorax (usually left) because of a posterolateral defect in the diaphragm. Infants usually present in the delivery room with respiratory distress, cyanosis, decreased breath sounds on the side of the hernia, and shift of the mediastinum to the side opposite the hernia. The infants are often difficult to resuscitate and require early intubation. The rapidity and severity of presentation with respiratory distress is dependent on the degree of pulmonary hypoplasia. The ipsilateral and to some extent contralateral lung are compressed in utero because of the hernia. Delivery room treatment is to intubate and ventilate and to decompress the gastrointestinal tract with a nasogastric tube. A chest x-ray will confirm the diagnosis.

Necrotizing Enterocolitis

Necrotizing enterocolitis (NEC) is the most common acquired gastrointestinal emergency in the neonatal intensive care unit. This disorder predominantly affects premature infants, although it is seen in term infants with polycythemia, congenital heart disease, and those undergoing exchange transfusions for hyperbilirubinemia. Several factors seem to be involved in the development of this condition: (1) intestinal ischemia, (2) infection, (3) immunologic immaturity of the gastrointestinal tract, and (4) feedings.

Both hypoxia and hypotension can decrease intestinal and, more specifically, mucosal blood flow in neonatal animals.[250] Numerous perinatal events could predispose the neonate to bowel ischemia, including asphyxia, respiratory distress, hypotension, patent ductus arteriosus, hypothermia, umbilical vessel catheterization, and exchange transfusion. These risk factors are present in most infants with NEC. Providing further support for the importance of ischemia is the intestinal pathology of transmural necrosis. However, there are infants without identifiable risk factors,[251] and, when patients with NEC are compared with controls, very few obvious individual risk factors are consistently associated with the occurrence of NEC.[252] It seems unlikely that bowel ischemia alone causes NEC.

Major support for the importance of infection comes from the epidemic nature of the disorder[253] and from the ability to abate epidemics by standard measures of infectious disease control such as cohorting of nurses and patients, isolation, and hand washing.[254] The importance of altered host defenses is supported by the protection against disease provided by the cellular elements of maternal milk in an experimental animal model of NEC[255,256] and by recent information that oral administration of IgA may decrease the incidence of disease in humans.[257]

Finally, the importance of how and what is fed to the premature neonate has been debated for a number of years.[253] Certainly most infants with NEC have been fed,[258] and milk does serve as a substrate for intestinal bacterial proliferation. However, the consensus of information from neonatal centers does not support the hypothesis that the volume or rate of feeding is implicated in the pathogenesis of NEC.[253] Although it is not conclusive that hypertonic feedings and oral medications can predispose to NEC, they are best avoided in the premature infant.

Clinically there is a varied spectrum of disease from a mild gastrointestinal disturbance to a rapid fulminant course characterized by intestinal gangrene, perforation, sepsis, and shock. The hallmark symptoms are abdominal distention, ileus, delayed gastric emptying, and bloody stools. The radiographic findings are bowel wall edema, pneumatosis intestinalis, biliary free air, and free peritoneal air. Associated symptoms include apnea, bradycardia, hypotension, and temperature instability.

NEONATAL HEMATOLOGY

Anemia

The normal hematocrit in a term infant ranges from 42 to 60 percent.[259] Anemia (defined as a hematocrit < 40 percent) can be caused by hemorrhage, hemolysis, or failure to produce red cells. Anemia presenting in the first 24 to 48 hours of life is usually the result of hemorrhage or hemolysis.[260] Hemorrhage can occur in utero (fetoplacental, fetomaternal, or twin to twin), perinatally (cord rupture, placenta previa, incision through placenta at cesarean section), or internally (intracranial hemorrhage, cephalohematoma, ruptured liver or spleen). When blood loss has been chronic (e.g., fetomaternal), infants will be pale at birth but well compensated and without signs of volume loss. The initial hematocrit will be low. Acute bleeding will present with signs of hypovolemia (tachycardia, poor perfusion, hypotension). The initial hematocrit can be normal or decreased, but after several hours of equilibration it will be decreased. Hemolysis is caused by blood group incompatibilities, enzyme–membrane abnormalities, infection, and disseminated intravascular coagulation.

Polycythemia

Elevated hematocrits occur in 2 to 5 percent of live births.[261,262] Although 50 percent of polycythemic infants are appropriate for gestational age (AGA), the proportion of polycythemic infants is greater in the SGA and LGA populations.[261] Causes of polycythemia include (1) twin to twin transfusion, (2) maternal to fetal transfusion, (3) intrapartum transfusion from the placenta, associated with fetal distress, (4) chronic

Table 21.16 Organ Related Symptoms of Hyperviscosity

Central nervous system	Irritability, jitteriness, seizures, lethargy
Cardiopulmonary	Respiratory distress caused by congestive heart failure or persistent pulmonary hypertension
Gastrointestinal	Vomiting, heme-positive stools, distention, necrotizing enterocolitis
Renal	Decreased urine output, renal vein thrombosis
Metabolic	Hypoglycemia
Hematologic	Hyperbilirubinemia, thrombocytopenia

intrauterine hypoxia (SGA infants, LGA infants of diabetic mothers), and (5) delayed cord clamping.[263]

The consequence of polycythemia is hyperviscosity, resulting in impaired perfusion of capillary beds. Therefore, clinical symptoms can be related to any organ system (Table 21.16). As viscosity measurements are not routinely performed at most institu-

Table 21.17 Differential Diagnosis of Neonatal Thrombotcytopenia

Diagnosis	Comments
Immune	Passively acquired antibody, e.g., idiopathic thrombocytopenic purpura, systemic lupus erythematosus, drug induced
	Isoimmune sensitization to PLA-1 antigen
Infections	Bacterial; congenital viral infections, e.g., cytomegalovirus, rubella
Syndromes	Absent radii; Fanconi's anemia
Giant hemangioma	
Thrombosis	
High-risk infant with respiratory distress syndrome, pulmonary hypertension, and so forth	Disseminated intravascular coagulation
	Isolated thrombocytopenia

tions, hyperviscosity is inferred from hematocrit because the major factor influencing viscosity in the newborn is red cell mass. All infants should be screened for polycythemia with either a cord blood hematocrit or a capillary heel stick hematocrit. Cord blood hematocrit greater than or equal to 57 percent[264] and capillary hematocrit of at least 70 percent are indicative of polycythemia. Confirmation of the diagnosis is a peripheral venous hematocrit of at least 64 percent.[264]

Neurologic sequelae have been associated with polycythemia/hyperviscosity. However, long-term studies suggest that the sequelae are usually of a mild nature.[265] It has not been demonstrated unequivocally that treatment in the neonatal period alters long-term outcome.[265-267] Thus treatment to lower hematocrit level with isovolemic partial exchange transfusion in the hopes of altering long-term outcome in an otherwise asymptomatic infant is contro-

versial. Treatment is indicated for the resolution of acute symptomatology.

Thrombocytopenia

Neonatal thrombocytopenia can be isolated or occur associated with deficiency of clotting factors. A differential diagnosis is presented in Table 21.17. The immune thrombocytopenias have important implications for perinatal care. In idiopathic thrombocytopenia purpura (ITP), maternal antiplatelet antibodies that cross the placenta lead to destruction of fetal platelets. Although there is a correlation between the degree of thrombocytopenia in mother and fetus,[268,269] the severity of thrombocytopenia in an individual fetus cannot be predicted with certainty. As there is a small but finite risk of intracranial hemorrhage if the delivery of these infants is traumatic, cesarean section is the route of choice for infants with a platelet count of less than $50,000/\mu l$.[269] In some

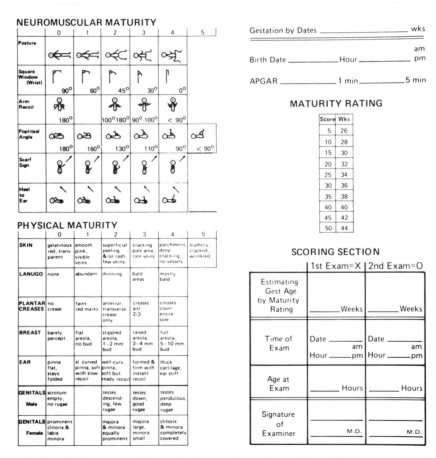

Fig. 21.17 Assessment of gestational age. (Adapted from Sweet,[323] with permission.)

cases, antenatal administration of prednisone to the mother has improved the fetal platelet count.[270] In alloimmune thrombocytopenia, maternal antibody to paternal platelet antigen on fetal platelets crosses the placenta and causes destruction of fetal platelets. As the maternal platelet count is normal, the diagnosis is suspected based on a history of a previously affected pregnancy. Intracranial hemorrhage is more common with this condition than in maternal ITP and can occur in the antenatal or intrapartum periods.[271] Preliminary work has suggested a role for intravenous gammaglobulin administered to the mother in prevention of this complication.[271,272] With both of these conditions, there is a role for percutaneous umbilical sampling to assess fetal platelet count. This information can be used to direct antepartum treatments and to aid in the decision to perform a cesarean section.

CLASSIFICATIONS OF NEWBORNS BY GROWTH AND GESTATIONAL AGE

In assessing the risk for mortality or morbidity in a given neonate, evaluation of birth weight and gestational age together provide the clearest picture. This requires an accurate assessment of the infant's gestational age. When large populations are considered, maternal dates remain the single best determinant of gestational age. However, in the individual neonate, especially when dates are uncertain, a reliable assessment of gestational age is necessary. A scoring system appraising gestational age on the basis of physical and neurologic criteria was developed by Dubowitz et al.[273] and later simplified by Ballard et al.[274] (Fig. 21.17). Infants can then be classified, using growth

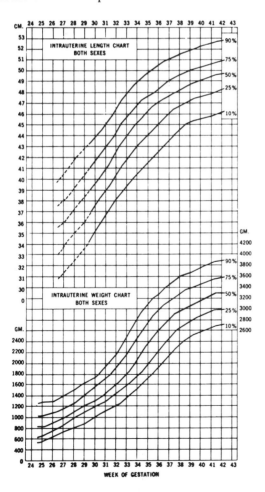
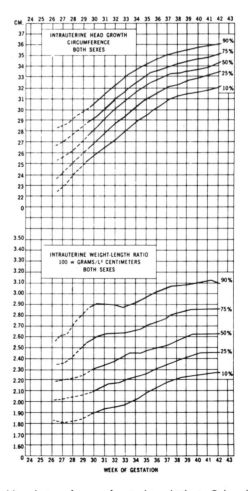

Fig. 21.18 Intrauterine growth curves for weight, length, and head circumference for singleton births in Colorado. (From Lubchenco et al.,[275] with permission.)

parameters and gestational age, by means of intra-uterine growth curves such as those developed by Lubchenco et al.[275] (Fig. 21.18). Infants born between 38 and 42 weeks are classified as term; less than 38 weeks, as preterm; and greater than 42 weeks, post-term. In each grouping, infants are then identified according to growth as AGA if birth weight falls between the 10th to 90th percentiles, SGA if birth weight is below the 10th percentile, and LGA if birth weight is above the 90th percentile. On the basis of a given infant's classification, the risk of mortality[276] (Fig. 21.19) can be assessed. Not only does mortality risk vary, but specific clinical problems can also be anticipated by an infant's birth weight/gestational age distribution as well.

There are numerous causes of growth retardation (see Ch. 27). Those operative early in pregnancy such as chromosomal aberrations, congenital viral infections, and some drug exposures induce symmetric retardation of weight, length, and head circumference. In most cases, the phenomenon occurs later in gestation and leads to more selective retardation of birth weight alone. Such factors include hypertension or other maternal vascular disease and multiple gestation.[277,278] Neonatal problems besides chromosomal abnormalities and congenital viral infections common in SGA infants include birth asphyxia, hypoglycemia, and polycythemia.

The most common identifiable conditions leading to excessive infant birth weight are maternal diabetes

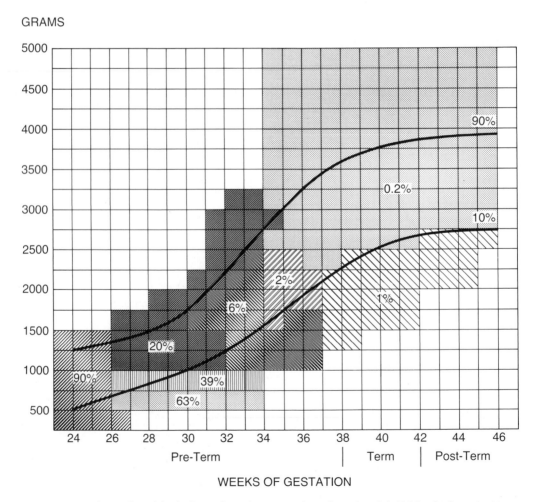

Fig. 21.19 Neonatal mortality risk by birth weight and gestational age based on 14,413 live births at the University of Colorado Health Sciences Center, 1974–1980. (From Koops et al.,[276] with permission.)

and maternal obesity.[277] Other conditions associated with macrosomia are erythroblastosis fetalis, other causes of fetal hydrops, and Beckwith syndrome. LGA infants are at particular risk for hypoglycemia and birth trauma.

NEONATAL JAUNDICE

The most common "problem" encountered in a term nursery population is jaundice. Neonatal hyperbilirubinemia occurs when the normal pathways of bilirubin metabolism and excretion are altered. To understand neonatal jaundice, brief consideration must be given to these pathways[279] (Fig. 21.20). The normal destruction of circulating red cells accounts for about 75 percent of the newborn's daily bilirubin production. The remaining sources include ineffective erythropoiesis and tissue heme proteins. Heme is converted to bilirubin in the reticuloendothelial system. Unconjugated bilirubin is lipid soluble and transported bound to albumin. Bilirubin enters the liver cells by dissociation from albumin in the hepatic sinusoids. Once in the hepatocyte, it is conjugated with glucuronic acid in a reaction catalyzed by glucuronyltransferase. The water-soluble conjugated bilirubin is secreted into the biliary tree for excretion via the gastrointestinal tract. The enzyme β-glucuronidase is present in small bowel and hydrolyzes some of the conjugated bilirubin. This unconjugated bilirubin can be reabsorbed into the circulation, adding to the total unconjugated bilirubin load (enterohepatic circulation).

Almost every newborn will develop a serum unconjugated bilirubin concentration of greater than 2 mg/dl during the first week of life. This transient hyperbilirubinemia has been called physiologic jaundice. Major predisposing factors of physiologic jaundice are (1) increased bilirubin load because of increased red cell volume with decreased cell survival, increased ineffective erythropoiesis, and the enterohepatic circulation; and (2) defective bilirubin conjugation. Also potentially involved are impaired hepatic uptake of bilirubin from the plasma and impaired bilirubin excretion. Clinically, physiologic jaundice should not be present in the first 24 hours of life. Total bilirubin should rise less than 5 mg/dl/day and peak at less than 12.9 mg/dl on days 3 to 4 in the term infant and at 15 mg/dl on days 5 to 7 in the premature

infant. Direct bilirubin should remain less than 2 mg/dl. Clinical jaundice should not persist more than 1 week in a term infant and 2 weeks in a premature.[279] Should any of these features be present, the etiology of the jaundice needs to be investigated.

Pathologic jaundice during the early neonatal period is indirect hyperbilirubinemia usually caused by overproduction of bilirubin. The leading cause in this group of patients is hemolytic disease, of which fetomaternal blood group incompatabilities (Rh and ABO) are the most common (see Ch. 29). Other causes of hemolysis include genetic disorders such as hereditary spherocytosis and drug-induced hemolysis. Etiologies of bilirubin overproduction include extravasated blood (bruising, hemorrhage), polycythemia, and exaggerated enterohepatic circulation of bilirubin because of mechanical gastrointestinal obstruction or reduced peristalsis usually from inadequate oral intake. Disease states involving decreased bilirubin clearance must be considered in the patients in whom no cause of overproduction can be identified. Causes of indirect hyperbilirubinemia in this category include (1) familial deficiency of glucuronyltransferase (Crigler-Najjar syndrome), (2) transient familial neonatal hyperbilirubinemia caused by an inhibitor of bilirubin conjugation in maternal serum (Lucey-Driscoll syndrome), (3) breast milk jaundice caused by an inhibitor of conjugation present in milk, and (4) hypothyroidism. Mixed or direct hyperbilirubinemia are rare during the first week of life.

A small percentage of breast-fed babies develop the syndrome of true breast milk jaundice. These infants have significant unconjugated hyperbilirubinemia, with concentrations rising progressively from day 4 of life, reaching a maximum of 12 to 20 mg/dl by days 10 to 15. There is then a slow decline, with bilirubin reaching normal values at 3 to 12 weeks of age. If breast-feeding is interrupted at any stage, a prompt decline in bilirubin values occurs within 48 hours. The etiology of breast milk jaundice is not entirely clear, but it is thought to be associated with milk possessing high lipoprotein lipase activity.[280] This results in higher levels of free fatty acids that interfere with bilirubin conjugation.[281] This entity is to be distinguished from jaundice in the breast-fed infant during the first week of life.[282] Breast-fed infants when compared with formula-fed infants have higher bilirubin levels. This is due to decreased intake over the first several days of life. Thus, rather than interrupting

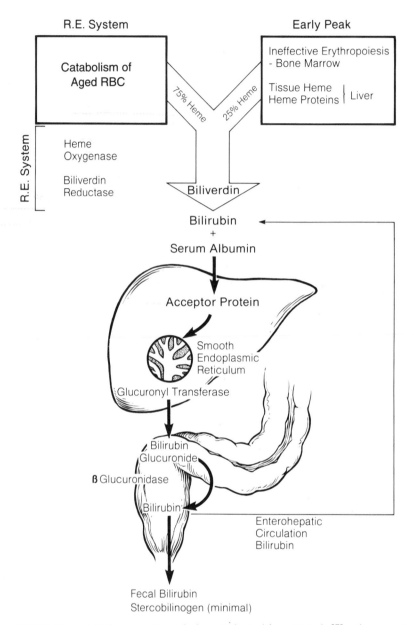

Fig. 21.20 Neonatal bile pigment metabolism. (Adapted from Maisels,[279] with permission.)

breast-feeding, the treatment is to increase the frequency of feeds to accelerate milk production.[283]

The overriding concern with neonatal hyperbilirubinemia is the development of bilirubin toxicity, causing the pathologic entity of kernicterus, the staining of certain areas of the brain (basal ganglia and hippocampus) by bilirubin. The clinical syndrome in term infants is marked by refusal to feed, high-pitched cry, hypertonicity, and opisthotonus. Survivors usually suffer sequelae, including athetoid cerebral palsy, high-frequency hearing loss, paralysis of upward gaze, and dental dysplasia.[284] The risk of kernicterus in a given infant is not well defined. The only group that one can speak of with any certainty are those infants with Rh isoimmunization in whom a level of 20 mg/dl has been associated with an increased risk of kernicterus.[285] This observation has been extended to the management of other neonates with hemolytic disease, although no definitive data exist regarding these infants. The risk is probably negligible for term infants without hemolytic disease even at levels higher than 20 mg/dl.[286] Prematures of 32 to 38 weeks gestation are probably safe up to levels of 20 mg/dl,[287] while for the smaller premature infant no meaningful data are available.[288] Finally, auditory evoked potential studies have clearly identified a reversible entry of bilirubin into the central nervous system.[289] The relevance of this finding to long-term outcome is unknown.

NURSERY CARE

Nurseries are classified based on level of care provided. Level I nurseries care for infants presumed healthy, with an emphasis on screening and surveillance. Level II nurseries can care for infants more than 30 weeks gestation, who weigh at least 1,200 g, and who require special attention short of the need for circulatory or ventilator support and major surgical procedures. Level III nurseries care for all newborn infants who are critically ill regardless of the level of support required. A perinatal center encompasses both high-risk obstetric services and level III nursery services.

Care of the normal newborn involves observation of transition from intra- to extrauterine life, establishing breast- or bottle-feeds, noting normal patterns of stooling and urination, and surveillance for neonatal problems. Signs suggestive of illness include temperature instability, change in activity, refusal to feed, pallor, cyanosis, jaundice, tachypnea and respiratory distress, delayed (beyond 24 hours) passage of first stool or void, and bilious vomiting. In addition, the following laboratory screens are performed: (1) blood type and direct and indirect Coombs' test on infants born to mothers with type O or Rh negative blood, (2) glucose screen in infants at risk for hypoglycemia, (3) hematocrit, (4) serologic test for syphilis, and (5) state-sponsored screen for inborn errors of metabolism (PKU, maple syrup urine disease, homocystinuria, galactosemia, sickle cell disease, hypothyroidism, cystic fibrosis).

Finally, babies routinely receive 1 mg IM of vitamin K to prevent vitamin K–deficient hemorrhagic disease of the newborn and either 1 percent silver nitrate or erythromycin ointment to prevent gonococcal ophthalmia neonatorum. The trend over the last

Table 21.18 Infant Criteria for Early Discharge

1. Delivery is vertex, single, sterile, and vaginal.
2. Apgar scores at 1 and 5 minutes are ≥7.
3. The infant is term (38–42 weeks) and weighs 2,700–4,000 g.
4. Minimum length of stay of 24 hours. A transition to normal thermoregulation in an open crib, completion of two successful feedings, evidence of stool and void, completion of neonatal screening for metabolic disease, and blood type and Coomb's test (Rh⁻ and O mothers) prior to discharge.
5. Vital signs within normal ranges at discharge: axillary temperature, 36.1°–37.2 degrees C; heart rate, 110–150/min; respiratory rate, 40–60/min
6. The infant has a normal neonatal hospital course and presents no signs or symptoms that require continuous observation:
   Blood dextrose maintained, >45 mg/dl
   Hematocrit, 45–65 percent
   ABO-incompatible infants must be held until 48 hours and released only if not requiring therapy for hemolysis.
7. Physical examination is completed by physician or trained physician's assistant.
8. Mother demonstrates understanding and ability to provide adequate care for her newborn; infant care education is provided on a one to one or classroom basis by the nursing staff prior to discharge.
9. Signed documentation by the mother that states her obligation to participate in follow-up care.

several years has been toward shorter hospital stays for well mothers and infants. Criteria for early discharge at the University of Colorado are presented in Table 21.18.[290] These criteria have been adapted from those of the American Academy of Pediatrics.[291,292] Early discharge can be safely carried out in indigent as well as middle-income populations.[290,293,294] Of considerable importance is the fact that most infants who manifest serious cardiorespiratory and infectious problems will do so in the first 6 hours of life.[294] Other problems such as jaundice and difficulties in breast-feeding typically occur later, but can usually be handled on an outpatient basis.

CARE OF THE PARENTS

Interest in maternal–infant bonding has grown in the last 20 years in part because of the observation of an excessive incidence of child abuse and nonorganic failure to thrive in infants who experienced a prolonged postdelivery separation from parents.[295] This circumstance had its roots in the historical approach to neonatal care, which emphasized infant isolation for prevention of infection. On the basis of this human experience as well as on studies of maternal–infant bonding in other species,[296] the pendulum has now shifted to permit liberal nursery-visiting policies.

Klaus and Kennell[297] outlined the steps in maternal–infant attachment as follows: (1) planning the pregnancy, (2) confirming the pregnancy, (3) accepting the pregnancy, (4) fetal movement, (5) accepting the fetus as an individual, (6) birth, (7) hearing and seeing the baby, (8) touching and holding the baby, and (9) caretaking. Numerous influences can affect this process. A mother's and father's actions and responses are derived from their own genetic endowment, their own interfamily relationships, cultural practices, past experiences with this or previous pregnancies, and, most importantly, how each was raised by his or her own parents.[297] Also critical is the in-hospital experience surrounding the birth—how doctors and nurses act, separation from the baby, and hospital practices.

The 60- to 90-minute period after delivery is a very important time. The infant is alert, active, and able to follow with his or her eyes,[298] allowing meaningful interaction to transpire between infant and parents. The infant's array of sensory and motor abilities evokes responses from the mother and initiates communication that may be helpful for attachment and induction of reciprocal actions. Whether a critical time period for these initial interactions exists is not clear, but improved mothering behavior does seem to occur with increased contact over the first 3 postpartum days.[299] The practical implications of this information are that labor and delivery should pose as little anxiety as possible for the mother, and parents and baby should have time together immediately after delivery if the baby's medical condition permits. Eye prophylaxis for gonococcal ophthalmitis should ideally be withheld until after the initial bonding has taken place. It can be performed safely within 1 hour of birth.

Mothers with high-risk pregnancies are at increased risk for subsequent parenting problems. It is important for both obstetrician and pediatrician alike to be involved prenatally, allowing time to prepare the family for anticipated aspects of the baby's care as well as providing reassurance that the odds are heavily in favor of a live baby who will ultimately be healthy. If one can before birth anticipate a need for neonatal intensive care (known congenital anomaly, refractory premature labor), maternal transport should be planned to a center with a unit that can care for the baby. In this way, a mother can be with her baby during its most critical care. Before delivery it is also very helpful to allow the parents to tour the unit their baby will occupy. This practice greatly reduces anxiety after the baby is born.

The single basic principle in dealing with parents of a sick infant is to provide essential information clearly and accurately to both parents, preferably when they are together. With improved survival rates, especially in prematures, most babies, despite early problems, will do well. It is therefore reasonable in most circumstances to be positive about the outcome. There is also no reason to emphasize problems that might occur in the future or to deal with individual worries of the physician. Questions, if asked, need to be answered honestly, but the list of parents' worries does not need to be voluntarily increased.

Before the parents' initial visit to the unit, a physician or nurse should describe what the baby and the equipment look like. When they arrive in the nursery, this can again be reviewed in detail. If a baby must be moved to another hospital, the mother should be given time to see and to touch her infant prior to transfer. The father should be encouraged to meet the baby at the receiving hospital so he can become comfortable with the intensive care unit. He can serve as a link between baby and mother with information and photographs.

As a baby's course proceeds, the nursery staff can help the parents to become comfortable with their infant. It is also important for the staff to discuss among themselves any problems that parents may be having as well as to keep a record of visits and phone calls. This approach will allow early intervention to deal with potential problems.

The birth of an infant with a congenital malformation provides another situation in which staff support is essential. Parents' reactions to the birth of a malformed infant follow a predictable course. For most, there is initial shock and denial, a period of sadness and anger, gradual adaptation, and finally an increased satisfaction with and ability to care for the baby. The parents must be allowed to pass through these stages and, in effect, to mourn the loss of the anticipated normal child.[300] Again, information needs to be provided clearly and accurately to both parents, including the prognosis for the particular problem.

The death of an infant or a stillborn is a highly stressful family event. This fact has been emphasized by Culberg,[301] who found that psychiatric disorders developed in 19 of 56 mothers studied 1 to 2 years after the deaths of their neonates. One of the major predispositions was a breakdown of communication between parents. The health care staff needs to encourage the parents to talk with each other, discuss their feelings, and display emotion. The staff should talk with the parents at the time of death and then several months later to review the findings of the autopsy, answer questions, and see how the family is doing.

OUTCOME OF NEONATAL INTENSIVE CARE

More sophisticated neonatal care has resulted in improved survival of very-low-birth-weight ($\leq 1,500$ g) infants, in particular those less than 1,000 g. Current survival rates are 90 percent or greater for infants 1,000 to 1,500 g (28 to 30 weeks gestation), 60 percent for infants 750 to 1,000 g (26 to 28 weeks gestation), and 20 percent for infants less than 750 g (24 to 26 weeks gestation). This improved survival comes with a price, as a variety of morbidities are seen in these infants. However, concern that improved survival would be associated with an increased rate of neurologic sequelae has been unfounded. Major neurologic morbidities seen in very-low-birth-weight infants include cerebral palsy (spastic dyplegia, quadriplegia, hemiplegia, or paresis), cognitive delay, and hydrocephalus. Stewart et al.[302] reviewed the world literature in 1980 and found approximately 10 per-

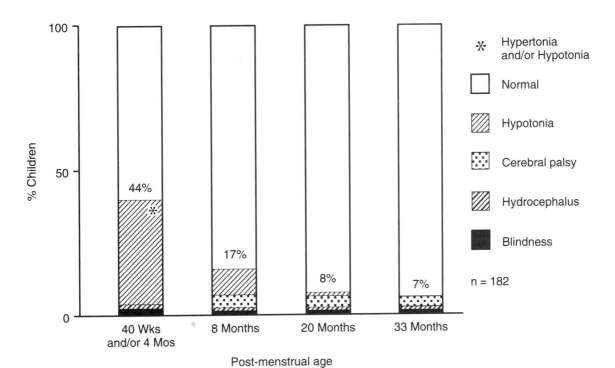

Fig. 21.21 Prevalence of neurologic abnormalities among very-low-birth-weight children born in Cleveland, Ohio, 1977–1978 at 4, 8, 20, and 33 months. (Adapted from Hack and Amiel-Tison,[307] with permission.)

cent of both the less than 1,500 g (15 percent of survivors) and less than 1,000 g (25 percent of survivors) population had major neurologic sequelae.[302] Since then, a number of centers have reported more recent data on the less than 1,000 g population. These studies have continued to demonstrate approximately 10 percent of the total population (15 to 30 percent of survivors) with major neurologic handicap.[303–306] The other feature that is very encouraging is that outcome improves with time; children look better at 5 years follow-up than at earlier examinations (Fig. 21.21).[307,308] Risk factors for neurologic morbidity include seizures, major intracranial hemorrhage, severe intrauterine growth retardation, need for mechanical ventilation, and poor early head growth.[309–312]

There are other morbidities that need to be considered as well. As the number of less than 1,000 g survivors has increased, a reemergence of retinopathy of prematurity has been seen. This disorder, caused by retinal vascular proliferation leading to hemorrhage, scarring, retinal detachment, and blindness, originally was thought to be due to inappropriate exposure to high concentrations of oxygen. It is now thought that the origin is multifactorial, with extreme prematurity evolving as a critical factor.[313] Incidence of acute proliferative retinopathy by birth weight is less than 10 percent in infants weighing more than 1,250 g, 15 percent in those 1,000 to 1,250 g, 40 percent in those 750 to 1,000 g, and 50 percent in those less than 750 g.[314] Severe retinopathy is evident in 5 percent of the infants 1,000 to 1,250 g, in 15 percent of the 750 to 1,000 g population, and 25 percent of the less than 750 g infants. Of the infants with severe retinopathy, 10 percent (4 percent of the total population) will go on to have severe visual problems. The other major neurosensory morbidity is hearing loss, which occurs in 2 percent of neonatal intensive care unit survivors.[315] Other sequelae of neonatal intensive care unit care include chronic lung disease, growth failure, short gut, and need for rehospitalization (as high as 60 percent in one series of <1,000 g infants, with the leading diagnosis being upper respiratory tract infection).[316,317] There is also a significant rate of postdischarge mortality that must be considered.[318]

REFERENCES

1. Inselman LS, Mellins RB: Growth and development of the lung. J Pediatr 98:1, 1981
2. Avery ME, Fletcher BD, Williams RG: The Lung and its Disorders in the Newborn Infant. 4th Ed. WB Saunders, Philadelphia, 1981
3. Hislop A, Reid LM: Formation of the pulmonary vasculature. p. 37. In Hodson WA (ed): Development of the Lung. Marcel Dekker, New York, 1977
4. Dunnill MS: Postnatal growth of the lung. Thorax 17:329, 1962
5. Campiche MA, Gautier A, Hernandez EI, Reymond A: An electron microscope study of the fetal development of human lung. Pediatrics 32:976, 1963
6. Buckingham S, Avery ME: Time of appearance of lung surfactant in the foetal mouse. Nature 193:688, 1962
7. Klaus M, Reiss OK, Tooley WM et al: Alveolar epithelial cell mitochondria as source of surface-active lung lining. Science 137:750, 1962
8. Orzalesi MM, Motoyama EK, Jacobson HN et al: The development of the lungs of lambs. Pediatrics 35:373, 1965
9. Spear GS, Vaeusorn O, Avery ME et al: Inclusions in terminal air spaces of fetal and neonatal human lung. Biol Neonate 14:344, 1969
10. Batenburg JJ, Van Golde LMG: Formation of pulmonary surfactant in whole lung and in isolated type II alveolar cells. p. 73. In Scarpelli EM, Cosmi EV (eds): Reviews in Perinatal Medicine. Vol. 3. Raven, New York, 1979
11. von Neergaard K: Neue auffassurgen uber einen grundbegriff der atommechanik die retraktionskraft der lunge, abhangig von der oberflachenspannung un den alveolen. Z Gesamte Exp Med 66:373, 1929
12. Mead J, Whittenberger JL, Radford EP Jr: Surface tension as a factor in pulmonary volume-pressure hysteresis. J Appl Physiol 10:191, 1957
13. Clements JA: Surface phenomena in relation to pulmonary function. Physiologist 5:11, 1962
14. Epstein MF, Farrell PM: The choline incorporation pathway: primary mechanism for de novo lecithin synthesis in fetal primate lung. Pediatr Res 9:658, 1975
15. Kotas RK, Farrell PM, Ulane RE, Chez RA: Fetal rhesus monkey lung development: lobar differences and discordances between stability and distensibility. J Appl Physiol 43:92, 1977
16. Jobe A: The role of surfactant in neonatal adaptation. Semin Perinatol 12:113, 1988
17. Clements JA, Tooley WH: Kinetics of surface-active material in the fetal lung. p. 349. In Hodson WA (ed):

Development of the Lung. Marcel Dekker, New York, 1977

18. Ekelund L, Burgoyne R, Enhorning G: Pulmonary surfactant release in fetal rabbits: immediate and delayed response to terbutaline. Am J Obstet Gynecol 147:437, 1983

19. Farrell PM, Hamosh M: The biochemistry of fetal lung development. Clin Perinatol 5:197, 1978

20. Ballard PL: Hormonal regulation of pulmonary surfactant. Endocrine Rev 10:165, 1989

21. Liggins GC: Premature delivery of foetal lambs infused with glucocorticoids. J Endocrinol 45:515, 1969

22. DeLemos RA, Shermeta DW, Knelson JH et al: Acceleration of appearance of pulmonary surfactant in the fetal lamb by administration of corticosteroids. Am Rev Respir Dis 102:459, 1970

23. Kotas RV, Avery ME: Accelerated appearance of pulmonary surfactant in the fetal rabbit. J Appl Physiol 30:358, 1971

24. Wang NS, Kotas RV, Avery ME, Thurlbeck WM: Accelerated appearance of osmiophilic bodies in fetal lungs following steroid injection. J Appl Physiol 30:362, 1971

25. Kotas RV, Kling OR, Block MF et al: Response of immature baboon fetal lung to intra-amniotic betamethasone. Am J Obstet Gynecol 130:712, 1978

26. Liggins GC, Howie RN: A controlled trial of antepartum glucocorticoid treatment for prevention of the respiratory distress syndrome in premature infants. Pediatrics 50:515, 1972

27. Block MF, Kling OR, Crosby WM: Antenatal glucocorticoid therapy for the prevention of respiratory distress syndrome in the premature infant. Obstet Gynecol 50:186, 1977

28. Papageorgiou AN, Desgranges MF, Masson M et al: The antenatal use of betamethasone in the prevention of respiratory distress syndrome: a controlled double-blind study. Pediatrics 63:73, 1979

29. Taeusch HW Jr, Frigoletto F, Kitzmiller J et al: Risk of respiratory distress syndrome after prenatal dexamethasone treatment. Pediatrics 63:64, 1979

30. Doran TA, Swyer P, MacMurray B et al: Results of a double-blind controlled study on the use of betamethasone in the prevention of respiratory distress syndrome. Am J Obstet Gynecol 136:313, 1980

31. Collaborative Group on Antenatal Steroid Therapy: Effect of antenatal dexamethasone administration on the prevention of respiratory distress syndrome. Am J Obstet Gynecol 141:276, 1981

32. Avery ME: The argument for prenatal administration of dexamethasone to prevent respiratory distress syndrome. J Pediatr 104:240, 1984

33. Collaborative Group on Antenatal Steroid Therapy: Effects of antenatal dexamethasone administration in the infant: long-term follow-up. J Pediatr 104:259, 1984

34. Boddy K, Dawes GS: Fetal breathing. Br Med Bull 31:3, 1975

35. Dawes GS: The central control of fetal breathing and skeletal muscle movements. J Physiol (Lond) 346:1, 1984

36. Kaplan M: Fetal breathing movements, an update for the pediatrician. Am J Dis Child 137:177, 1983

37. Boddy K, Dawes GS, Fisher R et al: Foetal respiratory movements, electrocortical and cardiovascular responses to hypoxaemia and hypercapnia in sheep. J Physiol (Lond) 243:599, 1974

38. Purves MJ: Respiratory sensitivity before and after birth. Acta Paediatr Scand 71:529, 1982

39. Harned HS Jr, Rowshan G, MacKinney LG, Sugioka K: Relationships of P_{O_2}, P_{CO_2}, and pH to onset of breathing of the term lamb as studied by a flow-through cuvette electrode assembly. Pediatrics 33:672, 1964

40. Harned HS Jr, MacKinney LG, Berryhill WS Jr, Holmes CK: Effects of hypoxia and acidity on the initiation of breathing in the fetal lamb at term. Am J Dis Child 112:334, 1966

41. Purves MJ, Biscoe TJ: Development of chemoreceptor activity. Br Med Bull 22:56, 1966

42. James LS, Weisbrot IM, Prince CE et al: The acid–base status of human infants in relation to birth asphyxia and the onset of respiration. J Pediatr 52:379, 1958

43. Harned HS Jr, Griffin CA III, Berryhill WS Jr et al: Role of carotid chemoreceptors in the initiation of effective breathing of the lamb at term. Pediatrics 39:329, 1967

44. Kitterman JA, Liggins GC, Clements JA, Tooley WH: Stimulation of breathing movements in fetal sheep by inhibitors of prostaglandin synthesis. J Dev Physiol 1:453, 1979

45. Kitterman JA, Liggins GC, Fewell JE, Tooley WH: Inhibition of breathing movements in fetal sheep by prostaglandins. J Appl Physiol 54:687, 1983

46. Harned HS Jr, Herrington RT, Ferreiro JI: The effects of immersion and temperature on respiration in newborn lambs. Pediatrics 45:598, 1970

47. Dawes GS: Foetal and Neonatal Physiology. Year Book, Chicago, 1968

48. Harned HS Jr, Herrington RT, Griffin CA III et al: Respiratory effects of division of the carotid sinus nerve in the lamb soon after the initiation of breathing. Pediatr Res 2:264, 1968

49. Wennergren G, Wennergren M: Neonatal breathing control mediated via the central chemoreceptors. Acta Physiol Scand 119:139, 1983

50. Jansen AH, Chernick V: Onset of breathing and control of respiration. Semin Perinatol 12:104, 1988

51. Burns BD: The central control of respiratory movements. Br Med Bull 19:7, 1963

52. Biscoe TJ, Purves MJ: Carotid body chemoreceptor activity in the newborn lamb. J Physiol (Lond) 190:443, 1967

53. Brady JP, Ceruti E: Chemoreceptor reflexes in the newborn infant: effects of varying degrees of hypoxia on the heart rate and ventilation in a warm environment. J Physiol (Lond) 184:631, 1966

54. Rigatto H, Brady JP, de la Torre Verduzco R: Chemoreceptor reflexes in preterm infants. II. The effect of gestational and postnatal age on the ventilatory response to inhaled carbon dioxide. Pediatrics 55:614, 1975

55. Agostoni E, Taglietti A, Agostoni AF, Setnikar I: Mechanical aspects of the first breath. J Appl Physiol 13:344, 1958

56. Karlberg P, Cherry RB, Escardó FE, Koch G: Respiratory studies in newborn infants. II. Pulmonary ventilation and mechanics of breathing in the first minutes of life, including the onset of respiration. Acta Paediatr Scand 51:121, 1962

57. Karlberg P: The adaptive changes in the immediate postnatal period, with particular reference to respiration. J Pediatr 56:585, 1960

58. Milner AD, Vyas H: Lung expansion at birth. J Pediatr 101:879, 1982

59. Karlberg P, Adams FH, Geubelle F, Wallgren G: Alteration of the infant's thorax during vaginal delivery. Acta Obstet Gynaecol Scand 41:223, 1962

60. Bosma J, Lind J: Upper respiratory mechanisms of newborn infants. Acta Paediatr Scand 51(Suppl 135):32, 1962

61. Jäykkä S: Capillary erection and lung expansion. Acta Paediatr Scand 46(Suppl 112), 1957

62. Klaus M, Tooley WH, Weaver KH, Clements JA: Lung volume in the newborn infant. Pediatrics 30:111, 1962

63. Humphreys PW, Normand ICS, Reynolds EOR, Strang LB: Pulmonary lymph flow and the uptake of liquid from the lungs of the lamb at the start of breathing. J Physiol (Lond) 193:1, 1967

64. Bland RD: Lung liquid clearance before and after birth. Semin Perinatol 12:124, 1988

65. Aherne W, Dawkins MJR: The removal of fluid from the pulmonary airways after birth in the rabbit, and the effect on this of prematurity and prenatal hypoxia. Biol Neonate 7:214, 1964

66. Mescher EJ, Platzker ACG, Ballard PL et al: Ontogeny of tracheal fluid, pulmonary surfactant, and plasma corticoids in the fetal lamb. J Appl Physiol 39:1017, 1975

67. Bland RD, McMillan DD, Bressack MA: Movement of water and protein in the fetal and newborn lung. Ann Rech Vet 8:418, 1977

68. Bland RD, Bressack MA, McMillan DD: Labor decreases the lung water content of newborn rabbits. Am J Obstet Gynecol 135:364, 1979

69. Peltonen T, Hirvonen L: Experimental studies on fetal and neonatal circulation. Acta Paediatr Scand 55(Suppl 161), 1965

70. Lind J, Wegelius C: Human fetal circulation: changes in the cardiovascular system at birth and disturbances in the post-natal closure of the foramen ovale and ductus arteriosus. Cold Spring Harbor Symp Quant Biol 19:109, 1954

71. Rudolph AM: The changes in the circulation after birth: their importance in congenital heart disease. Circulation 41:343, 1970

72. Heymann MA, Creasy RK, Rudolph AM: Quantitation of blood flow patterns in the foetal lamb in utero. p. 129. In Combine KS, Cross KW, Dawes GS, Nathanielsz PW (eds): Foetal and Neonatal Physiology. Cambridge University Press, Cambridge, 1973

73. Teitel DF: Circulatory adjustments to postnatal life. Semin Perinatol 12:96, 1988

74. Heymann MA, Iwamoto HS, Rudolph AM: Factors affecting changes in the neonatal systemic circulation. Annu Rev Physiol 43:371, 1981

75. Naeye RL: Arterial changes during the perinatal period. Arch Pathol Lab Med 71:121, 1961

76. Dawes GS: Changes in the circulation at birth. Anesthesiology 26:522, 1965

77. Moss AJ, Emmanoulides G, Duffie ER Jr: Closure of the ductus arteriosus in the newborn infant. Pediatrics 32:25, 1963

78. Gentile R, Stevenson G, Dooley T et al: Pulse Doppler echocardiographic determination of time of ductal closure in normal newborn infants. J Pediatr 98:443, 1981

79. Heymann MA, Rudolph AM: Control of the ductus arteriosus. Physiol Rev 55:62, 1975

80. Clyman RI: Ontogeny of the ductus arteriosus response to prostaglandins and inhibitors of their synthesis. Semin Perinatol 4:115, 1980

81. Klopfenstein HS, Rudolph AM: Postnatal changes in the circulation and responses to volume loading in sheep. Circ Res 42:839, 1978

82. Behrman RE, Lees MH: Organ blood flows of the fetal, newborn and adult rhesus monkey. Biol Neonate 18:330, 1971

83. Phibbs RH: Delivery room management of the newborn. p. 212. In Avery GB (ed): Neonatology. Pathophysiology and Management of the Newborn. 3rd Ed. JB Lippincott, Philadelphia, 1987

84. Shelley HJ: Carbohydrate reserves in the newborn infant. Br Med J 1:273, 1964

85. Dawes GS, Mott JC, Shelley HJ: The importance of cardiac glycogen for the maintenance of life in foetal lambs and newborn animals during anoxia. J Physiol (Lond) 146:516, 1959

86. Behrman RE, Lees MH, Peterson EN et al: Distribution of the circulation in the normal and asphyxiated fetal primate. Am J Obstet Gynecol 108:956, 1970

87. James LS: Acidosis of the newborn and its relation to birth asphyxia. Acta Paediatr Scand 49(Suppl 122):17, 1960

88. Adamsons K Jr, Behrman R, Dawes GS et al: Resuscitation by positive pressure ventilation and Tris-hydroxymethylaminomethane of rhesus monkeys asphyxiated at birth. J Pediatr 65:807, 1964

89. Cross KW: Resuscitation of the asphyxiated infant. Br Med Bull 22:73, 1966

90. Gupta JM, Tizard JPM: The sequence of events in neonatal apnea. Lancet 2:55, 1967

91. American Heart Association and American Academy of Pediatrics: Textbook of Neonatal Resuscitation. American Heart Association, Washington, DC, 1987

92. Apgar V: A proposal for a new method of evaluation of the newborn infant. Anesth Analg 32:260, 1953

93. Hull D: Lung expansion and ventilation during resuscitation of asphyxiated newborn infants. J Pediatr 75:47, 1969

94. Gregory GA, Gooding CA, Phibbs RH, Tooley WH: Meconium aspiration in infants — a prospective study. J Pediatr 85:848, 1974

95. Carson BS, Losey RW, Bowes WA, Simmons MA: Combined obstetric and pediatric approach to prevent meconium aspiration syndrome. Am J Obstet Gynecol 126:712, 1976

96. Vidyasagar D, Yeh TF, Harris V, Pildes RS: Assisted ventilation in infants with meconium aspiration syndrome. Pediatrics 56:208, 1975

97. Ting P, Brady JP: Tracheal suction in meconium aspiration. Am J Obstet Gynecol 122:767, 1975

98. Linder N, Aranda JV, Tsur M et al: Need for endotracheal intubation and suction in meconium-stained neonates. J Pediatr 112:613, 1988

99. MacDonald HM, Mulligan JC, Allen AC, Taylor PM: Neonatal asphyxia. I. Relationship of obstetric and neonatal complications to neonatal mortality in 38,405 consecutive deliveries. J Pediatr 96:898, 1980

100. Brown JK, Purvis RJ, Forfar JO, Cockburn F: Neurologic aspects of perinatal asphyxia. Dev Med Child Neurol 16:567, 1974

101. Drage JS, Kennedy C, Schwartz BK: The Apgar score as an index of neonatal mortality: a report from the collaborative study of cerebral palsy. Obstet Gynecol 24:222, 1964

102. Nelson KB, Ellenberg JH: Apgar scores as predictors of chronic neurologic disability. Pediatrics 68:36, 1981

103. Robertson C, Finer N: Term infants with hypoxic-ischemic encephalopathy: outcome at 3.5 years. Dev Med Child Neurol 27:473, 1985

104. Perlman JM, Tack ED: Renal injury in the asphyxiated newborn infant: relationship to neurologic outcome. J Pediatr 113:875, 1988

105. Freeman JM, Nelson KB: Intrapartum asphyxia and cerebral palsy. Pediatrics 82:240, 1988

106. Freeman JM (ed): Prenatal and Perinatal Factors Associated with Brain Disorders. Publication No. 85-1149, NIH, Bethesda, MD, 1985

107. Nelson KB, Ellenburg JH: Antecedents of cerebral palsy: multivariate analysis of risk. N Engl J Med 315:81, 1986

108. Volpe JJ: Hypoxic-ischemic encephalopathy: clinical aspects. p. 236. In Volpe JJ (ed): Neurology of the Newborn. 2nd Ed. WB Saunders, Philadelphia, 1987

109. Volpe JJ: Intraventricular hemorrhage and brain injury in the premature infant: neuropathology and pathogenesis. Clin Perinatol 16:361, 1989

110. Pasternak JF, Groothuis DR, Fischer JM, Fischer DP: Regional cerebral blood flow in the newborn beagle pup: the germinal matrix is a "low-flow" structure. Pediatr Res 16:499, 1982

111. Goddard J, Lewis RM, Armstrong DL, Zeller RS: Moderate, rapidly induced hypertension as a cause of intraventricular hemorrhage in the newborn beagle model. J Pediatr 96:1057, 1980

112. Andrew M, Castle V, Saigal S et al: Clinical impact of neonatal thrombocytopenia. J Pediatr 110:457, 1987

113. McDonald MM, Johnson ML, Rumack CM et al: Role of coagulopathy in newborn intracranial hemorrhage. Pediatrics 74:26, 1984

114. Volpe JJ: Neonatal intraventricular hemorrhage. N Engl J Med 304:886, 1981

115. Partridge JC, Babcock DS, Steichen JJ, Han BK: Optimal timing for diagnostic cranial ultrasound in low-birth-weight infants: detection of intracranial hemorrhage and ventricular dilation. J Pediatr 102:281, 1983

116. Papile L-A, Burstein J, Burstein R, Koffler H: Incidence and evolution of subependymal and intra-

ventricular hemorrhage: a study of infants with birth weights less than 1500 gm. J Pediatr 92:529, 1978

117. Volpe JJ: Intraventricular hemorrhage and brain injury in the premature infant. Diagnosis, prognosis, and prevention. Clin Perinatol 16:387, 1989

118. Guzzetta F, Shackelford GD, Volpe S et al: Periventricular echodensities in the premature newborn: critical determinant of neurologic outcome. Pediatrics 78:995, 1986

119. Szymonowicz W, Yu VYH, Bajuk B, Astbury J: Neurodevelopmental outcome of periventricular hemorrhage and leukomalacia in infants 1250 g or less at birth. Early Hum Dev 14:1, 1986

120. Williamson WD, Desmond MM, Wilson GS et al: Survival of low-birth-weight infants with neonatal intraventricular hemorrhage: outcome in the preschool years. Am J Dis Child 137:1181, 1983

121. Liechty EA, Gilmor RL, Bryson CQ, Bull MJ: Outcome of high risk neonates with ventriculomegaly. Dev Med Child Neurol 25:162, 1983

122. Shankaran S, Koepke T, Woldt E et al: Outcome after posthemorrhagic ventriculomegaly in comparison with mild hemorrhage without ventriculomegaly. J Pediatr 114:109, 1989

123. Shinnar S, Molteni RA, Gammon K et al: Intraventricular hemorrhage in the premature infant: a changing outlook. N Engl J Med 306:1464, 1982

124. Sinha S, Davies J, Toner N et al: Vitamin E supplementation reduces frequency of periventricular hemorrhage in very preterm babies. Lancet 1:466, 1987

125. Benson JWT, Hayward C, Osborne JP et al: Multicentre trial of ethamsylate for prevention of periventricular hemorrhage in very low birth weight infants. Lancet 1:1297, 1986

126. Morales WJ, Koerten J: Prevention of intraventricular hemorrhage in very low birth weight infants by maternally administered phenobarbital. Obstet Gynecol 68:295, 1986

127. Shankaran S, Cepeda EE, Ilagan N et al: Antenatal phenobarbital for the prevention of neonatal intracerebral hemorrhage. Am J Obstet Gynecol 154:53, 1986

128. Pomerance JJ, Teal JG, Gogolok JF et al: Maternally administered antenatal vitamin K: effect on neonatal prothrombin activity, partial thromboplastin time, and intraventricular hemorrhage. Obstet Gynecol 70:235, 1987

129. Volpe JJ: Neonatal seizures: current concepts and revised classification. Pediatrics 84:422, 1989

130. Volpe JJ: Neonatal seizures. p. 129. In Volpe JJ (ed): Neurology of the Newborn. 2nd Ed. WB Saunders, Philadelphia, 1987

131. Arey JB, Dent J: Causes of fetal and neonatal death with special reference to pulmonary and inflammatory lesions. J Pediatr 42:205, 1953

132. Valdes-Dapena MA, Arey JB: The causes of neonatal mortality: an analysis of 501 autopsies on newborn infants. J Pediatr 77:366, 1970

133. Rubin A: Birth injuries: incidence, mechanisms, and end results. Obstet Gynecol 23:218, 1964

134. Zelson C, Lee SJ, Pearl M: The incidence of skull fractures underlying cephalohematomas in newborn infants. J Pediatr 85:371, 1974

135. Volpe JJ: Neonatal intracranial hemorrhage: pathophysiology, neuropathology, and clinical features. Clin Perinatol 4:77, 1977

136. Cyr RM, Usher RH, McLean FH: Changing patterns of birth asphyxia and trauma over 20 years. Am J Obstet Gynecol 148:490, 1984

137. Eng GD: Brachial plexus palsy in newborn infants. Pediatrics 48:18, 1971

138. Brans YW, Cassady G: Neonatal spinal cord injuries. Am J Obstet Gynecol 123:918, 1975

139. Crothers B, Putnam MC: Obstetrical injuries of the spinal cord. Medicine (Baltimore) 6:41, 1927

140. Gresham EL: Birth trauma. Pediatr Clin North Am 22:317, 1975

141. Mitchell SC, Korones SB, Berendes HW: Congenital heart disease in 56,109 births: incidence and natural history. Circulation 43:323, 1971

142. Lambert EC, Canent RV, Hohn AR: Congenital cardiac anomalies in the newborn: a review of conditions causing death or severe distress in the first month of life. Pediatrics 37:343, 1966

143. Fox WW, Duara S: Persistent pulmonary hypertension in the neonate: diagnosis and management. J Pediatr 103:505, 1983

144. Rudolph AM: High pulmonary vascular resistance after birth. 1. Pathophysiologic considerations and etiologic classification. Clin Pediatr 19:585, 1980

145. Murphy JD, Rabinovitch M, Goldstein JD, Reid LM: The structural basis of persistent pulmonary hypertension of the newborn infant. J Pediatr 98:962, 1981

146. Goldberg SJ, Levy RA, Siassi B, Betten J: The effects of maternal hypoxia and hyperoxia upon the neonatal pulmonary vasculature. Pediatrics 48:528, 1971

147. Levin DL, Hyman AI, Heymann MA, Rudolph AM: Fetal hypertension and the development of increased pulmonary vascular smooth muscle: a possible mechanism for persistent pulmonary hypertension of the newborn infant. J Pediatr 92:265, 1978

148. Levin DL: Morphologic analysis of the pulmonary vascular bed in congenital left-sided diaphragmatic hernia. J Pediatr 92:805, 1978

149. Short BL, Miller MK, Anderson KD: Extracorporeal membrane oxygenation in the management of respiratory failure in the newborn. Clin Perinatal 14:737, 1987

150. Avery ME, Gatewood OB, Brumley G: Transient tachypnea of the newborn. Am J Dis Child 111:380, 1966

151. Bancalari E, Berlin JA: Meconium aspiration and other asphyxial disorders. Clin Perinatol 5:317, 1978

152. Bada HS, Alojipan LC, Andrews BF: Premature rupture of membranes and its effect on the newborn. Pediatr Clin North Am 24:491, 1977

153. Siegel JD, McCracken GH Jr: Sepsis neonatorum. N Engl J Med 304:642, 1981

154. Ablow RC, Driscoll SG, Effman EL et al: A comparison of early-onset group B streptococcal neonatal infection and the respiratory-distress syndrome of the newborn. N Engl J Med 294:65, 1976

155. Usher RH, Allen AC, McLean FH: Risk of respiratory distress syndrome related to gestational age, route of delivery, and maternal diabetes. Am J Obstet Gynecol 111:826, 1971

156. Avery ME, Mead J: Surface properties in relation to atelectasis and hyaline membrane disease. Am J Dis Child 97:517, 1959

157. Brumley GW: Lung development and lecithen metabolism. Arch Intern Med 127:413, 1971

158. Merritt TA, Farrell PM: Diminished pulmonary lecithin synthesis in acidosis: experimental findings as related to the respiratory distress syndrome. Pediatrics 57:32, 1976

159. Chen J, Clements JA, Cotton E et al: The pulmonary hypoperfusion syndrome. Pediatrics 35:733, 1965

160. Boyle RJ, Oh W: Respiratory distress syndrome. Clin Perinatol 5:283, 1978

161. Kitterman JA, Edmunds LH Jr, Gregory GA et al: Patent ductus arteriosus in premature infants: incidence, relation to pulmonary disease and management. N Engl J Med 287:473, 1972

162. Friedman WF, Hirschklau MJ, Printz MP et al: Pharmacologic closure of patent ductus arteriosus in the premature infant. N Engl J Med 295:526, 1976

163. Jacob J, Gluck L, Di Sessa T et al: The contribution of PDA in the neonate with severe RDS. J Pediatr 96:79, 1980

164. Northway WH Jr, Rosan RC, Porter DY: Pulmonary disease following respirator therapy of hyaline membrane disease. N Engl J Med 276:357, 1967

165. O'Brodovich HM, Mellins RB: Bronchopulmonary dysplasia: unresolved neonatal acute lung injury. Am Rev Respir Dis 132:694, 1985

166. Saigal S, O'Brodovich H: Long-term outcome of pre-term infants with respiratory disease. Clin Perinatol 14:635, 1987

167. Sauve RS, Singhal N: Long term morbidity of infants with bronchopulmonary dysplasia. Pediatrics 76:725, 1985

168. Stahlman M, Hedvall G, Dolanski E et al: Six year follow up of clinical hyaline membrane disease. Pediatr Clin North Am 20:433, 1973

169. Morley CJ, Miller N, Bangham AD, Davis JA: Dry artificial lung surfactant and its effect on very premature babies. Lancet 1:64, 1981

170. Halliday HL, McReid M, Meban C et al: Controlled trial of artificial surfactant to prevent respiratory distress syndrome. Lancet 1:476, 1984

171. Hallman M, Merritt TA, Jarvenpaa A-L et al: Exogenous human surfactant for treatment of severe respiratory distress syndrome: a randomized prospective clinical trial. J Pediatr 106:963, 1985

172. Kwong MS, Egan EA, Notter RH, Shapiro DL: Double-blind clinical trial of calf lung surfactant extract for the prevention of hyaline membrane disease in extremely premature infants. Pediatrics 76:585, 1985

173. Enhorning G, Shennan A, Possmayer F et al: Prevention of neonatal respiratory distress syndrome by tracheal instillation of surfactant: a randomized clinical trial. Pediatrics 76:145, 1985

174. Merritt TA, Hallman M, Bloom BT et al. Prophylactic treatment of very premature infants with human surfactant. N Engl J Med 315:785, 1986

175. Gitlin JD, Soll RF, Parad RB et al: Randomized controlled trial of exogenous surfactant for the treatment of hyaline membrane disease. Pediatrics 79:31, 1987

176. Raju TNK, Bhat R, McCulloch KM et al: Double-blind controlled trial of single-dose treatment with bovine surfactant in severe hyaline membrane disease. Lancet 1:651, 1987

177. Ten Centre Study Group: Ten centre trial of artificial surfactant (artificial lung expanding compound) in very premature babies. Br Med J 294:991, 1987

178. Collaborative European Multicenter Study Group: Surfactant replacement therapy for severe neonatal respiratory distress syndrome: an international randomized clinical trial. Pediatrics 82:683, 1988

179. Kendig JW, Notter RH, Cox C et al: Surfactant replacement therapy at birth: final analysis of a clinical trial and comparisons with similar trials. Pediatrics 82:756, 1988

180. Hobar JD, Soll RF, Sutherland JM et al: A multicenter randomized placebo-controlled trial of surfactant therapy for respiratory distress syndrome. N Engl J Med 320:959, 1989

181. Klaus M, Fanaroff A, Martin RJ: The physical environ-

ment. p. 96. In Klaus MH, Fanaroff AA (eds): Care of the High-Risk Neonate. 3rd Ed. WB Saunders, Philadelphia, 1986

182. Sinclair JC: Metabolic rate and temperature control. p. 354. In Smith CA, Nelson NM (eds): The Physiology of the Newborn Infant. 4th Ed. Charles C Thomas, Springfield, IL, 1976

183. Brück K: Temperature regulation in the newborn infant. Biol Neonate 3:65, 1961

184. Adamsons K Jr, Gandy GM, James LS: The influence of thermal factors upon oxygen consumption of the newborn human infant. J Pediatr 66:495, 1965

185. Adamsons K Jr, Towell ME: Thermal homeostasis in the fetus and newborn. Anesthesiology 26:531, 1965

186. Dawkins MJR, Hull D: Brown adipose tissue and the response of new-born rabbits to cold. J Physiol (Lond) 172:216, 1964

187. Aherne W, Hull D: The site of heat production in the newborn infant. Proc R Soc Med 57:1172, 1962

188. Karlberg P, Moore RE, Oliver TK Jr: The thermogenic response of the newborn infant to noradrenaline. Acta Paediatr Scand 51:284, 1962

189. Hey EN: The relation between environmental temperature and oxygen consumption in the new-born baby. J Physiol (Lond) 200:589, 1969

190. Scopes JW: Metabolic rate and temperature control in the human body. Br Med Bull 22:88, 1966

191. Hey E: The care of babies in incubators. p. 171. In Gairdner D, Hull D (eds): Recent Advances in Paediatrics. 4th Ed. Churchill, London, 1971

192. Hey EN, Katz G, O'Connell B: The total thermal insulation of the new-born baby. J Physiol (Lond) 207:683, 1970

193. Hey EN, Katz G: Evaporative water loss in the new-born baby. J Physiol (Lond) 200:605, 1969

194. Hey EN, Katz G: The optimum thermal environment for naked babies. Arch Dis Child 45:328, 1970

195. Hey EN, O'Connell B: Oxygen consumption and heat balance in the cot-nursed baby. Arch Dis Child 45:335, 1970

196. Hey EN, Mount LE: Heat losses from babies in incubators. Arch Dis Child 42:75, 1967

197. Silverman WA, Sinclair JC, Agate FJ Jr: The oxygen cost of minor changes in heat balance of small newborn infants. Acta Paediatr Scand 55:294, 1966

198. Dahm LS, James LS: Newborn temperature and calculated heat loss in the delivery room. Pediatrics 49:504, 1972

199. Du JNH, Oliver TK Jr: The baby in the delivery room: a suitable microenvironment. JAMA 207:1502, 1969

200. Gandy GM, Adamsons K Jr, Cunningham N, et al: Thermal environment and acid–base homeostasis in human infants during the first few hours of life. J Clin Invest 43:751, 1964

201. Silverman WA, Fertig JW, Berger AP: The influence of the thermal environment upon the survival of newly born premature infants. Pediatrics 22:876, 1958

202. Buetow KC, Klein SW: Effect of maintenance of "normal" skin temperature on survival of infants of low birth weight. Pediatrics 34:163, 1964

203. Day RL, Caligiuri L, Kamenski C, Ehrlich F: Body temperature and survival of premature infants. Pediatrics 34:171, 1964

204. Wheldon AE, Hull D: Incubation of very immature infants. Arch Dis Child 58:504, 1983

205. Glass L, Silverman WA, Sinclair JC: Effect of the thermal environment on cold resistance and growth of small infants after the first week of life. Pediatrics 41:1033, 1968

206. Wu PYK, Hodgeman JE: Insensible water loss in preterm infants: changes with postnatal development and non-ionizing radiant energy. Pediatrics 54:704, 1974

207. Oliver TK Jr, Karlberg P: Gaseous metabolism in newly born infants: the effects of environmental temperature and 15% oxygen in the inspired air. Am J Dis Child 105:427, 1963

208. Scopes JW, Ahmed I: Indirect assessment of oxygen requirements in newborn babies by monitoring deep body temperature. Arch Dis Child 41:25, 1966

209. Burnard ED, Cross KW: Rectal temperature in the newborn after birth asphyxia. Br Med J 2:1197, 1958

210. Cree JE, Meyer J, Hailey DM: Diazepam in labour: its metabolism and effect on the clinical condition and thermogenesis of the newborn. Br Med J 4:251, 1973

211. Mann TP, Elliott RIK: Neonatal cold injury due to accidental exposure to cold. Lancet 1:229, 1957

212. Ziegler EE, O'Donnell AM, Nelson SE, Fomon SJ: Body composition of the reference fetus. Growth 40:329, 1976

213. Sinclair JC, Driscoll JM Jr, Heird WC, Winters RM: Supportive management of the sick neonate: parenteral calories, water, and electrolytes. Pediatr Clin North Am 17:863, 1970

214. Sinclair JC, Silverman WA: Intrauterine growth in active tissue mass of the human fetus, with particular reference to the undergrown baby. Pediatrics 38:48, 1966

215. Leake RD: Perinatal nephrobiology: a developmental perspective. Clin Perinatol 4:321, 1977

216. Ogra PL, Greene HL: Human milk and breast feeding: an update on the state of the art. Pediatr Res 16:266, 1982

217. AAP Committee on Nutrition: Nutritional needs of low birth weight infants. Pediatrics 75:976, 1985

218. Hanning RM, Zlotkin SH: Amino acid and protein needs of the neonate: effects of excess and deficiency. Semin Perinatol 13:131, 1989

219. Goldman HI, Freudenthal R, Holland B, Karelitz S: Clinical effects of two different levels of protein intake on low-birth-weight infants. J Pediatr 74:881, 1969

220. Omans WB, Barness LA, Rose CS, Gjorgy P: Prolonged feeding studies in premature infants. J Pediatr 59:951, 1961

221. Goldman HI, Goldman JS, Kaufman I, Liebman OB: Late effects of early dietary protein intake on low-birth-weight infants. J Pediatr 85:764, 1974

222. Fomon S: Infant Nutrition. 2nd Ed. WB Saunders, Philadelphia, 1974

223. Auricchio S, Rubino A, Murset G: Intestinal glycosidase activities in the human embryo, fetus, and newborn. Pediatrics 35:944, 1965

224. Boellner SW, Beard AG, Panos TC: Impairment of intestinal hydrolysis of lactose in newborn infants. Pediatrics 36:542, 1965

225. Ehrenkranz, RA: Mineral needs of the very low birth weight infant. Semin Perinatol 13:142, 1989

226. Greene HL, Hambidge KM, Schanler R, Tsang RC: Guidelines for the use of vitamins, trace elements, calcium, magnesium and phosphorus in infants and children receiving total parenteral nutrition. Am J Clin Nutr 48:1324, 1989

227. Hanson LA, Winberg J: Breast milk and defense against infection in the newborn. Arch Dis Child 47:845, 1972

228. Chandra RK: Prospective status of the effect of breast feeding on incidence of infection and allergy. Acta Paediatr Scand 68:691, 1979

229. Schanler RJ: Human milk for preterm infants: nutritional and immune factors. Semin Perinatal 13:69, 1989

230. Atkinson SA, Bryan H, Anderson GH: Human milk feeding in premature infants: protein, fat, and carbohydrate balances in the first two weeks of life. J Pediatr 99:617, 1981

231. Lemons JA, Maye L, Hall D, Simmons M: Differences in the composition of preterm and term human milk during early lactation. Pediatr Res 16:113, 1982

232. Rowe JC, Wood DH, Rowe DW, Raisz LG: Nutritional hypophosphatemic rickets in a premature infant fed breast milk. N Engl J Med 300:293, 1979

233. Committee on Drugs: The transfer of drugs and other chemicals into human breast milk. Pediatrics 72:375, 1983

234. La Leche League International: The Womanly Art of Breastfeeding. 2nd Ed. La Leche League International, Franklin Park, IL., 1963

235. Lawrence RA: Breast-Feeding: a Guide for the Medical Profession. 3rd Ed. CV Mosby, St. Louis, 1989

236. Milley JR, Simmons MA: Metabolic requirements for fetal growth. Clin Perinatol 6:365, 1979

237. Senior B: Neonatal hypoglycemia. N Engl J Med 289:790, 1973

238. Cornblath M, Reisner SH: Blood glucose in the neonate and its clinical significance. N Engl J Med 273:378, 1965

239. Pagliara AS, Karl IE, Haymond M, Kipnis DM: Hypoglycemia in infancy and childhood. Part 1. J Pediatr 82:365, 1973

240. Lubchenco LO, Bard H: Incidence of hypoglycemia in newborn infants classified by birth weight and gestational age. Pediatrics 47:831, 1971

241. Pildes RS: Infants of diabetic mothers. N Engl J Med 289:902, 1973

242. Robert MF, Neff RK, Huball JP et al: Association between maternal diabetes and the respiratory-distress syndrome in the newborn. N Engl J Med 294:357, 1976

243. Miller E, Hare JW, Cloherty JP: Elevated maternal hemoglobin A_{1c} in early pregnancy and major congenital anomalies in infants of diabetic mothers. N Engl J Med 304:1331, 1981

244. Cornblath M, Wybregt SH, Baens GS, Klein RI: Symptomatic neonatal hypoglycemia: studies of carbohydrate metabolism in the newborn infant. VIII. Pediatrics 33:388, 1964

245. Lucas A, Morley R, Cole TJ: Adverse neurodevelopmental outcome of moderate neonatal hypoglycemia. Br Med J 297:1304, 1988

246. Anonymous: Brain damage by neonatal hypoglycemia. Lancet 1:882, 1989

247. Conrad PD, Sparks JW, Osberg I et al: Clinical application of a new glucose analyzer in the neonatal intensive care unit: comparison with other methods. J Pediatr 114:281, 1989

248. Reyes HM, Meller JL, Loeff D: Management of esophageal atresia and tracheoesophageal fistula. Clin Perinatol 16:79, 1989

249. Meller JL, Reyes HN, Loeff DS: Gastroschisis and omphalocoele. Clin Perinatol 16:113, 1989

250. Touloukian RJ, Posch JN, Spencer R: The pathogenesis of ischemic gastroenterocolitis of the neonate: selective gut mucosal ischemia in asphyxiated neonatal piglets. J Pediatr Surg 7:194, 1972

251. Kliegman RM, Fanaroff AA: Neonatal necrotizing enterocolitis: a nine-year experience. I. Epidemiology and uncommon observations. Am J Dis Child 135:603, 1981

252. Kliegman RM, Hack M, Jones P, Fanaroff AA: Epi-

demiologic study of necrotizing enterocolitis among low-birth-weight infants: absence of identifiable risk factors. J Pediatr 100:440, 1982

253. Kliegman RM, Fanaroff AA: Necrotizing enterocolitis. N Engl J Med 310:1093, 1984

254. Book LS, Overall JC Jr, Herbst JJ et al: Clustering of necrotizing enterocolitis. Interruption by infection-control measures. N Engl J Med 297:984, 1977

255. Barlow B, Santulli TV, Heird WC et al: An experimental study of acute neonatal enterocolitis—the importance of breast milk. J Pediatr Surg 9:587, 1974

256. Pitt J, Barlow B, Heird WC: Protection against experimental necrotizing enterocolitis by maternal milk. I. Role of milk leukocytes. Pediatr Res 11:906, 1977

257. Eibl MM, Wolf HM, Furnkranz H, Rosenkranz A: Prevention of necrotizing enterocolitis in low birth weight infants by IgA–IgG feeding. N Engl J Med 319:1, 1988

258. Santulli TV, Schullinger JN, Heird WC et al: Acute necrotizing enterocolitis in infancy: a review of 64 cases. Pediatrics 55:376, 1975

259. Oski FA, Naiman JL: Normal blood values in the newborn period. p. 1. In Oski FA, Naiman JL (eds): Hematologic Problems in the Newborn. 3rd Ed. WB Saunders, Philadelphia, 1982

260. Oski FA, Naiman JL: Anemia in the neonatal period. p. 56. In Oski FA, Naiman JL (eds): Hematologic Problems in the Newborn. 3rd Ed. WB Saunders, Philadelphia, 1982

261. Wirth FH, Goldberg KE, Lubchenco LO: Neonatal hyperviscosity. I. Incidence. Pediatrics 63:833, 1979

262. Stevens K, Wirth FH: Incidence of neonatal hyperviscosity at sea level. J Pediatr 97:118, 1980

263. Black VD, Lubchenco LO: Neonatal polycythemia and hyperviscosity. Pediatr Clin North Am 29:1137, 1982

264. Ramamurthy RS, Berlanga M: Postnatal alteration in hematocrit and viscosity in normal and polycythemic infants. J Pediatr 110:929, 1987

265. Black VD, Camp BW, Lubchenco LO et al: Neonatal hyperviscosity association with lower achievement and IQ scores at school age. Pediatrics 83:662, 1989

266. Black VD, Lubchenco LO, Koops BL et al: Neonatal hyperviscosity: randomized study of effect of partial plasma exchange on long term outcome. Pediatrics 75:1048, 1985

267. Van der Elst CW, Molteno CD, Malan AF, de V Heese H: The management of polycythemia in the newborn infant. Early Hum Devel 4:393, 1980

268. Terito M, Finklestein J, Oh W et al. Management of autoimmune thrombocytopenia in pregnancy and the neonate. Obstet Gynecol 41:579, 1973

269. Scott JE, Cruikshank DP, Kochenour NK et al: Fetal platelet counts in the obstetric management of immunologic thrombocytopenic purpura. Am J Obstet Gynecol 136:495, 1980

270. Karpatkin M, Porges RF, Karpatkin S: Platelet counts in infants of women with autoimmune thrombocytopenia: effect of steroid administration to the mother. N Engl J Med 305:936, 1981

271. Bussel JB: Management of infants of mothers with immune thrombocytopenic purpura. J Pediatr 113:497, 1988

272. Bussel JB, Berkowitz RL, McFarland JG et al: Antenatal treatment of neonatal alloimmune thrombocytopenia. N Engl J Med 319:1374, 1988

273. Dubowitz LMS, Dubowitz V, Goldberg C: Clinical assessment of gestational age in the newborn infant. J Pediatr 77:1, 1970

274. Ballard JL, Kazmaier K, Driver M: A simplified assessment of gestational age. Pediatr Res 11:374, 1977

275. Lubchenco LO, Hansman C, Boyd E: Intrauterine growth in length and head circumference as estimated from live births at gestational ages from 26 to 42 weeks. Pediatrics 37:403, 1966

276. Koops BL, Morgan LJ, Battaglia FC: Neonatal mortality risk in relation to birth weight and gestational age: update. J Pediatr 101:969, 1982

277. Lubchenco LO: The High Risk Infant. WB Saunders, Philadelphia, 1976

278. Jones MD Jr, Battaglia FC: Intrauterine growth retardation. Am J Obstet Gynecol 127:540, 1977

279. Maisels MJ: Neonatal jaundice. p. 534. In Avery GB (ed): Neonatology: Pathophysiology and Management of the Newborn. 3rd Ed. JB Lippincott, Philadelphia, 1987

280. Luzeau R, Levillain P, Odievre M, Lemonnier A: Demonstration of lipolytic activity in human milk that inhibits the glucuro-conjugation of bilirubin. Biomedicine 21:258, 1974

281. Bevan BR, Holton JB: Inhibition of bilirubin conjugation in rat liver slices by free fatty acids, with relevance to the problem of breast milk jaundice. Clin Chim Acta 41:101, 1972

282. Lascari AD: "Early" breast feeding jaundice: clinical significance. J Pediatr 108:156, 1986

283. DeCarvalho M, Klaus MH, Merkatz RB: Frequency of breast feeding and serum bilirubin concentration. Am J Dis Child 136:737, 1982

284. Perlstein MA: The late clinical syndrome of posticteric encephalopathy. Pediatr Clin North Am 7:665, 1960

285. Hsia DY, Allen FH Jr, Gellis SS, Diamond LK: Erythroblastosis fetalis. VIII. Studies of serum bilirubin in relation to kernicterus. N Engl J Med 247:668, 1952

286. Watchko JF, Oski FA: Bilirubin 20 mg/dl = vigintiphobia. Pediatrics 71:660, 1983

287. Shiller JG, Silverman WA: "Uncomplicated" hyperbilirubinemia of prematurity. Am J Dis Child 101:587, 1961

288. Levine RL: Bilirubin: worked out years ago? Pediatrics 64:380, 1979

289. Perlman M, Fainmesser P, Sohmer H et al: Auditory nerve–brainstem evoked responses in hyperbilirubinemic neonates. Pediatrics 72:658, 1983

290. Conrad PD, Wilkening RB, Rosenberg AA: Safety of newborn discharge in less than 36 hours in an indigent population. Am J Dis Child 143:98, 1989

291. AAP Committee on Fetus and Newborn: Criteria for early infant discharge and follow-up evaluation. Pediatrics 65:651, 1980

292. American Academy of Pediatrics, American College of Obstetricians and Gynecologists: Guidelines for Perinatal Care. 2nd Ed. Elk Grove Village, IL, 1988

293. Pittard WB III, Geddes K: Newborn hospitalization: a closer look. J Pediatr 112:257, 1988

294. Britton HL, Britton JR: Efficacy of early newborn discharge in a middle class population. Am J Dis Child 138:1041, 1984

295. Klein M, Stern L: Low birth weight and the battered child syndrome. Am J Dis Child 122:15, 1971

296. Klaus MH, Kennell JH: Mothers separated from their newborn infants. Pediatr Clin North Am 17:1015, 1970

297. Klaus M, Kennell J: Care of the parents. p. 147. In Klaus MH, Fanaroff AA (eds): Care of the High Risk Neonate. 3rd Ed. WB Saunders, Philadelphia, 1986

298. Brazelton TB, Scholl ML, Robey JS: Visual responses in the newborn. Pediatrics 37:284, 1966

299. Klaus MH, Jerauld R, Kreger NC: Maternal attachment: importance of the first post-partum days. N Engl J Med 286:460, 1972

300. Solnit AJ, Stark MH: Mourning and the birth of a defective child. Psychoanal Study Child 16:523, 1961

301. Cullberg J: Mental reactions of women to perinatal death. p. 326. In Morris N (ed): Psychosomatic Medicine in Obstetrics and Gynecology. S Karger, New York, 1972

302. Stewart AL, Reynolds EOR, Lipscomb AP: Outcome for infants of very low birth weight: survey of world literature. Lancet 1:1038, 1981

303. Bowman E, Yu VYH: Continuing morbidity in extremely low birth weight infants. Early Hum Dev 18:165, 1989

304. Kitchen W, Ford G, Orgill A et al: Outcome in infants with birth weight 500 to 999 gm: a regional study of 1979 and 1980 births. J Pediatr 104:921, 1984

305. Buckwald S, Zorn, WA, Egan EA: Mortality and follow up data for neonates weighing 500 to 800 g at birth. Am J Dis Child 138:779, 1984

306. Kraybill EN, Kennedy CA, Teplin SW, Campbell SK: Infants with birth weights less than 1001 g: survival, growth, and development. Am J Dis Child 138:837, 1984

307. Hack M, Amiel-Tison C: The outcome of neonatal intensive care. p. 378. In Klaus MH, Fararoff AA (eds): Care of the High Risk Neonate. 3rd Ed. WB Saunders, Philadelphia, 1986

308. Kitchen WH, Ford GW, Rickards AL et al: Children of birth weight <1000 g: changing outcome between ages 2 and 5 years. J Pediatr 110:283, 1987

309. Watkins A, Szymonowicz W, Jin X, Yu VYH: Significance of seizures in very low birth weight infants. Dev Med Child Neurol 30:162, 1988

310. Fitzhardinge PM, Kalman E, Ashby S, Pape KE: Present status of the infant of very low birth weight treated in a referral neonatal intensive care unit in 1974. Ciba Found Symp 59:139, 1978

311. Georgieff MK, Hoffman JS, Pereira GR et al: Effect of neonatal caloric deprivation on head growth and 1-year developmental status in preterm infants. J Pediatr 107:581, 1985

312. Bozynski MEA, Nelson MN, Matalon TAS et al: Prolonged mechanical ventilation and intracranial hemorrhage: impact on developmental progress through 18 months in infants weighing 1,200 grams or less at birth. Pediatrics 79:670, 1987

313. Lucey JF, Dangman B: A reexamination of the role of oxygen in retrolental fibroplasia. Pediatrics 73:82, 1984

314. Valentine PH, Jackson JC, Kalina RE, Woodrum DE: Increased survival of low birth weight infants: impact on the incidence of retinopathy of prematurity. Pediatrics 84:442, 1989

315. Kramer SJ, Vertes DR, Condon M: Auditory brainstem responses and clinical followup of high risk infants. Pediatrics 83:385, 1989

316. Hack M, Caron B, Rivers A, Fanaroff AA: The very low birth weight infant: the broader spectrum of morbidity during infancy and early childhood. JDBP 4:243, 1983

317. Hack M, DeMonterice D, Merkatz IR et al: Rehospitalization of the very low birth weight infant: a continuum of perinatal and environmental morbidity. Am J Dis Child 135:263, 1981

318. Allen DM, Buehler JW, Samuels RN, Brann AW: Mortality in infants discharged from neonatal intensive care units in Georgia. JAMA 261:1763, 1989

319. Ballard PL: Glucocorticoid receptors in the fetal lung.

p. 436. In Hodson WA (ed): Development of the Lung. Marcel Dekker, New York, 1977

320. Netter FH: The Ciba Collection of Medical Illustrations. The Respiratory System. Vol. 7. Ciba-Geigy, Summit, NJ, 1979

321. Avery ME, Said S: Surface phenomena in lungs in health and disease. Medicine (Baltimore) 44:503, 1965

322. Perelman RH, Engle MJ, Farrell PM: Perspectives on fetal lung development. Lung 159:53, 1981

323. Sweet AY: Classification of the low-birth-weight infant. p. 69. In Klaus MH, Fanaroff AA (eds): Care of the High-Risk Neonate. 3rd Ed. WB Saunders, Philadelphia, 1986

324. Nelson NM: Respiration and circulation after birth. p. 117. In Smith CA, Nelson NM (eds): The Physiology of the Newborn Infant. 4th Ed. Charles C Thomas, Springfield, IL, 1976

Chapter 22

Postpartum Care

Watson A. Bowes, Jr.

POSTPARTUM INVOLUTION

The Uterus

The crude weight of the pregnant uterus at term (excluding the fetus, placenta, membranes, and amniotic fluid) is approximately 1,000 g.[1] The weight of the nonpregnant uterus is between 50 and 100 g. It is not known how rapidly this 10-fold involution in organ weight occurs, but within 2 weeks after birth the uterus has usually returned to the pelvis, and by 6 weeks it is usually normal size, as estimated by palpation.

The involution of the uterus after childbirth has been studied for more than 100 years. The gross anatomic and histologic characteristics of the involutional process are based on the study of autopsy, hysterectomy, and endometrial biopsy specimens. Williams[2] studied 18 hysterectomy specimens from sterilization operations performed from postpartum days 7 through 20. Sharman[3] investigated 10 postmortem uteri (days 1 through 12) and 626 endometrial biopsy specimens obtained from 285 women (day 5 through the ninth month). Anderson and Davis[4] reported findings from 32 uteri, 2 postmortem and 30 hysterectomy specimens (day of delivery through 20 weeks postpartum).

Immediately after delivery, the decrease in endometrial surface contributes to the shearing off of the placenta at the decidual layer. The average diameter of the placenta is 18 cm; in the immediate postpartum uterus the average diameter of the site of placental attachment measures 9 cm. The placental site in the first 3 days after delivery is infiltrated with granulocytes and mononuclear cells, a reaction that extends into the endometrium and superficial myometrium. By the seventh day, there is evidence of the regeneration of endometrial glands, often appearing atypical, with irregular chromatin patterns, misshapen and enlarged nuclei, pleomorphism, and increased cytoplasm. By the end of the first week, there is also evidence of the regeneration of endometrial stroma, with mitotic figures noted in gland epithelium; by postpartum day 16, the endometrium is fully restored.

Decidual necrosis begins on the first day, and, by the seventh day, a well-demarcated zone can be seen between necrotic and viable tissue. An area of viable decidua remains between the necrotic slough and the deeper endomyometrium. Sharman[3] described the nonnecrotic decidual cells as participating in the reconstruction of the endometrium, a not unlikely role inasmuch as they were originally endometrial connective tissue cells to which they ultimately revert in the involutional process. By the sixth week, it is rare to find decidual cells.

The immediate inflammatory cell infiltrate of polymorphonuclear leukocytes and lymphocytes persists for about 10 days, presumably serving as an antibacterial barrier. The leukocyte response diminishes rapidly after the tenth day, and plasma cells are seen for the first time. The plasma cell and lymphocyte response may last as long as several months. In fact, endometrial stromal infiltrates of plasma cells and lymphocytes are the sign (and may be the only sign) of a recent pregnancy.

Hemostasis immediately after birth is accomplished by arterial smooth muscle concentration and compression of vessels by the involuting uterine muscle. Vessels in the placental site are characterized during the first 8 days by thrombosis, hyalinization, and endophlebitis in the veins and by hyalinization and obliterative fibrinoid endarteritis in the arteries. The mechanism for hyalinization of arterial walls, which is not completely understood, may be related to the previous trophoblastic infiltration of arterial walls that occurs early in pregnancy. Many of the thrombosed and hyalinized veins are extruded with the slough of the necrotic placental site, but hyalinized arteries remain for extended periods as stigmata of the placental site.

Restoration of the endometrium in areas other than the placental site occurs rapidly, with the process being completed by day 16 after delivery. The gland epithelium does not undergo the reactivity or the pseudoneoplastic appearance noted in placental site glands.[4]

The postpartum uterine discharge or lochia begins as a flow of blood lasting several hours, rapidly diminishing to a reddish-brown discharge through the third or fourth day postpartum. This is followed by a transition to a mucopurulent, somewhat malodorous discharge, lochia serosa, requiring the change of several perineal pads per day. The median duration of lochia serosa is 22 days.[5] However, 15 percent of women will have lochia serosa at the time of the 6-week postpartum examination. In the majority of patients the lochia serosa is followed by a yellow-white discharge, lochia alba. Breast-feeding or the use of oral contraceptive agents does not affect the duration of lochia. Not infrequently there is a sudden but transient increase in uterine bleeding between 7 and 14 days postpartum. This corresponds to the slough of the eschar over the site of placental attachment. Although it can be profuse, this bleeding episode is usually self-limited, requiring nothing more than reassurance of the patient. If it does not subside within 1 or 2 hours, the patient should be evaluated for possible retained placental tissue.

Ultrasound is useful in the management of abnormal postpartum bleeding. The empty uterus with a clear midline echo is quite easy to distinguish from the uterine cavity expanded by clot (sonolucent) or retained tissue (echodense). Serial ultrasound examinations of postpartum patients showed that in 20 to 30 percent there was some retained blood or tissue within 24 hours postdelivery. By the fourth postpartum day, only about 8 percent of patients showed endometrial cavity separation, a portion of which eventually had abnormal postpartum bleeding because of retained placental tissue.[6] In cases of abnormal postpartum bleeding, ultrasound examination efficiently detects patients who have retained tissue and who will therefore benefit from uterine evacuation and curettage. Those who have an empty uterine cavity will respond to therapy with oxytocin or methylergonovine.[7]

The Cervix

During pregnancy, the cervical epithelium increases in thickness, and the cervical glands show both hyperplasia and hypertrophy. Within the stroma, a distinct decidual reaction occurs. These changes are accompanied by a substantial increase in the vascularity of the cervix.[8] During labor and delivery, edema and interstitial hemorrhage occur. Colposcopic examination performed after delivery has demonstrated ulceration, laceration, and ecchymosis of the cervix.[9] Regression of the cervical epithelium begins within the first 4 days after delivery, and by the end of the first week edema and hemorrhage within the cervix are minimal. Vascular hypertrophy and hyperplasia persist throughout the first week postpartum. By 6 weeks postpartum, most of the antepartum changes have resolved, although round cell infiltration and some edema may persist for several months.[10]

The Fallopian Tube

The epithelium of the fallopian tube during pregnancy is characterized by a predominance of nonciliated cells, a phenomenon that is maintained by the balance between the high levels of progesterone and estrogen.[11] After delivery, in the absence of progesterone and estrogen, there is further extrusion of nuclei from nonciliated cells, and diminution in height of both ciliated and nonciliated cells. Andrews[11] demonstrated that the number and height of ciliated cells can be increased in the puerperium by treatment with estrogen.

Fallopian tubes removed between postpartum days 5 and 15 demonstrated inflammatory changes of acute salpingitis in 38 percent of cases, but no bacteria were found. The specific cause of the inflammatory change is unknown.[11] In patients treated with diethylstilbestrol (DES) for lactation suppression, no inflammatory changes in the fallopian tubes were found, suggesting that the number and activity of the ciliated cells are important factors in preventing inflammation. Furthermore, there were no correlations between the presence of histologic inflammation of the fallopian tubes and puerperal fever or other clinical signs of salpingitis.

Ovarian Function

It has long been recognized that women who breast-feed their infants will be amenorrheic for long periods of time, often until the infant is weaned. Several studies, using a variety of methods to indicate ovulation, have demonstrated that ovulation occurs as early as 27 days after delivery, with the mean time being approximately 70 to 75 days in nonlactating women.[12-14] Among those women who are breastfeeding their infants, the mean time to ovulation is about 190 days.

Menstruation resumes by 12 weeks postpartum in 70 percent of women who are not lactating, and the mean time to the first menstruation is 7 to 9 weeks.[15] In one study of lactating women, it was 36 months before 70 percent began to menstruate. The duration of anovulation depends on the frequency of breast-feeding, the duration of each feed, and the proportion of supplementary feeds.[16] The risk of ovulation within the first 6 months postpartum in a woman exclusively breast-feeding is 1 to 5 percent.

The hormonal basis for puerperal ovulation suppression in lactating women appears to be the persistence of elevated serum prolactin levels.[17] Prolactin levels fall to the normal range by the third week postpartum in nonlactating women, but remain elevated into the sixth week postpartum in lactating patients. Estrogen levels fall immediately after delivery in both lactating and nonlactating women and remain depressed in lactating patients. In those who are not lactating, estrogen levels begin to rise 2 weeks after delivery and are significantly higher than in lactating women by postpartum day 17. Follicle-stimulating hormone (FSH) levels are identical in breast-feeding and nonbreast-feeding women. It is therefore assumed that the ovary does not respond to FSH stimulation in the presence of increased prolactin levels.

Thyroid Function

Thyroid size and function throughout pregnancy and the puerperium have been quantitated with ultrasonography and thyroid hormone levels.[18] Thyroid volume increases approximately 30 percent during pregnancy and regresses to normal size gradually over a 12-week period. Thyroxine and triiodothyronine, which are both elevated throughout pregnancy, and triiodothyronine resin uptake, which is decreased during pregnancy, return to normal within 4 weeks postpartum. It is now recognized that the postpartum period is a time when women are at increased risk of developing autoimmune thyroiditis followed by hypothyroidism.[19]

Cardiovascular System and Coagulation

Blood volume increases throughout pregnancy to levels in the third trimester about 35 percent above nonpregnant values.[20] The greatest proportion of this increase consists of an increase of plasma volume that begins in the first trimester and amounts to an additional 1,200 ml of plasma, representing a 50 percent increase by the third trimester. Red blood cell (RBC) volume increases by about 250 ml.

Immediately after delivery, plasma volume is diminished by approximately 1,000 ml because of blood loss. By the third postpartum day, plasma volume has increased by 900 to 1,200 ml because of a shift of extracellular fluid into the vascular space.[21] The total blood volume by the third postpartum day, however, declines to 16 percent of the predelivery value.[22] Ueland[22] found that blood volume changes in the puerperium were the same regardless of the method of delivery, but patients who delivered vaginally had a 5 percent increase in hematocrit, whereas those who had a cesarean delivery had a 6 percent decrease in hematocrit. The rate at which RBC volume returns to prepregnancy levels is unknown, but when measured at 8 weeks postpartum it is found to be within the normal range.[23]

Pulse rate increases throughout pregnancy, as does stroke volume and cardiac output. Immediately postdelivery, these remain elevated or rise even higher for 30 to 60 minutes. Data are lacking about the rate at which cardiac hemodynamics return to normal levels, but normal values of cardiac output are found when measurements are made 8 to 10 weeks postpartum.[24] Following delivery there is a transient rise of approximately 5 percent in both diastolic and systolic blood pressures throughout the first 4 days postpartum.[25] In 12 percent of otherwise normotensive patients, the diastolic blood pressure will exceed 100 mmHg. Monheit et al.[26] reviewed data about the cardiovascular changes of the puerperium and stated that the rate of return to the normal physiologic status is hyperbolic, with most of the regression occurring early.

Ygge[27] studied blood coagulation and fibrinolysis in 10 normal pregnant women during the 4 weeks before delivery, during labor and delivery, and 2 weeks postpartum. Compared with antepartum values, there was a rapid decrease in platelets in some patients and no change or an increase in others. However, 2 weeks after delivery all patients demonstrated an increase in platelet count.

Fibrinolytic activity increased in the first 1 to 4 days after delivery and returned to normal in 1 week. Fibrinogen concentration gradually diminished over the 2-week postpartum period studied. The changes in the coagulation system together with vessel trauma and immobility account for the increased risk of thromboembolism noted in the puerperium, especially when operative delivery has occurred.

The Urinary Tract and Renal Function

It is generally accepted that the urinary tract becomes dilated during pregnancy, especially the renal pelves and the ureters above the pelvic brim. These findings, demonstrated 50 years ago by Baird,[28] affect the collecting system of the right kidney more than that of the left. It has now been shown that these changes are due predominantly to compression of the ureters by adjacent vasculature and, to a lesser extent, by compression from the enlarged uterus. Ureteral tone above the pelvic brim, which in pregnancy is higher than normal, diminishes in the lateral recumbent po-

sition and returns to nonpregnant levels immediately after cesarean delivery.[29]

The intravenous urography studies performed by Dure-Smith[30] demonstrated the ureteral and calyceal dilatation that occurs in pregnancy, presumably because of pressure from the iliac artery. His studies also suggest that subtle anatomic changes take place in the ureters that persist long after the pregnancy has ended. Ultrasound studies of the urinary tract also document the enlargement of the collecting system throughout pregnancy.[31] A study of serial ultrasound examinations of the urinary tract in 20 women throughout pregnancy included a single postpartum examination 6 weeks after delivery.[32] The overall trend was that of dilatation of the collecting system throughout pregnancy, estimated by measurements of the separation of the pelvis–calyceal echo complex, from a mean of 5.0 mm (first trimester) to 10 mm (third trimester) in the right kidney and from 3.0 mm to 4.0 mm in the left collecting system. Measurements in all but two patients had returned to 0 at the time of the 6-week postpartum examination. Cietak and Newton[33] performed serial nephrosonography on 34 patients throughout pregnancy and the puerperium. Twenty-four patients were followed for 12 weeks postpartum. In all patients there was no evidence of hydronephrosis at 6 or 12 weeks postpartum. However, more than 50 percent of patients at 12 weeks postpartum demonstrated persistence of urinary stasis, described as a slight separation of the renal pelvis. The authors interpret this finding as evidence of hyperdistensibility and suggest that pregnancy has a permanent effect on the size of the upper renal tract.

Early urodynamic studies of the bladder suggested that a state of bladder hypotonia occurs in the immediate postpartum period.[34] More recent studies, in which water cystometry and uroflowmetry were performed within 48 hours of delivery and again 4 weeks postpartum, demonstrated a slight but significant decrease in bladder capacity (from 395.5 to 331 ml) and volume at first void (from 277 to 224 ml) in the study interval. Nevertheless, all the urodynamic values studied were within normal limits on both occasions. The results were not affected by the weight of the infant or by an episiotomy. However, prolonged labor and the use of epidural anesthesia appeared to diminish postpartum bladder function transiently.[35]

The most detailed study of renal function in normal pregnancy is that of Sims and Krantz,[36] who studied 12 patients with serial renal function tests throughout pregnancy and for up to 1 year after delivery. Glomerular filtration, which increased by 50 percent early in pregnancy and remained elevated until delivery, returned to normal nonpregnant levels by postpartum week 8. Endogenous creatinine clearance, similarly elevated throughout pregnancy, also returned to normal by the eighth postpartum week. Renal plasma flow increased by 25 percent early in pregnancy, gradually diminished in the third trimester (even when measured in the lateral recumbent position), and continued to decrease to below-normal values in the postpartum period for up to 24 weeks. Normal values were finally established by 50 to 60 weeks after delivery. The reason for the prolonged postpartum depression of the renal plasma flow is not clear.

The rate at which changes in renal function return to normal is not known, because studies within the first 6 weeks postpartum are rare. Renal plasma flow decreases by postpartum day 5, while other measures of renal function continue to be elevated at this time.[37]

Management of the Puerperium

The immediate puerperium for most parturients is spent in the hospital. The duration of confinement for patients with uncomplicated vaginal births is 2 days. For patients with an uncomplicated postoperative course following cesarean delivery the postpartum stay is 4 or 5 days. With prospective payment for hospitalization, it is likely that the duration of postpartum hospitalization will be shortened even further.

If a patient has adequate support at home (i.e., help with housekeeping and meal preparation), there is little value in an extended hospital stay, provided the mother is adequately educated about infant care and feeding, family planning, and identification of danger signs in either the infant or herself. For mothers who do not have adequate support at home and who are insecure about infant care and feeding, additional postpartum confinement may be essential to provide adequate education and to achieve some measure of maternal self-confidence. We have found that patient education can be achieved most efficiently and effectively by the use of several short, single-concept videotapes, which are shown on the inhospital television circuit three times each day. One of the showing times is in the evening so that spouses can be informed as well.

In addition to the video presentations, the patients are given ample opportunity to discuss specific questions or concerns with a nurse or physician. It is also important to provide a new mother time and a sympathetic listener so that she can express her feelings and ask questions about her labor and delivery experience.[38]

The time from delivery until complete physiologic involution and psychological adjustment has been called "the fourth trimester."[39] Patients should understand that the lochia will persist for 3 to 8 weeks and that on days 7 to 14 there is likely to be an episode of heavy vaginal bleeding, which occurs when the placental eschar sloughs. Tampons are permissible if they are comfortable upon insertion and are changed frequently and if there are no perineal, vaginal, or cervical lacerations, which preclude insertion of a tampon until healing has occurred.

Physical activity, including walking up and down stairs, lifting heavy objects, riding in or driving a car, and performing muscle-toning exercises can be resumed without delay if the delivery has been uncomplicated. The most troublesome complaint is lethargy and fatigue. Consequently, every task or activity should be a brief one in the first few days of the puerperium. Mothers whose lethargy persists beyond several weeks must be evaluated, especially as regards thyroid dysfunction. An increasing number of reports of transient postpartum thyrotoxicosis followed by hypothyroidism has appeared. These episodes are characterized by goiter formation, the presence of antithyroid antibodies, and eventual resolution.[40,41]

Sexual activity may be resumed when the perineum is comfortable and when bright red bleeding has subsided. The desire and willingness to resume sexual activity in the puerperium varies greatly among women, depending on the site and state of healing of perineal or vaginal incisions and lacerations, the amount of vaginal atrophy secondary to breast-feeding, and the return of libido.[42] In a study of 50 parturients, Ryding[43] found that 20 percent had little desire for sexual activity 3 months after delivery, and an additional 21 percent had complete loss of desire or aversion to sexual activity. This variation in attitude, desire, and willingness must be acknowledged when counseling women about the resumption of sexual activity.

Many patients will be returning to work situations outside the home after their pregnancies. Frequently the physician must complete insurance or employer forms to establish maternity leave for patients. Six weeks is regarded as the normal period of "disability" following delivery,[44] although some mothers return to work sooner than 6 weeks.

A follow-up examination is frequently scheduled for 6 weeks postpartum. For many patients, an appointment sooner than this (approximately 2 weeks postpartum) or a home visit by a visiting nurse or nurse midwife will be more productive in detecting problems and providing support for a mother. Late puerperal infections, postpartum depression, and problems with infant care and feeding occur long before the 6-week postpartum visit.

Perineal Care

Many women who give birth have an episiotomy or spontaneous laceration of the perineum or vagina. In the United States, episiotomies are more often performed as midline than as mediolateral incisions. Provided that the incision or the laceration does not extend beyond the transverse perineal muscle, that there is no hematoma or extensive ecchymosis, and that a satisfactory repair has been accomplished, there is little need for perineal care beyond routine cleansing with a bath or shower. Analgesia can be accomplished in most patients with nonsteroidal antiinflammatory drugs such as ibuprofen. These drugs have been shown to be superior to acetaminophen or propoxyphene for episiotomy pain and uterine cramping.[45] Furthermore, because of a low milk:maternal plasma drug concentration ratio, a short half-life, and transformation into glucuronide metabolites, ibuprofen is safe for nursing mothers.

A patient who has had a mediolateral episiotomy or who has a third- or fourth-degree extension of a midline episiotomy, an extensive spontaneous second-degree laceration, or extensive perineal bruising may experience considerable perineal pain. Occasionally, the pain and periurethral swelling will prevent the patient from voiding, making urethral catheterization necessary. When a patient complains of inordinate perineal pain, the first and most important step is to reexamine the perineum, vagina, and rectum to detect and drain a hematoma or to identify a perineal infection. Perineal pain may be the first symptom of the very rare but potentially fatal complications of angioedema, necrotizing fasciitis, and fatal perineal cellulitis.[46-48]

In cases of immoderate perineal pain, sitz baths will provide additional pain relief. Although hot sitz baths have long been customary therapy for perineal pain, Droegemueller[49] outlined the rationale for using cold or "iced" sitz baths (which is similar to that for the treatment of athletic injuries, for which considerable success has been achieved with cold therapy) in these situations. Cold provides immediate pain relief as a result of decreased excitability of free nerve endings and decreased nerve conduction. Further pain relief comes from local vasoconstriction, which reduces edema, inhibits hematoma formation, and decreases muscle irritability and spasm. Patients who have alternated using hot and cold sitz baths usually prefer the cold.

The technique for administering a cold sitz bath is to first have the patient sit in a tub of water at room temperature, to which ice cubes are then added. This avoids the perceived or actual unpleasantness of sudden immersion in ice water. The patient remains in the ice water for 20 to 30 minutes.

Frequently what appears to be severe perineal pain is, in fact, the pain of prolapsed hemorrhoids. Witch hazel compresses, suppositories containing corticosteroids, or local anesthetic sprays or emollients may be helpful. Occasionally a thrombus will occur in a prolapsed hemorrhoid. It is a simple task to remove the thrombus through a small scalpel incision using local anesthesia. Dramatic relief of pain usually follows this procedure.

Patients with perineal incisions or lacerations should be advised to postpone sexual intercourse for 3 weeks or until there is no perineal discomfort. Tampons may be inserted whenever the patient is comfortable doing so. However, to avoid any risk of toxic shock syndrome, the use of tampons should be confined to the daytime to prevent leaving a tampon in the vagina for prolonged periods.

Maternal – Infant Attachment

The reaction of parents to a newborn infant is generally that of joy and exclamation and enlivens the atmosphere in even the most sterile and clinical of circumstances. The total concentration of the parents, especially the mother, on the infant and its welfare and the complete disregard for the surrounding environment and events is evident to even the most untrained observer of this scene. Klaus et al.[50] were among the first investigators to study and quantitate this phenomenon and to bring attention to the importance of the first few hours of maternal–infant association. Their studies as well as those of other investigators, including Robson and Powell,[51] have contributed substantially to major changes in hospital policies dealing with patients in labor and delivery and during the postpartum confinement. It is now recognized that there should be opportunities for parents to be with their newborns even from the first few moments after birth and as frequently as possible during the first days thereafter. These associations are usually characterized by fondling, kissing, cuddling, and gazing at the infant, which are manifestations of maternal commitment and protectiveness toward her infant. Separation of mother and infant in the first hours after birth has been shown to diminish or delay the development of these characteristic mothering behaviors,[52] a problem that is intensified when medical, obstetric, or newborn complications require intensive care for either the mother or her newborn infant.

Robson and Powell[51] summarized the literature on early maternal attachment and emphasized how difficult it is to accomplish good research studies about this phenomenon. While it is generally agreed that early association of the mother and infant is beneficial and not to be interfered with unnecessarily, there are still doubts about the long-term implications, if any, of a lack of early maternal–infant association. Is there, in fact, a "sensitive period" during which maternal–infant attachment must occur to prevent permanent, untoward consequences in the relationship? If attachment or "bonding," as the term has been popularized, does not occur in these early hours, will it result in parenting deficiencies and lead to child abuse and neglect or to other forms of maldevelopment of the child? In their monograph summarizing their investigations about parent–infant attachment, Klaus and Kennel[53] warn against drawing any such far-reaching conclusions. Although favoring the theory of a "sensitive period" soon after birth, during which close parent–infant interaction facilitates subsequent attachment and beneficial parenting behavior, these investigators concur that humans are highly adaptable and state that "there are many failsafe

routes to attachment." This appears to be the prevailing view among experts at this time.

The modern hospital maternity ward should enhance and encourage parent–infant attachment by such policies as flexible visiting hours for the father, encouragement of the infant rooming with the mother, and supportive attitudes about breast-feeding. These policies also allow the nursing staff to observe parenting behavior and to identify inept, inexperienced, or even malicious behavior toward the infant. Some situations may call for more intensive follow-up by visiting nurses, home-health visitors, or social workers to provide further support for the family during the posthospital convalescence.

The role of postpartum home visits for enhancing parenting behavior is controversial. Gray et al.[54] found this approach quite beneficial. Siegel et al.[55] studied the effect of early and prolonged inhospital mother–infant contact and a postpartum visitation program on attachment and parenting behavior. They found that early and prolonged maternal–infant contact in the hospital had a significant effect on enhancing subsequent parenting behavior, but the postpartum home visitations had no impact.

The development of the qualities associated with good parenting depends on many things. Certainly it does not depend solely on what transpires in the few hours surrounding the birth experience. There is evidence that specific identification of an infant with its mother's voice begins in utero during the third trimester.[56] Furthermore, the parents' own experience as children, as well as their intellectual and emotional attitudes about children, must play a large role in their own parenting behavior. Areskog et al.[57] showed that women who expressed fear of childbirth during the antenatal period had more complications and more pain in labor and also had more difficulties in attachment to their infants. Consequently, the peripartum period provides opportunities to enhance parenting behavior and to identify families in which follow-up after birth may be necessary to ensure the most favorable child development.[58]

In summary, the postpartum ward should be an environment that provides parents ample opportunity to interact with their newborn infants. Personnel, including nurses, nurses' aides, and physicians, caring for mothers and infants should be alert to signs of abnormal parenting (e.g., refusal of the mother to care for the infant, the use of negative or abusive names in describing or referring to the infant, inordinate delay in naming the infant, or obsessive and unrealistic concerns about the infant's health). These or other signs that maternal–infant attachment is delayed or endangered are as deserving of frequent follow-up during the postpartum period as any of the traditional medical or obstetric complications.

LACTATION AND BREAST-FEEDING

One of the important objectives of the puerperium is to enhance the maternal–infant interaction as regards nutrition of the infant. After several decades during which interest in breast-feeding languished in Western cultures, there has been renewed interest and enthusiasm for what is clearly the most reasonable means of feeding most newborn infants.[59] Between 1971 and 1981, the number of mothers breast-feeding their infants at the time of discharge from the hospital doubled. Furthermore, the duration of breast-feeding, measured at age 6 months, increased at a faster rate than did the incidence of breast-feeding in the hospital. Although the increase in breast-feeding is seen in all demographic groups, it is greatest in the upper-income and more highly educated groups. The increase in the popularity of breast-feeding is due in part to an increasing awareness of the advantages of this means of infant feeding. The litany of benefits includes improved infant nutrition, increased resistance to infection, decreased expense, and increased convenience.[60]

Successful breast-feeding depends to a great extent on the motivation of the mother and on the support she receives from family, friends, and health-care providers. Undoubtedly the mother's experience as a child contributes to her attitudes about childbearing and infant feeding.[61] Nevertheless, additional knowledge about breast-feeding may be gained during prenatal care from well-informed, enthusiastic, and supportive physicians and nurses, by reading from one of several lay books on breast-feeding, and by participating in classes on prepared childbirth. A variety of hospital practices, including the use of audiovisual aids, telephone hotlines, and in-service training for personnel, have been shown to increase the incidence of successful breast-feeding.[62]

The prenatal physical examination may identify problems that will affect breast-feeding. These include inverted nipples, which can be corrected in part by wearing of breast shields, or *Monilia* vaginal infections, which should be treated to avoid thrush in the infant, and painful *Monilia* infection of the nipples.

The Term Infant

Hospital routines should not interfere with reasonable breast-feeding practices. Allowing the infant to nurse in its wakeful period immediately after birth when the mouthing movements and rooting reflex are active will give the mother confidence and promote milk production and letdown. Furthermore, early suckling not only provides the infant with the important immunologic and antiinfective properties of colostrum, but also has been shown to enhance successful breast-feeding.[63]

Rooming-in allows the parents to become accustomed to demand feeding and provides the mother with opportunities to seek help from the nursing staff while she enhances her breast-feeding skills. Although the rooting and suckling reflexes are intact in a healthy newborn, successful breast-feeding is a learned talent for mother and infant. Neifert and Seacat[64] recommend that the infant be allowed to suckle for 5 minutes per breast per feeding the first day, 10 minutes the second day, and 15 minutes or more per breast per feeding thereafter. If suckling is interrupted before initiation of the letdown reflex, breast engorgement is encouraged and nipple soreness will increase.

The initial breast engorgement that occurs on the second to fourth postpartum day is due to lymphatic and vascular congestion, interstitial edema, and increased tension in the milk ducts. It is best managed with 24-hour demand feedings and, in stubborn cases, the use of oxytocin nasal spray to promote milk letdown. Hot compresses before nursing will facilitate letdown, and cold compresses between feedings may provide additional relief.

A common problem is nipple confusion, in which an infant accepts an artificial nipple but refuses the mother's nipple. This can be avoided by not offering supplemental fluids and by informing the mother of methods to make her nipple more protractile. Breast engorgement enhances this problem, but with patience it usually resolves within 24 to 48 hours.

Nipple soreness, another common complaint during the immediate puerperium, can be relieved by rotating breasts and the infant's position every 5 minutes while nursing; using frequent, shorter feedings rather than prolonged feeding times; avoiding irritating soaps, wet nursing pads, or other applications; and exposing the nipples for air drying followed by the application of hydrous lanolin. In cases of persistent nipple soreness or of sudden appearance of nipple soreness after lactation has been established, *Monilia* infection of the nipple must be considered.[64] The infection, which often occurs in association with thrush or *Monilia* diaper rash, can be documented by culture; it responds promptly to applications of nystatin cream.

An empathetic and caring nursing staff is essential to successful breast-feeding by the mother who is attempting it for the first time. In such cases, it is helpful if discharge from the hospital is postponed until milk letdown has occurred and the mother has gained confidence in her breast-feeding skills. In the hospital, education and patient confidence can be facilitated with a brief videotape presentation about breast-feeding, which anticipates some of the problems that might be encountered and offers helpful solutions. After discharge from the hospital, the mother should have 24-hour access to persons who can answer her questions about any difficulties she encounters with nursing. We have found it helpful to encourage the patients to call the postpartum ward and discuss the matter with one of the nurses. (This will require timely inservice instruction for the postpartum nurses about breast-feeding.) This has the advantage of allowing the new mother to talk with people who have recently been counseling her about breast-feeding and who are available on a 24-hour basis. Also helpful are books such as the readily available text by Neville and Neifert.[65] In many areas, the local chapter of the La Leche League will offer valuable advice to women who encounter problems with breast-feeding.

Maternal Nutrition During Lactation

Casey and Hambidge[66] recently reviewed the impact of lactation on the nutritional status of the mother. A healthy mother breast-feeding a healthy infant will produce approximately 600 to 900 ml breast milk per day and will provide her infant with approximately 520 kcal/day. This requires about 600 kcal/day (including the energy required to produce the milk),

which must be made up from the mother's diet or her body stores. For this purpose, the well-nourished woman stores about 5 kg fat throughout pregnancy, which can be called on during lactation to make up any nutritional deficit.

The daily allowances of nutrients recommended for the mother during lactation by the U.S. National Research Council[67] are listed below.

Calories	2,500
Protein	64 g
Vitamin A	1,200 μg retinol equiv.
Vitamin D	10 μg
Vitamin E	11 mg (α-tocopherol equiv.)
Thiamine	1.5 mg
Riboflavin	1.7 mg
Niacin	18 mg (niacin equiv.)
Folacin	500 μg
Vitamin B$_6$	2.5 mg
Vitamin B$_{12}$	4.0 μg
Ascorbic acid	100 mg
Calcium	1,200 mg
Phosphorus	1,200 mg
Magnesium	450 mg
Iron	18 mg
Zinc	25 mg
Iodine	200 μg

With the exception of iron and calcium, almost all of the other nutrients are provided in a well-balanced American diet. Even in situations in which there is obvious nutritional deprivation, the quantity and quality of breast milk seems to suffer very little. The composition of breast milk, however, can be influenced to some extent by the mother's diet. The protein content of breast milk is altered very little by the mother's diet, but the fat content is quite susceptible to dietary manipulation. Women who have diets in which the fat is largely of animal origin produce milk with high stearic acid content and low linoleic acid levels, whereas women with diets high in polyunsaturated fatty acids produce milk with high levels of linoleate. The importance of these differences on the subsequent health of breast-fed infants is unknown.

Levels of some but not all vitamins in breast milk can be influenced by maternal intake, but there is little evidence that breast milk in the otherwise well-nourished mother is vitamin deficient. Consequently, the need for vitamin supplementation for the lactating woman on a normal diet is not well established. Some vegetarians may have diets deficient in vitamin B_{12}, and vitamin B_{12} deficiency has been documented in a breast-fed infant of a vegetarian mother.[68] Also, infants of dark-skinned mothers who have had inadequate exposure to sunlight may become vitamin D deficient. This can be avoided by brief daily exposure to sunlight.[69]

Frequently, women inquire about the advisability of dieting and weight loss during lactation. Because of the increased metabolic rate and the increased energy requirements of lactating women, the appetite increases, leading to an increase in caloric intake. However, a persistent weight loss can be achieved through very modest diet restrictions without an untoward effect on the health of either the mother or the infant. Whichelow[70] found that lactating mothers who were losing weight had an average daily intake of 2,509 kcal, whereas women who were not losing weight consumed 2,946 kcal.

Contraindications to Breast-Feeding

There are very few contraindications to breast-feeding. Reduction mammoplasty with autotransplantation of the nipple simply makes breast-feeding impossible.

Puerperal infections including acute mastitis can be managed quite successfully while the mother continues to breast-feed. There is the possibility of transmitting in the breast milk certain viral infections, including cytomegalovirus, herpes simplex, and hepatitis B virus (HBV). Yet the morbidity of cytomegalovirus infection contracted by a healthy term neo-

nate is sufficiently low that potentially infected mothers should not be discouraged from breast-feeding. Withstanding one possible case of viral transmission in the breast milk,[71] the source of neonatal herpes infection is surface contact with the virus; consequently, instruction of the mother in proper handwashing and care of possibly contaminated articles of clothing is sufficient to protect the infant and to permit continued breast-feeding. As regards HBV infection, McGregor and Neifert[72] recommend that breast-feeding not be encouraged in women with acute hepatitis, hepatitis B/e antigenemia (HB_eAg), or other markers of heightened infectivity such as titers of HB_sAg over 1:1,000. However, breast-feeding is permissible in women without active HBV disease and certainly in the uncommon circumstance of an HB_sAg-positive newborn. Thus most mothers with HBV infection before or during pregnancy can be supported in their decision to breast-feed.

Certain medications render breast-feeding inadvisable. These include cyclophosphamide, choramphenicol, tetracycline, diagnostic and therapeutic radioactive substances, and lithium carbonate[73] (see Ch. 11). Most medications taken by the mother will enter the breast milk.[74] Because of the short duration for which most medications are prescribed, however, and the minimal amounts of drug that reach the breast milk (usually in concentrations similar to or less than in maternal plasma), it is usually safe to recommend that the infant continue nursing. The pharmacokinetics of most drugs ingested by breast-feeding women are such that administration of the drug at the time of or immediately after the infant nurses will result in the lowest amount of drug in the milk at the subsequent feeding. If there is any doubt about the effect of a specific drug taken by a mother and whether she should continue breast-feeding, one should consult a recent reference about the effect of drugs in the nursing infant.[74,75]

Breast Milk for the Premature Infant

There are substantial data confirming the psychological, nutritional, and immunologic advantages to using a mother's breast milk to feed her premature infant. Very small preterm infants will not gain weight as readily on breast milk as on formula, because the concentration of protein is less in breast milk.[76] For this reason, there may be the need to supplement breast milk with protein and with some electrolytes as well. While the quantity of protein in breast milk is not as great as that in formula, the quality of the protein is such that prematures fed breast milk appear to have fewer metabolic problems (azotemia, hyperaminoacidemia, and metabolic acidosis). Furthermore, the immunologically active constituents of breast milk (lactoferrin, lysozyme, lactoperoxidase, complement, leukocytes, and specific immunoglobulins) undoubtedly account for the lower incidence of infectious complications found in prematures fed breast milk.[77]

In addition to the nutritional and immunologic advantages of breast milk for the premature infant, there are the important psychological benefits for the mother. Women who give birth to preterm infants often have a sense of guilt and failure. By providing breast milk, the mother becomes an active part of the infant's daily care, which gives her a renewed sense of worth and importance.

In situations in which breast milk will be used for a premature infant, the mother must be instructed in the various methods of milk expression, collection, preservation, and transport. Hand expression is satisfactory in some cases, but in most situations a pump is more efficient and less time-consuming. The Egnell or Medela electric pumps, which simulate the physiologic sucking action of the infant, are available in many nurseries and can be leased from surgical supply companies or rental outlets. Often the local chapter of the La Leche League will provide information on the availability of electric pumps. Hand pumps can also be used. Most intensive care nurseries and many postpartum wards provide written instructions about milk expression and collection techniques. Occasionally it is difficult to maintain an adequate milk supply using artificial expression. Hopkins et al.[78] have demonstrated that in mothers who have delivered prematurely milk volume is inversely related to the delay in initiation of milk expression. Optimal milk production is associated with five or more milk expressions per day and pumping durations that exceeded 100 minutes per day. Also, nasal oxytocin (Syntocinon) can be helpful in augmenting milk letdown.

Breast milk can be refrigerated for 24 hours at 1 degree to 5 degrees C or frozen at -18 degrees to -23 degrees C for up to 3 months. Further details of milk expression, collection, storage, and transport

for use in the feeding of premature infants are well reviewed by Neifert.[79]

Complications of Breast-Feeding

The most common complication of breast-feeding is puerperal mastitis. This condition, which is characterized by fever, myalgias, and an area of pain and redness in either breast, usually has its onset before the end of the second postpartum week, but there is also an increase in its incidence in the fifth and sixth weeks postpartum. Niebyl et al.[80] reported 20 women in whom sporadic (nonepidemic) puerperal mastitis developed. The women were treated with penicillin V, ampicillin, or dicloxacillin and allowed to continue breast-feeding their infants. No abscesses developed. This experience is similar to that of others[81] who have found that in sporadic puerperal mastitis breast-feeding need not be discontinued. In fact, the combination of a penicillinase-resistant penicillin and continued breast-feeding will promptly result in resolution of the infection in 96 percent of cases.

From time to time, a patient will report problems with adequate milk production, sometimes called lactation failure. This problem is usually due to infrequent suckling, which can be corrected by decreasing the interval between feedings and by enhancing milk letdown with oxytocin nasal spray. If the milk supply is inadequate in spite of these measures, endogenous suppression of prolactin may be the problem, as in the unusual situation of retained placental fragments inhibiting lactogenesis as described by Neifert et al.[82] Removal of the retained placental tissue by curettage will result in prompt resumption of milk production. In the absence of any obvious source of prolactin inhibition (e.g., ergot preparations, pyridoxine, or diuretics), pharmacologic enhancement of lactation should be considered. Metoclopramide[83] and sulpiride[84] have both been shown to enhance milk production, presumably by blocking dopamine receptors and stimulating prolactin secretion. Metoclopramide is commercially available (Reglan); given in doses of 10 mg three or four times a day, it may be helpful in stubborn cases of lactation failure.

Lactation Suppression

For those patients who for personal or medical reasons will not breast-feed, some means of lactation suppression may be considered. The topic has been reviewed by Kochenour.[85] The safest method is simply to avoid suckling or other means of milk expression, and the natural inhibition of prolactin secretion will result in breast involution. In 30 to 50 percent of patients, this will be associated with 24 to 48 hours of breast engorgement and pain.[86,87] Breast support, ice packs, and analgesic medications are all helpful in ameliorating these symptoms.

For a number of years, a variety of estrogenic compounds or combinations of estrogen and androgen were given to suppress lactation. Estrogens may actually enhance prolactin secretion. However, it is likely that the net effect of lactation suppression is due to estrogen interference with prolactin binding within breast tissue.[88] Androgens, on the other hand, have been shown to reduce serum prolactin levels.[89] The most effective hormonal regimen for lactation suppression is a combination of testosterone enanthate (90 mg) and estradiol valerate (4 mg) given during or immediately after labor. Although this therapy suppresses both breast engorgment and pain in about 85 percent of patients, 40 percent of patients will experience rebound lactation. Another concern regarding hormonal lactation suppression is its effect on the risk of puerperal thromboembolism. Antithrombin III levels have been shown to be decreased by the administration of estrogen in the puerperium.[90–92] Furthermore, there has been an association between an increased incidence of puerperal thromboembolism and estrogen therapy for lactation suppression.[93,94] Although there has been no direct association between the estrogen–androgen combination therapy and thromboembolism, there is waning enthusiasm for hormonal lactation suppression because of the theoretic concerns about coagulation abnormalities, the large amount of testosterone administered, and the high incidence of rebound lactation.

Currently, the preferred method of pharmacologic lactation suppression is bromocriptine. This ergot derivative is a dopamine receptor agonist with prolonged action that inhibits the release of prolactin. The most effective regimen for lactation suppression is 2.5 mg twice a day for 14 days. This results in suppression of engorgement and pain in 90 percent or more of patients.[95,96]

Bromocriptine is effective even after lactation is established, and antithrombin III levels are not depressed by this drug.[95] These two attributes make bromocriptine a more reasonable choice for lactation suppression than the hormone regimens. However, 23 percent of patients have side effects, including symptomatic hypotension, nausea, and vomiting, and 18 to 40 percent have rebound breast secretion, congestion, or engorgement following the termination of therapy.[97] Furthermore, there have been reports of puerperal hypertension, stroke, seizures and myocardial infarctions in association with the use of bromocriptine prescribed for lactation suppression.[98–101] While these events are rare and a causal relationship with bromocriptine has not been established, the manufacturers' prescription recommendations include instructions to avoid the use of this medication in patients with hypertensive complications of pregnancy and to monitor blood pressure periodically during the time the patient is using the drug. Consequently, it can be questioned whether it is prudent to use a medication for 2 weeks that has this incidence of side effects, possibly rare life-threatening complications, and the requirement for blood pressure monitoring during the therapy as a treatment for puerperal breast engorgement, which, although painful, is never fatal and in most instances resolves within 72 hours.

PREGNANCY PREVENTION AND BIRTH CONTROL

The immediate postpartum period is a convenient time in which to discuss family planning with patients. Ideally, these conversations begin during the prenatal visits, but once delivery has occurred most patients are disposed to serious considerations about future pregnancies. The period of anovulation infertility lasts from 5 weeks in nonlactating women to 8 weeks or more in women who breast-feed their infants without supplementation.[13] Robson et al.[102] found that most women have resumed intercourse by 3 months, and for many resumption of an active sexual life begins much earlier. Consequently, it is important that a decision be made about pregnancy prevention before the patient leaves the hospital.

A patient should be apprised of the various options of pregnancy prevention and birth control in terms that she and her partner can understand. This may be done by individual instruction from nurses, physicians, or physician assistants or by a variety of single-concept films or videotapes. Many such films are available, but some hospitals or physician groups prefer to produce their own films for their specific patient populations. The decision about family planning methods will depend on the patient's motivation, the number of children, the religious background of the couple, the state of the mother's health, and whether she is breast-feeding. It cannot be assumed because a woman has used a method of contraception effectively before the current pregnancy that she will need no counseling thereafter. Debrovner and Winikoff[103] found that more than one-half of patients change contraceptive techniques between pregnancies.

Natural Methods

Natural methods of pregnancy prevention, recently reviewed by Flynn,[104] depend on the couple anticipating the fertile (periovulation) period of the menstrual cycle and not having intercourse during this time. For contraceptive purposes, the menstrual cycle can be regarded as having three phases. Phase I is from the onset of menstruation until the time of preovulation. This phase varies in length and is regarded as the relatively infertile phase. Phase II is the fertile phase, extending from several days preovulation to 48 hours postovulation. Phase III is the absolutely infertile phase, which is from 48 hours after ovulation until the onset of menstrual bleeding. The length of this phase is more consistent, lasting 10 to 16 days.

The most successful methods for a couple to determine the phase of the cycle is to test the cervical mucus or to measure the basal body temperature. Before the fertile phase, the cervical mucus is scant, thick, tacky, and breaks quickly when stretched between the thumb and forefinger. During the fertile phase, the cervical mucus is not only more abundant, but thick and clear; and it also stretches much more without breaking. During the postovulatory phase, the mucus again becomes scant, thick, and opaque, having the characteristics of phase I mucus. This happens rather abruptly; 3 days after it has occurred, the couple can assume they are in the absolutely infertile phase. The basal body temperature method makes use of the biphasic temperature elevation that occurs at the time of ovulation. A special basal body temperature thermometer with an expanded scale should be used and the temperature taken after a period of

sleep before daily activity or the intake of food and water. A sustained temperature rise of 0.2 to 0.6 degree C indicates ovulation has occurred. The postovulatory infertile period is regarded as the morning of the third sustained temperature rise until the onset of menstrual bleeding.

The natural methods of pregnancy prevention are most reliable if intercourse is confined to the postovulatory infertile phase. The Pearl index (the number of pregnancies per 100 women-years) for this method of contraception in Western cultures is reported as being between 4 and 5. This method requires a highly motivated couple who have learned the method well, and in these situations it can be quite effective.

The natural family planning methods cannot be utilized until regular menstrual cycles have resumed. In the first weeks or months following birth, provided there is little or no supplemental feeding for the infant, breast-feeding will provide 98 percent contraceptive protection for up to 6 months. At 6 months, or if menses returns, or if breast-feeding ceases to be full or nearly full before the sixth month, the risk of pregnancy increases.[105]

Barrier Methods

Barrier methods of contraception and vaginal spermicides have recently grown in popularity. The diaphragm has a long and colorful history as a contraceptive device. It is alleged that Casanova recommended that women cover the cervix with half of a lemon after first squeezing its juice into the vagina. The modern diaphragm, after long being used in Europe and England, was finally introduced and manufactured in this country in the 1920s by the Holland-Rantos Company.[106]

The failure rate for the diaphragm varies from 2.4 to 19.6 per 100 women-years. Because this method of contraception requires substantial motivation, instruction, and experience, it is more effective in older women who are familiar with the technique. Vessey and Wiggins[107] found a failure rate of 2.4 per 100 women-years among diaphragm users who were over 25 years old and who had a minimum of 5 months experience using it. This pregnancy rate is comparable to that reported for intrauterine device users.

The proper size of the diaphragm should be determined at the 6-week postpartum visit, even in patients who previously used this form of contraception. In women who are breast-feeding, anovulation leads to vaginal dryness and tightness, which may make the proper fitting of a diaphragm more difficult than in women who are not lactating. The diaphragm should be used with one of the spermicidal lubricants, all of which contain the detergent nonoxynol-9. This substance was shown by Chvapil et al.[108] to be absorbed from skin and mucous membranes in animals. However, there are no data about whether it is secreted in significant levels in human breast milk, and recent studies have not confirmed any higher rate of malformations in populations using it.[109]

The use of condoms alone or in combination with spermicides is often advised for women who wish to postpone a decision about sterilization or oral contraceptive therapy until the postpartum visit. Pregnancy rates for the condom are reported to be from 1.6 to 21 per 100 women-years, depending on the age and motivation of the population studied.[110]

The currently popular vaginal sponge is probably no more effective than other barrier or spermicidal methods.[111]

Steroid Contraceptive Medications

The combined estrogen–progestin preparations have proved to be the most effective method of contraception, with pregnancy rates reported as less than 0.5 per 100 women-years. During the 20 years since this type of contraception was introduced, the combinations of estrogen and progestin have been modified to reduce side effects and complications. Most compounds include 35 μg or less of estrogen and varying amounts of progestins. Cardiovascular complications, including hypertension, venous thrombosis, stroke, and myocardial infarction, have been substantially reduced with the reduction in estrogen content. The cardiovascular complications are found predominantly in women who smoke.[122] In nonsmoking women the risk–benefit ratio is clearly in favor of using oral contraceptive agents. This is particularly true when the additional benefits of these agents are considered, which include lowered risks of benign breast disease, ovarian and endometrial cancer, iron-deficiency anemia, toxic shock syndrome, pelvic inflammatory disease, and ectopic pregnancy.[113]

In patients who are not breast-feeding, oral contraceptive agents can be taken as early as 2 weeks after delivery. Beginning sooner than this probably involves increased risk of puerperal thromboembolism. Von Kaulla et al.[90] demonstrated decreased antithrombin III levels associated with oral contraceptive therapy in the immediate puerperium.

The effect of oral contraceptive agents on lactation is controversial. Controlled studies of the combined-type oral contraceptive agents with doses of ethinyl estradiol or mestranol of 50 μg or more demonstrated a suppressive effect on lactation. Progestin-only medications do not diminish lactation performance. These reports have been well summarized by Buchanan.[114] Combined-type contraceptive agents also decrease the protein, fat, lactose, calcium, and phosphorous concentrations of breast milk, but not to the degree to impair the growth of breast-fed infants.

Currently, the standard of care dictates the use of oral contraceptive agents containing 35 μg or less of ethinyl estradiol or its equivalent. Diaz et al.[115] studied the effect on lactation and infant growth of a low-dose combination oral contraceptive containing 0.03 mg ethinyl estradiol and 0.15 mg levonorgestrel. The medication was begun after all women were fully nursing 1 month after delivery. Among those women taking the oral contraceptive medications, there was a small but significant decrease in lactation performance and in the weight gain of their infants as compared with controls. In women whose motivation to breast-feed is marginal, the slight inhibition of lactation induced by oral contraceptive agents may be sufficient to discourage them from continuing to nurse their infants.

An occasional patient will benefit from the contraceptive effect of monthly injections of 150 mg of intramuscular medroxyprogesterone acetate.[116] Although this has been used widely in other countries, it lacks Food and Drug Administration approval in the United States. Breakthrough bleeding and a concern about serum lipid abnormalities limit its use to those situations in which effective contraception cannot be accomplished with other methods because of the lack of patient compliance.

Intrauterine Devices

Intrauterine devices (IUDs) are among the oldest forms of birth control, their history dating back at least as far as Hippocrates. Mishell[117] and Piotrow et al.[118] published helpful reviews of the current literature about this topic.

The biologic action of IUDs is a matter of concern to those who might object to the method if the principal action is to prevent implantation of the blastocyst. The recent investigations of Alvarez et al.[119] convincingly support the concept that the principal mode of action of IUDs is by a method other than destruction of live embryos. These authors, using techniques to recover ova from the genital tracts of women using no contraception and of women using IUDs, found fertilized eggs in one-half of women using no contraception but none in women using IUDs even though all patients had intercourse within the fertile period.

In 1986 all of the nonprogesterone-containing IUDs were withdrawn from the market in the United States because of the financial burden of defense in liability cases. Recently, a copper-containing, T-shaped IUD was reintroduced by the Population Council's Center for Biomedical Research and marketed under the name of ParaGard.[120]

The pregnancy rate with an IUD is reported to be between 1 and 6 per 100 women-years, with expulsion rates being 4 to 18 and removal for medical reasons being 12 to 16 per 100 women during the first year of use.[121] Addition of bioactive materials such as copper or progesterone to the IUD has not significantly reduced pregnancy rates but has reduced the risk of expulsion or abnormal bleeding.

The major side effects and complications are syncope, uterine perforation, abnormal uterine bleeding, uterine and pelvic infection, and ectopic pregnancy.[118] Syncope is a result of the vagal response that occurs in some women at the time of IUD insertion. Patients with a history of syncope or severe menstrual pain may be at greater risk from a complication, and the use of sedatives, analgesics, or atropine should be considered. These reactions are less common when the IUD is inserted in the puerperium, because functionally the cervix is slightly dilated.

Uterine perforation occurs in 0 to 8 per 1,000 insertions and is highest when the insertion is performed from 1 to 8 weeks after delivery. This is an important consideration when the insertion of the device is planned for the 6-week postpartum visit. If there is any doubt about adequate involution of the uterus, IUD insertion should be postponed for 2 to 3 additional weeks. However, Mishell and Roy[122] dem-

onstrated no increase in perforations with the use of the copper-T inserted 4 to 8 weeks postpartum. A withdrawal type of insertion appears to reduce the risk of this complication.

Bleeding and uterine cramping occur in 8 to 10 percent of women using an IUD and account for 4 to 15 removals of the device per 100 women in the first year of use. The cause of these symptoms is unknown, although they may be due to the local production of proteolytic enzymes and prostaglandins within the endometrium adjacent to the IUD. A variety of methods have been used to treat this complication, including the use of hormones, vitamins, and prostaglandin inhibitors, but there are no data establishing the effectiveness of any of these measures.

The relative risk of pelvic infection in IUD users ranges from 1.7 to 9.3. A variety of microorganisms have been implicated, including actinomycosis in some cases. Prompt removal of the device and antibiotic therapy are recommended when there is any evidence of salpingitis. However, in parous women who have used the IUD, the risk of infertility caused by pelvic infection is no greater than in patients who have never used an IUD.[123]

Although the overall risk of ectopic pregnancy is lower in women using the IUD when compared with women using no contraception, the chances that a pregnancy will be ectopic is 7 to 10 times higher in the IUD user.

There has been some enthusiasm for insertion of the IUD during the immediate postpartum period. Surprisingly, this practice is associated with fewer perforations than are insertions between 1 and 8 weeks. Not surprising, however, is the finding that much higher expulsion rates are noted (10 to 21 percent).[124]

The IUD has been found to be a satisfactory method of birth control in women who are breast-feeding. Cole et al.[125] reported a multicenter study showing that breast-feeding did not increase the risk of expulsion or other complications regardless of the time of insertion of the device.

Sterilization

Sterilization is the most frequently used method of fertility regulation in the world.[126] The puerperium is a convenient time for tubal ligation procedures to be performed in women who desire sterilization. The procedure can be performed at the time of a cesarean delivery or within the first 24 to 48 hours after delivery. In some hospitals the operation is performed immediately after delivery in uncomplicated patients, especially when epidural anesthesia was given for labor analgesia. With the use of small paraumbilical incision, the procedure seldom prolongs the patient's hospitalization more than 1 day beyond the ordinary length of stay.

The failure rate of postpartum sterilization procedures varies somewhat with the type of tubal ligation performed, but overall it is in the range of 0.5 to 1.0 percent. In the United States, the Pomeroy or Parkland procedures are those most commonly performed. In either case, a portion of fallopian tube from its middle third is removed, leaving the cut ends ligated together in a single structure, as in the Pomeroy procedure, or separately, as in the Parkland operation.[127] The somewhat more complicated Uchida procedure involves opening the serosa, which has been infiltrated with saline, removing a segment of the muscularis, and burying the proximal-stump fallopian tube beneath the serosa. Uchida[128] also described removing the distal portion of the tube, including the fimbria, although this is not always done. Using this procedure, Uchida reported an extraordinarily low failure rate (0 in 20,000), but there have been reports by others of pregnancies occurring after a Uchida tubal ligation.[129] At the time of a cesarean delivery, an Irving procedure can be performed, which involves removing a segment from the middle third of the tube and then burying the proximal stump in a small tunnel created in the anterior surface of the uterus.[130] This procedure requires a slightly larger incision if done after vaginal delivery. In some cases, Falope rings or Hulka clips are applied to the tubes through the standard paraumbilical incision.

There are also reports of immediate postpartum sterilization with the laparoscope,[131] but this method lacks widespread enthusiasm. The relaxed abdominal wall and the easy accessibility of the fallopian tubes endows the minilaparotomy with the advantages of convenience and speed without the possible risks of visceral injury that might occur with the trocar of the laparoscope. It seems to be the preferred technique for puerperal sterilization.

Perhaps more important than the type of procedure is the decision about the timing of the procedure or whether it should be performed at all. Puerperal sterilization as compared with interval sterilization is associated with increased incidence of guilt and regret.[132,133] With increasing frequency, couples are postponing tubal ligation procedures until 6 to 8 weeks after delivery.[126] This provides time to ensure that the infant is healthy and to review all the implications of the decision. In most patients, laparoscopic tubal ligation can be accomplished as an outpatient procedure with a minimum of morbidity or disruption of family routines.

The risks of tubal ligation procedures, whether performed in the puerperium or as an interval procedure, include the short-term problems of anesthetic accidents, hemorrhage, injury of the viscera, and infection. These complications are infrequent, and deaths from the procedure occur in 2 to 12 per 100,000 procedures. Long-term complications are less well defined and more controversial. About 10 to 15 percent of patients will have irregular menses and increased menstrual pain after tubal sterilization. This so-called post-tubal syndrome is sufficiently severe in some cases to require hysterectomy. Well-controlled prospective studies, however, have failed to provide convincing evidence that these symptoms occur more commonly after tubal sterilization than in control patients of the same age and previous menstrual history.[134,135]

There has also been concern about poststerilization depression.[136] Because depression is common in women of childbearing age and is even more common in the puerperium, it is difficult to know whether sterilization procedures are independent risk factors for depression. It is obvious, however, that the loss of fertility associated with a sterilization procedure will have important conscious and subconscious implications for many women. It is therefore not surprising that some patients manifest what appear to be transient grief reactions in response to tubal ligation. The loss of libido that may occur in such situations may be frightening to some women and equally disturbing to their partners. Reassurance that such reactions are temporary and are not necessarily symptoms of a seriously disturbed psyche is an important means of support during this crisis. Husbands must be aware of the dynamics of this situation to avoid a sense of estrangement.

Obstetricians must remember that vasectomy is often a more advisable and desirable alternative for a couple considering sterilization.[126] It can be performed as an outpatient procedure under local anesthesia with insignificant loss of time from work. Furthermore, almost all the failures (about 3 to 4 per 1,000 procedures) can be detected by a postoperative semen analysis. This is a decided advantage over the tubal ligation, wherein the failures are discovered only when a pregnancy occurs. Furthermore, vasectomy is less expensive and overall is associated with fewer complications. Contrary to previous concerns, recent studies have demonstrated that men who have had vasectomies are at no greater risk of autoimmune or cardiovascular disease.[137]

Reversal procedures following tubal and vas sterilization have become more common as the number of sterilization procedures increases among young parents of low parity. Success as measured by the occurrence of pregnancy following tubal reanastomosis varies from 40 to 85 percent, depending on the type of tubal ligation performed and on the length of functioning tube that remains.[126] Success rates for vas reanastamosis vary from 37 to 90 percent, with higher success rates being associated with shorter intervals from the time of vas ligation.[126]

Hysterectomy has been advocated as a means of sterilization that has the advantage of protecting the patient from future uterine or cervical cancer. Although the procedure is occasionally indicated in cases of intractable postpartum hemorrhage, uterine rupture, or for documented uterine or cervical disease, the morbidity of cesarean or puerperal hysterectomy operations is sufficiently great to preclude their consideration for elective sterilization.[138]

POSTPARTUM PSYCHOLOGICAL REACTIONS

The psychological reactions experienced by women following childbirth include the common, relatively mild, and transient "maternity blues" (50 to 70 percent incidence), more prolonged affective disorders

regarded as true postpartum depression (10 to 15 percent incidence), and frank puerperal psychosis (0.14 to 0.26 percent incidence). Although the specific etiology of these psychological disorders is unknown, they are not necessarily a continuum or progressively severe manifestations of a single underlying disorder.

Maternity Blues

The most common of the psychological manifestations of the puerperium is the transient state of tearfulness, anxiety, irritation, and restlessness, variously described as "maternity blues" or "postpartum blues." As it occurs in up to 70 percent of parturients,[139] it might well be considered a normal involutional phenomenon. The symptoms may appear on any day within the first week after delivery and usually have resolved by postpartum day 10. Occasional patients will note transient recurrence of the symptoms, especially weeping, for several weeks after delivery. Stein[140] has published a thorough review of current knowledge about this syndrome.

There appear to be no obstetric, social, economic, or personality correlates for maternity blues. While it is tempting to ascribe the symptoms of this syndrome to the changes in steroid hormone levels that occur immediately following delivery, no such correlation has been found.[141] However, lower than expected tryptophan levels have been documented in association with the depressive symptoms in the immediate postpartum period, suggesting a role for neurotransmitters in the elaboration of puerperal mood changes.[142] This is not an illogical association, and additional work may provide more details about the relationship.

Patients suffering from maternity blues manifest a wide range of symptoms, including weeping, depression, restlessness, elation, mood lability, headache, confusion, forgetfulness, irritability, depersonalization, insomnia, and negative feelings toward their infants. Not every patient experiences all these symptoms. Investigators who have studied the syndrome have differed in their criteria and definitions of the disorder, to some extent accounting for the varying incidence of maternity blues reported.

Because the syndrome is transient and of short duration, no therapy is indicated. Anticipatory explanation and a sympathetic and understanding attitude on the part of family members and those caring for the patient are all that are required for this troublesome and common complaint.

Postpartum Depression

Pitt[143] was one of the first to document carefully the incidence of neurotic depression in the puerperium. He found that 11 percent of the patients studied at 28 weeks gestation and at 6 weeks postpartum developed new cases of depression during the postpartum period. Depressive disorders variously characterized occur in 3 to 34 percent of parturients up to 1 year following birth.[144] In a recent study of 128 women randomly selected and interviewed on several occasions during their pregnancies and for 1 year after birth, Watson et al.[144] used a standardized psychiatric interview devised by Goldberg et al.[145] Eight patients (6 percent) were found to have psychiatric disorders when first interviewed (before 24 weeks gestation). Twenty patients (16 percent) had psychiatric disorders identified at 6 weeks postpartum, 15 of which were classified as affective (depressive) disorders. All but three of the cases of postpartum depression occurred either in women who experienced life situations other than the pregnancy that accounted for the depression or in women who had a previous history of significant depressive reactions. In other words, in the experience of these investigators, it was unusual to find postpartum depression occurring in a patient with an otherwise psychologically uncomplicated pregnancy and past history. They also confirmed a lack of association between postnatal depression and social class, marital status, or parity.

In an earlier study, Kaumar and Robson[146] obtained repeated psychiatric interviews from 119 primipara throughout and after pregnancy. At 12 weeks postpartum, these investigators found that 16 patients demonstrated psychiatric disorders, 113 of which were new episodes of depression. Unlike Watson et al.,[144] these observers found little overlap between antenatal and postnatal psychiatric disorders.

There have been several attempts to utilize questionnaires or interview techniques to identify the antepartum patient who is at high risk of developing postpartum major depression. Although no specific series of questions for the prediction of postpartum depression has been rigorously validated or widely used in obstetric practice, the work of Posner et al.[147] suggests that one or more of the following 12 characteristics should alert the caretakers that a patient is at increased risk for postpartum major depression:

1. Is under 20 years of age
2. Is unmarried
3. Is medically indigent
4. Comes from a family of six or more children
5. Was separated from one or both parents in childhood or adolescence
6. Received poor parental support and attention in childhood
7. Had limited parental support in adulthood
8. Has poor relationship with husband or boyfriend
9. Has economic problem with housing and/or income
10. Is dissatisfied with amount of education
11. Shows evidence of emotional problem, past or present
12. Has low self-esteem

It is appropriate that questions addressing some of these risk factors as well as the simple inquiry "are you happy?" be incorporated into the antenatal history.

Garvey and Tollefson[148] point out the high risk of recurrence (50 to 100 percent) of postpartum depression in subsequent pregnancies and the 20 to 30 percent risk of postpartum depression in women who have had a previous depressive reaction not associated with pregnancy. Consequently, it is important to inquire about psychiatric illness when taking the prenatal history.

In a review of the literature regarding postpartum neurotic disorders, Kumar[149] found no convincing evidence for specific correlations between these disorders and levels of hormones or neurotransmitters. Nevertheless, there is some evidence that tryptophan, the amino acid precursor of the neurotransmitter serotonin, is related to mood changes in the puerperium.[150] It is unlikely that the puerperal psychological disorders will eventually be linked to specific neurotransmitter abnormalities.

The signs and symptoms of postpartum depression are not different from those in the nonpregnant patient, but they may be difficult to differentiate from normal involutional phenomena (e.g., weight loss, sleeplessness) or from the transient "maternity blues." However, in addition to the more common symptoms of depression, the postpartum patient may manifest a sense of incapability of loving her family and manifest ambivalence toward her infant.

There is recent evidence that some cases of major depression are associated with thyroid dysfunction.[151] Because of the increasing incidence of thyroid dysfunction occurring in the puerperium, it is worth considering clinical and laboratory evaluation of thyroid function in those patients who manifest symptoms of postpartum depression.

In a brief but helpful review of current literature regarding postpartum depression, Garvey and Tollefson[148] recommend that the standard tricyclic antidepressants be used for the treatment of this disorder. The most common error in therapy is the use of inadequate doses of these medications. Garvey and Tollefson recommend using imipramine, with an initial nighttime dose of 50 mg to be increased to 100 mg by night 3 and to 150 mg by night 5. If after 2 weeks there is no improvement, the single bedtime dose is increased to 200 mg and after another 2 weeks to 300 mg if there is no response. If the response is still inadequate, a plasma imipramine level should be drawn to detect the occasional patient who rapidly metabolizes the drug. If therapeutic plasma levels have been achieved and there is no response, a second-generation tricyclic antidepressant should be considered. Therapy should be continued for 6 to 12 months and the patient followed carefully thereafter for a relapse of symptoms. During this time, breast-feeding should be discontinued, because the tricyclic antidepressants are transferred to breast milk and the consequences of chronic ingestion of these compounds by neonates are unknown. It is advisable to seek psychiatric consultation for patients with depressive reactions sufficiently severe to recommend long-term use of the medication.

Vandenbergh[152] emphasizes the importance of the family in the therapy of postpartum depression. Being physically and emotionally drained from the stresses of pregnancy and childbirth and further burdened by the incessant demands of her infant, the postpartum patient may be unable to meet the demands of her husband and the other children. This will compound her feeling of self-worthlessness. Helping the husband and other family members to understand the nature of the patient's illness and mobilizing resources to provide the patient with help with her home chores and the care of the other children will help to prevent her sense of entrapment and isolation. If a patient is at high risk of developing postpartum depression or if suspicious signs and symptoms develop during the immediate postpartum period, it is mandatory that the postpartum visits be scheduled sooner than the traditional 6 weeks. Vandenberg[151] notes that the moderately depressed mother will often experience such guilt and embarrassment secondary to her sense of failure in her mothering role that she will be unable to call her physician or admit the symptoms of her depression. Consequently, ample time must be set aside to explore in depth even the slightest symptom or sign of depression. Home visits in this situation may be appropriate to assess the patient's parenting skills and to determine how she is coping with the increased responsibilities of her new situation.

Postpartum Psychosis

Schizophrenia and manic–depressive reactions are seen with uncommon frequency in the puerperium, suggesting that there is a psychosis specific to the postpartum condition. In a study of all patients giving birth in 1966 and 1967 in Southampton, England, Nott[153] documented a significant increase in psychiatric referrals for specific psychoses in the 16 weeks after delivery. This confirmed the observation by Kendell et al.,[154] who found a significant increase in admissions to psychiatric hospitals during the puerperium as compared with the antepartum or the nonpregnant state. There is considerable debate as to whether the psychotic reactions that occur in the puerperium represent a unique psychiatric entity. This question is critically reviewed by Brockington et al.[155]

The signs and symptoms in general do not differ from those of acute, nonpuerperal psychosis, but the frequency of symptoms differs substantially. Most patients with puerperal psychosis are manic–depressive, with confusion and disorientation prominent features of the clinical presentation. Furthermore, the psychotic reactions occurring in the puerperium appear to have a more favorable prognosis than the nonpuerperal psychosis. The duration of the illness is frequently only 2 or 3 months.

During the immediate postpartum period, the early signs of depression may be difficult to distinguish from "maternity blues," but if suicidal thoughts or attempts occur, or if frankly delusional thoughts are expressed, the diagnosis of postpartum psychosis can be made.[152]

Clearly, all patients with puerperal psychosis require hospitalization for at least initial evaluation and institution of therapy. However, specific therapeutic management of puerperal psychotic disorders is a matter of controversy. Brockington et al.[155] points out the lack of properly conducted treatment trials in these disorders. Although electroconvulsive therapy, tricyclic antidepressants, neuroleptics, and lithium carbonate have all been recommended for specific subgroups of puerperal psychosis, none has been proved to enhance recovery. Whatever therapy for these conditions is instituted, it should be conducted or supervised by a psychiatrist.

MANAGING PERINATAL GRIEVING

For the most part, perinatal events are happy ones and are occasions for rejoicing. But there are those situations in which a patient and her family experience a loss associated with a pregnancy; these are situations in which special attention must be given to the grieving patient and her family.

The most obvious case of perinatal loss are those in which a fetal or neonatal death has occurred. Other more subtle losses can be associated with a significant amount of grieving, such as the birth of a critically ill or malformed infant, an unexpected hysterectomy performed for intractable postpartum hemorrhage, or even a planned postpartum sterilization procedure. Grief will occur with any significant loss, be it the actual death of an infant[156] or the loss of an idealized child in the case of the birth of a handicapped infant.[157]

Mourning is as old as the human race, but the clinical signs and symptoms of grief and their psychological ramifications as they relate to loss suffered by women during their pregnancies have been given special consideration in recent years. In studying the relatives of servicemen who died in World War II, Lindemann[158] recognized five manifestations of normal grieving. These include somatic symptoms of sleeplessness, fatigue, digestive symptoms, and sighing respirations; preoccupation with the image of the deceased; feelings of guilt; hostility and anger toward others; and disruption of the normal pattern of daily life. He also described the characteristics of what is now recognized as pathologic grief, which may occur if acute mourning is suppressed or interrupted. Some of the manifestations of this so-called morbid grief reaction are overactivity without a sense of loss, appearance or exacerbations of psychosomatic illness, alterations in relationships to friends and relatives, furious hostility toward specific persons, lasting loss of patterns of social interaction, activities detrimental to personal social and economic existence, and agitated depression.

Kennel et al.[159] studied the reaction of 20 mothers to the loss of their newborn infants. Characteristic signs and symptoms of mourning occurred in all the patients, even in situations in which the infant was nonviable. Similar grief reactions occurred in most of the parents of 101 critically ill infants who survived after referral to a regional neonatal intensive care unit.[160] This study, by Benfield et al.,[160] demonstrated that separation from a seriously ill newborn is sufficient to provoke typical grief reaction.

It is important that the characteristics of the grieving patient be recognized and understood by health professionals caring for such patients; otherwise, substantial misunderstanding and mismanagement of the patient will occur. For example, if the patient's reaction of anger and hostility is not anticipated, a nurse or physician may take personally statements or actions by the patient or her family and avoid the patient at the very time she needs the most consolation and support. Because of their own discomfort with the implications of death, physicians, nurses, and others on the postpartum unit often find it uncomfortable to deal with patients whose fetus or infant has died. As a consequence, there is a reluctance to discuss the death with the patient and a tendency to rely on the use of sedatives or tranquilizers to deal with the patient's symptoms of grief.[161-163] What is actually beneficial at such a time is a sympathetic listener and an opportunity to express and discuss feelings of guilt, anger, and hopelessness and the other symptoms of mourning.

It is not surprising that postpartum depression is more common and more severe in families that have suffered a perinatal loss. Rowe et al.[164] found that 6 of 26 mothers who experienced a perinatal loss had morbid grief reactions. Interestingly, the prolonged grief response occurred more commonly in those women who became pregnant within 5 months of the death of the infant. This finding suggests that in counseling women after the loss of an infant, one should avoid the traditional advice of encouraging the family to embark soon on another pregnancy as a "replacement" for the infant who died. Just how long the normal grief reaction lasts is not known, and surely it varies with different families. Lockwood and Lewis[165] studied 26 patients who had suffered a stillbirth; they followed several patients for as long as 2 years. Their data suggest that grief in this situation is usually resolved within 18 months, invariably with a resurgence of symptoms at the first anniversary of the loss.

Somatic symptoms of grief, such as anorexia, weakness, and fatigue, are now well recognized; other psychobiologic manifestations are also reported. Spontaneous abortion and infertility increase among couples who attempt to conceive after the loss of an infant.[166] Schleifer et al.[167] found significant suppression of lymphocyte stimulation in the spouses of women with advanced breast carcinoma. Although the most intense suppression was noted within the month after bereavement, a modified response was noted for as long as 14 months. These investigators suggest that this may account for the increase in morbidity and mortality associated with bereavement.

The regionalization of perinatal health care has resulted in a large proportion of the perinatal deaths occurring in tertiary centers. In some of these centers teams of physicians, nurses, social workers, and pastoral counselors have evolved to aid specifically in the management of families suffering a perinatal loss.[168–170] While this approach ensures an enlightened, understanding, and consistent approach to bereaved families, it suggests that the support of a grieving patient is a highly complex endeavor, to be accomplished only by a few specially trained individuals who care for postpartum patients. Kowalski[171] has listed the following guidelines for managing perinatal loss:

1. Keep the mother informed; be honest and forthright
2. Recognize and facilitate anticipatory grieving
3. Encourage the mother's major support person to remain with her throughout labor and delivery
4. Support the couple in seeing or touching the infant
5. Describe the infant in detail, particularly for couples who choose not to see
6. Encourage the mother to make as many choices about her care as possible
7. Teach the couple about the grieving process
8. Show infants during postpartum hospitalization on request
9. Allow photographs of the infant
10. Prepare the couple for hospital paperwork, such as autopsy requests, death certificates, and disposal of the body
11. Discuss funeral or memorial services
12. Help the couple to think about informing siblings
13. Assist the couple in deciding how to tell friends of the death and in packing away the baby's things
14. Discuss subsequent pregnancy
15. Use public health nurse referrals or schedule additional office visits

Clearly, management of grief is not solely a postpartum responsibility. This is particularly true when a prenatal diagnosis is made of fetal death or fetal abnormality. A continuum of support is essential as the patient moves from the prenatal setting, to labor and delivery, to the postpartum ward, and finally to her home. Relaxation of many of the traditional hospital routines may be necessary to provide the type of support these families need. For example, allowing a loved one to remain past visiting hours, providing a couple a private setting to be with their deceased infant, or allowing unusually early discharge with provisions for frequent phone calls and follow-up visits will often facilitate the resolution of grief.

It is also important to realize that the fathers of

infants who die have somewhat different grief responses than do the mothers. In a study of 28 fathers who had lost infants, Mandell et al.[172] found their grief characterized by the necessity to keep busy with increased work, feelings of diminished self-worth, self-blame, and limited ability to ask for help. Stoic responses are typical of men and may obstruct the normal resolution of grief.

REFERENCES

1. Hytten FE, Cheyne GA: The size and composition of the human pregnant uterus. J Obstet Gynaecol Br Commonw 76:400, 1969

2. Williams JS: Regeneration of the uterine mucosa after delivery, with especial reference to the placental site. Am J Obstet Gynecol 22:664, 1931

3. Sharman A: Postpartum regeneration of the human endometrium. J Anat 87:1, 1953

4. Anderson WR, Davis J: Placental site involution. Am J Obstet Gynecol 102:23, 1968

5. Oppenheimer LS, Sheriff EA, Goodman JDS et al: The duration of lochia. Br J Obstet Gynaecol 93:754, 1986

6. Lipinski JK, Adam AH: Ultrasonic prediction of complications following normal vaginal delivery. J Clin Ultrasound 9:17, 1981

7. Chang YL, Madrozo B, Drukker BH: Ultrasonic evaluation of the postpartum uterus in management of postpartum bleeding. Obstet Gynecol 58:227, 1981

8. Glass M, Rosenthal AH: Cervical changes in pregnancy, labor and puerperium. Am J Obstet Gynecol 60:353, 1950

9. Coppleson M, Reid BL: A colposcopic study of the cervix during pregnancy and the puerperium. J Obstet Gynaecol Br Commonw 73:575, 1966

10. McLaren HC: The involution of the cervix. Br Med J 1:347, 1952

11. Andrews MC: Epithelial changes in the puerperal fallopian tube. Am J Obstet Gynecol 62:28, 1951

12. Cronin TJ: Influence of lactation upon ovulation. Lancet 2:422, 1968

13. Perez A, Uela P, Masnick GS et al: First ovulation after childbirth: the effect of breast feeding. Am J Obstet Gynecol 114:1041, 1972

14. Sharman A: Ovulation after pregnancy. Fertil Steril 2:371, 1951

15. Sharman A: Menstruation after childbirth. J Obstet Gynaecol Br Emp 58:440, 1951

16. Gray RH, Campbell ON, Apelo R et al: Risk of ovulation during lactation. Lancet 335:25, 1990

17. Bonnar J, Franklin M, Nott PN et al: Effect of breastfeeding on pituitary–ovarian function after childbirth. Br Med J 4:82, 1975

18. Rasmusen NG, Hornnes PJ, Hegedüs L: Ultrasonographically determined thyroid size in pregnancy and postpartum: the goitrogenic effect of pregnancy. Am J Obstet Gynecol 160:1216, 1989

19. Jausson R, Dahlberg PA, Winsa B et al: The postpartum period constitutes an important risk for the development of clinical Graves disease in young women. Acta Endocrinol 116:321, 1987

20. Walters WAW, Limm VL: Blood volume and haemodynamics in pregnancy. Clin Obstet Gynaecol 2:301, 1975

21. Landesman R, Miller MM: Blood volume changes during the immediate postpartum period. Obstet Gynecol 21:40, 1963

22. Ueland K: Maternal cardiovascular dynamics. VIII. Intrapartum blood volume changes. Am J Obstet Gynecol 126:671, 1976

23. Paintin DB: The size of the total red cell volume in pregnancy. J Obstet Gynaecol Br Commonw 69:719, 1962

24. Walters WAW, MacGregor WG, Hills M: Cardiac output at rest during pregnancy and the puerperium. Clin Sci 30:1, 1966

25. Walters BNH, Thompson ME, Lea E, DeSwiet M: Blood pressure in the puerperium. Clin Sci 71:589, 1986

26. Monheit AG, Cousins L, Resnik R: The puerperium: anatomic and physiologic readjustments. Clin Obstet Gynecol 23:973, 1980

27. Ygge J: Changes in blood coagulation and fibrinolysis during the puerperium. Am J Obstet Gynecol 104:2, 1969

28. Baird D: The upper urinary tract in pregnancy and puerperium, with special reference to pyelitis of pregnancy. J Obstet Gynaecol Br Emp 42:733, 1935

29. Rubi RA, Sala NC: Ureteral function in pregnant women. III. Effect of different positions and of fetal delivery upon ureteral tonus. Am J Obstet Gynecol 101:230, 1968

30. Dure-Smith P: Pregnancy dilatation of the urinary tract. Radiology 96:545, 1970

31. Peake SL, Roxburgh HB, Langlois SL: Ultrasonic assessment of hydronephrosis of pregnancy. Radiology 146:167, 1983

32. Fried AM, Woodring JH, Thompson DJ: Hydroneph-

rosis of pregnancy: a prospective sequential study of the course of dilatation. J Ultrasound Med 2:255, 1983

33. Cietak KA, Newton JR: Serial qualitative maternal nephrosonography in pregnancy. Br J Radiol 58:399, 1985

34. Bennetts FA, Jud GE: Studies of the postpartum bladder. Am J Obstet Gynecol 42:419, 1941

35. Kerr-Wilson RHJ, Thompson SW, Orr JW Jr et al: Effect of labor on the postpartum bladder. Obstet Gynecol 64:115, 1984

36. Sims EAH, Kratz KE: Serial studies of renal function during pregnancy and the puerperium in normal women. J Clin Invest 37:1764, 1958

37. DeAlvarez RR: Renal glomerulotubular mechanisms during normal pregnancy. Am J Obstet Gynecol 75:931, 1958

38. Affonso DD: Missing pieces: a study of postpartum feeling. Birth Family J 4:159, 1980

39. Jennings B, Edmundson M: The postpartum period: after confinement: the fourth trimester. Clin Obstet Gynecol 23:1093, 1980

40. Fein H, Goldman JM, Weintraub BD: Postpartum lymphocytic thyroiditis in American women: a spectrum of thyroid dysfunction. Am J Obstet Gynecol 138:504, 1980

41. Amino N, Mori H, Iwatani Y et al: High prevalence of transient postpartum thyrotoxicosis and hypothyroidism. N Engl J Med 306:849, 1983

42. Reamy K, White SE: Sexuality in pregnancy and the puerperium: a review. Obstet Gynecol Surv 40:1, 1985

43. Ryding E-L: Sexuality during and after pregnancy. Acta Obstet Gynecol Scand 63:679, 1984

44. American College of Obstetrics and Gynecologists: Pregnancy, Work, and Disability. Technical Bulletin No. 58. ACOG, Washington, DC, 1980.

45. Windle ML, Booker LA, Rayburn WF: Postpartum pain after vaginal delivery: a review of comparative analgesic trials. J Reprod Med 34:891, 1989

46. Shy KK, Eschenback DA: Fatal perineal cellulitis from episiotomy site. Obstet Gynecol 54:292, 1979

47. Stiller RJ, Kaplan BM, Andreoli JW Jr: Hereditary angioedema and pregnancy. Obstet Gynecol 64:133, 1984

48. Ewing TL, Smale LE, Elliot FA: Maternal deaths associated with postpartum vulvar edema. Am J Obstet Gynecol 134:173, 1979

49. Droegemueller W: Cold sitz baths for relief of postpartum perineal pain. Clin Obstet Gynecol 23:1039, 1980

50. Klaus MH, Jerauld R, Kreger NC et al: Maternal attachment: importance of the first postpartum days. N Engl J Med 286:460, 1972

51. Robson KM, Powell E: Early maternal attachment. p. 155. In Brockington IF, Kumar R (eds): Motherhood and Mental Illness. Academic Press, San Diego, 1982

52. McClellan MS, Cabianca WC: Effects of early mother–infant contact following cesarean birth. Obstet Gynecol 56:52, 1980

53. Klaus M, Kennel J: Parent–Infant Bonding. CV Mosby, St. Louis, 1982

54. Gray J, Cutler C, Dean J et al: Prediction and prevention of child abuse and neglect. Child Abuse Neglect 1:45, 1977

55. Siegel E, Bauman KE, Schaefer ES et al: Hospital and home support during infancy: impact on maternal attachment, child abuse and neglect and health care utilization. Pediatrics 66:183, 1980

56. DeCasper AJ, Fifer W: Of human bonding: newborns prefer their mother's voices. Science 208:1174, 1980

57. Areskog B, Uddenberg N, Kjessler B: Experience of delivery in women with and without antenatal fear of childbirth. Gynecol Obstet Invest 16:1, 1983

58. Bibring GL, Dwyer TF, Huntington DS et al: A study of psychological processes in pregnancy of the earliest mother–child relationship. I. Some propositions and comments. Psychoanal Study Child 16:9, 1961

59. Martinez GA, Dodd DA: Milk feeding patterns in the United States: first 12 months of life. Pediatrics 71:166, 1983

60. Jelliffe DB, Jelliffe EFP: "Breast is best": modern meanings. N Engl J Med 297:912, 1977

61. Entwisle DR, Doering SG, Reilly TW: Sociopsychological determinants of women's breast-feeding behavior: a replication and extension. Orthopsychiatry 52:244, 1982

62. Winikoff B, Myers D, Laukaran VH, Stone R: Overcoming obstacles to breast-feeding in a large municipal hospital: applications of lessons learned. Pediatrics 80:423, 1987

63. Salariya EM, Easton PM, Carter JL: Duration of breast feeding after early initiation and frequent feeding. Lancet 2:1141, 1978

64. Neifert MR, Seacat JM: Medical management of successful breast-feeding. Pediatr Clin North Am 33:743, 1986

65. Neville MC, Neifert MR: Lactation: Physiology, Nutrition, and Breast-Feeding. Plenum Press, New York, 1983

66. Casey CE, Hambidge KM: Nutritional aspects of human lactation. p. 199. In Neville MC, Neifert MR

(eds): Lactation: Physiology, Nutrition, and Breast-Feeding. Plenum Press, New York, 1983

67. National Research Council, Food and Nutrition Board: Recommended Dietary Allowances. 9th Ed. National Academy of Sciences, Washington, DC, 1980

68. Higginbottom MC, Sweetman L, Nyhan WL: A syndrome of methylmalonic acidemia, homocystinuria, megaloblastic anemia and neurologic abnormalities in a vitamin B_{12} deficient breast-fed infant of a strict vegetarian. N Engl J Med 299:317, 1978

69. O'Connor P: Vitamin D deficiency in rickets in two breast-fed infants who were not receiving vitamin D supplementation. Clin Pediatr 16:361, 1977

70. Whichelow MJ: Success and failure of breast-feeding in relation to energy intake. Proc Nutr Soc 35:62A, 1975

71. Dunkle LM, Schmidt RR, O'Connor DP: Neonatal herpes simplex infection possibly acquired via maternal breast milk. Pediatrics 63:250, 1979

72. McGregor JA, Neifert MR: Maternal problems in lactation. p. 333. In Neville MC, Neifert MR (eds): Lactation: Physiology, Nutrition and Breast-Feeding. Plenum Press, New York, 1983

73. Bowes WA Jr: The effect of medications on the lactating mother and her infant. Clin Obstet Gynecol 23:1073, 1980

74. Peterson RG, Bowes WA Jr: Drugs, toxins, and environmental agents in breast milk. p. 367. In Neville MC, Neifert MR (eds): Lactation: Physiology, Nutrition, and Breast-Feeding. Plenum Press, New York, 1980

75. Briggs GG, Bodendorfer TW, Freeman RK, Yaffe SJ: Drugs in Pregnancy and Lactation: A Reference Guide to Fetal and Neonatal Risk. Williams & Wilkins, Baltimore, 1984

76. Atkinson SA, Bryan MH, Anderson GH: Human milk feeding in premature infants: protein, fat, and carbohydrate balances in the first two weeks of life. J Pediatr 99:617, 1981

77. Haywood AR: The immunology of breast milk. p. 249. In Neville MC, Neifert MR (eds): Lactation: Physiology, Nutrition, and Breast-Feeding. Plenum Press, New York, 1983

78. Hopkins JM, Schanler RJ, Garza C: Milk production by mothers of premature infants. Pediatrics 81:815, 1988

79. Neifert MR: The infant problems in breast-feeding. p. 273. In Neville MC, Neifert MR (eds): Lactation: Physiology, Nutrition, and Breast-Feeding. Plenum Press, New York, 1983

80. Niebyl JR, Spence MR, Parmley TH: Sporadic (non-epidemic) puerperal mastitis. J Reprod Med 20:97, 1978

81. Thomsen AC, Espersen T, Maigaard S: Course and treatment of milk statis, noninfectious inflammation of the breast, and infectious mastitis in nursing women. Am J Obstet Gynecol 149:492, 1984

82. Neifert MR, McDonough SL, Neville MC: Failure of lactogenesis associated with placental retention. Am J Obstet Gynecol 140:477, 1981

83. Sousa PSR: Metoclopramide and breast feeding. Br Med J 1:512, 1975

84. Aono T, Shigi T, Aki T et al: Augmentation of puerperal lactation by oral administration of sulpiride. J Clin Endocrinol Metab 48:478, 1979

85. Kochenour NK: Lactation suppression. Clin Obstet Gynecol 23:1045, 1980

86. Morris JA, Creasy RK, Hohe PT: Inhibition of puerperal lactation: double-blind comparison of chlorotrianisene, testosterone enanthate with estradiol valerate and placebo. Obstet Gynecol 36:107, 1970

87. Martin KE, Wolst MD: A comparative controlled study of hormones in the prevention of postpartum breast engorgement and lactation. Am J Obstet Gynecol 80:128, 1960

88. Neville MC, Berga SE: Cellular and molecular aspects of the hormonal control of mammary function. p. 141. In Neville MC, Neifert MR (eds): Lactation: Physiology, Nutrition, and Breast-Feeding. Plenum Press, New York, 1983

89. Weinstein D, Ben-David M, Polishuk WZ: Serum prolactin and the suppression of lactation. Br J Obstet Gynaecol 83:679, 1976

90. Von Kaulla E, Droegemueller W, Aok N et al: Effect of estrogens on postpartum hypercoagulability and antithrombin III activity. Am J Obstet Gynecol 113:920, 1972

91. Niebyl JR, Bell WR, Schaaf ME et al: The effect of chlorotrianisene as postpartum lactation suppression on blood coagulation factors. Am J Obstet Gynecol 134:518, 1979

92. Howie PW, Evans K, Forbes CD et al: The effects of stilbestrol and quinestrol upon coagulation and fibrinolysis during puerperium. Br J Obstet Gynaecol 82:968, 1975

93. Daniel DG, Campbell H, Turnbull AC: Puerperal thromboembolism and suppression of lactation. Lancet 2:287, 1967

94. Jeffcoate TNA, Miller J, Roose RF et al: Puerperal thromboembolism in relation to the inhibition of lactation by oestrogen therapy. Br Med J 4:19, 1968

95. Nilsen PA, Meling AB, Abildgaard U: Study of the suppression of lactation and the influence on blood clotting with bromocriptine (CB 154) (Parlodel): a double blind comparison with diethylstilbestrol. Acta Obstet Gynecol Scand 55:39, 1976

96. Duchesne C, Leke R: Bromocriptine mesylate for prevention of lactation. Obstet Gynecol 57:464, 1981

97. Sandoz Pharmaceuticals: Drug Information Brochure re. Parlodel (Bromocriptine Mesylate). Sandoz Pharmaceuticals, East Hanover, NJ, 1987

98. Willis J (ed): Postpartum hypertension, seizures, and strokes reported with bromocriptine. FDA Drug Bull 14:3, 1984

99. Katz M, Kroll I, Pak I et al: Puerperal hypertension, stroke, and seizures after suppression of lactation with bromocriptine. Obstet Gynecol 66:822, 1985

100. Iffy L, TenHove W, Frisoli G: Acute myocardial infarction in the puerperium in patients receiving bromocriptine. Am J Obstet Gynecol 155:371, 1986

101. Ruch A, Duhring JL: Postpartum myocardial infarction in a patient receiving bromocriptine. Obstet Gynecol 74:448, 1989

102. Robson KM, Brant H, Kumar R: Maternal sexuality during first pregnancy after childbirth. Br J Obstet Gynaecol 88:882, 1981

103. Debrovner CH, Winikoff B: Trends in postpartum contraceptive choice. Obstet Gynecol 63:65, 1984

104. Flynn AM: Natural methods of family planning. Clin Obstet Gynaecol 11:661, 1984

105. Family Health International: Breastfeeding as a family planning method. Lancet 2:1204, 1988

106. Wortman J: The diaphragm and other intravaginal barriers—a review. Popul Rep H:58, 1976

107. Vessey M, Wiggins P: Use-effectiveness of the diaphragm in a selected family planning clinic population in the United Kingdom. Contraception 9:15, 1974

108. Chvapil M, Eskelson CD, Shiffel V et al: Studies on nonoxynol-9 intravaginal absorption distribution, metabolism and excretion in rats and rabbits. Contraception 22:325, 1980

109. Shapiro S, Slone D, Kaufman DW et al: Birth defects and vaginal spermicides. JAMA 247:2381, 1982

110. Mills A: Barrier contraception. Clin Obstet Gynaecol 11:641, 1984

111. Edelman PA, McIntyre SL, Harper J: A comparative trial of the Today contraceptive sponge and diaphragm. Am J Obstet Gynecol 150:869, 1984

112. Kay CR: The Royal College of General Practitioners' oral contraceptive study: some recent observations. Clin Obstet Gynaecol 11:759, 1984

113. Ory HW: The noncontraceptive health benefits from oral contraceptive use. Fam Plann Perspect 14:182, 1982

114. Buchanan R: Breastfeeding: aid to infant health and fertility control. Popul Rep J O:49, 1975

115. Diaz S, Peralta G, Juez C et al: Fertility regulation in nursing women: III. Short-term influence of low-dose combined contraceptive upon lactation and infant growth. Contraception 27:1, 1983

116. Schwaille PC: Experience with Depo-Provera as an injectable contraceptive. J Reprod Med 13:113, 1974

117. Mishell DR Jr: Intrauterine devices. Clin Obstet Gynaecol 11:679, 1984

118. Piotrow PT, Rinehart W, Schmidt JC: IUDs—update on safety, effectiveness, and research. Popul Rep 8:49, 1979

119. Alvarez T, Brache V, Fernandez E et al: New insights on the mode of action of intrauterine contraceptive devices in women. Fertil Steril 49:768, 1988

120. Willis J (ed): Copper T 380A IUD marketed in U.S. FDA Drug Bull 18:19, 1988

121. U.S. Department of Health, Education and Welfare: Second Report on Intrauterine Contraceptive Devices. The Medical Device and Drug Advisory Committees on Obstetrics and Gynecology. Food and Drug Administration, Washington, DC, 1978

122. Mishell DR Jr, Roy S: Copper intrauterine contraceptive device event rate following insertion 4 to 8 weeks postpartum. Am J Obstet Gynecol 143:29, 1982

123. Daling JR, Weiss NS, Metch BJ et al: Primary tubal infertility in relation to use of an IUD. N Engl J Med 312:937, 1985

124. Cole LP, Edelman DA, Potts DM et al: Postpartum insertion of modified intrauterine devices. J Reprod Med 29:677, 1984

125. Cole LP, McCann MF, Higgins JE et al: Effects of breast feeding on IUD performance. Am J Public Health 73:384, 1983

126. Newton JR: Sterilization. Clin Obstet Gynecol 11:603, 1984

127. Pritchard JA, MacDonald PC, Gant NF: Williams Obstetrics. 17th Ed. Appleton-Century-Crofts, East Norwalk, CT, 1985

128. Uchida H: Uchida tubal sterilization. Am J Obstet Gynecol 121:153, 1975

129. Benedetti TJ, Miller FC: Uchida tubal sterilization failure: a report of four cases. Am J Obstet Gynecol 132:116, 1978

130. Irving FC: A new method of insuring sterility following cesarean section. Am J Obstet Gynecol 8:335, 1924

131. Aranda C, Prada C, Broutin A et al: Laparoscopic

sterilization immediately after term delivery: preliminary report. J Reprod Med 14:171, 1963

132. Sim M, Emens JM, Jordon JA: Psychiatric aspects of female sterilization. Br Med J 3:220, 1973

133. Emens JM, Olive JE: Timing of female sterilization. Br Med J 2:1126, 1978

134. Vessey M, Huggins G, Lawless M et al: Tubal sterilization: findings in a large prospective study. Br J Obstet Gynaecol 90:203, 1983

135. Bhiwandiwala PP, Mumford SD, Feldblum PJ: Menstrual pattern changes following laparoscopic sterilization with different occlusion techniques: a review of 10,004 cases. Am J Obstet Gynecol 145:684, 1983

136. Bledin KD, Brice B: Psychological conditions in pregnancy and the puerperium and their relevance to postpartum sterilization: a review. Bull WHO 61:533, 1983

137. Walker MW, Jick H, Hunter JR: Vasectomy and non-fatal myocardial infarction. Lancet 1:13, 1981

138. Haynes DM, Martin BJ: Cesarean hysterectomy: a twenty-five year review. Am J Obstet Gynecol 46:215, 1975

139. Yalom I, Lunde D, Moos R et al: Postpartum blues syndrome. Arch Gen Psychiatry 18:16, 1968

140. Stein G: The maternity blues. p. 119. In Brockington IF, Kumar R (eds): Motherhood and Mental Illness. Academic Press, London, 1982

141. Nott PN, Franklin M, Armitage et al: Hormonal changes and mood in the early puerperium. Br J Psychiatry 128:379, 1976

142. Handley SL, Sunn TL, Waldron S et al: Tryptophan, cortisol and puerperal mood. Br J Psychiatry 136:498, 1980

143. Pitt B: Atypical depression following childbirth. Br J Psychiatry 114:1325, 1968

144. Watson JP, Elliot SA, Rugg AJ et al: Psychiatric disorders in pregnancy and the first postnatal year. Br J Psychiatry 144:453, 1984

145. Goldberg DP, Cooper B, Eastwood MR et al: A standardized psychiatric interview for use in community surveys. Br J Prevent Soc Med 24:18, 1970

146. Kumar R, Robson K: Neurotic disturbance during pregnancy and the puerperium: preliminary report of a prospective survey of 119 primiparae. p. 40. In Sand M (ed): Mental Illness in Pregnancy and the Puerperium. Oxford University Press, London, 1978

147. Posner NA, Unterman RR, Williams KN: Postpartum depression: the obstetrician's concerns. p. 69. In Inwood DG (ed): Recent Advances in Postpartum Psychiatric Disorders. American Psychiatric Press, Inc., Washington, DC, 1985

148. Garvey MJ, Tollefson GD: Postpartum depression. J Reprod Med 29:113, 1984

149. Kumar R: Neurotic disorders in childbearing women. p. 71. In Brockington IF, Kumar R (eds): Motherhood and Mental Illness. Academic Press, San Diego, 1982

150. Handley SL, Dunn TL, Baker JM et al: Mood changes in puerperium and plasma tryptophan and cortisol concentrations. Br Med J 2:18, 1977

151. Nemeroff CB, Simon JS, Haggerty JJ Jr, Evans DL: Antithyroid antibodies in depressed patients. Am J Psych 142:7, 1985

152. Vandenberg RL: Postpartum depression. Clin Obstet Gynecol 23:1105, 1980

153. Nott PN: Psychiatric illness following childbirth in Southampton: a case register study. Psychol Med 12:557, 1982

154. Kendell RE, Rennie D, Clark JA et al: The social and obstetric correlates of psychiatric admission in the puerperium. Psychol Med 11:341, 1981

155. Brockington IF, Winokus G, Dean C: Puerperal psychosis. p. 37. In Brockington IF, Kumar R (eds): Motherhood and Mental Illness. Academic Press, London, 1982

156. Leppert PC, Pahlka BS: Grieving characteristics after spontaneous abortion: a management approach. Obstet Gynecol 64:119, 1984

157. Drotar D, Baskiewicz A, Irvin N et al: The adaptation of parents to the birth of an infant with a congenital malformation: a hypothetical model. Pediatrics 56:710, 1975

158. Lindemann E: Symptomatology and management of acute grief. Am J Psych 101:141, 1944

159. Kennel JH, Slyter H, Claus MKH: The mourning response of parents to the death of a newborn. N Engl J Med 83:344, 1970

160. Benfield DG, Leib SA, Reuter J: Grief response of parents after referral of the critically ill newborn to a regional center. N Engl J Med 294:975, 1976

161. Giles PFH: Reactions of women to perinatal death. Aust NZ J Obstet Gynaecol 10:207, 1970

162. Zahourek R, Jensen J: Grieving and the loss of the newborn. Am J Nurs 73:836, 1973

163. Seitz PM, Warrick LH: Perinatal death: the grieving mother. Am J Nurs 74:2028, 1974

164. Rowe J, Clyman R, Green C et al: Follow-up of families who experience perinatal death. Pediatrics 62:166, 1978

165. Lockwood S, Lewis IC: Management of grieving after stillbirth. Med J Aust 2:308, 1980

166. Mandell F, Wolf LC: Sudden infant death syndrome and subsequent pregnancy. Pediatrics 56:774, 1975

167. Schleifer SJ, Keller SE, Camerimo M et al: Suppression of lymphocyte stimulation following bereavement. JAMA 250:374, 1983

168. Lake M, Knuppel R, Murphy J et al: The role of a grief support team following stillbirths. Am J Obstet Gynecol 61:497, 1983

169. Furlong R, Hobbins J: Grief in the perinatal period. Obstet Gynecol 61:497, 1983

170. Condon JT: Management of established pathological grief reaction after stillbirth. Am J Psychiatry 143:987, 1986

171. Kowalski K: Managing perinatal loss. Clin Obstet Gynecol 23:1113, 1980

172. Mandell F, McAnulty E, Race RM: Observations of paternal response to sudden unanticipated infant deaths. Pediatrics 65:221, 1980

SECTION 5
Complicated Pregnancies

Fetal Wastage

Joe Leigh Simpson

Not all conceptions result in a liveborn infant. Many of these losses are not even appreciated clinically, and an additional 10 to 15 percent of clinically recognized pregnancies are lost during the first trimester. The phenomenon of pregnancy loss may also be recurrent. Of married women in the United States, 4 percent have experienced two fetal losses and 3 percent have experienced three or more losses.[1] This chapter considers the causes of fetal wastage and management of couples experiencing repetitive losses.[2-4]

SPECTRUM OF LOSSES THROUGHOUT PREGNANCY

Preclinical Losses

Frequency and Timing

Pregnancy is not generally recognized clinically until 5 to 6 weeks after the last menstrual period. However, prior to this time β-human chorionic gonadotropin (β-hCG) assays can detect pregnancies. Performing β-hCG assays on ovulating women attempting pregnancy allows us to determine frequency of preclinical pregnancy losses. In earlier studies, differences in preclinical loss rates differed greatly.[5-7] This was presumably the result of vicissitudes of β-hCG assays, specifically cross-reactivity with luteinizing hormone (LH). Wilcox et al.[8] performed daily urinary hCG assays beginning around the expected time of implantation. Of all pregnancies, 31 percent (61/198) were lost. The preclinical loss rate was 22 percent

(43/198), whereas the clinically recognized loss rate was 12 percent (19/155).

The relatively lower loss rates observed by Wilcox et al.[8] are consistent with data by Mills and colleagues.[9] In this National Institutes of Child Health and Human Development (NICHD) collaborative study, women were identified before pregnancy, and serum β-hCG assays performed 28 to 35 days after the previous menses. The fetal loss rate (preclinical and clinical) in normal women was only 16.1 percent. Some of these losses would probably be classified as preclinical, but most were clinical. That the total loss rate was slightly lower than that of Wilcox et al.[8] would be expected because in the collaborative study surveillance of the cohort was initiated several days later. It follows that the fourth week of gestation (second week of embryonic development) is a time of relatively high embryonic mortality.

Morphologic and Cytogenetic Findings

The one proven explanation for early losses is morphologic and genetic abnormalities in the early embryo. Decades ago Hertig and Rock[10-12] examined the fallopian tubes, uterine cavities, and endometria of women undergoing elective hysterectomy. All women were of proven fertility; their mean age was 33.6 years. Coital times were recorded prior to hysterectomy. Eight preimplantation embryos (less than 6 days from conception) were recovered. Four of these embryos were morphologically abnormal. The four abnormal embryos presumably would not have implanted or, if implanted, would not have survived very long thereafter (Fig. 23.1). Nine of 26 implanted embryos (6 to 14 embryonic days) were morphologically abnormal (Fig. 23.2).

Although currently not possible in the United States, cytogenetic analysis of early human preimplantation embryos has been performed in Europe. In aggregate, chromosomal abnormalities are estimated to exist in approximately 25 percent of in vitro fertilized embryos.[13-16] One can thus conclude that chromosomal abnormalities are not only frequent in morphologically normal embryos but logically even more frequent in morphologically abnormal embryos. It follows that cytogenetic abnormalities would be expected to be very frequent in the morphologically abnormal embryos recovered by Hertig and Rock.[12]

Consistent with this conclusion are studies in the mouse by Gropp.[17,18] Mice heterozygous for various Robertsonian translocations were mated to produce various monosomies and trisomies. By selective mating and sacrifice of pregnant females at varying gestational ages, both survivability and phenotypic characteristics of the various aberrant complements could be determined. In mice, as in humans, autosomal monosomy proved inviable. Most monosomies aborted around implantation (4 to 5 days after conception) (Fig. 23.3). Most trisomies survived only until immediately after implantation; only a few trisomies survived longer. These findings are analogous to those observed in aneuploid human fetuses.

Clinically Recognized Losses

Frequency and Timing

Clinically recognized fetal loss rates of 12 to 15 percent are well documented in both retrospective and prospective cohort studies. Traditionally, such losses were recognized after 8 weeks gestation on the basis of such clinical criteria as passage of tissue (products of conception), opening of the cervical os, uterine contractions, or bleeding. Studies utilizing ultrasonography have now made it clear that fetal demise occurs prior to the time overt clinical signs are manifested. Fetal viability ceases weeks before maternal symptoms appear; thus, most fetuses aborting clinically at 10 to 12 weeks actually died weeks previously.

Two sources of data have led to the preceding conclusion. First, in studies of obstetrical registrants routinely undergoing ultrasonography, few viable pregnancies are lost after 8 weeks gestation. For example, Wilson et al.[19] studied 734 women in whom an ultrasonographically normal pregnancy was documented at their first obstetric visit (7 to 12 weeks). The loss rate between the initial visit and 20 weeks was 2.4 percent. Loss rates were influenced greatly by maternal age. The loss rate was 4.5 percent in 133 women greater than 35 years old, 2.5 percent among those aged 30 to 35 years, and 1.5 percent in those under 30 years. Similar findings were observed by others.[20-22]

Second, cohort studies have been performed in pregnant women ascertained early in pregnancy.

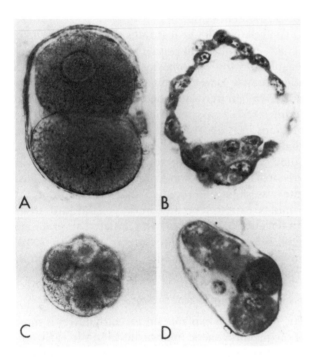

Fig. 23.1 Four views of three preimplanted embryos. (A) Normal two-cell embryo about 30 hours old. (B) Section of 107-cell normal blastocyte about 5 days old, showing inner (embryonic) and outer (abembryonic) masses. (C) Defective, necrotic blastomeres. (D) Another view of (C) showing necrotic blastomeres at left. (A, B, D from Hertig et al.[137] with permission. C from Hertig and Rock,[138] with permission.)

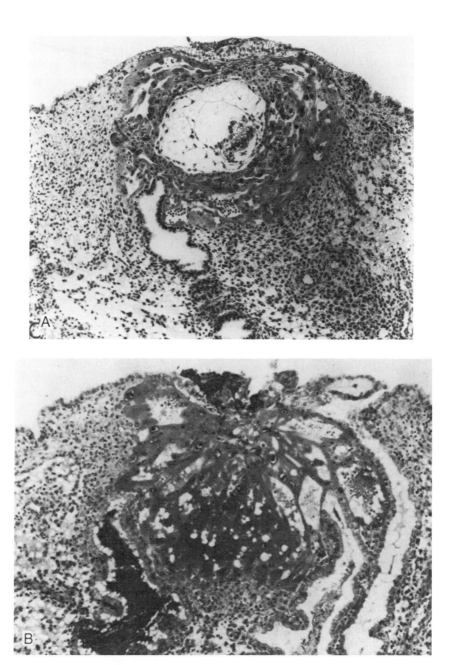

Fig. 23.2 Cross section of endometrium containing a normal 11-day-old embryo (A) compared to an abnormal 14-day-old embryo (B). (From Hertig and Rock,[139] with permission.) In the abnormal embryo no embryonic disc is present and only syncytiotroblasts are identifiable. (From Hertig and Rock,[138] with permission.)

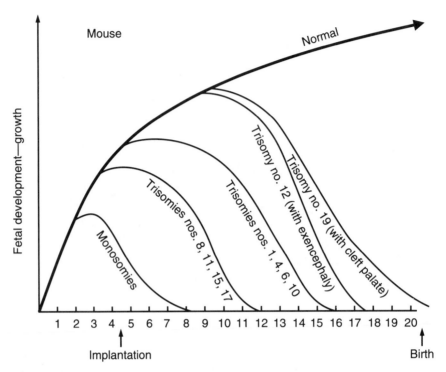

Fig. 23.3 Timing for loss of murine autosomal monosomy and murine autosomal trisomy. (From Gropp,[17] with permission.)

These are essential because studies of obstetric registrants potentially suffer from methodologic shortcomings. Precise information concerning timing of conception is unavailable, and the potential for selection bias exists. Women registering at 7 to 10 weeks gestation could be unusually health conscious and thus at low risk for abortion. Conversely, they could have valid reasons to be concerned about their pregnancy, thus being at high risk and being likely to seek care earlier than women in the general population. In the collaborative study by NICHD,[9] Simpson et al.[23] recruited women prior to conception. Among control subjects were 220 ultrasonographically proven normal pregnancies of 8 weeks gestation. The subject loss rate subsequently in pregnancy in the 220 women was 3.2 percent, similar to data reported from studies of obstetric registrants.

Most fetal demise occurring after 8 weeks appears to occur in the next 2 gestational months. Tabor et al.[24] reported background losses of only 0.7 percent

in 30- to 34-year-old women confirmed by ultrasound to have viable pregnancies at 16 weeks.

Cytogenetic Findings

At least 50 percent of clinically recognized pregnancy losses result from a chromosomal abnormality.[25-28] One unresolved difficulty is lack of information concerning the status of abortuses whose tissue fails to grow in culture. Could culture failures be disproportionately represented by chromosomal abnormalities? On the other hand, cytogenetically normal abortuses might preferentially fail to grow because they were infected. That the former is probable can be deduced from the study of Guerneri et al.,[29] who found a very high (77 percent) frequency of chromosomal abnormalities in women studied immediately after ultrasound diagnosis of fetal demise. Tissue for analysis was obtained by chorionic villus sampling, rather than reliance on recovery of spontaneously expelled products. Thus, a very high proportion (90 percent) of specimens proved informative. Johnson et al.[30] made similar observations on a smaller sample.

The frequency of chromosomal errors in fetal losses recognized to have been viable earlier in pregnancy but lost between 16 and 28 weeks is not precisely known. However, the rate is less than that of fetuses lost earlier in pregnancy. In the second trimester, one also observes chromosomal abnormalities more similar to those observed in liveborn infants: trisomies 13, 18, and 21; monosomy X; and sex chromosomal polysomies.[28,31]

The frequency of chromosomal abnormalities in third trimester losses (traditionally designated stillborn infants) is approximately 5 percent.[32,33] Again, this frequency is far less than that observed in earlier abortuses but higher than in liveborns (0.6 percent).

Pathologic Findings in First Trimester Abortuses

Autosomal Trisomy

Autosomal trisomies comprise the largest (53 percent) single class of chromosomal complements in cytogenetically abnormal spontaneous abortions. Frequencies of specific trisomies are listed in Table 23.1. Trisomy for every chromosome except chromosome 1 has been reported, and trisomy for that chromosome has been observed in an eight-cell embryo.[34] The most common trisomy is trisomy 16. Some but not all trisomies show a maternal age effect, a relationship that is especially impressive for double trisomies.

Trisomy for two autosomes (double trisomy) occurs and is lethal early in development.

Polyploidy

Polyploidy is the presence of more than two haploid chromosomal complements. Triploidy ($3N = 69$) and tetraploidy ($4N = 92$) occur often in abortuses.

Triploid abortuses are usually 69,XXY or 69,XXX, resulting from dispermy.[35,36] An association exists between triploidy and hydatidiform mole. A partial mole is said to exist if molar tissue and fetal parts coexist. By contrast, the more common complete hydatidiform mole is 46,XX, of androgenetic origin.[37,38]

Tetraploid conceptuses are uncommon, rarely progressing further than 2 to 3 weeks of embryonic life.

Monosomy X

Monosomy X is the single most common chromosomal abnormality in spontaneous abortions, accounting for 15 to 20 percent of abnormal specimens (Fig. 23.4). Although liveborn 45,X individuals usually lack germ cells, 45,X abortuses have germ cells, albeit rarely developing beyond the stage of the primordial germ cell. Thus, pathogenesis of germ cell failure in 45,X involves not failure of germ cell development, but rather more rapid attrition than that occurring in 46,XX embryos.[39,40] This observation makes plausible those few pregnancies occurring in 45,X individuals.[41]

Monosomy X usually occurs as a result of paternal sex chromosome loss.[42] This observation is consistent with, but does not explain, the inverse maternal age effect characteristic of 45,X.

Structural Chromosomal Rearrangement

Structural chromosomal rearrangements account for 1.5 percent of all abortuses (Table 23.1). Such abnormalities may either arise de novo during gametogenesis or be inherited from a parent carrying a "balanced" translocation or inversion. Phenotypic consequences depend on the duplicated or deficient chromosomal segments. Although not a common cause of sporadic losses, inherited rearrangements are an important cause of repeated fetal wastage.

Sex Chromosomal Polysomy (X or Y)

The complements 47,XXY and 47,XYY each occur in about 1 per 800 liveborn male births; 47,XXX occurs in 1 per 800 female births. X or Y polysomies are only slightly more common in abortuses, being observed in 0.6 percent of abortus specimens (1.3 percent of chromosomally abnormal abortuses).

Neural Tube Defects and Other Polygenic/Multifactorial Traits

Those 50 percent of first trimester abortuses that do not show chromosomal abnormalities could have undergone fetal demise as a result of other genetic etiologies: Mendelian or polygenic/multifactorial. Some excellent anatomic studies have shown[43,44] many structural abnormalities. However, lack of cytogenetic data on the dissected specimens makes it impos-

Table 23.1 Chromosomal Complements in Spontaneous Abortions Recognized Clinically in the First Trimester

Complement		Percentages
Normal		
46,XX or 46,XY		54.1
Triploidy		7.7
69,XXX	2.7	
69,XYX	0.2	
69,XXY	4.0	
Other	0.8	
Tetraploidy		2.6
92,XXX	1.5	
92,XXYY	0.55	
Not stated	0.55	
Monosomy X		8.6
Structural abnormalities		1.5
Sex chromosomal polysomy		0.2
47,XXX	0.05	
47,XXY	0.15	
Autosomal monosomy (G)		0.1
Autosomal trisomy		22.3
Chromosome		
No. 1	0	
No. 2	1.11	
No. 3	0.25	
No. 4	0.64	
No. 5	0.04	
No. 6	0.14	
No. 7	0.89	
No. 8	0.79	
No. 9	0.72	
No. 10	0.36	
No. 11	0.04	
No. 12	0.18	
No. 13	1.07	
No. 14	0.82	
No. 15	1.68	
No. 16	7.27	
No. 17	0.18	
No. 18	1.15	
No. 19	0.01	
No. 20	0.61	
No. 21	2.11	
No. 22	2.26	
Double trisomy		0.7
Mosaic trisomy		1.3
Other abnormalities or not specified		0.9
		100.0

(Pooled data from Simpson and Bombard.[134])

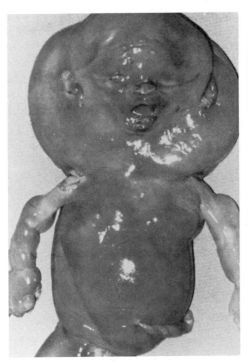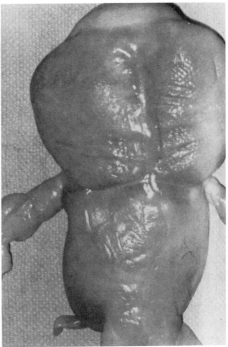

Fig. 23.4 Photograph of 45,X abortus. (From Simpson and Bombard,[134] with permission.)

sible to determine the precise role of noncytogenetic mechanisms in early embryonic maldevelopment. The generalized growth retardation so ubiquitously observed in early embryos could also reflect chromosome abnormalities.

Pathologic Findings in Later Fetal Losses

Anatomic defects due to polygenic/multifactorial factors (i.e., isolated anatomic defects) or Mendelian causes are responsible for losses throughout gestation.[43,44] However, these causes appear to be responsible for a relatively greater proportion of later fetal losses.[44–46] Although anatomic anomalies are observed frequently, lack of concomitant cytogenetic data makes it nearly impossible to delineate the precise role of noncytogenetic mechanisms in late fetal losses. A problem is determining the extent to which an ostensibly isolated anatomic defect in a late fetal death actually augurs multiple system defects suggestive of an underlying cytogenetic abnormality or mutant gene. One defect that almost certainly is not cytogenetic is neural tube defect, whose prevalence in abortuses is about 1 percent.[47]

GENETIC COUNSELING AND RECURRENCE RISKS

The obstetrician faced with a couple experiencing spontaneous abortion has several obligations: (1) inform them of the frequency of fetal wastage (12 to 15 percent of clinically recognized pregnancies) and its etiology (at least 50 percent cytogenetic); (2) indicate recurrence risks; and (3) determine the necessity of a formal evaluation for repetitive abortions.

Patient Education

The first obligation, education, can be fulfilled by summarizing the salient facts described previously and briefly recounting etiologies responsible for fetal losses (discussed later). Of additional relevance here is that abortion rates are positively correlated with advancing maternal age. Women over age 40 have twice the likelihood of experiencing a fetal loss of women in their third decade.[48] This increase is not solely the result of increased trisomic abortions. There have been claims of a relationship between fetal losses and gravidity,[49] but this apparent association is probably only a secondary effect of advanced maternal age.

Recurrence Risks

For decades, obstetricians believed in the concept of "habitual abortion." After three but not fewer fetal losses, the risk of subsequent losses was believed to rise sharply. Such beliefs were based on calculations made in 1938 by Malpas,[50] who concluded that after three abortions the likelihood of a subsequent one was 80 to 90 percent. Occurrence of three consecutive spontaneous abortions was said to confer on a woman the designation of "habitual aborter." Although these risk figures were later proved incorrect, they were in the interim unfortunately used as "controls" for clinical trials evaluating various treatment plans. This practice led to unwarranted acceptance of certain interventions, the most famous of which was diethylstilbestrol (DES) treatment.

In 1964, Warburton and Fraser[51] showed the likelihood of recurrent abortion to be only 25 to 30 percent, given a couple with at least one liveborn. This held irrespective of whether a woman had previously experienced one, two, three, or even four spontaneous abortions (Table 23.2). Thus, the concept of a subclass of habitual aborters (i.e., women with three prior abortions) was essentially refuted. Because Warburton and Fraser limited their study to women having liveborn infants, other studies were necessary. Poland et al.[52] thus calculated that the likelihood of fetal loss was 46 percent if a woman had at least one fetal loss (spontaneous abortus, stillborn infant, or early neonatal death) but no liveborn infants; women with liveborn infants had lower risks of abortion, as had already been shown by Warburton and Fraser.[51] Women who smoke cigarettes or drink alcohol moderately are probably at higher risk.[53] Recurrence risks are slightly higher if the abortus is cytogenetically normal than if cytogenetically abnormal.[54] Regan[55] also observed lower risks (5 percent) in nulliparous women and those with no prior losses; women whose previous pregnancy was lost had a 20 percent risk, and those with three losses had an even higher risk.

Irrespective, overall prognosis is quite favorable (60 to 70 percent likelihood of successful pregnancies) for most couples who have experienced repeated losses. Indeed, Vlaanderen and Treffers[56] reported successful pregnancies in each of 21 women having unexplained prior repetitive losses but subjected to no intervention.

Necessity of Formal Evaluation

Although every couple experiencing a fetal loss should be counseled and informed of recurrence risks, not every couple requires formal evaluation. Those experiencing their first or second early loss need not be studied in detail. However, any couple experiencing an anomalous stillborn or liveborn offspring should undergo cytogenetic studies, unless the infant itself was known to have a normal complement. Otherwise, parental chromosomal rearrangements (i.e., translocations, inversions) should be excluded.

Infertile couples who are in their fourth decade may choose to be evaluated after only two losses. After three losses, all couples should be offered formal evaluation. Once a couple enters evaluation, they should undergo all tests standard for a given practitioner. There is no scientific basis for performing some studies after three losses but deferring other studies until after four losses.

ETIOLOGY AND CLINICAL EVALUATION OF REPETITIVE ABORTIONS

Translocations

Structural chromosomal abnormalities are generally accepted as one explanation for repetitive abortions. The most common structural rearrangement encountered is a translocation (Fig. 23.5). Individuals

---

Table 23.2 Recurrence Risks for Counseling Women with Repeated Spontaneous Abortions

	Prior Abortions	Risk (Percentage)[a]
Women with liveborn infants	0	12
	1	24
	2	26
	3	32
	4	26
Women without liveborn infants	2 or more	40–45

[a] Recurrence risks are slightly higher in older women and those who smoke or drink alcohol. (Data from Warburton and Fraser[51] and Poland et al.[52])

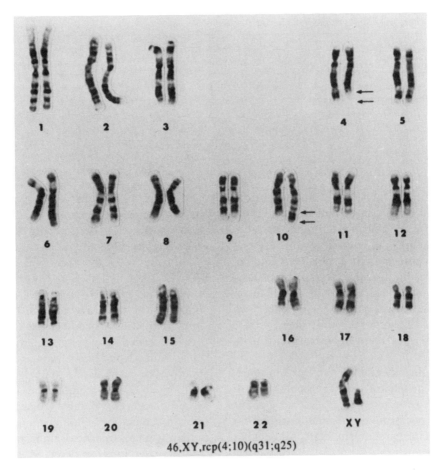

46,XY,rcp(4;10)(q31;q25)

Fig. 23.5 Balanced translocation detected in a woman experiencing multiple spontaneous abortions. (From Simpson and Tharapel,[135] with permission.)

with balanced translocations are phenotypically normal, but abortuses or abnormal liveborns may show chromosomal duplications or deficiencies as a result of normal meiotic segregation. About 60 percent of the translocations detected are reciprocal, and 40 percent are Robertsonian. Females are about twice as likely as males to show a balanced translocation (Table 23.3).[57]

The clinical significance of translocations can be illustrated by recalling the translocation between chromosomes 14 and 21. If a child has Down syndrome as a result of such a translocation, for example, 46,XX-14+(14q;21q), the rearrangement will prove to have originated de novo in 50 to 75 percent of cases. That is, it will not exist in either parent. The likelihood of Down syndrome recurring in progeny of parents whose offspring had a de novo translocation is minimal. On the other hand, the risk is significant in the 25 to 50 percent of families in which individuals have Down syndrome as the result of a balanced parental translocation, such as parental complement 45,XX-14,-21,+(14q;21q). Although the theoretical risk of having a child with Down syndrome is 33 percent, empirical risks are considerably less. The likelihood is only 2 percent if the father carries the translocation and about 10 percent if the mother carries the translocation.[58] For Robertsonian (centric-fusion) translocations other than t(14q;21q), empirical risks are lower. In t(13q;14q), risks for liveborn with trisomy 13 are 1 percent or less.

Reciprocal translocations do not involve centromeric fusion. Empirical data for specific transloca-

Table 23.3 Parental Translocations in Recurrent Abortions

Repeated Spontaneous Abortions with or without Normal Liveborn		Repeated Spontaneous Abortions with Stillborn or Abnormal Liveborn		Repeated Spontaneous Abortions without Subcategorization	
Female	Male	Female	Male	Female	Male
89/3723	57/3651	20/432	7/409	100/3074	65/3069
2.4%	1.6%	4.6%	1.7%	3.3%	2.1%

(Pooled data from Simpson et al.[57])

tions are not usually available, but useful generalizations can be made on the basis of pooled data derived from many different translocations. Studies of sperm chromosomes[59] theoretically could provide data specific for a given translocation in a specific individual, but they are not readily available. Irrespective, theoretical risks for abnormal offspring (unbalanced translocations) are greater than empirical risks. Overall, the risk is 12 percent for offspring of female heterozygotes and 12 percent for offspring of male heterozygotes.

Of relevance is that prevalence rates for translocations reported by myself and other gynecologists are lower than those reported by some other geneticists.[57] Routinely performing cytogenetic studies on all couples experiencing recurrent fetal losses yields a relatively lower frequency of translocations, namely about 1 to 2 percent of couples in our experience (Table 23.3). Investigations restricting their studies to couples experiencing not only abortions but also stillborn infants or anomalous liveborn infants find a higher proportion of translocations (Table 23.3). An unanswered question is whether prevalence rates are influenced by numbers of previous losses.

Detecting a chromosomal rearrangement can profoundly affect subsequent pregnancy management. If a rearrangement is detected, antenatal cytogenetic studies should be offered in subsequent pregnancies. In addition, the frequency of unbalanced fetuses is lower if parental balanced translocations are ascertained through repetitive abortions (3 percent) than if translocations are ascertained through an anomalous liveborn (nearly 20 percent).[58,60]

A few translocations preclude the possibility of normal liveborn infants. This unfortunate prognosis exists if a translocation involves homologous chromosomes [e.g., t(13q13q) or t(21q21q)]. If the father

carries such a structural rearrangement, artificial insemination may be appropriate. If the mother carries the rearrangement, donor ovum techniques or donor embryo transfer should be considered.

Inversions

A second parental chromosomal rearrangement responsible for repetitive pregnancy loss is an inversion. In this intrachromosomal rearrangement the order of genes is reversed. Analogous to translocations, individuals heterozygous for an inversion should be normal if their genes are merely rearranged. However, individuals with inversions suffer abnormal reproductive consequences as a result of normal meiotic phenomena, namely crossing-over in their gametes that yields unbalanced gametes. Pericentric inversions are detected in perhaps 0.1 percent of females and 0.1 percent of males experiencing repeated spontaneous abortions. Paracentric inversions are even more rare.

Counseling a couple about an inversion is complex.[60] Inversions involving only a small portion of the total chromosomal length paradoxically may be less significant clinically because the large duplications or large deficiencies that follow crossing-over are usually lethal. By contrast, inversions involving only 30 to 60 percent of the total chromosomal length are relatively more likely to be characterized by duplications or deficiencies compatible with survival.[61]

Overall, females with a pericentric inversion have an 8 percent risk of abnormal liveborns; males have a 5 percent risk.[60] Pericentric inversions ascertained through phenotypically normal probands are less likely to lead to abnormal liveborns, whereas certain inversions carry higher risks.

Few data are available on recurrence risks for paracentric inversions. There is probably little if any risk for unbalanced products at amniocentesis because recombinants are usually lethal. On the other hand, abortions and abnormal liveborns have been observed within the same kindred, for which reason antenatal cytogenetic studies should be offered.

Recurrent Aneuploidy

Known to be responsible for most sporadic abortions, numerical chromosomal abnormalities (aneuploidy) may also be responsible for recurrent fetal losses. Such reasoning is based on observations that the complements of successive abortuses in a given family are more likely to be either recurrently normal or recurrently abnormal (Table 23.4). That is, abortuses in a given family show nonrandom distribution with respect to chromosomal complements. If the complement of the first abortus is abnormal, the likelihood is 80 percent that the complement of the second abortus also will be abnormal. The recurrent abnormality usually is trisomy.

These data suggest that certain couples are predisposed toward chromosomally abnormal conceptions. Warburton et al.[62] argue that corrections for maternal age render the ostensible nonrandom distribution nonsignificant; although cognizant of the argument, I would still counsel increased risks compared to those of normal women of comparable age. If couples are predisposed to recurrent aneuploidy, they may logically be at increased risk for aneuploid liveborns. The trisomic autosome in a subsequent pregnancy may not always confer lethality but rather may be compatible with life (e.g., trisomy 21). Indeed, several

studies suggest that the risk of liveborn trisomy 21 following an aneuploid abortus is about 1 percent.[63]

If information concerning fetal chromosomal status is lacking, antenatal diagnosis may or may not be appropriate for couples having repetitive abortions. Risks for abnormal offspring are probably increased, but the low yet finite risk of amniocentesis or chorionic villus sampling is surely more troublesome to these couples than to those who have achieved pregnancies more uneventfully.

Luteal Phase Defects

Implantation in an inhospitable endometrium is a plausible explanation for spontaneous abortion. The hormone usually hypothesized to be abnormal is progesterone, deficiency of which might fail to prepare the estrogen primed endometrium for implantation. The term luteal phase deficiency (LPD) is used to describe the endometrium's manifesting an inadequate progesterone effect. Progesterone secreted by the corpus luteum is necessary to support the endometrium until the trophoblast produces sufficient progesterone to maintain pregnancy, an event occurring around 7 menstrual weeks (5 weeks after conception). Potential pathogenic mechanisms underlying LPD are diverse: decreased gonadotropin-releasing hormone (GNRH), decreased follicle-stimulating hormone (FSH), inadequate LH, inadequate ovarian steroidogenesis, and endometrial receptor defects.

LPD is believed by many to be a common cause of recurrent pregnancy loss, although its frequency has

Table 23.4 Recurrent Aneuploidy: The Relationships among Karyotypes of Successive Abortuses

Complement of First Abortus	Complement of Second Abortus					
	Normal	Trisomy	Monosomy	Triploidy	Tetraploidy	De Novo Rearrangement
Normal	142	18	5	7	3	2
Trisomy	31	30	1	4	3	1
Monosomy X	7	5	3	3	0	0
Triploidy	7	4	1	4	0	0
Tetraploidy	3	1	0	2	0	0
De novo rearrangement	1	3	0	0	0	0

(Data from Warburton et al.[62])

actually never been determined. It has been stated that LPD occurs in 35 percent of patients experiencing recurrent losses[64]; however, this estimate is derived from patients first ascertained on the basis of prior losses and then subjected to endometrial biopsy.[65] In no study have subjects without losses (controls) been studied concurrently to determine whether an LPD exists in fertile populations. Indeed, when biopsy specimens were obtained from regularly menstruating fertile women with no history of abortions in up to 10 serial cycles, the frequencies of LPD were 51.4 percent in any single cycle and 26.7 percent in sequential cycles.[66]

Assessing both the frequency and the validity of LPD is difficult because uniform diagnostic criteria are lacking. LPD was originally diagnosed on the basis of an endometrial biopsy's lagging at least 2 days behind the actual postovulation date, as determined by counting backward from the next menstrual period (assuming 14 days from ovulation to menses). Nuances of histologic dating and monthly variations in the menstrual cycle occur, presumably accounting for much of the 40 percent of "luteal phase defect" observed in normal women if the diagnosis is based on only one endometrial biopsy. In fact, the original reports of Noyes, Hertig, and Rock showed a mean error of 1.81 days in dating.[67] These investigators suggested that an endometrial biopsy is "out of phase" only if it lags 3 or more days behind the actual postovulation date. Not surprisingly, interobserver variation in interpreting endometrial biopsy results is frequent. Endometrial biopsy results ($N = 62$) read by five different pathologists resulted in differences in interpretation that would have altered management in approximately one-third of patients.[68] Reading coded endometrial biopsy slides a second time, the same pathologist agreed with the initial diagnosis in only 25 percent of samples.[69] At a minimum, at least two out-of-phase biopsies are necessary to make the diagnosis of LPD.

Diagnosis based on one[70] or more[71] progesterone concentrations in the luteal phase has been suggested. Horta et al.[72] measured progesterone in women having a history of three spontaneous abortions. Ten of 15 subjects had lower luteal progesterone concentrations than 15 healthy nonpregnant control women; all 10 went on to abort their pregnancies during the first trimester. However, in patients with two or more spontaneous abortions, low progesterone in the luteal phase is only 71 percent predictive of a LPD diagnosed on the basis of an abnormal endometrial biopsy.[70] Other studies showed recurrence risks to be slightly higher after cytogenetically normal abortuses.[73]

Progesterone receptors measured in the luteal endometrium have also proved unsuccessful in predicting pathologic dating.[74,75] One study showed lower progesterone receptor concentrations in the endometrium of women with LPD, but a large overlap with normal women was observed.[76] Another study showed both higher progesterone receptor concentrations and low serum progesterone in patients with an out-of-phase endometrial biopsy.[77] However, perturbations in endometrial receptors have not yet been correlated with actual pregnancy loss.

The lack of consensus concerning diagnostic criteria for LPD points to the necessity of a randomized study to document efficacy of therapeutic regimens, principally vaginal progesterone. Unfortunately, no such study is reported. A reasonable study often cited as support for efficacy of treatment is that of Tho et al.,[78] in which 23 of 100 women with repetitive spontaneous abortions showed "documented" luteal phase defects on the basis of "out-of-phase" endometrial biopsies. All 23 women were treated with progesterone suppositories, and 21 completed their pregnancies. A quasi-control group consisted of 37 other women who had no ostensible etiology for their losses. Twenty-two of these 37 were treated with "empirical" progesterone; 15 were not. Seventy-three percent of the treated women had successful pregnancies, compared to 47 percent of untreated women. Among 65 patients with recurrent abortions, Daya and Ward[65] found that 26 patients (40 percent) had both two consecutive out-of-phase biopsies and low progesterone levels. All were treated with progesterone, and only 3 (19 percent) of 16 later pregnancies aborted. Again, no controls were studied.

The study most suggestive that LPD is a valid entity was conducted on 33 infertile women whose LPD was documented by two out-of-phase biopsies.[79] (This study involved infertile women rather than those with recurrent abortions.) The investigators observed no abortions in the 14 women who conceived after an endometrial biopsy corrected by progesterone treatment was documented. Of the 16 women whose biopsy was not corrected, there were four pregnancies; all ended in spontaneous abortion.[79]

Given the controversy, I believe that treatment for LPD should be initiated only if the diagnosis is firmly established and only if couples are apprised of (unproven) claims of progesterone teratogenicity (see Ch. 11). Recommended treatment consists of exogenous progesterone, usually vaginal progesterone suppositories 25 mg twice daily beginning with the basal body temperature elevation and continuing at least 6 to 8 weeks. A few workers have suggested that hCG be administered empirically to women with unexplained repetitive losses, presumably to treat LPD.[80] Clomiphene citrate has also been used.

Thyroid Abnormalities

Decreased conception rates and fetal losses are associated with overt hypothyroidism or hyperthyroidism. However, subclinical thyroid dysfunction is not an explanation for repeated losses.[81] Therapy should be initiated only if hypothyroidism or hyperthyroidism is documented.

Diabetes Mellitus

Although spontaneous abortion rates were once believed to be no higher among patients with diabetes mellitus than among controls, a prospective collaborative study conducted by Mills and colleagues[9] recently showed that women whose diabetes is less well controlled are at increased risk. Metabolic data were gathered from the fifth week of gestation; information was collected allowing a variety of confounding variables to be taken into account. Women whose glycosylated hemoglobin was greater than 4 SD above the mean showed higher pregnancy loss rates than those showing lower glycosylated hemoglobin levels (Table 23.5). Miodnovic and colleagues[82–84] have accumulated data consistent with these findings, as have Greene et al.[85] Thus, poorly controlled diabetes mellitus should be considered one cause for early pregnancy loss. However, well-controlled or subclinical diabetes is probably not a cause of early pregnancy loss.

Intrauterine Adhesions (Synechiae)

Intrauterine adhesions could obviously interfere with implantation or early embryonic development. Adhesions may follow overzealous uterine curettage during the postpartum period, intrauterine surgery (e.g., myomectomy), or endometritis. Curettage is the usual explanation; adhesions are most likely to develop if it is performed 3 or 4 weeks post partum. Individuals with uterine synechiae usually manifest hypomenorrhea or amenorrhea, but 15 to 30 percent have repeated abortions. If adhesions are detected in a woman experiencing repetitive losses, lysis of adhesions under direct hyperoscopic visualization should be performed. Postoperatively, an intrauterine device (IUD) or inflated Foley catheter may be inserted into the uterus to discourage reapposition of healing uterine surfaces. Estrogen administration should also be initiated. Approximately 50 percent of subjects conceive after surgery, but the frequency of abortions remains high.[86]

Incomplete Müllerian Fusion

Müllerian fusion defects are an accepted cause of second trimester abortions. The pregnant uterus may be unable to accommodate the growing fetus, and the placenta may implant on a poorly vascularized septum. The prevalence of abortions in patients with such defects may be as high as 20 to 35 percent,[87] with loss rates higher in septate and bicornuate uteri than in unicornuate uterus or uterus didelphys. Hysterosalpingography and hysteroscopy are of great value in determining configuration of the uterine cavity (Fig. 23.6). Ultrasound may also be helpful.

First trimester abortions are probably due to müllerian fusion defects far less often. Abortions occurring after ultrasonographic confirmation of a viable pregnancy at 8 or 9 weeks may be attributed to uterine fusion defects whenever the latter are present. However, losses not recognized clinically until 10 to 12 weeks gestation and not having confirmation of prior viability are statistically more likely to represent missed abortions in which fetal demise occurred prior to 8 weeks. Women with second trimester abortions who have a müllerian fusion anomaly may benefit from uterine reconstruction, but reconstructive sur-

Table 23.5 Hyperglycemia and Fetal Losses

Initial Glycosylated Hemoglobin[a]		Deviation from Control	Mean Glycosylated Hemoglobin in First Trimester	
N	Loss Rate	Mean	N	Loss Rate
137	9.5%	<2 SD	137	10.3%
131	14.5%	2–4 SD	121	15.2%
112	21.4%	>4 SD	112	20.2%

[a] Relationship of diabetic control to fetal loss rates, assessed by (1) initial glycosylated hemoglobin obtained at 6 or 7 weeks gestation and (2) mean weekly first trimester glycosylated hemoglobin.
(Data from Mills et al.[9])

gery is not always advisable if losses are restricted to the first trimester.

Leiomyomas

Leiomyomas are usually multiple and seldom solitary. Although leiomyomas are frequent, relatively few affected women develop symptoms requiring medical or surgical therapy.

That leiomyomas cause pregnancy wastage is plausible but probably relatively uncommon. The coexistence of uterine leiomyomas and reproductive losses need not necessarily imply a causal relationship. Location of leiomyomas is probably more important than size. Submucous leiomyomas are the type most likely to cause abortion. Several mechanisms could be postulated: (1) thinning of the endometrium over the surface of a submucous leiomyoma, thus predisposing a fertilized ovum to implantation in a poorly

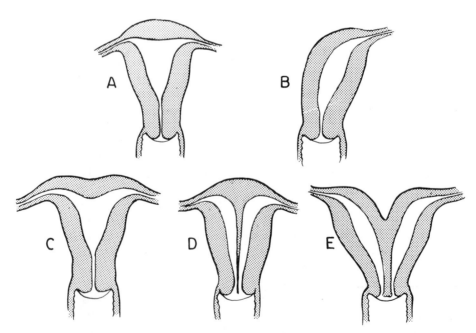

Fig. 23.6 Diagrammatic representation of some müllerian fusion anomalies. (A) Normal uterus, fallopian tubes, and cervix. (B) Uterus unicornis (absence of one uterine horn). (C) Uterus arcuatus (broadening and medial depression of a portion of the uterine septum). (D) Uterus septus (persistence of a complete uterine septum). (E) Uterus bicornis unicollis (two hemiuteri, each leading to same cervix). (From Simpson,[136] with permission.)

decidualized site; (2) rapid growth under the hormonal milieu of pregnancy, thus compromising blood supply of the leiomyoma and resulting in necrosis ("red degeneration") that in turn leads to uterine contractions and fetal expulsion; and (3) encroachment of leiomyomas on the space required by the developing fetus, leading to premature delivery through mechanisms analogous to those operative in incomplete müllerian fusion. Relative lack of space can also lead to fetal deformations (i.e., positional abnormalities arising in a genetically normal fetus).

Myomectomy may occasionally be warranted for women experiencing repetitive second trimester abortions. Ideally, surgery should be reserved for those whose abortuses were both phenotypically and karyotypically normal and in which viability until at least 9 to 10 weeks was documented.

Incompetent Internal Cervical Os

A functionally intact cervix and lower uterine cavity is obviously necessary for successful intrauterine pregnancy. Cervical incompetence is characterized by painless dilatation and effacement, usually during the mid-second or early third trimester. This condition frequently is preceded by traumatic events, such as cervical amputation, cervical lacerations, forceful cervical dilatation, or conization. The various operations proposed for correcting cervical incompetence are discussed in Chapter 25.

Infections

Infections are accepted causes of late fetal wastage and logically may be responsible for early fetal loss as well.

Microorganisms associated with spontaneous abortion include variola, vaccinia, *Salmonella typhi*, *Vibrio fetus*, malaria, cytomegalovirus, *Brucella*, *Toxoplasma*, *Mycoplasma hominis*, *Chlamydia trachomatis*, and *Ureaplasma urealyticum*. Transplacental infection occurs with each of these microorganisms, and sporadic losses could plausibly be caused by any. As an example, Sompolinsky et al.[88] studied spontaneous mid-trimester abortuses. *Ureaplasma*, *M. hominis*, or both were isolated from 32 placentas and 24 fetuses. Among 28 mid-trimester-induced abortions, these organisms were recovered from only one placenta and no abortuses. On the other hand, confounding factors may exist: Did the infection arise only secondarily

after demise for a noninfectious etiology? What was the cytogenetic and endocrine status of the pregnancy? Could the agents used to treat the infection actually cause the loss, or even fever per se?

Of the organisms mentioned, *Ureaplasma urealyticum* is most frequently implicated in repetitive abortion. Stray-Pedersen et al.[89] studied 46 women with histories of three or more consecutive losses of unknown etiology. Endometrial *Ureaplasma* was recovered significantly more often among women with repetitive abortions (28 percent) than among female controls (7 percent). Of 43 women in the former group, 13 harbored *Ureaplasma* in both cervix and endometrium. In 12 others, the organism was recovered only in the cervix, a circumstance less likely to cause abortions, given that *Ureaplasma* is ubiquitous in the vagina. All 43 women and their husbands were then treated with doxycycline, with subsequent cultures confirming eradication of *Ureaplasma*. Nineteen of the 43 women became pregnant. Of these 19, 3 experienced another spontaneous abortion and 16 had normal full-term infants. Only five full-term pregnancies among 18 women with untreated *Ureaplasma* were observed.

Empirical antibiotic therapy has been said to be beneficial to couples experiencing repeated losses, consistent with a role for infectious agents in repetitive abortions. Among repetitive aborters who were treated with tetracycline for 4 weeks, Toth et al.[90] reported recurrent fetal losses in only 10 percent. By contrast, 38 percent of aborters who elected not to receive tetracycline experienced further fetal loss. However, the two groups are not necessarily comparable, having self-selected different modes of treatment.

In conclusion, culturing the endometrium for *Ureaplasma urealyticum* seems reasonable; women having such an infection should be treated. Alternatively, tetracycline therapy is so innocuous that it is not unreasonable to prescribe doxycycline empirically (250 mg orally four times a day for 10 days, for both husband and wife) prior to pregnancy.

Antifetal Antibodies

Perturbations of the immune system can be responsible for fetal wastage. However, the nature of the immunologic process responsible for maintaining pregnancy has proved to be complex. Several different immunologic mechanisms may play a role.

One immunologic mechanism is that in which an otherwise normal mother produces antibodies against her fetus on the basis of genetic dissimilarities. Fetal loss is well documented in Rh-negative (D-negative) women having anti-D antibodies. An example more apropos to early pregnancy loss involves anti-P antibodies.[91] Most individuals are genotype Pp or PP, but an occasional female is homozygous pp. If a woman of genotype pp mates with a Pp or PP male, offspring may be Pp. If the mother develops anti-P antibodies, Pp fetuses are rejected early in gestation. Plasmapheresis may be efficacious.[92]

Autoimmune Disease

Association of pregnancy loss and certain autoimmune disease is generally accepted.[93] Individuals having lupus anticoagulant (LAC) antibodies and anticardiolipin antibodies have a specifically increased likelihood of fetal wastage. These two antibodies have closely related specificities and may be members of the same family of autoantibodies. Of the two, anticardiolipin antibody may be the more sensitive indicator; however, it may also be less specific.[94] LAC has been associated with subplacental clotting and fetal losses in all trimesters, as well as with poor reproductive history in general.[95] The abortifacient mechanism is thus presumably decidual. Incidentally, LAC antibody is actually a misnomer. In vitro it is an anticoagulant, but in vivo it increases the likelihood of thrombosis.

On the basis of a literature survey of 242 untreated pregnancies in 65 women, Scott et al.[96] state that the frequency of mid-trimester fetal death in women who show LAC or anticardiolipin antibodies is 91 percent. They[96] reported that 83 percent of 162 prior pregnancies in such women were lost in their experience. Increased frequency of other pregnancy complications (e.g., growth retardation, preeclampsia) also occurred. Treatment with prednisone and low-dose aspirin has been advocated.[97]

Although a relationship between anticardiolipin or LAC antibodies and second and third trimester losses seems reasonably well established, the situation is less clear for earlier pregnancy losses. Unander et al.[98] studied 99 women having three or more abortuses, 68 having no liveborns. Increased anticardiolipin anti-bodies were found in 42, but no control data were provided. The proportions of antibodies in "primary" and "secondary" aborters were the same. Howard et al.[99] detected LAC in 9 of 29 (31 percent) women having "three spontaneous miscarriages or stillbirths," and Cowchock et al.[100] observed anticardiolipin antibodies in 13.1 percent of 61 women with repeated abortuses. However, in the first controlled study, frequencies of LAC and anticardiolipin antibodies were 9 and 11 percent, respectively, neither different from control subjects.[101]

A relationship between other autoimmune phenomena (antisperm antibodies, antibodies to other nuclear antigens) and early losses could exist, but data are even more arguable than those for LAC and anticardiolipin antibodies.

In conclusion, evaluation of repetitive pregnancy losses in clinically asymptomatic women probably dictates a search for both LAC (activated thromboplastin time or platelet neutralization tests) and anticardiolipin antibodies (immunoassay). Prednisone and aspirin therapy treatment are best restricted to couples with second or third trimester losses.

Alloimmune Disease (Shared Parental Antigens)

During pregnancy, fetal rejection is apparently eschewed because the maternal immune system mitigates against the phenomenon through blocking or suppressive factors that protect the fetus. Parodoxically, blocking antibodies appear to develop or at least be enhanced if paternal antigens differ from maternal antigens. (Presumably the fetus inherits the antigen from its father, thus differing from its mother.) Such reasoning has been assumed to be the explanation for long-standing recognition that pregnant women frequently develop antipaternal antileukocytotoxic antibodies. About 20 percent of women develop these antibodies after their first pregnancy, and about 65 percent of multiparous women have such antibodies.[102,103]

Circumstantial support that parental *histoincompatibility* is beneficial in humans can be cited. Only 16.6 percent of women with multiple abortions have antipaternal antileukocytotoxic antibodies, in contrast to 64 percent of multiparous women and 20 percent of primiparous women.[104] Fifty percent of women with three or more recurrent abortions show no blocking factors, as demonstrated by failure to exhibit a mixed lymphocyte reaction when their lymphocytes are exposed to their spouse's lymphocytes.[105] Blocking antibodies have been observed in parous women but are lacking in some women having only abortuses.[106-109] Experimental support for a beneficial effect of maternal–fetal incompatibility in animals can also be cited: (1) increased placental size in mouse fetuses resulting from matings in which paternal and maternal histocompatibility antigens differ and (2) higher implantation frequencies in histoincompatible murine zygotes.[110]

On the other hand, not all investigators have observed increased human leukocyte antigen (HLA) sharing, depressed mixed lymphocyte reaction (MLR), or decreased blocking antibodies.[111] Some couples sharing HLA-DR antigens have experienced no spontaneous abortions, despite ten or more pregnancies.[112] In virtually all studies, critical information concerning whether the abortus actually inherited the paternal antigen shared by its mother and father is lacking. Furthermore, blocking antibodies develop only late in pregnancy. Thus, lack of these antibodies probably does not reflect inability to become pregnant per se.[113] Indeed, Sargent et al.[114] rarely detected cytotoxic antibodies (T-cell and B-cell): in only 1 of 16 successful pregnancies (through 17 weeks) and in 0 of 9 pregnancies ending in abortion.

An alternative interpretation of how some but not all couples sharing HLA antigens show deleterious effects involves postulating that normal pregnancy requires maternal–fetal histocompatibility not for HLA-DR but rather for another closely linked locus. This hypothesis is consistent with HLA antigens' failing to be expressed on trophoblasts. Moreover, the blocking antibodies said to be present in normal pregnancies but absent in women experiencing spontaneous abortion are directed against neither HLA-A, -B, -C, nor -DR.[115] Faulk and McIntyre[116,117] postulate that immune regulation is stimulated by placental antigens called trophoblast lymphocyte cross-reactive (TLX) antigens. Couples experiencing repetitive spontaneous abortions are said to share "TLX antigens" more often than couples without pregnancy wastage.

Another possibility is that the deleterious effect of parental antigen sharing could only be an ostensible explanation for repetitive abortion. The same data could be explained entirely on a nonimmunologic basis, by postulating existence of a lethal recessive gene near the HLA (or TLX) locus. Murine embryos homozygous for certain alleles at the T/t locus die at various stages of embryogenesis. Whether a T/t-like complex exists in humans is arguable. If it does exist, and further if it is linked to HLA, deleterious parental HLA sharing between mother and father (and hence between mother and fetus) could merely secondarily reflect homozygosity for the postulated gene.

If fetal rejection results from diminished fetal–maternal immunologic interaction, it follows that immunotherapy to enhance interaction at the few potentially differing loci is not unreasonable. The basis for the original attempts were reports that blood transfusions prior to kidney transplantation decreased allograft rejection.[118] Thus, women lacking blocking antibodies but sharing HLA antigens with their spouse have been immunized with either paternal leukocytes, third party leukocytes, or trophoblast membranes.

Potential efficacy of immunotherapy is highly controversial; it is reviewed in detail in a recent monograph.[119] Suffice to say that only a single, large prospective randomized trial is published.[120,121] In that trial 209 couples with repeated abortions were studied. Of those, 104 women had no antibody against paternal lymphocytes and no other apparent cause for the losses. A paired sequential trial was conducted, during which the experimental group received purified lymphocytes derived from their husbands. Seventeen of 22 (77 percent) women so injected had a successful pregnancy, compared to 10 of 27 (37 percent) controls given their own cells. Ostensible improvement in outcome in the immunized group compared to that of the nonimmunized group is tempered by lower successes in the control group than expected a priori (Table 23.2 shows that the expected rate is 60 to 70 percent). Unwitting selection biases could thus exist, possibly aggravated by relatively small sample sizes. Ongoing controlled studies are in progress in several centers.

Given the uncertainty concerning the role of immunologic factors in repetitive abortions, what constitutes a standard of care? It is surely worthwhile to discuss immunologic factors, particularly if no other explanation exists. However, immunologic evaluation should be initiated only by those physicians prepared to pursue a truly thorough approach. Merely determining HLA status without other studies is not recommended. Most obstetricians/gynecologists should probably refer couples desiring immunologic evaluation to colleagues having special expertise.

Drugs, Chemicals, and Noxious Agents

Various exogenous agents have been implicated in fetal losses. Indeed, women are exposed frequently to relatively low doses of ubiquitous agents. Unfortunately, adequate data are not available to determine definitively the role of these exogenous factors in early pregnancy losses. However, risks are probably low.

Exposure outcomes are usually deduced on the basis of case–control studies. That is, women who aborted claimed exposure to the agent in question more often than controls. However, case–control studies suffer certain inherent biases, as reviewed in Chapter 11. The primary bias is that controls have less incentive to recall antecedent events than subjects experiencing an abnormal outcome (recall bias). Because most corporations attempt to limit exposure of women in the reproductive age group to potentially dangerous chemicals, exposures are usually unwitting and, hence, poorly documented. Moreover, pregnant workers usually come into contact with many agents concurrently, making it nearly impossible to determine the effects of any single agent.

Given these caveats physicians should thus be cautious about attributing pregnancy loss to exogenous agents. On the other hand, common sense dictates that exposure to potentially noxious agents should be minimized.

X-Irradiation

Irradiation and antineoplastic agents are accepted abortifacients; in fact, they have established the principle that exogenous factors during embryogenesis cause fetal loss. Of course, therapeutic radiographs or chemotherapeutic drugs are administered during pregnancy only to seriously ill women whose pregnancies often must be terminated for maternal indications. Although exposure doses are far lower, it is prudent for pregnant hospital workers to avoid handling chemotherapeutic agents. Similarly, diagnostic radiographs (less than 10 rad) place a woman at little to no increased risk.

Cigarette Smoking

Smoking during pregnancy has been associated with spontaneous abortion. Kline et al.[53] found increased abortion rates in smokers, independent of maternal age and independent of alcohol consumption. A modest dose–response curve led Alberman et al.[122] to conclude that smokers showed a nonsignificantly higher proportion of abortuses with normal karyotypes. If verified, this observation would suggest that smoking affects the conceptus directly.

Alcohol

Association of alcohol consumption and fetal loss seems likely, at least in high exposure ranges. In one study,[53] 616 women suffering spontaneous abortions were compared with 632 women delivering at 28 gestational weeks or more. Among women whose pregnancies ended in spontaneous abortion, 17 percent drank at least twice per week; only 8.1 percent of controls consumed similar quantities of alcohol. Harlap and Shiono[123] also found a slightly increased risk for abortion in women who drank in the first trimester. The increase did not reach statistical significance, but it could not be explained on the basis of smoking, prior abortion, age, or other risk factors. On the other hand, Halmesmärki et al.[124] found that alcohol consumption was nearly identical in women who did and did not experience an abortion: 13 percent of aborters and 11 percent of control women consumed on average three to four drinks per week. Alcohol consumption was also similar in their spouses.

Contraceptive Agents

Obstetricians/gynecologists are well aware that conception with an intrauterine device in place increases the risk of fetal loss. However, if the device was removed prior to pregnancy, there is no increased risk of spontaneous abortion. Likewise, use of oral contraceptives before or during pregnancy has also not been associated with fetal loss.[125] Spermicide exposure, either prior to or after conception, similarly does not appear to increase the rate of spontaneous abortion despite earlier claims to the contrary.[125]

Environmental Chemicals

Among chemical agents claimed to be associated with fetal losses are anesthetic gases, arsenic, aniline, benzene, ethylene oxide, formaldehyde, and lead.[126,127] Many environmental toxicologists accept these agents as proven abortifacients, even in lower exposures. However, deleterious effects related to exposure to these agents by pregnant workers are far from established. Nonetheless, limiting exposure is prudent. The same holds true for exposure by health care workers to chemotherapeutic agents.

Of topical concern is a recent study claiming an association between pregnancy loss and video display terminal exposure of greater than 20 h/wk.[128] However, the general consensus is to the contrary.[129] Also of obstetric interest are studies explicitly showing no increased risk for either pregnant laboratory workers[130] or pregnant pharmaceutical industry workers.[131]

Trauma

Women commonly attribute pregnancy losses to trauma, such as a fall or blow to the abdomen. However, fetuses are actually well protected from external trauma by intervening maternal structures and amniotic fluid. Attributing a loss to all save truly traumatic events (e.g., gunshot wound in the uterus) should be avoided.

Psychological Factors

That impaired psychological well-being predisposes to early fetal losses has been claimed but never proved. Certainly neurotic or mentally ill women experience losses just as normal women do. Whether the frequency of losses is higher in the former is unknown because potential confounding factors have almost never been taken into account.

Investigations that have received considerable attention are those of Stray-Pederson et al.[132,133] Pregnant women who previously experienced repetitive abortions received increased attention but no specific medical therapy ("tender loving care"). Such women ($N = 16$) were more likely (85 percent) to complete their pregnancy than 42 other women not offered such close attention (36 percent successful outcome). A potential pitfall in this study was that only women living close to the university were eligible for the increased attention. Women living farther away served as "control." Unfortunately, "controls" may have differed from the experimental group in other ways as well.

Any ostensible beneficial effect of psychological well-being may be either more apparent than real or secondary to other factors. Empathy is always an admirable trait for physicians, but lack thereof need not necessarily lead to fetal losses.

Severe Maternal Illness

Many debilitating maternal diseases have been implicated in early abortion. Pathogenesis is not necessarily independent of mechanisms discussed previously, especially endocrinologic or immunologic.

Maternal diseases frequently cited as associated with fetal wastage include Wilson's disease, maternal phenylketonuria, cyanotic heart disease, hemoglobinopathies, and inflammatory bowel disease. Actually, any life-threatening disease would be expected to be associated with an increased abortion rate. Seriously ill women rarely become pregnant, but the disease process may worsen after onset of pregnancy. Overall, relatively few fetal losses are the result of severe maternal disease, and still fewer unexplained early repetitive losses are.

RECOMMENDED EVALUATION FOR RECURRENT PREGNANCY LOSSES

The following recommendations can be offered in evaluating couples experiencing recurrent pregnancy losses.

1. Couples experiencing only one first trimester abortion should be counseled but ordinarily not evaluated systematically. One might mention the beneficial effects of abortion in eliminating abnormal conceptuses, and the appropriate recurrence risks: (1) 25 to 30 percent in the presence of a prior liveborn, (2) 40 to 50 percent in the

absence of a prior liveborn, and (3) slightly higher percentages for older women or those who smoke or drink alcohol. If a specific medical illness exists, treatment is obviously appropriate. Intrauterine adhesions should be lysed, preferably under hysteroscopic visualization. Otherwise, no further evaluation need be undertaken, even if uterine anomalies or leiomyomas are detected. On the other hand, occurrence of an anomalous stillborn warrants evaluation irrespective of the number of early pregnancy losses.

2. Investigation may or may not be initiated after two spontaneous abortions, depending on the patient's age or desires. After three spontaneous abortions, evaluation is usually indicated. After discussing recurrence risks, one should (1) obtain a detailed family history, (2) perform a complete physical examination if not previously done, and (3) order the tests summarized in the following discussion.

3. Chromosomal studies should be performed on all couples having repetitive losses. Antenatal chromosomal studies should be offered if a balanced chromosomal rearrangement is detected in either parent.

4. It would be impractical and expensive to karyotype all abortuses. However, if a woman under evaluation aborts again, it is almost irresistible to avoid karyotyping that abortus. Detection of a trisomic abortus suggests the phenomenon of recurrent aneuploidy, justifying prenatal studies in future pregnancies. Performing prenatal cytogenetic studies solely on the basis of repeated losses is arguable but most reasonable among women aged 30 to 34 years.

5. To exclude LPDs, timed endometrial biopsies should be performed late in the luteal phase in two or more cycles. Results should be correlated with the date of ovulation. If histologic dating reveals an endometrium 2 or more days less than expected, the diagnosis can be made, subject to the diagnostic limitations discussed previously. Progesterone therapy may be indicated. If it is initiated, the patient should be informed about its unproven efficacy.

6. Other endocrine causes for repeated fetal losses save poorly controlled diabetes mellitus (hyperglycemia) seem unlikely. It is reasonable to assess thyroid and carbohydrate function, but not exhaustively in the absence of clinical symptoms.

7. The endometrium should be cultured for *Ureaplasma urealyticum,* or alternatively the couple treated empirically with doxycycline (250 mg four times/day for 10 days) before pregnancy.

8. An abortion occurring after fetal viability is documented by ultrasound (8 to 10 weeks gestation) dictates investigation for a uterine anomaly or submucous leiomyomas. The uterine cavity should be explored by hysteroscopy or hysterosalpingography. If a müllerian fusion defect (septate or bicornuate uterus) is detected in a woman experiencing one or more mid-trimester spontaneous abortions, surgical correction may be warranted. This holds true especially for the septate uterus. A large submucous leiomyoma may also justify myomectomy. Cervical incompetence should be managed by surgical cerclage during the next pregnancy.

9. To exclude autoimmune disease, at a minimum LAC and anticardiolipin antibody should be assessed. Women experiencing mid-trimester losses may benefit from treatment with steroids and aspirin, but the same does not necessarily hold when these antibodies are detected in asymptomatic women having first trimester pregnancy losses. No unanimity concerning evaluation and treatment for antisperm antibodies or other autoantibodies exists.

10. The propriety of immunologic evaluations and especially immunotherapy for couples sharing HLA antigens or showing blunted maternal response to paternal antigens is controversial. Determining parental HLA types but performing no other immunologic evaluation is not recommended. Detailed immunologic evaluation should be restricted to centers performing the gamut of immunologic tests; couples desiring evaluation for an immunologic basis for fetal wastage preferably should be referred to such centers.

11. One should discourage exposure to cigarettes

and alcohol yet remain cautious in ascribing cause and effect in individual cases. Similar counsel holds true for exposures to industrial toxins.

REFERENCES

1. U.S. Department Health and Human Services: Reproductive impairments among married couples. p. 5. In U.S. Vital and Health Statistics Series 23, No. 11. National Center for Health Statistics. Hyattsville, Md., 1982

2. Simpson JL: Incidence and timing of pregnancy losses: relevance to evaluating safety of early prenatal diagnosis. Am J Med Genet 35:165, 1990

3. Simpson JL, Golbus MS: Genetics in Obstetrics and Gynecology. 2nd Ed. WB Saunders, Philadelphia, (in press)

4. Simpson JL, Carson SA: Genetic and nongenetic causes of spontaneous abortion. In Sciarra JJ (ed): Gynecology and Obstetrics. JB Lippincott, Philadelphia (in press)

5. Miller JF, Williamson E, Glue J: Fetal loss after implantation: a prospective study. Lancet 2:554, 1980

6. Edmonds DK, Lindsey KS, Miller JR et al: Early embryonic mortality in women. Fertil Steril 38:447, 1982

7. Whitaker PG, Taylor A, Lind T: Unsuspected pregnancy loss in healthy women. Lancet 1:1126, 1983

8. Wilcox AJ, Weinberg CR, O'Connor JF et al: Incidence of early pregnancy loss. N Engl J Med 319:189, 1988

9. Mills JL, Simpson JL, Driscoll SG et al: NICHD-DIEP Study: incidence of spontaneous abortion among normal women with insulin-dependent diabetic women whose pregnancies were identified within 21 days of conception. N Engl J Med 319:1617, 1988

10. Hertig AT, Rock J, Adams EC: Description of human ova within the first 17 days of development. Am J Anat 98:435, 1956

11. Hertig AT, Rock J, Adams EC, Menkin MC: Thirty-four fertilized human ova, good, bad and indifferent, recovered from 210 women of known fertility: a study of biologic wastage in early human pregnancy. Pediatrics 25:202, 1959

12. Hertig AT, Rock J: Searching for early human ova. Gynecol Invest 4:121, 1973

13. Angell RR, Aitken JR, van-Look PFGA et al: Chromo-some abnormalities in human embryos after in vitro fertilization. Nature 303:336, 1983

14. Plachot M, Junca AM, Mandelbaum J et al: Chromosome investigations in early life: human preimplantation embryos. Hum Reprod 2:29, 1987

15. Papadopoulos G, Templeton AA, Fisk N, Randall J: The frequency of chromosome anomalies in human preimplantation embryos after in-vitro fertilization. Hum Reprod 4:91, 1989

16. Plachot M: Genetics of human oocytes. In Proceedings XII International Federation of Fertility Societies. Marrakesh, Morocco (in press)

17. Gropp A: Chromosomal animal model of human disease: fetal trisomy and development failure. p. 17. In Berry L, Poswillo DE (eds): Teratology. Springer-Verlag, Berlin, 1975

18. Gropp AL: Fetal mortality due to aneuploidy and irregular meiotic segregation in the mouse. p. 225. In Boué A, Thibault C (eds): Les Accidents Chromosomiques de la Reproduction. INSERM, Paris, 1973

19. Wilson RD, Kendrick V, Wittman BK et al: Risk of spontaneous abortion in ultrasonographically normal pregnancies. Lancet 2:920, 1984

20. Christiaens GCML, Stoutenbeek PH: Spontaneous abortion in proven intact pregnancies. Lancet 2:572, 1984

21. Gilmore DH, McNay MB: Spontaneous fetal loss rate in early pregnancy. Lancet 1:107, 1985

22. Cashner KA, Christopher CR, Dysert GA: Spontaneous fetal loss after demonstration of a live fetus in the first trimester. Obstet Gynecol 70:827, 1987

23. Simpson JL, Mills JL, Holmes LB et al: Low fetal loss rates after demonstration of a live fetus in the first trimester. JAMA 258:2555, 1987

24. Tabor A, Philip J, Madsen M et al: Randomized controlled trial of genetic amniocentesis in 4606 low-risk women. Lancet 1:1287, 1986

25. Kajii T, Ohama K, Nikawa N et al: Banding analysis of abnormal karyotype in spontaneous abortion. Am J Hum Genet 25:539, 1973

26. Boué J, Boué A, Lazar P: Retrospective and prospective epidemiological studies of 1500 karyotyped spontaneous human abortions. Teratology 12:11, 1975

27. Hassold T: A cytogenetic study of repeated spontaneous abortions. Am J Hum Genet 32:723, 1980

28. Stray-Pederson B, Stray-Pederson S: Etiologic factors and subsequential reproductive performance in 195 couples with a prior history of habitual abortion. Am J Obstet Gynecol 148:140, 1984

29. Guerneri S, Bettio D, Simoni G et al: Prevalence and distribution of chromosome abnormalities in a sample of first trimester internal abortions. Hum Reprod 2:735, 1987

30. Johnson M, Drugan A, Koppich FC et al: Postmortem CVS: a better method for cytogenetic evaluation of fetal loss than culture of abortus material. Am J Hum Genet 45:A262, 1989

31. Ruzicska P, Cziezel A: Cytogenetic studies on midtrimester abortuses. Humangenetik 10:273, 1971

32. Kuleshov NP: Chromosome anomalies of infants dying during the perinatal period and premature newborn. Hum Genet 34:151, 1976

33. Bauld R, Sutherland CR, Bain AD: Chromosome studies in investigation of stillbirths and neonatal deaths. Arch Dis Child 49:782, 1974

34. Watt JL, Templeton AA, Messinis I et al: Trisomy 1 in an eight cell human pre-embryo. J Med Genet 24:60, 1987

35. Kajii T, Nikawa N: Origin of triploidy and tetraploidy in man: cases with chromosome markers. Cytogenet Cell Genet 18:109, 1977

36. Jacobs PA, Angell RR, Buchanan IM et al: The origin of human triploids. Ann Hum Genet 42:49, 1978

37. Lawler SD, Rickhall VJ, Fisher RA et al: Genetic studies of complete and partial hydatidiform moles. Lancet 2:580, 1979

38. Beatty RA: The origin of human triploidy: an integration of qualitative and quantitative evidence. Am Hum Genet 41:299, 1978

39. Singh RJ, Carr DH: The anatomy and histology of XO embryos and fetuses. Anat Rec 155:369, 1966

40. Jirasek JE: Principles of reproductive embryology. p. 51. In Simpson JL (ed): Disorders of Sex Differentiation: Etiology and Clinical Delineation. Academic Press, San Diego, 1976

41. Simpson JL: Pregnancies in women with chromosomal abnormalities. p. 439. In Shulman JD, Simpson JL (eds): Genetic Diseases in Pregnancy. Academic Press, New York, 1981

42. Chandley AC: The origin of chromosome aberrations in man and their potential for survival and reproduction in the adult human populations. Ann Genet 24:5, 1981

43. Nishimura H, Tokamo K, Tanimura T, Yasuda M: Normal and abnormal development of human embryos: first report of the analysis of 1213 intact embryos. Teratology 1:281, 1968

44. Opitz JM: Prenatal and perinatal death: the future of development pathology. Pediatr Pathol 7:363, 1987

45. Craft H, Brazy JE: Autopsy: high yield in neonatal population. Am J Dis Child 140:1260, 1986

46. Meier RP, Manchester DK, Shikes RH et al: Perinatal autopsy: its clinical value. Obstet Gynecol 67:349, 1986

47. Byrne J, Warburton D: Neural tube defects in spontaneous abortion. Am J Med Genet 25:327, 1986

48. Stein Z, Kline J, Susser E et al: Maternal age and spontaneous abortion. p. 107. In Porter IH, Hook EB (eds): Human Embryonic and Fetal Death. Academic Press, San Diego, 1980

49. Roman E, Alberman E: Spontaneous abortion, gravidity, pregnancy order, age and pregnancy interval. p. 129. In Porter IH, Hook EB (eds): Human Embryonic and Fetal Death. Academic Press, San Diego, 1980

50. Malpas P: A study of abortion sequences. J Obstet Gynaecol Br Emp 45:932, 1938

51. Warburton D, Fraser FC: Spontaneous abortion risks in man: data from reproductive histories collected in a medical genetics units. Am J Human Genet 16:1, 1964

52. Poland BJ, Miller JR, Jones DC et al: Reproductive counseling in patients who have had a spontaneous abortion. Am J Obstet Gynecol 127:685, 1977

53. Kline J, Shrout P, Stein ZA et al: Drinking during pregnancy and spontaneous abortion. Lancet 2:176, 1980

54. Boué A, Gallano P: A collaborative study of the segregation of inherited chromosome structural arrangements in 1356 prenatal diagnoses. Prenat Diagn 4:45, 1973

55. Regan L: A prospective study of spontaneous abortion. p. 23. In Beard RW, Sharp F (eds): Early Pregnancy Loss: Mechanisms and Treatment. The Royal College of Obstetricians and Gynaecologists, London, 1988

56. Vlaanderen W, Treffers PE: Prognosis of subsequent pregnancies after recurrent spontaneous abortion in first trimester. Br Med J 295:92, 1987

57. Simpson JL, Meyers CM, Martin AO et al: Translocations are infrequent among couples having repeated spontaneous abortions but no other abnormal pregnancies. Fertil Steril 51:811, 1989

58. Daniel A, Hook EB, Wulf G: Risks of unbalanced progeny at amniocentesis to carriers of chromosome rearrangements: data from United States and Canadian Laboratories. Am J Med Genet 33:14, 1989

59. Martin RH: Invited editorial: Segregation analysis of translocations by the study of human sperm chromosome complements. Am J Hum Genet 44:461, 1989

60. Boué A, Gallano P: A collaborative study of the segregation of inherited chromosome structural arrangements in 1356 prenatal diagnoses. Prenat Diagn 4:45, 1984

61. Sutherland GR, Gardiner AJ, Carter RF: Familial pericentric inversion of chromosome 19 inv (19) (p13q13) with a note on genetic counseling of pericentric inversion carries. Clin Genet 10:53, 1976

62. Warburton D, Kline J, Stein Z et al: Does the karyotype of a spontaneous abortion predict the karyotype of a subsequent abortion? Evidence from 273 women with two karyotyped spontaneous abortions. Am J Hum Genet 41:465, 1987

63. Alberman ED: The abortus as a predictor of future trisomy 21. p. 69. In De la Cruz FF, Gerald PS (eds): Trisomy 21 (Down Syndrome). University Park Press, Baltimore, 1981

64. Jones GS: The luteal phase defect. Fertil Steril 27:351, 1976

65. Daya S, Ward S: Diagnostic test properties of serum progesterone in the evaluation of luteal phase defects. Fertil Steril 49:168, 1988

66. Davis OK, Berkley AS, Cholst IN et al: The incidence of luteal phase defect in normal, fertile women, determined by serial endometrial biopsy. Fertil Steril 51:582, 1989

67. Noyes RW, Hertig ATR, Rock J: Dating the endometrial biopsy. Fertil Steril 1:3, 1950

68. Scott RT, Synder RR, Strickland DM et al: The effect of interobserver variation in dating endometrial history on the diagnosis of luteal phase defects. Fertil Steril 50:888, 1988

69. Li TC, Dockery P, Rogers AW, Cooke ID: How precise is histologic dating of endometrium using the standard dating criteria. Fertil Steril 51:759, 1989

70. Daya S, Ward S, Burrows E: Progesterone profiles in luteal phase defect cycles and outcome of progesterone treatment in patients with recurrent spontaneous abortions. Am J Obstet Gynecol 158:225, 1988

71. Wu CH, Minassian SS: Integrated luteal progesterone: an assessment of luteal function. Fertil Steril 48:937, 1987

72. Horta JLH, Fernandez JG, DeSoto LB: Direct evidence of luteal insufficiency in women with habitual abortions. Obstet Gynecol 49:705, 1977

73. Brodie BL, Wentz AC: An update on the clinical relevance of luteal phase inadequacy. Semin Reprod Endocrinol 7:138, 1989

74. McRae MA, Blasco L, Lyttle CR: Serum hormones and their receptors in women with normal and inade-

quate corpus luteum function. Fertil Steril 42:58, 1984

75. Jacobs MH, Balasch J, Gonzalez-Merlo JM et al: Endometrial cytosol and nuclear progesterone receptors in luteal phase defect. Clin Endocrinol Metab 64:472, 1987

76. Spiritos NJ, Yurewicz EC, Moghissi KS et al: Pseudocorpus luteum insufficiency: a study of cytosol progesterone receptors in human endometrium. Obstet Gynecol 65:535, 1985

77. Saracoglu OF, Aksel S, Yeoman RR et al: Endometrial estradiol and progesterone receptors in patients with luteal phase defects and endometriosis. Fertil Steril 43:851, 1985

78. Tho PT, Byrd JR, McDonough PC: Etiologies and subsequent reproductive performance of 100 couples with recurrent abortions. Fertil Steril 32:389, 1979

79. Daly DC, Walters CA, Soto-Albers CE et al: Endometrial biopsy during treatment of luteal phase defects is predictive of therapeutic outcome. Fertil Steril 40:305, 1983

80. Harrison RE: Early recurrent pregnancy failure: treatment with human chorionic gonadotropin. p. 421. In Beard RW, Sharp F (eds): Early Pregnancy Loss: Mechanisms and Treatment. Royal College of Obstetricians and Gynaecologists, London, 1988

81. Montero M, Collea JV, Frasier D, Mestman J: Successful outcome of pregnancy in women with hypothyroidism. Ann Intern Med 94:31, 1981

82. Miodnovic M, Lavin JP, Knowles HC et al: Spontaneous abortion among insulin dependent diabetic women. Am J Obstet Gynecol 150:372, 1984

83. Miodovnik M, Mimouni F, Tsang RL et al: Glycemic control and spontaneous abortion in insulin dependent diabetic women. Obstet Gynecol 68:366, 1986

84. Miodovnik M, Skillman C, Holroyde JC et al: Elevated maternal glycohemoglobin in early pregnancy and spontaneous abortion among insulin dependent diabetic women. Am J Obstet Gynecol 153:439, 1985

85. Greene MF, Hare JW, Cloherty JP et al: First trimester hemoglobin A1 and risk for major malformation and spontaneous abortion in diabetic pregnancy. Teratology 39:225, 1989

86. Schenker J, Margelioth E: Intrauterine adhesions: an updated appraisal. Fertil Steril 37:593, 1982

87. Heinonen P, Saarikoski S, Pystynen P: Reproductive performance of women with uterine anomalies: an evaluation of 182 cases. Acta Obstet Gynecol Scand 61:157, 1982

88. Sompolinsky D, Solomon F, Elikina L et al: Infections

with mycoplasma and bacteria: individual midtrimester abortion and fetal loss. Am J Obstet Gynecol 121:610, 1975

89. Stray-Pedersen B, Eng J, Reikvan TM: Uterine T-mycoplasma colonization in reproductive failure. Am J Obstet Gynecol 130:307, 1978

90. Toth A, Lesser ML, Brooks-Toth CW et al: Outcome of subsequent pregnancies following antibiotic therapy after primary or multiple spontaneous abortions. Surg Gynecol Obstet 163:243, 1986

91. Levine P: ABO, P and MN blood group determinants in neoplasm foreign to the host. Semin Oncol 5:25, 1978

92. Rock JA, Shirey RS, Braine HG et al: Plasmapheresis for the treatment of repeated early pregnancy wastage associated with anti-P. Obstet Gynecol 66:57S, 1985

93. Branch DW, Ward K: Autoimmunity and pregnancy loss. Semin Reprod Endocrinol 7:168, 1989

94. Lockshin MD, Druzin ML, Goei S et al: Antibody to cardiolipin as a predictor of fetal distress or death in pregnant patients with systemic lupus erythematosus. N Engl J Med 313:152, 1985

95. Elias M, Eldor A: Thromboembolism in patients with "lupus" type circulating anticoagulant. Arch Intern Med 1244:510, 1984

96. Scott JR, Rote NS, Branch DW: Immunologic aspects of recurrent abortions and fetal death. Obstet Gynecol 70:645, 1987

97. Branch DW, Scott JR, Kochenour NK et al: Obstetric complications associated with the lupus anticoagulant. N Engl J Med 313:1322, 1985

98. Unander AM, Norberg R, Hohn L et al: Anti-cardiolipin antibodies and complement in ninety-nine women with habitual abortions. Am J Obstet Gynecol 156:114, 1987

99. Howard MA, Firkin BG, Healy DL, Choong SC: Lupus anticoagulant in women with multiple spontaneous miscarriage. Am J Hematol 26:175, 1987

100. Cowchock S, Smith JB, Gocial B: Antibodies to phospholipids and nuclear antigens in patients with repeated abortions. Am J Obstet Gynecol 155:1002, 1986

101. Petri M, Golbus M, Anderson R et al: Antinuclear antibody, lupus anticoagulant, and anticardiolipin antibody in women with idiopathic habitual abortion. Arthritis Rheum 30:601, 1987

102. Beard RW, Baude P, Mowbray JF et al: Protective antibodies and spontaneous abortion. Lancet 1:1090, 1983

103. Gill TH III: Immunogenetics of spontaneous abortions in humans. Transplantation 35:1, 1983

104. Thomas ML, Harger JH, Wegener DK et al: HLA sharing and spontaneous abortion. Am J Obstet Gynecol 151:1053, 1983

105. Beer AE, Quebbeman JF, Semprini AE: Immunopathological factors contributing to recurrent and spontaneous abortion in humans. p. 90. In Bennet MJ, Edmonds DK (eds): Spontaneous and Recurrent Abortions. Blackwell, Oxford, 1987

106. Rocklin RE, Kitzmiller JL, Carpenter CB et al: Absence of an immunologic blocking factor from the serum of women with chronic abortion. N Engl J Med 295:1209, 1976

107. Rocklin RE, Kitzmiller JL, Garvoy MR: Further characterization of an immunologic blocking factor that develops during pregnancy. Clin Immunol Immunopathol 22:305, 1982

108. Stimson WH, Strachan AF, Shepard A: Studies on the maternal immune response to placental antigens: absence of a blocking factor from the blood of abortion-prone women. Br J Obstet Gynaecol 86:41, 1979

109. Fitzet D, Bousquet J: Absence of a factor blocking cellular cytotoxicity in the serum of women with recurrent abortion. Br J Obstet Gynaecol 90:453, 1983

110. Beer AE, Billingham RF: The Immunology of Mammalian Reproduction. Prentice-Hall, Englewood, NJ, 1976

111. Oksenberg JR, Persitz E, Amar A et al: Maternal-paternal histocompatability: lack of association with habitual abortion. Fertil Steril 42:389, 1984

112. Ober CL, Martin AO, Simpson JL et al: Shared HLA antigens and reproductive performance among Hutterites. Am J Hum Genet 35:994, 1983

113. Regan L, Braude PR: Is antipaternal cytotoxic antibody a valid marker in the management of recurrent abortion? Lancet 2:1280, 1987

114. Sargent IL, Wilkins T, Redman CWG: Maternal immune responses to the fetus in early pregnancy and recurrent miscarriage. Lancet 2:1099, 1988

115. Power DA, Mason RJ, Stewart GM et al: The fetus as an allograft: evidence for protective antibodies to HLA-linked paternal antigens. Lancet 2:701, 1983

116. Faulk WP, McIntyre JA: Trophoblast survival. Transplantation 32:1, 1981

117. Faulk WO, Coulam CB, McIntyre JA: The role of trophoblast antigens in repetitive spontaneous abortions. Semin Reprod Endocrinol 7:182, 1989

118. Norman DJ, Barry JM, Fischer S: The beneficial effect of pretransplant third-party blood transfusions on allograft rejection in HLA identical sibling kidney transplants. Transplantation 41:125, 1986

119. Beard RW, Sharp F (eds): Early pregnancy loss: mechanism and treatment. In Proceedings of the Eighteenth Study Group of the Royal College of Obstetricians

and Gynaecologists. Royal College of Obstetricians and Gynaecologists, London, 1988

120. Mowbray JF, Gibbing C, Liddell H et al: Controlled trial of treatment of recurrent spontaneous abortion by immunization with paternal cells. Lancet 1:941, 1985

121. Mowbray JR, Underwood JL, Michel M et al: Immunization with paternal lymphocytes in women with recurrent miscarriage. Lancet 2:679, 1987

122. Alberman ED, Creasy M, Elliott M et al: Maternal effects associated with fetal chromosomal anomalies in spontaneous abortions. Br J Obstet Gynecol 83:621, 1976

123. Harlap S, Shino PH: Alcohol, smoking and incidence of spontaneous abortions in the first and second trimester. Lancet 2:173, 1980

124. Halmesmäki E, Valimaki M, Roine R et al: Maternal and paternal alcohol consumption and miscarriage. Br J Obstet Gynaecol 96:188, 1989

125. Simpson JL: Relationship between congenital anomalies and contraception. Adv Contracept 1:3, 1985

126. Fija-Talamanaca I, Settimi L: Occupational factors and reproductive outcome. p. 61. In Hafez ESE (ed): Spontaneous Abortion. MTP Press, Lancaster, United Kingdom, 1984

127. Barlow S, Sullivan FM: Reproductive Hazards of Industrial Chemicals: An Evaluation of Animal and Human Data. Academic Press, San Diego, 1982

128. Goldhaber MK, Polen MR, Hiatt RA: The risk of miscarriage and birth defects among women who use visual display terminals during pregnancy. Am J Indust Med 13:695, 1988

129. Blackwell R, Chang A: Video display terminals and pregnancy: a review. Br J Obstet Gynaecol 95:446, 1988

130. Heidam LZ: Spontaneous abortions among laboratory workers: a follow up study. J Epidemiol Community Health 38:36, 1984

131. Taskinen H, Lindbohm M-L, Hemninki K et al: Spontaneous abortions among women working in the pharmaceutical industry. Br J Indust Med 43:199, 1984

132. Stray-Pedersen B, Stray-Pedersen S: Etiologic factors and subsequent reproductive performance in 195 couples with a prior history of habitual abortion. Am J Obstet Gynecol 148:140, 1984

133. Stray-Pedersen B, Stray-Pedersen S: Recurrent abortion: the role of psychotherapy. p. 433. In Beard RW, Sharp F (eds): Early Pregnancy Loss: Mechanism and Treatment. Royal College of Obstetricians and Gynaecologists, London, 1988

134. Simpson JL, Bombard AT: Chromosomal abnormalities in spontaneous abortion: frequency, pathology and genetic counseling. p. 51. In Edmonds K, Bennett MJ (eds): Spontaneous and Recurrent Abortion. Blackwell, London, 1987

135. Simpson JL, Tharapel AT: Principles of cytogenetics. In Philip E, Barnes J (eds): Scientific Foundations of Obstetrics and Gynaecology, 4th Ed. Heinemann Medical Books, London (in press)

136. Simpson JL: Disorders of Sexual Differentiation, Etiology and Clinical Delineation. Academic Press, 1976

137. Hertig AT, Rock J, Adams EC, Mulligan WJ: On the implantation stages of the human ovum: a description of four normal and four abnormal specimens ranging from the second to the fifth day of development. Contrib Embryol 35:199, 1954

138. Hertig AT, Rock J: A series of potentially abortive ova recovered from fertile women prior to the first missed menstrual period. Am J Obstet Gynecol 58:968, 1949

139. Hertig AT, Rock J: On the development of the early human ovum with special reference to the trophoblast of the previllous stage: a description of seven normal and five pathologic ova. Am J Obstet Gynecol 47:149, 1944

Chapter 24

Ectopic Pregnancy

Alan H. DeCherney and David B. Seifer

Ectopic pregnancy is an unqualified disaster in human reproduction as illustrated by its contribution to maternal mortality, as well as its permanent debilitating effect on future fertility. It has become a public health problem of epidemic proportions.

INCIDENCE

The incidence of ectopic pregnancy is rising exponentially in the United States. Between 1970 and 1987, the number of reported cases more than quadrupled from 17,800 to approximately 88,000 with an increase from 1 in 200 live births to 1 in 43.[1] Only one-half of women who have sustained an ectopic pregnancy eventually deliver a liveborn infant. Up to 25 percent suffer a repeat ectopic pregnancy.[2] Ectopic pregnancies are responsible for approximately 10 percent of all maternal mortality (Fig. 24.1).[3] The chances for mortality seem to correlate with lower socioeconomic status.[2,4]

When scrutinizing the increased ratio of ectopic pregnancies to live births, one must realize that during the past decade changes in both the numerator and the denominator have occurred, some real and some spurious. Certainly, there has been an increase in the number of ectopic pregnancies as a whole. This increase is hypothesized to be due to (1) more adequate treatment of pelvic inflammatory disease, which in the past would have rendered the patient sterile; (2) the use of the intrauterine device (IUD); (3) an increase in surgical procedures for the treatment of fallopian tube disease; and (4) a greater number of elective sterilizations.[5] The artifactual change in the numerator is related to improved diagnostic techniques. Ectopic pregnancies that would have been mislabeled as unexplained abdominal pain or bleeding in the past are recognized today because pregnancy tests have become more sensitive. In regard to the denominator, earlier reports presented the incidence of ectopic pregnancy per live births. For each patient who elects to have a therapeutic abortion, a procedure that has been performed more frequently over the past decade, the denominator in the ratio of ectopic pregnancies to live births is reduced.

The vast majority of ectopic pregnancies (96 percent) are tubal, while 2 percent are uterine ectopic pregnancies (i.e., interstitial). The remaining 2 percent include cervical, abdominal, and ovarian pregnancies (Fig. 24.2).[6–8] Most tubal pregnancies are found in the distal two-thirds of the tube. A small portion of ectopic pregnancies are isthmic, located in the proximal portion of the extrauterine part of the tube (Fig. 24.3). This type of pregnancy represents a distinct surgical entity. The heterotopic pregnancy, defined as a combined intrauterine and extrauterine gestation, is an uncommon and perplexing problem. This rare event occurs in approximately one in 3,899 to 15,000 pregnancies.[9] The incidence of bilateral

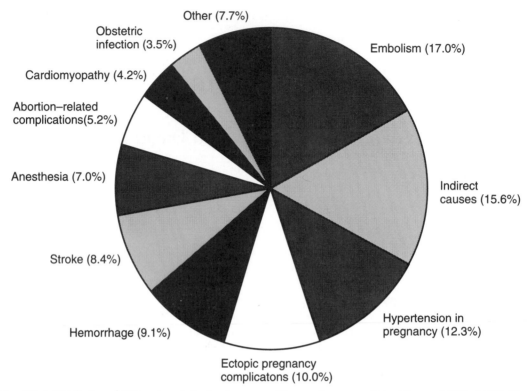

Fig. 24.1 Distribution of 601 maternal deaths, by cause, 19 reporting areas, United States, 1980–1985. (From Koonin et al.[104])

ectopic pregnancy is unknown, although isolated cases have been reported in the literature.[10,11]

PHYSIOLOGY AND ANATOMY OF THE TUBAL ECTOPIC PREGNANCY

Whether aberrations in tubal motility or hormonal stimulation cause ectopic pregnancy remains quite controversial. An understanding of normal tubal physiology is necessary to appreciate how these factors might contribute to an ectopic pregnancy.

The tube represents more than a conduit for sperm, ovum, and zygote. Fertilization occurs in the ampulla, as does early zygote development. Fimbrial mucosa and its accompanying cilia are important for ovum pickup and transport as well as for maintenance of the growing zygote.[12,13]

Laufer proposed that disjunctive hormonal pro-

duction by the cumulus oophorus cells leads to an ectopic pregnancy by adversely altering tubal motility.[14] Over a 20-year period, Gemzell found a 2.7 percent incidence of ectopic pregnancy in patients treated with human menopausal gonadotropins as compared with a 1.2 percent incidence in a control group.[15] No other evidence of tubal pathology was observed in these patients. Gemzell and co-workers hypothesized that high levels of estradiol predisposed to ectopic pregnancy, since 5 of the 10 patients in whom an ectopic pregnancy developed had been hyperstimulated. McBain confirmed these findings in women undergoing ovulation induction.[16]

The fertilized ovum apparently reaches the uterus about 80 hours after follicular rupture, spending approximately 72 hours in the ampulla followed by rapid transport through the isthmus.[17] Budowick emphasized an important anatomic relationship in the propagation of an ectopic pregnancy.[18] These

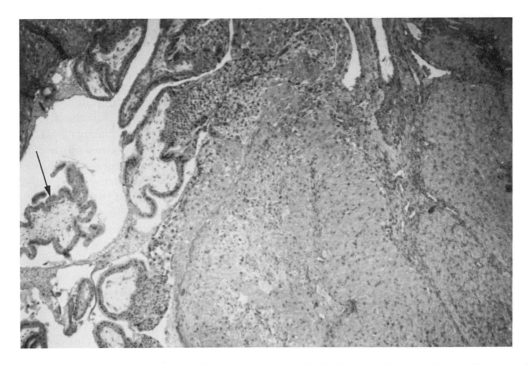

Fig. 24.2 An ovarian ectopic pregnancy. Villi (arrow) can be identified adjacent to the corpus luteum. (Courtesy of Dr. James Wheeler, Department of Surgical Pathology, Hospital of the University of Pennsylvania.)

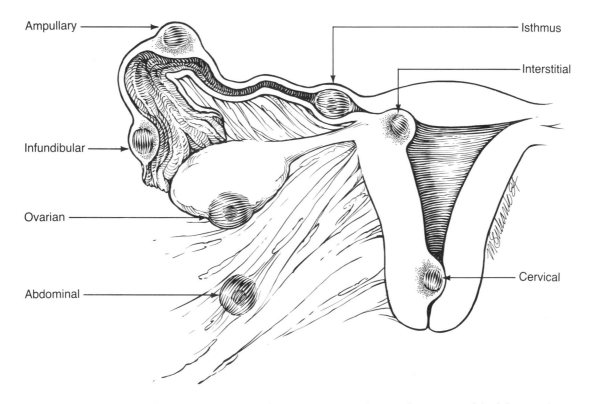

Fig. 24.3 Potential location of ectopic pregnancies. The majority occur in the ampullary portion of the fallopian tube.

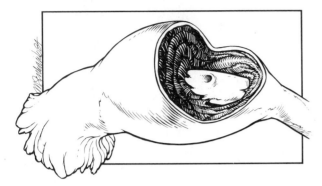

Fig. 24.4 A small defect in the endothelium of the ampullary portion of the fallopian tube is demonstrated with propagation of trophoblastic tissue and clot in the loose adventitious tissue between the serosa and the endothelium of the fallopian tube, as described by Budowick et al.[18]

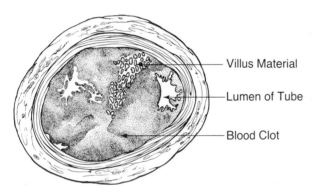

Villus Material

Lumen of Tube

Blood Clot

Fig. 24.5 The intact epithelium of the ampullary portion of the tube is noted. The villus material lies outside the tubal lumen.

workers hypothesized that trophoblastic tissue erodes easily and early through the epithelium of the endosalpinx in the ampullary portion of the tube (Fig. 24.4). This path represents the course of least resistance, since the tissue between the lumen of the tube and the serosa is composed of loose adventitia. The pregnancy then propagates at this site, which contains villus and embryonic tissue as well as clot (Fig. 24.5). Most importantly, the tubal lumen and its epithelium remain virtually unscathed in this type of ectopic pregnancy. Expansion usually occurs laterally or superiorly. If the growing pregnancy extends into the broad ligament, however, its blood supply is compromised, creating a more serious condition. Eventually, villi erode into the blood vessels, resulting in

vigorous bleeding. This process is quite different from the slow accumulation of blood that earlier resulted in an organized clot within the tube.

Sixty-five percent of patients with *unruptured* ectopic pregnancies may have a positive culdocentesis. This finding reflects extravasation of blood into the peritoneal cavity from between the serosal layer and the fimbrial endothelial tissue. In contrast, 85 percent of patients with ruptured ectopic pregnancies have a positive culdocentesis. The amount of blood is always greater in these cases.[5]

An isthmic ectopic pregnancy represents a very different anatomic process. In this portion of the tube, the tissue between the epithelium of the lumen of the tube and serosa is compact, composed mostly of muscularis (Fig. 24.6). This tissue helps squeeze the zygote into the uterine cavity and must overcome the resistance provided by the uterine musculature. Un-

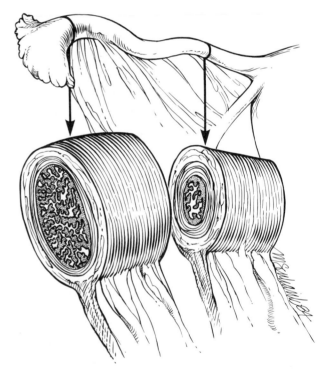

Fig. 24.6 The ampullary portion of the tube has minimal muscularis, permitting early egress of the zygote into the space between serosa and tubal epithelium. In the isthmic portion of the tube, however, the muscularis is quite well developed and dense, forcing the ectopic pregnancy to grow within the lumen of the tube itself.

like the ampullary ectopic pregnancy described previously, propagation of an isthmic ectopic pregnancy occurs within the tubal lumen. Therefore, the lumen is destroyed, necessitating a different surgical procedure.

ETIOLOGY OF ECTOPIC PREGNANCY

POSSIBLE ETIOLOGIES AND CONTRIBUTING FACTORS FOR ECTOPIC PREGNANCY

Diethylstilbestrol (DES) exposure

Endometriosis

Infection

Infertility

Intrauterine device (IUD)

Previous abdominal surgery

Previous ectopic pregnancy

Previous infertility surgery

Previous tubal sterilization

Transmigration of gamete and zygote

The etiology of ectopic pregnancy is quite variable and poorly understood. Certain risk factors have been identified and are believed to contribute to the impairment of migration of the fertilized ovum to the uterus, including (1) pelvic inflammatory disease (PID), which is found in approximately 50 percent of cases of ectopic pregnancy; (2) tubal endometriosis, which is rare; or (3) previous tubal surgery.[19] Ten percent of pregnancies after tubal surgery are ectopic, yet no clear distinction as to cause and effect is evident. Whether the causative factor is the healing process after tuboplasty or the antecedent damage to the tube is puzzling.

Pelvic Inflammatory Disease

A documented increase in sexually transmitted infections has been reported over the decade. The offending organisms seem to be most often *Chlamydia tra-chomatis* and *Neisseria gonorrhoeae*.[20] Westrom[21] has strengthened this circumstantial relationship between sexually transmitted disease and ectopic pregnancy, noting that patients with a documented episode of PID have a sevenfold increase in the rate of tubal pregnancies compared with women from normal control populations. Svensson et al.[22] examined 112 women with ectopic pregnancies and noted IgG antibodies to *C. trachomatis* in 75 percent of those studied compared to 21 percent of women with intrauterine pregnancies. These findings strongly suggest that previous chlamydial salpingitis may be a major etiologic factor in ectopic pregnancy. Corroborating data have been presented by Hartford et al.,[23] who found higher IgG titers for *C. trachomatis* in patients undergoing surgery for ectopic pregnancy.

Pelvic infection leads to inflammatory changes and damages the normal ciliary mechanism of tubal transport. Using the electron microscope to study biopsied material from sites of ectopic implantation, Vasquez et al.[24] demonstrated a marked decrease in the density of the cilia. Patton et al.,[25] also using electron microscopy, described flattened mucosal folds, extensive deciliation and degeneration of secretory epithelial cells, as well as decreased ciliary beat frequency in fallopian tubes of infertile women suspected of having previous chlamydial salpingitis. Draper et al.[26] found microdiverticula in the fallopian tubes of guinea pigs infected with gonorrhea. Certainly, the zygote could become entrapped in such a blind pouch. This work has been corroborated by Persaud,[27] who injected radiopaque materials into fallopian tubes removed in conjunction with the surgical treatment of an ectopic pregnancy and found a 49 percent incidence of tubal diverticula compared with a 10 percent incidence in controls.

Other factors tangentially related to PID in the etiology of ectopic pregnancy include previous therapeutic abortions, salpingitis isthmica nodosa, and previous abdominal surgical procedures.[28]

Previous Therapeutic Abortion

Levin et al. showed an increase in the relative risk for ectopic pregnancy from 1.3 after one abortion to 2.6 after two or more.[28] This finding has been confirmed by a case–control study conducted in Greece.[29] In reviewing the data from 4,004 women who had undergone previous therapeutic abortions, Chung et al.[30] observed a 0.57 percent incidence of ectopic pregnancy, as compared with 0.49 percent among controls. The study also illustrated that those women who underwent abortions associated with infection or with retained products of conception had an associated fivefold increase in subsequent ectopic pregnancies.

Intrauterine Device

The general consensus seems to be that the IUD does not cause ectopic pregnancy.[31,32] Yet Vessey et al.[33] found a 1.2-fold increase in the ectopic pregnancy rate among IUD wearers. Ory[34] described the major risk factor as length of use. Whether the salpingitis associated with IUD use is a cause of ectopic pregnancy or whether the IUD prevents intrauterine pregnancies but not ectopic pregnancies remains a subject of investigation.

Previous Sterilization Procedures

Several investigators have described an increased rate of ectopic pregnancy associated with postsurgical sterilization.[35-39] Most likely, a tubotubal fistula or uteroperitoneal fistula leads to implantation of the resulting pregnancy in the blind portion of the distal tube. Ectopic pregnancies seem to occur more frequently after sterilization by coagulation techniques. The closer the tubal disruption is to the uterine cornua, the greater the likelihood of an ectopic pregnancy.[37]

The Preembryo as a Cause of Ectopic Pregnancy

Although much emphasis has been placed on the role of tubal dysfunction as a cause of ectopic pregnancy, some workers have also considered the preembryo, with the hypothesis that an abnormal preembryo would dictate abnormal implantation. The incidence of abnormal karyotypes in ectopic pregnancies ranges from 17.4 to 44 percent. Therefore, chromosomal abnormalities seem to be no more frequent in ectopic pregnancies than in intrauterine gestations that are aborted.[40,41] On the other hand, some investigators have proposed poor oxygenation of the preembryo, and not merely ectopic implantation, as a cause of structural changes in the karyotype.[42]

DIAGNOSIS OF ECTOPIC PREGNANCY

The timely diagnosis of ectopic pregnancy demands that well-established clinical signs and symptoms and procedures, such as culdocentesis, be combined with more sophisticated and precise testing, such as β-human chorionic gonadotropin (β-hCG) determinations and ultrasound. Although often overlooked, laparoscopy has made a major contribution to the prompt and accurate diagnosis of ectopic pregnancy. In the past, surgeons were reluctant to perform laparotomy unless the finding of an ectopic pregnancy was ensured. Most ectopic pregnancies had presented after they had ruptured, at approximately 10 weeks gestation. The introduction of laparoscopy and its more liberal use permitted the detection of ectopic pregnancies at 8 to 10 weeks gestation. Combining more sophisticated testing with laparoscopy has allowed the diagnosis of ectopic pregnancy to be made between 5 and 6 weeks gestation in most cases. Since rupture of the tube usually occurs after 10 weeks, such catastrophic events should rarely be seen with the modern management of tubal ectopic gestations.

Signs and Symptoms

It has been demonstrated that abdominal pain and irregular vaginal bleeding are common presenting symptoms in ectopic pregnancy.[43-45] Of 328 patients presenting for admission with ectopic pregnancy, 94 percent had pain, 89 percent had missed a menstrual period, 80 percent had vaginal bleeding, and only 20 percent demonstrated signs suggestive of early shock.[43] An abdominal mass is palpable in only one-half of patients with an ectopic pregnancy.[44-46] Passage of a decidual cast (Fig. 24.7) in association with vaginal bleeding increases the likelihood of an ectopic pregnancy. The Arias-Stella phenomenon (Fig. 24.8) may be found in the endometrium in association with ectopic pregnancies. However, the phenomenon is also seen in 70 to 80 percent of therapeutic and spontaneous abortions[47] and is therefore not specific enough to be helpful.

Culdocentesis continues to be a valuable test crucial to the management of ectopic pregnancy. A patient who has a copious amount of blood in the cul-

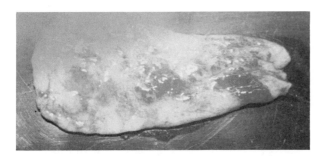

Fig. 24.7 Decidual cast of the uterine cavity. (From DeCherney et al.,[5] with permission.)

de-sac, as demonstrated by culdocentesis, should be taken to the operating room immediately. A patient who has only a small amount of blood (less than 3 to 5 ml) might be judiciously observed for a short period while the results of other diagnostic tests are gathered.

Chronic ectopic pregnancy is a definitive entity that may represent up to 60 percent of all ectopic pregnancies.[48] Diagnosis may be difficult because normal anatomic landmarks are distorted by the formation of adhesions resulting from the chronic inflammatory process. Chronic ectopic pregnancies also present a management quandary. Difficulty is

encountered in acting on the patient with declining β-hCG levels. The major question that must be addressed in most chronic ectopic pregnancies is, Will they resolve on their own, or will surgical intervention be indicated to prevent both catastrophic hemorrhage and permanent adhesion formation and tubal damage?

Diagnostic Procedures

The use of newer diagnostic tests, primarily β-hCG levels and ultrasound imaging, has had a major impact on maternal outcome in ectopic pregnancy, decreasing morbidity and mortality rates and increasing the use of conservative rather than radical surgical procedures. Such improvement is a direct result of earlier and more precise diagnosis. Older studies demonstrated that at least 80 percent of ectopic pregnancies had ruptured at the time of definitive surgery.[6] Today this figure has been reduced to 20 percent.[5,49,50]

Determination of β-hCG levels has proved the most important new test. In the past, the sensitivity of urinary pregnancy tests as well as interference from luteinizing hormone (LH) made the diagnosis of ectopic gestation difficult and confusing. The advent of

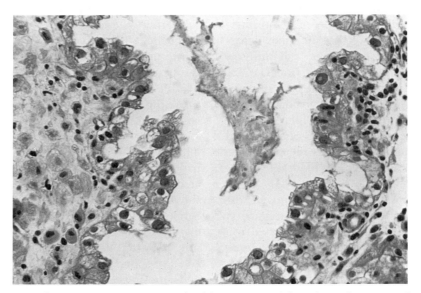

Fig. 24.8 Arias–Stella reaction. Hypersecretory glandular reaction with large hyperchromatic nuclei and cytoplasmic vacuolation. (From DeCherney et al.,[5] with permission.)

a radioimmunoassay (RIA) and radioreceptor assay for the β-subunit of hCG eliminates some of these problems. Sensitivity as low as 5 mIU/ml is now possible with RIA.[51-57] Therefore, a negative β-hCG result rules out an ectopic pregnancy in almost 100 percent of cases.[55] β-hCG testing also has another distinct advantage: In a normal intrauterine pregnancy, hormone levels should double every 2.4 days with a predictable slope of increase. Almost all pregnancies that fail to achieve this slope are abnormal, and most ectopic pregnancies are found in this group. Overall, approximately two-thirds of patients with an ectopic pregnancy have an abnormal progression of β-hCG levels. The remaining one-third demonstrate a normal increase.

At approximately 5 weeks gestation by menstrual age, an intrauterine gestational sac can first be appreciated on transvaginal ultrasound.[49,58] The presence of a pseudogestational sac similar in appearance to the gestational sac observed in a normal intrauterine pregnancy has been well documented.[59,60] An ectopic pregnancy may on occasion be detected by visualizing an adnexal mass or fetal activity within the fallopian tube. Complex sonographic adnexal masses were noted in 83 percent of ectopic pregnancies and in 94 percent of ectopic pregnancies when a mass was associated with cul-de-sac fluid.[61] Subramanyam et al.[62] have used the following ultrasound criteria alone to detect an ectopic pregnancy: absence of an intrauterine gestational sac, diffusely echogenic adnexal mass with areas of high-intensity echoes, and diffusely echogenic hematoma in the pouch of Douglas. The diagnosis of ectopic pregnancy on the basis of ultrasound findings of an empty uterus and adnexal mass can also be quite misleading, approaching no better than 50 percent accuracy.[63] The ability of ultrasound to estimate the amount of blood in the cul-de-sac, which would eliminate the need for culdocentesis, has yet to be evaluated.

Transvaginal ultrasonography has proved extremely useful in the diagnosis of ectopic pregnancy. Using a 5-MHz vaginal probe, Stiller evaluated 139 patients at risk for ectopic pregnancy.[64] Of the 22 ectopic pregnancies, 14 (64 percent) were accurately diagnosed at the time of the initial examination on the basis of the criteria of visualization of a gestational sac located outside the uterus in the absence of an intrauterine gestational sac. In these 22 cases, a yolk sac was seen in 13, a fetal pole in 3, and free peritoneal fluid or blood clots in 9. An additional 4 patients without an intrauterine or extrauterine gestational sac were definitively diagnosed as having an ectopic pregnancy because their β-hCG level exceeded the discriminatory zone in this study of 1,300 mIU/ml. Overall, 18 of 22 (82 percent) ectopic pregnancies were definitively identified at the time of the initial evaluation. Transvaginal ultrasonography also accurately diagnosed 103 of 117 (88 percent) of the intrauterine pregnancies at the initial assessment. In the 18 patients in whom a diagnosis could not be made when they were first seen, serial measurements of β-hCG and repeat ultrasound studies were performed. In this group, 4 women were subsequently found to have an ectopic gestation, 4 were observed to have an early intrauterine pregnancy, and 10 had complete abortions.

Timor-Tritsch has reported his experience using transvaginal ultrasonography for the evaluation of 202 patients with suspected ectopic pregnancies.[65] The diagnosis of an ectopic gestation was confirmed in 83 women. Only one false positive and one false negative case result were observed. Fetal cardiac activity was identified in the tube in 23 percent of cases. Timor-Tritsch has emphasized the importance of the tubal ring in establishing the diagnosis of ectopic pregnancy. The tubal ring represents the usually unruptured, thickened tubal wall and contains either the gestational sac or blood clots (Figs. 24.9 and 24.10). Care must be exercised to avoid confusing the tubal ring with the corpus luteum of pregnancy, ovarian follicles, small bowel, or other tubal pathology.

The one-third of patients who have normally rising β-hCG values represent a distinct problem. Do these patients have a normal intrauterine pregnancy or an ectopic pregnancy? When and at what level of β-hCG should an intrauterine sac be seen? At Yale University School of Medicine, this critical level has been documented to be approximately 6,500 mIU/ml.[45,50] Bryson[57] reported that the combination of β-hCG titers and ultrasound provides almost 100 percent accuracy in diagnosing ectopic pregnancies. Absence of an intrauterine sac when the hCG titer is greater than

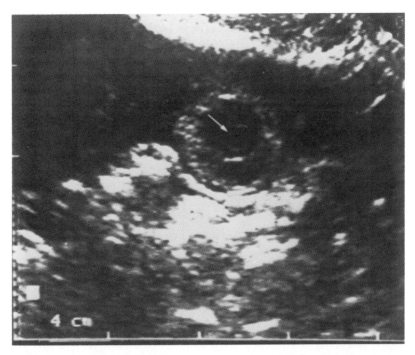

Fig. 24.9 Transvaginal ultrasonography (TVS) demonstrating cross section of a tubal ring containing a 5-week unruptured ectopic pregnancy. The faint outline of the yolk sac (arrow) can be seen. (From Timor-Tritsch et al.,[65] with permission.)

6,500 mIU/ml is as ominous as an abnormal increase in hCG levels and connotes either an ectopic pregnancy or an abnormal intrauterine pregnancy. The definitive diagnosis can only be made by examining intrauterine tissue by biopsy or curettage. The diagnostic evaluation using both β-hCG levels and ultrasound is outlined in Fig. 24.11.[8] Several points, however, require clarification. The "discriminating zone" varies, depending on the type of ultrasound employed. When using a transabdominal approach, the discriminating zone is approximately 6,500 mIU/ml at 42 days of gestation, as compared to a discriminating zone of approximately 1,300 to 1,400 mIU/ml at 35 days of gestation using a transvaginal probe.[58] Furthermore, it is important to note that the quantitative β-hCG values mentioned in this discussion are derived from the International Reference Preparation (IRP). Another reference established by the World Health Organization is the Second International Standard (2nd IS hCG). hCG concentrations are calibrated approximately twice as high when using the IRP as compared to using the 2nd IS hCG.[66]

SURGICAL MANAGEMENT OF ECTOPIC PREGNANCY

In order to determine the best operative procedure for the patient with an ectopic pregnancy, the clinician must consider the specific needs of the patient and the known success or failure rates for alternative surgical techniques. Obviously, a conservative salpingostomy is performed for the patient who wishes to preserve her fertility. On the other hand, the patient undergoing surgery for a third ectopic pregnancy may be better served by salpingectomy and subsequent in vitro fertilization. Deciding which surgical procedure will be performed also depends on gross anatomic distortion. An ectopic pregnancy that has ruptured into the broad ligament carries a poor prognosis for further fertility. Not only is the normal anatomy disrupted but pelvic blood supply is com-

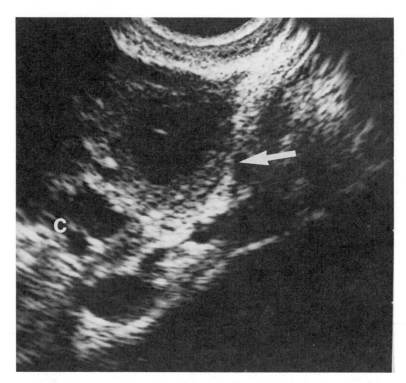

Fig. 24.10 TVS reveals cross section of an unruptured ampullary ectopic pregnancy at 8 weeks gestation (arrow). Blood clots (c) can be identified in the cul-de-sac. (Courtesy of Dr. Michael Blumenfeld, Department of Obstetrics and Gynecology, The Ohio State University, Columbus, Ohio.)

promised, leading to postoperative adhesion formation and scarring.

In the past, regardless of the surgical procedure employed, the overall success rate was poor. Fifty percent of patients did not achieve a viable pregnancy, and approximately 15 percent suffered a second ectopic pregnancy.[3,50,67] After two tubal ectopic pregnancies, between 33 and 50 percent of patients conceived, and approximately 10 to 25 percent had repeat ectopic pregnancies.[68,69] However, more recent data suggest that conservative surgery can result in substantially better reproductive outcomes.

Salpingectomy versus Salpingo-Oophorectomy

During the early 1950s Jeffcoate[70] recommended salpingo-oophorectomy as the surgical procedure of choice for an ectopic pregnancy. Thus, all ovulations would occur on the side of the remaining "normal" tube. This approach has been termed a paradoxical oophorectomy. Although this strategy had some theo-

retical basis, in practice it did not significantly improve subsequent fertility. Conception rates are equal after salpingostomy or salpingectomy alone. Furthermore, since the goal is to save as much ovarian tissue as possible, salpingo-oophorectomy is no longer recommended.

Salpingectomy versus Conservative Tubal Surgery

Recently, the debate as to whether salpingectomy or conservative tubal surgery is warranted in uncomplicated ectopic pregnancies has been renewed. In reviewing the data, one must first eliminate from the salpingostomy group cases in which (1) normal anatomy has clearly been destroyed, (2) the patient is unstable, and (3) there is no desire for further fertility. Today, early diagnosis is common and provides smaller unruptured ectopic pregnancies more suitable for conservative surgical treatment. In addition, microsurgical techniques developed for the treatment of chronic tubal disease (e.g., lavage versus

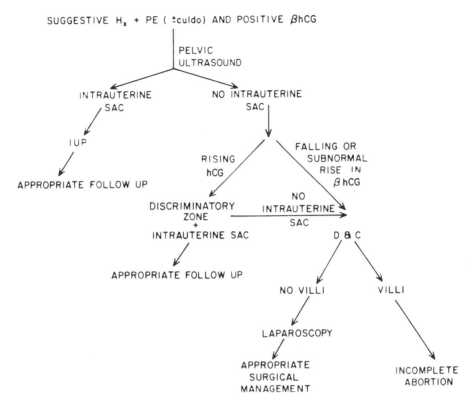

SUGGESTIVE H$_x$ + PE (±culdo) AND POSITIVE βhCG

PELVIC ULTRASOUND

INTRAUTERINE SAC

NO INTRAUTERINE SAC

IUP

APPROPRIATE FOLLOW UP

RISING hCG

FALLING OR SUBNORMAL RISE IN β hCG

DISCRIMINATORY ZONE + INTRAUTERINE SAC

NO INTRAUTERINE SAC

D & C

APPROPRIATE FOLLOW UP

NO VILLI

VILLI

LAPAROSCOPY

APPROPRIATE SURGICAL MANAGEMENT

INCOMPLETE ABORTION

Fig. 24.11 Paradigm illustrating the management of an ectopic pregnancy using β-hCG and ultrasound and the liberal use of laparoscopy. This paradigm will aid in defining an abnormal pregnancy but not in specifically diagnosing an ectopic pregnancy before inspection of the fallopian tube itself or examination of tissue after dilatation and curettage. (From DeCherney et al.,[5] with permission.)

sponging, microelectrocoagulation or laser coagulation, small-gauge nonreactive suture material, and careful handling of tissues) may now be applied to the ectopic pregnancy.[71] Nevertheless, one must question whether salvaging an already damaged tube does not simply increase the repeat ectopic pregnancy rate. In early studies comparing conservative to radical surgical procedures in the management of ectopic pregnancy, Timonen and Nieminen[72] found a pregnancy rate of 53 percent and an ectopic rate of 21 percent following conservative surgery, compared with 49 percent and 12.5 percent, respectively, after radical surgery. These data suggest a slight increase in repeat ectopic pregnancies after conservative surgery. Other workers have been unable to document this difference, and it appears that the repeat ectopic pregnancy rate is approximately the same.[50,65,73–75] On the other hand, conservative surgery did not ap-

pear to increase intrauterine pregnancy rates. Most recently, Langer et al.[74] reported the reproductive outcomes of 118 patients who had undergone conservative surgery for unruptured tubal pregnancies. After conservative therapy, 142 pregnancies were observed, of which 127 (89.4 percent) were intrauterine. The intrauterine pregnancies occurred in 83 patients, or 70.3 percent of the total population, and resulted in 75 live births. Fifteen repeat tubal pregnancies were observed, for a recurrence rate of 12.7 percent. At the time of the initial surgery, 65 patients were noted to have a normal contralateral tube. In this population, 81.5 percent subsequently had an intrauterine pregnancy, 76.1 percent a live birth, and 7.7 percent a recurrent tubal gestation. When the contralateral tube was absent or severely damaged, 57.1 percent of the patients experienced an intrauterine pregnancy and 47.6 percent had a live birth; 28.5

percent suffered a recurrent tubal pregnancy. Expression of the tubal implantation, or "milking" was performed in 33 patients. In this group, 60.6 percent subsequently had an intrauterine pregnancy and 57.5 percent a live birth. None of these patients suffered a recurrent tubal gestation. These results are extremely encouraging and support the use of conservative therapy in the patient with a tubal pregnancy. With further application of microsurgical techniques, these findings will probably be confirmed by other workers (Table 24.1).

TECHNIQUES OF CONSERVATIVE SURGERY

Techniques for conservative surgery in ectopic pregnancy can best be divided into three separate procedures based on the concept that the tube is anatomically and physiologically three different organs: fimbrial-infundibular, ampullary, and isthmic.

Fimbrial-Infundibular

Fimbrial-infundibular pregnancies represent so-called tubal abortions. They can be managed conservatively in two ways. First, one may merely pluck the pregnancy out of the distal end of the tube. This technique demands partial extrusion of the ectopic

Table 24.1 Overall Pregnancy Rate Utilizing Conservative Surgery for the Treatment of Tubal Ectopic Pregnancy

Investigators	Cases (N)	IUP (%)	Repeat Ectopic Pregnancies (%)
DeCherney and Kase[50]	49	39.6	11.6
Timonen and Nieminen[72]	240	38	15.7
Bruhat et al. (laparoscopy)[73]	25	72	12
DeCherney et al.[68] (laparoscopy)[83]	16	50	0
Langer et al.[74]	142	89.4	12.7

pregnancy from the tube before surgery. The second commonly used procedure in managing distal tubal ectopic pregnancies involves so-called milking of the fallopian tube. This procedure involves extrusion of the pregnancy through the distal end of the tube by a squeezing-compressing technique. Early experience showed this method to be the least satisfactory way to deal with ectopic pregnancies. Despite more positive results recently presented by Langer,[72] simple reflection certainly suggests that this method is contrary to all the rules of improved gynecologic surgical technique.[73] In addition, since the ectopic pregnancy has extra luminal growth, one can imagine the enhanced destruction of normal tubal architecture that must result from such vigorous maneuvers. This technique may also increase the chances for persistent trophoblastic growth.

Ampullary

Ampullary ectopic pregnancies are approached surgically by making a linear incision on the antimesenteric side of the tube. The incision can be made with either electrocautery, scalpel, or carbon dioxide or argon laser (Fig. 24.12). The products of conception are extruded, and hemostasis is achieved either by pinpoint electrocautery or by a running whip stitch of 6-0 Vicryl suture. This technique is employed if the tube is allowed to heal by secondary intention.[50] If the tube is to be closed primarily, the closure should be completed in two layers, muscularis and then serosa, with the finest-gauge suture material the surgeon is comfortable using. On occasion, it is difficult to control the bleeding, and one must ligate vessels within the broad ligament, as suggested by Schinfeld and Swolin.[76,77] A question often arises as to whether the operating microscope may be helpful. This instrument has not been found to provide adjunctive therapy of any merit.[71]

It is important not to débride the base of the pregnancy even though there is a tendency to remove most of the remaining trophoblastic tissue. The residual trophoblast does not present a problem. If one follows β-hCG levels postoperatively, there seems to be no difference in the fall of the titers when compar-

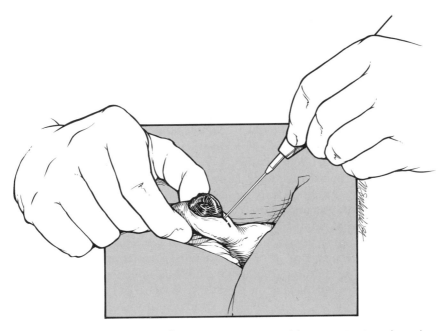

Fig. 24.12 Surgical approach to an ampullary ectopic pregnancy. A linear incision is made on the antimesenteric side of the fallopian tube at the point of maximal bulge. This can be done with electrocautery or the laser. This specific technique should be reserved for ampullary ectopic pregnancies only.

ing cases in which the tubes are left intact and those in which the tube has been removed.[78,79] These prolonged postoperative titers merely represent clearance of the β-hCG hormone. However, as more experience with linear salpingostomy via laparotomy and laparoscopy[77] accumulates and ectopic pregnancies are being treated earlier, there has been an increasing trend noted in the occurrence of persistent ectopic pregnancy following conservative surgery.[80–82] Therefore, it is of critical importance to follow serial β-hCG titers every 6 to 7 days after conservative surgery until nondetectable levels are noted.

A somewhat different approach to laparotomy and linear salpingostomy is the performance of these procedures utilizing the laparoscope.[73,83,84] Careful selection of cases is of utmost importance. A linear salpingostomy is executed on the antimesenteric side of the tube at the point of maximal bulge with either electrocautery or carbon dioxide or argon laser. Bleeding is controlled by laser or electrocautery, and the tube is allowed to heal by secondary intention. Results utilizing this technique in carefully selective

cases have been satisfactory and equal to other conservative techniques (see Table 24.1).

CRITERIA TO BE MET BEFORE LAPAROSCOPIC TREATMENT OF A TUBAL ECTOPIC PREGNANCY

Unruptured ampullary ectopic pregnancy, with conceptus usually less than 3 cm in diameter

Ectopic pregnancy in easily accessible site

Stable vital signs

Skill and experience of the operator with the laparoscope

Isthmic

The third form of ectopic pregnancy, an ectopic pregnancy that occurs in the isthmic portion of the fallopian tube, requires a different surgical approach. In an isthmic gestation, the pregnancy grows in the tubal lumen itself, thereby destroying the tubal endothelial architecture. Linear salpingostomy would not be the procedure of choice, since the lumen has been destroyed and healing would result in occlusion.[85] In fact, isthmic ectopic pregnancies are the only group in which a tubal fistula may result if the tube is allowed to heal by secondary intention after a linear salpingostomy (Fig. 24.13). The procedure of choice for an isthmic ectopic pregnancy is segmental resection.[86] The anastomosis can be performed either primarily or at a future procedure. Although favorable results have been reported with primary anastomosis, it would seem that this is the least optimal time to operate because of tissue hyperemia, edema, and potential for infection due to the presence of old blood. Primary anastomosis does have one important advantage: The tubal lumen is distended, making the anastomosis technically easier.

The overall philosophy in utilizing conservative surgical techniques for ectopic pregnancy must be aimed toward simplicity. Such procedures are usually performed in an emergency setting, and the gynecologic surgeon may lack the technical skills needed for microsurgery. All cases should receive the usual regimen of adjunctive therapy for tubal surgery, including prophylactic antibiotics, and measures to prevent adhesions such as the use of Hyskon (32 percent dextran-70 in dextrose) should be employed.

What procedure should be selected for the patient with recurrent ectopic pregnancies? This clinical dilemma occurs in 10 to 15 percent of patients who have had previous ectopic pregnancies.[45,87,88] Although the conception rate is less than 50 percent

after two previous tubal ectopic pregnancies, the intrauterine pregnancy rate is respectable and permits subsequent conservative procedures.[68,69] Nevertheless, this decision must be carefully weighed because the repeat ectopic pregnancy rate is high.

Consideration of the disposition of the contralateral tube is important for a number of reasons. Should other tubal pathology that might impair fertility be corrected at the time of surgery for the ectopic pregnancy? No, since the same unfavorable situation exists in this instance as it does for primary anastomosis. Should patency of the tube be assessed at the time of surgery for an ectopic pregnancy? Again, no. One may incorrectly conclude that the tube is obstructed because it is edematous, and there may be decidual reaction around the cornua. Furthermore, the risk of introducing infection in this situation must be seriously considered.

Does conservative surgery work at all? Could it be that those patients who conceive after linear salpingostomy are actually conceiving by utilizing the contralateral tube for zygote transport? DeCherney et al.[89] and Valle and Lifchez[90] examined the results in patients with only one fallopian tube who had a conservative surgical procedure performed for an ectopic pregnancy. Their overall findings in 45 patients included a pregnancy rate of approximately 50 percent and a repeat ectopic pregnancy rate of 20 percent. These data support the conclusion that a conservative procedure can be effective. Recurrent ectopic pregnancies are evenly divided between ipsilateral and contralateral tubes when both tubes are present.[5]

SALPINGECTOMY

Radical surgery, salpingectomy, is carried out by cross-clamping the superior position of the broad ligament and removing the damaged tube. Although many surgeons have recommended a small cornual resection, there is no evidence that a deep cornual resection is warranted. Data to document a significant number of pregnancies in the remaining stump are lacking. The raw surfaces created should be covered over by peritoneum. Most surgeons elect to perform a modified Coffey suspension, tacking the round ligament to the posterior surface of the uterus

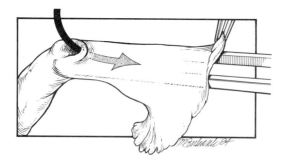

Fig. 24.13 Tubal fistula noted after a linear salpingostomy performed in the isthmic portion of the fallopian tube for an ectopic pregnancy.

with multiple interrupted sutures over the defect created in the broad ligament by division of the mesosalpinx.[91]

NONOPERATIVE MANAGEMENT OF ECTOPIC PREGNANCY

A ruptured ectopic pregnancy constitutes an acute emergency. Newer diagnostic and operative techniques, however, may permit a certain period of contemplative management in the unruptured ectopic pregnancy. Some data do exist as to how often an ectopic pregnancy, left untreated, would resolve spontaneously. Mashiach et al.[92] diagnosed an ectopic pregnancy by laparoscopy in four women. These women were discharged without surgical intervention, and only one returned requiring laparotomy. Unfortunately, this report did not address the damage to normal tubal architecture that might occur when a chronic ectopic pregnancy is left to resolve spontaneously. Recently, 13 asymptomatic patients with falling hCG titers were identified by laparoscopy as having a tubal pregnancy. None received surgical intervention and all were observed. Twelve of 13 patients had apparent reabsorption of the ectopic pregnancy without an eventful course.[93] Additional experience with this approach was described in 14 women with an ampullary ectopic pregnancy confirmed by laparoscopy.[94] Nine patients had spontaneous resolution and 4 eventually required surgery. Hysterosalpingogram (HSG) following spontaneous resolution of these nine ectopic pregnancies demonstrated patency in 6 patients. Thus, limited preliminary data may indicate that expectant management may have its place in carefully selected patients who can be followed with close surveillance.

An adjunct to expectant nonsurgical therapy is the use of chemotherapy to enhance destruction of trophoblastic tissue. This approach should probably be reserved for specific cases. Tanaka et al.[95] demonstrated that administration of methotrexate during an interstitial pregnancy resulted in bilateral tubal patency. After Tanaka's article, enthusiasm for this approach led to reports of use of methotrexate for the treatment of cervical,[96] cornual,[97] and persistent ectopic pregnancies.[98] Sauer et al.[99] and Ichinoe et al.[100] have described the largest clinical experience published to date, including 21 patients who under-

went treatment with a single course of methotrexate (1.0 mg/kg intramuscularly, 4 doses) accompanied by citrovorum factor (0.1 mg/kg). Twenty of 21 patients had resolution of their ectopic pregnancy. On the basis of these data, Sauer et al.[99] suggested that methotrexate could be recommended to treat unruptured ectopic pregnancies less than or equal to 3 cm in diameter. Ichinoe et al.[100] reported 23 patients treated with intramuscular injections of methotrexate (0.4 mg/kg/day for 5 days) every 2 weeks. All but one of 23 patients demonstrated resolution of the ectopic pregnancy, and 10 of 19 showed patent oviducts by HSG or laparoscopy. Reported side effects of methotrexate have included elevated liver enzymes, bone marrow suppression, stomatitis, and dermatitis. At present, more than 76 patients have received methotrexate resulting in a greater than 90 percent resolution of ectopic pregnancy without clinical complications.[101,102] This management may also be considered for patients with an ectopic pregnancy and coexisting hyperstimulation syndrome after induction of ovulation with hCG.

Rh IMMUNIZATION

Rh-negative women may become sensitized after an ectopic pregnancy. Yet, many of these patients are not treated postoperatively to prevent the subsequent development of erythroblastosis fetalis. The American College of Obstetricians and Gynecologists recommends that each patient with an ectopic pregnancy be given 50 μg of Rh immunoglobulin.[103]

SUMMARY

In conclusion, the management of ectopic pregnancy has undergone significant modification over the years. In many cases, it is no longer an acute emergency and is diagnosed earlier in gestation. Newer diagnostic tests, including β-hCG levels, transvaginal ultrasound, and laparoscopy, are largely responsible for these changes. The more frequent detection of an unruptured ectopic pregnancy has dictated the application of conservative surgical procedures that seem to be effective. The combination of microsurgical techniques and other conservative surgical procedures may increase pregnancy rates and perhaps yield a slight decline in repeat ectopic gestations. No technique will totally eliminate repeat ectopic pregnancies, because whatever the etiology (e.g., cellular damage due to infection), the effects are usually bilateral. Ultimately, reconstructive surgery will also reach a limit as to what can be accomplished to salvage fertility for these unfortunate patients.

Overall, women who have suffered an ectopic pregnancy still have a dismal reproductive future. Approximately 50 percent will have a viable intrauterine pregnancy, and 10 to 15 percent will have a repeat ectopic pregnancy. In vitro fertilization offers hope to some patients who have been rendered sterile or infertile after an ectopic pregnancy.

REFERENCES

1. Centers for Disease Control: Ectopic pregnancy—United States, 1987. MMWR 39:401, 1990
2. Thorburn J, Philipson M, Lindblom B: Fertility after ectopic pregnancy in relation to background factors and surgical treatment. Fertil Steril 49:595, 1988
3. Dorfman SF: Deaths from ectopic pregnancy, United States, 1979 to 1980. Obstet Gynecol 62:334, 1983
4. Budnick LD, Pakter J: Ectopic pregnancy in New York City. Am J Public Health 72:580, 1982
5. DeCherney AH, Maheux R: Modern management of tubal pregnancy. p. 61. In Leventhal JM et al: Current Problems in Obstetrics and Gynecology. Year Book, Chicago, 1983
6. Breen JL: A 21 year study of 654 ectopic pregnancies. J Obstet Gynecol 106:1004, 1970
7. Hallat JG: Primary ovarian pregnancy: a report of twenty-five cases. Am J Obstet Gynecol 143:55, 1982
8. Gerin-Lajoie L: Ovarian pregnancy. Am J Obstet Gynecol 62:920, 1951
9. Bello G, Schonholz D, Mosirpur J et al: Combined pregnancy: the Mount Sinai Experience. Obstet Gynecol Surv 41:603, 1986
10. Abrams RA, Kanter AE: Bilateral simultaneous extrauterine pregnancy. Am J Obstet Gynecol 56:1198, 1948
11. Willice R, LeMaire WJ, McLeon AGW: Bilateral tubal pregnancy with an unusual complication. South Med J 16:375, 1973
12. Pauerstein CJ, Eddy CA: The role of oviduct in reproduction: our knowledge and our ignorance. J Reprod Fertil 55:223, 1979
13. Croxatto HB, Ortiz MES: Egg transport in the fallopian tube. Gynecol Invest 6:215, 1975
14. Laufer N, DeCherney AH, Haseltine FP et al: Steroid secretion by the human egg-corona-cumulus complex in culture. J Clin Endocrinol Metab 58:1153, 1984
15. Gemzell G, Guillome J, Wang CF: Ectopic pregnancy following treatment with human gonadotropins. Am J Obstet Gynecol 143:761, 1982
16. McBain JC, Evans JH, Pepperell RJ et al: An unexpectedly high rate of ectopic pregnancy following the induction of ovulation with human pituitary and chorionic gonadotropin. Br J Obstet Gynaecol 87:5, 1980
17. Cheviakoff S, Diaz S, Carril M et al: Ovum transport in women. p. 416. In Harper MJK, Pauerstein CJ, Adams CE et al (eds): Ovum Transport and Fertility Regulation. Scriptor, Copenhagen, 1976
18. Budowick M, Johnson TRB, Genadry R et al: The histopathology of the developing tubal ectopic pregnancy. Fertil Steril 34:169, 1980
19. Marchbanks PA, Annegers JF, Coulam CB et al: Risk factors for ectopic pregnancy: a population-based study. JAMA 259:1823, 1988
20. Mardh PA, Ripa KT, Svensson L et al: *Chlamydia trachomatic* infections in patients with salpingitis. N Engl J Med 296:1377, 1977
21. Westrom L, Bengtsson LP, Mardh PA: Incidence, trends and risks of ectopic pregnancy in a population of women. Br Med J 282:15, 1981
22. Svensson L, Mardh PA, Ahlgren M et al: Ectopic pregnancy and antibodies to *Chlamydia trachomatis*. Fertil Steril 44:313, 1985
23. Hartford SL, Silva PD, diZerega GS: Serologic evidence of prior chlamydial infection in patients with tubal ectopic pregnancy and contralateral tubal disease. Fertil Steril 47:118, 1987
24. Vasquez G, Winston RML, Brosens IA: Tubal mucosa and ectopic pregnancy. Br J Obstet Gynecol 90:468, 1983
25. Patton DL, Moore DE, Spadoni LR et al: A comparison of the fallopian tube's response to overt and silent salpingitis. Obstet Gynecol 73:622, 1989
26. Draper DL, Donegan EA, James JF et al: In vitro modeling of acute salpingitis caused by *Neisseria* gonorrhea. Am J Obstet Gynecol 138:996, 1980
27. Persaud V: Etiology of tubal ectopic pregnancy. Obstet Gynecol 36:257, 1970
28. Levin AA, Schoenbaum SC, Stubblefield PG et al: Ec-

topic pregnancy and prior induced abortion. Am J Public Health 72:253, 1982

29. Panayotou PP, Kaskarelis DB, Miettinen OS et al: Induced abortion and ectopic pregnancy. Am J Obstet Gynecol 114:508, 1972

30. Chung CS, Smith RG, Steingoff PG et al: Induced abortion and ectopic pregnancy in subsequent pregnancies. Am J Epidemiol 115:879, 1982

31. Hallat JG: Ectopic pregnancy associated with the intrauterine device: a study of seventy cases. Am J Obstet Gynecol 125:754, 1976

32. Malhotra N, Chaundhury RR: Current status of intrauterine devices. II: Intrauterine devices and pelvic inflammatory disease and ectopic pregnancy. Obstet Gynecol Surv 37:1, 1982

33. Vessey MP, Yeates D, Flavel R: Risk of ectopic pregnancy and duration of use of an intrauterine device. Lancet 2:501, 1979

34. Ory HW: Women's health study: ectopic pregnancy and intrauterine contraceptive devices: new perspectives. Obstet Gynecol 57:137, 1981

35. DeStefano F, Peterson HB, Layde PM et al: Risk of ectopic pregnancy following tubal sterilization. Obstet Gynecol 60:326, 1982

36. Honore LH, O'Hara KE: Failed tubal sterilization as an etiologic factor in ectopic tubal pregnancy. Fertil Steril 29:509, 1978

37. McCausland A: High rate of ectopic pregnancy following laparoscopic tubal coagulation failures. Am J Obstet Gynecol 136:97, 1980

38. Wolf GC, Thompson NJ: Female sterilization and subsequent ectopic pregnancy. Obstet Gynecol 55:17, 1980

39. Davis MR: Recurrent ectopic pregnancy after tubal sterilization. Obstet Gynecol 68:suppl. 3, 445, 1986

40. Poland BJ, Dill FJ, Styblo C: Embryonic development in ectopic human pregnancy. Teratology 14:315, 1976

41. Elias S, LeBeau M, Simpson JL et al: Chromosome analysis of ectopic human conceptuses. Am J Obstet Gynecol 141:698, 1981

42. Maas DHA, Storey BT, Mastroianni L Jr: Oxygen tension in the oviduct of the rhesus monkey (Macaca mulatta). Fertil Steril 27:1312, 1976

43. Thorburn JEK, Janson PO, Lindstedt G: Early diagnosis of ectopic pregnancy. Acta Obstet Gynecol Scand 62:543, 1983

44. Alsuleiman SA, Grimes EM: Ectopic pregnancy: a review of 147 cases. J Reprod Med 27:101, 1982

45. DeCherney AH, Minkin AJ, Spangler S: Contempo-

rary management of ectopic pregnancy. J Reprod Med 26:519, 1981

46. Brenner PF, Roy S, Mishell DR Jr: Ectopic pregnancy: a study of 300 consecutive surgically treated cases. JAMA 243:673, 1980

47. Silverberg SG: Arias-Stella phenomenon in spontaneous and therapeutic abortion. Am J Obstet Gynecol 112:777, 1972

48. Cole T, Corlett RC Jr: Chronic ectopic pregnancy. Obstet Gynecol 59:63, 1982

49. DeCherney AH, Romero R, Polan ML: Ultrasound in reproductive endocrinology. Fertil Steril 37:323, 1982

50. DeCherney AH, Kase N: The conservative surgical management of unruptured ectopic pregnancy. Obstet Gynecol 54:451, 1979

51. Kauppila A, Rantakyla P, Huhtaniemi I et al: Trophoblastic markers in the differential diagnosis of ectopic pregnancy. Obstet Gynecol 55:560, 1980

52. Lundstrom V, Bremme K, Eneroth P et al: Serum beta-human chorionic gonadotropin levels in the early diagnosis of ectopic pregnancy. Acta Obstet Gynecol Scand 58:231, 1979

53. Ackerman R, Deutsch S, Krumholz B: Levels of human chorionic gonadotropin in unruptured and ruptured ectopic pregnancy. Obstet Gynecol 60:13, 1982

54. Pelosi MA: Use of the radioreceptor assay for human chorionic gonadotropin in the diagnosis of ectopic pregnancy. Acta Obstet Gynecol Scand 152:149, 1981

55. Schwartz RO, DiPietro DL: Beta-hCG as a diagnostic aid for suspected ectopic pregnancy. Surg Gynecol Obstet 56:197, 1980

56. Braunstein GD, Rasor J, Adler D et al: Serum human chorionic gonadotropin levels throughout normal pregnancy. J Obstet Gynecol 126:678, 1976

57. Bryson SCP: Beta-subunit of human chorionic gonadotropin, ultrasound, and ectopic pregnancy: a prospective study. Am J Obstet Gynecol 146:163, 1983

58. Fossum GT, Davajan V, Kletzky OH: Early detection of pregnancy with transvaginal ultrasound. Fertil Steril 49:788, 1988

59. Nyberg DA, Laing FC, Filly RA et al: Ultrasonographic differentiation of the gestational sac of early intrauterine pregnancy from the pseudogestation sac of ectopic pregnancy. Radiology 146:755, 1983

60. Shapiro B, Cullen M, Taylor K et al: Transvaginal ultrasonography for the diagnosis of ectopic pregnancy. Fertil Steril 50:425, 1988

61. Romero R, Kadar N, Castro D et al: The value of

adnexal sonographic findings in the diagnosis of ectopic pregnancy. Am J Obstet Gynecol 158:52, 1988

62. Subramanyam BR, Raghavendra BN, Balthazar EJ et al: Hematosalpinx in tubal pregnancy: sonographic pathologic correlation. AJR 14:361, 1982

63. Kelly MT, Santos-Ramos R, Duenhoelter JH: The value of sonography in suspected ectopic pregnancy. Obstet Gynecol 53:703, 1979

64. Stiller RJ, deRegt RH, Blair E: Transvaginal ultrasonography in patients at risk for ectopic pregnancy. Am J Obstet Gynecol 161:930, 1989

65. Timor-Tritsch IE, Monteagudo A: Transvaginal ultrasonography in obstetrical care: a new frontier. Obstet Gynecol Rep 2:210, 1990

66. Hussa, RO: The Clinical Marker hCG. Praeger, New York, 1987

67. Schenker JG, Evron S: New concepts in the surgical management of tubal pregnancy and the subsequent postoperative results. Fertil Steril 40:709, 1983

68. DeCherney AH, Silidker JS, Mezer HC et al: Reproductive outcome following the ectopic pregnancies. Fertil Steril 43:82, 1985

69. Tulandi T: Reproductive performance of women after two tubal ectopic pregnancies. Fertil Steril 50:164, 1988

70. Jeffcoate TNA: Salpingectomy or salpingo-oophorectomy. Br J Obstet Gynaecol 135:74, 1955

71. DeCherney AH, Polan ML, Kort H et al: Microsurgical technique in the management of tubal ectopic pregnancy. Fertil Steril 34:324, 1980

72. Timonen S, Nieminen U: Tubal pregnancy, choice of operative method of treatment. Acta Obstet Gynecol Scand 46:327, 1967

73. Bruhat MA, Manhes H, Mage G et al: Treatment of ectopic pregnancy by means of laparoscopy. Fertil Steril 33:411, 1980

74. Langer R, Raziel A, Ron-El R et al: Reproductive outcome after conservative surgery for unruptured tubal pregnancy—a 15-year experience. Fertil Steril 53:227, 1982

75. Seigler AM, Wang CF, Westoff C: Management of unruptured tubal pregnancy. Obstet Gynecol 36:599, 1981

76. Schinfeld JS, Reedy G: Mesosalpingeal vessel ligation for conservative treatment of ectopic pregnancy. J Reprod Med 28:823, 1983

77. Swolin K: A tubal surgeon's recommendations for the surgical treatment of ectopic pregnancy. J Reprod Med 25:38, 1980

78. Kamrava MM, Taymor ML, Berger MJ et al: Disappearance of human chorionic gonadotropin following removal of ectopic pregnancy. Obstet Gynecol 62:486, 1983

79. Steier JA, Bergsjo P, Myking OL: Human chorionic gonadotropin in maternal plasma after induced abortion, spontaneous abortion and removed ectopic pregnancy. Obstet Gynecol 64:391, 1984

80. DiMarchi J, Kosasa T, Kobara T et al: Persistent ectopic pregnancy. Obstet Gynecol 70:555, 1987

81. Seifer DB, Gutman JN, Doyle MB et al: Persistent ectopic pregnancy following laparoscopic linear salpingostomy. Obstet Gynecol 76:1121, 1990

82. Seifer DB, Diamond MP, DeCherney AH: Persistent ectopic pregnancy. Obstet Gynecol Clin North Am 18:145, 1991

83. DeCherney AH, Diamond M: Laparoscopic salpingostomy for ectopic pregnancy. Obstet Gynecol 70:948, 1987

84. DeCherney AH, Romero R, Naftolin F: Surgical management of unruptured ectopic pregnancy. Fertil Steril 35:21, 1981

85. DeCherney AH, Naftolin F, Graebe R: Isthmic ectopic pregnancy: segmental resection and anastomosis to conserve fertility. Fertil Steril 41:45S, 1984

86. DeCherney AH, Boyers S: Isthmic ectopic pregnancy: segmental resection as the treatment of choice. Fertil Steril 44:307, 1985

87. Hallat JG: Repeat ectopic pregnancy: a study of 123 consecutive cases. Am J Obstet Gynecol 122:520, 1975

88. Schoen JA, Nowak RJ: Repeat ectopic pregnancy: a 16-year clinical study. Obstet Gynecol 45:542, 1975

89. DeCherney AH, Maheux R, Naftolin F: Salpingostomy for ectopic pregnancy in the sole patent oviduct: reproductive outcome. Fertil Steril 37:619, 1982

90. Valle JA, Lifchez AS: Reproductive outcome following conservative surgery for tubal pregnancy in women with a single fallopian tube. Fertil Steril 39:316, 1983

91. Novy MJ: Surgical alternatives for ectopics: is conservative treatment best? Contemp Obstet Gynecol 21:91, 1983

92. Mashiach S, Carp HJA, Serr DM: Nonoperative management of ectopic pregnancy: a preliminary report. J Reprod Med 27:127, 1982

93. Garcia AJ, Aubert JM, Sama J, Josimovich JB: Expectant management of presumed ectopic pregnancies. Fertil Steril 48:395, 1987

94. Fernandez H, Rainhorn JD, Papiernik E et al: Spontaneous resolution of ectopic pregnancy. Obstet Gynecol 71:171, 1988

95. Tanaka T, Hayashi H, Kutsuzawa T: Treatment of in-

terstitial ectopic pregnancy with methotrexate: report of a successful case. Fertil Steril 37:851, 1982

96. Farabow W, Fulton J, Fletcher V et al: Cervical pregnancy treated with methotrexate. NC Med J 44:91, 1983

97. Brandes MC, Youngs DD, Goldstein DP et al: Treatment of cornual pregnancy with methotrexate: case report. Am J Obstet Gynecol 155:655, 1986

98. Higgins KA, Schwartz MB: Treatment of persistent trophoblast tissue after salpingostomy with methotrexate. Fertil Steril 45:427, 1986

99. Sauer MV, Gorrill MJ, Rodi IA et al: Nonsurgical management of unruptured ectopic pregnancy: an extended clinical trial. Fertil Steril 48:752, 1987

100. Ichinoe K, Wake N, Shinkai N et al: Nonsurgical therapy to preserve oviduct function in patients with tubal pregnancies. Am J Gynecol 156:484, 1987

101. Ory SJ, Villanueva AL, Sand PK et al: Conservative treatment of ectopic pregnancy with methotrexate. Am J Obstet Gynecol 154:1299, 1986

102. Ory SJ: Ectopic pregnancy current evaluation and treatment. Mayo Clinic Proc 64:874, 1989

103. American College of Obstetricians and Gynecologists: Prevention of D isoimmunization. ACOG Tech Bull 147, 1990

104. Koonin LM, Atrash HK, Rochat RW et al: Maternal mortality surveillance, United States, 1980–85. In: CDC Surveillance Summaries. MMWR 37:19, 1988

Chapter 25

Preterm Birth

Denise M. Main and Elliott K. Main

Despite the many medical and social advances of the past 40 years, the incidence of preterm deliveries has remained almost constant in the United States. One would have hoped that the introduction of tocolytic therapy, the improvements in the diagnosis of multiple gestation and placenta previa by ultrasound, the marked decrease in untreated syphilis (a major cause of prematurity in the past), and government-funded medical assistance and nutritional supplementation programs would have decreased the incidence of prematurity dramatically. Unfortunately, the national preterm delivery rate remains over 9 percent of all live births.

Indeed, the problem of preterm delivery has become magnified as other causes of perinatal morbidity and mortality have decreased. At least 75 percent of neonatal deaths not caused by congenital malformations result from preterm delivery. Although the relative risk of neonatal death is much higher than that of lasting morbidity, prematurity disproportionately contributes to developmental delay, visual and hearing impairment, chronic lung disease, and cerebral palsy.[1] For example, an infant born weighing less than 1,500 g is approximately 200 times more likely to die in infancy and, if a survivor, 10 times more likely to be neurologically impaired than a peer born weighing more than 2,500 g. Even in seemingly intact preterm survivors, school failure and family disruption are more common. Given the high rates of these complications and their close association with birth weight, it becomes very apparent that significant overall improvements in infant, child, and family health are very dependent on preventing preterm birth.

DEFINITIONS AND STATISTICS

To address this major medical and social issue, it is first necessary to review definitions. The classic term prematurity refers to birth weight less than 2,500 g. In its place are often substituted preterm to describe infants born before 37 weeks gestation (259 days from the first day of the mother's last menstrual period [LMP]) and low birth weight (LBW) to include infants regardless of gestational age who weigh less than 2,500 g at birth. Very low birth weight (VLBW) typically refers to infants weighing less than 1,500 g at birth.

Because of difficulty in accurately assigning gestational age, many studies have used a birth weight definition, equating a birth weight of less than 2,500 g with preterm birth. Although birth weight and gestational age are closely related, interchanging the two measures can lead to significant errors; 2,500 g is not the mean weight for 37 weeks gestation but rather for 35 weeks gestation. If LBW criteria alone are used, one-half of all babies born at 35 weeks gestation would be classified as term. Similarly, only 54 percent of LBW infants are preterm.[2]

Birth weight is influenced by a number of important factors in addition to gestational age, including race, parity, fetal sex, and environmental conditions such as altitude. The mean birth weight mentioned above is that reported by Brenner and associates[3] (Fig. 25.1). It is based on a racially mixed population near sea level in North Carolina. Ideally, each medical center should generate a birth weight versus gestational age chart for its own population. In the absence of such data, a published chart based on a similar population can be used.

The incidences of LBW and VLBW deliveries have remained almost constant since 1950, as illustrated in Figure 25.2. Over 69 per 1,000 liveborn infants are LBW, with 12 per 1,000 liveborns weighing less than 1,500 g. Rates of LBW and VLBW newborns in non-whites are consistently about twice as high as corresponding rates in whites (Fig. 25.3). Even when corrected for age and educational level, black women continue to deliver more LBW infants than do white women. In fact, the incidence of LBW and VLBW infants per 1,000 liveborn infants in nonwhites actually increased during the 1950s and 1960s, attributed in part to the increase in hospital deliveries for black women, with more LBW deliveries reported. A slight decline in the incidence of LBW newborns occurred during the 1970s. The major portion of this decrease resulted from a decrease in term LBW infants rather than in preterm LBW infants.[4] This improvement in term LBW has occurred equally in white and non-white populations. Data from 1980 to 1985 show no change, despite the availability of tocolysis (Fig.

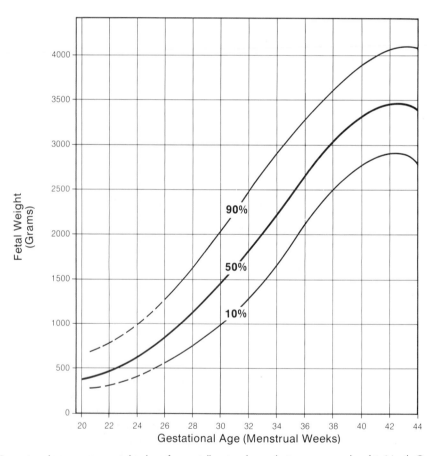

Fig. 25.1 Gestational age versus weight chart for racially mixed population near sea level in North Carolina. (Adapted from Brenner et al.,[3] with permission.)

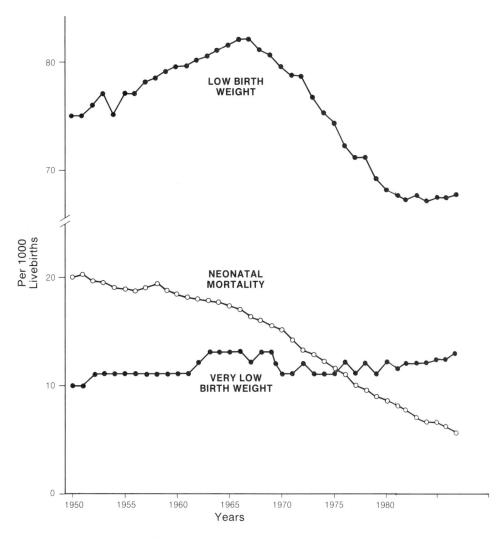

Fig. 25.2 Incidence of low birth weight, very low birth weight, and neonatal mortality per 1,000 live births in the United States for 1950–1987.

25.4).[5] The former analysis is based on data obtained from the annual volumes of *Vital Statistics of the United States,* which is clearly subject to the limitations of the initial data collection. Gestational age is computed from the date the LMP began as reported on birth certificates by 38 to 48 states, depending on the year studied.

Using the same data base, it is possible to calculate preterm delivery rates. Not surprisingly, there have also been minimal changes in this index. In 1970, the overall incidence of delivery at less than 37 completed weeks gestation was 93 per 1,000 live births. In 1987, the overall preterm delivery rate was 101 per 1,000 live births.[2] Blacks experienced a preterm delivery rate of 177 per 1,000 live births in 1970 and 178 per 1,000 in 1987 compared with 78 per 1,000 in 1970 and 85 per 1,000 in 1987 for whites. In addition, during this period, the gestational age at time of preterm delivery has been stable, with blacks experiencing a higher percentage of very early deliveries than whites (see Table 25.1 for 1987 data). Of the black infants born before 37 weeks gestation, 24.2 percent

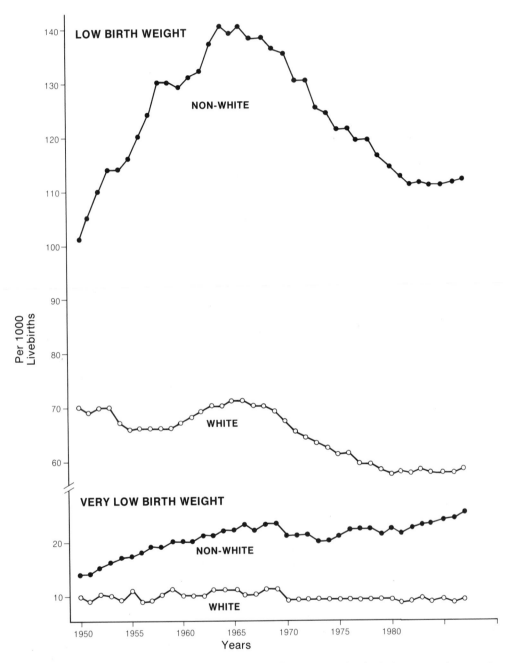

Fig. 25.3 Incidence of low birth weight and very low birth weight per 1,000 live births by race in the United States for 1950–1987.

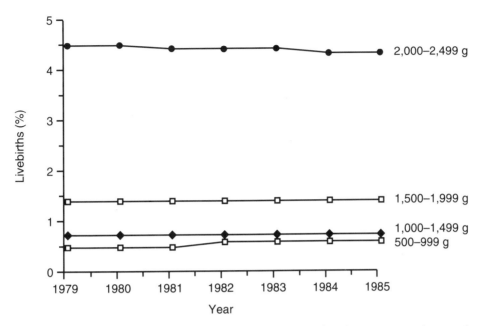

Fig. 25.4 Annual percentages of live births by 500-g categories for births less than 2,500 g in the United States for 1979–1985. (From Leveno et al.,[5] with permission.)

were less than 32 weeks gestation. In contrast, only 16.6 percent of the white preterm babies were born before 32 weeks gestation.

Neonatal Mortality

Despite the relative stability in the rate of preterm and LBW infants born in the United States since 1950, there has been a dramatic decrease in neonatal mortality, as shown in Figure 25.2. Much of this decrease can be attributed to improvements in the neonatal and perinatal care of preterm infants. Despite the marked improvement in neonatal survival over the past 40 years, the United States still compares relatively unfavorably with other developed countries

with respect to neonatal mortality. In 1986, 20 countries reported lower national neonatal mortality rates than the United States. Birth weight–specific neonatal mortality rates from the United States, however, are comparable with or lower than those of most developed countries. For example, a 28-week, 1,000-g newborn has a better chance of survival if born in Massachusetts than in Sweden.[6] Thus the major reason for the poor international rank in neonatal mortality listings in the United States is its unfavorable birth weight distributions. Any major improvement in the international standing of the United States awaits reduction in the proportion of high-risk LBW neonates.

Gestational Age-Specific Neonatal Mortality

A person's a person no matter how small.
From *Horton Hears a Who,* Dr. Seuss, 1954

Obstetricians must repeatedly make decisions regarding the management of VLBW preterm fetuses. One of the most important determinants of good neonatal outcome is the assessment of potential viability.

Table 25.1 Live Births by Period of Gestation (Weeks) and Race — 1987

	20–27	28–31	32–35	36
All women	7.3	11.4	48.2	33.1
White	6.2	10.4	47.9	35.5
Black	10.2	14.0	48.6	27.2

(Adapted from U.S. Department of Health and Human Services.[2])

Paul and colleagues[7] have shown that infants misjudged to be previable experience significantly higher mortality rates than do infants of the same weight and gestational age who are correctly estimated to be viable and receive intensive intrapartum care.

Neonatal survival data are often best presented for obstetricians in terms of best obstetric estimation of gestational age (Fig. 25.5). In part, this is because accurate in utero assessment of birth weight is difficult, especially in the presence of preterm rupture of membranes or preterm labor.[8] In addition, a recent nationwide Dutch study found obstetric estimate of gestational age to be a better predictor of neonatal mortality than actual birth weight.[9]

Over the past few decades, as neonatal and perinatal care has improved, the answer to the question "What is the lower limit of viability?" has been a progressively earlier gestational age. A handful of recent reports describe infants born at 22 weeks gestation who survive to hospital discharge, although these are rare, remarkable cases (and often involve larger than expected babies!). Survival at 23 weeks is also rare,

with rates ranging from 0 to 8 percent.[10–17] By 24 weeks gestation, survival becomes a reasonable possibility, with approximately 15 to 20 percent of all liveborns at this gestation surviving to hospital discharge. Recent series from tertiary centers often reveal that 50 to 60 percent of 25-week gestation neonates survive as do up to 85 percent of 26- to 28-week gestation neonates. By 29 weeks, survival is often in excess of 90 percent. Significant progress in survival rates have occurred between the early and late 1980s, especially for the 24- to 28-week fetus.[10,11] Application of aggressive obstetric and neonatal techniques to 22- and 23-week gestation infants, however, has minimally affected survival, suggesting a significant viability threshold of approximately 24 weeks gestation (and/or 600 g estimated birth weight).[10]

The survival figures cited above include all liveborn infants born at the reporting institutions, even those not successfully transferred from the delivery room to the nursery. Not surprisingly, higher survival rates are reported when only neonatal unit admissions are analyzed. Other variables such as infant sex (more girls survive than boys) and race (blacks weighing less

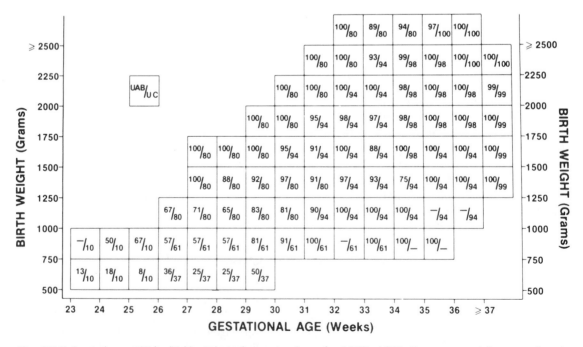

Fig. 25.5 Survival rates (%) by birth weight and gestational age for 1979–1981. Data in upper left corner of each square are from the University of Alabama at Birmingham; data in lower right corner are from the University of Colorado. (From Goldenberg et al.,[274] with permission.)

than 3,000 g do better than whites) influence survival significantly as well (Fig. 25.6). Several reviewers have demonstrated significant survival differences not explained by the above listed demographic factors.[18,19] Thus, when available, it is always best to use local statistics when evaluating patients.

Some investigators report improved survival rates for infants born at tertiary centers when compared with liveborn infants of comparable size and age transferred to neonatal centers after delivery[20] (Fig. 25.7). Others suggest no difference in long-term survival based on hospital level at delivery but some reduction in short-term neonatal morbidity with delivery at a tertiary center.[21] Part of the difficulty in comparing outcomes between inborn and outborn neonates is that maternal antepartum diagnoses differ between women transferred prior to delivery and those whose babies are transferred following birth.[22] Infants of women transferred prior to the onset of labor appear to do better than do those

transferred because of labor.[23] This may reflect an improved survival rate (though worse long-term neurologic morbidity rate) for growth-retarded, extremely preterm infants.[23] Multiple gestation newborns experience both lower survival and higher long-term morbidity.[23]

Gestational Age-Specific Neonatal Morbidity

Preterm infants are at risk for specific diseases relating to the immaturity of various organ systems. Common complications in these very premature infants include respiratory distress syndrome (RDS), bronchopulmonary dysplasia (BPD), patent ductus arteriosus (PDA), necrotizing enterocolitis (NEC), apnea, intraventricular hemorrhage (IVH), and retrolental fibroplasia (RLF). Extremely preterm infants are at greatest risk. There is wide interinstitutional variation in the frequency of these sequelae, which may reflect in part differences in definitions as well as clinical practices.[18]

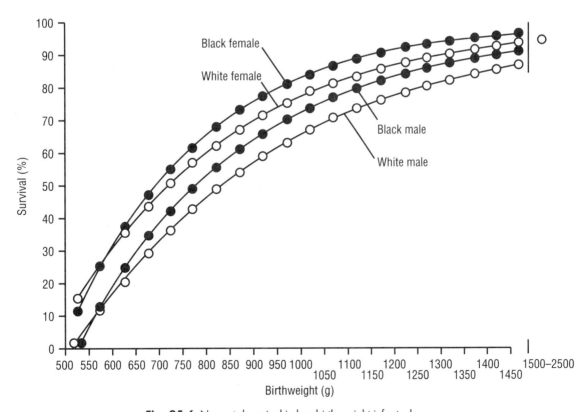

Fig. 25.6 Neonatal survival in low-birth-weight infants, by race.

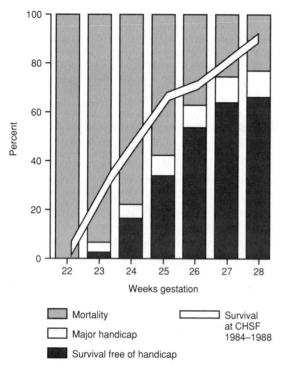

Fig. 25.7 Neonatal outcome at 22 to 28 weeks gestation at the Children's Hospital of San Francisco.

Long-Term Morbidity

During the 1950s, preterm infants were found to be at increased risk for serious neurodevelopmental handicaps such as severe mental retardation (IQ or DQ [developmental quotient] < 70), significant cerebral palsy, major seizure disorders, blindness, and deafness. Since then, concern about long-term neurologic sequelae has focused on progressively smaller infants of increasingly earlier gestational age. The rate of serious long-term disability increases with decreasing birth weight, but within each birth weight group the proportion of survivors who have serious handicaps has not changed significantly since the introduction of neonatal intensive care.[19] For infants born between 1975 and 1985, 26 percent of surviving infants with birth weights below 800 g, 17 percent of survivors with birth weights between 750 and 1,000 g, and 11 percent of survivors with birth weights between 1,000 and 1,500 g have major handicaps at 1 or 2 years of age. More moderate impairment defined as an IQ between 70 and 80 has been reported in an additional 41 percent of neonates born at less than 800 g, 31 percent born between 750

and 1,000 g, and 16 percent between 1,000 and 1,500 g birth weight.[19]

Studies of neurologic outcome are of necessity reviews of prior neonatal practices. Most outcome studies are based on 1 to 2 years of careful follow-up examinations, which may overestimate neurologic impairment. Longer term longitudinal studies are needed to identify problems with school performance or behavior. In this regard, several studies with longer periods of follow-up are worrisome; for example, a 10-year follow-up study of survivors weighing less than 1,000 g at birth revealed that 64 percent required special education.[24] Furthermore, hyperactive behavior is much more common in LBW infants compared with term controls. One study found that one-third of less than 1,500-g birth weight infants were hyperactive.[25] The less than 1,000-g group was not more affected than the 1,000- to 1,500-g group. Children described as hyperactive score less well on mental development tests at age 2 years than at age 1, suggesting that this behavior disorder affects test performance. Poor nonwhite children who are preterm are at particularly great risk to show a decrease in cognitive development over time, demonstrating the additive effects of perinatal and social risk factors.[26]

Investigators have sought to identify risk factors that might predispose to poor neurologic outcome. Few factors have been found to be predictive of neurologic damage. Factors implicated by some investigators include intraventricular hemorrhage, seizures, and long-term failure to regain birth weight.[27] One study found male infants to have more than twice the impairment rate of females.[28]

Preterm infants may also be at greater risk of experiencing other non-neurologic morbidity, such as chronic pulmonary disease or severe illness in general.[1] Besides the prolonged hospitalization at birth, a substantial portion of VLBW infants are rehospitalized during the first year of life.[29] Although much less well studied, there is concern that preterm birth disrupts maternal–infant bonding, which can have a major impact on family function.[1]

FACTORS ASSOCIATED WITH INCREASED PRETERM DELIVERY

A large number of epidemiologic studies have attempted to identify women at high risk to experience preterm delivery. Reproducible risk factors include low socioeconomic status, nonwhite race, maternal age of 18 years or less or of 40 years or more, low prepregnancy weight, and smoking.[30,31] For example, black college-educated women have fewer preterm infants than do black women who have not completed high school. At any given educational level, however, white women experience fewer preterm births than do blacks (Table 25.2). A further demonstration of the confounding association of low socioeconomic status with prematurity is that Mexican-Americans of comparable low socioeconomic class to blacks have far fewer preterm births.[2]

Maternal smoking level correlates very significantly with perinatal mortality, preterm delivery, premature preterm rupture of membranes, and bleeding during pregnancy.[32]

The impact of maternal employment on preterm delivery is controversial. Employed women as a whole do not deliver more preterm infants than do women without paid employment.[33] However, occupations associated with great fatigue and long work hours may predispose to preterm delivery, especially for women who have a history of prior poor pregnancy outcomes.[34]

One study of female obstetric residents suggested an increased risk of intrauterine growth retardation.[35] In a national sample of all residents, preterm labor and preeclampsia were increased, but preterm delivery and growth retardation were similar to the controls.[36]

Coitus and/or orgasm have been linked to prematurity in some studies[37,38] but not in others.[39,40] All of these studies have major design flaws, leaving open the question of a relationship between preterm delivery and sexual activity.

Women who do not seek prenatal care are significantly more likely to deliver before term regardless of social class. It is unclear whether there are intrinsic differences between women who obtain prenatal care and those who do not or whether some feature of prenatal care helps to minimize prematurity. Socially disadvantaged women appear to gain the most from prenatal care.[41] One study suggests that women who report major life event stresses during the third trimester of pregnancy are more likely to experience preterm labor.[42] In these cases, it is proposed that increased maternal catecholamine release secondary to maternal stress leads to uterine irritability. Although stress may be etiologic in some cases of preterm labor, it is difficult to evaluate inasmuch as the impact of life events is mediated by social support and mental health, factors that have not been adequately controlled in the obstetric literature.

Maternal nutritional status and weight gain in pregnancy are commonly assumed to relate to neonatal birth weight and preterm delivery. Certainly, extremes of malnutrition and starvation lead to a decrease in birth weight.[43,44] What remains unclear is the relationship between a variety of nutritional supplements and pregnancy outcome in women of all socioeconomic strata in the United States.[43] For example, additional protein supplementation in pregnancy in New York City was associated with a significant *increase* in neonatal mortality and a nonsignificant *decrease* in birth weight (32 g less than controls).[45] Of interest are the roles of copper and zinc balance in pregnancy. Low maternal serum zinc levels have been associated with preterm labor and low maternal and/or neonatal copper levels with preterm rupture of membranes.[46,47] However, further research is needed before supplementation with these trace metals can be recommended, especially because they may affect the balance of other metals such as iron and calcium. An interesting association between a woman's own low birth weight and the low birth weight of her offspring suggests that a mother's intrauterine growth and nutrition may be critical to her ability to bear full-term appropriately sized infants.[48] This association may explain in part the persistence of higher preterm delivery rates for well-educated black women.

The incidence of preterm birth correlates strongly with prior obstetric outcome. The history of one previous preterm birth is associated with a recurrence risk of 17 to 40 percent, with the risk increasing with the number of preterm births and decreasing with the number of term deliveries.[49–51] There is also a clear

Table 25.2 Low-Birth-Weight Rate by Race and Education: United States — 1987

| Race | Years of School Completed by Mother | | | | |
	0 – 8	9 – 11	12	13 – 15	16 +
White	8.2	8.5	5.5	4.7	4.2
Black	14.0	14.9	12.4	10.9	9.3

increase in subsequent preterm deliveries in women who have experienced one or more second-trimester abortions.[49] One spontaneous or legally induced first-trimester abortion does not increase the risk for prematurity.[50,52-54] There is still debate whether multiple first-trimester–induced abortions are associated with a higher preterm delivery rate, with some investigators finding such an association[54] and others not.[52]

Women with uterine malformations are also at greater risk for preterm delivery. The risk varies with the abnormality. Women with unicornuate or bicornuate uteri have worse pregnancy outcomes than do women with a complete uterine septum (Table 25.3).[55] Cerclage placement and metroplasty may improve pregnancy outcome in selected patients. Uterine myomata have been associated with increased antepartum bleeding and preterm labor.[56] The location of the myomata is an important consideration, with submucosal and subplacental being the most worrisome.

Cervical incompetence, whether secondary to trauma from a prior obstetric or gynecologic procedure, a result of diethylstilbestrol (DES) exposure in utero, or of unknown etiology, classically leads to painless second-trimester cervical dilatation and abortion. Once dilatation has occurred, preterm labor and/or rupture of membranes can occur, often making it difficult to establish the etiology of the preterm birth. Because of differences in definition and populations, the absolute contribution of this entity

to preterm delivery is unclear, with estimates of its incidence ranging from 1 in 1,000 to 1 in 54 deliveries. Diagnostic criteria and therapy for this condition are discussed in greater detail later in this chapter.

Between 1 and 1.5 million fetuses were exposed to DES between the late 1940s and 1971. Multiple studies have shown these women to be at increased risk for preterm delivery (15 to 28 percent of pregnancies) and spontaneous abortions (20 to 40 percent).[57] Furthermore, exposed women with genital malformations (T-shaped or other uterine abnormality, cervical incompetence, vaginal and/or cervical structural abnormalities) are more likely to experience preterm births and spontaneous abortions than are exposed women who do not have such structural changes.

Current pregnancy complications including placenta previa or abruptio, polyhydramnios or oligohydramnios, first-trimester bleeding, and multiple gestation have been associated with preterm delivery.[30,31] The only other placental abnormality that may predispose to preterm labor is a marginal insertion of the umbilical cord into the placenta. Women with cervical examination changes in dilatation and/or effacement are susceptible to spontaneous early births. A number of medical complications such as severe hypertension and worsening vascular compromise from diabetes can lead to preterm delivery for either maternal or fetal indications.

There is speculation that some cases of preterm labor may result from the fetus "perceiving" that intrauterine conditions are unfavorable. It has been hypothesized that fetal stress may increase fetal adrenal steroid production and lead to the onset of labor. Although this concept is poorly defined and reported, it behooves the obstetrician to take care to document fetal well-being before and during aggressive tocolytic therapy. Fetuses with congenital anomalies, especially when associated with oligohydramnios or polyhydramnios, often are born prior to term.

A growing body of evidence suggests that maternal genital tract infection and/or colonization may be among the most important preventable causes of preterm births.[58,59] Young, poor, nonwhite women are at increased risk for both sexually transmitted diseases and prematurity. The association between chorioamnionitis and preterm birth is well established, especially in the presence of preterm rupture of membranes. An increased rate of preterm delivery has

Table 25.3 Reproductive Performances of Patients With Uterine Abnormalities[a]

Anomaly	Abortion (%)	Preterm Delivery (%)	Term Delivery (%)	N
Unicornuate	47	20	33	15
Didelphys	32	24	44	25
Bicornuate complete	17	66	17	6
Bicornuate partial	28	20	52	92
Arcuate	28	14	58	46
Complete septum	17	3	79	29
Partial septum	31	12	58	52

[a] Results of 265 pregnancies in 182 patients, which include 19 patients with metroplasty. (Modified from Heinonen et al.,[55] with permission.)

been associated with group B streptococci, *Neisseria gonorrhoeae, Chlamydia trachomatis, Ureaplasma urealyticum, Treponema pallidum, Trichomonas vaginalis,* and *Gardnerella vaginalis.* However, the relative contribution of these organisms to prematurity and the potential benefits of antibiotic therapy remain unresolved.

Immediate Causes of Preterm Birth

Broadly categorized, there are four main obstetric diagnoses that result in preterm delivery. These are preterm labor, preterm premature rupture of the membranes (PPROM), maternal medical or obstetric complications, and fetal distress or demise. Meis et al.[60] recently studied the relative contributions of these factors as indicators for all low-birth-weight deliveries in a nine-county region in North Carolina. Using two samples of approximately 1,500 women each, one group receiving public assistance and the other having private insurance, this study showed significant differences in the obstetric factors leading to preterm, low-birth-weight deliveries (Fig. 25.8). PPROM and medical complications (both maternal and fetal) occurred significantly more often in the public pay (predominantly black) sample. Other investigators have suggested that more births under

1,000 g result from nonpreventable conditions than do births of larger low-birth-weight infants.[61]

Identifying Women Likely To Deliver Before Term by Risk-Scoring Indices

Identifying women at high risk to experience preterm labor is a necessary first step in preventing preterm births. Such identification both permits the physician to monitor the selected patient more carefully and lowers the threshold for intervention should problems arise during pregnancy. Several risk-scoring systems have been developed based on the factors outlined above to identify women likely to deliver preterm or LBW infants. Of these, the system devised by Papiernik and Kaminski[30] and modified by Creasy et al.[62] has been the most extensively applied. It was prospectively validated in New Zealand, although only 30 percent of women classified as high risk actually delivered prior to term.[62] When applied in the United States, however, similar screening systems have been disappointing.[63] Sensitivities have generally been under 50 percent and positive predictive values less than 20 percent. Thus there is a need for more objective, sensitive, and widely applicable indicators for those women likely to deliver preterm infants.

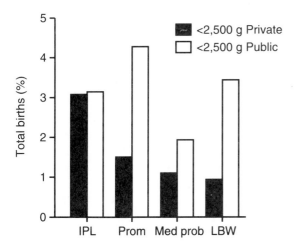
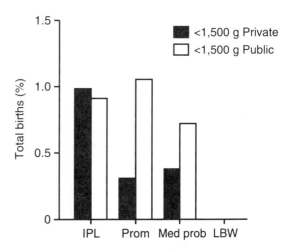

Fig. 25.8 Causes of preterm birth in obstetric patients with private insurance versus those with public assistance. (A) Birth weight under 2,500 g. (B) Birth weight under 1,500 g. IPL, idiopathic preterm labor; PROM, premature rupture of membranes; MedProb, medical complications, LBW, low birthweight. (Data from Meis et al.[60])

Biochemical and Biophysical Indices

Uterine activity may be an important predictor of preterm labor. Caldeyro-Barcia and Poseiro[64] demonstrated that women experience contractions at increasing frequency over a number of weeks before actual labor. Women destined to labor before term experience increased uterine contractility earlier in gestation than do those who labor first after 37 weeks gestation.[65] One study suggests that it is possible to identify women at significantly increased risk for preterm labor by monitoring them for 1 hour per week for uterine activity.[66] Women without known medical risks for preterm labor and who contracted over six times in at least 1 hour period between 28 and 32 weeks gestation had a 32 percent chance of developing preterm labor. In contrast, women who remained below the uterine contraction threshold experienced a significantly lower preterm labor rate (4 percent, respectively).[66] Although encouraging, this approach needs to be tested prospectively in larger samples before it can be widely applied.

Women with cervical dilatation of at least 2 cm at 26 to 30 weeks gestation are at significantly increased risk (27 percent chance) to deliver an infant weighing less than 2 kg.[67] Several studies have also demonstrated that women with more subtle cervical change are at somewhat increased risk to deliver prior to term.[68-70] On review, it is somewhat disappointing to note that more subtle cervical findings, although statistically significant in large samples, also have low positive predictive values and sensitivities.

A more recent observation is that women with vaginal pH readings of more than 4.5 appear to be at increased risk to experience PPROM or preterm labor.[71,72] This finding may be a reflection of the known association between bacterial vaginosis and anaerobic organisms and both preterm labor and PPROM. Further prospective studies are needed to determine if this potentially simple measurement may be a useful adjunct to risk screening.

Approaches to the Prevention of Preterm Birth

Assuming that at least a proportion of the women at risk for preterm deliveries can be identified, are there additional approaches above routine prenatal care that can prevent preterm labor and birth in these high-risk patients? A number of treatment regimens have been proposed, including the use of progesterone supplementation, prophylactic β-mimetic agents, the liberal use of cerclage, and the prescription of bed rest. None has clearly been shown to be of prophylactic benefit. In addition, intensive patient education programs and home uterine activity monitoring have been promoted to aid in the early diagnosis of preterm labor. These approaches are discussed here except for cerclage, which is covered in a later section of this chapter.

Parenteral progesterone, usually 17α-hydroxyprogesterone caproate (Delalutin), has been used for prophylaxis against preterm labor. Studies by Johnson and colleagues[73] suggested that 250 mg Delalutin given intramuscularly weekly decreased the incidence of preterm births in treated women who had either two or more prior preterm deliveries or miscarriages. Because of the small number of patients studied and the better results in the initial randomly controlled study as compared with the later, nonrandomized study, these reports are usually considered tentative. Initial concern about the teratogenicity of these agents has not been confirmed[74] (see Ch. 11). A more recent report from Israel described 160 patients who had at least two pregnancies immediately prior to the index pregnancy, which resulted in preterm birth or miscarriage.[75] Those receiving 250 mg Delalutin weekly had a significantly lower preterm labor rate than that of controls (29 vs. 59 percent) and a significantly lower rate of preterm births (16 vs. 38 percent). In addition, all of these women were treated with cerclages, and many received tocolytics. A study of an active-duty military population in the United States receiving 1,000 mg Delalutin IM weekly failed to demonstrate any reduction in preterm delivery rates compared with a placebo group.[76] Overall, the active-duty population was at higher risk than were military dependents, but still at relatively low risk. Of the 80 treated patients, 6.3 percent experienced preterm labor compared with 5.7 percent of the 88 controls.

The prophylactic use of β-mimetic agents before the onset of preterm labor has not been extensively evaluated, especially in singleton gestations. One study of 38 primigravid patients with preterm cervical dilatation demonstrated no benefit from a low-dose

(40 mg/day) prophylactic course of ritodrine.[77] These agents are commonly used without cervical change (i.e., prophylactically) in this country. As Leveno et al.[5] recently summarized, the large-scale use of ritodrine has not been associated with either a reduction in preterm or low-birth-weight deliveries or a shift to less preterm or larger low-birth-weight deliveries. Because of the lack of clearly demonstrated benefit and the potential for tachyphylaxis with β-mimetics, it is our recommendation that they should not be used before the onset of true preterm labor.

Reduced activity or bed rest in the late second and early third trimesters is commonly recommended as a means of potentially decreasing preterm births. This therapy is often prescribed for women with multiple gestations, although most studies do not demonstrate a prolongation of gestation.[78,79] Surprisingly, despite its common usage, there are no studies of its efficacy in high-risk singleton pregnancies. Furthermore, there is very little agreement as to what actually constitutes "reduced activity."

A pilot study suggested that educating women at high risk for preterm birth about the signs and symptoms of preterm labor and following these women closely with weekly or biweekly pelvic examinations enabled them to present earlier in the course of preterm labor.[80] Because of earlier, more successful therapy with tocolytics, the incidence of preterm births was decreased after the institution of this approach. Randomized controlled trials utilizing this approach, however, have failed to demonstrate benefit.[81-83] Most of these more rigorously designed studies have been performed with indigent populations. As noted earlier, preterm deliveries in poorer women are less likely to result from preterm labor, the main focus of this intervention strategy. In contrast, one large regional evaluation of this approach has suggested benefit in private pay but not public assistance patients.[84] Nonetheless, the lack of demonstrated benefit in the most rigorously controlled studies suggests limited utility of this aggressive outpatient management scheme.

An indirect extension of this approach is the utilization of daily home uterine activity monitoring of high-risk patients. As noted earlier, women destined to labor before term exhibit higher uterine contraction rates earlier in gestation than do women who first labor at term.[64,65] Even women carefully educated regarding the signs and symptoms of preterm contractions fail to identify the majority of monitor-detected uterine activity.[85]

Usually, patients enrolled in a home uterine activity monitoring program are selected because of very high risk for preterm labor because of prior preterm labor and delivery, a multiple gestation, or known uterine malformation. In addition to monitoring for contractions during two 1-hour periods daily, they receive extensive telephone education and support from trained nurses. Several randomized controlled trials have demonstrated significant pregnancy prolongation in women participating in this program compared with women receiving more traditional high-risk care.[86,87] In contrast, at least one randomized study comparing daily monitoring plus nursing support with daily telephone nursing support alone failed to demonstrate added value of the monitor.[88] A still unpublished randomized trial has found significant benefit to using the monitor alone without nursing support over standard outpatient care.[88a] Thus the majority of studies suggest a benefit when home uterine activity monitoring is used in conjunction with nursing support for select very high risk patients.

TREATMENT OF PRETERM LABOR

You got to know when to hold 'em,
Know when to fold 'em,
Know when to walk away,
Know when to run.

From Kenny Rogers' "The Gambler"
    1978 United Artists Music and Records Group Inc.

The challenge of treating preterm labor clearly illustrates one of the central dilemmas in obstetrics today: How does one balance the risks and benefits of modern intensive and sometimes invasive perinatal therapies? Or, more to the point, how does one decide when the baby (or mother) would be better off with a controlled delivery and optimal neonatal care rather than with "heroic" therapeutic interventions? The risks to the fetus of preterm birth were outlined in previous sections, and how closely linked they are to gestational age was emphasized. The benefits and risks of tocolytic drugs used in treating preterm labor are discussed in this section.

It is necessary to begin a general discussion of tocolytic drugs by pointing out that preterm birth rates have remained stable despite the use of millions of tablets and ampules of these powerful medications. This has been true in West Germany, where these drugs were first introduced, and it appears to be the case in the United States as well.[5] This should not be a surprise, as it is known that only 33 to 50 percent of preterm births are caused by preterm labor without rupture of membranes. Of this population, a large number are ineligible for tocolytic therapy because of advanced cervical dilatation or contraindications to drug use. A further proportion fail to reach term despite tocolytic therapy.

Evaluation of research and actual clinical use of tocolytic drugs has been significantly hampered by the difficulty in defining basic terms: What is success (or failure) when using tocolytic drugs? Is success reaching 37 weeks of gestation? Or 34 to 35 weeks, at which point nearly all babies do well? Or 48 hours to allow corticosteroid administration? Or, should success be reflected in improved perinatal morbidity/mortality data? Outcome data from 16 randomized placebo-controlled trials of β-mimetic tocolytics are summarized in Table 25.4.[89] As shown, these tocolytic agents are relatively more successful in delaying delivery for a short time than until term. Perhaps because of relatively small sample sizes, no cumulative reduction in neonatal morbidity or mortality could be shown.[89]

Definition of Preterm Labor

A second and even more fundamental problem is defining who is actually in preterm labor. What frequency and strength of contractions and how much cervical change should be required before treatment begins? The current most widely used definition is six to eight contractions per 1 hour or 4 contractions in 20 minutes, associated with cervical change.[90] The amount of cervical change and whether it represents change from a previous examination or only while under observation is not standardized. The less cervical change, the higher the "success" rate of tocolytic (and "placebo") therapy. This frames the clinical dilemma: Does one treat early with less clear evidence of preterm labor, "overtreat" but with high probability of success? Or, does one wait until there is significant change in the cervix, confirming the diagnosis, but at which point the chance of success will be reduced? Therefore, an area of important current research is whether there are patterns of uterine activity (frequency and intensity) that are sufficiently predictive of preterm labor to indicate when tocolytic therapy can be begun before cervical change, without overtreating large numbers.

Table 25.4 Outcome After Treatment With Tocolytic and Placebo

Outcome Measured	Treatment		Odds Ratio	Confidence Intervals	P (two-tailed)
	Tocolytics (%)	Placebo (%)			
No.	~462	~380			
Delivery <24 hr of trial entry	13.6	36.4	0.29	0.21–0.41	<0.00001
Delivery <48 hr of trial entry	27.1	40.1	0.59	0.42–0.83	0.003
Delivery <37 weeks	54.4	63.8	0.71	0.53–0.96	0.025
Birth weight <2,500 g	48.5	58.9	0.75	0.55–1.02	NS
RDS or severe respiratory difficulty	17.7	18.7	1.07	0.71–1.61	NS
Perinatal death	7.4	7.1	0.96	0.55–1.68	NS

(From King et al.,[89] with permission.)

Placebo Results

Most controlled studies of tocolytic drugs have compared the effect of the drug with hospitalization, bed rest, and intravenous fluids as "placebo." The high success rate reported in all such studies for the "placebo" group, often 50 percent, has led to despair over the definition of preterm labor. It should not be forgotten, however, that patients who are successfully "treated" with hydration and sedation constitute a high-risk group for returning in active preterm labor, a 30 percent risk, with more than one-half of these patients delivering preterm infants.[91] Hydration has not been shown to be of any benefit in evaluation of preterm uterine contractions[92] and may increase the risk of pulmonary edema if tocolytics are given subsequently.

Biochemistry of Myometrial Contractility and Tocolytic Action

Before drugs used to inhibit preterm labor are discussed, the key elements of myometrial activity and the site(s) of action of the various tocolytic agents are reviewed. Figure 25.9 summarizes the current knowledge of the regulatory mechanisms of uterine smooth muscle contractility. The following represents a condensation of material covered in two excellent reviews by leaders in the field.[93,94] The key process in actin–myosin interaction, and thus contraction, is myosin light-chain phosphorylation. This reaction is controlled by myosin light-chain kinase (MLK). The activity of tocolytic agents can be explained on the basis of their effects on the factors regulating the activity of this enzyme, notably calcium and cAMP (Fig. 25.9A). Calcium is essential for the activation of MLK and binds to the kinase as calmodulin–calcium complex. Intracellular calcium levels are regulated by two general mechanisms: (1) influx across the cell membrane and (2) release from intracellular storage sites.

The entry of calcium into cells occurs by at least two mechanisms. Depolarization leads to calcium influx through specific calcium channels that are voltage dependent. This is the site of action of the calcium channel blockers. Calcium can also enter through voltage-independent mechanisms, most notably the calcium–magnesium–ATPase system. Magnesium ions may interact here and also may compete with calcium for the voltage-dependent channels.

Intracellularly, calcium is stored in the sarcoplasmic reticulum and in mitochondria. cAMP and progesterone promote calcium storage at these sites, while prostaglandin $F_{2\alpha}$ ($PGF_{2\alpha}$) and oxytocin stimulate its release (Fig. 25.9B).

MLK is also regulated by cAMP. cAMP directly inhibits MLK function via phosphorylation. Levels of cAMP are increased by the action of adenylate cyclase, which in turn is stimulated by β-adrenergic agents. Therefore, β-mimetic tocolytics act through adenylate cyclase to increase cAMP, which inhibits MLK activity both by direct phosphorylation and by reducing intracellular free calcium (by inhibiting calcium release from storage vesicles) (Fig. 25.9C). β-Mimetics also interact with surface receptors on the trophoblast, leading to increased cAMP, which in this tissue increases production of progesterone.[95] Hormonal production is a lengthy process, and significant production is not seen for at least 18 hours.

For the myometrium to contract in a coordinated and effective manner (i.e., labor, whether term or preterm), individual smooth muscle cells must be functionally interconnected and able to communicate with their neighbors. The key element of this coordination and hence one of the keys for labor is the gap junction. The formation of gap junctions, along with other associated cellular events such as changes in the concentrations of receptors of oxytocin is regulated by estrogens and progesterone.[93] The pharmacology, side effects, and relative utility of tocolytic agents are now reviewed.

β-Mimetic Tocolytics

Pharmacology

Sympathomimetic or adrenergic drugs act through either α- or β-receptors. Stimulation of α-receptors leads to contraction of smooth muscles, while β-receptor stimulation carries the opposite effect, leading to smooth muscle relaxation at all sites: vascular, gastrointestinal, and uterine. β-Receptors are present in other tissues (e.g., the heart), which leads to the side effects of beta-mimetics. During the late 1960s, it was discovered that β-receptors could be further divided into β_1- and β_2-subtypes. β_1-Receptors are largely re-

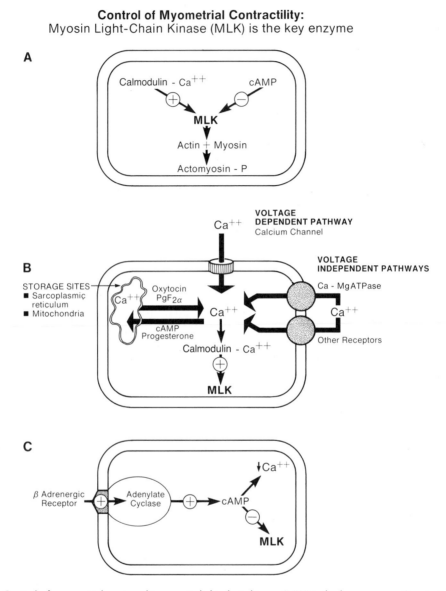

Control of Myometrial Contractility:
Myosin Light-Chain Kinase (MLK) is the key enzyme

Fig. 25.9 Control of myometrial contractility: myosin light-chain kinase (MLK) is the key enzyme. See text for details.

sponsible for the cardiac effects, while β_2-receptors mediate the smooth muscle relaxation as well as hepatic glycogen production and islet cell release of insulin. Table 25.5 displays the physiologic consequences of β_1- and β_2-stimulation in more detail.

β-Mimetics are all structurally related to epinephrine, with two carbons separating a benzene ring from an amino group. Relative β_2-activity appears to be associated with large alkyl substitutions on the amino group while maintaining hydroxyl groups at the 3 or 5 position on the benzene ring.[96] Figure 25.10 shows the chemical structures of the β-mimetics currently used for tocolytic therapy in the United States. It should be noted that when drugs are referred to as β_2-selective or β_2-specific, whether they be agonist or blocker, the selectivity is only relative and not absolute. First, β-receptors are not distributed on an "either/or" basis, but rather some tissues

Table 25.5 Physiologic Effects of β-Adrenergic Stimulation

β₁-Receptor Mediated	β₂-Receptor Mediated
Cardiac	Smooth muscle
Heart rate	Uterine activity
Stroke volume	Bronchiolar tone
	Vascular tone
	Intestinal motility
Renal	Renal
Renal blood flow	Renin
	Aldosterone
Metabolic	Metabolic
Lipolysis (ketones)	Insulin
Bicarbonate	Glycogen release (glucose)
Intracellular potassium	Skeletal muscle lactate

have a higher ratio of β_2- to β_1-receptors or vice versa. For example, the heart is primarily stimulated by β_1-agonists, but 14 percent of its β-receptors are β_2. Second, not all β_2-specific drugs are perfectly selective and will stimulate β_1-receptors to a certain extent. This is particularly true when serum drug concentrations are elevated.

Pharmacokinetics of Ritodrine

The therapeutic blood level of ritodrine has not been clearly established but appears to vary according to the degree of uterine activity rather than to cervical dilatation or status of the membranes.[97] Ritodrine is conjugated in the liver to inactive glucuronic and sulfuric esters. Both unconjugated and conjugated drugs are then excreted in the urine. Actual serum ritodrine levels vary greatly at a given infusion rate; for example, at an infusion rate of 50 μg/min, ritodrine levels may vary from 15 to 35 ng/ml from one patient to another.[97] The variability in serum levels among individuals at the same infusion rates appears to be related to differences in hepatic blood flow or serum concentrations of protein rather than maternal weight.[98] Concentrations of 80 ng/ml or more are commonly required initially to inhibit preterm labor. Ritodrine crosses the placenta readily, and fetal concentrations average 30 percent of maternal levels after a 2-hour infusion and are equal to those of the mother after longer infusions. In kinetics studies, it appears that serum ritodrine levels reach 75 percent of maximum levels within 20 minutes of a constant

intravenous infusion.[98] From clinical experience, it appears that the useful half-life of ritodrine is approximately 2 hours. Oral administration of 10 mg ritodrine produces peak serum levels at 20 to 80 minutes after ingestion. The decline in serum levels after oral use follows a two-compartment model with an initial half-life of 1.3 hours.[99] Maximum serum levels reached are 6.6 ± 2.9 ng/ml after 10 mg orally and 13.4 ± 5.2 ng/ml after 20 mg.

Dosage of Ritodrine

DOSAGE AND ADMINISTRATION OF RITODRINE HYDROCHLORIDE

Intravenous infusion

Monitor maternal heart rate and blood pressure, uterine activity, and fetal heart rate

Initial dose, 50 to 100 μg/min; then increase dose by 50 μg/min every 10 minutes until contractions stop or unacceptable side effects develop

Reduce the dose if side effects are poorly tolerated

Maximum dose: 350 μg/min

Discontinue ritodrine if labor persists at the maximum dose

If labor is successfully arrested, continue the infusion for at least 12 hours before beginning oral therapy

Oral therapy

Initial dose, 10 mg administered 30 minutes before stopping infusion; then 10 mg every 2 hours, or 20 mg every 4 hours, for 24 hours; if the uterus remains quiescent, 10 to 20 mg every 4 to 6 hours until further inhibition of labor is not indicated

Maximum dose: 120 mg/day

If labor recurs during oral administration, infusion may be repeated if the patient is qualified

---

The currently recommended protocol for intravenous therapy starts at 0.1 mg (100 μg)/min and is increased by 0.05 mg (50 μg) every 10 minutes up to a maximum of 0.35 (350 μg)/min. The rate is increased

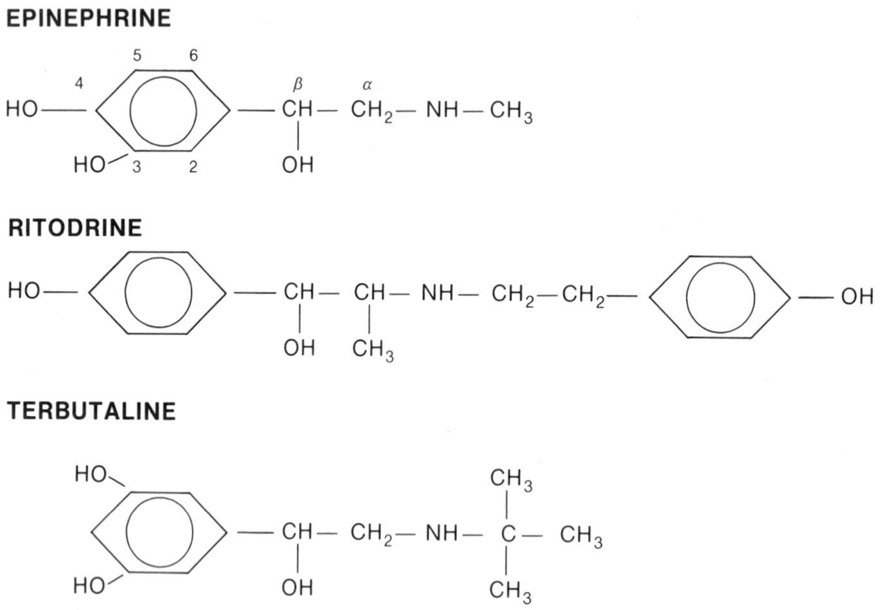

EPINEPHRINE

RITODRINE

TERBUTALINE

Fig. 25.10 Structure of epinephrine and β-agonist drugs currently used in the United States. β_2-Activity appears to be dependent on large alkyl substitutions on the amino group while maintaining hydroxyl groups at the 3 or 5 position on the benzene ring.

unless contractions cease, side effects occur, or the maximum rate is reached. The infusion is then maintained at that level for 12 hours after the cessation of contractions.[100]

Caritis et al.[97] at the University of Pittsburgh have had much experience correlating serum drug levels with side effects. These investigators noted that side effects occur most often when the infusion rate and concentration of ritodrine are increasing. The rate of change in the infusion rate or drug concentration appears to be more important than absolute drug level. Caritis and colleagues[98] have proposed an alternative protocol, which in their hands has fewer side effects but equal efficacy. The basic principle is to use as little drug as necessary, starting at 50 μg/min and increasing by 50 μg/min every 20 minutes only if contractions are more frequent than every 10 minutes. In addition, once labor is stopped, the infusion rate is maintained for only 1 hour and is then reduced every 20 minutes to the lowest rate that will inhibit contractions adequately. This rate is then maintained for 12 hours. The maximum dose may be exceeded for a short time in some patients, if the maternal pulse

is less than 110 bpm, as some of these individuals are exhibiting rapid clearance of the drug.

After intramuscular injection, ritodrine causes a dose-related increase in heart rate and blood pressure and a dose-related decrease in diastolic blood pressure. After a 10-mg injection, the maximal changes in heart rate, systolic blood pressure, and diastolic blood pressure are 22, 10, and 19 percent, respectively.[101] The single intramuscular injection of 5 to 10 mg of ritodrine results in labor-inhibiting concentrations with clinically insignificant cardiovascular effects. Thus the intramuscular route is preferable for women who are being transferred to another hospital.

As many patients experience a recurrence of preterm labor in the first days after intravenous therapy, treatment with oral β-mimetics has been recommended. Creasy et al.[102] showed that such a program will reduce the number of patients who need subsequent courses of intravenous tocolytics. Their study, however, failed to demonstrate any improvement in birth weight or gestational age at birth. There is little evidence that oral tocolytics are effective beyond the

---

> ### ALTERNATIVE INTRAVENOUS RITODRINE PROTOCOL TO MINIMIZE SIDE EFFECTS
>
> Begin infusion at 50 μg/min (0.05 mg/min)
>
> Increase by 50 μg/min every 20 minutes
>
> Maximum dose: 350 μg/min
>
> If contractions are less frequent than every 10 minutes, wait another 20 minutes before increasing dose
>
> Once labor is stopped, maintain infusion rate for 1 hour; then reduce every 20 minutes to the lowest rate that inhibits contractions adequately
>
> Continue this maintenance rate for 12 hours
>
> Potassium replacement is unnecessary on routine basis

first week after intravenous therapy. In fact, there are theoretic concerns, such as the development of tachyphylaxis, that can be raised against long-term β-mimetic therapy. Nonetheless, if the patient continues to have contractions, it is difficult to stop administration of a tocolytic drug.

The current recommended dosage for oral ritodrine is 20 mg every 4 hours following the first 24-hour period, during which 10 mg should be given every 2 hours. The pharmacokinetics of orally administered ritodrine reveal that blood levels in pregnant women after a 20-mg oral dose are low, but there is no difference between the fasting and fed states.[99] The maximal dosage of 120 mg/day is unlikely to sustain labor inhibition adequately in many women, and the recommended oral dose may need to be increased. Smaller or less frequent dosage cannot be recommended because of a lack of documented effectiveness and the drug's relatively short half-life. Many centers have found an elevated maternal pulse rate of 90 to 105 bpm to be a useful index of the drug's tocolytic effect. Maternal pulse rate may also be helpful in adjusting the dosage of ritodrine.

Terbutaline

Pharmacokinetics

There is only limited information regarding the pharmacokinetics of terbutaline in pregnant women. Serum levels range from 10 to 14 ng/ml following a 1-hour infusion of 0.010 mg (10 μg)/min. Of importance, at infusion rates above 5 μg/min this drug can be accumulated with raised serum levels and increased symptoms,[98] probably reflecting the longer half-life of terbutaline over ritodrine. Drug levels are 30 percent lower in pregnant patients than in nonpregnant volunteers. The onset of action is rapid with both intravenous bolus (1 to 2 minutes) and subcutaneous administration (3 to 5 minutes).

Oral administration of 5 mg gives an adequate blood level of 3 to 4 ng/ml at 1 hour, coinciding with the timing for bronchodilatation and tocolytic effects.[103] The half-life of terbutaline permits a dosing schedule of 5 mg every 4 to 6 hours.

Dosage of Terbutaline

As the labeling of terbutaline for tocolysis has not been approved by the Food and Drug Administration (FDA) (see the discussion of this issue later), there is no standard protocol for its use. Excessive dosages were used during the late 1970s (up to 80 μg/min at some centers), probably accounting for many of the reported cardiovascular side effects. Currently recommended protocols begin with 2.5 μg/min and increase by 2.5 μg/min every 20 minutes in a manner similar to ritodrine until a maximum of 17.5 to 20 μg/min is reached.[104]

Terbutaline allows the additional option of subcutaneous administration, with the usual dose being 250 μg (0.25 mg) every 3 hours.[105] This flexibility may allow some patients to avoid repeated intravenous tocolytic therapy, but the most appropriate role for subcutaneous administration is undefined.

Pulsatile Subcutaneous Pump Administration of Terbutaline

Both whole-animal and isolated human myometrial studies suggest that contractions resume after only several hours of *continuous* intravenous therapy with high-dose β-mimetic therapy. However, in the same studies, the myometrium remains quiescent longer with *pulsatile* administration of lower doses of the same tocolytic agent.[106] Because of the presumed delay in β-adrenergic receptor desensitization by pulsatile administration, recent attention has been focused on intermittent tocolytic dosing schedules. In the United States, this is most commonly accomplished by subcutaneous pump administration of terbutaline.

In 1988, Lam and colleagues[107] published a feasibility report of nine patients who had failed oral terbutaline therapy and who required hospital readmission for intravenous tocolysis. All were then started on low-dose terbutaline pump administration. Pregnancy prolongation averaged 9.2 ± 4.3 weeks. The minimal gestational age at delivery was 37.3 weeks. No maternal or fetal complications were noted. Lam has also presented improved pregnancy prolongation in women randomized to subcutaneous terbutaline over oral terbutaline following intravenous tocolysis. Further studies are needed to validate this potentially promising approach.

A needle is inserted into the thigh or abdomen and requires changing every 3 days. Dosage typically includes both a continuous basal rate (usually 0.05 to 0.08 mg/hr), which is titrated to abolish high-frequency, low-amplitude activity, and bolus doses of approximately 0.25 mg given up to eight times per day to cover times of increased uterine contractions.[108]

Oral terbutaline is given at 5 mg every 4 to 6 hours. In a double-blinded randomized comparison between terbutaline 5 mg every 4 hours and ritodrine 20 mg every 4 hours, terbutaline was significantly more effective.[104] Therefore oral terbutaline could be considered a reasonable and much less expensive alternative to ritodrine for maintenance oral therapy. One concern with oral long-term terbutaline therapy is the commonly seen worsening of glucose tolerance. Therefore most patients on chronic therapy should have their 50 gram oral glucose screening test for gestational diabetes mellitus repeated (see later discussion of hyperglycemia as a β-mimetic complication.)

β-Mimetic Complications

β-Mimetic therapy for preterm labor has been associated with a series of maternal deaths, largely from pulmonary edema (PE), but the drugs appear to have acceptable margins of safety if (1) the interaction between the pharmacology of β-mimetic drugs and the physiology of pregnancy is well understood, (2) there is careful attention to detail in the care of patients receiving these drugs, and (3) the potential for serious complications with these drugs is respected and contraindications are strictly observed. Symptomatic side effects are frequent with high-dose therapy. About 20 to 30 percent of patients experience nausea, and more than 50 percent of patients develop tachycardias greater than 120 bpm. Other maternal adverse effects of β-mimetic therapy are outlined in Table 25.6.[104,109]

Pulmonary Edema

PE is the most serious complication of tocolytic therapy and is one that can often be prevented. A recent review is recommended for a detailed discussion.[110] The reason for its frequent occurrence can be understood by reviewing the physiologic factors predisposing to PE in normal pregnancy that add to the stress of β-mimetic therapy, especially in the face of certain medical factors.

It had been assumed by many that the PE is secondary to volume overload/left heart failure. However, evaluation of cardiac function with either Swan-Ganz

Table 25.6 Maternal Complications of Parenteral β-Mimetic Tocolytic Therapy

	Approx. Incidence (%)
Hypokalemia (transient, <24 hr) <3.0 mEq/L	40–60
Hyperglycemia (transient, <24 hr) >140 mg/dl >200 mg/dl	20–50 Rare
Shortness of breath	5–20
Chest pain	5–16
Cardiac dysrhythmia	2–4
ECG "ischemia" changes	1–10
Hypotension	1–4
Pulmonary edema	<1–5

catheters or echocardiography has failed to demonstrate left ventricular failure in all but a few cases of PE, most of which were associated with underlying hypertension.[111] Noncardiogenic causes that may be important are decreased colloid oncotic pressure and increased pulmonary vascular permeability, especially when premature labor is associated with amnionitis. In one study, tocolysis for preterm labor was associated with a higher incidence of PE in the presence of maternal infection (21 percent) than when it was absent (1 percent).[112]

Of note, nearly all patients with PE were receiving either physiologic saline solutions or Ringer's lactated solution, which further decreases colloid oncotic pressure and expands vascular volume.[111] In any case, patients treated with β-mimetics should be considered as having a compromised cardiovascular system and, like the 70-year-old patient on a gynecology service, she should not receive large amounts of saline or Ringer's lactated solution.

In reviewing the reported cases and in our experience, it is uncommon for PE to develop in the first 24 hours of β-mimetic therapy unless one of the extra predisposing factors (listed above) is present. In fact, more than 90 percent of reported cases of PE occur after 24 hours of β-mimetic therapy. Glucocorticoids have often been associated with PE in this setting, and many investigators consider them a predisposing factor. However, betamethasone and dexamethasone have essentially no mineralocorticoid activity, and their association with maternal PE may be coincidental: The patients with the most cervical change receive the highest doses of β-mimetics and corticosteroids. There are now many cases of PE reported without concomitant use of corticosteroids.[110] Recommendations to avoid PE related to tocolytic treatment are outlined as follows.

Myocardial Ischemia and Cardiac Dysrhythmias

Symptomatic cardiac dysrhythmias and symptomatic myocardial ischemia have occurred during tocolytic therapy. Myocardial infarction with resultant maternal death has been reported.[109] Ischemia appears to be localized to the subendocardial region. The subendocardial oxygen supply : demand ratio can be reduced by two factors that are known to be operative during pregnancy and β-mimetic therapy: the placental arterial–venous fistula that diminishes aortic diastolic blood pressure and the induced tachycardia resulting in a shortened diastole, which is the time for myocardial perfusion. If a patient develops chest pain during therapy, one should discontinue the β-mimetic and administer oxygen. With severe pain, therapy with nitrates may be necessary. Premature ventricular contraction, premature nodal contraction, and atrial fibrillation have been noted in association with β-mimetic therapy.[109] These usually respond well to discontinuation of the drug and oxygen administration.

The most important steps to prevent these cardiac complications are (1) excluding patients with prior cardiac disease and (2) limiting infusion rates so that maternal pulse does not exceed 130 bpm. We and others have not found baseline electrocardiograms (ECGs) or routine ECGs during treatment to be helpful. A baseline ECG rarely uncovers abnormalities; there is a very poor correlation between symptoms of myocardial ischemia and ECG changes in these patients.[113,114] In fact, enzyme (creatinine phosphokinase) evidence of myocardial injury in association with tocolytic-induced ECG changes has not been documented.[115] Nonetheless, if a patient does not quickly respond to oxygen and discontinuation of β-mimetic therapy, an ECG is in order.

Hypotension

Hypotension is rarely as significant a problem with ritodrine or terbutaline as it was with isoxsuprine, a β-mimetic agent used during the 1970s. There is evidence of a mild (5 to 10 mmHg) fall in diastolic blood pressure with the current drugs. Importantly, however, the extensive peripheral vasodilatation makes it difficult for the patient to mount a normal, vasoconstrictive response to hypovolemia. This is one of the reasons β-mimetics are dangerous in the face of antepartum hemorrhage. Another is that the important early signs of excessive blood loss such as maternal and fetal tachycardia are masked by these drugs.[109]

Hyperglycemia and Hypokalemia

β-Mimetic agents compound the problems of patients with overt or gestational diabetes mellitus. Increased glycogenolysis with resultant hyperglycemia, increased lactic acid release from skeletal muscles, and ketone formation from fat stores, as well as a fall in bicarbonate, markedly increase the risk of ketoacidosis.[116] We therefore avoid the use of these drugs in women with diabetes. If it is absolutely necessary to use β-mimetics, we concomitantly use an intravenous insulin infusion. In the nondiabetic woman, β-mimetics will cause a significant increase in serum glucose level, although rarely over 180 mg/dl.[104]

β-Mimetics also lead to potassium flux from plasma into cells, thereby causing a fall in serum measurements without a change in excretion. Hence there is no change in total body potassium. We recommend measurement of glucose and potassium before initiating therapy and on several occasions during the first 24 hours of treatment. This will ensure that the unrecognized gestational diabetic and the occasional normal patient in whom significant hyperglycemia ($>$180 mg/dl) develops will not be missed. After 24 hours of therapy, both the serum glucose and potassium levels will have begun to return to baseline even without specific therapy.[117] No potassium replacement is needed unless the serum potassium level falls below 2.5 mEq/L.

Chronic administration of β-mimetic tocolytics can have significant effects on glucose tolerance. Main et al.[117] noted a clear deterioration in glucose tolerance with over a 1-week use of oral terbutaline. Up to 63 percent of pregnant women on terbutaline may have an abnormal 1-hour 50-g glucose screening test. Of interest, a similar study of ritodrine showed no such effects.[118]

Neonatal Side Effects

Hypoglycemia and ileus have been reported with β-mimetics.[119] On a positive note, some reports link β-mimetic drugs with improved neonatal lung function and with a decreased incidence of RDS. These effects are not uniformly found and are not of the magnitude of those associated with corticosteroids. With all tocolytic drugs, β-mimetics, and magnesium sulfate, adverse neonatal effects are greatest when the fetus is born close to a period of high-dose parenteral therapy.[120] This must caution against use of these drugs when there is advanced cervical dilatation and delivery appears inevitable.

Contraindications for β-Mimetic Tocolytic Therapy

Conditions that should be considered absolute contraindications to β-mimetic therapy are summarized as follows.

ABSOLUTE CONTRAINDICATIONS TO THE ADMINISTRATION OF β-MIMETIC AGENTS

Maternal cardiac disease (structural, ischemia, or dysrhythmias)

Eclampsia or preeclampsia

Significant antepartum hemorrhage of any etiology

Chorioamnionitis

Fetal mortality or significant abnormality

Significant fetal growth retardation

Uncontrolled maternal diabetes mellitus

Maternal medical conditions that would be seriously affected by the pharmacologic properties of the β-adrenergic agonists such as hyperthyroidism, uncontrolled hypertension, hypovolemia

Any obstetric or medical condition that contraindicates prolongation of pregnancy

---

Situations in which the patient is at increased risk for β-mimetic complications (relative contraindications) are listed below. Careful risk–benefit evaluation needs to be performed on an individual basis in these cases.

CONDITIONS OF INCREASED RISK/RELATIVE CONTRAINDICATIONS

Multiple gestation
Preterm rupture of membranes
Febrile patient
Maternal diabetes (well controlled)
Maternal chronic hypertension
Patients receiving potassium-depleting diuretics
History of severe migraine headaches

Magnesium Sulfate

It has long been known that strips of uterine muscle have reduced contractility in the presence of magnesium ion. It was not until the early 1970s, however, that magnesium sulfate began to be used clinically in the United States for the inhibition of preterm labor.[121,122] The mechanism of tocolytic activity of magnesium is unclear. It has been suggested that it acts by competition with calcium either at the motor end plate, reducing excitation, or at the cell membrane, reducing calcium influx into the cell at depolarization.

Magnesium sulfate must be administered parenterally in order to elevate serum levels out of the normal range. The therapeutic dosage and therapeutic serum levels have not been formally established but empirically are similar to those used for intravenous treatment of preeclampsia: a 4-g loading dose given over 20 minutes, followed by an infusion of 2 g/hr, dropping to 1 g/hr once contractions cease. Elliott[123] and others have suggested a 6-g loading dose and infusions of 3 g/hr to ensure blood levels of greater than 5 mg/dl in the early hours of treatment, but formal pharmacokinetics studies have not been conducted.

Madden et al.[124] were unable to show that serum levels correlated with successful tocolytic therapy. In 101 episodes of preterm labor treated with magnesium sulfate, no difference was found in the proportions of tocolytic success when serum levels were less than 6 mg/dl, compared with when levels were more than 6 mg/dl. Mean serum magnesium levels in patients with successful tocolysis were similar to those in patients in whom tocolysis failed. The investigators concluded that serum magnesium levels alone should not serve as the endpoint of therapy and that the drug should be titrated on the basis of clinical efficacy or maternal toxicity.

Excess magnesium is rapidly excreted by the kidney, provided there is normal renal function. Should there be any evidence of renal impairment, such as oliguria or a serum creatinine level over 0.9 mg/dl, magnesium therapy should be approached cautiously, the patient followed with serum levels, and doses adjusted accordingly. Magnesium sulfate should not be used in patients with myasthenia gravis.

Efficacy

Intravenous magnesium sulfate appears to have tocolytic success at a level comparable to that of β-mimetics. Elliott[123] reported his experience with 274 singleton pregnancies in preterm labor with intact membranes. The time gained after initiation of therapy depended on cervical dilatation (Table 25.7).

Others have reported somewhat less impressive results, especially when the cervix is dilated to 2 cm or more.[121] In small studies, magnesium sulfate was better than alcohol[121] but not different from ritodrine.[125]

Beall et al.[126] randomized patients to ritodrine, terbutaline, or magnesium sulfate as the initial intravenous tocolytic. Failure rates were similar (approximately 30 percent) between the magnesium and β-mimetic groups, but the reasons for failure were quite different. Few of the patients receiving magnesium failed because of drug intolerance (side effects). Most of the failures were secondary to persistent contractions necessitating a switch to a β-mimetic. Of interest, the secondary drug also had high success rates, supporting the concept of sequential therapy.

In two other studies ritodrine and magnesium sulfate had equivalent efficacy.[127,128] When both drugs were used together, the incidence of side effects rose significantly.

Magnesium has a relatively low rate of symptomatic side effects, and its cost is low. It has therefore become the tocolytic agent of choice in a number of major centers. There can be, however, major and life-threatening complications with magnesium therapy, including chest pain and PE. In the largest clinical experience, 355 patients reported by Elliott,[123] side effects were noted in 7 percent (Table 25.8). Four patients (1.1 percent) developed PE, a rate similar to that seen with β-mimetics. It should be pointed out that Elliott used higher magnesium sulfate doses than other investigators, and it is not clear that maternal fluids were restricted.

Summary

Magnesium sulfate has emerged as a legitimate alternative for β-mimetic therapy, particularly for patients who have contraindications for β-mimetic use and have limited cervical change. It must be remembered that the benefits of tocolytic therapy are not as great as originally suggested, which requires the physician

Table 25.7 Tocolytic Effect of Intravenous Magnesium Sulfate[a]

Initial Dilatation of Cervix (cm)	Percentage of Patients Reaching	
	48 hours	7 days
0–2	87	64
3–4	64	56

[a] A noncontrolled report of experience with 274 singleton patients with intact membranes.
(From Elliott,[123] with permission.)

Table 25.8 Adverse Effects of Magnesium Sulfate Tocolytic Therapy in 355 Patients

Side Effect	Percentage
Pulmonary edema	1.1
Chest pain	1.1
Severe nausea or flushing	3.6
Drowsiness or blurred vision	0.8
Total	6.6

(From Elliott,[123] with permission.)

to be doubly aware of the potential for drug complications and ways of avoiding them.

Other Agents With Tocolytic Activity

Indomethacin

Because prostaglandins appear to be part of the final pathway of smooth muscle contraction, prostaglandin synthetase inhibitors have theoretical appeal as tocolytic agents. Indomethacin has been the most widely used drug of this class and has proved highly effective in several studies in the United States[129] and in Israel.[130,131] Indomethacin is well tolerated by the mother but should be avoided in patients with peptic ulcer disease. It is well absorbed orally or per rectum. The usual dose is a 50 mg loading dose by mouth or 50 to 100 mg per rectum if the patient cannot tolerate the oral dose. Subsequently, 25 to 50 mg is administered orally every 4 to 6 hours, depending on the response.

The fundamental problem with indomethacin and the other currently available prostaglandin synthesis inhibitors is the lack of specificity in their action. They act by inhibiting the ubiquitous cyclooxygenase enzyme. This enzyme controls the synthesis of all prostanoids, including prostaglandins, prostacyclins, and thromboxanes. The products have varied effects on multiple organ systems and play important roles in maintaining fetal circulation.

Three side effects of indomethacin have been of concern. Constriction of the ductus arteriosus is usually transient and has not been reported to cause long-term adverse effects on the infant.[132-134] Oligohydramnios resulting from decreased fetal urinary output is dose related and reversible. Primary pulmonary hypertension in the neonate has been associated with prolonged (>48 hours) indomethacin therapy.[135,136]

In a recent study utilizing fetal echocardiography, 7 of 14 fetuses whose mothers were receiving indomethacin for tocolysis demonstrated significant ductal constriction.[137] Three fetuses had tricuspid regurgitation. All constrictions resolved within 24 hours after the drug was stopped, and no primary pulmonary hypertension was noted in the neonates. The fetal ductus is more sensitive to indomethacin as term approaches and thus the authors recommended the drug not be used beyond 34 weeks gestation.

Indomethacin therapy for patent ductus arteriosus in the newborn causes a reversible decrease in fetal urine output, and presumably this is the etiology of the decreased amniotic fluid volume observed in utero.[138-140] There is no evidence of a change in renal blood flow or altered fetal renal artery velocity waveforms.[141] However, prostaglandins antagonize the peripheral action of antidiuretic hormone, and perhaps this is the mechanism of decreased fetal urine output with indomethacin administration.[142]

Primary pulmonary hypertension has been reported in infants who received chronic therapy, but rarely under 34 weeks gestation. No cases of primary pulmonary hypertension in the newborn have been reported with 24 to 48 hours of therapy, whereas the incidence appears to be in the 5 to 10 percent range with long-term therapy.[143] Ductal constriction in utero causes increased pulmonary blood flow and, with time, increased pulmonary arterial smooth muscle and constriction of pulmonary arterioles. After birth, persistent pulmonary hypertension leads to patent ductus arteriosus, which may require indomethacin for closure.

Several series have now been reported in which patients with polyhydramnios have been treated successfully with indomethacin,[144-147] and it may be the drug of choice in patients with concomitant polyhydramnios and preterm labor.

Calcium Channel Blockers

Inhibitors of intracellular calcium entry have potent effects on the contraction of smooth muscle. Currently, they are being used quite successfully in the treatment of a wide variety of cardiovascular diseases, including certain types of hypertension, angina, and arrhythmias. Two randomized controlled trials comparing nifedipine to intravenous ritodrine have demonstrated at least comparable efficacy.[148,149] Nifedipine has milder effects on maternal pulse, diastolic blood pressure, and serum glucose and electrolytes than does ritodrine.[150] Maternal symptoms are infrequent but include flushing, headache, dizziness, and nausea. One case report describes skeletal muscle blockade when used in conjunction with magnesium sulfate,[151] so this combination therapy should be avoided.

Adverse neonatal effects from maternal nifedipine

use have not been described. However, several animal studies have reported reduction in uteroplacental blood flow, fetal bradycardia, and hypoxic myocardial depression with other calcium channel blockers, including verapamil, nicardipine, and diltiazem. A report of Doppler assessment of fetal and uteroplacental circulation during nifedipine use in 11 women for treatment of preterm labor is encouraging.[152] No changes in middle cerebral artery, renal artery, ductus arteriosus, umbilical artery, or maternal vessels were noted between pretreatment values and values obtained after 5 hours of therapy.

Because of the relatively limited published information available about nifedipine, its use is restricted in many centers. When administered as a tocolytic agent, nifedipine is usually given as a 10- to 20-mg dose every 6 hours orally. Patients in active preterm labor may be given a loading dose of 10 mg sublingually every 20 minutes for up to three doses, followed by oral administration every 6 hours.

Alcohol

Alcohol is of historic interest as a tocolytic agent.[153] Now that there are multiple alternatives, the serious side effects of intravenous alcohol (intoxication, dehydration, hangover, risk of obtundation and aspiration, and elevated maternal and fetal lactate levels) preclude its use in modern obstetrics.

Controversial Issues in Tocolytic Treatment

Several topics of controversy are addressed in this section, with the understanding that absolute answers are not currently available. The difficult issue of the use of tocolytic agents when membranes have ruptured preterm is discussed in the section on premature rupture of the membranes (PROM).

Are Antibiotics a Useful Adjunctive Treatment for Women With Preterm Labor and Intact Membranes?

At least 11 studies have been done to determine the frequency of occult intraamniotic infections in women with preterm labor. On average, 16 percent of the 367 women evaluated had positive amniotic fluid cultures (study means ranged from 3 to 48 percent).[59] Women at earlier gestational ages and those who fail tocolysis are more likely to have positive cultures. The most common organisms isolated are anaerobic, including fusobacteria (25 percent); *Bacte-*

roides, not *fragilis,* (20 percent); *Ureaplasma* (9 percent); and *Gardnerella vaginalis* (5 percent).

Women with preterm labor and intact membranes have been randomized to receive either an antibiotic or placebo. In two studies utilizing erythromycin, ampicillin, or clindamycin, significant pregnancy prolongation occurred in the treated patients.[154,155] In the third study comparing ampicillin and erythromycin to placebo, no significant benefit was apparent from treatment.[156] More studies are needed to confirm the value of adjunctive antibiotic therapy in afebrile women with preterm labor and intact membranes. Whether treatment should be elected and the optimal agent, dose, and duration of treatment remain unclear.

Combination Therapy: Are Two Tocolytics Better Than One?

As all intravenous tocolytics have significant failure rates, especially in the face of advanced preterm labor, several groups have asked whether combination therapy may offer advantages.

One randomized trial compared ritodrine treatment alone with combination ritodrine–magnesium sulfate therapy and found improved pregnancy prolongation with combination therapy.[157] However, almost one-half of patients in both groups had tachycardia in excess of 140 bpm. Another group compared ritodrine with ritodrine–magnesium sulfate and was forced to halt the study when nearly one-half the 24 patients receiving combination therapy developed cardiovascular symptoms.[158] This study did use higher doses of magnesium sulfate than are more commonly recommended, 8.4 g in the first hour, 4.8 g in the second hour, then 2.4 g/hr thereafter. There are physiologic concerns regarding this combination, as both β-mimetics and magnesium sulfate can have similar effects on the cardiovascular system —an increase in cardiac output and cardiac performance with decreased peripheral vascular resistance.

We therefore prefer to discontinue the use of one parenteral tocolytic before initiating another and have had good results with "substitution" rather than "combination." There is actually good support in the literature for sequential therapy. Beall and associates[126] randomized patients to ritodrine, terbutaline, or magnesium sulfate therapy. Initial success rates were comparable at approximately 70 percent for either ritodrine or magnesium sulfate. Most failures with ritodrine were due to maternal side effects, while most failures with magnesium sulfate were because of persistent contractions. Almost 90 percent of women who failed the initial agent responded favorably to the alternative.

A combination that may have more benefit in the future is that of β-mimetics and calcium channel blockers, which is currently under study in several centers. It should be recalled that patients who break through intravenous tocolytics have a high incidence of underlying amnionitis and partial abruption. Therefore these diagnoses should be considered before multidrug therapy is instituted.

"Approved" or "Unapproved" Drugs?

The FDA has stated that the use of approved drugs for nonlabeled indications may be entirely appropriate based on medical advances extensively reported in the medical literature[159]:

The appropriateness or the legality of prescribing approved drugs for uses not included in their official labeling is sometimes a cause of concern and confusion among practitioners.

Under the Federal Food, Drug, and Cosmetic (FD&C) Act, a drug approved for marketing may be labeled, promoted, and advertised by the manufacturer only for those uses for which the drug's safety and effectiveness have been established and which FDA has approved. . . .

The FD&C Act does not, however, limit the manner in which a physician may use an approved drug. Once a product has been approved for marketing, a physician may prescribe it for uses or in treatment regimens or patient populations that are not included in approved labeling. Such "unapproved" or, more precisely, "unlabeled" uses may be appropriate and rational in certain circumstances, and may, in fact, reflect approaches to drug therapy that have been extensively reported in medical literature. . . .

Before such advances can be added to the approved labeling, however, data substantiating the effectiveness of a new use or regimen must be submitted by the manufacturer to FDA for evaluation. This may take time and, without the initiative of the drug manufacturer of the product that is involved, may never occur. For that reason, accepted medical practice often in-

cludes drug use that is not reflected in approved drug labeling.

How Long Should a Patient Remain on Oral Tocolytics and Which Oral Tocolytic Should Be Used?

The literature regarding the effectiveness of oral tocolytics is surprisingly sparse, considering the widespread use of these agents. Creasy et al.[102] studied 55 patients who received oral ritodrine or placebo following parenteral therapy until 31 to 38 weeks gestation and could not document an improvement in birth weight, gestational age, or infant outcome. The only benefit noted was the prevention of recurrent episodes of preterm labor. Brown and Tejani[160] evaluated 46 patients receiving either terbutaline (5 mg every 6 hours) or placebo until 38 weeks and did find improvement in time gained in utero. In a double-blind randomized direct comparison between oral ritodrine and terbutaline, Caritis et al.[104] found terbutaline (5 mg every 4 hours) statistically and clinically superior to ritodrine (20 mg every 4 hours) when looking at prolongation of pregnancy and rate of recurrent preterm labor. Of interest is that this study achieved these excellent results in the terbutaline group with only 5 days of oral therapy. A shorter period of treatment has several advantages besides the obvious one of cost. The occurrence of tachyphylaxis is real in patients on these drugs and worth avoiding, especially should one need to re-treat recurrent preterm labor. Second, as a matter of general principle, it is preferable to limit the duration of fetal exposure to any drug. In summary, oral tocolytic treatment may be of benefit following parenteral use, but the choice of drug and duration of therapy are currently not established.

Through What Gestational Age Should Parenteral Tocolytics Be Used?

This question can be examined from both a risk–benefit and a cost–benefit standpoint. There is an approximately 50 percent placebo success rate and a failure rate of 10 to 20 percent, so that at most only 30 to 40 percent of patients who receive tocolytics actually benefit from them. Therefore, if the chance of effective tocolytic activity is only one out of three, the rate of side effects, albeit low, becomes a more major concern.

The risks of being born preterm are now well established, and it is clear that these risks are related to gestational age. Comparing statistics from many neonatal centers across the country, it appears that at 34 weeks gestation (mean weight of 2,200 to 2,400 g), the survival data are very close to those at term, within 1 to 1.5 percent of the survival rate beyond 37 weeks. Furthermore, in a tertiary care center, while there is certainly additional neonatal morbidity at 34 to 36 weeks, it is usually of the less severe variety—mild RDS, hyperbilirubinemia, or poor feeding—and rarely a cause of long-term sequelae. Therefore, because of the small but real maternal risks and the limited neonatal benefits, we recommend limiting the use of intravenous tocolytic agents to gestational ages below 35 weeks. Thirty-three to 35 weeks represent a "gray zone," and pulmonary immaturity should be documented.

Cost–benefit studies are useful not only for health care planning but also as a measure of short-term morbidity. In such a study, Korenbrot et al.[161] could not document either an improvement in survival rate or lower cost, adding both maternal and neonatal charges in patients treated with tocolytic agents versus untreated mothers beyond 33 weeks gestation.

Glucocorticoids for Enhancement of Fetal Pulmonary Maturation

It has been known for over 25 years that antepartum administration of glucocorticoids accelerates the appearance of pulmonary surfactant in fetal animals.[162] In the 20 years since the landmark trial of Liggins and Howie,[163] there have been 11 other prospective randomized controlled trials of glucocorticoids before preterm delivery. This intense scrutiny makes corticosteroid therapy among the best studied of any of the obstetric interventions. Eleven of the 12 randomized trials demonstrated reduced RDS with an overall reduction of over 50 percent (summary odds ratio of 0.49).[164] A recent meta-analysis of these trials[164] also demonstrated overall reductions in neonatal death, cerebral hemorrhage, and necrotizing enterocolitis. Any obstetrician who continues to have doubts concerning antenatal glucocorticoid efficacy should carefully study that review. The technique of meta-analysis also allows for more careful analysis of some of the more controversial areas in glucocorticoid therapy. These are summarized in Table 25.9 using odds ratios

Table 25.9 Meta-Analysis of Randomized Trials of Corticosteroids Used Before Preterm Delivery

Outcome	Odds Ratio	95% Confidence Interval
RDS	0.49^a	0.41–0.60
Overall		
Before 31 wks	0.38^a	0.24–0.60
After 34 wks	0.62	0.29–1.30
Male infants	0.43^a	0.29–0.64
Female infants	0.36^a	0.23–0.57
Neonatal death	0.59^a	0.47–0.75
Maternal infection	1.11	0.81–1.51
Neonatal/fetal infection	0.83	0.54–1.26
RDS after PROM	0.55^a	0.40–0.75
Neonatal infection	1.61	0.87–2.98

^{a} Highly significant when compared with placebo.

together with 95 percent confidence intervals. The odds ratio is the ratio of the odds of an undesired outcome (e.g., RDS) versus a desired outcome (e.g., no RDS) among those allocated to corticosteroids, to the odds of undesired outcome versus desired outcome among the controls. Should the 95 percent confidence interval include 1.0, the difference is also compatible with chance variation. An odds ratio of 0.6 suggests that the risk of the undesired outcome is reduced by 40 percent. For example, the data suggest that corticosteroids also reduce the risk of periventricular hemorrhage and necrotizing enterocolitis by between 10 and 80 percent.

Infants benefited most if they were born 24 hours to 7 days after therapy, but babies born outside this time frame also were aided. Infants did better at all gestational ages at which RDS occurs, and the overall data revealed no evidence that fetal gender influences the protective effect of corticosteroids[164] (odds ratio for males, 0.43; females, 0.36). The separate analysis of corticosteroid administration after PROM also indicated a significant reduction in respiratory morbidity.[164]

Several groups have reported a reduction in the incidence of IVH, PDA, NEC, and abnormal neurologic examinations in association with steroid use.[165,166] It is not clear whether these are direct benefits or come about through the reduction in RDS and/or concomitant ventilator usage.[166]

Why then is there remaining controversy regarding the use of corticosteroids to promote fetal lung maturation? Some American centers reviewed their own experience and decided that "unstressful labor and atraumatic delivery" gave as good an outcome as prenatal glucocorticoids.[167] With these reported "good" outcomes, often compared with data reported by other centers and other times, and because of concern about the limited long-term follow-up and short-term infectious complications, these centers opted not to use corticosteroids to improve perinatal survival. We would suggest that the question should be rephrased from "Do our babies do as well as those in other institutions who use steroids?" to "Could our babies do even better if they received steroids prenatally?" All sides can agree from the literature that (1) diagnosis and incidence of RDS is not uniform, (2) obstetric factors can be of major importance and are often overlooked in the reporting of trials, and (3) glucocorticoids are not a perfect therapy.

The two largest prospective randomized trials of glucocorticoids are the extended Liggins study[165] and the Collaborative Group on Antenatal Steroid Therapy.[168] It is useful to review their data, summarized in Table 25.10.

The infants in the initial trial of Liggins and Howie have been followed for 6 years, 1 year into school, and have shown no impairment in cognitive and psychosocial development or on physical, including pulmonary, examination.[169] Likewise, the Collaborative Group[170] has published a 3-year follow-up study on its

infants, with no detectable growth, physical, motor, or developmental deficiencies noted.

The major short-term side effect of concern is the risk of infection for both the mother and infant. Neither of the two largest studies mentioned above[165,168] noted any increased incidence of neonatal or maternal infections. There may be some excess risk in mothers and infants when steroids are given in the face of preterm rupture of the membranes (see discussion below). Increased fetal jeopardy in pregnancies complicated by proteinuric hypertension was suggested by the original Liggins[165] study but has not been confirmed in subsequent series.[171,172]

Another complication of prenatal glucocorticoid therapy is short-term impairment of maternal glucose tolerance, particularly in the insulin-dependent diabetic. To prevent ketoacidosis, these patients may require short-term management with insulin infusions for several days and should be observed carefully.

Mechanisms of Steroid Action

It has been proposed that glucocorticoids reduce the incidence of RDS through multiple mechanisms. Responses to steroids can be observed in lung structure, function (pressure volume studies), and biochemical parameters. Clearly, high doses of steroids induce many enzyme systems, several of which are important for surfactant production such as choline phosphotransferase.[173] Glucocorticoids also have a role in the regulation of the intracellular storage and/or secretion of surfactant by the type II pneumocyte.

Adjunctive Treatment Approaches To Minimize Neonatal Lung Disease

Clinical studies show a significant reduction but not elimination of RDS after steroid therapy. This has led to alternative treatment approaches to enhance pulmonary maturation. The two most promising are maternal adjunctive treatment with thyroid-releasing hormones (TRH) and neonatal treatment with surfactant.

A number of whole-animal and tissue culture experiments have demonstrated that fetal thyroxine or maternal TRH administration accelerates both functional and morphologic lung maturation.[174-176] Studies have also revealed a further synergistic interaction between glucocorticoids and thyroid hormones. Two recently completed randomized human trials be-

Table 25.10 Glucocorticoids and the Prevention of RDS: Data From the Two Largest Randomized Trials[a]

No. of Weeks	Study	Steroid % RDS (N)	Control % RDS (N)	p Value
30–32	Liggins	8.7 (23)	56.0 (25)	0.001
32–34	Liggins	0 (50)	12.9 (31)	0.04
30–34	Collaborative	10.6 (66)	25.4 (63)	0.03
>34	Liggins	5.5 (73)	5.4 (74)	NS
	Collaborative	5.0 (64)	6.2 (80)	NS

[a] These data represent singleton infants who delivered from 1 to 7 days after steroid administration. In the Liggins[165] study, doses of 12 mg betamethasone were given 24 hours apart. In the Collaborative study,[168] four doses of 6 mg dexamethasone were given 12 hours apart.

tween glucocorticoid treatment alone and glucocorticoid plus TRH treatment have recently been completed.[177,178] In these trials the incidence and severity of RDS were not reduced by the combined therapy. However, infants whose mothers received TRH experienced shorter times on the ventilator and reduced rates of chronic lung disease.[177,178] No significant immediate maternal or fetal complications were noted, and the incidences of other major complications of premature infants were not altered.[179] While these preliminary results show promise, it is not yet known who will benefit, when to use this combination therapy, and how to maximize its benefits.

Several centers have demonstrated a reduction in severity of acute RDS with the intratracheal administration of surfactant (Chap. 21).[180] Single-dose administration, however, has failed to improve significantly clinical status later in the neonatal period or to reduce neonatal mortality.[180] Further studies are needed to evaluate the role of human versus calf serum surfactant and multiple- versus single-dose treatment regimens. There appears to be an additive benefit of antenatal steroid administration *and* postnatal surfactant treatment over postnatal surfactant treatment alone.[181]

CERVICAL INCOMPETENCE

The second fault in women which hindered conception is when the seed is not retained or the orifice of the womb is so slack that it cannot rightly contract itself to keep in the seed; which chiefly is caused by abortion, or hard labor in childbirth, whereby the fibers of the womb are broken in pieces one from another and they, and the inner orifice of the womb over much slackened.

(From Cole and Culpepper, *Practice of Physick*, 1658).

Diagnosis

Cervical incompetence, or premature cervical dilatation, is an important cause of second-trimester pregnancy loss and is marked by gradual, painless dilatation and effacement of the cervix with bulging and later rupture of the membranes. This history in a prior pregnancy is critical for establishing the diag-

nosis. Short labors with the delivery of an immature fetus or loss of the pregnancy at progressively earlier gestational ages in successive pregnancies is characteristic of the incompetent cervix.

The most common cause of cervical incompetence is prior trauma to the cervix, particularly from prior obstetric or gynecologic procedures. The current practice of using tapered cervical dilators and pretreating nulliparous patients with laminaria before dilatation and extraction or dilatation and curettage has greatly reduced cervical trauma. Recent evidence indicates that prior first-trimester termination is not a risk factor if (1) it was done after 1973, (2) it was performed by an experienced operator, (3) it was performed using local anesthesia only, and (4) laminaria were used in nulliparas.[182] The role of cone biopsy in the development of subsequent cervical incompetence remains controversial.[183,183a]

Congenital structure changes in the cervix can occur in association with other uterine malformations or after DES exposure. In our experience at the University of Pennsylvania[184] with DES-exposed women, cervical incompetence has not been common unless there were associated and significant uterine, cervical, or vaginal changes. Therefore, unless these abnormalities are present, we have followed DES-exposed patients expectantly with frequent vaginal examinations rather than perform a prophylactic cerclage. However, 5 of 21 women thus followed developed PROM and experienced perinatal deaths. Others have recommended ultrasonic evaluation and selective cerclage.[185] Certainly, DES exposure in conjunction with a cervical shortening or abnormality is a particularly high-risk situation that generally merits cerclage.

It has been recognized that there may be a congenital predisposition toward cervical incompetence. Patients with a higher concentration of smooth muscle in the cervix, relative to a deficit of collagen fibers, are at increased risk for cervical incompetence.[186]

It should be recalled that only a distinct minority, 15 to 20 percent in most series, of second-trimester miscarriages can be traced to cervical incompetence. Unfortunately, there are no objective criteria for establishing the diagnosis of cervical incompetence. The use of dilators or balloons to determine cervical resistance and/or hysterosalpingograms to measure the width of the cervical canal between pregnancies have not been sensitive or specific. During the past several years, there has been interest in applying ultrasound to diagnose cervical incompetence during pregnancy.[187] However, examinations are required frequently, and there is a high rate of false-positive and false-negative results. Larger prospective studies are needed before ultrasonography can be used routinely in the management of these patients.

Another approach that we have utilized in women who have a somewhat suggestive but not classic history of cervical incompetence is to perform weekly or biweekly cervical examinations during the second trimester. Only those patients who have significant cervical change undergo a cerclage. In several studies, however, the observation of cervical dilatation in the late second trimester was common and not predictive of premature delivery. An additional problem with this approach is that treatment after 20 weeks or with advanced cervical dilatation is less successful.[188]

ETIOLOGY OF INCOMPETENT CERVIX

Trauma
    Mechanical dilatation of cervix
    Cone biopsy (extensive), cervical amputation
    Obstetric lacerations (spontaneous precipitous labor, operative delivery)

Congenital
Associated with uterine anomalies
DES exposure: more common with cervical, vaginal, or uterine changes
? Increased muscular composition of cervix
? Family history

Cerclage Technique

Since the early 1950s, obstetricians have sought an effective surgical technique to strengthen the cervix and thereby prevent premature cervical dilatation. In 1950, Lash and Lash[188a] described a repair in the nonpregnant patient that involved partial excision of the cervix, presumably removing the areas of weakness. However, this technique was associated with a high incidence of subsequent infertility. In 1955,

Shirodkar[189] reported successful management of cervical incompetence with the use of a submucosal band, first of fascia lata and later of Mersilene, placed at the level of the internal os. This procedure, which could be performed during pregnancy, required anterior displacement of the bladder and a fair amount of submucosal dissection. The Shirodkar cerclage was also difficult to remove so that most successful pregnancies were delivered via cesarean section.

Several years later, McDonald[190] described the use of a purse-string technique that could easily be performed during pregnancy. This approach involves either four or five "bites" as high on the cervix as possible. A metal catheter is used to help identify the posterior extent of the bladder. The knot is placed anteriorly to facilitate removal. This operative technique is illustrated in Figure 25.11. The optimal choice for the suture material has not been established, but obviously a permanent suture is required. We use a single 5-mm Mersilene band double-headed with blunt needles. A major advantage of the wide band is a reduced likelihood of pulling through the cervix later in pregnancy. Others in our institution and elsewhere prefer one or two purse-string stitches with either monofilament Nylon, Polydek, or silk. The McDonald procedure has proved to be as effective as the Shirodkar technique[191] and requires considerably less dissection. Therefore we consider it to be the method of choice. In the setting of advanced dilatation with bulging membranes, the technique of overfilling the bladder with 1,000 cc of saline commonly elevates the membranes out of the operative field and is quite helpful.[192] For patients who have a very short or amputated cervix, or who have failed a vaginal suture, a transabdominal cerclage may be necessary. For a more thorough discussion of this uncommonly indicated procedure, the reader is referred to the recent review of Marx.[193]

After the cerclage, patients should decrease their physical activity and have periods of bed rest during the day. Sexual activity is usually prohibited. The status of the cervix is followed by weekly or biweekly pelvic examinations. If there is progressive cervical shortening, activity can be further decreased. Monitoring may indicate contractions that are not recognized by the patient. The cerclage is removed electively at 37 weeks gestation, a procedure that can usually be accomplished in the office.

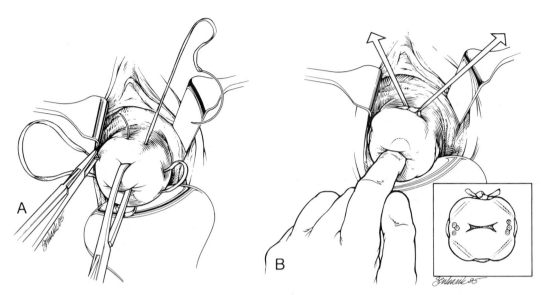

Fig. 25.11 Placement of sutures for McDonald cervical cerclage. (A) We use a double-headed Mersilene band with four "bites" in the cervix, avoiding the vessels. (B) The suture is placed high up on the cervix close to the cervical–vaginal junction, approximating the level of the internal os.

Timing

The best results have been obtained with a cerclage performed before 18 weeks and before cervical dilatation. In the presence of preexisting cervical abnormalities, shortening, or large lacerations, we consider placing the sutures as early as 12 weeks gestation after ultrasonic demonstration of fetal cardiac activity.

In most cases, a cerclage would not be performed after 26 weeks gestation. The great risk of inducing PROM or preterm labor and the ability to prolong gestation with bed rest rule against surgical intervention in such cases.

Risks and Morbidity

Cervical injury at the time of delivery is the most commonly reported morbidity from a McDonald cerclage. While fibrous scar tissue may form at the site of the stitch, producing an abnormal labor curve, a recent study has shown that most patients will have a normal labor curve after a cerclage.[193a] A fibrous "band" may rupture, leading to a cervical laceration (1 to 13 percent), or never dilate (cervical dystocia, 2 to 5 percent), requiring cesarean birth.[183] The cervical laceration may rarely extend to the broad ligament or corpus of the uterus, requiring extensive repair or hysterectomy.

Later in the pregnancy, displacement of the suture also can occur (3 to 12 percent). A second cerclage has a much lower success rate.[183] Use of a Mersilene band may decrease this problem. Other serious common complications of cerclage are PROM (1 to 9 percent) and chorioamnionitis (1 to 7 percent). The risk depends on the timing during gestation and on whether there is cervical dilatation. For elective cerclage at the beginning of the second trimester, the risk of infection appears to be under 1 percent. On the other hand, a cerclage done when the cervix is dilated more than 3 cm with a protruding bag of waters carries at least a 30 percent risk of PROM and/or chorioamnionitis.[188,194] Certainly, cerclage is quite risky under these circumstances and should be considered only in the special case of a clearly previable fetus. The parents must be fully informed of the risks of the procedure and the likelihood of imminent abortion if conservative therapy is followed.

"Success" Rate of Cervical Cerclage

There has never been a randomized prospective study documenting the benefit of cerclage for women with a "classic" history of cervical incompetence. The utility of cerclage was established in the era before randomized trials became standard. Success, defined as fetal survival, is impressive. In every study since 1965 of reasonable size (≥ 100 patients), 80 to 90 percent of the pregnancies have resulted in viable live births.[183] To "prove" efficacy, the investigators used the patients as their own controls and compared their postcerclage outcome with fetal survival before cerclage. Their precerclage survival rate ranged from 13 to 38 percent. This comparison, while alluring, has major inadequacies. First, past obstetric and neonatal practices are compared with current practice. Second and more important, the underlying assumption is that women with one to two previous preterm losses are at very high risk to have another, that is, that the problem is by definition repetitive.

There are no data on the recurrence rate in a carefully defined group at high risk for cervical incompetence. We do have data for previous preterm birth as a whole. After one such birth, 85 percent of patients will deliver at term in the next pregnancy, and after two consecutive preterm births 70 percent will spontaneously be "cured." Similarly, there are several series of "recurrent" second-trimester losses. The subsequent live birth rate in these series is consistently 70 to 75 percent.[195] Therefore, in all but the strongest history of cervical incompetence, the usefulness of cerclage must be viewed as unproven.

This is of importance in light of recent attempts to expand the role of cerclage to patients with "atypical" histories for cervical incompetence or histories that clearly have an element of preterm labor.[196] Two prospective randomized trials of cerclage included patients at moderate or high risk of preterm birth but excluded those with classic indications for cerclage.[197,198] In both trials, which included a total of more than 700 women, there was no benefit from cervical cerclage. In a recent report of a prospective, randomized study of 905 women in which the obstetrician was "uncertain" as to whether to place a cerclage, a 13 percent delivery rate prior to 33 weeks was observed in women treated with a cerclage versus an 18 percent rate in controls ($p = 0.03$).[199] There were similar statistically significant reductions in birth weight under 1,500 g and in neonatal death. While this is encouraging, one must note how well the controls did, indicating a relatively low overall benefit in this group of "obstetrically uncertain" cervical incompetence.

In summary, we believe that there is a group of patients who do have cervical incompetence as an etiology for second- and early third-trimester loss, but this group is small. McDonald cerclage is easy to perform and safe when done electively at 12 to 16 weeks gestation but does carry delayed risks that may not manifest themselves until delivery. Finally, the benefits of cerclage are probably overstated when current outcome is compared retrospectively with the results in prior pregnancies.

PREMATURE RUPTURE OF THE MEMBRANES

PROM is most commonly defined as leakage of amniotic fluid through the cervix, beginning at least 1 hour prior to the onset of labor. We limit the discussion to issues involving the diagnosis, etiology, implications, and management of PPROM, that is, PROM occurring before 37 weeks gestation.

Diagnosis

Most commonly, the patient presents with a history of a large gush of fluid from the vagina followed by persistent, uncontrolled leakage. Importantly, some patients will only report small, intermittent leakage. Therefore any history of passing fluid through the vagina during pregnancy should be evaluated by a sterile speculum examination of the vagina to collect fluid for confirmatory tests. It is extremely important that digital examination of the cervix be avoided until delivery is anticipated within 24 hours. Schutte and colleagues[200] have demonstrated a significant increase in neonatal infection and neonatal mortality when a digital examination precedes delivery by more than 24 hours in the presence of PROM.

When a sterile speculum examination is performed soon after PROM, one frequently finds a collection or "pool" of fluid that can be tested for pH with nitrazine paper. Since amniotic fluid is slightly alkaline, with a pH of ~ 7.15, vaginal secretions containing amniotic fluid will usually result in pH changes in the blue-green range, 6.5 to 7.5. Nitrazine testing is accurate in 90 to 98 percent of cases.[201] False-positive values can result from vaginal infections that raise vaginal pH, especially *T. vaginalis,* the presence of blood, or cervical mucus. False-negative reactions are more frequent when only a scant amount of fluid is present.

An additional test that is commonly used relies on

the property of amniotic fluid to "fern." When placed on a clean slide and allowed to air dry, amniotic fluid produces a microscopic arborization or "fern" pattern. Figure 25.12 demonstrates a typical fern pattern. This crystallization is due to the interaction of amniotic fluid proteins and salts and accurately confirms PROM in 85 to 98 percent of cases. False-positive tests can result from the collection of cervical mucus, which also "ferns" but usually in a more coarse pattern. The fern test is unaffected by meconium, changes in vaginal pH, and blood:amniotic fluid ratios of up to 1:5.[202,203] The fern pattern in samples heavily contaminated with blood is atypical and appears more "skeletonized." [203]

In cases highly suggestive by history but negative or equivocal by the above tests, it is often helpful to place the patient in a semiupright position for approximately 1 hour to encourage the pooling of secretions. During this time, the woman may be monitored to rule out fetal distress and uterine contractions. A repeat sterile speculum examination for nitrazine and fern evaluation is often diagnostic at this point. Another useful adjunct to the diagnosis is an ultrasound evaluation of amniotic fluid volume. While nonspecific, a finding of decreased fluid supports a history of ruptured membranes. This evaluation is also important to assess fetal size and position.

A number of other tests that can be performed on small volumes of vaginal secretions have been described. One of the more promising tests relies on the slide measurement of α-fetoprotein (AFP).[204] This test is particularly useful for pregnancies of less than 35 weeks gestation, because amniotic fluid AFP is higher in the second and early third trimesters of pregnancy than at term. Maternal urine, serum, and seminal fluid do not demonstrate positive slide values for AFP.

Other tests include the measurement of glucose and fructose, which are much lower in amniotic fluid than in cervical mucus; and the measurement of diamine oxidase, which is present in amniotic fluid and absent in vaginal secretions, but requires a scintillation counter for determination and a change in the color of amniotic fluid from clear to white following heating for 1 minute with an alcohol burner.[205–207] These may be of use in select cases in which the diagnosis of PROM remains elusive despite the repetitive performance of the more common tests.

Several investigators have recommended that an amniocentesis be performed to inject a dilute solution of a dye (e.g., Evans blue T-1824 or sodium fluorescein)[208] into the amniotic cavity. Methylene blue should not be used, because it has been associated with hemolytic anemia and hyperbilirubinemia in the infant. Dye studies are seldom indicated in our opinion, even if the diagnosis of PROM remains inconclusive. There is a small but real risk of trauma to the fetus from the amniocentesis, especially in the presence of oligohydramnios, as well as concern that the procedure may introduce infection or lead to rupture of otherwise intact membranes. In addition, it is possible to obtain a false-positive result from an extraovular leakage of dye.

Etiology

The etiology of PPROM is unknown. The fetal membranes are made up of a thin layer of amnion and a thicker outer layer of chorion that is directly opposed to maternal decidual tissue. Interspersed between the amnion and chorion is a collagen-rich connective tissue zone that serves in part to replenish the amnion. By 26 weeks gestation, the amnion is composed of a single layer of cuboidal cells. The chorionic cells are usually four to six layers in thickness. The amnion has

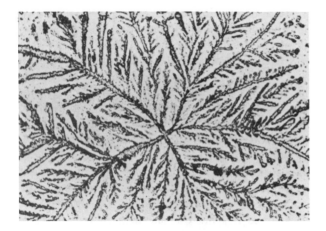

Fig. 25.12 Demonstration of amniotic fluid arborization pattern. (From Reece et al.,[202] with permission.)

greater tensile strength than the chorion, although both membrane layers together withstand greater bursting pressures than they do separately.

The amount of physical stress tolerated by the membranes decreases as pregnancy progresses. Membranes supported by a closed cervix require much greater pressures to rupture than do membranes covering an open area of 3 to 4 cm in diameter.[208] As gestational age advances, the relative concentration of collagen decreases as well.[209] All these factors help to maintain preterm membrane integrity but facilitate rupture of membranes in labor at term.

Why then do some membranes rupture early? The answer to this important question is incomplete. However, most studies suggest that local defects within the membranes may predispose to rupture.[210-214] Bourne[210] stained the fetal membranes through the cervix with Trypan blue dye and demonstrated that the site of rupture is usually immediately above the cervix, an area of membranes that is poorly supported physically and nutritionally. Histologic work has confirmed that, at term, intact membranes excised at the time of cesarean section show localized areas of weakness over the internal os and also in the area directly across from the placental site.[211] A possible explanation for these areas of weakness involves serial damage to the membranes from uterine contractions and fetal growth. The membranes respond to physical stress in part as an "elastic" substance with full return to prior configuration and in part as a "viscous" substance with persistent deformation and thinning after application and removal of a stress.[212] Other explanations include changes in collagen content in membranes that rupture prematurely compared with gestational age-matched control membranes.[209,213] The interaction of a variety of proteases and proteolytic enzymes affects membrane elasticity and may also contribute to PPROM.[214]

Many investigators suspect that PROM, especially PPROM, may result from a variety of genital pathogens that cause subclinical and asymptomatic infections. It is postulated that these organisms may ascend through the cervix and weaken the fetal membranes. Support for this hypothesis is threefold.

First, histologic studies of membranes following PPROM often demonstrate significant bacterial contamination diffusely along the choriodecidual inter-face with minimal involvement of the amnion. This suggests spread of the organisms along the maternal–fetal surfaces before membrane rupture.[59]

Second, a number of investigators have associated increased rates of isolation of specific genital tract pathogens with the presence of PROM. The organisms statistically associated with PROM in one study but not uniformly confirmed in others include *B. fragilis,* other anaerobes, *N. gonorrhoeae, C. trachomatis, T. vaginalis,* and group B β-hemolytic streptococci.[59] In most of these cases, the suspected pathogen was isolated twice as often in women with PROM. For example, PROM occurred in 15.3 percent of women colonized with group B streptococci compared with 7 percent of women not colonized, a highly statistically significant association in this report involving 6,706 parturients.[215] Whether this increased relative risk truly reflects the actions of the organism under study, other organisms, or associated socioeconomic factors remains unclear.

Third, there is an increased risk of maternal, fetal, and neonatal infection in the presence of PPROM. Many of these infections are evident soon after the membranes have ruptured. In these cases, it is thought that subclinical infection may actually precede and contribute to PROM. With preterm as opposed to term PROM, the frequency of infection does not appear to increase as the period between amniotic fluid leakage and delivery lengthens.

Certain social and obstetric factors have also been associated with PROM. Using a large data base from Ontario, Meyer and Tonascia[32] reported that smokers were three times more likely than nonsmokers to experience PROM before 34 weeks gestation. In addition, heavier smokers in this study experienced more PROM than lighter smokers. In his analysis of data from the Perinatal Collaborative Project, Naeye[216] found an association between term PROM and smoking but none between PPROM and smoking. Furthermore, he was unable to demonstrate that heavy smokers were at greater risk than were light smokers. However, a recent case-control study by Hadley et al. has demonstrated both smoking and a history of previous preterm PROM to be significant risk factors.[216a]

Naeye[216] also observed an association between preterm deliveries caused by PROM and the combination of coitus within 9 days of delivery and the histologic diagnosis of chorioamnionitis. In the absence of chorioamnionitis, the association with coitus and PPROM persisted but with a much lower relative risk. This relationship has not been confirmed by other investigators.

Women who have suffered PROM in a prior pregnancy are at increased risk to experience it again. A 21 percent recurrence rate for PPROM was reported by Naeye.[216] Bleeding in pregnancy also predisposes to membrane rupture.[217] Whether multiple induced abortions increase the risk of PROM is unclear, but such an association is suggested in at least one recent study.[52]

Maternal Risks

Whether a cause or result of PPROM, intrauterine infection is a potentially serious complication to the mother. Intrauterine infection, defined as the presence of a positive amniotic fluid culture regardless of the presence or absence of clinical evidence of infection, occurs on average in 28 percent of women with PPROM (range, 14.6 to 43.3 percent).[59] Although most instances of amnionitis respond well to antibiotic administration and delivery, maternal deaths from sepsis can occur.[218] In one study, amnionitis was more common at 23 to 31 weeks gestation than at 32 to 34 weeks gestation.[208] This may reflect the more limited antibacterial properties of amniotic fluid from preterm pregnancies and may place these patients at greater risk of amnionitis.

Placental abruption occurs in 5 to 6 percent of cases of PPROM, a much higher rate than for controls.[219,220] Approximately one-fourth of the abruptions are diagnosed within the first 24 hours following PROM, and these may be related to rapid decompression of uterine volume. Those occurring later in the course of expectant management appear to be associated with more severe oligohydramnios[219] or with prior bleeding.[220]

Fetal and Neonatal Risks

Not surprisingly, infection is a major potential complication for the fetus and neonate as well as for the mother. The same vaginal organisms that lead to maternal infection can result in congenital pneumonia, sepsis, or meningitis. However, the presence of obvious culture-documented amnionitis usually does not result in neonatal infection. In published series, the range of neonatal sepsis in cases of PPROM with or without clinical amnionitis has ranged from 2 to 19 percent and the range of neonatal deaths caused by infection from 1 to 7 percent. The frequency of neonatal infection varies considerably with gestational age, fetal sex, race, and maternal antepartum course, as well as the definition used by the investigators. Studies requiring positive cultures for diagnosis tend to detect lower sepsis rates than those combining clinical course, radiographic findings, and neonatal bacterial colonization for diagnosis. In general, maternal and neonatal infections are more common in low socioeconomic populations.

A number of other potential fetal complications can result from PPROM. There is a higher risk of frank or occult cord prolapse, particularly if the fetus is not in a cephalic presentation. Furthermore, regardless of presentation, the risks of fetal distress in labor leading to cesarean delivery are significantly higher with PPROM than with isolated preterm labor (7.9 vs. 1.5 percent).[221] The most common fetal heart rate tracing leading to operative delivery is severe variable decelerations.[221]

Pulmonary hypoplasia is an additional concern, particularly when fetal membranes are ruptured prior to 26 weeks gestation. In two recent series, one-third of babies born following PROM before 26 weeks gestation but delivered after 26 weeks gestation developed pulmonary hypoplasia.[222,223] Fetuses exposed to extreme oligohydramnios are more likely to experience this complication. Skeletal deformities, presumably related to compression following oligohydramnios, also are quite common. Twenty-seven percent of fetuses with PROM prior to 26 weeks who experienced prolonged rupture before delivery developed skeletal deformations.[223]

The adverse complications from PROM must be balanced against the risks from prematurity. In this respect, PROM may offer preterm infants an advantage. Mead[224] evaluated the effect of PROM on fetal lung maturity. He found 14 studies that suggested a reduction in RDS following PROM and 11 investigations that failed to demonstrate such an association. Some of the many confounding variables contributing to discrepancies in study results include wide gestational age categories, unequal sex distribution, difficulty in distinguishing congenital pneumonia from

RDS, failure to control for route of delivery and degree of asphyxia, and small sample size. Furthermore, the duration of the time from PROM to delivery necessary to have such a beneficial effect, if it is actually present, and the gestational ages at which this effect exists are unclear.

Natural History

Because of the significant risks of preterm birth, particularly at early gestational ages, many clinicians advocate a conservative approach to the management of PPROM, that is, expectant, observational management. Without any medical intervention, what is the natural course of PPROM? The duration of PROM is inversely related to the gestational age at time of membrane rupture. When PROM occurs prior to 26 weeks gestation, 30 to 40 percent of cases will gain at least one additional week before delivery and 20 percent will gain over 4 weeks.[222] By contrast, 70 to 80 percent of patients who experience PROM between 28 to 34 weeks gestation deliver within the first week after PROM and more than one-half of these within the first 4 days.[225] At term, 80 percent of women go into labor within the first 24 hours after rupture of the membranes.

Management

Weighing Risks of PROM and Prematurity

The management of PPROM remains one of the most controversial areas in obstetrics. In general, the management options include a conservative approach of "letting nature take its course," a recourse to immediate delivery, or aggressive schemes to attempt to delay delivery and/or accelerate fetal lung maturation. The choice of which therapeutic modality is most appropriate is based on balancing the relative risks from PROM, specifically infection and asphyxia from cord compression or prolapse, against the risks of prematurity. There is almost universal agreement that delivery should be expeditiously undertaken regardless of the gestational age when clinical chorioamnionitis is diagnosed. Traditional obstetric indications for cesarean section, such as fetal distress, are used to determine mode of delivery in this situation.

In the absence of overt infection, the relative risks from PROM versus those from prematurity vary significantly with gestational age and population char-

acteristics. In general, the risks of preterm birth outweigh the risks of infection and cord compression below 30 to 32 weeks gestation, while the risks from PROM outweigh prematurity after 34 to 35 weeks gestation.[226] Exactly where the relative risk ratio shifts depends in part on the population. For example, blacks often have higher risks of infection and lower rates of respiratory distress. Thus each medical center should establish a management scheme on the basis of its own neonatal outcome data.

Because of the central role of gestational age in determining the relative risks inherent in the different approaches, it is crucial to assess gestational age accurately. In this regard, it is important to remember that biparietal diameter measurements by ultrasound are much less accurate in the presence of PROM, with errors leading to both over- and underestimations of fetal age.[227,228] Determination of the femur length may be a more reliable index of gestational age in these situations.

Use of Amniocentesis

Another controversial area is the use of amniocentesis to detect the presence of infection and to assess fetal lung maturity. When advocated, this approach is usually recommended for the intermediate group of women whose gestations are complicated by PROM between 30 and 34 weeks gestation.[226] Even advocates of amniocentesis recommend this procedure only when there is an adequate pocket of fluid and an area for needle insertion that is free from the placenta and cord. Placing the patient in the Trendelenburg position for several hours prior to the amniocentesis may increase intrauterine retention of fluid and facilitate the procedure.

Although debated, most investigators who recommend amniocentesis perform it in the first 24 hours after membrane rupture. Bacterial cultures are more likely to be positive when the amniocentesis is performed relatively early, within the first 48 hours after PROM, rather than later, supporting the theory that subclinical infections often precede PPROM.[229]

Garite and colleagues[225] reported their experience with 98 amniocenteses performed in the presence of PROM between 28 to 34 weeks gestation. None of the patients demonstrated signs of clinical amnionitis, and none were in labor. A mature lecithin/sphingomyelin (L/S) ratio of at least 1.8 : 1 was found in 39 percent of samples. An additional 13 percent had Gram stains of unspun amniotic fluid that demonstrated the presence of bacteria. Thus approximately one-half of these asymptomatic women were delivered expeditiously because of amniotic fluid findings. Other investigators have reported similar rates of positive findings on Gram stain.

However, is amniocentesis really necessary and of benefit to these women? Important issues regarding the decision for or against performing an amniocentesis revolve around the safety of the procedure for mother and fetus and the utility of the information obtained.

Some reassurance regarding the relative safety of amniocentesis in the presence of PPROM has been provided. Yeast et al.[230] performed a retrospective chart review of 138 patients with PROM at 28 to 34 weeks gestation who were not in labor or clinically infected. Amniocentesis was performed in 91 women compared with 46 women for whom amniocentesis was considered impossible because of the absence of a fluid pocket or placenta-free window. There was no difference in time to onset of labor between the two groups. Review of the neonatal records failed to demonstrate any evidence of fetal injury from the amniocentesis needle. Only one maternal complication was recorded, and that was a small hematoma of the superior broad ligament noted at cesarean section. Although reassuring, this study must be interpreted cautiously. The sample size is relatively small, and the retrospective nature of the study excludes careful assessments of the placenta and cord. Other investigations of third-trimester amniocenteses have demonstrated perforation of maternal epigastric and uterine vessels and significant intraperitoneal and uterine hematomas.[231] A literature review reported the risk of fetal injury to be between 0.6 and 2.0 percent and that of placenta and cord injury to be 0.3 to 1.1 percent.[231] Therefore potential risks from the procedure must be explained to the patient.

Free-flowing vaginally collected amniotic fluid can be used to check for phosphatidylglycerol.[232,233] One case report suggests that bacterial contaminants in vaginally collected fluid may produce phosphatidylglycerol, thus creating a false impression of fetal lung maturity.[234] Although often reliable, vaginally collected amniotic fluid will sometimes provide false-low or false-elevated L/S values.[232,233] One report suggests that breech presentation may lower the L/S value because the vaginally collected fluid contains a large amount of fetal urine.[235]

There is debate in the literature regarding the utility of tests for fetal lung maturity in PPROM. One question raised is whether a mature L/S ratio accurately predicts good neonatal outcome, particularly in pregnancies under 32 weeks gestation. Garite et al.[225] reported a low incidence of RDS with a mature L/S ratio regardless of gestational age,[225] while others are more cautious about neonatal outcome in very preterm infants, even with pulmonary maturity documented by amniocentesis. A further question is whether a straight gestational age cutoff, usually between 33 and 35 weeks, is as good a predictor of neonatal morbidity and mortality.

Amniotic fluid obtained by amniocentesis can be used to screen for asymptomatic amnionitis. A number of investigators have confirmed that a Gram stain of unspun amniotic fluid is a fairly accurate predictor of impending chorioamnionitis. Approximately 10^5 organisms per milliliter is needed before a Gram stain will be positive. Thus not all culture-positive fluids have positive Gram stains, though virtually all positive Gram stains result from culture-positive fluids. The presence of white blood cells (WBCs) in amniotic fluid has not proven helpful in predicting infection.

Similarly, WBC counts from peripheral blood are not reliably predictive of the presence or absence of chorioamnionitis. In contrast, several investigators report that C-reactive protein may identify women with subclinical or overt infection.[236] Others have reported considerable overlap between C-reactive protein in infected and noninfected pregnancies.[237] Because of its low specificity, most centers do not consider this test clinically useful.

Recently, several investigators have suggested that ultrasound assessment may be as accurate a predictor of subsequent clinically apparent maternal or neonatal infection as amniocentesis and Gram stain and culture results.[238–240] Vintzileos et al.[238] compared amniotic fluid volume and amniocentesis performed on admission in 54 pregnancies and found each to be similarly efficacious. Qualitative amniotic fluid volume (vertical measurement of largest pocket <1 cm) had a sensitivity of 50 percent, specificity of 93 percent, positive predictive value of 66.6 percent, and negative predictive value of 86.6 percent. Amniocentesis had a sensitivity of 58 percent, specificity of 88 percent, positive predictive value of 58 percent, and negative predictive value of 88 percent.[238] The same investigators have suggested that daily biophysical profiles with delivery for a persistently low score (7 or less on two examinations 2 hours apart) leads to a lower rate of neonatal sepsis than management based on amniocentesis.[239] Goldstein et al[240] studied fetal behavior and intra-amniotic infection defined as positive amniotic fluid cultures. All fetuses demonstrating an episode of fetal activity (breathing and body movements) of more than 30 seconds in a 30-minute period had negative cultures, while the absence of fetal breathing and less than 50 seconds of gross body movements in 30 minutes identified only women with infection. In patients with some fetal breathing lasting less than 30 seconds but body movements of more than 50 seconds, 64 percent of cultures were positive. Others have found absent fetal breathing to be somewhat less predictive of adverse outcome.[241]

Thus it appears that there are imperfect means with which to identify women who will develop clinically significant infections following PROM. No one has demonstrated that delivery of afebrile, asymptomatic women improves either neonatal or maternal outcome. In large part this is because most infants born to clinically infected mothers are themselves not infected. Furthermore, not all women with positive tests develop clinical amnionitis. Therefore many obstetricians still await clinical signs of infection or fetal distress in the presence of PROM before intervening.

Use of Corticosteroids

As summarized earlier in this chapter, maternally administered corticosteroids appear to accelerate fetal lung maturation. A number of randomized trials of corticosteroids in the presence of PROM have revealed conflicting results. Two recent meta-analyses[164,242] that aggregated data from published randomized trials suggest overall benefit and no increase in neonatal infections or other morbidity from corticosteroid use with PROM. It is therefore now our policy to administer these agents to women with PROM who are at less than 32 weeks gestation and

between 32 and 34 weeks gestation if lung immaturity is documented.

Use of Tocolytics

Should tocolytic agents be used in patients with preterm PROM? This is yet another controversial question in the management of PPROM. Tocolytic use was discouraged by the report from the National Institutes of Health Collaborative Study on Antenatal Steroids that noted an association between tocolytic use in PROM and a higher rate of RDS.[243] In 1987, Garite et al.[244] reported a randomized trial of intravenous ritodrine administered between 25 and 30 weeks gestation at the start of labor (N = 39) versus placebo (N = 40). Twenty-three of the 39 women randomized to tocolytic therapy actually received the treatment while the others were delivered because of suspected chorioamnionitis, advanced labor, or fetal distress. There was no significant improvement in pregnancy prolongation or morbidity in this study. Weiner et al.[245] randomized 109 patients with PROM at up to 34 weeks gestation to intravenous tocolysis once three contractions per hour were detected versus bed rest. There were no differences in outcome in patients over 28 weeks gestation. However, five patients under 28 weeks who received tocolytics had a significantly longer latency period than did 12 patients treated with bed rest alone. In a retrospective comparison, Bourgeois et al.[246] compared women with PROM at less than 34 weeks gestation treated prophylactically with tocolytics versus those treated only after the start of labor. They suggested increased benefit from the early treatment approach. Thus the available evidence for the use of tocolytics in the presence of PPROM is far from compelling.

Use of Antibiotics

In contrast to the equivocal results obtained with tocolytic therapy, several randomized trials of antibiotics in the presence of PPROM have demonstrated benefit in terms of pregnancy prolongation and/or fetal morbidity.[247-251] Antibiotics used included ampicillin, mezlicillin, ampicillin, gentamicin, and erythromycin. The optimal agent, dose, and duration of treatment remain unclear. Given the distribution of pathogens, however, it appears appropriate to cover both β-hemolytic streptococci and anaerobes. Further trials are continuing in this area.

Expectant Management of PROM

As can be determined from the preceding sections, the optimal management for PPROM is far from completely decided. The absence of benefit and potential for harm from more aggressive approaches have led many obstetricians to elect an expectant approach to PPROM. This too can present complications unless carefully managed. It is crucial that women with PROM be monitored closely to detect cord compression and cord prolapse. In addition, maternal temperature and uterine tenderness should be assessed. It is of critical importance to avoid digital examination of the cervix unless delivery is anticipated within 24 hours of examination.

Management of PROM Preceding Fetal Viability

When PROM occurs before 25 weeks gestation, the likelihood of intact neonatal survival is low. In 53 pregnancies complicated by PROM between 16 and 25 weeks gestation, 25 percent of the fetuses survived the neonatal period.[222] Almost 60 percent of the mothers had complications, most commonly infectious, but none developed lasting sequelae. In another 118 cases of PROM between 16 to 26 weeks gestation, the total perinatal mortality was 67.7 percent.[218] Only 13.3 percent of the infants with PROM at 23 weeks or less survived while 50 percent of those with PROM at 24 to 26 weeks survived. Sixty-seven percent of the infants were developmentally normal on follow-up. Maternal morbidity was high and included one death from sepsis. Because of the relatively low chance of successful outcome and the high rate of infectious complications, it is important that the patient be carefully informed of the risks of expectant management.

CONDUCT OF LABOR AND DELIVERY FOR THE PRETERM INFANT

Fetal Monitoring

No other fetus benefits more from fetal monitoring than does the very premature. Careful and intensive fetal surveillance of these fetuses has been associated with significantly improved outcome in every major

study.[252,253] This is in contrast to the finding in the same studies that routine monitoring is only of borderline benefit to the normal term infant. Electronic fetal monitoring is not the only option. Recently, Luthy et al.[254] showed that attentive nursing care (one on one) with auscultation every 15 minutes gives perinatal mortality results statistically no different from those with electronic fetal monitoring. However, they subsequently showed that electronic fetal monitoring gives better information about fetal and neonatal well-being and improved predictability regarding fetal status.[255] Ominous heart rate tracings have the same associations with fetal acidosis as they do later in gestation, but prompt cesarean delivery can minimize their effect on perinatal morbidity and mortality.[256,257]

Fetal Heart Rate

Mean fetal heart rate falls continuously, from 160 bpm at 22 weeks gestation, to 140 bpm at term. This is apparently due to a gradual increase in parasympathetic tone. At no age after 26 to 28 weeks should the normal baseline heart rate be above 170 bpm.

Variability

Changes in fetal heart rate variability in the preterm fetus carry the same significance for risk of acidosis as in term infants. Zanini et al.[256] clearly demonstrated that, for any periodic change in premature infants, fetal pH is significantly less if variability is absent.

Resistance to Hypoxia

Some have reported an apparent tolerance in premature infants to prolonged periods of hypoxia both in utero and in the neonatal nursery. This has led to a concept of "plasticity," or the ability of the premature brain to absorb insults and "bounce back." While this idea may have some validity, particularly in considering prognosis, it is dangerous to use it when managing patients in labor. Premature infants do sustain hypoxic–ischemic insults and have higher rates of cerebral palsy. Therefore we must move toward immediate correction or delivery when ominous patterns occur during labor.

Anesthesia and Analgesia

There is no one method of anesthesia or analgesia in labor with a preterm fetus that is superior for all conditions. Here we must stress the most important goal of intensive perinatal care: to provide the neonatologist with the least traumatized, least depressed, and least acidotic fetus consistent with maternal health.

Epidural anesthesia offers the advantage of pelvic floor and outlet muscle relaxation, minimizing an important source of resistance to the soft premature fetal head. Of concern, however, is the higher rate of hypotension associated with this method. Hypotension can largely be avoided by adequate preloading with a crystalloid and more gradual onset of the block. Paracervical block is undesirable because of the high risk of bradycardia, secondary either to transplacental passage of the anesthetic agent causing direct myocardial depression or to local uterine vascular vasospasm with diminished uteroplacental perfusion. The use of parenteral narcotics, even early in labor, is generally minimized because of concern for respiratory depression and because of the uncertain speed of preterm labor. However, the role of narcotics and other central nervous system (CNS) depressants has been reevaluated, with attention focused on the "brain-protective" action of these drugs.[258] The ability to extrapolate data from a research laboratory with monkeys to the labor floor may be limited. Thus the concept of narcotic-induced prevention of serious neurologic damage remains an interesting research hypothesis. Not using analgesia or anesthesia also has the risk of maternal hyperventilation. Furthermore, maternal self-control is crucial for proper conduct of the second stage of labor.

Each choice of anesthesia for cesarean delivery has its own advantages and disadvantages. For such an operative delivery, the epidural technique requires a deeper, more intense block, involving more spinal segments than vaginal delivery. This further increases the risk of hypotension (able to be lessened, as discussed above). In addition, preloading the mother with large volumes of dextrose-containing fluid can further increase fetal acidosis.[259] General anesthesia is quicker to administer in an emergency situation and usually involves less changes in uteroplacental perfusion. However, it does entail greater risks to the mother, can lead to fetal depression if the surgery is difficult, and deprives the mother of perhaps her only chance to see and bond with a sick premature infant during its first hours of life.

Labor

The course of labor in preterm gestation is significantly shorter than that of term pregnancy. Of particular importance are the rapidity of the active phase and the short second stage of labor. These need to be considered as one follows the labor to ensure the fetus does not have a precipitous delivery without control of the fetal head. Multiparous women can have particularly short active phases, with 30 to 90 minutes not uncommon.

Delivery

The two predominant goals for the intrapartum management of the preterm infant are (1) avoidance of asphyxia and (2) avoidance of birth trauma. The critical role of asphyxia is demonstrated by a study from Michael Reese Hospital (Fig. 25.13).[260] In 136 neo-

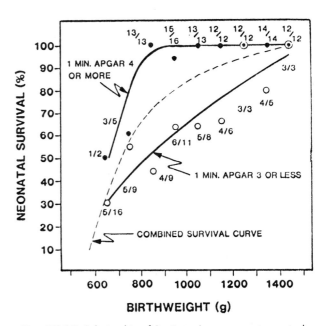

Fig. 25.13 Relationship of 1-minute Apgar score to survival in very-low-birth-weight infants. (From Myers et al.,[260] with permission.)

nates of less than 32 weeks gestation, the 1-minute Apgar score was highly correlated with survival. Babies with 1-minute Apgar scores of 4 or more had a 95 percent survival, while infants with a score of 3 or less had only a 56 percent survival rate. The implication from this and other studies is that initial condition at birth substantially affects survival. How then can one "optimize" the birth process for the VLBW (<1,500 g) infant?

Episiotomy

A generous episiotomy is recommended by many investigators, based on common sense, to minimize the forces of outlet perineal resistance on the small soft head. In fact, these forces are probably much less than those of the cervix and muscles of the vagina through which the fetus has already passed. Data demonstrating improved outcome associated with the use of episiotomy are very difficult to find.[261] When delivering a VLBW infant, we perform an early episiotomy if there is perineal resistance. Few multiparous women will be in this group.

"Prophylactic" Forceps

An analysis of the National Collaborative Perinatal Project data found that the premature infants (<2,500 g birth weight) who had the best outcome were the ones delivered by low forceps.[262] Thus credence was given to the concept that "prophylactic" forceps protected the fragile fetal head. Recent studies, albeit with smaller numbers, have not been able to show this benefit.[261,263] In fact, O'Driscoll et al.[264] suggested that forceps may be harmful. He has presented a series of preterm infants with traumatic intracranial hemorrhages, all of which were delivered with outlet forceps.[264] Therefore it does not seem appropriate to expedite delivery prophylactically with forceps when more than minimal traction will be needed. It also should be noted that current "premie" forceps were designed for infants weighing 1,500 to 1,900 g and appear clearly too large for the under 1,000-g fetus. The most important point is to pay careful attention to controlling the often rapid second stage to avoid the head "bursting" through

the perineum. With this approach we rarely use "prophylactic" forceps.

Cesarean Section

The optimal method of delivery for the VLBW infant continues to be a source of debate. Unfortunately, most studies in this area have significant faults. They are typically retrospective reviews of outcome with little attempt made to compare characteristics of infants who were delivered vaginally to those who were delivered by cesarean section. Thus the role of confounding variables cannot be eliminated and may be of overriding importance, particularly in the studies of vertex infants.

That the VLBW nonvertex infant does better after a cesarean birth is widely believed but has not yet been proven in a prospective randomized study. There are intuitive reasons for desiring to avoid trapping of the aftercoming head, an infrequent but disastrous complication, as well as other manipulations that could lead to trauma and hypoxia. Most retrospective studies have confirmed a benefit from cesarean section. Main et al. presented the largest such series, 216 breeches of 750 to 1,500 g birth weight delivered over 4 years. The mortality rate in the cesarean section group was 29 percent, significantly less than the 58 percent mortality rate for breech infants born vaginally ($p < 0.001$).[265] This advantage remained after correction for hospital setting, birth weight, and presence of growth retardation.[265] However, in this study, as in many others, the smallest VLBW breeches were more apt to have been delivered vaginally and their higher mortality rate may have had as much to do with their size as with their method of delivery. Other studies with somewhat smaller numbers of VLBW breeches found trends toward improvement with cesarean birth that did not reach statistical significance or lost significance when confounding variables were considered.[266,267,267a] Therefore, while we feel comfortable with the current American trend toward cesarean delivery of all VLBW nonvertex infants, we have to acknowledge that these data are not conclusive enough to take a dogmatic position.

A critical technical point cannot be overstressed. One does not want to avoid a traumatic vaginal delivery only to struggle and have a difficult cesarean birth because of an undeveloped lower uterine segment or an inadequate incision.[267] Clearly, the operation must be carried out in a way that will fulfill its purpose, atraumatic delivery. While some have recommended routine use of a low vertical or classic incision, we believe that the exact uterine incision can depend on the fetal position and on the anatomy of the individual patient. If the lower uterine segment is wide enough for a large "smile" incision and the fetus is in the lower one-third of the uterus, a transverse incision may still be reasonable.

Routine cesarean delivery of VLBW vertex infants can no longer be supported. Several large studies have failed to note improvement in perinatal morbidity or mortality with cesarean birth for indications other than classic obstetric ones.[267a,268,269] The trend favoring cesarean section seen in some studies disappears after adjustment for confounding factors.[270]

A current focus of interest is whether labor and/or delivery cause neonatal intracranial hemorrhage (ICH). Kosmetatos et al.[271] suggested that cesarean-delivered VLBW infants had a significantly reduced incidence of ICH. This was immediately followed by four studies that could not find such an advantage.

More recently, data have been presented suggesting that it is not the route of delivery but the presence of active labor that is critical in the development of ICH.[272] Most studies, when corrected for gestational age, presentation, and labor complications, fail to support this finding. One recent study[273] carefully separates out "high-risk" VLBW labor (e.g., preeclampsia, vaginal bleeding, abnormal heart rate tracing) from "low-risk" VLBW (e.g., preterm labor, incompetent cervix). Cesarean section was of no value in the low-risk group, but was associated with highly significantly improved survival rates in the high-risk group. Thus we can identify situations requiring delivery in the face of a long closed cervix that may tilt analysis in VLBW fetuses away from a long and potentially morbid induction of labor toward elective cesarean birth. However, we must acknowledge that studies to date have not provided clear evidence that this approach is of great benefit to the infant and mother.

With these caveats, we close by summarizing the key elements for providing optimal care of the preterm fetus:

1. Prevention of preterm birth has not yet been accomplished. It is clear that preterm birth has multiple etiologies and therefore is unlikely to yield to a single intervention. In evaluating new therapies, the need for randomized controlled trials is self-evident.

2. Tocolytics and glucocorticoids are late therapies in the problem of preterm birth. In fact, knowing when to use and when not to use tocolytics is of critical importance.

3. The focus of intrapartum care of VLBW fetuses is to give the infant to the neonatologist in the best possible condition. There is inadequate evidence to recommend routine cesarean birth for all VLBW vertex infants.

REFERENCES

1. McCormick MC: The contribution of low birthweight to infant mortality and childhood morbidity. N Engl J Med 312:82, 1985

2. U.S. Department of Health and Human Services, Public Health Service, National Center for Health Statistics: Vital Statistics of the United States 1987. Vol. I. USDHHS, Hyattsville, MD, 1990

3. Brenner WE, Edelman DA, Hendricks CH: A standard of fetal growth for the United States of America. Am J Obstet Gynecol 126:555, 1976

4. Kessel S, Villar J, Berendes H, Nugent R: The changing pattern of low birth weight in the United States. JAMA 251:1978, 1984

5. Leveno KJ, Little BB, Cunningham FG: The national impact of ritodrine hydrochloride for inhibition of preterm labor. Obstet Gynecol 76:12, 1990

6. Guyer B, Wallach L, Rosen S: Birth-weight-standardized neonatal mortality rates and the prevention of low birth weight: how does Massachusetts compare with Sweden? N Engl J Med 306:1230, 1982

7. Paul R, Koh K, Monfared A: Obstetric factors influencing outcome in infants weighing from 1,001 to 1,500 grams. Am J Obstet Gynecol 133:503, 1979

8. Main DM, Hadley CB: The role of ultrasound in the management of preterm labor. Clin Obstet Gynecol 31:1:53, 1988

9. Verloove-Vanhorick SP, Verwey RA, Brand R et al: Neonatal mortality risk in relation to gestational age and birthweight: results of a national survey of pre-

term and very-low-birth-weight infants in the Netherlands. Lancet 1:55, 1986

10. Hack M, Fanaroff AA: Outcomes of extremely-low-birth-weight infants between 1982 and 1988. N Engl J Med 321:1642, 1989

11. Ferrara TB, Hoekstra RE, Gaziano E et al: Changing outcome of extremely premature infants (≤26 weeks gestation and ≤750 gm): survival and follow-up at a tertiary center. Am J Obstet Gynecol 161:1114, 1989

12. Nwaesei CG, Young DC, Byrne JM et al: Preterm birth at 23 to 26 weeks gestation: is active obstetric management justified? Am J Obstet Gynecol 157:890, 1987

13. Wood B, Katz V, Bose C et al: Survival and morbidity of extremely premature infants based on obstetric assessment of gestational age. Obstet Gynecol 74:889, 1989

14. Heinonen K, Hakulinen A, Jokela V: Survival of the smallest: time trends and determinants of mortality in a very preterm population during the 1980s. Lancet 2:204, 1988

15. Milligan JE, Shennan AT, Hoskins EM: Perinatal intensive care: where and how to draw the line. Am J Obstet Gynecol 148:499, 1984

16. Wariyar U, Richmond S, Hey E: Pregnancy outcome at 24–31 weeks gestation: neonatal survivors. Arch Dis Child 64:678, 1989

17. Resnick MB, Carter RL, Ariet M et al: Effect of birthweight, race, and sex on survival of low birthweight infants in neonatal intensive care. Am J Obstet Gynecol 161:184, 1989

18. Horbar JD, McAuliffe TL, Adler SM et al: Variability in 28-day outcomes for very low birth weight infants: an analysis of 11 neonatal intensive care units. Pediatrics 82:554, 1988

19. Ehrenhaft PM, Wagner JL, Herdman RC: Changing prognosis for very low birth weight infants. Obstet Gynecol 74:528, 1989

20. Lumley J, Kitchen WH, Roy RND et al: The survival of extremely-low-birthweight infants in Victoria: 1982–1985. Med J Aust 149:242, 1988

21. Lubchenco LO, Butterfield LJ, Delaney-Black V et al: Outcome of very-low-birth-weight infants: does antepartum versus neonatal referral have a better impact on mortality, morbidity, or long-term outcome? Am J Obstet Gynecol 160:539, 1989

22. Delaney-Black V, Lubchenco LO, Butterfield LJ et al: Outcome of very low birthweight infants: are populations of neonates inherently different after antenatal versus neonatal referral? Am J Obstet Gynecol 160:545, 1989

23. Yu VYH, Wong PY, Bajuk B et al: Outcome of extremely low birthweight infants. Br J Obstet Gynaecol 93:162, 1986

24. Nickel R, Bennett F, Lamson F: School performance of children with birth weights of 1,000 g or less. Am J Dis Child 136:105, 1982

25. Astbury J, Orgill A, Bajuk B et al: Determinants of developmental performance of very low birthweight survivors at one and two years of age. Dev Med Child Neurol 25:709, 1983

26. Resnick MB, Stralka K, Carter RL et al: Effects of birthweight and sociodemographic variables on mental development of neonatal intensive care unit survivors. Am J Obstet Gynecol 162:374, 1990

27. Yu VYH, Downe L, Astbury J et al: Perinatal factors and adverse outcome in extremely low birthweight infants. Arch Dis Child 61:554, 1986

28. Brothwood M, Wolke D, Gamsu H et al: Prognosis of the very low birthweight baby in relation to gender. Arch Dis Child 61:559, 1986

29. McCormick MC, Shapiro S, Starfield BH: Rehospitalization during the first year of life for high risk survivors. Pediatrics 66:991, 1980

30. Papiernik E, Kaminski M: Multifactorial study of the risk of prematurity at 32 weeks of gestation. J Perinat Med 2:30, 1974

31. Main DM: The epidemiology of preterm birth. Clin Obstet Gynecol 31:3:521, 1988

32. Meyer M, Tonascia J: Maternal smoking, pregnancy complications, and perinatal mortality. Am J Obstet Gynecol 128:494, 1977

33. Murphy J, Dauncey M, Newcombe R et al: Employment in pregnancy: prevalence, maternal characteristics, perinatal outcome. Lancet 1:1163, 1984

34. Mamelle N, Laumon B, Lazar P: Prematurity and occupational activity during pregnancy. Am J Epidemiol 119:309, 1984

35. Grunebaum AG, Minkoff H, Blake D: Pregnancy among obstetricians: a comparison of births before, during, and after residency. Am J Obstet Gynecol 157:79, 1987

36. Klebanoff MA, Shiono PH, Rhoads GG: Outcomes of pregnancy in a national sample of resident physicians. N Engl J Med 323:1040, 1990

37. Naeye R: Coitus and associated amniotic-fluid infections. N Engl J Med 301:1198, 1979

38. Goodlin R, Keller D, Raffin M: Orgasm during late pregnancy. Obstet Gynecol 38:916, 1971

39. Mills J, Harlap S, Harley E: Should coitus late in pregnancy be discouraged? Lancet 2:136, 1981

40. Klebanoff M, Nugent R, Rhoads G: Coitus during pregnancy: is it safe? Lancet 2:914, 1984

41. Greenberg R: The impact of prenatal care in different social groups. Am J Obstet Gynecol 145:797, 1983

42. Newton R, Hunt L: Psychosocial stress in pregnancy and its relation to low birthweight. Br Med J 288:1191, 1984

43. Graham G: Poverty, hunger, malnutrition, prematurity, and infant mortality in the United States. Pediatrics 75:117, 1985

44. Lind T: Would more calories per day keep low birthweight at bay? Lancet 1:501, 1984

45. Rush D, Stein Z, Susser MA: A randomized controlled trial of prenatal nutritional supplementation in New York City. Pediatrics 65:683, 1980

46. Kiilholma P, Gronroos M, Erkkola R et al: The role of calcium, copper, iron and zinc in preterm delivery and premature rupture of fetal membranes. Gynecol Obstet Invest 17:194, 1984

47. Artal R, Burgeson R, Fernandez F et al: Fetal and maternal copper levels in patients at term with and without premature rupture of membranes. Obstet Gynecol 53:608, 1979

48. Klebanoff M, Graubard B, Kessel S et al: Low birthweight across generations. JAMA 252:2423, 1984

49. Bakketeig LS, Hoffman HJ: Epidemiology of preterm birth: results from a longitudinal study of births in Norway. p. 67. In Elder MG, Hendricks CH (eds): Preterm Labor. Butterworths, London, 1981

50. Keirse M, Rush R, Anderson A et al: Risk of preterm delivery in patients with previous preterm delivery and/or abortion. Br J Obstet Gynaecol 85:81, 1978

51. Funderburk S, Guthrie D, Meldrum D: Suboptimal pregnancy outcome among women with prior abortions and premature births. Am J Obstet Gynecol 126:55, 1976

52. Linn S, Schoenbaum S, Monson R et al: The relationship between induced abortion and outcome of subsequent pregnancies. Am J Obstet Gynecol 146:136, 1983

53. Hogue C, Cates W, Tietze C: The effects of induced abortion on subsequent reproduction. Epidemiol Rev 4:66, 1982

54. Chung C, Smith R, Steinhoff P et al: Induced abortion and spontaneous fetal loss in subsequent pregnancies. Am J Public Health 72:548, 1982

55. Heinonen P, Saarikoski S, Pystynen P: Reproductive performance of women with uterine anomalies. Acta Obstet Gynecol Scand 61:157, 1982

56. Rice JP, Kay HH, Mahony BS: The clinical significance of uterine leiomyomas in pregnancy. Am J Obstet Gynecol 160:1212, 1989

57. Stillman R: In utero exposure to diethylstilbestrol: adverse effects on the reproductive tract and reproductive performance in male and female offspring. Am J Obstet Gynecol 142:905, 1982

58. Gravett M: Causes of preterm delivery. Semin Perinatol 8:246, 1984

59. Romero R, Mazor M: Infection and preterm labor. Clin Obstet Gynecol 31:3:553, 1988

60. Meis PJ, Ernest JM, Moore ML: Causes of low birthweight births in public and private patients. Am J Obstet Gynecol 156:1165, 1987

61. Amon E, Anderson GD, Sibai BM et al: Factors responsible for preterm delivery of the immature newborn infant ($\leq$1,000 gm). Am J Obstet Gynecol 156:1143, 1987

62. Creasy R, Gummer B, Liggins G: System for predicting spontaneous preterm birth. Obstet Gynecol 55:692, 1980

63. Main DM, Gabbe SG: Risk scoring for preterm labor: where do we go from here? Am J Obstet Gynecol 157:789, 1987

64. Caldeyro-Barcia R, Poseiro J: Physiology of the uterine contractions. Clin Obstet Gynecol 3:386, 1960

65. Nageotte MP, Dorchester W, Porto M et al: Quantitation of uterine activity preceding preterm, term, and post-term labor. Am J Obstet Gynecol 158:1254, 1988

66. Main DM, Katz M, Chiu G et al: Intermittent weekly contraction monitoring to predict preterm labor in low-risk women: a blinded study. Obstet Gynecol 72:757, 1988

67. Leveno KJ, Cox K, Roark M: Cervical dilatation and prematurity revisited. Obstet Gynecol 68:434, 1986

68. Blondel B, LeCoutour X, Kaminski M et al: Prediction of preterm delivery: is it substantially improved by routine vaginal examinations? Am J Obstet Gynecol 162:1042, 1990

69. Copper RL, Goldenberg RL, Davis RO et al: Warning symptoms, uterine contractions, and cervical examination findings in women at risk of preterm delivery. Am J Obstet Gynecol 162:748, 1990

70. Stubbs TM, Van Dorsten JP, Miller MC: The preterm cervix and preterm labor: relative risks, predictive values, and change over time. Am J Obstet Gynecol 155:829, 1986

71. Ernest JM, Meis PJ, Moore ML et al: Vaginal pH: a marker of preterm premature rupture of the membranes. Obstet Gynecol 74:734, 1989

72. Gleeson RP, Elder AM, Turner MJ et al: Vaginal pH in pregnancy in women delivered at and before term. Br J Obstet Gynaecol 96:183, 1989

73. Johnson J, Lee P, Zachary A et al: High-risk

prematurity—progestin treatment and steroid studies. Obstet Gynecol 54:412, 1979

74. Wilson J, Brent R: Are female sex hormones teratogenic? Am J Obstet Gynecol 141:567, 1981

75. Yemini M, Borenstein R, Dreazen E et al: Prevention of premature labor by 17 alpha-hydroxyprogesterone caproate. Am J Obstet Gynecol 151:574, 1985

76. Hauth J, Gilstrap L, Brekken A et al: The effect of 17 alpha-hydroxyprogesterone caproate on pregnancy outcome in an active-duty military population. Am J Obstet Gynecol 146:187, 1983

77. Walters W, Wood C: A trial of oral ritodrine for the prevention of premature labour. Br J Obstet Gynaecol 84:26, 1977

78. Crowther CA, Neilson JP, Verkuyl DAA et al: Preterm labour in twin pregnancies: can it be prevented by hospital admission? Br J Obstet Gynaecol 96:850, 1989

79. Saunders MC, Dick JS, Brown IM et al: The effects of hospital admission for bed rest on the duration of twin pregnancy: a randomised trial. Lancet 2:793, 1985

80. Herron M, Katz M, Creasy R: Evaluation of a preterm birth prevention program: preliminary report. Obstet Gynecol 59:452, 1982

81. Main DM, Richardson DK, Hadley CB et al: Controlled trial of a preterm labor detection program: efficacy and costs. Obstet Gynecol 74:873, 1989

82. Mueller-Heubach E, Reddick D, Barnett B et al: Preterm birth prevention: evaluation of a prospective controlled randomized trial. Am J Obstet Gynecol 160:1172, 1989

83. Goldenberg RL, Davis RO, Copper RL et al: The Alabama preterm birth prevention project. Obstet Gynecol 75:933, 1990

84. Buescher PA, Meis PJ, Ernest JM et al: A comparison of women in and out of a prematurity prevention project in a North Carolina perinatal care region. Am J Public Health 78:264, 1988

85. Newman RB, Gill PJ, Wittiech P et al: Maternal perception of prelabor uterine activity. Obstet Gynecol 68:765, 1986

86. Hill WC, Fleming AD, Martin RW et al: Home uterine activity monitoring is associated with a reduction in preterm birth. Obstet Gynecol 76:13S, 1990

87. Morrison JC, Martin JN Jr, Martin RW et al: Prevention of preterm birth by ambulatory assessment of uterine activity: a randomized study. Am J Obstet Gynecol 156:536, 1987

88. Iams JD, Johnson FF, O'Shaughnessy RW: A prospective random trial of home uterine activity monitoring in pregnancies at increased risk of preterm labor. Am J Obstet Gynecol 159:595, 1988

88a. Sunderji S, Gall S, Mou S et al: Earlier detection of preterm labor: Multicenter prospective randomized clinical trial of home uterine activity monitoring. Am J Obstet Gynecol 164:259, 1991

89. King JF, Grand A, Keirse MJN et al: Betamimetics in preterm labour: an overview of randomised controlled trials. Br J Obstet Gynaecol 95:211, 1988

90. Gonik B, Creasy RK: Preterm labor: its diagnosis and management. Am J Obstet Gynecol 154:3, 1986

91. Valenzuela G, Cline S, Hayashi R: Follow-up of hydration and sedation in the pretherapy of premature labor. Am J Obstet Gynecol 147:396, 1983

92. Pircon RA, Strassner HT, Kirz DS et al: Controlled trial of hydration and bed rest versus bed rest alone in the evaluation of preterm uterine contractions. Am J Obstet Gynecol 161:775, 1989

93. Huszar G, Naftolin F: The myometrium and uterine cervix in normal and preterm labor. N Engl J Med 311:571, 1984

94. Roberts J: Current understanding of pharmacologic mechanisms in the prevention of preterm birth. Clin Obstet Gynecol 27:592, 1984

95. Caritis SN, Hirsch RP, Zeleznik AJ: Adrenergic stimulation of placental progesterone production. J Clin Endocrinol Metab 56:969, 1983

96. Weiner N: Norepinephrine, epinephrine and the sympathomimetic amines. p. 143. In Gilman AG, Goodman LS, Gilman A (eds): The Pharmacological Basis of Therapeutics. 6th Ed. Macmillan, New York, 1980

97. Caritis S, Lin LS, Toig G et al: Pharmacodynamics of ritodrine in pregnant women during preterm labor. Am J Obstet Gynecol 147:752, 1983

98. Caritis SN, Venkataramanan R, Darby MJ et al: Pharmacokinetics of ritodrine administered intravenously: recommendations for changes in the current regimen. Am J Obstet Gynecol 162:429, 1990

99. Caritis SN, Venkataramanan R, Cotroneo M et al: Pharmacokinetics of orally administered ritodrine. Am J Obstet Gynecol 161:32, 1989

100. Barden T, Peter J, Merkatz I: Ritodrine hydrochloride: a betamimetic agent for use in preterm labor. Obstet Gynecol 56:1, 1980

101. Caritis SN, Venkataramanan R, Cotroneo M et al: Pharmacokinetics and pharmacodynamics of ritodrine after intramuscular administration to pregnant women. Am J Obstet Gynecol 162:1215, 1990

102. Creasy R, Golbus M, Laros R et al: Oral ritodrine maintenance in the treatment of preterm labor. Am J Obstet Gynecol 137:212, 1980

103. Berg G, Lindberg C, Ryder G: Terbutaline in the treatment of preterm labor. Eur J Respir Dis 65(Suppl. 134):219, 1984

104. Caritis S, Toig G, Heddinger L et al: A double-blind study comparing ritodrine and terbutaline in the treatment of preterm labor. Am J Obstet Gynecol 150:7, 1984

105. Stubblefield P, Heyl P: Treatment of premature labor with subcutaneous terbutaline. Obstet Gynecol 59:457, 1982

106. Casper RF, Lye SJ: Myometrial desensitization to continuous but not to intermittent β-adrenergic agonist infusion in the sheep. Am J Obstet Gynecol 154:301, 1986

107. Lam F, Gill P, Smith M: Use of the subcutaneous terbutaline pump for long-term tocolysis. Obstet Gynecol 72:810, 1988

108. Lam F: Miniature pump infusion of terbutaline—an option in preterm labor. Contemp Ob/Gyn 52, 1989

109. Benedetti T: Maternal complications of parenteral beta-sympathomimetic therapy for premature labor. Am J Obstet Gynecol 145:1, 1983

110. Hawker F: Pulmonary oedema associated with beta₂-sympathomimetic treatment of premature labour. Anaesth Intens Care 12:143, 1984

111. Philipsen T, Eriksen PS, Lynggard F: Pulmonary edema following ritodrine-saline infusion in premature labor. Obstet Gynecol 58:304, 1981

112. Hatjis CG, Swain M: Systemic tocolysis for premature labor is associated with an increased incidence of pulmonary edema in the presence of maternal infection. Am J Obstet Gynecol 159:723, 1988

113. Hendricks SK, Keroes J, Katz M: Electrocardiographic changes associated with ritodrine-induced maternal tachycardia and hypokalemia. Am J Obstet Gynecol 154:921, 1986

114. Ying Y-K, Tejani N: Angina pectoris as a complication of ritodrine hydrochloride therapy in premature labor. Obstet Gynecol 60:385, 1982

115. Mordes D, Kreutner K, Metzger W et al: Dangers of intravenous ritodrine in diabetic patients. JAMA 248:973, 1982

116. Young D, Toofanian A, Leveno K: Potassium and glucose concentrations without treatment during ritodrine tocolysis. Am J Obstet Gynecol 98:105, 1983

117. Main EK, Main DM, Gabbe SG: Chronic oral terbutaline tocolytic therapy is associated with maternal glucose intolerance. Am J Obstet Gynecol 157:644, 1987

118. Main DM, Main EK, Strong SE et al: The effect of oral ritodrine therapy on glucal tolerance in pregnancy. Am J Obstet Gynecol 152:1031, 1985

119. Epstein M, Nicholls E, Stubblefield P: Neonatal hypoglycemia after beta-sympathomimetic tocolytic therapy. Pediatrics 94:449, 1979

120. Lipsitz P: The clinical and biochemical effects of excess magnesium in the newborn. Pediatrics 47:501, 1971

121. Steer C, Petrie R: A comparison of magnesium sulfate and alcohol for the prevention of premature labor. Am J Obstet Gynecol 129:1, 1977

122. Spisso K, Harbert G, Thiagarajah S: The use of magnesium sulfate as the primary tocolytic agent to prevent premature delivery. Am J Obstet Gynecol 142:840, 1982

123. Elliott J: Magnesium sulfate as a tocolytic agent. Am J Obstet Gynecol 147:277, 1983

124. Madden C, Owen J, Hauth JC: Magnesium tocolysis: serum levels versus success. Am J Obstet Gynecol 162:1177, 1990

125. Tchilinguirian N, Najem R, Sullivan G et al: The use of ritodrine and magnesium sulfate in the arrest of premature labor. Int J Gynaecol Obstet 22:117, 1984

126. Beall MH, Edgar BW, Paril RH et al: A comparison of ritodrine, terbutaline, and magnesium sulfate for the suppression of preterm labor. Am J Obstet Gynecol 153:854, 1985

127. Hollander DI, Nagey DA, Pupkin MJ: Magnesium sulphate and ritodrine hydrochloride: a randomized comparison. Am J Obstet Gynecol 156:631, 1987

128. Wilkens IA, Lynch L, Mehaleb KE et al: Efficacy and side effects of magnesium sulphate and ritodrine as tocolytic agents. Am J Obstet Gynecol 159:685, 1988

129. Niebyl J, Blake D, White R et al: The inhibition of premature labor with indomethacin. Am J Obstet Gynecol 136:1014, 1980

130. Zuckerman H, Shalev E, Gilad G et al: Further study of the inhibition of premature labor by indomethacin. Part I. J Perinat Med 12:19, 1984

131. Zuckerman H, Shalev E, Gilad G et al: Further study of the inhibition of premature labor by indomethacin. Part II. J Perinat Med 12:25, 1984

132. Levin D, Mills L, Parkey M et al: Constriction of the fetal ductus arteriosus after administration of indomethacin to the pregnant ewe. J Pediatr 94:647, 1979

133. Niebyl JR, Witter FR: Neonatal outcome after indomethacin treatment for preterm labor. Am J Obstet Gynecol 155:747, 1986

134. Dudley DKL, Hardie MJ: Fetal and neonatal effects of indomethacin used as a tocolytic agent. Am J Obstet Gynecol 151:181, 1985

135. Manchester D, Margolis H, Sheldon R: Possible association between maternal indomethacin therapy and

primary pulmonary hypertension of the newborn. Am J Obstet Gynecol 126:467, 1976

136. Csaba I, Sulyok E, Ertl T: Relationship of maternal treatment with indomethacin to persistence of fetal circulation syndrome. J Pediatr 92:484, 1978

137. Moise KJ, Huhta JC, Sharif DS et al: Indomethacin in the treatment of premature labor: effects on the fetal ductus arteriosus. N Engl J Med 319:327, 1988

138. Kirshon B, Moise KJ, Wasserstrum N et al: Influence of short-term indomethacin therapy on fetal urine output. Obstet Gynecol 72:51, 1988

139. Hickok DE, Hollenbach KA, Reilley SF et al: The association between decreased amniotic fluid volume and treatment with nonsteroidal anti-inflammatory agents for preterm labor. Am J Obstet Gynecol 160:1525, 1989

140. Wurtzel D: Prenatal administration of indomethacin as a tocolytic agent: effect on neonatal renal function. Obstet Gynecol 76:689, 1990

141. Mari G, Moise KJ, Deter RL et al: Doppler assessment of the renal blood flow velocity waveform during indomethacin therapy for preterm labor and polyhydramnios. Obstet Gynecol 75:199, 1990

142. Anderson RJ, Berl T, McDonald KM et al: Prostaglandins: effects on blood pressure, renal blood flow, sodium and water excretion. Kidney Int 10:205, 1976

143. Besinger RE, Niebyl JR, Keyes WG et al: A randomized comparative trial of indomethacin and ritodrine for the longterm treatment of preterm labor. Am J Obstet Gynecol 164:981, 1991

144. Cabrol D, Landesman R, Muller J et al: Treatment of polyhydramnios with prostaglandin synthetase inhibitor (indomethacin). Am J Obstet Gynecol 157:422, 1987

145. Mamopoulos M, Assimakopoulos E, Reece AE et al: Maternal indomethacin therapy in the treatment of polyhydramnios. Am J Obstet Gynecol 162:1225, 1990

146. Kirshon B, Mari G, Moise KJ: Indomethacin therapy in the treatment of symptomatic polyhydramnios. Obstet Gynecol 75:202, 1990

147. Lange IR, Harman CR, Ash KM et al: Twin with hydramnios: treating premature labor at source. Am J Obstet Gynecol 160:552, 1989

148. Read MD, Wellby DE: The use of a calcium antagonist (nifedipine) to suppress preterm labor. Br J Obstet Gynaecol 93:933, 1986

149. Ferguson JE, Dyson DC, Schutz T et al: A comparison of tocolysis with nifedipine or ritodrine: analysis of efficacy and maternal, fetal and neonatal outcome. Am J Obstet Gynecol 163:105, 1990

150. Ferguson JE, Dyson DC, Holbrook H et al: Cardiovas-cular and metabolic effects associated with nifedipine and ritodrine tocolysis. Am J Obstet Gynecol 161:788, 1989

151. Snyder SW, Cardwell MS: Neuromuscular blockade with magnesium sulfate and nifedipine. Am J Obstet Gynecol 161:35, 1989

152. Mari G, Kirshon B, Moise KJ et al: Doppler assessment of the fetal and uteroplacental circulation during nifedipine therapy for preterm labor. Am J Obstet Gynecol 161:1514, 1989

153. Lauersen N, Merkatz I, Tejani N et al: Inhibition of premature labor: a multicenter comparison of ritodrine and ethanol. Am J Obstet Gynecol 127:837, 1977

154. McGregor JA, French JI, Reller B et al: Adjunctive erythromycin treatment for idiopathic preterm labor: results of a randomized, double-blinded, placebo-controlled trial. Am J Obstet Gynecol 154:98, 1986

155. Morales WJ, Angel JF, O'Brien WF et al: A randomized study of antibiotic therapy in idiopathic preterm labor. Obstet Gynecol 72:829, 1988

156. Newton ER, Dinsmoor MJ, Gibbs RS: A randomized, blinded, placebo-controlled trial of antibiotics in idiopathic preterm labor. Obstet Gynecol 74:562, 1989

157. Hatjis CG, Swain M, Nelson LH: Efficacy of combined administration of magnesium sulfate and ritodrine in the treatment of premature labor. Obstet Gynecol 69:317, 1987

158. Ferguson JE, Hensleigh PA, Kredenster D: Adjunctive use of magnesium sulfate with ritodrine for preterm labor tocolysis. Am J Obstet Gynecol 148:166, 1984

159. Use of approved drugs for unlabeled indications. FDA Drug Bull 12(1):4, 1982

160. Brown S, Tejani N: Terbutaline sulfate in the prevention of recurrence of premature labor. Obstet Gynecol 57:22, 1981

161. Korenbrot C, Aalto L, Laros R: The cost effectiveness of stopping preterm labor with beta-adrenergic treatment. N Engl J Med 310:691, 1984

162. Kikkawa Y, Motoyama EK, Gluck L: Study of the lungs of fetal and newborn rabbits. Am J Pathol 52:177, 1968

163. Liggins GC, Howie RN: A controlled trial of antepartum glucocorticoid treatment for prevention of the respiratory distress syndrome in premature infants. Pediatrics 50:515, 1972

164. Crowley P, Chalmers I, Keirse MJ: The effects of corticosteroid administration before preterm delivery: an overview of the evidence from controlled trials. Br J Obstet Gynaecol 97:11, 1990

165. Liggins GC: The prevention of RDS by maternal beta-

methasone administration. p. 97. In Moore TD: Lung Maturation and the Prevention of Hyaline Membrane Disease. Report of the Seventieth Ross Conference on Pediatric Research. Ross Laboratories, Columbus, OH, 1976

166. Clyman R, Ballard P, Sniderman S et al: Prenatal administration of betamethasone for prevention of patent ductus arteriosus. J Pediatr 98:123, 1981

167. Quirk J, Raker R, Petrie R et al: The role of glucocorticoids, unstressful labor, and atraumatic delivery in the prevention of respiratory distress syndrome. Obstet Gynecol 134:768, 1979

168. Collaborative Group on Antenatal Steroid Therapy: Effect of antenatal dexamethasone administration on the prevention of respiratory distress syndrome. Am J Obstet Gynecol 141:276, 1981

169. MacArthur G, Howie R, Dezoete J et al: School progress and cognitive development of 6-year-old children whose mothers were treated antenatally with betamethasone. Pediatrics 70:99, 1982

170. Collaborative Group on Antenatal Steroid Therapy: Effects of antenatal dexamethasone administration in the infant: long-term follow-up. J Pediatr 104:259, 1984

171. Nochimson D, Petrie R: Glucocorticoid therapy for the induction of pulmonary maturity in severely hypertensive gravid women. Am J Obstet Gynecol 133:449, 1979

172. Ricke PS, Elliott JP, Freeman R: Use of corticosteroids in pregnancy-induced hypertension. Obstet Gynecol 55:206, 1980

173. Gross I, Ballard PL, Ballard RA et al: Corticosteroid stimulation of phosphatidyl choline synthesis in cultured fetal rabbit lung: evidence for de novo protein synthesis mediated by glucocorticoid receptors. Endocrinology 112:829, 1983

174. Ballard P: Combined hormonal treatment and lung maturation. Semin Perinatol 8:283, 1984

175. Devaskar U, Nitta K, Szewezyk K et al: Transplacental stimulation of functional morphologic fetal lung maturation: effect of thyrotropin-releasing hormone. Am J Obstet Gynecol 157:460, 1987

176. Oulton M, Rasmusson MG, Yoon RY et al: Gestation-dependent effects of the combined treatment of glucocorticoids and thyrotropin-releasing hormone on surfactant production by fetal rabbit lung. Am J Obstet Gynecol 160:961, 1989

177. Morales WJ, O'Brien WF, Angel JL et al: Fetal lung maturation: the combined use of corticosteroids and thyrotropin-releasing hormone. Obstet Gynecol 73:111, 1989

178. Ballard RA, Ballard PL, Creasy R et al: Prenatal thyrotropin-releasing hormone plus corticosteroid decreases chronic lung disease in very low birthweight infants. Clinical Research Abstract, Western Meeting, Carmel, CA, February 6–9, 1990

179. Ballard RA, Ballard PL, Creasy R et al: Prenatal treatment with thyrotropin-releasing hormone plus corticosteroid: absence of maternal, fetal or neonatal side effects. Clinical Research Abstract, Western Meeting, Carmel, CA, February 6–9, 1990

180. Horbar JD, Soll RF, Sutherland JM et al: A multicenter randomized, placebo-controlled trial of surfactant therapy for respiratory distress syndrome. N Engl J Med 320:959, 1989

181. Farrell EE, Silver RK, Kimberlin LV et al: Impact of antenatal dexamethasone administration on respiratory distress syndrome in surfactant-treated infants. Am J Obstet Gynecol 161:628, 1989

182. Schuly KF, Grimes DA, Cates W Jr: Measures to prevent cervical injury during suction curettage abortion. Lancet 1:1182, 1983

183. Harger JH: Cervical cerclage: patient selection, morbidity, and success rates. Clin Perinatol 10:321, 1983

183a. Jones JM, Sweetnam P, Hibbard BM: The outcome of pregnancy after cone biopsy of the cervix: a case control study, Br J Obstet Gynaecol 86:913, 1979

184. Ludmir J, Landon MB, Gabbe SG et al: Management of the diethylstilbestrol-exposed pregnant patient: a prospective study. Am J Obstet Gynecol 157:665, 1987

185. Michaels WH, Thompson HO, Schreiber FR et al: Ultrasound surveillance of the cervix during pregnancy in diethylstilbestrol-exposed offspring. Obstet Gynecol 73:230, 1989

186. Buckingham JC, Buethe RA, Danforth DN: Collagen-muscle ratio in clinically normal and clinically incompetent cervices. Am J Obstet Gynecol 91:231, 1965

187. Brook I, Feingold M, Schwartz A et al: Ultrasonography in the diagnosis of cervical incompetence in pregnancy—a new diagnostic approach. Br J Obstet Gynaecol 88:640, 1981

188. Charles D, Edwards W: Infectious complications of cervical cerclage. Am J Obstet Gynecol 141:1065, 1981

188a. Lash AF, Lash SR: Habitual abortion: The competent internal os of the cervix. Am J Obstet Gynecol 59:68, 1950

189. Shirodkar VN: A method of operative treatment for habitual abortions in the second trimester of pregnancy. Antiseptic 52:299, 1955

190. McDonald IA: Suture of the cervix for inevitable abortion. J Obstet Gynaecol Br Emp 64:346, 1957

191. Harger J: Comparison of success and morbidity in cer-

vical cerclage procedures. Obstet Gynecol 56:543, 1980

192. Scheerer LJ, Lam F, Bartolucci L et al: A new technique for reduction of prolapsed fetal membranes for emergency cervical cerclage. Obstet Gynecol 74:408, 1989

193. Marx PD: Transabdominal cervicoisthmic cerclage: a review. Obstet Gynecol Surv 44:7:518, 1989

193a. Weissman A, Jakobi P, Zahi S, Zimmer EZ: The effect of cervical cerclage on the course of labor. Obstet Gynecol 76:168, 1990

194. Olatunbosun O, Dyck F: Cervical cerclage operation for a dilated cervix. Obstet Gynecol 57:166, 1981

195. Harger JH, Archer DF, Marchese SM et al: Etiology of recurrent pregnancy losses and outcome of subsequent pregnancies. Obstet Gynecol 62:574, 1983

196. Crombleholme W, Minkoff H, Delke I et al: Cervical cerclage: an aggressive approach to threatened or recurrent pregnancy wastage. Am J Obstet Gynecol 146:168, 1983

197. Rush RW, Issacs S, McPherson K et al: A randomized controlled trial of cervical cerclage in women at high risk of spontaneous preterm delivery. Br J Obstet Gynaecol 91:724, 1984

198. Lazar P, Gueguen S, Dreyfus J et al: Multicentred controlled trial of cervical cerclage in women at moderate risk of preterm delivery. Br J Obstet Gynaecol 91:731, 1984

199. MacNaughton MC, Chalmers IG, Chamberlain GVP et al: Interim report of the Medical Research Council/ Royal College of Obstetricians and Gynaecologists multicentre randomized trial of cervical cerclage. Br J Obstet Gynaecol 95:437, 1988

200. Schutte M, Treffers P, Kloosterman G et al: Management of premature rupture of membranes: the risk of vaginal examination to the infant. Am J Obstet Gynecol 146:395, 1983

201. Smith R: A technic for the detection of rupture of the membranes: a review and preliminary report. Obstet Gynecol 48:172, 1976

202. Reece EA, Chervenak F, Moya F et al: Amniotic fluid arborization: effect of blood, meconium, and pH alterations. Obstet Gynecol 64:248, 1984

203. Rosemond RL, Lombardi SJ, Boehm FH: Ferning of amniotic fluid contaminated with blood. Obstet Gynecol 75:338, 1990

204. Rochelson B, Richardson D, Macri J: Rapid assay — possible application in the diagnosis of premature rupture of the membranes. Obstet Gynecol 62:414, 1983

205. Gorodeski I, Paz M, Insler V et al: Diagnosis of rupture of the fetal membranes by glucose and fructose measurements. Obstet Gynecol 53:611, 1979

206. Gahl W, Kozina T, Fuhrmann D et al: Diamine oxidase in the diagnosis of ruptured fetal membranes. Obstet Gynecol 60:297, 1982

207. Iannetta O: A new simple test for detecting rupture of the fetal membranes. Obstet Gynecol 63:575, 1984

208. Kitzmiller J: Preterm premature rupture of the membranes. p. 298. In Fuchs F, Stubblefield PG (eds): Preterm Birth Causes, Prevention and Management. Macmillan, New York, 1984

209. Skinner S, Campos G, Liggins G: Collagen content of human amniotic membranes: effect of gestation length and premature rupture. Obstet Gynecol 57:487, 1981

210. Bourne G: The Human Amnion and Chorion. Lloyd-Luke Medical Books, London, 1960

211. Ibrahim M, Bou-Resli M, Al-Zaid N, Bishay L: Intact fetal membranes: morphological predisposal to rupture. Acta Obstet Gynecol Scand 62:481, 1983

212. Lavery J, Miller C: Deformation and creep in the human chorioamniotic sac. Am J Obstet Gynecol 134:366, 1979

213. Al-Zaid NS, Gumaa KA, Bou-Resli MN et al: Premature rupture of fetal membranes changes in collagen type. Acta Obstet Gynecol Scand 67:291, 1988

214. Lonky NM, Hayashi RH: A proposed mechanism for premature rupture of membranes. Obstet Gynecol Surv 43:1:22, 1988

215. Regan J, Chao S, James LS: Premature rupture of membranes, preterm delivery, and group B streptococcal colonization of mothers. Am J Obstet Gynecol 141:184, 1981

216. Naeye R: Factors that predispose to premature rupture of the fetal membranes. Obstet Gynecol 60:93, 1982

216a. Hadley CB, Main DM, Gabbe SG: Risk factors for preterm premature rupture of the fetal membranes. Am J Perinatol 7:374, 1990

217. Joffe M: Association of syndromes predisposing to low birthweight. Early Hum Dev 10:107, 1984

218. Moretti M, Sibai BM: Maternal and perinatal outcome of expectant management of premature rupture of membranes in the midtrimester. Am J Obstet Gynecol 159:390, 1988

219. Vintzileos AM, Campbell WA, Nochimson DJ et al: Preterm premature rupture of the membranes: a risk factor for the development of abruptio placentae. Am J Obstet Gynecol 156:1235, 1987

220. Gonen R, Hannah ME, Milligan JE: Does prolonged preterm premature rupture of the membranes predis-

pose to abruptio placentae? Obstet Gynecol 74:347, 1989

221. Moberg L, Garite T, Freeman R: Fetal heart rate patterns and fetal distress in patients with preterm premature rupture of membranes. Obstet Gynecol 64:60, 1984

222. Taylor J, Garite T: Premature rupture of membranes before fetal viability. Obstet Gynecol 64:615, 1984

223. Nimrod C, Varela-Gittings F, Machin G et al: The effect of very prolonged membrane rupture on fetal development. Am J Obstet Gynecol 148:540, 1984

224. Mead PB: Management of the patient with premature rupture of membranes. Clin Perinatol 7:243, 1980

225. Garite T, Freeman R, Linzey E et al: Prospective randomized study of corticosteroids in the management of premature rupture of the membranes and the premature gestation. Am J Obstet Gynecol 141:508, 1981

226. Garite T: Premature rupture of the membranes: the enigma of the obstetrician. Am J Obstet Gynecol 151:1001, 1985

227. O'Keeffe DF, Garite TJ, Elliott JP et al: The accuracy of estimated gestational age based on ultrasound measurement of biparietal diameter in preterm premature rupture of the membranes. Am J Obstet Gynecol 151:309, 1985

228. Bottoms SF, Welch RA, Zador IE et al: Clinical interpretation of ultrasound measurements in preterm pregnancies with premature rupture of the membranes. Obstet Gynecol 69:358, 1987

229. Zlatnik F, Cruikshank D, Petzold C, Galask R: Amniocentesis in the identification of inapparent infection in preterm patients with premature rupture of the membranes. J Reprod Med 29:656, 1984

230. Yeast J, Garite T, Dorchester W: The risks of amniocentesis in the management of premature rupture of the membranes. Am J Obstet Gynecol 149:505, 1984

231. Galle P, Meis P: Complications of amniocentesis. J Reprod Med 27:149, 1982

232. Dombroski R, MacKenna J, Brame K: Comparison of amniotic fluid maturity profiles in paired vaginal and amniocentesis specimens. Am J Obstet Gynecol 140:461, 1981

233. Shaver DC, Spinnato JA, Whybrew D et al: Comparison of phospholipids in vaginal and amniocentesis specimens of patients with premature rupture of membranes. Am J Obstet Gynecol 156:454, 1987

234. Schumacher RE, Parisi VM, Steady HM et al: Bacteria causing false positive test for phosphatidylglycerol in amniotic fluid. Am J Obstet Gynecol 151:1067, 1985

235. Feijen H, Dony J, Martin C: The L/S ratio in vaginally

collected amniotic fluid: a misleading result in a breech presentation. Eur J Obstet Gynecol Reprod Biol 18:77, 1984

236. Evans M, Hajj S, Devoe L et al: C-reactive protein as a predictor of infectious morbidity with premature rupture of membranes. Am J Obstet Gynecol 138:648, 1980

237. Fisk NM, Fysh J, Child AG et al: Is C-reactive protein really useful in preterm premature rupture of the membranes? Br J Obstet Gynaecol 94:1159, 1987

238. Vintzileos AM, Campbell WA, Nochimson DJ et al: Qualitative amniotic fluid volume versus amniocentesis in predicting infection in preterm premature rupture of the membranes. Obstet Gynecol 67:579, 1986

239. Vintzileos AM, Bors-Koefoed R, Pelegano JF et al: The use of fetal biophysical profile improves pregnancy outcome in premature rupture of the membranes. Am J Obstet Gynecol 157:236, 1987

240. Goldstein I, Romero R, Merrill S et al: Fetal body and breathing movements as predictors of intraamniotic infection in preterm premature rupture of membranes. Am J Obstet Gynecol 159:363, 1988

241. Kivikoski AI, Amon E, Vaalamo PO et al: Effect of third-trimester premature rupture of membranes on fetal breathing movements: a prospective case–control study. Am J Obstet Gynecol 159:1474, 1988

242. Ohlsson A: Treatments of preterm premature rupture of the membranes: a meta-analysis. Am J Obstet Gynecol 160:890, 1989

243. Curet L, Rao V, Zachman R et al: Association between ruptured membranes, tocolytic therapy, and respiratory distress syndrome. Am J Obstet Gynecol 148:263, 1984

244. Garite TJ, Keegan KA, Freeman RK et al: A randomized trial of ritodrine tocolysis versus expectant management in patients with premature rupture of membranes at 25 to 30 weeks of gestation. Am J Obstet Gynecol 157:388, 1987

245. Weiner CP, Renk K, Klugman M: The therapeutic efficacy and cost-effectiveness of aggressive tocolysis for premature labor associated with premature rupture of the membranes. Am J Obstet Gynecol 159:216, 1988

246. Bourgeois FJ, Harbert GM, Andersen WA et al: Early versus late tocolytic treatment for preterm premature membrane rupture. Am J Obstet Gynecol 159:742, 1988

247. Amon E, Lewis SV, Sibai BM et al: Ampicillin prophylaxis in preterm premature rupture of the membranes: a prospective randomized study. Am J Obstet Gynecol 159:539, 1988

248. Morales WJ, Angel JL, O'Brien WF et al: Use of ampi-

cillin and corticosteroids in premature rupture of membranes: a randomized study. Obstet Gynecol 73:721, 1989

249. Christmas JT, Cox SM, Gilstrap LC et al: Expectant management of preterm ruptured membranes: effect of antimicrobial therapy on interval to delivery. Abstract 15 presented at the 10th Annual Meeting of the Society of Perinatal Obstetricians, Houston, TX, 1990

250. McGregor JA, French JI: Double-blind, randomized, placebo controlled, prospective evaluation of the efficacy of short course erythromycin in prolonging gestation among women with preterm rupture of membranes. Am J Obstet Gynecol (in press), 1991

251. Johnston MM, Sanchez-Ramos L, Vaughn AJ et al: Antibiotic therapy in preterm premature rupture of membranes: a randomized, prospective, double-blind trial. Am J Obstet Gynecol 163:743, 1990

252. Hon E, Zanini D, Quilligan E: The neonatal value of fetal monitoring. Am J Obstet Gynecol 122:508, 1975

253. Neutra RR, Fienberg SE, Greeland S, Friedman EA: Effect of fetal monitoring on neonatal death rates. N Engl J Med 299:324, 1978

254. Luthy DA, Shy KK, van Belle G et al: A randomized trial of electronic fetal monitoring in preterm labor. Obstet Gynecol 69:687, 1987

255. Larson EB, van Belle G, Shy KK et al: Fetal monitoring and predictions by clinicians: observations during a randomized clinical trial in very low birth weight infants. Obstet Gynecol 74:584, 1989

256. Zanini B, Paul R, Huey J: Intrapartum fetal heart rate: correlation with scalp pH in the preterm fetus. Am J Obstet Gynecol 136:43, 1980

257. Bowes W, Gabbe S, Bowes C: Fetal heart rate monitoring in premature infants weighing 1,500 gm or less. Am J Obstet Gynecol 137:791, 1980

258. Myers R, Myers S: Use of sedative, analgesic and anesthetic drugs during labor and delivery: bane or boon? Am J Obstet Gynecol 133:83, 1979

259. Kenepp N, Shelley W, Gabbe S et al: Fetal and neonatal hazards of maternal hydration with 5% dextrose before cesarean section. Lancet 1:1150, 1982

260. Myers S, Paton J, Fisher D: Neonatal survival of the tiny infant: the challenge. Presented at the Annual Meeting, Society of Perinatal Obstetricians, 1985

261. Barrett J, Boehm F, Vaughn W: The effect of type of delivery on neonatal outcome in singleton infants of birth weight of 1,000 g or less. JAMA 250:625, 1983

262. Bishop E, Israel S, Briscoe C: Obstetric influences on the premature infant's first year of development: a report from the Collaborative Study of Cerebral Palsy. Obstet Gynecol 26:628, 1965

263. Schwartz D, Miodovnik M, Lavin J: Neonatal outcome among low birth weight infants delivered spontaneously or by low forceps. Obstet Gynecol 62:283, 1983

264. O'Driscoll K, Meagher D, MacDonald D et al: Traumatic intracranial haemorrhage in firstborn infants and delivery with obstetric forceps. Br J Obstet Gynaecol 88:577, 1981

265. Main D, Main E, Maurer M: Cesarean section versus vaginal delivery for the breech fetus weighing less than 1,500 grams. Am J Obstet Gynecol 146:580, 1983

266. Westgren LMR, Songster G, Paul RH: Preterm breech delivery: another retrospective study. Obstet Gynecol 66:481, 1985

267. Haesslein I, Goodlin R: Delivery of the tiny newborn. Am J Obstet Gynecol 134:192, 1979

267a. Malloy MH, Rhoads GG, Schramm W, Land G: Increasing cesarean section rates in very low-birth-weight infants, effect on outcome. JAMA 262:1475, 1989

268. Kitchen W, Ford GW, Doyle LW et al: Cesarean section or vaginal delivery at 24 to 28 weeks gestation: comparison of survival and neonatal and two-year morbidity. Obstet Gynecol 66:149, 1985

269. Malloy MH, Rhoads GG, Schramm W et al: Increasing cesarean section rates in very low birthweight infants: effect on outcome. JAMA 262:1475, 1989

270. Olshan A, Shy K, Luthy D et al: Cesarean birth and neonatal mortality in very low birth weight infants. Obstet Gynecol 64:267, 1984

271. Kosmetatos N, Dinton C, Williams M et al: Intracranial hemorrhage in the premature: its predictive features and outcome. Am J Dis Child 134:855, 1980

272. Anderson GD, Bada HS, Sibai BM et al: The relationship between labor and route of delivery in the preterm infant. Am J Obstet Gynecol 158:1382, 1988

273. Dietl J, Arnold H, Mentzel H et al: Effect of cesarean section on outcome in high- and low-risk very preterm infants. Arch Gynecol Obstet 246:91, 1989

274. Goldenberg RL et al: Survival of infants with low birth weight and early gestational age, 1979 to 1981. Am J Obstet Gynecol 149:508, 1984

Chapter 26

Multiple Gestations

Usha Chitkara and Richard L. Berkowitz

The phenomenon of twinning has fascinated human-kind throughout recorded history. Twins have often been regarded as being inherently "different" from singletons, and societal responses to their birth have ranged from awe to fear. Researchers have been interested in exploiting their uniqueness in an attempt to separate the influence of genetic and environmental factors on both fetal and postpartum development.[1] Obstetricians have long been aware that pregnancies complicated by twinning are by their very nature at higher risk than those of most singletons. Finally, parents and future siblings are often overjoyed or overwhelmed when they are told that twins are expected but are virtually never neutral in their response.

Twins are either monozygotic (MZ) or dizygotic (DZ). In the former case a single fertilized ovum splits into two distinct individuals after a variable number of divisions. Such twins are almost always genetically identical and therefore of the same sex. On rare occasions mutations can cause genetic discordance resulting in phenotypic and chromosomal dissimilarities between MZ twins. On the other hand, when two separate ova are fertilized, DZ twins result. These individuals are as genetically distinct as any other children born to the same couple. Sets of DZ twins may be of the same or opposite sex. Dizygotic half-siblings have been reported in which two ova were fertilized by different fathers, and it has been hypothesized that monovular dispermic fertilization may occur. These latter situations are very uncommon,

however. In most cases, DZ twins are genetically dissimilar true siblings, and MZ twins are genetically identical.

The frequency of MZ twins is fairly constant throughout the world at a rate of approximately 4 per 1,000 births. This rate does not seem to vary with maternal characteristics such as age or parity. DZ twinning, however, is associated with multiple ovulation, and its frequency varies between races and within countries and is affected by several identifiable factors. In general the frequency of DZ twins is low in Asians, intermediate in whites, and high in blacks. In the United States, the overall incidence of twins is approximately 12 per 1,000 births, and two-thirds are DZ.[1] The Yorubas of Western Nigeria, however, have a frequency of 45 twins per 1,000 births, of whom about 90 percent are DZ.[2]

The frequency of DZ births is affected by maternal age, increasing from a rate of 3 in 1,000 in women under age 20 to 14 in 1,000 at ages 35 to 40. Above age 40 the rate declines. The frequency of DZ twinning also increases with parity independent of maternal age.[1]

The different rates of DZ twinning may be due to racial or individual variations in pituitary gonadotropin production. In several animal species, such as cattle, swine, and sheep, polyovulation in response to uteroplacental or pituitary gonadotropins is commercially exploited. Infertility patients treated with menopausal urinary gonadotropins (Pergonal) or clomiphene citrate are well known to have a dose-dependent increase in multiple births when compared with women who conceive without these agents. Although DZ twins predominate in these patients, triplets and higher numbers of conceptuses may also occur. The use of in vitro fertilization and embryo transfer has further increased the incidence of multiple pregnancies. Two series of in vitro fertilization pregnancies suggest that the incidence of multiple gestations in these patients may be as high as 22 percent.[3,4]

The cause of MZ twinning is unclear. Benirschke and Kim[5] state that it is probably an uncommon occurrence among other mammals. In two species of armadillo, however, polyembryony regularly follows implantation of a single blastocyst. Oxygen deprivation has been experimentally shown to enhance fission in fish embryos, and some teratogens have been associated with increased MZ twinning rates in laboratory animals, but there is currently no satisfactory explanation for the fact that MZ twins occur in humans with such a constant frequency around the world.

PLACENTATION

Twin placentas are described in terms of their membranes (Fig. 26.1). The sac of a singleton pregnancy consists of an outer chorion and an inner amnion. Both DZ twins develop within similar sacs because both blastocysts generate their own placentas. If these blastocysts are not implanted proximal to each other, two separate placentas result, each of which has a chorion and an amnion. Should they implant side by side, intimate fusion of the placental discs occurs, but these placentas are always diamniotic and dichorionic, and vascular anastomoses rarely occur. Although MZ twins may also have placentas with two amnions and two chorions, this generally is not the case. Some MZ placentas have a single chorion that usually surrounds two amnions, but occasionally only a single amnion exists as well. Regardless of whether these monochorial placentas are diamniotic or monoamniotic, they are always a single disc and only occur in MZ twins. Triplets and quadruplets have been delivered with monochorial placentas that were all shown to be MZ. Almost all monochorial placentas

have blood vessel communications between the fetal circulations.

The type of placenta that develops in a MZ pregnancy is determined by the time at which cleavage of the fertilized ovum occurs. If twinning is accomplished during the first 2 to 3 days, it precedes the setting aside of cells that eventually become the chorion. In that case, two chorions and two amnions are formed. After approximately 3 days, however, twinning cannot split the chorionic cavity, and from that time on a monochorial placenta must result. If the split occurs between the third and eighth days a diamniotic monochorial placenta develops. Between the eighth and thirteenth days, the amnion has already been formed, and the placenta is therefore monoamniotic and monochorionic. Embryonic cleavage between the thirteenth and fifteenth days results in conjoined twins within a single amnion and chorion; beyond that point, the process of twinning cannot occur.

The frequency of placental types within a population is influenced by the rate of DZ twinning. In the United States approximately 80 percent of twin placentas are dichorionic and 20 percent are monochorionic. In Nigeria, where DZ twinning is much more common, the frequency of dichorionic placentas approaches 95 percent.[5]

Because monochorial placentas can only occur in MZ pregnancies, study of the membranes establishes zygosity in 20 percent of cases in the United States. In approximately 35 percent of cases the twins are of opposite sex and therefore necessarily DZ. This leaves only 45 percent of cases (twins of like sex having dichorionic placentas), in which further studies are necessary to determine zygosity. Cameron[6] found that this 45 percent breaks down into 8 percent MZ and 37 percent DZ. He states, "The percentage of monozygotic dichorionic pairs is inversely proportional to the completeness of the genotyping." In other words, the more genotypic markers that are studied, the greater the likelihood of demonstrating dizygosity. Cameron used six blood group markers, four red blood cell enzymes, and placental alkaline phosphatase in order to determine zygosity.

The often cited Weinberg's rule states that in a population of twins the estimated number of MZ pairs is almost exactly equal to the total minus twice the number of twins of unlike sex. The assumption

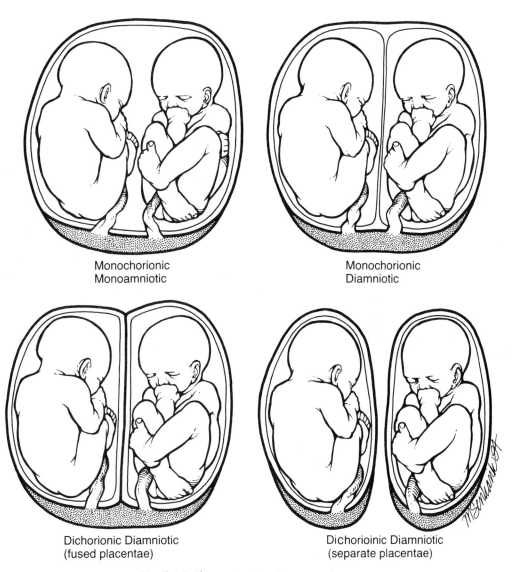

Monochorionic
Monoamniotic

Monochorionic
Diamniotic

Dichorionic Diamniotic
(fused placentae)

Dichorioinic Diamniotic
(separate placentae)

Fig. 26.1 Placentation in twin pregnancies.

underlying this rule is that among DZ pairs the sex of one twin is independent of that of the other, resulting in almost exactly equal numbers of like and unlike sexed pairs. The small difference anticipated from exact equality is due to the fact that the sex ratio is not precisely 0.5. This rule has been questioned by several authorities, who present evidence that in DZ populations there seems to be a higher frequency of like-sex than opposite-sex twins at birth.[7] Cameron's data would favor the latter view.

PERINATAL MORBIDITY AND MORTALITY

Numerous reports have documented that perinatal morbidity and mortality are greater in twins than in singletons. A collaborative study of 6,503 sets of twins delivered at 32 different hospitals between 1961 and 1972 has been published.[8] The overall perinatal mortality in this series was 124 per 1,000 births. When only those twins weighing more than 1,000 g were considered, the perinatal loss was 62 per 1,000 births, which was approximately three times greater than that of comparable singletons at the same institutions.

A high incidence of low-birth-weight infants is the major cause of the increased perinatal mortality rate in twins. Both preterm delivery and intrauterine growth retardation (IUGR) contribute to this problem. In addition to prematurity and retarded growth in utero, however, twins have an increased frequency of congenital anomalies, placenta previa, abruptio placenta, preeclampsia, cord accidents, and malpresentations.

Because of advances in both maternal–fetal medicine and neonatal care, a general decline in perinatal mortality has been reported over the past decade from centers around the world. In general, this overall trend has been noted to occur in multiple gestations as well. Desgranges et al.[9] report a perinatal mortality rate of 95 per 1,000 in 213 twins delivered between 1969 and 1973 as compared with 56 per 1,000 in 221 twins delivered between 1974 and 1979 at the Hôpital Notre-Dame in Montreal. During these periods, there was essentially no change in the fetal death rates (28 per 1,000 versus 32 per 1,000), but the neonatal mortality rate fell from 68 per 1,000 to 24 per 1,000. The frequency of anomalies during the entire period was 23 per 1,000, and these accounted for 18 percent of all deaths. The average length of pregnancy in both study periods was identical, and the improved neonatal outcome was found to be due to increased survival rates in neonates weighing 1,000 to 1,500 g at birth.

With the routine use of antenatal fetal heart rate testing, Rattan and colleagues[10] noted a marked reduction in the fetal mortality after 32 weeks at the University of South Florida, when 153 twins delivered between 1975 and 1979 were compared with 160 twins delivered between 1980 and 1983. The rate of stillbirths fell from 23 per 1,000 in the former period to 0 per 1,000 in the latter.

Despite these encouraging trends, the problems associated with multiple gestations continue to place these infants at higher risk than their singleton counterparts. Hawrylyshyn et al.[11] reported an overall perinatal mortality rate of 91 per 1,000 births in 177 twin pairs delivered between 1975 and 1979 in Toronto. The number of cases in each year was fairly small, but there was no demonstrable decline in perinatal mortality rate during the study period. In this series, more than 70 percent of the deaths occurred before 30 weeks gestation. Those deaths took place either in utero or during the neonatal period in association with respiratory distress syndrome (RDS), intracerebral hemorrhage, or necrotizing enterocolitis. These workers conclude that if obstetricians are to have a major impact on the perinatal survival of twins, they must concentrate on the period between 25 and 30 weeks.

In multifetal gestations with three or more fetuses the most important complication again is premature delivery with its concomitant increase in perinatal morbidity and mortality. Accurate knowledge of the outcome of these pregnancies is limited. All of the published series to date contain relatively small numbers of triplets, even smaller numbers of quadruplets, and virtually no information other than isolated case reports regarding the outcome of pregnancies with quintuplets and higher-order births. Among the three fairly large series that were published prior to 1983, Holcberg et al.[12] reported a perinatal mortality rate of 312 per 1,000 among 31 triplet pregnancies managed in their institution between 1960 and 1979. Ron-El et al.[13] reported a perinatal mortality rate of 185 per 1,000 in their series of 29 triplet and 6 quadruplet gestations managed between 1970 and 1978. Loucopoulos and Jewelewicz, in a series of 27 triplets, 7 quadruplets, and 1 quintuplet cared for from 1965 to 1981, noted a perinatal mortality rate of 148 per 1,000.[14]

Major improvements in perinatal and neonatal care over the past two decades have resulted in significantly better survival rates for triplets and perhaps higher-order pregnancies. This is clearly reflected in the results of some of the larger series of multiple gestations that have recently been published. Lipitz et al.[15] reported a perinatal mortality rate of 93 per 1,000 among 78 triplet gestations managed in their institution between 1975 and 1988. Gonen et al.,[16] presenting their data on 30 multiple gestations (24 triplets, 5 quadruplets, and 1 quintuplet) from 1978 to 1988, reported a perinatal mortality rate of 51.5 per 1,000, and the experience of Newman et al.[17] with 198 triplet pregnancies delivered between 1985 and 1988 was similar.

A recent review of the subject by Alvarez and Berkowitz[18] concludes that although perinatal mortality rates have decreased, the risk of prematurity in multifetal gestations has not changed significantly over the past 20 to 30 years. The average gestational age at delivery for triplets consistently seems to be 33 to 35 weeks. Approximately 75 percent of these patients deliver prior to 37 weeks, and at least 20 percent deliver prior to 32 weeks. The number of reported patients with four or more fetuses is currently too small for a meaningful analysis of perinatal morbidity and mortality rates. However, one can assume that at best the outcome in those pregnancies is the same as with triplets, and it probably is worse.

DIAGNOSIS

It is obviously impossible to offer specialized antepartum care if the twins are undiagnosed until the intrapartum period. An often quoted statistic in the older literature is that 50 percent of twins are not diagnosed until the time of delivery.[19] Because of the current widespread use of diagnostic ultrasound, this is certainly no longer true. The number of twins in the United States diagnosed during the antenatal period is currently unknown, but there must be substantial variations from one institution to another, depending on the degree to which ultrasound is used. In a report from Yale-New Haven Hospital,[20] 91 percent of 385 twin sets delivered between 1977 and 1981 were diagnosed before the onset of labor.

Multiple gestations should be suspected whenever (1) the uterus seems to be larger than dates, (2) hydramnios or unexplained anemia develops, (3) auscultation of more than one fetal heart is suspected, or (4) the pregnancy has occurred after ovulation induction or in vitro fertilization. They may be diagnosed serendipitously at the time of ultrasound scanning before a genetic amniocentesis or as a result of an elevated serum α-fetoprotein (AFP) level in mass screening programs.

An argument often used in support of universal ultrasound screening for all pregnant women during the second trimester is that it would result in the early diagnosis of multiple pregnancies with almost 100 percent accuracy.[21] Persson and Kullander[22] reported the results of this type of screening program, which has been in effect at the Malmo General Hospital in Sweden since 1973. Originally the program began with a single scan performed in the thirtieth week, but currently all women are offered examinations at both 17 and 33 weeks. This hospital has the only maternity unit serving a city of 240,000 inhabitants, and compliance with the program has been 96.4 percent. Between 1974 and 1982, 98 percent of 254 multiple gestations were detected by ultrasound screening. There were no false-positive diagnoses, but 2 percent of the multiple gestations were missed on the first examination. When data from a comparable number of twins delivered in their hospital between 1970 and 1974 are contrasted with those from 1975 and 1982, Persson and Kullander report that perinatal mortality rate fell from 107 per 1,000 to 34 per 1,000, major morbidity (e.g., cerebral palsy, mental retardation, late motor development, and hearing defects) decreased from 9.6 to 3.6 percent, and frequency of delivery prior to 38 weeks dropped from 34 to 15.8 percent. The marked improvement in these figures is obviously due to multiple factors, but early diagnosis is among them.

Separate gestational sacs can be identified ultrasonically as early as 6 weeks from the first day of the last menstrual period. Using transabdominal scanning an embryo within each sac should be visible by 7 weeks, and beating fetal hearts should be seen by 7.5 to 8 weeks.[23] With good equipment the fetal cranial pole is also identifiable during this period, but the intracranial landmarks used for accurate biparietal diameter measurements are usually not seen until 14 to 16 weeks. Increasing sophistication in the development and use of endovaginal scanning has made it possible to visualize these developmental landmarks 1 to 2 weeks earlier than with abdominal scanning techniques so that the embryonic pole and fetal heart can be seen by 6 weeks, and the intracranial landmarks are visible by 10 to 12 weeks gestation.[24] The earliest reported diagnosis of twins was strongly suspected 10 days after ovulation and confirmed 23 days later.[25] This patient was given clomiphene citrate and hCG to induce ovulation. Two follicles measuring 2.8 and 3.0 cm, respectively, were noted in the right ovary the day the human chorionic gonadotropin (hCG) was administered. Two days later, an ultrasound examination revealed that both follicles had collapsed. Ten days after ovulation, the plasma progesterone level was found to be significantly above the upper limit of normal for a singleton, and the twin pregnancy was

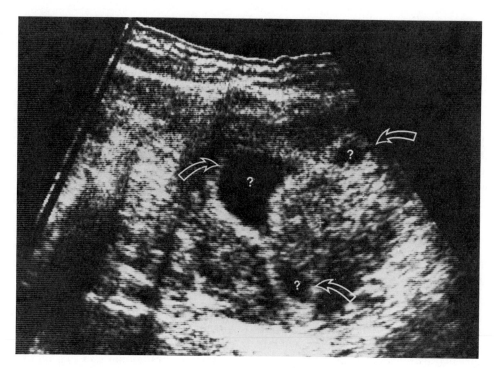

Fig. 26.2 The scanning plane may artifactually transect a sac in such a fashion as to give the impression of multiple sacs. In this case, the three gestational sacs were all part of the single normal larger one. (From Jeanty and Romero,[23] with permission.)

ultrasonically visualized 47 days from the onset of the last menstrual period.

In general, the ultrasonic diagnosis of multiple gestations within the first trimester is relatively straightforward. It is mandatory, however, to visualize separate fetuses (Fig. 26.2). Retromembranous collections of blood or fluid or a prominent fetal yolk sac should not be confused with a twin gestation. Demonstration of the viability of each fetus at the time of the examination requires visualization of independent cardiac activity. Unfortunately, mistakes regarding the number of fetuses present can be made when scans are hastily interpreted. This is particularly true in the third trimester but may also occur in the first and second trimester, especially with four or more fetuses. It must be remembered that an ultrasound image, unlike a flat plate of the abdomen, does not provide a composite overview. The image displayed is only a tomographic slice through the area being studied. It is therefore possible to display two circular structures that may represent different fetal heads or, alternatively, the head and thorax of the same fetus in a tucked position. Misinterpretation in this setting has resulted in the incorrect diagnosis of twins when only one fetus was present. On the other hand, rapid and careless scanning may result in failure to detect a second fetus whose head is deeply engaged in the pelvis or pushed up under the maternal ribs. If a multiple gestation is suspected, the ultrasonologist must be painstakingly thorough in examining the entire uterine cavity. A scan should not be completed until the orientation of all the visualized fetal parts is understood.[26]

EARLY WASTAGE IN MULTIPLE GESTATIONS

As a result of ultrasound studies performed during the first trimester, there is evidence to suggest that the incidence of multiple gestations in humans is higher than is usually appreciated and that a significant amount of early wastage occurs in these preg-

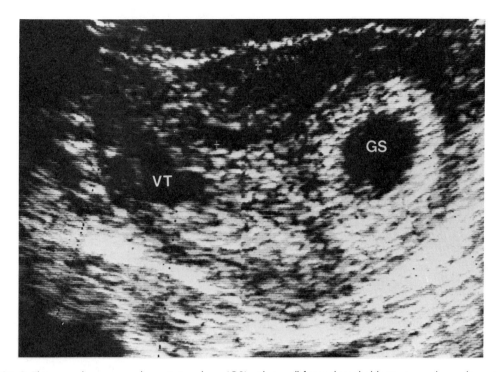

Fig. 26.3 This scan shows an early gestational sac (GS) with a well-formed trophoblastic rim and an adjacent vanishing twin (VT). (From Jeanty et al.,[187] with permission.)

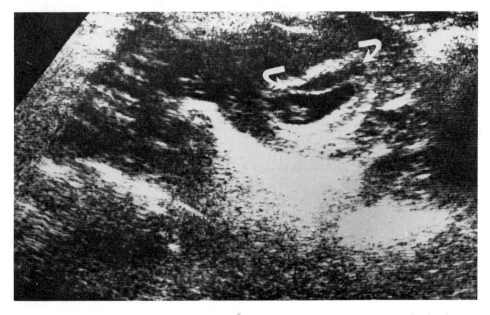

Fig. 26.4 Vanishing twin with an incomplete trophoblastic rim (arrows) adjacent to a normally developing embryo. (From Jeanty and Romero,[23] with permission.)

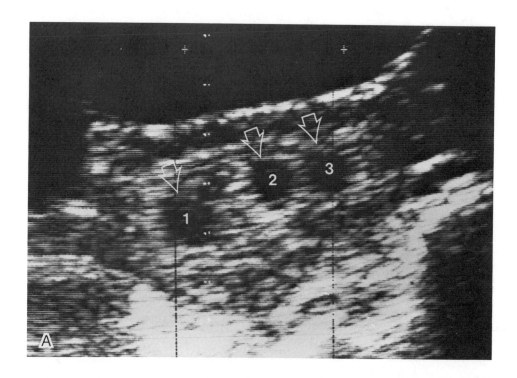

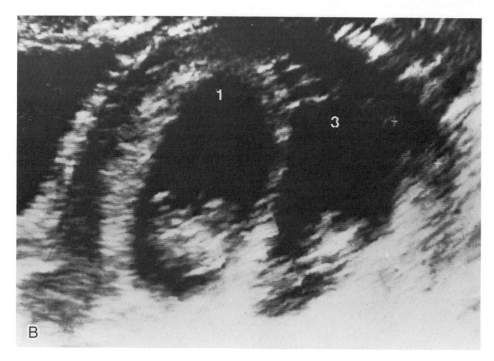

Fig. 26.5 (A) Three gestational sacs seen early in the first trimester. (B) Two weeks later, the second sac has disappeared, and only the two lateral ones remain. (From Jeanty et al.,[187] with permission.)

nancies. This has led to the concept of the "vanishing twin" (Figs. 26.3 and 26.4). Landy et al.[27] reviewed nine series that have addressed this phenomenon. The series vary in regard to the populations studied, timing of the ultrasonography, and number of scans performed. Frequencies of twin "disappearance" in patients scanned before 14 weeks gestational age reportedly range from 13 to 78 percent. The higher rates were found in studies performed before 10 weeks gestation.

One explanation for the disappearance of a gestational sac is reabsorption, which has been documented to occur in both human singleton and multiple pregnancies (Fig. 26.5). This phenomenon has been ultrasonically described in human multiple gestations between 7 to 12 weeks. The true incidence of reabsorption of one or more gestational sacs is unknown, but it apparently can occur without adverse effects on a coexisting fetus.

Another explanation for sac disappearance is the presence of a blighted ovum or anembryonic pregnancy. Robinson and Caines[28] define a blighted ovum as a gestational sac having a volume of 2.5 cc or more, in which no fetus can be identified on ultrasound examination. It should be noted that the sac need not be totally anechoic because disorganized echoes may be present in some cases. Several studies have reported that the only apparent complication of regression of a blighted ovum is slight vaginal bleeding. Regardless of whether vaginal bleeding accompanies regression of a blighted ovum, a coexisting normal pregnancy has a good prognosis for carrying to term. Robinson and Caines report that 8 of 11 patients with a blighted ovum and normal appearing co-twin delivered appropriately grown singletons at term, 1 delivered an infant whose size was appropriate for gestational age (AGA) at 36 weeks, and 1 delivered a morphologically normal but growth-retarded stillborn at 35 weeks. The eleventh patient in this group aborted "a fresh fetus" at 25 weeks. Experience with patients undergoing elective first trimester reduction of multifetal pregnancies suggests that the clinical course and outcome of those pregnancies are similar to those observed with the naturally occurring phenomenon of a blighted or "disappearing" co-twin.[29–31]

Landy et al.[27] point out that pathologic evidence to confirm "disappearance" rates as high as 78 percent is lacking. Examination of the placenta and membranes after delivery of a singleton thought to be a surviving twin rarely shows evidence of the one that disappeared. It is also true that examination of the products of an abortion is usually not helpful in verifying the presence of a sac that has "vanished." The difficulty encountered in obtaining positive pathologic confirmation of the diagnosis, however, does not mean that it is incorrect. On the other hand, false diagnoses are certainly possible as a result of poor ultrasound studies. If equipment with inferior resolution is used, or if the types of artifacts described earlier are misread as being second sacs, the presence of multiple gestations may be overdiagnosed. Particular attention should be paid to the fact that pressure from the scanning transducer can create an hourglass appearance in a normal single sac that may be incorrectly interpreted as demonstrating two separate sacs.

Aside from first trimester bleeding there are no reported maternal complications associated with the disappearance of a fetus.[27] The associated overall abortion rates in reported series range from 7 to 37 percent. However, in two studies when a vanished sac was associated with vaginal bleeding during the first trimester, spontaneous abortions occurred in 26 percent (5 of 19)[32] and 92 percent (11 of 12) of cases.[33]

Landy et al.[27] conclude that the phenomenon of the vanishing twin truly seems to exist. Although on the basis of current information it is impossible to determine the exact prevalence of this occurrence, their data suggest that a reasonable figure for its incidence may be as high as 21 percent.[34] These investigators caution, however, that it is necessary to make "an accurate, faultless diagnosis" of multiple gestation in the first trimester before sharing this information with the mother, because of its inevitable emotional and social impact.

GROWTH AND DEVELOPMENT

Normal individual twins grow at the same rate as singletons up to 30 to 32 weeks gestation. After that time, they do not gain weight as rapidly as singletons of the same gestational age.[35] Daw and Walker[36] stated that after 32 weeks the combined weight gain of both twins is approximately equivalent to that gained by a singleton for the remaining portion of the pregnancy. The retardation in each twin's somatic growth is thought to be related to "crowding" in utero. The implication of this concept is that at some point in the third trimester the placenta can no longer keep pace with the nutrient requirements of both developing fetuses. This process occurs even earlier than 30 weeks when more than two fetuses are present.

A study of specimens obtained by induced abortion performed between 8.5 and 21 weeks showed the relationship between body weight and length in twins to be the same as that in singletons.[37] This finding supports the concept that twins are not growth retarded during the first half of pregnancy. Fenner et al.[38] have provided some insight into the other end of the gestational age spectrum by studying 146 twins admitted to their neonatal unit with gestational ages at birth ranging from 30 weeks to term. When data from these infants were plotted on Lubchenco's growth charts for singletons, these workers found that the twins' birth weights dropped below the mean for singletons by 32 weeks but remained within the low normal range until week 36, after which time they fell progressively below the tenth percentile. Twin birth lengths and head circumferences, however, remained within the low normal range for singletons throughout the entire pregnancy. The disparity between relatively normal head size and body length in associated with somatic deprivation is compatible with the concept of asymmetric growth retardation. The latter is a mechanism whereby in mildly growth retarded fetuses head growth is preferentially favored at the expense of increases in body weight.[39] These studies suggest that alterations in twin growth occur primarily in the third trimester, worsen as gestational age progresses, and are usually asymmetric in nature.

In the large collaborative study conducted by Kohl and Casey[8] birth weights differed by 500 to 999 g in 18 percent of the twin sets and were in excess of 1,000 g in 3 percent. Obviously these discrepancies in birth weight could be due, in part, to constitutional factors. Because DZ twins are genetically distinct individuals, it is not surprising that they should be programmed to have very different weights at birth. There are, however, several pathologic situations in which twins may be born with substantial weight differences. These include the twin-to-twin transfusion syndrome, the combination of an anomalous fetus with a normal co-twin, and growth retardation affecting only one twin because of local placental factors.[26] IUGR, on the other hand, can affect both twins relatively equally, in which case they are both small but not discordant in size. Detection of differences in size in utero therefore suggests that IUGR may be present but is not diagnostic of that condition. Conversely, the demonstration that twin fetuses have similar sizes does not rule out abnormal growth. It therefore is necessary to assess each twin individually if abnormal growth in utero is to be detected.

ASSESSING FETAL GROWTH WITH ULTRASOUND

In addition to being an extremely effective and non-invasive method for diagnosing the presence of twins ultrasound is the most accurate method whereby their developmental progress can be followed. Duff and Brown[40] demonstrated that urinary estriol values are of little help in assessing fetal well-being in multiple gestations. Ultrasonic scanning on a regular basis permits ongoing assessment of individual growth.

Are Singleton Nomograms Applicable to Twins?

The first question to be asked is whether ultrasound nomograms devised for singletons can be used to follow twins. Conflicting data regarding this issue exist in the published literature. Some investigators have found twins to have smaller biparietal diameters (BPDs) than those of singletons at all gestational ages,[41] whereas others have found mean BPD values corresponding to those of singletons until the third trimester but demonstrating progressive slowing in growth of the twin BPDs thereafter.[42-46] When, however, values for 18 sets of concordant twins with verified menstrual dates were compared with values from singletons that were AGA at birth, Crane et al.[47] found that the two groups had mean BPD values that were essentially identical throughout gestation. These investigators conclude that normal twin BPD growth is similar to that of AGA singletons at all stages of gestation, and the conflicting results of earlier studies are due to the inclusion of discordant twins with

IUGR in the study group. A similar conclusion was reached by Graham et al.,[48] who studied 104 twins with concordant growth, excellent gestational age assessment, and delivery after 36 weeks, finding almost identical results when BPD and femur length (FL) values were compared with those from a selected population of singletons. Other investigators[46,49] also found no significant difference in BPD between uncomplicated singleton and twin pregnancies, suggesting that charts derived from singleton pregnancies may be reliably used for estimation of gestational age of twins.

Neonatal anthropometric data obtained from concordant twins suggest that although there is significant reduction of birth weights of twins in late pregnancy, head circumference and body lengths are generally similar to those of normal singletons at corresponding gestational age.[45,47] These findings are consistent with ultrasound observations showing twin FL growth patterns similar to those of singletons throughout gestation[44,48,50] but a reduction in the abdominal circumference growth in twins after 32 weeks.[44,45]

The Significance of Divergent BPDs

In 1976 Dorros[51] reported a case in which BPD values in a set of twins were discordant by 7 to 10 mm on three examinations performed between 38 and 41 weeks. At delivery one infant was found to be severely growth retarded; the other was AGA. The placenta had an infarct covering approximately 20 percent of the total surface area and was located near the origin of the growth retarded twin's umbilical cord. Several series have subsequently shown that as the difference between twin BPDs increases, the likelihood that the smaller fetus will be growth retarded increases. Leveno et al.[52] reported that a comparison of BPD differences of 4 mm or less with those of 5 mm or greater showed an increase in the number of pairs with one growth retarded twin from 7 to 22 percent. Houlton[53] noted an overall increase in small for gestational age (SGA) infants from 40 to 71 percent in a comparison of BPD differentials below 6 mm with those of 6 mm or greater.

Crane et al.[47] defined discordancy in utero as an intrapair difference in BPD of 5 mm or more and a fall in BPD below 2 SD for gestational age on their normal twin curve. Twelve sets of twins met this criteria for discordancy, 9 of whom were subsequently shown to have a difference in birth weight of more than 25 percent. Those cases in which significant BPD differences in utero did not correlate with major birth weight discrepancies were thought to be due to artifactual flattening of one BPD in association with abnormal fetal presentations and/or crowding in utero. Crane et al. suggested that head circumferences (HCs) be measured if BPD intrapair differences exceed 5 mm. Since head circumference is less likely to be affected by molding in utero, an intrapair HC difference of less than 5 percent suggests that true discrepancy does not exist.

In a study by Chitkara et al.[54] BPD intrapair differentials of 5 mm or greater did correlate with an increased incidence of significant birth weight differences, but estimated fetal weight (EFW) and abdominal circumference measurements were better predictors of this outcome. Other observers[55,56] have not found differences between twin BPDs to correlate at all with birth weight differentials.

This compilation of confusing and seemingly conflicting data can probably be summarized as follows: Significant differences in twin BPDs may reflect the fact that one twin is growth retarded; however, the finding may be purely artifactual. Measurements of the HC and other parameters, along with serial examinations, help distinguish between these alternatives in most cases. Nevertheless, although major intrapair BPD differences may reflect IUGR in one fetus, they are not the only criterion that should be used to look for abnormal development in utero because they will not be present when both twins are growth retarded.

The Use of Multiple Parameters to Assess IUGR and Growth Discordance

How then should growth in utero be followed in multiple pregnancies? BPD alone, as an isolated variable, is a poor predictor of IUGR in twins. Neilson[57] retrospectively analyzed 66 twin pregnancies with good dates by plotting BPD values on a singleton nomogram. Only 56 percent of the 43 SGA neonates were found to have abnormal BPD growth, and 49 percent of the fetuses with abnormal BPD curves were found not to be growth retarded at delivery. In a subsequent prospective study of 31 twin pregnancies, Neilson[58] made an initial scan for dating before 20 weeks and a "second stage" examination between 34 and 36 weeks. At the second examination, fetal size was assessed by calculating the product of crown–rump length (CRL) and trunk area (TA), plotted on a nomogram devised for singletons. In this series, 19 of the 62 neonates were SGA and all of them fell below the tenth percentile on the CRL and TA nomogram. In addition, 23 percent of the AGA babies were in the abnormal zone. Interestingly, the numbers calculated for each fetus did not prove useful in predicting weight differences within twin pairs at delivery.

Our experience[54] and that of others[45,59–61] suggests that a survey of multiple parameters on serial ultrasound examinations provides the most accurate assessment of the size of each individual fetus in twin gestations. The highest accuracy for predicting either appropriate or retarded growth is obtained from EFW. Among individual parameters, abdominal circumference (AC) is the single most sensitive measurement in predicting both IUGR and growth discordancy.[54,60,61] Recent studies suggest that an intrapair difference in AC measurement of 2 cm or more can be effectively used as a screening test for discordant fetal growth and IUGR in the smaller twin.[60,61] On the other hand, individual measurements of BPD, HC, or FL are relatively poor predictors for either IUGR or growth discordancy.[54,60,61]

Probably the most important conclusions that can be drawn from these various studies are that it is technically feasible to measure multiple ultrasound parameters in twin pregnancies and that consideration of as many variables as possible maximizes the effectiveness of an ultrasonic assessment of fetal size. The same general principles can be applied to the assessment of growth in triplet births and higher-order multiple gestations. Another point that should be stressed is that growth is a dynamic process and therefore patients with multiple gestations should be followed with serial scans. Since growth retardation is a process that usually occurs during the third trimester and the predictive accuracy of any fetal measurement in utero is inversely proportional to the scan–delivery interval, we recommend that women with twins be scanned every 3 to 4 weeks after the twenty-

sixth week, and more frequently if IUGR or growth discordance is suspected.

ULTRASONOGRAPHIC PREDICTION OF AMNIONICITY AND CHORIONICITY

The risk for many of the complications occurring in multiple gestation depends on whether the placentation is monochorionic or dichorionic. The incidence of IUGR and fetal death is higher in monochorionic (MC) than dichorionic (DC) twins, and the twin-to-twin transfusion syndrome (TTS) occurs only in MC twins. Antenatal knowledge of the type of placentation and chorionicity is not only helpful but in some cases critical for determining optimal management. This is true when deciding whether IUGR in one fetus of a twin gestation is due to TTS or uteroplacental insufficiency and when contemplating selectively terminating one abnormal twin or performing an elective first trimester multifetal pregnancy reduction procedure. In these latter situations if the gestation is monochorionic a shared placental circulation could result in death or damage to a surviving fetus.

The sonographic prediction of chorionicity and amnionicity should be systematically approached by determining the number of placentas visualized and the sex of each fetus and then by assessing the membranes that divide the sacs. The pregnancy is clearly dichorionic if two separate placental discs are seen or if the twins are of different sex. When a single placenta is present and the twins are of the same sex, careful sonographic examination of the dividing membrane usually results in a correct diagnosis. In dichorionic diamniotic (DC/DA) pregnancies the dividing membrane appears "thick,"[62–65] has a measured diameter of 2 mm or more,[66] and has either three or four layers that can be identified[67,68] (Fig. 26.6). With a monochorionic diamniotic (MC/DA) pregnancy only two layers of membranes are identified and the membrane appears to be "thin and hairlike"[67] (Fig. 26.7). D'Alton et al. caution that a floating MC/DA membrane may fold back on itself and give a false impression of having four layers. These investigators suggest that inspection of the membranes near their placental insertion reduces this artifact.[68] Significant magnification of the image is helpful in counting the number of layers. Determina-

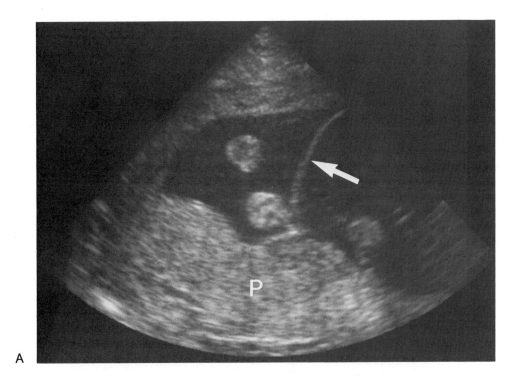

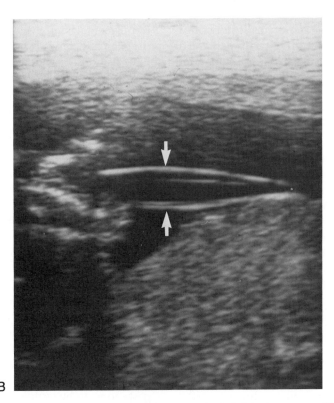

Fig. 26.6 (A) The dividing membrane (arrow) is thick, suggestive of a DC/DA placentation. (B) Visualization of four layers in the dividing membrane suggests DC/DA placentation.

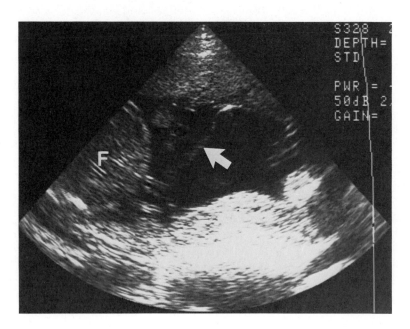

Fig. 26.7 The dividing membrane (arrow) is thin and hair-like, suggestive of MChorionic/DA placentation.

tion of membrane thickness allows correct identification of DC or MC gestation in 80 to 90 percent of cases.[62-64] Counting the number of layers adds a few extra minutes to the total scanning time but increases the predictive accuracy to almost 100 percent.[67,68]

In some pregnancies with MC/DA placentation, the dividing membranes may not be sonographically visualized because they are very thin. In other cases they may not be seen because severe oligohydramnios causes them to be closely apposed to the fetus in that sac. This results in a "stuck twin" appearance, in which the trapped fetus remains firmly held against the uterine wall despite changes in maternal position[63] (Fig. 26.8). Diagnosis of this condition confirms the presence of a DA gestation, which should be distinguished from a MA gestation in which dividing membranes are absent. In the latter situation free movement of both twins, and occasionally entanglement of their umbilical cords, can be demonstrated.[69]

DOPPLER STUDIES IN MULTIPLE GESTATION

Advances in Doppler ultrasound technology within the past decade have made it possible to evaluate fetoplacental hemodynamics in normal and abnormal pregnancies. Several studies in singleton pregnancies have demonstrated that abnormal Doppler velocimetry in the umbilical artery (UA) and other fetal vessels is often associated with fetal IUGR, pregnancy complications, and adverse perinatal outcome.[70-73] Although some investigators favor continuous wave systems, we think that Doppler studies in multiple gestations are best performed using a pulsed Doppler duplex system, in order to be certain that the vessel being studied belongs to a targeted fetus.

In 32 uncomplicated twin pregnancies in which both fetuses were AGA, Giles et al.[74] found that the UA systolic/diastolic (S/D) ratios were similar to those of normal singleton AGA fetuses. Their findings were confirmed by Gerson et al.,[75] who prospectively studied 65 normal twin pregnancies between 20 and 39 weeks gestation. These authors reported that UA S/D ratios in normal twins decrease with advancing gestation and that the relationship between S/D ratio and gestational age is the same in singleton and normal AGA twins. These studies and our own observations suggest that the S/D ratios in fetuses of a twin gestation can be evaluated as if two singleton fetuses were being assessed.

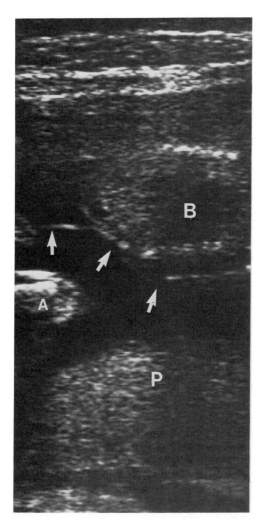

Fig. 26.8 Twin gestation with severe oligohydramnios in sac of twin B. The separating membrane (arrows) is closely apposed to this fetus and was visualized with difficulty. Sac of twin A showed severe polyhydramnios. P, placenta.

Fetal growth retardation in singleton pregnancies is often associated with abnormal Doppler study results, which may precede documentation of the IUGR by sonographic biometry or abnormalities in other tests of fetal well-being.[73] These observations are consistent with histologic evidence that abnormal UA wave forms may reflect vascular lesions in the placenta that can be presumed to increase resistance to blood flow through the umbilical arteries.[76] Similar

alterations in UA S/D ratios have been documented in some growth retarded twins. In their study of 76 twin pregnancies, Giles et al.[74] had 33 patients in whom one or both twins were SGA; in 78 percent of these pregnancies at least one fetus had an elevated S/D ratio. Farmakaides et al.[77] performed Doppler studies in 43 twin pregnancies and tried to predict growth discordancy by examining S/D ratio differences in each twin pair. They found that a ratio difference of 0.4 or more between the twins was predictive of a weight difference of more than 349 g with a sensitivity of 73 percent and a specificity of 82 percent. Similar observations were reported by Saldana et al.[78] These investigators found that an S/D ratio difference 0.4 or more was a better predictor than ultrasound for birth weight discordancy in the SGA/AGA twin pairs but was poor in predicting discordant weight in the SGA/SGA, AGA/AGA, and AGA/large for gestational age (LGA) twin pairs. They also suggested that to obtain maximal information, the absolute S/D ratios as well as differences in these ratios must be carefully evaluated in all cases.

Opinions regarding the usefulness of routinely performing Doppler studies in all twin pregnancies vary. Two recent studies illustrate this controversy. The first, by Giles et al.,[79] described the clinical management and pregnancy outcome in a study group of 112 women with twin gestations in whom results of two or more Doppler studies were made available to the patients' obstetricians. These results were compared with those of a group of 95 patients in whom Doppler studies were performed but not reported to the clinicians. In the study group the first test was performed at 28 to 32 weeks gestation, and this was repeated 4 to 5 weeks later if the initial study result was normal. If, however, a Doppler evaluation finding was abnormal, further studies were repeated as often as once a week, along with nonstress tests and sonographic studies. Patients were delivered if their nonstress test results were persistently abnormal or serial sonographic studies showed failure of fetal growth. In this series a significant reduction in perinatal mortality and morbidity was noted in the study group. It is interesting that the improvement in outcome was achieved without any appreciable differences in gestational age at delivery or mode of delivery between the two study groups. The second study[80] was a prospective evaluation of 89 twin pregnancies that attempted to determine the predictive value of umbilical artery Doppler studies in identifying twin fetuses destined to be SGA at birth. Serial Doppler recordings were made from each twin once a month from 22 weeks gestation until delivery, but the results were not made available to the patients' clinicians. Thirty-two of the 178 infants in this series were SGA at birth, but results of only 24 of the 82 Doppler studies performed in the growth retarded fetuses were abnormal, giving an overall sensitivity of 29 percent and a positive predictive value of 34 percent. This study, therefore, did not confirm the relatively high predictive value of Doppler studies for SGA twins reported by other investigators.[74,77]

From our review of the current literature, we are not convinced that Doppler studies should be routinely performed as part of the antepartum surveillance of women with mutiple gestations. However, when IUGR is suspected in one or more fetuses, Doppler velocimetry is a useful adjunct in assessing and following these pregnancies.

Our routine for the surveillance of patients with multiple gestations is as follows:

1. Initial ultrasound evaluation is performed at 18 to 20 weeks gestation. This includes standard biometry to confirm gestational age and size of each fetus, assessment of amniotic fluid volume in each sac, evaluation of each fetus's anatomy to rule out morphologic anomalies, and attempt to determine chorionicity by examining fetal gender, number of placentas, and thickness as well as number of layers in the membrane separating the sacs.
2. If the first study is normal, subsequent scans for fetal growth are made at 24 to 26 weeks and every 3 to 4 weeks thereafter as long as fetal growth and amniotic fluid volume in each sac remain normal.
3. If there is evidence of IUGR, discordant fetal growth, or discordant fluid volumes, fetal surveillance is intensified and includes frequent nonstress testing along with biophysical profile and Doppler velocimetry studies. Absent diastolic, or reversed diastolic, flow often predicts imminent death in utero, and serious considera-

tion should be given to delivering patients with these findings if the healthy fetus is mature enough to be able to tolerate an elective delivery.

ABNORMALITIES ASSOCIATED WITH MULTIPLE GESTATION

Twin-Twin Transfusion Syndrome

Benirschke and Kim[5] state that, as a group, MZ monochorial twins have greater disparity in weight than dichorial twins. A comparison of DZ and dichorial MZ twins with MZ twins having a monochorial placenta shows this effect on birth weight to be due entirely to type of placentation and not zygosity. This finding is best explained by the twin-to-twin transfusion syndrome.

To our knowledge, the twin-to-twin transfusion syndrome in humans has only been reported in association with monochorionic placentas. On very rare occasions, vascular communications may exist between dichorial placentas, even in the case of DZ twins as evidenced by the occurrence of blood group chimeras,[81] but these anastomoses are the rule rather than the unusual exception among monochorionic twins. The potential for the transfusion syndrome is present when the arterial circulation of one twin is in communication with the venous circulation of the other through arteriovenous shunts in a "common villous district"[5] (Figs. 26.9 and 26.10). In this situation, one fetus becomes a donor that transfuses its co-twin. The donor becomes anemic and growth retarded. Although occasionally it may become hydropic as a result of high-output failure, more frequently this twin is significantly smaller than the other. The recipient, on the other hand, becomes polycythemic and can suffer from congestive heart failure as a result of circulatory overload. Thromboses of peripheral vessels may also develop in association with the hypertransfused state.

The perinatal mortality rate associated with the transfusion syndrome may be as high as 70 percent. Two recent studies[82,83] suggest that three antenatal factors that almost invariably predict a fatal outcome in these pregnancies are (1) early gestational age at diagnosis with delivery before 28 weeks, (2) severe hydramnios requiring therapeutic amniocentesis, and (3) fetal hydrops. If hydramnios develops early,

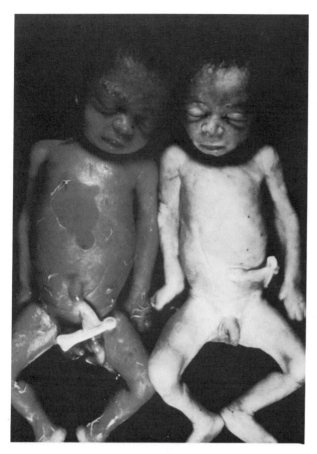

Fig. 26.9 Stillborn male twins at 31 weeks gestation, secondary to the twin-to-twin transfusion syndrome. The plethoric twin on the left weighed 1,670 g and the anemic growth retarded twin on the right weighed 1,300 g.

premature labor often occurs before the third trimester.

Nance[81] states that if the birth weights of MZ twins differ by less than 20 percent, the difference usually does not persist during later development. If, however, the weights are discrepant by more than 25 percent, differences in height, and in some cases developmental delay, may persist into adult life.

The twin-to-twin transfusion syndrome can be ultrasonically detected in utero.[84] When severe, the syndrome usually manifests itself clinically as a result of hydramnios that is almost always found to exist in the sac of the larger twin. Sonographic criteria that provide an almost unequivocal antenatal diagnosis of

twin-twin transfusion syndrome include (1) presence of same sex twins with a single placenta; (2) thin (two layer) separating membrane between the sacs; (3) significantly discordant fetal growth (although this is not inevitably present); (4) discordant amniotic fluid volume with polyhydramnios in the sac of the larger recipient, and possibly a "stuck twin" appearance as a result of oligohydramnios in the donor's sac; (5) evidence of hydrops or cardiac failure in either fetus but more frequently in the larger twin.

When twins of unequal size are discovered on ultrasound examination, it is important to distinguish the transfusion syndrome from a pregnancy in which one fetus is growth retarded but the other is developing normally. In the latter situation the normal twin is usually surrounded by an appropriate quantity of amniotic fluid and oligohydramnios may or may not be present in the other sac. In the transfusion syndrome, however, hydramnios and ultrasonic evidence of hydrops are often noted in association with the larger twin, while the donor is smaller than it should be and not simply smaller than its larger sibling. This latter point may be useful in ruling out a third uncommon situation, namely that of a normal fetus and a larger hydropic co-twin who is anomalous or erythroblastotic.

Reports of Doppler studies in fetuses with the twin-to-twin transfusion syndrome are conflicting. Farmakaides et al.[77] reported two cases in which umbilical artery waveforms of the twins were discordant and concluded that a simultaneous observation of high- and low-resistance S/D ratios was highly suggestive of this diagnosis. On the other hand, in eight cases in which the diagnosis was documented or strongly suspected, Giles et al.[74] found no difference in interpair S/D ratios. Pretorius et al.[85] also reported eight cases of twin-twin transfusion syndrome and found no consistent pattern of umbilical artery Doppler S/D ratios. The mortality rate in this latter study was very high; five of eight pregnancies ended in fetal or neonatal death of both twins. In all five instances of perinatal loss, one or both of the twins had either absent or reversed diastolic flow. These investigators concluded that although evidence of greatly increased placental resistance (i.e., absent or reversed diastolic flow) is not helpful in identifying the donor from the recipient twin, it invariably predicts a poor outcome.

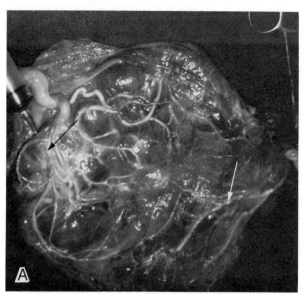
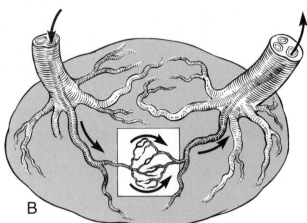

Fig. 26.10 (A) The placenta of a pregnancy complicated by the twin-to-twin transfusion syndrome. Milk has been injected into an artery on the "donor" side of the placenta (black arrow). It can be seen returning through the venous circulation on that side but is also evident in the venous circulation of the "recipient" (white arrow). (B) The arteriovenous shunt shown in (A).

Congenital Anomalies in Multiple Gestations

There is general agreement that anomalies occur more frequently in twins than in singletons, but controversy exists regarding the degree of difference. A large series from Czechoslovakia[86] reported a rate of anomalies of 1.4 percent for singletons, 2.71 percent for twins, and 6.1 percent for triplets. Among cases of twins in which anomalies were detected, both twins were affected in 14.8 percent. There were no cases of triplets in which all three infants were affected. Hendricks[87] found the frequency of anomalies to be more than 3 times higher in twins than in singletons, whereas in Kohl and Casey's[8] series the frequency was 1.5 to 2 times higher. Other studies cited by Benirschke and Kim[5] report smaller increases.

The diagnosis of a variety of morphologic abnormalities in multiple gestations has been made in utero with ultrasound. It is possible to detect anomalies of one or both fetuses or conversely to rule out specific disorders in twins who are known to be at increased risk for them. As is true for singletons, however, an ultrasonic diagnosis can only be made when a potentially detectable anatomic abnormality has become manifest at the time the fetus is studied. Neilson et al.[88] describe four cases in which anomalies in one or both twins were heralded by elevated serum AFP values. In all these patients, the abnormalities were detected by ultrasound. They also reported one case in which an elevated serum AFP value was found to be due to an intrauterine death of one twin in association with a healthy co-twin.

Anomalies Related to Twinning

Some anomalies such as acardia and conjoining are directly related to the twinning process. Acardia is a malformation that occurs in one of MZ twins, triplets, or even quintuplets with a frequency of approximately 1 per 30,000 deliveries[5] (Fig. 26.11). These extremely malformed fetuses either have no heart at all (holoacardia) or only some rudimentary cardiac tissue (pseudoacardia) in association with other multiple developmental abnormalities. Aside from a single case report[89] to the contrary, these patients always have monochorial placentas and vascular anastomoses that sustain the life of the acardiac monster. Because of their isosexual status and monochorial relationship, they are considered to be MZ and there-

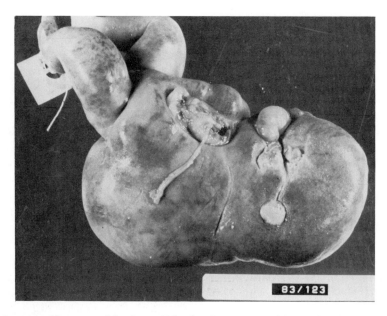

Fig. 26.11 Acardiac twin. (Courtesy of Dr. James Wheeler, Department of Surgical Pathology, Hospital of the University of Pennsylvania, Philadelphia, PA.)

fore represent the ultimate of discordance in the development of genetically identical individuals.

Controversy exists regarding the etiology of this condition. Kaplan and Benirschke[90] believe that reversal of flow through the acardiac twin secondary to at least one artery-to-artery and one vein-to-vein connection in the placenta leads to the anomaly of twin reversed arterial perfusion (TRAP) sequence. Retrograde fetal perfusion has been documented to occur by Doppler studies in two cases.[91,92] Other authors,[81,89] however, believe that acardia is a primary defect in cardiac development and that although the placental vascular anastomoses are necessary for survival of the affected twin, they are not responsible for the abnormalities.

There is also a high incidence of chromosomal abnormalities in these pregnancies. In 6 of the 12 acardiac cases reported by Van Allen et al.[93] an abnormal karyotype was found in the perfused twin and a normal karyotype in the pump twin. The remaining six perfused twins were chromosomally normal.

Antenatal diagnosis by ultrasound of an acardiac fetus co-existing with a normal co-twin is fairly straightforward. The anomalous twin may appear to be an amorphous mass or may show a wide range of abnormalities that depend on which organ system has

failed to develop. The lower extremities and body are typically more completely developed, and the most severe abnormalities involve the upper body. Frequently the heart is absent or rudimentary, and a single umbilical artery is present in approximately half the cases. As mentioned previously, a retrograde pattern of fetal perfusion can be demonstrated to occur through the umbilical arteries by Doppler studies.

Nance[81] presents evidence to suggest that a group of birth defects involving midline structures, including symmelia, exstrophy of the cloaca, and midline neural tube defects, may be associated in some way with the twinning process. Symmelia is a rare severe defect that results from fusion of the preaxial halves of the developing hindlimb buds. This produces a single lower extremity with a knee that flexes in the opposite direction from normal. The incidence of this condition is 100 times higher in MZ births than in singletons. MZ twins have also been shown to have a higher frequency of neural tube defects than singletons,[94] and they are often discordant for the abnormality. Nance suggests that the MZ twinning process, with its attendant opportunities for asymmetry, cytoplasmic deficiency, and competition in utero, may favor the discordant expression of midline neurologic defects in these twins. He also cites evidence that 10 percent of all cases of exstrophy of the cloaca occur in like-sex twins. In each of these instances, it is unclear whether the occurrence of a malformation somehow initiates the twinning process or whether a common factor predisposes to both events. Discordance is often, but not always, a feature of these midline defects in MZ twins.

Conjoined twins occur with a frequency of about 1 per 50,000 deliveries and in approximately 1 per 600 twin births.[95-97] The most famous conjoined twins were Chang and Eng Bunker, who were born in Siam in 1811. These xiphopagus twins (i.e., joined by a band of tissue extending from the umbilicus to the xiphoid cartilage) lived unseparated for 63 years. P. T. Barnum exhibited them extensively for a number of years. At the age of 31, they married two sisters, who bore them a total of 26 children. They died within hours of each other.[95-97]

The precise etiology of conjoined twinning is unknown, but the most widely accepted theory is that incomplete division of an MZ embryo occurs at approximately 13 to 15 days post ovulation. Most conjoined twins are female: the ratio of females to males is reported as 2:1 or 3:1. The majority of these infants are delivered prematurely and are stillborn.[96] They are classified according to their site of union. The most common location is the chest (thoracopagus) (Fig. 26.12), followed by the anterior abdominal wall from the xiphoid to the umbilicus (xiphopagus), the buttocks (pygopagus), the ischium (ischiopagus), and the head (craniopagus).[96] Organs may be shared to varying degrees in different sets of twins. Major congenital anomalies of one or both twins are not uncommon and must be carefully searched for before definitive therapy is attempted. The success of surgical separation depends on the degree of union, the absence of major anomalies, and the presence of separate hearts.

In 1950 Gray et al.[98] proposed a set of radiographic criteria for diagnosing ventrally fused twins. These include the twins' facing each other with their heads at the same level and thoracic cages in close proximity, loss of the usual flexion of the fetal spines and occasionally hyperextension of the cervical spines, and no change in position of the twins relative to each other in response to external manipulations or spontaneous fetal movement. Hydramnios is said to be

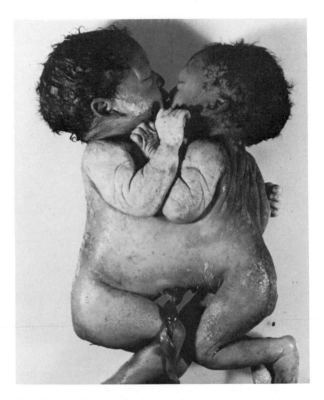

Fig. 26.12 Conjoined twins attached at the chest of thoracopagus, the most common form of conjoined twins. They originate at the primitive streak stage of the embryonic plate (13 to 15 days). (Courtesy of Dr. James Wheeler, Department of Surgical Pathology, Hospital of the University of Pennsylvania, Philadelphia, PA.)

present in almost one-half the reported cases of conjoined twins. Amniography or fetography has been helpful in establishing the diagnosis radiographically because these procedures outline the fetal body contours and occasionally demonstrate a shared gastrointestinal tract.[99] Ultrasound, however, has become the safest and most reliable way to make this diagnosis in utero. At least eight reports in which this condition has been antenatally detected with ultrasound have been published.[99-106] Gore et al.[102] state that since fetal soft tissues are so well visualized with today's sonographic equipment, invasive imaging procedures such as amniography should no longer be necessary.

Once the antenatal diagnosis has been established, the mode of delivery can be planned. Vaughn and Powell[96] point out that dystocia, previously thought to be rare, since the union between conjoined twins is usually soft and pliable, may be a frequent and serious complication if vaginal delivery is attempted at term. When dystocia occurs in this setting, intrauterine surgical separation may be required that could result in devastating consequences for the fetuses and significant trauma to the mother. Craniopagus twins do not develop this type of dystocia, since it can be anticipated that they will deliver "in series" rather than "in parallel." It is therefore recommended that most conjoined twins be delivered by cesarean section at term or if they present in premature labor and are potentially salvageable. If they are considered to have a poor chance of surviving and are small enough to pass through the birth canal without damaging the mother, vaginal delivery may be the option of choice. Compton[107] states, however, that with near term size twins, cesarean section seems indicated even if the fetuses are dead. This conclusion is based on the premise that maternal morbidity from elective cesarean section is predictably lower than that associated with failed partial vaginal delivery necessitating emergency cesarean section.

CHROMOSOMAL ANOMALIES IN TWINS

Most known chromosomal anomalies have been reported in twins.[108] DZ twins are usually discordant for these anomalies, and surprisingly, MZ twins may be as well. Such MZ twins are known as heterokaryotypes, and, in these cases it is assumed that a maldistribution of chromosomal material occurred at about the same time as the twinning process itself (postzygotic non-disjunction). Phenotypically dissimilar MZ twins may have similar chromosome mosaicisms in lymphocyte cultures due to the shared fetal circulation in a MC placenta but show different karyotypes in fibroblast cultures.[109,110] Since most cytogenetic studies are performed on lymphocytes, it is likely that some heterokaryotypic twins have gone unrecognized.

The incidence of Down syndrome is no more common in twins than in singletons. Although most pregnancies with one affected fetus are DZ, there have been rare cases of MZ twins discordant for trisomy 21.[111] Concordance for Down syndrome in DZ twins is unusual, but several investigators have reported a somewhat higher concordance rate in DZ pairs than would be expected, even allowing for maternal age.[112,113] This suggests that some women may have a unique predisposition to this chromosomal anomaly.

DEATH OF ONE TWIN IN UTERO

The death of one twin in utero is not an exceptionally rare event. Hanna and Hill[114] report a frequency of 2.2 percent over an 8-year period at their institution and cite a Swiss study in which the frequency was 6.8 percent over a period of almost 10 years. When only one twin dies in utero, it may become a fetus papyraceous. In that condition, the fluid is reabsorbed from the dead twin's body and the latter is compressed into the adjacent membranes by the growth of the living fetus. Benirschke and Kim[5] observed that this process can occur with any kind of placentation and that it is occasionally seen as a result of the twin-to-twin transfusion syndrome.

When a dead twin remains undelivered, a legitimate medical concern is the potential for disseminated intravascular coagulation (DIC) in the mother. DIC is well known to complicate some cases of retained dead fetuses in singleton pregnancies.[115] This is usually a chronic process that develops slowly in response to the release of thromboplastic material from the degenerating fetus into the maternal circulation. Although most cases of this type of DIC have been reported in the setting of a singleton gestation, it can occur after the death of one fetus in a multiple gestation.[116]

Romero and colleagues[117] have reported a case in which death of one twin in utero was detected at 26 weeks gestation (Fig. 26.13). Three and a half weeks later, the patient's fibrinogen level had fallen from an initial value of 370 to 95 mg/dl. In response to an intravenous infusion of heparin, the hypofibrinogemia was reversed. After a total of 25 days of therapy, the heparin was stopped and the patient delivered vaginally a 2,040-g infant with Apgar scores of 9 and 9 and a macerated 350-g stillborn at 36 weeks. Successful reversal of maternal antepartum DIC with the use of heparin has also been documented in two other patients. In each case the pregnancy was prolonged by 10 weeks and outcome was normal for the surviving twin.[116,118] These cases demonstrate that in selected situations it may be possible to treat the chronic maternal coagulopathy associated with a re-

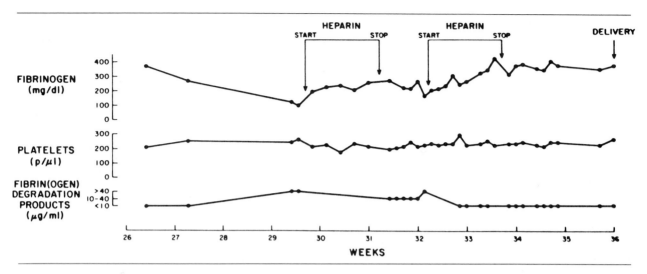

Fig. 26.13 Effect of heparin therapy after 26 weeks gestation on the platelet count and the plasma concentrations of fibrinogen and fibrin/fibrinogen degradation products in a pregnancy complicated by the death of one twin in utero. (From Romero et al.,[117] with permission.)

tained dead twin to allow a premature living co-twin to continue to develop in utero. Fortunately, however, this is usually not necessary because the incidence of this complication must be very low. In our experience with 25 cases in which death of an anomalous twin fetus was selectively induced during the second trimester, none of the patients developed evidence of clinical DIC. Similar experiences have been reported by other groups in another 34 pregnancies.[119-122] Therefore, as Hanna and Hill[114] have suggested, when death in utero of one twin is detected before 34 weeks, conservative management is the wisest course. This should include weekly maternal clotting profiles and serial assessments of fetal growth and well-being. Since no coagulation disorders have been observed after spontaneous or induced first trimester death of one or more fetuses in a multiple gestation, monitoring of coagulation factors may not be necessary when losses occur prior to 13 weeks.

It should be noted that normal maternal fibrinogen levels or successful reversal of a consumption coagulopathy within the maternal circulation does not ensure that the surviving fetus will be unaffected by the process. If vascular anastomoses exist within a monochorial placenta, the shared circulation may permit embolization of thromboplastic material from the dead fetus directly into its living sibling. This phenom-

enon has been cited as the cause of intrauterine DIC and bilateral cortical necrosis,[123] multicystic encephalomalacia,[124] and other structural abnormalities[125-127] in liveborn MZ twins with stillborn macerated co-twins. By contrast, because of the virtual absence of shared circulations, this should be a far less likely occurrence in the case of DZ twins or MZ twins with dichorionic placentas. Carlson and Towers[128] presented a series of 17 multiple gestations in which one fetus had died and also reviewed the literature on this subject. They concluded that there is a 17 percent chance that the "surviving twin" in a MC gestation will either die or suffer major morbidity, whereas these possibilities are unlikely to occur in the surviving twin in a DC gestation. In addition, in their series they observed a high occurrence of lesser morbidities, including abnormal fetal heart rate test results, cesarean section for fetal distress, IUGR, and hyperbilirubinemia, in the surviving infant, and the incidence of these complications was similar in MC and DC twin pregnancies.

SELECTIVE TERMINATION OF AN ANOMALOUS FETUS

The diagnosis of discordancy for a major genetic disease before the time limit for legal termination of pregnancy in the second trimester places the parents in an extremely difficult position. Traditional choices in this setting are to terminate the pregnancy and sacrifice one normal child or to continue the pregnancy with the certain knowledge that one child will be afflicted with a devastating condition. A third choice is to perform selective termination of the affected fetus, anticipating healthy survival of the normal twin. Technical difficulties associated with this latter procedure in DZ twin gestations have, to a large extent, been resolved since its first description over a decade ago.[129] However, several issues pertaining to technical, medical, ethical, and psychological problems related to this procedure must be carefully considered and discussed with the parents.

Several techniques that have been successfully used to perform selective terminations in the second trimester include cardiac puncture with exsanguination,[129,130] removal of the affected twin at hysterotomy,[131] cardiac puncture with intracardiac injection of calcium gluconate,[120] air embolization through the umbilical vessels with fetoscopic guidance,[119] and intracardiac injection of potassium chloride.[132] The latter approach has gained acceptance because of its safety and is currently preferred for both selective termination procedures in the second trimester and elective reduction of fetal numbers in the first trimester.[29–31,121,122,132]

Immediate problems and complications associated with selective termination procedures include selection of the wrong fetus, technical inability to accomplish the objective of the procedure, premature rupture of the membranes, infection, and loss of the entire pregnancy. Before initiating the procedure, it is critical that the abnormal fetus be correctly identified. When the indication for selective termination is an abnormal karyotype diagnosed by amniocentesis or chorionic villus sampling, a sonographically identifiable marker may or may not be present. If the gender of the twins is different, or the affected fetus has a gross morphologic anomaly, such as hydrocephaly or omphalocele, the abnormal twin can be easily identified by sonography. However, in the absence of such visible signs, one must rely on the information provided by the original diagnostic procedures, which frequently have been performed elsewhere and several days or weeks before the patient presents herself to have the termination performed. In those cases in which accurate localizing information is lacking, fetal blood sampling and rapid karyotype determination should be performed to reidentify the abnormal fetus before selective termination is attempted. Furthermore, in all cases a sample of fetal tissue must be obtained from the terminated twin to confirm that the correct fetus has been selected.

In our series of 25 patients who underwent this procedure, the abnormal fetus was correctly identified in all cases. Four of the first 6 patients in this series lost their entire pregnancy secondary to complications of the procedure (i.e., infection or preterm delivery). Among the last 19 patients, however, there were no cases of infection or perinatal loss. Eleven of these women (58 percent) delivered at or beyond 37 weeks gestation; 3 (16 percent) between 32 and 36 weeks; and 5 (26 percent) between 28 and 31 weeks. There were no perinatal deaths, and all of the 19 infants are alive and healthy except one, who delivered at 28 weeks and developed sequelae of severe hyaline membrane disease and an intraventricular hemorrhage after birth.

In considering selective termination of an abnormal twin, particular caution must be exercised in excluding the possibility of a MC gestation. Vascular connections between fetal circulations occur in approximately 70 percent of MZ twins. In this situation, a lethal agent injected into the anomalous fetus may enter the circulation of its normal sibling and result in death or permanent damage.[121] To prevent this possibility it has been suggested that pericardial tamponade with an innocuous agent such as normal saline might be attempted.[133] However, even if this were successful it is possible that the normal twin could exsanguinate into the vasculature of the dead twin because of a marked decrease in peripheral resistance of the shared circulations.[121] To date all reported attempts at selective termination in MC pregnancies have led to the death of the second twin within a short time, with the exception of four cases: three in which the affected fetus was surgically removed by hysterotomy[121,134,135] and another in which pericardial tamponade with injection of normal saline was achieved.[133]

In summary, the therapeutic option of selective termination requires significant technical competence, a need to verify the diagnosis on the fetus that is terminated, and thorough counseling prior to the procedure. When everything has been considered, selective termination may be the best choice for a particular set of parents in this unenviable predicament, but detailed and truly informed consent is mandatory.

FIRST TRIMESTER MULTIFETAL PREGNANCY REDUCTION

The increasingly successful use of ovulatory drugs, in vitro fertilization, and related therapies has resulted in a growing incidence of multifetal pregnancies with three or more fetuses. Because of a high risk of perinatal morbidity and mortality from premature delivery in these pregnancies, first trimester reduction[29-31] of the number of fetuses has been advocated as a method to improve outcome. The original method of transcervical aspiration of gestational sacs described by Dumez et al.[136] has largely been abandoned. Currently, the method of choice consists of injecting a small dose of potassium chloride into the fetal thorax under real-time sonographic guidance, using either a transabdominal[29-31,122] or transvaginal approach.[137]

A recent report from our institution presented the outcome of 85 cases of transabdominal multifetal pregnancy reduction.[31] These procedures were all performed between 9.5 and 13 weeks gestation. The pregnancies consisted of 28 triplets, 47 quadruplets, 4 quintuplets, 4 sextuplets, 1 septuplet, and 1 nontuplet. Eighty of these pregnancies were reduced to twins, 4 to triplets, and in one case, in which a large uterine septum was present, to a single fetus. In this series 45 women delivered viable fetuses, 8 lost their entire pregnancy, and 32 pregnancies were ongoing uneventfully at the time the report was written. The mean gestational age at delivery was 35.7 weeks for those patients delivering viable fetuses. In these 45 cases, 16 delivered at or after 37 weeks, 16 between 34.5 and 37 weeks, 9 between 32 and 34.5 weeks, and 4 before 32 weeks. There were no instances of perinatal deaths, and the neonatal outcome was excellent in all cases except for one twin delivered electively at 29 weeks because of severe pregnancy induced hypertension, who developed chronic sequelae of severe hyaline membrane disease.

The experience cited above, as well as that reported in other series,[30,122] indicates that first trimester pregnancy reduction is technically feasible and results in the delivery of healthy infants close to term in the majority of cases. Although we believe that most people would agree that perinatal morbidity and mortality are likely to improve when pregnancies with four or more fetuses are reduced to smaller numbers, the advantages of reducing triplets to twins are far more controversial. We do not think that a first trimester reduction from three to two fetuses can be justified on the basis of improving perinatal mortality rate. However, since virtually all published series indicate that at least 20 percent of triplet pregnancies are likely to deliver before 32 weeks, a reduction in the morbidity associated with severe prematurity may result from reducing three fetuses to two. Until more detailed data are available from triplet pregnancies managed conservatively under modern circumstances, it is not possible to know whether multifetal pregnancy reduction does truly reduce perinatal morbidity in these cases.

PROBLEMS RELATED TO PLACENTATION

Benirschke and Kim[5] note that prolapse of the cord and rupture of a vasa previa with fetal exsanguination are more common in twins than in singletons. They attribute the latter to the fact that a velamentous cord insertion occurs in 7 percent of twin placentas as opposed to 1 percent of singleton placentas. Robinson et al.[138] found that 7.1 percent of 72 pregnancies having a velamentous insertion of the cord had associated deformational defects of the neonate. This is defined as an alteration in shape and/or structure of a part of the fetus that has differentiated normally (e.g., clubfoot). These workers speculate that competition for space between the developing fetus and the placenta due to mechanical factors that cause crowding in utero leads to fetal structural defects of a deformational nature and also alters the direction in which the placenta can grow. The latter situation secondarily causes velamentous insertion to occur when the bulk of the placental tissue is forced to grow laterally, leaving the umbilical cord, which initially was located centrally, in an area that eventually becomes atrophic chorion laeve. The increased incidence of velamentous cord insertions in twin pregnancies may result from competition for space when two blastocysts happen to implant in close proximity. In support of this theory is the observation that velamentous insertions are more common in the most closely approximated twin placentas.

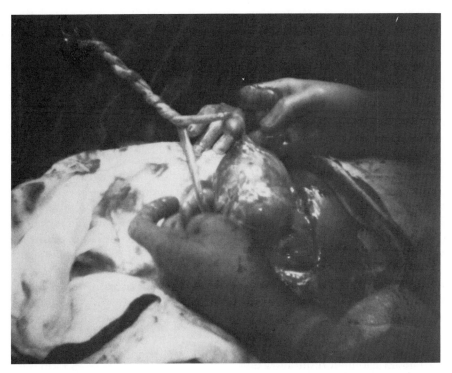

Fig. 26.14 Entangled cords found at cesarean section in a case of MC/MA twins.

MA twins are rare and have a high risk of fetal mortality. In a study from 1935, the survival rate of both twins was 16 percent; more recent series report double survival rates of 40 percent.[139] The high fetal mortality rate associated with a single amniotic sac is due to prematurity, vascular anastomoses in the placenta, and, most commonly, entanglement of the umbilical cords (Fig. .26.14). The latter is said to occur in as many as 70 percent of MA twins. Cord entanglement has been detected ultrasonically at 19 weeks in a case of MA twins discordant for an open neural tube defect.[140] Inability to visualize a membrane separating two sacs in a twin gestation is suggestive of a MA pregnancy but is not diagnostic because occasionally the membrane can remain undetected even though it is present. Townsend and Filly[141] suggest that the observation of entangled umbilical cords in the absence of a membrane separating twin fetuses provides a reliable sign for the sonographic diagnosis of MA twin gestation. They point out, though, that it is essential to trace both cords into the entangled mass before making this diagnosis. Another uncommon mishap that can result from this type of placentation

is inadvertent clamping of the undelivered twin's cord after delivery of the first twin. McLeod and McCoy[142] present just such a case in which a tight cord around the neck of twin A was clamped and divided and then found to belong to twin B. After abdominal manipulation, the second twin was rapidly delivered by forceps, and both neonates survived. These workers suggest that whenever possible, division of a cord around the first twin's neck should be prevented. They end their paper with the reminder that if the wrong cord has been severed, "immediate extraction of the second twin is essential."

AMNIOCENTESIS IN MULTIPLE GESTATIONS

When Should Both Sacs Be Tapped?

There are some situations in which it is obviously necessary to perform amniocentesis on each twin sac. Genetic studies must be performed on fluid surrounding both twins because, if DZ, they are genetically distinct individuals. Twins at risk of erythroblastosis fetalis must also have each sac tapped for optical density determinations, since one twin may be Rh-positive and the other Rh-negative.[143] It should be noted that twins in Rh sensitized pregnancies have been successfully transfused in utero.[144]

The issue of pulmonary maturity studies in twins is more complex. Two series have found a close correlation between lecithin/spingomyelin (L/S) ratios in amniotic fluid samples from twin sets. Spellacy et al.[145] found no significant difference in fluids obtained from both sacs when L/S ratios were studied in 14 pregnancies. Sims and colleagues[146] also found the L/S ratios of both sacs to be closely related in 20 set of twins. Obladen and Gluck,[147] however, noted significant discrepancies in postnatal phospholipid profiles of tracheal effluent in eight pairs of twins, six of whom were delivered vaginally.

Wilkinson et al.[148] reported a case of quadruplets delivered at 30 weeks by cesarean section in which the presenting baby had amniotic fluid and pharyngeal aspirate L/S ratio values that were on the borderline of maturity, whereas those of the other three infants were clearly immature and almost identical to each other. The firstborn infant had mild respiratory distress; the other three developed severe hyaline membrane disease. None of the neonates experienced birth asphyxia or postnatal hypothermia, and all the pharyngeal aspirates were collected within 10 minutes of birth. These investigators cite an earlier publication from their group, in which the firstborn of triplets and quadruplets had also been found to have higher pharyngeal L/S ratios and less severe respiratory distress than those of their siblings delivered subsequently. This relationship was found regardless of whether the firstborn was delivered vaginally after spontaneous labor or was the presenting fetus and was delivered by cesarean section.

Norman et al.[149] studied 30 African women with twins, all of whom had both sacs tapped immediately before delivery by cesarean section. Twenty-four of these patients were not in labor at the time of their delivery, and no significant intrapair differences in L/S ratio were found in this group. Six women who were in labor, however, were found to have a significant increase in the L/S ratio of their presenting twin when compared with its sibling. In addition, both free and unconjugated glucocorticoids were found to be increased in the amniotic fluid of the presenting twin after labor had begun, but no significant difference

was noted within twin sets when labor had not commenced. These latter reports suggest that the onset of labor in multiple pregnancy may be determined by the fetus with the most mature lungs, which apparently is often the one presenting.

It is possible that one twin may be significantly more stressed in utero than the other. The concept of accelerated lung maturation in response to antenatal stress has become widely accepted.[150] It is therefore certainly conceivable that one twin may be pulmonically mature, although the other is not. Leveno et al.[151] presented a series of 42 twin pregnancies delivered by cesarean section in whom amniocentesis on each sac was performed immediately before delivery. The cesarean sections were performed for a variety of indications, and no mention is made of the presence or absence of labor. In this group of patients, there were four instances in which one twin had an L/S ratio less than 2, while its sibling's value was 2 or greater. The pair with the greatest difference had L/S ratios of 0.7 and 3.5. However, only one of these eight neonates developed hyaline membrane disease, and that was a twin whose L/S ratio was 1.4 while its sibling's was 2.2. Interestingly, in this series there were seven pairs in whom only one fetus was growth retarded; IUGR was not found to increase the L/S ratio significantly in these cases. Similarly, Norman et al.[149] compared the L/S ratios from each sac before the onset of labor in eight sets of twins with only one growth retarded fetus and were unable to find significant differences.

It appears that the stress associated with IUGR may not be sufficient to cause a significant difference in lung maturity when only one twin is affected. There has been a case report,[152] however, that raises the possibility that the stress associated with premature rupture of membranes (PROM) for more than 16 hours in a presenting fetus may give it a pulmonary advantage over its co-twin with intact membranes. It is likely that other stressful processes could affect twins in an unequal manner and result in major differences related to pulmonary surfactant production.

We believe it is reasonable to assume that in most cases of nonlaboring patients with twins, an L/S ratio from one sac accurately reflects the status of both fetuses. If one twin appears to be abnormal for any reason, however, or if the patient is in premature labor, both sacs should be tapped to assess pulmonary maturity. Should the operator elect to tap only one sac in these situations, it should be that of the twin who appears to be normal in the former case, and that of the second twin in the latter. The stressed twin or the presenting twin in these two instances can be assumed to have an L/S ratio at least as mature as that of its sibling and probably more so.

The Technique of Tapping Multiple Sacs

Elias et al.[153] reported that they were successful in obtaining fluid from both amniotic sacs in 19 of 20 pregnancies during the second trimester. These workers used ultrasound to identify the lie of each fetus and then introduced an amniocentesis needle into one sac using a standard insertion technique. After aspirating some fluid they introduced a blue dye, to serve as a marker, and then removed the needle. A different needle was then inserted and the aspiration of untinged fluid indicated that the second sac had been successfully entered. Several points should be stressed:

1. The usual precautions applying to all cases of amniocentesis must certainly be followed when multiple sacs are to be tapped. A thorough ultrasound examination should precede the amniocentesis, at which time the viability of all fetuses

should be verified, their gestational ages and relative sizes assessed, the position of the placenta(s) and dividing membranes noted (Figs. 26.15 and 26.16), and a search for gross fetal, uterine, and adnexal pathology performed. It is particularly important to note the position of one fetus relative to the other(s) and to label appropriately a drawing in the patient's chart as well as the aspirated fluids so that at a later date it will be possible to correlate a particular fetus with its fluid specimen. This is mandatory if, in the case of genetic studies, selective termination is to be considered.

2. Direct ultrasonic visualization of the needle tip during its insertion allows for much greater precision in guiding the needle to an optimal sampling site. It also reduces the potential for traumatizing the fetus. Jeanty et al.[154] published a description of how this can easily be accomplished.

3. Use of a marker dye is very helpful in performing amniocentesis on more than one sac, but methylene blue has been associated with fetal hemolysis when injected intra-amniotically.[155] It is therefore recommended that either indigo carmine or Evans blue be utilized rather than methylene blue. Whatever dye is used, it should not be red, to prevent confusion in the event of a bloody tap.

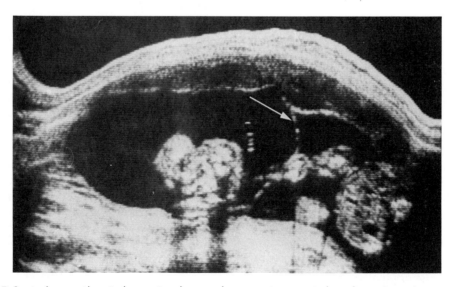

Fig. 26.15 Sagittal scan with a single anterior placenta demonstrating a vertical membrane (arrow) separating the two sacs.

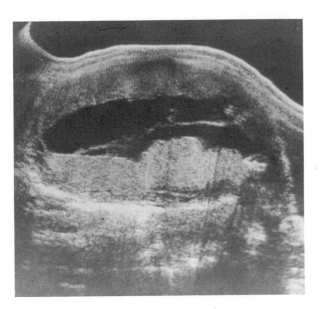

Fig. 26.16 Sagittal scan revealing individual anterior and posterior placentas with the membranes running horizontally between the two sacs.

4. When failure to see a separating membrane between the sacs suggests the possibility of a MA twin gestation, use of a marker dye alone may not definitively rule out this diagnosis since aspiration of colored fluid on a second needle insertion may represent re-entry into the first sac. Under these circumstances a technique described by Tabsh[156] may be useful in differentiating a single MA sac from separate DA sacs where the membrane is simply not being visualized. Leaving the needle in place after an initial sample of fluid is withdrawn, 0.1 ml of air drawn into the syringe through a micropore filter is mixed with 0.5 ml of marker dye and 5 ml of aspirated amniotic fluid. This mixture is then injected back into the sac under firm, gentle pressure in order to create microbubbles within the amniotic fluid. The microbubbles serve as ultrasonic contrast agents within the first sac and should demarcate it from a second sac if one is present. A site for needle insertion into the second sac can then be selected. Aspiration of colorless fluid confirms that a second sac has been entered, whereas fluid colored with dye indicates that the original sac has been re-entered. If the microbubbles are seen around both fetuses, a diagnosis of MA twins can be confirmed.

MANAGEMENT OF MULTIPLE GESTATIONS

The Antepartum Period

Specialized antenatal care cannot be offered to women with multiple gestations unless they are known to be carrying more than one fetus. In areas in which universal ultrasound screening is not performed, the early diagnosis of twins depends on maintaining a high index of suspicion whenever uterine size appears to be larger than dates. Once suspected, twins can be easily diagnosed by performing a thorough ultrasound examination. After confirmation of a multiple gestation, the issue arises as to which, if any, of the various methods used in an attempt to improve perinatal outcome in these patients is worthy of consideration.

The value of *bed rest* in the hospital for a patient carrying twins is controversial. Marivate and Norman[2] cite five studies that reported a reduction in perinatal mortality and prematurity rates and two others that found no difference in those variables when patients with twins routinely admitted to the hospital were compared with those treated on an outpatient basis. Two prospective randomized trials published in 1984 and 1985 found no benefit from late hospital admission,[157,158] and in the latter study preterm delivery was more common among the hospitalized group.

Hawrylyshyn et al.[11] reported that in their series of 175 consecutive twin deliveries, bed rest after 30 weeks had no effect on perinatal mortality. Since 70 percent of the perinatal deaths in their study occurred before gestational week 30, these workers concluded that elective hospitalization must include the period from 25 to 30 weeks to exert any significant impact on both the survival and the quality of survival of twins. In support of this concept, it should be noted that Chervenak et al.[20] found that 81 percent of the perinatal mortality in their series of 385 twin pregnancies occurred before gestational week 29.

Two recent studies evaluated the role of early routine hospital admission for twin gestations and came to similar conclusions. The first was a multicenter randomized study from Australia in which 11 hospitals participated.[159] Of 141 women with twins in the study, 72 were assigned to outpatient care and 69 were hospitalized from gestational weeks 26 to 30. No differences between the groups could be demonstrated in the frequencies of major maternal complications, preterm delivery, or mean birth weights at delivery. Surprisingly, in fact, there was a trend toward greater frequency of preterm delivery and admission of neonates to the neonatal intensive care unit (NICU) in the group admitted to the hospital. Leveno et al.[160] similarly observed no differences in pregnancy outcome between 134 patients with twin gestations who were hospitalized from gestational weeks 24 to 32 and 177 patients who were not routinely hospitalized.

Bed rest in the hospital is expensive and disrupts normal family life. Since there is no evidence to suggest that it is universally beneficial, it is probably wise to reserve this for patients with multiple gestations having identifiable risk factors for the occurrence of preterm labor or abnormal fetal growth in utero.

Prophylactic administration of tocolytic agents to women with twins has been tried with varying degrees of success. Marivate and Norman[2] cite one report in which pregnancy prolongation and increased birth weight were associated with this approach and three other series that found no improvement in these variables when prophylactic tocolysis was administered to patients with twins. Since an increased incidence of maternal cardiovascular complications has been reported in women with multiple gestations who have been treated with β-agonists,[161] it seems prudent to restrict the use of these agents to women who have demonstrated that they are in premature labor.

Results of studies using prophylactic *cervical cerclage* in women with multiple gestations have been disappointing.[2] Since this surgical procedure may be associated with adverse sequelae for both the mother and her fetuses, it is recommended that cerclage placement be limited to women with either a strong suggestive history or objectively documented cervical incompetence.

Houlton et al.[162] evaluated the effectiveness of a *cervical assessment score*, based on the length of the cervical canal in centimeters minus the dilatation of the internal os in centimeters, to predict the onset of labor in a series of women with twins. These workers found a significant relationship between a cervical score of 0, or a decrease in cervical score, and the onset of labor within the subsequent 14 days. Similar

effectiveness of this scoring system was reported by Nielson et al.[163] in a more recent study. On the other hand, O'Connor et al.[164] found that routine cervical assessment and uterine activity measurements were not helpful in predicting premature delivery. Nevertheless, Marivate and Norman[2] suggest that the use of the simple scoring system described permits the selection of a group of patients with twins at increased risk for premature delivery.

Another concept related to early detection of preterm labor involves *ambulatory home monitoring of uterine contractions* with a mobile tocodynamometer, the efficacy of which has been demonstrated in singleton pregnancies at risk for preterm labor. Although the efficacy of this method for detecting preterm labor in multiple gestations has not yet been evaluated with prospective randomized trials, clinical studies suggest that this may be a useful adjunct in the intensified antepartum surveillance of these patients.[17] These women may benefit maximally from prophylactic bed rest in the hospital and aggressive early tocolysis for documented premature labor. A randomized prospective study would shed some light on the efficacy of this approach, but to our knowledge this has not yet been performed.

The value of *special twin clinics* has been described by several investigators.[2,164] In these clinics, where all women known to be carrying twins are seen at regular intervals by the same medical team, several advantages accrue. Patients have the opportunity in this type of clinical setting to develop rapport with a small group of caregivers. This should result in an increased awareness of their special problems and may increase compliance with therapeutic directives. The patients can also talk with other women who are expecting twins and learn that their antenatal experiences are not unique. Furthermore, the medical personnel become more adept at detecting early signs of the special problems associated with twin pregnancies. Finally, and perhaps most importantly, the team of caregivers has the opportunity to develop an antenatal management protocol that is maximally effective for their population of patients.

The value of performing *serial ultrasound studies* to evaluate the growth and development of each fetus in a multiple gestation has been mentioned earlier in this chapter. It should also be noted that assessment of fetal well-being by simultaneous nonstress heart rate testing in twin pregnancies seems both feasible and efficacious. Devoe and Azor[165] reported 24 sets of twins who underwent 120 simultaneously recorded nonstress tests (NSTs) in the third trimester. Technical problems in obtaining readable tracings were encountered in only 15 percent of cases. Reactive NSTs were found to be associated with a good prognosis if delivery occurred within 1 week, whereas nonreactive NSTs were less specific but in some cases reflected significant distress in utero. These investigators concluded that NSTs in twins, whether reactive or nonreactive, appear to be prognostically comparable to those previously reported in singleton third trimester pregnancies. They point out, however, that contraction stress tests (CSTs) are of more limited applicability in twin gestations. The two major problems encountered when contractions are stimulated in these patients are the technical difficulties associated with obtaining two interpretable external fetal heart rate tracings and the potential for initiating premature labor.

Prior to 1983, three relatively large series were published describing the management of pregnancies in which three or more fetuses were involved. Ron-El et al.[13] reported their experience with 29 triplet and 6 quadruplet pregnancies in Tel Aviv between 1970 and 1978. Seven of these pregnancies were conceived spontaneously, and the other 19 followed the administration of fertility drugs. Hospitalization was recommended at the beginning of the third trimester or with the onset of complications. Patients were given prophylactic oral tocolysis beginning in the second trimester and intravenous β-agonist therapy if premature contractions occurred. Depot hydroxyprogesterone caproate was administered twice weekly from mid-second trimester until pulmonary maturity was demonstrated. Dexamethasone was administered when premature contractions were documented. Cervical cerclage was performed in women with prepregnancy evidence of cervical incompetence or when signs of painless cervical dilatation were recognized during prenatal examinations. The cesarean section rate was 44 percent, and the mean birth weight was 1,830 ± 536 g. The overall perinatal mortality rate was 185 per 1,000.

In another series from Israel, Holcberg et al.[12] describe the outcome of 31 triplet pregnancies managed between 1960 and 1979 at their institution in Beersheba. Twenty-one of these pregnancies were conceived spontaneously, and 10 followed the induction of ovulation. Triplet gestation was diagnosed earlier in the group with induced ovulation, and their period of hospitalization before delivery was longer than that of the group that conceived spontaneously. The most frequent antenatal complications for the entire group were preterm delivery (97 percent), pregnancy-induced hypertension (46 percent), and anemia (29 percent). Thirteen percent of patients required postpartum blood transfusions for excessive bleeding from an atonic uterus. The overall perinatal mortality rate was 312 per 1,000. The only neonatal death occurring in an infant born after 31 weeks was due to congenital malformations incompatible with life. Three of the total of nine stillborns occurred in a MC/MA pregnancy delivered during the thirty-sixth week. The cords of these infants were all found to be thoroughly entangled. The incidence of cesarean section was 32 percent. In this series, patients in whom ovulation had been induced fared significantly better than those who conceived spontaneously. The birth weights were higher, the duration of pregnancy was longer, and the incidence of pregnancy-induced hypertension and perinatal death was lower. Holcberg et al. attribute these differences in outcome to the earlier diagnosis and longer hospitalizations mentioned previously.

Loucopoulos and Jewelewicz[14] reported the outcome of 35 pregnancies involving 27 sets of triplets, 7 sets of quadruplets, and 1 set of quintuplets at the Sloane Hospital for Women in New York between 1965 and 1981. Six of the patients conceived triplets spontaneously, and the remainder became pregnant after the use of ovulatory agents. Bed rest was advised as soon as the diagnosis of multifetal pregnancy was made and hospitalization was planned at 28 to 30 weeks unless complications occurred earlier. Betamethasone was administered electively at 26 to 28 weeks and repeated weekly thereafter. Oral phenobarbital administration, at a dose of 30 mg three times a day, was begun at the same time in an attempt to reduce the degree of neonatal hyperbilirubinemia. Tocolytic agents were not routinely used, and cervical cerclage was not performed. The cesarean section rate was 42 percent, and the mean birth weight was 1,815 ± 628 g. The overall perinatal mortality rate was 148 per 1,000.

Among four recent studies evaluating various management protocols in multiple gestations involving three or more fetuses, the report of Goldman et al.[166] assessed the efficacy of elective cerclage. Of 27 multiple pregnancies, 12 with triplets and 3 with quadruplets received elective cerclage, whereas 10 triplet and 2 quadruplet gestations did not. These investigators found that the cerclage group achieved a significantly longer mean gestation, higher birth weights, higher Apgar scores, lower rates of RDS, and a significantly lower perinatal mortality rate. Lipitz et al.,[15] however, reporting their experience with 78 triplets managed between 1975 and 1988, concluded that there was no benefit of elective cervical cerclage either in prolonging gestation or in decreasing fetal loss. Of these patients 86 percent delivered prematurely; the mean gestational age at delivery was 33.2 weeks. The perinatal and neonatal mortality rates were 93 per 1,000 and 51 per 1,000 live births, respectively. A higher proportion of low Apgar scores and respiratory disorders occurred in the third infant in patients delivered vaginally. These investigators recommend cesarean section as the preferred mode of delivery in triplet pregnancies.

Gonen et al.[16] reported the outcome and follow-up data of 30 multiple gestations (24 triplets, 5 quadruplets, and 1 quintuplet) managed over a 10-year period from 1978 to 1988. In their study, the early neonatal mortality rate was 31.6 per 1,000, late neonatal mortality rate was 21 per 1,000, and perinatal mortality rate was 51.5 per 1,000 live births. The incidence of RDS was 43 percent, bronchopulmonary dysplasia 6 percent, retinopathy of prematurity 3 percent, intraventricular hemorrhage 4 percent, and cerebral palsy 2 percent. Follow-up on 84 infants for a period of 1 to 10 years showed that 75 percent of them were free of any neurologic or developmental handicap, 22 percent had mild functional delay, one was mildly handicapped, and one was moderately handicapped. Although all patients were not managed with the same protocol, the investigators concluded that the most likely determinants of the excellent outcome in this series were early diagnosis, meticulous antenatal care, early hospitalization, frequent evaluation of fetal well-being, delivery by cesarean section, presence of a trained neonatologist for each neonate at the time of delivery, and resources of a highly skilled NICU.

A recent publication[17] reviews the outpatient antepartum management and pregnancy outcome of 198 women who delivered triplets between 1985 and 1988. The study involved 24 centers, with individual patients managed at the discretion of obstetricians in both private and academic practices. All patients were managed with the assistance of ambulatory perinatal nursing to provide outpatient surveillance. Uterine activity was monitored twice a day with a portable tocodynamometer and daily telephone contact, along with around-the-clock availability of the nursing staff providing a liaison between the patient and her physician. Modified bed rest was prescribed for almost all patients, but prophylactic tocolytic agents or betamethasone were used at the discretion of the individual physician. Although patients were hospitalized for either preterm labor or other medical complications, the average stay for antepartum hospitalization was only 15 days in this series. The mean gestational age and birth weight at delivery were 33.6 ± 3 weeks and $1,871 \pm 555$ g, respectively. The corrected perinatal survival rate was 95 percent, leading the investigators to conclude that routine hospitalization is unnecessary for patients with triplets, and intensive outpatient surveillance is justifiable and is associated with excellent outcomes in these pregnancies.

The Intrapartum Period

A number of factors must be considered when evaluating a laboring patient with twins or reviewing series that present delivery outcomes in women with multiple gestations. These variables include the gestational age and estimated weights of fetuses, their positions relative to each other, the availability of real-time ultrasound on the labor floor and in the delivery room, and the capability of monitoring each twin independently during the entire intrapartum period. Older series may not be applicable to current practice because our ability to monitor both twins closely during labor and delivery has increased considerably in recent years.

All combinations of intrapartum twin presentations can be classified into three groups: twin A vertex, twin B vertex; twin A vertex, twin B nonvertex; and twin A nonvertex, twin B either vertex or nonvertex. In a series of 362 twin deliveries presented by Chervenak et al.[167] these presentations were found in

42.5, 38.4, and 19.1 percent of cases, respectively. These data were similar to the findings of other investigators.[8,19]

In the series by Chervenak et al.[167] 81.2 percent of the vertex-vertex twin gestations were delivered vaginally. These investigators, and several others cited in their paper, believe that when both twins present in vertex presentation, a cesarean section should only be performed for the same indications applied to singletons. This recommendation implies that both twins can be monitored during labor.

Currently, cesarean section seems to be the delivery method of choice when the presenting twin is in a nonvertex position, as there are no studies documenting the safety of vaginal delivery for this group. External cephalic version of the presenting twin would be difficult, if not impossible, in these patients. Furthermore, if the second twin is in a vertex presentation and faces its sibling the potential for locking exists. Khunda[168] states that frequency of locking is approximately 1 per 1,000 twin deliveries, with an associated fetal mortality rate of 31 percent. This condition occurs most commonly in breech-vertex presentations when the fetal chins overlie each other. It is usually not recognized until the body of the presenting infant is out of the vagina and the aftercoming head cannot be delivered. Eventually it becomes clear that entry of the first twin's head into the pelvis is being obstructed by that of the second twin. Sevitz and Merrell[169] published a case in which a vaginal delivery was accomplished and one twin survived after intravenous administration of a β-mimetic agent to a women whose twins had locked during delivery. The more devastating consequences of this disorder, however, have been aptly described by Nissen.[170] Finally, it is possible that the second twin could complicate the delivery of the first in more subtle ways, such as by deflexing its head. It may eventually be shown that in some circumstances fears regarding a vaginal delivery when the leading twin presents in a nonvertex position are unwarranted, but this has not yet been convincingly demonstrated.

The management of that subset of women whose twins are in vertex-breech or vertex-transverse lies is particularly controversial. Chervenak et al.[167] cite 11 references in which depressed Apgar scores and increased perinatal mortality rates associated with vaginal breech delivery of the second twin have led some of these investigators to recommend cesarean section whenever twin B is in a nonvertex lie. Conflicting data have been reported, however. Acker et al.[171] found no perinatal deaths when 74 nonvertex first or second twins weighing more than 1,499 g were delivered by cesarean section or when 76 nonvertex second twins with similar birth weights were delivered vaginally. Furthermore, no statistically significant difference was found in low 5-minute Apgar scores when these two groups were compared.

Chervenak and colleagues[172] presented the intrapartum management of 93 vertex-breech and 42 vertex-transverse twin sets. Seventy-eight percent of the vertex-breech group and 53 percent of the vertex-transverse group were delivered vaginally. Seventy-six second twins were delivered vaginally by breech extraction, 16 of whom had birth weights of less than 1,500 g. Within that group there were 6 neonatal deaths, 4 intraventricular hemorrhages, and a 67 percent occurrence of depressed 5-minute Apgar scores. It should be noted that there were also 7 neonatal deaths and 4 intraventricular hemorrhages in the firstborn fetuses of the same pregnancies, all of whom were delivered in vertex presentation. At birth weights above 1,500 g, however, there were no neonatal deaths or documented intraventricular hemorrhages and only three cases (5 percent) of 5-minute Apgar scores of less than 7 in the group of second twins delivered vaginally by breech extraction. Chervenak et al. state that their data do not prove that vaginal breech delivery of the low-birth-weight second twin is more damaging than delivery by cesarean section. Nevertheless, because of the documented ill effects of vaginal delivery on low-birth-weight singleton breech infants[173,174] and the absence of evidence that being a second twin gives these infants an advantage relative to their singleton counterparts, vaginal breech delivery was not advised for second twins weighing less than 1,500 g. On the other hand, if a second twin weighs between 1,500 and 3,500 g and the criteria for vaginal delivery of a singleton breech are met, this series suggests that vaginal breech delivery is an acceptable option.

The same group has reported their experience with 25 external cephalic versions performed on 14 transverse and 11 breech malpositioned second twins.[175] Version to vertex presentation was successful in 71 percent and 73 percent of cases, respectively. Among the 25 attempted cases only 2 neonates had 5-minute Apgar scores below 7. However, in a study reported by Gocke et al.[176] the success rate for external cephalic version of the second twin was only 46 percent. Their study analyzed 136 sets of vertex-nonvertex twins with birth weights greater than 1,500 g in whom delivery of the second twin was managed by primary cesarean section, external version, or primary breech extraction. A primary attempt at delivery of the second twin by external version was performed on 41 twins, 55 underwent attempted breech extraction, and 40 patients had a primary cesarean section. No differences were noted in the incidence of neonatal mortality or morbidity among the three modes of delivery. External version was associated not only with a higher failure rate than breech extraction but also with a higher rate of fetal distress, cord prolapse, and compound presentation. These investigators, therefore, suggest that primary breech extraction of the second nonvertex twin weighing more than 1,500 g is a reasonable alternative to either cesarean section or external version.

Analyzing their own extensive experience along with a review of the published literature, Chervenak et al.[167] have made the following recommendations for patients presenting with twins in vertex/nonvertex lies. During the intrapartum period, a sonographic EFW for twin B should be determined. With current methods[177] there is a 10 percent standard deviation in the sonographic estimation of fetal weight, so that 95 percent of the time estimates are accurate to within ±20 percent. Therefore, using a cutoff for EFW of 2,000 g is unlikely to result in the birth of a neonate weighing less than 1,500 g. On the basis of the arguments cited, these investigators believe that a birth weight in excess of 1,500 g is sufficient for a vaginal breech delivery but a lesser weight is not. Regardless of the EFW, they suggest that an attempt be made to convert the second twin to a vertex presentation by performing an external version after the first twin has been delivered. If this proves successful, a vaginal delivery can be anticipated. If the attempted version is unsuccessful and the EFW is between 2,000 and 3,500 g, a breech extraction can be performed unless the other criteria for a singleton vaginal breech delivery are not satisfied. By contrast, if the EFW is less than 2,000 g or the criteria for a singleton vaginal breech delivery are not met, a cesar-

ean section should be performed after the failed external version. Evrard and Gold[178] discuss the reluctance of some obstetricians ever to consider a combined vaginal-abdominal approach to delivering twins but point out that there are some situations in which it is appropriate. Other workers have made reference to this form of delivery in a small number of patients in their twin series.[167,179]

In commenting on their series of triplets, quadruplets, and quintuplets, Loucopoulos and Jewelewicz[14] state, "The mode of delivery does not seem to play any particular role insofar as outcome is concerned. Continuous fetal surveillance, speed, and atraumatic delivery are the hallmarks of successful intrapartum management. In experienced hands, vaginal delivery should be attempted unless there is a medical indication for cesarean section." They caution, however, that general anesthesia should be used if one is contemplating vaginal delivery since the absence of adequate uterine relaxation could make an internal version or extraction impossible and thereby increase the risk of neonatal injury. It is fair to point out that great skill with external versions and/or breech deliveries might be required in order to achieve the atraumatic but speedy delivery called for by these investigators. In our opinion, only an experienced obstetrician with demonstrated expertise in these maneuvers should even consider attempting the vaginal delivery of a patient who is known to have three or more viable fetuses. For these pregnancies elective cesarean section is really considered the safest mode of delivery with the best outcome for each infant.

Time Interval between Deliveries

Another variable that many investigators have considered important in the outcome of twin pregnancies is the interval between their deliveries. After delivery of the first twin, uterine inertia may develop, the second twin's cord may prolapse, and partial separation of its placenta may render the second twin hypoxic. In addition, the cervix can clamp down, making rapid delivery of the second twin extremely difficult if fetal distress develops. Many reports have suggested that the interval between deliveries should ideally be within 15 minutes, and certainly not more than 30 minutes.[5,8,19,180,181] Most of the data in support of this view, however, were obtained before the advent of intrapartum fetal monitoring.

Rayburn et al.[179] reported the outcome of 115 second twins delivered vaginally at or beyond 34 weeks gestation after the vertex delivery of their siblings. The second twin was visually monitored ultrasonically on some occasions, and continuous monitoring of the fetal heart was performed in all cases. Oxytocin was used if uterine contractions subsided within 10 minutes after delivery of the first twin. In this series 70 second twins delivered within 15 minutes of the first twin, 28 within 16 to 30 minutes, and 17 more than 30 minutes later. The longest interdelivery interval was 134 minutes. All these infants survived and none of them had a traumatic delivery. All 17 of the neonates delivering beyond 30 minutes had 5-minute Apgar scores of 8 and 10. In those cases with delivery intervals in excess of 15 minutes, the birth weight differential was not in excess of ± 200 g when first and second twins were compared. In the series reported by Chervenak et al.[175] the fetal heart rate of the second twin was monitored with ultrasound visualization throughout the period between twin deliveries and no difference in the occurrence of low 5-minute Apgar scores was noted in relation to the length of the interdelivery interval.

It seems apparent that although some second twins may require rapid delivery, others can be safely followed with fetal heart rate surveillance and remain undelivered for substantial periods of time. This less hurried approach when twin B is not in distress may reduce the incidence of both maternal and fetal trauma associated with difficult deliveries performed to meet arbitrary deadlines.

There are obviously situations in which expeditious delivery of the second twin is desirable shortly after the birth of the first, but this is not always the case. Several extraordinary examples attest to this fact. Mashiach et al.[182] reported a case of a woman with a triplet pregnancy in a uterus didelphys, with fetuses A and B in the right uterine horn and fetus C in the left horn. A missed abortion of fetus A was noted at 22 weeks. At 27 weeks the right horn began to contract and a macerated fetus A was delivered vaginally, but the passage of fetus B was obstructed by the vertex of fetus C. A cesarean section was then performed on the right uterine horn and a 1,080-g infant, who died in 2 weeks, was delivered. Since the left horn was not contracting, it was left intact. At 37 weeks, 72 days after the first two deliveries, an elective cesarean section was performed, and a 2,490-g healthy infant was delivered, who went home with the mother on the seventh postpartum day. These workers cite several other examples of significant delays in the delivery of twins who were located in separate uterine horns.

Woolfson et al.[183] reported the case of a woman with a single normally shaped uterus who delivered a 570-g first twin vaginally as a breech at 25 weeks. This infant died of respiratory distress in 5 days. The first twin's placenta was retained within the uterus, and the cervical os closed to less than 3 cm after delivery. The cord was cut at the level of the cervix, and prophylactic antibiotics were administered. The patient was followed with serial maternal clotting profiles and ultrasound examinations of the remaining fetus. At 32 weeks, after 53 days in the hospital following delivery of the first twin, labor resumed and spontaneous rupture of the membranes occurred. A cesarean section was performed, and a 1,600-g infant with Apgar scores of 7 and 9 was delivered. The placentas weighed 310 and 110 g, and the patient's postoperative course was uneventful. These investigators cite four other reports in which intervals varying from 14 to 84 days were reported in twin deliveries wherein tocolytics, cervical cerclage, or simple observation was the mainstay of management.

Another such case, recently reported by Feichtinger et al.,[184] achieved 12 additional weeks and delivery of a healthy second twin, following delivery and death of the first twin at 21 weeks gestation. This patient presented with preterm labor and ruptured membranes at 21 weeks. A cerclage suture that had been prophylactically placed at 12 weeks gestation was removed to allow delivery of a nonviable twin A. There was no evidence of placental separation; the sac of twin B was intact, and its heart rate monitoring was normal. A Shirodkar type of cerclage was then placed, and the patient was treated with tocolytics, intravenous antibiotics, and vaginal antiseptic suppositories. Her subsequent antepartum course after discharge from the hospital at 24 weeks was apparently unremarkable, until readmission for preterm labor and uneventful delivery at 33 weeks gestation. The infant weighed 1,750 g and had an uncomplicated neonatal course.

It must be recognized that these cases represent

spectacular successes. This type of management, however, should not be considered "standard of care." If an individual case is considered for such a treatment protocol, the potential risks, which may be considerable, along with the benefits must be discussed in detail and fully informed consent obtained from the patient.

Ultrasound and the Intrapartum Management of Multiple Gestations

The value of ultrasound in diagnosing multiple gestations, performing amniocentesis on multiple sacs, and following the growth and development of twins in utero has been extensively discussed in the literature, but little has been written about its usefulness during labor and delivery.

On admission to the delivery floor, the position of each twin can be quickly and accurately assessed and viability of both fetuses confirmed by direct visualization of their hearts. Knowledge of the presentation of each twin permits the establishment of a management protocol regarding the anticipated route of delivery. If a vaginal delivery is to be attempted, the weights of both twins can be rapidly assessed using the method of Shepard et al.[177] This information is particularly important for the second twin because if it is thought to weigh less than 1,500 g or more than 3,500 g, a vaginal breech delivery may not be attempted. It is also possible to rule out extension of the head when a fetus is in breech presentation, by using the method described by Berkowitz and Hobbins.[185] Ballas et al.[186] cited an incidence of more than 70 percent for spinal cord transection when 11 breeches with extended heads were delivered vaginally, compared with no cord injuries when 9 infants with deflexed heads were delivered by cesarean section. Although these data were derived from singleton breeches, there is no reason to believe that they could not apply to twins as well.

As has been mentioned repeatedly in the discussion of the intrapartum management of twins, both fetuses must be monitored electronically throughout labor to assure their well-being. A scalp electrode can easily be attached to the presenting part of twin A, and the second twin can be monitored with an external Doppler transducer. In practice, however, it is often difficult to find the optimal spot from which to monitor the second twin. By using real-time ultrasound twin B's heart can be precisely located and the Doppler transducer placed accordingly. If movement of the second twin results in loss of a readable tracing, the transducer can be repositioned after real-time ultrasound has revealed the new position of twin B's heart.

When a patient with twins is taken to the delivery room, the real-time scanner should accompany her. After delivery of the first infant, real-time examination immediately and precisely establishes the position of the second. Visualization of the fetal heart allows twin B to be monitored for evidence of bradycardia until one fetal pole settles into the pelvis, membranes are ruptured, and a scalp electrode is applied. Although visual monitoring of the heart does not provide subtle information such as a loss of baseline variability, it does permit early detection of significant deviations from the normal fetal heart rate range.

In addition to monitoring heart rate, visualization of the second twin permits both external and internal manipulations to be performed in a more controlled fashion. Externally, it is often possible to guide the vertex over the inlet by directing pressure from the ultrasound transducer over the fetal head while pushing the buttocks toward the fundus with the other hand.[185] If this is unsuccessful, internal versions can be made less difficult by visualizing the operator's hand within the uterus and directing it toward the fetal feet. This technique can reduce the confusion often experienced when a fetal small part is blindly caught and it is unclear whether it belongs to an upper or a lower extremity.

CONCLUSION

The patient carrying more than one fetus presents a formidable challenge to the obstetrician. The high perinatal morbidity and mortality rates traditionally associated with multiple gestations are due to many factors, some of which can still not be altered. The extraordinary advances in technology of the past 10 to 20 years, however, have given us new insights into some problems peculiar to twins as well as some tools with which to detect those problems. Early diagnosis of multiple gestations and follow-up with serial studies hold the potential for administering specialized regimens to selected patients, and this should have a major impact on the outcome of some pregnancies.

REFERENCES

1. Hrubec Z, Robinette CD: The study of human twins in medical research. N Engl J Med 310:435, 1984
2. Marivate M, Norman RJ: Twins. Clin Obstet Gynaecol 9:723, 1982
3. Kurachi K, Aono T, Susuki M et al: Results of HMG (Hurregon)—hCG therapy in 6,096 treatment cycles of 2,166 Japanese women with anovulatory infertility. Eur J Obstet Gynecol Reprod Biol 19(1):43, 1985
4. Australian In-Vitro Fertilization Collaborative Group: In-vitro fertilization pregancies in Australia and New Zealand. Med J Aust 148:429, 1988
5. Benirschke K, Kim CK: Multiple pregnancy. N Engl J Med 288:1276, 1973
6. Cameron AH: The Birmingham twin survey. Proc R Soc Med 61:229, 1968
7. James WH: Is Weinberg's differential rule valid? Acta Genet Med Gemellol 28:69, 1979
8. Kohl SG, Casey G: Twin gestation. Mt Sinai J Med 42:523, 1975
9. Desgranges MF, De Muylder X, Moutquin JM et al: Perinatal profile of twin pregnancies: a retrospective review of 11 years (1969–1979) at Hôpital Notre-Dame, Montreal, Canada. Acta Genet Med Gemollol 31:157, 1982
10. Rattan PK, Knuppel RA, O'Brien WF: Intrauterine fetal death in twins after thirty-two weeks of gestation, abstracted. Proceedings of the Society of Perinatal Obstetricians Annual Meeting, San Antonio, February 1984
11. Hawrylyshyn PA, Barkin M, Bernstein A, Papsin FR: Twin pregnancies—a continuing perinatal challenge. Obstet Gynecol 59:463, 1982
12. Holcberg G, Biele Y, Jewenthal H, Insler V: Outcome of pregnancy in 31 triplet gestations. Obstet Gynecol 59:472, 1982
13. Ron-El R, Caspi E, Schreyers P et al: Triplet and quadruplet pregnancies and management. Obstet Gynecol 57:458, 1981
14. Loucopoulos A, Jewelewicz R: Management of multifetal pregnancies: sixteen years' experience at the Sloane Hospital for Women. Am J Obstet Gynecol 143:902, 1982
15. Lipitz S, Reichman B, Paret G et al: The improving outcome of triplet pregnancies. Am J Obstet Gynecol 161:1279, 1989

16. Gonen R, Heyman E, Asztalos EV et al: The outcome of triplet, quadruplet, and quintuplet pregnancies managed in a perinatal unit: obstetric, neonatal, and follow-up data. Am J Obstet Gynecol 162:454, 1990
17. Newman RB, Hamer C, Clinton Miller M: Outpatient triplet management: a contemporary review. Am J Obstet Gynecol 161:547, 1989
18. Alvarez M, Berkowitz RL: Multifetal gestation. Clin Obstet Gynecol 33:79, 1990
19. Farooqui MO, Grossman JH, Shannon RA: A review of twin pregnancy and perinatal mortality. Obstet Gynecol Surv 28:144, 1973
20. Chervenak FA, Youcha S, Johnson RE et al: Antenatal diagnosis and perinatal outcome in a series of 385 consecutive twin pregnancies. J Reprod Med 29:727, 1984
21. Cetrulo CL, Ingardia CJ, Sbarra AJ: Management of multiple gestation. Clin Obstet Gynecol 23:533, 1980
22. Persson PH, Kullander S: Long-term experience of general ultrasound screening in pregnancy. Am J Obstet Gynecol 146:942, 1983
23. Jeanty P, Romero R (eds): What does an early gestation look like? p. 34. In Obstetrical Ultrasound. McGraw-Hill, New York, 1984
24. Blumenfeld Z, Rottem S, Elgali S et al: Transvaginal sonographic assessment of early embryological development. In Timor-Tritsch IE, Rottem S (eds): Transvaginal Sonography. Elsevier Science, New York, 1988
25. Smith DH, Picker RH, Saunders DM: Twin pregnancy suspected before implantation. Obstet Gynecol 56:252, 1980
26. Berkowitz RL: Ultrasound in the antenatal management of multiple gestations. p. 69. In Hobbins JC (ed): Diagnostic Ultrasound in Obstetrics. Churchill Livingstone, New York, 1979
27. Landy HJ, Keith L, Keith D: The vanishing twin. Acta Genet Med Gemellol 31:179, 1982
28. Robinson HP, Caines JS: Sonar evidence of early pregnancy failure in patients with twin conceptions. Br J Obstet Gynaecol 84:22, 1977
29. Berkowitz RL, Lynch L, Chitkara U et al: Selective reduction of multifetal pregnancies in the first trimester. N Engl J Med 318:1043, 1988
30. Khalil M, Tabsh A: Transabdominal multifetal pregnancy reduction: report of 40 cases. Obstet Gynecol 75:739, 1990
31. Lynch L, Berkowitz RL, Chitkara U, Alvarez M: First-trimester transabdominal multifetal pregnancy reduction: a report of 85 cases. Obstet Gynecol 75:735, 1990
32. Finberg HJ, Birnholz JC: Ultrasound observations in

multiple gestation with first trimester bleeding. The blighted twin. Radiology 132:137, 1979

33. Varma TR: Ultrasound evidence of early pregnancy failure in patients with multiple conceptions. Br J Obstet Gynaecol 86:290, 1979

34. Landy HJ, Weiner S, Corson SL et al: The "vanishing twin": ultrasonographic assessment of fetal disappearance in the first trimester. Am J Obstet Gynecol 155:14, 1986

35. McKeown T, Record RG: Observations on foetal growth in multiple pregnancy in man. J Endocrinol 8:386, 1952

36. Daw E, Walker J: Growth differences in twin pregnancy. Br J Clin Pract 29:150, 1975

37. Iffy L, Lavenhar MA, Jakobovits A, Kaminetzky HA: The rate of early intrauterine growth in twin gestation. Am J Obstet Gynecol 146:970, 1983

38. Fenner A, Malm T, Kusserow U: Intrauterine growth of twins. Eur J Pediatr 133:119, 1980

39. Winick M, Brasel JA, Velasco EG: Effects of prenatal nutrition upon pregnancy risk. Clin Obstet Gynecol 16:184, 1973

40. Duff GB, Brown JB: Urinary estriol excretion in twin pregnancies. J Obstet Gynaecol Br Commonw 81:695, 1974

41. Leveno KJ, Santos-Ramos R, Duenhoelter JH et al: Sonar cephalometry in twins: a table of biparietal diameters for normal twin fetuses and a comparison with singletons. Am J Obstet Gynecol 135:727, 1979

42. Bleker OP, Kloosterman GJ, Huidekoper BL, Breur W: Intrauterine growth of twins as estimated from birthweight and the fetal biparietal diameter. Eur J Obstet Reprod Biol 7(2):85, 1977

43. Schneider L, Bessis R, Tabaste JL et al: Echographic survey of twin foetal growth: a plea for specific charts for twins. p. 137. In Nance WE (ed): Twin Research: Clinical Studies: Alan R Liss, New York, 1977

44. Grumbach K, Coleman BG, Arger PH et al: Twin and singleton growth patterns compared using ultrasound. Radiology 158:237, 1986

45. Socol ML, Tamura RK, Sabbagha RE et al: Diminished biparietal diameter and abdominal circumference growth in twins. Obstet Gynecol 64:235, 1984

46. Scheer K: Ultrasound in twin gestations. J Clin Ultrasound 2:197, 1975

47. Crane JP, Tomich PG, Kopta M: Ultrasonic growth patterns in normal and discordant twins. Obstet Gynecol 55:678, 1980

48. Graham D, Shah Y, Moodley S et al: Biparietal diameter femoral length growth in normal twin pregnancies, abstracted. Proceedings of the Society of Perinatal Obstetricians Annual Meeting, San Antonio, February 1984

49. Shah YG, Graham D, Stinson SK et al: Biparietal diameter growth in uncomplicated twin gestation. Am J Perinatol 4:229, 1987

50. Haines CJ, Langlois SL, Jones WR: Ultrasonic measurement of fetal femoral length in singleton and twin pregnancies. Am J Obstet Gynecol 155:838, 1986

51. Dorros G: The prenatal diagnosis of intrauterine growth retardation in one fetus of a twin gestation. Obstet Gynecol, Suppl., 48:46, 1976

52. Leveno KJ, Santos-Ramos R, Duenhoelter JH et al: Sonar cephalometry in twin pregnancy: discordancy of the biparietal diameter after 28 weeks' gestation. Am J Obstet Gynecol 138:615, 1980

53. Houlton MCC: Divergent biparietal diameter growth rates in twin pregnancies. Obstet Gynecol 49:542, 1977

54. Chitkara U, Berkowitz GS, Levine R et al: Twin pregnancy: routine use of ultrasound examinations in the prenatal diagnosis of IUGR and discordant growth. Am J Perinatol 2:49, 1985

55. Divers WA, Hemsell DL: The use of ultrasound in multiple gestations. Obstet Gynecol 53:500, 1979

56. Persson PH, Grennert L: The intrauterine growth of the biparietal diameter of twins. Acta Genet Med Gemellol 28:273, 1979

57. Neilson JP: Detection of the small-for-dates twin fetus by ultrasound. Br J Obstet Gynaecol 88:27, 1981

58. Neilson JP: Detection of the small-for-gestational age twin fetus by a two-stage ultrasound examination schedule. Acta Genet Med Gemellol 31:235, 1982

59. Yarkouni S, Reece EA, Holford T et al: Estimated fetal weight in the evaluation of growth in twin gestations: a prospective longitudinal study. Obstet Gynecol 69:636, 1987

60. Storlazzi E, Vintzileos AM, Campbell WA et al: Ultrasonic diagnosis of discordant fetal growth in twin gestations. Obstet Gynecol 69:363, 1987

61. Brown CEL, Guzick DS, Leveno KJ et al: Prediction of discordant twins using ultrasound measurement of biparietal diameter and abdominal perimeter. Obstet Gynecol 70:677, 1987

62. Barss VA, Benacerraf BR, Frigoletto FD: Ultrasonographic determination of chorion type in twin gestation. Obstet Gynecol 66:779, 1985

63. Mahony BS, Filly RA, Callen PW Amnionicity and chorionicity in twin pregnancies: prediction using ultrasound. Radiology 155:205, 1985

64. Hertzberg BS, Kurtz AB, Choi HY et al: Significance of membrane thickness in the sonographic evaluation of twin gestations. AJR 148:151, 1987

65. Townsend RR, Simpson GF, Filly RA: Membrane

thickness in ultrasound prediction of chorionicity of twin gestations. J Ultrasound Med 7:327, 1988

66. Winn HN, Gabrielli S, Reece EA et al: Ultrasonographic criteria for the prenatal diagnosis of placental chorionicity in twin gestations. Am J Obstet Gynecol 161:1540, 1989

67. D'Alton ME, Dudley DKL: Ultrasound in the antenatal management of twin gestation. Semin Perinatol 10:30, 1986

68. D'Alton ME, Dudley DK: The ultrasonographic prediction of chorionicity in twin gestation. Am J Obstet Gynecol 160:557, 1989

69. Nyberg DA, Filly RA, Golbus MS et al: Entangled umbilical cords: a sign of monoamniotic twins. J Ultrasound Med 3:29, 1984

70. Trudinger BJ, Giles WB, Cook CM: Flow velocity waveforms in the maternal uteroplacental and fetal umbilical placental circulations. Am J Obstet Gynecol 152:155, 1985

71. Campbell S, Pearce JMF, Hackett G et al: Qualitative assessment of uteroplacental blood flow: early screening test for high-risk pregnancies. Obstet Gynecol 68:649, 1986

72. Fleischer A, Schulman H, Farmakides G et al: Uterine artery Doppler velocimetry in pregnant women with hypertension. Am J Obstet Gynecol 154:806, 1986

73. Berkowitz GS, Chitkara U, Rosenberg J et al: Sonographic estimation of fetal weight and Doppler analysis of umbilical artery velocimetry in the prediction of intrauterine growth retardation: a prospective study. Am J Obstet Gynecol 158:1149, 1988

74. Giles WB, Trudinger BJ, Cook CM: Fetal umbilical artery flow velocity-time waveforms in twin pregnancies. Br J Obstet Gynaecol 92:490, 1985

75. Gerson A, Johnson A, Wallace D et al: Umbilical arterial systolic/diastolic values in normal twin gestation. Obstet Gynecol 72:205, 1988

76. Giles WB, Trudinger BJ, Baird PJ: Fetal umbilical artery flow velocity waveforms and placental resistance: pathological correlation. Br J Obstet Gynaecol 92:31, 1985

77. Farmakides G, Schulman H, Saldana LR et al: Surveillance of twin pregnancy with umbilical arterial velocimetry. Am J Obstet Gynecol 153:789, 1985

78. Saldana LR, Eads MC, Schaefer TR: Umbilical blood waveforms in fetal surveillance of twins. Am J Obstet Gynecol 157:712, 1987

79. Giles WB, Trudingr BJ, Cook CM, Connelly A: Umbilical artery flow velocity waveforms and twin pregnancy outcome. Obstet Gynecol 72:894, 1988

80. Hastie SJ, Danskin F, Neilson JP, Whittle MJ: Predic-

tion of the small for gestational age twin fetus by Doppler umbilical artery waveform analysis. Obstet Gynecol 74:730, 1989

81. Nance WE: Malformations unique to the twinning process. Prog Clin Biol Res 69A:123, 1981

82. Bebbington MW, Wittmann BK: Fetal transfusion syndrome: antenatal factors predicting outcome. Am J Obstet Gynecol 160:913, 1989

83. Gonsoulin W, Moise KJ, Kirshon B et al: Outcome of twin-twin transfusion diagnosed before 28 weeks of gestation. Obstet Gynecol 75:214, 1990

84. Wittman BK, Baldwin VJ, Nichol B: Antenatal diagnosis of twin transfusion syndrome by ultrasound. Obstet Gynecol 58:123, 1981

85. Pretorius DH, Manchester D, Barkin S et al: Doppler ultrasound of twin transfusion syndrome. J Ultrasound Med 7:117, 1988

86. Onyskowova A, Dolezal A, Jedlicka V: The frequency and the character of malformations in multiple birth (a preliminary report). Teratology 4:496, 1971

87. Hendricks CH: Twinning in relation to birth weight, mortality, and congenital anomalies. Obstet Gynecol 27:47, 1966

88. Neilson JP, Hood VD, Cupples W: Ultrasonic evaluation of twin pregnancies associated with raised serum alpha-fetoprotein levels. Acta Genet Med Gemellol 31:229, 1982

89. Gewolb IH, Freedman RM, Kleinman CS, Hobbins JC: Prenatal diagnosis of a human pseudoacardiac anomaly. Obstet Gynecol 61:657, 1983

90. Kaplan C, Benirschke K: The acardiac anomaly: new case reports and current status. Acta Genet Med Gemellol 28:51, 1979

91. Pretorius DH, Leopold GR, Moore TR et al: Acardiac twin: report of Doppler sonography. J Ultrasound Med 7:413, 1988

92. Benson CB, Bieber FR, Genest DR, Doubilet PM: Doppler demonstration of reversed umbilical blood flow in an acardiac twin. J. Clin Ultrasound 17:291, 1989

93. Van Allen MI, Smith DW, Shepard TH: Twin reversed arterial perfusion (TRAP) sequence: a study of 14 twin pregnancies with acardius. Semin Perinatol 7:285, 1983

94. Windham GC, Bjerkedal T, Sever LE: The association of twinning and neural tube defects: studies in Los Angeles, California, and Norway. Acta Genet Med Gemellol 31:165, 1982

95. Harper RG, Kenigsberg K, Sia CG: Xiphopagus conjoined twins: a 300-year review of the obstetric, morphopathologic, neonatal and surgical parameters. Am J Obstet 137:617, 1980

96. Vaughn TC, Powell C: The obstetrical mangement of conjoined twins. Obstet Gynecol, suppl., 53:67, 1979

97. Wedberg R, Kaplan C, Leopold G et al: Cephalothoracopagus (Janiceps) twinning. Obstet Gynecol 54:392, 1979

98. Gray CM, Nix HG, Wallace AJ: Thoracopagus twins: prenatal diagnosis. Radiology 54:398, 1950

99. Apuzzio JJ, Ganesh V, Landau I, Pelosi M: Prenatal diagnosis of conjoined twins. Am J Obstet Gynecol 148:343, 1984

100. Austin E, Schifrin BS, Pomerance JJ et al: The antepartum diagnosis of conjoined twins. J Pediatr Surg 15:332, 1980

101. Fagan CJ: Antepartum diagnosis of conjoined twins by ultrasonography. AJR 129:921, 1977

102. Gore RM, Filly RA, Parer JT: Sonographic antepartum diagnosis of conjoined twins. JAMA 247:3351, 1982

103. Morgan CL, Trought WS, Sheldon G et al: B-scan and real time ultrasound in the antepartum diagnosis of conjoined twins and pericardial effusion. AJR 130:578, 1978

104. Schmidt W, Herberling D, Kubli F: Antepartum ultrasonographic diagnosis of conjoined twins in early pregnancy. Am J Obstet Gynecol 139:961, 1981

105. Wilson RL, Shaub MS, Cetrulo CJ: The antepartum findings of conjoined twins. J Clin Ultrasound 5:35, 1977

106. Wood MJ, Thompson HE, Robertson FM: Real-time ultrasound diagnosis of conjoined twins. J Clin Ultrasound 9:195, 1981

107. Compton HL: Conjoined twins. Obstet Gynecol 37:27, 1971

108. Benirschke K, Kim CK: Multiple pregnancy. N Engl J Med 288:1329, 1973

109. Uchida IA, deSa DJ, Whelan DT: 45↑/46XX mosaicism in discordant monozygotic twins. Pediatrics 71:413, 1983

110. Potter AM, Taitz LS: Turner's syndrome in one of monozygotic twins with mosaicism. Acta Pediatr Scand 61:473, 1972

111. Rogers JG, Voullaire L, Gold H: Monozygotic twins discordant for trisomy 21. Am J Med Genet 11:143, 1982

112. Macdonald AD: Mongolism in twins. J Med Genet 1:39, 1964

113. Avni A, Amir J, Wilunsky E et al: Down's syndrome in twins of unlike sex. J Med Genet 20:94, 1983

114. Hanna JH, Hill JM: Single intrauterine fetal demise in multiple gestation. Obstet Gynecol 63:126, 1984

115. Pritchard JA, Ratnoff OD: Studies of fibrinogen and other hemostatic factors in women with intrauterine death and delayed delivery. Surg Obstet Gynecol 101:467, 1955

116. Skelly H, Marivate M, Norman R et al: Consumptive coagulopathy following fetal death in a triplet pregnancy. Am J Obstet Gynecol 142:595, 1982

117. Romero R, Duffy TP, Berkowitz RL et al: Prolongation of a preterm pregnancy complicated by death of a single twin in utero and disseminated intravascular coagulation. N Engl J Med 310:772, 1984

118. Angel JL, O'Brien WF: Management of the dead fetus syndrome with a surviving twin. Clin Decis Obstet Gynecol 1:6, 1987

119. Rodeck CH, Mibeshan RS, Abramowicz J, Campbell S: Selective fetocide of the affected twin by fetoscopic air embolism. Prenat Diagn 2:189, 1982

120. Antsaklis A, Politis J, Karagiannopoulos C, Kaskarelis D: Selective survival of only the healthy fetus following prenatal diagnosis of thalassaemia major in binovular twin gestation. Prenat Diagn 4:289, 1984

121. Golbus MS, Cunningham N, Goldberg JD et al: Selective termination of multiple gestations. Am J Med Genet 34:339, 1988

122. Wapner RJ, Davis G, Johnson A et al: Selective reduction of multifetal pregnancies. Lancet 335:90, 1990

123. Moore CM, McAdams AJ, Sutherland J: Intrauterine disseminated intravascular coagulation: a syndrome of multiple pregnancy with a dead twin fetus. J Pediatr 74:523, 1969

124. Yoshioka H, Kadomoto Y, Mino M et al: Multicystic encephalomalacia in liveborn twin with a stillborn macerated co-twin. J Pediatr 95:798, 1979

125. Benirschke K: Twin placenta in perinatal mortality. NY State J Med 61:1499, 1961

126. Hoyme HE, Higginbottom MC, Jones KL: Vascular etiology of disruptive structural defects in monozygotic twins. Pediatrics 67:288, 1981

127. Schinzel AAGL, Smith DW, Miller JR: Monozygotic twinning and structural defects. J Pediatr 95:921, 1979

128. Carlson NJ, Towers CV: Multiple gestation complicated by the death of one fetus. Obstet Gynecol 73:685, 1989

129. Aberg A, Mitelman F, Cantz M, Gehler J: Cardiac puncture of fetus with Hurler's disease avoiding abortion of unaffected co-twin. Lancet 2:990, 1978

130. Kerenyi TD, Chitkara U: Selective birth in twin pregnancy with discordancy for Down's syndrome. N Engl J Med 304:1525, 1981

131. Beck L, Terinde R, Rohrborn G et al: Twin pregnancy, abortion of one fetus with Down's syndrome by sectio

parva, the other delivered mature and healthy. Eur J Obstet Gynaecol Reprod Biol 12:267, 1981

132. Chitkara U, Berkowitz RL, Wilkins IA et al: Selective second-trimester termination of the anomalous fetus in twin pregnancies. Obstet Gynecol 73:690, 1989

133. Wittman BK, Farquharson DF, Thomas WDS: The role of feticide in the management of severe twin transfusion syndrome. Am J Obstet Gynecol 155:1023, 1986

134. Robie GF, Payne GG, Morgan MA: Selective delivery of an acardiac acephalic twin. N Engl J Med 320:512, 1989

135. Urig MA, Simpson GF, Elliott JP, Clewell WH: Twin-twin transfusion syndrome: the surgical removal of one twin as a treatment option. Fetal Ther 3:185, 1988

136. Dumez Y, Oury JF: Method for first trimester selective abortion in multiple pregnancy. Contrib Gynecol Obstet 15:50, 1986

137. Gonen Y, Blankier J, Casper RF: Transvaginal ultrasound in selective embryo reduction for multiple pregnancy. Obstet Gynecol 75:720, 1990

138. Robinson LK, Jones KL, Benirschke K: The nature of structural defects associated with velamentous and marginal insertion of the umbilical cord. Am J Obstet Gynecol 146:191, 1983

139. Colburn DW, Pasquale SA: Monoamniotic twin pregnancy. J Reprod Med 27:165, 1982

140. Nyberg DA, Filly RA, Golbus MS, Stephens JD: Entangled umbilical cords: a sign of monoamniotic twins. J Ultrasound Med 3:29, 1984

141. Townsend RR, Filly RA: Sonography of nonconjoined monoamniotic twin pregnancies. J Ultrasound Med 7:665, 1988

142. McLeod FN, McCoy DR: Monoamniotic twins with an unusual cord complication. Br J Obstet Gynaecol 88:774, 1981

143. Beischer NA, Pepperell RJ, Barrie JU: Twin pregnancy and erythroblastosis. Obstet Gynecol 34:22, 1969

144. Ellis MI, Coxon A, Noble C: Intrauterine transfusion of twins. Br Med J 1:609, 1970

145. Spellacy WN, Cruz AC, and Buhi WC, Birk SA: Amniotic fluid L/S ratio in twin gestation. Obstet Gynecol 50:68, 1977

146. Sims CD, Cowan DB, Parkinson CE: The lecithin sphingomyelin (L/S) ratio in twin pregnancies. Br J Obstet Gynaecol 83:447, 1976

147. Obladen M, Gluck L: RDS and tracheal phospholipid composition in twins: independent of gestational age. J Pediatr 90:799, 1977

148. Wilkinson AR, Jenkins PA, Baum JD: Uterine position and fetal lung maturity in triplet and quadruplet pregnancy. Lancet 2:663, 1982

149. Norman RJ, Joubert SM, Marivate M: Amniotic fluid phospholipids and glucocorticoids in multiple pregnancy. Br J Obstet Gynaecol 90:51, 1983

150. Gluck L, Kulovich MV: Maturation of the fetal lung, RDS, and amniotic fluid. In Villee CA, Villee DB, Zuckerman J (eds): Respiratory Distress Syndrome. Academic Press, San Diego, 1973

151. Leveno KJ, Quirk JG, Whalley PJ et al: Fetal lung maturation in twin gestation. Am J Obstet Gynecol 148:405, 1984

152. Wender DF, Kandall C, Leppert PC, Berkowitz RL: Hyaline membrane disease in twin B following prolonged rupture of membranes for twin A. Conn Med 45:83, 1981

153. Elias S, Gerbie AB, Simpson JL et al: Genetic amniocentesis in twin gestations. Am J Obstet Gynecol 138:169, 1980

154. Jeanty P, Rodesch F, Romero R et al: How to improve your amniocentesis technique. Am J Obstet Gynecol 146:593, 1983

155. McEnerney JK, McEnerney LN: Unfavorable neonatal outcome after intraamniotic injection of methylene blue. Obstet Gynecol, suppl., 61:35, 1983

156. Tabsh K: Genetic amniocentesis in multiple gestation: a new technique to diagnose monoamniotic twins. Obstet Gynecol 75:296, 1990

157. Hartikainen-Sorri AL, Jouppila P: Is routine hospitalization needed in antenatal care of twin pregnancy? J Perinat Med 12:31, 1984

158. Saunders MC, Dick JS, Brown IM: The effects of hospital admission for bed rest on the duration of twin pregnancy: a randomized trial. Lancet 2:793, 1985

159. MacLennan AH, Green RC, O'Shea R et al: Routine hospital admission in twin pregnancy between 26 and 30 weeks' gestation. Lancet 335:267, 1990

160. Leveno KJ, Andrews WW, Gilstrap LC et al: Impact of elective hospitalization on outcome of twin pregnancy, abstracted. Proceedings of the Society of Perinatal Obstetricians, Houston, Texas, January 1990

161. Katz M, Robertson PA, Creasy RK: Cardiovascular complications associated with terbutaline treatment for preterm labor. Am J Obstet Gynecol 139:605, 1981

162. Houlton MCC, Marivate M, Philpott RH: Factors associated with preterm labour and changes in the cervix before labour in twin pregnancy. Br J Obstet Gynaecol 89:190, 1982

163. Neilson JP, Verkuyl AA, Crowther CA, Bannerman C: Preterm labor in twin pregnancies: prediction by cervical assessment. Obstet Gynecol 72:719, 1988

164. O'Connor MC, Arias E, Royston JP, Dalrymple IJ: The merits of special antenatal care for twin pregnancies. Br J Obstet Gynaecol 88:222, 1981

165. Devoe LD, Azor H: Simultaneous nonstress fetal heart rate testing in twin pregnancy. Obstet Gynecol 58:450, 1981

166. Goldman GA, Dicker D, Peleg A, Goldman JA: Is elective cerclage justified in the management of triplet and quadruplet pregnancy? Aust NZ J Obstet Gynaecol 29:9, 1989

167. Chervenak FA, Johnson RE, Youcha S: Intrapartum management of twin gestation. Obstet Gynecol 65:119, 1985

168. Khunda S: Locked twins. Obstet Gynecol 39:453, 1972

169. Sevitz H, Merrell DA: The use of a beta-sympathomimetic drug in locked twins. Br J Obstet Gynaecol 88:76, 1981

170. Nissen Ed: Twins: collision, impaction, compaction, and interlocking. Obstet Gynecol 11:514, 1958

171. Acker D, Lieberman M, Holbrook H et al: Delivery of the second twin. Obstet Gynecol 59:710, 1982

172. Chervenak FA, Johnson RE, Berkowitz RL et al: Is routine cesarean section necessary for vertex-breech and vertex-transverse twin gestations? Am J Obstet Gynecol 148:1, 1984

173. Duenhoelter JH, Wells CE, Reisch JS: A paired controlled study of vaginal and abdominal delivery of the low birth weight breech fetus. Obstet Gynecol 54:310, 1979

174. Goldenberg RL, Nelson KG: The premature breech. Am J Obstet Gynecol 127:240, 1977

175. Chervenak FA, Johnson RE, Berkowitz RL, Hobbins JC: Intrapartum external version of the second twin. Obstet Gynecol 62:160, 1983

176. Gocke SE, Nageotte MP, Garite T et al: Management of the nonvertex second twin: primary cesarean section, external version, or primary breech extraction. Am J Obstet Gynecol 161:111, 1989

177. Shepard MJ, Richards VA, Berkowitz RL, et al: An evaluation of the two equations for predicting fetal weight by ultrasound. Am J Obstet Gynecol 142:47, 1982

178. Evrard JR, Gold EM: Cesarean section for delivery of the second twin. Obstet Gynecol 57:581, 1981

179. Rayburn WF, Lavin JP, Miodovnik M, Varner MW: Multiple gestation: time interval between delivery of the first and second twins. Obstet Gynecol 63:502, 1984

180. Ferguson WF: Perinatal mortality in multiple gestations: a review of perinatal deaths from 1609 multiple gestations. Obstet Gynecol 23:861, 1964

181. Spurway JH: The fate and management of the second twin. Am J Obstet Gynecol 83:1377, 1962

182. Mashiach S, Ben-Rafael Z, Dor J, Serr DM: Triplet pregnancy in uterus didelphys with delivery interval of 72 days. Obstet Gynecol 58:519, 1981

183. Woolfson J, Fay T, Bates A: Twins with 54 days between deliveries: case report. Br J Obstet Gynaecol 90:685, 1983

184. Feichtinger W, Breitenecker G, Frohlich H: Prolongation of pregnancy and survival of twin B after loss of twin A at 21 weeks' gestation. Am J Obstet Gynecol 161:891, 1989

185. Berkowitz RL, Hobbins JC: Delivering twins with the help of ultrasound. Contemp Obstet Gynecol 19:128, 1982

186. Ballas S, Toaff R, Jaffa AJ: Deflexion of the fetal head in breech presentation. Obstet Gynecol 52:653, 1978

187. Jeanty P, Rodesch F, Verhoogen C et al: The vanishing twin. Ultrasonics 2:25, 1981

Chapter 27

Intrauterine Growth Retardation

Steven G. Gabbe

Abnormal intrauterine growth has been recognized for over 20 years. In 1954, Clifford described the dysmature, wasted fetus associated with prolonged pregnancy[1] (Fig. 27.1). Lubchenco et al.,[2] Usher and McLean,[3] and others[4,5] laid the groundwork for the recognition of the growth-retarded infant through population studies that established the relationship between gestational age and weight. Gruenwald highlighted the important differences among the neonate with low birth weight secondary to prematurity, the infant born too soon, and the infant who was small when compared with other newborns of the same gestational age, the infant born too small.[6] These babies were clearly identified as being at high risk for perinatal morbidity and mortality. This chapter presents the varied etiologies of the growth retardation syndromes, discusses recent advances in the detection and management of this problem, and reviews the available information on the long-term prognosis for infants who have suffered from impaired intrauterine growth.

DEFINITION

Intrauterine growth retardation (IUGR) is not a common problem, complicating 3 to 7 percent of all pregnancies. However, IUGR is the second most important cause of perinatal mortality after preterm delivery.[7] Approximately 20 percent of all stillborn infants are growth retarded. The perinatal mortality rate for growth-retarded infants may be 6 to 10 times greater than that for a normally grown population, 120/1,000 for all cases of growth retardation and 100/1,000 if anomalous infants are excluded. The incidence of intrapartum asphyxia in cases complicated by IUGR has been reported to be 50 percent.[8] These infants also suffer an increased incidence of hypoglycemia, hypocalcemia, polycythemia, and hypothermia in the neonatal period, as shown below.

IMMEDIATE NEONATAL MORBIDITY IN IUGR

Birth asphyxia

Meconium aspiration

Hypoglycemia

Hypocalcemia

Hypothermia

Polycythemia, hyperviscosity

Thrombocytopenia

Pulmonary hemorrhage

Malformations

Sepsis

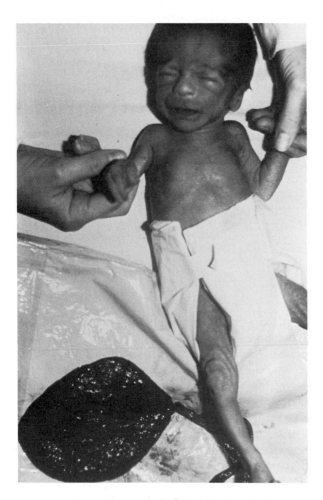

Fig. 27.1 A growth-retarded infant exhibiting subcutaneous wasting.

Obstetricians must be aware of IUGR as a distinct diagnostic entity if the elevated perinatal morbidity and mortality rates are to be reduced. Early observers appreciated the need to separate low-birth-weight babies who were premature but normally grown from those who had failed to achieve the size expected for their gestational age. They recognized the disproportionate morbidity and mortality rates of these growth-retarded infants. Infants who at birth are below the tenth percentile in weight for their gestational age are considered growth retarded if one refers to the growth curves established by Lubchenco and Babson. This definition, birth weight below the

tenth percentile, although arbitrary, has been most widely used in describing IUGR.

Using the tenth percentile cutoff, approximately 70 percent of the infants designated as growth retarded are normally or constitutionally small, so-called light for gestational age or small for gestational age (SGA).[9] These neonates are *not* at increased risk for poor outcome. However, this group below the tenth percentile also includes infants who are truly growth retarded in terms of their growth potential, and these babies may suffer markedly increased perinatal morbidity and mortality. Usher has pointed out that when restricting the cutoff weight for IUGR to 2 SDs below the mean, only infants below the third percentile are considered growth retarded. The major aim of defining this syndrome should be the accurate description of a group of infants who have increased morbidity and mortality. Using the third percentile may overlook some growth-retarded infants, and the tenth percentile cutoff includes normal infants who may be monitored unnecessarily.

Some perinatologists have suggested that weight and gestational age alone are inadequate to describe the full spectrum of infants who are growth retarded.[10,11] They have proposed using a ponderal index, the ratio of soft tissue mass to the skeletal frame as measured by crown to heel length and often defined as birth weight × 100 (crown–heel length).[11] Infants with a ponderal index below the third percentile for gestational age or a crown–rump length less than the 1.5 percentile for gestational age are included in the growth-retarded group.

In summary, growth retardation should be considered a spectrum of abnormal growth patterns that may vary from patient to patient. Altman has stressed that the term IUGR should be reserved for those fetuses for whom there is clear evidence that growth has faltered.[12] A multiparous woman whose first two babies weighed 3,500 g at 40 weeks gestation may deliver a 2,700-g infant at the same gestational age in her third pregnancy. Although not growth retarded by birth weight percentile for gestational age, this infant's small size may reflect impaired growth.

The biologic significance of any definition of IUGR can only be measured by discovering which parameters predict most accurately infants at risk for short- and long-term impairment. The prognostic value of the third and tenth percentiles still remains to be determined. Until a definition of growth retardation is uniformly applied by perinatologists using growth curves that are appropriate for their own patient populations, we will be unable to determine how effectively we have detected and treated IUGR.[13,14]

ETIOLOGY

The definitions that have been reviewed permit only postpartum identification of the growth-retarded infant. Indeed, absolute identification of IUGR has largely remained a postpartum event, particularly in the case of the constitutionally small infant. When considering the definition and detection of IUGR, one must also review the etiologies of IUGR and their appropriate therapies. As Dawes has pointed out, "Small for dates . . . as a label is inadequate. It is only the first step in analysis—the acknowledgment of partial ignorance. [We] need to find out why, and to discover whether that condition can be prevented, and whether it can be cured either antenatally or postnatally." [15] Clinicians have become more aware of IUGR, and, with that awareness, their ability to monitor intrauterine fetal growth and assess fetal well-being has improved. Although knowledge of the regulation and aberrations of normal fetal growth remains rudimentary, some important clinical correlations have been established (Table 27.1).

Intrauterine infection, though long recognized as a cause of growth retardation, accounts for less than 10 percent of all cases. Herpes, cytomegalovirus, rubella, and toxoplasmosis are well documented, and other intrauterine infections are strongly suspected (Ch. 40). The infectious process produces early disruption of fetal growth during the stage of cell hyperplasia and is, therefore, associated with a poor prognosis for normal development. For the agents associated with IUGR, prevention of the infection is the most important therapy.

Chromosomal abnormalities and congenital malformations have both been associated with less than 10 percent of cases of IUGR. Abnormalities in cell replication and reduced cell number produce a pattern of impaired growth that is early in onset and

Table 27.1 Factors Associated with IUGR

Fetal
  Congenital infection
  Congenital malformation
Placental
  Decreased placental mass
    Abruption
    Infarction
    Prolonged gestation
    Twins
  Intrinsic placental disease
    Poor implantation site
    Malformation
    Vascular disease
  Decreased placental flow
    Maternal vascular disease
    Postural hypotension
    Hyperviscosity
Maternal
  Decreased nutrient availability
    Starvation
    Ileojejunal bypass
  Decreased oxygen availability
    High altitude
    Hemoglobinopathy
    Cyanotic heart disease
    Smoking
  Drug ingestion
    Ethanol
    Hydantoin
    Coumarin
  Prior poor pregnancy outcome

symmetrical (Table 27.2). In general, the earlier the insult and the longer its duration, the poorer the prognosis. Growth retardation has been observed in 53 percent of cases of trisomy 13 and 64 percent of cases of trisomy 18.[16] Congenital anomalies such as

Table 27.2 Etiologies of IUGR

Symmetrical	Asymmetrical
Congenital infection	Maternal vascular disease
Cytogenetic abnormality	
Congenital malformation	
Maternal drug ingestion	
Maternal smoking	
Maternal alcohol abuse	

renal agenesis represent a related situation.[17] It has been assumed that these infants are small because they have a congenital malformation. However, Spiers has suggested that early growth retardation itself may set the stage for a variety of congenital malformations.[18] Pedersen and Molsted-Pedersen observed that some fetuses of insulin-dependent diabetic mothers, particularly those whose diabetes was not well controlled, were found to be growth retarded at 7 to 14 weeks gestation. These infants were also more likely to have a major malformation at delivery or exhibit abnormalities in gross motor and language and speech development at 4 to 5 years of age.[19,20]

An absolute or relative decrease in placental mass affects the quantity of substrate the fetus receives and has been recognized ultrasonographically to antedate fetal growth retardation.[21] Thus, a circumvallate placenta, partial placental abruption, placenta accreta, placental infarction, or hemangioma may result in growth retardation. An elevated maternal serum α-fetoprotein level in the second trimester has been associated with IUGR and may be due to abnormal placentation.[22] In the prolonged pregnancy, a relative decrease in placental mass and function in relation to increased fetal size may limit further fetal growth.[23] An intrinsic placental abnormality has been identified in some cases of growth retardation including the presence of a single umbilical artery. Placental location has also been linked to growth retardation. Placenta previa without bleeding has been suggested as a risk factor, because the low implantation site may not be optimal for nutrient transfer.[24]

Twin gestation represents a relative decrease in placental mass in relation to fetal mass and is, therefore, often associated with IUGR (Ch. 26). In 1966, Gruenwald observed that the growth curve of twins deviated from that of singletons with a progressive fall of growth after 32 weeks.[25] This finding implies relative placental insufficiency as opposed to intrinsic fetal compromise and suggests that the longer the twin pregnancy continues, the greater the retardation of intrauterine growth with "catch-up" growth observed after birth. Thus, twins represent a group of fetuses at high risk for IUGR as confirmed by an incidence of 17.5 percent in one study.[26] Although

twins have an increased incidence of perinatal mortality that relates primarily to prematurity and subsequent respiratory distress syndrome (RDS), growth retardation represents the second most prevalent cause of morbidity for these infants.

Decreased uteroplacental blood flow with its associated reduction in transfer of nutrients to the fetus is responsible for the majority of clinically recognized cases of IUGR. Maternal vascular disease, whether chronic hypertension, preeclampsia, or diabetes with vasculopathy, has been associated with impaired fetal growth.[27-29] In preeclampsia, failure of trophoblastic invasion of maternal spiral arterioles by 20 to 22 weeks gestation and intimal thickening accompanied by fibrinoid degeneration of the media of these arterioles result in luminal narrowing and, therefore, decreased blood flow through the placental bed.[30] Such cases are marked by asymmetric IUGR, maintenance of normal fetal head growth, and reduction in the size of the fetal liver, heart, thymus, spleen, pancreas, and adrenal glands (Table 27.2). Doppler flow studies have now demonstrated increased flow in the internal carotid artery with reduced flow in the descending aorta and renal arteries of the growth-retarded human fetus.[31,32] Decreased placental blood flow from postural maternal hypotension and maternal hyperviscosity with sludging has also been reported to cause IUGR. Some patients with hypertension have been noted to demonstrate a reduction in the normal expansion of blood volume seen in pregnancy. This contracted circulating blood volume has been correlated with IUGR. A reduction in maternal oxygenation in women living at high altitude or those with cyanotic heart disease or parenchymal lung disease may be responsible for IUGR. Those hemoglobinopathies and anemias that impair maternal and fetal oxygenation have also been linked to limited fetal growth.[33]

Poor maternal weight gain has long been recognized as a risk factor for growth retardation. Controversy still exists about the contribution maternal malnutrition can make to IUGR. Studies of the offspring of women pregnant during the siege of Leningrad in 1942 and the Dutch famine in 1945 indicate little effect on fetal growth by such dietary restriction.[34] In Holland, despite a maternal intake of 600 to 900 calories daily for 6 months, the average birth weight fell only 240 g. However, investigation in Guatemalan Indian tribes has indicated that protein malnutrition before 26 weeks growth can result in symmetrical growth retardation.[35] Protein restriction after 26 weeks did not limit fetal growth. The degree of malnourishment observed in Guatemala or during the Dutch famine would not ordinarily be found in the United States. However, pregnant women may be subject to poor nutrition through limited gastrointestinal absorption imposed by Crohn's disease or ulcerative colitis. These conditions have not been generally associated with increased numbers of growth-retarded infants. Massively obese women who have undergone ileojejunal bypass are reported to have smaller infants than average, but they do not usually fall below the tenth percentile in birth weight.

Glucose is a critical fetal nutrient, and if its supply is restricted, growth retardation may result. Using cord blood sampling, Economides observed significantly lower maternal and fetal glucose levels in cases of growth retardation and speculated that the major cause of fetal hypoglycemia in these cases was reduced glucose supply from the mother due to impaired placental perfusion.[36] Khouzami observed a significant association between maternal hypoglycemia on a 3-hour oral glucose tolerance test (GTT) and subsequent birth of non-low-birth-weight but growth-retarded babies.[37] More recently, Langer demonstrated that a ''flat'' GTT was associated with a 20-fold increase in IUGR in normotensive patients. He suggests that the 3-hour GTT may be used as a screening test to identify women at high risk for IUGR.[38]

Maternal drug ingestion may produce IUGR by a direct effect on fetal growth as well as through inadequate dietary intake. Smoking produces a symmetrically growth-retarded fetus through reduced uterine blood flow and impaired fetal oxygenation.[39] The consumption of alcohol and the use of coumarin or hydantoin derivatives are now well known to produce particular dysmorphic features in association with impaired fetal growth. Mills et al. have demonstrated a significant increase in the risk of IUGR with the consumption of one to two drinks daily.[40] Maternal use of cocaine has been associated with not only IUGR but also reduced head circumference growth.[41]

In 1971, Lobl et al. reported data suggesting that advanced maternal age was a factor in the etiology of IUGR.[42] More recently, Berkowitz et al. found no evidence that the first births of women between 30 and 34 or those over 35 were at increased risk for growth retardation.[43] Miller and Merritt have also demonstrated that if one controls for underlying medical complications, maternal age is not related to restricted fetal growth.[44]

Prior poor pregnancy outcome is clearly correlated with the subsequent delivery of a growth-retarded infant.[45] Galbraith et al.[46] and Tejani[47] have shown that prior birth of an IUGR infant is the obstetric factor most often associated with the subsequent birth of a growth-retarded infant. The study populations did include women with underlying medical problems. Tejani and Mann in a retrospective study of 83 multigravidas who had delivered IUGR infants noted that the perinatal wastage from their 200 prior pregnancies was 41 percent.[48] This striking figure, which includes spontaneous abortions as well as neonatal and intrauterine deaths, points to the significance of poor obstetric history as a risk factor for IUGR. Women whose first pregnancy results in a growth-retarded infant have a 1 in 4 risk of delivering a second infant below the tenth percentile. After two pregnancies complicated by IUGR, there is a fourfold increase in the risk for a subsequent growth-retarded infant.[45] When all indices of risk have been applied, the one-third of the population considered at highest risk accounts for two-thirds of the infants identified as growth retarded. Two-thirds of pregnancies, although not judged to be ''at risk'' for IUGR, yield one-third of neonates below the tenth percentile.[46] Most of these babies are constitutionally small.

In summary, a framework does exist for considering the causes of growth retardation. Is the fetus abnormal? The delivery system disrupted? The maternal supply line compromised? These questions categorize the source of the problem without explaining the mechanism by which the growth process is disturbed. Even when one is aware of these clinical associations, the sum of the many factors affecting the growth of an individual fetus is unpredictable. Although we cannot predict a precise outcome for any patient, we can look at a group of pregnant women and decide which of them are at risk by virtue of the many associated conditions discussed previously.

DIAGNOSIS

During the past decade, great strides have been made in detecting the growth-retarded fetus and have served as the basis for plans designed to reduce the associated perinatal morbidity and mortality. In the past, clinical parameters such as maternal weight gain and measurement of fundal height were used to reflect fetal growth. Belizan et al. observed that curvilinear fundal height measurements in centimeters from the symphysis pubis could be closely correlated with gestational age: a lag of 4 cm or more suggests growth retardation.[49] However, Persson reported a sensitivity of 27 percent and a positive predictive value of only 18 percent using carefully performed fundal height measurements to detect IUGR.[50] Fundal height measurements should be viewed as a screening technique and yield most accurate predictions when applied to a high-risk population. As noted earlier, low maternal weight gain has been associated with fetal growth retardation. Yet the clinician sees many instances of normally grown infants whose mothers gained little weight and growth-retarded babies whose mothers exhibited normal weight gain.

The application of ultrasound technology to obstetrics has offered the opportunity to monitor fetal growth reliably.[9] In 1971, Campbell and Dewhurst first established serial cephalometry as a useful tool in the detection of the growth-retarded fetus.[51] Two patterns of altered head growth were described. In "late flattening," or asymmetrical growth retardation, which represents approximately two-thirds of all cases of IUGR, the biparietal diameter (BPD) increases normally until late pregnancy and then lags behind. However, this falloff in BPD growth occurs *after* other signs of IUGR such as oligohydramnios and decreased abdominal circumference growth. In the "low-profile" or symmetrical type, impaired head growth occurs much earlier in gestation. The asymmetrical pattern is often associated with maternal hypertension, whereas symmetrical IUGR is characteristic of pregnancies complicated by intrauterine infection, chromosomal abnormalities, or teratogenic drugs. Not surprisingly, serial BPD measurements alone most often fail to detect asymmetrical or brain sparing IUGR.

In an attempt to increase detection of the fetus with asymmetrical growth retardation, head circumference (HC) to abdominal circumference (AC) ratios were assessed (Figs. 27.2 and 27.3).[52,53] In the normally growing fetus, the HC/AC ratio exceeds 1.0 before 32 weeks gestation, is approximately 1.0 at 32 to 34 weeks gestation, and falls below 1.0 after 34 weeks gestation. In fetuses affected by asymmetrical growth retardation, the HC remains larger than that of the body (Fig. 27.2). The HC/AC ratio is then elevated. The AC is smaller because fetal liver volume is reduced as a result of decreased glycogen storage. In symmetrical IUGR, both the HC and the AC are reduced, and the HC/AC ratio remains normal (Fig. 27.3). Using the HC/AC ratio, 85 percent of growth-retarded fetuses are detected, with a reduction in false-negative diagnoses. Thus, a single set of measurements, even when determined in the latter part of pregnancy, can be very helpful in evaluating the status of intrauterine growth.

In some cases, measurement of the HC may be difficult as a result of fetal position. One can then compare the femur length (FL), which is relatively spared in asymmetrical IUGR, to the AC.[54] The FL/AC is 22 at all gestational ages from 21 weeks to term and so can be applied without knowledge of the number of weeks gestation. An FL/AC ratio greater than 23.5 suggests IUGR.

Decreased amniotic fluid volume has been associated clinically with IUGR and may be the earliest sign detected on ultrasonography, preceding an elevation in HC/AC ratio and lagging fetal growth (Fig. 27.4). Decreased perfusion of the fetal kidneys and reduced urine production explain this observation.[32] In an early study, Manning reported that a vertical pocket of amniotic fluid measuring 1 cm or more reflected an adequate fluid volume.[55] Of fetuses with fluid pockets less than 1 cm, 96 percent were actually

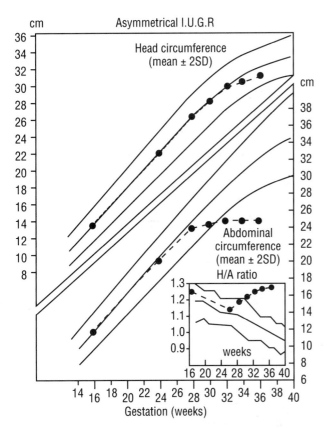

Fig. 27.2 Growth chart in a case of asymmetrical IUGR. Although head circumference is preserved, abdominal circumference growth falls off early in the third trimester. For this reason, the H/A ratio shown in the lower right corner of the graph becomes elevated. IUGR, intrauterine growth retardation. (From Chudleigh and Pearce,[109] with permission.)

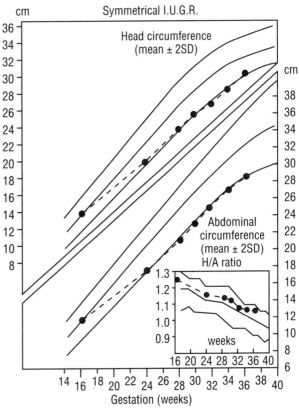

Fig. 27.3 Growth chart in a case of symmetrical IUGR. Note the early onset of both head circumference and abdominal circumference growth retardation. For this reason, the H/A ratio shown in the lower right corner remains normal. IUGR, intrauterine growth retardation. (From Chudleigh and Pearce,[109] with permission.)

growth retarded. Only 5 of 91 cases with an adequate amount of amniotic fluid exhibited IUGR. The patient with an uncertain gestational age who presents late in pregnancy poses a difficult diagnostic dilemma because interpretation of BPD and HC/AC ratios must be related to accurate gestational age. Measuring an amniotic fluid pocket, such as the FL/AC ratio, does not rely on knowledge of the gestational age. More recently, Manning and his colleagues have broadened their criteria.[56] A 2-cm vertical pocket is considered normal; 1 to 2 cm is marginal, and less than 1 cm is decreased. Using this definition, they observed a 6 percent incidence of IUGR with a pocket

2 cm or larger, 20 percent with a pocket 1 to 2 cm, and 39 percent with a pocket less than 1 cm. One may also use the amniotic fluid index (Fig. 27.4) to quantitate amniotic fluid volume (Ch. 12), although this technique requires a knowledge of gestational age. The overall clinical impression of reduced amniotic fluid on ultrasonography may be most important.

Advanced placental grade, a grade 3 placenta observed early in the third trimester, has been correlated with IUGR (Fig. 27.5).[57] Like amniotic fluid volume and FL/AC ratio, placental grade is gestational-age-independent. More recent studies have

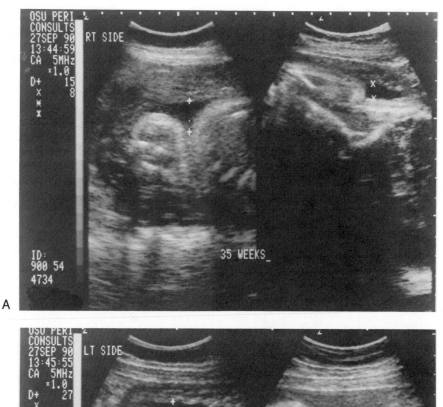

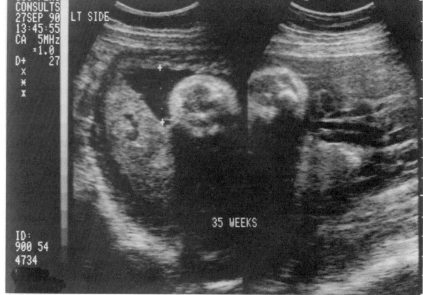

Fig. 27.4 (A & B) Amniotic fluid index (AFI) performed at 35 weeks on a patient whose fundal height measured 30 cm. Findings consistent with asymmetrical growth retardation were observed, including estimated fetal weight of 1,500 g, head circumference/abdominal circumference ratio of 1.15, and AFI of 5.0 cm, as illustrated. At 35 weeks, the fiftieth percentile for the AFI is 14.0 cm; the fifth percentile is 11.9 cm. Note that one amniotic fluid pocket greater than 2.0 cm was found.

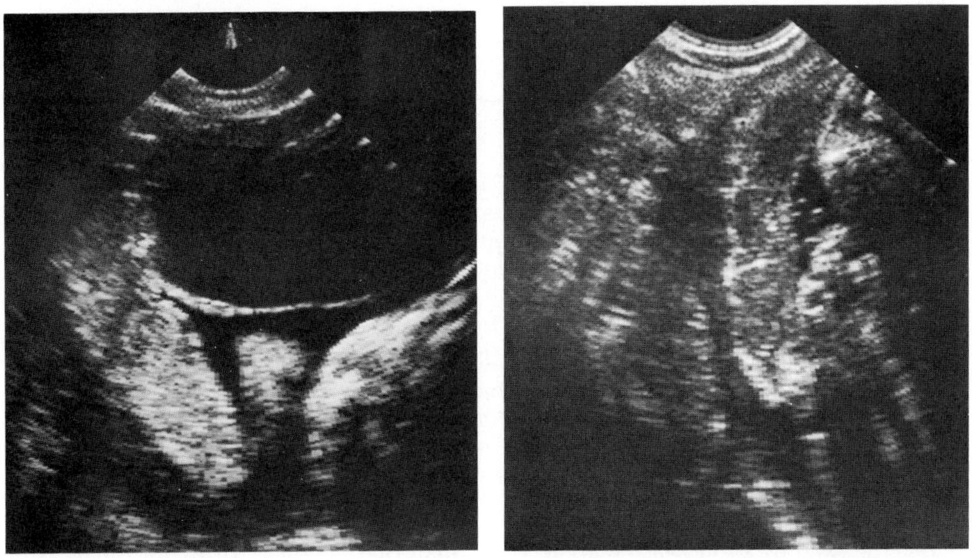

Placenta Baby A

Placenta Baby B

Fig. 27.5 Placental morphology in twins. Twin B, who was growth retarded, demonstrated a grade 3 placenta; that of twin A was grade 0. (From DiGaetano and Gabbe,[110] with permission.)

found a positive predictive value for IUGR with advanced placental grade of less than 20 percent.[58]

In late pregnancy, symmetrical IUGR may be difficult to distinguish from incorrect dates. Some investigators have observed that growth of the transcerebellar diameter is spared in the symmetrically growth-retarded fetus and can be used to date the pregnancy.[59] Not all studies have confirmed this relationship.[60]

An accurate ultrasonographic assessment of fetal weight is essential in detecting and following patients suspected of having growth-retarded infants.[61] Using a multifractional equation and a measurement of AC, a weight can be predicted and related to BPD. Formulas that incorporate the FL may increase the accuracy of in utero weight estimation for the fetus with IUGR.[62]

Overall, the three most predictive ultrasonographic criteria for the diagnosis of IUGR are decreased amniotic fluid volume, elevated HC/AC ratio, and estimated fetal weight below the tenth percentile.[58] In a frequently quoted study, Benson et al. evaluated the predictive value of a variety of ultrasound parameters using the data derived from a large number of published reports (Table 27.3).[58] The calculations were based on a population with a 10 percent incidence of growth retardation. Even those parameters that were thought to be most sensitive accurately predicted the presence of IUGR in only 50 percent of cases. The specificity for these ultrasound criteria was approximately 90 percent, which is not surprising, considering that, by definition, only 10 percent of the infants were growth retarded. Despite the low sensitivities and poor positive predictive values derived by Benson, more recent ultrasound studies utilizing a variety of fetal parameters presently permit the recognition of the growth-retarded fetus in 75 to 85 percent of cases.[9,63-65] Nevertheless, when the obstetrician uses ultrasound data to develop a plan of management, he or she must consider the accuracy with which gestational age has been established and the clinical setting. In this way, unnecessary interventions resulting in the delivery of a normal but constitutionally small infant may be prevented.

A practical approach for the detection of the growth-retarded fetus includes a careful history to determine those patients with significant risk factors. In this at-risk population, an ultrasound examination should be performed at 16 to 18 weeks to establish

Table 27.3 Diagnostic Value of Ultrasound in Detecting IUGR[a]

Measure	Sensitivity	Specificity	Predictive Value	
			Positive	Negative
Placental grade	62	64	16	94
AFV	24–80	72–98	21–55	92–97
BPD				
Small	24–88	62–94	21–44	92–98
Poor growth	75	84	35	97
FL/AC	34–49	78–83	18–20	92–98
HC/AC	82	94	62	98
EFW	89	88	45	99

[a] Estimated values if a 10 percent prevalence of IUGR is assumed (Bayes' theorem).

Abbreviations: AFV, amniotic fluid volume; BPD, biparietal diameter; FL/AC femur length/abdominal circumference ratio; HC/AC, head circumference/abdominal circumference ratio; EFW, estimated fetal weight.

(Modified from Benson et al.,[58] with permission.)

gestational dates, followed by a follow-up scan at 34 weeks to evaluate fetal growth. In low-risk patients, a lag in fundal height measurement should signal the need for an ultrasound study.

MANAGEMENT

In developing a plan for the management of suspected growth retardation, one must remember the major etiologic groups described previously. Most infants thought to be growth retarded are constitutionally small and require no intervention. Unfortunately, this diagnosis is usually made retrospectively. Approximately 15 percent exhibit symmetrical growth retardation due to an early fetal insult for which there is no effective therapy. Here, an accurate diagnosis is essential. Finally, approximately 15 percent have asymmetrical growth retardation or extrinsic growth failure due to placental disease or reduced uteroplacental blood flow. In such cases, antepartum fetal monitoring and carefully timed delivery may be critical.

Once growth retardation is suspected, a well-organized approach to management should be undertaken. The clinician should evaluate and treat problems that may be contributing to growth retardation. Therapy of growth retardation is often nonspecific but should be directed at the underlying cause of poor fetal growth if one can be determined. When a maternal medical problem such as inflammatory bowel disease is contributing to poor growth, specific therapy should be instituted. Alleviation of hypoxia, therapy of high blood pressure and anemia, and hyperalimentation are three examples. Nicolaides et al. administered 55 percent oxygen by face mask to mothers whose pregnancies were complicated by severe growth retardation, oligohydramnios, and decreased blood flow in the fetal descending aorta.[66] Ten minutes of maternal hyperoxygenation raised the fetal Po_2 to normal or near-normal in five of six cases. These preliminary studies suggest that maternal hyperoxygenation may permit prolongation of the pregnancy if the hypoxic fetus is too immature to survive. When placental infarction has been implicated as the underlying etiology, Moe has reported subcutaneous heparin therapy to have a favorable influence on pregnancy outcome.[67] Certainly, mothers should be counseled to stop smoking and alcohol ingestion. Nonspecific therapies include bed rest in the left lateral decubitus position to increase placental blood flow. Although an inadequate diet has not been clearly established as a cause of growth retardation in this country, dietary supplementation may be helpful.

Serial evaluations of fetal growth should be instituted as soon as the diagnosis of growth retardation is confirmed or for patients in whom suspicion of growth retardation is high. In the clinic setting, special effort should be made to have the same examiner

Table 27.4 Utilization of Ultrasonography in the Diagnosis and Evaluation of IUGR

Parameter	Results	Diagnosis	Plan
BPD	Appropriate for dates (within 2 weeks of dates)	No IUGR	Repeat only if indicated by clinical parameters (e.g., lagging fundal growth)
EFW	Above 10th percentile		
HC/AC ratio	In normal range		
Amniotic fluid volume	Normal		
BPD	Appropriate for dates (within 2 weeks of dates)	Probable asymmetrical IUGR	Repeat ultrasound examination every 2–3 weeks if not delivered
EFW	Below 10th percentile		Start antepartum surveillance and continue until delivery
HC/AC ratio	Above 95th percentile		
Amniotic fluid volume	Low		
BPD	2 weeks or more; smaller than expected for menstrual dates	Probable symmetrical IUGR	Repeat ultrasound examination every 2–3 weeks if not delivered
EFW	Below 10th percentile		Start antepartum surveillance and continue until delivery
HC/AC ratio	In normal range		
Amniotic fluid volume	Normal or low		If IUGR present before 20 weeks, scan for anomalies and consider fetal karyotype

Abbreviations: BPD, biparietal diameter; EFW, estimated fetal weight; HC/AC, head to abdominal ratio.
(Modified from Grannum,[69] with permission.)

see the patient each visit to measure the fundal height and assess fetal weight. Ultrasound examinations should be scheduled every 2 to 3 weeks and should include determinations of the BPD, HC/AC, fetal weight, and amniotic fluid volume. Arrest of head growth is of great concern, especially in light of the most recent data available on ultimate developmental potential for the growth-retarded infant.[68] Lack of head growth over a 2-week period should alert the physician to evaluate critically the mother's condition, as well as the results of other antepartum testing for that patient. Clear documentation of arrested head growth over a 4-week period is alarming, and the feasibility and safety of delivery should be reviewed. Grannum has developed a helpful outline for the diagnosis and evaluation of the growth-retarded fetus with ultrasonography (Table 27.4).[69]

Ultrasound should be used not only to document abnormal growth but also to detect lethal congenital malformations such as renal agenesis (Fig. 27.6). In cases of symmetrical growth retardation, amniocentesis, placental biopsy, or cord blood sampling should be considered to rule out a chromosomal abnormality such as trisomy 13, 18, or 21 (Table 27.5).[16] Trisomy 18 may present with growth retardation and polyhydramnios. If the diagnosis of a lethal anomaly can be made with certainty, an unnecessary cesarean section for fetal distress may be prevented.

Fetal well-being should also be assessed regularly, once the diagnosis of growth retardation is entertained. These infants have increased incidence of intrauterine demise, presumably from cord compression as well as placental insufficiency. Monitoring these infants should help to decrease their stillbirth rate by detecting the compromised fetus and allowing timely intervention. Twice weekly nonstress tests

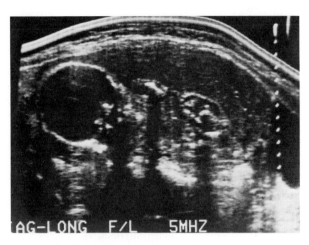

Fig. 27.6 Oligohydramnios due to renal agenesis. (From Di-Gaetano and Gabbe,[110] with permission.)

(NSTs) should be instituted as soon as the diagnosis of growth retardation is suspected. Experience with the NST in cases of growth retardation has confirmed that a reactive NST correlates highly with a fetus that is not in immediate danger of intrauterine demise.[70] Visser and associates performed antepartum fetal heart rate monitoring immediately before cordocentesis in 58 growth-retarded and 29 appropriately grown fetuses.[71] In the appropriately grown fetuses, blood PO_2 and pH values were within the normal range for gestation in 27 cases demonstrating a reactive heart rate pattern and 2 in which the tracing was nonreactive. In contrast, abnormal antepartum heart rate patterns were found in 15 of the 19 growth-retarded fetuses with hypoxemia, acidemia, or both. The best heart rate marker for fetal hypoxemia was a pattern characterized by repetitive decelerations. In that group, only 2 fetuses demonstrated normal PO_2 and pH values. In *none* of the cases with a reactive heart rate pattern was the growth-retarded fetus acidemic. However, many growth-retarded fetuses with a normal heart rate pattern were found to have fetal PO_2 values in the lower range of normal. Overall, antepartum fetal heart rate patterns in both normal and growth-retarded fetuses were found to correlate well with fetal oxygenation. The appearance of spontaneous decelerations during the NST may reflect oligohydramnios and cord compression and has been associated with a high perinatal mortality rate.[72]

Nonreactive NST results are often falsely positive

and should be further evaluated with a biophysical profile or contraction stress test (CST) before any management decision is made. A negative CST result, even when the CST is performed early in the third trimester, is an indication of adequate placental respiratory reserve.[73] Conversely, positive CST results occur in 30 percent of the pregnancies complicated by proven growth retardation. In a study by Lin et al., 30 percent of growth-retarded infants had nonreactive NST results and 40 percent had positive CST results. Ninety-two percent of IUGR infants with a nonreactive positive pattern exhibited perinatal morbidity.[74] However, a 25 to 50 percent false-positive rate has been associated with the CST by some investigators.[73] Therefore, information from antepartum fetal heart rate testing must always be reviewed in concert with the gestational age of the fetus, as well as other indices of fetal well-being and fetal growth.

Maternal monitoring of fetal activity has been used extensively in Great Britain, Scandinavia, and Israel for the assessment of pregnancies complicated by IUGR. In a study of 50 cases, Matthews clearly showed the predictive value of fetal activity charting for growth-retarded fetuses subsequently demonstrating distress in labor.[75] The techniques available for monitoring fetal movement are reviewed in Chapter 13.

Doppler Velocimetry

Doppler flow studies, particularly of the umbilical artery, have been applied to identify patients at risk for IUGR and to assess the condition of the fetus thought to be growth retarded. These studies have also contributed to our understanding of the pathophysiology of IUGR. As noted earlier, Wladimiroff

Table 27.5 Chromosomal Abnormalities and IUGR

	Ultrasound Findings Present		
IUGR	Anomaly	Hydramnios	Abnormal Karyotype
X			12/180 (7%)
X	X		18/57 (32%)
X		X	6/22 (27%)
X	X	X	7/15 (47%)

(From Eydoux et al.,[16] with permission.)

observed an increase in the pulsatility index of the umbilical artery associated with a reduced pulsatility index in the internal carotid artery, suggesting "brain sparing" in cases of asymmetrical growth retardation.[31] An increase in the pulsatility index in the fetal renal artery was observed by Veille, consistent with decreased renal blood flow.[32] Earlier studies by Giles et al. demonstrated that the small arterial vessel count in the tertiary stem villi of the placenta is significantly lower in patients with high umbilical artery systolic to diastolic (S/D) ratios than in those with normal S/D ratios.[76] These observations suggest that the increased resistance to flow as demonstrated by a high S/D ratio may be due to obliteration of the small muscular arteries in the tertiary stem villi. Rochelson et al. also noted a significant reduction in the small muscular artery count and the small muscular artery/villus ratio in the placentas of trisomic fetuses.[77] Abnormal umbilical artery Doppler waveforms could be closely correlated with reduced small muscular artery counts. This study suggests that growth retardation in the fetus with a chromosomal abnormality may be due to not only poor intrinsic growth potential but abnormalities in placental morphology and fetal–placental blood flow. More recently, Fok et al. demonstrated that the percentage of abnormal arterial vessels in the placentas of 14 growth-retarded fetuses could be correlated with the Doppler resistance index.[78] In studies of uterine artery blood flow, Schulman found that women with hypertensive disorders who had an elevated uterine artery S/D ratio (greater than 2.6) and/or diastolic notching were more likely to have pregnancies complicated by IUGR and intrauterine fetal death.[79] He noted that the changes in uterine artery flow patterns might precede those observed in the umbilical artery and antedate fetal growth retardation.

Doppler flow studies may reveal the likelihood of significant perinatal morbidity and mortality in cases of IUGR. Soothill et al. measured umbilical venous Po_2, Pco_2, pH, and plasma lactate levels in 29 growth-retarded fetuses.[80] They found significant negative correlations between the severity of fetal hypoxia, hypercapnea, acidosis, and hyperlacticemia and the mean velocity of flow in the fetal aorta. Hackett et al. reported that fetuses with absent end diastolic flow in the fetal aorta were significantly more growth retarded and required delivery at an earlier

gestational age than those in whom end diastolic flow was observed.[81] These fetuses were also more likely to suffer perinatal death, necrotizing enterocolitis, and hemorrhage. Absent end diastolic velocity in the umbilical artery has repeatedly been associated with poor perinatal outcome (Fig. 27.7). In a study of 31 fetuses with absent end diastolic velocity in the umbilical artery, Brar and Platt noted that over 80 percent were growth retarded.[82] There were 10 perinatal deaths, for a perinatal mortality rate of 32 percent. Of note, 5 fetuses showed improvement in umbilical artery waveforms in response to bed rest. Brar warned that it appeared premature to intervene in a pregnancy solely on the basis of such abnormal waveforms because antepartum improvement could occur. McGowan et al. reported similar findings in a study of 15 singleton preterm pregnancies evaluated on the day of delivery.[83] Absent end diastolic velocity in the umbilical artery was associated with a high incidence of early delivery, growth retardation, oligohydramnios, pregnancy-induced hypertension, cesarean section for fetal distress, and low Apgar scores. These fetuses usually had evidence of acute or chronic hypoxia.

Can Doppler flow studies be used to predict the pregnancy at risk for fetal growth retardation? In one of the first studies to address this question, Campbell and his colleagues evaluated uterine artery waveforms in 126 consecutive pregnancies during the second trimester.[84] They reported a sensitivity of 68 percent, specificity of 69 percent, positive predictive value of 42 percent, and negative predictive value of 87 percent in identifying pregnancies complicated by growth retardation, uteroplacental insufficiency, and pregnancy-induced hypertension. Steel used continuous wave Doppler ultrasound to evaluate the uteroplacental circulation in 1,014 nulliparous women between 16 and 22 weeks gestation.[85] If the initial Doppler determination was abnormal, a repeat study was performed at 24 weeks gestation. Persistently abnormal waveforms were observed in 118 women, or 12 percent of the study population. Hypertension was significantly more frequent among these women (29/118, 25 percent) than among women with normal Doppler waveforms (45/896, 5 percent). Furthermore, hypertension in women with abnormal waveforms was more likely to be severe: 10 percent had proteinuria and 13 percent demonstrated IUGR.

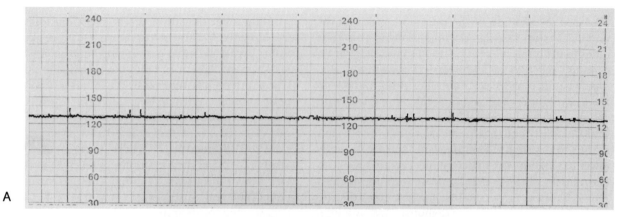

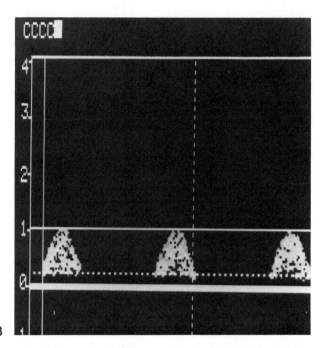

Fig. 27.7 (A) External fetal heart rate tracing, showing a baseline heart rate of 130 bpm with absent variability. (B) Umbilical artery Doppler study revealing absent end diastolic flow. A 25-year-old primigravid patient was seen at 28 weeks 3 days gestation for hypertension and suspected growth retardation. Gestational age had been established by first-trimester ultrasound. The patient's blood pressure was found to be 140/90 mmHg with no edema or proteinuria. Ultrasonography revealed a fetus in a breech presentation with an estimated fetal weight of 650 g, below the tenth percentile for gestational age. Amniotic fluid volume was reduced. Magnesium sulfate was begun, and corticosteroids were administered. On the third hospital day, the fetal heart rate tracing, which was initially normal, showed absent heart rate variability (Fig. A). Doppler flow studies revealed absent end diastolic flow in the umbilical artery (Fig. B). A primary cesarean section was then performed; a 620-g male infant with Apgar scores of 6 at 1 minute and 8 at 5 minutes was delivered. The umbilical artery cord pH was 7.23, with a base excess of −8. The infant was initially intubated but was weaned to room air by the twelfth hour of life. The infant had no significant morbidity.

IUGR was not observed in any patient with normal waveforms. Although the positive predictive value of the test was poor, 10 percent for hypertension with proteinuria, sensitivity was high for hypertension associated with either proteinuria (63 percent) or IUGR (100 percent).

Other investigators have not found the assessment of Doppler waveforms to be of value in screening for pregnancies at risk for growth retardation and hypertensive complications. Benson and Doubilet reviewed 15 studies in which Doppler criteria were used to predict the presence of IUGR.[86] Analysis of the data using a prevalence rate of 10 percent revealed positive predictive values of 17 to 57 percent. These results are not as good as those observed using sonographic estimates of fetal growth. Berkowitz et al. also noted that although the umbilical S/D ratio was abnormal significantly earlier in gestation than the sonographic estimate of fetal weight, sonographic biometry proved to be a more sensitive technique for the prenatal detection of IUGR.[65]

In summary, Doppler velocimetry, particularly of the umbilical artery, may improve our understanding of the pathophysiology of fetal growth retardation and identify the fetus with IUGR at greatest risk for morbidity and mortality.[87] The value of Doppler flow studies in predicting those patients whose pregnancies will subsequently be complicated by preeclampsia and/or fetal growth retardation remains to be determined.

DELIVERY

Proper timing of delivery is often the critical management issue when dealing with the growth-retarded fetus. Frigoletto has emphasized, "The majority of fetal deaths occur after the 36th week of gestation and before labor which leads to the conclusion that many deaths could be prevented by accurate recognition of growth retardation and appropriately timed and conducted intervention."[88] The crux of management is to balance the hazards of prematurity with the threat of intrauterine demise. Careful consideration should be given to the reliability of the information on which the gestational age of the fetus has been established, the fetal growth curve, and the results of antepartum fetal monitoring.

Amniocentesis may be an important adjunct to this decision-making process. Gluck and Kulovich's observation that the stressed fetus may demonstrate advanced pulmonary maturity has been confirmed by several investigators.[89] This advanced maturity is reflected not only by a lecithin/sphingomyelin (L/S) ratio greater than 2.0 before 34 weeks but also by the presence of phosphatidylglycerol (PG) prior to 35 weeks. Amniocentesis, therefore, can give information about fetal stress as well as an indication of the risk for RDS should the fetus require delivery. The L/S ratio may also provide information that allows more accurate dating of the pregnancy. A surprisingly low L/S ratio would suggest an earlier gestational age rather than fetal growth retardation. In cases of symmetrical growth retardation, a late amniocentesis may also be employed to obtain amniotic fluid for a fetal karyotype.

To review, if growth retardation is suspected or anticipated, twice weekly NSTs and daily maternal assessment of fetal activity should be instituted. Ultrasound examinations to assess fetal growth should be scheduled every 2 to 3 weeks. As long as studies show continued fetal head growth and test results remain reassuring, no intervention is required. If the patient fails an NST, a CST or a biophysical profile must follow. If the CST result is positive or the fetal biophysical profile score is 6 with oligohydramnios or 4 or less, delivery should be considered (Ch. 13). An assessment of fetal lung maturity should be made if possible. In the face of a mature L/S ratio and ominous antepartum test results, delivery should be effected. If the patient has an immature L/S ratio and abnormal test findings, then consideration can be given to steroid administration with continuous heart rate monitoring until delivery or until antepartum test results improve. If amniotic fluid cannot be obtained for an L/S ratio as a result of oligohydramnios and the clinical picture supports the diagnosis of severe IUGR, early delivery should be considered. In these difficult cases, the pediatricians who will care for the baby should be included in the decision-making process.

Because a large proportion of growth-retarded infants suffer intrapartum asphyxia, intrapartum management demands continuous fetal heart rate monitoring. Cord blood sampling has demonstrated that these fetuses may exhibit increased lactic acid levels, polycythemia, hypoglycemia, and acidosis before labor.[90] During labor, a tracing without late decelerations is predictive of a good outcome in cases complicated by IUGR. However, with late decelerations, the incidence of asphyxia in growth-retarded infants is far greater than in normally grown infants. Therefore, earlier intervention may be indicated.[91] As many growth-retarded fetuses require preterm delivery, an unfavorable cervix is not uncommon and can preclude internal fetal heart rate monitoring. In the face of an inadequate external tracing, cesarean section may be necessary. Even if the external heart rate tracing is acceptable, the safety of prolonged induction when the fetus is at great risk for intrapartum asphyxia can be questioned.

NEONATAL OUTCOME

Neonatal morbidity must be anticipated when the growth-retarded fetus is delivered (see boxlist, p. 923). These infants suffer more frequently from meconium aspiration than do appropriately grown infants. Gasping in utero in response to asphyxia appears to contribute to this problem. Meconium aspiration is rarely seen before 34 weeks gestation and is, therefore, largely a problem of the mature growth-retarded infant. At delivery, careful suctioning of the nasopharynx and oropharynx with the DeLee catheter decreases the incidence of this complication.[92] Further clearing of the airway can be accomplished at delivery by direct laryngoscopy and aspiration by an experienced pediatrician. Because immediate attention to the many neonatal problems experienced by these infants is essential, a neonatologist should be present in the delivery room when an infant suspected of being growth retarded is to be delivered.

Hypoglycemia is a frequent problem in growth-retarded infants, a result not only of inadequate glycogen reserves secondary to intrauterine malnutrition but also of a gluconeogenic pathway that is less responsive to hypoglycemia than that of the normally grown infant.[93] This metabolic problem is compounded by an increased demand for glucose and

may be further compromised by limited oral intake. Hypoglycemia should be anticipated in all growth-retarded infants and frequent blood glucose monitoring instituted. Hypocalcemia, another well-recognized problem in growth-retarded babies, may be due to relative hypoparathyroidism, a result of acidosis associated with intrauterine asphyxia.[94] Hyperphosphatemia secondary to tissue breakdown may also contribute. Frequent calcium monitoring is essential as symptoms are nonspecific and similar to those associated with hypoglycemia.

Polycythemia is observed three to four times more frequently in the growth-retarded infant than in weight-matched controls. Polycythemia results from hypoxia, which leads to increased production of red blood cells, and from transfer of blood volume from the placental circulation to the fetal circulation in the face of intrauterine asphyxia.[93] Thus, these infants produce more red blood cells that are shunted to them if hypoxia occurs during labor. Polycythemia leads to increased red blood cell breakdown accounting in part for the high incidence of hyperbilirubinemia in these infants. Polycythemia is a criterion for, but does not necessarily lead to, hyperviscosity, which can result in capillary bed sludging and thrombosis. Multiple organ systems can be affected, leading to pulmonary hypertension, cerebral infarction, and necrotizing enterocolitis.

Hyponatremia resulting from impaired renal function is also frequently reported in growth-retarded infants. The renal complications associated with IUGR may be attributed to asphyxia, which can produce central nervous system injury leading to inappropriate antidiuretic hormone (ADH) secretion.[93]

Hypothermia is another common problem for the growth-retarded infant and results from decreased body fat stores secondary to intrauterine malnourishment.[93] Hypothermia, if unrecognized and untreated, contributes to the metabolic deterioration of the already unstable growth-retarded infant.

There is good evidence to suggest that RDS and intraventricular hemorrhage (IVH) occur less frequently in growth-retarded premature infants than in normally grown premature infants of comparable gestational ages. Procianoy and colleagues demonstrated that RDS occurred in 74 percent of appropriately grown infants but was diagnosed in only 5 percent of growth-retarded infants. Similarly, appropriately grown neonates had a 42 percent incidence of IVH hemorrhage, whereas this complication was detected in just 11 percent of growth-retarded infants.[95]

The past two decades have seen tremendous advances in the overall management of the low-birth-weight infant. Obstetricians are more aware of the syndrome of IUGR, and improved techniques for the detection of impaired intrauterine growth and the assessment of well-being are now available. Technology required for the neonatal care of these infants advances each year.

Have improvements in obstetric and pediatric care favorably affected the outcome for the growth-retarded infant? The perinatal mortality rate for those infants who receive optimal intrapartum and neonatal management is decreased when compared to that for age-matched controls who did not have intensive care.[96] The ultimate growth potential for these infants also appears to be good. Although Babson's data in 1970 indicated that only partial "catch-up growth" could be expected in growth-retarded term infants,[97] the degree of catch-up growth observed in several longitudinal studies made since that time suggests that these infants can be expected to have normal growth curves. In the 8-year follow-up of children weighing less than 1,500 g at birth by Kitchen et al., 75 percent of growth-retarded infants achieved a height and weight above the tenth percentile. Of infants whose birth weight fell below the third percentile, 60 percent had reached the twenty-fifth percentile for weight at 8 years. In Kitchen and associates' study, however, 50 percent of the children with small head circumferences still had head circumferences below the tenth percentile at the 8-year follow-up visit in spite of their growth in height and weight.[98]

Similarly, the study of preterm infants with IUGR by Vohr et al. showed a pattern of catch-up to normal levels by 2 years of age.[99] Low studied this same weight group but for only 1 year and confirmed that the differences between the growth-retarded and appropriately grown groups disappeared at 12 months of age.[100] Kumar noted that in infants whose birth weights were less than 1,250 g, at 1 year 46 percent of the growth-retarded infants remained less than the third percentile for weight and 38 percent remained less than the third percentile for height.[101] Perhaps longer follow-up would reveal the catch-up growth that has been observed in other studies. In general, those infants suffering growth retardation near the time of delivery do tend to catch up. However, those neonates with earlier onset and more long-standing growth retardation in utero continue to lag behind.

The issue of long-term neurologic sequelae remains unresolved. In 1972, Fitzhardinge and Stevens, evaluating a group of 96 growth-retarded infants, noted that between 50 percent of males and 36 percent of females had poor school performance and overall 25 percent had minimal cerebral dysfunction. Major neurologic deficits were much less frequent.[102] Other studies have shown low birth weight and short gestation to be risk factors for cerebral palsy. However, the vast majority of children with cerebral palsy are not growth retarded. Commey and Fitzhardinge studied a group of outborn infants, most but not all of whom weighed less than 1,500 g, and found that 49 percent had developmental handicaps at 2 years. Twenty-one percent had major neurologic sequelae. They attributed this poor neurologic outcome to hypoxic insults sustained in the intrapartum or immediate neonatal period.[103] Their study population was admittedly skewed since only the sickest infants were transferred to their care. The large number of severe neurologic deficits observed in this group of infants in whom more than 90 percent had no intrapartum fetal monitoring underscores the tremendous impact that recognition and prevention of intrapartum asphyxia can have on ultimate outcome.

The positive effect of intrapartum surveillance is reflected in the data of Low et al.[100] In a study of 88 growth-retarded infants, they reported no severe neurologic sequelae. They did detect a lag in mental development that was significant in the growth-retarded babies when compared to appropriately grown controls, especially in the group with birth weights less than 2,300 g. This study correlates well with Lipper's data on low-birth-weight babies. She observed that growth-retarded infants with head circumference below the tenth percentile have two to three times the number of serious neurologic sequelae of their normocephalic counterparts.[104] The study by Kumar et al. of infants with a mean birth weight of 1,066 g showed that 30 percent of these very-low-birth-weight growth-retarded premature infants had major neurologic problems.[101]

The pattern that emerges from evaluation of these data emphasizes that neurologic outcome depends on the degree of growth retardation, its time of onset, and the immaturity of the infant at birth. An early intrauterine insult, between 10 to 17 weeks gestation, could limit neuronal cellular multiplication and would obviously have a profound effect on neurologic function.[105] In the third trimester, brain development is characterized by glial multiplication, dendritic arborization, establishment of synaptic connections, and myelinization, all of which continue during the first 2 years of life. Recovery after a period of impaired growth in the third trimester is, therefore, more likely to occur. Thus, the preterm appropriately grown infant has more normal neurologic development and fewer severe neurologic deficits than its preterm growth-retarded counterpart. Developmental milestones and neurologic development of mature infants with IUGR and mature infants of normal birth weight are similar. Presumably, this also reflects heightened physician awareness of the growth-retarded infant that allows detection, appropriate antepartum management, and intrapartum therapy.[106,107] The premature growth-retarded infant suffers from increased susceptibility to intrauterine asphyxia and all of the neonatal complications of the premature, as well as those of the infant with IUGR. If growth retardation is associated with lagging head growth before 26 weeks, even mature infants have significant developmental delay at 4 years of age.[108] Ideally continued improvement in neonatal intensive care and greater familiarity with the complex physiology of these compromised infants will be reflected in a falling incidence of neurologic deficits and more normal neurologic development in the infant with IUGR.

Despite increased awareness of the IUGR syndrome and improved ability to observe intrauterine growth and evaluate fetal well-being in utero, understanding of this disease remains limited. Continued assessment of the underlying physiology and the effi-cacy of therapy are necessary if perinatal morbidity and mortality are to be decreased.

REFERENCES

1. Clifford SH: Postmaturity with placental dysfunction. J Pediatr 44:1, 1954
2. Lubchenco LO, Hansman C, Boyd E: Intrauterine growth in length and head circumference as estimated from live births at gestational ages from 26 to 42 weeks. Pediatrics 37:403, 1966
3. Usher R, McLean F: Intrauterine growth of live-born Caucasian infants at sea level: standards obtained from measurements in 7 dimensions of infants born between 25 and 44 weeks of gestation. J Pediatr 74:901, 1969
4. Battaglia FC, Lubchenco LO: A practical classification of newborn infants by weight and gestational age. J Pediatr 71:159, 1967
5. Babson SG, Behrman RE, Lessel R: Fetal growth: live-born birth weights for gestational age of white middle class infants. Pediatrics 45:937, 1970
6. Gruenwald P: Chronic fetal distress and placental insufficiency. Biol Neonate 5:215, 1963
7. Wolfe HM, Gross TL: Increased risk to the growth retarded fetus. p. 111. In Gross TM, Sokol RJ (eds): Intrauterine Growth Retardation. Year Book Medical Publishers, Chicago, 1989
8. Low JA, Boston RW, Pancham SR: Fetal asphyxia during the intrapartum period in intrauterine growth-retarded infants. Am J Obstet Gynecol 113:351, 1972
9. Ott WJ: The diagnosis of altered fetal growth. Obstet Gynecol Clinics North Am 15:237, 1988
10. Miller HC, Hassanein K: Maternal factors in "fetally malnourished" black newborn infants. Am J Obstet Gynecol 118:62, 1974
11. Daikoku NH, Johnson JWC, Graf C et al: Patterns of intrauterine growth retardation. Obstet Gynecol 54:211, 1979
12. Altman DG, Hytten FE: Assessment of fetal size and fetal growth. p. 111. In Chalmers I, Enkin M, Kearse MJNC (eds): Effective Care in Pregnancy and Childbirth. Vol. 1. Oxford University Press, Oxford, 1989
13. Seeds JW: Impaired fetal growth: definition and clinical diagnosis. Obstet Gynecol 64:303, 1984
14. Goldenberg RL, Cutter GR, Hoffman HJ et al: Intrauterine growth retardation: standards for diagnosis. Am J Obstet Gynecol 161:271, 1989
15. Dawes GS: Size at birth. p. 1. CIBA Foundation Sym-

posium 27. Associated Scientific Publishers, Amsterdam, 1974

16. Eydoux P, Choiset A, LePorrier N et al: Chromosomal prenatal diagnosis: study of 936 cases of intrauterine abnormalities after ultrasound assessment. Prenatal Diagn 9:255, 1989

17. Wald NJ, Cuckle HS, Boreham J et al: Birth weight of infants with spina bifida cystica. Br J Obstet Gynaecol 87:578, 1980

18. Spiers PS: Does growth retardation predispose the fetus to congenital malformation? Lancet 1:312, 1982

19. Pedersen JF, Molsted-Pedersen L: Early fetal growth delay detected by ultrasound marks increased risk of congenital malformation in diabetic pregnancy. Br Med J 283:269, 1981

20. Petersen MB, Pedersen SA, Greisen G et al: Early growth delay in diabetic pregnancy: relation to psychomotor development at age 4. Br Med J 296:598, 1988

21. Hoogland HJ, de Haan J, Martin CB Jr: Placental size during early pregnancy and fetal outcome: a preliminary report of a sequential ultrasonographic study. Am J Obstet Gynecol 138:441, 1980

22. Robinson L, Grau P, Crandall BF: Pregnancy outcomes after increasing maternal serum alpha-fetoprotein levels. Obstet Gynecol 74:17, 1989

23. Baur R: Morphometry of the placental exchange area. Adv Anat Embryol Cell Biol 53:3, 1977

24. Chapman MG, Furness ET, Jones WR et al: Significance of the ultrasound location of placental site in early pregnancy. Br J Obstet Gynaecol 86:846, 1979

25. Gruenwald P: Growth of the human fetus. II: Abnormal growth in twins and infants of mothers with diabetes, hypertension, or isoimmunization. Am J Obstet Gynecol 94:1120, 1966

26. Houlton MCC, Marivate M, Philpott RH: The prediction of fetal growth retardation in twin pregnancy. Br J Obstet Gynaecol 88:264, 1981

27. Long PA, Abell DA, Beischer NA: Fetal growth retardation and preeclampsia. Br J Obstet Gynaecol 87:13, 1980

28. Katz AE, Davison JM, Hayslett JP et al: Pregnancy in women with kidney disease. Kidney Int 18:192, 1980

29. Zulman JI, Talal N, Hoffman GS et al: Problems associated with the management of pregnancies in patients with systemic lupus erythematosus. J Rheumatol 7:327, 1980

30. DeWolf F, Brosens I, Renaer M: Fetal growth retardation and the maternal arterial supply of the human placenta in the absence of sustained hypertension. Br J Obstet Gynaecol 87:678, 1980

31. Wladimiroff JW, Wijngaard JAGW, Degani S et al: Cerebral and umbilical arterial blood flow velocity waveforms in normal and growth-retarded pregnancies. Obstet Gynecol 69:705, 1987

32. Veille JC, Kanaan C: Duplex Doppler ultrasonographic evaluation of the fetal renal artery in normal and abnormal fetuses. Am J Obstet Gynecol 161:1502, 1989

33. Pritchard JA, Scott DE, Whalley PJ et al: The effects of maternal sickle cell hemoglobinopathies and sickle cell trait on reproductive performance. Am J Obstet Gynecol 117:662, 1973

34. Smith CA: Effects of maternal undernutrition upon the newborn infant in Holland (1944–1945). Am J Obstet Gynecol 30:229, 1947

35. Lechtig A, Yarbrough C, Delgado H et al: Effect of moderate maternal malnutrition on the placenta. Am J Obstet Gynecol 123:191, 1975

36. Economides DL, Nicolaides KH: Blood glucose and oxygen tension levels in small-for-gestational-age fetuses. Am J Obstet Gynecol 160:385, 1989

37. Khouzami VA, Ginsburg DS, Daikoku NH et al: The glucose tolerance test as a means of identifying intrauterine growth retardation. Am J Obstet Gynecol 139:423, 1981

38. Langer O, Damus K, Maiman M et al: A link between relative hypoglycemia-hypoinsulinemia during oral glucose tolerance tests and intrauterine growth retardation. Am J Obstet Gynecol 155:711, 1986

39. Haworth JC, Ellestad-Sayed JJ, King J et al: Fetal growth retardation in cigarette-smoking mothers is not due to decreased maternal food intake. Am J Obstet Gynecol 137:719, 1980

40. Mills JL, Graubard BI, Harley EE et al: Maternal alcohol consumption and birth weight: how much drinking during pregnancy is safe? JAMA 252:1875, 1984

41. Little BB, Snell LM, Klein VR et al: Cocaine abuse during pregnancy: maternal and fetal implications. Obstet Gynecol 74:157, 1989

42. Lobl M, Welcher DW, Mellits ED: Maternal age and intellectual function of offspring. Johns Hopkins Med J 128:347, 1971

43. Berkowitz GS, Skovron ML, Lapinski RH et al: Delayed childbearing and the outcome of pregnancy. N Engl J Med 322:659, 1990

44. Miller H, Merritt TA: Fetal Growth in Humans. Year Book Medical Publishers, Chicago, 1979

45. Wolfe HM, Gross TL, Sokol RJ: Recurrent small for gestational age birth: perinatal risks and outcomes. Am J Obstet Gynecol 157:288, 1987

46. Galbraith RS, Karchman EJ, Piercy WN et al: The clin-

ical prediction of intrauterine growth retardation. Am J Obstet Gynecol 133:231, 1979

47. Tejani NA: Recurrence of intrauterine growth retardation. Obstet Gynecol 59:329, 1982

48. Tejani N, Mann LI: Diagnosis and management of the small for gestational age fetus. p. 943. In Frigoletto FD (ed): Clinical Obstetrics and Gynecology. Harper & Row, Hagerstown, MD, 1977

49. Belizan JM, Villar J, Nardin JC et al: Diagnosis of intrauterine growth retardation by a simple clinical method: measurement of uterine height. Am J Obstet Gynecol 131:643, 1978

50. Persson B, Stangenberg M, Lunell NO et al: Prediction of size of infants at birth by measurement of symphysis fundus height. Br J Obstet Gynaecol 93:206, 1986

51. Campbell S, Dewhurst CJ: Diagnosis of the small-for-dates fetus by serial ultrasonic cephalometry. Lancet 2:1002, 1971

52. Crane JP, Kopta MM: Prediction of intrauterine growth retardation via ultrasonically measured head/abdominal circumference ratios. Obstet Gynecol 54:597, 1979

53. Seeds JW: Impaired fetal growth: ultrasonic evaluation and clinical management. Obstet Gynecol 64:577, 1984

54. Hadlock FP, Deter RL, Harrist RB et al: A date-independent predictor of intrauterine growth retardation: femur length/abdominal circumference ratio. AJR 141:979, 1983

55. Manning FA, Hill LM, Platt LD: Qualitative amniotic fluid volume determination by ultrasound: antepartum detection of intrauterine growth retardation. Am J Obstet Gynecol 193:254, 1981

56. Manning FA, Lange IR, Morrison I, Harman CR: Determination of fetal health: methods for antepartum and intrapartum fetal assessment. Curr Probl Obstet Gynecol 7:1, 1983

57. Kazzi GM, Gross TL, Sokol RJ et al: Detection of intrauterine growth retardation: a new use for sonographic placental grading. Am J Obstet Gynecol 145:733, 1983

58. Benson CB, Doubilet PM, Saltzman DH: Intrauterine growth retardation: predictive value of US criteria for antenatal diagnosis. Radiology 160:415, 1986

59. Reece EA, Goldstein I, Pilu G et al: Fetal cerebellar growth unaffected by intrauterine growth retardation: a new parameter for prenatal diagnosis. Am J Obstet Gynecol 157:632, 1987

60. Hill LM, Guzick D, Rivello D et al: The transverse cerebellar diameter cannot be used to assess gestational age in the small for gestational age fetus. Obstet Gynecol 75:329, 1990

61. Sabbagha RE, Minogue J, Tamura RK et al: Estimation of birth weight by use of ultrasonographic formulas targeted to large-, appropriate-, and small-for-gestational-age fetuses. Am J Obstet Gynecol 160:854, 1989

62. Guidetti DA, Divon MY, Braverman JJ et al: Sonographic estimates of fetal weight in the intrauterine growth retardation population. Am J Perinatol 6:457, 1989

63. Divon MY, Guidetti DA, Braverman JJ et al: Intrauterine growth retardation—a prospective study of the diagnostic value of real-time sonography combined with umbilical artery flow velocimetry. Obstet Gynecol 72:611, 1988

64. Hassan MM, Bottoms SF, Mariona FG et al: The use of clinical, biochemical, and ultrasound parameters for the diagnosis of intrauterine growth retardation. Am J Perinatol 4:19, 1987

65. Berkowitz GS, Chitkara U, Rosenberg J et al: Sonographic estimation of fetal weight and Doppler analysis of umbilical artery velocimetry in the prediction of intrauterine growth retardation: a prospective study. Am J Obstet Gynecol 158:1149, 1988

66. Nicolaides KH, Bradley RJ, Soothill PW et al: Maternal oxygen therapy for intrauterine growth retardation. Lancet 1:942, 1987

67. Moe N: Anticoagulant therapy in the prevention of placental infarction and perinatal death. Obstet Gynecol 58:481, 1981

68. Hobbins JC, Berkowitz RL, Grannum P: Diagnosis and antepartum management of intrauterine growth retardation. J Reprod Med 21:319, 1978

69. Grannum PAT: Ultrasonic measurements for diagnosis. p. 123. In Gross TM, Sokol RJ (eds): Intrauterine Growth Retardation. Year Book Medical Publishers, Chicago, 1989

70. Flynn AM, Kelly J, O'Conor M: Unstressed antepartum cardiotocography in the management of the fetus suspected of growth retardation. Br J Obstet Gynaecol 86:106, 1979

71. Visser GHA, Sadovsky G, Nicolaides KH: Antepartum heart rate patterns in small-for-gestational-age third-trimester fetuses: correlations with blood gas values obtained at cordocentesis. Am J Obstet Gynecol 162:698, 1990

72. Pazos R, Vuolo K, Aladjem S et al: Association of spontaneous fetal heart rate decelerations during antepar-

tum nonstress testing and intrauterine growth retardation. Am J Obstet Gynecol 144:574, 1982

73. Gabbe SG, Freeman RD, Goebelsmann U: Evaluation of the contraction stress test before 33 weeks' gestation. Obstet Gynecol 52:649, 1978

74. Lin CC, Devoe LD, River P et al: Oxytocin challenge test and intrauterine growth retardation. Am J Obstet Gynecol 140:282, 1981

75. Matthews DD: Maternal assessment of fetal activity in small-for-dates infants. Obstet Gynecol 45:488, 1975

76. Giles WB, Trudinger BJ, Baird PJ: Fetal umbilical artery flow velocity waveforms and placental resistance: pathological correlation. Br J Obstet Gynaecol 92:31, 1985

77. Rochelson B, Kaplan C, Guzman E et al: A quantitative analysis of placental vasculature in the third-trimester fetus with autosomal trisomy. Obstet Gynecol 75:59, 1990

78. Fok RY, Pavlova Z, Benirschke K et al: The correlation of arterial lesions with umbilical artery Doppler velocimetry in the placentas of small-for-dates pregnancies. Obstet Gynecol 75:578, 1990

79. Schulman H: The clinical implications of Doppler ultrasound analysis of the uterine and umbilical arteries. Am J Obstet Gynecol 157:889, 1987

80. Soothill PW, Bilardo CM, Nicolaides KH et al: Relation of fetal hypoxia in growth retardation to mean blood velocity in the fetal aorta. Lancet 2:118, 1986

81. Hackett GA, Campbell S, Gamsu H et al: Doppler studies in the growth retarded fetus and prediction of neonatal necrotising enterocolitis, haemorrhage, and neonatal morbidity. Br Med J 294:13, 1987

82. Brar HS, Platt LD: Antepartum improvement of abnormal umbilical artery velocimetry: does it occur? Am J Obstet Gynecol 160:36, 1989

83. McCowan LM, Erskine LA, Ritchie K: Umbilical artery Doppler blood flow studies in the preterm, small for gestational age fetus. Am J Obstet Gynecol 156:655, 1987

84. Campbell S, Pearce JMF, Hackett G et al: Qualitative assessment of uteroplacental blood flow: early screening test for high risk pregnancies. Obstet Gynecol 68:649, 1986

85. Steel SA, Pearce JM, McParland P et al: Early Doppler ultrasound screening in prediction of hypertensive disorders of pregnancy. Lancet 335:1548, 1990

86. Benson CB, Doubilet PM: Doppler criteria for intrauterine growth retardation: predictive values. J Ultrasound Med 7:655, 1988

87. Berkowitz GS, Mehalek KE, Chitkara U et al: Doppler umbilical velocimetry in the prediction of adverse outcome in pregnancies at risk for intrauterine growth retardation. Obstet Gynecol 71:742, 1988

88. Frigoletto FD: Evaluation and management of deferred fetal growth. p. 922. In Frigoletto FD (ed): Clinical Obstetrics and Gynecology. Harper & Row, Hagerstown, MD, 1977

89. Gluck L, Kulovich MV: Lecithin/sphingomyelin ratios in amniotic fluid in normal and abnormal pregnancy. Am J Obstet Gynecol 115:539, 1973

90. Soothill PW, Nicolaides KH, Campbell S: Prenatal asphyxia, hyperlacticaemia, hypoglycaemia, and erythroblastosis in growth retarded fetuses. Br Med J 294:1051, 1987

91. Lin C-C, Moawad AH, Rosenow PJ et al: Acid-base characteristics of fetuses with intrauterine growth retardation during labor and delivery. Am J Obstet Gynecol 137:573, 1980

92. Carson BS, Losey RW, Bowes WA Jr et al: Combined obstetric and pediatric approach to prevent meconium aspiration syndrome. Am J Obstet Gynecol 126:712, 1976

93. Oh W: Considerations in neonates with intrauterine growth retardation. p. 989. In Frigoletto FD (ed): Clinical Obstetrics and Gynecology. Harper & Row, Hagerstown, MD, 1977

94. Tsang RC, Oh W: Neonatal hypocalcemia in low birth-weight infants. Pediatrics 45:773, 1970

95. Procianoy RS, Garcia-Prats FA, Adams JM et al: Hyaline membrane disease and intraventricular haemorrhage in small for gestational age infants. Arch Dis Child 55:502, 1980

96. Kitchen WH, Richards A, Ryan MM et al: A longitudinal study of very low-birthweight infants. II: Results of controlled trial of intensive care and incidence of handicaps. Dev Med Child Neurol 21:582, 1979

97. Babson SG: Growth of low-birthweight infants. J Pediatr 77:11, 1970

98. Kitchen WH, McDougass AB, Naylor FD: A longitudinal study of very low-birthweight infants. III: Distance growth at eight years of age. Dev Med Child Neurol 22:1633, 1980

99. Vohr BR, Oh W, Rosenfield AG et al: The preterm small-for-gestational age infant: a two-year follow-up study. Am J Obstet Gynecol 133:425, 1979

100. Low JA, Galbraith RS, Muir D et al: Intrauterine growth retardation: a preliminary report of long-term morbidity. Am J Obstet Gynecol 130:534, 1978

101. Kumar SP, Anday EK, Sacks LM et al: Follow-up studies of very low birthweight infants (1,250 grams or

less) born and treated within a perinatal center. Pediatrics 66:438, 1980

102. Fitzhardinge PM, Steven EM: The small-for-date infant. II: Neurological and intellectual sequelae. Pediatrics 50:50, 1972

103. Commey JOO, Fitzhardinge PM: Handicap in the preterm small-for-gestational age infant. J Pediatr 94:779, 1979

104. Lipper E, Lee K-S, Gartner LM et al: Determinants of neurobehavioral outcome in low birthweight infants. Pediatrics 67:502, 1981

105. Dobbing J: The later development of the brain and its vulnerability. p. 565. In Davis JA, Dobbing J (eds): Scientific Foundations of Paediatrics. WB Saunders, Philadelphia, 1974

106. Breart G, Poisson-Salomon A-S: Intrauterine growth retardation and mental handicap: epidemiological evidence. Bailliere's Clin Obstet Gynaecol 2:91, 1988

107. Wennergren M, Wennergren G, Vilbergsson G: Obstetric characteristics and neonatal performance in a four-year small for gestational age population. Obstet Gynecol 72:615, 1988

108. Fancourt R, Campbell S, Harvey D et al: Follow-up study of small-for-dates babies. Br Med J 1:1435, 1976

109. Chudleigh P, Pearce JM: Obstetric Ultrasound. Churchill Livingstone, Edinburgh, 1986

110. DiGaetano AF, Gabbe SG: Intrauterine growth retardation. In Leventhal JM (ed): Current Problems in Obstetrics and Gynecology. Year Book Medical Publishers, Chicago, 1983

Chapter 28

Prolonged Pregnancy

Roger K. Freeman and David C. Lagrew, Jr.

Post-term or postdate pregnancy is a common problem facing those who practice obstetrics. Previously, the diagnosis of postdate pregnancy was often the result of poor dating. Today, there are fewer postdate patients because of better dating through the use of first and second trimester ultrasound. Because this group now contains fewer patients with poor dating, these patients as a whole are at higher risk for complications associated with post-term pregnancy.

Comprehensive management of postdate pregnancy involves both fetal testing and consideration for delivery, with the choice for each individual pregnancy dependent on several clinical factors. If the management choice is fetal testing, there are different methods available for selection. If delivery is chosen, the clinician must determine the timing, route, and method. This chapter will address specific problems related to intrapartum management, examine neonatal issues that pose special problems for the pediatrician and neonatologist, and develop an approach to the management of these challenging and complex clinical dilemmas.

BACKGROUND

Post-term pregnancy has not always been of universal concern. Until the development of accurate dating techniques there was controversy over whether it was physiologically possible for pregnancy to exceed the forty-second week. Despite a description of postmaturity by Ballantyne as early as the turn of the century,[1] the American medical community viewed the problem with less concern than the European. As recently as the early 1960s, American obstetricians were skeptical of McClure-Brown's data showing a twofold increase in fetal mortality when the patient reached 42 weeks gestation.[2] Conversely, American pediatricians agreed more with the British position that post-term pregnancy presented fetal danger, in part, because of Clifford's postmaturity classification system (1952), which helped define the degree of affliction these children suffered.[3] The accumulation of other pediatric data supported Clifford's conclusions,[4] and gradually evidence began to suggest that both fetus and neonate were at increased risk. In the late 1960s and 1970s, the American obstetric literature recognized these increased risks, and with the advent of ultrasound dating, it became clear that gestations could truly exceed 42 weeks.

British authors recommended routine induction of labor between 42 and 43 weeks gestation to prevent poor outcome. They demonstrated beneficial perinatal results from such aggressive management.[2] Subsequent to this recommendation, investigators attempted without success to demonstrate the efficacy of routine inductions. A large study by Lucas et al., involving more than 60,000 post-term pregnancies, did not show improvement in fetal and neonatal outcome from routine induction.[5] Other studies suggested that elective induction increased the cesarean section rate.[6] During this time, however, the fetus could not be evaluated prior to or during labor; therefore, the risks of induction were imposed on many fetuses with inadequate uteroplacental reserve. In addition, fetuses with uteroplacental insufficiency and oligohydramnios underwent prolonged inductions without intrapartum monitoring. Some researchers theorized that the better statistical results in Great Britain were actually the result of closer intrapartum attention with frequent auscultation of the fetal heart rate by nurse/midwives during labor.

DEFINITION AND INCIDENCE

Most authors define a postdate or post-term pregnancy as that which has reached 42 weeks of amenorrhea. Note that this definition relates to the length of the pregnancy. The incidence of perinatal mortality increases after 40 weeks gestation and rises twofold by 42 weeks gestation, making this an appropriate point for concern (Fig. 28.1).[2]

The appropriate diagnosis of post-term pregnancy depends on accurate dating. Approximately 50 percent of patients deliver by their estimated date of confinement, and about 35 to 40 percent deliver within the following 2 weeks (Fig. 28.2). Saito et al. estimate that two-thirds of patients thought to be postdate from menstrual history actually deliver at normal ovulatory ages.[7] Rayburn et al. calculate the incidence of patients reaching 42 weeks gestation as varying from 3 to 12 percent.[8] With accurate gestational age estimation, the lower range is more appropriate.[8] Early prenatal examination and ultrasound clearly increase the probability of accurate dating.

Morbidity and Mortality

The rate of maternal, fetal, and neonatal complications increases exponentially with gestational age.[2-4] The primary maternal risk is cesarean section, with its increased incidence of postpartum infection, hemorrhage from uterine atony, prolonged hospitalization, wound complications, and pulmonary emboli. Eden et al. found the cesarean section rate more than doubled when passing the forty-second week compared to gestations at 38 to 40 weeks.[9] He attributed this primarily to the incidence of cephalopelvic disproportion resulting from larger infants. Some cesarean sections are due to the attempted induction of patients with unripe cervices. Of note, few postdate cesarean sections are performed for fetal distress, the overall incidence of fetal distress being minimally elevated over the term population.[10]

Maternal complications include trauma and postpartum hemorrhage from the vaginal delivery of large babies.[11] Vaginal side wall and cervical lacerations and fourth degree extensions are all more common with instrumented deliveries of macrosomic infants. These complications carry the potential for urinary retention, fistula formation, hemorrhage, infection, and wound breakdown.

Neonatal complications from the postdate pregnancy include postmaturity with placental insufficiency, birth trauma from macrosomia, and meconium aspiration syndrome.[11a] Each of these may result in acute and chronic injury to the child. Although the incidence of fetal demise has declined with improved perinatal management, perinatal mortality increases past term.[12] While the attendant risks have been lowered in postdate pregnancy, they have not been eliminated.

Most early work in postdate pregnancy focused on the poorly grown postmature infant, the incidence of which reaches 10 percent by the forty-third week.[8] Postmaturity represents the clinical condition of the infant in a prolonged gestation. Clifford described the postmature fetus as fragile, withered, and meconium stained with long nails. These fetuses are at increased risk for intrauterine death. The postmature neonate suffers hypoglycemia, heat instability, and meconium aspiration.[3] Growth retardation subsequent to postmaturity is the result of uteroplacental insufficiency from a small, aging, deteriorating placenta.[11] First the placenta deprives the fetus of support for anabolic processes. Fetal weight is reduced as the fetus uses energy stores in the adipose tissue and liver. Diminished fetal plasma volume leads to oligohydramnios. With further deterioration the placenta loses respiratory function, and the fetus faces asphyxial damage with possible stillbirth.

Fortunately, long-term problems appear to arise less often with postmaturity than other forms of

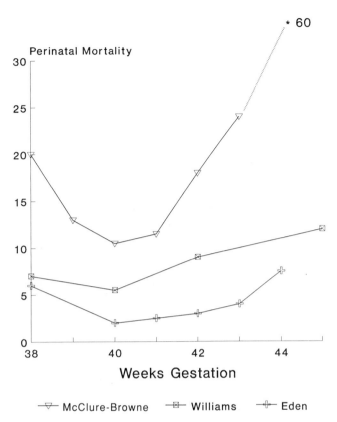

Fig. 28.1 Comparison of perinatal mortality rates versus gestational age through the past three decades. (McClure-Browne[2] data collected in 1958, Williams[57] in 1970–1976, and Eden[6] in 1983–1985.)

growth retardation.[12] Mannino reported that these infants regain normal weight quickly and exhibit few long-term neurologic problems.[12] Unlike the deprivation of other forms of fetal dysmaturity, postmaturity has a rapid onset and is of short duration.

Although fetal growth can cease with postmaturity, a number of fetuses, particularly males, continue growing and exceed 4,000 g (Fig. 28.3). Secher et al.[13] showed that most infants continue interval growth after 40 weeks. Continuing growth in a longer gestation leads to macrosomia. About 25 to 30 percent of post-term neonates weigh more than 4,000 g, a percentage rate that is three times greater than that of term newborns.[9,14] Large infants frequently undergo prolonged labors and difficult deliveries and have an increased risk of birth trauma. The incidence of shoulder dystocia reaches 1.9 times that of average

size infants.[9] Macrosomic infants are also subject to asphyxia. Callenbach and Hall found that long-term neurologic damage was as prevalent in larger post-term infants as in dysmature post-term infants.[15] This differs from data presented by Shime, who suggests that poor neurologic outcome is more likely in small infants.[16] Collectively, these data support the contention that antenatal surveillance is necessary in all post-term pregnancies regardless of growth.

The post-term infant is likely to have meconium stained fluid and be at risk for meconium aspiration syndrome. The 25 to 30 percent incidence of meconium staining is about double the incidence at term.[9,14] Meconium passage results from increased hypoxic stimulation to the parasympathetic system or is a function of the mere presence of a more mature, active vagal reflex. The diminished amniotic fluid

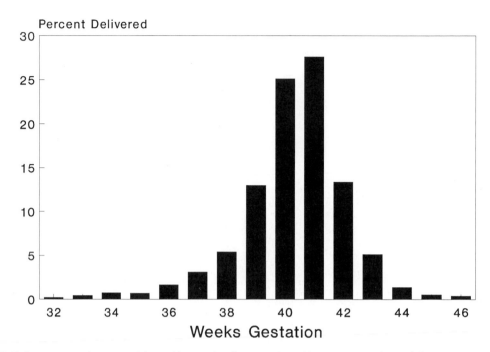

Fig. 28.2 Percentage of patients delivered by weeks of amenorrhea. More recent studies with better gestational age assessment have decreased the percentage of 42 weeks and beyond to less than 10 percent. (Data from Treloar et al.[58])

causes the meconium to be thicker and more likely to obstruct airways. Aspiration into the alveoli can cause significant respiratory embarrassment and death.

MANAGEMENT

Recent changes in obstetric care have affected the management recommendations of post-term pregnancy. Post-term pregnancies identified by accurate gestational age assessment are more likely to have complications. Poorly dated patients diluted risks in previous studies. Obstetric management must reflect this higher risk and warrants an aggressive delivery policy and fetal surveillance. The increased number of large infants also changes management recommendations. Many authors feel that induction of labor prevents further growth and fetal deprivation.[17] Although studies of routine induction have shown no improvement in maternal or neonatal outcome, most

were conducted before the development of improved techniques for cervical ripening.

Diagnosis

The accurate diagnosis of a post-term pregnancy can be made only by proper dating. Accurate diagnosis allows concentration of management on the highest-risk patients. A major problem of determining gestational age is that all methods of estimating it lose accuracy in the third trimester, when fetal growth diminishes. Therefore, we must determine an accurate estimated delivery date before the third trimester. Since we cannot predict those women who will be undelivered by 42 weeks gestation, we must accurately date *all* prenatal patients.

The obstetrician should review clinical parameters in all patients since they are helpful in establishing gestational age at minimal cost. Anderson et al. found that last menstrual period was the best clinical predictor of gestational age.[18] Seventy-one percent of his

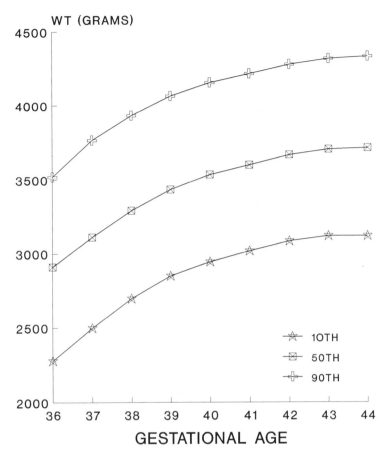

Fig. 28.3 Birthweight for male fetuses in California 1970–1976. Note the increasing numbers of infants greater than 4,000 g after term. (From Williams et al.,[57] with permission.)

patients could recall the exact date of the last period, 25 percent an approximate date, and 4 percent no date. Estimate gestational age by comparing the regularity, date, amount, and length of menses. The use of oral contraceptives may explain delayed ovulation. An early pelvic examination may be helpful in confirming these dates. Other clinical parameters include date of first pregnancy test, first fetal heart tones (11 to 12 weeks with Doppler, 19 to 20 weeks with fetoscope), fundal height at umbilicus (20 weeks), and quickening.

Ultrasound has become the gold standard for the determination of gestational age. Routine first and second trimester ultrasound decreases the incidence of post-term pregnancy.[19] Ultrasound is clearly bene-

ficial in patients without known or reliable clinical data. In patients with regular menses, basal body temperature records, or timed insemination, ultrasound is of less value.

Ultrasound is most accurate in early gestation. Measurement of crown–rump length in early pregnancy correlates with accurate dates within 3 to 5 days.[20] The crown–rump length becomes less accurate in determining gestational age after 12 weeks because the fetus begins to curve. Crane showed that second trimester biparietal diameter and femur length measurements were as predictive of gestational age as late crown–rump length.[21] A screening ultrasound at 16 to 18 weeks also allows a review of fetal anatomy. In the second trimester, the accuracy of ultrasound is

±1.5 weeks. The most cost-effective ultrasound dating, therefore, is between 16 to 20 weeks.

Sonographic accuracy lessens in the third trimester as bone growth rate decreases. At this gestational age, ultrasound predicts gestational age only within 3 to 4 weeks; therefore, it is of little help in confirming gestational age unless other dating parameters are poor. Never use a third trimester ultrasound to disprove a postdate pregnancy. Such dating may cause inappropriate intervention or inaction leading to poor outcome.

The Choice: Expectant Management versus Induction of Labor

The first major decision in management depends on the certainty of the dates. The accuracy of the estimation of gestational age is important when planning intervention. Treat patients with unsure dates in a less aggressive fashion when considering delivery if the cervix is not favorable for induction. In these patients, the same protocol for antenatal surveillance should be followed as in well-dated pregnancies. There are two basic schemes of management for well-dated post-term patients (Fig. 28.4).

Patients with a ripe cervix may benefit from the induction of labor. However, these cases constitute a minority of postdate pregnancies. Harris et al. found that only 8.2 percent of pregnancies at 42 weeks had a ripe cervix as judged by a Bishop score above 7.[22] There are two major reasons for inducing labor in patients with a ripe cervix. First, some fetuses continue growing after term, become macrosomic, and are at increased risk for cephalopelvic disproportion and birth trauma. Second, although antenatal surveillance with appropriate methods markedly reduces stillbirths, it is not perfect. In 1/1,000 patients, antepartum monitoring fails to predict poor outcome.[23] Therefore, if the cervix is ripe, delivery probably provides the safest alternative for both mother and baby. Induction with a ripe cervix is appropriate after 41 weeks gestation has passed and spontaneous labor has not ensued.

With confirmed dates and an unripe cervix, there are two alternatives in management. The most established method is to initiate antepartum surveillance while awaiting spontaneous labor[24] and/or spontaneous cervical ripening. The other approach is to administer prostaglandin gel for cervical ripening and proceed with induction.[25]

There are problems with both management schemes that must be considered. The purpose of expectant management and testing is to await cervical ripening or spontaneous labor. However, clinical trials with expectant management conversely show an increase in the cesarean section rate compared to that at term.[23] In comparison to cervical ripening with prostaglandin, Dyson found that expectant management has a higher overall cesarean rate.[25] He attributed this finding to the increasing incidence of larger babies as well as fetal distress.

Although prostaglandin ripening of the cervix has not been extensively studied in the postdate pregnancy, it also appears to have shortcomings. Dyson et al. found that 50 percent of patients in whom the gel did not ripen the cervix required cesarean delivery.[25] In addition, uterine hyperstimulation can occasionally be seen with prostaglandin gel. Therefore, fetuses with worrisome antenatal surveillance are poor candidates for ripening. Other factors may also play a role. Boyd et al. found uterine dysfunction and an increased cesarean section rate in primigravid post-term pregnancies, independent of the induction of labor and the size of the infant.[26]

Cervical Ripening with Prostaglandin

Routine induction with oxytocin in post-term patients does not appear to improve outcome because an unripe cervix is present in up to 80 percent of patients reaching 42 weeks gestation.[22,27] Prostaglandin E_2 gel applied locally to the cervix produces softening, dilatation, and shortening. The clinical effects are shortened labor, reduced number of failed inductions, and decreased need for artificial amniotomy.[25] Dyson used both 3.0-mg intravaginal and 0.5-mg intracervical prostaglandin E_2 gel in post-term gestations. He randomized 302 patients to prostaglandin ripening versus expectant management with antenatal surveillance. The gel group delivered on average 4 days sooner and had less meconium stained fluid, meconium aspiration syndrome, dysmaturity, and fetal distress. The nulliparous patients also had a decreased cesarean section rate. Although there were fewer macrosomic infants (19 versus 28.2 percent), this difference was not statistically significant. The

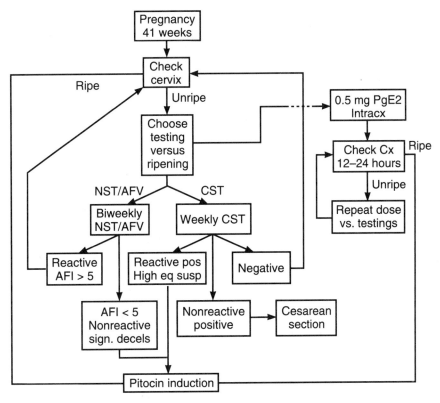

Fig. 28.4 Postdate pregnancy management flow chart. The scheme depicts the various decision making processes involved in the management of the post-term pregnancy with respect to delivery. The decision whether to use intracervical prostaglandin should be based on clinical data regarding patient safety and ripeness of the cervix. It has been our practice to attempt a trial of induction in well-dated pregnancies at 43 weeks gestation.

efficacy of this method is being studied in larger multi-institutional trials.[17]

The protocol for prostaglandin ripening may be used in patients with an unripe cervix at 41 weeks gestation. The gel is given on the afternoon or evening before the scheduled induction. Before administration, obtain a reassuring fetal heart rate and uterine activity pattern. Ripening with prostaglandin may not be advisable if there are abnormal decelerations, elevated baseline fetal heart rate, or poor variability. Another contraindication is frequent or prolonged uterine contractions. Carefully place 0.5 mg of prostaglandin E_2 gel intracervically after checking the cervix. Observe the patient on the fetal heart rate monitor for approximately 2 hours or until uterine activity has subsided. Fifteen percent of patients in Dyson's study began spontaneous labor and did not require

oxytocin induction. The next morning, oxytocin induction may be initiated with standard protocols if the cervix has ripened. If the cervix remains unfavorable, a second dose of prostaglandin may be considered. Expectant management with fetal surveillance is another option at this time.

Expectant Management with Antenatal Surveillance

Most management schemes require some form of antenatal surveillance of fetal well-being. There is no uniform agreement about the best method or time to initiate testing. Make your individual decision on the basis of which test has the lowest failure rate, is most cost-effective, and has a reasonable intervention rate in your population.

Previously most testing schemes have suggested beginning testing at 42 weeks gestation since this represented the highest-risk population and a manageable proportion of patients. The general trend in the United States has been to begin testing during 41 weeks gestation. This practice appears to be reasonable in light of the increased incidence of perinatal mortality after 40 weeks gestation. Porto et al. demonstrated an increase in positive contraction stress test results from 40 to 42 weeks gestation.[28] Since cost-effectiveness becomes an issue, fetal movement charting may be a reasonable alternative prior to the forty-first week.

Most antepartum testing in the United States is done with the nonstress test (NST). This test is simple and brief and requires relatively inexpensive equipment. The NST yields few equivocal results and interventions are rarely necessary for abnormal test results.[29] The major concern about this modality is falsely reassuring results. Weekly NSTs appear to have a false negative rate of 6.1/1,000 with false negatives defined as a stillbirth within a week of a reassuring test result.[30] Boehm et al. decreased the false negative rate by twice weekly testing from 6.1 to 1.9/1,000.[30] Randomized studies have failed to show that following patients with a weekly NST is better than having no fetal surveillance at all.[31,32] Therefore, to improve detection of the compromised fetus, perform NSTs twice weekly.

Consider spontaneous decelerations significant. Phelan et al. demonstrated that most poor perinatal outcome was confined to patients with decelerations on their NST.[33] Small et al. showed improvement in fetal and neonatal outcome with the induction of labor for significant decelerations on a NST.[34] Unfortunately, this aggressive policy increased the intervention rate from 0.97 to 31.8 percent.

Another surveillance choice is the contraction stress test (CST). The major benefit of the CST is that negative results appear to predict fetal well-being for 7 days. Weekly CSTs are effective in preventing stillbirth and have a false negative rate of only 0.71/1,000.[23] The CST is performed with inexpensive equipment and has an acceptable intervention rate for an abnormal test result of 10.4 percent.[10] Nipple stimulation techniques have significantly reduced testing time while not sacrificing accuracy.[35] The major problem of the CST is the high rate of equivocal results.[23,29]

The major benefit of the CST for primary surveillance in the post-term pregnancy is that after a reactive negative CST result the patient does not require repeat testing for 7 days. In contrast, patients with equivocal test results require repeat testing in 24 hours. The equivocal test result is the major disadvantage of the CST since up to 35.5 percent of tests have equivocal results in post-term patients.[10] For positive and highly suspicious test results, attempted delivery is indicated. If the CST result is reactive but positive, attempt a trial of labor, since up to 66 percent of such patients are delivered vaginally.[23] Should the CST result be nonreactive and positive, the patient should have constant electronic fetal monitoring while preparations are made for cesarean section. If the fetus remains nonreactive during monitoring, perform a cesarean section.[23]

With clinically significant oligohydramnios, cord compression, manifested by variable decelerations, may occur. Variable decelerations should be evaluated by an estimate of amniotic fluid volume.

The introduction of real-time ultrasound has provided a new vista of fetal biophysical observations to assess fetal status. Manning and others have used the combination of fetal movement, fetal tone, amniotic fluid volume, fetal breathing, and heart rate reactivity to assess fetal status.[36] This biophysical profile (BBP) was initially used on a weekly basis to evaluate post-term pregnancies. Weekly testing yielded results similar to those of the weekly NST with false negative rates of approximately 7/1,000.[36] Johnson et al. showed improved efficacy by twice weekly testing and aggressive intervention for diminished fluid volume.[37] They followed 307 patients with such surveillance without a demise. Intervention for abnormal results was an acceptable 10.4 percent of patients followed with BPP.

Realizing that a reactive fetus invariably demonstrates fetal tone and movement, another group of investigators have introduced the modified BPP. This twice weekly test uses the NST and amniotic fluid volume (NST/AFV) to predict outcome. Eden et al. introduced this approach in a series of 109 post-term patients and observed no stillbirths.[38] Subsequent work by Clark et al. appears to confirm these initial results in a group of 6,000 consecutive patients without a demise. In this study, approximately 40 percent of patients were post-term.[39] The intervention rate was 23.9 percent in Eden's group and in Clark's patients 3 percent for all diagnoses. The incidence of intervention appears to depend on the definition of oligohydramnios and the strategy followed in the presence of significant decelerations. The NST/AFV test has a small number of equivocal results. Although these initial data appear promising, further experience with this modality will be needed to establish the efficacy and intervention rate.

The assessment of amniotic fluid volume can be performed by using several techniques. Subjective estimation by skilled sonographers has been shown to correlate with findings at delivery.[40] However, this method makes serial observation difficult since observers vary. The utilization of AFV estimates is also hampered by our poor understanding of amniotic fluid dynamics. Clement et al. described six post-term pregnancies in which the AFV dropped abruptly within 24 hours.[41] One stillbirth occurred. Identification of these cases of oligohydramnios with rapid onset raises some theoretical concern about the use of AFV as a "chronic" marker in the postdate pregnancy.

Semiquantitative techniques to assess AFV have been proposed by various authors. Initial BPP methods utilized the deepest vertical pocket to assign numeric values to fluid volume. The thresholds for abnormal AFV varied from a vertical pocket of less than 1 to less than 3 cm. Chamberlain et al. found that the perinatal mortality rate in fetuses with no more than a 1-cm pocket was 187.5/1,000 overall and 109.4/1,000 after excluding anomalies.[42] These data included all gestational ages. Oligohydramnios was observed in only 0.85 percent of the total population.[42] Johnson found that only 3.7 percent (11/293) of post-term fetuses develop this degree of oligohydramnios.[37] Six of the 11 fetuses had meconium below the cords, and 3 required admission to the neonatal intensive care unit.[37] In the group with a 1- to 2-cm pocket or marginally decreased fluid, only 1 of 9 neonates was admitted to the intensive care unit. Crowley and O'Herlihy observed that 19.4 percent of post-term patients had a pocket less than 3 cm.[43] Eleven percent of Crowley's patients with decreased fluid had a cesarean section for fetal distress compared to 0.75 percent in the group with normal fluid.[43] The 3-cm cutoff appears to lead to a large number of interventions.

Another method for assessing AFV is the amniotic fluid index (AFI). This method uses real-time ultrasound to measure the vertical fluid pocket depths in centimeters in each uterine quadrant. Measurements are then totaled to yield the AFI. Phelan et al. found a mean AFI of 14.1 ± 3.5 ($\pm$SD) at 42 weeks gestation.[44] Less than 5 cm is considered low, 5 to 8 cm borderline, and greater than 8 cm normal.[45] This method can be performed rapidly and can be taught to technicians and nurses with minimal ultrasound experience. If the patient remains undelivered by 43 weeks gestation, it has been our policy to attempt induction of labor. This approach should only be followed in well-dated gestations. To our knowledge, however, there are no data in the literature that have proved that this protocol will improve outcome.

Intrapartum Management

Careful intrapartum management is also important to guarantee continued fetal and neonatal well-being. The major complications in the intrapartum period are meconium staining, macrosomia, and fetal intolerance to labor. The key to proper management is the timely recognition of problems with prompt reaction and skilled actions.

Meconium staining is four times more common in post-term pregnancy than in term gestations. Before the institution of suctioning techniques, meconium aspiration syndrome was the leading cause of mortality in infants over 2,500 g. Clifford based his staging system for the prediction of clinical outcome in dysmature post-term infants largely on the degree of meconium staining present.[3] There are two primary reasons that meconium is more common in such post-term pregnancies. First, the greater the length of time in utero, the more chance for activation of the mature vagal system with excretion of meconium. Second, hypoxia is more likely to occur in the infant who shows the stigmata of dysmaturity and placental insufficiency. The other factor that increases the rate of perinatal morbidity associated with meconium in post-term pregnancies is the diminished amniotic fluid volume. With oligohydramnios, there is less dilution of meconium and the tenacious meconium is more likely to cause airway obstruction.

Always suspect meconium at any post-term delivery. On rupture of membranes carefully inspect the fluid for staining. When minimal fluid is encountered at the time of membrane rupture, suspect that thick meconium may be present. Amnioinfusion in one study diluted meconium, improved 1-minute Apgar scores, and decreased the number of infants with meconium below the cords.[46] Instillation of normal saline solution through an intrauterine pressure catheter is a relatively benign procedure and may reduce variable decelerations.[47]

Meconium aspiration syndrome may be prevented by aggressive suctioning at the time of delivery of the head. Most cases of aspiration appear to occur when the infant takes its first few breaths. Carson et al. showed that thorough suctioning of the nasopharynx and oropharynx before delivery of the shoulders could prevent aspiration.[48] This technique should be combined with neonatal tracheal aspiration when meconium is present at or below the vocal cords.[49] Although these techniques have been shown to reduce significantly the likelihood of meconium aspiration syndrome, they cannot prevent the disease completely. Autopsy data on stillborn infants have demonstrated the presence of meconium in the bronchial airways.[50]

Another important aspect of management is preventing birth trauma associated with macrosomia. Suspect macrosomia in all post-term gestations. Estimate fetal weight immediately prior to or in the early stages of labor on all post-term pregnancies that are candidates for vaginal delivery. The sizes of the infant and of the maternal pelvis are important in attempting to prevent birth trauma. A significant finding in primiparous patients is the failure of the vertex to engage.

Estimation of fetal weight is difficult in the post-term pregnancy, but the use of ultrasound has improved accuracy. If clinical estimates indicate that the fetus is large or the maternal pelvis is small, an ultrasound estimated fetal weight may be helpful. Ultrasonic weight predictions generally fall within 20 percent of the actual birthweight.[51] Chervenak found ultrasonic estimation of fetal weight to have a sensitivity of 60.5 percent and specificity of 90.7 percent for predicting a birthweight over 4,000 g.[52]

There are several precautions one must remember in patients with suspected macrosomia. Avoid mid-pelvic operative vaginal delivery, particularly with a prolonged second stage. Benedetti and Gabbe noted that the risk of shoulder dystocia was increased from 0.16 to 4.57 percent in patients with a prolonged second stage who underwent mid-pelvic delivery for the delivery of a macrosomic infant.[53] Notify pediatrics and anesthesia staff so they may prepare for delivery. Someone skilled in the various maneuvers to relieve shoulder dystocia should be present for the delivery. Finally, consider primary cesarean section for suspected macrosomia in patients with an estimated fetal weight greater than 4,500 g, a marginal pelvis, or a previous difficult vaginal delivery with the same or smaller size infant.

Intrapartum asphyxia is also more common in the post-term pregnancy; therefore, close observation of the fetal heart rate is necessary. Factors that cause fetal distress are placental deterioration, long labor, and oligohydramnios. The incidence of cesarean section for fetal distress increases from 5.4 to 13.1 percent in post-term patients who develop oligohydramnios.[54]

Cord compression is more likely in these gestations since the oligohydramnios is combined with a thin, easily compressible umbilical cord.[55] As noted, cord compression can be prevented with a normal saline amnioinfusion, which can reduce severe variable decelerations.[47] These patterns alone do not require immediate intervention as long as the fetal heart rate variability and baseline remain within normal limits. Variable decelerations result primarily from cord compression, not hypoxia. Variable decelerations should be followed, however, for evidence of coexisting hypoxia. A slow return to baseline, blunting of the shape of the deceleration, and overshoot are signs for concern with variable decelerations (see Fig. 15.18).

Late decelerations indicate more direct evidence of fetal hypoxia. If they are intermittent, manage late decelerations conservatively by changing maternal position and oxygen administration. If vaginal delivery is not imminent, cesarean section should be considered when late decelerations are frequent and persistent. If persistent late decelerations are associated with decreased variability or an elevated baseline fetal heart rate, rapid delivery is indicated (see Fig. 15.21). Fetal sleep cycles may be differentiated from true depression by the use of fetal scalp stimulation or pH sampling.[56] Clark showed the virtual absence of acidosis in fetuses whose heart rate rose in response to scalp stimulation.[56]

CONCLUSION

Although postdate pregnancy increases the risks for both fetus and mother, satisfactory outcome can be expected with appropriate pregnancy dating, fetal surveillance, intervention when necessary, and careful intrapartum and neonatal management.

REFERENCES

1. Ballantyne JW: The problem of the postmature infant. J Obstet Gynaecol Br Emp II:6,521

2. McClure-Browne JC: Postmaturity. Am J Obstet Gynecol 85:573, 1963

3. Clifford SH: Postmaturity—with placental dysfunction. J Pediatr 44:1, 1954

4. Zwerdling MA: Factors pertaining to prolonged pregnancy and its outcome. J Pediatr 40:202, 1967

5. Lucas WE, Anctil AO, Callagan DA: The problem of postterm pregnancy. Am J Obstet Gynecol 91:241, 1965

6. Gibb DM, Cardozo LD, Studd JW et al: Prolonged pregnancy: is induction of labour indicated? A prospective study. Br J Obstet Gynaecol 89:292, 1982

7. Saito M, Yazawa K, Hashiguchi A: Time of ovulation and prolonged pregnancy. Am J Obstet Gynecol 112:31, 1972

8. Rayburn WF, Motley ME, Stempel LE: Antepartum prediction of the postmature infant. Obstet Gynecol 160:148, 1982

9. Eden RD, Seifert LS, Winegar A: Perinatal characteristics of uncomplicated postdate pregnancies. Obstet Gynecol 69:296, 1987

10. Lagrew DC, Freeman RK, Dorchester: Antepartum surveillance in postterm pregnancy with the contraction stress test. Society of Perinatal Obstetricians Abstract, Las Vegas, February, 1988

11. Sack RA: The large infant: a study of maternal, obstetrical, fetal, and newborn characteristics, including a long-term pediatric follow up. Am J Obstet Gynecol 104:195, 1969

11a. Vorherr H: Placental insufficiency in relation of postterm pregnancy and fetal postmaturity. Am J Obstet Gynecol 123:67, 1975

12. Mannino F: Neonatal complications of postterm gestation. J Reprod Med 33:271, 1988

13. Secher NJ, Hansen PK, Lenstrup C et al: Birth weight for gestational age charts based on early ultrasound estimation of gestational age. Br J Obstet Gynaecol 93:128, 1986

14. Freeman RK, Garite TJ, Modanlou H et al: Postdate pregnancy: utilization of contraction stress testing for primary fetal surveillance. Am J Obstet Gynecol 140:128, 1981

15. Callenbach JC, Hall RT: Morbidity and mortality of advanced gestational age: post-term or postmature. Obstet Gynecol 53:721, 1978

16. Shime J, Librach CL, Gare DJ et al: The influence of prolonged pregnancy on infant development at one and two years of age: a prospective controlled study. Am J Obstet Gynecol 154:341, 1986

17. Dyson DC: Fetal surveillance vs. labor induction at 42 weeks in postterm gestation. J Reprod Med 33:262, 1988

18. Anderson HF, Johnson TRB, Flora JD et al: Gestational age assessment. II. Prediction from combined clinical observations. Am J Obstet Gynecol 140:770, 1981

19. Grennert L, Persson P, Gennser G et al: Benefits of ultrasound screening of a pregnant population. Acta Obstet Gynecol Scand suppl., 78:5, 1978

20. Robinson HP, Fleming JEE: A critical evaluation of sonar "crown–rump" length measurements. Br J Obstet Gynaecol 82:702, 1975

21. Kopta MM, May RR, Crane JP: A comparison of the reliability of the estimated date of confinement predicted by crown–rump length and biparietal diameter. Am J Obstet Gynecol 145:562, 1983

22. Harris BA, Huddleston JF, Sutliff G et al: The unfavorable cervix in prolonged pregnancy. Obstet Gynecol 62:171, 1983

23. Lagrew DC, Freeman RK: Contraction stress test in assessment and care of the fetus. p. 351. In Eden RD, Boehm FH (eds): Assessment and Care of the Fetus: Physiologic, Clinical, and Medicolegal Principles. Appleton & Lange, East Nowalk, CT, 1990

24. Lagrew DC, Freeman RK: Management of postdate pregnancy. Am J Obstet Gynecol 154:8, 1986

25. Dyson DC, Miller PD, Armstrong MA: Management of prolonged pregnancy: induction of labor versus antepartum fetal testing. Am J Obstet Gynecol 156:928, 1987

26. Boyd ME, Usher RH, McLean FH et al: Obstetric consequences of postmaturity. Am J Obstet Gynecol 158:334, 1988

27. Katz Z, Yemini M, Lancet M et al: Non-aggressive management of post-date pregnancies. Eur J Obstet Gynecol Reprod Biol 15:71, 1983

28. Porto M, Merrill PA, Lovett SM et al: When should antepartum testing begin in post-term pregnancy? Society of Perinatal Obstetricians, San Antonio, Texas, January 1986

29. Lagrew DC, Freeman RK: Fetal monitoring in the prolonged pregnancy. p. 123. In Spencer J (ed): Fetal Monitoring. Royal Postgraduate Medical School, University of London, 1989

30. Boehm FH, Salyer S, Shah DM et al: Improved outcome of twice weekly nonstress testing. Obstet Gynecol 67:566, 1986

31. Lumley J, Lester A, Anderson E et al: A randomized trial of weekly cardiotocography in high risk obstetrical patients. Brit J Obstet Gyn 90:101, 1983

32. Kidd L, Panel N, Smith R: Non-stress antenatal cardiotocography—a prospective randomized clinical trial. Br Obstet Gynaecol 92:115, 1985

33. Phelan JP, Platt LD, Yeh SY et al: Continuing role of the nonstress test in the management of postdates pregnancy. Obstet Gynecol 64:624, 1984

34. Small ML, Phelan JP, Smith CV et al: An active management approach to the postdate fetus with a reactive nonstress test and fetal heart rate decelerations. Obstet Gynecol 70:636, 1987

35. Huddleston JF, Sutliff G, Robinson D: Contraction stress test by intermittent nipple stimulation. Obstet Gynecol 63:669, 1984

36. Manning FA, Platt LD, Sipos L: Antepartum fetal evaluation: development of a fetal biophysical profile. Am J Obstet Gynecol 136:787, 1980

37. Johnson JM, Harman CR, Lange IR et al: Biophysical profile scoring in the management of the postterm pregnancy: an analysis of 307 patients. Am J Obstet Gynecol 154:269, 1986

38. Eden RD, Gergely RZ, Schifrin BS et al: Comparison of antepartum testing schemes for the management of the postdate pregnancy. Am J Obstet Gynecol 144:683, 1982

39. Clark SL, Sabey P, Jolley K: Nonstress testing with acoustic stimulation and amniotic fluid volume assessment: 5973 tests without unexpected fetal death. Am J Obstet Gynecol 160:694, 1989

40. Goldstein RB, Filly RA: Sonographic estimation of amniotic fluid volume. J Ultrasound Med 7:363, 1988

41. Clement D, Schifrin BS, Kates RB: Acute oligohydramnios in postdate pregnancy. Am J Obstet Gynecol 157:884, 1987

42. Chamberlain PF, Manning FA, Morrison T et al: Ultrasound evaluation of amniotic fluid volume. Am J Obstet Gynecol 150:245, 1984

43. Crowley P, O'Herlihy C: The value of ultrasound measurement of amniotic fluid volume in the management of prolonged pregnancies. Br J Obstet Gynaecol 91:444, 1984

44. Phelan JP, Ahn MY, Smith CV et al: Amniotic fluid index measurements during pregnancy. J Reprod Med 32:601, 1987

45. Rutherford SE, Phelan JP, Smith CV et al: The four quadrant assessment of amniotic fluid volume: an adjunct to antepartum fetal heart rate testing. Obstet Gynecol 70:353, 1987

46. Wenstrom KD, Parsons MT: The prevention of meconium aspiration in labor using amnioinfusion. Obstet Gynecol 73:647, 1989

47. Miyazaki FS, Taylor NA: Saline amnioinfusion for relief of variable or prolonged decelerations. Am J Obstet Gynecol 146:670, 1983

48. Carson BS, Losey RW, Bowes WA: Combined obstetric and pediatric approach to prevent meconium aspiration syndrome. Am J Obstet Gynecol 126:712, 1976

49. Bloom RD, Copley C: Meconium in amniotic fluid. Lesson 2. p. 17. In American Heart Association Textbook of Neonatal Resuscitation.

50. Brown BL, Gleicher N: Intrauterine meconium aspiration. Obstet Gynecol 57:26, 1981

51. Shepard MJ, Richards VA, Berkowitz RL: An evaluation of two equations for predicting fetal weight by ultrasound. Am J Obstet Gynecol 142:47, 1982

52. Chervenak JL, Divon MY, Hirsch J et al: Macrosomia in the postdate pregnancy: is routine ultrasonographic screening indicated? Am J Obstet Gynecol 161:753, 1989

53. Benedetti TJ, Gabbe SG: Shoulder dystocia: a complication of fetal macrosomia and prolonged second stage of labor with mid-pelvic delivery. Obstet Gynecol 52:526, 1978

54. Leveno KJ, Quirk JG, Cunningham FG et al: Prolonged pregnancy: observations concerning the causes of fetal distress. Am J Obstet Gynecol 150:465, 1984

55. Silver RK, Dooley SL, Tamura RK et al: Umbilical cord size and amniotic fluid volume in prolonged pregnancy. Am J Obstet Gynecol 157:716, 1987

56. Clark SL, Gimovsky ML, Miller FC: Fetal heart rate response to scalp blood sampling. Am J Obstet Gynecol 144:706, 1982

57. Williams RL, Creasy RK, Cunningham GC et al: Fetal growth and perinatal viability in California. Obstet Gynecol 59:624, 1982

58. Treloar AE, Behn BG, Cowan DW: Analysis of gestational interval. Am J Obstet Gynecol 99:34, 1967

Chapter 29

Isoimmunization in Pregnancy

D. Ware Branch and James R. Scott

This chapter reviews the causes and management of isoimmunization in pregnancy. Included are Rh isoimmunization, sensitization caused by other erythrocyte antigens, ABO incompatibility, and platelet isoimmunization. Rh isoimmunization is emphasized because it remains a leading cause of fetal or neonatal death from hemolytic disease. Also, to a great extent, the principles of pathophysiology and management discussed in relation to Rh isoimmunization apply to the other causes of isoimmunization. Under Rh isoimmunization, the following are discussed: the genetics and biochemistry of the Rh antigen, the causes of Rh isoimmunization, the use of Rh-immune globulin, and the management of the Rh-isoimmunized pregnancy. Throughout this chapter, the traditional term sensitization is used interchangeably with isoimmunization.

HISTORY OF ERYTHROBLASTOSIS FETALIS

In 1932, Diamond et al.[1] concluded from personal observation that erythroblastosis fetalis was associated with fetal edema, neonatal hyperbilirubinemia, and neonatal anemia. In 1938, Darrow[2] proposed that these related conditions were caused by the passage of maternal antibodies across the placenta and that the antibodies led to destruction of the fetal erythrocytes. One year later, Levine and Stetson[3] observed the presence of atypical agglutinins in the serum of a woman who had just delivered a hydropic stillborn infant; these agglutinins were found to be active against her husband's erythrocytes even though he ostensibly was of the same blood group as the mother. Levine and Stetson suggested that an immunizing property in the blood or tissues of the fetus must have been inherited from the father and passed into the maternal circulation, causing her to develop the agglutinin. This was the first suggestion that erythroblastosis fetalis was an isoimmune disorder, and within 3 years the role of isoimmunization (rhesus incompatibility) in the pathogenesis of erythroblastosis was established.[4] Five years later, in 1944, Halbrecht[5] related neonatal jaundice to ABO incompatibility.

Although many erythrocyte antigens have subsequently been described, only a few proved to be clinically important causes of maternal isoimmunization leading to hemolysis of fetal and neonatal cells. Platelet isoimmunization was also described. This was shown not to be a cause of fetal or neonatal hemolysis but instead of neonatal thrombocytopenia and, in severe cases, morbid hemorrhage or death.

With the number of cases of fetal or neonatal hemolytic disease resulting from Rh antigen incompatibility decreasing as a result of the widespread use of Rh-immune globulin prophylaxis, the importance of the "minor antigens" of the erythrocyte membrane as a cause of isoimmunization has increased. Platelet isoimmunization is also a relatively uncommon clinical problem; however, as with isoimmunization to the minor erythrocyte antigens, appropriate obstetric management is crucial for optimal perinatal outcome.

GENETICS AND BIOCHEMISTRY OF THE Rh ANTIGEN

Nomenclature

In 1940, Landsteiner and Wiener[6] announced that they had produced rabbit immune sera to rhesus monkey erythrocytes that, even after adsorption, agglutinated the majority (85 percent) of human erythrocytes; they designated this newly discovered property of serum the Rh factor. Agglutinated cells were called Rh+. Of course, it is now recognized that the "Rh factor" is an antibody directed against an erythrocyte surface antigen of the rhesus blood group system.

Since the discovery of the Rh blood group system, development of an adequate nomenclature has been hampered by its high degree of polymorphism. Five major antigens can be identified with known typing sera, and there are many variant antigens. Unfortunately, three different systems of nomenclature have been suggested. Two of these, the Fisher-Race system and the Wiener system, were established during the 1940s and are the ones most frequently used in the literature. The HLA-like system of Rosenfield and colleagues was proposed in 1962.[7] In obstetrics, the Fisher-Race nomenclature is best known. Although this system has some limitations in terms of our current understanding of genetics and in its classification of the numerous variant antigens, it is well suited to understanding the inheritance of the Rh antigen and the clinical management of Rh isoimmunization.[8]

The Fisher-Race nomenclature assumes the presence of three genetic loci, each with two (major) alleles. The antigens produced by these alleles were originally identified by specific antisera and have been lettered C, c, D, E, and e. No antiserum specific for a "d" antigen has been found, and thus the use of the letter *d* indicates the absence of a discernible allelic product. The designations anti-C, anti-c, anti-D, anti-E, and anti-e have been adopted to indicate specific antisera. An Rh gene complex is designated by the three appropriate letters; thus, eight gene complexes could exist (listed in decreasing order of fre-

Table 29.1 Frequency of Phenotypes and Genotypes in the White Population

Phenotype	Population Frequency (%)	Frequency Within	
		Genotype	Phenotype (%)
CcDe	35	CDe/cde (R^1/r)	94
		CDe/cDe (R^1/R^0)	6
		cDe/Cde (R^0/r')	<1
CDe	20	CDe/CDe (R^1/R^1)	95
		CDe/Cde (R^1/r')	5
ce	16	cde/cde (r/r)	100
CcDEe	13	CDe/cDE (R^1/R^2)	89
		CDe/cdE (R^1/r'')	7
		cDE/Cde (R^2/r')	2
		CDE/cde (R^z/r)	1
		CDE/cDe (R^z/R^0)	<1
cDEe	10	cDE/cde (R^2/r)	93
		cDE/cDe (R^2/R^0)	6
		cDe/cdE (R^0/r'')	1
cDE	3	cDE/cDe (R^2/R^0)	86
		cDE/cdE (R^2/r'')	14
cDe	2	cDe/cde (R^0/r)	97
		cDe/cDe (R^0/R^0)	3
Cce	1	Cde/cde (r'/r)	100

quency in the white population): CDe, cde, cDE, cDe, Cde, cdE, CDE, and CdE. Genotypes are indicated as pairs of gene complexes, such as CDe/cde. Certain genotypes, hence certain phenotypes, are more common in the population than others (Table 29.1).[9] The genotypes CDe/cde and CDe/CDe are most common among whites, resulting in 55 percent of the white population being of phenotypes CcDe and CDe. The genotype CdE has actually never been demonstrated.[8] Although the alleles are always written in the order C(c), D(d), E(e), Fisher has shown that the actual order of the genes on chromosome No. 1 is D(d), C(c), E(e).[8]

According to the Fisher-Race concept, the Rh antigen complex is the final expression of a group of at least five possible antigens (C, D, E, c, e). The vast majority of instances of Rh isoimmunizations causing transfusion reactions or serious hemolytic disease of the fetus and newborn are the result of incompatibility with respect to the D antigen. For this reason, common convention holds that Rh-positive indicates the presence of the D antigen and Rh-negative indicates the absence of D antigen on erythrocytes.

Working at the same time as Fisher and Race, Wiener developed a system of nomenclature based on the assumption of only one genetic locus.[10] In the Wiener system, the eight genotypes are designated (in decreasing order of frequency in the white population) R^1, r, R^2, R^0, r′, r″, R^Z, and r^Y (Table 29.1).

In 1973, Rosenfield and co-workers[7] suggested that no previously described model could explain the vast quantitative differences observed in the expression of Rh antigens. Furthermore, they pointed out that such modern genetic concepts as the operon model of gene function with nonlinked regulator genes were poorly accommodated by the simple Mendelian model of Fisher and Race. Rosenfield therefore proposed an updated system of nomenclature that numbered the antigens observed as in the human leukocyte antigen (HLA) system.

Unique Rh antibodies have been used to identify nearly three dozen antigenic variants in the Rh blood group system. Two of the most common (albeit still infrequent in absolute terms) are the C^W antigen and the D^u antigen. The latter is a heterogeneous group of clinically important D antigen variants, most often found in blacks. The erythrocytes of D^u-positive individuals appear to express an incomplete form of the normal D antigen. Such erythrocytes can be shown to bind anti-D typing sera but, in some cases, only by sensitive indirect antiglobulin methods. At least some D^u antigens are capable of causing sensitization in an Rh-negative mother. And some D^u variants are significantly different, antigenically speaking, from the normal D antigen. Rarely this has resulted in a D^u-positive mother's becoming sensitized to her D-positive fetus.

Genetic Expression

The genetic locus for the Rh antigen is on the short arm of chromosome 1. This location was originally determined by linkage studies and later confirmed by somatic cell hybridization.[11] In 1974, Marsh and associates were able to localize the Rh gene complex to the distal end of the short arm of chromosome 1.[12] The three loci of the gene complex appear to be very closely linked because recombination has been observed in only one or two families.[13]

The expression of the Rh antigen on the erythrocyte membrane is genetically controlled, not only in terms of the structure of the antigen but also in terms of the number of specific Rh-antigen sites (e.g., D, E, C, c, or e). Several genetic factors have been shown to alter the number of specific Rh-antigen sites. These include the gene dosage, the relative position of the alleles, and the presence or absence of regulator genes.

Studies indicate that a relatively constant amount of Rh antigen is available on the surface of the red cell, totaling about 1 to 2×10^5 sites per cell.[14] For example, erythrocytes that contain only D antigen (_D_/_D_) have been estimated to have about 155,000 antigen sites per cell (range 110,000 to 202,000) by using radiolabeled anti-D.[14] With similar techniques, the total number of Rh-antigen sites on the erythrocytes of CDe/cDE individuals has been estimated to be 152,000.[15] Of these sites, the average cell carries about 10,000 to 30,000 D-antigen sites.[16]

Gene dosage has an effect on the number of specific Rh-antigen sites expressed. Individuals homozygous for a particular genotype possess up to twice as many antigenic sites as heterozygous individuals.[14] For example, the erythrocytes of individuals homozygous for the c allele have twice as many c-antigen sites (80,000) as the erythrocytes of heterozygotes. Similar observations have been made in regard to the other alleles (E, e, and C).[14,15]

An effect of allelic interaction on Rh-antigen sites has been described. Erythrocytes of individuals of genotype CDe/cde express less D antigen than those of individuals of genotype cDE/cde.[17] Thus, the presence of the C antigen seems to affect the expression of the D antigen. Similarly, individuals of genotype CDe/cDE express less C antigen than those of genotype CDe/cde.[9] In addition, genes other than those coding for the Rh antigen per se may affect the final antigenic expression; two independently segregating regulator genes have been described.[7]

Biochemistry and Immunology

The Rh antigens on human erythrocytes are polypeptides embedded in the lipid phase of the erythrocyte membrane, distributed throughout the membrane in a nonrandom fashion.[18] The molecular weight of the D antigen is 28,000 to 33,000 daltons.[19] The final tertiary structure and antigenic expression of the protein are dependent on its association with a membrane lipid and in this context may be thought of as a protein–lipid complex, or proteolipid.[19,20] The antigen appears very early in the gestational life, having been demonstrated on the red blood cells of a 52-day-old embryo.[21] The antigen is also expressed early in the erythroid series. By using ^{125}I-labeled anti-D, pronormoblasts have been shown to contain D antigen.[22]

At least three, and perhaps as many as seven, different D-antigen epitopes have been discovered using human monoclonal anti-D antibodies.[16] One fascinating and plausible hypothesis suggests that the different epitopes are part of the same protein–lipid complex but are more or less expressed according to the depth to which the polypeptide portion is embedded in the membrane lipid bilayer.[16] It is tempting to speculate that some of the immunologic variation in the Rh blood group system (and, hence, fetal hemolytic disease) is explained by the variable expression of the D-antigen epitopes and the specificity of the antibodies formed against them.

The precise function of the Rh antigen is unknown, but recent evidence suggests that the antigen interacts with a membrane adenosine triphosphatase (ATPase).[20] In this role, the antigen probably functions as part of a proton or cation pump that serves to control volume or electrolyte flux across the erythrocyte membrane. Consistent with this hypothesis, Rh_{null} erythrocytes, which appear to lack the Rh antigen, have increased osmotic fragility and abnormal shapes.[23]

CAUSES OF Rh ISOIMMUNIZATION

For Rh isoimmunization to develop, at least three circumstances must hold:

1. The fetus must have Rh-positive erythrocytes, and the mother must have Rh-negative erythrocytes.
2. A sufficient number of fetal erythrocytes must have gained access to the maternal circulation.
3. The mother must have the immunogenic capacity to produce antibody directed against the D antigen.

Incidence of Rh-Incompatible Pregnancy

The highest proportion of Rh-negative individuals is found among the Basques of France and Spain. Between 25 and 40 percent of these people are Rh-negative. Overall, about 15 percent of white Americans and 5 to 8 percent of black Americans are Rh-negative. All people of eastern Asia (including American Indians) were likely Rh-positive before mixing with Europeans. Currently, less than 3 percent of Eskimos and American Indians are Rh-negative, but the figure may be higher in some subpopulations. Five to 10 percent of American Hispanics, whose genetic background is Asian and Spanish, are Rh-negative. In the white population, an Rh-negative woman stands a roughly 85 percent chance of mating with an Rh-positive man. Sixty percent of Rh-positive men are heterozygous and 40 percent are homozygous at the D locus. Given that one-half of conceptions due to heterozygous men will be Rh-positive, the overall chance of an Rh-positive man producing an Rh-positive fetus is 70 percent. Thus, without knowing the father's blood type, an Rh-negative woman has about a 60 percent chance of bearing an Rh-positive fetus (0.85×0.70). Among whites, the net result is that about 10 percent of pregnancies are Rh-incompatible. However, sufficient fetomaternal hemorrhage and the subsequent maternal antibody response do not occur in every case: fewer than 20 percent of the incompatible pregnancies eventuate in maternal sensitization. In the era before Rh-immune globulin prophylaxis, about 1 percent of pregnant women had anti-D antibody.

Fetomaternal Hemorrhage

In 1941, Levine and co-workers[4] first proposed that the transplacental passage of fetal erythrocytes led to the isoimmunization of the mother. During the mid-1950s, fetal erythrocytes were first demonstrated in the maternal circulation.[24] Since then, numerous studies have confirmed the presence of fetal erythrocytes in the maternal circulation during pregnancy and in the immediate postpartum period. Fetomaternal hemorrhage sufficient to cause isoimmunization is most common at the time of delivery, occurring in about 15 to 50 percent of births.[24–27] In more than half of these delivery-associated fetomaternal bleeds, the amount of fetal blood entering the maternal circulation is 0.1 ml or less.[27,28] But in 0.2 to 1 percent of cases, the estimated volume of fetomaternal hemorrhage is 30 ml or more.[25,29,30] Parity does not appear to be an important predisposing factor in the risk of fetomaternal hemorrhage. Certain clinical factors, such as cesarean delivery, multiple gestation, bleeding placenta previa or abruptio, manual removal of the placenta, or intrauterine manipulation, may increase the chance of substantial hemorrhage. However, the majority of excessive fetomaternal hemorrhages occur in association with uncomplicated vaginal deliveries.[30,31]

The amount of fetomaternal hemorrhage necessary to cause isoimmunization is still a subject of controversy and doubtlessly varies with the immunogenic capacity of the Rh-positive erythrocytes and the immune responsiveness of the mother. As little as 0.1 ml of Rh-positive erythrocyte has been shown to sensitize some Rh-negative volunteers.[27] Indeed, about 3 percent of the women found to have an estimated 0.1 ml of fetal erythrocytes in their circulation after an Rh-incompatible delivery can be expected to develop anti-D antibodies within 6 to 12 months.

Overall, about 16 percent of Rh-negative women become isoimmunized by their first Rh-incompatible (ABO-compatible) pregnancy if not treated with Rh-immune globulin.[28] Half these women respond with the production of sufficient anti-D antibody to be detectable within the first 6 months after delivery; in the remainder, anti-D is not detected until early in the second incompatible pregnancy. In this latter group, although sensitization likely occurred during the first pregnancy, the primary immune response is too slight for detectable antibody levels to develop. Not all Rh-negative women bearing Rh-positive infants become sensitized, but after several incompatible pregnancies, the risk of sensitization approaches 50 percent. Even without labor or the obvious disruption of the choriodecidual junction, antepartum fetomaternal hemorrhage occurs in sufficient volume to result in isoimmunization in a small percentage of cases. In one large series, fetomaternal hemorrhage was detected in 6.7 percent of first trimester determinations, 15.9 percent of second trimester determinations, and 28.9 percent of third trimester determinations.[24] Overall, about 1 to 2 percent of untreated Rh-negative mothers become sensitized before delivery.[32] However, sensitization rarely occurs before the third trimester.

Fetomaternal hemorrhage leading to isoimmunization has been described with abortion and tubal pregnancy.[33–36] Fetal Rh antigens are present by the thirty-eighth day after conception and, assuming that 0.1 ml of fetal blood is required to cause isoimmunization, a fetomaternal hemorrhage leading to sensitization could occur by the seventh week after the last menses.[37] In one case, significant numbers of fetal red blood cells were demonstrated in the maternal circulation after an elective termination of a 6-week pregnancy.[38]

Estimates of the incidence and the amount of fetomaternal hemorrhage after abortion have varied. An extensive review in 1969 discovered that 4.5 to 25.5 percent of spontaneous abortions resulted in detectable fetomaternal hemorrhage.[26] Indeed, for the unsensitized Rh-negative woman, spontaneous first trimester abortion carries a 3 to 4 percent risk of isoimmunization.[39] Induced abortions are even more likely to produce detectable fetomaternal hemorrhage (in 6.5 to 26.5 percent of cases); the overall risk of sensitization is about 5 percent.[36] Saline injection termination and hysterotomy are also associated with significant fetomaternal hemorrhage.[35,36]

Ectopic pregnancy can result in isoimmunization in the susceptible woman.[33] The risk of significant fetomaternal hemorrhage may actually be greater in ruptured tubal pregnancy because of the possible absorption of fetal erythrocytes into the maternal circulation across the peritoneum.[40]

Amniocentesis in the second and third trimester is associated with fetomaternal hemorrhage in 15 to 25 percent of cases, even with ultrasonographic localization of the placenta.[41,42] Isoimmunization after amniocentesis has also been described.[43] Chorionic villus sampling has been associated with fetomaternal hemorrhage of sufficient amount to induce Rh immunization.[44]

Maternal Immunologic Response

At least two characteristics of the individual affect whether isoimmunization will occur in the susceptible Rh-negative woman. First, as many as 30 percent of Rh-negative individuals appear to be immunologic "nonresponders" who do not become sensitized even when challenged with large volumes of Rh-positive blood.[45,46] Second, ABO incompatibility exerts a protective effect against the development of Rh sensitization.[47]

Levine and Stetson[3] are credited with first having recognized the association between ABO incompatibility and the lower-than-expected incidence of Rh isoimmunization. Fetomaternal ABO incompatibility is now well accepted as being protective against isoimmunization.[47,48] Two mechanisms have been proposed. The first suggests that the ABO incompatible fetal cells are more rapidly cleared from the maternal circulation so that trapping of the antigen in the spleen, where sensitization can be initiated, does not occur. Indeed, it has been shown that, although the chance of fetomaternal hemorrhage at the time of delivery is not altered in ABO-incompatible pregnancies, the number of fetal cells detectable in the maternal circulation is less, thus suggesting rapid clearance.[25,26] A second mechanism for the protective effect of ABO incompatibility suggests that maternal anti-A or anti-B antibodies damage or alter the fetal Rh antigen so that it is no longer immunogenic.[48]

Whatever the mechanism, ABO incompatibility diminishes the risk of isoimmunization from 10 percent to about 1.5 to 2 percent after the delivery of an Rh-positive fetus.[49] This effect is most pronounced in matings in which the mother is O and the father is A, B, or AB.[50]

THE USE OF Rh-IMMUNE GLOBULIN

The principle that passively administered antibody prevents active immunization by its specific antigen is termed antibody-mediated immune suppression (AMIS) and was well known to immunologists for decades before being applied to the prevention of Rh disease. During the early 1960s, Freda et al. in the United States and Finn and co-workers in Great Britain simultaneously undertook to evaluate AMIS in humans. Both groups achieved a high degree of protection from isoimmunization by administering anti-D immune globulin (Rh-immune globulin) to Rh-negative male volunteers who had been infused with Rh-positive red cells.[51,52] A study initiated by Pollack et al.[53] in 1963 established that 300 μg of Rh-immune globulin would reliably prevent isoimmunization in male volunteers who had received 10 ml of Rh-positive cells. By extrapolation of the data, Pollack et al.[53] showed that 20 μg Rh-immune globulin per ml of fetal erythrocytes was required to prevent isoimmunization; thus, the "20 μg/1 ml" rule was established.

Early trials using AMIS to prevent isoimmunization in Rh-negative women delivering Rh-positive infants were excitingly successful.[54–56] The administration of Rh-immune globulin within 72 hours of delivery reduced isoimmunization to less than 1.5 percent in the Rh-negative women who were followed through a subsequent incompatible pregnancy. This represented a 7- to 10-fold decrease in isoimmunization compared with the controls. Although 300 μg or more of Rh-immune globulin was used, it has subsequently been shown that a dose of 100 to 150 μg is probably adequate;[56,57] nonetheless, the standard approved dose in North America remains 300 μg.

The 72-hour time limit set for the postpartum administration of Rh-immune globulin is an artifact of the early male prisoner volunteer studies,[58] in which prison officials would only allow the investigators to visit the volunteers at 3-day intervals; thus, the use of Rh-immune globulin at intervals of more than 3 days after a challenge with Rh-positive cells was never extensively evaluated. However, to be effective, Rh-immune globulin must be given before the primary immune response is established. The time required to mount a primary immune response doubtlessly varies from case to case, and it is prudent to administer Rh-immune globulin as soon as possible after delivery. If for some reason the neonatal Rh status is unknown by the third day after delivery, it is preferable to administer Rh-immune globulin to an Rh-negative mother, rather than to continue to wait for the neonatal results. Finally, if a Rh-negative mother who is a candidate for Rh-immune prophylaxis is mistakenly not treated within the recommended 72 hours following delivery, she should still be given Rh-immune globulin as late as 14 to 28 days after delivery in an effort to prevent sensitization.

Antepartum Prophylaxis

Early trials showed that 1 to 2 percent of susceptible women become sensitized in spite of postpartum Rh-immune prophylaxis. Most of these "prophylaxis failures" result from antepartum fetomaternal hemorrhage. In an effort to address this problem, Bowman and colleagues in Canada began an antepartum Rh-prophylaxis trial in 1968.[59] This trial, which used 300 μg of Rh-immune globulin given at 28 weeks and 34 weeks gestation, reduced the rate of antenatal sensitization from 1.8 to 0.1 percent. Subsequently, it was shown that 300 μg of Rh-immune globulin given only at 28 weeks gestation is nearly as effective.[60] Reviewing several large studies, the 1979 McMaster University Conference on the prevention of Rh disease confirmed that the antepartum administration of Rh-immune globulin could reduce the risk of antepartum isoimmunization by more than one-half.[32] In more than 18,000 control cases, the incidence of antepartum sensitization was 1.05 percent, whereas in more than 10,000 treated cases, it was only 0.17 percent. In spite of this, the use of antepartum prophylaxis remains controversial because of uncertainty concerning cost-effectiveness of large-scale antepartum prophylaxis. Writing in favor of antepartum prophylaxis, Kochenour and Beeson[61] estimated in 1982 that the cost of Rh-immune globulin antepartum prophylaxis per isoimmunization that was avoided at the University of Utah was $1,334. This figure compares very favorably with the cost involved in treating even one sensitized pregnancy. In 1985, Bowman contended that the cost of antepartum prophylaxis (estimated to be about $3,300 per case of sensitization prevented) was little, if any, argument against its use.[62]

Mechanism

The precise mechanism of AMIS is not clearly understood. There are three theories: (1) antigen deviation, (2) antigen blocking–competitive inhibition, and (3) central inhibition. The hypothesis that AMIS works by diversion of the antigen from the immunologic apparatus that is responsible for antibody formation was first suggested by Race and Sanger.[53] Support for this theory came from an observation of increased clearance of ^{51}Cr-labeled Rh-positive red cells in Rh-negative volunteers who were treated with Rh-immune globulin. This increased clearance was presumed to be caused by intravascular hemolysis that resulted in the destruction or alteration of the Rh antigen so that it did not incite the formation of anti-D antibody. However, it is now known that IgG anti-D does not cause intravascular hemolysis of Rh-positive cells; instead, the intact, antibody-coated cells are removed from the circulation by the spleen or lymph nodes,[63] the very site of antibody formation.

Antigen deviation could also occur by phagocytosis of the antibody-coated Rh-positive cells; this phenomenon could, and presumably does, occur in the spleen and lymph nodes. But as Pollack[64] pointed out, (1) macrophage ingestion and processing of antigen are essential to immunization and (2) passive immunization that is directed against red cell antigens has been shown to be specific. Contrariwise, if antigen deviation through phagocytosis were the primary mechanism of AMIS, one would think that all red cell antigens would be destroyed. For these reasons, antigen deviation is probably not the mechanism of AMIS.

Antigen blocking by anti-D antibody is also not the probable mechanism for AMIS: antibody preparations that lack the Fc portion have been shown to bind avidly to antigen, yet they do not suppress the immune response.[65] In addition, Pollack[64] showed that in the usual doses of anti-D used to effect immune suppression, less than 20 percent of the Rh antigen is bound.

The most plausible mechanism for AMIS is that of central inhibition, as proposed by Gorman[66] and elaborated on by Pollack.[64] In the scenario set forth by Pollack,[64] fetal erythrocytes coated with exogenously administered anti-D are filtered out of the circulation by the spleen and lymph nodes. The increase in the local concentrations of anti-D bound to the D antigen appears to "suppress" the primary immune response by interrupting the commitment of B cells to IgG-producing plasma cell clones. Exactly how this suppression is effected is poorly understood, but the binding of antibody–antigen complexes (anti-D–D antigen complexes) by immune effector cells results in the release of cytokines that inhibit the proliferation of B cells specific for the antigen. The process appears to be dependent on the presence of Fc receptor on the IgG; Fab' fragments do not inhibit AMIS.

MANAGEMENT OF THE UNSENSITIZED, Rh-NEGATIVE PREGNANT WOMAN

At the first prenatal visit of any pregnancy, the patient should have blood drawn for determination of the ABO blood group, Rh type, and antibody screen (Table 29.2). It is essential that these determinations be made in each subsequent pregnancy. Previous maternal typing is not an acceptable substitute.

If the patient is Rh-negative, is D^u-negative, and has no demonstrable antibody detected, she is a candidate for Rh-immune globulin prophylaxis at 28 weeks gestation and again immediately post partum.

Table 29.2 The Management of an Unsensitized Rh-negative, D^u-negative Pregnant Patient

Time in Gestation	Laboratory and Management
Early prenatal visit (<20 wks)	ABO blood group, Rh type, antibody screen (indirect Coombs test)
28 Weeks	Repeat antibody screen 　If result negative (no anti-D), administer Rh-immune globulin, 300 μg 　If result positive (anti-D present), manage as Rh-immunized pregnancy
Post partum	Repeat antibody screen Screen for excessive fetomaternal hemorrhage 　If antibody screen result negative (no anti-D) and estimated fetomaternal hemorrhage <30 ml^a, administer Rh-immune globulin, 300 μg, if neonate Rh- or D^u-positive 　If antibody screen result negative (no anti-D) and estimated fetomaternal hemorrhage >30 ml^a, administer Rh-immune globulin, 300 μg per 30 ml estimated fetal blood, if neonate Rh- or D^u-positive 　If antibody screen result positive (anti-D present), manage next pregnancy as Rh-immunized

^{a} Screening for excessive fetomaternal hemorrhage is controversial from the standpoint of cost-effectiveness. The most recent ACOG Technical Bulletin regarding Rh immune globulin (ACOG Technical Bulletin 147) does not recommend screening for excessive fetomaternal hemorrhage.

Before the administration of a full 300-μg dose of Rh-immune globulin at 28 weeks gestation, a second antibody screen should be performed to ensure that the patient is not actively producing anti-D. If anti-D is discovered, then the patient should be considered Rh-sensitized and the pregnancy managed accordingly (discussed later).

After antepartum prophylaxis at 28 weeks gestation, it was originally recommended that an antibody screen be repeated at 35 to 36 weeks to ensure that isoimmunization (anti-D titer greater than 1:4) had not occurred. However, the risk of isoimmunization after antepartum prophylaxis is negligible, and it is extremely unlikely that the rare case would require active intervention before delivery. Thus, a repeat antepartum antibody screen at 35 to 36 weeks gestation is probably not necessary.

When the Rh-negative, unsensitized patient is admitted for delivery care, an antibody screen is routinely performed (as for any patient admitted for delivery). If the antibody screen result is negative and the newborn is Rh-positive or D^u-positive, the mother is a candidate for prophylaxis. Because up to 1 percent of deliveries result in a fetomaternal hemorrhage of greater than 30 ml (the largest volume of fetal blood adequately covered by a standard 300-μg dose of Rh-immune globulin), patients should be screened for "excessive" (>30 ml of whole blood) fetomaternal hemorrhage immediately post par-

tum.[67] An erythrocyte rosette test has been shown to be particularly sensitive in detecting excessive fetomaternal hemorrhage,[30] but many laboratories continue to use an acid elution method. If the volume of hemorrhage is found to be greater than 30 ml whole blood, a dose of Rh-immune globulin calculated at 10 μg/ml of whole blood should be administered.

Infrequently, an Rh-negative woman is found to have a "weak" Rh antibody detectable only by very sensitive techniques.[67a] The majority of such women are not Rh-immunized and should be given prophylactic Rh-immune globulin according to the usual protocol.

The issue of D^u-positivity may confuse the proper use of Rh-immune globulin prophylaxis. The D^u-positive mother who delivers an Rh-positive infant is not at significant risk of Rh sensitization, probably because the D^u antigen is actually a weakly expressed D antigen. Thus, for practical purposes, D^u-positive mothers may be treated as if they were Rh-positive. However, infrequently a woman previously typed as Rh-negative is unexpectedly found to be D^u-positive during pregnancy or after delivery. In this situation, the clinician should be suspicious that the patient's "new" D^u-positive status is actually due to a large number of fetal cells in the maternal circulation. Appropriate studies should be undertaken, and if fetomaternal hemorrhage is found, the mother should be treated with Rh-immune globulin.

Table 29.3 Other Uses of Rh-Immune Globulin

Indication	Dose of Rh-Immune Globulin
First trimester spontaneous or induced abortion	50 μg
First trimester chorionic villus sampling	50 μg
Ectopic pregnancy	300 μg
Amniocentesis or second trimester chorionic villus sampling	300 μg
Fetomaternal hemorrhage	10 μg/estimated ml of whole fetal blood

Because of the risk of significant fetomaternal hemorrhage with abortion or ectopic pregnancy, Rh-immune globulin prophylaxis is indicated if the patient is Rh-negative and unsensitized. If the pregnancy loss occurs at 12 weeks gestation or less, a 50-μg dose of Rh-immune globulin is adequate to cover the entire fetal blood volume[68] (Table 29.3). If the gestational age is unknown or beyond 12 weeks, a full 300-μg dose of Rh-immune globulin is indicated.

An Rh-negative, unsensitized patient who shows antepartum bleeding or suffers an unexplained second or third trimester fetal death should be evaluated for the possibility of massive fetomaternal hemorrhage. If fetal cells are found in the maternal circulation, Rh-immune globulin is indicated at a dose of 10 μg per estimated milliliter of whole fetal blood (Table 29.3).

A common indication for antenatal Rh-immune globulin is the performance of chorionic villus sampling or amniocentesis in an Rh-negative, unsensitized patient. For first trimester procedures, 50 μg of Rh-immune globulin is protective. However, for second or third trimester procedures, a full 300-μg dose is indicated even if the procedure is not associated with detectable hemorrhage (Table 29.3). When amniocentesis is performed within 72 hours of delivery, as for the determination of fetal pulmonary maturity, Rh-immune globulin may be withheld and administered immediately post partum only if the infant is found to be Rh-positive or D^u-positive.

Since the availability of Rh-immune globulin in the United States in the late 1960s, great inroads have been realized in reducing the incidence of Rh isoimmunization. By 1979, the Connecticut Rh registry found that only 1.2 percent of Rh-negative pregnant patients were sensitized.[69] Antepartum sensitizations and failures of postpartum prophylaxis accounted for more than half of these cases. The now widespread use of antepartum Rh-immune globulin prophylaxis has greatly reduced antepartum sensitizations. However two significant problems remain: (1) postpartum prophylaxis failures[70] and (2) failure to administer Rh-immune globulin when it is indicated.[70,71] Routine use of postpartum screening programs to detect "excessive" fetomaternal hemorrhage will likely prevent the majority of postpartum prophylaxis failures. It is the responsibility of the health care system, the physicians in particular, to administer Rh-immune globulin prophylaxis to all patients in whom it is indicated.

THE Rh-ISOIMMUNIZED PREGNANCY: ASSESSMENT OF THE FETUS

Any patient with an anti-D antibody titer greater than 1:4 should be considered Rh-sensitized and the pregnancy managed accordingly. The eventual goal of management is to minimize the fetal and neonatal risk of morbidity and mortality. Patients (fetuses) can be roughly categorized into those unlikely to require intrauterine intervention and able to be delivered when they achieve pulmonary maturation and those likely to have moderate to severe hemolytic disease requiring intrauterine transfusion and early delivery. An accurate assignment of gestational age using menstrual dates and ultrasound is crucial to optimal management of the Rh-isoimmunized pregnancy; in part, the timing of amniocentesis, cordocentesis, and delivery depends on proper assignment.

Determination of the Fetal Antigen Status

When first confronted with an Rh-immunized pregnant woman, one should consider the probability that the fetus might be Rh-negative and therefore not need expensive and potentially risky procedures. If the woman might have become sensitized during a pregnancy fathered by another partner or by a mismatched blood transfusion, determining the paternal Rh antigen status is reasonable since the father of the current pregnancy might be Rh-negative. If he is Rh-negative (and one is sure that he is the father of the fetus), further intervention is not required. If the father is Rh-positive, the probability that he is heterozygous for the D antigen can be determined by using Rh antisera to deduce the most likely genotype. Of course, if the man has fathered Rh-negative children, he is an obligate heterozygote. If there is a reasonable probability that the father of the fetus is heterozygous for the D antigen, one author has recommended fetal blood sampling at 18 to 20 weeks gestation to determine the fetal D antigen status.[72] Such an approach seems rational for the patient in whom cordocentesis and probable transfusion is planned on the basis of obstetric history. However, patients with either no previous affected infant or infants with only mild to moderate hemolysis present a somewhat different risk–benefit dilemma. One should individualize cases, weighing the risks of cordocentesis against the risks of serial amnioceteses. Cordocentesis is slightly more likely than amniocentesis to cause fetal death, and insertions of the needle through the placenta may be associated with a fetomaternal hemorrhage large enough to cause an increase in the maternal anti-D titer.[73]

Antibody Titer in Maternal Sera

In the first sensitized pregnancy, the level of the anti-D antibody titer in the maternal serum determines the need for amniocentesis. Several workers have noted the absence of severe erythroblastosis or perinatal death when the antibody levels remain below a certain "critical titer."[48,74,75] This titer varies from laboratory to laboratory but is usually in the 1 : 16 to 1 : 32 range. Freda[75] found no perinatal deaths caused by hemolytic disease when the anti-D titer within 1 week of delivery was 1 : 16 or less. Queenan[48] reported only one perinatal death with maternal anti-D titers of 1 : 32 or less. However, the reliability and method of antibody titration vary greatly from one laboratory to another. As the number of sensitized pregnancies diminishes, the familiarity of laboratory personnel with titration techniques also decreases. Because of this potential problem, an anti-D titer of 1 : 8 or greater is usually considered an indication for amniocentesis to manage the sensitized pregnancy. If the initial anti-D titer is less than 1 : 8, and if the patient does not have a history of a previously affected infant, the pregnancy may be followed with both anti-D titers every 2 to 4 weeks and serial ultrasound assessment of the fetus.

Beyond using the "critical titer" to establish the need for amniocentesis, anti-D titers are not particularly useful in the management of most Rh-isoimmunized pregnancies; indeed, titers may remain stable throughout gestation in as many as 80 percent of the severely affected pregnancies.[75] Possible explanations for this observation include the following: (1) the binding constant of anti-D varies from individual to individual, (2) the Rh-antigen expression on the fetal erythrocyte membrane varies from individual to individual,[16] and (3) the ability of the fetus to replace erythrocytes without compromising liver function varies from individual to individual.

Obstetric History

A well-documented obstetric history can be an important management guide in an Rh-isoimmunized patient. Studies made prior to the advent of intrauterine therapy clearly showed that fetal hemolytic disease tends to be either as severe, or more severe, in subsequent pregnancies. A history of previous intrauterine or neonatal death from hemolytic disease carries a particularly grave prognosis.[74,76] If a mother has had a hydropic fetus, the chance that the next Rh-incompatible fetus will become hydropic (if left untreated) is more than 80 percent. Only occasionally will an Rh-incompatible fetus be less severely affected than its previous sibling.

In general, hemolysis and hydrops develop at the same time or somewhat earlier in subsequent pregnancies; this may be used as a rough guide as to when to initiate fetal studies and transfusions. However, the history is not particularly helpful if the previous pregnancy was the first sensitized pregnancy because relatively few fetuses in the first sensitized pregnancy develop hydrops.

Amniotic Fluid Analysis

In 1956, Bevis[77] reported that the spectrophotometrically determined bilirubin concentration of the amniotic fluid in Rh-sensitized pregnancies correlated with the severity of fetal hemolysis. Bilirubin is a byproduct of fetal hemolysis that reaches the amniotic fluid primarily by excretion into fetal pulmonary and tracheal secretions and diffusion across the fetal membranes and the umbilical cord. The now classic work of Liley in 1961[78] demonstrated that antenatal determinations of the bilirubin concentrations in amniotic fluid could be used to predict the severity of hemolytic disease. Using a policy of selected induction based on amniotic fluid spectrophotometric findings, Liley reduced perinatal mortality in Rh-sensitized pregnancies from 22 to 9 percent over a 5-year period. This was accomplished primarily by avoiding the preterm delivery of mildly affected fetuses.

A spectrophotometric scan of normal amniotic fluid beyond the mid-second trimester is nearly linear, with a slightly increased light absorbance in the lower wavelengths. Amniotic fluid from a fetus with hemolysis contains bilirubin and demonstrates an increased absorbance in the range from 375 to 525 nm, with a peak at about 450 nm. The deviation in light absorbance (optical density) at 450 nm from the expected straight line is referred to as ΔOD_{450}, expressed in optical density (Fig. 29.1). Before 26 weeks gestation, normal amniotic fluid contains a small amount of bilirubin; thus, ΔOD_{450} determinations obtained during this period need to be cautiously interpreted.

According to the original management scheme devised by Liley,[79] the amniotic fluid of an Rh-isoimmunized pregnancy was spectrophotometrically analyzed first at 29 to 32 weeks and then again at 33 to 35 weeks. The OD_{450} values were then plotted (Fig. 29.2). On the basis of clinical outcome, Liley divided the graph into three prognostic zones: upper zone (zone 3), middle zone (zone 2), and lower zone (zone 1). The ΔOD_{450} values of severely affected fetuses fell in the upper zone, and those of unaffected or mildly affected fetuses fell in the lower zone. The ΔOD_{450} values in the middle zone were associated with a range of hemolytic disease from mild to severe, depending primarily on the trend defined by the amniotic fluid bilirubin determinations. There is a tendency for amniotic fluid bilirubin to decrease as pregnancy advances; thus, the boundaries of the zones slope downward as gestational age increases. In turn, this means that a given ΔOD_{450} value is more likely indicative of significant fetal hemolysis at 33 weeks gestation than at 26 weeks gestation.

Liley[80] later modified his original graph by subdividing the upper and middle zones. The ΔOD_{450} values falling in the upper subdivision of each zone were associated with worse prognoses. However, because of the wide range of infant affliction represented in the middle zone, Liley carefully emphasized

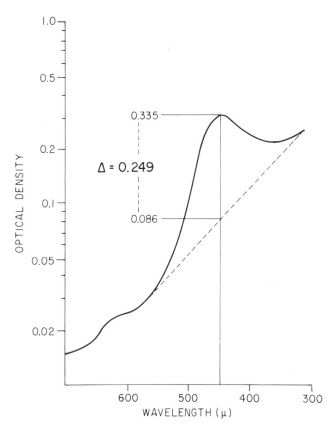

Fig. 29.1 Spectrophotometric scan of amniotic fluid taken from an Rh-sensitized pregnancy with fetal hydrops. The heavy solid line represents the actual spectrophotometric scan of the bilirubin-containing fluid. The interrupted line shows where the scan would be traced if there had been no increase in bilirubin in the fluid. The difference between the optical density at the peak of the heavy solid line at 450 nm and the interrupted line at 450 nm is the OD_{450}.

the need for repeating the amniotic fluid analyses to establish the ΔOD_{450} trend. Queenan[81] subsequently analyzed serial amniotic fluid ΔOD_{450} values in patients delivered of unaffected (Rh-negative), mildly affected (cord hemoglobin greater than 14 g), severely affected (cord blood hemoglobin less than 10 g), and stillborn infants. These ΔOD_{450} values described a clear downward trend in unaffected and mildly affected infants, and values from the severely affected fetuses showed a mixed pattern of somewhat higher values. The amniotic fluid ΔOD_{450} values from infants who died in utero from erythroblastosis showed upward trends except in a single case that was

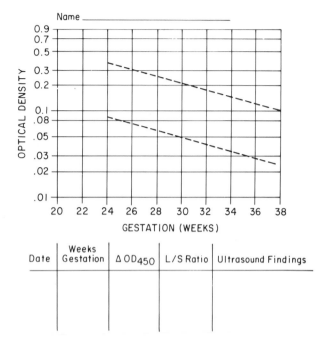

Fig. 29.2 Liley graph used at the University of Utah Medical Center.

complicated by polyhydramnios. Thus, a horizontal or rising trend is ominous and indicates the need for intervention by either intrauterine transfusion or delivery.

The usefulness of the late-second and early-third trimester amniotic fluid ΔOD_{450} determinations for the management of Rh-immunized pregnancies has been confirmed by years of experience in many centers. However, several practical caveats deserve mention. First, a single ΔOD_{450} value is often insufficient for management purposes: the ΔOD_{450} trend, as established by serial amniocenteses, provides more reliable information about fetal status. Second, relying solely on the ΔOD_{450} values occasionally leads to the false impression that a mildly or moderately involved fetus is severely anemic or vice versa. In a recent report, MacKenzie et al. found that fully 21 percent of the ΔOD_{450} values were misleading in terms of predicting the degree of fetal anemia.[82] Fi-

nally, the fairly common practice of extrapolating Liley's original graph for use prior to 26 weeks gestation has proved to be controversial, if not erroneous. Nicolaides et al. showed that two-thirds of severely anemic fetuses (fetal hemoglobin < 6 g/dl) at 18 to 25 weeks gestation had ΔOD_{450} values in the middle or lower zone, incorrectly suggesting only mild to moderate anemia.[83] On the other hand, other investigators contend that although there is overlap, second trimester ΔOD_{450} values are quite useful in determining which fetuses are severely anemic.[84]

Fetal Blood Analysis

Direct fetal vascular access via fetoscopic or ultrasound-guided vascular puncture was developed in the 1970s, thus enabling direct assessment of the degree of fetal anemia and fetal intravascular transfusion.[85-87] Fetal blood sampling also allows determination of the presence or absence of the offending antigen on the fetal erythrocytes, provided the antigen status or zygosity of the father is unknown.[72,88] As care of isoimmunized pregnancies is becoming concentrated at a few tertiary centers, so also is the expertise for fetal blood sampling. As a result, direct fetal blood sampling is now a first step in the analysis of the fetus at risk for severe hemolytic disease. MacKenzie and colleagues have confirmed the utility of fetal blood sampling in the management of Rh-isoimmunized pregnancies.[82] In 51 consecutive sensitized pregnancies, 11 fetuses were found by blood sampling to be Rh-negative and thus required no further evaluation. Of the continuing pregnancies, the fetal hematocrit and the amniotic fluid ΔOD_{450} value were in agreement in 79 percent of cases. However, the amniotic fluid ΔOD_{450} value underestimated the degree of fetal anemia in 11 percent of comparisons and overestimated it in 10 percent.

Concerns about the morbidity or mortality associated with fetal blood sampling continue to limit enthusiasm for it as a method of monitoring fetuses at risk for mild to moderate hemolysis. In experienced hands, the attributable fetal loss rate is about 0.5 to 1 percent.[88,89] Moreover, transplacental needle passage is associated with some degree of fetomaternal hemorrhage in over 50 percent of cases.[73] A potentially dangerous increase in the maternal anti-D titer occurs when the volume of hemorrhage is over 1 ml.

Ultrasound and Doppler Studies

Ultrasonographic examination of the fetus has become an extremely important adjunct in the management of the Rh-sensitized pregnancy, primarily as a guide to amniocenteses and intrauterine transfusions. Several ultrasound findings have been advocated as indicators of fetal anemia and therefore useful as noninvasive measures to follow the progression of fetal hemolysis. Evidence of cardiac failure, such as cardiac enlargement, pericardial effusion, pleural effusion, ascites, and subcutaneous edema, appear late, when fetal anemia is severe. Indeed, at 18 to 24 weeks gestation sonographic evidence of fetal ascites predicts a fetal hematocrit less than 15 percent.[87,90] Ultrasound parameters suggested to be sensitive for lesser degrees of fetal anemia include increased placental thickness,[91] increased umbilical vein diameter,[92] appearance of a pericardial effusion,[93] and bowel wall edema.[94] However, none of these has proved to be reliable in distinguishing mild from severe disease, even in experienced hands.[90,95] Recently, it has been suggested that the measurement of the fetal liver length may reliably predict lesser degrees of fetal anemia,[96,97] but these findings need independent confirmation.

Doppler ultrasound determination of blood velocity waveforms is another noninvasive method suggested for assessment of fetal anemia. Increased blood velocities in the umbilical vein[98] and the fetal descending aorta[99,100] have been associated with fetal anemia. There is a fairly good correlation between the actual fetal hemoglobin/hematocrit and the value calculated by using arterial flow-velocity measurements. The most impressive data are those of Nicolaides et al.,[100] who studied 68 isoimmunized pregnancies. The investigators found that in isoimmunized pregnancies the fetal hemoglobin deficit was positively correlated with the deviation from normal of the aortic mean velocity ($r = 0.464$). The results were best for nonhydropic fetuses, in which there was a linear positive correlation ($r = 0.60$). For hydropic fetuses, the correlation was not as good, presumably because some cases of severe anemia are associated with cardiac decompensation that results in decreased flow velocities. However, it is as yet too early to use Doppler studies alone to follow isoimmunized pregnancies. There is a large overlap in aortic velocities between normal and anemic fetuses,[100] and one prospective analysis found that Doppler studies are not reliable enough for management purposes.[101] Doppler echocardiographic study of the fetus has likewise proved of little aid to fetal management.[102]

Ultrasound and Doppler ultrasound technology are advancing at a rapid pace. These noninvasive tools may one day be used to determine accurately and reliably the degree of fetal anemia and, thus, to direct fetal management. But at present, these tools cannot be recommended in lieu of amniotic fluid ΔOD_{450} determinations or fetal blood sampling for determining the need for intrauterine transfusion or delivery in Rh-immunized pregnancies. This is not to say that sonography is without value. At our institution we rely on once or twice weekly ultrasound evaluations of the fetus with suspected or proven moderate-to-severe hemolysis to detect early evidence of hydrops and to follow the response to transfusion.

Determining the Need for Intrauterine Transfusion

About half of susceptible infants of Rh-immunized pregnancies do not require intrauterine transfusion or extensive extrauterine therapy. Such fetuses are considered to have mild to moderate hemolytic disease. In general, a prognosis of mild to moderate fetal hemolysis is suggested when (1) the involved pregnancy is the first sensitized pregnancy or (2) previously delivered Rh-positive infants have been mildly to moderately affected (no hydrops; mild to moderate anemia). In such cases, we perform ultrasound examinations of the fetus every 2 to 4 weeks from 18 weeks gestation until delivery (see Fig. 29.3). If the fetus shows no evidence of hydrops, we use amniotic fluid ΔOD_{450} determinations for the initial management, performing the first at 24 to 28 weeks gestation. The timing of repeat amniocenteses and determination of the need for intrauterine transfusion or delivery are based on the ΔOD_{450} values and trend. If the values fall within the low zone or the lower half of the middle zone, amniocentesis is re-

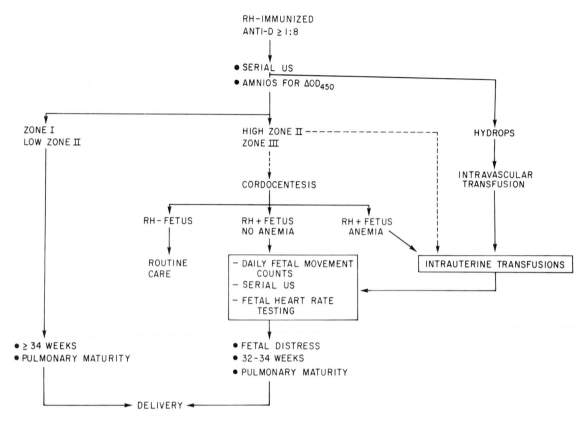

Fig. 29.3 Flow diagram outlining the management of Rh-immunized pregnancies at the University of Utah Medical Center.

peated every 10 days to 3 weeks, depending on the ΔOD_{450} trend. Severe anemia requiring intrauterine transfusion should be suspected when the ΔOD_{450} values rise into the upper quarter of the middle zone before 30 weeks gestation or into zone 3 before 30 and 32 weeks gestation. Depending on the clinical situation, a single ΔOD_{450} value in zone 3 also may be taken as an indication of severe anemia prior to 32 to 34 weeks gestation. If at any time the fetus has evidence of hydrops by ultrasound, one can assume a fetal hematocrit less than 15 percent,[87,90] and provisions for fetal blood sampling and transfusion should be made immediately. As shown by the broken line in Figure 29.3, the need for cordocentesis in the management of nonhydropic fetuses with ΔOD_{450} values indicative of severe anemia (and requiring intrauterine transfusion) is controversial. Experienced practitioners have described excellent perinatal outcomes

using either intraperitoneal[103-105] or intravascular[106] transfusions. The optimum management in an individual case will be determined by the experience and expertise of the physicians involved.

When the obstetric history suggests that the fetus is at risk for moderate to severe hemolysis and hydrops, we are more likely to begin the search for fetal hemolysis earlier in the pregnancy (18 to 22 weeks gestation). In this situation, cordocentesis to determine the fetal hematocrit (and antigen status) is a reasonable first step, since ΔOD_{450} values are less reliable in the mid-second trimester.[81] Nevertheless, some experienced practitioners continue to use serial ΔOD_{450} values and serial sonography to follow and treat these cases. Again, the optimum management in an individual case will be determined by the experience and expertise of the physicians involved.

The presence of fetal hydrops is to be taken as

evidence of severe fetal anemia and indication for immediate intravascular transfusion (with or without concomitant intraperitoneal transfusion).

INTRAUTERINE TRANSFUSION IN THE Rh-ISOIMMUNIZED PREGNANCY

In 1963, Liley reported the first successful intrauterine transfusion,[78] and a new therapeutic modality was created, one that provided obstetricians with a much-needed alternative to preterm delivery in severe erythroblastosis fetalis. The administration of erythrocytes to the involved fetus accomplishes two goals: (1) correcting fetal anemia and consequently improving fetal oxygenation and (2) reducing extramedullary hematopoietic demand, leading to a fall in portal venous pressure and improved hepatic function.

Originally, intrauterine transfusions were done by the intraperitoneal route, and this approach was the mainstay of transfusion therapy until the last decade. In 1981, Rodeck et al.[85] reported the successful intravenous transfusion of two erythroblastotic fetuses using a fetoscopic technique. Although the fetoscopic approach was quite successful,[86] introduction of the transfusion needle by ultrasound guidance (without the fetoscope) has become the most popular technique.[107–109] The umbilical vein is the most commonly used vessel, usually at its insertion into the placenta.

Intrauterine Intraperitoneal Transfusion

Immediately prior to the procedure, an intravenous line is placed in the mother, who is sedated with a parenterally administered narcotic and a short-acting benzodiazepine. We also administer an antiemetic and a prophylactic antibiotic. Using real-time ultrasound, fetal position and condition, placental location, and disposition of the amniotic fluid are determined. Intraperitoneal access is best accomplished with the fetus on its side or back. Some workers have suggested external manipulation of the fetus for positioning.[110,111] The fetal bladder and pelvic bones serve as useful landmarks. Peritoneal access is ideally

accomplished through the lateral or anterolateral abdominal wall. Care must be taken to avoid the umbilical cord and its insertion into the fetal abdomen.

After a site for needle insertion is chosen on the maternal abdomen, the area is prepared and draped in a sterile fashion. Using aseptic technique, an 18- or 20-gauge needle is directed under real-time guidance into the fetal peritoneum, ideally just cephalad and lateral to the fetal bladder. When it is felt that the needle tip has entered the fetal peritoneal cavity, saline solution or a small air bubble is introduced through the needle to verify its location within the peritoneal cavity (Fig. 29.4). Although we usually instill the blood through the needle, Bowman suggests using an epidural catheter for the actual transfusion.[112] About 30 cm of the size 16 catheter is passed down the needle. When the catheter is clearly seen in the fetal peritoneal cavity, the needle is then withdrawn from the maternal abdomen, leaving the catheter threaded for transfusion.

After verification that the needle tip or catheter is in the fetal peritoneal cavity, the transfusion is performed at a rate no faster than 5 to 10 ml/min. Using real-time ultrasonography, it is often possible to see the influx of red cells into the peritoneal cavity. Type O-negative, leukocyte-poor packed erythrocytes cross-matched with the maternal serum are used. The desired hematocrit for the packed cells is 75 to 80 percent. The transfusion is carried out manually with a 20- to 30-ml syringe connected to the transfusion line with a three-way stopcock.

The volume of blood in milliliters to be transfused is calculated by subtracting 20 from the gestational age in weeks and then multiplying it by 10. Thus, a 28-week fetus would receive 80 ml of blood. This simple formula is intended to provide a reasonable amount of blood to the fetus without creating undue intraperitoneal pressure. When fetal ascites is present, some of this fluid should be gently aspirated before transfusion. Bowman has suggested that no more than twice the volume of the proposed transfusion should be removed, with a maximum being 150 ml.[28] The rate of absorption of the transfused blood from the peritoneal cavity into the bloodstream is said to be about 12 percent per day in the nonhydropic fetus. However, in our experience, little or

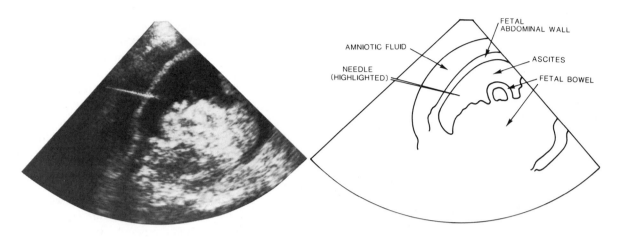

Fig. 29.4 Ultrasonographic study showing intrauterine transfusion needle in the fetal peritoneal cavity.

none of the transfused blood is detectable by ultrasonographic examination 3 days after transfusion in cases in which the fetus is not hydropic. If the fetus is hydropic, absorption is variable and certainly not predictable. In some cases it is adequate,[28] but in others absorption is quite poor.

It is important that the fetal heart rate be monitored periodically during the procedure in case fetal bradycardia occurs during transfusion. Bradycardia early in the procedure presages fetal death.[112] Late in the procedure, a fall in the fetal heart rate may indicate vena caval compression by an increased intraperitoneal pressure. Monitoring can be done easily with real-time ultrasound.

According to Bowman, one can estimate the residual donor hemoglobin in the fetus after the transfusion.[112] His estimation assumes that 55 percent of the transfused hemoglobin enters the fetal circulation after intraperitoneal transfusion and that the daily red cell loss is about 1/120 of the total. The amount of remaining donor hemoglobin may be estimated by the following calculation:

Remaining donor hemoglobin (g/dl) =

$$\frac{0.55 \times a}{85 \times b} \times \frac{120 - c}{120}$$

where a is donor transfusion hemoglobin in g/dl, b is the estimated fetal weight, and c is the number of days since transfusion. According to Bowman, the goal is to keep the donor hemoglobin in the fetus above 10 g/dl. This necessarily requires that the first and second transfusions be performed about 10 days apart. The timing of subsequent transfusions is calculated according to the preceding formula, which predicts a repeat intraperitoneal transfusion about every 4 weeks. Thus, the basic intraperitoneal transfusion schedule puts the second transfusion about 10 days after the first and a repeat every 4 weeks thereafter.

Intravascular Transfusion

Preparation of the patient is the same as for fetal intraperitoneal transfusion. The approach to the umbilical cord is determined with real-time ultrasound. A 20- or 22-gauge needle is used, and the progress of the needle tip is followed and guided by using continuous real-time ultrasound. When the placenta is anterior, we prefer to use the transplacental approach into the umbilical vein (Fig. 29.5). Otherwise, we attempt to enter the vessel by traversing the amniotic fluid and puncturing the cord near its insertion into the placenta. If the fetus is particularly active (in spite of the sedation administered to the mother) or the needle passes through an area occupied by the fetal extremities, the fetus can be paralyzed immediately on entry into the vessel by injecting pancuronium bromide, 0.05 to 0.1 mg/kg of estimated fetal weight. As with intraperitoneal transfusion, O-negative, leukocyte-poor packed erythrocytes cross-matched with

ANTERIOR or FUNDAL PLACENTA
Needle (highlighted)

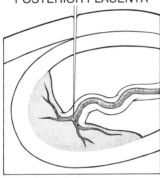

Umbilical
vein
Placenta

POSTERIOR PLACENTA

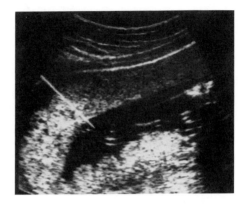

Fig. 29.5 Technique for intravascular fetal transfusion.

the maternal serum are used. When vascular access is attained, a small amount of blood is withdrawn into one to three heparinized 1-ml syringes and the hematocrit immediately determined. One sample should be used to determine the fetal antigen status if it is still in doubt.

With modern ultrasound, there is usually little doubt about the proper placement of the needle tip in the fetal circulation. A low fetal hematocrit confirms correct needle placement. We determine the volume of blood to be transfused according to a method derived from the work of Nicolaides et al.[113] Our goal is to achieve a post-transfusion hematocrit of 40 to 45 percent. The initial fetal hematocrit, the hematocrit of the donor blood, and the gestational age are used in conjunction with the graphs shown in Figure 29.6

to determine the amount of blood to be infused. When the infusion is started, it is crucial to note ultrasound "turbulence" streaming along the vessel. This confirms that the needle tip is still within the vessel. We infuse blood at a rapid rate of about 10 ml/min. Before withdrawal of the needle, a post-transfusion sample is drawn for measurement of the hematocrit.

After intravascular transfusion, the decline in the donor hematocrit is dependent on the life span of the donor erythrocytes, the rate of fetal growth, and the ratio of fetal to donor erythrocytes (since the fetal erythrocytes are subject to hemolysis). The latter is most influential between the first and second intravascular transfusion, during which time the ratio of fetal cells to donor cells is greatest. MacGregor and colleagues[114] have shown that the following equations

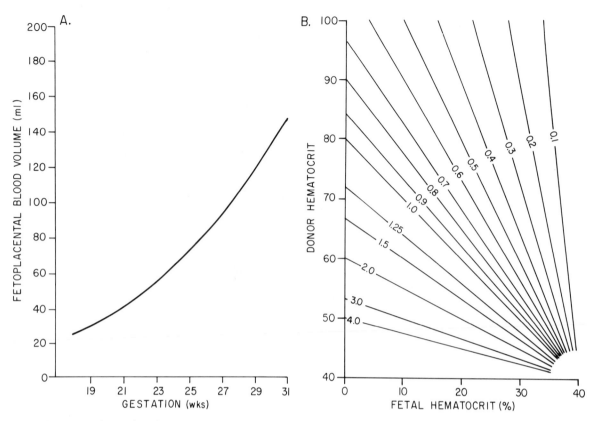

Fig. 29.6 Graphs used to determine rapidly the volume of blood to be transfused intravascularly to achieve a post-transfusion hematocrit of 40 to 45 percent. First, the estimated fetoplacental blood volume (EFBV) is determined by using the gestational age and graph A. Second, the pretransfusion fetal hematocrit and the donor blood hematocrit are used in conjunction with graph B to derive the multiplying factor. This factor is then multiplied by the EFBV to determine the amount of blood to be transfused. For example, at 26 weeks gestation, the EFBV is found on the abscissa of graph A to be 85 ml. If the pretransfusion hematocrit is 20 percent and the donor blood hematocrit is 80 percent, the multiplying factor derived from graph B is 0.5. Multiplying this number by the EFBV (0.5 × 85 ml) shows that about 42 ml should be transfused. (Adapted from Nicolaides et al.,[113] with permission.)

may be used to predict the fetal hematocrit after transfusion:

(a) Predicted HCT =
$$\frac{(\text{HCT f} - \text{HCT i}) \times (\text{EFW}_1/\text{EFW}_2) \times (120 - \text{days elapsed})}{120}$$

(b) Predicted HCT =
$$\frac{\text{HCT f} \times (\text{EFW}_1/\text{EFW}_2) \times (120 - \text{days elapsed})}{120}$$

where HCT f is the post-transfusion hematocrit, HCT i is the initial (pretransfusion) hematocrit, EFW$_1$ is the

ultrasonographically estimated fetal weight at the index transfusion, the EFW$_2$ is the ultrasonographically estimated fetal weight at the subsequent transfusion. Equation (a) is used to predict the fetal hematocrit after the first transfusion. Equation (b) is intended to predict the fetal hematocrit between subsequent transfusions. After the first transfusion, the decline in the fetal hematocrit is about 1.5 percent per day (SD = 1.6 percent); after subsequent transfusions, the decline in fetal hematocrit is about 1.2 percent per day (SD = 0.6 percent). Using intravascular transfusions for the management of severe fetal hemolysis, one should time subsequent transfusions to keep the fetal hematocrit above 25 to 30 percent. Although most authors suggest simply transfusing the fetus, some perform in utero exchange transfusions because of the fear that an overall increase in blood volume would compromise the fetal cardiac capacity.[115,116] These fears are probably unfounded.[117]

Intraperitoneal Versus Intravascular Transfusion

Direct intravascular transfusion has two distinct advantages over intraperitoneal transfusion. The first is that intravascular access allows the degree of fetal anemia to be measured. In turn, this allows the amount of blood required for the fetus to reach an acceptable hematocrit to be calculated with fair precision, rather than estimated as with intraperitoneal transfusion. Second, intravascular transfusion provides immediate correction of the fetal anemia. This appears to be particularly helpful in fetal hydrops, a problem for which intraperitoneal transfusion frequently proves ineffective. There are now numerous reports of the reversal of hydrops after intravascular transfusion.[109,118] Also, intravascular transfusion prevents the occasional problem of the fetus's developing hydrops soon after the first intraperitoneal transfusion because the amount of blood absorbed does not keep pace with the rate of developing anemia.

On the other hand, using intravascular transfusions alone increases the total number of procedures required because the volume of blood transfused at each procedure is smaller than that given via the intraperitoneal route. Also, fully 80 percent of blood transfused into the peritoneal cavity of nonhydropic fetuses appears in the fetal circulation,[119] a figure considerably higher than previously thought. Perhaps intravascular *exchange* transfusion may allow a longer interval between intravascular transfusions by replacing a greater volume of the fetal cells with donor cells at the time of the procedure.[116]

Intravascular transfusion is more effective than intraperitoneal transfusion in treating hydropic fetuses and in many cases is lifesaving. A recently published case–control comparison suggests that the intravascular approach is actually safer for the fetus than the intraperitoneal approach.[106] It may be that a combined approach will prove effective and allow the fewest number of procedures.[119,120] A recently completed study shows that, when compared to intravascular transfusions alone, combined intravascular and

intraperitoneal transfusion achieves a significantly longer interval between transfusions and maintains higher fetal hematocrits.[120] The authors performed intraperitoneal transfusions immediately after the intravascular transfusions. The amount of blood transfused intravascularly was calculated as described in this chapter, and the amount of blood subsequently transfused intraperitoneally was calculated according to the following equation:

$$V_{IPT} = V_{IVT} \frac{(\text{desired HCT} - \text{HCT f})}{(\text{HCT f} - \text{HCT i})}$$

where V_{IPT} is the volume of blood to be transfused intraperitoneally, V_{IVT} is the volume of blood transfused intravascularly, HCT f is the fetal hematocrit after the intravascular transfusion, and HCT i is the initial (pretransfusion) value. The desired fetal hematocrit is arbitrarily set between 50 to 60 percent. Using the estimated decline in fetal hematocrit and clinical parameters to decide on the timing of the next transfusion, the investigators performed only 3.2 procedures per patient. The mean fall in the hematocrit was slightly less than 1 percent per day. As with intravascular transfusion, the goal of the combined approach should be to keep the fetal hematocrit above 25 to 30 percent.

Transfusion-Related Risks

Series using cases from the 1970s and early 1980s suggest that the risk of death attributable to intraperitoneal transfusion is about 4 percent per procedure and that a transplacental approach bears three times the risk of other approaches.[112] Because multiple procedures are required, the risk of fetal death runs about 10 percent per case.[112]

Fewer data regarding the risk of fetal mortality with intravascular transfusions are available. The mortality rate per procedure is probably about 2 percent,[117,121] and the reported overall attributable fetal mortality ranges from about 1 to over 12 percent.[106,108,112,116,121] No study has compared the risks associated with intravascular and intraperitoneal transfusions by experienced practitioners using modern technology and techniques. The pertinent technology has improved dramatically during the evolution of intravascular transfusions, especially in the area of ultrasound and neonatal care. Comparisons of fetal outcomes using intravascular transfusion to historical cases managed with intraperitoneal transfusions are subject to several biases. These notwithstanding, Harman et al. recently reported that management with intravascular transfusions resulted in fewer procedural implications and attributable fetal losses than management with intraperitoneal transfusions in matched, historical cases.[106]

Other risks of intrauterine transfusion include intrauterine infection, rupture of the membranes, and fetomaternal hemorrhage. We feel that infection can be largely prevented through the use of prophylactic antibiotics.

Other Therapies

Alternatives to intrauterine transfusion have been sought for the treatment of fetal hemolysis. Most of these have been aimed at modifying the maternal immune response so as to decrease the severity of erythroblastosis. Two of these, promethazine[122,123] and oral ingestion of Rh-positive erythrocytes,[124,125] are of historical interest only. Neither proved to be of benefit.

Plasmapheresis to reduce the level of maternal anti-D has also been tried in the treatment of severe Rh isoimmunization. Although the removal of several liters of plasma per week results in a transient reduction in the anti-D titer during or immediately after treatment, a chronic, significant reduction in antibody titer is difficult, if not impossible, to achieve by this technique.[126–128] Some studies suggest a benefit to plasmapheresis,[129,130] but these results are difficult to interpret because of the concomitant use of other treatments and the lack of controls. Furthermore, all studies of plasmapheresis in which several or more liters of plasma were removed weekly demonstrated an increase in anti-D titers or in concentration soon after plasmapheresis was stopped. This "rebound" phenomenon has been attributed to the removal of the negative feedback influence on further anti-D production by high circulating titers of anti-D antibody.[131] Repeated "small-volume" plasmapheresis may prevent antibody rebound.[131] The potential usefulness of plasmapheresis must be tempered by its potential for serious consequences for the mother and fetus. There are two case reports documenting maternal sepsis in Rh-sensitized patients undergoing plasmapheresis.[127,129] In view of the lack of a clearly documented benefit, plasmapheresis is not currently used at most centers.

The successful use of intravenous high-dose immunoglobulin (IgG) in platelet isoimmunization has led to its trial use in the treatment of severe Rh isoimmunization. The supposed mechanism of action is via either Fc receptor blockade in the fetal reticuloendothelial system (limiting the removal and destruction of anti-D coated erythrocytes in the fetal spleen and liver) or blockade of Fc-mediated antibody placental transport (limiting the transplacental passage of anti-D to the fetus). The apparent success of IgG therapy in ameliorating severe Rh disease[132–134] presents exciting possibilities. The IgG has been given to the mother in doses of 0.4 g/kg/day for 5 days, with the assumption that significant amounts cross the placenta and thereby have a beneficial effect on the fetus. However, placental transport of exogenous IgG may be limited before 32 weeks gestation.[135] Introduction of the IgG directly into the fetal circulation via cordocentesis may turn out to be the most effective route of administration prior to 32 weeks gestation. Further studies and treatment of more patients will be necessary to verify the tentative conclusion that IgG therapy has a place in the management of severe Rh immunization.

Timing of Delivery

During the early 1960s, it was recognized that preterm delivery markedly reduced the incidence of perinatal death in Rh-sensitized pregnancies,[76,136] primarily as a result of a decrease in the incidence of intrauterine death. However, severely affected fetuses continued to die in utero or from complications of prematurity. Fortunately, refinements in the technique of intrauterine transfusion have made possible the prolongation of intrauterine life until a gestational age compatible with extrauterine survival is reached. Also, the availability of phospholipid analysis of the amniotic fluid to determine fetal pulmonary maturity has greatly clarified the timing of delivery in relation to neonatal risk. Finally, the vast improvements in neonatal care over the past two decades have also led to excellent survival rates, with acceptable morbidity rates, for the preterm infant.

If the history and antenatal studies indicate mild fetal hemolysis, fetal pulmonary maturity is awaited before undertaking delivery by induction of labor, usually at 34 to 37 weeks gestation. If the cervix is not ripe, intracervical prostaglandin gel for cervical ripening is used prior to induction.

Rather than subject the fetus to the risk of intrauterine transfusion, severely sensitized pregnancies are delivered after 32 weeks gestation at our institution. This policy is based on a greater than 95 percent overall neonatal survival rate after 32 weeks gestation in our neonatal intensive care unit. There were no neonatal deaths in 29 erythroblastotic fetuses delivered after 29 weeks gestation from 1978 to 1982. Overall survival may have increased further since then with the addition of surfactant therapy to neonatal treatment. But in the interest of limiting morbidity, some investigators recommend the judicious use of intrauterine transfusion after 32 weeks gestation when pulmonary phospholipid studies at 32 to 33 weeks indicate that the fetus is immature.[112] Delivery is then accomplished between 34 to 36 weeks gestation. Regardless of the usual institutional practices, individual case circumstances need to be carefully weighed when making the decision as to when the fetus should be delivered.

Perinatal Outcome

Perinatal survival in severe Rh isoimmunization has improved steadily with the improvements in intrauterine transfusion techniques and neonatal intensive care. In 1968, Queenan[137] reported a 34 percent survival rate in 591 fetuses treated with intraperitoneal transfusion. In this series, the earlier a fetus required transfusion, the poorer the outcome. Fetuses transfused before 25 weeks gestation suffered a 91 percent perinatal mortality rate. Other workers reported that evidence of hydrops, such as ascites noted at the time of the first intrauterine transfusion, presaged a very poor outcome.[138] However, by 1971 more optimistic results were published; one series reported an overall perinatal survival rate of 40 percent in 56 fetuses requiring intrauterine (intraperitoneal) transfusion.[139] By 1978, Bowman claimed an overall perinatal survival rate of 70 percent.[28] In addition, the survival rate of fetuses with hydrops was an impressive 50 percent. More recently, Bowman and Manning[104] and Scott et al.[103] reported perinatal survival rates of more than 80 percent using intraperitoneal transfusion.

Table 29.4 Perinatal Survival Rates with Intrauterine Transfusion

Author	Survival Rate
Intraperitoneal	
Bowman et al.[104]	20/22 (86%)
Scott et al.[103]	16/20 (80%)
Watts et al.[105]	30/35 (86%)
Total	66/77 (86%)
Intravascular	
Nicolaides et al.[140]	20/21 (95%)
Berkowitz et al.[141]	13/17 (76%)
Grannum et al.[142]	21/26 (82%)
Ronkin et al.[143]	8/8 (100%)
Barass et al.[131]	12/14 (86%)
Poissonnier et al.[116]	84/107 (78%)
Total	158/193 (82%)

The use of intravascular transfusion has not dramatically improved the overall perinatal survival rate among infants with severe hemolytic disease (Table 29.4),[104,105,116,121,140–143] but it may improve the outcome for fetuses who are hydropic at the time of initial presentation. In one large series,[116] intravascular transfusion was used to achieve a survival rate of over 60 percent among 47 fetuses with hydrops. Smaller series have also achieved high survival rates.[118,121]

SENSITIZATION CAUSED BY MINOR ANTIGENS

The success of Rh-immune prophylaxis has focused attention on the relative importance of maternal sensitization to the erythrocyte antigens other than the D antigen.[144] Traditionally these erythrocyte antigens were called "minor," "atypical," or "irregular" antigens. They were only infrequently the cause of maternal immunization or fetal or neonatal hemolytic disease. However, today maternal antibodies to the minor antigens are detected as frequently as or more frequently than anti-D antibody. An analysis of recent cases of maternal sensitization to erythrocyte antigens in northern England found antibodies to the minor antigens to be more than five times as common as antibodies to the D antigen (3 vs. 0.5 per 1,000 births).[71]

The overall incidence of the atypical erythrocyte antibodies varies within any population; however, incidence is higher in multiparas and in patients who have been transfused. Most are probably the result of incompatible red cell transfusions. Queenan et al.[145] reported an incidence of irregular antibodies of 1.62 percent for 18,378 consecutive obstetric patients screened at New York Hospital from 1960 through 1967. Polesky[146] detected irregular antibodies in 2.44 percent of 43,000 women screened. Fortunately, some of the more frequently identified atypical antibodies, such as anti-Le[a], anti-Le[b], and anti-I, do not cause hemolytic disease of the newborn. Le[a] and Le[b], the Lewis antigens, are not true erythrocyte antigens: they are antigens secreted by tissues other than the red cells that are acquired by erythrocytes by adsorption.[147] Fetal erythrocytes acquire very little antigen in utero and thus react weakly with anti-Lewis antibodies.

Of the atypical antibodies that can cause fetal or neonatal hemolysis, older series found anti-Kell, anti-E, and anti-C to be most common. Tovey's recent study found the most common potentially serious antibodies to be (in decreasing order of frequency) anti-E, anti-Kell, anti-c, anti-c + E, and anti-Fy[a] (Duffy).[71] A complete list of irregular antibodies and antigens as compiled by Weinstein is given in Table 29.5. The reports of their association with hemolytic disease of the newborn and the management proposed are shown as well.

Several investigators have suggested that the fetal anemia associated with anti-Kell sensitization is qualitatively different from that of Rh disease.[148,149] Specifically, it appears that the Δ OD$_{450}$ values may not be as elevated for a given degree of fetal anemia.[149] One explanation for this is that the primary cause of anemia in Kell sensitization is the suppression of fetal erythropoiesis rather than hemolysis.[117] Management of Kell sensitization in pregnancy should include the more liberal use of cordocentesis, rather than dependence on the amniotic fluid bilirubin levels, to determine the degree of fetal anemia.

Once an atypical antibody is detected in a pregnant woman, consideration should be given to determining the paternal antigen status, especially if the sensitization might be due to transfusion. As regards the Kell antigen, over 90 percent of individuals are Kell-antigen-negative and only 0.2 percent are homozygous. Over 95 percent of whites and 80 percent of blacks are Duffy-antigen-negative. On the other hand, 80 percent of men are c-antigen-positive, and nearly half are homozygous. For the majority of atypical antibodies, it appears reasonable to determine the fetal antigen status via cordocentesis at 18 to 22 weeks gestation in order to decide whether special antenatal management is in order.

ABO INCOMPATIBILITY

Twenty to 25 percent of pregnancies are ABO-incompatible: that is, the mother's serum contains anti-A or anti-B, whereas the fetus's erythrocytes contain the respective antigen. As a result ABO incompatibility is a common cause of hemolytic disease of the newborn, accounting for over 60 percent of all cases.[150] Fortunately, the disease is always manifested as no worse than moderate neonatal anemia and mild to moderate neonatal hyperbilirubinemia. Less than 1 percent of cases require exchange transfusion.[151] ABO incompatibility has never clearly been shown to be a cause of fetal hemolysis and can generally be regarded as a pediatric rather than an obstetric problem.[152]

There are several reasons why ABO incompatibility rarely results in severe hemolytic disease. Individuals with group A or B blood types produce predominantly IgM anti-B or anti-A, which cross the placenta poorly. Also, there are fewer A and B antigen sites on the fetal erythrocyte than on the adult erythrocyte; thus, less antibody can bind to fetal red cell membranes. Finally, maternal and fetal tissues other than erythrocytes contain the A and B antigens, and some investigators believe that anti-A or anti-B antibodies are absorbed by these sites so that less of the antibodies are available for erythrocyte binding.[150]

The A and B antigens are "naturally occurring" antigens: that is, they occur widely in nature unassociated with erythrocyte membranes. Therefore, A or B sensitization does not require prior exposure to red cells through pregnancy or by transfusion, and it is not unusual for ABO-hemolytic disease to affect the firstborn child. Clinically apparent hemolytic disease of the newborn resulting from ABO incompatibility is mostly confined to the situation wherein the mother is type O and the infant is type A or B,[150] because group O individuals produce anti-A and anti-B that is

Table 29.5 Atypical Antibodies and Their Relationship to Fetal Hemolytic Disease

Blood Group System	Antigens Related to Hemolytic Disease	Hemolytic Disease Severity	Proposed Management
Lewis	Not a proven cause of hemolytic disease of the newborn		
I	Not a proven cause of hemolytic disease of the newborn		
Kell	K	Mild to severe with hydrops fetalis	Amniotic fluid bilirubin studies
	k	Mild	Expectant
	Ko	Mild	Expectant
	Kp^a	Mild	Expectant
	Kp^b	Mild	Expectant
	Js^a	Mild	Expectant
	Js^b	Mild	Expectant
Rh (non-D)	E	Mild to severe with hydrops fetalis	Amniotic fluid bilirubin studies
	C	Mild to severe with hydrops fetalis	Amniotic fluid bilirubin studies
	c	Mild to severe with hydrops fetalis	Amniotic fluid bilirubin studies
Duffy	Fy^a	Mild to severe with hydrops fetalis	Amniotic fluid bilirubin studies
	Fy^b	Not a cause of hemolytic disease of the newborn	
	By^3	Mild	Expectant
Kidd	Jk^a	Mild to severe	Amniotic fluid bilirubin studies
	Jk^b	Mild	Expectant
	Jk^3	Mild	Expectant
MNSs	M	Mild to severe	Amniotic fluid bilirubin studies
	N	Mild	Expectant
	S	Mild to severe	Amniotic fluid bilirubin studies
	s	Mild to severe	Amniotic fluid bilirubin studies
	U	Mild to severe	Amniotic fluid bilirubin studies
	Mi^a	Moderate	Amniotic fluid bilirubin studies
MSSs	Mt^a	Moderate	Amniotic fluid bilirubin studies
	Vw	Mild	Expectant
	Mur	Mild	Expectant
	Hil	Mild	Expectant
	Hut	Mild	Expectant
Lutheran	Lu^a	Mild	Expectant
	Lu^b	Mild	Expectant

(continued)

Table 29.5 (continued)

Blood Group System	Antigens Related to Hemolytic Disease	Hemolytic Disease Severity	Proposed Management
Diego	DI^a	Mild to severe	Amniotic fluid bilirubin studies
	Di^b	Mild to severe	Amniotic fluid bilirubin studies
Xg	Xg^a	Mild	Expectant
P	pp$_1$pk$_{(Tj^a)}$	Mild to severe	Amniotic fluid bilirubin studies
Public antigens	Yt^a	Moderate to severe	Amniotic fluid bilirubin studies
	Yt^b	Mild	Expectant
	Lan	Mild	Expectant
	En^a	Moderate	Amniotic fluid bilirubin studies
	Ge	Mild	Expectant
	Jr^a	Mild	Expectant
	Co^a	Severe	Amniotic fluid bilirubin studies
	Co^{a-b-}	Mild	Expectant
Private antigens	Batty	Mild	Expectant
	Becker	Mild	Expectant
	Berrens	Mild	Expectant
	Biles	Moderate	Amniotic fluid bilirubin studies
	Evans	Mild	Expectant
	Gonzales	Mild	Expectant
	Good	Severe	Amniotic fluid bilirubin studies
	Heibel	Moderate	Amniotic fluid bilirubin studies
	Hunt	Mild	Expectant
	Jobbins	Mild	Expectant
	Radin	Moderate	Amniotic fluid bilirubin studies
	Rm	Mild	Expectant
	Ven	Mild	Expectant
	Wright^a	Severe	Amniotic fluid bilirubin studies
	Wright^b	Mild	Expectant
	Zd	Moderate	Amniotic fluid bilirubin studies

(Modified from Weinstein,[144] with permission.)

predominantly of the IgG class and can therefore cross the placenta to bind to the fetal erythrocytes.

In most cases, ABO hemolytic disease manifests itself as mild to moderate hyperbilirubinemia during the first 24 hours of life. It is rarely associated with significant anemia. Because high levels of bilirubin can cause kernicterus, phototherapy or exchange transfusion may be indicated, according to the degree of hyperbilirubinemia.

Because ABO incompatibility is likely to occur in subsequent pregnancies, the delivery of an affected newborn should be clearly documented in the patient's record. However, since significant fetal hemolysis does not occur, screening for anti-A or anti-B antibodies in the mother's serum and analysis of the amniotic fluid for bilirubin are not required.

NONIMMUNE HYDROPS FETALIS

Hydrops fetalis not due to erythrocyte antibodies is termed nonimmune hydrops fetalis (NIHF). Sonographically and grossly, NIHF is indistinguishable from hydrops due to erythroblastosis fetalis (Fig. 29.7). Because of the effectiveness of Rh-immune in nature, most cases of fetal hydrops seen today are nonimmune in nature. The incidence of NIHF ranges from 1 in 2,500 to 3,500 births.[153,154]

NIHF is associated with a wide variety of fetal conditions. In one large series, Hutchinson et al.[153] found a high incidence of major anomalies (41 percent), including congenital heart disease, cystic adenomatoid malformation of the lung, and renal dysplasia. Holzgreve et al. found that the most common "causes" of NIHF were cardiac anomalies (22 percent), chromosomal abnormalities (14 percent), multiple anomalies (12 percent), and hematologic abnormalities (10 percent).[155] We recently reviewed all cases of antenatally diagnosed NIHF at our institution and found 60 cases over an 8-year period. Nearly one-quarter of our cases were due to chromosomal abnormalities, and 18 percent were associated with multiple anomalies. In contrast to the findings of many others, we found that less than 2 percent of cases of NIHF were due to *isolated* cardiac defects. Fetal cardiac dysrhythmias such as supraventricular

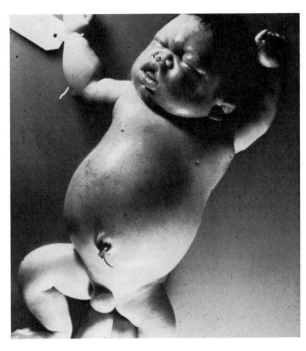

Fig. 29.7 Hydropic stillborn fetus. Nonimmune hydrops fetalis resulted from homozygous α-thalassemia. (Courtesy of Dr. James Wheeler, Department of Surgical Pathology, Hospital of the University of Pennsylvania, Philadelphia, PA.)

tachycardia have also been associated with nonimmune hydrops fetalis.

The perinatal mortality rate observed in cases of NIHF is at least 50 percent; our own experience and several series suggest a mortality rate of over 90 percent.[153,156] An outline for the evaluation of NIHF is shown in Table 29.6.

NIHF resulting from human parvovirus B19 deserves special comment in the context of this chapter. In children, human parvovirus B19 causes a mild viral exanthem known as erythema infectiosum (fifth disease). In otherwise normal adults, parvovirus infection can result in a rubella-like disease characterized by a transient maculopapular rash, arthralgias, and malaise. In many cases, the symptoms are so mild that they are ignored by the patient.

More recently, a more serious consequence of human parvovirus has been recognized. Parvovirus B19 appears to precipitate aplastic crises in patients

Table 29.6   Evaluation of Nonimmune Hydrops Fetalis

Test	Possible Diagnosis
Maternal studies	
Complete blood count	α-Thalassemia carrier
Kleihauer-Betke test	Fetomaternal hemorrhage
TORCH screen, RPR	Congenital infections
Medical history	Hereditary diseases, metabolic diseases, infections, medications
Fetal studies (amniocentesis/ cordocentesis)	
Karyotype	Chromosomal abnormalities
Hematocrit	Fetal anemia (e.g., from fetomaternal hemorrhage)
Viral cultures	Cytomegalovirus, herpes simplex virus, parvovirus, other viruses
Total plasma IgM	Congenital infections
Hemoglobin electrophoresis	α-Thalassemia
Specific metabolic tests	Metabolic disorders
Fetal sonography	Anomalies, tumors, cardiac dysrhythmias

with chronic hemolytic anemias because the virus infects and destroys erythroid progenitor cells, thus impairing effective erythropoiesis. Severe anemia may occur in the fetus following congenital infection by an analagous mechanism. As in the adult, the virus has a predilection for the erythroid precursor cells and causes erythroid failure.[156a] In the fetus, as in the adult with chronic hemolysis, erythrocytes have a relatively short life span. Moreover, fetal erythropoiesis is stressed by a substantial physiologic expansion of the fetal red cell mass in the second trimester. For these reasons, impairment or arrest of fetal erythrogenesis by human parvovirus B19 may result in severe fetal anemia with hydrops, especially if the congenital infection occurs in the second trimester. Since the fetal infection appears to be transient in most cases, support of the anemic fetus by transfusion may be reasonable. Successful management of infected, hydropic fetuses by serial intravascular transfusion has been reported.[156b,156c] The physician should note, how-

ever, that only about one-third of maternal parvovirus infections result in congenital infection, and most infected fetuses do not require intrauterine therapy and appear normal at birth.[156d]

PLATELET ISOIMMUNIZATION

Neonatal thrombocytopenia, resulting from maternal isoimmunization, is uncommon and occurs about once in every 1,000 to 5,000 births.[157,158] It is analogous to Rh isoimmunization in that the mother forms IgG antibodies to antigens present on the fetal and paternal platelets. These antibodies cross the placenta and lead to an increase in platelet destruction by way of the sequestration in the reticuloendothelial system.[159] There is a wide variation in the severity of neonatal isoimmune thrombocytopenia. Some infants present with only mild petechiae; others manifest extensive, severe hemorrhage. The attributable perinatal mortality rate is 5 to 13 percent.[157,159] Most of the mortality is due to intracranial hemorrhage, which more recent large series have shown occurs in 9 to 14 percent of affected infants.[159,160]

Hemorrhagic complications usually appear in the immediate neonatal period, but fetal thrombocytopenia is often detected by 20 to 22 weeks gestation[161,162] and intracranial bleeding occurring in utero has been reported in numerous cases.[163–166] The in utero intracranial hemorrhage appears typically to result in porencephalic cysts.[165] The frequency of in utero intracranial hemorrhage in isoimmune thrombocytopenia is not firmly established, but a recent report of 88 cases found evidence of in utero intracranial hemorrhage in five infants (6 percent).[160]

Unlike those affected by Rh isoimmunization, firstborn children are often affected with isoimmune thrombocytopenia. In the series reviewed by Pearson et al.,[157] 20 percent of the affected infants were born of primigravidas. A more recent review found that the firstborn infant was the initially affected infant in nearly 60 percent of cases.[159] This suggests that fetal platelets gain access to the maternal circulation more easily than do fetal erythrocytes.

The P1[A1] platelet antigen is the most common cause of neonatal isoimmune thrombocytopenia.

Sensitive antibody detection techniques show that $P1^{A1}$ isoimmunization is responsible for more than 80 percent of cases of platelet isoimmunization.[159,160,167] However, about 20 percent of cases have no maternal antiplatelet antibody detectable by the usually available techniques. In these cases, the diagnosis is one of exclusion. Only 3 percent of individuals lack the $P1^{A1}$ antigen; thus, the finding that a normal mother of a thrombocytopenic infant has $P1^{A1}$-negative platelets is strong evidence that isoimmunization is the cause of the thrombocytopenia. Seven other antigens have been reported to cause isoimmunization and neonatal thrombocytopenia: $DUZO^a$, $P1^{E2}$, Ko^a, Bak^a, Pen (Yuk), Br^a, and $P1^{A2}$.[159,160] It is also reported that anti-HLA antibodies may cause neonatal isoimmune thrombocytopenia.[168] Maternal HLA type may influence susceptibility to platelet isoimmunization to $P1^{A1}$ antigens; HLA-B8 and HLA-DR3 are associated with isoimmunization.[169]

The therapy of neonatal isoimmune thrombocytopenia is directed at preventing hemorrhage in the fetus and neonate. For several reasons, antenatal treatment has been a focus of attention in the last 6 years. First, it is now clear that the fetus may be severely thrombocytopenic and may spontaneously hemorrhage in utero. Second, previous birth of an affected infant predicts a 75 to 97 percent chance of similar or worse neonatal thrombocytopenia in the next pregnancy.[159] Finally, the availability of cordocentesis allows fetal platelet count determinations and individualized fetal therapy. Although maternally administered adrenocorticosteroids may improve the fetal platelet count in cases of idiopathic thrombocytopenic purpura,[170] there is little evidence that adrenocorticosteroids improve the fetal platelet count in isoimmune thrombocytopenia. Given the risks of steroid therapy, these drugs cannot be recommended in such cases.

In utero therapy has been suggested for thrombocytopenic fetuses at risk for hemorrhage (i.e., a low intrauterine platelet count and/or a sibling with thrombocytopenia and hemorrhage). Both fetal platelet transfusions and maternally administered high-dose immune globulin appear to raise the fetal platelet count in utero, and each therapy has its supporters. According to one scheme of management,[171,172] the diagnosis of fetal thrombocytopenia is made via cordocentesis at 20 to 22 weeks gestation and the patient with an affected fetus is advised to rest carefully until approximately 37 weeks. At that time, another fetal platelet count is performed and carefully washed maternal platelets are transfused into the fetus via cordocentesis according to the following formula:

$$V = EFBV \frac{(\text{desired FPC} - \text{pretransfusion FPC})}{\text{count of platelet concentrate}}$$

where V is the volume of platelet concentrate to be transfused, EFBV is the estimated fetal blood volume, and FPC is the fetal platelet count.[172] This approach, with a single fetal platelet transfusion immediately prior to delivery, is the most reasonable management for fetuses considered to be at low risk for hemorrhage in utero.

Another group of investigators has suggested treatment of affected fetuses at risk for hemorrhage in utero with weekly intrauterine platelet transfusions beginning in the second trimester to prevent spontaneous fetal hemorrhage in the second and early third trimesters.[173] Their case report demonstrated the short life span of platelets transfused in utero, with counts always dropping from post-transfusion levels over 150,000 cells/μl to fewer than 50,000 cells/μl immediately prior to the weekly transfusion. However attractive from a therapeutic standpoint, this approach will likely be limited by the morbidity and mortality rates associated with frequent cordocentesis and the difficulty and risks of repeated plateletpheresis. Fetal intracranial hemorrhage is rare before the third trimester, and it has been suggested that weekly intrauterine platelet transfusions might be limited to the third trimester, with delivery as soon as pulmonary maturity is documented.[174,175]

Maternally administered high-dose immunoglobulin (IgG) has recently been touted as a low-risk, noninvasive therapy for fetal isoimmune thrombocytopenia.[175] This approach is based on the observation that isoimmune thrombocytopenia may be effectively treated by giving the neonate intravenous IgG.[177–179] The mechanism of action is thought to be Fc-receptor blockade in the reticuloendothelial system, thus inhibiting the uptake of IgG coated platelets by reticuloendothelial cells. By analogy, intravenous IgG administered to the mother may treat fetal isoimmune thrombocytopenia if sufficient IgG crosses the placenta. Bussel et al. treated seven pregnant women who had previously delivered an infant with isoimmune thrombocytopenia (platelet counts < 30,000 cells/μl) with 1.0 g of IgG administered intravenously once each week from 20 to 26 weeks gestation until delivery.[176] Six of the fetuses had cordocentesis at 20 to 22 weeks gestation to prove the diagnosis of fetal thrombocytopenia; five of the six had platelet counts less than 40,000 cells/μl. Five patients also received dexamethasone daily. All treated cases were delivered of healthy infants with platelet counts greater than 30,000 cells/μl at birth, and the investigators concluded that high-dose IgG administered to the mother during pregnancy prevents neonatal isoimmune thrombocytopenia (with or without dexamethasone). In all cases, the treated infants had higher platelet counts than their untreated siblings. However, the treatment does not always appear to be successful because three infants had platelet counts of 50,000 cells/μl or less at birth. Moreover, in three other case reports maternally administered high-dose IgG had no effect on the fetal platelet count,[172,180,181] although only one used the regimen proposed by Bussel et al.[181] One problem with maternally administered IgG is that it may not cross the placenta effectively prior to 32 weeks gestation.[135] Further work is needed to establish whether IgG administered to the mother actually treats fetal thrombocytopenia in the second and early third trimesters because the treatment is quite expensive, costing well over $1,000 per weekly course. Although research results have not been published to date, delivery of the IgG directly into the fetal circulation via cordocentesis may turn out to be the most effective and least expensive method of therapy.

Cesarean delivery is generally considered the preferred method in cases of isoimmune thrombocytopenia because it is assumed to be the least traumatic. However, this point has never been proved and would appear to be moot if the fetal platelet count immediately prior to delivery is normal.

The newborn who is actively bleeding or is at significant risk of hemorrhage because of severe thrombocytopenia should be transfused with carefully washed maternal (antigen-negative) platelets. This requires anticipatory preparation of maternal platelets prior

to elective delivery. The response is typically excellent, boosting the neonatal platelet count to an acceptable level in over 95 percent of cases.[159] In an unexpected emergency, donor platelets may be tried, but at least two-thirds of cases do not respond with a significant rise in the platelet count.[159] Intravenous IgG has been used successfully to treat neonatal isoimmune thrombocytopenia[177-179] and is fast becoming part of the standard treatment regimen, with or without platelet transfusion. The beneficial effect may take up to 24 hours,[179] but repeated daily infusions of 0.4 to 1 g/k of IgG sustain the neonatal platelet count in the normal range. Corticosteroids may also be beneficial, and several investigators suggest using them in conjunction with other therapies.

SUMMARY

The incidence of serious isoimmunization leading to fetal or neonatal death has fallen dramatically since the introduction of Rh-immune globulin during the late 1960s. However, with the decreased incidence, there has evolved a decreased awareness of the prevention and management of isoimmunization in pregnancy. Today, Rh isoimmunization is virtually a preventable disease, and the unsensitized patient who is at risk should be identified early in pregnancy and appropriately treated with Rh-immune globulin. A few Rh-negative patients nevertheless become sensitized because of antepartum sensitization or postpartum prophylaxis failure, but these problems are being addressed with the use of antepartum prophylaxis and detection of excessive fetomaternal hemorrhage. However, pregnancy associated sensitization caused by the minor antigens is not preventable by immunoprophylaxis. Thus, proper surveillance for maternal antibodies that cause hemolytic disease of the newborn is the obligation of every physician who cares for pregnant women. If isoimmunization is detected, appropriate diagnostic studies must be carried out to determine the severity of fetal involvement and the need for intervention with intrauterine transfusions or delivery.

REFERENCES

1. Diamond LK, Blackfan KD, Baty JM: Erythroblastosis

fetalis and its association with universal edema of the fetus, icterus gravis neonatorum and anemia of the newborn. J Pediatr 1:269, 1932

2. Darrow RR: Icterus gravis (erythroblastosis) neonatorum: examination of etiologic considerations. Arch Pathol Lab Med 25:378, 1938

3. Levine P, Stetson RE: An unusual case of intragroup agglutination. JAMA 113:126, 1939

4. Levin P, Burnham L, Katzin EM et al: The role of isoimmunization in the pathogenesis of erythroblastosis fetalis. Am J Obstet Gynecol 42:925, 1941

5. Halbrecht I: Role of hemagglutinins anti-A and anti-B in the pathogenesis of jaundice of the newborn (icterus neonatorum precox). Am J Dis Child 68:248, 1944

6. Landsteiner K, Wiener AS: An agglutinable factor in human blood recognized by immune sera for rhesus blood. Proc Soc Exp Biol Med 43:223, 1940

7. Rosenfield RE, Allen FH, Rubenstein P: Genetic model for the Rh blood-group system. Proc Natl Acad Sci USA 70:1303, 1973

8. Race RR, Sanger R: Blood Groups in Man. 6th Ed. Blackwell Scientific Publications, Oxford, 1975

9. Rote NS: Pathophysiology of Rh isoimmunization. Clin Obstet Gynecol 25:243, 1982

10. Wiener AS: The Rh series of allelic genes. Science 100:595, 1944

11. Marsh W, Kimball LF: Mapping assignment of the Rh and Duffy blood group genes to chromosome 1. Mayo Clin Proc 52:145, 1977

12. Marsh WL, Chaganti RSK, Mayer K et al: Mapping human autosomes: evidence supporting assignment of rhesus to the short arm of chromosome number 1. Science 183:966, 1974

13. Stroup M: Rh system: genetics and function. Mayo Clin Proc 52:141, 1977

14. Hughes-Jones NC, Gardner B, Lincoln PJ: Observations on the number of available c, D, and E antigen sites on red cells. Vox Sang 21:210, 1971

15. Skov F, Hughes-Jones NC: Observations on the number of available C antigen sites on red cells. Vox Sang 33:170, 1977

16. Gorick BD, Thompson KM, Melamed MD, Hughes-Jones NC: Three epitopes on the human Rh antigen D recognized by ^{125}I-labelled human monoclonal IgG antibodies. Vox Sang 55:165, 1988

17. Masouredis SP: Relationship between Rho(D) genotype and quantity of I[131] anti-Rho(D) bound to red cells. J Clin Invest 39:1450, 1960

18. James NT, James V: Nearest neighbor analysis on the distribution of Rh antigens on erythrocyte membranes. Br J Haematol 40:657, 1978

19. Bloyd C, Blanchard D, Lambin P et al: Human monoclonal antibody against Rh(D) antigen: partial characterization of the Rh(D) polypeptide from human erythrocytes. Blood 69:1491, 1987

20. Brown PJ, Evans JP, Sinor LT et al: The rhesus antigen: a dicyclohexylcarbodiimide-binding proteolipid. Am J Pathol 110:127, 1983

21. Bergstrom H, Nilsson LA, Nilsson L et al: Demonstration of Rh antigens in a 38-day-old fetus. Am J Obstet Gynecol 99:130, 1967

22. Reardon A, Masouredis SP: Blood group D antigen content of nucleated red cell precursors. Blood 50:981, 1977

23. Lauf PK, Clinton HJ: Increased potassium transport and ouabain binding in human Rh null red blood cells. Blood 48:457, 1976

24. Cohen F, Zuelzer WW, Gustafson DC et al: Mechanisms of isoimmunization. I: The transplacental passage of fetal erythrocytes in homospecific pregnancies. Blood 23:621, 1964

25. Lloyd LK, Miya F, Hebertson RM et al: Intrapartum fetomaternal bleeding in Rh-negative women. Obstet Gynecol 56:285, 1980

26. Woodrow JC: Transplacental hemorrhage. Series Haematol 3:15, 1970

27. Zipursky A, Israels LG: The pathogenesis and prevention of Rh immunization. Can Med Assoc J 97:1245, 1967

28. Bowman JM: The management of Rh-isoimmunization. Obstet Gynecol 52:1, 1978

29. Sebring ES, Polesky HF: Detection of fetal maternal hemorrhage in Rh immune globulin candidates: a rosetting technique using enzyme-treated Rh$_2$Rh$_2$ indicator erythrocytes. Transfusion 22:486, 1982

30. Stedman CM, Baudin JC, White CA, Cooper ES: Use of the erythrocyte rosette test to screen for excessive fetomaternal hemorrhage in Rh-negative women. Am J Obstet Gynecol 154:1363, 1986

31. Ness PM, Baldwin ML, Niebyl JR: Clinical high-risk designation does not predict excess fetal–maternal hemorrhge. Am J Obstet Gynecol 156:154, 1987

32. Davey MG, Zipursky A: McMaster Conference on Prevention of Rh Immunization. Vox Sang 36:50, 1979

33. Aborjaily AN: Rh sensitization after tubal pregnancy. N Engl J Med 281:1076, 1969

34. Litwak O, Taswell HF, Banner EA et al: Fetal erythrocytes in maternal circulation after spontaneous abortion. JAMA 214:531, 1970

35. Matthews CD, Matthews AEB, Gilbey BE: Antibody development in rhesus-negative patients following abortion. Lancet 2:318, 1969

36. Queenan JT, Shah S, Kubarych SF et al: Role of in-

duced abortion in rhesus immunization. Lancet 1:815, 1971

37. Ascari WQ: Abortion and maternal Rh immunization. Clin Obstet Gynecol 14:625, 1971

38. Leong M, Duby S, Kinch RA: Fetal–maternal transfusion following early abortion. Obstet Gynecol 54:424, 1979

39. Freda VJ, Gorman JG, Galen RS et al: The threat of Rh immunization from abortion. Lancet 2:147, 1970

40. Katz J, Marcus RG: The risk of Rh isoimmunization in ruptured tubal pregnancy. Br Med J 3:667, 1972

41. Harrison R, Campbell S, Craft I: Risks of fetomaternal hemorrhage resulting from amniocentesis with and without ultrasound placental localization. Obstet Gynecol 48:557, 1976

42. Mennuti MT, Brummond W, Crombleholme WR et al: Fetal maternal bleeding associated with genetic amniocentesis. Obstet Gynecol 55:48, 1980

43. Henry G, Wexler P, Robinson A: Rh-immune globulin after amniocentesis for genetic diagnosis. Obstet Gynecol 48:557, 1976

44. Blackemore KJ, Baumgarten A, Shoenfeld-Dimaio M et al: Rise in maternal serum alpha-protein concentration following chorionic villus sampling. Am J Obstet Gynecol 155:988, 1986

45. Pollack W, Ascari WQ, Crispen JF et al: Studies on Rh prophylaxis after transfusion with Rh-positive blood. Transfusion 11:340, 1971

46. Pollack W, Ascari WQ, Kochesky RJ et al: Studies on Rh prophylaxis. I: Relationship between doses at anti-Rh and size of antigenic stimulus. Transfusion 11:333, 1971

47. Nevanlinna HR, Vainio T: The influence of mother–child ABO incompatibility on Rh immunization. Vox Sang 1:26, 1956

48. Queenan JT: Modern Management of the Rh Problem. 2nd Ed. Harper & Row, Hagerstown, MD, 1977

49. Woodrow JC: The immune response in the mother. Series Haematol 3:27, 1970

50. Ascari WQ, Levin P, Pollack W: Incidence of maternal Rh immunization by ABO compatible and incompatible pregnancies. Br Med J 1:399, 1969

51. Clarke CA, Donohoe WTA, Finn R et al: Further extraperitoneal studies on the prevention of Rh haemolytic disease. Br Med J 1:979, 1963

52. Freda VJ, Gorman JG, Pollack W: Successful prevention of experimental Rh sensitization in man with anti-Rh gamma 2-globulin antibody preparation. Transfusion 4:26, 1964

53. Pollack W, Gorman JG, Freda VJ: Rh immune suppression: past, present, and future. p. 9. In Frigoletto FD, Jewett JR, Konugres AD (eds): Rh Hemolytic Dis-

ease: New Strategy for Eradication. GK Hall, Boston, 1982

54. Hamilton EG: Prevention of Rh isoimmunization by injection of anti-D antibody. Obstet Gynecol 30:812, 1967

55. Pollack W, Singer HO, Gorman JG et al: The prevention of isoimmunization to the Rh factor by passive immunization with Rh D immune globulin. Haematology 2:1, 1968

56. Chown B, Duff AM, James J et al: Prevention of primary Rh immunization: first report of the Western Canadian Trial. Can Med Assoc J 100:1021, 1969

57. Mollison PL, Barron SL, Bowley C, et al: Controlled trial of various anti-D dosages in suppression of Rh sensitization following pregnancy. Br Med J 2:75, 1974

58. Freda VJ, Gorman JG, Pollack W et al: Prevention of Rh hemolytic disease—ten years clinical experience with Rh immune globulin. N Engl J Med 292:1014, 1975

59. Bowman JM, Chown B, Lewis M, Pollack JM: Rh_0-isoimmunization during pregnancy. Can Med Assoc J 118:623, 1978

60. Bowman JM, Pollock JM: Antenatal Rh prophylaxis: 28 weeks' gestation service program. Can Med Assoc J 118:627, 1978

61. Kochenour NK, Beeson JH: The use of Rh-immune globulin. Clin Obstet Gynecol 25(2):283, 1982

62. Bowman JM: Controversies in Rh prophylaxis: who needs Rh immune globulin and when should it be used? Am J Obstet Gynecol 151:289, 1985

63. Mollison PL: The reticulo-endothelial system and red cell destruction. Proc R Soc Med 55:915, 1962

64. Pollack W: Recent understanding for the mechanism by which passively administered antibody suppresses the immune response to Rh antigen in unimmunized Rh-negative women. Clin Obstet Gynecol 25:255, 1982

65. Chan PL, Sinclair NR: Regulation of the immune response. VI: Inability of F(ab)2 antibody to terminate established immune responses and its ability to interfere with IgG antibody-mediated immunosuppression. Immunology 24:289, 1973

66. Gorman JG, Freda VJ, Pollack W: Prevention of rhesus haemolytic disease. Lancet 2:181, 1965

67. Oberman HA (ed): Standards for Blood Banks and Transfusion Services. 10th Ed. American Association of Blood Banks, Washington, DC, 1981

67a. Bowman JM, Pollock JM, Biggins KR: Antenatal studies and the management of hemolytic disease of the newborn. Meth Hematol 17:163, 1988

68. Keith LG, Berger GS: The risk of Rh immunization associated with abortion, spontaneous and induced. p.

111. In Frigoletto FD, Jewett JF, Konugres AA (eds): Rh Hemolytic Disease: New Strategy for Eradication. GK Hall, Boston, 1982

69. Gustafson J: Connecticut Rh Registry: ten years' experience. p. 79. In Frigoletto FD, Jewett JF, Konugres AA (eds): Rh Hemolytic Disease: New Strategy for Eradication. GK Hall, Boston, 1982

70. Baskett TF, Parsons ML, Peddle LJ: The experience and effectiveness of the Nova Scotia Rh Program, 1964–84. Can Med Assoc J 134:1259, 1986

71. Tovey LAD: Haemolytic disease of the newborn—the changing scene. Br J Obstet Gynecol 93:960, 1986

72. Reece EA, Copel JA, Scioscia AL et al: Diagnostic fetal umbilical blood sampling in the management of isoimmunization. Am J Obstet Gynecol 159:1057, 1988

73. Nicolini U, Kochenour NK, Greco P et al: Consequences of fetomaternal hemorrhage after intrauterine transfusion. Br Med J 297:1379, 1988

74. Allen H, Diamond LK, Jones AR: Erythroblastosis fetalis. IX: Problems of stillbirth. N Engl J Med 251:453, 1954

75. Freda VJ: The Rh problem in obstetrics and a new concept of its management using amniocenteses and spectrophotometric scanning of amniotic fluid. Am J Obstet Gynecol 92:341, 1965

76. McElin TW, Buckingham JC, Danforth DN: The outcome and treatment of Rh-sensitized pregnancies. Am J Obstet Gynecol 84:4678, 1962

77. Bevis DCA: Blood pigments in haemolytic disease of the newborn. J Obstet Gynaecol Br Emp 63:65, 1956

78. Liley AW: Liquor amnii analysis in the management of pregnancy complicated by rhesus sensitization. Am J Obstet Gynecol 82:1359, 1961

79. Liley AW: Intrauterine transfusion of foetus in haemolytic disease. Br Med J 2:1107, 1963

80. Liley AW: Errors in the assessment of hemolytic disease from amniotic fluid. Am J Obstet Gynecol 86:485, 1963

81. Queenan JT: Current management of the Rh-sensitized patient. Clin Obstet Gynecol 25:293, 1982

82. MacKenzie IA, Bowell PF, Castle BM et al: Serial fetal blood sampling for the management of pregnancies complicated by severe rhesus (D) isoimmunization. Br J Obstet Gynecol 95:735, 1988

83. Nicolaides KH, Rodeck Ch, Mibashan RS, Kemp JR: Have Liley charts outlived their usefulness? Am J Obstet Gynecol 155:90, 1986

84. Ananth U, Queenan JT: Does midtrimester $\Delta\text{-OD}_{450}$ of amniotic fluid reflect the severity of Rh disease? Am J Obstet Gynecol 161:47, 1989

85. Rodeck CH, Holman CA, Karnicki J et al: Direct intravascular fetal blood transfusion by fetoscopy in severe rhesus isoimmunization. Lancet 1:625, 1981

86. Rodeck CH, Nicolaides KH, Warsof SL et al: The management of severe rhesus isoimmunization by fetoscopic intravascular transfusion. Am J Obstet Gynecol 150:749, 1984

87. Nicolaides KH, Rodeck CH, Millar DS, Mibashan RS: Fetal haematology in rhesus isoimmunization. Br Med J 290:661, 1985

88. Daffos F, Capella-Pavlovsky M, Forestier F: Fetal blood sampling during pregnancy with use of a needle guided by ultrasound: a study of 606 consecutive cases. Am J Obstet Gynecol 153:655, 1985

89. Daffos F, Forestier F, Kaplan C, Cox W: Prenatal diagnosis and management of bleeding disorders with fetal blood sampling. Am J Obstet Gynecol 158:939, 1988

90. Chitkara U, Wilkins I, Lynch L et al: The role of sonography in assessing severity of fetal anemia in Rh and Kell-isoimmunized pregnancies. Obstet Gynecol 71:393, 1988

91. Grannum PA: Ultrasound examination of the placenta. Clin Obstet Gynecol 10:459, 1983

92. DeVore GR, Mayden K, Tortora M et al: Dilatation of the umbilical vein in rhesus hemolytic anemia: a predictor of severe disease. Am J Obstet Gynecol 141:464, 1981

93. DeVore GR, Acherman RJ, Cabal LA et al: Hypoalbuminemia: The etiology of antenatally diagnosed pericardial effusion in rhesus hemolytic disease. Am J Obstet Gynecol 142:1056, 1982

94. Benacerraf BR, Frigoletto FD: Sonographic sign for the detection of early fetal ascites in the management of severe isoimmune disease without intrauterine transfusion. Am J Obstet Gynecol 152:1039, 1985

95. Nicolaides KH, Fontanarosa M, Gabbe SG, Rodeck CH: Failure of ultrasonographic parameters to predict the severity of fetal anemia in rhesus isoimmunization. Am J Obstet Gynecol 158:920, 1988

96. Vintzileos AM, Campbell WA, Storlazzi E et al: Fetal liver ultrasound measurements in isoimmunized pregnancies. Obstet Gynecol 68:162, 1986

97. Roberts AB, Mitchell JM, Pattison NS: Fetal liver length in normal and isoimmunized pregnancies. Am J Obstet Gynecol 161:42, 1989

98. Kirkinen P, Jouppila P: Umbilical vein blood flow in rhesus isoimmunization. Br J Obstet Gynecol 90:640, 1983

99. Rightmire DA, Nicolaides KH, Rodeck CH, Campbell S: Fetal blood velocities in Rh isoimmunization: relationship to gestational age and to fetal hematocrit. Obstet Gynecol 68:233, 1986

100. Nicolaides KH, Bilardo CM, Campbell S: Prediction of fetal anemia by measurement of the mean blood velocity in the fetal aorta. Am J Obstet Gynecol 162:209, 1990

101. Copel JA, Grannum PA, Green JJ et al: Pulsed Doppler flow-velocity waveforms in the prediction of fetal hematocrit of the severely isoimmunized pregnancy. Am J Obstet Gynecol 161:341, 1989

102. Copel JA, Grannum PA, Green JJ et al: Fetal cardiac output in the isoimmunized pregnancy: a pulsed Doppler–echocardiographic study of patients undergoing intravascular intrauterine transfusion. Am J Obstet Gynecol 161:361, 1989

103. Scott JR, Kochenour NK, Larkin RM et al: Changes in the management of severely Rh-immunized patients. Am J Obstet Gynecol 149:336, 1984

104. Bowman JM, Manning FA: Intrauterine fetal transfusions: Winnipeg, 1982. Obstet Gynecol 61:201, 1983

105. Watts DH, Luthy DA, Benedetti TJ et al: Intraperitoneal fetal transfusion under direct ultrasound guidance. Obstet Gynecol 71:84, 1988

106. Harman CR, Bowman JM, Manning FA, Menticoglou SH: Intrauterine transfusion — intraperitoneal versus intravascular approach: a case–control comparison. Am J Obstet Gynecol 162:1053, 1990

107. Bang J, Bock J, Trolle D: Ultrasound guided fetal intravenous transfusion for severe rhesus haemolytic disease. Br Med J 284:373, 1982

108. Berkowitz RL, Chitkara U, Goldberg JD et al: Intrauterine intravascular transfusions for severe red blood cell isoimmunization: ultrasound-guided percutaneous approach. Am J Obstet Gynecol 155:574, 1986

109. Seeds JW, Bowes WA: Ultrasound-guided fetal intravascular transfusion in severe rhesus isoimmunization. Am J Obstet Gynecol 154:1105, 1986

110. Berkowitz RL, Hobbins JC: Intrauterine transfusion utilizing ultrasound. Obstet Gynecol 57:33, 1981

111. Clewell WH, Dunne MG, Johnson ML, Bowes WA: Fetal transfusion with real-time ultrasound guidance. Obstet Gynecol 57:516, 1981

112. Bowman JM: Hemolytic disease (erythroblastosis fetalis). p. 613. In Creasy RK, Resnik R (ed): Maternal Fetal Medicine: Principles of Practice. 2nd Ed. WB Saunders, Philadelphia, 1989

113. Nicolaides KH, Clewell WH, Mibashan RS, et al: Fetal haemoglobin measurement in the assessment of red cell isoimmunization. Lancet 1:1073, 1988

114. MacGregor SN, Socol ML, Pielet BW et al: Prediction of hematocrit decline after intravascular fetal transfusion. Am J Obstet Gynecol 161:1491, 1989

115. Grannum PA, Copel JA, Plaxe SC et al: In utero exchange transfusion by direct intravascular injection in severe erythroblastosis fetalis. N Engl J Med 314:1431, 1986

116. Poissonnier H-M, Brossard Y, Demedeiros N et al: Two hundred intrauterine exchange transfusions in severe blood incompatibilities. Am J Obstet Gynecol 161:709, 1989

117. Rodeck CH, Letsky E: How the management of erythroblastosis fetalis has changed. Br J Obstet Gynaecol 96(7):759, 1989

118. Socol ML, MacGregor SN, Pielet BW et al: Percutaneous umbilical transfusion in severe rhesus isoimmunization: resolution of fetal hydrops. Am J Obstet Gynecol 157:1369, 1987

119. Pattison N, Roberts A: The management of severe erythroblastosis fetalis by fetal transfusion: survival of transfused adult erythrocytes in the fetus. Obstet Gynecol 74:901, 1989

120. Nicolini U, Kochenour NK, Greco P et al: When to perform the next intrauterine transfusion in patients with Rh allo-immunization: combined intravascular and intraperitoneal transfusion allows longer intervals. Fetal Ther 4:14, 1989

121. Barass VA, Benacerraf BR, Frigoletto FD et al: Management of isoimmunized pregnancy by use of intravascular techniques. Am J Obstet Gynecol 159:932, 1988

122. Gusdon JP, Moore V, Myrvik QN et al: Promethazine HCl as an immunosuppressant. J Immunol 108:1340, 1972

123. Gusdon JP: The treatment of erythroblastosis with promethazine hydrochloride. J Reprod Med 26:454, 1981

124. Bierme SJ, Blanc M, Abbal M, Fournie A: Oral Rh treatment for severely immunized mothers. Lancet 1:604, 1979

125. Bierme SJ, Blanc M, Fournie A et al: Desensitization by oral antigen. p. 249. In Frigoletto FD, Jewett JF, Konugres AA (eds): Rh Hemolytic Disease: New Strategy for Eradication. GK Hall, Boston, 1982

126. Bowman JM, Peddle LJ, Anderson C: Plasmapheresis in severe Rh isoimmunization. Vox Sang 15:272, 1968

127. Clarke CA, Bradley J, Elson CJ et al: Intensive plasmapheresis as a therapeutic measure in rhesus-immunized women. Lancet 1:793, 1970

128. Powell LC: Intense plasmapheresis in the pregnant Rh-sensitized woman. Am J Obstet Gynecol 101:153, 1968

129. Fraser ID, Bennett MO, Bothamley JE et al: Intensive antenatal plasmapheresis in severe rhesus isoimmunization. Lancet 1:6, 1976

130. Graham-Pole J, Barr W, Willoughby MLN: Continuous-flow plasmapheresis in management of severe rhesus disease. Br Med J 1:1185, 1974

131. Rubinstein P: Repeated small volume plasmapheresis in the management of hemolytic disease of the newborn. p. 111. In Frigoletto FD, Jewett JF, Konugres

AA (eds): Rh Hemolytic Disease: New Strategy for Eradication. GK Hall, Boston, 1982

132. Berlin G, Selbing A, Ryden G: Rhesus haemolytic disease treated with high-dose intravenous immunoglobulin. Lancet 1:1153, 1985

133. de la Camara C, Arrieta R, Gonzalez A et al: High-dose intravenous immunoglobulin as the sole prenatal treatment for severe Rh immunization. N Engl J Med 318:519, 1988

134. Scott JR, Branch DW, Kochenour NK, Ward K: Intravenous immunoglobulin treatment of pregnant patients with recurrent pregnancy loss caused by antiphospholipid antibodies and Rh immunization. Am J Obstet Gynecol 159:1055, 1988

135. Sidiropoulos D, Herrmann U, Morell A et al: Transplacental passage of intravenous immunoglobulin in the last trimester of pregnancy. J Pediatr 109:505, 1986

136. Boggs TR: Survival rates in Rh sensitizations. Pediatrics 33:758, 1964

137. Queenan JT: Intrauterine transfusion: a cooperative study. Am J Obstet Gynecol 104:397, 1969

138. Wade MF, Ogden JA, Anderson GG et al: Intrauterine fetal transfusion: experience with 101 transfusions in 48 mothers. Am J Obstet Gynecol 105:962, 1969

139. Bowes WA: Intrauterine transfusion: indications and results. Clin Obstet Gynecol 14:561, 1971

140. Nicolaides KH, Soothill PW, Rodeck CH, Clewell W: Rh disease: intravascular fetal blood transfusion by cordocentesis. Fetal Ther 1:185, 1986

141. Berkowitz RL, Chitkara U, Wilkins IA et al: Intravascular monitoring and management of erythroblastosis fetalis. Am J Obstet Gynecol 158:83, 1988

142. Grannum PAT, Copel JA, Moya JA et al: The reversal of hydrops fetalis by intravascular transfusion in severe isoimmune fetal anemia. Am J Obstet Gynecol 158:914, 1988

143. Ronkin S, Chayen B, Wapner RJ et al: Intravascular exchange and bolus transfusion in the severely isoimmunized fetus. Am J Obstet Gynecol 160:407, 1989

144. Weinstein L: Irregular antibodies causing hemolytic disease of the newborn: a continuing problem. p. 321. In Pitkin RM, Scott JR (eds): Clinical Obstetrics and Gynecology. Vol. 25. No. 2. Harper & Row, Philadelphia, 1982

145. Queenan JT, Smith BD, Haber JM et al: Irregular antibodies in the obstetric patient. Obstet Gynecol 34:767, 1969

146. Polesky HF: Blood group antibodies in prenatal sera. Minn Med 50:601, 1967

147. Giblett ER: Blood group antibodies causing hemolytic disease of the newborn. Obstet Gynecol 7:1044, 1964

148. Berkowitz RL, Beyta Y, Sadovsky E: Death in utero due to Kell sensitization without excessive elevation of the OD_{450} value in amniotic fluid. Obstet Gynecol 60:746, 1982

149. Caine ME, Mueller-Heubach E: Kell sensitization in pregnancy. Am J Obstet Gynecol 154:85, 1986

150. Cook LN: ABO hemolytic disease. Clin Obstet Gynecol 25:333, 1982

151. Zipursky A, Pollock J, Neelands P et al: The transplacental passage of foetal red blood cells and the pathogenesis of Rh immunization during pregnancy. Lancet 2:489, 1963

152. Zlatnick FJ: Non-Rh_o(D) hemolytic disease of the newborn: an obstetric viewpoint. Semin Perinatol 1:169, 1977

153. Hutchinson AA, Drew JH, Yu VYH et al: Nonimmunologic hydrops fetalis: a review of 61 cases. Obstet Gynecol 59:347, 1982

154. Maidman JE, Yeager C, Anderson V et al: Prenatal diagnosis and management of non-immunologic hydrops fetalis. Obstet Gynecol 56:571, 1980

155. Holzgreve W, Curry CJR, Golbus MS et al: Investigation of nonimmune hydrops fetalis. Am J Obstet Gynecol 150:805, 1984

156. Etches PC, Lemons JA: Nonimmune hydrops fetalis: report of 22 cases including three siblings. Pediatrics 64:326, 1979

156a. Anand A, Gray ES, Brown T et al: Human parvovirus infection in pregnancy and hydrops fetalis. N Engl J Med 316:183, 1987

156b. Schwarz TF, Roggendorf M, Hottentrager B et al: Human parvovirus B19 infection in pregnancy. Lancet 2:566, 1988

156c. Peters MT, Nicolaides KH: Cordocentesis for the diagnosis and treatment of human fetal parvovirus infection. Obstet Gynecol 75:501, 1990

156d. Public Health Laboratory Service Working Party on Fifth Disease: Prospective study of human parvovirus (B19) in pregnancy. Br Med J 300:1166, 1990

157. Pearson HA, Shulman NR, Marder VJ, Cone TE: Isoimmune neonatal thrombocytopenic purpura: clinical and therapeutic considerations. Blood 23:154, 1964

158. Resnikoff-Etievant MF: Management of alloimmune neonatal and antenatal thrombocytopenia. Vox Sang 55:193, 1988

159. Shulman NR, Jordan JV: Platelet immunology. p. 476. In Colman RW, Hirsh J, Marder VJ et al (eds): Hemostasis and Thrombosis: Basic Principles and Clinical Practice. JB Lippincott, Philadelphia, 1987

160. Mueller-Eckhardt C, Grubert A, Weisheit M et al: 384 cases of suspected neonatal alloimmune thrombocytopenia. Lancet 1:363, 1989

161. Daffos F, Forestier F, Kaplan C, Cox W: Prenatal diag-

nosis and management of bleeding disorders with fetal blood sampling. Am J Obstet Gynecol 159:939, 1988

162. Bussel JB, Berkowitz RL, McFarland JH et al: Antenatal treatment of neonatal alloimmune thrombocytopenia. N Engl J Med 319:1374, 1988

163. Zalneraitis EL, Young RSK, Kirshnamoorthy KS: Intracranial hemorrhage in utero as a complication of isoimmune thrombocytopenia. J Pediatr 95:611, 1979

164. Naidu S, Messmore H, Caserta V, Fine M: CNS lesions in neonatal isoimmune thrombocytopenia. Arch Neurol 40:552, 1983

165. Herman JH, Jumbelic MI, Ancona RJ, Kickler TS: In utero cerebral hemorrhage in alloimmune thrombocytopenia. Am J Pediatr Hematol Oncol 8:312, 1986

166. Burrows RF, Caco CC, Kelton JG: Neonatal alloimmune thrombocytopenia: spontaneous in utero hemorrhage. Am J Hematol 28:98, 1988

167. von dem Borne AEG, van Leeuwen EF, von Reisz LE et al: Neonatal alloimmune thrombocytopenia: detection and characterization of the responsible antibodies by the platelet immunofluorescence test. Blood 57:649, 1981

168. Sternbach MS, Malette M, Nadon F, Guevin RM: Severe alloimmune neonatal thrombocytopenia due to specific HLA antibodies. Curr Stud Hematol Blood Transfus 52:97, 1986

169. Resnikoff-Etievant MF, Kaplan C, Muller JY et al: Allo-immune thrombocytopenias, definition of a group at risk: a prospective study. Curr Stud Hematol Blood Transfus 55:119, 1988

170. Karpatkin M, Porges RF, Karpatkin S: Platelet counts in infants of women with autoimmune thrombocytopenia. N Engl J Med 305:936, 1981

171. Daffos F, Forestier F, Muller JY et al: Prenatal treatment of alloimmune thrombocytopenia. Lancet 2:632, 1984

172. Kaplan C, Daffos F, Forestier F et al: Management of alloimmune thrombocytopenia: antenatal diagnosis and in utero transfusion of maternal platelets. Blood 72:340, 1988

173. Nicolini U, Rodeck GH, Kochenour NK et al: In-utero platelet transfusions for alloimmune thrombocytopenia. Lancet 2:506, 1988

174. Mueller-Eckhardt C, Kiefel V, Jovanovic V et al: Prenatal treatment of fetal alloimmune thrombocytopenia. Lancet 2:910, 1988

175. Management of alloimmune neonatal thrombocytopenia. Editorial, Lancet 1:137, 1989

176. Bussel JB, Berkowitz RL, McFarland JG et al: Antenatal treatment of neonatal alloimmune thrombocytopenia. N Engl J Med 319:1374, 1988

177. Derycke M, Drysus M, Ropert JC, Tchernia G: Intravenous immunoglobulin for neonatal isoimmune thrombocytopenia. Arch Dis Child 60:667, 1985

178. Sidiropoulos D, Straume B: Treatment of neonatal isoimmune thrombocytopenia with intravenous immunoglobulin. Blut 48:383, 1984

179. Massey GV, McWilliams NB, Mueller DG et al: Intravenous immunoglobulin in treatment of neonatal isoimmune thrombocytopenia. J Pediatr 111:133, 1987

180. Water AH, Ireland R, Mibashan RS et al: Fetal platelet transfusions in the management of alloimmune thrombocytopenia. Thromb Haemost 58:323, 1987

181. Mir N, Samson D, House MJ, Kovar IZ: Failure of antenatal high-dose immunoglobulin to improve fetal platelet count in neonatal alloimmune thrombocytopenia. Vox Sang 55:188, 1988

SECTION 6
Pregnancy and Co-existing Disease

Hypertension

Baha M. Sibai and Garland D. Anderson

Hypertension complicates about 7 percent of all pregnancies. The incidence varies among different hospitals, regions, and countries. The term *hypertensive disorders of pregnancy* refers to all forms of hypertension seen during gestation. The three most common forms are preeclampsia, acute pregnancy-induced hypertension, and chronic essential hypertension. Preeclampsia is responsible for approximately 70 percent of cases.[1] The hypertensive disorders of pregnancy constitute a wide range of disorders that may cause minor problems or life-threatening emergencies for both the mother and her fetus.[2] Although mild preeclampsia that develops at term has been associated with little risk of hypertension in subsequent pregnancies, severe preeclampsia at 28 weeks gestation suggests that a woman is at high risk of serious complications in future pregnancies.

The terminology used to classify the hypertensive disorders of pregnancy has been confusing and inconsistent, making comparison of studies difficult and often impossible.[3] For many years, the hypertensive disorders of gestation were labeled toxemia of pregnancy. This term was used because it was felt that this wide variety of disorders had as a common etiologic agent a circulating toxin. We now know this to be untrue.

DEFINITIONS

The Committee on Terminology of the American College of Obstetricians and Gynecologists (ACOG) has classified the hypertensive disorders of pregnancy as follows.[4]

Preeclampsia-Eclampsia

The so-called classic triad of preeclampsia includes hypertension, proteinuria, and edema. The diagnosis of preeclampsia is based on blood pressure criteria, as well as proteinuria or edema or both. Blood pressure must increase by at least 30 mmHg systolic or 15 mmHg diastolic. Readings of 140/90 mmHg after 20 weeks gestation, if prior blood pressure is unknown, are considered sufficiently elevated for the diagnosis of preeclampsia. The elevation must be present on two measurements taken 6 hours apart. The Committee defines either an increase in mean arterial pressure of 20 mmHg or, if the prior blood pressure is unknown, a mean arterial pressure of 105 mmHg as an indication of hypertension. Mean arterial pressure is one-third the pulse pressure plus the diastolic pressure. Edema is diagnosed as clinically evident swelling. However, fluid retention can also be manifest as a rapid increase in weight without evidence of edema.

Proteinuria is defined as a concentration of 0.1 g/L or more in at least two random urine specimens collected 6 hours or more apart or 0.3 g in a 24-hour collection. In mild preeclampsia, the diastolic blood pressure remains below 100 mmHg. The criteria for severe preeclampsia are as follows.

CRITERIA FOR SEVERE PREECLAMPSIA

Blood pressure ≥ 160 mmHg systolic or ≥ 110 mmHg diastolic, recorded on at least two occasions at least 6 hours apart with patient at bed rest

Proteinuria ≥ 5 g in 24 hours (3+ or 4+ on qualitative examination)

Oliguria (≤ 400 ml in 24 hours)

Cerebral or visual disturbances

Epigastric pain

Pulmonary edema or cyanosis

Impaired liver function of unclear etiology

Thrombocytopenia

(From American College of Obstetricians and Gynecologists,[4] with permission.)

Eclampsia is the occurrence of seizures unattributable to other causes.

Chronic Hypertension

Chronic hypertension is defined as hypertension present before the pregnancy or diagnosed before the twentieth week of gestation. The Committee defines hypertension as blood pressure greater than 140/90 mmHg. Hypertension that persists for more than 42 days post partum is also classified as chronic hypertension. There are many causes of primary and secondary hypertension in pregnancy.

CHRONIC HYPERTENSION

Primary essential hypertension

Secondary hypertension
  Renal
    Acute glomerulonephritis
    Chronic nephritis
    Lupus nephritis
    Diabetic nephropathy
  Endocrine
    Cushing syndrome
    Primary aldosteronism
    Pheochromocytoma
    Thyrotoxicosis
  Neurologic disorders
    Quadriplegia

Chronic Hypertension with Superimposed Preeclampsia

Women with chronic hypertension may also show the development of superimposed preeclampsia. The Committee recommends that the diagnosis be made on the basis of an elevation of blood pressure (30 mmHg systolic or 15 mmHg diastolic or 20 mmHg mean arterial pressure) together with the appearance of proteinuria or generalized edema.

Transient Hypertension

Transient hypertension is the development of elevated blood pressure during pregnancy or in the first 24 hours post partum without other signs of preeclampsia or preexisting hypertension. The blood pressure must return to normal within 10 days after delivery.

Despite these diagnostic criteria, problems remain in classifying the hypertensive disorders of pregnancy.[5] Generalized edema is common in normal pregnancy, although it does not occur as frequently and is not as marked as when associated with preeclampsia. Dexter and Weiss reported edema of the hands, face, or both in 64 of 100 consecutive women examined during the third trimester of normotensive uncomplicated pregnancies.[6] Other studies have found a similar incidence of edema.[7] The Nelson classification, widely used in the British Commonwealth, does not include edema as a diagnostic criterion in the classification of preeclampsia.[7] ACOG did not insist on proteinuria as a diagnostic sign because it usually appears late. For example, proteinuria may not occur until after the convulsion in 5 to 10 percent of eclamptic women. The renal lesion characteristic of preeclampsia is almost never seen in the absence of proteinuria.[8] At long-term follow-up, the incidence of hypertension is much higher in women who have had hypertension in pregnancy without proteinuria than those who have had both hypertension and proteinuria.[9]

In 1986, Davey and MacGillivray[10] proposed a new clinical definition and classification of the hypertensive disorders of pregnancy that are based only on signs of hypertension and proteinuria and disregard etiology and pathology. This classification proposed new definitions of hypertension and proteinuria based on standardized methods of measurements and was intended to define clinical entities by which all cases of hypertension and proteinuria developing ante partum, intra partum, or post partum may be classified. This classification was endorsed by the International Society for the Study of Hypertension in Pregnancy. However, this classification is cumbersome and most diagnoses are determined in retrospect. Thus, it has no value for clinical management, but it may be useful for comparing the results of reports from all over the world. In addition, this classification generated considerable controversy regarding its potential clinical usefulness.[11-13]

PREECLAMPSIA

Preeclampsia is a form of hypertension that is unique to human pregnancy. Very rarely it has been reported in subhuman primates.[14] The incidence ranges between 14 and 20 percent in primigravidas and between 5.7 and 7.3 percent in multiparas.[15,16] The incidence is significantly increased in patients with twin pregnancies and in those with previous preeclampsia.[17] For patients with twin pregnancies, both incidence and severity are significantly higher than in those with singleton pregnancies.[18]

The etiology of preeclampsia is unknown. Many theories have been suggested, but most of them did not withstand the test of time. Some of the theories that are still under consideration are listed in the boxlist below.

THEORIES ASSOCIATED WITH THE ETIOLOGY OF PREECLAMPSIA

Abnormal trophoblast invasion

Coagulation abnormalities

Vascular endothelial damage

Cardiovascular maladaptation

Immunologic phenomena

Genetic predisposition

Dietary deficiencies or excesses

Pathophysiology

During normal pregnancy impressive physiologic changes occur in the uteroplacental vasculature in general and in the cardiovascular system in particular. These changes are most likely induced by the interaction of the fetal allograft with maternal tissue. The development of mutual immunologic tolerance in the first trimester is thought to lead to important morphologic and biochemical changes in the systemic and uteroplacental maternal circulation.

Uterine Vascular Changes

The human placenta receives its blood supply from numerous uteroplacental arteries that are developed by the action of migratory interstitial and endovascular trophoblast into the walls of the spiral arteries, transforming the uteroplacental arterial bed into a low-resistance, low-pressure, high-flow system. The conversion of the spiral arteries of the nonpregnant uterus into the uteroplacental arteries has been termed "physiologic changes" by Brosens.[19] In a normal pregnancy, these trophoblast-induced vascular changes extend all the way from the intervillous space to the origin of the spiral arteries from the radial arteries in the inner one-third of the myometrium. It is suggested that these vascular changes are effected in two stages: "the conversion of the decidual segments of the spiral arteries by a wave of endovascular trophoblast migration in the first trimester and the myometrial segments by a subsequent wave in the second trimester."[19] This process is reportedly associated with extensive fibrinoid formation and degeneration of the muscular layer in the arterial wall. These vascular changes result in the conversion of approximately 100 to 150 spiral arteries into distended, tortuous, and funnel-shaped vessels that communicate through multiple openings into the intervillous space.

In contrast, pregnancies complicated by preeclampsia and/or by small for gestational age (SGA) infants demonstrate inadequate maternal vascular response to placentation. In these pregnancies, the vascular changes described are usually restricted only to the decidual segments of the uteroplacental arteries. Hence, the myometrial segments of the spiral arteries are left with their musculoelastic architecture, thereby rendering them responsive to hormonal influences.[20] Additionally, the number of well-developed arteries is smaller than that found in normotensive pregnancies. The authors postulate that this defective vascular response to placentation is due to inhibition of the second wave of endovascular trophoblast migration that normally occurs from about gestational week 16 onward. These pathologic changes may have the effect of curtailing the increased blood supply required by the fetoplacental unit in the later stages of pregnancy, and they may be responsible for the decreased uteroplacental blood flow seen in most cases of preeclampsia. These conclusions were recently supported by Frusca and associates.[21] These authors studied placental bed biopsy specimens obtained during cesarean section from normal pregnancies ($N = 14$), preeclamptic pregnancies ($N = 24$), and chronic hypertensive pregnancies only ($N = 5$). Biopsy findings from the preeclamptic group demonstrated abnormal vascular changes in all of them and 18 with acute atherotic changes. On the other hand, 13 of the 14 biopsy specimens from normotensive pregnancies had normal vascular physiologic changes, whereas the specimens from the hypertensive patients showed all three types of physiologic changes. In addition, they found that the

mean birthweight was significantly lower in the group with atherosis than in the other group without such findings. However, it is important to note that these vascular changes are not a consistent finding in spiral arteries of hypertensive pregnancies and were demonstrated in a significant proportion of normotensive pregnancies complicated by fetal growth retardation.[20,22]

Using electron microscopy, Shanklin and Sibai[23] studied the ultrastructural changes in placental bed and uterine boundary vessels in 33 preeclamptic and 12 normotensive pregnancies. They found extensive ultrastructural endothelial injury in both the placental site and the nonplacental site in all the specimens from preeclamptic women, but not in the normotensives. The injury appeared to affect the endothelial mitochondria, a finding that suggests a possible metabolic link in the pathophysiology. The endothelial injury ranged from swelling to complete erosion, and the swelling was associated with enlargement of endothelial nuclei resulting in reduction of the lumen. In some cases, the erosion was complete with associated deposition of heavy fibrin (Fig. 30.1). In addition, there was no correlation between the type or degree of endothelial damage and the level of maternal hypertension.

Hemostatic Changes

Preeclampsia is associated with vasospasm, activation of the coagulation system, and abnormal hemostasis. There is good evidence from several studies that preeclampsia is accompanied by endothelial injury, increased platelet activation with platelet consumption in the microvasculature, and excessive clotting activity.[24,25] Saleh et al.[24] evaluated the hemostatic system before and 24 to 48 hours after delivery in 26 control pregnancies, 15 with mild preeclampsia and 18 with severe preeclampsia. They found that preeclampsia was associated with high fibronectin, low antithrombin III, and low α_2-antiplasmin levels. They suggested that these findings reflected endothelial injury (high fibronectin), clotting (low antithrombin III), and fibrinolysis (low α_2-antiplasmin). In addition, they found that after delivery, fibronectin levels decreased in the preeclamptic group while α_2-antiplasmin levels increased in all groups. They concluded, "Vascular endothelial injury plays a central role in the hemostatic changes associated with pre-

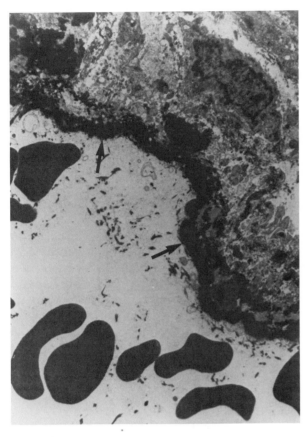

Fig. 30.1 Compacted heavy fibrin deposition (arrows) and loose luminal fibrin replacing extensively eroded endothelium, nonplacental site region, uterine boundary zone, preeclampsia. (Original electron microscopic magnification ×2500). (From Shanklin and Sibai,[23] with permission.)

eclampsia." In a subsequent report,[25] the authors evaluated hemostasis in various hypertensive disorders of pregnancies. They found elevated fibronectin, low antithrombin III, and reduced α_2-antiplasmin in patients with pure preeclampsia, as well as chronic hypertension with superimposed preeclampsia. In addition, they found that fibronectin levels had better correlation with preeclampsia than either antithrombin III or α_2-antiplasmin. They suggested that fibronectin might be useful for diagnosing superimposed preeclampsia in women with chronic hypertension. Elevated fibronectin levels have also been reported in preeclampsia in other studies.[26] In addition, two reports found elevated fibronectin

values in patients prior to the development of preeclampsia.[27,28]

Some authors have suggested that endothelial cell injury plays a central role in the pathophysiology of preeclampsia.[29–31] Rodgers et al.[29] reported that serum from preeclamptic women is cytotoxic to endothelial cells in vitro. In addition, they found that the cytotoxic activity in serum of preeclamptic women was reduced after 24 to 48 hours following delivery. In a subsequent report,[30] the authors found that mitogenic activity was significantly increased in the sera of preeclamptic women before delivery as compared to that of normotensive pregnant control subjects. In addition, the mitogenic activity diminished rapidly post partum. They suggested that vasospasm in preeclampsia may result from potent vasoconstrictors released at sites of endothelial cell injury. More recently,[31] the same group proposed that "poorly perfused placental tissue releases a factor(s) into the systemic circulation that injures endothelial cells."

Antithrombin III is a plasma proteinase inhibitor and is a major plasma inhibitor of thrombin. Weiner and Brand[32] reported that the level of plasma antithrombin III activity remains unaltered during normal pregnancy but is reduced in patients with preeclampsia. In a subsequent report, Weiner et al.[33] evaluated the use of antithrombin III measurement as a diagnostic test for preeclampsia in pregnancies complicated by hypertension. Women with chronic hypertension had only normal values, whereas those with either preeclampsia or superimposed preeclampsia had significantly lower levels than the normotensive group. There are currently about 20 reports dealing with this subject in preeclampsia; however, the findings have been inconsistent. In general, the evidence supports reduced antithrombin III activity in preeclampsia that reflects consumption secondary to enhanced clotting.

β-Thromboglobulin and platelet Factor IV are platelet-specific proteins. Their presence in the plasma indicates platelet aggregation and degranulation secondary to platelet activation and aggregation in vivo. Wallenburg and Rotmans[34] found enhanced reactivity of the platelet thromboxane pathway in hypertensive pregnancies and normotensive pregnancies complicated by fetal growth retardation. They suggested that this enhanced reactivity might be responsible for the increased platelet activation and consumption in such pregnancies. Higher levels of plasma β-thromboglobulin have been reported in patients with preeclampsia than in normotensive patients. Socol et al.[35] measured plasma β-thromboglobulin and platelet Factor IV in 11 patients with preeclampsia, 11 with superimposed preeclampsia, and 10 normotensive control subjects. They found higher plasma levels of β-thromboglobulin but normal platelet Factor IV in the preeclamptic groups.

Thrombin is an enzyme that converts fibrinogen to fibrin. It is inactivated by antithrombin III, resulting in generation of thrombin–antithrombin III complexes. An increased level of this complex suggests enhancement of thrombin generation. deBoer et al.[36] investigated plasma levels of the coagulation inhibitors antithrombin III, protein C, protein S, and thrombin–antithrombin III complexes. They observed reduced protein C levels but normal protein S levels in preeclamptic compared to normotensive pregnancies. In addition, they observed increased thrombin–antithrombin III complex levels in the preeclamptic group. The levels of these complexes correlated with platelet count and antithrombin III levels. Thus, they suggested that enhanced thrombin generation in preeclampsia may result from increased platelet activation and consumption. Gilabert et al.[37] evaluated protein C, protein S, and antithrombin III in normal pregnancy and severe preeclamptic states. They found reduced protein C and antithrombin III levels but normal protein S in severe preeclampsia.

Changes in Prostanoids

Several studies have described the various prostaglandins and their metabolites throughout pregnancy. They have measured the concentrations of these substances in plasma, serum, amniotic fluid, placental tissues, urine, or cord blood. The data have been conflicting and inconsistent, reflecting differences in methodology. This subject was recently reviewed by Friedman.[38] In general, the data suggest that the production of both prostacyclin (prostaglandin I_2 [PGI_2]) and thromboxane A_2 (TXA_2) is increased during pregnancy, with the balance in favor of PGI_2.

Reproductive tissues produce large amounts of both prostanoids, and during pregnancy production increases in both maternal and fetoplacental tis-

sues.[39] Prostacyclin is produced by the vascular endothelium as well as in the renal cortex. It is a potent vasodilator and inhibitor of platelet aggregation. TXA_2 is produced by the platelets and trophoblast. It is a potent vasoconstrictor and platelet aggregator. Hence, these eicosanoids have opposite effects and play a major role in regulation of vascular tone and vascular blood flow. Prostacyclin is chemically unstable, with a half-life of 3 minutes in blood at 37 degrees C. It is usually quantified by measuring its stable degradation product 6-keto-$PGF_{1\alpha}$. TXA_2 has a biologic half-life of about 30 seconds at 37 degrees C; hence it is usually measured as its stable hydrolysis product, thromboxane B_2 (TXB_2).

Changes in prostaglandin production and/or catabolism in uteroplacental and umbilical tissues have been reportedly associated with the development of preeclampsia, although the reports have been inconsistent.[38] These discrepancies may reflect some of the inherent problems in the measurement of prostaglandins and the diagnosis of preeclampsia. Recently, an imbalance in prostanoid production or catabolism has been suggested as responsible for the pathophysiologic changes in preeclampsia.[40] However, the role of prostaglandins in the etiology of preeclampsia remains unclear.

Goodman et al.[41] investigated PGI_2 biosynthesis during pregnancy by measuring urinary excretion of various dimer metabolites with the use of specific gas chromatography–mass spectrometry assays. They found that normal pregnant women had a fivefold increase in urinary excretion of these dimer metabolites in comparison to nonpregnant women. In addition, patients with pregnancy induced hypertension (PIH) had a significant 50 percent reduction in urinary dinor excretion in comparison to normotensive patients. Recently, Fitzgerald et al.[42] prospectively determined PGI_2 biosynthesis in pregnant women at risk for developing PIH by measurement of the urinary metabolite 2,3-dinor-6-keto-$PGF_{1\alpha}$. The study groups included 12 women who developed PIH, 22 women with hypertension during labor, 9 women with chronic hypertension, and 24 women who remained normotensive throughout gestation. They found a significant increase in prostacyclin biosynthesis in all study groups during pregnancy. However, patients who ultimately developed PIH exhibited a lesser increment and the difference persisted throughout gestation. In addition, they found that measurement of the urinary dinor metabolites was a better predictor of subsequent development of PIH than the more invasive angiotensin infusion test. Thus, the authors suggested a pathophysiologic role for altered prostacyclin biosynthesis in women with PIH.

In contrast to the preceding urinary findings in preeclampsia, the data regarding maternal plasma findings of either PGI_2 or TXA_2 metabolites have been highly variable and inconsistent.[38,43] The most consistent finding was an increase in TXA_2/PGI_2 ratio. In addition, Moodley et al.[44] found significantly lower levels of 6-keto-PGF_{1_α} in central venous blood from 21 primigravid women with diagnosed eclampsia.

Several studies have reported abnormal prostanoid production in either fetal or placental tissues. These findings were recently reviewed by Friedman,[38] as well as Walsh and Parisi.[43] The evidence suggests that umbilical artery production of PGI_2 is reduced and capacity of umbilical vessels to synthesize PGI_2 and TXA_2 is impaired. In addition, there is agreement in the literature that in preeclampsia, placental production of PGI_2 is reduced while that of TXA_2 is increased, leading to an increased TXA_2/PGI_2 ratio. Walsh[40,43] measured the simultaneous production rates of PGI_2 and TXA_2 in normal and preeclamptic patients. He found that the production of TXA_2 by placentas from preeclamptic patients was three times as high as that in placentas from normotensive pregnancies, whereas PGI_2 production was less than half. In addition, he found that the ratio of the placental production rate of TXA_2 to PGI_2 was seven times higher in preeclamptic than normotensive pregnancy. He suggested that this imbalance would account for the major clinical symptoms seen in preeclampsia (Fig. 30.2).[40]

Several investigators compared prostacyclin or TXA_2 levels in amniotic fluid of normotensive and preeclamptic–eclamptic patients. The findings of six such studies suggest that TXA_2 values are normal and PGI_2 values are abnormal only in patients with severe disease.[45,46]

The preceding data suggest that the pathogenesis of preeclampsia may be related to abnormal prostaglandin production and/or metabolism in the uteroplacental and umbilical vasculature. However, it

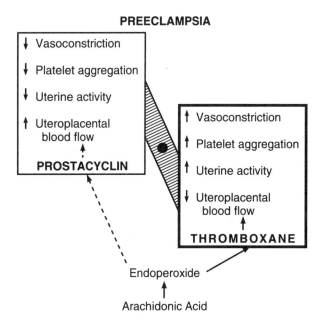

Fig. 30.2 Comparison of the balance in the biologic actions of prostacyclin and thromboxane in normal pregnancy with the imbalance of increased thromboxane and decreased prostacyclin in preeclamptic pregnancy. The heavy type and box for thromboxane suggest an exacerbation of its actions in preeclampsia, whereas the lighter type and box for prostacyclin suggest a diminution of its actions. (From Walsh,[40] with permission.)

should be noted that the increased TXA_2/PGI_2 ratio observed by various investigators in different maternal and fetal tissues may be an effect rather than a cause of preeclampsia.

Diagnosis

Preeclampsia is a clinical syndrome that embraces a wide spectrum of signs and symptoms that have been clinically observed to develop alone or in combination. Elevation of the blood pressure is the traditional hallmark of the diagnosis of the disease. However, recent evidence suggests that in some patients the disease may manifest itself in the form of either a capillary leak (edema, proteinuria) or a spectrum of abnormal hemostasis with multiple organ dysfunction. These latter patients usually present with clinical manifestations that are not typical of preeclampsia (e.g., hypertension is absent).

The diagnosis of preeclampsia and determination of the severity of the disease process are generally based on maternal blood pressure measurements as ascertained by a variety of medical personnel who regularly measure blood pressure in prenatal clinics, local physicians' offices, and in-hospital units. Several factors may influence measurement of the blood pressure by means of a sphygmomanometer: accuracy of the equipment used, size of cuff, duration of rest period before recording, posture of patient, and Korotkoff phase used (phase IV or phase V) for diastolic blood pressure measurements.[10,47] The effects of these factors on measurements of blood pressure have been recently summarized by Sibai.[47] In these reports, the authors recommend that all blood pressure values be recorded with the woman in a sitting position (ambulatory patient) or in a semireclining position (hospitalized patient). The right arm should be consistently in a roughly horizontal position at heart level. For diastolic blood pressure measurements, both phases (muffling sound and disappearance sound) should be recorded, but phase IV (muffling) should be used for diagnosis. This is very important since the level measured at phase IV is about 5 to 10 mmHg higher than that measured at phase V. In addition, the standard deviation in diastolic pressure at phase V is very high because of the hyperdynamic circulation during pregnancy.[48]

Rise in blood pressure has been used as the criterion for the diagnosis of PIH by several authors. This definition is usually unreliable since a gradual increase in blood pressure from second to third trimester is seen in most normotensive pregnancies. Mac-

Gillivray et al.[49] reported that 73 percent of primigravid patients with normotensive pregnancies demonstrate an increase in diastolic blood pressure of more than 15 mmHg at some stage during the course of their pregnancy. In addition, 57 percent of these patients demonstrate an increase of more than 20 mmHg during the course of pregnancy. Redman and Jeffries[50] analyzed different thresholds of raised diastolic blood pressure in 16,211 singleton pregnancies to determine the best way of diagnosing preeclampsia. They found that elevation in diastolic blood pressure of at least 25 mmHg and a maximum reading of at least 90 mmHg constituted the most useful criteria.

Villar and Sibai[15] prospectively studied blood pressure changes during the course of pregnancy in 700 young primigravidas. One hundred thirty-seven patients (19.6 percent) had preeclampsia. The pregnancy outcome according to blood pressure findings is summarized in Table 30.1. The sensitivity and positive predictive values for preeclampsia of a threshold increase in diastolic blood pressure 15 mmHg or greater on two occasions were 39 and 32 percent, respectively. The respective values for a threshold increase in systolic pressures were 22 and 33 percent. In addition, the use of a threshold increase criterion is dependent on at least two observations during the course of pregnancy that will be influenced by at least three factors: gestational age at time of first observation, frequency of blood pressure measurements, and the two observations to be selected. Thus, these criteria are inadequate to diagnose preeclampsia as such. However, they may be useful in association with the presence of pathologic edema, proteinuria, or

Table 30.1 Pregnancy Outcome According to Threshold Increase in Systolic or Diastolic Pressures on Two Occasions during the Third Trimester

Blood Pressure Criteria	Normotensive Number (%)	Preeclampsia Number (%)
Increase in diastolic ≥15 mmHg	113 (68)	53 (32)
Increase in systolic ≥30 mmHg	60 (67)	30 (33)
Threshold increase in both	32 (58)	23 (42)

(Modified from Villar and Sibai,[15] with permission.)

other associated symptoms of preeclampsia, such as persistent headache, visual symptoms, or epigastric pain. It is important to emphasize that the presence of these symptoms is more important than the absolute level of blood pressure in establishing the diagnosis of preeclampsia.

Prediction of Preeclampsia

A review of the world literature reveals that more than 100 clinical, biophysical, and biochemical tests have been recommended to predict or identify the patient at risk for the future development of the disease.[47] A summary of these clinical tests is listed below.

CLINICAL TESTS USED TO PREDICT PREECLAMPSIA

Average MAP-2[a] $\geq$ 85 – 90 mmHg

MAP at 20 weeks $\geq$ 90 mmHg

Rollover test at 28 – 32 weeks

Combination of the above

Isometric exercise test

Angiotensin infusion test at 26 – 30 weeks

Doppler velocimetry of uterine and umbilical vessels at 18 – 26 weeks

---

[a] MAP-2 = mean arterial pressure in the second trimester.

The value of mean arterial pressure in the second trimester (MAP-2) in predicting preeclampsia was investigated by Chesley and Sibai[51] as well as by Villar and Sibai.[15] The sensitivity of the test in various reports ranged from 0 to 99 percent, and the specificity varied from 53 to 97 percent. The value of the rollover test in predicting preeclampsia was evaluated in 14 reports. The sensitivity ranged from 0 to 93 percent, and the specificity ranged from 54 to 91 percent. In addition, the results of the pooled data for the various tests and the lack of agreement between serial tests suggest that none of these clinical tests is sufficiently reliable for use as a screening test in clinical practice. At our institution, none of these tests is used for screening purposes.

There are reports describing the predictive value of substances that can be measured in maternal plasma, serum, or urine. Some of the substances evaluated were cations, hormones, prostaglandin metabolites, various parameters of coagulation and hemostasis, and uric acid.[47] These reports differed in their methodology, included a heterogeneous group of patients with all forms of hypertension, parity, and gestational ages at time of sampling. Comparison and evaluation are, therefore, limited, explaining the wide scatter of results and lack of agreement among the findings by various authors. Hence, none of these substances has proved sufficiently reliable for use as a screening test.

Prevention of Preeclampsia

There are numerous reports and clinical trials describing the use of various methods to prevent or reduce the incidence of preeclampsia. Since the etiology of the disease is unknown, these methods were used in an attempt to correct theoretical abnormalities in preeclampsia. (Some of the methods used are summarized below.)

METHODS USED TO PREVENT PREECLAMPSIA

High-protein, low-salt diet

Nutritional supplementation
  Calcium
  Magnesium
  Zinc
  Fish and evening primrose oil

Antihypertensive drugs including diuretics

Antithrombotic agents
  Low-dose aspirin
  Dipyridamole
  Combination low-dose aspirin/dipyridamole
  Heparin

(From Sibai,[47] with permission.)

No efficacy of high-protein or low-salt diets has ever been documented.

Calcium Supplementation

Several epidemiologic studies and a few clinical supplementation trials have suggested a relationship between calcium, magnesium, and/or zinc intake and PIH. It has been shown that there is an inverse association between calcium intake and maternal blood pressure and the incidences of preeclampsia and eclampsia in epidemiologic studies. The findings of these studies were recently reviewed by Belizan and associates.[52] The blood pressure lowering effect of calcium was thought to be mediated by alterations in plasma renin activity and parathyroid hormone. In addition, calcium supplementation during pregnancy was shown to reduce angiotensin II vascular sensitivity in such pregnancies. Kawasaki et al.[53] compared pregnancy outcome in 22 women given calcium supplementation (600 mg calcium aspartate daily) from 20 weeks until delivery to the outcome in 72 women who did not receive such supplementation. These women were judged to be at risk for preeclampsia. They found that calcium supplementation was associated with a significant reduction in vascular sensitivity to angiotensin II infusions. The incidences of preeclampsia were 4.5 percent in the calcium supplemented group and 21.2 percent in the nonsupplemented group. The authors concluded that oral calcium supplementation can prevent the development of preeclampsia. This is a surprising finding since the amount of elemental calcium ingested by the supplemented group (156 mg daily) is far below the normal daily requirements of 1,200 to 1,600 mg/d. In addition, the study was not well controlled.

Villar et al.[54] studied 52 normotensive pregnant women who were randomly assigned in a double-blind fashion to receive either a placebo ($N = 27$) or calcium carbonate containing 1,500 mg of elemental calcium ($N = 25$) from 26 weeks gestation till delivery. The women in the calcium supplemented group had an average systolic and diastolic blood pressure value at term 4 to 5 mmHg lower than the respective value in the placebo group. The incidences of PIH at term were 4 percent in the calcium group and 11.1 percent in the placebo group. Although this is an interesting finding, the small sample size makes it difficult to draw any definite conclusions.

Lopez-Jaramillo et al.[55] reported a double-blind controlled trial involving 106 young nulliparous pregnant women who were randomized to receive either calcium gluconate containing 2 g of elemental calcium or placebo daily starting at 24 weeks gestation. Fourteen women (6 in calcium group and 8 in the placebo group) were excluded from the analysis. The incidences of PIH were 4.1 percent in the calcium supplemented group ($N = 49$) and 27.9 percent in the placebo group ($N = 43$). In addition, the calcium supplemented group demonstrated a significant decrease in both systolic and diastolic blood pressures during the course of pregnancy. Moreover, this group also had a significant increase in serum ionized calcium levels. The authors concluded that calcium supplementation during the third trimester is effective in reducing the incidence of PIH.

Magnesium Supplementation

Serum magnesium levels are usually lower during pregnancy than in the nonpregnant state and rapidly return to prepregnancy concentrations after delivery. The relationship between dietary magnesium deficiency and hypertension has been the subject of several experimental and observational studies.[56] Dietary magnesium deficiency during pregnancy has been implicated in the pathogenesis of preeclampsia, fetal growth retardation, and preterm delivery.[56,59] In addition, in patients with preeclampsia magnesium levels were reported to be lower than or similar to those in normotensive pregnancies. Since parenteral magnesium sulfate is the drug of choice in preeclampsia, some authors suggested an etiologic relationship between magnesium deficiency and preeclampsia.[57,58]

In a retrospective study, Conradt et al.[58] compared the pregnancy outcome in 4,023 low-risk pregnancies to that in 882 high-risk pregnancies. The high-risk group was treated with β-sympathomimetic agents in combination with various doses of magnesium aspartate hydrochloride. The incidence of preeclampsia in the high-risk treated group was 0 percent; it was 2 percent in the no treatment group. In addition, the incidence of fetal growth retardation was significantly reduced in the treated group. The authors concluded that routine supplementation with magnesium during pregnancy prevents preeclampsia and fetal growth retardation.

Spatling and Spatling[59] reported a double-blind study involving 568 women who were randomized to receive either 14 mmol magnesium-aspartate-hydrochloride ($N = 278$) or aspartic acid as placebo ($N = 290$). The supplementation was given daily starting at 16 weeks gestation or earlier and was continued throughout pregnancy. The incidences of preeclampsia were similar in the two groups; however, the magnesium supplemented group had a lower incidence of both preterm delivery and number of newborns admitted to the intensive care unit.

Sibai et al.[56] studied 400 young primigravidas who were enrolled at 13 to 24 weeks gestation to receive either 365 mg of elemental magnesium (as magnesium aspartate hydrochloride) or aspartic acid placebo. The magnesium supplemented group had significantly higher serum magnesium levels. However, there were no significant differences between the two groups in the incidence of preeclampsia, fetal growth retardation, or preterm delivery. In addition, magnesium supplementation did not influence the course of either systolic or diastolic blood pressure during the course of pregnancy.

Zinc Supplementation

Dietary zinc deficiency during pregnancy has been reportedly associated with poor pregnancy outcome.[60] In addition, reduced plasma zinc levels as well as lowered placental zinc levels have been reported in pregnancies complicated by preeclampsia.[61] Hunt et al.[62] studied the effect of zinc supplementation on the outcome of pregnancy in 213 low-income Mexican women. The patients were randomly allocated in a double-blind fashion to receive either placebo capsules or capsules containing 20 mg zinc/d. The incidence of pregnancy-induced hypertension was significantly reduced in the zinc supplemental group (2 vs. 16 percent). In addition, they found no other differences in pregnancy outcome between the two groups.

Mohamed and associates[63] studied pregnancy outcome in 494 women enrolled in a zinc supplementation trial (246 were given 20 mg/d zinc supplementation; 248 received placebo). They found no

differences between the two groups in weight gain, blood pressure, or incidence of preeclampsia (4.6 percent in the zinc group vs. 1.3 percent in the control group). In addition, they found no differences in terms of neonatal birthweight, fetal growth retardation, or incidence of preterm delivery.

At the present time, there are no adequate data to prove a strong association between prevention of preeclampsia and any nutritional supplementation. Thus, routine supplementation of all pregnant women with these nutrients is not recommended.

Antithrombic Agents

Preeclampsia is associated with vasospasm and activation of the coagulation–hemostasis systems. Enhanced platelet activation plays a central role in the above changes with resultant abnormality in the thromboxane/prostacyclin balance. Hence, several authors have used pharmacologic manipulation to alter the ratio in an attempt to prevent or ameliorate the course of preeclampsia.

Aspirin inhibits the synthesis of prostaglandins by irreversibly acetylating and inactivating cyclo-oxygenase. In vitro, platelet cyclo-oxygenase is more sensitive to inhibition by very low doses of aspirin (<80 mg) than vascular endothelial cyclo-oxygenase. Therefore, treatment with low doses of aspirin could alter the balance of prostacyclin and thromboxane.[64] This biochemical selectivity of low-dose aspirin appears to be related to its unusual kinetics, which result in presystemic acetylation of platelets exposed to higher concentrations of aspirin in the portal circulation. Sibai et al.[65] found that effective inhibition of thromboxane generation by platelets (98 percent decrease from baseline) can be achieved after 1 week of therapy with 80 mg of daily aspirin during pregnancy. In addition, they found that a 60-mg dose resulted in 60 percent decrease in platelet thromboxane generation after 1 week and 97 percent decrease after 2 weeks of therapy.

Beaufils and associates[66] studied 102 patients at risk for preeclampsia, fetal growth retardation, or fetal demise. Fifty-two women were treated with aspirin 150 mg/d plus dipyridamole 300 mg/d from 12 weeks gestation until delivery. The other 50 patients served as controls. The authors reported absent preeclampsia and fetal deaths in the treatment group, whereas there were six cases of preeclampsia and five fetal deaths in the control group. The incidences of fetal growth retardation were 8.3 percent among the treated group and 28.8 percent among the controls. However, the study results are questionable in that the two groups were not randomized and differed in parity and degree of preexisting chronic hypertension or renal disease.

Wallenburg et al.[67] studied 207 primigravidas who were screened by angiotensin II infusions at 28 weeks gestation. Forty-six patients had positive test results and thus were judged to be at increased risk for preeclampsia. These 46 patients were randomized to receive either a placebo ($N = 23$) or aspirin 60 mg/d ($N = 23$). Two patients in the aspirin group were later excluded for poor compliance. At 33 to 35 weeks gestation, a venous blood sample was drawn for determination of thrombin-induced production of malondialdehyde (MDA) by platelets. This dose caused 90 percent inhibition of platelets' MDA synthesis. The aspirin treated group had no preeclampsia or severe PIH; the placebo treated group had three cases of severe PIH, seven of preeclampsia, and one of eclampsia. The incidences of fetal growth retardation were 19 percent in the aspirin group and 39 percent in the control group.

Benigni et al.[68] studied 33 women at risk for preeclampsia who were randomly assigned to receive 60 mg of aspirin ($N = 17$) or placebo ($N = 16$) daily from 12 weeks gestation until delivery. The authors reported that low-dose aspirin selectively suppressed maternal platelet TXB_2 production without affecting vascular prostacyclin. In addition, they found that low doses of aspirin were associated with longer gestational ages and higher neonatal birthweights. There were three cases of pregnancy-induced hypertension in the placebo group only.

Schiff et al.[69] studied 791 pregnant women at risk for preeclampsia who were screened by the rollover test at 28 to 29 weeks gestation. Sixty-nine patients had positive test results, and 65 were randomized to receive either 100 mg of aspirin daily ($N = 34$) or a matching placebo ($N = 31$). The incidence of pregnancy-induced hypertension was significantly lower in the aspirin treated group (11.8 vs. 35.5 percent). In addition, the incidence of preeclampsia was 2.9 percent in the aspirin treated group, whereas it was 22.6 percent in the placebo group. They concluded that low daily doses of aspirin in the third trimester reduce the incidence of pregnancy-induced hypertension and preeclampsia.

Currently, large clinical trials are underway all over the world to assess the safety and effectiveness of low-dose aspirin in preventing preeclampsia and its complications. Thus, the use of low-dose aspirin for preventing preeclampsia should await the results of these clinical trials.

Organ System Involvement

Women with preeclampsia may exhibit a symptom complex ranging from minimal blood pressure elevation to derangements of multiple organ systems. The renal, hematologic, and hepatic systems are most likely to be involved.

Renal Function

Renal plasma flow and glomerular filtration rate (GFR) increase during normal pregnancy.[70] These changes are responsible for the fall in serum creatinine, urea, and uric acid concentrations. In preeclampsia, vasospasm and glomerular capillary endothelial swelling (glomerular endotheliosis) lead to a reduction in GFR ranging from 25 percent in mild cases to 50 percent in severe cases.[71] Serum creatinine is rarely elevated in preeclampsia, but uric acid is commonly increased.[72]

The clinical significance of elevated uric acid levels in preeclampsia/eclampsia has been confusing. In a study of 332 women with preexisting hypertension, plasma urate levels were found to be a better indicator of fetal prognosis than blood pressure. Uric acid levels above 5 mg/dl were associated with poor perinatal outcome.[73] However, in a comparison of 69 eclamptic women who had uric acid levels of less than 6.0 mg/dl with those who had values above 10.0 mg/dl, Pritchard and Stone[74] found no significant difference between the two groups for blood pressure, perinatal outcome, or incidence of hypertension in subsequent pregnancies.

Hepatic Function

The liver is not primarily involved in preeclampsia, and hepatic involvement is seen in only 10 percent of women with severe preeclampsia.[75,76] Fibrinogen deposition has been found along the walls of hepatic sinusoids in preeclamptic patients with no laboratory or histologic evidence of liver involvement.[77] When liver dysfunction occurs in preeclampsia, mild elevation of serum transaminase is most common. Bilirubin is rarely increased in preeclampsia, but, when it is elevated, the indirect fraction predominates. Elevated liver enzymes are part of the syndrome of hemolysis, elevated liver enzymes, and low platelets (HELLP).

Hepatic rupture is a dramatic complication of preeclampsia. It carries a maternal mortality rate of 70 percent.[78] In such cases, surgical intervention has been recommended. Henney et al.[79] suggested that hepatic rupture is biphasic. In phase 1, necrosis, intrahepatic hemorrhage, and subcapsular hemorrhage may occur; they can be managed conservatively. Once phase 2 is reached with rupture of Glisson's capsule, surgery is mandated if the lives of the mother and her fetus are to be saved. Nine cases of liver hematoma diagnosed by ultrasonography, computed tomography (CT) scan, or laparotomy have been managed conservatively, with all surviving.[80,81] None of these patients had suffered hepatic rupture, however.

Hematologic Changes

Fibrinogen levels in women with mild, moderate, or severe preeclampsia, in the absence of placental abruption, are usually the same as those observed in normal pregnancy.[82] Fibrinogen levels were found to be normal in women with preeclampsia who had glomerular endotheliosis identified by renal biopsy.[83]

Thrombin time is frequently prolonged in preeclampsia.[84] Since these women have normal fibrinogen levels and no significant elevation of serum fibrin degradation products, however, there may be a qualitative alteration of the fibrinogen molecule or so-called dysfibrinogenemia. Although changes in the coagulation system may occur, they are not usually of clinical significance. When a group of 104 preeclamptic women were compared with 61 normal women, no differences in coagulation parameters were found between the two groups.[85] With vasospasm and disruption of vascular endothelium, however, platelet deposition may occur, leading to thrombocytopenia. Gibson et al.[85] reported thrombocytopenia ($<150 \times 10^3/mm^3$) in 18 percent of preeclamptic women and in 39 percent of women with eclampsia. Sibai et al.[86] observed thrombocyto-

penia in 17 percent and disseminated intravascular coagulopathy (DIC) in 7.3 percent of 303 women with severe preeclampsia. Twelve of the 22 with DIC had abruptio placentae.

HELLP Syndrome

Recent reports have described the syndrome of hemolysis, elevated liver enzymes, and low platelets in severe preeclampsia. There is considerable debate regarding the definition, diagnosis, incidence, etiology, and management of this syndrome.[87] Patients with such findings were previously described by many investigators. Goodlin[88] labeled this syndrome (*e*dema, *p*roteinuria, *h*ypertension) EPH gestosis type B; he claimed that this clinical presentation had been reported in the obstetric literature a century earlier. Weinstein[76] considered it a unique variant of preeclampsia and coined the term HELLP syndrome for this entity.

A review of the literature highlights the differences in the degree of abnormal laboratory findings and the criteria used to diagnose HELLP syndrome. Thrombocytopenia (platelet count $<100 \times 10^3/\mu l$) has been the most consistent finding among the various reports. However, some investigators have included only those values determined before delivery, whereas others report platelet counts obtained both ante partum and post partum. In addition, considerable differences in the levels of serum glutamic oxaloacetic transaminase (SGOT) and bilirubin have been considered abnormal; several reports have not even included these data. Hemolysis has been defined as the presence of an abnormal peripheral smear with burr cells and schistocytes.[89]

In view of the diagnostic problems described previously, Sibai[89] recommended that uniform and standardized laboratory values be used to diagnose this syndrome. He suggested that lactic dehydrogenase (LDH) and bilirubin values be included in the diagnosis of hemolysis. In addition, the degree of abnormality of liver enzymes should be defined as a certain number of standard deviations from the normal value for each hospital population. Furthermore, the rate of change in either liver enzymes or platelet count may be as important as the absolute value in establishing the diagnosis. Our laboratory criteria to establish the diagnosis are as follows.

LABORATORY VALUES USED TO DIAGNOSE HELLP SYNDROME

Hemolysis
    Abnormal peripheral blood smear
    Increased bilirubin greater than or equal to 1.2 mg/dl
    Increased lactic dehydrogenase greater than 600 IU/L

Elevated liver enzymes
    Increased SGOT greater than 72 IU/L
    Increased lactic dehydrogenase as above

Low platelets
    Platelet count less than $100 \times 10^3/\mu l$

The reported incidence of HELLP syndrome in preeclampsia has ranged from 2 to 12 percent.[87] The true incidence remains unknown, however, considering the differences in diagnostic criteria used. The syndrome appears to be most common in white patients. The incidence of HELLP syndrome is also higher in preeclamptic patients who have been managed conservatively.

The typical presentation is that of a white multiparous patient with a maternal age of 25 years or above. The patient is usually seen remote from term complaining of epigastric or right upper-quadrant pain (90 percent); some have nausea or vomiting (50 percent), and others have nonspecific viral-syndrome-like symptoms. The majority of patients (90 percent) give a history of malaise for the past few days before presentation; some may present with hematuria or gastrointestinal bleeding. Hypertension and proteinuria may be absent or slightly abnormal.[90,91] Physical examination demonstrates right upper-quadrant tenderness (80 percent) and significant weight gain with edema (60 percent). Hypertension may be absent (20 percent), mild (30 percent), or severe (50 percent), depending on the duration of signs and symptoms. Severe hypertension is usually more common in patients who develop the syndrome during conservative management of preeclampsia. It is important to emphasize that some of these patients may have a variety of signs and symptoms, none of which is diagnostic of severe preeclampsia. Thus, Sibai recommended that all pregnant women having any of these symptoms should have a complete blood count and platelet and liver enzyme determinations irrespective of maternal blood pressure.[89]

Preeclamptic women presenting with HELLP syndrome are often misdiagnosed as having various medical and surgical diseases, such as idiopathic thrombocytopenic purpura, thrombotic thrombocytopenic purpura (TTP), hemolytic uremic syndrome, gallbladder disease, viral hepatitis, pyelonephritis, acute fatty liver of pregnancy, kidney stones, glomerulonephritis, and gastroenteritis.[89]

Management of preeclamptic patients presenting with the HELLP syndrome is highly controversial. Some investigators[76,92] recommend immediate delivery, whereas others[93,94] suggest a more conservative approach intended to prolong pregnancy in patients remote from term. The cases studied in these reports are highly variable with a wide range of abnormal laboratory findings and gestational age at time of presentation. It is therefore difficult to compare or draw

---

THERAPEUTIC MODALITIES USED TO TREAT OR REVERSE HELLP SYNDROME

Plasma volume expansion
    Bed rest
    Crystalloids
    Albumin 5–25%

Antithrombotic agents
    Low-dose aspirin
    Dipyridamole
    Heparin
    Antithrombin III
    Prostacyclin infusions

Immunosuppressive agents
    Steroids

Miscellaneous
    Fresh-frozen plasma infusions
    Exchange plasmapheresis
    Dialysis

(From Sibai,[89] with permission.)

Table 30.2 Perinatal Outcome in HELLP Syndrome

	Number[a]	Percentage
Stillbirths	22	19.3
Neonatal deaths	16	17.4
Perinatal deaths	38	33.3
Gestational age (wk)		
≤30	47	41.2
31–36	46	40.4
>36	21	18.4
SGA	36	31.6

[a] N = 112 births.
(From Sibai et al.,[89] with permission.)

any conclusions from these findings. (The accompanying boxlist describes some of the modalities reported in the literature that were used to treat or reverse the presence of this syndrome.[89])

There is general agreement that pregnancies complicated by preeclampsia and the HELLP syndrome are associated with poor maternal and perinatal outcomes.[87] The reported perinatal mortality rate has ranged from 7.7 to 60 percent and maternal mortality from 0 to 24 percent. Maternal morbidity is common. Most of these patients have required transfusions of blood and blood products and are at increased risk for the development of acute renal failure, pulmonary edema, ascites, pleural effusions, and hepatic rupture. Moreover, these pregnancies are associated with high incidences of abruptio placenta and DIC.

Sibai et al.[87] reported on 112 patients with severe preeclampsia–eclampsia in which the diagnosis of HELLP syndrome had been made before delivery. The incidence of this syndrome was significantly higher in white women, multigravidas, and those who had been misdiagnosed or treated conservatively. The overall perinatal outcome is summarized in Table 30.2. There were two maternal deaths, and two patients had sustained ruptured subcapsular hematomas of the liver but survived. The incidence of abruptio placenta was 20 percent, 42 (38 percent) had DIC, and 104 (93 percent) required blood and/or blood products to correct hypovolemia or coagulopathy.

The HELLP syndrome may develop ante partum or post partum. Analysis of 304 cases studied by Sibai[89] revealed that 209 (69 percent) had evidence of the syndrome ante partum, whereas 95 (31 percent) developed the manifestations post partum. Among the antepartum group, 8 (4 percent) developed the syndrome at 17 to 20 weeks gestation and 23 (11 percent) at 21 to 26 weeks gestation, for a total of 15 percent during the second trimester. This group included 1 maternal death, 1 ruptured subcapsular hematoma of the liver, 5 cases of acute renal failure, and 12 cases of DIC. This finding underscores the importance of suspecting the presence of this syndrome in all pregnant women who complain of right upper-quadrant pain, malaise, nausea, or vomiting during this period.

In the postpartum period, the time of onset of the manifestations ranged from a few hours to 6 days, with the majority developing within 48 hours post partum. Seventy-five (79 percent) of the 95 patients had evidence of preeclampsia prior to delivery. However, 20 (21 percent) had no such evidence either ante partum or intra partum. It is the authors' experience that patients in this group are at increased risk for the development of pulmonary edema and acute renal failure. The differential diagnosis in these patients should include exacerbation of systemic lupus erythematosus, TTP, and hemolytic uremic syndrome.

Patients with the HELLP syndrome who are remote from term should be referred to a tertiary care center, and initial management should be as for any patient with severe preeclampsia. The first priority is to assess and stabilize maternal condition, particularly coagulation abnormalities. The next step is to evaluate fetal well-being by using the nonstress test and biophysical profile. Then, a decision must be made as to whether or not immediate delivery is indicated. Amniocentesis may be performed in patients at less than 34 weeks gestation without risk of bleeding complications. In the absence of laboratory evidence of DIC and fetal lung maturity, the patient may be given two doses of steroids to accelerate fetal lung maturity and then delivered 24 hours after the last dose. During this time, both maternal and fetal conditions should be monitored very closely. In addition, the presence of this syndrome is not an indication for immediate delivery by cesarean section. It is the authors' opinion that such an approach might prove detrimental to both mother and fetus. Patients presenting with well-established labor should be allowed to deliver vaginally as indicated. In addition, labor may be initiated with oxytocin in those with favorable cervix.

Hemodynamic Changes in Preeclampsia

Women with severe preeclampsia frequently have a reduction in total blood volume. They are, therefore, much less tolerant of increased blood loss at delivery than are women with normal pregnancies. Vascular sensitivity to vasoactive substances such as angiotensin II and catecholamines is increased. The increased pressor response to angiotensin II may antedate the clinical onset of preeclampsia by several months.[95] Peripheral vascular resistance and left ventricular work are both increased as a result of generalized arteriolar vasospasm. Central venous pressure (CVP) is usually low (1 to 5 cmH$_2$O); pulmonary capillary wedge pressure (PCWP) is in the low normal range (0 to 10 mmHg). There is also a poor correlation between PCWP and CVP.[96] There is considerable controversy regarding the findings of hemodynamic monitoring in women with severe preeclampsia or eclampsia. In 1984, Hankins et al.[97] reviewed the findings in six published reports and classified them according to therapy prior to insertion of the Swan–Ganz catheter. The authors reported findings that ranged from a low-output, high-resistance state to a high-output, low-resistance state. In addition, the PCWP was reported to be either low, normal, or high.

FACTORS THAT MAY INFLUENCE THE REPORTED HEMODYNAMIC CHANGES IN PREECLAMPSIA

Severity and duration of disease process

Presence of underlying cardiac or renal disease

Presence or absence of labor

Gestational age and parity

Therapeutic interventions prior to measurements

Various methods used for measuring cardiac output

Dynamic fluctuation of cardiovascular system

The differences reflect differences in patient populations as well as the wide variety of treatment modalities used (see the accompanying box).

Cotton et al.[98] reported the hemodynamic profile of 45 women with severe preeclampsia–eclampsia. The hemodynamic measurements were obtained invasively after the administration of magnesium sulfate and a minimal amount of fluids. The study group included a heterogenous group of patients: 32 were primigravida, 14 had eclampsia, 2 had pulmonary edema, 6 had chronic hypertension, and 13 were in labor. The mean gestational age was 25.4 ± 0.6 weeks (range 27 to 41.5 weeks). The mean cardiac index was 4.14 L/min/m^2, the mean pulmonary capillary wedge pressure was 10 ± 1 mmHg (range 4 to 30), and the mean systemic vascular resistance was 1,496 ± 64 dynes · sec/cm^5. In addition, they found disparity between the CVP and the PCWP. They concluded that the majority of these patients have normal to high cardiac indices and pulmonary wedge pressures accompanied by normal or hyperdynamic left ventricular function.

Wallenburg[99] reported hemodynamic findings in 44 untreated nulliparous preeclamptic patients, in 22 preeclamptic patients who had received various therapies prior to the measurements, and in 7 normotensive pregnant controls. He found that the majority of untreated preeclamptic patients had low cardiac output, low pulmonary wedge pressure, and high systemic vascular resistance. On the other hand, in the 22 preeclamptic patients who had received various therapies, he found a wide range of hemodynamics. In the untreated group, the median cardiac index was 3 L/min/m^2 (range 2 to 4.7) and the median PCWP was 4 mmHg (range 1 to 13). The median central venous pressure was 1 mmHg (range −2 to 6). He concluded that the hemodynamic profile of the preeclamptic nulliparous patients is characterized by severe volume depletion that is reflected by low output, low PCWP, and high systemic vascular resistance. Similar findings were reported recently by Belfort et al.,[100] who studied the hemodynamic changes in 10 untreated patients with severe preeclampsia. The mean cardiac index in the study was 3 L/min/m^2 (range 1.47 to 3.95), the mean PCWP was 5 mmHg (range 0 to 10), and the mean central venous pressure was 2 mmHg (range 0 to 5). Again, these findings

Table 30.3 Comparison of the Hemodynamic Profile of Preeclamptic Patients in the Mabie[101] Study versus the Dutch Study

	Mabie et al.[101] (N = 15)	Wallenburg[99] (N = 44)
Heart rate	88 (65–110)[a]	90 (60–130)
Mean arterial pressure (mmHg)	126 (100–150)	120 (95–143)
Mean pulmonary artery pressure (mmHg)	16 (8–22)	9 (3–18)
Pulmonary capillary wedge pressure (mmHg)	8 (3–13)	4 (0–13)
Central venous pressure (mmHg)	5 (0–10)	1 (−2–6)
Cardiac index (L/min/m^2)	4.1 (3.1–5.2)	3 (2.0–4.7)
Stroke index (ml/beat/m^2)	45 (33–65)	35 (20–57)
System vascular resistance index (dynes.sec.cm^{-5}/m^2)	2,416 (1,660–3,310)	2,970 (2,100–4,585)
Resistance index (dynes.sec.cm^{-5})	122 (62–207)	82 (25–133)

[a] Data from the Mabie study are presented as median and range.
(Data from Mabie et al.[101] and Wallenburg.[99])

reflect a state of volume depletion. Thus, the authors of these two studies recommended plasma volume expansion prior to the use of vasodilators in the management of such patients. They also cautioned that the use of vasodilators such as hydralazine without prior correction of the hypovolemia might result in severe maternal hypotension.

Mabie et al.[101] reported the hemodynamic findings in 49 severe preeclamptic–eclamptic patients. The authors noted different hemodynamic profiles in those with pulmonary edema as compared to those without this complication. In 41 patients without edema, all patients had normal to elevated cardiac index and systemic vascular resistance and 93 percent had normal to elevated PCWP. In a subgroup of these patients without treatment except for magnesium sulfate (N = 15), the hemodynamic profile was also variable. Table 30.3 summarizes the findings in this study as compared to other reports.

In summary, the hemodynamic findings in preeclampsia are highly variable. As a practical point, patients are often transferred to a tertiary care center several hours after initial therapy has been started. In addition, the clinical diagnosis of preeclampsia is often suspect, particularly remote from term. On the other hand, there is definite evidence to suggest that CVP does not correlate with PCWP in such pregnancies. Hence, CVP monitoring should not be used to gauge the use of fluid therapy in managing these pregnancies.

Doppler Velocimetry Studies

There are numerous reports describing the use of the uteroplacental flow velocity waveforms (FVWs) in the prediction, diagnosis, and management of preeclampsia. Campbell et al.[102] reported that measurements of uteroplacental FVWs at 16 to 18 weeks gestation yielded a useful screening test to predict the future development of PIH, fetal growth retardation, and fetal asphyxia. They noted that an abnormal uteroplacental artery Doppler finding at 16 to 18 weeks predicted 64 percent of the hypertensive pregnancies. Adruini et al.[103] evaluated the uteroplacental FVW in 64 high-risk pregnancies studied at 18 to 20 weeks gestation. The 22 patients who subsequently developed PIH showed higher resistance index values than the normotensive group. The sensitivity of this measurement was 64 percent, specificity was 84 percent, and positive predictive value was 70 percent. The authors suggested that this screening test can be useful to identify those patients who will remain normotensive.

Fleischer et al.[104] studied 71 women with hypertensive disorders of pregnancy. They found that when the systolic to diastolic ratio (S/D) exceeded 2.6 and there was a notch in the uterine artery FVW, then the pregnancy was commonly complicated by either poor perinatal outcome or preeclampsia. The positive and negative predictive values of such a finding were 93 and 91 percent, respectively. In a subsequent report, Ducey et al.[105] suggested using Doppler velocimetry

Table 30.4 Fetal and Neonatal Parameters versus Doppler-Derived Patterns: Systolic to Diastolic Ratio (S/D)[a]

	Normal in Both $N = 66$	Abnormal Umbilical Only $N = 27$	Abnormal Uterine Only $N = 12$	Abnormal in Both $N = 31$
Birthweight (g)	$3,261 \pm 522$	$2,098 \pm 811$	$2,464 \pm 722$	$1,627 \pm 697$
Gestational age (wk)	39 ± 2	35.7 ± 3.2	36.3 ± 3	33.3 ± 2.7
Delivery <37 wk (%)	11	61	67	84
C/S for fetal distress (%)	8	39	8	62

[a] S/D ratios in umbilical and uterine arteries. C/S, cesarean section.
(Adapted from Ducey et al.,[105] with permission.)

in the clinical evaluation of all pregnant women with hypertension. In this report, the authors studied 136 pregnant hypertensive women with Doppler velocimetry of both the uterine and the umbilical arteries. They found that patients with both normal uterine and umbilical artery ratios had an excellent perinatal outcome, whereas those with both abnormal uterine and umbilical artery ratios had a poor perinatal outcome (Table 30.4).

In contrast, Havretty and associates[106] found no differences in uteroplacental FVWs between 32 patients with PIH and 32 carefully matched women with normotensive pregnancies. Gudmundsson and Marsal[107] studied FVWs weekly from the umbilical and arcuate arteries in 58 hospitalized women with preeclampsia. The maximum FVW was analyzed for pulsility index, and the results from the final examination were related to pregnancy outcome. They found that an umbilical artery FVW was a better predictor of fetal growth retardation than the arcuate artery FVW. Cameron et al.[108] studied Doppler FVWs in the fetal aorta and umbilical artery in 41 patients with hypertension in pregnancy. They found the highest number of abnormal patterns in both vessels in patients with severe disease. They also noted that the Doppler assessment finding was often abnormal before the nonstress test or the biophysical profile.

In summary, the data regarding examination of the uteroplacental circulation for the prediction and diagnosis of preeclampsia are contradictory. As a result, Redman[109] suggested that this method should not be used in clinical practice. During the past 3 years, we have been evaluating the usefulness of Doppler examination of the uteroplacental and fetal circulations in the diagnosis and management of hypertensive disorders of pregnancy. We believe that it is very difficult to interpret the results obtained from the uteroplacental circulation because of its anatomic complexity. On the other hand, evaluation of fetal vessels is very helpful in identifying those pregnancies that may require frequent monitoring with traditional tests of fetal well-being such as the nonstress test and biophysical profile. In general, the presence or loss of end-diastolic frequencies or reverse flow patterns in the umbilical artery is usually associated with poor perinatal outcome.[110]

The Management of Preeclampsia

Once the diagnosis of preeclampsia has been made, definitive therapy in the form of delivery is the desired goal, since it is the only cure for the disease. The ultimate goal of therapy must always be safety of the mother first, followed by delivery of a live mature newborn who will not require intensive and prolonged neonatal care. The decision for immediate delivery versus expectant management is usually dependent on one or more of the following: severity of the disease process, fetal gestational age, maternal condition, fetal condition, and Bishop score. In the United States, management of these patients usually involves bed rest in the hospital for the duration of pregnancy since this approach enhances the likelihood of fetal survival and diminishes the frequency of progression to severe disease. In many such instances, this treatment arrests the clinical course of the disease or at least improves it long enough to achieve fetal maturity without jeopardizing maternal safety. The success rate of this expectant management depends on fetal gestational age and on the state to which the disease has progressed at the time of hospitalization. Hospitalization may appear expensive, but such care prolongs gestation and reduces the higher cost incurred by delivery of a premature infant who requires prolonged neonatal intensive care.

Women with preeclampsia who have a favorable cervix at, or near, term should receive intravenous magnesium sulfate to prevent convulsions and undergo induction of labor. When the cervix is unfavorable or the patient is not near term, she can be hospitalized and observed closely, if her blood pressure has returned to normal after hospitalization. A management plan for patients with mild preeclampsia is summarized in Figure 30.3.[111]

Patients are allowed to eat a regular hospital diet without salt restriction, and their activity is not restricted to complete bed rest. Diuretics and antihypertensive drugs are not prescribed and sedatives are not used. Our experience indicates that spontaneous diuresis ensues within the first 48 hours of hospitalization in the majority of these patients. The diuresis is usually accompanied by a decrease in weight and improvement in maternal blood pressure. All patients undergo serial evaluation of maternal and fetal well-being until delivery. The frequency of testing usually depends on the fetal gestational age and maternal response after hospitalization. This evaluation is very important since patients may develop thrombocytopenia and abnormal liver enzymes with minimal blood pressure elevations.[90] In addition, these patients are at increased risk for the development of convulsions and abruptio placenta, and the fetus is at risk for intrauterine growth retardation.

If the patient becomes normotensive in the absence of significant proteinuria, outpatient observation may be considered in a select group of patients. This form of management is appropriate in a reliable patient only during the early stages of the disease when

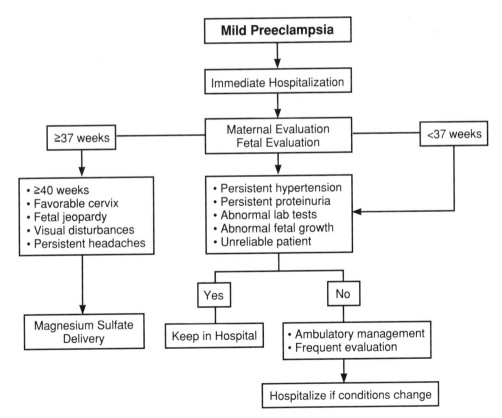

Fig. 30.3 Recommended management of mild preeclampsia at University of Tennessee, Memphis.

the fetus is immature and in the absence of evidence of fetal jeopardy. A typical regimen for these patients consists of bed rest at home, daily urine dipstick measurements of proteinuria, and home blood pressure monitoring by a nurse. The patient is instructed to keep fetal movement counts and is warned of symptoms of impending eclampsia. In addition, she is evaluated in the antepartum testing area for maternal and fetal well-being at least two times per week. If there is any evidence of disease progression and/or if acute hypertension or proteinuria develops, then prompt hospitalization is indicated. If there are signs of worsening maternal or fetal disease at any time during hospitalization, then delivery is indicated.

The results of conservative treatment of 576 primigravid women with singleton pregnancies in whom preeclampsia developed have been reported by Gilstrap et al.[112] Women with mild disease were admitted to a high-risk pregnancy unit; patients with severe disease were initially observed in the labor and delivery suite. If after 24 hours there was no improvement, patients with severe disease were delivered. If improvement did occur, they were transferred to the high-risk pregnancy unit, where blood pressure was determined four times each day, and were weighed three times each week. The women were allowed to ambulate as desired, but their activity was markedly decreased as compared with their usual home activity. They were given a general hospital diet (approximately 2,400 cal/d), and the only supplement was 65 mg elemental iron. Morning urine samples were measured three times weekly for protein content. Renal function was monitored by 24-hour creatinine clearance. Ultrasonography was used to assess gestational age serially in those women thought to have growth-retarded fetuses. Antepartum testing was performed only in women suspected of having growth-retarded fetuses and those who complained of decreased fetal movement.

Factors influencing delivery before term were persistent or severe hypertension, exacerbation of hypertension, rapid weight gain, decrease in GFR, appearance of significant proteinuria, definite evidence of fetal growth retardation, and symptoms including headache, scotomata, and epigastric pain. These factors were rarely identified without either worsening of persistent mild hypertension or recurrence of hypertension in a woman who became normotensive

after admission. Only 34 women (6 percent) had a poor response with persistent hypertension and were delivered within 1 week of admission. Most patients (81 percent) remained normotensive for the remainder of the pregnancy.

Pregnancy was continued in women with a good response until they went into spontaneous labor or until the cervix was considered favorable for oxytocin induction at or near term. Mean birthweight was 2,824 g, and only 8.4 percent of infants were SGA. There were four perinatal deaths, for a perinatal mortality rate (PMR) of 9 in 1,000.

Thirty-four women left the high-risk unit against medical advice. Four suffered stillbirths 18 to 55 days later, and all had severe hypertension: the PMR in these patients was 129 in 1,000.

Sibai et al.[113] evaluated pregnancy outcome in 200 young primigravidas who were hospitalized with mild preeclampsia at 26 to 35 weeks gestation. All patients had persistent elevations of blood pressure ($\geq$140/90 mmHg) 24 hours after hospitalization, proteinuria ($>$300 mg/24 hr), and elevated uric acid. The 200 women were randomly allocated to treatment with either labetalol hydrochloride or to hospitalization only. The average number of days of pregnancy prolongation was similar in both groups (21 days). There were no differences between the two groups in gestational age at delivery, birthweight, or cord blood gas measurements. However, the incidence of SGA infants was significantly higher in the labetalol-treated group (18 vs. 9 percent). Table 30.5 compares

Table 30.5 Pregnancy Outcome in Hospitalized Women with Mild Preeclampsia

	Gilstrap et al.[112] $N = 545$ No. (%)	Sibai et al.[113] $N = 200$ No. (%)
Gestational age at hospitalization (wks)	25–38	26–35
Average pregnancy prolongation (days)	24	21
Mean birthweight (g)	2,824	2,258
Fetal growth retardation	48 (8.4)	27 (13.5)
Perinatal deaths	5 (0.9)	1 (0.5)
Abruptio placenta	5 (1)	2 (1)
Eclampsia	1 (0.5)	0

pregnancy outcomes in hospitalized patients from Parkland Memorial Hospital, Dallas, and E. H. Crump Women's Hospital, Memphis.

The antepartum use of antihypertensive drugs for mild preeclampsia remote from term is highly controversial. There are many clinical reports (controlled and uncontrolled) describing the use of various drugs in an attempt to prolong gestation and improve perinatal outcome in these pregnancies. The majority of these studies was retrospective, few included a control group, and most did not have adequate sample size. Moreover, none of these studies demonstrated a better perinatal outcome when compared with studies that included only hospitalization for preeclampsia.[113]

Rubin et al.[114] compared the use of atenolol with use of a placebo in a randomized trial of 120 women with mild to moderate preeclampsia. The mean gestational age at entry of the study was 33.8 weeks, and the mean blood pressure was 140/95 mmHg. Atenolol was given daily in a dose of 100 to 200 mg. Unfortunately, about one-third of the patients were excluded from the study for various reasons and the two groups were not well matched, as most patients in the placebo group were primigravidas. The authors reported a significant reduction in the incidence of patients who progressed to severe disease, incidences of proteinuria, and a number of readmissions for hypertension in the atenolol-treated group. In addition, the use of atenolol was associated with better perinatal outcome and lower neonatal morbidity due to prematurity.

Wichman et al.[115] compared the use of metoprolol with placebo in 52 women with mild PIH. Metoprolol was used in a dose of 50 mg twice daily in 26 patients, and the other 26 received placebos. The authors found no differences between the two groups in perinatal outcome. This study did not have adequate sample size to provide differences in perinatal outcome.

Labetalol is a nonselective β-blocker with some α_1-blocking effects. Recent clinical studies suggest that this drug is ideal for managing preeclampsia remote from term. Walker et al.[116] reported 70 patients with mild PIH treated with either labetalol or bed rest. Patients given labetalol exhibited significant reductions in severe hypertension, proteinuria, and platelet consumption. There were no adverse side effects in either the mothers receiving labetalol or their in-

fants. Pickles and associates[117] reported the fetal outcome in a randomized double-blind controlled trial of labetalol ($N = 70$) versus placebo ($N = 74$) in women with mild pregnancy-induced hypertension. Labetalol was used in a dose of 100 mg to 200 mg three times daily. They found some reduction in preterm delivery and neonatal complications in the labetalol-treated group. There were no perinatal deaths in either group. They concluded that labetalol was a safe and effective drug in the management of these pregnancies.

In summary, the evidence in the literature does not support any benefit from the use of antihypertensive drugs in pregnancies with mild preeclampsia.

Severe Preeclampsia

The clinical course of severe preeclampsia is usually characterized by progressive deterioration in both maternal and fetal conditions. In these cases, the ultimate goals of therapy must always be safety of the mother first and then consideration for optimum perinatal outcome. Since the only cure for severe preeclampsia is delivery, there is universal agreement to deliver all patients if the disease develops beyond 34 weeks gestation, or if there is evidence of fetal lung maturity and/or fetal jeopardy prior to that time. In this situation, appropriate management should include parenteral medication to prevent convulsions, control of maternal blood pressure within a safe range, and then induction of labor to initiate delivery. If delivery of a preterm infant (< 36 weeks) is anticipated at a level I or level II hospital, the mother should be transferred to a tertiary care center with proper neonatal intensive care facilities.

There is disagreement about the best way to manage patients who have severe disease before 34 weeks gestation. Some institutions consider delivery the definitive therapy for all cases, regardless of gestational age; others recommend prolonging pregnancy in all patients remote from term until development of fetal lung maturity, fetal or maternal jeopardy, or gestational age of 36 weeks or greater.

In general, the maternal and perinatal outcomes are poor when women with severe preeclampsia are managed conservatively. Martin and Tupper[118] described the results of conservative management in 55 women with severe preeclampsia. Patients were treated with bed rest, oral phenobarbital 60 to 120 mg four times a day and magnesium sulfate if there was hyperreflexia or if maternal blood pressure exceeded 170/110 mmHg. Conservative therapy was continued if there was a favorable response to the initial treatment. Antihypertensive agents were used when systolic blood pressure rose above 180 mmHg or diastolic was greater than 120 mmHg. Evidence of fetal lung maturity or maternal or fetal compromise was an indication for delivery.

The pregnancies were continued for a mean duration of 19.2 days. Twelve women (22 percent) required antihypertensive therapy (hydralazine or methyldopa) with or without a diuretic. Ten patients went into spontaneous labor. Of the remaining 45 women, the primary indications for delivery were fetal lung maturity, worsening maternal disease, and a positive contraction stress test or nonreactive nonstress test result. Thirty of the neonates (56.6 percent) were severely growth retarded (below the 2.5th percentile), and 9 were asphyxiated. There were 3 stillbirths and 2 neonatal deaths for a PMR of 89 in 1,000. Only 9 women were at less than 30 weeks gestation when hospitalized (mean gestational age 27.6 weeks). These patients were delivered at a mean gestational age of 31.6 weeks (range 30.7 to 34.6 weeks) and had 3 perinatal deaths, for a PMR of 333 in 1,000.

Odendaal and co-workers[119] described the results of conservative management in 129 patients with severe preeclampsia before 34 weeks. The patients were treated with bed rest, magnesium sulfate, and various antihypertensive drugs. The average gestational age of these pregnancies was 29.4 weeks, and the average period of pregnancy prolongation was 11 days. There were 22 stillbirths (9 mid-trimester) and 20 neonatal deaths, for a mortality rate of 31.6 percent. Abruptio placenta was responsible for 36 percent of the intrauterine deaths. Forty-five of the women had a gestational age of less than 28 weeks at time of diagnosis and 11 less than 24 weeks (all resulting in perinatal deaths). In the remaining 34 patients with gestations between 24 and 28 weeks, 14 (41 percent) survived.

Sibai et al.[120] reported the results of conservative management in 60 women in whom severe preeclampsia developed at 18 to 27 weeks gestation. Thirty-four women were managed in other centers and subsequently referred to our perinatal unit. The patients were initially managed with parenteral mag-

nesium sulfate for 24 to 72 hours, and then with antihypertensive drugs to keep diastolic pressure below 100 mmHg. Antepartum fetal evaluation was rarely used in that study.

The incidence of serious complications in these mothers was extremely high (Table 30.6). None of the 3 women with renal failure required dialysis, and all had normal renal function at the time of discharge from the hospital. In 2 women, hypertensive encephalopathy developed post partum and required infusion of nitroprusside to control hypertension. One woman suffered an intracerebral hemorrhage due to a ruptured aneurysm at the bifurcation of the right internal carotid artery. The aneurysm was clipped, and the patient had no further complications. One of the maternal transfers was found to have a ruptured subcapsular hematoma of the liver 4 days after conservative treatment of preeclampsia at 23.5 weeks gestation. The postoperative course after surgical evacuation of the hematoma was complicated by pulmonary edema and acute renal tubular necrosis. She was discharged without renal or hepatic deficits 17 days after admission.

Fetal outcome was also poor. The 60 pregnancies resulted in 31 stillbirths and 21 neonatal deaths, for a PMR of 87 percent. There was only one perinatal survival (3.3 percent) among the 31 patients who had severe preeclampsia at or before 25 weeks, whereas the perinatal survival rate was 24 percent (7 of 29) in the group who had severe preeclampsia between 26 and 27 weeks. The average period of pregnancy prolongation in these 60 pregnancies was 11 days, and the mean gestational age at delivery was 27.7 weeks.

Table 30.6   Severe Preeclampsia in Mid-Trimester ($N = 60$)

Maternal Complication	Incidence	
	N	%
Abruptio placenta	13	21.7
Thrombocytopenia	12	20.0
HELLP[a]	10	16.7
Eclampsia	10	16.7
Disseminated intravascular coagulation	5	8.3
Acute renal failure	3	5.0

[a] HELLP = hemolysis, elevated liver enzymes, and low platelet count.

In addition, the neonatal morbidity rate was significantly high.

Occasionally, women with severe preeclampsia have marked improvement in blood pressure and protein excretion shortly after hospitalization. These patients should be admitted to the labor and delivery area for close observation of maternal and fetal status. They should receive intravenous magnesium sulfate to control convulsions and bolus doses of hydralazine (5 to 10 mg) intravenously as needed to keep diastolic pressure below 100 mmHg. Women with persistent severe hypertension or other signs of maternal or fetal deterioration during the observation period should be delivered within 24 hours, irrespective of fetal gestational age or lung maturity. We perform amniocentesis if the gestational age is between 33 and 34 weeks; if the lecithin/sphingomyelin ratio indicates immaturity, we administer glucocorticoids.

Corticosteroids have been suggested as safe and effective drugs for preventing respiratory distress syndrome (RDS), treating thrombocytopenia, and improving perinatal outcome in severe preeclampsia. A review of the literature reveals substantial differences in methodology and drug selection among investigators who advocate the use of steroids for preeclampsia. This subject was recently reviewed by Gonzalez-Ruiz and Sibai.[121] A patient may be considered suitable for steroid therapy if there is no evidence of maternal or fetal jeopardy and if delivery is not expected to occur within 48 hours. We limit the use of steroids to patients whose fetuses have documented fetal lung immaturity at 33 to 34 weeks and to most patients with gestational ages between 26 and 32 weeks. Maximum benefit is achieved when steroid therapy is given in appropriate doses and the last dose is administered at least 24 hours before delivery. Different regimens of steroids have been suggested for preventing RDS, but we prefer betamethasone given as 12 mg as soon as possible and the dose repeated 24 hours later.

For pregnancies at 28 to 32 weeks, the management is dependent on clinical response during the observation period. Some of these women (especially those with normal hematologic and hepatic laboratory findings) demonstrate marked diuresis with improvement in blood pressure and proteinuria. If the patient's diastolic blood pressure remains below 100 mmHg after a 24-hour period of observation in the labor and delivery area, magnesium sulfate is then discontinued and the patient is followed very closely in the hospital. Hospitalization includes frequent evaluation of maternal and fetal well-being. Such pregnancies should be managed at tertiary care centers. It is our experience that the majority of these patients require delivery within 2 weeks after hospitalization. However, some patients may continue the pregnancy for more than 2 weeks. We believe that an additional 2 weeks in utero at these gestational ages significantly reduces such neonatal morbidity as RDS, intraventricular hemorrhage, and necrotizing enterocolitis. Our management plan for women with severe preeclampsia is summarized in Figure 30.4.

For the past 5 years, we have used a new protocol for the management of severe preeclampsia prior to 28 weeks.[122] If the gestation is 24 weeks or less, we recommend termination of pregnancy with prostaglandin E_2 vaginal suppositories. If the gestation is more than 24 weeks, the patients are counseled about the risks and benefits of continuing the pregnancy. If they elect to continue with the pregnancy, they are given intravenous magnesium sulfate for at least 24 hours, and blood pressure is then aggressively controlled. These patients undergo intensive evaluation of maternal and fetal status on a daily basis. Pregnancy is then continued until the development of either maternal or fetal jeopardy (Fig. 30.5). Maternal evaluation should include daily platelet count and measurement of liver enzymes; fetal evaluation should include antepartum fetal heart testing in combination with the biophysical profile on a daily basis. Maternal hypertension may be treated with either methyldopa, labetalol, or nifedipine.

During the past 5 years, we have managed about 120 such patients with this protocol. For a gestational age between 24 and 28 weeks, the average duration of pregnancy prolongation is 2 weeks and the perinatal survival rate is about 70 percent.

We believe that all women who meet the blood pressure criteria for preeclampsia should receive intravenous magnesium sulfate to prevent eclamptic convulsions. Our rationale for this approach is the observation that in most series of eclampsia, 20 percent of the women had only minimal blood pressure elevation, frequently without edema or proteinuria.

Magnesium sulfate is administered by a controlled

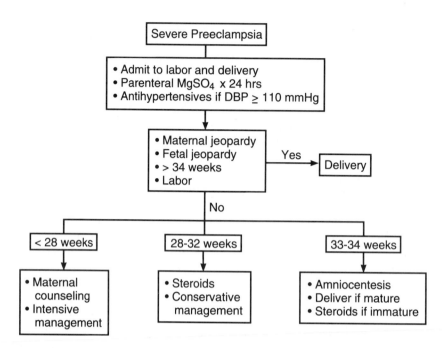

Fig. 30.4 Recommended management for severe preeclampsia at University of Tennessee, Memphis. DBP, diastolic blood pressure.

continuous intravenous infusion with a loading dose of 6 g in 100 ml over 15 to 20 minutes. We believe that the intravenous route for magnesium therapy permits more precise control of the patient's blood level and prevents the pain of intramuscular injections. Maintenance therapy is given at a rate of 2 g in 100 ml of fluid/hr. Serum magnesium levels are obtained 4 to 6 hours later, with the rate of infusion adjusted to keep serum magnesium levels between 4.8 and 9.6 mg/dl (4 to 6 mEq/L). Treatment is continued for 24 hours post delivery.

The magnesium ion goes beyond intracellular fluid and enters bones and cells as well.[123] Magnesium circulates largely unbound to protein and is excreted in the urine.[124] Therefore, an accurate record of maternal urine output must be maintained. In patients with normal renal function, the half-life for magnesium excretion is about 4 hours. In the therapeutic range (4.8 to 9.6 mg/dl), magnesium sulfate slows neuromuscular conduction and depresses central nervous system (CNS) irritability.

For this reason, maternal respiratory rate, deep tendon reflexes, and state of consciousness must be frequently monitored to detect magnesium toxicity (Table 30.7). An ampule of calcium gluconate, 1 g (10 ml of 10 percent solution), should be drawn up in a syringe and clearly labeled and be kept at the bedside in case of magnesium toxicity. If magnesium toxicity is suspected, the infusion of magnesium sulfate should be discontinued. If respiratory depression occurs, the calcium gluconate should be given intravenously over 3 minutes. If respiratory arrest develops, the patient should receive mechanical ventilatory support as needed.

The mechanism of action of magnesium ions is highly controversial. Some believe its action is peripheral at the neuromuscular junction with little if any central effects.[125,126] Others believe that the main action of magnesium is central, with a minimal neuromuscular blocking effect.[127,128] Pritchard[128] cites the short time necessary to effect a remarkable clinical response in women with severe preeclampsia–eclampsia as strong evidence of central nervous system action. Also, the therapeutic levels are much lower than those needed to produce complete neuromuscular blockade (15 to 17 mg/dl).

We carefully monitor the amount of intravenous fluid used in women with preeclampsia or eclampsia.

Management of Severe PIH in the Second Trimester

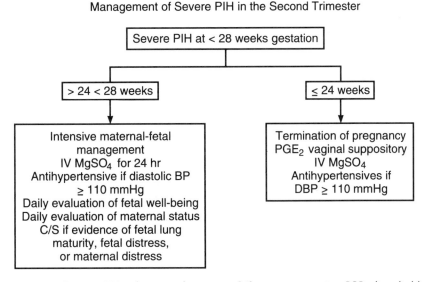

Fig. 30.5 Management of severe PIH in the second trimester. C/S, cesarean section; DBP, diastolic blood pressure.

Intake and output should be assessed hourly. We give 5 percent dextrose in Ringer's lactate solution at 50 to 125 ml/hr. A Foley catheter should be inserted to permit accurate evaluation of urine output. We are particularly cautious with women with chronic hypertension or renal disease. Frequently in the active phase of labor, urine output may drop below 30 ml/hr. In those cases in which the cervix is continuing to dilate, we have not given a fluid challenge or diuretics. Typically in these women, urine output increases to 30 ml/hr after 2 to 3 hours. Our goal is to maintain the urine output at 30 ml/hr. If output drops below 100 ml in 4 hours, the dose of magnesium sulfate and intravenous fluids should be reduced accordingly.

Table 30.7 Magnesium Toxicity

Loss of patellar reflex	8–12 mg/dl
Feeling of warmth, flushing	9–12 mg/dl
Somnolence	10–12 mg/dl
Slurred speech	10–12 mg/dl
Muscular paralysis	15–17 mg/dl
Respiratory difficulty	15–17 mg/dl
Cardiac arrest	30–35 mg/dl

Another cause of decreased urine output is a drop in maternal blood pressure due to the repeated injections of hydralazine. Hydralazine has a relatively long duration of action and, when multiple bolus injections of hydralazine are used to control blood pressure, the diastolic blood pressure may be reduced more than intended, that is, below 90 mmHg. This frequently reduces urine output for 2 to 3 hours. One of the potential problems when attempting to limit intravenous fluids to 125 ml/hr is that high concentrations of drugs must be used if the woman is receiving intravenous magnesium sulfate, oxytocin, and hydralazine.

To control severe maternal hypertension intra partum, we use bolus injections of hydralazine of 5 to 10 mg every 20 to 30 minutes to lower the diastolic blood pressure to the 90- to 100-mmHg range. This requires monitoring of blood pressure every 5 minutes for at least 30 minutes after the drug is given. An alternative regimen is to use bolus injections of labetalol hydrochloride of 20 to 50 mg. Unlike hydralazine, labetalol does not cause maternal tachycardia, flushing, or headaches. We have found this drug to be safe and effective in the management of these patients.[129] Other potent antihypertensive medications such as sodium nitroprusside, diazoxide, or nitroglycerine are rarely needed in the management of these patients. Diuretics such as furosemide are not used except in the presence of pulmonary edema.[130]

Maternal analgesia can be provided by the intermittent use of small doses (25 to 50 mg) of intravenous meperidine or segmental epidural analgesia. Local infiltration anesthesia with or without pudendal block or epidural anesthesia can be used for all cases of vaginal delivery for patients with mild disease. In addition, continuous epidural anesthesia or balanced general anesthesia can be used for all cesarean sections. The use of epidural anesthesia for patients with severe preeclampsia–eclampsia is controversial. It is important to emphasize that the administration of epidural anesthesia requires the availability of personnel with special expertise in obstetric anesthesia. In addition, in selected cases it requires the availability of central hemodynamic monitoring, since infusions of large amounts of crystalloids or colloids are usually used as precautionary measures before its administration. Moreover, the use of conduction anesthesia is contraindicated in the presence of fetal distress or coagulopathy.

On the other hand, significant hypertension and tachycardia are frequently observed after laryngoscopy and endotracheal intubation in patients undergoing general anesthesia. Transient but severe hypertension after tracheal intubation can result in significant increase in maternal intracranial pressures with the dangers of cerebral edema and hemorrhage and increased afterload with the dangers of pulmonary edema. These responses can be prevented or attenuated by the use of labetalol prior to endotracheal intubation. Labetalol should be used in a dose of 20 mg intravenously followed by 10-mg increments up to a total dose of 1 mg/kg.[131]

For patients with the HELLP syndrome, the use of pudendal block or epidural anesthesia is contraindicated since these patients are at risk of bleeding into these areas. In case of cesarean section, platelet transfusions are usually indicated to correct severe thrombocytopenia. Our policy is to transfuse 10 U of platelets in all patients with a platelet count less than $50 \times 10^3/\mu l$ prior to intubation. Generalized oozing from the operative site is very common, and to minimize the risk of hematoma formation, we recommend that a subfascial drain be used, the bladder flap be left open, and the wound be left open with sutures in situ

above the fascia. These wounds can be successfully closed within 72 hours. Failure to adhere to these recommendations results in a 25 percent incidence of hematoma formation.[89]

Recently, some investigators have recommended the use of invasive hemodynamic monitoring in managing patients with severe preeclampsia. Clark and Cotton[132] reported that indications for such monitoring should include pulmonary edema, persistent oliguria unresponsive to fluid challenge, intractable severe hypertension, and, in some cases, necessity of epidural anesthesia. Other authors[99,100] recommended using Swan-Ganz catheters to monitor fluid therapy and response to antihypertensive drugs. These investigators recommended plasma volume expansion with colloid plasma substitute to increase cardiac index and pulmonary capillary wedge pressure prior to the use of epidural or vasodilator drugs in an attempt to prevent potential severe hypotension. In addition, Mabie et al.[133] suggested that invasive hemodynamic monitoring is very helpful in the diagnosis and management of pulmonary edema in markedly obese hypertensive women.

We believe that the use of invasive hemodynamic monitoring is rarely indicated in the management of these patients. Its use for the preceding indications is empirical, and its benefit has not been conclusively proved. We believe that only a select group of women with pulmonary edema may benefit from invasive hemodynamic monitoring.

If the patient is already in spontaneous labor, continuous electronic fetal heart rate and uterine activity monitoring should be instituted in all cases. If labor is not well established, and in the absence of fetal malpresentation or distress, intravenous oxytocin should be administered to induce labor. This approach is used in all patients with a favorable cervix and all with gestational age 32 weeks or more irrespective of cervical status. In patients with an unripe cervix and gestational age less than 32 weeks, elective cesarean section is the method of choice for delivery of all patients with severe preeclampsia–eclampsia. This approach is based on our experience of a high incidence of intrapartum complications such as abruptio placenta and fetal distress in these patients.

At delivery, blood loss may be greater than that expected in normal patients. Magnesium sulfate may impair uterine contractility after delivery. Women with severe preeclampsia or eclampsia have contracted blood volume and tolerate blood loss poorly. These patients should have blood typed and cross-matched and available in the delivery area. A sudden drop in blood pressure following delivery may be due to hypovolemia.

After delivery, the patient should be kept in the recovery room under close observation for about 12 to 24 hours, during which magnesium sulfate should be continued. Most patients show evidence of resolution of the disease process within 24 hours. However, some patients, especially those with the HELLP syndrome or severe disease in the mid-trimester, may require intensive monitoring for several days. Such patients will require magnesium sulfate administration for more than 24 hours. These patients are at increased risk for the development of pulmonary edema from fluid overload, fluid mobilization, and compromised renal function.[130]

Maternal and Perinatal Outcome with Preeclampsia

Perinatal outcome in preeclampsia is usually dependent on one or more of the following factors: gestational age at onset of preeclampsia and at time of delivery, severity of disease process, presence of multiple gestation, and presence of underlying hypertensive or renal disease.[134] For patients with mild disease at term, the PMR, incidence of fetal growth retardation, and neonatal morbidity rate are similar to those of normotensive pregnancies. At the E. H. Crump Women's Hospital in Memphis, the perinatal mortality rate in these pregnancies is 1/1,000 and the incidence of fetal growth retardation is only 4 percent.

Long et al.[16] reported the pregnancy outcome in 2,434 singleton pregnancies with preeclampsia during a 7-year period (1971 to 1978). They found that patients with preterm preeclampsia (< 37 weeks) had a worse perinatal outcome than those with preeclampsia at 37 weeks or later. In the preterm group, the perinatal mortality rate was 10.5 percent, the incidence of fetal growth retardation was 18.2 percent, and the incidence of abruptio placenta was 4.5 percent. In contrast, for women with term preeclampsia, the respective incidences were 0.6, 5.6, and 0.4 percent. In a subsequent report, Long and Oats[18] reported that in patients with twin pregnancy, preeclampsia tends to develop earlier in gestation and maternal disease is usually more severe than it is in

singleton pregnancies. Thus, the perinatal outcome for twins in preeclampsia is worse than that in singleton pregnancy.

Pregnancies complicated by severe preeclampsia are usually associated with high perinatal mortality and morbidity rates. This increase in perinatal risk is mainly related to extreme prematurity, fetal growth retardation, abruptio placenta, and perinatal asphyxia. Sibai et al. reported pregnancy outcome in 303 such pregnancies. There were 28 stillbirths and 15 neonatal deaths, for an uncorrected PMR of 145 in 1,000. The corrected PMR was 135; 20 percent were SGA. There were marked differences in perinatal outcome between patients with and without preexisting chronic hypertension and between those developing the disease before or after 36 weeks gestation.

Severe preeclampsia is a major cause of maternal mortality and morbidity. Complicated or mismanaged cases are responsible for most deaths. Patients with onset in mid-trimester and those with HELLP syndrome and pulmonary edema are at significant risk for maternal mortality and morbidity (Table 30.8).

Counseling Women Who Have Had Preeclampsia in Prior Pregnancies

There appears to be a strong familial predisposition for preeclampsia. The incidence of severe preeclampsia was compared in the first pregnancy of sisters of primigravidas with and without preeclampsia.[135] In 273 primigravidas whose sisters did not have preeclampsia, the incidence of severe preeclampsia was 4.5 percent. The incidence of severe preeclampsia was 13.8 percent for women whose sisters had severe preeclampsia during their first pregnancies. The incidence of severe preeclampsia in the mothers and mothers-in-law of women in whom preeclampsia developed during their first pregnancies has been examined as well: it was 15.9 percent in the 126 mothers of primigravidas who had severe preeclampsia as compared to 4.4 percent in the 136 mothers-in-law. The incidence in a control group of primigravidas was 3.1 percent. The incidence of mild preeclampsia was higher in the mothers than in the mothers-in-law of these women, but this difference was not significant.

Kilpatrick and associates found an association between susceptibility to preeclampsia within families

Table 30.8 Maternal Complications in Preeclampsia

Complications	Midtrimester (%)	HELLP Syndrome (%)	Pulmonary Edema (%)
Abruptio placenta	21.7	20.0	32.4
Disseminated intravascular coagulation	8.3	38.0	48.6
HELLP	16.7	100.0	42.3
Acute renal failure	5.0	8.0	27.0
Encephalopathy	3.7	1.8	16.2
Ruptured liver	1.7	1.8	5.4
Pulmonary edema	5.0	4.5	100.0
Maternal deaths	0	1.8	10.5

and frequency of human leukocyte antigen DR4 (HLA-DR4).[136] The authors studied pregnancy outcome in sisters of 56 women who had proteinuric preeclampsia. The incidence of preeclampsia in the first pregnancy of the sisters was 11 percent compared to 2 percent in the maternity hospital, for a relative risk of 6.0. In addition, they found that the frequency of HLA-DR4 was higher in sisters with preeclampsia (44 percent) than in sisters with normotensive pregnancies (19 percent), and more of them shared HLA-DR4 with their spouses. They concluded that susceptibility to preeclampsia is associated with HLA-DR4.

We have examined the pregnancy outcomes and incidences of preeclampsia in subsequent pregnancies, as well as the incidence of chronic hypertension and diabetes in women who had severe preeclampsia (287 women) or eclampsia (119 women) in their first pregnancies (age 11 to 25 years), compared with 409 women (age 12 to 25 years) who remained normotensive during their first pregnancies. The two groups were well matched for age, race, height, and gestational age at delivery and for obstetric complications other than hypertension. Each woman had at least one subsequent pregnancy (range 1 to 11) and was followed for a minimum of 2 years (range 2 to 24). There was no significant difference in the incidence of diabetes mellitus in the two groups (1.3 vs. 1.5 percent). The incidence of chronic hypertension was significantly higher in the preeclampsia group (14.8 vs. 5.6 percent; $p < 0.001$). This difference became even greater for those women followed for more than 10 years (51 vs. 14 percent; $p < 0.001$). The incidence of severe preeclampsia was also significantly higher in

the second pregnancies (25.9 vs. 4.6 percent) as well as in the subsequent pregnancies (12.2 vs. 5.0 percent) of women with preeclampsia.[137]

Prior pregnancy outcome may be useful in counseling women who have had preeclampsia in a previous pregnancy. The risk of having preeclampsia in a second pregnancy ranges from 25 to 60 percent. For patients with severe preeclampsia in the mid-trimester, the incidence of recurrent preeclampsia is about 60 percent; half develop again in the mid-trimester. In addition, subsequent pregnancies are associated with high perinatal mortality and morbidity rates. These patients should be instructed to seek prenatal care early in pregnancy and should receive frequent prenatal visits. In addition, they should be counseled of the increased risk of chronic hypertension and the possibility of undiagnosed underlying renal disease.

Ihle et al.[138] evaluated renal function at 6 weeks to 6 months post partum in 178 women with a clinical diagnosis of preeclampsia. The onset of preeclampsia was at 24 to 36 weeks in 84 patients and at 37 weeks or later in 94 patients. Maternal evaluation consisted of urine microscopy, electrolytes, 24-hour urine for clearance and proteinuria, intravenous pyelography, and renal biopsy when indicated. They found a high incidence of renal disease (90 percent) in those with early onset preeclampsia and in multiparous patients. They suggested that women with early onset preeclampsia have renal evaluation after delivery.

Patients with preeclampsia and the HELLP syndrome can receive oral contraceptives without any risk of developing the syndrome again.[87] In addition, the recurrence risk for this syndrome in subsequent pregnancies is very small. Sibai[89] followed 59 patients with previous HELLP syndrome through 80 subsequent pregnancies. Only 2 patients (3.4 percent) had recurrent HELLP syndrome in subsequent pregnancies. Two patients had prior ruptured subcapsular liver hematoma, and both had uneventful subsequent pregnancies.

ECLAMPSIA

Eclampsia is the occurrence of convulsions or coma unrelated to other cerebral conditions with signs and symptoms of preeclampsia. Early writings of both the Egyptians and the Chinese warned of the dangers of convulsions encountered during pregnancy.[139] Hippocrates noted that headaches, convulsions, and drowsiness were ominous signs associated with pregnancy. The term *eclampsia* appeared in a treatise on gynecology written by Varandaeus in 1619.[6] Clonic spasms associated with pregnancy were described by Pew in 1694. In 1772, De la Motte recognized that prompt delivery of pregnant women with convulsions favored their recovery. Stroganoff, in 1900, reported a 5.4 percent maternal mortality rate as compared to the figures of 17 to 29 percent for European clinics and 21 to 49 percent for American clinics of the same period.[140] Stroganoff placed his patients in a darkened room and administered chloroform, chloral hydrate, and morphine to produce profound sedation and narcosis. Modifications were made in this regimen; eventually, magnesium sulfate was popularized by Pritchard and Zuspan as the drug of choice for eclampsia.

Pathophysiology

Although great advances have been made in treating eclampsia, the pathophysiologic events leading to convulsions remain unknown. Several theories have been advanced but are unproved. There is a functional derangement of multiple organ systems, such as the central nervous, hematologic, hepatic, renal, and cardiovascular systems. The degree of dysfunction depends not only on other medical or obstetric factors that may be present but on whether there has been a delay in the treatment of preeclampsia or iatrogenic complicating factors as well.

Renal function is impaired by reduced GFR, de-

creased renal plasma flow, and reduced clearance of uric acid. Liver damage consisting of periportal necrosis with hepatocellular damage is frequently found in women who have died from eclampsia.[141] In addition, a high incidence of cerebral edema or hemorrhage is found at autopsy. These organ system derangements may be summarized as follows:

ORGAN SYSTEM DERANGEMENTS IN ECLAMPSIA

Cardiovascular
- Generalized vasospasm
- Increased peripheral vascular resistance
- Increased left ventricular stroke work index
- Decreased central venous pressure
- Decreased pulmonary wedge pressure

Hematologic
- Decreased plasma volume
- Increased blood viscosity
- Hemoconcentration
- Coagulopathy

Renal
- Decreased glomerular filtration rate
- Decreased renal plasma flow
- Decreased uric acid clearance

Hepatic (at autopsy)
- Periportal necrosis
- Hepatocellular damage
- Subcapsular hematoma

Central nervous system (at autopsy)
- Cerebral edema
- Cerebral hemorrhage

Women in whom eclampsia develops exhibit a wide spectrum of signs and symptoms, ranging from extremely high blood pressure, 4+ proteinuria, generalized edema, and 4+ patellar reflexes to minimal blood pressure elevation, absence of proteinuria or edema, and normal reflexes.

Eclampsia usually begins as a gradual process, starting with rapid weight gain and ending with the onset of generalized convulsions or coma. Excess weight gain (with or without clinical edema) of more than 2 lb/wk during the last trimester may be the first warning sign (Fig. 30.6).[6] Hypertension is the hallmark of eclampsia, and excess weight gain and/or edema is not necessary for the diagnosis.[142,143] In about 20 percent of cases, hypertension may be "relative" (120/80 mmHg), signified by any rise in blood pressure that is 30 mmHg systolic or 15 mmHg diastolic above the first trimester blood pressure reading. Eclampsia is usually associated with significant proteinuria (> 2+ on dipstick). In a recent series of 67 eclamptic women, headache (82.5 percent), visual disturbances (44.4 percent), and right upper quadrant/epigastric pain (19 percent) were the most common premonitory symptoms before convulsions.[142] Of interest was the absence of edema (32 percent), proteinuria (21 percent), and hyperreflexia (20 percent) in 200 eclamptic women studied by the author.[143]

Convulsions may occur ante partum, intra partum, or post partum. One-half of cases of eclampsia usually occur before the onset of labor; the other 50 percent are equally divided between the intrapartum and postpartum periods. Analysis of 254 cases of eclampsia managed at our institution revealed that it developed before delivery in 180 patients (71 percent) and after delivery in 74 (29 percent). Although rare, atypi-

cal eclampsia may occur before 20 weeks gestation and more than 48 hours after delivery[144,145] (see p. 1029). Convulsions developed in 40 patients more than 48 hours after delivery. Fourteen patients (5.5 percent) experienced convulsions before 27 weeks gestation (6 before 21 weeks gestation); eclampsia developed in 115 (45 percent) at 37 to 41 weeks.

Eclampsia is primarily a disease of the young primigravida, but its incidence is also increased in women more than 35 years of age. The highest incidence occurs in the low-income nonwhite primigravida. The incidence has ranged from 1 : 147 to 1 : 3,448 pregnancies,[146,147] with an incidence of 3.6 percent in twin gestations.[18] The incidence depends on the socioeconomic status of the patient population and the number of maternal referrals to the hospital. At the University of Mississippi Medical Center, the incidence of eclampsia was 1 : 147 for 1955 to 1960 and 1 : 254 for 1971 to mid-1973.[146] Of interest, only 7.2 percent of these patients received prenatal care in the medical center's prenatal clinics. The incidence of eclampsia at the E. H. Crump Women's Hospital is now 1 : 320 deliveries. This figure is the same as that reported for 1960 to 1970.[142] However, two significant changes have occurred during this period: (1) the incidence of primigravidas has increased from 20 to 40 percent

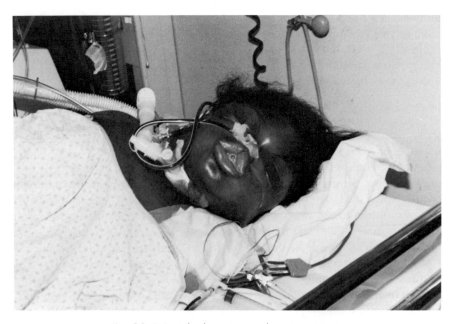

Fig. 30.6 Facial edema in an eclamptic patient.

Table 30.9 Incidence of Eclampsia

Institution	Patient Population	Incidence
University of Tennessee (Memphis)		
1960–1970	All	1:300
1977–1989	All	1:320
1977–1989	Registered prenatals	1:688
University of Mississippi		
1955–1960	All	1:147
1971–mid-1973	All	1:254
University of Virginia		
1938–1963	All	1:235
1970–1976	All	1:623
Parkland Memorial Hospital		
1955–1975	All	1:766
Athens General Hospital (Athens, Georgia)		
1966–1975	All	1:1,228

and (2) the hospital has an increased number of referrals (approximately 2,000 women annually). Forty percent of women treated for eclampsia at our hospital have received prenatal care in our clinics; 23 percent have had no prenatal care. Table 30.9 shows the incidence of eclampsia reported from several institutions.

Cerebral Manifestation of Eclampsia

Cerebral blood flow is autoregulated within a wide range of blood pressure. Loss of autoregulation has been suggested as the first step in acute hypertensive encephalopathy, leading to abnormally high cerebral perfusion. Experimentally induced hypertensive encephalopathy in animals shows alternating segments of constriction and dilatation in cortical arterioles.[148] The dilated ischemic segments become increasingly permeable, leading to extravasation of fluid and local edema formation, which causes compression of vessels and reduced blood flow as it accumulates. Other changes that would be anticipated are petechial hemorrhages, patchy vessel wall necrosis, and generalized edema. CT scans in patients with hypertensive encephalopathy show ill-defined areas of diminished density in the white matter.[149]

There are several case reports and a few large studies describing the CT scan findings in complicated cases of eclampsia. The abnormal pattern reported was either edema, hemorrhage, or ill-defined areas of diminished density in the white matter. Cerebral edema by CT scan evaluation was reported by Beeson and Duda,[150] Gaitz and Bramford,[151] Kirby and Jaindl,[152] and Dunn et al.[153] These authors recommended using mannitol and/or dexamethasone to treat such patients. Beck and Menesez[154] described a case of eclampsia in which CT scan evaluation demonstrated the presence of periventricular subependymal hemorrhage. They suggested obtaining CT scan evaluation in patients with eclampsia and focal neurologic signs. Sibai et al.[155] studied 20 women who had suffered eclamptic convulsions. Three patients had transient neurologic deficits, three experienced transient cortical blindness, and one was in a deep comatose state. The other 13 women had atypical eclampsia. All CT scans were normal. Similar findings were reported by Pritchard et al.[156]

Richards et al.[157] performed CT scans in 20 unconscious eclamptic patients. Changes compatible with cerebral edema were demonstrated in 75 percent of patients, and cerebral hemorrhage was present in 9 percent. Brown et al.[158] studied CT scans in 49 women with eclampsia. They found abnormal findings in 14 (29 percent).

Magnetic resonance imaging (MRI) appears superior to other processes for defining intracranial anatomy and pathophysiology. Its application in eclampsia has been reported by Crawford and associates, who found higher sensitivity relative to CT in its ability to detect CNS lesions.[159] We have performed MRI in 15 eclamptic women; changes compatible with ischemic changes or edema were demonstrated in 5 (33 percent) of the patients.

Abnormal electroencephalogram (EEG) findings have been reported in women with eclampsia. Pritchard and Stone[74] noted that 17 of 29 women who had eclampsia were considered to have an abnormal EEG in the puerperium. Most common were changes compatible with a recent convulsive state. We have performed EEGs on 65 women with eclampsia.[155] Initial EEGs were obtained within 48 hours of hospitalization and then serially during the next 6 months. Three women also had normal cerebral arteriograms. Forty-nine of the 65 patients with eclampsia (75 percent) had abnormal findings. We previously reported that 7 of 14 women with preeclampsia (50 percent) and 2 of 13 normotensive women (15 percent) had abnormal EEG results. All patients had adequate serum magnesium levels (4.5 to 11 mg/dl). Five of the 65 women demonstrated seizure activity on EEG with serum magnesium levels in the therapeutic range. It appears that magnesium suppresses seizure activity by a mechanism other than the one that alters the EEG. All the abnormalities noted on EEG are nonspecific and have been reported in other conditions, such as polycythemia, hypoxia, renal disease, hypocalcemia, hypercalcemia, and water intoxication.[160]

EEG abnormalities have been reported to be directly related to the severity of maternal hypertension in eclampsia; some abnormal EEG results become normal after lowering of blood pressure to the normotensive range. We found no correlation between the degree of blood pressure elevation and EEG abnormalities and consider it unlikely these abnormal EEG changes were due to hypertensive encephalopathy alone.[160]

Management of Labor and Delivery in Eclampsia

The woman with eclampsia should undergo continuous intensive monitoring. She should not be left alone in a darkened room. The guard rails should be up on the bed and a padded tongue blade kept at the bedside. A large-bore peripheral intravenous line should be in place. No other anticonvulsants should be left at the bedside except a syringe containing 2 to 4 g magnesium sulfate. Control of convulsions with magnesium sulfate is outlined later. We agree with Pritchard[156] that no more than 8 g magnesium sulfate

should be given over a short period to control convulsions.

No single test or set of laboratory determinations is useful in predicting maternal or neonatal outcome in women with eclampsia. Alterations in tests of renal or hepatic function occur frequently. A significant disturbance in the integrity of the coagulation system is unlikely. We previously recommended only a complete blood count (including blood smear and platelet count), clot observation, and serum creatinine in women with eclampsia.[161] Liver function tests were obtained only in women with upper abdominal pain. However, because of an increase in the number of women with HELLP syndrome and eclampsia as well as those with serious medical problems, we have expanded the laboratory tests ordered in eclamptic women to include determinations of fibrinogen, electrolytes, and arterial blood gases.

Once convulsions have been controlled and the woman has regained consciousness, her general medical condition is assessed. When she is stable, induction of labor with oxytocin is initiated. Delivery is the treatment for eclampsia. Fetal heart rate and intensity of uterine contractions should be closely monitored. If labor is not well established, and in the absence of fetal malpresentation or fetal distress, oxytocin may be used to induce labor in all patients beyond 32 weeks gestation, irrespective of cervical dilatation or effacement. The same approach is used in patients with a gestational age below 32 weeks if the cervix is favorable for induction. However, women with an unfavorable cervix and a gestational age of less than 32 weeks are stabilized with magnesium sulfate and are then delivered electively by cesarean section. This approach is based on our previous experience with high intrapartum complication rates in eclampsia that develops before 32 weeks gestation.[162] These complications include a high incidence of fetal growth retardation (30 percent), abruption (23 percent), and fetal distress during labor (65 percent).

In a review of 10 women who had undergone electronic internal fetal monitoring during an eclamptic convulsion, 6 had fetal bradycardia (fetal heart rate below 120 beats/min) that varied in duration from 30 seconds to 9 minutes.[163] The interval from onset of the seizure to the fall in fetal heart rate was 5 minutes. Transitory fetal tachycardia occurred frequently after the prolonged bradycardia. In addition, loss of beat-to-beat variability with transitory late decelerations occurred during the recovery phase.

Uterine hyperactivity demonstrated by both increased uterine tone and increased frequency of uterine contractions occurs during an eclamptic seizure. The duration of the increased uterine activity varies from 2 to 14 minutes.

Fetal outcome is generally good after an eclamptic convulsion. The mechanism for the transitory fetal distress may be a decrease in uterine blood flow caused by intense vasospasm and uterine hyperactivity. The absence of maternal respiration during the convulsion may also be a factor contributing to these fetal heart rate changes. Since the fetal heart rate pattern usually returns to normal after a convulsion, other conditions should be considered if an abnormal pattern persists. It may take longer for the heart rate pattern to return to baseline in an eclamptic woman whose fetus is preterm and growth-retarded. Placental abruption may occur after the convulsion and should be considered if uterine hyperactivity remains or bradycardia persists.

Treatment of Eclamptic Convulsions

Eclamptic convulsions are a life-threatening emergency and require proper care in order to minimize morbidity and mortality. Observing the development of an eclamptic convulsion is frightening. Initially, the patient's face becomes distorted and there is protrusion of the eyes. This is followed by a congested facial expression. Foam often exudes from the mouth. The woman usually bites her tongue unless it is protected. Respirations are absent throughout the seizure. Typically, the convulsion, which can be divided into two phases, continues for 60 to 75 seconds. The first phase, which lasts 15 to 20 seconds, begins with facial twitching, which proceeds to the body's becoming rigid and having generalized muscular contractions. The second phase lasts approximately 60 seconds; the muscles of the body alternately contract and relax in rapid succession. This phase begins with the muscles of the jaw and rapidly involves the eyelids, other facial muscles, and then all the muscles of the body. Coma follows the convulsion, and the woman usually remembers nothing of the recent events. If she has repeated convulsions, some degree of consciousness returns after each convulsion. She may enter a combative state and be very agitated and difficult to control. Rapid and deep respirations usually begin as soon as the convulsions end. Maintenance of oxygenation is usually not a problem after a single convulsion; the risk of aspiration is low in the well-managed patient.

Several steps should be taken in managing an eclamptic convulsion.

1. *Do not attempt to shorten or abolish the initial convulsion:* Because eclampsia is so frightening, the natural tendency is to do something to abolish the convulsion. Drugs such as diazepam should not be given in an attempt to stop or shorten the convulsion, especially if the patient does not have an intravenous line in place and someone skilled in intubation is not immediately available. Diazepam causes phlebitis and venous thrombosis and should not be given without secure intravenous access. In addition, no more than 5 mg should be given over a 60-second period. Rapid administration of diazepam may lead to apnea or cardiac arrest or both.[164]

2. *Prevent maternal injury during the convulsion:* A padded tongue blade should be inserted between the patient's teeth to prevent biting of the tongue. Care should be taken to avoid stimulating the gag reflex with the blade. Its only purpose is to prevent the patient from biting her tongue. Place the woman on her left side and then suction the foam and secretions from her mouth. That serious maternal injuries may occur during eclamptic seizures is well demonstrated in the report from Magee-Women's Hospital, Pittsburgh, Pennsylvania.[165] Among the 52 women with eclampsia, one had a dislocated shoulder, fractured humerus, and multiple facial contusions from a fall in the emergency room following a convulsion. Two other women had severe airway obstruction.

3. *Maintain adequate oxygenation:* After the convulsion has ceased, the patient begins to breathe again and oxygenation is rarely a problem. Difficulty with oxygenation may occur in women who have had repetitive convulsions or have received drugs in an attempt to abolish the convulsions.

Such women should have a chest radiograph to rule out aspiration pneumonia.

4. *Minimize the risk of aspiration:* Aspiration should be a rare occurrence with eclamptic convulsions. It may be caused by forcing the padded tongue blade to the back of the throat, stimulating the gag reflex with resultant vomiting and aspiration. At our hospital, all women who have had aspiration as a result of eclamptic convulsions had received many drugs in an attempt to control their convulsions. The lungs should always be auscultated after the convulsion has ended, to ensure they are clear.

5. *Give adequate magnesium sulfate to control the convulsions:* As soon as the convulsion has ended, a large secure intravenous line should be inserted and a loading dose of magnesium sulfate given intravenously. In our institution, we use a 6-g intravenous loading dose given over *15 to 20 minutes.* In addition to providing a good initial serum magnesium level, the serum magnesium level does not fall below the therapeutic range for several hours after the initial 6-g loading dose as often happens when using a 4-g loading dose. If the patient has a convulsion after the loading dose, another bolus of 2 g magnesium sulfate can be given intravenously over 3 to 5 minutes. Approximately 10 to 15 percent of women have a second convulsion after receiving the intravenous loading dose of magnesium sulfate. Pritchard reported that 10 of 83 women who had eclampsia treated before delivery again suffered convulsions shortly after an initial injection of magnesium sulfate, 4 g intravenously and 10 g intramuscularly.[156] However, most remained free of seizures after an additional 2 g intravenous magnesium sulfate.

We use serum magnesium levels in the clinical management of the eclamptic woman. If the initial level, obtained 4 hours after the loading dose, is high (over 10 mg/dl), we reduce the 2-g maintenance dose of magnesium sulfate. This occasionally occurs in women with renal compromise. Similarly, in the rare patient with a brisk urine output, we give a maintenance dose of 3 g/hr to keep levels in the therapeutic range.

In a series by Sibai,[166] of 262 eclamptic women, 36 (14 percent) had an additional convulsion after receiving magnesium sulfate. An occasional patient has recurrent convulsions while receiving therapeutic doses of magnesium sulfate. In these cases, a short-acting barbiturate such as sodium amobarbital can be given in a dose of up to 250 mg intravenously over 3 to 5 minutes. We treated one patient who had recurrent convulsions with a serum magnesium level of 9.4 mg/dl and who had also received sodium amobarbital. She was given an intravenous sodium pentothal drip and experienced no further seizures.

Magnesium toxicity was responsible for the only death in Pritchard and co-workers' series of eclamptic women[156] and nearly led to a maternal death at the University of Tennessee.[161] In both cases, the patients were supposed to have received a loading dose of 4 g magnesium sulfate but, because of an error in preparing the drug, received 20 g magnesium sulfate over a few minutes. We believe that having both 1-g and 5-g vials of magnesium sulfate on the labor and delivery floor could contribute to an error in making the necessary dilution. Therefore, we now stock only 5-g vials of magnesium sulfate.

Rarely, a woman may have an eclamptic seizure, lapse into a coma, and die. Magnesium toxicity should be considered in those women who do not regain consciousness. A case of magnesium sulfate toxicity details the features of this serious complication.[167] Within a few minutes of starting what was supposed to be a magnesium loading dose, 4 g magnesium sulfate in 250 ml saline, the patient went into cardiorespiratory arrest. Immediate resuscitation, including intubation, was performed. Approximately one-half the loading dose had been given. An intracerebral accident or eclampsia was thought to be the etiology of the coma; the loading dose was continued and maintenance therapy started. Initial blood gas findings were normal, and the electrocardiogram (ECG) result was normal 15 minutes after the arrest. Mechanical ventilatory support was required. The patient's vital signs were stable, but her pupils were nonreactive. Serum electrolytes, glucose, blood urea nitrogen (BUN), and creatinine were normal. Results of CT of the head and cerebral angiograms were normal. A magnesium level of 35 mg/dl was reported 3.5

hours later from a blood sample taken via femoral venipuncture at the time of arrest. The magnesium sulfate infusion was stopped immediately. During the first 5 hours after the cardiorespiratory arrest, 1,344 mg of magnesium was excreted in the urine. Twelve hours after the arrest, an uncomplicated low vertical cesarean section was performed for a breech presentation. The 3,160-g male infant had Apgar scores of 8 and 9 at 1 and 5 minutes. Maternal and cord blood magnesium at delivery was 5.8 mg/dl. Both mother and baby were discharged from the hospital with no apparent residual effects. Of interest, the patient reported she could hear and see what was occurring around her, but she could not make any movements while she had the endotracheal tube in place. Figure 30.7 presents the maternal magnesium levels in this case.

6. *Maternal acidemia should be corrected:* We obtain a blood gas reading on every patient who has had an eclamptic convulsion. Blood oxygenation and

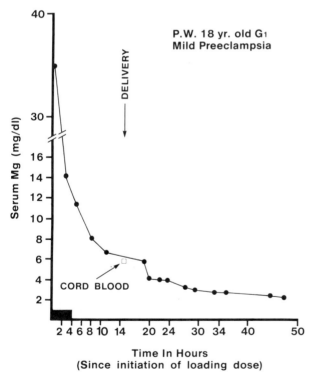

Fig. 30.7 A patient with magnesium toxicity. (From McCubbin et al.,[167] with permission.)

pH results should be in the normal range. Patients who have had repeated convulsions may be acidotic, and a low Po_2 may indicate aspiration pneumonitis. Sodium bicarbonate is not given unless the pH is below 7.10. Abnormal blood gases may be the result of respiratory depression.

7. *Avoid polypharmacy:* Polypharmacy is extremely hazardous in the woman with eclampsia, as addition of diazepam or phenytoin may lead to respiratory depression or respiratory arrest.

In many centers outside the United States, magnesium sulfate is rarely used to prevent or treat eclamptic convulsions. As a result, the ideal anticonvulsant in these centers is yet to be found.[166] During the past 60 years numerous anticonvulsive drugs have been introduced and replaced because of dissatisfaction with the results obtained with their use. These drugs have included bromethol, chloral hydrate, paraldehyde, phenothiazines, lytic cocktails, barbiturates, diazepam, chlordiazepoxide, and clonazepam. The overzealous use of these drugs in eclampsia has been associated with significant maternal–neonatal CNS and respiratory depression.[160,168] The use of large doses of diazepam (> 30 mg) during labor is associated with loss of beat-to-beat fetal heart rate variability and significant neonatal morbidity (respiratory depression, apnea, hypotonia, cold stress, poor sucking). The use of the barbiturate chlormethiozole (which is commonly used in Europe and Australia) in anticonvulsive doses may depress maternal laryngeal reflexes, thus increasing the likelihood of aspiration during convulsion. In addition, the use of intravenous phenobarbital has the potential of producing laryngospasm and circulatory and respiratory depression. Moreover, none of these drugs has been proved to be superior to or as effective as magnesium sulfate in treating eclamptic convulsions.

Recently, phenytoin has been advocated for the prevention and treatment of eclamptic convulsions. Slater et al.[168] evaluated a regimen of phenytoin based on maternal weight in 26 patients (7 had severe preeclampsia, 17 had mild disease, and 2 had eclampsia). They reported no seizures after the initiation of phenytoin (750 to 1,250 mg intravenously at a rate of ≤ 25 mg/min) and noted no major maternal or neonatal side effects.

Ryan et al.[169] investigated the safety, efficacy, and

pharmacokinetics of phenytoin. They reported that an appropriate regimen should include a loading dose of 15 mg/kg pregnancy weight to be administered as 10 mg/kg initially and 5 mg/kg 2 hours later. This loading dose was to be followed by a maintenance dose of 200 mg orally or intravenously every 8 hours to start 12 hours after a second bolus. The maintenance dose was continued for 3 to 5 days after delivery. This regimen requires obtaining frequent monitoring of phenytoin and albumin levels. They reported this regimen to be effective and safe in 80 such patients studied. One of the 80 patients developed convulsions after receiving an inadequate dose. They recommended the use of phenytoin as a logical alternative to magnesium sulfate.

Others have compared the use of phenytoin to magnesium sulfate in preeclampsia–eclampsia.[170–172] Two patients with eclampsia randomized to phenytoin developed subsequent convulsions. They found that phenytoin was better tolerated and associated with fewer side effects than magnesium sulfate.

On the other hand, the widespread use of phenytoin for severe preeclampsia–eclampsia in the United Kingdom was questioned by Tufnell et al.[173] They reported that 3 (17 percent) of 18 preeclamptic–eclamptic women developed a further convulsion after the administration of the recommended dose. Phenytoin serum levels were measured in 2 of the 3 patients and were in the therapeutic range in both. This report was followed by two letters to the editor in support of and against the use of this therapy.[174,175] Slater et al.[174] stated that they have extended their series to include 70 patients with preeclampsia–eclampsia who were treated with phenytoin. They reported the development of convulsions in 2 of 8 eclamptic women after the initiation of phenytoin infusions. Sibai[166] reported the development of convulsions in 4 of 7 eclamptic women after receiving loading doses of phenytoin.

Laboratory Findings in Eclampsia

Women who have eclampsia have contracted blood volumes. Pritchard and Stone[74] found no significant increase in blood volume or red blood cell (RBC) volume in 13 women with antepartum eclampsia who were not bleeding, as compared to their nonpregnant values. Seven of these women had a normal pregnancy after having had eclampsia; in those pregnan-

cies, blood volumes increased 40.7 percent and RBC volume 31.8 percent over their nonpregnant values. A significant number of patients with eclampsia have thrombocytopenia. Pritchard et al.[176] observed a mean platelet count of $202 \times 10^3/\mu l$ in 95 women with eclampsia, compared to $278 \times 10^3/\mu l$ in controls. Twenty-eight of the 95 eclamptic women had low platelet counts, which were below 100×10^3, and 3 had counts below $50 \times 10^3/\mu l$. Sibai et al.[161] found a mean platelet count of $269 \times 10^3/\mu l$ in 67 eclamptic women, as compared to $266 \times 10^3/\mu l$ in pregnant controls. However, 10 of the 62 eclamptic women had platelet counts more than 2 SDs below the normal mean. In neither series was there evidence of DIC or demonstrable microangiopathic hemolytic anemia.

We have reviewed the coagulation factors in eclamptic women we have treated during the past 8 years. In addition, laboratory values were examined with regard to the presence or absence of placental abruption. Mean platelet counts and fibrinogen levels were only slightly lower in the eclamptic women with placental abruption. However, a higher percentage of the women with placental abruption had lower platelet counts and fibrinogen, as compared to those who did not have placental abruption. Hematocrits were significantly higher than those in a group of pregnant controls.

Creatinine clearances were found to be markedly impaired in a group of Egyptian eclamptic women as compared to values in pregnant controls, 48.5 ± 9.9 ml/min versus 110.4 ± 32.5 ml/min.[177] Pritchard and Stone[74] found a mean BUN of 12.0 mg/dl in 69 eclamptic women with a range of 5 to 28 mg/dl. Six of the women had had an initial BUN over 20 mg/dl. We have found the serum creatinine to be elevated more than 2 SDs in 73 of 149 women (49.5 percent) with eclampsia. The incidence was higher in eclamptic women with abruptio placenta.

Liver function test results are abnormal in many women with eclampsia.[74] LDH was elevated in 74 percent of eclamptic patients. Shukla et al.[178] also reported elevation of the hepatic fraction of LDH in women with eclampsia. Both alkaline phosphatase and SGOT may be increased. Total bilirubin levels are rarely elevated. We found liver function tests in eclamptic women with right upper-quadrant pain more likely to be abnormal (Table 30.10).

Table 30.10 Liver Function Tests in Eclamptic Women with Right Upper Quadrant Pain

Laboratory Test > 2SD	Incidence[a]	
	With RUQ Pain	Without RUQ Pain
SGOT	9/12(75)	3/42(7)
LDH	12/12(100)	27/44(61)
Alkaline phosphatase	12/12(100)	6/44(14)
Total bilirubin	5/12(42)	1/44[b](2)

[a] Numbers in parentheses are percentages.

[b] Patient had sickle cell disease.

Atypical Eclampsia

Eclampsia occurring before 20 weeks gestation or after 48 hours post partum is exceedingly rare, and, for lack of a better term, has been called atypical eclampsia. Eclampsia occurring before 20 weeks gestation has usually been reported with molar or hydropic degeneration of the placenta. Chesley et al.[179] observed 35 cases of probable eclampsia associated with molar degeneration of the placenta in a review of the literature through 1944. In 26 of these patients, eclampsia occurred during the first half of gestation. Six of the women had a coexistent fetus. Two cases of eclampsia have been reported without molar degeneration of the placenta during the first half of gestation.[180,181] In one woman who had Rh isoimmunization, eclampsia developed at 16 weeks gestation. The placenta revealed cystic hydropic degeneration of the villi. No molar changes were present.

In two Memphis hospitals, which delivered 45,000 patients between August 1977 and March 1981, only three women without molar degeneration were treated for eclampsia during the first half of pregnancy.[144] Two of these women showed evidence of chronic hypertension or renal disease. The third patient was a young primigravida without evidence of underlying medical disorders. In all these women, gestational age was confirmed by ultrasonographic measurements and postmortem examination of the fetus and placenta. None of the women had a history of seizure disorder, and none had evidence of neurologic deficit either during admission or at follow-up visits; two had subsequent pregnancies without convulsions.

Although rare, eclampsia can occur during the first half of gestation. Eclamptic women may be misdiagnosed as having hypertensive encephalopathy or a seizure disorder. Women in whom convulsions develop in association with hypertension and proteinuria during the first half of pregnancy should be considered to have eclampsia. They should be treated with parenteral magnesium sulfate to control convulsions, with termination of pregnancy as the definitive goal.

Late postpartum eclampsia is eclampsia that occurs more than 48 hours after delivery. Of the 186 women we have treated for eclampsia during the past 8 years, eclampsia developed in 25 more than 48 hours post partum (13.4 percent). A review of the clinical course of late postpartum eclampsia has been reported.[182] Twelve of the 17 women described in that report had been treated for preeclampsia and received standard intravenous magnesium sulfate therapy. The mean duration of magnesium sulfate therapy was 32 hours (range 24 to 72 hours). Several women were at home when the convulsions developed. In addition, 2 were receiving intravenous magnesium sulfate at the time of the convulsions (serum magnesium levels 5.2 and 9.1 mg/dl). Thirteen were primigravidas, and 4 were multigravidas. The clinical characteristics of these women are summarized in Table 30.11. All the women had experienced headaches and visual disturbances (blurred vision and scotomas for 1 to 3 days before the onset of convulsions). The most striking finding in these women was the brisk diuresis that

Table 30.11 Clinical Picture in Women with Late Postpartum Eclampsia

Symptoms/Signs	Incidence	
	N	%
Severe headaches[a]	17	100
Visual disturbances[a]	17	100
Diastolic blood pressure (90 to 130 mmHg)	17	100
Hyperuricemia	17	100
Immediate marked diuresis	17	100
Hyperreflexia with clonus	13	76
Proteinuria	5	29
Edema	4	25

[a] Occurred 1 to 3 days before convulsions.

occurred immediately after the convulsion. Urinary outputs of 500 to 1,000 ml during the first hour after the seizure were common. Because of the unusual time of occurrence of eclampsia in these women, neurologic consultations were obtained. CT scans showed no abnormalities in 10 of the women. Of 9 women who had lumbar punctures, all had normal findings. Two of the women had unilateral upper extremity paresis that resolved.

Of interest is the high rate of occurrence of late postpartum eclampsia in Nigerian women. In a report of 25 cases of postpartum eclampsia, 17 (68 percent) occurred more than 48 hours post partum.[183] Uric acid levels were elevated in these women with eclampsia before delivery or during the immediate postpartum period.

Obviously, eclampsia can occur more than 48 hours post partum. Women in whom it develops more than 48 hours post partum with the typical clinical findings of eclampsia should be treated with magnesium sulfate to control seizures. Because of the late onset of the convulsions, other diagnoses should be considered. No further neurologic evaluation is necessary for women who present with the typical clinical course of late postpartum eclampsia.

Maternity Morbidity and Mortality in Eclampsia

Pritchard et al.[156] reported only one maternal death in 245 women treated for eclampsia at Parkland Hospital, Dallas, Texas, from 1955 to 1983, a maternal mortality rate of 0.4 percent. This death was caused by magnesium toxicity. Endotracheal intubation was not accomplished promptly in this short and very obese woman; as a result, respiratory arrest, cardiorespiratory arrest, and death ensued. Three other women had respiratory depression. In 91 women cared for since 1975 by Pritchard, 2 showed the development of pulmonary edema.[156] In neither case was intravenous fluid therapy considered excessive. This series is impressive for both the extremely low mortality rate and the low incidence of maternal complications.

One maternal death occurred in our series of 264 patients with eclampsia. The patient had five convulsions before arriving at our hospital and went into cardiorespiratory arrest in the parking lot. The patient was resuscitated, and her seizures were controlled with magnesium sulfate. However, she did not regain consciousness after cardiac arrest. She underwent a cesarean section for fetal distress with the delivery of a 3,090-g infant with normal Apgar scores. The child had no serious problems in the nursery and was discharged in good condition. DIC developed after the operation. The postoperative course was complicated by sepsis, continuing convulsions, and pulmonary insufficiency. An EEG on the second postoperative day demonstrated absent cortical activity. A CT scan failed to demonstrate either intracerebral hemorrhage or cerebral edema. The patient remained comatose and died 8 weeks post partum. Table 30.12 lists the maternal complications observed in eclamptic patients at Parkland and E. H. Crump Women's Hospitals.

Harbert et al.[184] reported on 168 women treated for eclampsia between 1939 and 1963. Delivery within an arbitrary time limit after control of the convulsion was not an essential part of therapy. Forty-seven of the 83 patients in whom eclampsia occurred before the spontaneous onset of labor were delivered within 48 hours of the first convulsive episode. In the other 36 patients with eclampsia before delivery, the interval between occurrence of the convulsion and spontaneous onset of labor ranged from 93 hours to 43 days. During the first 6 years of the study, eight maternal deaths occurred. From December 1944 to termination of the study in 1963, 108 women with eclampsia were managed without another maternal death. The uncorrected PMR was 216/1,000. The corrected PMR was 280/1,000 (14 fetal deaths and 3 neonatal deaths) in 60 patients delivered 72 hours or longer after admission.

Lopez-Llera and Horta[185] reviewed 365 cases of eclampsia in Mexican women during a 9-year period ending in 1973. There were 49 deaths, for a mortality rate of 13.5 percent. Several factors were found to increase the risk of maternal death in eclampsia:

1. *Gestational age at which eclampsia occurred:* Eight of 28 women (28.5 percent) in whom eclampsia had developed before 28 weeks gestation died. In women in whom the onset of eclampsia occurred after 30 weeks gestation, there were 41 maternal deaths (12.2 percent) ($p < 0.02$).
2. *Age at which eclampsia occurred:* The 73 teenagers with eclampsia had a maternal mortality rate of 5.5 percent as compared to the 89 women over

Table 30.12 Maternal Complications of Eclampsia

Complication	Parkland Hospital 1955–1983 (N = 245)		E. H. Crump Hospital 1977–1985 (N = 186)	
	N	%	N	%
Seizure following MgSO₄ therapy	10/83	(12)	28	(15)
Magnesium intoxication,	4	(1.6)	3	(1.6)
requiring intubation	3	(1.2)	0	(0)
Pulmonary edema	2/91	(2.2)	9	(4.8)
Azotemia requiring dialysis	0/245	(0)	2	(1.1)
Second antihypertensive drug needed to control blood pressure	0	(0)	4	(2.1)
Intracranial hemorrhage	0	(0)	0	(0)
Maternal death	1	(0.4)	1	(0.5)

30 years of age, who had a mortality rate of 20 percent ($p < 0.005$). Further analysis of maternal deaths gives a maternal mortality rate of 8.9 percent for the 118 women aged 15 to 24 years ($p < 0.02$), 19.5 percent for the 118 women aged 25 to 34 years, and 18.6 percent for the 43 women aged 35 to 46 years.

3. *Twin pregnancies:* The series included 18 twin pregnancies. The maternal mortality rate in these multiple gestations was double the figure for the entire group of eclamptic women.

In our experience, primigravid women with eclampsia have a lower incidence of serious complications than multigravid women (Table 30.13). This is

Table 30.13 Relationship of Parity to Complications Associated with Eclampsia

Complication	Primigravida (N = 157)		Multigravida (N = 29)	
	N	%	N	%
HELLP	14	8.9	5	17.2
DIC	4	2.5	5	17.2
Renal failure	4	2.5	4	13.8
Postpartum hemorrhage	21	13.4	5	17.2
Pulmonary edema	5	3.2	4	13.8

Abbreviations: HELLP, hemolysis, elevated liver enzymes, and low platelets; DIC, disseminated intravascular coagulopathy.

probably attributable to the higher incidence of chronic hypertension and underlying renal disease in the multigravid women rather than to any effect of eclampsia per se. In particular, we believe that careful attention should be given to intravenous fluid therapy in multigravid women with eclampsia. In our experience, pulmonary edema is much more likely to develop. Likewise, the incidence of renal failure is much higher in multigravid women with eclampsia than primigravid women with eclampsia.

In our series, maternal transfers and patients who had received no prenatal care had higher complication rates (Table 30.14). More than 90 percent of women with eclampsia who had no prenatal care were first seen in the emergency room of another hospital. Many were treated by a physician who was seeing his or her first case of eclampsia. Referral often occurred before the women had received adequate treatment with magnesium sulfate.

Perinatal Outcome in Eclampsia

The main risks to the fetus of the eclamptic woman are abruptio placenta, prematurity, intrauterine growth retardation, and hypoxic episodes during the convulsions.[186,187]

Abruptio placenta is a significant perinatal risk in women in whom eclampsia develops before delivery. Pritchard et al.[156] reported a 5.5 percent incidence of abruptio placenta in this setting. Abruption was the contributing factor in the death of three stillborn fetuses who weighed more than 2,000 g. Abdella et

Table 30.14 Maternal Complications from Eclampsia: 1977–1985[a]

Complication	Maternal Transfer and No Prenatal Care (N = 111)		Prenatal Care at University (N = 75)		Total (N = 186)	
	N	%	N	%	N	%
Abruptio placenta	18	(16.2)	3	(4)	21	(11.3)
Pulmonary edema	6	(5.4)	3	(4)	9	(4.8)
Cardiorespiratory arrest	6	(5.4)	2	(2.7)	8	(4.3)
Acute renal failure	7	(6.3)	1	(1.3)	8	(4.3)
Aspiration	4	(3.6)	0		4	(2.2)
Pleural effusion	2	(1.8)	0		2	(1.1)
Maternal death	1	(0.9)	0		1	(0.5)

[a] This study was performed at E. H. Crump Women's Hospital, Memphis, Tennessee.

al.[188] reported abruptio placenta in 13 of 55 women (23.6 percent) in whom eclampsia developed before delivery at the University of Tennessee. In these patients, there were three stillbirths and three neonatal deaths for a PMR of 460/1,000. We have now managed 134 women with eclampsia before delivery. The incidence of abruptio placenta was 15 percent (20 of 134 cases), and the PMR for women in whom abruptio placenta developed was 422/1,000. One other study has reported a PMR of 45 percent in women who have eclampsia and in whom abruptio placenta develops.[189]

Neonatal Outcome in Eclampsia

Brazy et al.[190] reported a high incidence of retarded fetal growth (39 percent less than tenth percentile and 96 percent less than fiftieth percentile) in 28 infants from pregnancies complicated by severe hypertension. Eight of these patients had eclampsia. In addition, 29 percent of the infants had symmetric growth retardation. The same investigators reported a high incidence of perinatal asphyxia, low Apgar scores, and hematologic abnormalities, including an increased incidence of thrombocytopenia, leukopenia, neutropenia, and DIC. They suggested the presence of a common pathologic process leading to the abnormal hematologic findings in both mother and infant.

Sibai et al.[162] followed 28 premature infants and 14 full-term infants of eclamptic mothers for up to 50 months. Eight of the 12 infants who were small for

age by weight at birth showed catch-up growth at an average of 20.6 months (range 2 to 48 months). In all, only 2 of the infants remained growth-retarded by weight, height, and head circumference; both were mentally retarded. A total of 3 infants had major neurologic deficits resulting in cerebral palsy and mental retardation on follow-up evaluation. General health continued to be a problem for the premature infants during the first year of life. Several had multiple hospitalizations for either pulmonary or neurologic complications.

Maternal Transport of the Eclamptic Patient

During the past 20 years, there has been a marked reduction in the number of eclamptic patients. Consequently, most obstetricians have little or no experience in the management of eclampsia. A recent survey of a random sample of obstetricians from all 50 states indicated that about 50 percent of obstetricians in private practice had not seen an eclamptic patient during the past year.

Because management of the eclamptic patient requires the availability of neonatal and obstetric intensive care units (ICUs) and personnel with special expertise, we believe that eclamptic patients should not be managed at level I hospitals. We recommend that eclamptic patients with term gestations be cared for only at level II or III hospitals with adequate facilities and with consultants from other specialties, if needed. For those eclamptic patients who are remote from term, referral should be made to a tertiary care center. We recommend that the following steps be taken before transfer of these critically ill patients:

1. The referring physician and/or nurse should consult the physician at the perinatal center about the referral and appropriate treatment. All maternal records including prenatal data and a detailed summary of the patient's condition should be sent with the patient.
2. Blood pressure should be stabilized and convulsions controlled.
3. Adequate prophylactic anticonvulsive medications should be given. An accepted regimen is 4 g intravenous magnesium sulfate as a loading dose, with a simultaneous intramuscular dose of 10 g.
4. Such patients should be sent in an ambulance with medical personnel in attendance for proper management in case of subsequent convulsions.

Can Eclampsia Be Prevented?

Eclampsia is generally considered a preventable complication of pregnancy. Zuspan[191] believes that the severe forms of preeclampsia should be preventable by appropriate prenatal care. He also contends that convulsions should not occur once the woman with preeclampsia is admitted to the hospital. Zuspan stresses that when eclampsia does occur, it is because of failure to diagnose preeclampsia, lack of surveillance of women at risk of development of preeclampsia–eclampsia, and inadequate treatment once preeclampsia develops. The low incidence of eclampsia in women managed with early and prolonged hospitalizations for mild preeclampsia has been documented by others.[112]

We recently reviewed 179 cases of eclampsia treated at the University of Tennessee between 1977 and 1985 in an attempt to determine the number of cases of preventable eclampsia. The seventeenth edition of Williams's *Obstetrics* was considered the standard in deciding the adequacy of prenatal care. This text recommends that all pregnant patients be seen every 2 weeks from 28 to 36 weeks gestation followed by weekly visits until term. It is recommended that magnesium sulfate be continued for 24 hours in the management of preeclamptic patients, since postpartum eclampsia rarely occurs beyond 24 hours after delivery.[192]

Table 30.15 Factors Associated with Eclampsia

Factor	Cases ($N = 179$)
Physician error	
Inadequate prenatal care	25
Failure of diagnosis or treatment	35
Patient error	
No prenatal care	39
Failure to keep prenatal appointment	15
Failure of magnesium sulfate therapy	
Convulsion while receiving magnesium sulfate	23
Magnesium levels below therapeutic range	9

All factors that may have been involved in the development of eclampsia are summarized in Table 30.15. Patients were then grouped into categories of physician error, patient failure, and failure of magnesium sulfate therapy.

Patient failure was thought to be a factor in 54 of the women in whom eclampsia developed (30 percent). Thirty-nine of these women did not receive prenatal care, and 15 patients failed to keep their last scheduled prenatal appointment. Thirty-four presented with eclampsia; the other 20 presented with preeclampsia.

Physician error was a factor in 60 cases of eclampsia (34 percent). Inadequate prenatal follow-up was found to be the case in 25 (20 percent) of the women who had prenatal care. Physician error was responsible for the development of eclampsia in 35 of the 100 women who had received appropriate prenatal care. These errors generally were a failure to diagnose preeclampsia or lack of treatment or inappropriate treatment once the diagnosis of preeclampsia was made.

Twenty-three women had eclamptic seizures while receiving magnesium sulfate. Three of the 23 were receiving the standard intramuscular regimen recommended by Pritchard; the others were receiving the standard intravenous regimen with maintenance doses of 1 to 3 g/hr. Nine had magnesium levels below the therapeutic range.

Fifty-six patients (31 percent) were judged to have nonpreventable eclampsia (Table 30.16). All 56 had appropriate prenatal care, were diagnosed and hos-

Table 30.16   Factors Involved in Unavoidable Eclampsia

Factor	All Cases of Eclampsia (N = 179)	Unavoidable Eclampsia (N = 56)
Abrupt onset	32	24
Late postpartum onset	22	16
Convulsion on magnesium sulfate	23	7[a]
Mild preeclampsia with good response[b]	—	6
Early onset (<21 weeks)	5	3

[a] Adequate serum magnesium levels.

[b] Normal blood pressure after hospitalization.

pitalized appropriately, and received adequate therapy with magnesium sulfate. Twenty-four patients in whom convulsions developed before their next appropriately-scheduled prenatal visit or persons in whom convulsions developed even though they were normotensive after hospitalization for mild preeclampsia remote from term were considered to have had abrupt onset of eclampsia. Twenty-two had convulsions before their next prenatal visit and 2 in the immediate postpartum period. None of these patients had any premonitory signs or symptoms of preeclampsia at the time of the last prenatal visit or during labor. Six women were hospitalized with the diagnosis of mild preeclampsia remote from term. They had a drop in blood pressure and diuresis within 48 hours of hospitalization, but convulsions developed 4 to 10 days after hospitalization. An additional 9 of the women had eclamptic convulsions more than 72 hours after delivery. The remaining 7 cases had convulsions with serum magnesium levels in the therapeutic range.

These findings are in agreement with those of Campbell and Templeton,[193] who studied factors leading to the development of eclampsia in 66 patients. These workers found that in 28 patients (42.4 percent), eclampsia was not preventable.

Clearly, a large number of the cases of eclampsia are avoidable. It appears, however, that approximately 30 to 40 percent cannot be prevented despite adherence to present standards of prenatal care. Forty of the 56 nonpreventable cases (71.4 percent) were due to development of convulsions before the next appropriately scheduled prenatal visit or oc-

curred more than 72 hours after delivery. Prevention of these cases would have required increased frequency of prenatal visits for all obstetric patients during the last trimester and prolongation of hospitalization for all women after delivery.

Counseling Women with Eclampsia and Their Relatives

Bryans et al.,[194] in their long-term follow-up study of women who had eclampsia treated at the Medical College of Georgia, found no increase in hypertension in these patients above that expected in the general female population. He concluded that preeclampsia–eclampsia did not cause hypertensive disease and was not a manifestation of subsequent essential hypertension in pregnant women. Chesley et al.[195] followed women who developed eclampsia at the Margaret Hague Hospital, New Jersey, from its opening in 1931 through 1951. He traced all but three of the women who survived to 1974. Chesley also concluded that eclampsia does not cause hypertension.[195] The average annual death rate was 5.11/1,000 with 31 deaths in the 187 white women who had eclampsia during their pregnancies. This was not significantly different from the number of deaths expected. However, 33 of 59 white women who had eclampsia as multiparas had died at an average rate of 21.3/1,000, which was significantly higher than the expected mortality rate. Eighty-two percent of the remote deaths were due to cardiovascular–renal disease in women who had eclampsia as multiparas.

Chesley reported that the prognosis for future pregnancies after eclampsia was good. Another 409 pregnancies occurred in the 158 women in whom eclampsia developed during their first pregnancy. Preeclampsia–eclampsia recurred in 34.5 percent of the women and in 20.6 percent of their subsequent pregnancies. When hypertension occurred in a future pregnancy, it was usually mild. Eclampsia developed in three women, for an incidence of 0.9 percent in pregnancies beyond 20 weeks gestation.

The sisters and daughters of eclamptic women are at increased risk for development of preeclampsia and eclampsia.[196] Chesley[197] reviewed the incidence of preeclampsia in the first pregnancies of daughters of eclamptic mothers. Preeclampsia developed in 63 of the 257 first pregnancies (24.9 percent). Eclampsia occurred in 7 of these pregnancies (2.7 percent). The outcome of the first pregnancy carried to viability of

Table 30.17 Counseling Women with Eclampsia and Their Relatives

Relationship to Eclamptic Women	> 20 weeks	Preeclampsia		Eclampsia	
		N	%	N	%
Eclamptic women[195,a]	340	70	20.6	3	0.9
Sister[199,a]	147	54	37.6	6	4.1
Daughter[196,b]	257	63	24.9	7	2.7
Daughter-in-law[197,b]	75	6	8.0	—	—

[a] All future pregnancies.

[b] First pregnancy.

sisters of eclamptic women was also studied. Preeclampsia occurred in 54 (37 percent) of first pregnancies, and eclampsia developed in 6 women (4.1 percent). The outcomes of these pregnancies are summarized in Table 30.17.[198] Because of the increased risk of preeclampsia–eclampsia in these women, their pregnancies should be closely monitored.

The incidence of severe preeclampsia is much higher in future pregnancies in women who have had eclampsia before 35 weeks gestation (31.2 percent) than in those with onset of eclampsia later in gestation (7.7 percent).[199] The incidence of growth retardation was 41.9 percent in the future pregnancies of the women who had the early onset of eclampsia as compared to an incidence of 11.4 percent in women with eclampsia after 35 weeks gestation. It remains our impression that women who develop eclampsia early in pregnancy have a significant risk of serious complications in future pregnancies.

CHRONIC HYPERTENSION

Pathophysiology

Patients with labile or borderline hypertension have several pathophysiologic alterations, including elevated cardiac output, central redistribution of blood volume, enhanced activity of the autonomic nervous system, increased left ventricular ejection rate, and normal total peripheral resistance.[200] However, patients with mild to moderate hypertension have normal cardiac output.[201] In these cases, the increase in blood pressure is due to an increase in total peripheral resistance. Because vascular resistance and arterial pressure are elevated, ventricular work load is

increased. The heart rate may be increased while stroke volume and left ventricular ejection rate are normal. Over time, the patient with moderate essential hypertension will show evidence of cardiac strain. Stroke volume remains normal or may start to fall. Myocardial contractility remains normal; ECG studies frequently show increased thickness of the left ventricular wall. In the absence of renal disease, plasma volume contraction is proportionate to the increase in diastolic blood pressure. When the diastolic blood pressure equals or exceeds 105 mmHg, decrease in plasma volume becomes more apparent.

Clinical evidence of end-organ damage characterizes severe essential hypertension. Cardiac enlargement is evident on chest radiograph and ECG. Total peripheral resistance becomes even higher and cardiac output may begin to fall. Stroke volume decreases and intravascular volume decreases still further. With the decrease in cardiac output and intravascular volume, plasma renin activity rises. These changes lead to a great increase in left ventricular tension, making myocardial contractions increasingly difficult. Pulmonary edema occurs if the patient is not treated.[202]

Benefits of Treating Hypertension

The Framingham, Massachusetts, study, an 18-year investigation of 5,127 men and women between 30 and 60 years of age, evaluated risk factors relating to cardiovascular disease in an entire community. Hypertension was a prominent factor in cardiovascular-related morbidity and mortality.[203] Mortality was increased twofold for subjects with blood pressure at entry above 160/95 mmHg compared to those with blood pressure below 140/90 mmHg. Hypertensive women compared to normotensive women had a greater increase in cardiovascular death than similar groups of men.

The Veterans Administration Cooperative Study of Antihypertensive Agents was a randomized study of treatment versus placebo for men without secondary hypertension with diastolic blood pressure between 90 and 129 mmHg.[204,205] The occurrence of morbidity due to cardiovascular complications was significantly higher in men with diastolic blood pressure of 105 mmHg or more. Those men who received antihypertensive therapy with initial diastolic blood pressures of 90 to 114 mmHg had a lower incidence of cardiovascular morbidity.

The Hypertensive Detection and Follow-up Program Cooperative Group studied more than 10,000 hypertensive patients between the ages of 30 and 69 in 14 urban centers.[206] The patients were assigned to a stepped-care program or advised to seek treatment from their regular source of care. The stepped-care group was given free transportation, medical care, and antihypertensive drugs. Waiting times were short, lost patients were recalled, and extensive patient education was provided. More than 70 percent of the patient population had diastolic blood pressures of 90 to 104 mmHg. A thiazide diuretic was given and an antihypertensive agent added when needed. The therapeutic goal was to lower the diastolic blood pressure below 90 mmHg or by 10 mmHg, whichever figure was lower. At the end of 5 years, the goal was reached in 43.6 percent of the referred care group compared with 64.9 percent of the stepped-care group. The 5-year mortality rate was 20 percent lower in the stepped-care group, with initial diastolic blood pressures of 90 to 104 mmHg, as was the incidence of morbid events.

We believe that nonpregnant women with mild chronic hypertension do not require antihypertensive therapy unless they have other high-risk factors for premature cardiovascular disease. Cardiovascular risk factors include a family history of early cardiovascular disease, smoking, diabetes mellitus, and elevated cholesterol. This high-risk group should receive antihypertensive treatment to maintain diastolic blood pressures below 90 mmHg. In addition, because of the proven benefit of antihypertensive therapy in patients with diastolic blood pressures exceeding 105 mmHg, we also institute antihypertensive therapy in this group.

Chronic Hypertension in Pregnancy

Pregnancies complicated by chronic hypertension are associated with increased perinatal mortality and morbidity.[207] These women are at increased risk for the development of superimposed preeclampsia and abruptio placenta.[208] These complications are responsible for most of the perinatal deaths as well as the increased incidence of fetal growth retardation and premature delivery in such pregnancies. The reported incidence of superimposed preeclampsia ranges from 10 to 50 percent, depending on the degree of hypertension at the onset of pregnancy. The incidence of abruptio placenta is likewise increased, depending on the severity of the hypertension and its duration. The reported incidence ranges from 0.45 percent in mild cases[209] to 10 percent in severe cases.[188] Other factors influencing the incidence of abruptio placenta include maternal age, parity, and geographic location of the reporting institution. In patients with uncomplicated mild chronic hypertension, perinatal outcome is similar to that in the general obstetric population.[207] By contrast, the perinatal mortality rate is markedly increased in patients with severe hypertension, in those with renal disease, and in those with preeclampsia and/or abruptio placenta.[210]

In addition to the perinatal risks described, these pregnancies are associated with increased maternal mortality and morbidity.[210,211] Most of the maternal risks are related to the development of either superimposed preeclampsia or abruptio placenta or both. Maternal mortality was not observed in recent reports including patients with mild disease but rose to 3 to 6 percent in patients with severe disease delivering during 1931 to 1950.[210,211] Maternal mortality is usually due to a malignant rise in blood pressure with consequent congestive heart failure and/or cerebrovascular accidents. There is also the potential risk that pregnancy might cause damage to the maternal cardiovascular and renal systems. These risks are dependent on maternal age, duration of hypertension, presence of associated medical complications, and severity of hypertension early in pregnancy.

Antihypertensive Therapy

The use of antihypertensive medications in pregnancy is highly controversial. Recent surveys on the management of such pregnancies from various

Table 30.18 First Drug of Choice in Treating Chronic Hypertension During Pregnancy

Drug	Frequency of Use (%)			
	United States	United Kingdom	Australia	Sweden
Methyldopa	71	91	70	N/A
Diuretics	13	72	1	19–31
Hydralazine	14	0	4	31–83
Propranolol	1	17	3	N/A
Other β-blockers	0	0	13	15–61

N/A = data not available.

countries[212–215] indicate considerable disagreement about the antihypertensive medications to be used as well as the level of diastolic blood pressure at which to initiate treatment. Tables 30.18 and 30.19 compare the frequencies with which various medications are used by obstetricians in the United States, Europe, and Australia. In these studies, there is considerable disagreement about the populations studied as well as the definition of superimposed preeclampsia. American investigators usually use strict criteria for the diagnosis of chronic hypertension. By contrast, European and Australian studies tend to include a heterogeneous group of patients with essential hypertension, pregnancy-induced hypertension, or chronic hypertension with superimposed preeclampsia. Furthermore, there are differences in the technique of taking the blood pressure of patients, including the position of the arm and the end point in selecting diastolic blood pressure (phase IV or V). Thus, it is difficult to compare the results and draw any conclusions regarding the clinical efficacy or benefits of the various medications selected.

The potential maternal benefits of using antihypertensive medications in pregnancy include prevention of exacerbation of the hypertensive state and possibly reduction in the incidence of superimposed preeclampsia or abruptio placenta. There is no evidence to suggest any maternal benefits from treating mild to moderate hypertension during pregnancy.[207] Although there are definite benefits to the mother from treating severe degrees of hypertension during pregnancy, including reduction in both maternal mortality and morbidity,[216] such therapy does not reduce the incidence of either superimposed preeclampsia or abruptio placenta.[211]

Most of the perinatal risks from chronic hypertension during pregnancy are related to superimposed preeclampsia and abruptio placenta. To prove any fetal benefits from the use of these medications, it is important to demonstrate that such therapy reduces the incidence of one or both of these complications.

Antihypertensive Drugs in Pregnancy

Many drugs are currently available for treating chronic hypertension in pregnancy. Some have been studied extensively; others have been used infrequently or are still under clinical trial. The drugs used most often in pregnancy are adrenoceptor blocking agents, thiazide diuretics, and hydralazine.

Table 30.19 Continuation of Prepregnancy Antihypertensive Drugs During Pregnancy

Drug	Frequency of Use (%)			
	United States	United Kingdom	Australia	Sweden
Methyldopa	95	87	95	33
Hydralazine	80	0	65	97
Propranolol	27	17	38	30
Other β-blockers	0	0	59	68

Adrenoceptor Blocking Agents

Adrenoceptors are classified into α- and β-types according to receptor affinity.

Adrenoceptors are further subclassified functionally into α_1-subtypes and as presynaptic or postsynaptic according to their location at adrenergic nerve terminals. α_1-Adrenoceptors are usually found at postsynaptic sites, whereas α_2-adrenoceptors are located at both presynaptic and postsynaptic sites. Stimulation of postsynaptic α_1- and α_2-adrenoceptors results in vasoconstriction, whereas blockade of these receptors results in vasodilatation. By contrast, stimulation of presynaptic α_2-receptors inhibits the release of norepinephrine, whereas blockade of such receptors results in increased release of this neurotransmitter. Thus, selectivity for the various α-adrenoceptor subtypes plays an important role in determining the effectiveness and side effects of the various antihypertensive drugs currently available.

β-Adrenoceptors are also divided into β_1- and β_2-subtypes and are further subdivided into presynaptic and postsynaptic subtypes. Stimulation of presynaptic β-receptors results in norepinephrine release, whereas their blockade inhibits release of this neurotransmitter. Stimulation of postsynaptic β_1-receptors results in increased heart rate and contractility, whereas stimulation of β_2-receptors results in vasodilatation, bronchodilation, uterine relaxation, and hyperglycemia.

Adrenoceptors are located both peripherally and centrally. Stimulation and blockade of these receptors at different sites produce opposite effects. For example, stimulation of centrally located α_2-receptors reduces blood pressure, whereas stimulation of these receptors peripherally increases blood pressure. By contrast, stimulation of centrally located β-receptors increases central sympathetic tone, whereas blockade of these receptors reduces sympathetic outflow. Thus, the degree of transfer across the blood–brain barrier of the various adrenoceptor blocking agents also influences their antihypertensive actions and side effects.

Methyldopa

The drug methyldopa is the agent most frequently used to treat hypertension during pregnancy. Three recent surveys from Britain,[212] Australia,[214] and the United States[215] revealed that methyldopa was most often the drug of choice (Tables 30.18 and 30.19). It lowers blood pressure by stimulation of central α_2-receptors via α-methylnorepinephrine, which is the active form of α-methyldopa. In addition, it might act as an α_2-blocker via a false neurotransmitter effect. Maternal side effects include dry mouth, lethargy, and drowsiness. Other side effects seen with prolonged use include hepatitis, hemolytic anemia, and a positive Coombs test.

Almost all controlled trials studying the treatment of chronic hypertension during pregnancy have used methyldopa alone or in combination. In addition, this drug has been the standard against which new antihypertensive agents are compared. Kincaid-Smith et al.[217] treated 32 severely hypertensive pregnant women with methyldopa at various stages of gestation. These investigators reported a perinatal loss of 9.3 percent, which was considered a favorable outcome as compared to predicted results. Several reports have since been published on pregnancy outcome of mild to moderate chronic hypertension using methyldopa alone or in combination with other antihypertensive medications. Table 30.20 summarizes some of these reports.[217–224] It was apparent from the first two clinical trials utilizing methyldopa[219–221] that its use was associated with a reduction in the incidence of mid-pregnancy abortions. Redman et al.[220] suggested that this beneficial effect was unrelated to blood pressure control but might be mediated through reduction of uterine tone brought about by the effects of methyldopa on fetal steroid production. Alternatively, this result might be due to the blockade of α-receptors in uterine smooth muscles. Although Redman[216] reported smaller head circumferences in male infants of patients treated between 16 and 20 weeks gestation, there were no untoward effects on long-term follow-up of these infants at 7.5 years of age.

The usual oral dosage of methyldopa is an initial loading dose of 1 g followed by a maintenance dose of 1 to 2 g/d given in four divided doses. The daily dosage can be increased to 4 g as needed. The plasma half-life of methyldopa is about 2 hours, and peak plasma levels occur within 2 hours after oral administration. The fall in blood pressure is maximal about 4 hours after an oral dose. Most of the drug is excreted via the kidney. If adequate blood pressure control is not achieved with the dosage, additional antihyper-

Table 30.20 Pregnancy Outcome in Studies Employing Methyldopa to Treat Chronic Hypertension

Investigator	No. of Patients	Preeclampsia (%)	PNM/1,000
Leather et al.[219,a]			
Control	24	—	83
Treated	23	—	0
Redman et al.[220,a]			
Control	107	4.7	19
Treated	101	6.0	10
Arias and Zamora[222]			
Control	29	44.8	0
Treated	29	13.8	0
Gallery et al.[223]			
Oxprenolol	26	7.6	0
Methyldopa	27	7.4	74
Fidler et al.[224]			
Oxprenolol	24	8.3	0
Methyldopa	22	9.1	0
Mabie et al.[218]			
Control	82	30.0	12
Treated	82	34.0	12

[a] Excluding spontaneous losses in mid-pregnancy miscarriages.

tensive agents, such as hydralazine, β-blockers, or diuretics, may be added.

Clonidine

Clonidine is a potent α_2-adrenoceptor central stimulant. Its potential side effects include rebound hypertension following abrupt discontinuation. Its safety and efficacy during pregnancy are unknown. Horvarth et al.[225] reported a randomized study in 100 pregnant hypertensive women comparing clonidine to methyldopa. They found clonidine to be safe and as effective as methyldopa.

Prazosin

Prazosin is a selective α_2-postsynaptic blocker. It reduces both systolic and diastolic blood pressures, while producing significantly less tachycardia and sodium retention than methyldopa. Prazosin causes vasodilatation of both the resistance and capacitance vessels, thereby reducing cardiac preload and afterload. In addition, it produces a decrease in plasma renin activity. Prazosin lowers blood pressure without reducing renal blood flow or GFR. It is metabolized in the liver and excreted almost completely in the bile. Thus, prazosin became the drug of choice for the

treatment of hypertension characterized by high plasma renin levels.[226]

The usual dose of prazosin is 1 mg twice daily; however, the drug has been used in doses as high as 20 mg/d. The median time to peak concentration in nonpregnancy is 2 hours, and the mean elimination half-life is 2 to 3 hours. Rubin et al.[227] studied the disposition and effect of orally administered prazosin in eight hypertensive pregnant women whose blood pressure was uncontrolled by atenolol during the third trimester. They found that prazosin was absorbed slowly but completely and that its half-life was about 3 hours. Lubbe et al.[228] assessed the pregnancy outcomes in 14 women receiving prazosin and oxprenolol. They reported no incidence of superimposed preeclampsia, and infant birthweights were higher than those in patients receiving either methyldopa or no medication. Lubbe and Hodge[229] evaluated pregnancy outcome in 25 women with severe essential hypertension treated with a combination of prazosin and oxprenolol. The average duration of therapy was 12 weeks, and the mean gestational age at the time of delivery was 38.4 weeks. The 26 births in this study included 3 stillbirths and 3 growth-retarded infants.

β-Blockers

The drugs in the category of β-blockers have different hemodynamic effects that depend on their receptor selectivity and presence of intrinsic sympathomimetic activity (ISA). The properties of some of these medications are summarized in the section Antihypertensive Agents. Drugs without ISA (i.e., propranolol, atenolol) reduce both cardiac output and heart rate in association with their antihypertensive effects. On the other hand, drugs with ISA reduce mean arterial blood pressure without influencing either cardiac output or heart rate. The mechanisms of action of these drugs are complex and highly controversial.[230–232]

β-Blockers were introduced during the 1960s and have been used extensively to treat thyroid disease, mitral valve prolapse, migraine headaches, and chronic hypertension. Side effects associated with their use in nonpregnant individuals include bronchial spasm, hypoglycemia, and cold extremities. The use of β-blockers in pregnancy has been associated with neonatal bradycardia, hypoglycemia, fetal growth retardation, altered adaptation to perinatal asphyxia, and neonatal respiratory depression.[233] However, most of these neonatal effects may be attributable to maternal disease rather than to the medications used.

There are numerous reports describing the management of hypertension during pregnancy with various β-blockers. This subject was recently reviewed by Rubin,[234] who concluded that these drugs are safe when used during pregnancy. In addition, he reported that their use was associated with better perinatal outcome than that achieved with either methyldopa or hydralazine. However, we believe it is almost impossible to draw any conclusions regarding the safety and efficacy of these drugs. It is difficult to compare the results of these studies because (1) they involved heterogeneous groups of patients with chronic hypertension, preeclampsia, and chronic hypertension with superimposed preeclampsia; (2) the β-blockers were used in association with other antihypertensive agents such as diuretics, hydralazine, methyldopa, or prazosin; and (3) the blood pressure value at the time of initiating therapy and the duration of treatment were highly variable.[235–238]

Propranolol is the β-blocker most commonly used during pregnancy. The usual dose is 40 to 240 mg/d. This drug is not a potent antihypertensive agent and is, therefore, frequently combined with a diuretic and/or vasodilator. Lieberman et al.[235] reported poor perinatal outcome in nine patients with moderate hypertension during the second trimester who were treated with both propranolol and a diuretic. Eliahou et al.[236] described 26 pregnancies treated with propranolol early in gestation. Fourteen patients received propranolol alone, and the other 12 women required additional antihypertensive medications. The 26 pregnancies resulted in three stillbirths and one spontaneous abortion, a 15 percent pregnancy loss. Two of the 22 liveborn infants were growth retarded. Tcherdakoff et al.[237] treated nine hypertensive pregnant women with propranolol in association with diuretics and hydralazine. Eight of the nine pregnancies ended in live births; one resulted in a stillbirth. Bott-Kanner et al.[238] employed propranolol with hydralazine in 13 patients with 15 pregnancies. One stillbirth occurred.

Several Australian and European reports describe the use of oxprenolol in pregnancy. In two independent controlled trials, oxprenolol was compared with methyldopa. Gallery et al.[223] reported no stillbirths or

neonatal deaths among 26 oxprenolol-treated patients, and the average birthweight in the methyldopa-treated group was lower. In contrast, Fidler et al.[224] found no difference in pregnancy outcome and neonatal birthweight between 25 hypertensive patients treated with oxprenolol and 22 similar patients treated with methyldopa. In addition, they found that the oxprenolol-treated group had a higher incidence of abnormal fetal heart rate tracings during labor. The difference in outcome between these two trials may be attributed to the level of blood pressure achieved in the groups treated with methyldopa. The average blood pressure during therapy with methyldopa was 115/70 mmHg in Gallery's study versus 132/88 mmHg in the patients studied by Fidler and co-workers. Consequently, the lower birthweights observed in Gallery's investigation may be related to reduced uteroplacental blood flow brought about by lowering maternal blood pressure to a normotensive range.

There are a few reports describing the use of atenolol during pregnancy. Thorley et al.[239] employed atenolol in 13 hypertensive pregnant women whose blood pressure was uncontrolled by methyldopa. The dose of atenolol used was 100 mg/d orally. The drug's plasma half-life was about 8 hours, and the levels of atenolol in cord blood were similar to maternal levels. All but one of the infants were delivered at or beyond 36 weeks gestation and all had 5-minute Apgar scores of 6 or greater. Thorley et al. concluded that atenolol was safe when used during pregnancy. Dubois et al.[240] reported 121 patients (125 pregnancies) treated with either pindolol ($N = 38$), atenolol ($N = 31$), or acebutolol ($N = 56$). There were two abortions and one stillbirth among the 125 pregnancies. Although there were no significant differences in Apgar scores among the three groups, the average neonatal birthweight in the atenolol-treated group was significantly lower. In addition, neonatal bradycardia was more pronounced with atenolol treatment. Liedholm[241] reviewed the pregnancy outcomes in 113 hypertensive women of whom 52 received atenolol alone and 34 received atenolol with hydralazine. He reported favorable pregnancy outcomes and minimal side effects in association with this agent.

Sandstrom[242] compared the use of metoprolol with hydralazine in hypertensive pregnant women previously treated with thiazide diuretics. Metoprolol was used with thiazides in 103 cases, metoprolol with hydralazine in 86 cases, and hydralazine with thiazides in 99 cases. The metoprolol-treated groups had a better perinatal outcome than did the hydralazine plus thiazide-treated group. However, the average birthweights and neonatal lengths were similar among the three treatment groups.

Labetalol is a nonselective β-blocker with some α_1-blocking effects. Michael[243] used labetalol in 85 pregnant patients with moderate to severe hypertension during the second trimester. The dose of labetalol ranged from 300 to 1,200 mg/d. Effective blood pressure control was achieved in all but 6 patients. Side effects were minimal; they included maternal hypotension, scalp tingling, lethargy, and rash. There were two stillbirths and two neonatal deaths, for an overall PMR of 6.6 percent. Michael concluded that labetalol was a safe and effective drug for managing hypertension in pregnancy. Redman[179] compared labetalol with methyldopa in the treatment of severe hypertension during pregnancy. Thirty-nine patients received labetalol (400 mg/d) and 35 methyldopa (1 g/d). No difference in pregnancy outcome was observed between the two groups. There is a good correlation between maternal and neonatal plasma levels of labetalol.[244,245]

Plouin et al.[246] compared labetalol to methyldopa in a randomized trial involving 176 pregnant women with mild to moderate hypertension. Four stillbirths occurred in women treated with methyldopa and one neonatal death occurred in the labetalol group. Blood pressure control was better with labetalol (supplementary therapy was needed in 21 percent of the methyldopa group versus 13 percent of the labetalol group). Mean birthweight, gestational age at delivery, and newborn parameters were similar.

Calcium Channel Blockers

There are few reports describing the use of calcium channel blockers alone or in combination with other drugs during pregnancy. Walters and Redman[247] used nifedipine in 21 women with severe hypertension during pregnancy or the puerperium. Blood pressure fell by an average of 26/20 mmHg at 20 minutes after oral administration. The main side effects were headache and flushing. No adverse fetal effects were noted. Constantine et al.[248] used slow-release nifedipine as part of combination therapy in 23 pregnant hypertensive women. Good blood pressure control was achieved in 20. The PMR was 130/1,000

with high rates of abnormal fetal heart rate testing, cesarean sections, and fetal growth retardation. The authors concluded that combination therapy with nifedipine should only be used in severe hypertension or in the context of a controlled clinical trial. Two other studies used nifedipine in association with atenolol in the management of severe hypertension in pregnancy. These authors reported good control of blood pressure and favorable effects on platelet count in patients with thrombocytopenia.[249,250]

Using indium-113 scintigraphy, Lindow and associates[251] found no change in uteroplacental blood flow after reduction of maternal blood pressure in 10 women with pregnancy-induced hypertension.[251] In addition, Hanretty et al.[252] reported that nifedipine does not adversely affect either uteroplacental or umbilical Doppler FVWs in severe preeclampsia.

Allen et al.[253] studied the acute effects of a single 20-mg oral dose of nitrenedipine in 10 women with pregnancy-induced hypertension. Maternal blood pressure fell significantly and remained under control for at least 4 hours. Maternal heart rate increased by 10 percent; fetal heart rate was unchanged. The drug's tocolytic properties may inhibit labor (see Ch. 25).

Angiotensin-Converting Enzyme Inhibitors

Three angiotensin-converting enzyme (ACE) inhibitors are available in the United States: captopril, enalapril, and lisinopril. They induce vasodilatation by inhibiting the enzyme that converts angiotensin I to angiotensin II. In addition, they increase the synthesis of vasodilating prostaglandins. Captopril causes abortions and fetal deaths in experimental animals by reducing uteroplacental blood flow.[254] In human pregnancy ACE inhibitor therapy has been associated with several fetal and neonatal complications: neonatal hypotension, fetal growth retardation, oligohydramnios, neonatal anuria and renal failure, and neonatal deaths.[254–261] Thus, it has been recommended that ACE inhibitors not be used in pregnancy.

Thiazide Diuretics

Thiazide diuretics are generally the first drugs selected in the treatment of nonpregnant hypertensive patients. Consequently, most women with chronic hypertension become pregnant while on diuretics. Initially, these drugs result in a reduction in both plasma and extracellular fluid volumes with a concomitant decrease in cardiac output. However, these changes tend to return to pretreatment levels within 4 weeks of therapy. These effects are followed by a long-term reduction in peripheral vascular resistance, which is thought to be related to reduced intracellular sodium concentration in vascular smooth muscle cells.[262]

There is considerable controversy regarding the benefits and risks of diuretics for treatment of chronic hypertension during pregnancy. In their review of the literature, Collins et al.[263] concluded that prophylactic thiazide therapy does not reduce the incidence of preeclampsia. Similar findings were reported by MacGillivray.[264] He found that patients receiving diuretics delivered infants who weighed less than those born to control pregnant patients. In addition, Gant et al.[265] found the short-term use of diuretics in pregnancy to reduce uteroplacental blood flow as measured by the metabolic clearance of dehydroepiandrosterone sulfate (DHEAS). Sibai et al.[262] noted that pregnant patients with chronic hypertension treated with diuretics have a marked reduction in plasma volume when compared to a control group not receiving these medications. However, plasma volume expansion was normal after the discontinuation of diuretics (Fig. 30.8). In a subsequent report, Sibai et al.[266] studied plasma volume findings in 20 hypertensive pregnant patients who were receiving diuretics prior to and early in pregnancy. Ten patients were continued on diuretics throughout gestation, and diuretics were discontinued in the remaining 10 patients. Plasma volume was significantly higher when patients discontinued the diuretics (Fig. 30.9). However, pregnancy outcome was similar for the two groups. Since plasma volume depletion is associated with poor perinatal outcome,[267] we have cautioned against the use of diuretics in pregnancies complicated by chronic hypertension.

Adverse maternal effects reported with the use of diuretics during pregnancy include hypokalemia, hyponatremia, hyperglycemia, elevated uric acid, hemorrhagic pancreatitis, and even death. Neonatal adverse effects are electrolyte imbalance, thrombocytopenia, and small size for gestational age.

Hydralazine

Hydralazine is the agent most commonly used to control severe hypertension in preeclampsia. In that situation it is usually given intravenously as a continuous

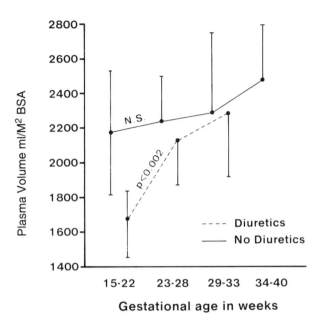

Fig. 30.8 Serial plasma volumes (mean ± 1 SD) throughout gestation in the two groups of hypertensive patients. (From Sibai et al.,[266] with permission.)

infusion or in small bolus injections. Hydralazine is a potent vasodilator that acts directly on vascular smooth muscle. After its intravenous use, the hypotensive effects of this drug develop gradually over 15 to 30 minutes, peaking at 20 minutes. The elimination half-life is about 3 hours. The usual bolus dose is 5 to 10 mg to be repeated every 20 to 30 minutes as needed. Its main side effects are fluid retention, tachycardia, and headache.

Because oral hydralazine is a weak antihypertensive drug when used alone, it is usually combined with a diuretic or methyldopa. Chesley considers hydralazine the drug of choice for treating severe chronic hypertension during pregnancy. In addition, it is the drug most often used by obstetricians in Sweden (Table 30.18). The usual oral dose is 10 mg given four times daily, but this can be increased to 75 mg given four times daily, for a maximum dose of 300 mg. A maternal lupus-like syndrome and neonatal thrombocytopenia are associated with the chronic administration of hydralazine.

Management of Chronic Hypertension during Pregnancy

The following is a detailed description of the management plan at the University of Tennessee Center for the Health Sciences. Our approach has been refined

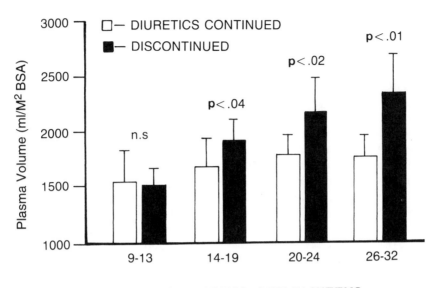

Fig. 30.9 Comparison of mean plasma volume findings for two groups of hypertensive patients. (From Sibai et al.,[262] with permission.)

over the past 11 years after an extensive experience during which approximately 1,800 patients with chronic hypertension have been delivered.

Patients are advised to seek prenatal care as early as possible. Prior to conception, they are told the potential harmful effects of the various antihypertensive medications. Early prenatal care helps document the severity of their hypertension and permits accurate determination of gestational age. Most patients are hospitalized at the time of their first prenatal visit. A careful physical examination and diagnostic tests are performed to determine the severity of the hypertension and its etiology. On the basis of this assessment, patients are classified into either a low-risk or a high-risk group. The factors that characterize patients in the high-risk category are summarized in the following discussion.

The patient is seen by a nutritionist who counsels her about diet, weight gain, and sodium intake during pregnancy. Many of these patients have been consuming up to 10 g sodium daily without being aware of this excess. Patients are advised to restrict their sodium intake to about 2 g/d. In addition, they are counseled about the harmful effects of smoking, stress, and caffeine on both maternal blood pressure and fetal well-being. Patients are instructed to rest during the day, especially after meals. Frequent prenatal visits play an important part in the management of these patients. They are usually seen once every 2 weeks during the first half of pregnancy and then weekly until delivery.

Laboratory evaluation includes serial measurements of hematocrit, serum creatinine, potassium, uric acid, creatinine clearance, and 24-hour urinary excretion of protein and sodium. Urine culture and sensitivity tests are performed at least once every trimester. Catecholamine determinations are usually made for patients presenting with severe hypertension early in gestation. Additional tests such as a chest radiograph and ECG are performed in patients classified as high-risk. In addition, screening for collagen vascular disease using fluorescent antinuclear antibodies is performed in patients having proteinuria early in pregnancy.

Fetal evaluation includes serial ultrasonography for fetal gestational age and growth and antepartum fetal heart rate testing starting at 34 weeks. For patients classified as high-risk, nonstress testing may begin as early as 26 weeks gestation. In addition, daily fetal movement counts, fetal biophysical profiles, and serial plasma volume determinations may be used to determine the optimum time for delivery.

The occurrence of pyelonephritis, exacerbation of hypertension, development of significant protein-uria, and/or increased uric acid level is considered an indication for hospitalization. It is our experience that a significant elevation in uric acid ($>$ 6 mg/dl) is an early sign of superimposed preeclampsia.

Our policy has been to avoid using antihypertensive medications in mild to moderate chronic hypertension. Diuretics are usually discontinued in all such patients who have been receiving them. In addition, all other antihypertensive medications are discontinued in patients classified as low-risk. In these women, pregnancy is allowed to continue until 41 weeks gestation with close fetal surveillance. However, in patients considered high-risk and those requiring antihypertensive medications, the pregnancy is not allowed to go beyond 40 weeks. The development of severe superimposed preeclampsia or fetal growth retardation or both is considered an indication for delivery irrespective of gestational age. In such patients amniocentesis is performed and, if needed, steroids are usually given to accelerate fetal lung maturation.

Management of Severe (High-Risk) Chronic Hypertension in Pregnancy

Little information about the perinatal outcome of pregnancies in women with severe chronic hypertension who are seen during the first trimester is known. In the past, concerns about the risk of acute renal, cardiac, or cerebrovascular accidents led many patients to have an abortion. Approximately 28 to 70 percent of obstetricians surveyed in Britain[212] and Australia[214] recommended early termination of these pregnancies. In the United States, Sibai and Watson[215] found that 20 percent recommended termination of pregnancy with normal renal function and 43 percent recommended termination of pregnancy in the presence of impaired renal function.

Chesley and Annitto[268] reported their experience with 301 pregnancies in 218 women with coexisting hypertensive disease during 1931 through 1944. There were six immediate maternal deaths (2 percent) and seven late puerperal deaths. All deaths occurred in women who had superimposed preeclampsia. Of the 308 pregnancies, only 12 women had severe hypertension before the pregnancy. Thirty percent of these pregnancies were complicated by

superimposed preeclampsia; the fetal loss rate in this subgroup of women was 50 percent, and the incidence of abruptio placenta was 10 percent. Increased fetal loss was also noted in women with higher initial blood pressures, in women with a second trimester rise in blood pressure, in women with decreased renal function in pregnancy, and in those who demonstrated higher pressure at the time of delivery.

Landesman et al.[210] evaluated the outcome of 144 women with severe hypertension defined as a blood pressure exceeding 179/109 mmHg who delivered at the New York Lying-In Hospital between 1943 and 1953. Forty-two (30 percent) of the 144 pregnancies ended in an abortion; one-half of these were elective terminations. In 102 women who continued their pregnancies, the rate of fetal loss was 28.4 percent (29 of 102). The total perinatal survival rate among these 144 women was 52 percent. Twenty-nine patients developed superimposed preeclampsia and suffered a fetal loss of 41 percent. The early onset of superimposed preeclampsia was a critical factor in predicting perinatal outcome. Sixty percent of the women with fetal deaths showed the development of superimposed preeclampsia before 29 weeks gestation, and all women with fetal deaths showed superimposed preeclampsia before 37 weeks gestation. By contrast, in only 17 percent of patients with liveborn infants did preeclampsia develop before 25 weeks gestation, and in 40 percent preeclampsia did not develop until after 36 weeks gestation. The incidence of infants weighing less than 2,500 g was 63.3 percent, compared to the total clinic population of 7.0 percent. In addition, 44.4 percent of the infants were thought to be growth-retarded. The 73 women with severe hypertension in whom preeclampsia did not develop had a better outcome. The fetal death rate was 23.3 percent, the incidence of infants below 2,500 g was 28.4 percent, and 29.6 percent were small for gestation. Two maternal deaths occurred in women in whom preeclampsia developed. One died of renal failure and the other of a cerebral hemorrhage.

Over the past 6.5 years, we have treated 44 women with severe hypertension who were seen during the first trimester of pregnancy.[211] Patients were hospitalized at the time of the initial prenatal visit for the evaluation of renal and cardiac function and control of their hypertension. Each woman had blood pressure elevation of at least 170/110 mmHg on two occasions more than 24 hours apart after hospitalization. The mean duration of hypertension was 9.0 ± 4.1 years. The initial mean systolic blood pressure was 182 ± 15 mmHg, and initial diastolic blood pressure 116 ± 7 mmHg.

Sixteen women were receiving antihypertensive agents other than methyldopa, 12 were taking diuretics, and 4 were on a β-blocker. We treated all these patients with methyldopa and added oral hydralazine when necessary to keep systolic blood pressure below 160 mmHg and/or diastolic blood pressure below 110 mmHg. When systolic blood pressure rose above 180 mmHg and/or diastolic blood pressure exceeded 120 mmHg, the patient was hospitalized and treated with a continuous infusion of hydralazine to achieve adequate blood pressure control. Superimposed preeclampsia was diagnosed in the presence of worsening hypertension plus proteinuria, at least 2 g in 24 hours, during the second and third trimesters in the absence of significant proteinuria (300 mg) during the first trimester. For those women with significant proteinuria during the first trimester, the diagnosis of superimposed preeclampsia was made in the presence of the preceding criteria plus a significant elevation in serum uric acid. Maternal complications are as follows.

Forty-two of the 144 women were hospitalized at least twice during the antepartum period. Fifteen of the 20 women who had significant deterioration in renal function were in the superimposed preeclampsia group. The mean serum creatinine at the end of pregnancy in these 20 patients was 1.68 ± 0.85 mg/dl (range 1.1 to 4.2 mg/dl), and the mean creatinine clearance was 62 ± 23 ml/min (range 22 to 100 ml/min). After delivery, renal function returned to the values recorded at the initial prenatal visit in 19 of 20 women.

As expected, acceptable blood pressure control was difficult to achieve in these patients. Ten of these women initially required intravenous hydralazine to maintain diastolic blood pressure below 100 mmHg. Even with large doses of methyldopa (up to 4 g/d) and hydralazine (up to 400 mg/d), intravenous hydralazine was required in 11 women after the initial hospitalization.

Of the 33 women with prior pregnancies, 10 had had poor pregnancy outcomes: five abortions and

Table 30.21 Pregnancy Outcome in Women with Severe Hypertension

Factor	With Preeclampsia[a] (N = 23)	Without Preeclampsia[a] (N = 21)
Gestational age (wk)	28.6 ± 2.4	36.5 ± 2.9
Birthweight (g)	827 ± 314	2632 ± 743
Placental weight (g)	232 ± 106	630 ± 183
<37 weeks gestation	23 (100%)	8 (38%)
Small for gestational age	18 (78%)	1 (5%)
Perinatal mortality	11 (48%)	0 (0%)

[a] $p < 0.0005$ for all categories studied.

eight stillbirths. Three of the 10 had experienced placental abruption, 2 had suffered eclampsia. In the present pregnancy, among 44 births there were ten fetal deaths and one neonatal death for a PMR of 25 percent. All perinatal losses occurred in fetuses weighing less than 800 g and below 29 weeks gestational age; all were in patients with superimposed preeclampsia. Six of the 11 perinatal deaths occurred in the 10 women with prior poor pregnancy outcome and 4 were in primigravid patients. The mean gestational age at delivery was 32.3 ± 4.7 weeks; 31 women delivered before 37 weeks gestation. The mean birthweight was 1,688 ± 1,068 g (range 310 to 3,600 g), and 19 (43 percent) infants were SGA. Most of the poor pregnancy outcomes could be related to preeclampsia (Table 30.21). Twenty of the 34 liveborn infants were admitted to the neonatal intensive care unit. One died within 24 hours of admission. The 19 surviving infants remained in the ICU an average of 39 ± 24 days (range 10 to 92 days). Follow-up is available in 17 of the babies, now 9 months to 4 years of age, discharged from the neonatal ICU. One infant who suffered an intraventricular hemorrhage and neonatal seizures has cerebral palsy, seizures, and retarded motor development at 18 months of age. The others are normal.

In women with severe hypertension during the first trimester, the decision to continue the pregnancy should not be made without extensive counseling. The woman must understand the potential for serious morbidity or mortality for her and the high fetal wastage. These women need intensive follow-up and may require multiple hospital admissions. Blood pressure is difficult to control, often demanding the use of multiple oral drugs as well as intravenous therapy. In our experience, the risk of superimposed preeclampsia is high (52 percent), and all of the perinatal mortality (25 percent) occurs in this group. Women with a prior poor pregnancy history are again likely to suffer a pregnancy loss (60 percent).

Management of Mild (Low-Risk) Chronic Hypertension

We have reported our recent experience caring for 211 women with mild chronic hypertension.[207] Each patient had a documented history of chronic hypertension before pregnancy and an elevation of blood pressure (at least 140/90 mmHg on two occasions more than 24 hours apart) before 20 weeks gestation. Most of these women were taking antihypertensive medications prior to pregnancy, including 23 on thiazide diuretics and 13 on methyldopa at their initial prenatal visit. Antihypertensive agents were discontinued in all patients and were restarted only for a significant elevation of blood pressure (systolic above 160 mmHg and diastolic above 110 mmHg). The 211 pregnancies resulted in 215 births, including four sets of twins. The PMR, 28.1/1,000, is the same as that of our general obstetric population for this period. All six perinatal deaths, two stillbirths, and four neonatal deaths involved fetuses less than 1,000 g or 29 weeks gestation.

As in patients with severe hypertension, the onset of superimposed preeclampsia was a key factor in predicting perinatal outcome (Table 30.22). In the absence of preeclampsia, the PMR was 5/1,000. In these patients, the incidence of SGA infants and abruptio placenta was less than that in our general obstetric population (Table 30.22).

The 21 women in whom preeclampsia developed had a poor pregnancy outcome. Their PMR was 240/1,000, and the incidence of fetal growth retardation was 32 percent.

Twenty-eight of the 211 women had an exacerbation of hypertension that required treatment with antihypertensive medications. Changes in MAP at 20 to 26 weeks gestation were predictive of a future requirement for antihypertensive medications (Fig. 30.10). MAP decreased during mid-trimester in 104 women (49 percent); only 4 required antihypertensive therapy. MAP was unchanged in 71 women (34 percent), and 11 (16 percent) required antihypertensive therapy. However, of 40 (17 percent) patients in whom MAP increased during the second trimester, 13 (32 percent) needed antihypertensive medications. Only 3 of 23 women who were taking thiazide diuretics and only 2 of 13 on methyldopa early in pregnancy required antihypertensive treatment later in pregnancy. Of the 175 women not on antihypertensive therapy at their initial prenatal visit, only 23 (13 percent) required these agents later in gestation. In fact, 32 of these women were normotensive during the third trimester.

We recently conducted a randomized clinical trial comparing the use of no treatment ($N = 100$) to methyldopa ($N = 100$) or labetalol ($N = 100$) in the management of mild chronic hypertension during pregnancy. All patients had a documented history of chronic hypertension and were enrolled during the first trimester. In the no treatment group, antihypertensive drugs were used only if the blood pressures exceeded 160 mmHg systolic or 110 mmHg diastolic. All patients were followed with ultrasound and antepartum fetal evaluation as needed. There were no differences among the three subgroups in terms of either superimposed preeclampsia (16 to 18 percent), abruptio placenta (1.3 to 2.1 percent), or fetal growth retardation (8 to 11 percent). In addition, there were no differences among the groups regarding gestational age at delivery, birthweights, placental weights, or incidence of preterm delivery. There was one stillbirth in the no treatment group, a mid-trimester loss at 23 weeks in the methyldopa group, and one still-

Table 30.22 Outcome in Women with Mild Chronic Hypertension

Outcome	With Preeclampsia ($N = 21$)[a]		Without Preeclampsia ($N = 190$)[b]	
	N	%	N	%
Premature (<37 weeks)	15	71.4	11	5.7
Small for gestational age	7	32.0	10	5.3
Abruptio placenta	2	9.5	1	0.5
Perinatal mortality rate	5	24.0	1	0.5

[a] 22 births.
[b] 193 births.

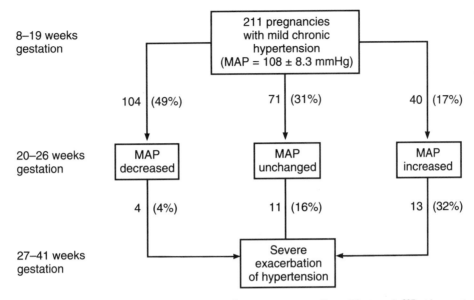

Fig. 30.10 Mean arterial blood pressure (MAP) during pregnancy. (From Sibai et al.,[207] with permission.)

birth in the labetalol group. Thus, it is concluded that antihypertensive therapy does not improve pregnancy outcome in women with essential mild chronic hypertension.

In summary, superimposed preeclampsia and abruptio placenta are responsible for most poor perinatal outcome in women with mild chronic hypertension. Antihypertensive drugs do not influence these complications. Diuretics reduce plasma volume expansion without influencing maternal blood pressure. As a result, we recommend that diuretics be discontinued in all women receiving them during pregnancy.

REFERENCES

1. Browne FJ: Chronic hypertension and pregnancy. Br Med J 2:283, 1947
2. Wellen I: The infant mortality in specific hypertensive disease of pregnancy and in essential hypertension. Am J Obstet Gynecol 66:36, 1953
3. Hughes EC (ed): Obstetric-Gynecologic Terminology. FA Davis, Philadelphia, 1972
4. American College of Obstetricians and Gynecologists Technical Bulletin No. 91. ACOG, Washington, DC, 1986
5. Chesley L: Hypertensive disorders in pregnancy. p. 751. In Gleicher N (ed): Principles of Medical Therapy in Pregnancy. Plenum, New York, 1985
6. Dexter L, Weiss S: Preeclamptic and eclamptic toxemia of pregnancy. Little, Brown, Boston, 1941
7. Nelson TR: A clinical study of preeclampsia. J Obstet Gynaecol Br Emp 62:48, 1955
8. Sheehan HL, Lynch JB: Pathology of Toxaemia of Pregnancy. Churchill Livingstone, Edinburgh, 1973
9. Berman S: Observations in the toxemia clinic. Boston Lying-in-Hospital, 1923–1930. N Engl J Med 203:361, 1930
10. Davey DA, MacGillivray I: The classification and definition of the tensive disorders of pregnancy. Am J Obstet Gynecol 158:892, 1988
11. Anonymous: Classification of hypertensive disorders of pregnancy. Lancet 1:935, 1989
12. Roberts JM: Classification of hypertensive disorders of pregnancy. Lancet 2:112, 1989
13. Lilford RJ: Classification of hypertensive disorders of pregnancy. Lancet 2:112, 1989
14. Beurel JN Jr: Eclampsia in lowland gorilla. Am J Obstet Gynecol 141:345, 1981
15. Villar MA, Sibai BM: Clinical significance of elevated mean arterial blood in second trimester and threshold increase in systolic or diastolic pressure during third trimester. Am J Obstet Gynecol 160:419, 1989

16. Long PA, Abell DA, Beischer NA: Parity and pre-eclampsia. Aust NZ J Obstet Gynaecol 19:203, 1979

17. Campbell DM, MacGillivray I, Carr-Hill R: Pre-eclampsia in second pregnancy. Br J Obstet Gynaecol 92:131, 1985

18. Long P, Oats J: Preeclampsia in twin-pregnancy—severity and pathogenesis. Aust NZ J Obstet Gynaecol 27:1, 1987

19. Brosens IA: Morphological changes in the uteroplacental bed in pregnancy hypertension. Clin Obstet Gynaecol 4:583, 1977

20. Kong TY, DeWolf F, Robertson WB, Brosens I: Inadequate maternal vascular response to placentation in pregnancies complicated by preeclampsia and by small-for-gestational age infants. Br J Obstet Gynaecol 93:1049, 1986

21. Frusca T, Morassi L, Pecorell S et al: Histological features of uteroplacental vessels in normal and hypertensive patients in relation to birthweight. Br J Obstet Gynaecol 96:835, 1989

22. Sheppard BL, Bonnar J: An ultrastructural study of uteroplacental spiral arteries in hypertensive and normotensive pregnancy and fetal growth retardation. Br J Obstet Gynaecol 88:695, 1981

23. Shanklin DR, Sibai BM: Ultrastructural aspects of preeclampsia. I: placental bed and uterine boundary vessels. Am J Obstet Gynecol 161:735, 1989

24. Saleh AA, Bottoms SF, Welch RA et al: Preeclampsia, delivery, and the hemostatic system. Am J Obstet Gynecol 157:331, 1987

25. Saleh AA, Bottoms SF, Norman G et al: Hemostasis in hypertensive disorders of pregnancy. Obstet Gynecol 71:719, 1988

26. Stubbs TM, Lazarchick J, Horger EO III: Plasma fibronectin levels in preeclampsia. A possible biochemical marker for vascular endothelial damage. Am J Obstet Gynecol 150:885, 1986

27. Lazarchick J, Stubbs TM, Remein L et al: Predictive value of fibronectin levels in normotensive gravid women destined to become preeclamptic. Am J Obstet Gynecol 154:1050, 1986

28. Ballenger V, Spitz B, Kieckens L et al: Predictive value of increased plasma levels of fibronectin in gestational hypertension. Am J Obstet Gynecol 161:432, 1989

29. Rodgers GM, Taylor RN, Roberts JM: Preeclampsia is associated with a serum factor cytotoxic to human endothelial cells. Am J Obstet Gynecol 159:908, 1988

30. Musci TJ, Roberts JM, Rodgers GM, Taylor RN: Mitogenic activity is increased in the sera of preeclamptic women before delivery. Am J Obstet Gynecol 159:1446, 1988

31. Roberts JM, Taylor RN, Musci TJ et al: Preeclampsia: an endothelial cell disorder. Am J Obstet Gynecol 161:1200, 1989

32. Weiner CP, Brandt J: Plasma antithrombin III activity: an aid in the diagnosis of preeclampsia–eclampsia. Am J Obstet Gynecol 142:275, 1982

33. Weiner CP, Kwaan HC, Xu C et al: Antithrombin III activity in women with hypertension with pregnancy. Obstet Gynecol 65:301, 1985

34. Wallenburg HCS, Rotmans N: Enhanced reactivity of the platelet thromboxane pathway in normotensive and hypertensive pregnancies with insufficient fetal growth. Am J Obstet Gynecol 144:523, 1982

35. Socol ML, Weiner CP, Louis G et al: Platelet activation in preeclampsia. Am J Obstet Gynecol 151:494, 1985

36. deBoer K, Tencate JW, Sturk A et al: Enhanced thrombin generation in normal and hypertensive pregnancy. Am J Obstet Gynecol 160:95, 1989

37. Gilabert J, Fernandez JA, Espana F et al: Physiological coagulation inhibitors (protein S, protein C and antithrombin III) in severe preeclamptic states and in users of oral contraceptives. Thromb Res 49:319, 1988

38. Friedman SA: Preeclampsia: a review of the role of prostaglandins. Obstet Gynecol 71:122, 1988

39. Ylikorkala O, Makila UM: Prostacyclin and thromboxane in gynecology and obstetrics. Am J Obstet Gynecol 152:318, 1985

40. Walsh SW: Preeclampsia: an imbalance in placenta prostacyclin and thromboxane production. Am J Obstet Gynecol 152:335, 1985

41. Goodman RP, Killam AP, Brash AR, Branch RA: Comparison of production during normal pregnancy and pregnancy complicated by hypertension. Am J Obstet Gynecol 142:817, 1982

42. Fitzgerald DJ, Entmann SS, Mulloy K, Fitzgerald GA: Decreased prostaglandin biosynthesis preceding the clinical manifestation of pregnancy-induced hypertension. Circulation 75:956, 1987

43. Walsh SW, Parisi VM: The role of arachidonic acid metabolites in preeclampsia. Semin Perinatol 10(4):335, 1986

44. Moodley J, Reddi K, Norman RJ: Decreased central venous concentration of immunoreactive prostaglandins E, F, and 6-keto-PGF$_{1\alpha}$ in eclampsia. Br Med J 288:1487, 1984

45. Brown HL, Klein L, Waitzman M: Plasma and amniotic fluid prostacyclin and thromboxane in mild pregnancy induced hypertension. Am J Perinatol 4(2):152, 1987

46. Moodley J, Kistnasarny MB, Reddi K et al: Amniotic fluid prostacyclin in African women with eclampsia. Clin Exp Hypertens Pregnancy B5(1):29, 1986

47. Sibai BM: Pitfalls in diagnosis and management of preeclampsia. Am J Obstet Gynecol 159:1, 1988

48. Wichman K, Ryden G, Wichman M: The influence of different positions and Korotkoff sounds on the blood pressure mean measurements in pregnancy. Acta Obstet Gynecol Scan, suppl., 118:25, 1984

49. MacGillivray I, Rose GA, Rowe D: Blood pressure survey in pregnancy. Clin Sci 72:395, 1969

50. Redman CWG, Jeffries M: Revised definition of preeclampsia. Lancet 1:809, 1988

51. Chesley LC, Sibai BM: Clinical significance of elevated mean arterial pressure in the second trimester. Am J Obstet Gynecol 159:275, 1988

52. Belizan JM, Villar J, Repke J: The relationship between calcium intake and pregnancy-induced hypertension: up-to-date evidence. Am J Obstet Gynecol 158:898, 1988

53. Kawasaki N, Matsui K, Nakamura T et al: Effect of calcium supplementation on the vascular sensitivity to angiotensin II in pregnant women. Am J Obstet Gynecol 153:576, 1985

54. Villar J, Repke J, Belizan JM, Pareja G: Calcium supplementation reduces blood pressure during pregnancy: results from a randomized clinical trial. Obstet Gynecol 70:317, 1987

55. Lopez-Jaramillo P, Narvaez M, Weigel RP, Yepez R: Calcium supplementation reduces blood pressure during pregnancy: results from a randomized clinical trial. Obstet Gynecol 70:317, 1989

56. Sibai BM, Villar MA, Bray E: Magnesium supplementation during pregnancy: a double-blind randomized controlled clinical trial. Am J Obstet Gynecol 161:115, 1989

57. Altura BM, Altura BT, Carella A: Magnesium deficiency induced spasm of umbilical vessels: relation to preeclampsia, hypertension, growth retardation. Science 221:376, 1983

58. Conradt A, Weidinger H, Algayer H: On the role of magnesium in fetal hypotrophy, pregnancy-induced hypertension and preeclampsia. Mag Bull 6:68, 1984

59. Spatling L, Spatling G: Magnesium supplementation in pregnancy: a double-blind study. Br J Obstet Gynaecol 95:120, 1988

60. Lazebnik N, Kuhnert BR, Kuhnert BM, Thompson KL: Zinc status, pregnancy complications and labor abnormalities. Am J Obstet Gynecol 158:161, 1988

61. Brophy MH, Harris NF, Crawford IL: Elevated copper and lowered zinc in the placentae of preeclampsia. Clin Acta 145:107, 1985

62. Hunt IF, Murphy NJ, Cleaver AE et al: Zinc supplementation during pregnancy: effects on selected blood constituents and on progress and outcome of pregnancy in low-income women of Mexican descent. Am J Clin Nutr 40:508, 1984

63. Mohamed K, James DK, Golding J, McCabe R: Zinc supplementation during pregnancy: a double blind randomized controlled trial. Br Med J 299:826, 1989

64. Spitz B, Magness RR, Cox SM et al: Low-dose aspirin. I: Effect on angiotensin II pressor responses and blood prostaglandin concentration in pregnant women sensitive to angiotensin II. Am J Obstet Gynecol 159:1035, 1988

65. Sibai BM, Mirro R, Chesney CM, Leffer C: Low dose aspirin in pregnancy. Obstet Gynecol 74:551, 1989

66. Beaufils M, Donsimoni R, Uzam S et al: Prevention of preeclampsia by early antiplatelet therapy. Lancet 2:840, 1985

67. Wallenburg HLS, Dekker GA, Makowitz JW: Low-dose aspirin prevents pregnancy-induced hypertension and preeclampsia in angiotensin-sensitive primigravidae. Lancet 1:1, 1986

68. Benigni A, Gregorini G, Frusca T et al: Effect of low-dose aspirin on fetal and maternal generation of thromboxane by platelets in women at risk for pregnancy-induced hypertension. N Eng J Med 321:357, 1989

69. Schiff E, Peleg E, Goldenberg M et al: The use of aspirin to prevent pregnancy-induced hypertension and lower the ratio of thromboxane A_2 to prostacyclin in relatively high risk pregnancies. N Eng J Med 321:351, 1989

70. Dunlop W, Davidson JM: The effect of normal pregnancy on renal handling of uric acid. Br J Obstet Gynecol 84:13, 1987

71. Chesley LC: Hypertension and renal diseases. p. 477. In Chesley LC (ed): Hypertensive Disorders in Pregnancy. 2nd ed. Appleton-Century-Crofts, East Norwalk, CT, 1978

72. Handler JS: The role of lactic acid in reduced excretion of uric acid in toxemia of pregnancy. J Clin Invest 39:1526, 1960

73. Redman CWG, Beilin LJ, Bonnar J: Plasma urate measurement in predicting fetal death in hypertensive pregnancies. Lancet 1:1370, 1976

74. Pritchard JA, Stone SR: Clinical and laboratory observations on eclampsia. Am J Obstet Gynecol 99:754, 1967

75. Steven MM: Pregnancy and liver disease. Gut 22:592, 1981

76. Weinstein L: Syndrome of hemolysis, elevated liver enzymes, and low platelet count: a severe consequence of hypertension in pregnancy. Am J Obstet Gynecol 142:159, 1982

77. Arias F, Mancill-Jimenez R: Hepatic fibrinogen deposits in preeclampsia—immunofluorescent evidence. N Engl J Med 11:294, 1976

78. Bis KA, Waxman B: Rupture of the liver associated with pregnancy: a review of the literature and report of 2 cases. Obstet Gynecol Surv 31:763, 1976

79. Henny CP, Lim AE, Brummelkamp WH et al: A review of the importance of acute multidisciplinary treatment following spontaneous rupture of the liver capsule during pregnancy. Surg Gynecol Obstet 156:593, 1983

80. Goodlin RC, Anderson JC, Hodgson PE: Conservative treatment of liver hematoma in the postpartum period. J Reprod Med 30:368, 1985

81. Manas KJ, Welsh JD, Rankin RA: Hepatic haemorrhage without rupture in preeclampsia. N Engl J Med 312:424, 1985

82. Galton M, Merritt K, Beller FK: Coagulation studies on the peripheral circulation of patients with toxemia of pregnancy: a study for evaluation of disseminated intravascular coagulation and toxemia. J Reprod Med 6:89, 1971

83. Morris RH, Vassalli P, Beller FK et al: Immunofluorescent studies of renal biopsies in the diagnosis of toxemia in pregnancy. Obstet Gynecol 24:32, 1964

84. Pritchard JA, Cunningham FG, Mason RA: Coagulation changes in eclampsia: their frequency and pathogenesis. Am J Obstet Gynecol 124:855, 1976

85. Gibson B, Huntger D, Nedme PB et al: Thrombocytopenia in preeclampsia and eclampsia. Semin Thromb Haemost 8:234, 1982

86. Sibai BM, Spinnato JA, Watson DL et al: Pregnancy outcome in 303 cases with severe preeclampsia. Obstet Gynecol 64:319, 1984

87. Sibai BM, Taslimi MM, El-Nazer A et al: Maternal-perinatal outcome associated with the syndrome of hemolysis, elevated liver enzymes, and low platelets in severe preeclampsia-eclampsia. Am J Obstet Gynecol 155:501, 1986

88. Goodlin RC: Hemolysis, elevated liver enzymes, and low platelets syndrome. Obstet Gynecol 64:449, 1984

89. Sibai BM: The HELLP syndrome—much ado about nothing? Am J Obstet Gynecol 162:311, 1990

90. Schwartz ML, Brenner WE: Pregnancy-induced hypertension presenting with life-threatening thrombocytopenia. Am J Obstet Gynecol 146:756, 1983

91. Aarnoudse JG, Houthoff HF, Weits J et al: A syndrome of liver damage and intravascular coagulation in the last trimester of normotensive pregnancy: a clinical and histopathological study. Br J Obstet Gynaecol 93:145, 1986

92. Kilam AP, Dillard SH, Patton RC et al: Pregnancy

induced hypertension complicated by acute liver disease and disseminated intravascular coagulation. Am J Obstet Gynecol 123:823, 1975

93. Mackenna J, Dover NL, Brame RG: Preeclampsia associated with hemolysis, elevated liver enzymes and low platelets—an obstetric emergency? Obstet Gynecol 62:751, 1983

94. Thiagarajah S, Bourgeois FJ, Harbert GM et al: Thrombocytopenia in preeclampsia: associated abnormalities and management principles. Am J Obstet Gynecol 150:1, 1984

95. Gant NF, Daley GL, Chands et al: A study of angiotensin II response throughout primigravid pregnancy. J Clin Invest 52:2682, 1973

96. Cotton DB, Gonik B, Dorman K et al: Cardiovascular alteration in severe pregnancy-induced hypertension: relationship of central venous pressure to capillary wedge pressure. Am J Obstet Gynecol 151:762, 1985

97. Hankins GDV, Wendel GS Sr, Cunningham FG, Leveno KJ: Longitudinal evaluation of hemodynamic changes in eclampsia. Am J Obstet Gynecol 150:506, 1984

98. Cotton DB, Lee W, Huhta JC, Dorman K: Hemodynamic profile of severe pregnancy-induced hypertension. Am J Obstet Gynecol 158:523, 1988

99. Wallenburg HS: Hemodynamics in hypertensive pregnancy. p. 66. In Rubin PC (ed): Handbook of Hypertension. Hypertension in Pregnancy. Vol. 10. Elsevier, Amsterdam, 1988

100. Belfort M, Dommissee J, Davey DA: Hemodynamic changes in gestational proteinuric hypertension: the effects of rapid volume expansion and vasodilator therapy. Br J Obstet Gynecol 96:634, 1989

101. Mabie WE, Ratts TE, Sibai BM: The hemodynamic profile of severe preeclamptic patients requiring delivery. Am J Obstet Gynecol 161:1443, 1989

102. Campbell S, Pearce JMF, Hackett G et al: Qualitative assessment of uteroplacental blood flow: early screening test for high risk pregnancies. Obstet Gynecol 68:649, 1986

103. Adruini D, Rizzo G, Romanini C, Mancuso S: Uteroplacental blood flow velocity waveforms as predictors of pregnancy-induced hypertension. Eur J Obstet Gynecol Reprod Biol 26:335, 1987

104. Fleischer A, Schulman H, Farmakides G et al: Uterine artery Doppler velocimetry in pregnant women with hypertension. Am J Obstet Gynecol 154:806, 1986

105. Ducey J, Schulman H, Farmakides G et al: A classification of hypertension in pregnancy based on Doppler velocimetry. Am J Obstet Gynecol 157:680, 1987

106. Havretty K, White MJ, Rubin PC: Doppler uteroplacental waveforms in pregnancy-induced hypertension: a reappraisal. Lancet 1:650, 1988

107. Gudmundsson S, Marsal K: Ultrasound Doppler evaluation of uteroplacental and fetoplacental circulation in preeclampsia. Arch Gynecol Obstet 243:199, 1988

108. Cameron AD, Nicholson SF, Nimrod CA et al: Doppler waveforms in fetal aorta and umbilical artery in patients with hypertension in pregnancy. Am J Obstet Gynecol 158:339, 1988

109. Redman CWG: Examination of the placental circulation by Doppler ultrasound: its place in management still to be defined. Br Med J 298:622, 1989

110. Fairlie F, Moretti M, Sibai BM, Walker JJ: Umbilical uteroplacental velocimetry in preeclampsia. Proceedings of the 10th Annual Meeting of the Society of Perinatal Obstetricians. Abstract 396. Houston, Texas, January 23–27, 1990

111. Sibai BM: Preeclampsia–eclampsia: valid treatment approaches. Contemp Obstet Gynecol 35(9):84, 1990

112. Gilstrap LC, Cunningham GF, Whalley PJ: Management of pregnancy-induced hypertension in the nulliparas patient remote from term. Semin Perinatol 2(1):73, 1978

113. Sibai BM, Gonzalez AR, Mabie WC, Moretti M: A comparison of labetalol plus hospitalization versus hospitalization alone in the management of preeclampsia remote from term. Obstet Gynecol 70:323, 1987

114. Rubin PC, Butters L, Clark DM et al: Placebo controlled trial of atenolol in treatment of pregnancy associated hypertension. Lancet 1:431, 1983

115. Wichman K, Ryden G, Kallwig BE: A placebo controlled trial of metroprolol in the treatment of hypertension in pregnancy. Scand J Clin Lab Invest 44:30, 1984

116. Walker JJ, Crooks A, Erwin L et al: Labetalol in pregnancy-induced hypertension: fetal and maternal effects. p. 591. In Riley A, Symonds EM (eds): The Investigation of Labetalol in the Management of Hypertension in Pregnancy. Excerpta Medica International Congress Series, Amsterdam, 1982

117. Pickles CJ, Symonds EM, Broughton-Pipkin F: The fetal outcome in a randomized double-blind controlled trial of labetalol versus placebo pregnancy-induced hypertension. Br J Obstet Gynaecol 96:38, 1989

118. Martin TR, Tupper WRC: The management of severe toxemia in patients less than 36 weeks gestation. Obstet Gynecol 54:602, 1979

119. Odendaal JH, Pattinson RC, Dutoit R: Fetal and neonatal outcome in patients with severe preeclampsia before 34 weeks. S Afr Med J 71:555, 1987

120. Sibai BM, Taslimi M, Abdella TN et al: Maternal peri-natal outcome of conservative management of severe preeclampsia in midtrimester. Am J Obstet Gynecol 152:32, 1985

121. Gonzalez-Ruiz AR, Sibai BM: Glucocorticoids for lung maturation in preeclampsia. Contemp Obstet Gynecol 29:147, 1987

122. Sibai BM: Definitive therapy for pregnancy-induced hypertension. Contemp Obstet Gynecol 31:51, 1988

123. Chesley LC: Parenteral magnesium sulfate and the distribution, plasma levels and excretion of magnesium. Am J Obstet Gynecol 133:1, 1979

124. Massey SG: Pharmacology of magnesium. Annu Rev Pharmacol Toxicol 133:1, 1977

125. Somjen G, Hilmy M, Stephen CR: Failure to anesthetize human subjects by intravenous administration of magnesium sulfate. J Pharmacol Exp Ther 154:652, 1966

126. Hibbard BJ, Rosen M: The management of severe preeclampsia and eclampsia. Br J Anaesth 49:3, 1977

127. Bargis LF, Gucer G: Effect of magnesium sulfate on epileptic foci. Epilepsia 19:81, 1978

128. Pritchard JA: The use of magnesium sulfate in pre-eclampsia-eclampsia. J Reprod Med 23:107, 1979

129. Mabie WC, Gonzalez AR, Sibai BM et al: A comparative trial of labetalol and hydralazine in the acute management of severe hypertension complicating pregnancy. Obstet Gynecol 70:328, 1987

130. Sibai BM, Mabie WE, Harvey CJ, Gonzalez AR: Pulmonary edema in severe preeclampsia-eclampsia: analysis of 37 consecutive cases. Am J Obstet Gynecol 159:650, 1988

131. Ramanathan J, Sibai BM, Mabie WC et al: The use of labetalol for attenuation of the hypertensive response to endotracheal intubation in preeclampsia. Am J Obstet Gynecol 159:650, 1988

132. Clark SL, Cotton DB: Clinical indications for pulmonary artery catheterization in the patient with severe preeclampsia. Am J Obstet Gynecol 158:650, 1988

133. Mabie WC, Ratts TE, Ramanathan KB, Sibai BM: Circulatory congestion in obese hypertensive women: a subset of pulmonary edema in pregnancy. Obstet Gynecol 72:553, 1988

134. Sibai BM: Preeclampsia-eclampsia: maternal perinatal outcomes. Contemp Obstet Gynecol 32:109, 1988

135. Sutherland A, Cooper DW, Howie PW et al: The incidence of severe preeclampsia among mothers and mothers-in-law of preeclamptics and controls. Br J Obstet Gynecol 88:785, 1981

136. Kilpatrick DC, Liston WA, Gibson F, Livingstone J: Association between susceptibility to preeclampsia within families and HLA DR4. Lancet 2:1063, 1989

137. Sibai BMN, El-Nazer A, Gonzalez-Ruiz AR: Severe preeclampsia-eclampsia among mothers and mothers-in-law of preeclamptics and controls. Br J Obstet Gynaecol 88:785, 1981

138. Ihle BU, Long P, Oats J: Early onset preeclampsia: recognition of underlying renal disease. Br Med J 249:79, 1987

139. Chesley LC: History. p. 17. In Chesley LC (ed): Hypertensive Disorders in Pregnancy. Appleton-Century-Crofts, East Norwalk, CT, 1978

140. Walker VN, Baker WS: A comparison study of antihypertensive drug therapy and modified Stroganoff method in the management of severe toxemia of pregnancy. Am J Obstet Gynecol 81:1, 1961

141. Sheehan HL, Lynch JB: Pathology of Toxemia of Pregnancy. Churchill Livingstone, Edinburgh, 1973

142. Sibai BM, McCubbin JH, Anderson GD et al: Eclampsia. I: Observation from 67 recent cases. Obstet Gynecol 58:609, 1981

143. Sibai BM: Eclampsia. p. 320. In Rubin PC (ed): Handbook of Hypertension-Hypertension in Pregnancy. Vol. 10. Elsevier, Amsterdam 1988

144. Sibai BM, Abdella TN, Taylor HA: Eclampsia in the first half of pregnancy: report of three cases and review of the literature. J Reprod Med 27:11, 1982

145. Sibai BM, Schneider JM, Morrison JC et al: The late postpartum eclampsia controversy. Obstet Gynecol 55:1, 1980

146. Ferraz EM, Sherline DM: Convulsive toxemia of pregnancy (eclampsia). South Med J 69:2, 1976

147. Moller B, Lindmark G: Eclampsia in Sweden, 1976–1980. Acta Obstet Gynecol Scand 65:307, 1986

148. Giese J: The Pathogenesis of Hypertensive Vascular Disease. Copenhagen, 1968

149. Rail DL, Perkin GD: Computerized tomographic appearance of hypertensive encephalopathy. Arch Neurol 37:310, 1980

150. Beeson JH, Duda EE: Computed axial tomography scan demonstrating of cerebral edema in eclampsia preceded by blindness. Obstet Gynecol 60:529, 1982

151. Gaitz JP, Bramford CR: Unusual computed tomographic scan in eclampsia. Arch Neurol 39:66, 1983

152. Kirby JC, Jaindl JJ: Cerebral CT scan findings in toxemia of pregnancy. Radiology 151:114, 1984

153. Dunn R, Lee W, Cotton DB: Evaluation of computerized axial tomography of eclamptic women with seizures refractory to magnesium sulfate. Am J Obstet Gynecol 155:267, 1986

154. Beck DW, Menesez AH: Intracerebral hemorrhage in a patient with eclampsia. JAMA 246:13, 1981

155. Sibai BM, Spinnato JA, Watson DL, Anderson GD: Eclampsia. IV: Neurologic findings and future outcome. Am J Obstet Gynecol 152:184, 1985

156. Pritchard JA, Cunningham FG, Pritchard SA: The Parkland Memorial Hospital protocol for treatment of eclampsia: evaluation of 245 cases. Am J Obstet Gynecol 148:951, 1984

157. Richards AM, Moodley J, Graham DI et al: Active management of the unconscious eclamptic patient. Br J Obstet Gynaecol 93:554, 1986

158. Brown ECL, Purdy P, Cunningham GF: Head computed tomographic scans in women with eclampsia. Am J Obstet Gynecol 159:915, 1988

159. Crawford S, Varner MW, Digre KB et al: Cranial magnetic resonance imaging in eclampsia. Obstet Gynecol 70:474, 1987

160. Sibai BM, Spinnato JA, Watson DL et al: Effects of magnesium sulfate on electroencephalographic findings in preeclampsia-eclampsia. Obstet Gynecol 64:261, 1984

161. Sibai BM, Anderson GD, McCubbin JH: Eclampsia. II: Clinical significance of laboratory findings. Obstet Gynecol 59:153, 1982

162. Sibai BM, Anderson GD, Abdella TN et al: Eclampsia. III: Neonatal outcome, growth and development. Am J Obstet Gynecol 146:307, 1983

163. Paul RH, Koh KS, Bernstein SG: Changes in fetal heart rate–uterine contraction patterns associated with eclampsia. Am J Obstet Gynecol 130:165, 1978

164. Physicians' Desk Reference. 44th Ed. p. 1828. Medical Economics, Oradell, NJ, 1990

165. Gedekoh RH, Hayashi TT, McDonald HM: Eclampsia at Magee-Women's Hospital, 1970 to 1980. Am J Obstet Gynecol 140:860, 1981

166. Sibai BM: Magnesium sulfate is the ideal anticonvulsant in preeclampsia-eclampsia. Am J Obstet Gynecol 162:1141, 1990

167. McCubbin JH, Sibai BM, Abdella TN et al: Cardiopulmonary arrest due to acute maternal hypermagnesemia. Letter to the editor. Lancet 1:1058, 1981

168. Slater RM, Wilcox FL, Smith WD et al: Phenytoin infusion in severe preeclampsia. Lancet 1:1417, 1987

169. Ryan G, Lange IR, Naugler MA: Clinical experience with phenytoin prophylaxis in severe preeclampsia. Am J Obstet Gynecol 161:1297, 1989

170. Donaldson JO: Does magnesium sulfate treat eclamptic convulsions? Clin Neuropharmacol 9:37, 1986

171. Kaplan PW, Lesser RP, Fisher RS et al: No, magnesium sulfate should not be used in treating eclamptic convulsions. Arch Neurol 45:1361, 1988

172. Repke JT, Friedman SA, Lim KH et al: A comparison of intravenous phenytoin and magnesium sulfate in preeclampsia. Society of Perinatal Obstetricians. Abstract 12. Houston, Texas, January 25–27, 1990

173. Tufnell DJ, O'Donovan P, Lilford RJ et al: Phenytoin in preeclampsia. Lancet 2:273, 1989

174. Slater RM, Wilcox FL, Smith WD, Maresh MJA: Phenytoin in preeclampsia. Letter to the editor. Lancet 2:1224, 1989

175. Tufnell DJ, O'Donovan P, Lilford RJ et al: Phenytoin in preeclampsia. Letter to the editor. Lancet 2:1224, 1989

176. Pritchard JA, Cunningham FG, Mason RA: Coagulation changes in eclampsia: their frequency and pathogenesis. Am J Obstet Gynecol 124:855, 1976

177. Fadel HE, Sammour DM, Mahran M et al: Creatinine clearance rate in preeclampsia and eclampsia. Obstet Gynecol 32:5, 1968

178. Shukla PK, Sharma D, Mandal RK: Serum lactate dehydrogenase in detecting liver damage associated with preeclampsia. Br J Obstet Gynaecol 85:40, 1978

179. Chesley LC, Cosgrove SA, Preece J et al: Hydatidiform mole, with special reference to recurrence and associated eclampsia. Am J Obstet Gynecol 52:311, 1946

180. Lindheimer MD, Spargo BH, Katz AI: Eclampsia during the 16th gestational week. JAMA 230:1006, 1974

181. Speck G: Eclampsia at the sixteenth week of gestation, with Rh isoimmunization and cystic degeneration of the placenta. Obstet Gynecol 15:70, 1960

182. Watson DL, Sibai BM, Shaver DC et al: Late postpartum eclampsia: an update. South Med J 76:1487, 1983

183. Agobe JT, Adewaze HO: Biochemical studies and delayed postpartum convulsions in Nigeria. p. 501. In Bomar J, MacGillivray I, Symonds EM (eds): Pregnancy Hypertension. University Park Press, Baltimore, 1980

184. Harbert GM, Claiborne HA, McGaughey HS et al: Convulsive toxemia. Am J Obstet Gynecol 10:336, 1968

185. Lopez-Llera M, Horta JLH: Maternal mortality rates in eclampsia. Am J Obstet Gynecol 124:149, 1976

186. Lopez-Llera M, Horta JLH: Perinatal mortality in preeclampsia. J Reprod Med 8:281, 1972

187. Neutra R: Fetal death in eclampsia. I: Its relation to low gestational age, retarded fetal growth and low birthweight. Br J Obstet Gynaecol 82:382, 1975

188. Abdella TN, Sibai BM, Hays JM et al: Relationship of hypertensive disease to abruptio placentae. Obstet Gynecol 63:365, 1984

189. Lopez-Llera M, de la Luz Espinosa MM, Arratia S: Eclampsia and placental abruption: basic patterns, management and morbidity. Int J Gynecol Obstet 27:335, 1988

190. Brazy JE, Grimm JK, Little VA: Neonatal manifestations of severe maternal hypertension occurring before the thirty-sixth week of pregnancy. J Pediatr 100:165, 1982

191. Zuspan FP: Problems encountered in the treatment of pregnancy induced hypertension. Am J Obstet Gynecol 131:591, 1978

192. Sibai BM, Abdella TN, Spinnato JA et al: Eclampsia. V: The incidence of nonpreventable eclampsia. Am J Obstet Gynecol 154:581, 1986

193. Campbell DM, Templeton AA: Is eclampsia preventable? p. 483. In Bonnar J, MacGillivray I, Symonds EM (eds): Pregnancy Hypertension. University Park Press, Baltimore, 1980

194. Bryans CI, Southerland WL, Zuspan FP: Eclampsia: a long-term follow-up study. Obstet Gynecol 21:6, 1963

195. Chesley LC, Cosgrove RA, Annitto JE: A follow-up study of eclamptic women. Am J Obstet Gynecol 83:1360, 1962

196. Chesley LC, Cosgrove RA, Annitto JE: Pregnancy in the sisters and daughters of eclamptic women. Pathol Microbiol (Basel) 24:662, 1961

197. Chesley LC, Annitto JE, Cosgrove RA: The familial factor in toxemia of pregnancy. Obstet Gynecol 32:303, 1968

198. Chesley LC: Hypertensive disorders in pregnancy. J Nurse Midwifery 30:2, 1985

199. Lopez-Llera M, Horta JLH: Pregnancy after eclampsia. Am J Obstet Gynecol 119:193, 1974

200. Sullivan L, Jay M: Hypertension and Pregnancy. Year Book Medical Publishers, Chicago, 1986

201. Frohlich ED: Hemodynamics of hypertension. p. 15. In Genest J, Koiw E, Kuchel O (eds): Hypertension. New York, McGraw-Hill, 1977

202. Hollander W: Role of hypertension in atherosclerosis and cardiovascular disease. Am J Cardiol 38:786, 1976

203. Kannel WB, Castelli WP, NcNamara PM et al: The Framingham Study: some factors affecting morbidity and mortality in hypertension. Milbank Mem Fund Q 47:116, 1969

204. Veterans Administrative Cooperative Study Group on Antihypertensive Agents: Effect of treatment on morbidity: results in patients with diastolic blood pressure averaging 115 through 129 mmHg. JAMA 213:1143, 1970

205. Veterans Administration Cooperative Study Group on Antihypertensive Agents: Effect of treatment on morbidity: results in patients with diastolic blood pressure averaging 90 through 114 mmHg. JAMA 213:1143, 1970

206. Hypertensive Detection and Follow-up Program Cooperative Group: Four-year findings of the Hypertensive Detection and Follow-up Program 1: reduction in mortality of persons with high blood pressure, including mild hypertension. JAMA 242:2562, 1979

207. Sibai BM, Abdella TN, Anderson GD: Pregnancy out-

come in 211 patients with mild chronic hypertension. Obstet Gynecol 61:571, 1983

208. Lin CC, Lindheimer MD, Riber P et al: Fetal outcome in hypertensive disorders of pregnancy. Am J Obstet Gynecol 142:255, 1982

209. Dunlop JC: Chronic hypertension and perinatal mortality. Proc R Soc Med 59:838, 1966

210. Landesman R, Holze E, Scherr L: Fetal mortality in essential hypertension. Obstet Gynecol 6:354, 1955

211. Sibai BM, Anderson GD: Intensive management of severe hypertension in the first trimester. Obstet Gynecol 67:517, 1986

212. Lewis PJ, Bulpitt CJ, Zuspan FP: A comparison of current British and American practice in the management of hypertension in pregnancy. J Obstet Gynaecol 1:78, 1980

213. Lindberg BS, Sandstrom B: How Swedish obstetricians manage hypertension in pregnancy: a questionnaire study. Acta Obstet Gynaecol Scando 60:327, 1981

214. Trudinger BJ, Rarik I: Attitudes to the management of hypertension in pregnancy: a survey of Australian Fellows. Aust NZ J Obstet Gynaecol 22:191, 1982

215. Sibai BM, Watson DL: How American obstetricians manage hypertension during pregnancy. Presented at the Annual Meeting of the American College of Obstetrics and Gynecology, Washington, DC, 1985

216. Redman CWG: Treatment of hypertension in pregnancy. Kidney Int 18:267, 1980

217. Kincaid-Smith P, Bullen M, Mills J: Prolonged use of methyldopa in severe hypertension in pregnancy. Br Med J 1:274, 1966

218. Mabie WC, Pernoll ML, Biswas MK: Chronic hypertension in pregnancy. Obstet Gynecol 67:197, 1986

219. Leather HM, Humphreys DM, Baker PB et al: A controlled trial of hypertensive agents in hypertension in pregnancy. Lancet 1:488, 1968

220. Redman CWG, Beilin LJ, Bonnar J et al: Fetal outcome in trial of antihypertensive treatment in pregnancy. Lancet 2:753, 1976

221. Redman CWG, Beilin LJ, Bonnar J: Treatment of hypertension in pregnancy with methyldopa: blood pressure control and side effects. Br J Obstet Gynaecol 84:419, 1977

222. Arias F, Zamora J: Antihypertensive treatment and pregnancy outcome in patients with mild chronic hypertension. Obstet Gynecol 53:489, 1979

223. Gallery EDM, Saunders DM, Hunyor N et al: Randomized comparison of methyldopa and oxprenolol for treatment of hypertension in pregnancy. Br Med J 1:1591, 1979

224. Fidler J, Smith V, Fayers P et al: Randomized controlled comparative study of methyldopa and oxprenolol in treatment of hypertension in pregnancy. Br Med J 286:1927, 1983

225. Horvath JS, Phippard A, Korda A et al: Clonidine hydrochloride: a safe and effective antihypertensive agent in pregnancy. Obstet Gynecol 66:634, 1985

226. McNair A, Rasmussen S, Neilsen PE: The antihypertensive side effect of prazosin on mild to moderate hypertension, changes in plasma volume, extracellular volume and glomerular filtration rate. Acta Med Scand 207:413, 1980

227. Rubin PC, Butters L, Low RA et al: Clinical pharmacological studies with prazosin during pregnancy complicated by hypertension. Br J Pharmacol 16:543, 1983

228. Lubbe WF, Hodge JV, Kellaway GSM: Antihypertensive treatment and fetal welfare in essential hypertension in pregnancy: a retrospective survey of experience with various regimes at National Women's Hospital, Auckland, 1970–80. NZ Med J 95:1, 1982

229. Lubbe WF, Hodge JV: Combined alpha- and beta-adrenoceptor antagonism with prazosin and oxprenolol in control of severe hypertension in pregnancy. NZ Med J 94:169, 1981

230. Veld AJM, Schalekamp MADH: Effects of 10 different beta-adrenoceptor antagonists on hemodynamics, plasma renin activity, and plasma norepinephrine in hypertension. J Cardiovasc Pharmacol, suppl. 5:530, 1983

231. Svendsen TL: Central hemodynamics of beta-adrenoceptor blocking drugs: beta$_1$, selectivity versus intrinsic sympathomimetic activity. J Cardiovasc Pharmacol, suppl. 5:21, 1983

232. van Zwieten PA, Timmermans PBMWM: Differential pharmacological properties of beta-adrenoceptor blocking drugs. J Cardiovasc Pharmacol, suppl. 5:1, 1983

233. Court DJ, Parer JT: On risks and benefits of propranolol and other beta blockers. Contemp Obstet 24:179, 1984

234. Rubin PC: Beta-blockers in pregnancy. N Engl J Med 305:1223, 1981

235. Lieberman BA, Stirrat GM, Cohen SL et al: The possible adverse effect of propranolol on the fetus in pregnancies complicated by severe hypertension. Br J Obstet Gynaecol 85:678, 1978

236. Eliahou HE, Silverberg DS, Reisen E et al: Propranolol for the treatment of hypertension in pregnancy. Br J Obstet Gynaecol 85:431, 1978

237. Tcherdakoff PH, Colliard M, Berrard E et al: Propranolol in hypertension during pregnancy. Br Med J 2:670, 1978

238. Bott-Kanner G, Schweitzer A, Reisner SH et al: Propranolol and hydralazine in the management of essential hypertension in pregnancy. Br J Obstet Gynecol 87:110, 1980

239. Thorley KJ, McAinsh J, Cruickshank JM: Atenolol in the treatment of pregnancy-induced hypertension. Br J Clin Pharmacol 12:725, 1981

240. Dubois D, Petitcolas J, Temperville B et al: Treatment of hypertension in pregnancy with beta-adrenoceptor antagonists. Br J Clin Pharmacol 13:375S, 1982

241. Liedholm H: Atenolol in the treatment of hypertension of pregnancy. Drugs 25:suppl. 2, 206, 1983

242. Sandstrom B: Clinical trials of adrenergic antagonists in pregnancy hypertension. Acta Obstet Gynecol Scand, suppl. 118:57, 1984

243. Michael CA: The evaluation of labetalol in the treatment of hypertension complicating pregnancy. Br J Clin Pharmacol, 8:suppl. 1, 127, 1982

244. Lardoux H, Gerard J, Blazquez G: Hypertension in pregnancy: evaluation of two beta blockers atenolol and labetalol. Eur Heart J, suppl. G:35, 1983

245. Michael CA: Use of labetalol in the treatment of severe hypertension during pregnancy. Br J Clin Pharmacol 8:2115, 1979

246. Plouin PF, Breat G, Milard F et al: Comparison of antihypertensive efficacy and perinatal safety of labetalol and methyldopa in the treatment of hypertension in pregnancy: a randomized controlled trial. Br J Obstet Gynaecol 95:868, 1988

247. Walters NJ, Redman CWG: Treatment of severe pregnancy-associated hypertension with calcium antagonist nifedipine. Br J Obstet Gynaecol 91:330, 1984

248. Constantine G, Beevers DG, Reynolds AL et al: Nifedipine as a second line antihypertensive drug in pregnancy. Br J Obstet Gynaecol 94:1136, 1987

249. Rubin PC, McCabe R, Low RA: Calcium channel blockage with nifedipine combined with atenolol in the management of severe preeclampsia. Clin Exp Hyper-Hyper Pregnancy B3:379, 1984

250. Greer IA, Walker JJ, Bjornsson S, Calder AA: Second line therapy with nifedipine in severe pregnancy induced hypertension. Clin Exp Hyper-Hyper in Pregnancy. B8:277, 1989

251. Lindow SW, Davies N, Davey DA, Smith JA: The effect of sublingual nifedipine on uteroplacental blood flow in hypertensive pregnancy. Br J Obstet Gynaecol 95:1276, 1988

252. Hanretty KP, Whittle MJ, Howie CA, Rubin PC: Effect of nifedipine on Doppler flow velocity waveforms in severe preeclampsia. Br Med J 299:1205, 1989

253. Allen J, Maigaard S, Forman A et al: Acute effects of nitrendipine in pregnancy-induced hypertension. Br J Obstet Gynaecol 94:222, 1987

254. Broughton Pipkin F, Symonds EM, Twiner SR: The effect of captopril upon mother and fetus in the chronically cannulated ewe and in the pregnant rabbit. J Physiol 323:415, 1982

255. Broughton Pipkin F, Baker PN, Symonds EM: ACE inhibitors in pregnancy. Lancet 2:96, 1989

256. Duminy PC, Burger P: Fetal abnormality associated with the use of captopril during pregnancy. S Afr Med J 60:805, 1981

257. Mochizuki M: Treatment of hypertension in pregnancy by a combined drug regimen including captopril. Clin Exp Hyper-Hyper in Pregnancy B5:69, 1986

258. Kreft-Jais C, Plouin PF, Tchobroutsky C et al: Angiotensin converting enzyme inhibitors in pregnancy: a survey of 22 patients given captopril and 9 given enalapril. Br J Obstet Gynaecol 95:420, 1988

259. Are ACE inhibitors safe in pregnancy? Lancet 2:482, 1989

260. Scott AA, Dilip MP: Neonatal renal failure: a complication of maternal antihypertensive therapy. Am J Obstet Gynecol 160:1223, 1989

261. Rosa FW, Bosco LA, Graham CF et al: Neonatal anuria with maternal angiotensin converting enzyme inhilutor. Obstet Gynecol 74:371, 1989

262. Sibai BM, Abdella TN, Anderson GD et al: Plasma volume findings in pregnant women with mild hypertension: therapeutic considerations. Am J Obstet Gynecol 145:539, 1983

263. Collins R, Yusuf S, Peto R: Overview of randomized trials of diuretics in pregnancy. Br Med J 190:17, 1985

264. McGillivray I: Sodium and water balance in pregnancy hypertension: the role of diuretics. Clin Obstet Gynaecol 4:459, 1977

265. Gant NF, Madden JD, Sitteri PK et al: The metabolic clearance rate of dehydroepiandrosterone sulfate. Am J Obstet Gynecol 123:159, 1975

266. Sibai BM, Grossman RA, Grossman HG: Effects of diuretics on plasma volume in pregnancies with long-term hypertension. Am J Obstet Gynecol 150:831, 1984

267. Sibai BM, Abdella TN, Anderson GD et al: Plasma volume determinations in pregnancies complicated by chronic hypertension and intrauterine fetal demise. Obstet Gynecol 60:174, 1982

268. Chesley LC, Annitto JE: Pregnancy in the patient with hypertensive disease. Am J Obstet Gynecol 53:372, 1947

Chapter 31

Cardiac and Pulmonary Disease

Mark B. Landon and Philip Samuels

HEART DISEASE

Cardiac disease complicates approximately 1 percent of all pregnancies. It remains the major nonobstetric cause of maternal death in the United States.[1] The cardiovascular changes that accompany pregnancy can impose a tremendous risk on women with certain categories of heart disease. Patients known to have only minimal limitation of their activity while nonpregnant can suddenly experience worsening symptoms during gestation. The fetus may also become jeopardized when maternal cardiac status deteriorates. Severe limitations on cardiac performance that result in the delivery of poorly oxygenated blood to the pregnant uterus can critically affect fetal growth and viability. Therefore the consideration of hemodynamic changes that occur during gestation becomes extremely important when planning therapy for the pregnant patient with heart disease. Before describing specific maternal cardiac diseases, it is best to begin by reviewing some of the basic circulatory adjustments of normal pregnancy.

Blood Volume

Expansion of maternal plasma volume accounts for most of the increase in blood volume found in pregnancy. Plasma volume rises to levels that are 50 percent above the nonpregnant mean by 32 weeks gestation (Table 31.1).[2] A patient with a multiple gestation may have significantly greater increments in plasma volume. Early investigators believed that plasma volume declined in later pregnancy. However, those studies were performed while patients remained supine. In the supine position, caval compression results in increased pooling of blood in the lower extremities and increased venous pressure. This proportionately increases filtration of plasma into the extracellular space.[3] Studies subsequently performed in the left lateral position have documented that plasma volume remains stable from 32 weeks gestation until delivery.

Primarily hormonal mechanisms seem to be responsible for the plasma volume expansion of normal pregnancy. Plasma renin activity rises sharply secondary to estrogen-augmented hepatic production of renin substrate. Progesterone competitively blocks the action of aldosterone at the renal tubule. Nevertheless, sodium and water are gradually retained, resulting in a 6 to 8 L expansion of total body water. Two-thirds of this increase, or 4 to 6 L, is distributed extracellularly.[4]

Red cell mass increases from 16 weeks gestation until term and may reach values that are 20 percent above the average nonpregnant mean. A dilutional anemia results during the second trimester because of the proportionately greater rise in plasma volume. Later in pregnancy, hemoglobin levels increase as erythropoiesis continues and plasma volume stabilizes. Blood volume increases an average of 40 per-

Table 31.1 Circulatory Adjustments During Normal Pregnancy

	Rise	Peak
Blood volume	Early 6 wk	↑ 40% (avg) by 32 wk
Plasma volume	Early 6 wk	↑ 50% (avg) by 32 wk
Red cell volume	Progressively after first trimester	↑ 20% by term

cent over nonpregnant levels.[5] The magnitude of this increment in blood volume may be correlated with birth weight in primigravid patients.

After delivery, blood volume declines significantly. Postpartum diuresis as well as the blood loss associated with delivery contribute to a rapid decline in plasma volume. The hematocrit will rise 2 to 3 percent in the week following vaginal delivery. In women who are not breast-feeding, blood volume usually returns to nonpregnant levels within 2 months.

Cardiac Output

Cardiac output rises approximately 30 to 50 percent over baseline values by 20 to 24 weeks gestation.[6] Marked fluctuations in resting output are observed with changes in maternal position. Cardiac output measured in the left lateral position falls during the last trimester of pregnancy. In supine subjects studied during the second half of gestation, cardiac output is significantly decreased, falling to values below those obtained in the immediate postpartum period.[7] This phenomenon is believed to result from venacaval compression by the gravid uterus. Normally, collateral vessels serve to ensure adequate return of blood to the right side of the heart. Women who fail to develop sufficient collateral circulation will experience hypotension should they remain supine for a prolonged period of time. This vasovagal-like syndrome has been termed the "supine hypotensive syndrome of pregnancy."[8] The characteristic symptoms of hypotension and bradycardia may be promptly relieved by placing the patient in the left lateral position.

The increased cardiac output observed early in pregnancy can be attributed to a larger stroke vol-

ume. As pregnancy advances, heart rate rises, while cardiac output remains unchanged or falls. It follows therefore that stroke volume must progressively decline (Fig. 31.1). The physiologic mechanism for the early increase in stroke volume has not been well explained. Burwell[8a] first suggested that the rise in cardiac output associated with pregnancy might occur in response to a decline in peripheral vascular resistance. He proposed that the circulation of the pregnant woman was similar to that found in patients with an arteriovenous fistula.

Volume changes alone are not responsible for the increased cardiac output found in pregnancy. Studies of the pulmonary vasculature reveal no change in pulmonary artery diastolic pressure during gestation.[9] This important index of cardiac function reflects left ventricular filling pressure. For end-diastolic volume to increase without a change in end-diastolic pressure, left ventricular enlargement must be present. Katz et al.,[10] using echocardiographic techniques, have demonstrated that the diameter of the left ventricle increases early in gestation. It has been postulated that ventricular distensibility may be affected by elevated levels of steroid hormones.[6] End-diastolic volume can thereby increase without an increased filling pressure, resulting in an increased stroke volume. Estrogens may alter contractile proteins within the myocardium, resulting in improved contractility and further increasing stroke volume and output.

The changes observed in cardiac output are not uniformly distributed. Early in gestation, renal blood flow increases to values 30 percent above the nonpregnant level. Uterine blood flow rises throughout pregnancy to a level of 500 cc/min in a term singleton pregnancy. The uterus and growing fetus receive a greater amount of cardiac output even before full placental development occurs. Measurements of uterine blood flow demonstrate the increase to be approximately 200 ml/min by midpregnancy. Blood flow to the skin is greatly increased and may permit dissipation of heat generated by the growing fetus.

Labor and Delivery

Labor produces sudden and often profound changes in the cardiovascular system. With each uterine contraction, systemic venous pressure increases as blood

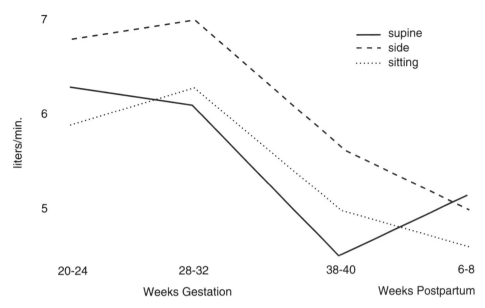

Fig. 31.1 Maternal cardiac output during pregnancy and postpartum. Cardiac output is greatest in the lateral recumbent position, peaking at 28 to 32 weeks gestation. In supine subjects near term, cardiac output falls to values lower than those obtained during the immediate postpartum period. (From Ueland et al.,[7] with permission.)

is returned from the engorged uterine veins. Right ventricular pressure rises, and cardiac output increases about 20 percent in the supine position. Mean arterial pressure rises and is followed by a reflex bradycardia. Because uterine contractions can result in significant compression of the aorta and iliac arteries, much of the increase in cardiac output is distributed to the upper extremities and head.

Anesthesia greatly influences the hemodynamic changes observed during labor. Epidural anesthesia may attenuate the normal increase in cardiac output and heart rate because it acts as an analgesic as well as a peripheral vasodilator, which reduces venous return to the heart. These changes result in a diminished preload or ventricular end-diastolic volume. Nonetheless, regional anesthesia can be used effectively in most patients with cardiac disease. It may, however, impose great risks on those with right to left shunting. Regional techniques may also be hazardous in patients with hypertrophic obstructive cardiomyopathy (IHSS).

Elective cesarean section may avoid some of the circulatory changes produced by uterine activity. Prior to surgery, both epidural and spinal anesthesia produce a fall in cardiac output and blood pressure.

Hypotension is generally corrected by employing left lateral uterine displacement and infusing appropriate intravenous fluids. Correction of hypotension with ephedrine is inadvisable in patients who cannot tolerate tachycardia.

Following vaginal delivery, because of the reduction in caval compression and an increase in blood volume, circulating cardiac output may rise dramatically. A bradycardia often ensues and lasts for a few days. After a cesarean section that is accompanied by an average blood loss in excess of 1,000 cc, cardiac output and blood pressure may temporarily decrease.

Diagnosis and Detection of Cardiac Disease

Pregnancy is often accompanied by physical changes that may be confused with underlying cardiac disease. Symptoms and clinical signs that are associated with heart disease are often present in a normal pregnancy. It is not unusual for patients to experience fatigue, shortness of breath, orthopnea, and peripheral edema, findings similar to those present in congestive heart failure. Palpitations may also be reported by a normal obstetric patient. The following symptoms, however, should alert the obstetrician to the presence of underlying cardiac disease: (1) any progressive limitation of physical activity because of worsening dyspnea, (2) chest pain that accompanies exercise or increased activity, and (3) syncope that is preceded by palpitations or physical exertion.

SIGNS AND SYMPTOMS OF CARDIAC DISEASE

History

    Progressive or severe dyspnea

    Dyspnea at rest

    Paroxysmal nocturnal dyspnea

    Angina or syncope with exertion

    Hemoptysis

Physical examination

    Loud systolic murmur or click

    Diastolic murmur

    Cardiomegaly including parasternal heave

    Cyanosis or clubbing

    Persistent jugular venous distension

    Features of Marfan syndrome

Electrocardiogram

    Arrhythmia

Physical examination of the heart and cardiovascular system reveals normal physiologic changes that, like many of the symptoms described above, suggest heart disease. Systolic outflow murmurs are observed in 90 percent of pregnant women. However, diastolic murmurs are noted in no more than 10 percent of patients and, when present, require further evaluation.[11] A third heart sound is often heard and is not a sign of abnormality. Venous distension and accompanying peripheral edema are found in the majority of pregnancies. While neck veins may become pronounced, normal venous pulsations should occur. If absent, further evaluation is required.

Interpreting the results of standard techniques used to investigate cardiac disease may be difficult in pregnancy. Chest x-rays will often demonstrate cardiomegaly and increased pulmonary vascular markings. Therefore more significant changes must be present to suggest hemodynamically significant cardiac disease. Electrocardiographic findings may aid in the preliminary diagnosis of valvular disease or anatomic defects if chamber hypertrophy is suggested. However, myocardial ischemia must not be confused with the ST–T segment depression and flattening of T waves in the precordial leads, which may be present in normal pregnant women.[11] Premature atrial and ventricular beats are also common in pregnancy.

Because it does not expose the mother and the fetus to radiation, echocardiography has become the preferred technique for the detection of cardiac abnormalities during pregnancy. Using M-mode echocardiography, Rubler et al.[12] have documented that the internal dimensions of the left ventricle, ejection fraction, and stroke volume are all increased in pregnant women after the first trimester. Echocardiography has also confirmed that cardiac output rises later in pregnancy in patients studied in the lateral recumbent position.

General Considerations in Management

The successful management of heart disease in pregnancy requires close cooperation between the cardiologist and the obstetrician. In the best circumstances, cardiac disease is identified *prior* to pregnancy, so that appropriate counseling regarding risks and outcome can be undertaken. Certain conditions, including Eisenmenger syndrome and primary pulmonary hypertension, have been associated with such high maternal mortality rates that pregnancy is not advised. Patients with mitral stenosis may elect to undergo cardiac catheterization and possible valve replacement earlier in their illness if contemplating pregnancy. In such patients, a porcine valve may be preferred because it reduces the need for anticoagulation.

It is important to define precisely the nature of a patient's cardiac disease. This information will enable the physician to assess the risks of pregnancy appropriately not only for the mother but for her fetus as well. A multifactorial pattern of inheritance has been suggested for most congenital heart disease. The risk ranges from 2 to 4 percent,[13] depending on the mother's malformation.

MATERNAL MORTALITY RISK ASSOCIATED WITH SPECIFIC CARDIAC DISEASES

Group I, mortality <1%

Atrial septal defect (uncomplicated)

Ventricular septal defect (uncomplicated)

Patient ductus arteriosus (uncomplicated)

Pulmonic/tricuspid disease

Corrected tetralogy of Fallot

Porcine valve

Mitral stenosis (mild)

Group II, mortality 5%–15%

Mitral stenosis with atrial fibrillation

Artificial valve

Mitral stenosis (moderate to severe)

Aortic stenosis

Coarctation of aorta (uncomplicated)

Uncorrected tetralogy of Fallot

Previous myocardial infarction

Group III, mortality 25%–50%

Pulmonary hypertension

Coarctation of aorta (complicated)

Marfan syndrome with aortic involvement

(Adapted from Clark,[133] with permission.)

The specific cardiac lesion present will also determine the need for antibiotic prophylaxis during labor and delivery. Although the efficacy of antibiotic prophylaxis against infective endocarditis has not been proven, the low risk of drug toxicity when weighed against the dangers of endocarditis makes such prophylaxis the recommended practice. Manual removal of the placenta is an absolute indication for antibiotic prophylaxis in patients with structural heart disease. For some patients, including those with prosthetic valves, mortality rates are particularly high should they become infected. Prophylaxis usually includes the intravenous administration of aqueous penicillin G and an aminoglycoside at the start of true labor, with continuation every 8 hours until one dose postdelivery has been given. Vancomycin may be substituted in patients who are allergic to penicillin (Table 31.2).

Antibiotic prophylaxis for rheumatic fever should be used in patients with a positive past history, especially if they demonstrate valvular disease. The American Heart Association recommends a monthly injection of 1.2 million units of benzathine penicillin G. Alternative regimens include daily oral administration of penicillin or erythromycin.

Anticoagulation may be required in individuals with prosthetic valves as well as those with arrhythmias who may be at risk for an arterial embolus. Patients with mitral stenosis and associated atrial fibrillation should also be anticoagulated. Pregnancy will influence the type of anticoagulation therapy to be used. Oral anticoagulants are contraindicated, as fetal exposure to coumadin during the first 2 months of gestation can result in a significant malformation rate. Heparin does not cross the placenta and is the preferred anticoagulant.

Careful assessment by both the cardiologist and obstetrician should ensure that the patient's hemodynamic status remains optimal during pregnancy. Weight, blood pressure, and pulse should be monitored and a detailed cardiovascular examination should be performed at each visit. It is important to consider conditions that may stress patients with significant cardiac disease such as anemia and infection. In a patient who demonstrates worsening symptoms, it is often necessary to institute changes in diet, activity, or medication. In doing so, one must carefully consider the effects on the fetus of such therapeutic decisions.

Occasionally, cardiac function in patients with valvular disease may deteriorate, and, when medical management fails, cardiac surgery may become necessary. This decision usually follows conservative treatment, including hospitalization, bed rest, diuresis, and correction of arrhythmias when present. If it must be performed, cardiac surgery should ideally be undertaken early in gestation, but preferably following early development. Open heart surgery has been associated with a low maternal mortality rate.[14] Fetal survival rates appear to be improving, following earlier experience in which fetal mortality was found to be as high as 33 percent. In 68 cases utilizing cardio-

Table 31.2 Recommended Regimen for Antibiotic Prophylaxis

For labor and delivery	Ampicillin 2.0 g IM or IV plus gentamicin 1.5 mg/kg IM or IV given in active labor; one follow-up dose may be given 8 hours later and postpartum
Oral regimen for minor or repetitive procedures in low risk patients	Amoxicillin 3.0 g orally 1 hour before procedure and 1.5 g 6 hours later
Penicillin-allergic patients	Vancomycin 1.0 g IV slowly over 1 hour, plus gentamicin 1.5 mg/kg IM or IV given 1 hour before procedure; may be repeated once 8 to 12 hours later

(Adapted from Shulman et al.,[134] with permission.)

pulmonary bypass, Becker[15] reported one maternal death and an 80 percent fetal salvage rate. It is recommended that perfusion hypothermia be avoided, as this may be responsible for the fetal bradycardia observed during cardiopulmonary bypass. Fetal heart rate and uterine monitoring have been used sparingly, but may help to guide the adjustment of blood flow and pressure while the pregnant patient is maintained on bypass.

Specific Cardiac Diseases

Despite the declining incidence of rheumatic fever in the United States, rheumatic heart disease remains the most common cardiac problem encountered in pregnancy. In Third World countries where congenital lesions often remain uncorrected, rheumatic fever is still common and may result in valvular disease in women of childbearing age. The prognosis for patients with rheumatic disease who receive optimal care is generally good. Szekely et al.[16] reported a maternal mortality rate of approximately 1 percent in 2,856 pregnancies over a 27-year period prior to 1970. In this series, no maternal deaths were reported after 1960. Patients at greatest risk are those who develop severe congestive failure or atrial arrhythmias.

Chesley[17] has studied the long-term effects of pregnancy in women with severe rheumatic heart disease. He compared the survival of 38 patients with 51 pregnancies to that of 96 patients who did not become pregnant after heart disease was diagnosed. Both groups were comparable with respect to mortality statistics, suggesting that, in patients who survive pregnancy, life expectancy is not shortened.

The improvement in pediatric surgical techniques and in neonatal intensive care over the past two dec-

ades will undoubtedly permit more patients with congenital heart disease to become pregnant. Patients who develop right to left shunting with increased pulmonary vascular pressure still exhibit maternal mortality rates approaching 50 percent. Prior surgical repair for patients with congenital heart disease does appear to make a significant difference in the outcome of their pregnancy. Whittemore and colleagues[18] examined this issue by comparing two subgroups of a total of 233 patients with congenital heart defects through 482 pregnancies. The percentage of pregnancies resulting in live births did not differ significantly between the surgically corrected and control groups (average live birth rate, 77 percent). Outcome as determined by birth weight and viability, however, was markedly improved in patients who underwent successful surgery for cyanotic lesions. As expected, the live birth rate was also dependent on the degree of cardiac impairment. This study also demonstrated a significantly higher incidence of congenital heart defects (16.1 percent) in infants born to affected mothers than has been previously reported.

Acquired Valvular Disease

Mitral Stenosis

Mitral stenosis is the most common form of rheumatic heart disease found in pregnancy. It can occur as an isolated lesion or can accompany aortic or right-sided valvular lesions. Mitral stenosis is usually a sequel of rheumatic fever. In patients who develop carditis, mitral insufficiency often precedes the development of stenosis. Symptoms may not appear for over a decade, at which time a reduction in cardiac output causes patients to become easily fatigued. Obstruction to left atrial outflow produces a rise in atrial pressure and eventually pulmonary capillary wedge pressure. Pulmonary congestive and right ventricular failure are seen 5 to 10 years after the onset of symptoms.[19] In symptomatic patients, the maternal mortality rate during pregnancy is sufficiently high to recommend surgical correction prior to pregnancy.

The augmented cardiac output of pregnancy, including tachycardia and increased circulatory volume, impose a tremendous stress on patients with significant mitral disease. Szekely and Snaith[20] estimated that symptoms of pulmonary congestion may develop in 25 percent of pregnant women. Dyspnea is often present by 20 weeks gestation, when resting cardiac output has reached its maximum.

Symptoms of reduced cardiac output should be treated with limitation of activity and, if the patient is volume overloaded, cautious diuresis. Control of arrhythmias, particularly atrial fibrillation, is essential. In hemodynamically stable patients, digitalis is initially used to slow the ventricular rate prior to cardioversion. As the size of the left atrium increases, there is a possibility that mural thrombus formation may occur. Thus a patient with mitral stenosis may initially present with systemic arterial embolization. In this case, anticoagulation employing heparin will be required.

If medical measures are unsuccessful in the treatment of symptoms, valve replacement or commisurotomy must be considered. Commisurotomy should ideally be performed in patients who do not have significant regurgitation and who have limited calcification of the mitral valve. No other valvular disease should be present. Szekely and Snaith[20] reported 69 cases of mitral commisurotomy in which two maternal deaths occurred. Six fetal deaths also followed the procedure. In 101 closed mitral commisurotomies recently performed in the United States, no maternal deaths and only three fetal losses were reported.[15] Valve replacement has become more popular with improved understanding of maternal and fetal physiology during cardiopulmonary bypass. Becker[15] reported 19 cases of mitral valve replacement during pregnancy in which the major indication for surgery was refractory congestive failure. All mothers survived, as did 15 fetuses (79 percent). This series included four patients with thrombosed prostheses and one case of infective endocarditis.

Labor and delivery is a hazardous process for the patient with mitral stenosis. Patients with significant disease require invasive monitoring (see Ch. 19). Pulmonary capillary wedge pressure and cardiac output are determined by the use of the Swan-Ganz catheter. The volume of fluids administered should be monitored carefully during both labor and the immediate postpartum period. Clark et al.[21] have emphasized that because pulmonary capillary wedge pressure does not accurately reflect left ventricular filling pressures in women with mitral stenosis, such patients often require high-normal wedge pressure to maintain cardiac output. Patients should labor in the semi-Fowler's position, and oxygen may be given. Ventricular rate must be monitored closely to avoid tachycardia, which can result in decreased cardiac output. It should be remembered that stenosis of the mitral valve is accompanied by a relatively fixed stroke volume that may not rise with an increase in heart rate. Rapid heart rates further decrease diastolic filling time and elevate left atrial pressure. Verapamil or digitalis may be required to slow the ventricular rate in cases of atrial arrhythmias. If sinus tachycardia becomes excessive (> 140 bpm), the use of anesthetics to alleviate pain or cautious use of propranolol may be employed. Patients who receive epidural anesthesia should be carefully observed for hypotension, which may precipitate tachycardia. Systemic vascular resistance is best maintained with the α-agonist metaraminol. The β-agonist component of ephedrine will result in tachycardia, and its use should therefore be avoided. In patients delivering vaginally, the second stage of labor, including intense Valsalva efforts, may be shortened by the use of outlet forceps or vacuum extraction. A large bolus of intravenous oxytocin should be avoided, as it may precipitate hypotension.

The most hazardous time for women with mitral stenosis is the postpartum period.[16] A rise in wedge pressure is common, and careful attention must be given to changes in cardiac output that accompany fluid shifts following delivery. Antibiotic prophylaxis is required in patients with mitral stenosis.

Aortic Stenosis

Aortic stenosis is a rare complication of pregnancy. Valvular thickening resulting from acute rheumatic disease does not typically occur for several decades following the initial attack. Most patients become symptomatic in the fifth or sixth decade of life. Once symptoms of angina, dyspnea, or syncope arise, progressive decompensation follows, with mortality rates approaching 50 percent within 5 years.[20]

Obstruction to left ventricular outflow and reduction in cardiac output are responsible for the symptomatology present. Physical exertion may result in relative ischemia of the cerebral and coronary vessels, producing syncope and angina. With long-standing aortic stenosis, left ventricular hypertrophy occurs as a compensatory mechanism. This further increases the oxygen requirements of the heart and the propensity for anginal episodes. A rise in left atrial pressure is needed to fill the hypertrophied left ventricle. This may be reflected in elevated pulmonary vascular pressures, leading to progressive dyspnea.

Mortality rates as high as 17 percent have been reported in pregnant patients with aortic stenosis.[22] There may not be a clear advantage to pregnancy termination. Arias and Pineda[22] reported two fatalities in five patients whose pregnancies were interrupted. Of note, these patients were probably among the most critically ill in their series. The high mortality rate associated with pregnancy termination may reflect the occurrence of hypovolemia, which decreases venous return and left ventricular filling. This effect is poorly tolerated in patients with aortic stenosis who require an adequate end-diastolic volume in the face of increased filling pressures and a fixed afterload or impedance to outflow.

For this reason, regional anesthetic techniques that can decrease preload or end-diastolic volume must be used with great caution during labor and delivery. Hypotension is avoided by the use of left lateral uterine displacement and appropriate fluid administration. A fall in blood pressure produces tachycardia, which can aggravate the condition of compromised patients. Tachycardia will decrease the ventricular filling time and further reduce cardiac output. Central monitoring employing a Swan-Ganz catheter is encouraged in all symptomatic patients, as well as in those who have physical or diagnostic signs suggesting significant valve obstruction. As hypovolemia poses a greater risk than fluid overload, wedge pressures should be maintained in the 16 to 18 mmHg range to protect against unexpected blood loss.

Antibiotic prophylaxis is recommended in laboring women with aortic stenosis.

Mitral Regurgitation

Mitral regurgitation may follow rheumatic fever or an episode of endocarditis. It is also observed in patients with idiopathic hypertrophic subaortic stenosis (IHSS) and mitral valve prolapse. A floppy mitral valve may be the most common cause of regurgitation in women of childbearing age.

Women with mitral regurgitation develop symptoms of left-sided failure later in life than do patients with pure mitral stenosis. A diminished ventricular output results in symptoms of fatigue and, eventually, dyspnea from pulmonary congestion. Elevation of pressure within the left atrium predisposes to fibrillation and mural thrombus formation. At the end stage of this disease, patients with elevated pulmonary arteriolar pressure will demonstrate signs of right-sided failure, including peripheral edema and hepatomegaly.

The hemodynamic changes of pregnancy are usually well tolerated in patients with minimal mitral insufficiency. Frequently, the typical decrescendo systolic murmur will be diminished during pregnancy, because the fall in peripheral vascular resistance reduces the amount of regurgitation flow across the mitral valve. Patients with long-standing disease may develop atrial enlargement and fibrillation. The risk for arrhythmias may be increased during pregnancy.[23] Reduction of left ventricular afterload may therefore become an important therapeutic maneuver in patients with impaired cardiac output. Patients with chronic disease, including those with a large left ventricle, may require inotropic support if the afterload is substantially reduced.

During labor and delivery, patients with mitral insufficiency may benefit from central monitoring to direct fluid and drug therapy. Pain during labor and delivery may be associated with an increase in blood pressure that is due to enhanced sympathetic activity. If systemic vascular resistance also rises, pulmonary congestion may follow. Epidural analgesia is recommended to prevent this occurrence. Regional anesthesia may impair venous return to the heart and often requires careful administration of intravenous fluids to maintain filling of the enlarged left ventricle. Patients with this lesion should also receive antibiotic prophylaxis during labor and delivery.

Aortic Regurgitation

Aortic regurgitation occurs approximately 10 years after the onset of rheumatic fever. In this setting, coexistent mitral disease is common. Occasionally, aortic regurgitation is seen with a congenital bicuspid valve or in association with a collagen vascular disease such as rheumatoid arthritis or systemic lupus erythematosus. Dilatation of the aortic root is responsible for regurgitation in patients with Marfan syndrome.

Most patients with aortic insufficiency experience symptoms of failure during the fourth or fifth decade of life. Progressive left ventricular dilatation results from a state of chronic volume overload. In compensated cases, left ventricular end-diastolic pressure remains normal for several years. Pregnancy is complicated by episodes of failure in less than 10 percent of cases.[20] Restriction of activity as well as treatment with digitalis and diuretics is employed should symptoms of cardiac failure develop. Patients with aortic regurgitation caused by endocarditis may require valve replacement. Heterograft valves are preferred in pregnancy because they do not require anticoagulation.[24]

As with mitral regurgitation, the decrease in systemic vascular resistance observed during pregnancy may reduce the amount of regurgitant flow and the intensity of the murmur. The stress of labor and delivery, however, may precipitate left-sided ventricular dysfunction. Afterload reduction using phentolamine or sodium nitroprusside has been successfully employed when vascular resistance remains high. Epidural anesthesia is recommended for vaginal delivery and may serve to prevent peripheral vasoconstriction. Mangano[25] emphasizes that bradycardia is poorly tolerated in patients with significant aortic regurgitation. Slowing of the heart rate increases the duration of ventricular diastole and regurgitation across the valve. Ideally, the maternal heart rate should be maintained between 80 and 100 bpm.[25]

Congenital Lesions

Left to Right Shunt

Left to right shunting may occur through an atrial septal defect (ASD), ventricular septal defect (VSD), or patent ductus arteriosus (PDA). Surgical correction of these lesions is often performed during infancy and childhood. However, some patients are first discovered to have such defects when pregnant. During pregnancy, right-sided and left-sided resistance decreases in a similar manner; therefore the degree of shunting is not significantly altered. Small defects are usually associated with a good pregnancy outcome. In patients who have developed pulmonary hypertension that has led to shunt reversal, as in Eisenmenger syndrome, maternal mortality rates of up to 50 percent have been reported. During pregnancy, left to right shunting may be increased following the expected increases in intravascular volume and cardiac output.

Ventricular Septal Defect. Small VSDs often close spontaneously in early life, and large defects discovered in childhood are most often surgically repaired. The small group of patients with uncorrected large VSDs are themselves growth retarded and may experience frequent respiratory infections.

Patients with small VSDs generally tolerate pregnancy well. The degree of left to right shunting is not significantly altered if baseline pulmonary vascular resistance is normal. Hemodynamic changes of pregnancy, including an increased circulating blood volume and tachycardia, may, however, increase left to right shunting to a critical level. Once pulmonary vascular resistance rises, right ventricular failure develops and reverse shunting with cyanosis may occur.

Increases in systemic vascular resistance, which accompany the stress of labor, may increase the degree of left to right shunting. Continuous epidural anesthesia is an effective method to relieve pain and lower systemic resistance. However, recognition that lowering of systemic pressure may not be tolerated by all patients is essential. Women with significant pulmonary hypertension exhibit a right to left shunt, and a further fall in arterial P_{O_2} will occur if systemic vascular resistance is markedly reduced. During labor, the development of cyanosis while a good cardiac output is maintained signals right to left shunting. Oxygen should be administered and steps taken to increase vascular resistance. A Swan-Ganz catheter should be inserted, if not already in place. During labor and delivery, patients with VSDs do require antibiotic prophylaxis. Careful newborn assessment of the offspring of affected mothers has revealed a 4 percent incidence of VSDs.[13]

Atrial Septal Defect. ASD is the most common congenital heart lesion found in the adult population. Interatrial shunting produces greater pulmonary blood flow relative to the systemic circulation. This change is generally well tolerated, unless pulmonary hypertension is present. Young women with an ASD are often asymptomatic or may experience mild fatigue. Atrial arrhythmias, pulmonary hypertension, and right-sided failure are complications that are not observed until the fourth or fifth decade of life.

No specific therapy is required in this group of pregnant women. Prophylactic antibiotics are often administered, although the risk of bacterial endocarditis is low, and routine anticoagulation is not recommended. Uncomplicated patients may be managed during labor and delivery without invasive monitoring. Epidural anesthesia is a well-accepted analgesic technique. It avoids marked increases in systemic vascular resistance that would augment left to right shunting.[23]

In advanced cases of ASD, shunting increases during pregnancy, right and left atrial pressure may rise, and atrial distention worsens. Associated supraventricular arrhythmias may then occur. Eventually, marked increases in pulmonary blood flow produce a rise in pulmonary vascular resistance, which leads to right-sided heart failure. These patients will require more intensive monitoring during pregnancy, labor, and delivery. Treatment to correct arrhythmias should be immediately instituted. With dysfunctional atrial contractions, incomplete atrial emptying occurs, increasing the potential for shunting. Hypotension may follow. Supraventricular tachycardia that acutely results in cardiac failure or hypotension is best treated with direct current cardioversion. Digitalization may also be necessary.

Patent Ductus Arteriosus. Most patients with PDA have their lesion corrected during childhood. As with an ASD, patients with a small ductus usually have a benign clinical course until middle age. Young patients will tolerate pregnancy well and specifically require only antibiotic prophylaxis during labor and delivery.

Large PDAs are associated with growth retardation, chronic respiratory infections, and congestive heart failure during childhood and early adulthood. These patients develop pulmonary hypertension that is associated with significant mortality during gestation.[20]

The increase in left ventricular volume and work that accompanies pregnancy results in left-sided failure, which further exacerbates preexisting pulmonary congestion. For this reason, therapeutic termination of pregnancy is generally indicated if significant right to left shunting is detected early in gestation.

Right to Left Shunts

Tetralogy of Fallot. Tetralogy of Fallot, a congenital anomaly, consists of right ventricular outflow obstruction, VSD, right ventricular hypertrophy, and an overriding aorta. Right to left shunting is usually present, resulting in cyanosis. In the past, patients with uncorrected tetralogy of Fallot rarely lived past childhood, making pregnancy with this condition extremely uncommon. Spontaneous abortions and intrauterine growth retardation were frequently observed.

The outcome for these patients has improved remarkably following corrective surgery. Singh et al.[26] reported 31 pregnancies in 27 patients with completely corrected lesions. All of these pregnancies ended in live births at term, and few maternal complications were reported. There was, however, a 20 percent incidence of growth retardation in the infants studied. Only one neonate was detected to have pulmonary atresia. Few maternal complications were reported in the study group.

Whittemore et al.[18] have confirmed both the safety and the improved outcome in pregnancy in patients with corrected cyanotic lesions. They reported an overall 78 percent live birth rate versus 55 percent in the uncorrected group. Cardiovascular complications were more common in the cyanotic group, although overall the incidence of congestive failure was low. Palliative surgery for tetralogy was also effective, and 13 of 18 pregnancies in these patients resulted in a liveborn infant.[18]

As many as 40 percent of patients with an uncorrected tetralogy will experience cardiac failure during pregnancy. Thus the uncorrected lesion can present a challenge to both the cardiologist and obstetrician. Symptoms of left-sided heart failure and endocarditis should be carefully reviewed. Obstetric management includes monitoring to detect possible fetal growth retardation. Cyanosis has been associated with miscarriage and preterm birth in these patients.

During labor and delivery, invasive monitoring will permit the prompt recognition of cardiac failure. The increase in cardiac output observed during labor may raise pulmonary vascular tone and increase shunting to the left side of the heart. Venous return should be carefully maintained, because a fall in blood volume may limit the ability of the right ventricular to perfuse the lungs. This will also depend on the degree of right ventricular obstruction. Continuous delivery of oxygen to the cyanotic mother is recommended.

In these patients, relief of pain during labor and delivery is best managed with systemic medications, inhalation analgesia, or pudendal block. Epidural or spinal anesthesia should be employed with caution because of the potential for hypotension resulting from decreases in vascular resistance and venous return. Ephedrine should be carefully administered in patients with right-sided failure, as it may produce a rise in pulmonary vascular resistance. In most cases, general anesthesia is preferred for cesarean section.

Complications may arise in the postpartum period, particularly if maternal blood volume is contracted. As systemic resistance falls, right to left shunting will be increased, and cyanosis will worsen. For this reason, it is essential that blood be made available for these patients.

Eisenmenger Syndrome. Eisenmenger syndrome is defined as right to left or bidirectional shunting at either the atrial or ventricular level, combined with elevated pulmonary vascular resistance. Maternal mortality ranges from 12 to 70 percent, and fetal mortality approaches 50 percent.[20] Gleicher et al.[27] have reported that at least 30 percent of fetuses will be growth retarded. Because of these risks, termination of pregnancy is strongly recommended in patients with Eisenmenger syndrome complicated by significant pulmonary hypertension.

The amount of right to left shunting observed in patients with this disorder will be dependent on the degree of pulmonary hypertension present. It will also be affected by the relationship between pulmonary and systemic vascular resistances. Right ventricular failure will also limit pulmonary blood flow and may increase right to left shunting.

These considerations make it imperative that Swan-Ganz monitoring be employed for management during labor and delivery. Efforts should be made to avoid central hypovolemia. This includes the use of uterine displacement to ensure adequate venous return to the heart. Controversy exists regarding the use of epidural anesthesia in patients with Eisenmenger syndrome. Theoretically, a fall in systemic vascular resistance could result in greater right to left shunting and cyanosis. Midwall and associates,[28] however, failed to demonstrate a change in shunt flow or pulmonary resistance in a single patient treated with epidural analgesia during labor and delivery. In that case report, oxygen proved to be an effective pulmonary vasodilator and resulted in increased peripheral oxygen saturation. Abboud and coworkers[29] have described the use of epidural morphine in a patient with pulmonary hypertension. This technique provides good analgesia with little effect on systemic blood pressure. Because the degree of pulmonary vascular reactivity probably varies in patients with Eisenmenger syndrome, it is best to make serial determinations of arterial oxygen concentrations when administering epidural anesthesia. Patients who manifest a fall in Po_2 despite oxygen support should probably not be managed with this anesthetic technique.

Coarctation of the Aorta

Patients with severe coarctation usually have their defect surgically corrected during infancy. Therefore, this lesion is infrequently encountered in pregnant women. Early studies reported a maternal mortality rate of 17 percent. Fortunately, maternal death is now a rare complication of this lesion.[30]

Patients at greatest risk are those with associated cardiac lesions or aneurysms of the aorta or circle of Willis. Classically, coarctation is recognized when a large difference in blood pressure is found between measurements in the upper extremities and legs. Because the constriction is often located at the level of the left subclavian artery, there may be isolated hypertension when blood pressure is determined in the right arm.

The risk of aortic dissection is probably overstated. However, antihypertensive therapy probably reduces whatever risk is present.[31] In suspected cases of dissection, vaginal delivery is not advised.

If significant obstruction of the aorta is present, left ventricular compromise may be exacerbated during pregnancy. Stroke volume is relatively fixed in these patients, so that normal compensatory mechanisms such as tachycardia may not be sufficient to maintain an adequate cardiac output. Hypotension during labor and postpartum should therefore be avoided. Appropriate precautions should be taken against infective endocarditis.

Surgical repair during pregnancy should be limited to cases of aortic dissection. Neurologic symptoms should be carefully elevated as well. It is not uncommon to find cerebral berry aneurysms in association with coarctation of the aorta. The risk that the newborn will also have this cardiac lesion is approximately 2 percent.[13]

Developmental Cardiac Lesions

Marfan Syndrome

Marfan syndrome is an autosomal dominant disorder of connective tissue marked by joint deformities, arachnodactyly, dislocations of the ocular lens, and cardiac manifestations, including weakness of the aortic root and wall. Mitral valve prolapse is found in 90 percent of cases. The prevalence of Marfan syndrome is 4 to 6 per 100,000. Certain families with Marfan syndrome appear to have formed frustes of this condition, in which there are significant skeletal deformities present in the absence of disease of the aorta or aortic valve.[32]

Patients with Marfan syndrome must receive genetic counseling and be made aware of the risks of pregnancy with their particular condition. The variability in the clinical expression of this disorder makes it imperative to study the cardiovascular system of these patients before counseling them about the dangers of pregnancy. Ultrasonographic measurement of the width of the aorta has been helpful in selecting patients at greatest risk for aortic dissection, although serial measurements of aortic root diameter may occasionally fail to detect a patient at risk for

dissection.[33] Pyeritz[34] has suggested that dilatation of the aorta greater than 40 mm is a contraindication to pregnancy. He reviewed 26 pregnancies complicated by Marfan syndrome in which there was only one maternal death. This resulted from endocarditis in a woman who had congestive heart failure and mitral insufficiency before conception. A review of the literature in that report substantiates that the mortality rate of up to 50 percent that has been associated with Marfan disease in pregnancy reflects cases in which significant maternal cardiovascular disease existed prior to conception.

Aortic dissection occurs frequently during pregnancy and may be influenced by superimposed hypertension. Symptoms of dissection include excruciating chest pain that migrates posteriorly. Occasionally, painless dissection is encountered that may be accompanied by hypertension and tachycardia. Hypotension follows if the dissection is large or if it ruptures. With ascending aortic arch involvement, a loud murmur of aortic insufficiency may be auscultated. Emergency surgical correction is required in patients with progressive dissection.

The management of patients with Marfan disease includes efforts to minimize both the hypertension and the contractile force transmitted to the aortic wall. β-Blockade using propranolol may be efficacious. Regional anesthesia for labor and delivery is generally well tolerated. If a patient requires surgical treatment for her cardiovascular disease, delivery by cesarean section is recommended. Cardiac surgery is preferably performed at a later date.[35] When administering general anesthesia, avoidance of agents that promote hypertension during induction is recommended. Antibiotic prophylaxis is suggested during labor and delivery.

Mitral Valve Prolapse

Mitral valve prolapse (MVP) is the most common congenital heart lesion found in young women of childbearing age. The incidence in the general population is approximately 7 percent. While there appears to be a genetic predisposition influencing development of this lesion, no clear pattern of inheritance exists. Histologic examination of the mitral valve leaflets reveals myxomatous degeneration. MVP is associated with skeletal deformities including pectus excavatum and a high-arched palate and is observed in Marfan syndrome, as noted above, and in Ehler-Danlos syndrome.

Most women with MVP have uneventful pregnancies. Rayburn and Fontana[36] reviewed the outcome of 42 pregnancies among 25 patients diagnosed by auscultatory and echocardiographic findings. In their series, cardiovascular complications were limited to one case of congestive heart failure that occurred in a preeclamptic patient treated with intravenous β-mimetics as well as glucocorticoids.

Debate still exists as to whether routine antibiotic prophylaxis is warranted during pregnancy in patients with MVP. Sugrue et al.[37] have advised that antibiotics are not necessary in most patients undergoing routine vaginal delivery. Other authors suggest treating only those patients who have mitral regurgitation. However, in pregnancy, defining a normal physiologic ejection murmur may not be possible, particularly in patients presenting during labor and delivery. Moreover, the click and murmur of MVP may vary with both left ventricular volume and contractility. Therefore, because of the relative safety of therapy, it is recommended that prophylactic antibiotics be administered until this issue is further resolved.

Idiopathic Hypertrophic Subaortic Stenosis

IHSS or asymmetric septal hypertrophy (ASH) is an autosomal dominant cardiac lesion that exhibits variable penetrance. As such, genetic counseling should be undertaken in affected individuals. Prenatal ultrasonographic diagnosis has been reported.[38] IHSS manifests as obstruction to left ventricular flow secondary to a hypertrophied interventricular septum and outflow tract. The symptoms at presentation with this lesion include dyspnea, angina, and syncope.

During ventricular systole, contraction of the myocardium results in narrowing of the outflow tract. Conditions that increase left ventricular end-diastolic volume will improve this condition. Pregnancy, which is marked by an increased circulating blood volume, may initially result in improvement in outflow tract obstruction. As gestation advances, the fall in systemic vascular resistance and diminished preload because of reduced venous return resulting from compression of the vena cava may exacerbate the symptoms found in patients with IHSS. Complications arising in pregnancy include ventricular failure

and supraventricular tachycardias.[39] These may be found in association with left atrial distention resulting from coexisting mitral regurgitation. Only one maternal death has been reported in a patient with IHSS.[40]

Management of patients with IHSS should include (1) avoidance of inotropic agents such as digitalis, which may exacerbate obstruction and precipitate failure; (2) maintenance of the left lateral decubitus position during labor; (3) restriction of the use of diuretics or drugs that decrease systemic vascular resistance; and (4) prompt recognition and treatment of arrhythmias.[41] Kolibash et al.[41] have suggested that β-blockade can be helpful when symptoms arise during pregnancy or labor. They advocated the use of forceps to minimize Valsalva efforts that might increase outflow obstruction.[41]

Other Cardiac Diseases

Peripartum Cardiomyopathy

Peripartum cardiomyopathy has classically been defined as congestive failure with cardiomyopathy found in the last month of pregnancy or in the first 5 months postpartum.[42,43] Symptoms of left-sided failure occur in association with a dilated hypocontractile heart in patients who have no previous history of cardiac disease. The overwhelming majority (82 percent) of patients present with cardiac symptoms in the first 3 months postpartum.[42] Most reports have documented the higher frequency of this lesion among older black multiparas.

The etiology of this disease is unknown despite multiple theories suggesting an autoimmune process, viral infections, and genetic predisposition. Histologic examination of the myocardium reveals muscular hypertrophy surrounded by interstitial edema and chronic inflammatory infiltrate.[44] These findings, which are suggestive of an infectious or immune-mediated myocarditis, have led investigators to believe that an acute viral infection possibly from Coxsackie B virus may be responsible for this disorder.[45] Melvin and associates[45] studied endomyocardial biopsy material obtained from three patients with postpartum congestive cardiomyopathy and found acute myocardial inflammatory changes. Two of the patients had histories of influenza-like infections, and one patient had antibody to Coxsackie B virus. The investigators postulated that viral myocardial infections could trigger an autoimmune myocarditis. They therefore treated these patients with steroids and azathioprine and later found that two of the patients had no residual fibrosis on biopsy. This management should probably be restricted to cases in which the diagnosis has been established by endomyocardial biopsy.

Primary therapy of peripartum cardiomyopathy should include bed rest, sodium restriction, digitalis, and diuretics.[46] Thromboembolic complications stemming from mural thrombi are not uncommon. Anticoagulation may be necessary, particularly in patients with massively enlarged cardiac chambers.

It is generally accepted that the clinical course of this disease can be predicted by the size of the heart several months after the diagnosis has been made. Approximately 50 percent of affected women will continue to have symptoms of failure and cardiomegaly beyond 6 months. These women should be advised against pregnancy because the incidence of recurrent disease is high, with mortality rates approaching 100 percent. In those with normal heart size, there still remains a risk for temporary worsening of cardiac function during pregnancy. Based on data from two studies, persistent cardiomegaly has been associated with a 5-year mortality rate exceeding 50 percent.[42,43]

Ischemic Cardiac Disease

Coronary artery disease is uncommon in women during the reproductive years. However, more women are delaying childbearing and more are smoking. For these reasons, the frequency of ischemic cardiac disease during pregnancy may be increasing. The incidence of myocardial infarction during pregnancy has been estimated to be 1 in 10,000.[47] This is likely to be an overestimate, as Hankins and colleagues[48] could document only 68 cases in the literature published prior to 1985. Arterial hypertension has been documented in one-third of women who suffer a myocardial infarction during pregnancy; however, mortality rates for these women do not appear to be greater than those without an elevation in blood pressure.[49] Whereas cigarette smoking and diabetes mellitus are other recognized risk factors for atherosclerosis, maternal age exceeding 35 years is the most consistent characteristic in pregnant women suffering a myocardial infarction.[48]

Coronary atherosclerosis is the predominant finding in pregnant women with a myocardial infarction; however, other causes of limited coronary blood flow can be observed. Coronary artery spasm and embolism may also limit oxygen availability to the myocardium and can produce angina as well as infarction. Beary et al.[50] noted normal coronary anatomy in two of five women who sustained an infarction and subsequently underwent coronary angiography during the postpartum period.

Chest pain suggesting myocardial ischemia requires medical attention, even in seemingly low-risk pregnant women. Anginal episodes should be evaluated with electrocardiography and exercise stress testing if clinical suspicion is high. Thallium nucleotide imaging of coronary blood flow is generally not performed during pregnancy because of the associated radiation exposure (estimated 780 mrad) with this procedure.[51] Two-dimensional echocardiography may be of some value in detecting wall motion abnormalities during chest pain. If myocardial ischemia is strongly suggested, then interruption of pregnancy should be considered. In women at less than 24 weeks gestation, this may provide rapid symptomatic improvement.[49] If pregnancy is continued and symptoms do not abate with cessation of smoking and prescribed rest, then medical therapy to prevent coronary artery spasm including nitrates, β-adrenergics, or calcium channel blockers should be initiated. Repeated severe anginal episodes may necessitate coronary angiography with consideration for angioplasty or even bypass surgery during pregnancy.[52]

Myocardial infarction is usually suggested by prolonged chest pain associated with diaphoresis, nausea, and dyspnea. It may or may not be related to physical exertion. Electrocardiographic changes and a rise in the serum creatine phosphokinase MB fraction have been documented in most cases during gestation.[48] Approximately two-thirds of women have had their infarction during the third trimester. In these women, the mortality rate has been reported to be 45 percent compared with 23 percent suffering an infarction during the first two trimesters.[48] Hankins and colleagues[48] have reported that approximately 20 percent of pregnant women die at the time of infarction, and mortality occurs in 50 percent of patients who deliver within 2 weeks of the event. In contrast, these investigators found no deaths among 34 women without recurrent infarction who delivered more than 2 weeks postinfarction. Unexplained fetal death was reported in five of these cases. The preponderance of infarctions during the third trimester and the increased risk of maternal mortality when delivery occurs within 2 weeks of infarction suggest that the hemodynamic burdens of late pregnancy and delivery are particularly hazardous to women with coronary artery disease.

The management of myocardial infarction during pregnancy is essentially the same as in the nonpregnant individual. Patients are admitted to the coronary or medical intensive care unit. Oxygen is administered, and pain should be minimized. Careful observation is undertaken for signs of congestive failure, arrhythmias, and further chest pain. These complications warrant consideration of pregnancy termination in women at less than 24 weeks gestation. As stated above, an effort should be made to allow a period of healing and recovery before initiating labor. In women with no symptoms, pregnancy can be allowed to progress to fetal maturity. During labor and delivery, pain should be minimized to decrease myocardial oxygen consumption. Conduction anesthesia is recommended and may reduce the normal anticipated increase in cardiac output.[48] Cesarean section is reserved for obstetric indications, as it does not improve maternal survival rates. There is continued debate as to whether women with a previous myocardial infarction should attempt pregnancy. Careful evaluation including thallium scanning and angiography may identify women at greatest risk, although there is insufficient data available with which to counsel this group of patients.

PULMONARY DISEASE

Tuberculosis

Tuberculosis is a pulmonary infection caused by the acid-fast bacillus *Mycobacterium tuberculosis*. There has been a decline in the frequency of tuberculosis in the United States over the past 50 years. Most obstetricians do not consider this diagnosis when a pregnant patient presents with lethargy and respiratory symptoms. However, as more women enter the United States from developing nations, there has been a resurgence of tuberculosis in the pregnant population, primarily in urban areas.

Pregnancy should not be a deterrent to the accurate diagnosis and treatment of tuberculosis. Tuberculin skin testing with subcutaneous administration of intermediate strength purified protein derivative (PPD) is the mainstay of testing for tuberculosis in the United States. This method, however, has several drawbacks. Only 80 percent of patients with a reactivation of tuberculosis will have positive skin tests. In addition, any patient who has previously received the bacillus Calmette-Guérin (BCG) vaccine will retain a positive tuberculin skin test for life. Although this vaccine is rarely used in the United States, it is administered routinely in countries where tuberculosis is endemic.

If a differential diagnosis of tuberculosis is entertained in a patient presenting with respiratory symptoms and lethargy, a chest x-ray with abdominal shielding should be obtained without hesitation. A chest x-ray should also be taken without delay if the patient's previously negative tuberculin skin test becomes positive, if it cannot be determined when a patient's skin test became positive, or if a patient has persistent respiratory or constitutional symptoms.[53] Many obstetricians are fearful and hesitate too long before obtaining chest x-rays during pregnancy. Without abdominal shielding, the radiation exposure to the fetus from a single chest x-ray is minimal, approximately 2.5 mrad. With abdominal shielding, the exposure is even less.[54,55] Nonetheless, chest x-rays should be delayed until after the first trimester if there is not a pressing indication.

The definitive diagnosis of tuberculosis is based on identifying *Mycobacterium tuberculosis* by culture or acid-fast stain of the sputum. First-morning sputum specimens obtained on 3 consecutive days are usually the best source for cultures and stain. If the patient is not able to produce a sputum sample voluntarily, production can be elicited by having the patient inhale aerosolized hypertonic saline. Any patient having a positive smear for acid-fast bacilli should be started on antituberculous chemotherapy while awaiting the results of cultures and drug sensitivity tests. One must often wait up to 6 weeks before final culture results are available.

When adequate treatment is implemented, tuberculosis appears to have no adverse effect on pregnancy, and, conversely, pregnancy does not alter the natural history of the disease.[56-58] One controversial study did find a 10-fold increase in spontaneous first-trimester pregnancy losses in patients with active tuberculosis.[59] In that study, however, the control group had a first-trimester miscarriage rate of only 2 percent, which is excessively low. Early in this century, abortion was recommended for patients with tuberculosis. Current data, however, strongly suggest that there is no maternal or fetal indication for pregnancy termination in the gravida with tuberculosis.

Highly effective chemotherapeutic agents have been developed for the treatment of tuberculosis (Table 31.3). Although the prognosis for tuberculosis during pregnancy is excellent, severe complications such as miliary, renal, and meningeal tuberculosis have developed.[60] Tuberculosis should therefore be taken seriously whenever it is diagnosed. Current standard therapy is isoniazid in a single daily dose of 300 mg and ethambutol in a dose of 15 mg/kg/day. This therapy should be continued for 18 to 24 months. Shorter courses of isoniazid and rifampin have been approved for use in pulmonary tuberculosis. The efficacy of this therapy during pregnancy, however, has not been statistically verified.[61]

Isoniazid prophylaxis is often recommended for patients under the age of 35 years who have recently converted their tuberculin skin test but do not have active disease and do have normal liver function. Such prophylaxis is discouraged during pregnancy but may be begun during the postpartum period. The major adverse effects of isoniazid include toxic hepatitis, peripheral neuropathy, and hypersensitivity reactions. Transient elevations of the serum transaminases are seen in approximately 20 percent of patients. Transaminase levels should therefore be monitored monthly. If they reach five times the upper limit of normal, the drug should be discontinued. If these guidelines are followed, serious isoniazid hepatitis can be avoided.[62]

Peripheral neuropathy appears to be related to a deficiency of pyridoxine, vitamin B_6. Patients taking isoniazid should receive a 20 to 50 mg supplement of pyridoxine daily to prevent this complication. Hypersensitivity reactions to isoniazid may take the form of an antinuclear antibody–positive, drug-induced systemic lupus erythematosus. Other less serious hypersensitivity manifestations may also be seen. Isoniazid has been studied extensively during pregnancy, and there appears to be no increase in congenital malformations.[63] Only one study noted a small excess of nonspecific congenital anomalies in patients taking this drug, but certainly no associated syndrome was observed.[64]

Ethambutol also appears safe for use during gestation and has not been associated with an increase in congenital anomalies.[63] In doses higher than those usually recommended (> 15 mg/kg/day), ethambutol can produce retrobulbar neuritis. This finding has not been observed in abortuses or in neonates of mothers receiving this medication.[65,66]

If possible, streptomycin should be avoided during pregnancy. In one report, more than 10 percent of the offspring of patients treated with streptomycin during pregnancy showed damage to cranial nerve VIII.[63] While other studies have also shown severe hearing loss as well as abnormal caloric tests and audiograms, none has found auditory nerve damage in

Table 31.3 Antituberculosis Agents

Drug	Dosage	Maternal Side Effects
Isoniazid	300 mg/day (single dose)	Toxic hepatitis, peripheral neuropathy (prevented with pyridoxine)
Ethambutol	15 mg/kg/day (single dose)	Optic neuritis
p-Aminosalicylic acid (PAS)	10–12 g/day (2 or 3 divided doses)	Gastrointestinal disturbance
Rifampin	600 mg/day (single dose)	Orange discoloration of body secretions, gastrointestinal disturbance, liver toxicity
Streptomycin	15 mg/kg/day (single dose)	Cranial nerve VIII toxicity, nephrotoxicity

as many as 10 percent of cases.[67] Drug levels were not meticulously monitored in the patients in those studies.

Rifampin inhibits DNA-dependent RNA polymerase. It readily crosses the placenta and could theoretically injure the fetus. One study reported a 3 to 4 percent incidence of severe congenital malformations associated with the use of rifampin during pregnancy.[63] This figure, however, is not significantly higher than the expected background rate of malformations. Nevertheless, rifampin should be used with caution during gestation and only when isoniazid and ethambutol cannot be given or when drug resistance is encountered.

p-Aminosalicylic acid (PAS) was once commonly used during pregnancy. Because it is associated with severe gastrointestinal side effects, it is no longer recommended for the gravida who is already prone to nausea and vomiting. Its use has not been associated with congenital malformations.

Transplacental passage of tuberculosis is extremely rare. Most perinatal infections occur when a mother with active tuberculosis handles her neonate.[67a] The risk to the child of contracting tuberculosis from a mother with active disease during the first year of life may be as high as 50 percent.[68] Daily administration of isoniazid chemoprophylaxis can be given to the newborn for the length of the mother's treatment.[69] This therapy, however, requires a great deal of compliance and motivation on the part of the parent to make certain that the child receives the medication. Another alternative is to administer BCG vaccine to the neonate.[68] After vaccination, the child must then be separated from the mother until it develops a positive PPD skin test. This approach, however, has the drawback of rendering the child tuberculin positive for life.

Sarcoidosis

Sarcoidosis is a granulomatous disease that can involve many organ systems. It most commonly affects the lungs and lymph nodes but may also affect the skin, eyes, liver, central nervous system, and heart. The hallmark histologic finding is the noncaseating granuloma. While the etiology of the disease is unknown, patients demonstrate excessive immunoglobulin levels and impaired delayed hypersensitivity, suggesting an immune cause. The disease is most commonly diagnosed between the ages of 20 and 40 years. The usual clinical presentation includes symmetric bilateral hilar lymphadenopathy discovered on a routine chest x-ray and palpable cervical adenopathy. The differential diagnosis must include Hodgkin's disease, other lymphomas, and tuberculosis. The only method for definitive diagnosis is lymph node biopsy usually performed during bronchoscopy or mediastinoscopy. In more advanced cases of sarcoidosis, there is a constant nonproductive cough and interstitial pulmonary disease. The Kveim test is positive in most patients with sarcoidosis presenting with lymph adenopathy. This test, however, is rarely used today and is mentioned here for historical purposes. Most patients with sarcoidosis will also have abnormal levels of angiotensin-converting enzyme.

Many patients with sarcoidosis require no treatment. Approximately two-thirds will improve spontaneously within 2 to 3 years of the initial diagnosis. These women usually have no clinical evidence of disease and only minor residual findings on chest x-ray. Of the remaining patients, most will experience a slow progression of the disease over many years with both exacerbations and remissions. Very few will suffer a rapid downhill course. It has been estimated that 0.05 percent of pregnancies are associated with sarcoidosis.[69] This means that in a large hospital that delivers 5,000 infants annually, two or three pregnant women may have sarcoidosis.

Pregnancy has no long-term adverse effect on the course of sarcoidosis. Similarly, sarcoidosis does not have a deleterious effect on perinatal outcome in asymptomatic patients. Therefore, sarcoidosis is not a contraindication to pregnancy. Most patients appear to improve during gestation.[70-72] This amelioration may be due to increased circulating levels of cortisol. During the puerperium, however, there may be a relapse of the illness, but such relapses are usually not serious.[72,73] In a recent paper, Haynes de Regt[74] reviewed 15 cases of proven sarcoidosis during a 10-year period at Downstate Medical Center. Eleven patients remained stable during pregnancy, while two experienced progression of the disease and two others died of complications. Factors that appear to indicate a poor prognosis included pulmonary parenchymal lesions on chest x-ray, advanced roentgenologic staging, advanced maternal age, low inflammatory activity, requirement of drugs other than steroids, and the presence of extrapulmonary sarcoidosis.[74]

In patients with known sarcoidosis, an attempt must be made early in gestation to identify renal or hepatic involvement. A recent report highlights a case in which sarcoidosis first presented as acute renal failure during pregnancy.[75] This evaluation should include a 24-hour urine collection for creatinine clearance and total protein excretion, liver function studies, and an ECG. Any patient presenting with an unknown skin rash and pulmonary symptoms should be evaluated for the possibility of sarcoidosis, as a recent case report demonstrated that sarcoidosis first appeared as pruritic white papules in a pregnant woman.[76] The pregnant patient with sarcoidosis should also undergo pulmonary function testing early in pregnancy and again near term. Arterial blood gas evaluation is necessary only when clinically indicated.

When medical treatment is necessary, glucocorticoids are the mainstay for sarcoidosis. Progressive deterioration of pulmonary function testing is the major indication for corticosteroids. Patients are usually started on 60 mg of prednisone daily. The dose is tapered once a remission has been established. During pregnancy, the amount of corticosteroid can often be reduced because of the aforementioned increased levels of circulating cortisol. The risk of postpartum relapse, however, requires that these women receive parenteral steroids during labor and increased doses of steroids immediately after delivery.

Pneumonia

Most bacterial pneumonia in pregnant women is due to *Streptococcus pneumoniae*. Most of these patients are smokers.[77] The clinical hallmarks of pneumococcal pneumonia include sudden onset, productive cough, purulent sputum, tachypnea, and shaking chills. The diagnosis should be made on the basis of chest x-ray, Gram stain of the sputum, and cultures of blood and sputum. The chest x-ray usually reveals lobar consolidation and air bronchograms. Gram stain shows numerous leukocytes and gram-positive diplococci.

Patients with pneumococcal pneumonia complicating pregnancy should be hospitalized and receive 600,000 units of aqueous penicillin G intravenously four times daily. Parenteral treatment should continue for several days after defervescence. The ther-

apy can then be changed to an oral penicillin or ampicillin (500 mg four times daily). The treatment should be continued for a total of 10 to 14 days. For patients who are allergic to penicillin, either a cephalosporin or erythromycin can be used. It should be noted, however, that 10 to 15 percent of patients who are allergic to penicillin will also react to cephalosporins. A vaccine consisting of the capsular antigens from *S. pneumoniae* has been used to prevent pneumococcal infections. Its effects on the pregnant patient, however, are unknown. Therefore it should not be used during pregnancy except in special circumstances, such as the patient about to undergo splenectomy.[78] In this instance, the benefit outweighs the risk.

Mycoplasma pneumonia is caused by *Mycoplasma pneumoniae,* a small organism lacking a cell wall. It therefore does not respond to therapy with penicillin or cephalosporins. This form of pneumonia is common in young adults. In contrast to the sudden onset of pneumococcal pneumonia, patients with mycoplasma pneumonia usually have a slow, gradual onset of symptoms with a nonproductive cough. The diagnosis is usually made clinically. On chest x-ray, infiltrates are diffuse and patchy and can be either unilateral or bilateral. Complement-fixing antibodies to mycoplasma and the presence of cold agglutinins can be used to confirm the clinical diagnosis of this disease. One must consider the diagnosis of mycoplasma pneumonia in any patient whose clinical symptoms are not responding to penicillin or to cephalosporins. During pregnancy, the treatment of mycoplasma pneumonia consists of the administration of erythromycin for 10 to 14 days. Tetracycline and its derivatives should be avoided.

Even with improved technology and antibiotics, Madinger and co-workers[79] feel that the maternal and fetal outcomes are not considerably improving in patients with pneumonia. They retrospectively reviewed 25 cases of pneumonia during pregnancy that occurred among 32,179 deliveries. Medical complications included bacteremia in 16 percent, empyema in 8 percent, atrial fibrillation in 4 percent, and respiratory failure necessitating intubation and ventilation in 20 percent. Preterm labor occurred in 44 percent of the patients and preterm delivery in 36 percent. One patient with cystic fibrosis died. Perinatal mortality included one stillbirth and two neonatal deaths. There is a significant correlation between underlying maternal disease, maternal medical complications, and preterm delivery in the gravida with pneumonia.[79]

Asthma

Asthma is the most common obstructive pulmonary disease that coexists with pregnancy. It is observed in 0.4 to 1.3 percent of pregnant women.[80,81] A study at Johns Hopkins Hospital reported a 1 percent incidence of asthma complicating pregnancy and a 0.15 percent incidence of severe asthma during gestation requiring hospitalization.[82] Pregnancy can have a varying effect on the course of asthma. Data compiled from nine studies published between 1953 and 1976 revealed that 49 percent of pregnant patients had no change in the course of their asthma, 29 percent showed improvement, and 22 percent showed exacerbation of their disease.[83–86] A more recent study from the United Kingdom demonstrated that asthma improved in 69 percent of pregnant women, worsened in 9 percent, and showed no change in 22 percent.[87] Juniper and colleagues[88] examined reasons for improvement of asthma during pregnancy. They studied airway compliance in asthmatic women at 3-month intervals prior to pregnancy and subsequently in each trimester of pregnancy. A twofold improvement in airway responsiveness during pregnancy was observed.[88] This improvement was not statistically related to changes in levels of progesterone or estriol.

Nonetheless, asthma continues to be a major problem for adolescents who become pregnant. Apter and co-investigators[89] studied 28 pregnancies in 21 adolescents at Northwestern University Medical School. There were 56 exacerbations of asthma, including 22 hospitalizations and 20 emergency room visits. In 64 percent of the pregnancies, systemic corticosteroids had to be administered on an inpatient or outpatient basis.[89] These investigators found that the two most frequent factors associated with exacerbations of asthma included respiratory tract infections (59 percent) and noncompliance with medical regimens (27 percent). Williams[90] noted that approximately one-third of patients with asthma reacted differently in subsequent pregnancies irrespective of the sex of the fetus.

Older studies have suggested that intrauterine growth retardation (IUGR), preterm birth, and peri-natal morbidity and mortality occurred more commonly in pregnancies associated with asthma.[86,91] No study demonstrates an increase in the rate of fetal malformations in the asthmatic patient. More recent data indicate that the risk of perinatal morbidity and mortality is minimally increased in the asthmatic patient, especially if adequate medical care is received. Sims and co-workers[92] observed a small increase in the number of small for gestational age newborns in mothers receiving oral steroid therapy. In the study of Apter et al.,[89] there was only one premature infant and no cases complicated by IUGR.

The goals in treating asthma during pregnancy are as follows: (1) reduction in the number of asthmatic attacks, (2) prevention of severe asthmatic attacks (status asthmaticus), and (3) assurance of adequate maternal and fetal oxygenation. Patients receiving allergen desensitization may continue this treatment throughout pregnancy.[93] The Centers for Disease Control (CDC) recommends that patients with chronic bronchial asthma receive yearly influenza immunization.[94] This is a killed vaccine and can be administered safely during pregnancy. The theophyllines, including aminophylline, remain the mainstay of therapy for the pregnant asthmatic. cAMP, which produces relaxation of the bronchi, is released when β_2-receptors are stimulated by agonists. cAMP is metabolized by phosphodiesterase. Theophyllines inhibit phosphodiesterase and therefore increase circulating levels of cAMP. Aminophylline crosses the placenta but has shown no harmful fetal effects.[95–97] Similarly, aminophylline will appear in breast milk but will not have significant effects on the neonate.

Many theophylline preparations are available. Elixirs are rapidly absorbed but must be taken often. Sustained-release capsules can be given two or three times daily but are absorbed more slowly. No single preparation holds an advantage over another. It is best for physicians to familiarize themselves with one or two preparations and use them. Smoking increases the clearance of aminophylline, and a higher dose will be needed in these patients. The goal of therapy is to keep the theophylline level between 10 and 20 μgm/ml at all times. A recent study by Gardner and co-workers[98] has shown that the clearance of theophylline during the first two trimesters of pregnancy was not significantly different from the clearance in nonpregnant women. In the third trimester, however, there was a statistically significant reduction in the clearance of theophylline. Theophylline clearance remained depressed even in the early postpartum period. It is important, therefore, to measure blood levels of theophylline at least monthly and to adjust the dosage accordingly. Levels should be checked more often in the third trimester. Theophylline toxicity is commonly manifested by nausea and vomiting, but increased levels of theophylline may also cause tachycardia and cardiac arrhythmias.

β-Sympathomimetic drugs are also indicated in the treatment of chronic bronchial asthma. These medications may be administered in the form of an inhaler or as an oral preparation. There is presently no evidence that β-mimetic drugs are teratogenic. Because most of these medications do not exhibit pure β_2-selectivity, cardiovascular side effects including tachycardia and arrhythmias are not unusual. Terbutaline is the most commonly prescribed oral β-mimetic agent. It is usually administered in a dosage of 2.5 to 5 mg four times daily in addition to a theophylline preparation. Aerosolized β-mimetic agents such as albuterol are more commonly used than are oral preparations. The aerosolized agents act locally and lack most systemic side effects.

Corticosteroids have an important role in the management of asthma during pregnancy. They should be administered without hesitation in patients who cannot be adequately managed using β-mimetic agents and theophylline preparations. Corticosteroid aerosols should be used whenever possible, as they are highly active topically but have little systemic activity. The most common side effect of corticosteroid aerosols, candidiasis of the upper airways and upper gastrointestinal tract, is observed in approximately 5 percent of patients.[99] It is more likely to occur with prolonged treatment and therefore should not be a problem if used only during pregnancy.

Systemic corticosteroids should be employed when the aerosolized forms are inadequate. Although administration of glucocorticoids to pregnant rabbits has been associated with cleft palate,[100] these medications are safe for use during pregnancy when indicated. In one literature review, 2 of 260 infants born to mothers taking steroids before 14 weeks gestation developed a cleft palate.[99] Many studies have since clearly demonstrated that the use of glucocorticoids is safe during gestation and is not associated with

congenital anomalies.[101-104] An increased incidence of IUGR in fetuses born to women taking 10 mg prednisone daily throughout pregnancy for a history of infertility has been reported.[105] Presumably these women were nonsmokers who did not have underlying chronic diseases that would be associated with IUGR.

Although fetal adrenal suppression may occur after maternal glucocorticoid ingestion, it is extremely rare. Schatz and colleagues[106] found no evidence of neonatal adrenal suppression in 71 infants born to mothers receiving a daily average of 8.2 mg of prednisone during gestation. In another report, neonatal adrenal insufficiency was not observed in infants whose mothers received up to 60 mg of prednisone daily throughout pregnancy.[107]

The lack of fetal and neonatal effects associated with maternal glucocorticoid ingestion is probably due to the small amount of administered glucocorticoid that actually reaches the fetal compartment. A fetus is exposed to only 10 to 30 percent of the prednisone ingested by the mother.[108,109] Most of the drug is inactivated by placental 11-β-ol-dehydrogenase. Of the small amount of prednisone that actually reaches the fetus, even a smaller fraction will be metabolized by the fetus to the active form of the drug, prednisolone. Ballard and co-workers[110] reported that one-sixth of a dose of hydrocortisone reaches the fetus and one-third of a dose of betamethasone enters the fetal circulation. It is apparent therefore that prednisone is the oral glucocorticoid of choice to treat maternal asthma while minimizing fetal exposure. When selecting a corticosteroid for use during pregnancy, it is important to look at the ratio of glucocorticoid to mineralocorticoid activity as well as the amount of drug that crosses the placenta. Methylprednisolone is an excellent choice. It has minimal mineralocorticoid effects and crosses the placenta poorly.

Status asthmaticus requires immediate therapeutic intervention. During this period of acute treatment, the patient should receive a 30 to 40 percent concentration of humidified oxygen, and she should be well hydrated. Subcutaneous catecholamines should be administered. Because it has both α- and β-agonist activity, epinephrine can theoretically decrease uterine blood flow and thus decrease fetal oxygenation during this critical period. In a pregnant sheep model, while epinephrine did reduce uterine blood flow, it did not impair fetal oxygenation. In humans, there is no evidence that using epinephrine for the treatment of acute asthma has deleterious effects on the fetus. Terbutaline, a β_2-agonist that is more selective than epinephrine, is a better first-line drug in pregnancy. In the emergent situation, however, epinephrine can be used if terbutaline is not immediately available. If the patient does not improve rapidly after the subcutaneous administration of catecholamines, intravenous aminophylline should be administered. In the patient who has not been taking an aminophylline preparation, a loading dose of 5 mg/kg should be given over 30 minutes followed by a maintenance infusion of 0.6 mg/kg hr. One must remember that individuals vary greatly in the rate at which they metabolize aminophylline. Blood levels must be determined frequently early in the course of intravenous therapy, and the infusion rate must be adjusted accordingly. Smokers metabolize aminophylline rapidly. Nebulized β-mimetic agents should also be administered during this time. Frequent assessment of arterial blood gases should be used to monitor the patient's response to therapy. If the patient does not improve over several hours, intravenous corticosteroids should be utilized. Methylprednisolone in a dose of 60 mg every 6 to 8 hours or hydrocortisone in a dose of 100 mg every 4 hours is usually administered until the asthma attack clears. In the unusual patient who is resistant to these measures and has a falling PO_2, endotracheal intubation should be considered. This procedure should only be undertaken under the guidance of a pulmonary specialist or anesthesiologist. Schreier and colleagues[111] reported two pregnant women who required intubation for respiratory failure complicating asthma during the third trimester. They demonstrated that maintenance of an adequate PO_2 was an essential component of therapy in these cases. In addition, they utilized a warm solution of metaproterenol in saline for bronchial irrigation and suction. They found that this served as a bronchoalveolar lavage and facilitated recovery.[111]

Acute asthma attacks are unusual during labor. Should they occur, however, they are treated in the usual fashion. Epidural anesthesia is preferred for labor, vaginal delivery, and cesarean section. General anesthesia carries the risks of atelectasis and subsequent chest infection.[112] If the patient has been receiving corticosteroids during pregnancy, increased dosages should be used for the stress of labor and delivery. Generally, 100 mg of hydrocortisone every 4 to 6 hours or 60 mg of methylprednisolone administered intravenously at 6- to 8-hour intervals during labor and for 24 hours after delivery should suffice. Thereafter the patient should resume her maintenance dose of oral glucocorticoids.

Pulmonary Embolus

Pulmonary embolus complicates between 0.09 and 0.7 per 1,000 pregnancies.[113,114] Prompt diagnosis and treatment are imperative as untreated pulmonary emboli during pregnancy carry a 12.8 percent mortality rate, while treatment lowers this to 0.7 percent.[115] If untreated, more than one-third of these patients will have recurrent emboli.[116] The vast majority of pulmonary emboli arise from thrombophlebitis of the deep femoral and pelvic veins. The reported incidence of deep venous thrombosis during pregnancy is 0.4 per 1,000.[113] This figure is six times more frequent than in nonpregnant women.[117]

It is now common for patients in preterm labor to be aggressively treated with prolonged bed rest and β-mimetic agents. This approach places these patients at increased risk for thrombophlebitis and pulmonary embolism. Gurz and Heiselman[118] report a case of a fatal pulmonary embolus that occurred during tocolysis. It is prudent therefore to administer prophylactic, low-dose heparin, to patients who are at prolonged bed rest.

The patient with an acute pulmonary embolus usually presents with chest pain and dyspnea. Occasionally, a pleural friction rub may be auscultated. The chest x-ray is often normal, but arterial blood gas values usually show a decreased PO_2 and a slightly more decreased PCO_2. Hypercapnea, however, bodes a poor outcome.[118] Massive pulmonary emboli are easily diagnosed. Hypotension and cardiovascular collapse often complicate such cases. In contrast, patients with small emboli may only have subtle signs and symptoms. It is imperative to establish the proper diagnosis in the patients, as these small clots may be the harbinger of a massive embolus. Two recent reports show that the sudden onset of blindness may be due to hypotension caused by pulmonary embolus in the absence of other symptoms.[119,120]

The diagnosis of pulmonary embolus must be established radiographically. Adequate technique is essential so that fetal exposure to ionizing radiation is minimized. Pulmonary perfusion and ventilation scans are useful in diagnosing pulmonary embolism only if the chest x-ray is normal. Calculations have shown that maximum fetal radiation exposure from this type of study is 50 mrem.[121] These isotopes are excreted through the maternal urinary tract. The fetus receives 85 percent of its radiation exposure from the maternal bladder. Brisk diuresis and frequent micturition should therefore theoretically lower fetal exposure.[121] If necessary, a Foley catheter can be used to empty the bladder.

If the ventilation/perfusion scan is equivocal or if the patient's chest x-ray is abnormal, selective pulmonary angiography should be immediately undertaken. In experienced hands, the procedure carries a morbidity of less than 1 percent. Abdominal shielding should be used during the procedure. The increased plasma volume and vasodilatation that occur during pregnancy should make the procedure faster and technically easier than in the nonpregnant patient. Ginsburg and colleagues[122] have carefully looked at radiation exposure from various procedures during pregnancy. Their review suggests that there is a small increase in the risk of childhood cancer following radiation exposures of less than 5 rads.[122] They feel that with careful use of available procedures, the diagnosis of venous thrombosis is possible with fetal exposure below 0.5 rads. Furthermore, in diagnosing pulmonary embolism, it is possible to keep fetal radiation exposure below 0.05 rads.[122] Because the risk to the fetus from such exposure is small in both relative and absolute terms, the diagnostic procedure should be undertaken without hesitation when necessary.

Once the diagnosis is established, therapy should be initiated without delay. Anticoagulation with heparin is the treatment of choice. Heparin, a large negatively charged protein with a molecular weight of 20,000 daltons, does not cross the placenta.[123] The main complication of heparin therapy is maternal bleeding. This can be reduced, however, with meticulous attention to dosage and frequent monitoring of the activated partial thromboplastin time (APTT). Hemorrhage, nevertheless, appears to complicate the course of between 8 and 33 percent of patients anticoagulated with heparin.[124] The anticoagulant activity of heparin can be quickly reversed with protamine sulfate. Other potential complications of hepa-

rin therapy include osteoporosis, alopecia, urticaria, bronchoconstriction secondary to histamine release, and profound thrombocytopenia.[125] Platelet counts should be checked twice weekly during the first 2 weeks of therapy and then monthly therafter, or immediately if signs of petechiae or purpura develop.

An initial heparin loading dose of 70 units/kg is administered intravenously, followed by a continuous infusion of 1,000 units per hour. This dose must be adjusted to keep the APTT approximately twice normal or the heparin titer at 0.2 to 0.4 units/ml. The required maintenance dose of heparin can show large interpatient variation. This regimen is continued for approximately 10 days in clinically stable patients.

For the remainder of pregnancy, patients should receive a moderate dose of subcutaneous heparin. A dose of 7,500 to 10,000 units of heparin administered every 8 to 12 hours is usually sufficient to keep the APTT about 1.5 times normal and the heparin titer approximately 0.1 to 0.2 units/ml.[126] Continuous subcutaneous pumps can also be used for this purpose on an outpatient basis. One must realize that the dosage must be individualized until the desired APTT is reached. With the increase in Factor VIII and most other coagulation factors that is normally seen in pregnancy, the subcutaneous dose may need to be increased rather frequently during gestation.[127] In the stable patient, therapy should be discontinued during labor and delivery but can be restarted several hours postpartum. During the postpartum period, the patient can be given coumadin, even if breast-feeding. Although coumadin does not appear in breast milk in significant amounts, its use during breast-feeding has been controversial. Anticoagulant therapy should be continued for 6 weeks postpartum, at which time coagulation factors should have returned to prepregnant levels.

Oral anticoagulants should not be used during gestation. These drugs are vitamin K antagonists that readily cross the placenta and are teratogenic when used in early pregnancy. In the first trimester, these drugs are associated with facial dysmorphisms, hypoplastic digits, stippled epiphyses, and mental retardation.[128-130] In midtrimester, optic atrophy, faulty brain development, and developmental retardation may occur.[128] In addition, the fetus is anticoagulated by these drugs which can result in severe fetal hemorrhage in the event of trauma or preterm labor.

Currently, heparin used throughout pregnancy appears to be safer than switching to oral anticoagulants during the second and early third trimesters. Even though it is more expensive and more inconvenient, the benefits of heparin therapy appear to outweigh the risks of using oral anticoagulants during gestation.

Recently, several studies have advocated the use of a surgical approach to thrombophlebitis and pulmonary emboli during pregnancy. Mogensen and co-workers[117] treated eight pregnant women with acute iliofemoral venous thrombosis by thrombectomy. All of the women did well and were treated with heparin postoperatively. These researchers surmised that even when thrombophlebitis occurs in early pregnancy there is no need for pregnancy termination. Blegvad and co-investigators[131] performed a pulmonary embolectomy successfully on a woman during the second trimester. The patient had severe right ventricular failure caused by obstruction of 85 percent of the pulmonary arterial circulation. Three months after embolectomy, she delivered a normal infant. Splinter and colleagues[132] report an open pulmonary embolectomy that was performed after cesarean section. Both mother and child recovered fully. In both cases, the embolectomy was carried out with the mother on cardiopulmonary bypass.[131,132] While these cases present interesting options, the role of surgical intervention in thromboembolic disease during pregnancy needs to be further delineated.

REFERENCES

1. Hibbard LT: Maternal mortality due to cardiac disease. Clin Obstet Gynecol 18:27, 1975
2. Scott DE: Anemia in pregnancy. Obstet Gynecol Annu 1:219, 1972
3. Chesley LC, Duffus GM: Posture and apparent plasma volume in late pregnancy. J Obstet Gynaecol Br Commonw 78:406, 1971
4. Lindheimer MD, Katz AI: Sodium and diuretics in pregnancy. N Engl J Med 288:891, 1973
5. Metcalfe J, Ueland K: Maternal cardiovascular adjustment to pregnancy. Prog Cardiovasc Dis 16:363, 1974
6. Metcalfe J, McAnulty JH, Ueland K: Cardiovascular physiology. Clin Obstet Gynecol 24:693, 1981
7. Ueland K, Novy MJ, Peterson EN, Metcalfe J: Maternal cardiovascular dynamics. IV. The influence of gestational age on the maternal cardiovascular response to posture and exercise. Am J Obstet Gynecol 104:856, 1969
8. Ken MG, Scott DB, Samuel E: Studies of the inferior cava in late pregnancy. Br Med J 1:532, 1964
8a. Burwell CS: The placenta as a modified arteriovenous fistula, considered in relation to the circulatory adjustments of pregnancy. Am J Med Sci 195:1, 1938
9. Barry WH, Crossman W: Cardiac catheterization. In Braunwald E (ed): Heart Disease: A Textbook of Cardiovascular Medicine. Vol. I. Philadelphia, WB Saunders, 1980
10. Katz R, Karliner JS, Resnik R: Effects of a natural volume overload state (pregnancy) on left ventricular performance in normal human subjects. Circulation 58:434, 1978
11. Oram S, Holt M: Innocent depression of the ST–T segment and flattening of the T-wave during pregnancy. J Obstet Gynaecol Br Commonw 68:765, 1961
12. Rubler S, Damini PM, Pinto ER: Cardiac size and performance during pregnancy estimated with echocardiography. Am J Cardiol 40:534, 1977
13. Nora JJ, Nora AH, Wexler P: Hereditary and environmental aspects as they affect the fetus and newborn. Clin Obstet Gynecol 24:851, 1981
14. Zitnak RS, Brandenburg RO, Sheldon R, Wallace RB: Pregnancy and open heart surgery. Circulation 39:257, 1969
15. Becker RM: Intracardiac surgery in pregnant women. Ann Thoracic Surg 36:463, 1983
16. Szekely P, Turner R, Snaith L: Pregnancy and the changing pattern of rheumatic heart disease. Br Heart J 35:1293, 1973
17. Chesley LC: Severe rheumatic cardiac disease and pregnancy: the ultimate prognosis. Am J Obstet Gynecol 136:552, 1980
18. Whittemore R, Hobbins JC, Engle MA: Pregnancy and its outcome in women with and without surgical treatment of congenital heart disease. Am J Cardiol 50:641, 1982
19. Rapaport E: Natural history of aortic and mitral valve disorders. Am J Cardiol 35:221, 1982
20. Szekely P, Snaith L: Heart Disease and Pregnancy. Churchill Livingstone, New York, 1974
21. Clark SL, Phelan J, Greenspoon J: Labor and delivery in the presence of mitral stenosis: central hemodynamic observations. Am J Obstet Gynecol 152:984, 1985
22. Arias F, Pineda J: Aortic stenosis and pregnancy. J Reprod Med 20:229, 1978
23. Sullivan JM, Ramanathan KB: Management of medical problems in pregnancy—severe cardiac disease. N Engl J Med 313:304, 1985

24. Larrea JP, Nunez L, Reque JA et al: Pregnancy and mechanical valve prosthesis: a high risk situation for the mother and fetus. Ann Thoracic Surg 36:459, 1983

25. Mangano DT: Anesthesia for the pregnant cardiac patient. p. 345. In Shnider SM, Levinson G (eds): Anesthesia for Obstetrics. Williams & Wilkins, Baltimore, 1987

26. Singh H, Bolton PJ, Oakley CM: Pregnancy after surgical correction of tetralogy of Fallot. Br Med J 285:168, 1982

27. Gleicher N, Midwall J, Hockberger D: Eisenmenger's syndrome and pregnancy. Obstet Gynecol Surv 34:721, 1979

28. Midwall J, Jaffin H, Herman MV, Kupersmith J: Shunt flow and pulmonary hemodynamics during labor and delivery in the Eisenmenger syndrome. Am J Cardiol 42:299, 1978

29. Abboud JK, Raya J, Noueihed R: Intrathecal morphine for relief of labor pain in a parturient with severe pulmonary hypertension. Anesthesiology 59:477, 1983

30. Deal K, Wooley CF: Coarctation of the aorta and pregnancy. Ann Intern Med 78:706, 1972

31. Benny PS, Prasao J, MacVicar J: Pregnancy and coarctation of the aorta: case report. Br J Obstet Gynaecol 87:1159, 1980

32. Pyeritz RE, McKusick VA: The Marfan syndrome: diagnosis and management. N Engl J Med 300:722, 1979

33. Rosenblum N, Grossman A, Gabbe SG: Failure of serial echocardiographic studies to predict dissection in a pregnant woman with Marfan's syndrome. Am J Obstet Gynecol 146:470, 1983

34. Pyeritz RE: Maternal and fetal complications of pregnancy in the Marfan syndrome. Am J Med 71:784, 1982

35. Mor-Yosef S, Younis J, Granat M et al: Marfan's syndrome in pregnancy. Obstet Gynecol Surv 43:382, 1988

36. Rayburn WF, Fontana ME: Mitral valve prolapse and pregnancy. Am J Obstet Gynecol 141:9, 1981

37. Sugrue D, Blake S, Troy P, MacDonald D: Antibiotic prophylaxis against infective endocarditis after normal delivery—is it necessary? Br Heart J 44:499, 1980

38. Stewart PA, Buis-Lein T, Verivey RA, Wladimiroff JW: Prenatal ultrasonic diagnosis of familial asymmetric septal hypertrophy. Prenat Diagn 6:249, 1986

39. Turner GD, McGarry K, Oakley CM: Management of pregnancy with hypertrophic cardiomyopathy. Br Med J 1:1749, 1979

40. Shah DM, Sunderji SG: Hypertrophic cardiomyopathy and pregnancy: report of a maternal mortality and review of literature. Obstet Gynecol Surv 40:444, 1985

41. Kolibash AJ, Ruiz DE, Lewis RP: Idiopathic hypertrophic subaortic stenosis in pregnancy. Ann Intern Med 82:791, 1975

42. Walsh JJ, Burch GE: Postpartal heart disease. Arch Intern Med 108:817, 1961

43. DeMakis JG, Rahimtoola SH: Peripartum cardiomyopathy. Circulation 44:964, 1971

44. DeMakis JG, Rahimtoola SH, Sutton GC: Natural course of peripartum cardiomyopathy. Circulation 44:1053, 1971

45. Melvin KR, Richardson PJ, Olsen EGJ et al: Peripartum cardiomyopathy due to myocarditis. N Engl J Med 307:731, 1982

46. Julian DG, Szekely P: Peripartum cardiomyopathy. Prog Cardiovasc Dis 27:223, 1985

47. Ginz B: Myocardial infarction in pregnancy. J Obstet Gynaecol Br Commonw 77:610, 1970

48. Hankins GDV, Wendal GD, Leveno KJ et al: Myocardial infarction during pregnancy: a review. Obstet Gynecol 65:139, 1985

49. Hussaini MH: Myocardial infarction during pregnancy: report of two cases with a review of the literature. Postgrad Med J 47:660, 1971

50. Beary JF, Summer WR, Bulkley BH: Postpartum acute myocardial infarction: a rare occurrence of uncertain etiology. Am J Cardiol 43:158, 1979

51. Goldmann ME, Mueller J: Coronary artery disease in pregnancy. p. 141. In Elkayam U, Gleicher N (eds): Cardiac Problems in Pregnancy. Alan R. Liss, New York, 1982

52. Majdan JF, Walinsley P, Cowchock SF et al: Coronary artery bypass surgery during pregnancy. Am J Cardiol 52:1145, 1983

53. Weinstein L, Murphy T: The management of tuberculosis during pregnancy. Clin Perinatol 1:395, 1974

54. Bonebarak CR, Noller KL, Loehnen CP et al: Routine chest roentgenography in pregnancy. JAMA 240:2747, 1978

55. Swartz HM, Reichling BA: Hazards of radiation exposure for pregnant women. JAMA 239:1907, 1978

56. Schaefer G, Zervoudakis IA, Fuchs FF, David S: Pregnancy in pulmonary tuberculosis. Obstet Gynecol 46:706, 1975

57. De March AP: Tuberculosis in pregnancy: five to ten year review of 215 patients in their fertile age. Chest 68:800, 1975

58. Maccato ML: Pneumonia and pulmonary tuberculosis in pregnancy. Obstet Gynecol Clin North Am 16:417, 1989

59. Bjerkedal T, Bahna SL, Lehmann EH: Course and outcome of pregnancy in women with pulmonary tuberculosis. Scand Respir Dis 56:245, 1975

60. Golvitch IM: Tuberculous meningitis in pregnancy. Am J Obstet Gynecol 110:1144, 1971

61. American Thoracic Society: Guidelines for short course tuberculosis chemotherapy. Am Rev Respir Dis 121:611, 1980

62. Byrd RB, Horn BR, Solomon DA, Griggs GA: Toxic effects of isoniazid in tuberculosis chemoprophylaxis. JAMA 241:1239, 1979

63. Sider DF, Layde PM, Johnson MW, Lyle HA: Treatment of tuberculosis during pregnancy. Am Rev Respir Dis 122:65, 1980

64. Heinonen OP, Slone D, Shapiro S: Birth Defects and Drugs in Pregnancy. Publishing Sciences Group, Littleton, MA, 1977

65. Sewitt T, Nebel L, Terracina S, Ankarman S: Ethambutol in pregnancy: observations on embryogenesis. Chest 66:25, 1974

66. Brobowitz ID: Ethambutol in pregnancy. Chest 66:20, 1974

67. Robinson GC, Cambon KG: Hearing loss in infants of tuberculous mothers treated with streptomycin in pregnancy. N Engl J Med 271:949, 1964

67a. Perinatal prophylaxis of tuberculosis. (Editorial). Lancet 336:1479, 1990

68. Kendig EL Jr: The place of BCG vaccine in the management of infants born of tuberculous mothers. N Engl J Med 281:520, 1969

69. Grossman JH III, Littner MD: Severe sarcoidosis in pregnancy. Obstet Gynecol 50(Suppl):81, 1976

70. Dines DE, Banner EA: Sarcoidosis during pregnancy: improvement in pulmonary function. JAMA 200:726, 1967

71. Mayock RL, Sullivan RD, Greening RR, Jones R: Sarcoidosis in pregnancy. JAMA 164:158, 1957

72. O'Leary JA: Ten year study of sarcoidosis in pregnancy. Am J Obstet Gynecol 84:462, 1962

73. Weinberger SE, Weiss ST, Cohen WR et al: Pregnancy and the lung. Am Rev Respir Dis 121:559, 1980

74. Haynes de Regt R: Sarcoidosis and pregnancy. Obstet Gynecol 70:369, 1987

75. Warren GV, Sprague SM, Corwin HL: Sarcoidosis presenting as acute renal failure during pregnancy. Am J Kidney Dis 12:161, 1988

76. Sahn EE: Pruritic white papules in pregnant woman: sarcoidosis. Arch Dermatol 123:1559, 1987

77. Hopwood HG: Pneumonia in pregnancy. Obstet Gynecol 25:875, 1965

78. Austrian R: Pneumococcal vaccine: development and prospects. Am J Med 67:546, 1979

79. Madinger NE, Greenspoon JS, Ellrodt AG: Pneumonia during pregnancy: has modern technology improved maternal and fetal outcome? Am J Obstet Gynecol 161:657, 1989

80. Greenberger PA, Patterson R: Management of asthma during pregnancy. N Engl J Med 312:897, 1985

81. De Swiet M: Diseases of the respiratory system. Clin Obstet Gynecol 4:287, 1977

82. Hernandez E, Angle CS, Johnson JWC: Asthma in pregnancy: current concepts. Obstet Gynecol 55:739, 1980

83. Turner ES, Greenberger PA, Patterson R: Management of the pregnant asthmatic patient. Ann Intern Med 93:905, 1980

84. Hiddleson HJH: Bronchial asthma and pregnancy. NZ Med J 63:521, 1964

85. Gordon M, Niswander KR, Berendes H, Kantor AG: Fetal morbidity following potentially anoxigenic obstetric conditions. VII. Bronchial asthma. Am J Obstet Gynecol 106:421, 1970

86. Schaefer G, Silverman F: Pregnancy complicated by asthma. Am J Obstet Gynecol 82:182, 1961

87. White RJ, Coutts II, Gibbs CJ, MacIntyre C: A prospective study of asthma during pregnancy and the puerperium. Respir Med 83:103, 1989

88. Juniper EF, Daniel EE, Roberts RS et al: Improvement in airway responsiveness and asthma severity during pregnancy: a prospective study. Am Rev Respir Dis 140:924, 1989

89. Apter AJ, Greenberger PA, Patterson R: Outcomes of pregnancy in adolescents with severe asthma. Arch Intern Med 149:2571, 1989

90. Williams DA: Asthma in pregnancy. Acta Allergy 22:311, 1967

91. Gordon M, Niswander KR, Berendes H, Kantor AG: Fetal morbidity following potentially anoxigenic obstetric conditions. VII. Bronchial asthma. Am J Obstet Gynecol 106:421, 1970

92. Sims CD, Chamberlin GVP, DeSwiet M: Lung function tests in bronchial asthma during and after pregnancy. Br J Obstet Gynaecol 88:434, 1976

93. Metzger WJ, Turner E, Patterson R: The safety of immunotherapy during pregnancy. J Allergy Clin Immunol 61:268, 1978

94. Centers for Disease Control: Prevention and control of influenza. MMWR 33:253, 1984

95. Greenberger P, Patterson R: Safety of therapy for allergic systems during pregnancy. Ann Intern Med 89:234, 1978

96. Weinstein AM, Dubin BD, Podleski WK et al: Asthma in pregnancy. JAMA 241:1161, 1979

97. Nelson MM, Forfar JO: Associations between drugs

administered during pregnancy and congenital abnormalities of the fetus. Br Med J 1:523, 1971

98. Gardner MJ, Schatz M, Cousins L et al: Longitudinal effects of pregnancy on the pharmacokinetics of theophylline. Eur J Clin Pharmacol 32:289, 1987

99. Bongiovanni AM, McPadden AJ: Steroids during pregnancy and possible fetal consequences. Fertil Steril 2:181, 1960

100. Fainstat TP: Cortisone-induced congenital cleft palate in rabbits. Endocrinology 55:502, 1954

101. Greenberger PA, Patterson R: Beclomethasone dipropionate for severe asthma during pregnancy. Ann Intern Med 98:478, 1983

102. Schatz M, Patterson R, Zeitz S et al: Corticosteroid therapy for the pregnant asthmatic patient. JAMA 233:804, 1975

103. Turner ES, Greenberger PA, Patterson R: Management of the pregnant asthmatic patient. Ann Intern Med 93:905, 1980

104. Greenberger P, Patterson R: Safety of therapy for allergic symptoms during pregnancy. Ann Intern Med 89:234, 1978

105. Reinisch JM, Simon NG, Karow WG, Gandelman R: Prenatal exposure to prednisone in humans and animals retards intrauterine growth. Science 202:436, 1978

106. Schatz M, Patterson R, Zeitz S et al: Corticosteroid therapy for the pregnant asthmatic patient. JAMA 233:804, 1975

107. Weinberger SE, Weiss ST, Coatan WR et al: Pregnancy and the lung. Am Rev Respir Dis 121:559, 1980

108. Beitins R, Baynard F, Ances IG et al: The transplacental passage of prednisone and prednisolone in pregnancy near term. J Pediatr 81:936, 1972

109. Levitz M, Jansen V, Dancis J: The transfer and metabolism of corticosteroids in the perfused human placenta. Am J Obstet Gynecol 132:363, 1978

110. Ballard PL, Granberg P, Ballard RA: Glucocorticoid levels in maternal and cord serum after prenatal beclomethasone therapy to prevent respiratory distress syndrome. J Clin Invest 56:1548, 1975

111. Schreier L, Cutler RM, Saigal V: Respiratory failure in asthma during the third trimester: report of two cases. Am J Obstet Gynecol 160:80, 1989

112. Marx GF: Obstetric anesthesia in the presence of medical complications. Clin Obstet Gynecol 17:165, 1974

113. Aaro LA, Jjergens JL: Thrombophlebitis associated with pregnancy. Am J Obstet Gynecol 109:1128, 1971

114. Treffers BL, Fluiderkoper GH, Weehink GH, Kloosterman GJ: Epidemiological observations of thromboembolic disease during pregnancy and in the puerperium in 56,022 women. Int J Gynaecol Obstet 21:327, 1983

115. VillaSanta U: Thromboembolic disease in pregnancy. Am J Obstet Gynecol 93:142, 1965

116. Barritt DW, Jorden SC: Anticoagulant drugs in the treatment of pulmonary embolism: a controlled trial. Lancet 1:1309, 1960

117. Mogensen K, Skibsted L, Wadt J, Nissen F: Thrombectomy of acute iliofemoral venous thrombosis during pregnancy. Surg Gynecol Obstet 169:50, 1989

118. Girz BA, Heiselman DE: Fatal intrapartum pulmonary embolus during tocolysis. Am J Obstet Gynecol 158:145, 1988

119. Stiller RJ, Leone-Tomaschoff S, Cuteri J, Beck L: Postpartum pulmonary embolus as an unusual cause of cortical blindness. Am J Obstet Gynecol 162:696, 1990

120. Stein LB, Robert RI, Marx J, Rossoff L: Transient cortical blindness following an acute hypotensive event in the postpartum period. NY State J Med 89:682, 1989

121. Macus CS, Mason GR, Kuperus JH, Mena I: Pulmonary imaging in pregnancy: maternal risk and fetal dosimetry. Clin Nucl Med 10:1, 1985

122. Ginsberg JS, Hirsh J, Rainbow AJ, Coates G: Risks to the fetus of radiologic procedures used in the diagnosis of maternal venous thromboembolic disease. Thromb Haemost 61:189, 1989

123. Qaso LA, Juergens JL: Thrombophlebitis associated with pregnancy. Am J Obstet Gynecol 109:1128, 1971

124. Gervin AS: Complications of heparin therapy. Surg Gynecol Obstet 140:789, 1975

125. Merrill LK, VerBurg DJ: The choice of long term anticoagulants for the pregnant patient. Obstet Gynecol 47:711, 1976

126. Baskin HF, Murray JM, Harris RE: Low dose heparin for the prevention of thromboembolic disease in pregnancy. Am J Obstet Gynecol 129:590, 1977

127. Spearing GS, Fraser I, Turner G, Dixon G: Long term self administered subcutaneous heparin in pregnancy. Br Med J 1:1457, 1978

128. Stevenson R, Burton DM, Ferlavto GJ, Taylor HA: Hazards of oral anticoagulants during pregnancy. JAMA 243:1549, 1980

129. Shavi WL, Hall JG: Multiple congenital anomalies associated with oral anticoagulants. Am J Obstet Gynecol 127:191, 1977

130. Harrod MJE, Sherrod PS: Warfarin embryopathy in siblings. Obstet Gynecol 57:673, 1981

131. Blegvad S, Lund O, Nielsen TT, Guldholt I: Emergency embolectomy in a patient with massive pulmonary embolism during second trimester pregnancy. Acta Obstet Gynecol Scand 68:267, 1989

132. Splinter WM, Dwane PD, Wigle RD, McGrath MJ: Anaesthetic management of emergency cesarean sec-

tion followed by pulmonary embolectomy. Can J Anaesth 36:689, 1989

133. Clark SL: Structural cardiac disease in pregnancy. In
Clark SL, Phelan JP, Cotton DB (eds): Critical Care

Obstetrics. Medical Economics Books, Oradell, NJ,
1987

134. Shulman ST, Amren DP, Bisno AL et al: Prevention of
bacterial endocarditis. Circulation 70(6):1125A, 1984

Chapter 32

Renal Disease

Philip Samuels

ALTERED RENAL PHYSIOLOGY IN PREGNANCY

Renal plasma flow (RPF) increases greatly during pregnancy.[1] It peaks in the first trimester and, although it decreases near term, remains higher than in the nonpregnant patient. This change is due in part to increased cardiac output and decreased renal vascular resistance. The glomerular filtration rate (GFR) increases by 50 percent during a normal gestation.[2] It rises early in pregnancy and remains elevated through delivery. The percentage increase in GFR is greater than the percentage increase in RPF. This elevation of the filtration fraction leads to a fall in the blood urea nitrogen (BUN) and serum creatinine values.

Because GFR increases to such a great degree, electrolytes, glucose, and other filtered substances reach the renal tubules in greater amounts. The kidney handles sodium efficiently, reabsorbing most of the filtered load in the proximal convoluted tubule. Glucose reabsorption, however, does not increase proportionately during pregnancy. The average renal threshold for glucose is reduced to 155 mg/dl from 194 mg/dl in the nonpregnant individual.[3] Glycosuria therefore can be seen in the normal gravida.

Urate is handled by filtration and secretion. Its clearance increases early in pregnancy, leading to lower serum levels of uric acid. In late pregnancy, urate clearance and serum urate levels return to their prepregnancy values. Serum urate levels are elevated in patients with preeclampsia. Whether this is due to decreased RPF, hemoconcentration, renal tubular dysfunction, or other renal circulatory changes remains uncertain.

ASYMPTOMATIC BACTERIURIA AND ACUTE PYELONEPHRITIS

The diagnosis of asymptomatic bacteriuria (ASB) is based on a clean catch voided urine culture revealing greater than 100,000 colonies/ml of a single organism.[4] Some investigators have suggested that two consecutively voided specimens should contain the same organism before making the diagnosis of bacteriuria.[5,6] Between 1.2 and 5 percent of young girls will demonstrate ASB at some time before puberty.[7] After puberty, with the onset of sexual activity, the prevalence of ASB may increase to 10 percent.[7] Of women with ASB, approximately 35 percent have bacteria arising from the kidneys rather than from the lower urinary tract.

It is important to diagnose and treat ASB in pregnancy. Left untreated, a symptomatic urinary tract infection (UTI) will develop in up to 40 percent of these patients.[8,9] Recognition and therapy for ASB can eliminate 70 percent of acute UTIs in pregnancy. Nonetheless, 2 percent of pregnant women with negative urine cultures develop symptomatic cystitis or pyelonephritis. This group accounts for 30 percent of the cases of acute UTI that develop during gestation. We advocate screening of all women for ASB at their first prenatal visit.

Escherichia coli is the organism responsible for most ASB. Patients can therefore be safely treated with nitrofurantoin, ampicillin, cephalosporins, and short-acting sulfa drugs. Sulfa compounds should be avoided near term, as they compete for bilirubin-binding sites on albumin in the fetus and newborn and could cause kernicterus. Nitrofurantoin should not be used in patients with glucose-6-phosphate dehydrogenase deficiency, as there is a risk for hemolytic crisis. If the fetus has this enzyme deficiency, it may also experience hemolysis. Therapy for ASB should be continued for 10 to 14 days after which time the patient should have another culture performed. Approximately 15 percent of patients will experience a reinfection and/or will not respond to initial therapy. Therapy should be reinstituted after careful microbial sensitivity testing. Patients with recurrent UTI during pregnancy and those with a history of pyelonephritis should undergo radiographic evaluation of the upper urinary tract. The procedure should be delayed until the patient is 2 months postpartum so that the anatomic and physiologic changes of pregnancy can regress. Of the women in the above categories, 20 percent will show a structural abnormality, but most will be insignificant.

Occasionally it is difficult to distinguish severe cystitis from pyelonephritis. Although the drugs used for treatment are similar, pyelonephritis requires intravenous antibiotics. Sandberg and co-investigators[10] studied symptomatic UTI in 174 women. They found that C-reactive protein was elevated in 91 percent of pregnant women with acute pyelonephritis and only 5 percent of women with cystitis. They also noted that the urine concentrating ability was lower in women with acute pyelonephritis. Because the erythrocyte sedimentation rate is normally elevated in pregnancy, they found that this was not a useful parameter for distinguishing pyelonephritis from cystitis.

Occurring in approximately 1 to 2 percent of all pregnancies, pyelonephritis is an important source of maternal morbidity. Recurrent pyelonephritis has been implicated as a cause of fetal death and intrauterine growth retardation (IUGR). There appears to be an association between acute pyelonephritis and preterm labor.[11,12] Fan and co-workers,[13] however, have shown that if pyelonephritis is aggressively treated, it does not increase the likelihood of preterm labor, premature delivery, or low-birth-weight infants.

Acute pyelonephritis must be treated on an inpatient basis, utilizing intravenous antibiotics. Empiric therapy should be begun as soon as the presumptive diagnosis is made. Therapy can be tailored to the specific organism after sensitivities have been obtained approximately 48 hours later. Because septicemia may occasionally result from pyelonephritis, blood cultures should be drawn. *E. coli* is the most common organism isolated in pyelonephritis. During gestation, the right side is most often affected, as engorged blood vessels may inhibit ureteral drainage of the kidney. Generally, a broad spectrum first-generation cephalosporin is the initial therapy of choice. Fan and co-investigators[13] reviewed 107 cases of pyelonephritis in 103 pregnant women. They report that 33 percent were resistant to ampicillin and 13 percent to first-generation cephalosporins. If such resistance is encountered or if the patient is allergic to cephalosporins, an aminoglycoside can safely be administered. Peak and trough aminoglycoside levels, however, should be monitored. The serum creatinine and BUN should be followed as well. During the febrile period, acetaminophen should be employed to keep the patient's temperature below 38 degrees C. Small doses of acetaminophen will not mask the fever and symptoms of a patient who is unresponsive to treatment.

Intravenous antibiotic therapy should be continued for 24 to 48 hours after the patient becomes afebrile and costovertebral angle tenderness disappears. After the cessation of intravenous therapy, treatment with appropriate oral antibiotics should be continued for 2 to 3 weeks. Upon termination of therapy, urine cultures should be obtained on a monthly basis. After an episode of acute pyelonephritis, antibiotic suppression should be implemented and continued for the remainder of pregnancy. Nitrofurantoin 100 mg once or twice daily is an acceptable regimen for suppression. In a study by Van Dorsten and colleagues,[14] the overall frequency of positive urine cultures following hospitalization for pyelonephritis was 38 percent. Nitrofurantoin suppression reduced the rate to 8 percent. Nitrofurantoin did not lower the rate of positive cultures if the inpatient antibiotic selection was inappropriate or if the culture was positive at time of discharge.[14]

Cunningham and co-workers[15] point out that pulmonary injury resembling adult respiratory distress syndrome (ARDS) can occur in patients with acute pyelonephritis. Clinical manifestations of this complication usually occur 24 to 48 hours after the patient is admitted for pyelonephritis.[15,16] Some of these patients will require endotracheal intubation and mechanical ventilation. In this series, there was no evidence that pulmonary edema was caused by intravenous fluid overload.[15] This ARDS-type picture probably results from endotoxin-induced alveolar capillary membrane injury.

Austenfeld and Snow[17] studied 64 pregnancies in 30 women who had previously undergone ureteral reimplantation for vesicoureteral reflux. During pregnancy, 57 percent of these women had one or more UTIs and 17 percent had more than one UTI or an episode of pyelonephritis.[17] More frequent urine cultures and aggressive therapy during pregnancy are recommended for this group of patients.

UROLITHIASIS

The prevalence of urolithiasis during pregnancy is 0.03 percent, with an incidence no higher than that of the general population.[18] Colicky abdominal pain, recurrent UTI, and hematuria suggest urolithiasis. If the diagnosis is suspected, intravenous pyelography should be undertaken, limiting this study to the minimum number of exposures necessary to make the diagnosis. Ultrasound can often be used to establish the diagnosis without radiation exposure. In any patient suspected or proved to have renal stones, serum calcium and phosphorous levels should be obtained to rule out hyperparathyroidism. Serum urate should also be determined.

Because of the physiologic hydroureter characteristic of pregnancy, most patients with symptomatic urolithiasis will spontaneously pass their stones. Treatment should be conservative, consisting of hydration and narcotic analgesia for pain relief.[19] Epidural anesthesia has been advocated to establish a segmental block from T11 to L2. While this approach may promote passage of the stone, it remains controversial. Lithotripsy is contraindicated during pregnancy.

Recurrent UTI with urease-containing organisms causes precipitation of calcium phosphate in the kidney that may lead to the development of staghorn calculi. Surgery is rarely indicated in these patients, especially during gestation. Patients with staghorn calculi should have frequent urine cultures, and bacteriuria should be treated aggressively. Recurrent infections can lead to chronic pyelonephritis with resultant loss of kidney function.

GLOMERULONEPHRITIS

Acute glomerulonephritis is an uncommon complication of pregnancy, with an estimated incidence of 1 per 40,000 pregnancies.[20] Poststreptococcal glomerulonephritis rarely occurs in adults. In this disorder, renal function tends to deteriorate during the acute phase of the disease, but usually later recovers.[21] Acute glomerulonephritis can be difficult to distinguish from preeclampsia. Periorbital edema, a striking clinical feature of acute glomerulonephritis, is often seen in pregnancy-induced hypertension. Hematuria, red blood cell (RBC) casts in the urine sediment, and depressed serum complement levels indicate glomerular disease. In poststreptococcal acute glomerulonephritis, antistreptolysin O titers rise.

Treatment of acute glomerulonephritis in pregnancy is similar to that of the nonpregnant patient. Blood pressure control is essential, and careful attention to fluid balance is imperative. Sodium intake should be restricted to 500 mg/day during the acute disease. Serum potassium levels must also be carefully monitored.

Packham and co-workers[22] extensively reviewed 395 pregnancies in 238 women with primary glomerulonephritis. Only 51 percent of infants were born after 36 weeks gestation. Excluding therapeutic abortion, 20 percent of fetuses were lost, 15 percent after 20 weeks gestation. IUGR was noted in 15 percent of the fetuses. Maternal renal function deteriorated in 15 percent of pregnancies and failed to resolve post partum in 5 percent.[22] Hypertension was recorded in 52 percent of the pregnancies, developing before 32 weeks gestation in 26 percent. This blood pressure elevation was not an exacerbation of previously diagnosed hypertension, as in only 12 percent of pregnancies was there noted to be antecedent hypertension. Eighteen percent of the women who developed de novo hypertension in pregnancy remained hypertensive post partum. Increased proteinuria was recorded in 59 percent of these pregnancies and was irreversible in 15 percent.[22] The highest incidence of fetal and maternal complications occurred in patients with primary focal and segmental hyalinosis and sclerosis. The lowest incidence of complications was observed in non-IgA diffuse mesangial proliferative glomerulonephritis.[22] The presence of severe vessel lesions on renal biopsy was associated with a significantly higher rate of fetal loss after 20 weeks gestation. Packham and co-workers[23] also studied 33 pregnancies in 24 patients with biopsy-proven membranous glomerulonephritis. Fetal loss occurred in 24 percent of pregnancies, preterm delivery in 43 percent, and a term liveborn in only 33 percent of patients. Hypertension was noted in 46 percent of these pregnant women. Thirty percent of patients had proteinuria in the nephrotic range in the first trimester.[23] The presence of heavy proteinuria during the first trimester correlated with a poor fetal and maternal outcome.[23] Jungers et al.[24] described 69 pregnancies in 34 patients with IgA glomerulonephritis. The fetal loss rate in this group was 15 percent. Preexisting hypertension was statistically associated with poor fetal outcome. Hypertension at the time of conception also correlated with a deterioration of maternal renal function during pregnancy. Hypertension in the first pregnancy was highly predictive of recurrence of hypertension in a subsequent pregnancy.[24] Kincaide-Smith and Fairley[25] analyzed 102 pregnancies in 65 women with IgA glomerulonephritis. They noted that hypertension occurred in 63 percent of pregnancies, with 18 percent being severe. They also observed a decrease in renal function in 22 percent of these women.[25]

CHRONIC RENAL DISEASE

Diagnosis

Chronic renal disease can be silent until its advanced stages. Because obstetricians routinely examine the patient's urine for the presence of protein, glucose, and ketones, they may be the first to detect chronic renal disease.

Any gravida with more than trace proteinuria should collect a 24-hour urine specimen for creatinine clearance and total protein excretion. This test is safe, inexpensive, and of only minor inconvenience to the patient. Creatinine clearance is greatly elevated in pregnancy and, during the first trimester, may exceed 150 ml/min. Before pregnancy, 24-hour urinary protein excretion should not exceed 0.15 g. During gestation, quantities up to 0.3 g per day may be normal. Moderate proteinuria (<2 g per day) is seen in glomerular disease, most commonly lipoid nephrosis, systemic lupus erythematosus, and glomerulonephritis.

Microscopic examination of the urine can reveal much about the patient's renal status. If renal disease is suspected, a catheterized specimen should be obtained. RBCs greater than 1 to 2 per high-power field or RBC casts are indicative of renal disease. RBCs usually indicate glomerular disease or collagen vascular disease. Less frequently, they suggest trauma or malignant hypertension. Increased numbers of white blood cells (WBCs) (>1 to 2 per HPF) or the appearance of WBC casts is usually indicative of acute or chronic infection. Cellular casts are found in the presence of renal tubular dysfunction, and hyaline casts suggest proteinuria. A single bacterium seen in an unspun catheterized urine specimen is suggestive of significant bacteriuria, and a follow-up culture should be performed.

The obstetrician can easily be misled when relying solely on the BUN and serum creatinine to assess renal function. A 70 percent decline in creatinine clearance, an indirect measure of GFR, can be seen before a significant rise in the BUN or serum creatinine occurs. In fact, little change in the serum creatinine or the BUN is seen until the creatinine falls to 50 ml/min. Below that level, small decrements in creatinine clearance can lead to large increases in the BUN and creatinine. A single creatinine clearance value less than 100 ml/min is not diagnostic of renal disease. An incomplete 24-hour urine collection is the most frequent cause of this finding. An abnormal clearance therefore should be repeated.

Serum urate is an often overlooked but helpful parameter in detecting renal dysfunction. Excretion of uric acid is dependent not only on glomerular filtration but also on tubular secretion. An elevated serum urate in the presence of a normal BUN and serum creatinine may therefore implicate tubular disease.

Effect of Pregnancy on Renal Function

Although baseline creatinine clearance is decreased in patients with chronic renal insufficiency, it should still increase during gestation. A moderate fall in creatinine clearance is often observed during late gestation in patients with renal disease. This decrease is typically more severe in patients with diffuse glomerular disease. It usually reverses after delivery.

The long-term effect of pregnancy on renal disease remains controversial. If the patient's serum creatinine is less than 1.5 mg/dl, pregnancy should have little effect on the long-term prognosis of the patient's kidney disease. Pregnancy, however, is associated with an increased incidence of pyelonephritis in patients with chronic renal disease. There are few data concerning the long-term effect of pregnancy on renal disease in women with true renal insufficiency. Occasionally, some patients with a baseline serum creatinine of more than 1.5 mg/dl will experience a significant decrease in renal function during gestation that does not improve during the postpartum period.[26,27] This deterioration occurs more frequently in women with diffuse glomerulonephritis. It is not possible, however, to predict which patients with renal insufficiency will experience a permanent reduction in renal function. If renal function significantly deteriorates during gestation, termination of pregnancy may not reverse the process. Abortion therefore cannot be recommended for all patients who become pregnant and whose baseline serum creatinine exceeds 1.5 mg/dl. Ideally, patients with chronic renal disease should be thoroughly counseled about the possible consequences of pregnancy before conception.

Severe hypertension is the greatest threat to the pregnant patient with chronic renal disease. Left uncontrolled, hypertension can lead to intracerebral hemorrhage as well as deteriorating renal function. In most pregnancies complicated by chronic renal dysfunction, some degree of hypertension is present.[26,28] Approximately 50 percent of these patients will have worsening hypertension as pregnancy progresses, and diastolic blood pressures of 110 mmHg or greater will develop in about 20 percent of cases.[29] Those patients with diffuse proliferative glomerulonephritis and nephrosclerosis are at greatest risk for the development of severe hypertension. Blood pressure control is the cornerstone for the successful treatment of chronic renal disease in pregnancy.

Worsening proteinuria is common during pregnancy complicated by chronic renal disease and often reaches the nephrotic range.[29] In general, massive proteinuria does not indicate an increased risk for mother or fetus.[30] Low serum albumin, however, has been correlated with low birth weight.[31] The development of massive proteinuria is not necessarily a harbinger of preeclampsia. Nevertheless, in late pregnancy it is often difficult to differentiate impending preeclampsia from worsening chronic renal disease.

Effect of Chronic Renal Disease on Pregnancy

More than 85 percent of women with chronic renal disease will have a surviving infant if renal function is well preserved. Earlier reports were more pessimistic, citing a 5.8 percent incidence of stillbirth, a 4.9 percent incidence of neonatal deaths, and an increase in second-trimester losses.[29] If hypertension is not controlled and if renal function is not well preserved, there is still a high likelihood of pregnancy loss.[22] Antepartum fetal surveillance and advances in neonatal care have made great strides in improving perinatal outcome in these patients. One study reported a total fetal loss rate of 13.8 percent including miscarriage, stillbirths, and neonatal deaths.[28]

The outlook for women with severe renal insufficiency, those with a baseline serum creatinine of more than 1.5 mg/dl, is less clear. This is due in part to the limited number of pregnancies in such patients as well as to the large number who undergo elective abortion. One study reported no surviving infants when the maternal BUN was greater than 60 mg/dl.[30] Other investigations, however, have found that about 80 percent of such pregnancies resulted in surviving infants.[28,32] Preterm births and IUGR remain important problems in these pregnancies. The reported incidence of preterm birth ranges from 20 to 50 percent.[29,33]

Surveillance and Treatment

A 24-hour urine collection for creatinine clearance and total protein excretion should be obtained as soon as the pregnancy is confirmed. These parameters should be monitored monthly. The patient should be seen once every 2 weeks until 32 weeks gestation and weekly thereafter. These are general guidelines, and more frequent visits may be necessary in individual cases.

Control of hypertension is critical in managing patients with chronic renal disease. Methyldopa, clonidine, β-blockers, and hydralazine can be used to treat blood pressure effectively as long as the dosages are monitored carefully. More evidence regarding the safety of calcium channel blockers is being accumulated, and these drugs soon may play a role in treating chronic hypertension during pregnancy. There is still controversy concerning the safety of angiotensin-converting enzyme inhibitors during pregnancy, and, if at all possible, these agents should be avoided.

Hydralazine can be added as a second drug in refractory patients. Concomitant treatment with a β-blocker is often necessary because of the reflex tachycardia associated with the use of hydralazine.

The use of diuretics in pregnancy is controversial.[34-36] For massive debilitating edema, a short course of diuretics can be helpful. Electrolytes must be monitored carefully. Salt restriction does not appear to be beneficial once edema has developed. Salt restriction, however, should be instituted without hesitation in pregnant women with true renal insufficiency.

Fetal growth should be assessed with serial ultrasonography, because IUGR is common in women with chronic renal disease. Antepartum fetal heart rate testing should be started at 28 weeks gestation.[37]

Obstetricians should have a low threshold for hospitalizing patients with chronic renal disease. Increasing hypertension and decreasing renal function warrant immediate hospitalization. A sudden deterioration of renal function may be due to infection, dehydration, electrolyte imbalance, or obstruction.

The timing of delivery must be individualized. Maternal indications for delivery include uncontrollable hypertension, the development of superimposed preeclampsia, and decreasing renal function after fetal viability has been reached. Fetal indications are dictated by the assessment of fetal growth and fetal well-being.

Renal biopsy is rarely indicated during pregnancy. It is never indicated after 34 weeks gestation when delivery of the fetus and subsequent biopsy would be a safer alternative. Excessive bleeding secondary to the greatly increased renal blood flow has been reported by some[38] but not all[39] observers. If coagulation indices are normal and blood pressure is well controlled, morbidity should be no greater than observed in the nonpregnant patient.[40] Packham and Fairley[41] report a series of 111 renal biopsies performed in 104 pregnant women over 20 years. The complication rate was 4.5%. The most likely clinical dilemma necessitating renal biopsy in a pregnant woman would be the development of nephrotic syndrome and increasing hypertension between 22 and 32 weeks gestation. In this case, renal biopsy may distinguish chronic renal disease from preeclampsia and impact significantly on the treatment plan.

Hemodialysis in Pregnancy

Patients on chronic hemodialysis can have successful pregnancies.[42-48] Many women with chronic renal failure, however, experience oligomenorrhea, and their fertility is often impaired.[49] These women commonly fail to use a method of contraception. It is therefore important that a serum β-hCG level be assessed whenever pregnancy is suspected.

As in all patients with impaired renal function, the most important aspect of care is meticulous control of blood pressure. During dialysis, wide fluctuations in blood pressure often occur. One case report describes fetal distress associated with hypotension during dialysis.[38] Sudden volume shifts therefore should be avoided.[48] In late pregnancy, continuous fetal heart rate monitoring should be carried out during dialysis. If possible, the patient should be positioned on her left side with the uterus displaced from the vena cava. During dialysis, one must pay particular attention to electrolyte balance. Pregnant patients are in a state of chronic compensated respiratory alkalosis, and large drops in serum bicarbonate should be prevented. Dialysates containing glucose and bicarbonate are preferred, and those containing citrates should be avoided.[48]

Patients should be counseled that a successful pregnancy will require longer and more frequent periods of dialysis.[43,48] Patients must also follow a careful diet ingesting at least 70 g of protein and 1.5 g of calcium daily. Weight gain should be limited to 0.5 kg between dialysis sessions.

Chronic anemia is often a problem in hemodialysis patients. The hematocrit should be kept above 25 percent, and transfusion with packed RBCs or erythropoietin therapy may be necessary to accomplish this objective.[43] Polyhydramnios appears to be a frequent complication in pregnant patients undergoing hemodialysis.[48,50]

The point at which to initiate hemodialysis is controversial. Cohen and co-investigators[45] feel that the early initiation of regular hemodialysis in patients with moderate renal insufficiency may improve pregnancy outcome. In two cases, when regular hemodialysis was begun in the second trimester, both patients carried to term, although the infants had IUGR.[45] Redrow and co-workers[46] report 14 pregnancies in 13 women undergoing dialysis. Ten of those pregnancies were successful. Five of eight pregnancies managed with chronic ambulatory peritoneal dialysis or chronic cycling peritoneal dialysis were successful. The investigators hypothesize several advantages for peritoneal dialysis. These include a more constant chemical and extracellular environment for the fetus, higher hematocrit levels, infrequent episodes of hypotension, and no heparin requirement. They also postulate that intraperitoneal insulin facilitates the management of blood glucose in diabetic patients and that intraperitoneal magnesium used in the dialysate reduces the likelihood of preterm labor.

Preterm birth does occur more frequently in patients undergoing dialysis.[51] Progesterone is removed during dialysis and at least one group has advocated that parenteral progesterone therapy should be administered to the patient undergoing dialysis.[52] In their review, Yasin and Doun[48] report a 40.7 percent incidence of premature contractions. Although it is tempting to perform a cesarean section when the patient approaches term, cesarean section should not be routine in these patients. It should be performed only for obstetric indications.

PREGNANCY IN THE RENAL TRANSPLANT RECIPIENT

Pregnancy following renal transplantation has become increasingly common. Many previously anovulatory patients begin ovulating postoperatively and regain fertility as renal function normalizes.[53] As in the case of women on hemodialysis, many transplant recipients have failed to realize they are pregnant until well into the second trimester.

Whenever possible, patients with allografts should wait 2 to 5 years after transplantation before becoming pregnant. By this time, renal function has equilibrated and the dose of immunosuppressive agents has been stabilized. It has been suggested that patients be free of significant hypertension and proteinuria before attempting pregnancy.[54] There should also be no evidence of allograft rejection. Most reported pregnancies have occurred in patients who have received allografts from cadaver donors. Whether the source of the allograft, either cadaver or living donor, influences maternal and/or perinatal outcome cannot yet be determined.

Upon learning they are pregnant, many women stop taking all medications. The importance of continuing immunosuppressive therapy cannot be emphasized strongly enough to renal allograft recipients. Glucocorticoids are metabolized in the placenta, with only limited amounts reaching the fetus. No studies have documented an increased rate of malformations. Adrenocortical insufficiency has been rarely reported in infants born to mothers taking glucocorticoids.[55] Nevertheless, a pediatrician should be present at the delivery and should be aware of this possibility.

Azathioprine cannot be activated in the fetus because of its lack of inosinate pyrophosphorylase.[56] Azathioprine has been shown to cause decreased levels of IgG and IgM as well as a smaller thymic shadow on chest x-ray in these neonates.[57] Chromosomal aberrations, which cleared within 20 to 32 months, have also been demonstrated in lymphocytes of infants exposed to azathioprine in utero.[58] The long-term implications of this treatment are not yet known. IUGR has been reported in infants born to mothers receiving azathioprine.[59] These risks are outweighed, however, by the disastrous consequences of allograft rejection that may occur if the patient stops her medication.

The fetal effects of cyclosporin are not yet delineated. Successful pregnancies have been associated with its use.[60-63] In fact, Salamalekis et al.[62] feel that there may be less teratogenic potential from cyclosporin A than from azathioprine.

During pregnancy, renal allograft recipients must be carefully watched for signs of rejection. Significant episodes of rejection may occur in as many as 9 percent of transplant recipients during gestation. This figure is no greater than that expected in the nonpregnant population. Unfortunately, the clinical hallmarks of rejection—fever, oliguria, tenderness, decreasing renal function—are not always exhibited by the pregnant patient. Occasionally, rejection may mimic pyelonephritis or preeclampsia, which occurs in approximately one-third of renal transplant patients. In these cases renal biopsy is indicated to distinguish rejection from preeclampsia. Rejection has been known to occur during the puerperium when maternal immune competence returns to its prepregnancy level.[64] Therefore it may be advisable to increase the dose of immunosuppressive medications in the immediate postpartum period.

Infection can be disastrous for the renal allograft. Therefore, urine cultures should be obtained at least monthly during pregnancy, and any bacteriuria should be aggressively treated. It is crucial to remember that the allograft is denervated, and the patient may experience no pain with pyelonephritis. The only symptoms may be fever and nausea.

Renal function, as determined by 24-hour creatinine clearance and protein excretion, should be assessed monthly. Approximately 15 percent of transplant recipients will exhibit a significant decrease in renal function in late pregnancy.[60] This condition usually, but not always, reverses after pregnancy. Proteinuria develops in about 40 percent of patients near term but most often disappears soon after delivery unless significant hypertension is present.

As in patients with chronic renal disease, serial ultrasonography should be used to assess fetal growth, and antepartum fetal heart rate testing should be started at 28 weeks gestation. Approximately 50 percent of renal allograft recipients will deliver preterm. Preterm labor, preterm rupture of membranes, and IUGR are common. Vaginal delivery should be accomplished when possible, and cesarean section should be reserved for obstetric indications. Allograft recipients may have an increased frequency of cephalopelvic disproportion from pelvic osteodystrophy,[65] resulting from prolonged renal disease with hypercalcemia or extended steroid use. The transplanted kidney, however, rarely obstructs vaginal delivery despite its pelvic location.

ACUTE RENAL FAILURE IN PREGNANCY

Acute renal failure (ARF) is defined as a urine output of less than 400 ml in 24 hours. To make the diagnosis, ureteral and urethral obstruction must be excluded. The incidence of ARF during pregnancy is approximately 1 per 10,000. It is seen most fre-

quently in septic first-trimester abortions and in cases of sudden severe volume depletion resulting from hemorrhage caused by placenta previa, placental abruption, or postpartum uterine atony.[66] It is also observed in the marked volume contraction associated with severe preeclampsia[67] and with acute fatty liver of pregnancy.[67,68]

The incidence of ARF in pregnancy has decreased over the years. Stratta and colleagues[69] reported 81 cases of pregnancy-related ARF between 1958 and 1987, accounting for 9 percent of the total number of ARF cases needing dialysis during that interval. In three successive 10-year periods (1958–1967, 1968–1977, 1978–1987), the incidence of pregnancy-related ARF fell from 43 percent to 2.8 percent of the total number of cases of ARF. The incidence changed from 1 in 3,000 to 1 in 15,000 pregnancies over the study period.[69] In these 81 ARF cases, 11.6 percent experienced irreversible renal damage, the majority of which occurred in cases of severe preeclampsia/eclampsia.[69]

Renal ischemia is the common denominator in all cases of ARF. With mild ischemia, quickly reversible prerenal failure results. With more prolonged ischemia, acute tubular necrosis occurs. This process is also reversible, as glomeruli are not affected. Severe ischemia, however, may produce acute cortical necrosis. This pathology is irreversible, although on occasion a small amount of renal function is preserved.[70] Stratta and colleagues[71] have reported 17 cases of ARF occurring over 15 years, and all were due to preeclampsia/eclampsia. Cortical necrosis occurred in 29.5 percent of the cases.[71] Whether or not ARF was associated with cortical necrosis did not appear to be related to chronologic age, parity, gestational age at which preeclampsia commenced, duration of preeclampsia prior to delivery, or eclamptic seizures. The only statistically significant factor associated with the appearance of cortical necrosis was placental abruption.[71] In another study, Turney and co-workers[72] demonstrated that acute cortical necrosis, which occurred in 12.7 percent of their patients with ARF, carried a 100 percent mortality within 6 years.

Sibai and colleagues[73] studied the remote prognosis in 31 consecutive cases of ARF in patients with hypertensive disorders of pregnancy. Eighteen of the 31 patients had "pure" preeclampsia, while 13 pregnancies had other hypertensive disorders and renal disease. Fifty percent of the 18 patients with pure preeclampsia required dialysis during hospitalization, and all 18 patients had acute tubular necrosis. Of the other 13 women, 42 percent required dialysis and three patients had bilateral cortical necrosis. The majority of pregnancies in both groups were complicated by placental abruption and hemorrhage.[73] All 16 surviving patients in the pure preeclampsia group had normal renal function on long-term follow-up. Conversely, 9 of the 11 surviving patients in the other group required long-term dialysis, and four ultimately died of end-stage renal disease.[73] Turney and colleagues[72] also performed follow-up examinations of their patients. They found that maternal survival was adversely affected by increasing age. Their 1-year maternal survival was 78.6 percent. Follow-up of survivors showed normal renal function up to 31 years after ARF.[72]

Clinically, patients with reversible ARF first experience a period of oliguria of variable duration. Polyuria then occurs. It is important to recognize that BUN and serum creatinine continue to rise early in the polyuric phase. During the recovery phase, urine output approaches normal. In these patients, it is important to monitor electrolytes frequently and to treat any imbalance carefully. The urine to plasma osmolality ratio should be determined early in the course of the disease. If the ratio is 1.5 or greater, prerenal pathology is likely, and the disorder tends to be of shorter duration and lesser severity. A ratio near 1.0 suggests acute tubular necrosis.

The main goal of treatment is the elimination of the underlying cause. Volume and electrolyte balance must receive constant scrutiny. To assess volume requirements, invasive hemodynamic monitoring is useful and lessens the need for clinical guesswork. This is especially true during the polyuric phase. Central hyperalimentation may also be required if renal failure is prolonged.

Acidosis frequently occurs in cases of ARF. Arterial blood gases therefore should be followed regularly. Acidosis must be treated promptly to prevent hyperkalemia, which may develop rapidly and can be fatal. Absolute restriction of potassium intake should be instituted immediately. Sodium bicarbonate, used to treat acidosis, may overload the patient with sodium and water. In this case, peritoneal or hemodialysis may be instituted. The main indications for dialysis in ARF of pregnancy are hypernatremia, hyperkalemia, severe acidosis, volume overload, and worsening uremia.

HEMOLYTIC UREMIC SYNDROME

The postpartum hemolytic uremic syndrome is a rare idiopathic disorder that must be considered when a patient shows signs of hemolysis and decreasing renal function in the postpartum period. This idiopathic syndrome was first described in 1968 and may occur as early as the first trimester and up to 2 months post partum.[74–77] In fact, it has even been reported following an ectopic pregnancy.[78] Most patients have no predisposing factors. Prodromal symptoms include vomiting, diarrhea, and a flu-like illness. Forty-nine cases have been reported with a 61 percent mortality rate.[76] These cases date back to 1968; with improved intensive care monitoring and treatment, the prognosis is now probably much better. Coratelli and co-workers[74] reported a case of hemolytic uremic syndrome that was diagnosed at 13 weeks gestation and confirmed by renal biopsy. Circulating endotoxin was detected and was progressively reduced by hemodialysis performed daily from the third to the ninth days of the disease. Complete normalization of renal function occurred by day 34. These investigators propose that initiation of early dialysis may play an important role in supporting patients through the disease process. They also feel that endotoxins are key pathogenic factors in the disorder.[74] Conversely, Li and co-workers[79] discovered hemolytic uremic syndrome in a patient recovering from an uncomplicated cesarean section. No endotoxins were found in the patient's serum, stool, or renal biopsy material. The patient underwent dialysis and recovered.[79] Conte and co-workers[80] suggest that plasma exchange in cases of acute renal failure caused by the postpartum hemolytic uremic syndrome can play a vital role in supporting the patient through the illness.

Disseminated intravascular coagulation (DIC) with hemolysis usually accompanies the renal failure. However, DIC is not the cause of the syndrome. Microscopically, the kidney shows thrombotic microangiopathy. The glomerular capillary wall is thick, and biopsy specimens taken later in the course of the disease show severe nephrosclerosis and deposition of the third component of complement (C_3).

Some researchers believe that this syndrome is due to decreased production of prostacyclin in the kidneys.[81,82] Prostacyclin infusions have been used to treat patients, but this therapy still remains experimental. One observer noted a decrease in antithrombin III in a patient with postpartum hemolytic uremic syndrome. This patient was successfully treated with an infusion of antithrombin III concentrate.[83]

REFERENCES

1. DeAlvarez R: Renal glomerulotubular mechanisms during normal pregnancy: I. Glomerular filtration rate, renal plasma flow and creatinine clearance. Am J Obstet Gynecol 75:931, 1958

2. Davidson J: Changes in renal function and other aspects of homeostasis in early pregnancy. J Obstet Gynaecol Br Commonw 81:1003, 1974

3. Christensen P: Tubular reabsorption of glucose during pregnancy. Scand J Clin Lab Invest 10:364, 1958

4. Kass E: Asymptomatic infections of the urinary tract. Trans Assoc Am Physicians 60:56, 1956

5. Norden C, Kass E: Bacteriuria of pregnancy—a critical reappraisal. Annu Rev Med 19:431, 1968

6. McFadyen I, Eykryn S, Gardner N et al: Bacteriuria of pregnancy. J Obstet Gynaecol Br Commonw 80:385, 1973

7. Kunin C: The natural history of recurrent bacteriuria in schoolgirls. N Engl J Med 282:1443, 1970

8. Savage W, Hajj S, Kass E: Demographic and prognostic characteristics of bacteriuria in pregnancy. Medicine (Baltimore) 46:385, 1967

9. Whalley P: Bacteriuria of pregnancy. Am J Obstet Gynecol 97:723, 1967

10. Sandberg T, Lidin-Janson G, Eden CS: Host response in women with symptomatic urinary tract infection. Scand J Infect Dis 21:67, 1989

11. Brumfitt W: The significance of symptomatic and asymptomatic infection in pregnancy. Contrib Nephrol 25:23, 1981

12. Gilstrap L, Leveno K, Cunningham F et al: Renal infection and pregnancy outcome. Am J Obstet Gynecol 141:709, 1981

13. Fan YD, Pastorek JG II, Miller JM Jr, Mulvey J: Acute pyelonephritis in pregnancy. Am J Perinatol 4:324, 1987

14. Van Dorsten JP, Lenke RR, Schifrin BS: Pyelonephritis in pregnancy: the role of in-hospital management and nitrofurantoin suppression. J Reprod Med 32:895, 1987

15. Cunningham FG, Lucas MJ, Hankins GD: Pulmonary injury complicating antepartum pyelonephritis. Am J Obstet Gynecol 156:797, 1987

16. Pruett K, Faro S: Pyelonephritis associated with respiratory distress. Obstet Gynecol 69:444, 1987

17. Austenfeld MS, Snow BW: Complications of pregnancy in women after reimplantation for vesicoureteral reflux. J Urol 140:1103, 1988

18. Harris R, Dunnihoo D: The incidence and significance of urinary calculi in pregnancy. Am J Obstet Gynecol 99:237, 1967

19. Strong D, Murchison R, Lynch D: The management of ureteral calculi during pregnancy. Surv Gynecol Obstet 146:604, 1978

20. Nadler N, Salinas-Madrigal L, Charles A, Pollack V: Acute glomerulonephritis during late pregnancy. Obstet Gynecol 34:277, 1969

21. Wilson C: Changes in renal function. p. 177. In Morris N, Browne J (eds): Nontoxemic Hypertension in Pregnancy. Little, Brown, Boston, 1958

22. Packham DK, North RA, Fairley KF et al: Primary glomerulonephritis and pregnancy. Q J Med 71:537, 1989

23. Packham D, North RA, Fairley KF et al: Membranous glomerulonephritis and pregnancy. Clin Nephrol 30:487, 1988

24. Jungers P, Forget D, Houillier P et al: Pregnancy in IgA nephropathy, reflux nephropathy, and focal glomerular sclerosis. Am J Kidney Dis 9:334, 1987

25. Kincaid-Smith P, Fairley KF: Renal disease in pregnancy: three controversial areas: mesangial IgA nephropathy, focal glomerular sclerosis (focal and segmental hyalinosis and sclerosis), and reflux nephropathy. Am J Kidney Dis 9:328, 1987

26. Bear R: Pregnancy in patients with renal disease: a study of 44 cases. Obstet Gynecol 48:13, 1976

27. Hou S: Pregnancy in women with chronic renal disease. N Engl J Med 312:839, 1985

28. Hou S, Grossman S, Madias N: Pregnancy in women with renal disease and moderate renal insufficiency. Am J Med 78:185, 1985

29. Katz A, Davison J, Hayslett J et al: Pregnancy in women with kidney disease. Kidney Int 18:192, 1980

30. Mackay E: Pregnancy and renal disease: a ten-year study. Aust NZ J Obstet Gynaecol 3:21, 1963

31. Studd J, Blainey J: Pregnancy and the nephrotic syndrome. Br Med J 1:276, 1969

32. Kincaid-Smith P, Fairley K, Bullen M: Kidney disease and pregnancy. Med J Aust 11:1155, 1967

33. Surian M, Imbasciati E, Banfi G et al: Glomerular disease and pregnancy. Nephron 36:101, 1984

34. Sibai B, Grossman R, Grossman H: Effects of diuretics on plasma volume in pregnancies with long term hypertension. Am J Obstet Gynecol 150:831, 1984

35. Crosland D, Flowers C: Chlorothiazide and its relationship to neonatal jaundice. Obstet Gynecol 22:500, 1963

36. Rodriguez S, Leikin S, Hiller M: Neonatal thrombocytopenia associated with ante-partum administration of thiazide drugs. N Engl J Med 270:881, 1964

37. Sanchez-Casajuz A, Famos I, Santos M: Monitorizacion fetal en el transcurso de hemodialissi durante el embarazo. Rev Clin Esp 149:187, 1978

38. Schewitz L, Friedman E, Pollak V: Bleeding after renal biopsy in pregnancy. Obstet Gynecol 26:295, 1965

39. Lindheimer M, Spargo B, Katz A: Renal biopsy in pregnancy-induced hypertension. J Reprod Med 15:189, 1975

40. Lindheimer M, Fisher K, Spargo B, Katz A: Hypertension in pregnancy: a biopsy study with long term follow-up. Contrib Nephrol 25:71, 1981

41. Packham D, Fairley KF: Renal biopsy: indications and complications in pregnancy. Br J Obstet Gynaecol 94:935, 1987

42. Ackrill P, Goodwin F, Marsh F et al: Successful pregnancy in patient on regular dialysis. Br Med J 2:172, 1975

43. Kobayashi H, Matsumoto Y, Otsubo O et al: Successful pregnancy in a patient undergoing chronic hemodialysis. Obstet Gynecol 57:382, 1981

44. Savdie E, Caterson R, Mahony J, Clifton-Bligh P: Successful pregnancies in women treated by haemodialysis. Med J Aust 2:9, 1982

45. Cohen D, Frenkel Y, Maschiach S, Eliahou HE: Dialysis during pregnancy in advanced chronic renal failure patients: outcome and progression. Clin Nephrol 29:144, 1988

46. Redrow M, Cherem L, Elliott J et al: Dialysis in the management of pregnant patients with renal insufficiency. Medicine 67:199, 1988

47. Hou S: Pregnancy in women requiring dialysis for renal failure. Am J Kidney Dis 9:368, 1987

48. Yasin SY, Doun SWB: Hemodialysis in pregnancy. Obstet Gynecol Surv 43:655, 1988

49. Lim V, Henriquez C, Sievertsen G, Prohman L: Ovarian function in chronic renal failure: evidence suggesting hypothalamic anovulation. Ann Intern Med 57:7, 1980

50. Nageotte MP, Grundy HO: Pregnancy outcome in women requiring chronic hemodialysis. Obstet Gynecol 72:456, 1988

51. Fine L, Barnett E, Danovitch G et al: Systemic lupus erythematosus in pregnancy. Ann Intern Med 94:667, 1981

52. Johnson T, Lorenz R, Menon K, Nolan G: Successful outcome of a pregnancy requiring dialysis: effects on serum progesterone and estrogens. J Reprod Med 22:217, 1979

53. Merkatz I, Schwartz G, David D et al: Resumption of female reproductive function following renal transplantation. JAMA 216:1749, 1971

54. Davison J, Lind T, Uldall P: Planned pregnancy in a renal transplant recipient. Br J Obstet Gynaecol 83:518, 1976

55. Penn I, Makowski E, Harris P: Parenthood following renal transplantation. Kidney Int 18:221, 1980

56. Saarikoski S, Sappala M: Immunosuppression during pregnancy: transmission of azathioprine and its metabolites from mother to the fetus. Am J Obstet Gynecol 115:1100, 1973

57. Cote C, Meuwissen H, Pickering R: Effects on the neonate of prednisone and azathioprine administered to the mother during pregnancy. J Pediatr 85:324, 1974

58. Price H, Salaman J, Laurence K, Langmaid H: Immunosuppressive drugs and the fetus. Transplantation 21:294, 1976

59. Scott J: Fetal growth retardation associated with maternal administration of immunosuppresive drugs. Am J Obstet Gynecol 128:668, 1977

60. Davison J, Lindheimer M: Pregnancy in women with renal allografts. Semin Nephrol 4:240, 1984

61. Lewis G, Lamont C, Lee H, Slapak M: Successful pregnancy in a renal transplant recipient taking cyclosporin A. Br Med J 186:603, 1983

62. Salamalekis EE, Mortakis AE, Phocas I et al: Successful pregnancy in a renal transplant recipient taking cyclosporin A: hormonal and immunological studies. Int J Gynaecol Obstet 30:267, 1989

63. Prieto C, Errasti P, Olaizola JI et al: Successful twin pregnancies in renal transplant recipients taking cyclosporine. Transplantation 48:1065, 1989

64. Parsons V, Bewick M, Elias J et al: Pregnancy following renal transplantation. J R Soc Med 72:815, 1979

65. Huffer W, Kuzela D, Popovtzer M: Metabolic bone disease in chronic renal failure. II. Renal transplant patients. Am J Pathol 78:385, 1975

66. Davison J: Renal disease. p. 236. In deSwiet M (ed): Medical Disorders in Obstetric Practice. Blackwell, Oxford, 1984

67. Pertuiset N, Grunfeld JP: Acute renal failure in pregnancy. Baillieres Clin Obstet Gynaecol 1:873, 1987

68. Grunfeld JP, Pertuiset N: Acute renal failure in pregnancy: 1987. Am J Kidney Dis 9:359, 1987

69. Stratta P, Canavese C, Dogliani M et al: Pregnancy-related acute renal failure. Clin Nephrol 32:14, 1989

70. Grunfeld J, Ganeval D, Bournerias F: Acute renal failure in pregnancy. Kidney Int 18:179, 1980

71. Stratta P, Canavese C, Colla L et al: Acute renal failure in preeclampsia–eclampsia. Gynecol Obstet Invest 24:225, 1987

72. Turney JH, Ellis CM, Parsons FM: Obstetric acute renal failure 1956–1987. Br J Obstet Gynaecol 96:679, 1989

73. Sibai BM, Villar MA, Mabie BC: Acute renal failure in hypertensive disorders of pregnancy: pregnancy outcome and remote prognosis in thirty-one consecutive cases. Am J Obstet Gynecol 162:777, 1990

74. Coratelli P, Buongiorno E, Passavanti G: Endotoxemia in hemolytic uremic syndrome. Nephron 50:365, 1988

75. Robson J, Martin A, Burkley V: Irreversible postpartum renal failure: a new syndrome. Q J Med 37:423, 1968

76. Segonds A, Louradour N, Suc J, Orfila C: Postpartum hemolytic uremic syndrome: a study of three cases with a review of the literature. Clin Nephrol 12:229, 1979

77. Wagoner R, Holley K, Johnson W: Accelerated nephrosclerosis and postpartum acute renal failure in normotensive patients. Ann Intern Med 69:237, 1968

78. Creasey GW, Morgan J: Hemolytic uremic syndrome after ectopic pregnancy: postectopic nephrosclerosis. Obstet Gynecol 69:448, 1987

79. Li PK, Lai FM, Tam JS, Lai KN: Acute renal failure due to postpartum haemolytic uraemic syndrome. Aust NZ J Obstet Gynaecol 28:228, 1988

80. Conte F, Mewroni M, Battini G et al: Plasma exchange in acute renal failure due to postpartum hemolytic-uremic syndrome: report of a case. Nephron 50:167, 1988

81. Remuzzi G, Misiani R, Marchesi D et al: Treatment of hemolytic uremic syndrome with plasma. Clin Nephrol 12:279, 1979

82. Webster J, Rees A, Lewis P, Hensby C: Prostacyclin deficiency in haemolytic uraemic syndrome. Br Med J 281:271, 1980

83. Brandt P, Jesperson J, Gregerson G: Post-partum haemolytic-uraemic syndrome successfully treated with antithrombin III. Br Med J 281:449, 1980

Chapter 33

Diabetes Mellitus and Other Endocrine Diseases

Mark B. Landon

DIABETES MELLITUS

The discovery of insulin in 1921 remains the most significant advancement in the treatment of pregnancy complicated by diabetes mellitus. Prior to that time, pregnancy in the diabetic woman was uncommon and was accompanied by high maternal and fetal mortality rates. Through improved understanding of the pathophysiology of diabetes in pregnancy as well as the development of techniques to prevent these complications, fetal and neonatal mortality have been reduced from approximately 65 percent before the discovery of insulin to 2 to 5 percent at the present time (Fig. 33.1). If optimal care is delivered to the diabetic woman, the perinatal mortality rate excluding major congenital malformations is equivalent to that observed in normal pregnancies.

Controversy still exists regarding the management of pregnancy complicated by diabetes. While the benefit of careful regulation of maternal glucose levels is generally well accepted, questions remain regarding those factors that contribute to intrauterine deaths and congenital malformations, as well as the significant neonatal morbidity observed in the infant of the diabetic mother (IDM). There is also debate concerning which methods are most predictive for the assessment of antepartum fetal well-being and maturity. Before reviewing these issues it is important to have an understanding of carbohydrate metabo-

lism and the pathophysiology of diabetes during pregnancy.

Pathophysiology

During normal pregnancy, maternal metabolism adjusts to provide adequate nutrition for both the mother and the growing fetoplacental unit. Early in pregnancy, glucose homeostasis is affected by increases in estrogen and progesterone, which lead to β-cell hyperplasia and increased insulin secretion.[1] With increased peripheral utilization of glucose, maternal fasting glucose levels will fall. Glycogen deposition increases in peripheral tissues, accompanied by a decrease in hepatic glucose production. Insulin-dependent diabetic patients therefore commonly experience periods of hypoglycemia in the first trimester. Additionally, maternal circulating levels of amino acids are reduced, while levels of fatty acids, triglycerides, and ketones are increased. Maternal mechanisms to offset this state of "accelerated starvation" include increased protein metabolism and accelerated renal gluconeogenesis.[2]

Lipids become an important maternal fuel as pregnancy advances. Early in pregnancy, fat storage increases. With the rise of human placental lactogen (hPL), a polypeptide hormone produced by the syncytiotrophoblast, lipolysis is stimulated in adipose tissue.[3] The release of glycerol and fatty acids reduces both maternal glucose and amino acid utilization and in doing so spares these fuels for the fetus.

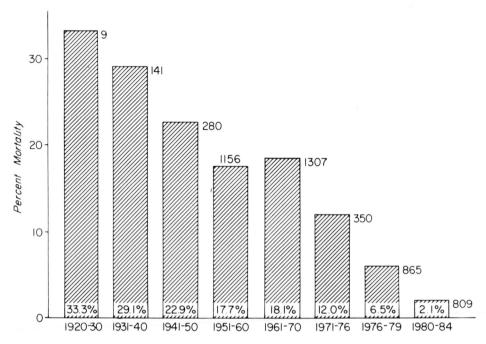

Fig. 33.1 Perinatal mortality in pregnancies complicated by insulin-dependent diabetes mellitus, classes B through R. Number at the top of column indicates total number of cases in each time period. (Adapted from Gabbe,[12] with permission.)

The actions of hPL are responsible in part for the "diabetogenic state" of pregnancy. In the normal pregnant woman, glucose hemostasis is maintained by the exaggerated rate and amount of insulin release that accompanies decreased sensitivity to insulin (Fig. 33.2).[4] Other hormones that appear to modify this response include elevated levels of free cortisol, estrogen, and progesterone. With placental growth, larger amounts of these contrainsulin factors are synthesized. A woman with overt diabetes cannot respond to this stress and requires additional insulin therapy as pregnancy progresses. Her increased insulin requirement, approximately 30 percent over the prepregnancy dose, is roughly equivalent to the endogenous increase seen in a normal gestation. If the pregnant woman has borderline pancreatic reserve, it is possible that her endogenous insulin production will be inadequate, particularly late in gestation. Diabetes will then be revealed for the first time. Unlike known insulin-requiring patients, obese gestational diabetes with β-cell reserve but presumed peripheral insulin resistance may experience large increases in both insulin secretion and requirement during pregnancy. These patients demonstrate increased levels of fasting triglycerides and elevated serum LDL and HDL levels.[5] With weight loss following pregnancy, most of these women will exhibit normal glucose homeostasis and will no longer require insulin.

Glucagon, which has both glycogenolytic and gluconeogenic actions, appears to contribute little to the "diabetogenic stress" of pregnancy. Levels of this hormone show a modest increase over nonpregnant values as pregnancy advances.[6] In normal pregnant women, glucagon levels appear to be suppressed in response to glucose administration. This phenomenon results in "facilitated anabolism," periods after meals marked by more prolonged hyperglycemia that counterbalance the "accelerated starvation" of the fasting state.

Maternal glucose appears to pass to the fetus by carrier-mediated facilitated diffusion. Fetal blood glucose levels usually remain 20 to 30 mg/dl lower than those of the mother. There is a close correlation between fetal glucose uptake and maternal blood levels.[7] The fetal level is normally maintained within narrow limits because maternal glucose hemostasis is

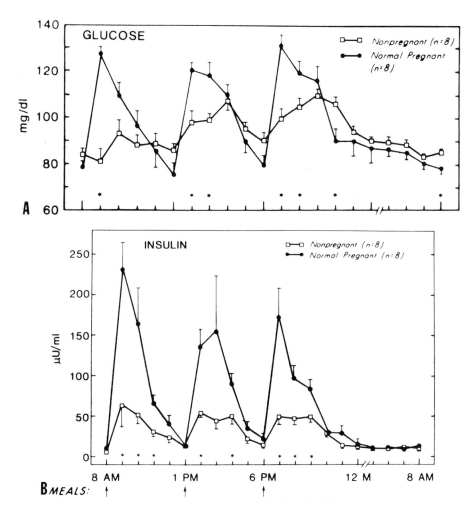

Fig. 33.2 Mean (±SEM) values for (A) glucose and (B) insulin at intervals of 1 hour from 8:00 A.M. to midnight and 2 hours thereafter in eight nonpregnant and eight normal pregnant women in the third trimester. Mealtimes are indicated by arrows along the abscissa. Pregnant women demonstrate a greater amplitude in plasma glucose excursion after meals. The increased postprandial insulin secretion is apparent. (From Phelps et al.,[189] with permission.)

so well regulated. Protein hormones such as insulin, glucagon, growth hormone, and hPL do not cross the placenta. Ketoacids appear to diffuse freely across the placenta and may serve as a fetal fuel during periods of maternal starvation.[8]

During pregnancy in the insulin-dependent diabetic woman, periods of hyperglycemia result in fetal hyperglycemia. Persistently elevated levels of glucose will stimulate the fetal pancreas, resulting in a β-cell hyperplasia and fetal hyperinsulinemia.[9] The latter appears to play the major role in inducing excessive fetal growth and probably contributes to the in-

creased risk of intrauterine death, respiratory distress syndrome, hypoglycemia, and other morbidity seen in the IDM.

Daily glucose excursions even in well-controlled diabetic women often exceed those of normal patients.[10] Fetal macrosomia appears to be primarily a consequence of fetal hyperinsulinemia induced by fetal hyperglycemia. Increased deposition of fat, protein, and glycogen leads to excessive birth weights in up to one-half of pregnancies complicated by diabetes (Fig. 33.3). It is hypothesized that glucose serves as the primary precursor for α-glycerophosphate

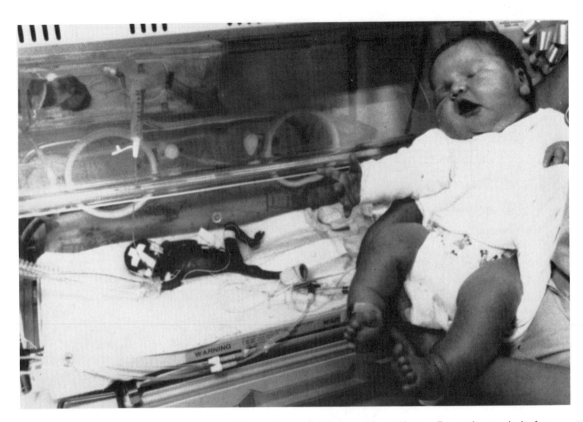

Fig. 33.3 Two extremes of growth abnormalities in infants of diabetic mothers. The small growth-retarded infant on the left weighed 470 g and is the offspring of a woman with nephropathy and hypertension, delivered at 28 weeks gestation. The neonate on the right is the 5,100-g baby of a woman with suboptimally controlled class C diabetes.

used in triglyceride synthesis.[11] Amino acids and possibly fatty acids may also stimulate fetal insulin secretion and therefore promote excessive fetal growth.

Perinatal Morbidity and Mortality

Fetal Death

In the past, sudden and unexplained stillbirth occurred in 10 to 30 percent of pregnancies complicated by insulin-dependent diabetes mellitus (IDDM).[12] Although relatively uncommon today, such losses still plague the pregnancies of patients who do not receive optimal care. Stillbirths have been observed most often after week 36 of pregnancy in patients with vascular disease, poor glycemic control, hydramnios, fetal macrosomia, or preeclampsia. In an effort to prevent intrauterine deaths, a strategy of scheduled preterm deliveries was established. This empiric approach reduced the number of stillbirths,

but errors in estimation of fetal size and gestational age as well as the functional immaturity characteristic of the IDM contributed to many neonatal deaths from hyaline membrane disease (HMD).

The precise cause of the excessive stillbirth rate in pregnancies complicated by diabetes remains unknown. Because extramedullary hematopoiesis is frequently observed in stillborn IDMs, chronic intrauterine hypoxia has been cited as a likely cause of these intrauterine fetal deaths. Maternal diabetes may produce alterations in red blood cell oxygen release and placental blood flow.[13]

Reduced uterine blood flow is thought to contribute to the increased incidence of intrauterine growth retardation in pregnancies complicated by diabetic vasculopathy. Investigations using radioactive tracers have also suggested a relationship between poor maternal metabolic control and reduced uteroplacental blood flow.[14] Ketoacidosis and preeclampsia, two factors known to be associated with an increased incidence of intrauterine deaths, may further decrease uterine blood flow. In diabetic ketoacidosis, hypovolemia and hypotension caused by dehydration may reduce flow through the intervillous space, whereas in preeclampsia narrowing and vasospasm of spiral arterioles may result.

Alterations in fetal carbohydrate metabolism also may contribute to intrauterine asphyxia.[15-17] There is considerable evidence linking hyperinsulinemia and fetal hypoxia. Hyperinsulinemia induced in fetal lambs by an infusion of exogenous insulin produces an increase in oxygen consumption and a decrease in arterial oxygen content.[18] Thus hyperinsulinemia in the fetus of the diabetic mother may increase fetal metabolic rate and oxygen requirements in the presence of several conditions such as hyperglycemia, ketoacidosis, preeclampsia, and maternal vasculopathy, which can reduce placental blood flow and fetal oxygenation.

Congenital Malformations

With the reduction in intrauterine deaths and a marked decrease in neonatal mortality related to HMD and traumatic delivery, congenital malformations have emerged as the most important cause of perinatal loss in pregnancies complicated by IDDM. In the past, these anomalies were responsible for approximately 10 percent of all perinatal deaths. At present, however, malformations account for 30 to 50 percent of perinatal mortality.[19] Neonatal deaths now exceed stillbirths in pregnancies complicated by IDDM, and fatal congenital malformations account for this changing pattern.

Most studies have documented a two- to fourfold increase in major malformations in infants of insulin-dependent diabetic mothers. In a prospective analysis, Simpson et al.[19] observed an 8.5 percent incidence of major anomalies in the IDDM population, while the malformation rate in a small group of concurrently gathered control subjects was 2.4 percent. Similar figures were obtained in the Diabetes in Early Pregnancy Study in the United States.[20] The incidences of major anomalies were 2.1 percent in 389 control patients and 9.0 percent in 279 IDDM women. In general, the incidences of major malformations in worldwide studies of offspring of IDDM mothers have ranged from 5 to 10 percent.

CONGENITAL MALFORMATIONS IN INFANTS OF DIABETIC MOTHERS

Cardiovascular
  Transposition of the great vessels
  Ventricular septal defect
  Atrial septal defect
  Hypoplastic left ventricle
  Situs inversus
  Anomalies of the aorta

Central nervous system
  Anencephaly
  Encephalocele
  Meningomyelocele
  Holoprosencephaly
  Microcephaly

Skeletal
  Caudal regression syndrome
  Spina bifida

Genitourinary
  Absent kidneys (Potter syndrome)
  Polycystic kidneys
  Double ureter

Gastrointestinal
  Tracheoesophageal fistula
  Bowel atresia
  Imperforate anus

The insult that causes malformations in IDM impacts on most organ systems and must act before 7 weeks gestation.[21] The congenital defect thought to be most characteristic of diabetic embryopathy is sacral agenesis or caudal dysplasia, an anomaly found 200 to 400 times more often in offspring of women with diabetes than in offspring of women without diabetes (Fig. 33.4).[22] Central nervous system malformations, particularly anencephaly, open spina bifida, and possibly holoprosencephaly are increased tenfold.[23] Cardiac anomalies, especially ventricular septal defects and complex lesions such as transposition of the great vessels, are increased fivefold.

It appears that a derangement in maternal metabolism, possibly in association with a greater genetic susceptibility, contributes to abnormal embryogenesis. Maternal hyperglycemia has been proposed by

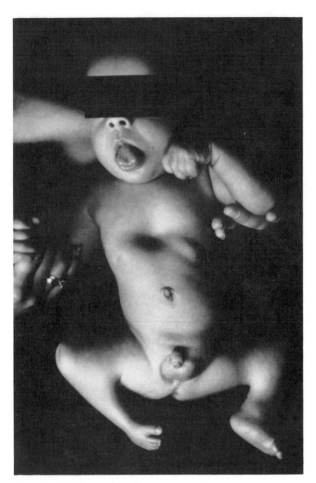

Fig. 33.4 Infant of a diabetic mother with caudal regression syndrome. The mother of this infant presented with class F diabetes at 26 weeks, in poor glycemic control. Ultrasound examination revealed absent lower lumbar spine and sacrum and hypoplastic lower extremities.

most investigators as the primary factor, but hyperketonemia and hypoglycemia also have been suggested.[24]

Several mechanisms have been proposed by which the above teratogenic factors produce malformations. Freinkel et al.[25] suggested that anomalies might arise from inhibition of glycolysis, the key energy-producing process during embryogenesis. They found that D-mannose added to the culture medium of rat embryos inhibited glycolysis and produced growth retardation and derangements of neural tube closure. Freinkel et al.[25] also stressed the sensitivity of

normal embryogenesis to alterations in these key energy-producing pathways, a process they labeled "fuel-mediated" teratogenesis. Goldman et al.[26] suggested that the mechanism responsible for the increased incidence of neural tube defects in embryos cultured in a hyperglycemic medium may involve a functional deficiency of arachidonic acid, because supplementation with arachidonic acid or myoinositol will reduce the frequency of neural tube defects in this experimental model.

Macrosomia

Excessive growth may predispose the IDM to shoulder dystocia, traumatic birth injury, and asphyxia. Newborn adiposity also may be associated with a significant risk for obesity in later life.[27]

Some have defined macrosomia as a birth weight in excess of 4,000 to 4,500 g, but others prefer categorizing infants as large for gestational age (a birth weight >90th percentile) using population-specific growth curves. According to these definitions, macrosomia has been observed in as many as 50 percent of pregnancies complicated by gestational diabetes mellitus (GDM) and 40 percent of IDDM pregnancies. Delivery of an infant weighing greater than 4,500 g occurred *10 times* more often in diabetic women than in a nondiabetic control population.[28]

Fetal macrosomia in the IDM is reflected by increased adiposity, muscle mass, and organomegaly. The disproportionate increase in the size of the trunk and shoulder compared with the head may contribute to the likelihood of a difficult vaginal delivery.[29] An increase in total body fat in the IDM has been supported by direct measurements as well as assessment of subcutaneous stores using skinfold thickness measurements.[30] The amount of subcutaneous fat present in the IDM may be an indication of the quality of diabetic control achieved during gestation.[31]

The concept that maternal hyperglycemia leading to fetal hyperglycemia and hyperinsulinemia results in excessive fetal growth and adipose deposition was first advanced by the Danish internist Pedersen.[9] Increased β-cell mass may be identified as early as the second trimester.[32] Evidence supporting the Pedersen hypothesis also has come from studies of amniotic fluid and cord blood insulin and C-peptide levels. Both are increased in the amniotic fluid of insulin-treated diabetic women at term.[33] In addition to glucose, other substrates can modify the fetal insulin secretory response. Of the major nutrients, it is likely that amino acids are important regulators of fetal insulin secretion.[34]

Hypoglycemia

Neonatal hypoglycemia, a blood glucose level below 40 mg/dl during the first 12 hours of life, results from a rapid drop in plasma glucose concentrations following clamping of the umbilical cord. The degree of hypoglycemia may be influenced by at least two factors: (1) maternal glucose control during the latter half of pregnancy and (2) maternal glycemia during labor and delivery. Maternal blood glucose levels greater than 90 mg/dl during delivery have been found to increase significantly the frequency of neonatal hypoglycemia.[35] Presumably, prior poor maternal glucose control can result in fetal β-cell hyperplasia, leading to exaggerated insulin release following delivery. IDMs exhibiting hypoglycemia have elevated cord C-peptide and free insulin levels at birth and an exaggerated pancreatic response to glucose loading.[36]

Respiratory Distress Syndrome

The precise mechanism by which maternal diabetes affects pulmonary development remains unknown. Experimental animal studies have focused primarily on the effects of hyperglycemia and hyperinsulinemia on pulmonary surfactant biosynthesis. An extensive review of the literature confirms that both of these factors are involved in delayed pulmonary maturation in the IDM.[37]

In vitro studies have documented that insulin can interfere with substrate availability for surfactant biosynthesis.[38,39] Smith[40] has postulated that insulin interferes with the normal timing of glucocorticoid-induced pulmonary maturation in the fetus. Cortisol apparently acts on pulmonary fibroblasts to induce synthesis of fibroblast-pneumocyte factor, which then acts on type II cells to stimulate phospholipid synthesis.[41] Carlson and co-workers[42] have shown that insulin blocks cortisol action at the level of the fibroblast by reducing the production of fibroblast-pneumocyte factor.

Clinical studies investigating the effects of maternal diabetes on fetal lung maturation have produced conflicting data. With the introduction of protocols that have emphasized glucose control and antepartum surveillance until lung maturity has been established, respiratory distress syndrome has become a less common occurrence in the IDM. Several studies agree that in well-controlled diabetic women delivered at term, the risk of respiratory distress syndrome is no higher than that observed in the general population.[43,44] In recent studies that have emphasized rigorous maternal glycemic control, respiratory distress syndrome virtually has been eliminated.

Calcium and Magnesium Metabolism

Neonatal hypocalcemia, serum levels below 7 mg/dl, occurs at an increased rate in the IDM when one controls for predisposing factors such as prematurity and birth asphyxia.[45] Hypocalcemia in the IDM has been associated with a failure to increase parathyroid hormone (PTH) synthesis following birth.[45] Decreased serum magnesium levels also have been documented in pregnant diabetic women as well as their infants. Mimouni et al.[46] described reduced amniotic fluid magnesium concentrations in women with IDDM. Their findings may be explained by a drop in fetal urinary magnesium excretion, which would accompany a relative magnesium-deficient state. Magnesium deficiency paradoxically then may inhibit fetal PTH secretion.

Hyperbilirubinemia and Polycythemia

Hyperbilirubinemia is frequently observed in the IDM. Neonatal jaundice has been reported in as many as 53 percent of pregnancies complicated by IDDM and in 38 percent of pregnancies with GDM.[47,48] Although several mechanisms have been proposed to explain these clinical findings, the pathogenesis of hyperbilirubinemia remains uncertain. In the past, the jaundice observed in the IDM often was attributed to prematurity. Investigators who have analyzed morbidity carefully, according to gestational age, however, have rejected this concept.[49]

Although severe hyperbilirubinemia may be observed independent of polycythemia, a common pathway for these complications most likely involves increased red blood cell production, stimulated by increased erythropoietin in the IDM. Presumably, the major stimulus for red cell production is a state of relative hypoxia in utero, as described previously. Although cord erythropoietin levels generally are normal in IDMs whose mothers demonstrate good glycemic control during gestation, Shannon et al.[50] and Ylinen et al.[48] found that HbA_{1c} values in late pregnancy were significantly elevated in mothers of hyperbilirubinemic infants.

Maternal Classification and Risk Assessment

In 1949, Priscilla White[51] noted that the patient's age at onset of diabetes, the duration of the disease, and the presence of vasculopathy significantly influenced perinatal outcome. Her pioneering work led to a classification system that has been widely applied to pregnant women with diabetes. A modification of this scheme is presented in Table 33.1. Counseling a patient and formulating a plan of management requires assessment of both maternal and fetal risks. The White classification facilitates this evaluation.

Class A_1 diabetes mellitus includes those patients who have demonstrated carbohydrate intolerance during a 100-g, 3-hour oral glucose tolerance test (GTT); however, their fasting and 2-hour postprandial glucose levels are less than 105 mg/dl and 120 mg/dl, respectively. These patients are generally managed by dietary regulation alone. If the fasting value of the GTT is elevated ($\geq$ 105 mg/dl) and/or 2-hour postprandial glucose levels exceed 120 mg/dl,

Table 33.1 Modified White Classification of Pregnant Diabetic Women

Class	Diabetes Onset Age (years)		Duration (years)	Vascular Disease	Insulin Need
Gestational diabetes					
A_1	Any		Any	0	0
A_2	Any		Any	0	+
Pregestational diabetes					
B	>20		<10	0	+
C	10–19	or	10–19	0	+
D	<10	or	>20	+	+
F	Any		Any	+	+
R	Any		Any	+	+
T	Any		Any	+	+
H	Any		Any	+	+

(Modified from White,[51] with permission.)

patients are designated class A_2. These women usually require insulin.

The second International Workshop Conference on Gestational Diabetes sponsored by the American Diabetes Association in cooperation with the American College of Obstetricians and Gynecologists recommended that the term *gestational diabetes* rather than *class A diabetes* be used to describe women with carbohydrate intolerance of variable severity with onset or recognition during the present pregnancy.[52] The term *gestational diabetes* fails to specify whether the patient requires dietary adjustment alone or treatment with diet and insulin. This distinction is important, because those patients who are normoglycemic while fasting have a significantly lower perinatal mortality rate.[53] They do not appear to experience an increased incidence of intrauterine deaths in late pregnancy. Gestational diabetics who require insulin are at greater risk for a poor perinatal outcome than are those controlled by diet alone. This observation probably reflects more marked maternal hyperglycemia and, in some cases, a delay in the institution of insulin therapy.

Patients requiring insulin are designated by the letters B, C, D, R, F, and T. Class B patients are those whose onset of disease occurs after age 20 years. They have had diabetes less than 10 years and have no vascular complications. Included in this subgroup of patients are those who have been previously treated with oral hypoglycemic agents.

Class C diabetes includes patients whose disease onset is between ages 10 and 19 years or who have had the disease for 10 to 19 years. Vascular disease is not present.

Class D represents women whose disease is of 20 years duration or more, or whose onset occurred before age 10 years, or who have benign retinopathy. The latter includes microaneurysms, exudates, and venous dilatation.

Nephropathy

Class F describes the 5 to 10 percent of patients with underlying renal disease. This includes those with reduced creatinine clearance and/or proteinuria of at least 400 mg in 24 hours measured during the first trimester. Several factors present prior to 20 weeks gestation appear to be predictive of perinatal outcome in these women (e.g., perinatal death or birth weight <1,100 g): (1) proteinuria more than 3.0 g/24 h, (2) serum creatinine more than 1.5 mg/dl, (3) anemia with hematocrit less than 25 percent, and (4) hypertension (mean arterial pressure >107 mmHg).

In a series of 27 class F women, if any one of the above factors was present early in gestation, over one-half of the pregnancies resulted in perinatal deaths or infants weighing less than 1,100 gm.[54] In contrast, when no risk factors were present, over 90 percent experienced a successful perinatal outcome.[54]

Several studies have failed to demonstrate a permanent worsening of diabetic renal disease as a result of pregnancy.[55,56] Kitzmiller and colleagues[55] reviewed 35 pregnancies complicated by diabetic nephropathy. Proteinuria increased in 69 percent, and hypertension developed in 73 percent. Following delivery, proteinuria declined in 65 percent of cases. In only two patients did protein excretion increase after gestation. Changes in creatinine clearance during pregnancy are variable in class F patients. Kitzmiller,[57] in reviewing 44 patients from the literature, noted that about one-third of women had an expected rise in creatinine clearance during gestation compared with one-third who had a decline of more than 15 percent by the third trimester. Of interest, most patients with a severe reduction in creatinine clearance (<50 ml/min) measured during the first trimester did not demonstrate a further reduction in clearance during pregnancy. However, a decline in renal function was evident in 20 to 30 percent of cases. Several investigators have confirmed that any deterioration of renal function after pregnancy is consistent with the natural course of diabetic nephropathy and is not related to pregnancy per se.[58]

With improved survival of diabetic patients following renal transplantation, a small group of kidney recipients have now achieved pregnancy (class T). Nine cases of pregnancy complicated by diabetes and prior renal transplantation have recently been described.[59] In this series, there was no episode of renal allograft rejection. Prednisone and azathioprine were administered throughout gestation. A single maternal death and two fetal deaths did occur in patients with preexisting peripheral vascular disease. Superimposed preeclampsia occurred in six patients. All seven surviving infants were delivered prior to term, with fetal compromise evident in six of these cases.

Retinopathy

Class R diabetes designates patients with proliferative retinopathy. There is no difference in the prevalence of retinopathy in women who have or have not been pregnant.[60] However, retinopathy may worsen significantly during pregnancy in spite of the major advances that have been made in diagnosis and treatment. Laser photocoagulation therapy during pregnancy with careful follow-up has helped to maintain many pregnancies to a gestational age at which neonatal survival is likely.

In a large series of 172 patients, including 40 cases with background retinopathy and 11 with proliferative changes, only one patient developed new onset proliferative retinopathy during pregnancy.[61] A review of the literature by Kitzmiller et al.[62] confirmed the observation that progression to proliferative retinopathy during pregnancy rarely occurs in women with background retinopathy or in those without any eye ground changes. Of the 561 women in these two categories, only 17 (3.0 percent) developed neovascularization during gestation. In contrast, 23 of 26 (88.5 percent) with untreated proliferative disease experienced worsening retinopathy during pregnancy.[62]

Moloney and Drury[63] have reported that pregnancy may increase the prevalence of some background changes. These investigators noted a characteristic increase in streak-blob hemorrhages and soft exudates, which often resolved between examination. Retinopathy progressed despite strict metabolic control. Phelps and colleagues[64] have related worsening retinal disease, as well as the magnitude of improvement in glycemia during early pregnancy, to plasma glucose at the first prenatal visit. Chang and colleagues[65] have also reported the development of proliferative changes with rapid normalization of glucose control. Whether improved control contributes to a deterioration of background retinopathy remains uncertain. Fortunately, most patients who require laser photocoagulation will respond to this therapy and should therefore be promptly treated. However, those women who demonstrate severe florid disc neovascularization which is unresponsive to laser therapy during early pregnancy may be at great risk for deterioration of their vision. Termination of pregnancy should be considered in this group of patients.

In addition to background and proliferative eye disease, Sinclair and colleagues[66] have described vas-oocclusive lesions associated with the development of macular edema during pregnancy. Cystic macular edema is most often found in patients with protein-uric nephropathy and hypertensive disease leading to retinal edema. Macular capillary permeability is a feature of this process. The degree of macular edema is directly related to the fall in plasma oncotic pressure present in these women. In the series of Sinclair et al.,[66] seven women with minimal or no retinopathy before becoming pregnant developed severe macular edema associated with preproliferative or prolifera-tive retinopathy during the course of their pregnan-cies. Although proliferation was controlled with pho-tocoagulation, the macular edema worsened until delivery in all cases and was often aggravated by pho-tocoagulation.[66] While both macular edema and reti-nopathy regressed after delivery in some patients, in others these pathologic processes persisted, resulting in significant visual loss.

Coronary Artery Disease

Class H diabetes refers to the presence of diabetes of any duration associated with ischemic myocardial disease. There is evidence that the small number of women who have coronary artery disease are at an increased risk for mortality during gestation.[67] This is especially true of women with a previous myocardial infarction or an infarction during pregnancy. For these cases, maternal mortality rates exceed 50 per-cent.[68] While there are a few reports of successful pregnancies following myocardial infarction in dia-betic women, cardiac status should be carefully as-sessed early in gestation or preferably prior to preg-nancy. If ECG abnormalities are encountered, echocardiography may be employed to assess ventric-ular function or modified stress testing may be under-taken.

Detection of Diabetes in Pregnancy

Ninety percent of the cases of diabetes that compli-cate pregnancy are GDM.[69] The detection of GDM is therefore an important diagnostic challenge. Patients with GDM represent a group with significant risk for

developing glucose intolerance later in life. It has been reported that 50 percent of these patients will become diabetic in the 15 years following preg-nancy.[70]

As noted above, GDM is a state restricted to preg-nant women whose impaired glucose tolerance is discovered during pregnancy. Because in most cases patients with GDM have normal fasting glucose levels, some challenge of glucose tolerance must be undertaken. Traditionally, obstetricians relied on his-torical and clinical risk factors to select those patients most likely to develop GDM. This group included patients with a family history of diabetes or those whose past pregnancies were marked by an unex-plained stillbirth or the delivery of a malformed or macrosomic infant. Obesity, hypertension, glycos-uria, and maternal age over 25 years were other indi-cations for screening. Glycosuria is common in preg-nancy and reflects a relative decrease in the tubular reabsorption of glucose. This finding is more likely to signal true carbohydrate intolerance if noted on a second voided fasting urine specimen. Interestingly, over one-half of all patients who exhibit an abnormal GTT lack the risk factors mentioned above. Coustan and colleagues[71] reported that in a series of 6,214 women, screening using historical risk factors and an arbitrary age cut-off of 30 years missed 35 percent of cases of GDM.

It is therefore recommended that *all* pregnant women be screened for gestational diabetes with a 50-g oral glucose load followed by a glucose determi-nation 1 hour later (Table 33.2).[72] The patient need not be fasting when this test is performed. However, sensitivity is improved if the test is performed in

Table 33.2   Detection of Gestational Diabetes — Upper Limits of Normalcy

Screening Test	Plasma (mg/dl)
50-g, 1-hour	130–140
Oral GTT[a]	
Fasting	105
1-Hour	190
2-Hour	165
3-Hour	145

[a] Diagnosis of gestational diabetes is made when any two values are met or exceeded.

the fasting state.[73] The sensitivity of this screening technique is approximately 80 percent, and its specificity approaches 90 percent. The test is generally performed at 24 to 28 weeks gestation. Patients whose plasma glucose level equals or exceeds 130 to 140 mg/dl should be evaluated with a 3-hour GTT. A normal glucose screen in early pregnancy does not necessarily rule out later development of GDM. A significant number of false negatives will result if screening thresholds for performing a GTT exceed 140 mg/dl. One can expect approximately 15 percent of patients with an abnormal screening value to have an abnormal 3-hour GTT. However, most patients whose 1-hour screening value exceeds 190 mg/dl will exhibit abnormal glucose tolerance.[74] In these women, it is preferable to check a fasting glucose level before administering a 100-g carbohydrate load.

The oral GTT rather than the intravenous test is preferred, because it is more physiologic and assesses the gastrointestinal factors involved in insulin secretion. Furthermore, the oral GTT appears to be more sensitive and has been well standardized. The normal values for the GTT are listed in Table 33.2. The patient must have two abnormal postprandial glucose determinations to be designated a gestational diabetic. In women whose GTT is normal but who have significant risk factors, including a previous history of GDM, a repeat test may be performed at 32 to 34 weeks gestation.[75]

Although elevated fasting values do indicate the presence of overt diabetes, glucose tolerance testing in the immediate postpartum period is unreliable in detecting previously unrecognized GDM. Similarly, postpartum glycohemoglobin levels, if elevated, seem to correlate with abnormal glucose tolerance.[76] Patients who have been identified as gestational diabetics should have a follow-up 75-g oral glucose tolerance test at 6 weeks gestation to determine if they have persistent carbohydrate intolerance (Table 33.3).

Treatment of the Insulin-Dependent Patient

Fetal glucose levels reflect those of the mother. Therefore the benefits of careful regulation of maternal glucose homeostasis will be apparent in improved perinatal outcomes. Self-monitoring of blood glucose combined with aggressive insulin therapy has made the maintenance of maternal normoglycemia (levels of 60 to 120 mg/dl) a therapeutic reality (Table 33.4). In most institutions, patients are taught to monitor their glucose control using glucose-oxidase–impregnated reagent strips and a glucose reflectance meter.[77] Glucose determinations are made in the fasting state before lunch and dinner and at bedtime. Postprandial and nocturnal values are also helpful.

During pregnancy, most insulin-dependent patients will require multiple insulin injections. A combination of intermediate-acting and regular insulin before breakfast and at dinnertime is the most commonly employed regimen. As a general rule, the amount of intermediate-acting insulin taken in the morning will exceed that of regular by a two to one ratio.[78] Patients usually receive two-thirds of their total insulin dose at breakfast and the remaining third

Table 33.3 Postpartum Evaluation for Carbohydrate Intolerance

1. 75-g oral glucose load, administered under conditions described for 100-g oral test
2. Venous plasma glucose measured fasting and at 30-minute intervals for 2 hours

Normal	Impaired Glucose Tolerance	Diabetes Mellitus
Fasting <115 mg/dl	<140 mg/dl	≥140 mg/dl
and	and	or
1/2, 1, and 1 1/2 hr <200 mg/dl	1 value ≥200 mg/dl	1 value ≥200 mg/dl
and	and	and
2 hr <140 mg/dl	≥140 to <200 mg/dl	≥200 mg/dl

(From National Institutes of Health Diabetes Data Group,[188] with permission.)

Table 33.4 Target Plasma Glucose Levels in Pregnancy

Time	mg/dl
Before breakfast	60–90
Before lunch, dinner, bedtime snack	60–105
After meals	≤120
2 A.M. to 6 A.M.	>60

at dinnertime. An alternative regimen is to administer separate injections of regular insulin at dinnertime and intermediate-acting insulin at bedtime to reduce the frequency of nocturnal hypoglycemia.[78] The latter may occur when the mother is in a relative fasting state while placental and fetal glucose consumption continue. All patients and their families should be instructed in the use of glucagon for treatment of serious hypoglycemia. Patients who have achieved good glycemic control during early pregnancy can be managed as outpatients. Early hospitalization is necessary for those pregnant women who are poorly controlled or unfamiliar with self-monitoring techniques.

The presence of maternal vasculopathy should be thoroughly assessed early in pregnancy. The patient should be evaluated by an ophthalmologist familiar with diabetic retinopathy. Baseline renal function is established by assaying a 24-hour urine collection for creatinine clearance and protein. An ECG and urine culture are also obtained.

Diet therapy is critical to successful regulation of maternal diabetes. A program consisting of three meals and several snacks is employed for most patients. Dietary composition should be 50 to 60 percent carbohydrate, 20 percent protein, and 25 to 30 percent fat with less than 10 percent saturated fats, up to 10 percent polyunsaturated fatty acids, and the remainder derived from monosaturated sources.[79] Caloric intake is established based on prepregnancy weight and weight gain during gestation. Weight reduction is not advised. Patients should consume approximately 35 kcal/kg ideal body weight. Obese women may be managed with an intake as low as 1,600 calories per day, although if ketonuria develops this allowance may be increased.

Patients who fail to maintain adequate control despite multiple insulin injections and dietary adjustment may be candidates for continuous subcutaneous insulin infusion (CSII) pump therapy. The initiation of this treatment almost always requires hospitalization. A basal infusion rate is established that is approximately 1 unit per hour. Bolus infusions are then given with meals and snacks. Multiple blood glucose determinations are made to prevent periods of hyper- and hypoglycemia. Many groups have now treated pregnant patients for varying periods of time with CSII. Glucose values may become normalized with minimal amplitude of daily excursions in a select group of pregnant diabetics. Episodes of hypoglycemia are usually secondary to errors in dose selection or failure to adhere to the required diet.[80] The risk of nocturnal hypoglycemia, which is markedly increased in the pregnant state, necessitates that great care be made in selecting candidates for CSII. Patients who fail to exhibit normal counterregulatory responses to hypoglycemia should probably be discouraged from using an insulin pump. While this technique may be valuable for a small group of pregnant women with diabetes mellitus, it has not been demonstrated to be superior to multiple-injection regimens. Coustan and colleagues[81] randomized 22 pregnant women to intensive conventional therapy with multiple-injection versus pump therapy. There were no differences between the two treatment groups with respect to outpatient mean glucose levels, glycosylated hemoglobin levels, or glycemic excursions.[81] In our experience over the past decade, we have found it necessary to institute pump therapy to achieve good glycemic control in only one patient. However, we have chosen to maintain women who have demonstrated good control using continuous infusion devices prior to pregnancy on this therapy throughout gestation.

After the initial hospitalization, patients are followed with outpatient visits at 1- to 2-week intervals. Following careful review of the patient's daily glucose values, adjustments in insulin dosage are made. The patient is instructed to contact her physician should periods of hypoglycemia or hyperglycemia occur. Fetal growth is evaluated by serial ultrasound examinations at 4- to 6-week intervals. In the third trimester, pregnancy-induced hypertension may become evident, necessitating hospitalization. This complication has been observed in up to 25 percent of diabetic pregnancies.[9] Ophthalmologic examinations are performed during each trimester and are repeated more often if retinopathy is detected. Ketonuria is common in normal pregnant women, especially during the third trimester, when fat stores may be mobilized as an important maternal energy source. The pregnant woman is more likely to exhibit ketonuria because calories from glucose and amino acids are diverted to the fetus, prompting the catabolism of maternal fat. This process does not appear to be deleterious to the fetus or mother.[31]

Ketonuria can also signal the presence of ketoacidosis in pregnancies complicated by diabetes mellitus. Ketoacidosis has been associated with an increased risk for intrauterine fetal death. To diagnose ketoacidosis, maternal arterial pH must be determined. The biochemical definition of diabetic ketoacidosis (DKA) includes a plasma glucose in excess of 300 mg/dl, plasma HCO_3 less than 15 mEq/L, and an arterial pH less than 7.30.[82] Serum acetone is positive at a 1:2 dilution.

The stress of infection is the most common precipitating factor in cases of DKA. Failure to administer insulin in a stable patient is rarely sufficient to bring on this crisis. The volume depletion that accompanies many infections through gastrointestinal and insensible water loss leads to increased hepatic production of ketoacids. This increased ketogenesis and gluconeogenesis may be secondary to a rise in glucagon and catecholamines. Dehydration results from the factors mentioned above, as well as through osmotic diuresis. Volume depletion may exacerbate DKA by reducing glomerular filtration and therefore glucose and ketone anion excretion.

Early recognition of signs and symptoms of DKA will improve both maternal and fetal outcome. Clinical signs of volume depletion follow the symptoms of hyperglycemia that include polydipsia and polyuria. Once the patient develops malaise, drowsiness, and hyperventilation, acidosis is usually present. During middle and late pregnancy, it is important to recognize that acidosis may be more severe than the clinical symptoms suggest. Pedersen[9] found that DKA may develop at relatively low levels of hyperglycemia (200 to 300 mg/dl). A simplified treatment plan for DKA in pregnancy follows.

Antepartum Fetal Surveillance

During the past 15 years, the understanding of the importance of maternal glycemic control in relation to fetal outcome has played a major role in reducing

---

MANAGEMENT OF DIABETIC KETOACIDOSIS DURING PREGNANCY

1. Laboratory Assessment
   Obtain arterial blood gases to document degree of acidosis present. Measure glucose, ketones, and electrolytes at 1–2-hour intervals

2. Insulin
   Low dose, intravenous
   Loading dose: 0.2–0.4 U/kg
   Maintenance: 2.0–10.0 U/hr

3. Fluids
   Isotonic NaCl
   Total replacement in first 12 hours = 4–6 L
   1.0 L in first hour
   500–100 ml/hr for 2–4 hours
   250 ml/hr until 80% replaced

4. Glucose
   Begin D5 normal saline when plasma level reaches 250 mg/dl

5. Potassium
   If initially normal or reduced, administer 40–60 mEq/L
   If elevated, give 20–30 mEq/L once levels begin to decline

6. Bicarbonate
   Add one ampule (44 mEq) to 1 L of 0.45 normal saline if pH is less than 7.10

---

perinatal mortality in pregnancies complicated by diabetes.[83] As previously noted, studies using a sheep model have demonstrated decreased oxygenation of the fetus in association with hyperinsulinemia and hyperglycemia.[16,18] Hyperglycemia and minimal hypoxemia may also induce lactic acidosis and fetal death in animal models.[15] Therefore programs of fetal surveillance are initiated in the third trimester, when the risk of sudden intrauterine death appears to be greatest. Well-controlled patients, as well as those without vasculopathy or significant hypertension, rarely have abnormal tests of fetal condition. Most importantly, the presence of reassuring antepartum testing allows the obstetrician to await further fetal

Table 33.5 Antepartum Fetal Surveillance in Low-Risk Insulin-Dependent Diabetes Mellitus[a]

Study	
Ultrasonography at 4–6-week intervals	Yes
Maternal assessment of fetal activity, daily at 28 weeks	Yes
Nonstress test (NST) weekly at 28 weeks	Yes
	Twice weekly at 34 weeks
Contraction stress test or biophysical profile if NST nonreactive	Yes
L/S, lung profile	Yes, if elective delivery planned prior to 39 weeks

[a] Low-risk IDDM: excellent control (60–120 mg/dl), no vasculopathy (classes B, C), no prior stillbirth.

maturation and avoid unnecessary premature intervention.

Estriol assays were the first tests widely employed for fetal monitoring in pregnancies complicated by diabetes mellitus. Rising estriol values were rarely associated with a sudden intrauterine death. However, urinary estriol assays do have a significant false-positive rate. Therefore management employing estriol testing alone could lead to a high rate of unnecessary intervention for presumed fetal distress.[84] Data from a number of studies has demonstrated limited clinical utility for the urinary estriol assay in pregnancies complicated by diabetes.[85]

The contraction stress test (CST) remains an important and valuable tool in the assessment of fetal well-being in pregnancies complicated by diabetes.[86] It has been repeatedly demonstrated that in a well-controlled patient, a negative CST predicts fetal survival for 1 week.[87,88] Positive CSTs, observed in approximately 10 percent of insulin-dependent diabetic patients, have been associated with an increased perinatal mortality rate, late decelerations during labor, low Apgar scores, respiratory distress syndrome, and growth retardation. The CST does have a significant false-positive rate of up to 60 percent.[88]

The nonstress test (NST) appears to be the preferred antepartum heart rate screening test in the management of patients with diabetes mellitus.[89] An NST that is nonreactive requires that a CST be performed. In most cases, heart rate monitoring is begun at approximately 32 to 34 weeks gestation and should be performed twice weekly (Tables 33.5 and 33.6). In patients with vascular disease or poor control, in whom the incidence of abnormal tests and intrauterine deaths is greater, testing is performed earlier in gestation and more frequently. An increased fetal

death rate within 1 week of a reactive NST has been reported for patients with insulin-dependent diabetes.[88,90] These reports confirm that, if the NST is to be used as the primary method of antepartum heart rate testing, it must be done at least twice weekly (Fig. 33.5).

Most recently, the fetal biophysical profile (BPP) rather than the CST has been used to evaluate the significance of a nonreactive NST result. Golde and colleagues[91] observed that 430 of 434 BPPs performed after a reactive NST were associated with reassuring scores of 8 or greater. Of 25 BPPs performed after a nonreactive NST result, 21 had scores of 8, and 4 had lower scores. In this series, even patients with low scores had good perinatal outcomes. The BPP did not appear to add more information about fetal condition if the NST result was reactive, but a score of 8 based on ultrasound parameters was as reliable in predicting good fetal outcome as was a reactive NST. In a study of 98 patients, Dicker and

Table 33.6 Antepartum Fetal Surveillance in High-Risk Insulin-Dependent Diabetes Mellitus[a]

Study	
Ultrasonography at 4-week intervals	Yes
Maternal assessment of fetal activity, daily at 28 weeks	Yes
Nonstress test (NST)	Minimum twice weekly
Contraction stress test or biophysical profile if NST nonreactive	Yes
L/S, lung profile at 37–38 weeks	Yes

[a] High-risk IDDM: poor control (macrosomia, hydramnios), vasculopathy (classes, D, F, R), prior stillbirth.

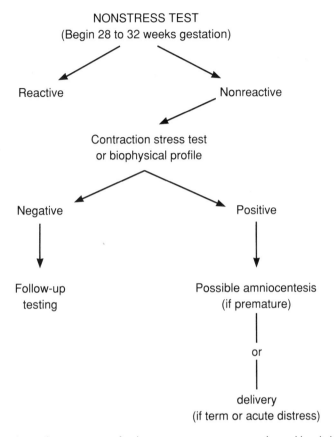

NONSTRESS TEST
(Begin 28 to 32 weeks gestation)

Reactive   Nonreactive

Contraction stress test
or biophysical profile

Negative   Positive

Follow-up   Possible amniocentesis
testing   (if premature)

or

delivery
(if term or acute distress)

Fig. 33.5 Scheme for antepartum fetal testing in pregnancy complicated by diabetes mellitus.

colleagues[92] confirmed that a normal BPP predicts normal Apgar scores in 99 percent of patients. In their series, only 2.9 percent of 978 BPPs were abnormal. Importantly, a total of 10 patients had an abnormal BPP just before delivery. In six of these cases, neonatal asphyxia or depression was present. Unfortunately, these investigators did not describe the metabolic status of their patients.

Johnson and associates[93] have also described their experience with the BPP in diabetic women. They performed twice-weekly tests in 50 women with insulin-dependent diabetes and weekly examinations in 188 women with GDM. There were no stillbirths in this series. The incidence of abnormal BPPs was low —only 8 of 238 tests (3.3%). The 230 fetuses with a normal score before delivery experienced minimal morbidity. In contrast, of eight patients with an abnormal score, 37.5 percent suffered significant neonatal morbidity. Although this study did not demon-

strate the superiority of the BPP over the NST alone, it did establish that the BPP may also be used for fetal surveillance with few unnecessary interventions, thereby allowing prolongation of pregnancy beyond 37 weeks in most of the patients studied.

Maternal monitoring of fetal activity is an easy and practical method that has proven useful in the monitoring of a variety of high-risk pregnancies (see Ch. 13). While this method has not been studied solely in pregnancies complicated by diabetes, it appears that assessment of fetal activity is comparable to heart rate testing. Patients may record fetal activity over a 12-hour period. They should appreciate at least 10 movements during this interval. If the length of time is found to increase before this number of movements is counted, or if less than 10 movements are recorded, heart rate testing is immediately performed. Patients may also count fetal movement for several 30-minute or 1-hour periods each day.

Ultrasound has been shown to be an extremely valuable tool in evaluating fetal growth, estimating fetal weight, and detecting hydramnios and malformations. A determination of maternal serum α-fetoprotein at 16 weeks gestation should be used in association with a detailed ultrasound study at 18 weeks to detect neural tube defects and other anomalies. In diabetic women, a maternal serum α-fetoprotein level greater than two multiples of the median increases the risk of neural tube defects and other anomalies. Fetal echocardiography is performed at 20 to 22 weeks gestation for the investigation of possible cardiac defects.

Ultrasound examinations are repeated at 4- to 6-week intervals to assess fetal growth. Antenatal detection of the macrosomic or growth-retarded fetus will facilitate selection of the optimal time and route of delivery in pregnancies complicated by diabetes. An increased rate of cephalopelvic disproportion and shoulder dystocia accompanied by significant risk of traumatic birth injury and asphyxia have been consistently associated with the vaginal delivery of large infants. The risk of such complications rises exponentially when fetal weight exceeds 4 kg and is greater for the fetus of a diabetic mother when compared with a similar-birth-weight fetus whose mother does not have diabetes.[94]

The macrosomic IDM is characterized by selective organomegaly, with increases in insulin-sensitive tissues including fat, muscle mass, and hepatomegaly. A disproportionate increase in the size of the trunk and shoulders is common in large-for-gestational-age (LGA) IDMs. Thus sonographic measurements of the fetal abdominal circumference (AC) have proven most helpful in predicting fetal macrosomia. Using an AC of more than the 90th percentile obtained within 2 weeks of delivery, Tamura et al.[95] correctly identified 78 percent of macrosomic fetuses. In a series of 201 gestational diabetic women reported by Bochner et al.,[96] 36 of 41 cases of macrosomia were identified by an AC above the 90th percentile at 30 to 33 weeks gestation. Despite a high false-positive rate, the risk of shoulder dystocia was 9.3 percent in the suspected LGA group versus 0.8 percent in the group with a normal AC measurement at 30 to 33 weeks.

We have found serial ultrasonography to be most useful in detecting growth abnormalities in diabetic pregnancies.[97] In our study of 79 diabetic women examined on at least three occasions during the third trimester, growth curves were similar for femoral length and head circumference for both normally grown and LGA fetuses. In contrast, growth of the AC was accelerated as early as 32 weeks in the LGA group. An AC growth velocity of at least 1.2 cm/wk detected LGA fetuses with 84 percent sensitivity and 85 percent specificity.

Doppler umbilical artery velocimetry has been proposed as a clinical tool for antepartum fetal surveillance in pregnancies at risk for placental vascular disease. Because women with insulin-dependent diabetes are at increased risk for the development of preeclampsia and fetal growth retardation, Doppler ultrasonography could be helpful in this population. In a serial study of 35 patients, umbilical artery waveforms were abnormal in 50 percent of fetuses of women with vascular disease compared with 12 percent of those without hypertension or nephropathy.[98] In women with vascular disease, increased placental resistance was correlated with fetal growth retardation. Umbilical artery waveform measurements were independent of glycemic control in this study. Although still somewhat investigational, umbilical and uterine artery Doppler studies may be helpful in the early identification of diabetic patients with vasculopathy who are at increased risk for fetal growth retardation.

Timing of Delivery

In the past, elective preterm delivery of the insulin-dependent patient to avoid an unexpected intrauterine fetal death was commonplace and often resulted in a high incidence of neonatal morbidity and mortality. With improved glycemic control and better methods of antepartum fetal surveillance, many patients are now delivered at term. Nevertheless, the rate of elective intervention still remains high in pregnancies complicated by diabetes. In most centers, elective delivery will be planned at 38 to 39 weeks gestation. It is important not only to use results of antepartum testing but also to recognize all the clinical features involving mother and fetus before a decision is made to intervene. This includes evaluation of the degree of glycemic control, hypertension, nephropathy, and the patient's ophthalmologic status.

Unless excellent gestational dating has been established in a well-controlled patient who has reached 39 weeks gestation, an amniocentesis should be performed prior to elective delivery to document fetal pulmonary maturity. The value of the lecithin/sphingomyelin ratio (L/S) has been questioned in diabetic pregnancies. Most series, however, report a low incidence of respiratory distress syndrome with a mature L/S ratio. In one study of 93 insulin-dependent patients, an L/S ratio of 2.0 or greater was associated with a 3 percent risk of respiratory distress syndrome, a result no different from that observed in the nondiabetic population. In three of the five cases of respiratory distress syndrome, delivery was performed before 37 weeks.[99] The presence of the acidic phospholipid phosphatidylglycerol (PG) is a final marker of fetal pulmonary maturation. Several studies have suggested that hyperinsulinemia may be associated with delayed appearance of PG and an increased incidence of respiratory distress syndrome. In one series, four infants who developed respiratory distress syndrome at delivery had L/S ratios between 2.0 and 3.0 but absent PG.[100] Reduced amounts of PG compared with phosphatidyinositol in amniotic fluid from gestations complicated by diabetes were also noted. Caution must therefore be used in planning the delivery of patients with a mature L/S and absent PG. *If antepartum assessment remains reassuring, delivery may be delayed for another week. In addition, the clinician must be familiar with the laboratory analysis of amniotic fluid in his or her institution and the neonatal outcome at various L/S ratios in the presence or absence of PG.*

When antepartum testing suggests fetal compromise, delivery must be considered. If amniotic fluid analysis yields a mature L/S ratio, delivery should be executed promptly. When the LS ratio is immature, the decision to proceed with delivery should be based on confirmation of deteriorating fetal condition by several positive test results. For example, if the results of both the NST and the CST or BPP indicate fetal compromise, delivery is indicated.

The route of delivery for the diabetic patient remains controversial. Delivery by cesarean section usually is favored when fetal distress has been suggested by antepartum heart rate monitoring. An elective delivery is scheduled if at 37 to 38 weeks gestation the fetus has a mature lung profile and is at significant risk for intrauterine demise because of the mother's poor metabolic control or a history of stillbirth. We now reserve elective cesarean section for cases in which the cervix cannot be ripened with prostaglandin gel or when fetal macrosomia is suspected. In well-controlled patients without vascular disease and an unfavorable cervix, we often delay intervention until week 40. Despite this approach, the cesarean section rate for women with classes B to R diabetes remains approximately 50 percent.

Labor, Delivery and the Puerperium

During labor, continuous fetal heart rate monitoring is mandatory. Labor is allowed to progress as long as normal rates of cervical dilatation and descent of the fetal vertex are documented. Despite attempts to select patients with obvious fetal macrosomia for delivery by elective cesarean section, arrest of dilatation or descent should alert the physician to the possibility of cephalopelvic disproportion.

Because neonatal hypoglycemia is related directly to maternal glucose levels during labor as well as to the degree of antepartum metabolic control, it is important to maintain maternal plasma glucose levels at approximately 100 mg/dl during labor. Neonatal hypoglycemia may result from β-cell stimulation in utero as a result of elevated blood glucose levels during labor. A continuous infusion of both insulin and glucose has proven most valuable to control maternal glycemia during labor and delivery. We withhold the usual morning insulin dose before an elective induction of labor. Ten units of regular insulin may be added to 1,000 ml of solution containing 5 percent dextrose. An infusion rate of 100 to 125 ml/hr will result in acceptable glucose control (70 to 140 mg/dl) in most cases. Glucose levels are monitored at the bedside each hour with a glucose reflectance meter.

Another simplified regimen has been devised by Jovanovic and Peterson.[78] In well-controlled patients, the usual dose of neutral protamine Hagedorn (NPH) insulin is given at bedtime, and the morning insulin dose is withheld. Once active labor begins or the glucose levels falls to less than 70 mg/dl, the infusion is changed from saline to 5 percent dextrose at a rate of 2.5 mg/kg/min. Glucose levels are monitored, and the infusion rate is adjusted accordingly. Regular insulin is administered if glucose values exceed 140 mg/dl. It is important to use a flow sheet that summarizes glucose values, insulin dosage, and other metabolic parameters during labor.

When cesarean section is to be performed, it should be scheduled for early morning. This simplifies intrapartum glucose control and allows the neonatal team to prepare for the care of the newborn. The patient should not eat or drink after midnight, and her usual morning insulin dose is withheld. Epidural anesthesia is preferred because it allows the anesthesiologist to detect early signs of hypoglycemia and also permits the mother to interact with her newborn infant. After surgery, glucose levels are monitored every 2 hours, and an intravenous solution of 5 percent dextrose is administered.

Postpartum insulin requirements are usually significantly lower than prepregnancy needs. The objective of "tight control" used in the antepartum period is relaxed for several days, and glucose values of 150 to 200 mg/dl are acceptable. Patients who delivered vaginally and who are able to eat a regular diet are given one-third to one-half of their end-of-pregnancy dose of NPH insulin the morning after delivery. An occasional patient may require little or no insulin during the first 24 to 48 hours postpartum. Frequent glucose determinations are used to guide the insulin dose. If the patient has been given supplemental regular insulin in addition to the morning NPH dose, the amount of NPH insulin on the following morning is increased to an amount equal to two-thirds of the additional regular insulin. Most patients are stabilized on this regimen within a few days after delivery.

Women with diabetes are encouraged to breastfeed. Dietary adjustments for breast-feeding are made as they are in nondiabetic patients. The insulin dose may be somewhat lower in lactating women because of the caloric expenditure associated with nursing.

Management of the Patient with GDM

Women with GDM generally do not need hospitalization for dietary instruction and management. Once the diagnosis is established, patients begin a dietary program of 2,000 to 2,500 calories daily with the exclusion of simple carbohydrates.[101] Obese women with GDM may be managed on as little as 1,700 to 1,800 kcal/day with less weight gain and no apparent reduction in fetal size.[102]

The single most important therapeutic intervention in pregnancy complicated by GDM is the careful monitoring of maternal glucose levels throughout the third trimester. Fasting and 2-hour postprandial glucose levels are monitored at least weekly. Some advocate self-monitoring of glucose to ascertain better the level of glycemic control achieved by diet therapy.[103] If the fasting plasma glucose level exceeds 105 mg/dl and/or postprandial values are greater than 120 mg/dl on several occasions, therapy with human insulin is begun.

Langer and Mazze[104] proposed that a repetitive fasting blood glucose of at least 95 mg/dl justifies insulin therapy to reduce the frequency of macrosomia. Coustan and Imarah[105] reported that "prophylactic" insulin given to patients who would normally be treated by diet alone may also reduce the frequency of macrosomia, cesarean section, and birth trauma. It has been suggested that insulin may reduce subtle degrees of postprandial hyperglycemia that can promote excessive fetal growth.[105] Alternatively, insulin may regulate maternal levels of other fetal insulin secretagogues such as branched-chain amino acids. In contrast to Coustan and Imarah's study, Persson and co-workers[106] performed a prospective randomized investigation of "prophylactic insulin" therapy. They noted similar rates of macrosomia and no differences in skinfold thicknesses in the offspring of diet- and diet-plus-insulin–treated GDM women. Until larger prospective randomized studies indicate the benefit of prophylactic insulin, insulin should be reserved for women who demonstrate significant fasting or postprandial hyperglycemia.

Patients with GDM who are well controlled are at low risk for intrauterine death. However, gestational diabetic women requiring insulin undergo fetal testing in a manner similar to uncomplicated insulin-dependent patients.[107] Antepartum fetal heart rate testing prior to term has been recommended in three groups of patients with GDM: (1) those who require insulin, (2) those with hypertension, and (3) those who have a history of prior stillbirth. Maternal assessment of fetal activity is begun at 28 weeks. Gestational diabetics may be safely followed until 40 weeks as long as fasting and postprandial glucose values remain normal. At 40 weeks, fetal surveillance is begun with nonstress testing. As with pregestational diabetic patients, ultrasound is employed to identify macrosomia and to help select the safest route of delivery.

Counseling the Diabetic Patient

Anomalies of the cardiac, renal, and central nervous systems arise during the first 7 weeks of gestation, a time when it is most unusual for patients to seek pre-natal care. Therefore, the management and counseling of women with diabetes in the reproductive age group should begin prior to conception. Unfortunately, it has been estimated that less than 20 percent of diabetic women in the United States seek prepregnancy care.[89]

Molsted-Pedersen[108] has demonstrated a reduced rate of major congenital malformations in patients optimally managed before conception in hospitals with special diabetes clinics. The rate of malformations fell from 19.4 to 8.5 percent in class D and F patients who attended a prepregnancy clinic. In Germany, Fuhrmann et al.[109] found that intensive treatment begun prior to conception in 307 diabetic women reduced the malformation rate to 1 percent. Nearly 90 percent of women in this study maintained mean glucose levels less than 100 mg/dl. In contrast, the incidence of anomalies in the offspring of 593 diabetic women who registered for care after 8 weeks gestation was 8.0 percent (47/593). Only 20 percent of those women had mean daily glucose levels of less than 100 mg/dl. Most recently, Mills et al.[20] have reported that diabetic women who registered prior to pregnancy had fewer infants with anomalies when compared with late registrants (4.9 vs. 9.0 percent). While the incidence of 4.9 percent remains higher than that in a normal control population (2 percent), normalization of glycemia was not established in the early-entry group.

Glycosylated hemoglobin levels obtained during the first trimester may be used to counsel diabetic women regarding the risk for an anomalous infant. In a retrospective study at the Joslin Clinic, Miller and colleagues[110] observed that elevated hemoglobin A_{1c} concentrations early in pregnancy could be correlated with an increased incidence of malformations. In 58 patients with elevated glycosylated hemoglobin levels, 13 malformed infants were noted. Their finding has been confirmed by Ylinen et al.,[111] who measured glycosylated hemoglobin before 15 weeks gestation in 142 pregnancies. In pregnancies complicated by fetal malformations, mean values were significantly higher than in pregnancies without malforma-tions. In the subgroup of patients with glycosylated hemoglobin values of more than 10 percent, fetal malformations were present in 6 of 17 cases. Overall, the risk of a major fetal anomaly may be as high as 1 in 4 or 1 in 5 when the glycosylated hemoglobin level is several percent above normal values. Regardless of the glycosylated hemoglobin value obtained, all patients require a careful program of surveillance as outlined earlier to detect fetal malformations. The risk for spontaneous abortion also appears increased with marked elevations in glycosylated hemoglobin. However, for diabetic women in good control, there appears to be no greater likelihood for miscarriage.[112]

With the increasing evidence that poor control is responsible for the congenital malformations seen in pregnancies complicated by diabetes, it is apparent that preconception counseling involving the patient and her family should be instituted. Physicians who care for young women with diabetes must be aware of the importance of such counseling. At this time, the nonpregnant patient may learn techniques for self-monitoring of glucose as well as the need for proper dietary management. Questions may be answered regarding risk factors for complications and the plan for general management of diabetes in pregnancy. Planning for pregnancy should optimally be accomplished over several months. Glycosylated hemoglobin measurements are performed to aid in the timing of conception. The patient should attempt to achieve a glycosylated hemoglobin level within 2 SD of the mean for the reference laboratory.[113a]

Contraception

There is no evidence that diabetes mellitus impairs fertility. Family planning is thus an important consideration for the diabetic woman. A careful history and complete gynecologic examination and counseling are required before selecting a method of contraception. Barrier methods continue to be safe and inexpensive methods of birth control. The diaphragm, used correctly with a spermicide, has a failure rate of less than 10 percent. Because there are no inherent risks with the diaphragm and other barrier methods, these have become the preferred interim method of contraception for insulin-dependent diabetic women.

Combined oral contraceptives (OC) are the most effective reversible method of contraception, with failure rates generally less than 1 percent. There is, however, continued controversy regarding their use in the diabetic woman. The serious side effects of pill use, including thromboembolic disease and myocardial infarction, may be increased in diabetic women using combined OCs. In a retrospective study, Steel and Duncan observed five cardiovascular complications in 136 diabetic women using primary low-dose pills.[113b] Three patients had cerebrovascular accidents, one had a myocardial infarction, and one had an axillary vein thrombosis. Several other women exhibited rapid progression of retinopathy. Other than Steel and Duncan's study, there is limited data concerning the safety of the combined OC pill in diabetic women. A recent report by Klein et al. noted no association of past use or number of years of use of oral contraceptive with severity of retinopathy or hypertension in 384 diabetic women.[113c] Nevertheless, many physicians refrain from using OCs in diabetic women and encourage other forms of contraception. Those who prescribe low-dose OCs to diabetic women should restrict them to patients without vascular complications or additional risk factors such as smoking or a strong family history of myocardial disease.

Women using OCs may demonstrate increased resistance to insulin as a result of a diminished concentration of insulin receptors.[113d] Although carbohydrate metabolism may be affected by the progestin component of the pill, disturbances in diabetic control are actually uncommon with its use. In Steel and Duncan's study, 81 percent of patients using the pill did not require a change in insulin dose.[113e] Triphasic OCs may also be used safely in women who have had GDM without other risk factors. Skouby demonstrated normal glucose tolerance and lipid levels in nonobese women who had GDM and were followed after six months of therapy.[113f] After the completion of childbearing, permanent sterilization including tubal ligation and vasectomy should be discussed with the patient as well as her partner.

THYROID DISEASE

Thyroid disorders are commonly found in women of childbearing age and have been estimated to occur in 0.2 percent of all pregnancies. While the euthyroid state appears to benefit pregnancy, the precise role of the thyroid gland in reproduction is poorly understood. In most series, untreated hypothyroidism has been associated with impaired fertility and pregnancy loss.[114] Successful management of the pregnant woman with thyroid disease requires an understanding of the potential effects on the mother and fetus of these disorders and their treatment.

Thyroid Function During Pregnancy and Laboratory Assessment

The thyroid gland appears to be functioning maximally during normal pregnancy. Basal metabolic rate, which in the past was employed as an indirect measurement of thyroid function, is elevated in pregnant women.

The activity of the thyroid gland as measured by radioactive uptake studies depends on the pool of circulating inorganic iodine. A greater uptake of radioactive iodine is observed in states such as pregnancy in which circulating levels of iodine are reduced. Early in pregnancy, increased glomerular filtration and renal excretion of iodine results in a decreased plasma inorganic iodine concentration.[115] Enlargement of the thyroid gland during gestation is believed to represent a compensatory mechanism to maintain gland activity despite the decrease in plasma inorganic iodine. This observation may explain the discrepancies between studies contrasting the appearance of goiter in pregnancy in different geographical locations.[116] Presumably, the availability of iodine in the diet can influence the incidence of goiter in pregnancy. Placental production of independent thyroid stimulators such as human chorionic thyrotropin is not believed to contribute greatly to an increase in gland size or activity.

Laboratory assessment of thyroid function is dramatically altered by the hormonal changes of pregnancy. The most significant finding is a rise in thyroxine-binding globulin (TBG) to levels twice normal by 12 weeks gestation. Hyperestrogenic states, including the use of oral contraceptives, also induce hepatic biosynthesis of TBG. The majority of thyroid hormone (>99%) is bound to TBG. Measurements of total serum thyroxine (T4) by radioimmunoassay or competitive protein-binding techniques include bound as well as the minute fraction of free T4. It is this free fraction that exerts its biologic activity. Free levels of T4 and triiodothyronine (T3) are not significantly elevated during pregnancy. Direct measurements of free levels of T3 and T4 are the most accurate method for assessing thyroid function in the face of increased TBG concentrations. However, the serum free thyroxine concentration is most often measured by nonequilibrium dialysis, which may be affected by large increases in TBG.[117] Because assays for free T3 and T4 are not widely available, an estimate of free hormone activity is generally obtained by employing the resin T3 uptake test (RT3U).

The RT3U serves as an indirect measurement of TBG concentration. The patient's serum is incubated along with radioiodine-labeled T3 as well as an ion exchange resin. The resin competes with TBG binding sites in the patient's serum for the tracer-labeled T3. Pregnancy and other conditions in which TBG is elevated produce more unoccupied binding sites and therefore *decreased* resin uptake of the radioiodine-labeled T3. In pregnancy complicated by hyperthyroidism, the RT3U is higher than normal. This reflects greater saturation of the patient's TBG with thyroid hormone, allowing the resin to bind more tracer.

It is useful to calculate the free thyroxine index (FT4I) based on the results obtained by the RT3U and total T4. The use of this formula attempts to correct for states of altered TBG concentrations, yet this index is not directly proportional to free hormone concentration. In clinical practice, an elevated FT4I is, however, consistent with hyperthyroidism just as a low value reflects hypothyroidism.

[Free thyroxine index (FT4I)
= Total T4 × (patient RT3U/normal RT3U)].

The most sensitive test for the detection of primary hypothyroidism is a measurement of serum thyroid-stimulating hormone (TSH) concentration. Serum TSH concentrations remain normal during pregnancy.[118] Elevated values in the presence of a normal FT4I value reflect pituitary stimulation of a marginally active gland. In this case, early thyroid failure may be diagnosed and treated. Normal TSH values in the face of a low FT4I most often reflect secondary hypothyroidism of central (hypothalamic–pituitary) origin (Fig. 33.6).

Fetal and Neonatal Thyroid Function

The fetal thyroid gland develops by 7 weeks gestation. However, synthesis of thyroid hormone does not begin until approximately 10 weeks, when colloid and follicle formation may be demonstrated, and the gland begins to concentrate iodide. It is at this time that the fetal thyroid may become vulnerable to both exogenous iodide, such as ^{131}I, as well as to antithyroid medications.[119]

The fetal hypothalamic–pituitary–thyroid system appears to function independently from that of the mother. The role of maternal thyroid hormone in early fetal development is unknown. Thyroxine and T3, as well as TSH, do not cross the placenta in significant amounts. Therefore fetal levels of these hormones do not correspond to maternal levels. Fetal TSH can be measured after the first trimester and by

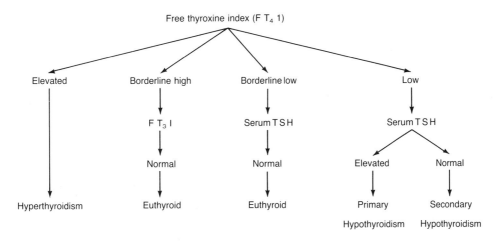

Fig. 33.6 Laboratory workup of thyroid disease in pregnancy. (From Mestman,[190] with permission.)

20 weeks rises abruptly, causing an increase in fetal T4 production.[120] Fetal T3 levels are quite low during the first two trimesters and then rise during the third trimester. This probably reflects maturity of the enzyme systems that deiodinate T4. Interestingly, prior to the third trimester, fetal thyroxine is principally metabolized to 3,3′,5′-triiodothyronine or reverse T3 (rT3). This hormone is found in large concentrations in the amniotic fluid, with peak levels occurring by midgestation.[121] The reason for this large production of rT3 remains unclear.

Following delivery, there is an abrupt increase in fetal TSH concentration that is believed to be secondary to a rise in hypothalamic thyrotropin-releasing hormone secretion.[122] T4 and T3 levels increase as a result of TSH secretion and enhanced monodeiodination of T4 to T3. rT3 levels then decline sharply. Peak T4 activity occurs by the second day of life, returning to normal adult concentrations by the end of the first week after delivery.[123]

Hyperthyroidism

Thyrotoxicosis is encountered in approximately 0.2 percent of pregnancies.[117] While menstrual irregularities have been observed in hyperthyroid women, fertility is generally not impaired. Most women with mild to moderate disease appear to tolerate pregnancy well. There is no clear evidence that pregnancy worsens the disease or makes it more difficult to treat. However, thyroid storm is a serious complication that may be encountered in undiagnosed or undertreated patients. Control of hyperthyroidism is essential for both fetal and maternal well-being. Uncontrolled disease is associated with an increased incidence of neonatal morbidity resulting from preterm birth and low birth weight.[124] There is debate as to whether pregnancy-induced hypertension is more common in hyperthyroid women.

Graves' disease is the most frequent cause of hyperthyroidism in pregnancy. Toxic nodular goiter, thyrotoxicosis factitia, and gestational trophoblastic disease are far less common etiologies. Patients with Hashimoto's disease may experience periods of hyperactive thyroid secretion before manifesting overt hypothyroidism.

The clinical diagnosis of hyperthyroidism in pregnancy may be difficult because of confusion with symptoms normally present during gestation. Pregnancy is a hypermetabolic state in which heat intolerance, nervousness, and mild tachycardia are common. In contrast, a resting tachycardia in excess of 100 bpm or weight loss despite good dietary intake should alert the physician to the possibility of hyperthyroidism. Ophthalmologic signs of Graves' disease, including exophthalmos, and lid lag (von Graefe's sign) are also helpful in making the diagnosis. The presence of hyperactive deep tendon reflexes, tremor, and eye signs, coupled with an obvious goiter, usually correlate with a positive laboratory diagnosis. Patients with hyperemesis may also have underlying hyperthyroidism.[125]

As noted earlier, laboratory testing for hyperthyroidism, particularly during pregnancy, requires calculation of FT4I. In rare cases, hyperthyroidism will be present with a normal FT4I but elevated free T3 levels (T3 thyrotoxicosis). This condition can be demonstrated by calculating the free triiodothyronine index (FT3I).[126]

Treatment of hyperthyroidism during pregnancy involves either antithyroid medications or surgery. Radioactive ablation employing ^{131}I is contraindicated. By 10 weeks gestation, the fetus may concentrate this radioisotope, resulting in hypothyroidism. A careful review of the patient's menstrual history and contraception practices should be undertaken before administering ^{131}I to any young woman.

Medical therapy for hyperthyroidism is generally preferred in the pregnant patient because it presents less risk than surgery. Propylthiouracil (PTU) and methimazole (Tapazole) are equally effective drugs that block thyroid hormone synthesis. Methimazole has been used less commonly because of a reported association with aplasia cutis of the scalp in newborns. Recent studies of offspring exposed to methimazole do not support this association.[127] It is recommended that the minimal amount of thioamide necessary to maintain the patient in a euthyroid state be used during pregnancy. The usual starting dose of PTU is approximately 300 mg per day in two or three divided doses. Patients must be closely followed for improvement in their symptoms, including weight gain and normalization of pulse, as well as a decline in serum T4 levels. These therapeutic effects do not usually occur until 2 to 4 weeks after the initiation of treatment. At that time, if the FT4I is falling, the dose of PTU may be reduced. Subsequent determinations of thyroid activity are made every 2 weeks, and, in some cases, the medication can be discontinued during the third trimester. Because disease may flare in the postpartum period, it is important to determine thyroid hormone levels prior to discharge from the hospital.

Minor side effects are frequently noted in patients receiving antithyroid medications. Approximately 5 percent will develop a purpuric rash, pruritus, or drug fever. Agranulocytosis is the most serious complication. Patients taking antithyroid drugs are instructed to seek immediate medical attention if early signs of neutropenia such as a sore throat and fever develop. In this setting, a leukocyte count should be performed immediately.

A major concern when using antithyroid medications during gestation is transplacental passage of these drugs and their effects on the fetus. However, fetal goiter and neonatal hypothyroidism appear to be rare complications of maternal therapy. In the past, T4 or T3 was given to mothers receiving PTU in the hope that it would protect the fetus from developing hypothyroidism. This practice is now discouraged, because transplacental passage of T4 and T3 is minimal. In addition, administration of thyroid hormones may make maternal thyrotoxicosis more difficult to control. In infants born to mothers receiving antithyroid medications, early diagnosis and treatment of hypothyroidism probably prevents neurologic sequelae. Transient mild hypothyroxinemia and elevated TSH values have been observed in neonates exposed to antithyroid medication in utero.[128,129] Therefore it is important to repeat abnormal neonatal blood studies several days after birth in this group of infants. Burrow and colleagues[130] have examined intellectual development in 28 children whose mothers received PTU during gestation. They compared intelligence quotients with those of siblings not exposed to antithyroid medication and found no difference among the groups.

Careful evaluation of the neonate for hyperthyroidism is equally important. It is estimated that 1 percent of pregnant women with Graves' disease will give birth to an infant with neonatal hyperthyroidism.[131] The onset of neonatal thyrotoxicosis may be delayed in women treated with antithyroid medication. The mother may not necessarily be hyperthyroid during pregnancy, as cases have been described of patients treated years before their pregnancy for Graves' dis-

ease. Thyroid stimulation of the fetus is believed to result from maternal passage of a thyroid-stimulating immunoglobulin, formerly referred to as long-acting thyroid stimulator (LATS). High levels of LATS-protector have also been observed in sera of mothers delivered of thyrotoxic infants.[131,132] Most cases of neonatal hyperthyroidism are transient, although, if progressive and unrecognized, central nervous system development may be impaired.

Thyroid Storm

Thyroid storm is an uncommon endocrinologic emergency that may occur in the undiagnosed as well as partially treated hyperthyroid patient. In pregnancy, rare cases may follow infection or surgery or may accompany labor and delivery. This clinical state of exaggerated hypermetabolism is characterized by hyperpyrexia (> 103 degrees F), tachycardia, and agitation. Cardiovascular complications in addition to sinus tachycardia include atrial arrhythmia and occasionally congestive heart failure.[133] Hypotension and cardiovascular collapse may ensue if the entity is not promptly recognized and properly treated. Peripheral catecholamine-mediated effects of thyroid excess are responsible for the presentation of this disorder, which may resemble amphetamine-induced psychosis. Treatment with propranolol is usually successful in counteracting the catecholamine excess present. This drug may be administered orally or intravenously in association with careful cardiac monitoring. Following stabilization of the patient's pulse, an oral maintenance of 20 to 80 mg every 6 hours is prescribed. Because large amounts of insensible water loss from perspiration may be present, adequate hydration is an essential component of the therapy for thyroid storm.

Reduction in thyroid hormone production is achieved initially by the administration of either intravenous sodium iodide (1 g in two divided doses of 500 mg over 24 hours) or oral saturated solution of potassium iodide (five drops every 6 hours). It should be remembered that these compounds may cross the placenta and block fetal thyroid hormone synthesis. PTU is begun immediately in doses up to 1,800 mg per day and is then tapered to a maintenance dosage. An additional benefit of PTU therapy is a reduction in the peripheral conversion of T4 to T3. Methimazole lacks this property and is therefore not used in the treatment of thyroid storm. Since there is some evidence that adrenocorticotropic hormone (ACTH) secretion is inadequate during this crisis, parenteral steroids have been advocated as well.[134] Glucocorticoids act synergistically with iodide and PTU to inhibit T4 release as well as peripheral conversion of T4 to T3.

Hypothyroidism

Hypothyroidism is rare in pregnancy because women with markedly reduced thyroid gland function are often infertile. Hypothyroidism is usually secondary to Hashimoto's disease, thyroid gland ablation by ^{131}I, surgery, or antithyroid medications. Iodine deficiency is rare in the United States. Secondary hypothyroidism from hypothalamic or pituitary failure is also uncommon.

The effect of hypothyroidism on pregnancy outcome has been widely debated. The rates of stillbirth and miscarriage appear to be increased in hypothyroid women. Davis and colleagues[135] have reported an increased incidence of preeclampsia, abruption, and fetal growth retardation in the setting of maternal hypothyroidism. Reports by Man et al.[136,137] have demonstrated a higher incidence of mental retardation and congenital anomalies in children whose mothers were believed to be hypothyroid during pregnancy. In these studies, the diagnosis of hypothyroidism was made on the basis of "hypothyroxinemia" as reflected by lower butanol-extractable iodine levels during pregnancy. These findings have not been supported by more recent investigators.[135] Today, the diagnosis of true hypothyroidism is confirmed by the presence of a low FT4I and an elevated serum TSH level.

The clinical diagnosis of hypothyroidism may be extremely difficult. Nonspecific symptoms such as lethargy and weakness are often present. Weight gain and cold sensitivity may accompany physical findings that include myxedematous changes, hair loss, and cool, dry skin.

Since the advent of radioimmunoassay, more documented cases of hypothyroidism in pregnancy have been reported. The outcomes of such pregnancies generally appear to be good provided that replacement therapy is instituted and patients are carefully followed. In one report, of 11 pregnancies occurring in 9 hypothyroid women, pregnancy outcome was not altered by the disease, and newborn follow-up at 2.7 years failed to reveal any developmental abnormalities.[138]

Therapy consists of sufficient replacement of thyroid medication to achieve a euthyroid state. The patient is generally begun on 0.05 to 0.1 mg daily of L-thyroxine (Synthroid) with the dose increased to a maximum of 0.2 mg daily over several weeks. Ideal replacement may be titrated by following the serum TSH concentration, which may take as long as 2 months to return to baseline.

Occasionally, a pregnant patient may present who is already taking thyroid replacement but does not have well-documented hypothyroidism. Proper evaluation of such patients would require discontinuing thyroid replacement for a period of at least 1 month before assaying serum TSH levels. The hypothalamic–pituitary–thyroid axis takes at least this long to recover after a period of chronic thyroid therapy. Because hypothyroidism may present a risk to mother and fetus, replacement therapy is generally not interrupted during pregnancy. In this setting, it is most appropriate to follow TSH and free thyroxine indices to determine the amount of medication required to keep the patient euthyroid. A definitive work-up for hypothyroidism may be made postpartum.

Postpartum Thyroid Dysfunction

Postpartum exacerbations of subclinical thyroid disease have been found in several studies. During pregnancy, a relative suppression of both humoral and cellular immunity may occur. Therefore, autoimmune thyroid disease may improve early in gestation. However, this condition, like many autoimmune disorders, may worsen after delivery.[139–141] Amino and colleagues[141] reported that 5.5 percent (28/507) of postpartum women experienced transient thyrotoxicosis or hypothyroidism 3 to 8 months after delivery. Most of the patients studied had antithyroid microsomal antibodies present in their serum, although they did not have a previous history of a thyroid disorder. Transient hyperthyroidism alone occurred in 2.5 percent of this patient population. Interestingly, the presentation of some of these patients mimicked postpartum psychosis. Approximately one-third of patients with transient thyrotoxicosis later developed hypothyroidism, confirming that Graves' disease and

Hashimoto's thyroiditis may present as a spectrum of thyroid disorders. In those patients documented to have postpartum hypothyroidism, the disease persisted in only one of eight cases. However, these patients were followed no longer than 1 year. In another series of six cases of primary hypothyroidism (lymphocytic thyroiditis) presenting in the postpartum periods, chronic thyroid dysfunction was documented in all cases followed up to 2 years after delivery.[141] Postpartum thyroiditis may recur with subsequent pregnancies.[142]

Solitary Thyroid Nodule

Because they are potentially malignant, solitary thyroid nodules require evaluation. Small masses in the thyroid gland are common and most often benign; therefore a complete evaluation is recommended before surgical excision. The suspicion of malignancy is heightened if the patient's past history includes neck irradiation or inherited medullary carcinoma. Most often, however, there are no predisposing factors.

Because radioisotope scanning is contraindicated during pregnancy, ultrasound is the preferred method for evaluating a thyroid nodule. Cystic lesions are usually benign. Thyroid function tests may be helpful in the evaluation of solid lesions, as these may occasionally represent a toxic adenoma. Recently, fine-needle aspiration has been shown to be a safe and reliable technique that may distinguish between benign and malignant disease with a high degree of accuracy.[143] If needle aspiration fails to reveal a malignancy, suppression therapy with thyroxine may be utilized. Many nodules will diminish in size when TSH production is inhibited. If this does not occur or if enlargement is observed, a malignancy is more likely. Definite enlargement of the mass or the presence of suspicious palpable nodes requires prompt surgical attention. Fortunately, most papillary adenocarcinomas of the thyroid are limited to the gland and are cured by surgical excision.

Parathyroid Disease: Calcium Metabolism During Pregnancy

During pregnancy, daily calcium intake must be increased to 1,200 mg/day, approximately one-third greater than the nonpregnant requirement. An increase in calcium intake is necessary during gestation to preserve maternal homeostasis, while fetal and placental growth occur. At term, it is estimated that 25 to 30 g of calcium will have accumulated in the fetus.[115] The fetal uptake of calcium is greatest late in gestation.

Levels of ionized calcium do not change appreciably in pregnancy. However, the total calcium concentration does fall progressively, reaching its nadir during the middle of the third trimester. Serum magnesium and phosphorous levels also decline during pregnancy (Fig. 33.7).[144] The decrease in total serum calcium is believed to reflect principally a fall in the protein bound portion of the ion. Almost one-half of all plasma calcium is bound to protein, albumin being the greatest carrier. Ionized or free amounts of cal-

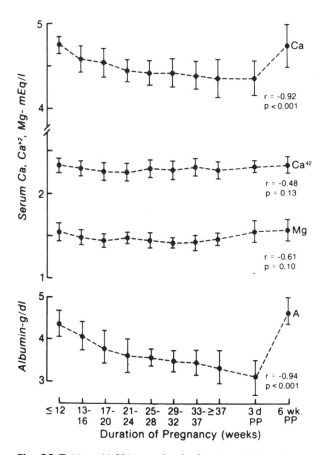

Fig. 33.7 Mean (±SD) serum levels of total and ionic calcium, magnesium, and albumin during pregnancy and the puerperium. The total calcium concentration in maternal serum declines during gestation, reaching a nadir during the third trimester and rising thereafter. (From Pitkin et al.[146] with permission.)

cium account for up to 45 percent, with the remainder forming complexes with phosphate and other anions. As albumin levels decrease and plasma volume expansion takes place, calcium levels decline to an average of 5 percent lower than nonpregnant values by the end of pregnancy. Increased glomerular filtration leading to greater calcium excretion as well as active placental transfer may also contribute to the fall in calcium levels observed during normal gestation.

Maternal gastrointestinal absorption of calcium is enhanced by increased levels of 1,25-dihydroxyvitamin D.[145] The mechanism responsible for this rise in vitamin D is uncertain, although it may result from the elevated PTH secretion that accompanies pregnancy. Pitkin et al.[146] have demonstrated a progressive increase in PTH levels in 30 patients studied longitudinally during pregnancy. Debate continues as to whether the "physiologic hyperparathyroidism of pregnancy" is secondary to the decline in maternal serum ionized calcium levels or primary in response to fetal demands for calcium. If the latter is true, then these maternal adjustments precede that period of pregnancy when fetal requirements are greatest. Nonetheless, the rise in maternal PTH does facilitate both calcium reabsorption from bone and renal hydroxylation of 25-hydroxyvitamin D. The pregnancy requirement for vitamin D is roughly 400 IU/day, the same as that of the nonpregnant woman. Studies on calcitonin secretion during pregnancy have produced conflicting data. A rise in calcitonin secretion during pregnancy might be protective against maternal osteopenia from excess PTH production. However, increased levels of this hormone have not been uniformly observed.[147,148]

The placenta plays an important role in calcium and phosphorous metabolism. Active transport of calcium to the fetus probably occurs, because newborn levels are in excess of those measured in the mother by 1 or 2 mg/dl.[149] While it has been suggested that PTH may facilitate placental transfer of calcium to the fetal compartment, it is important to note that PTH and calcitonin do not cross the placenta. While 25-hydroxyvitamin D is transferred across the placenta, passage of 1,25-dihydroxyvitamin D is unlikely.[150]

PTH has been identified in the fetus as early as 10 weeks gestation. However, most reports suggest that the state of chronic hypercalcemia in utero suppresses parathyroid function during fetal life. At birth, with cessation of the maternal supply of calcium, fetal calcium levels begin to fall. Both PTH and 1,25-dihydroxyvitamin D levels increase and are probably involved in the stabilization of neonatal calcium levels by the first week of life.[151]

Hyperparathyroidism

Hyperparathyroidism occurs infrequently during pregnancy, with fewer than 90 cases reported prior to 1982.[152] Undoubtedly, more cases will be detected through the widespread use of automated assays for serum calcium determinations. Primary hyperparathyroidism usually results from a parathyroid adenoma, although hyperplasia of the glands is found in 10 to 20 percent of cases. This condition does not seem to affect fertility and is more common in women than men by a 3 : 1 ratio. Approximately one-fourth of all cases are found in the reproductive age group.

Patients with hyperparathyroidism and mild hypercalcemia may present with rather nonspecific symptoms, including generalized fatigue, muscle weakness, constipation, and abdominal or back pain. Hypercalcemia may impair renal concentrating ability, leading to polyuria and polydipsia. The presence

Clinical Features of Hyperparathyroidism
Fatigue
Muscle weakness
Abdominal pain
Bone pain, fractures
Polyuria
Polydipsia
Nephrolithiasis
Pancreatitis
Peptic ulcer disease
Hypocalcemic tetany of the newborn
Constipation

of bone pain and fractures, as well as nephrolithiasis, usually signifies progressive disease. Rarely, patients may present with pancreatitis or peptic ulcer disease.

Establishing the laboratory diagnosis of hyperparathyroidism during pregnancy may be difficult. As noted above, total serum calcium is reduced in a normal pregnancy. However, serum calcium is usually elevated and phosphate levels reduced in hyperparathyroidism. Occasionally, it may be helpful to measure the serum level of ionized calcium. Marked phosphaturia secondary to a reduction in tubular reabsorption of phosphate when accompanied by hypercalcemia suggests hyperparathyroidism. PTH levels, which normally increase in pregnancy, are usually elevated out of proportion to the serum calcium level.[144] When PTH levels are not elevated, other causes of hypercalcemia, including malignancy, hypervitaminosis D, sarcoidosis, milk alkali syndrome, and thyroid disease, must be considered.

Hyperparathyroidism during pregnancy is associated with increased perinatal morbidity and mortality. The review of Shangold et al.[152] of 159 pregnancies in 63 women revealed that 84 resulted in normal liveborn term infants, 7 were interrupted by elective abortion, 13 terminated in spontaneous abortion, and 11 ended in intrauterine fetal death. The incidence of preterm births and growth retardation did not appear greater than that in the normal population. All four neonatal deaths followed episodes of tetany. Overall, some morbidity was observed in 45 percent of these infants, including 35 cases of neonatal tetany. Recent analysis of collected case reports has revealed a decline in the frequency of stillbirths, neonatal deaths, and tetany during the past three decades. In the last 10 years, the incidence of stillbirths and neonatal deaths has fallen to 2 percent. Neonatal tetany is observed in 15 percent of cases. The fall in perinatal mortality probably reflects detection and better management of maternal disease.

Hypocalcemic tetany in the newborn often leads to the diagnosis of maternal hyperparathyroidism. Reduced serum calcium levels in the neonatal period are believed to result from chronic maternal hypercalcemia and resultant fetal hypercalcemia, which suppresses fetal PTH synthesis. After delivery, the fetus exhibits relative hypoparathyroidism and is unable to mobilize calcium. Neonatal tetany may occur at birth or appear after a period of several days. Severe hypo-

calcemia may also lead to seizures in the newborn. It is possible that other factors such as diminished end-organ response to PTH or defective 1,25-dihydroxyvitamin D synthesis may also be responsible for some cases of neonatal tetany.[153] In any event, the neonatologist must be informed of the birth of potentially affected infants.

Because of the high rate of perinatal complications observed in hyperparathyroidism, many authorities recommend prompt surgical excision of abnormal parathyroid tissue at the time of diagnosis. Parathyroidectomy, although traditionally performed in the second trimester, may in selected cases be a reasonable treatment option in late pregnancy.[154] In the review cited above, surgery was performed in 16 cases. Fourteen women were cured by the procedure, and 12 of these subsequently had a successful pregnancy. Surgical therapy is indicated in patients with severe disease (i.e., those with markedly elevated levels of serum calcium and progressive symptoms including bone disease and nephrocalcinosis). Occasionally, such patients will present in hypercalcemic crisis (calcium level of at least 12 mg/dl), requiring emergency medical intervention. In these cases, medical control of hypercalcemia should be undertaken prior to surgery. Therapy in these cases includes careful administration of intravenous isotonic saline along with a loop diuretic such as furosemide, which inhibits tubular reabsorption of calcium. Thiazides should be avoided, as they result in calcium retention. Mithramycin, which has been used effectively in hypercalcemic cancer patients, is contraindicated during pregnancy, as its effects are not fully known.

The treatment of hyperparathyroidism during pregnancy must be individualized. The patient's symptoms, the severity of her disease, and the gestational age are factors that will influence therapy. Medical treatment may be successfully employed for short periods of time, particularly if delivery can be accomplished. Montoro et al.[155] reported two pregnant patients treated with oral phosphate whose infants remained normocalcemic throughout the neonatal period. Patterson[154] described a pregnant woman treated with oral phosphosoda who became profoundly hypokalemic in the absence of diarrhea.[154] Phosphate therapy is best reserved for patients with relatively mild disease and normal renal function. It should be remembered that soft tissue calcification may develop in patients with renal insufficiency whose excretion of phosphate is reduced.

Hypoparathyroidism

Hypoparathyroidism is an uncommon entity that usually results from inadvertent removal of the parathyroid gland during thyroid surgery. It has also been found in association with various autoimmune endocrine diseases, including Addison's disease, chronic lymphocytic thyroiditis, and premature ovarian failure. Pseudohypoparathyroidism is a condition in which the glands are normal. However, end-organ refractoriness to PTH is observed.

The diagnosis of hypoparathyroidism is usually suggested by a history of prior neck surgery and is confirmed by the presence of low serum calcium levels and elevated serum phosphate. Hypocalcemia produces nonspecific symptoms of weakness, lethargy, and bone pain. With severe depression of serum calcium, however, irritability and tetany may develop. Tetany may be demonstrated by the appearance of carpopedal spasm (Trousseau's sign) following the inflation of the blood pressure cuff above the systolic pressure for a period of several minutes. It may also be elicited by tapping the facial nerve, which causes twitching of the upper lip (Chvostek's sign).

In pregnancy, the principal concern associated with this disorder is inadequate transfer of calcium to the fetus, with the subsequent development of secondary hyperparathyroidism in the fetus and newborn. Bone demineralization and subperiosteal resorption as well as osteitis fibrosa cystica have been described in infants born to hypoparathyroid mothers.[156,157]

Therapy is aimed at supplying adequate calcium to elevate maternal concentration to the normal range. Maternal treatment consists of supplemental calcium in daily doses of 1 to 4 g, as well as 100,000 to 150,000 IU of vitamin D. During pregnancy, because of profound physiologic changes in calcium homeostasis, careful monitoring of maternal calcium levels must be performed. In recent years, a short-acting vitamin D, 1,25-dihydroxycholicalciferol (Calcitriol), has been found to be fairly predictable in its response in pregnant women. The recommended dose is 2 to 3 μg/day.[158] However, during pregnancy, the dosage of Calcitriol must often be increased to maintain normal serum calcium levels.

During labor and delivery, calcium levels, if low, may be normalized by an intravenous infusion of calcium gluconate. Hyperventilation, which results in tetany, may aggravate this condition and should therefore be discouraged. Because maternal transfer of calcium to the fetus ceases following delivery, it is important to lower the dose of supplemental calcium to prepregnancy levels. In nonlactating women, levels of calcium may rise dramatically if calcium and Calcitriol intake is not reduced. In women who breastfeed, however, little adjustment in the amount of the vitamin D supplementation would appear necessary. There is a single report of a woman with hypoparathyroidism who experienced significant reduction in vitamin D requirements with lactation.[159]

PITUITARY DISEASE

Prolactin-Producing Adenomas

With widely available radioimmunoassays for serum prolactin and improved techniques for radiologic diagnosis, an increasing number of prolactin-secreting pituitary adenomas are now being detected in women. Spontaneous ovulation is uncommon when a pituitary tumor is present. Therefore most patients with this disorder will present with amenorrhea–galactorrhea or anovulatory cycles and infertility. With the use of ovulation induction and suppression of prolactin synthesis by dopaminergic agents such as bromocriptine, pregnancy has become increasingly common in patients with prolactinomas.

The pituitary gland normally increases in size during pregnancy. Much of the gland enlargement is thought to be secondary to hyperplasia of the lactotropic cells of the anterior pituitary that are stimulated by estrogen. Although this stimulus may result in the enlargement of adenomas during pregnancy,[160] most patients with a microadenoma, a pituitary tumor less than 1 cm in size, have an uneventful pregnancy.[161–163] In those few patients who do become symptomatic, regression usually follows delivery.

The vast majority of women with prolactin-secreting adenomas will require ovulation induction to conceive. Nonpregnant patients who present with amenorrhea–galactorrhea and hyperprolactinemia (a prolactin level of at least 20 ng/ml) should be investigated for the presence of a pituitary adenoma. While serum prolactin levels have been correlated with the presence of pituitary adenomas, in a patient considering pregnancy with hyperprolactinemia of any degree a thorough radiologic investigation is warranted. Debate continues regarding the appropriate sequence of the work-up for this disorder, though it appears that computerized tomography (CT) and more recently magnetic resonance imaging (MRI) have replaced coned-down sella turcica radiographs and polytomography as the procedure of choice to evaluate the size of the pituitary gland.

Once a pituitary tumor is diagnosed, it may be prudent to reevaluate the gland for growth after several months before attempting ovulation induction. Macroadenomas, tumors measuring 1 cm or more, should be definitively treated with surgery or radiation, as over one-third of these patients may develop symptoms during pregnancy.[160,163]

Evaluation for possible prolactin-secreting tumors is made difficult during pregnancy by the physiologic rise in serum prolactin that accompanies normal gestation. At term, serum prolactin levels may reach values 20 times normal. Furthermore, prolactin levels do not always rise during pregnancy in women with prolactinomas, and they do not always rise with pregnancy-induced tumor enlargement.[164] Therefore, radiologic diagnosis is necessary for the pregnant patient who develops severe headaches or a visual field defect.

Management of the pregnant patient with a previously diagnosed prolactinoma requires careful attention by a team of physicians, including the obstetrician, endocrinologist, and ophthalmologist. The development of headaches may reflect tumor enlargement and impingement on the diaphragmatic sella or adjacent dura. Visual disturbances result from optic nerve compression. If the optic chiasm is compressed by superior extension, bitemporal hemianopsia may develop. Visual field and ophthalmologic examinations should therefore be performed in symptomatic patients.[163] While the limitations of serum prolactin levels have been discussed, marked elevations outside of the pregnant range for a given gestational age may signal rapid tumor enlargement.

Gemzell and Wang[160] reviewed the course of 85 women during 91 pregnancies with previously un-treated microadenomas and reported that only 5 percent experienced complications. Four of the five pregnancies associated with symptoms of headache and visual disturbance showed resolution following delivery. One patient who had a visual field defect noted early in pregnancy subsequently underwent a transphenoidal hypophysectomy after a cesarean section for a triplet gestation at 36 weeks.

Maygar and Marshall[161] report that symptoms seem to occur more frequently in the first trimester than in the second or third, noting a median time at onset of 10 weeks gestation. However, the likelihood of developing visual symptoms did not differ in each trimester. In their series, symptoms requiring therapy occurred in over 20 percent of the 91 patients who had untreated tumors, but in only 1 percent of women with previously treated adenomas.

Molitch[163] reviewed 16 series of 246 cases of pregnancy and prolactin-secreting pituitary microadenomas. Only 4 of the 246 women (1.6 percent) had symptoms of tumor enlargement, and 11 (4.5 percent) had asymptomatic enlargement on radiologic examination. In no case was surgical intervention necessary. Molitch[163] also reviewed 45 cases of women with macroadenomas, of which 7 (15.5 percent) experienced symptomatic tumor enlargement. Surgery was required in four of these women during pregnancy. The risk of developing symptoms is probably related to the size of the tumor at the onset of pregnancy. Further data are necessary to define which group of patients with a microadenoma should be treated with bromocriptine for a prolonged period of time prior to conception.

Therapy for complications arising during pregnancy is influenced by both gestational age and the severity of symptoms. If fetal maturity is present, induction of labor or cesarean section should be accomplished. Cesarean section is generally performed for obstetric indications. Earlier in gestation, if radiologic evidence suggests tumor enlargement, therapy should not be delayed. Treatment employing bromocriptine has been successful in several symptomatic patients and has become the preferred therapy during pregnancy.[164] This drug appears to be safe in early pregnancy, as evidenced by its use for induction of ovulation in large groups of hyperprolactinemic women without an increased incidence of congenital malformations.[165,166] Other treatment modalities employed during pregnancy include transphenoidal surgery[161-163] and, in one case, hydrocortisone therapy.[155] Complications of transphenoidal surgery are infection, hypopituitarism, hemorrhage, and transient diabetes insipidus. The risk of these complications is probably not increased during pregnancy.

Following delivery, radiologic assessment of tumor size and a serum prolactin assay should be performed at the first postpartum visit. Breast-feeding is not contraindicated in the presence of a prolactin-secreting microadenoma.[162] Because serum prolactin levels may remain elevated while nursing, caution must be used in interpreting these results. Counseling patients regarding future pregnancies requires establishing that progression of tumor growth has not occurred. Gemzell and Wang[160] concluded that, in 16 patients with untreated pituitary adenomas, symptoms did not seem to occur with increasing frequency in subsequent pregnancies.

Diabetes Insipidus

Diabetes insipidus is a rare disorder with fewer than 100 cases complicating pregnancy reported in the literature. The disease results from inadequate or absent antidiuretic hormone (ADH; or vasopressin) production by the posterior pituitary gland. The etiology of diabetes insipidus is often unknown, although in most cases it follows pituitary surgery or destruction by tumor of the normal pituitary architecture. Massive polyuria, resulting from failure of the renal tubular concentrating mechanism, and a dilute urine, specific gravity less than 1.005, are characteristic of diabetes insipidus. To combat dehydration and the intense thirst produced by this syndrome, patients consume large quantities of fluid. The diagnosis of diabetes insipidus relies on the demonstration of continued polyuria and relative urinary hyposmolarity when a patient is water restricted. The administration of intramuscular vasopressin to such a patient will result in water retention and an appropriate increase in urine osmolality. This response is not observed in patients with nephrogenic diabetes insipidus, a state in which free water clearance is increased because of the renal tubule's insensitivity to ADH. Other conditions that cause polyuria, such as diabetes mellitus, hyperparathyroidism with hypercalcemia, and chronic renal tubular disease, must also be considered in the differential diagnosis. However, these can usually be distinguished from central diabetes insipidus by appropriate laboratory investigation.

Hime and Richardson[167] reviewed 67 cases of diabetes insipidus complicating pregnancy and noted that 58 percent of cases seemed to deteriorate during gestation. In an attempt to explain this phenomenon, Durr[168] has suggested that the increased glomerular filtration seen in pregnancy may increase the requirement of ADH. Patients with mild disease may also worsen during pregnancy because of a diminished response of the renal tubule to ADH, possibly as a result of progesterone antagonism.[169] Impaired liver function including fatty liver of pregnancy has been observed with diabetes insipidus during pregnancy, suggesting that several factors may explain worsening of this condition.[169]

Synthetic vasopressin, in the form of L-deamino-8-D-arginine vasopressin (DDAVP), is the treatment of choice. This drug is given intranasally in doses of approximately 0.1 mg up to three times daily. Oxytocic activity is rarely observed. Burrow and colleagues[170] have reported the successful use of DDAVP in pregnancy and the puerperium and suggest that this drug is safe for both mother and fetus.

Spontaneous labor and lactation seem to occur in most cases of diabetes insipidus. While older reports suggest an increased number of dysfunctional labors in affected patients, oxytocin release appears to be independent of vasopressin secretion.[171]

Pituitary Insufficiency

In 1937, Sheehan[172] described postpartum ischemic necrosis of the anterior pituitary. This form of hypopituitarism is usually observed in patients who have experienced severe postpartum hemorrhage with hypotensive shock. Lymphocytic hypophysitis as well as destruction of the gland from tumor invasion, surgery, or radiotherapy may also accompany pregnancy, although fertility is often compromised in such patients. Antepartum pituitary infarction has been described as a rare complication of insulin-dependent diabetes mellitus.[173] In these cases, insulin requirements may fall dramatically.

Patients with Sheehan syndrome may exhibit varying degrees of hypopituitarism so that specific assays of tropic hormones as well as stimulation and suppression tests may be necessary to establish the diagnosis. During pregnancy, because of normal physiologic changes, adjustments must be made in interpreting both hormone levels and responses to various stimuli. An average delay of 7 years has been observed between the onset and the diagnosis of this disorder. A history of hypovolemic shock and antecedent postpartum hemorrhage has been recorded as a precipitating event in up to 79 percent of cases.[174] The characteristic clinical picture begins with failure to lactate. However, this may not be observed in all cases. Some patients may present with late-onset disease and progress to loss of axillary and pubic hair, oligomenorrhea, or amenorrhea with senile vaginal atrophic changes, as well as signs and symptoms of hypothyroidism. Patients with these findings are usually infertile, although the frequency of pregnancy with this disorder is difficult to ascertain. In a review of 19 patients with Sheehan syndrome documented by endocrinologic studies or postmortem examination, 39 pregnancies occurred after the onset of hypopituitarism.[174] Eleven of these women required hormonal therapy to establish a pregnancy, and replacement therapy was used during 15 (38 percent) of the 39 pregnancies. The treated group had a live birth rate of 87 percent compared with 54 percent in untreated patients, suggesting that early diagnosis and proper therapy result in a more favorable outcome.

The treatment of pituitary insufficiency involves replacement of those hormones necessary to maintain normal metabolism and respond to stress. Thyroid hormone may be provided as L-thyroxine in doses of 0.1 to 0.2 mg daily. Corticosteroids are essential for those patients who manifest any degree of adrenal insufficiency. The maintenance dosage of cortisone acetate is provided as 25 mg every morning and 12.5 mg every evening or as prednisone 5 mg and 2.5 mg, respectively. Mineralocorticoid replacement is rarely necessary, because adrenal production of aldosterone is not solely dependent on ACTH stimulation. The dose of glucocorticoids should be increased during the stress of labor and delivery.

ADRENAL DISEASE

Cushing Syndrome

Cushing syndrome, which is characterized by excess glucocorticoid production, is usually secondary to inappropriate hypersecretion of ACTH by a pituitary adenoma. Primary adrenal disease resulting from an adrenal tumor has been reported to be more common during pregnancy than in the nonpregnant state. However, adrenal hyperplasia still causes most cases of Cushing syndrome in pregnancy.[175] Other etiologies include neoplastic ectopic ACTH production, nodular adrenal hyperplasia, or excessive doses of exogenous corticosteroids.

Women with Cushing syndrome are usually infertile, making de novo cases rare in pregnancy. Most occur in patients who have been previously or partially treated. The clinical features of this disorder may be difficult to distinguish from many signs and symptoms that accompany normal pregnancy. Weakness, weight gain, edema, striae, hypertension, and impaired glucose tolerance may be observed both during gestation and in Cushing syndrome. The early onset of hypertension with easy bruising and proximal myopathy should strongly suggest the diagnosis and prompt further evaluation.

Laboratory diagnosis includes the demonstration of elevated serum cortisol levels without diurnal variation, as well as a failure to suppress cortisol secretion with the administration of dexamethasone. Assays for ACTH are of variable accuracy and may confuse the diagnosis. During gestation, there is normally a rise in total and free cortisol. Therefore laboratory results must be compared with established norms for pregnancy. Diurnal variation in cortisol production is maintained in normal pregnancy, although free plasma cortisol levels at term may be twice those of nonpregnant women. Furthermore, even in normal pregnant patients, cortisol secretion may not be suppressed with low doses (1 mg) of dexamethasone.[175] Most patients with adrenocortical hyperplasia will demonstrate a reduction in plasma and urinary corticosteroids with an 8-mg dose (2 mg every 6 hours for 2 days). If such suppression fails, an adrenal tumor, autonomous adrenal nodule, or ectopic ACTH production must be considered.

Pregnancy outcome in Cushing syndrome is marked by a high rate of preterm delivery and stillbirths in cases not electively terminated.[175-178] It has been suggested that maternal hyperglycemia may be a contributing factor to the intrauterine deaths observed.

Koerten and colleagues[178] reviewed 33 cases of Cushing syndrome in pregnancy and concluded that maternal complications are more common with adrenal adenomas than with hyperplasia. In that review, every patient with an adenoma developed hypertension if the pregnancy progressed beyond the first trimester. Seven of 16 patients (47 percent) developed pulmonary edema and one died. In contrast, only 1 of the 12 patients with adrenal hyperplasia demonstrated hypertensive disease. The overall prematurity rate (delivery after 20 weeks) was 20 of 33 cases (61 percent); stillbirths occurred in four cases.

Management of the pregnant patient with cortisol excess includes first identifying the source of the hormone production and then instituting proper therapy. Patients with pituitary disease are most often treated surgically if a tumor can be well defined. Surgical removal of adrenal adenomas can be accomplished through a posterior incision. Bevan and colleagues[179] examined maternal and fetal outcomes based on the timing of surgical therapy. Fetal loss occurred in 1 of 11 patients (9 percent) treated during gestation versus 8 of 26 (31 percent) in whom definitive therapy was delayed. Because the incidence of adrenal adenoma and carcinoma appears to be increased in pregnant patients with Cushing syndrome, prompt investigation employing abdominal CT or MRI is warranted, particularly if failure to suppress excess cortisol production with high levels of dexamethasone is observed. Again, surgery is indicated if an adrenal tumor is discovered.

Primary Aldosteronism

Few cases of primary aldosteronism during pregnancy have been reported. The diagnosis is suggested in a patient with hypertension, hypokalemia, and metabolic alkalosis. Because aldosterone secretion is increased during pregnancy, the diagnosis can be difficult to establish. Failure to replete serum potassium may also suppress aldosterone secretion, thus obscuring the diagnosis.[180] Amelioration of hypertension and hypokalemia during gestation has been attributed to high levels of progesterone, which may block the action of aldosterone. In spite of this, patients often present with severe hypertension and superimposed preeclampsia. The management for patients without toxemia is controversial. While prompt surgical excision of underlying adrenal adenomas has been suggested by early case reports, Lotgering and associates[181] have described successful medical therapy from midgestation, consisting of spironolactone, an aldosterone antagonist, as well as other antihypertensive medications.

Adrenal Insufficiency

Adrenal insufficiency may be primary (Addison's disease) or secondary to pituitary failure or adrenal suppression resulting from steroid replacement. Adrenal crisis, an acute life-threatening condition, may accompany stressful conditions such as labor, the puerperium, or surgery. Unfortunately, the diagnosis of hypoadrenalism is often made with difficulty, particularly in those patients who possess enough adrenal reserve to sustain normal daily activity. In pregnancy, adrenal crisis during the postpartum periods may lead to the diagnosis of adrenal insufficiency for the first time.[182]

The clinical presentation of Addison's disease during gestation is similar to that in the nonpregnant state. Fatigue, weakness, anorexia, nausea, hypotension, hypoglycemia, and increased skin pigmentation are hallmarks for this endocrinopathy. Mineralocorticoid deficiency leads to renal sodium loss with resultant depletion of the intravascular volume. A small cardiac silhouette on chest x-ray is often associated with a state of reduced cardiac output and, eventually, circulatory collapse. Hypoglycemia, which is often common in early pregnancy, may be exacerbated by glucocorticoid deficiency.

The diagnosis of adrenal insufficiency is based on specific laboratory findings. Plasma cortisol levels are decreased. However, because cortisol-binding globulin is elevated in pregnancy, even low normal cortisol values may actually reflect a state of adrenal insufficiency.[183]

Stimulation of the adrenal gland by synthetic ACTH may be helpful in establishing a diagnosis.[184] Following the intravenous administration of 0.25 mg of Cortrosyn, plasma cortisol should be increased at least twofold over baseline values. Failure to respond to this stimulus suggests primary adrenal insufficiency. This test may be used in pregnancy because little ACTH crosses the placenta. Measurement of serum ACTH may also be of benefit in distinguishing primary adrenal insufficiency from hypopituitarism.

Pregnancy usually proceeds normally in treated patients. Maintenance replacement of adrenocortical hormones is provided by cortisone acetate 25 mg orally each morning and 12.5 mg in the evening. As an alternative, prednisone may be substituted in doses of 5 mg and 2.5 mg, respectively. Mineralocorticoid deficiency is treated with fludrocortisone acetate (Florinef) in a dose of 0.05 to 0.1 mg per day. The use of a mineralocorticoid requires careful observation for symptoms of fluid overload. The presence of edema, excess weight gain, and electrolyte imbalance often requires an adjustment in the dose of mineralocorticoid.

Adrenal crisis is a rare, life-threatening disturbance that demands immediate medical attention. Treatment in an intensive care setting is recommended. As noted, women with undiagnosed Addison's disease may present with a crisis during the puerperium. Symptoms include nausea, vomiting, and profound epigastric pain accompanied by hypothermia and hypotension. Treatment initially consists of glucocorticoid and fluid replacement. Intravenous hydrocortisone should be given in a dose of 100 mg, followed by repeat doses every 6 hours for a period of up to several days. Mineralocorticoid replacement is indicated in cases of refractory hypotension or hyperkalemia.

All patients with adrenal insufficiency should wear an identifying bracelet. Emergency medical kits have also been prepared to help these patients when they travel. Women with Addison's disease require an increase in steroid replacement during periods of infection or stress and during labor and delivery.

Pheochromocytoma

Pheochromocytoma is a rare catecholamine-producing tumor that is uncommonly associated with pregnancy. The tumors arise from chromaffin cells of the adrenal medulla or sympathetic nervous tissue, including remnants of the organs of Zuckerkandl, neural crest tissue that lies along the abdominal aorta. In pregnancy, as in the nonpregnant states, the tumor is located in the adrenal gland in 90 percent of cases.[185] The incidence of malignancy, which can be diagnosed only when metastases are present, is approximately 10 percent. Schenker et al.[186] have reported mortality rates of 55 percent with postpartum diagnosis versus 11 percent if diagnosed during pregnancy. Fetal loss can exceed 50 percent.

In pregnancy, pheochromocytoma may present as a hypertensive crisis marked by cerebral hemorrhage or severe congestive heart failure. Pheochromocy-

toma can be easily confused with other medical diseases. The signs and symptoms of pheochromocytoma can mimic those of severe pregnancy-induced hypertension. Hypertension, headache, abdominal pain, and blurring of vision are common to both entities (Table 33.7). However, the presence of paroxysmal hypertension, particularly before 20 weeks gestation, as well as orthostasis and the absence of significant proteinuria and edema may be helpful in the differential diagnosis. Thyrotoxicosis may also resemble this disease. However, significant diastolic hypertension is rarely observed with hyperthyroidism. Unexplained circulatory collapse, which may occur after delivery, should also warrant evaluation for a possible pheochromocytoma.

The definitive diagnosis depends on laboratory measurement of catecholamines and their metabolites in a 24 hours urine collection. Elevated metanephrine excretion appears to be the most sensitive and specific finding, although isolated elevated vanillylmandelic acid excretion may be present.[185] The use of certain medications such as α-methyldopa (Aldomet) will interfere with these assays.

Pharmacologic testing may establish this diagnosis in the nonpregnant patient. The phentolamine (Regitine) tests is based on the observation that marked α-adrenergic blockade will produce a fall in blood pressure in many patients with pheochromocytoma. This test is *not* advised during pregnancy, as it has been associated with both maternal and fetal deaths.[187] Nonetheless, it is of extreme importance that the diagnosis be established. Approximately 90 percent of maternal deaths caused by pheochromocytoma occur in those patients who were undiag-

Table 33.7 Symptoms and Signs in 89 Cases of Pheochromocytoma in Pregnancy

	Percent
Paroxysmal or sustained hypertension	82
Headaches	66
Palpitation	36
Sweating	30
Blurred vision	17
Anxiety	15
Convulsion-dyspnea	10

(Adapted from Schenker and Crowers,[185] with permission.)

nosed prior to delivery.[66] In patients with symptoms suggesting pheochromocytoma and with laboratory findings that support the diagnosis, an effort should be made using radiologic techniques to localize the tumor. CT of the abdomen or MRI are the procedures of choice. In the nonpregnant state, selective venous catheterization of the adrenals may be performed. The tumor is bilateral in about 10 percent of cases, including those encountered during gestation.

Prior to surgery, the patient should be stabilized on either oral doses of phenoxybenzamine or intravenous phentolamine in an effort to reduce the catecholamine-mediated effects. Careful evaluation of fluid status with central monitoring is essential when using these preparations. β-Blockade employing propranolol or similar agents should be reserved for treatment of tachyarrhythmias and should not be instituted prior to α-blockade, as hypertensive crisis may ensue.

Schenker and Chowers[185] recommend prompt surgical removal of any pheochromocytoma detected during pregnancy, regardless of gestational age. In their series, fetal loss exceeded 50 percent and was not improved with early diagnosis. In patients detected during the third trimester, maternal stabilization with medical therapy has been successfully accomplished, thereby allowing further fetal maturation.[187] Cesarean section is preferred, as it minimizes the potential catecholamine surges associated with labor and vaginal delivery. Adrenal exploration may also be performed at the time of cesarean section. Careful follow-up of these patients is advised because the tumors may recur and are potentially malignant.

REFERENCES

1. Kalkhoff RK, Kissebah AH, Kim HJ: Carbohydrate and lipid metabolism during normal pregnancy: relationship to gestational hormone action. p. 3. In Merkatz IR, Adam PAJ (eds): The Diabetic Pregnancy: a Perinatal Perspective. Grune & Stratton, New York, 1979

2. Freinkel N, Metzger BE, Mitzan M et al: Accelerated starvation and mechanisms for the conservation of maternal nitrogen during pregnancy. Isr J Med Sci 8:426, 1972

3. Kaplan SL: Human chorionic somatomammotropin secretion, biologic effects and physiologic significance. p. 75. In Jaffe RB (ed): The Endocrine Milieu of Pregnancy, Puerperium and Childhood. Ross Laboratories, Columbus, OH, 1974

4. Yen SSC: Endocrine regulation of metabolic homeostasis during pregnancy. Clin Obstet Gynecol 16:130, 1973

5. Hollingsworth DR, Grundy SM: Pregnancy-associated hypertriglyceridemia in normal and diabetic women: differences in insulin-dependent, non-insulin-dependent, and gestational diabetes. Diabetes 31:1092, 1981

6. Spellacy WN: Maternal and fetal metabolic interrelationships. p. 42. In Sutherland HW, Stowers JM (eds): Carbohydrate Metabolism in Pregnancy and the Newborn. Churchill Livingstone, New York, 1975

7. Beard RW, Turner RC, Oakley N: Fetal response to glucose loading. Postgrad Med J 47:68, 1971

8. Felig P: Maternal and fetal fuel homeostasis in human pregnancy. Am J Clin Nutr 26:998, 1973

9. Pedersen J: The Pregnant Diabetic and Her Newborn. 2nd Ed. Williams & Wilkins, Baltimore, 1977

10. Rigg L, Cousins L, Hollingsworth D et al: Effects of exogenous insulin on excursions and diurnal rhythms of plasma glucose in pregnant diabetic patients with and without residual beta-cell function. Am J Obstet Gynecol 136:537, 1980

11. Szabo AJ, Opperman W, Hanover B et al: Fetal adipose tissue development: relationship to maternal free fatty acid levels. p. 167. In Camerini-Davalos RA, Coles HS (eds): Early Diabetes in Early Life. Academic Press, San Diego, 1975

12. Gabbe SG: Management of diabetes in pregnancy: six decades of experience. p. 37. In Pitkin RM, Zlatnik F (eds): The Yearbook of Obstetrics and Gynecology. Year Book Medical Publishers, Chicago, 1980

13. Madsen H: Fetal oxygenation in diabetic pregnancy. Dan Med Bull 33:64, 1986

14. Nyland L, Lunell NO, Lewander R et al: Uteroplacental blood flow in diabetic pregnancy: measurements with indium 113m and a computer linked gamma camera. Am J Obstet Gynecol 144:298, 1982

15. Kitzmiller JL, Phillippe M, von Oeyen P et al: Hyperglycemia, hypoxia, and fetal acidosis in rhesus monkeys, abstracted. Presented at the 28th Annual Meeting of The Society for Gynecologic Investigation, St. Louis, MO, March 1981

16. Phillips AF, Dubin JW, Matty PJ et al: Arterial hypoxemia and hyperinsulinemia in the chronically hyperglycemic fetal lamb. Pediatr Res 16:653, 1982

17. Shelley JH, Bassett JM, Milner RDG: Control of carbohydrate metabolism in the fetus and newborn. Br Med Bull 31:37, 1975

18. Carson BS, Phillips AF, Simmons MA et al: Effects of a sustained insulin infusion upon glucose uptake and

oxygenation of the ovine fetus. Pediatr Res 14:147, 1980

19. Simpson JL, Elias S, Martin AO et al: Diabetes in pregnancy, Northwestern University Series (1977–1981). I. Prospective study of anomalies in offspring of mothers with diabetes mellitus. Am J Obstet Gynecol 146:263, 1983

20. Mills JL, Knopp RH, Simpson JP et al: Lack of relations of increased malformation rates in infants of diabetic mothers to glycemic control during organogenesis. N Engl J Med 318:671, 1988

21. Mills JL, Baker L, Goldman A: Malformations in infants of diabetic mothers occur before the seventh gestational week: implications for treatment. Diabetes 28:292, 1979

22. Kucera J: Rate and type of congenital anomalies among offspring of diabetic women. J Reprod Med 7:61, 1971

23. Reece EA, Hobbins JC: Diabetic embryopathy: pathogenesis, prenatal diagnosis and prevention. Obstet Gynecol Surv 41:325, 1986

24. Sadler TW, Horton WE Jr: Mechanisms of diabetes-induced congenital malformations as studied in mammalian embryo culture. p. 51. In Jovanovic L, Peterson CM, Fuhrmann K (eds): Diabetes in Pregnancy: Teratology, Toxicity and Treatment. Praeger, New York, 1986

25. Freinkel N, Lewis NJ, Akazama S et al: The honeybee syndrome: implication of the teratogenicity of mannose in rat-embryo culture. N Engl J Med 310:223, 1984

26. Goldman AS, Baker L, Piddington R et al: Hyperglycemia-induced teratogenesis is mediated by a functional deficiency of arachidonic acid. Proc Natl Acad Sci USA 82:8227, 1985

27. Pettit DJ, Bennett PH, Knowler WC et al: Gestational diabetes mellitus and impaired glucose tolerance during pregnancy: long term effects on obesity and glucose tolerance in the offspring. Diabetes 34(suppl 2):119, 1985

28. Spellacy WN, Miller S, Winegar A et al: Macrosomia — maternal characteristics and infant complications. Obstet Gynecol 66:158, 1985

29. Modanlou HD, Komatsu G, Freeman RK et al: Large-for-gestational age neonates: anthropometric reasons for shoulder dystocia. Obstet Gynecol 60:417, 1982

30. Brans YW, Shannon DL, Hunter MA et al: Maternal diabetes and neonatal macrosomia. II. Neonatal anthropometric measurements. Early Hum Dev 8:297, 1983

31. Whitelaw A: Subcutaneous fat in newborn infants of diabetic mothers: an indication of quality of diabetic control. Lancet 1:15, 1977

32. Reiher H, Furhmann K, Noack S et al: Age-dependent insulin secretion of the endocrine pancreas in vitro from fetuses of diabetic and nondiabetic patients. Diabetes Care 6:446, 1983

33. Falluca F, Garguilo P, Troili F et al: Amniotic fluid insulin, C-peptide concentrations and fetal morbidity in infants of diabetic mothers. Am J Obstet Gynecol 153:534, 1985

34. Milner RD, Hill DH: Fetal growth control: the role of insulin and related peptides. Clin Endocrinol 21:415, 1984

35. Soler NG, Soler SM, Malins JM: Neonatal morbidity among infants of diabetic mothers. Diabetes Care 1:340, 1978

36. Kuhl C, Anderson GE, Hartil J et al: Metabolic events in infants of diabetic mothers during first 24 hours after birth. Acta Paediatr Scand 71:19, 1982

37. Bourbon JR, Farrell PM: Fetal lung development in the diabetic pregnancy. Pediatr Res 19:253, 1985

38. Hallman M, Wermer D: Effects of maternal insulin or glucose infusion on the fetus: study on lung surfactant phospholipids, plasma myoinositol, and fetal growth in the rabbit. Am J Obstet Gynecol 142:817, 1982

39. Smith BT, Giroud CJP, Robert M et al: Insulin antagonism of cortisol action on lecithin synthesis by cultures of fetal lung cells. J Pediatr 87:953, 1975

40. Smith BT: Pulmonary surfactant during fetal development and neonatal adaptation: hormonal control. p. 357. In Robertson B, Van Golde LMB, Batenburg JJ (eds): Pulmonary Surfactant. Elsevier, Amsterdam, 1985

41. Post M, Barsoumian A, Smith BT: The cellular mechanisms of glucocorticoid acceleration of fetal lung maturation. J Biol Chem 261:2179, 1986

42. Carlson KS, Smith BT et al: Insulin acts on the fibroblast to inhibit glucocorticoid stimulation of lung maturation. J Appl Physiol 57:1577, 1984

43. Gabbe SG, Lowensohn RI, Wu PY et al: Current patterns of neonatal morbidity and mortality in infants of diabetic mothers. Diabetes Care 1:335, 1978

44. Gabbe SG, Lowensohn RI, Mestan J et al: Lecithin/sphingomyelin ratio in pregnancies complicated by diabetes mellitus. Am J Obstet Gynecol 128:757, 1977

45. Tsang RC, Chen I-W, Friedman MA et al: Parathyroid function in infants of diabetic mothers. J Pediatr 86:399, 1975

46. Mimouni F, Miodovnik M, Tsang RC et al: Decreased amniotic fluid magnesium concentration in diabetic pregnancy. Obstet Gynecol 69:12, 1987

47. Widness JA, Cowett RM, Coustan DR et al: Neonatal morbidities in infants of mothers with glucose intolerance in pregnancy. Diabetes 34(suppl 2):61, 1985

48. Ylinen K, Raivio K, Teramo K: Haemoglobin A1c predicts the perinatal outcome in insulin-dependent diabetic pregnancies. Br J Obstet Gynaecol 88:961, 1981

49. Stevenson DK, Bartoletti AL, Offstrander CR et al: Pulmonary excretion of carbon monoxide in the human infant as an index of bilirubin production. II. Infants of diabetic mothers. J Pediatr 94:956, 1979

50. Shannon K, Davis JC, Kitzmiller JL et al: Erythropoiesis in infants of diabetic mothers. Pediatr Res 30:161, 1986

51. White P: Pregnancy complicating diabetes. Am J Med 7:609, 1949

52. Summary and Recommendations of the Second International Workshop–Conference on Gestational Diabetes. Diabetes 34(Suppl 2):123, 1985

53. Gabbe SG, Mestman JH, Freeman RK et al: Management and outcome of class A diabetes mellitus. Am J Obstet Gynecol 127:465, 1977

54. Main EK, Main DM, Landon MB, Gabbe SG: Factors predicting perinatal outcome in pregnancies complicated by diabetic nephropathy (class F). Sixth Annual Meeting, Society of Perinatal Obstetricians, San Antonio, February 1986

55. Kitzmiller JL, Brown ER, Phillippe M et al: Diabetic nephropathy and perinatal outcome. Am J Obstet Gynecol 141:741, 1981

56. Reece EA, Coustan DR, Hayslett JP et al: Diabetic nephropathy: pregnancy performance and fetomaternal outcome. Am J Obstet Gynecol 159:56, 1988

57. Kitzmiller JP: Diabetic nephropathy. p. 489. In Reece EA, Coustan DR (eds): Diabetes Mellitus in Pregnancy: Principles and Practice. Churchill Livingstone, New York, 1988

58. Hayslett JP, Reece EA: Effects of diabetic nephropathy on pregnancy. Am J Kidney Dis 9:344, 1987

59. Ogburn PL Jr, Kitzmiller JL, Hare JW et al: Pregnancy following renal transplantation in class T diabetes mellitus. JAMA 255:911, 1986

60. Carstensen LL, Frost-Lansen K, Fulgeberg S, Nerup J: Does pregnancy influence the prognosis of uncomplicated insulin-dependent diabetes? Diabetes Care 5:1, 1982

61. Horvat M, Maclear H, Goldberg L, Crock CW: Diabetic retinopathy in pregnancy: a 12 year prospective study. Br J Ophthalmol 64:398, 1980

62. Kitzmiller JL, Gavin LA, Gin GD et al: Managing diabetes and pregnancy. Curr Probl Obstet Gynecol Fertil 11:113, 1988

63. Moloney JBM, Drury MI: The effect of pregnancy on the natural course of diabetic retinopathy. Am J Ophth 93:745, 1982

64. Phelps RL, Sakol P, Metzger BE et al: Changes in diabetic retinopathy during pregnancy: correlations with regulation of hyperglycemia. Arch Ophthalmol 104:1806, 1986

65. Chang S, Fuhrmann M, and the Diabetes in Early Pregnancy Study Group: Pregnancy, retinopathy, normoglycemia: a preliminary analysis. Diabetes 34(Suppl):3A, 1985

66. Sinclair SH, Nesler C, Foxman B et al: Macular edema and pregnancy in insulin dependent diabetes. Am J Ophthalmol 97:154, 1984

67. Silfen SL, Wapner RJ, Gabbe SG: Maternal outcome in class H diabetes mellitus. Obstet Gynecol 55:749, 1980

68. Hare JW: Maternal complications. p. 96. In Hare JW (ed): Diabetes Complicating Pregnancy: The Joslin Clinic Method. Alan R. Liss, New York, 1989

69. Freinkel N: Gestational diabetes 1979: philosophical and practical aspects of a major health problem. Diabetes Care 3:399, 1980

70. O'Sullivan JB: Body weight and subsequent diabetes mellitus. JAMA 248:949, 1982

71. Coustan DR, Nelson C, Carpenter NW et al: Maternal age and screening for gestational diabetes: a population based study. Obstet Gynecol 73:557, 1989

72. Summary and Recommendations of the Third International Workshop–Conference on Gestational Diabetes. Diabetes (in press).

73. Coustan DR. Widness JA, Carpenter MW et al: Should the fifty-gram, one-hour plasma glucose screening test be administered in the fasting or fed state? Am J Obstet Gynecol 154:1031, 1986

74. Carpenter MW, Coustan DR: Criteria for screening tests of gestational diabetes. Am J Obstet Gynecol 144:768, 1982

75. Jovanovic L, Peterson CM: Screening for gestational diabetes, optimum timing and criteria for retesting. Diabetes 34(Suppl 2):21, 1985

76. Widness JA, Schwartz HC, Zeller WP et al: Glycohemoglobin in postpartum women. Obstet Gynecol 57:414, 1981

77. Landon MB, Gabbe SG: Glucose monitoring and insulin administration in the pregnant diabetic patient. Clin Obstet Gynecol 28:496, 1985

78. Jovanovic L, Peterson CM: Management of the pregnant, insulin-dependent diabetic woman. Diabetes Care 3:63, 1980

79. The American Diabetes Association: Principles of nutrition and dietary recommendations for individuals with diabetes mellitus. Diabetes 28:1027, 1979

80. Rudolf MCJ, Coustan DR, Sherwin RS et al: Efficacy of insulin pump in the home treatment of pregnancy diabetics. Diabetes 30:891, 1981

81. Coustan DR, Reece EA, Sherwin RS et al: A random-

ized clinical trial of the insulin pump vs intensive conventional therapy in diabetic pregnancies. JAMA 255:631, 1986

82. Kitabchi AE, Young R, Sacks H, Morris L: Diabetic ketoacidosis: reappraisal of therapeutic approach. Annu Rev Med 30:339, 1979

83. Landon MB, Gabbe SG: Antepartum fetal surveillance and delivery timing in diabetic pregnancies. Clin Diabetes 8:1, 1990

84. Fern PE, Grunert GM, Lewis SB: Urinary estriols: are they of value in normoglycemic diabetic pregnancy? Diabetes Care 5:316, 1982

85. Dooley SL, Depp R, Socol ML et al: Urinary estriols in diabetic pregnancy: a reappraisal. Obstet Gynecol 64:459, 1984

86. Gabbe SG, Mestman JH, Freeman RK et al: Management and outcome of diabetes mellitus classes B–R. Am J Obstet Gynecol 129:723, 1977

87. Evertson LR, Gauthier RJ, Collea JV: Fetal demise following negative contraction stress tests. Obstet Gynecol 130:424, 1978

88. Barret JM, Salyer SL, Boehm FH: The non-stress test: an evaluation of 1,000 patients. Am J Obstet Gynecol 141:153, 1981

89. Landon MB, Gabbe SG, Sachs L: Management of diabetes mellitus and pregnancy: a survey of obstetricians and maternal–fetal specialists. Obstet Gynecol 75:635, 1990

90. Miller JM, Horger EO: Antepartum heart rate testing in diabetic pregnancy. J Reprod Med 30:515, 1985

91. Golde SH, Montoro M, Good-Anderson B et al: The role of non-stress tests, fetal biophysical profile, and CSTs in the outpatient management of insulin-requiring diabetic pregnancies. Am J Obstet Gynecol 148:269, 1984

92. Dicker D, Feldberg D, Yeshaya A et al: Fetal surveillance in insulin-dependent diabetic pregnancy: predictive value of the biophysical profile. Am J Obstet Gynecol 159:800, 1988

93. Johnson JM, Lange IR, Harman CR et al: Biophysical profile scoring in the management of the diabetic pregnancy. Obstet Gyneol 72:841, 1988

94. Acker DB, Sachs BP, Friedman EA: Risk factors for shoulder dystocia. Obstet Gynecol 66:762, 1985

95. Tamura RK, Sabbagha RE, Depp R et al: Diabetic macrosomia: accuracy of third trimester ultrasound. Obstet Gynecol 67:828, 1986

96. Bochner CJ, Medearis AL, Williams J et al: Early third trimester screening in gestational diabetes to determine the risk of macrosomia and labor dystocia at term. Am J Obstet Gynecol 157:703, 1987

97. Landon MB, Mintz MG, Gabbe SG: Sonographic evaluation of fetal abdominal growth: predictor of the large-for-gestational age infant in pregnancies complicated by diabetes mellitus. Am J Obstet Gynecol 160:115, 1989

98. Landon MB, Gabbe SG, Bruner JP, Ludmir J: Doppler umbilical artery velocimetry in pregnancy complicated by insulin dependent diabetes mellitus. Obstet Gynecol 73:961, 1989

99. Gabbe SG, Lowensohn RI, Mestman JH et al: The lecithin/sphingomyelin ratio in pregnancies complicated by diabetes mellitus. Am J Obstet Gynecol 128:757, 1977

100. Hallman H, Teramo K: Amniotic fluid phospholipid profile as a prediction of fetal maturity in diabetic pregnancies. Obstet Gynecol 54:703, 1979

101. Hollingsworth DR, Ney DM: Dietary management of diabetes during pregnancy. p. 285. In Reece EA, Coustan DR (eds): Diabetes Mellitus in Pregnancy: Principles and Practice. Churchill Livingstone, New York, 1988

102. Algert S, Shragg P, Hollingsworth DR: Moderate caloric restriction in obese women with gestational diabetes. Obstet Gynecol 65:487, 1985

103. Goldberg J, Franklin B, Lasser L et al: Gestational diabetes: impact of home glucose monitoring on neonatal birth weight. Am J Obstet Gynecol 154:546, 1986

104. Langer O, Mazze RM: The relationship between large for gestational age infants and glycemic control in women with gestational diabetes. Am J Obstet Gynecol 159:1478, 1988

105. Coustan DR, Imarah J: Prophylactic insulin treatment of gestational diabetes reduced the incidence of macrosomia, operative delivery, and birth trauma. Am J Obstet Gynecol 150:836, 1984

106. Persson B, Stangenberg M, Hasson U, Nordlander E: Gestational diabetes mellitus: comparative evaluation of two treatment regimens, diet versus insulin and diet. Diabetes 34(Suppl 2):101, 1985

107. Landon MB, Gabbe SG: Antepartum fetal surveillance in gestational diabetes mellitus. Diabetes 34(Suppl 2):50, 1985

108. Molsted-Pedersen L: Pregnancy and diabetes, a survey. Acta Endocrinol 94(Suppl)238:13, 1980

109. Fuhrmann K, Reiher H, Semmler K et al: Prevention of congenital malformations in infants of insulin-dependent diabetic mothers. Diabetes Care 6:219, 1983

110. Miller E, Hare JW, Cloherty JP et al: Elevated maternal HbA$_1$ in early pregnancy and major congenital anomalies in infants of diabetic mothers. N Engl J Med 304:1331, 1981

111. Ylinen K, Aula P, Stenman UH et al: Risk of minor and major fetal malformations in diabetics with high hae-

moglobin A_{1c} values in early pregnancy. Br Med J 289:345, 1984

112. Mills J, Simpson JL, Driscoll SG et al: Incidence of spontaneous abortion among normal and insulin-dependent diabetic women whose pregnancies were identified within 21 days of conception. N Engl J Med 319:1617, 1988

113a. Freinkel N: Diabetic embryopathy and fuel-mediated organ neteratogenesis: lessons from animal models. Horm Metab Res 20:463, 1988

113b. Steel JM, Duncan LJP: Serious complications of oral contraception in insulin dependent diabetes. Contraception 17:291, 1978

113c. Klein BEK, Moss SE, Klein R: Oral contraceptives in women with diabetes. Diabetes Care 13:895, 1990

113d. DePiaro R, Forte F, Bertoli A et al: Changes in insulin receptors during oral contraception. J Clin Endocrinol Metab 52:29, 1982

113e. Steel JM, Duncan LJP: The effect of oral contraceptives on insulin requirements in diabetic women. Br J Fam Plann 3:77, 1978

113f. Skouby S, Kuhl C, Molsted-Pederson L et al: Triphasic oral contraception: metabolic effects in normal women and those with previous gestational diabetes. Am J Obstet Gynecol 153:495, 1985

114. Potter JD: Hypothyroidism and reproductive failure. Surg Gynecol Obstet 150:251, 1980

115. Mestman JH: Thyroid and parathyroid disease in pregnancy. p. 489. In Quilligan EJ, Kretchmer N (eds): Fetal and Maternal Medicine. Wiley, New York, 1980

116. Burrow GN, Polackwich R, Donabedian R: The hypothalamic–pituitary–thyroid axis in normal pregnancy. p. 1. In Fisher DA, Burrow GN (eds): Perinatal Thyroid Physiology and Disease. Raven Press, New York, 1975

117. Burrow GN: The management of thyrotoxicosis in pregnancy. N Engl J Med 313:562, 1985

118. Harada A, Hershman JM, Reed AW et al: Comparison of thyroid stimulators and thyroid hormone concentrations in the sera of pregnant women. J Clin Endocrinol Metab 48:793, 1979

119. Evans TC, Kretzchman RM, Hodges RE, Song CW: Radioiodine uptake studies of human fetal thyroid. J Nucl Med 8:157, 1967

120. Greenberg AH, Czernichow P, Reba RC et al: Observations on the maturation of thyroid function in early fetal life. J Clin Invest 49:1790, 1970

121. Landau H, Sack J, Fruch TH et al: Amniotic fluid 3,3′,5′-triiodothyroidism. J Clin Endocrinol Metab 50:799, 1980

122. Lombardi G, Lupoli G, Scopasa F et al: Plasma immunoreactive thyrotropin releasing hormone (TRH) values in normal newborns. J Endocrinol Invest 1:69, 1978

123. Oddie TH, Fisher DA, Bernard B, Lam RW: Thyroid function at birth in infants 30 to 45 weeks gestation. J Pediatr 90:803, 1977

124. Mestman JH, Manning PR, Hodgman J: Hyperthyroidism and pregnancy. Arch Intern Med 134:434, 1974

125. Bouillon R, Nalsens M, VanAssche FA: Hyperthyroxinemia: a cause for hyperemesis gravidarum. Am J Obstet Gynecol 143:922, 1982

126. Wallace EZ, Gandhi VS: Triiodothyronine thyrotoxicosis in pregnancy. Am J Obstet Gynecol 130:106, 1978

127. Van Dyke CP, Heydendael RJ, DeKleine MJ: Methimazole, carbimazole, and congenital skin defects. Ann Intern Med 106:60, 1987

128. Momotani N, Jaeduk N, Oyanagi H et al: Antithyroid drug therapy for Graves' disease during pregnancy: optimal regimen for fetal status. N Engl J Med 315:1, 1986

129. Cheron RG, Kaplan MG, Larsen PR et al: Neonatal thyroid function after propylthiouracil therapy for maternal Graves' disease. N Engl J Med 304:525, 1981

130. Burrow GN, Klatskin EH, Genel M: Intellectual development in children whose mothers received propylthiouracil during pregnancy. Yale J Biol Med 51:151, 1978

131. Munro DS, Dirmikis SM, Humphries H et al: The role of thyroid stimulating immunoglobulin of Graves' disease in neonatal thyrotoxicosis. Br J Obstet Gynaecol 85:837, 1988

132. Zakarija M, McKenzie JM: Pregnancy-associated changes in the thyroid-stimulating antibody of Graves' disease and the relationship to neonatal hyperthyroidism. J Clin Endocrinol Metab 57:1036, 1983

133. Davis LE, Lucas MJ, Hankins GDV et al: Thyrotoxicosis complicating pregnancy. Am J Obstet Gynecol 160:63, 1989

134. Lowy C: Endocrine emergencies in pregnancy. Clin Endocrinol Metab 9:569, 1989

135. Davis LE, Leveno KL, Cunningham FG: Hypothyroidism complicating pregnancy. Obstet Gynecol 72:108, 1988

136. Man EB, Holden RH, Jones WS: Thyroid function in human pregnancy. VII. Development and retardation of four year old progeny of euthyroid and hypothyroxinemic woman. Am J Obstet Gynecol 109:12, 1971

137. Man EB, Jones WS, Holden RH, Mellita ED: Thyroid function in human pregnancies. VIII. Retardation of progeny aged 7 years: relationships to maternal age

and maternal thyroid function. Am J Obstet Gynecol 111:905, 1971

138. Montoro MN, Collea JA, Frasier SN, Mestman JH: Successful outcome of pregnancy in women with hypothyroidism. Ann Intern Med 94:31, 1981

139. Amino N, Miyai K, Kuro R et al: Transient postpartum hypothyroidism: fourteen cases with autoimmune thyroiditis. Ann Intern Med 87:155, 1977

140. Fein HG, Goldman JM, Weintraub BD: Postpartum lymphocytic thyroiditis in American women: a spectrum of thyroid dysfunction. Am J Obstet Gynecol 138:504, 1980

141. Amino N, Mori H, Iwatani Y et al: High prevalence of transient postpartum thyrotoxicosis and hypothyroidism. N Engl J Med 306:849, 1982

142. Walfish PG, Chan JYC: Postpartum hyperthyroidism. Clin Endocrinol Metab 14:417, 1985

143. VanHerk AJ, Rich P, Ljung BE et al: The thyroid nodule. Ann Intern Med 96:221, 1982

144. Pitkin RM: Calcium metabolism in pregnancy and the perinatal period: a review. Am J Obstet Gynecol 151:99, 1985

145. Reddy GS, Norman AW, Willis DM: Regulation of vitamin D metabolism in normal human pregnancy. J Clin Endocrinol Metab 56:363, 1983

146. Pitkin RM, Reynolds WA, Williams GA, Harris GK: Calcium metabolism in pregnancy: a longitudinal study. Am J Obstet Gynecol 133:781, 1979

147. Whitehead M, Lane G, Young O: Interrelationships of calcium-regulating hormones during normal pregnancy. Br Med J 3:10, 1981

148. Drake TS, Kaplan RA, Lewis TA: The physiologic hyperparathyroidism of pregnancy: is it primary or secondary? Obstet Gynecol 53:746, 1979

149. Schauberger CW, Pitkin RM: Maternal–perinatal calcium relationships. Obstet Gynecol 53:75, 1979

150. Delvin EE, Glorieux FH, Salle BL et al: Control of vitamin D metabolism in preterm infants: fetomaternal relationships. Arch Dis Child 57:754, 1982

151. Steichen JJ, Tsang RC, Gratton TL et al: Vitamin D homeostasis in the perinatal period: 1,25-dihydroxyvitamin D in maternal, cord, and neonatal blood. N Engl J Med 302:315, 1989

152. Shangold MM, Dor N, Welt SI et al: Hyperparathyroidism and pregnancy: a review. Obstet Gynecol Surv 37:217, 1982

153. Monteleone JA, Lee JB, Tashjean AH, Cantor HE: Transient neonatal hypocalcemia, hypomagnesemia, and high serum parathyroid hormone with maternal hyperparathyroidism. Ann Intern Med 82:670, 1975

154. Patterson R: Hyperparathyroidism in pregnancy. Obstet Gynecol 70:457, 1987

155. Montoro MM, Collea JV, Mestman JH: Management of hyperparathyroidism in pregnancy with oral phosphate therapy. Obstet Gynecol 55:431, 1989

156. Stuart C, Aceto T, Kuhn JP, Terplan K: Intrauterine hyperparathyroidism. Am J Dis Child 133:67, 1979

157. Graders D, LeRoit HD, Karplus M et al: Congenital hyperparathyrodism and rickets secondary to maternal hypoparathyroidism and vitamin D deficiency. Isr J Med Sci 17:705, 1981

158. Salle BL, Berthezene F, Glorieux FH: Hypoparathyroidism during pregnancy: treatment with Calcitriol. J Clin Endocrinol Metab 52:810, 1981

159. Cundy T, Haining SA, Guilland-Cumming DF et al: Remission of hypoparathyroidism during lactation: evidence for a physiological role for prolactin in the regulation of vitamin D metabolism. Clin Endocrinol 26:667, 1987

160. Gemzell C, Wang CF: Outcome of pregnancy in women with pituitary adenoma. Fertil Steril 31:363, 1979

161. Maygar DM, Marshall JR: Pituitary tumors and pregnancy. Am J Obstet Gynecol 132:739, 1978

162. Jewelewicz R, VanDeWiele RL: Clinical course and outcome of pregnancy in twenty-five patients with pituitary microadenomas. Am J Obstet Gynecol 136:339, 1980

163. Molitch ME: Pregnancy and the hyperprolactinemic woman. N Engl J Med 312:21, 1984

164. Divers W, Yen SSC: Prolactin producing microadenomas in pregnancy. Obstet Gynecol 62:425, 1983

165. Turkalj I, Braun P, Krup P: Surveillance of bromocriptine in pregnancy. JAMA 247:1589, 1982

166. Jewelewicz R, Zimmerman EA, Carmel PW: Conservative management of a pituitary tumor during pregnancy following induction of ovulation with gonadotropins. Fertil Steril 28:35, 1977

167. Hime MC, Richardson JA: Diabetes insipidus and pregnancy: case reports, incidence and review of the literature. Obstet Gynecol Surv 33:375, 1978

168. Durr JA: Diabetes insipidus in pregnancy. Am J Kidney Dis 9:276, 1978

169. Barron WM, Cohen LM, Ulland LA et al: Transient vasopressin-resistant diabetes insipidus of pregnancy. N Engl J Med 310:442, 1984

170. Burrow GN, Wassenar W, Robertson GL, Sehl H: DDAVP treatment of diabetes insipidus during pregnancy and the postpartum period. Acta Endocrinol 97:23, 1981

171. Shangold MM, Freeman R, Kumaresan P et al: Plasma oxytocin concentrations in a pregnant woman with total vasopressin deficiency. Obstet Gynecol 61:662, 1983

172. Sheehan HL: Postpartum necrosis of the anterior pituitary. J Pathol Bacteriol 45:189, 1937

173. Dorfman SG, Dillaplain RP, Gambrell RD: Antepartum pituitary infarction. Obstet Gynecol 53:215, 1979

174. Grimes HG, Brooks MH: Pregnancy in Sheehan's syndrome: report of a case and review. Obstet Gynecol Surv 35:481, 1980

175. Anderson KJ, Walters WAW: Cushing's syndrome and pregnancy. Aust NZ J, Obstet Gynaecol, 16:225, 1976

176. Grimes EM, Fayez JA, Miller GL: Cushing's syndrome and pregnancy. Obstet Gynecol 42:550, 1973

177. Check JH, Caro JF, Kendall B et al: Cushing's syndrome in pregnancy: effect of associated diabetes on fetal and neonatal complications. Am J Obstet Gynecol 133:846, 1979

178. Koerten JM, Morales WJ, Washington SR, Castaldo TW: Cushing's syndrome in pregnancy: a case report and literature review. Am J Obstet Gynecol 154:626, 1986

179. Bevan JS, Gough MH, Gillmer MDG et al: Cushing's syndrome in pregnancy: the timing of definitive treatment. Clin Endocrinol 27:225, 1987

180. Merrill RH, Dombroski RA, MacKenna JM: Primary hyperaldosteronism during pregnancy. Am J Obstet Gynecol 160:785, 1984

181. Lotgering FK, Derkx FMH, Wallenburg HCS: Primary hyperaldosteronism in pregnancy. Am J Obstet Gynecol 155:986, 1986

182. Brent F: Addison's disease and pregnancy. Am J Surg 79:645, 1950

183. Carr BR, Parker CR, Madden JD et al: Maternal plasma adrenocorticotropin and cortisol relationships throughout human pregnancy. Am J Obstet Gynecol 139:416, 1981

184. O'Shaughnessy RW, Hackett KJ: Maternal Addison's disease and fetal growth retardation. J Reprod Med 29:752, 1984

185. Schenker JG, Crowers I: Pheochromocytoma and pregnancy: review of 89 cases. Obstet Gynecol Surv 26:739, 1971

186. Schenker JG, Granat M: Pheochromocytoma and pregnancy—an update and appraisal. Aust NZ J Obstet Gynaecol 22:1, 1982

187. Venuto R, Burstein P, Schmeider R: Pheochromocytoma: antepartum diagnosis and management with tumor resection in the puerperium. Am J Obstet Gynecol 150:431, 1984

188. National Institutes of Health Diabetes Data Group: Classification and diagnosis of diabetes mellitus and other categories of glucose intolerance. Diabetes 28:1039, 1979

189. Phelps RL, Metzger BE, Freinkel N: Carbohydrate metabolism in pregnancy. Am J Obstet Gynecol 140:730, 1981

190. Mestman J: Management of thyroid disease in pregnancy. Clin Perinatol 7:376, 1980

Chapter 34

Hematologic Diseases

Philip Samuels

IRON DEFICIENCY ANEMIA

During a singleton pregnancy, maternal plasma volume gradually expands by approximately 50 percent (1,000 ml). The total red blood cell (RBC) mass also increases, but only by approximately 300 ml (25%), and this starts later in pregnancy.[1] It is not surprising, therefore, that hemoglobin and hematocrit levels usually fall during gestation. These changes are not necessarily pathologic but usually represent a physiologic alteration of pregnancy. By 6 weeks postpartum, in the absence of excessive blood loss during the puerperium, hemoglobin and hematocrit levels have returned to normal.

Approximately 50 percent of pregnant women are anemic with a hematocrit less than 32 percent. The incidence of anemia changes with epidemiologic differences in the population studied. Approximately 75 percent of anemias that occur during pregnancy are secondary to iron deficiency.[1] Ho and coinvestigators[2] performed elaborate hematologic evaluations of 221 normal full-term gravidas in Taiwan. None of the studied patients received an added hematinic during gestation. Of these previously nonanemic patients, 23 (10.4%) developed clinical anemia after a full-term pregnancy. Of the 23, 11 (47.8%) developed florid iron deficiency anemia, while another 11 developed moderate iron depletion. In 22 of 23 anemic patients, therefore, the anemia was secondary to iron deficiency.[2] The remaining patient was diagnosed as

having folate deficiency. Among the 198 nonanemic gravidas at term, 92 (46.5%) showed evidence of iron depletion even though they had a normal hematocrit.[2]

To distinguish the normal physiologic changes of pregnancy from pathologic iron deficiency anemia, one must understand the iron requirements of pregnancy (Table 34.1) and the proper use of hematologic laboratory parameters. In the adult woman, iron stores are located in the bone marrow, liver, and spleen in the form of ferritin. Ferritin comprises approximately 25 percent (500 mg) of the 2-g iron stores found in the normal woman. Approximately 65 percent of storage iron is found in the circulating RBCs.[1,3–5] If the dietary iron intake is poor, the interval between pregnancies is short, or, delivery is complicated by hemorrhage, iron deficiency anemia readily develops.

The first pathologic change to occur in iron deficiency anemia is the depletion of bone marrow, liver, and spleen iron stores. The serum iron falls, as does the percentage saturation of transferrin. The total iron-binding capacity rises, as this is a reflection of unbound transferrin. A fall in the hematocrit follows. Microcytic hypochromic RBCs are released into the circulation. Should iron deficiency be combined with folate deficiency, normocytic and normochromic RBCs will be observed on peripheral smear.

Care must be taken when using laboratory parameters to establish the diagnosis of iron deficiency anemia during gestation. A serum iron concentration less

Table 34.1   Iron Requirements for Pregnancy and the Puerperium

Event	Elemental Iron
Increased red blood cell mass	450 mg
Fetus and placenta	360 mg
Vaginal delivery	190 mg
Lactation	1 mg/day

than 60 μg/dl with less than 16 percent saturation of transferrin is suggestive of iron deficiency. An increase in total iron-binding capacity, however, is not reliable, as 15 percent of pregnant women without iron deficiency will show an increase in this parameter.[6] Serum ferritin levels normally decrease mildly during pregnancy. A significantly reduced ferritin concentration is also indicative of iron deficiency anemia and is the best parameter with which to judge the degree of iron deficiency. If a patient has been iron deficient for an extended period of time and begins taking iron, her serum iron level can rise before she has repleted her iron stores. The ferritin level will indicate the status of her iron stores. If hematologic parameters remain confusing, bone marrow aspiration, which can be performed safely during gestation, will provide the definitive diagnosis. This procedure, however, is rarely necessary.

Whether all women should receive prophylactic iron during pregnancy remains moot. In pregnancy, iron absorption from the duodenum increases, providing 1.3 to 2.6 mg of elemental iron daily in patients with ideal dietary habits.[7,8] In patients who do not show clear signs of iron deficiency anemia, it is uncertain whether prophylactic iron leads to increased hemoglobin levels at term.[9] Iron prophylaxis is safe, and, with the exception of dyspepsia and constipation, side effects are few. One 325-mg tablet of ferrous sulfate daily provides adequate prophylaxis. It contains 60 mg of elemental iron, 10 percent of which is absorbed. If the iron is not needed, it will not be absorbed and will be excreted in the stool. The standard generic iron tablets and the amount of elemental iron they provide are listed in Table 34.2.

One iron tablet three times daily is recommended for the pregnant patient with iron deficiency anemia.

To ensure maximum absorption, iron should be ingested about 30 minutes before meals. When taken in this manner, however, dyspepsia and nausea are more common. Therapy, therefore, must be individualized to maximize patient compliance. If isolated iron deficiency anemia is present, one should see a dramatic reticulocytosis approximately 2 weeks after the initiation of therapy. Because iron absorption is pH dependent, taking iron with ascorbic acid (vitamin C) may increase duodenal absorption. Conversely, taking iron with antacids will decrease absorption.

Folate Deficiency

Folic acid, a water-soluble vitamin, is found in green vegetables, peanuts, and liver. Folate stores are located primarily in the liver and are usually sufficient for 6 weeks. After 3 weeks of a diet deficient in folate, the serum folate level falls. Two weeks later, hypersegmentation of neutrophils occurs. After 17 weeks without folate ingestion, RBC folate levels drop. In the next week a megaloblastic bone marrow develops. During pregnancy, folate deficiency is the most common cause of megaloblastic anemia, as vitamin B_{12} deficiency is extremely rare. The daily folate requirement in the nonpregnant state is approximately 50 μg, but this rises three- to fourfold during gestation.[10] Fetal demands increase the requirement, as does the decrease in the gastrointestinal absorption of folate during pregnancy.[11]

Clinical megaloblastic anemia seldom occurs before the third trimester of pregnancy. If the patient is at risk for folate deficiency or has mild anemia, an attempt should be made to detect this disorder before megaloblastosis occurs. Historically, the disorder was detected by counting the number of lobes in the patient's neutrophils. In most folate-deficient patients, 5 percent of the neutrophils exhibit five or more

Table 34.2   Elemental Iron Available From Common Iron Preparations

Preparation	Elemental Iron (mg)
Ferrous gluconate, 325 mg	37–39
Ferrous sulfate, 325 mg	60–65
Ferrous fumarate, 325 mg	107

lobes.[12] Today, serum folate and RBC folate levels are the best tests for folate deficiency.[13]

Folate deficiency rarely occurs in the fetus and is not a cause of significant perinatal morbidity. Maternal morbidity, however, may result from the anemia, especially if the patient additionally suffers significant blood loss during the puerperium. Most prenatal vitamins that require physician prescription contain 1 mg of folic acid. Most nonprescription prenatal vitamins contain 0.8 mg of folic acid. These amounts are more than adequate to prevent and treat folate deficiency. Women with significant hemoglobinopathies, patients receiving phenytoin or other anticonvulsants, and women carrying a multiple gestation may require more than 1 mg supplemental folate daily. If the patient is folic acid deficient, her reticulocyte count will be depressed. Within 3 days after the administration of sufficient folic acid, reticulocytosis usually occurs. Leukopenia and thrombocytopenia, which accompany megaloblastosis, are rapidly reversed. The hematocrit may rise as much as 1 percent per day after 1 week of folate replacement.

Iron deficiency is a frequent concomitant of folic acid deficiency. If a patient with folate deficiency does not develop a significant reticulocytosis within 1 week after administration of sufficient replacement therapy, appropriate tests for iron deficiency should be performed.

Hemoglobinopathies

Hemoglobin is a tetrameric protein composed of two pairs of polypeptide chains with a heme group attached to each chain.[14] The normal adult hemoglobin A_1 comprises 95 percent of hemoglobin. It consists of two α-chains and two β-chains. The remaining 5 percent of hemoglobin usually consists of hemoglobin A_2 (containing two α-chains and two δ-chains) and hemoglobin F (with two α-chains and two γ-chains). In the fetus, hemoglobin F (fetal hemoglobin) declines during the third trimester of pregnancy, reaching its permanent nadir several months after birth. Hemoglobinopathies arise when there is a change in the structure of a peptide chain or a defect in the ability to synthesize a specific polypeptide chain. The patterns of inheritance are often straightforward. The prevalence of the most common hemoglobinopathies is shown in Table 34.3.

Table 34.3 Hemoglobinopathies

Hemoglobinopathy	Frequency in Adult Blacks
Sickle cell trait	1 : 12
Sickle cell disease	1 : 708
Hemoglobin C trait	1 : 41
Hemoglobin C disease	1 : 4,790
Hemoglobin SC disease	1 : 757
Hemoglobin S/β thalassemia	1 : 1,672

Hemoglobin S

Hemoglobin S, an abnormal hemoglobin, is present in patients with sickle cell disease (hemoglobin SS) and sickle cell trait (hemoglobin AS). A single substitution of valine for glutamic acid at the sixth position in the β-polypeptide chain causes a significant change in the physical characteristics of this hemoglobin. At low oxygen tensions, RBCs containing hemoglobin S assume a sickle shape. Sludging in small vessels occurs, resulting in microinfarction of the affected organs. Sickle cells have a lifespan of 5 to 10 days, compared with 120 days for a normal RBC. Sickling is triggered by hypoxia, acidosis, or dehydration. Infants with sickle cell anemia show no signs of the disease until the concentration of hemoglobin F falls to adult levels. Some patients do not experience symptoms until adolescence.

Approximately 1 of 12 adult blacks in the United States is heterozygous for hemoglobin S and, therefore, has sickle cell trait (hemoglobin AS) and carries the affected gene. These individuals generally have 35 to 45 percent hemoglobin S and are asymptomatic. The child of two individuals with sickle cell trait has a 50 percent probability of inheriting the trait and a 25 percent probability of actually having sickle cell disease. One of every 625 black children born in the United States is homozygous for hemoglobin S, and the frequency of sickle cell disease among adult blacks is 1 in 708.[15] All at-risk patients should be screened for hemoglobin S at their first prenatal visit. Patients with a positive screen should undergo hemoglobin electrophoresis. Women identified as having sickle cell trait (hemoglobin AS) are not at increased risk for poor perinatal outcome. The spouse, however, should be tested, and if both are carriers of a hemoglobinopathy prenatal diagnosis should be offered.

Prenatal diagnosis can be performed by DNA analysis with the polymerase chain reaction and Southern blotting.[16,17] Hemoglobin S can also be identified by hemoglobin electrophoresis of fetal blood.[17]

Painful vasoocclusive episodes involving multiple organs are the clinical hallmark of sickle cell anemia. The most common sites for these episodes are the extremities, joints, and abdomen. Vasoocclusive episodes can also occur in the lung, resulting in pulmonary infarction. Analgesia, oxygen, and hydration are the clinical foundation for treating these painful crises.

Sickle cell disease can affect virtually all organ systems. Osteomyelitis is common, and osteomyelitis caused by *Salmonella* is found almost exclusively in these patients. The risk of pyelonephritis is increased. Sickling may also occur in the renal medulla, where oxygen tension is reduced, resulting in papillary necrosis. These patients also exhibit renal tubular dysfunction and hyposthenuria. Because of chronic hemolysis and decreased RBC survival, patients with sickle cell anemia often demonstrate some degree of jaundice. Biliary stasis commonly occurs during crises, and cholelithiasis is seen in about 30 percent of cases.[18,19] Because of chronic anemia, high output cardiac failure can occur. Left ventricular hypertrophy and cardiomegaly are not uncommon.

Many pregnancies complicated by sickle cell anemia are associated with poor perinatal outcomes. The rate of spontaneous abortion may be as high as 25 percent.[20-22] Perinatal mortality rates of up to 40 percent were reported in the past, but the current estimate is approximately 15 percent.[21-26] Powars and coworkers[27] studied 156 pregnancies in 79 women with sickle cell anemia. In this group, the perinatal mortality rate was 52.7 percent before 1972 and 22.7 percent after that time. Much of this poor perinatal outcome is related to preterm birth. Approximately 30 percent of infants born to mothers with sickle cell disease have birth weights below 2,500 g.[21] It has been hypothesized that sickling in the uterine vessels may lead to decreased fetal oxygenation and intrauterine growth retardation.[28] In the past, it was thought that increased levels of hemoglobin F in the mother spared her from increased painful crises during pregnancy and may also have a protective effect on the neonate. However, in a recent study by Anyaegbunam and colleagues,[29] hemoglobin F levels were inversely correlated with birth weight percentile.

Stillbirth rates of 8 to 10 percent have been described in patients with sickle cell anemia.[21] These fetal deaths happen not only during crises but also can occur unexpectedly. Careful antepartum fetal testing must therefore be utilized, including serial ultrasonography to assess fetal growth. In another study, Anyaegbunam and coworkers[30] studied Doppler flow velocimetry in patients with hemoglobinopathies. They showed abnormal systolic/diastolic ratios for the uterine or umbilical arteries in 88 percent of patients with hemoglobin SS compared with 7 percent of patients with hemoglobin AS and 4 percent of patients with hemoglobin AA. However, only 8 patients with hemoglobin SS were studied compared with 40 patients with hemoglobin AS and 48 women with hemoglobin AA.[30] Although this is statistically significant, more investigations must be done before Doppler velocimetry is applied routinely as a part of antenatal testing for all patients with sickle cell disease.

Although maternal mortality is rare in patients with sickle cell anemia, maternal morbidity is great. Infections are common, occurring in 50 to 67 percent of women with hemoglobin SS. Most are urinary tract infections (UTI), which can be detected by frequent urine cultures. Patients with hemoglobin AS are also at greater risk for a UTI and should be screened as well. Pulmonary infection and infarction are also common. Patients with sickle cell anemia should receive pneumococcal vaccine before pregnancy. Any infection demands prompt attention, because fever, dehydration, and acidosis will result in further sickling and painful crises. The incidence of pregnancy-induced hypertension is increased in patients with sickle cell anemia and may complicate almost one-third of pregnancies in these patients.[24] Painful crises also appear to be more common during gestation.[31,32]

The care of the pregnant patient with sickle cell anemia must be individualized and meticulous. These patients will benefit from care in a center experienced in treating the multitude of problems that can complicate such pregnancies. From early gestation, good dietary habits should be promoted. A folate supplement of at least 1 mg/day should be administered as soon as pregnancy is confirmed. Although hemoglobin and hematocrit levels are decreased, iron supplements need not be routinely given. Serum iron and ferritin levels should be checked monthly and iron supplementation started only when these levels are diminished. Abudu and coworkers[33] found that serum ferritin values were significantly higher in pregnant women with hemoglobin SS disease than in those with hemoglobin AA. They concluded that the physiologic changes of pregnancy in patients with hemoglobin SS did not result in an iron deficiency state and that the use of prophylactic iron supplementations in these patients appears unjustified.

The role of prophylactic transfusions in the gravida with sickle cell anemia is more controversial and questionable today than when the first edition of this book was published. This therapy, which replaces the patient's sickle cells with normal RBCs, can both improve oxygen carrying capacity and suppress the synthesis of sickle hemoglobin. A previous study showed a sevenfold reduction in perinatal mortality in patients receiving prophylactic transfusions.[34] In the same group of patients, there was a significant decrease in fetal growth retardation and preterm births. Morrison and coworkers[35] have also previously reported reduced perinatal wastage and maternal morbidity using a regimen of exchange transfusion. In contrast, workers at Johns Hopkins believe that meticulous prenatal care gives results as favorable as those obtained with prophylactic transfusion.[20] Many patients in that series, however, did require transfusion for painful crises and anemia. The most recent study by Koshy and coinvestigators[36] followed 72 pregnant patients with sickle cell anemia, one-half of whom received prophylactic transfusions and one-half transfusions only for medical or obstetric emergencies. There was no significant difference in perinatal outcome between the offspring of mothers who received prophylactic transfusions and those who did not. Two risk factors were identified as harbingers of an unfavorable outcome: (1) the occurrence of a perinatal death in a previous pregnancy and (2) twins in the present pregnancy. Even though there was no difference in perinatal morbidity and mortality, prophylactic transfusion did appear to decrease significantly the incidence of painful crises. The investigators concluded that the omission of prophylactic red blood cell transfusion will not harm pregnant patients with sickle cell disease or their offspring.[36]

Keidan and coworkers[37] performed a prospective study to see which patients might benefit most from transfusion. Although the number of patients was small, the conclusions reached in this study are interesting. These investigators devised a "sicklecrit," which was the product of the packed corpuscular volume and the percentage of hemoglobin S. They also looked at erythrocyte filterability through pores of 5 μm diameter. Using these methods, they hoped to assess blood rheology in large and small vessels, respectively, to monitor the effects of exchange transfusion in sickle cell disease.[37] This preliminary work may prove helpful in deciding which patients will benefit from prophylactic transfusion. Tuck and coworkers[38] delineated the risks involved with exchange transfusion. In a study of 51 pregnancies transfused between 1978 and 1984, 22 percent developed atypical red cell antibodies and 14 percent had immediate minor transfusion reactions. These data showed no significant difference in maternal or fetal outcome between patients who were transfused prophylactically and those who were not.[38]

If one chooses to perform prophylactic transfusion, the goal is to maintain a percentage of hemoglobin A above 20 percent at all times and preferably above 40 percent, as well as to maintain the hematocrit above 25 percent. Morrison et al.[35] recommend that prophylactic transfusion begin at 28 weeks gestation. Buffy-coat-poor washed RBCs are used to reduce the risk of isosensitization. Other risks of transfusion therapy include hepatitis, acquired immune deficiency syndrome (AIDS), transfusion reactions, and hemochromatosis. Human immunodeficiency virus (HIV) antibody testing and new tests for non-A, non-B hepatitis have made transfusion safer.

Either booster or exchange transfusions can be used for prophylaxis, painful crises, or other indications. Exchange transfusions are preferable because they result in less stress on the cardiovascular system, thus decreasing the possibility of congestive heart failure. Exchange transfusions also raise the percentage of hemoglobin A more efficiently. If only booster transfusions are utilized, diuretics should probably be administered to prevent fluid overload. The technique for prophylactic exchange transfusion is shown below. In the exchange transfusion, the patient is first given 500 ml of crystalloid. A 500-ml phlebotomy is then performed, followed by transfusion of 2 units of buffy-coat-poor washed and packed RBCs. This procedure is repeated 6 to 8 hours later.[35] The following morning a hematocrit and hemoglobin electrophoresis are performed. If the hematocrit is less than 35 percent or if the hemoglobin A level is below 40 percent, the procedure is repeated until the desired levels are reached.[35]

TECHNIQUE FOR PARTIAL EXCHANGE TRANSFUSION

1. Perform baseline studies: hemoglobin, hematocrit, reticulocyte count, hemoglobin electrophoresis.
2. Type and crossmatch 4 units of buffy-coat-poor, washed, packed RBCs.
3. Infuse 500 ml normal saline (60 minutes).
4. Remove 500 ml by phlebotomy (30 minutes).
5. Infuse 2 units packed RBCs (90 minutes).
6. Repeat entire procedure.
7. Allow 12 hours for equilibration.
8. Obtain hematocrit and hemoglobin electrophoresis.
9. Discharge patient if hematocrit is > 35 percent and hemoglobin A > 40 percent.
10. Repeat procedure.
    a. When hematocrit is < 25 percent
    b. When hemoglobin A is < 20 percent
    c. If crisis occurs
    d. If labor ensues

(Adapted from Morrison et al.,[93] with permission.)

A vaginal delivery is preferred for patients with sickle cell anemia. Cesarean section should be reserved for obstetric indications. Patients should labor in the left lateral recumbent position and receive supplemental oxygen. While adequate hydration should be maintained, fluid overload must be avoided. Conduction anesthesia is recommended, as it provides excellent pain relief and can be used for a cesarean section, if necessary.

Hemoglobin SC Disease

Hemoglobin C is another β-chain variant in which lysine is substituted for glutamic acid in the sixth position. Clinically significant hemoglobin SC disease occurs in 1 in 833 adult blacks in the United States.[15] Women with both S and C hemoglobin suffer less morbidity in pregnancy than do patients with only hemoglobin S.[20-22] As in sickle cell disease, however, there is an increased incidence of early spontaneous abortion and pregnancy-induced hypertension.[20-23]

Because patients with SC disease can have only mild symptoms, the hemoglobinopathy may remain undiagnosed until they suffer a crisis during pregnancy. These crises may be marked by sequestration of a large volume of RBCs in the spleen accompanied by a dramatic fall in hematocrit.[39,40] Because these patients have increased splenic activity, they may be mildly thrombocytopenic throughout pregnancy. During gestation, patients with hemoglobin SC should receive the same program of prenatal care outlined for women with hemoglobin SS. The role of prophylactic transfusions for hemoglobin SC is more controversial than for hemoglobin SS. Clearly, symptomatic patients should be transfused when necessary.

THALASSEMIA

Thalassemia results from a defect in the rate of globin chain synthesis. Any of the polypeptide chains can be affected. The disease may range from minimal suppression of synthesis of the affected chain to its complete absence. Either α- or β-thalassemia can occur. Heterozygous patients are often asymptomatic. Thalassemia can be detected by prenatal diagnosis. Wainscoat and coworkers[41] were able to offer prenatal diagnosis to 19 of 25 families with a potential for β-thalassemia using linkage analysis of restriction fragment length polymorphisms (RFLP). Cao and colleagues[42] reported their experience with prenatal diagnosis of β-thalassemia in 1,000 pregnancies followed at least 12 months after birth. Fetal blood sampling was carried out by placental aspiration, which yielded a sufficient amount of blood in 99 percent of cases. The fetal mortality rate associated with the fetal blood sampling, however, was 6.3 percent.

Homozygous α-thalassemia results in the formation of tetramers of β-chains known as hemoglobin Bart. This hemoglobinopathy can result in hydrops fetalis. Ghosh and coinvestigators[43] reported their experience with 26 Chinese women who were at risk of giving birth to a fetus with homozygous α-thalassemia. Six of the 26 fetuses were affected. In two of the six cases, progressive fetal ascites appeared before 24 weeks gestation. These pregnancies were terminated and the diagnoses confirmed. In the remaining four cases, there was evidence of intrauterine growth retardation by 28 weeks gestation. At later gestational ages, an increase in the transverse cardiac diameter was seen in the affected fetuses.[43] Woo and colleagues[44] reported that umbilical artery velocimetry reveals a hyperdynamic circulatory state in fetuses that are hydropic because of α-thalassemia. In a study from Taiwan, Hsieh et al.[45] demonstrated that umbilical vein blood flow measurements can help to distinguish hydrops fetalis caused by hemoglobin Bart from hydrops fetalis having other causes. The umbilical vein diameter, blood velocity, and blood flow in fetuses with hemoglobin Bart were usually higher than those in fetuses with hydrops fetalis having other etiologies.

β-Thalassemia is the most common form of thalassemia. Patients with the heterozygous state are usually asymptomatic. They are detected by an increase in their level of hemoglobin A_2. In the homozygous state, synthesis of hemoglobin A_1 may be completely suppressed. This condition is characterized by an increase in both hemoglobin F and hemoglobin A_2. The homozygous state of β-thalassemia is known as thalassemia major, or Cooley's anemia. Patients with this disorder are transfusion dependent and have marked hepatosplenomegaly and bone changes secondary to increased hematopoiesis. These individuals usually die of infectious or cardiovascular complications before they reach childbearing age. Successful full-term pregnancies have been reported.[46] The few patients who do become pregnant generally exhibit severe anemia and congestive heart failure. Prenatal care is dependent on transfusion therapy similar to that used in the care of the patient with sickle cell anemia.

Heterozygous β-thalassemia has different forms of expression. Patients with thalassemia minima have microcytosis but are asymptomatic. Those with thalassemia intermedia exhibit splenomegaly and significant anemia and may become transfusion dependent during pregnancy. Their anemia can be significant enough to produce high-output cardiac failure.[47] These patients should be managed with a treatment program similar to that followed for patients with sickle cell anemia. As in the case of sickle hemoglobinopathies, iron supplementation should only be given if necessary, as indiscriminate use of iron can lead to hemochromatosis. White and coworkers[48] have shown that patients with a β-thalassemia usually have a much higher ferritin concentration than normal patients and those who are α-thalassemia carriers. In β-thalassemia carriers, the incidence of iron deficiency anemia is four times less common than it is in α-thalassemia carriers and normal patients.[48] Van der Weyden and coworkers[49] have convincingly shown that red cell ferritin and plasma ferritin can be used in combination to determine if a patient has a potential for iron overload. Although iron is not necessary, folic acid supplementation appears important in β-thalassemia carriers. Leung and coinvestigators[50] showed that the daily administration of folate significantly increased the predelivery hemoglobin concentration in both nulliparous and multiparous patients.

As in the case of sickle cell anemia, antepartum fetal evaluation is essential in patients with thalassemia who are anemic. Asymptomatic thalassemia carriers need no special testing. However, patients with thalassemia should undergo frequent ultrasonography to assess fetal growth, as well as nonstress testing to evaluate fetal well being.

Occasionally, individuals will inherit two hemoglobinopathies, such as sickle cell thalassemia (hemoglobin S Thal). The prevalence of this disorder among adult blacks in the United States is $1:1,672$.[51] The clinical course is variable. If minimal suppression of β-chains occurs, patients may be free of symptoms. However, with total suppression of β-chain synthesis, a clinical picture similar to that of sickle cell anemia will develop. The course of these patients during pregnancy is quite variable and their therapy must be individualized.

Immune Thrombocytopenic Purpura

In patients with immune thrombocytopenic purpura (ITP), the decrease in the circulating platelet count is secondary to peripheral destruction and sequestration of platelets resulting from the production of antiplatelet antibodies and the clearance of these complexes by the reticuloendothelial system. Patients with ITP may demonstrate increased levels of platelet-associated IgG, IgM, and C_3 as well as increased levels of antiplatelet IgG.[52,53] These platelet-associated immunoglobulins presumably damage the platelets, rendering them more susceptible to phagocytosis or sequestration in the reticuloendothelial system. The bone marrow in ITP will demonstrate an increased number of megakaryocytes.

ITP usually has its onset before age 30 years and is more common in women. It may be the harbinger of systemic lupus erythematosus or another autoimmune disease. Because idiosyncratic reactions to drugs are also a cause of thrombocytopenia, a careful drug history is necessary before diagnosing ITP. Thrombocytopenia is also occasionally an early sign of preeclampsia.

The major goal in treating patients with ITP is the prevention of bleeding episodes. Many patients require no therapy. Glucocorticoids are the mainstay of therapy. Patients are maintained on the minimum dose of glucocorticoid necessary to prevent petechiae. Ballem and coinvestigators[54] advocate using the maternal bleeding time as an indication for treatment. They recommend that anyone with a bleeding time greater than 20 minutes should be treated with glucocorticoids. By limiting treatment in this fashion, side effects during pregnancy can be minimized. The mechanism of action of glucocorticoids is unclear, but these medications probably inhibit phagocytosis by the reticuloendothelial system or prevent antibody binding.[53] For patients who do not respond to steroids, splenectomy should be considered.[55] When necessary, it can be safely carried out during gestation. Splenectomy is successful in raising the platelet count in about 75 percent of cases. Nonetheless, these patients still have the ability to produce antiplatelet antibodies.[56] In those patients not responding to splenectomy, the destruction of platelets continues in the liver and bone marrow.[55,57] Until recently, cytotoxic agents have been used in such cases. However, platelet counts can now be raised using high doses of intravenous gammaglobulins.[58-65] The usual dose is 400 mg/kg per day for 5 days. By the third day, there is usually a significant increase in platelet count. Because the length of time the platelet count remains elevated is variable, this therapy is only a temporary measure, which is useful in preparing a patient for a planned cesarean section or splenectomy. It may also help stop an acute bleeding event. No adverse fetal effects have been reported

with gammaglobulin therapy. Plasmaphoresis to remove circulating antiplatelet IgG has also been used as an emergent measure. It appears to work best in patients with acute disease.[66] Platelet transfusions are of little help, except in the case of severe hemorrhage or intraoperative bleeding. In ITP, the transfused platelets are destroyed soon after infusion. Excessive bleeding at surgery is not generally seen unless the platelet count falls below $50,000/\mu l$. Danazol can be used to raise the platelet count, but only in the postpartum period.

For the obstetrician, the greatest dilemma in management of a patient with ITP is selection of the route of delivery. Transplacental passage of circulating antiplatelet IgG may depress the fetal platelet count. If the fetal platelet count is above $50,000/\mu l$, there appears to be little danger of significant fetal bleeding. In the severely thrombocytopenic fetus, cesarean section might be less traumatic.

Can we accurately identify the fetus at risk? Unfortunately, the maternal platelet count is a poor indicator of the fetal platelet count.[56,68-71] Maternal platelet-associated IgG also fails to predict the fetal platelet count.[56,72] In a recent paper by Samuels and colleagues,[72] two factors were identified that select infants at risk for neonatal thrombocytopenia: a maternal history of ITP and an elevated titer of indirect, circulating antiplatelet IgG. They further demonstrated that thrombocytopenia limited to late pregnancy is a rather common phenomenon, and these patients are at minimal risk for developing severe neonatal thrombocytopenia.[72] In a patient who has a normal platelet count early in or prior to pregnancy and has no history of a bleeding diathesis, the risk of the fetus developing severe thrombocytopenia is negligible. In those mothers with a history of ITP, platelet antibody testing can identify which fetuses are at risk for being thrombocytopenic. In the study of Samuels et al., 18 of 70 (26%) fetuses whose mothers had a past history of ITP and who had circulating antiplatelet IgG were born with platelet counts less than $50,000/\mu l$. Therefore, mothers with a past history of ITP and circulating antiplatelet IgG warrant either cesarean section or a fetal platelet determination prior to vaginal delivery.[72] In Figure 34.1 a scheme for delivery of the thrombocytopenic gravida with a platelet count above $75,000/\mu l$ is shown.

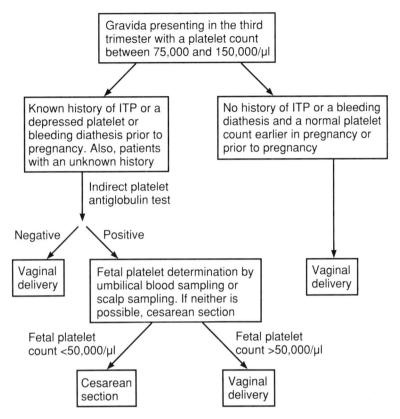

Fig. 34.1 Flowchart of method to determine delivery of the gravida with a platelet count between 75,000 and 150,000 μl.

The fetal platelet count can be assessed by obtaining an intrapartum fetal scalp sample after amniotomy.[67] If the platelet count is more than 50,000/μl the patient may be allowed to labor. Christiaens and Helmerhorst[73] reported 15 cases in which fetal scalp sampling was utilized. Falsely low platelet counts were found in almost one-half of the samples. In two of these 15 cases, this could have altered obstetric management.[73] Furthermore, scalp sampling is not possible in patients with an unfavorable cervix or who have not undergone amniotomy. More recently, the fetal platelet count has been assessed by percutaneous umbilical blood sampling.[74,75] Moise and coworkers[74] report their experience with 22 fetuses who underwent 26 umbilical cord punctures to assess the fetal platelet count. Blood could not be obtained from one fetus. Platelet counts less than 150,000/μl were found in five cases, but none were below 50,000/μl. Persistent

fetal bradycardia necessitating cesarean section occurred in two (9.7%) cases. Percutaneous umbilical blood sampling appears to be safe in most mothers with thrombocytopenia. However, limited experience exists regarding hemostasis in the umbilical cord of a fetus with a platelet count below 50,000/μl. This technique requires further study. Interestingly, one case of twins with discordant platelet counts has been reported in a mother with ITP.[76] Therefore, if fetal sampling is indicated, both twins should probably undergo evaluation.[76]

Thrombocytopenia will develop during the neonatal period in up to 70 percent of infants born to mothers with ITP.[77] This phenomenon is usually mild and peaks 4 to 6 days after delivery.[77] The platelet count gradually rises as passively acquired antiplatelet antibody levels drop. Breast-feeding has been associated with a drop in the neonatal platelet count,[78] which may result from passage of maternal antiplatelet IgG into colostrum. Whether breast-feeding is advisable should be determined on an individual basis.

Neonatal Alloimmune Thrombocytopenia

In neonatal alloimmune thrombocytopenia, a rare disorder, the mother lacks a specific platelet antigen and develops antibodies to this antigen. If the fetus inherits this antigen from its father, maternal antibody can cross the placenta, resulting in severe neonatal thrombocytopenia. The mother, however, will have a normal platelet count. Deaver and coinvestigators[79] reviewed 58 cases of neonatal alloimmune thrombocytopenia. The overall mortality rate was 9 percent, and the total incidence of suspected intracranial hemorrhage was 28 percent. The mortality rate was 24 percent in the firstborn infant and only 5 percent in subsequent offspring. The improved outcome in the latter group appeared to be related to more frequent utilization of cesarean section and to earlier use of corticosteroids in these children because obstetricians and pediatricians were expecting the disease.[79] Transfusion of maternal platelets into the neonate also improved outcome in these cases. The most common antibodies noted in these patients are anti-PLA 1 and BAK antibodies.[80] After birth or in utero the child can be transfused with the mother's platelets since she lacks the antigen that would lead to platelet destruction by circulating antibodies. Bussel and colleagues[81] have demonstrated that the antenatal use of intravenous immunoglobulin may help to prevent thrombocytopenia in infants at risk for neonatal alloimmune thrombocytopenia. These investigators administered 1 g/kg per week to at risk mothers and observed no toxicity. In two mothers who had previously given birth to an infant with intracranial hemorrhage, the platelet count was normalized in the subsequent pregnancy.

von Willebrand's Disease

von Willebrand's disease is an inherited disorder of coagulation and has a prevalence of 1/10,000. It is an autosomal dominant disorder, although a rare autosomal recessive form has been identified. von Willebrand's disease is characterized by a decrease or defect in the von Willebrand's portion of the Factor VIII complex. von Willebrand's factor, also known as the *ristocetin cofactor,* plays a significant role in platelet aggregation. There are several variants of von Willebrand's disease. These are delineated by the portion of von Willebrand's factor that is decreased or absent. The most common form, type I, is characterized by a quantitative decrease in the entire von Willebrand's factor. In type IIB, the only clinical symptom in pregnancy may be thrombocytopenia. This diagnosis, therefore, should be considered in the gravida presenting with isolated thrombocytopenia during pregnancy.[82,83]

The clinical severity of von Willebrand's disease is quite variable. Menorrhagia, easy bruising, gingival bleeding, and epistaxis are common. Some patients may be entirely asymptomatic until they have severe bleeding after surgery or trauma.

Classically the bleeding time is prolonged in patients with von Willebrand's disease as a result of diminished platelet aggregation. Occasionally, the activated partial thromboplastin time (APTT) will also be abnormal. In pregnancy, clotting factors including the Factor VIII complex increase, and the patient's bleeding time may improve as gestation progresses.[84,85] This is especially true for type IA von Willebrand's disease. In type IB, the patient may not correct her bleeding time.[86] Heavy bleeding may be encountered in patients with von Willebrand's disease undergoing elective or spontaneous first-trimester abortion because the levels of factor VIII have not yet risen. von Willebrand's disease does not appear to affect fetal growth or development. Postpartum hemorrhage may be a serious problem. The concentration of factor VIII C appears to determine the risk of hemorrhage. If the factor VIII C level is greater than 50 percent of normal and the patient has a normal bleeding time, she should not bleed excessively at vaginal delivery.[85-89] The clinical course during labor is quite variable. In a study by Chediak and coworkers,[90] bleeding complications were seen in six of eight (75%) pregnancies. Five of the newborns had von Willebrand's disease, one of whom was born with a scalp hematoma. Conti and associates,[91] conversely, reported no bleeding complications during the puerperium in five women with von Willebrand's disease.

Factor VIII levels appear to correlate with bleeding during the puerperium. Therefore, in those patients who do not normalize their bleeding time and whose concentration of factor VIII C is below 50 percent at term, transfusion with cryoprecipitate should be considered before vaginal delivery.[89] Cryoprecipitate is the treatment of choice, as it contains all forms of both factor VIII C and the ristocetin cofactor. Commercial preparations of factor VIII lack the high-molecular-weight forms of the ristocetin cofactor. Each unit of cryoprecipitate is contained in a volume of approximately 40 ml. Cryoprecipitate promotes a slow rise in factor VIII C. One should wait about 24 hours after administering cryoprecipitate before checking the response in factor VIII activity.

If a cesarean section is to be performed, factor VIII C levels should be 80 percent of normal, and the bleeding time should be in the normal range.[88] If these criteria are not met, cryoprecipitate should be administered preoperatively. The amount of cryoprecipitate administered must be individualized for each patient. One report has recommended administering 15 to 20 units of cryoprecipitate twice daily for the first 2 or 3 days followed by 8 to 10 units twice daily for the next 4 to 5 days.[92] After delivery, Factor VIII complex levels fall to the prepregnant levels within a period of 48 to 72 hours. The levels of ristocetin cofactor drop to the prepregnant levels even more quickly. The obstetrician must remember the dangers of delayed postpartum hemorrhage in the patient with von Willebrand's disease. Caldwell et al.[92] recommend that a patient should be treated for a full week to prevent late postpartum hemorrhage.

REFERENCES

1. Pitkin RM: Nutritional influences during pregnancy. Med Clin North Am 61:3, 1977
2. Ho CH, Yuan CC, Yeh SH: Serum ferritin, folate and cobalamin levels and their correlation with anemia in normal full-term pregnant women. Eur J Obstet Gynecol Reprod Biol 26:7, 1987
3. DeLeeuw NKM, Lowenstein L, Hsieh YS: Iron deficiency and hydremia of normal pregnancy. Medicine 45:291, 1966
4. Chopa J, Noe E, Matthew J et al: Anemia in pregnancy. Am J Public Health 57:857, 1967
5. Holly RG: Dynamics of iron metabolism in pregnancy. Am J Obstet Gynecol 93:370, 1965
6. Carr MC: Serum iron/TIBC in the diagnosis of iron deficiency anemia during pregnancy. Obstet Gynecol 38:602, 1971
7. Zuspan FP, Long WN, Russell JK et al: Anemia in pregnancy. J Reprod Med 6:13, 1971
8. Pritchard JA: Changes in the blood volume during pregnancy and delivery. Anesthesiology 26:393, 1965
9. Fenton V, Cavill I, Fisher J: Iron stores in pregnancy. Br J Haematol 37:145, 1977
10. Rothman D: Folic acid in pregnancy. Am J Obstet Gynecol 108:49, 1970
11. Giles C, Ball EW: Iron and folic acid deficiency in pregnancy. Br Med J 1:656, 1965
12. Hibbard BM, Hibbard ED: Neutrophil hypersegmentation and defective folate metabolism in pregnancy. J Obstet Gynaecol Br Commonw 78:776, 1971
13. Ek J: Plasma and red cell folate values in newborn infants and their mothers in relation to gestational age. J Pediatr 97:288, 1980
14. Lambert EK, Bloom RN, Kosby M: Pregnancy in patients with hemoglobinopathies and thalassemias. J Reprod Med 19:193, 1977
15. Motulsky AG: Frequency of sickling disorders in US blacks. N Engl J Med 288:31, 1973
16. Lynch JR, Brown JM: The polymerase chain reaction: current and future clinical applications. J Med Genet 27:2, 1990
17. Posey YF, Shah D, Ulm JE et al: Prenatal diagnosis of sickle cell anemia: hemoglobin electrophoresis versus DNA analysis. Am J Clin Pathol 92:347, 1989
18. Barret-Connor E: Cholelithiasis in sickle cell anemia. Am J Med 45:889, 1968
19. Cameron JL, Moddrey WC, Ziridema GD et al: Biliary tract disease in sickle cell anemia: surgical considerations. Ann Surg 174:702, 1971
20. Charache S, Scott J, Niebyl J, Bonds D: Management of sickle cell disease in pregnant patients. Obstet Gynecol 55:407, 1980
21. Fort AT, Morrison JC, Berreras L et al: Counseling the patient with sickle cell disease about reproduction: pregnancy outcome does not justify the maternal risk. Am J Obstet Gynecol 111:391, 1971
22. Freeman MG, Ruth GJ: SS disease and SC disease—obstetric considerations and treatment. Clin Obstet Gynecol 12:134, 1969
23. Curtis EM: Pregnancy in sickle cell anemia, sickle cell-hemoglobin C disease, and variants thereof. Am J Obstet Gynecol 77:1312, 1959
24. Horger EO III: Sickle cell and sickle cell-hemoglobin disease during pregnancy. Obstet Gynecol 39:873, 1972
25. Milner PF, Jones BR, Dobler J: Outcome of pregnancy

in sickle cell anemia and sickle cell–hemoglobin C disease. Am J Obstet Gynecol 138:239, 1980

26. Fessas P, Loukopoulos D: Beta thalassaemias. Clin Hematol 3:411, 1974

27. Powars DR, Sandhu M, Niland-Weiss J et al: Pregnancy in sickle cell disease. Obstet Gynecol 67:217, 1986

28. Fiakpui EF, Moron EM: Pregnancy in sickle hemoglobins. J Reprod Med 11:28, 1973

29. Anyaegbunam A, Billett HH, Langer O et al: Maternal hemoglobin F levels may have an adverse effect on neonatal birth weight in pregnancies with sickle cell disease. Am J Obstet Gynecol 161:654, 1989

30. Anyaegbunam A, Langer O, Brustman L et al: The application of uterine and umbilical artery velocimetry to the antenatal supervision of pregnancies complicated by maternal sickle hemoglobinopathies. Am J Obstet Gynecol 159:544, 1988

31. Perkins RP: Inherited disorders of hemoglobin synthesis and pregnancy. Am J Obstet Gynecol 111:130, 1971

32. Baum KF, Dunn DT, Maude GH, Serjeant GR: The painful crisis of homozygous sickle cell disease: a study of the risk factors. Arch Intern Med 147:1231, 1987

33. Abudu OO, Macaulay K, Oluboyede OA: Serial evaluation of iron stores in pregnant Nigerians with hemoglobin SS or SC. J Natl Med Assoc 82:41, 1990

34. Cunningham FG, Pritchard JA, Mason R: Pregnancy and sickle cell hemoglobinopathies: results with and without prophylactic transfusions. Obstet Gynecol 62:419, 1983

35. Morrison JC, Schneider JM, Whybrew WD et al: Prophylactic transfusions in pregnant patients with sickle hemoglobinopathies: benefit versus risk. Obstet Gynecol 56:274, 1980

36. Koshy M, Burd L, Wallace D et al: Prophylactic red-cell transfusions in pregnant patients with sickle cell disease: a randomized cooperative study. N Engl J Med 319:1447, 1988

37. Keidan AJ, Marwah SS, Bareford D et al: Laboratory tests for monitoring prophylactic exchange transfusion in pregnancy. Clin Lab Haematol 10:243, 1988

38. Tuck SM, James CE, Brewster EM et al: Prophylactic blood transfusion in maternal sickle cell syndromes. Br J Obstet Gynaecol 94:121, 1987

39. Fullerton WT, Hendrickse J, Williams W et al: Hemoglobin SC: clinical course. p. 215. In Jonxis JHP (ed): Abnormal hemoglobins in Africa: A Symposium. Blackwell Scientific Publications, Oxford, 1965.

40. Solanki DL, Kletter GG, Castro O: Acute splenic sequestration crises in adults with sickle cell disease. Am J Med 80:985, 1986

41. Wainscoat JS, Work S, Sampietro M et al: Feasibility of prenatal diagnosis of beta thalassaemia by DNA polymorphisms in an Italian population. Br J Haematol 62:495, 1986

42. Cao A, Falchi AM, Tuveri T et al: Prenatal diagnosis of thalassemia major by fetal blood analysis: experience with 1,000 cases. Prenat Diagn 6:159, 1986

43. Ghosh A, Tan MH, Liang ST et al: Ultrasound evaluation of pregnancies at risk for homozygous alpha-thalassaemia-1. Prenat Diagn 7:307, 1987

44. Woo JS, Liang ST, Lo RL, Chan FY: Doppler blood flow velocity waveforms in alpha-thalassemia hydrops fetalis. J Ultrasound Med 6:679, 1987

45. Hsieh FJ, Chang FM, Huang HC et al: Umbilical vein blood flow measurement in nonimmune hydrops fetalis. Obstet Gynecol 71:188, 1988

46. Mordel N, Birkenfeld A, Goldfarb AN, Rachmilewitz EA: Successful full-term pregnancy in homozygous beta-thalassemia major: case report and review of the literature. Obstet Gynecol 73:837, 1989

47. Necheles T: Obstetric complications associated with haemoglobinopathies. Clin Hematol 2:497, 1973

48. White JM, Richards R, Jelenski G et al: Iron state in alpha and beta thalassaemia trait. J Clin Pathol 39:256, 1986

49. Van der Weyden MB, Fong H, Hallam LJ, Harrison C: Red cell ferritin and iron overload in heterozygous beta-thalassemia. Am J Hematol 30:201, 1989

50. Leung CF, Lao TT, Chang AM: Effect of folate supplement on pregnant women with beta-thalassaemia minor. Eur J Obstet Gynecol Reprod Biol 33:209, 1989

51. Schmidt RM: Laboratory diagnosis of hemoglobinopathies. JAMA 224:1276, 1973

52. Cines DB, Schreiber AD: Immune thrombocytopenia. N Engl J Med 300:106, 1979

53. McMillan R: Chronic idiopathic thrombocytopenic purpura. N Engl J Med 304:1135, 1981

54. Ballem PJ, Buskard N, Wittmann BK et al: ITP in pregnancy: use of the bleeding time as an indicator for treatment. Blut 59:132, 1989

55. DiFino SM, Lachant NA, Kirshner JJ, Gottlieb AJ: Adult idiopathic thrombocytopenic purpura. Am J Med 69:430, 1980

56. Cines D, Dusek B, Tomaski A et al: Immune thrombocytopenic purpura and pregnancy. N Engl J Med 306:826, 1982

57. Karpatkin S: Autoimmune thrombocytopenic purpura. Blood 56:329, 1980

58. Fehr J, Hoffman V, Kappeler V: Transient reversal of thrombocytopenia in idiopathic thrombocytopenia

purpura by high dose intravenous gammaglobulin. N Engl J Med 306:1254, 1982

59. Newland AC, Treleaven JG, Minchinton RM et al: High dose intravenous IgG in adults with autoimmune thrombocytopenia. Lancet 1:84, 1983

60. Carroll RR, Noyes WD, Kilchers CS: High dose intravenous immunoglobulin therapy in patients with immune thrombocytopenia purpura. JAMA 249:1748, 1983

61. Mizunuma H, Takahashi Y, Taguchi H et al: A new approach to idiopathic thrombocytopenia purpura during pregnancy by high dose immunoglobulin G infusion. Am J Obstet Gynecol 148:216, 1984

62. Rose VL, Gordon LI: Idiopathic thrombocytopenic purpura in pregnancy: successful management with immunoglobulin infusion. JAMA 254:2626, 1985

63. Gounder MP, Baker D, Saletan S et al: Intravenous gammaglobulin therapy in the management of a patient with idiopathic thrombocytopenic purpura and a warm autoimmune erythrocyte panagglutinin during pregnancy. Obstet Gynecol 67:741, 1986

64. Fabris P, Quaini R, Coser P et al: Successful treatment of a steroid-resistant form of idiopathic thrombocytopenic purpura in pregnancy with high doses of intravenous immunoglobulins. Acta Haematol 77:107, 1987

65. Davidson BN, Rayburn WF, Bishop RC et al: Immunoglobulin therapy for autoimmune thrombocytopenia purpura during pregnancy: a report of two cases. J Reprod Med 32:107, 1987

66. Weir AB III, Poon M, McGowan EI: Plasma exchange in idiopathic thrombocytopenia purpura. Arch Intern Med 140:1101, 1980

67. Scott JR, Cruikshank DP, Kochenour NK et al: Fetal platelet counts in the obstetric management of immunologic thrombocytopenic purpura. Am J Obstet Gynecol 136:495, 1990

68. Territo M, Finklestein J, Oh W et al: Management of autoimmune thrombocytopenia in pregnancy and in the neonate. Obstet Gynecol 41:579, 1973

69. O'Reilly RA, Taber B-Z: Immunologic thrombocytopenic purpura and pregnancy. Obstet Gynecol 51:590, 1978

70. Murray JM, Harris RE: The management of the pregnant patient with idiopathic thrombocytopenia purpura. Am J Obstet Gynecol 126:449, 1976

71. Laros RK Jr, Sweet RL: Management of idiopathic thrombocytopenic purpura during pregnancy. Am J Obstet Gynecol 122:182, 1975

72. Samuels P, Bussel JB, Braitman LE et al: Estimation of the risk of thrombocytopenia in the offspring of pregnant women with presumed immune thrombocytopenic purpura. N Engl J Med 323:229, 1990

73. Christiaens GC, Helmerhorst FM: Validity of intrapartum diagnosis of fetal thrombocytopenia. Am J Obstet Gynecol 157:864, 1987

74. Moise KJ Jr, Carpenter RJ Jr, Cotton DB et al: Percutaneous umbilical cord blood sampling in the evaluation of fetal platelet counts in pregnant patients with autoimmune thrombocytopenic purpura. Obstet Gynecol 72:346, 1988

75. Scioscia AI, Grannum PA, Copel JA, Hobbins JC: The use of percutaneous umbilical blood sampling in immune thrombocytopenic purpura. Am J Obstet Gynecol 159:1066, 1988

76. Moise KJ Jr, Cotton DB: Discordant fetal platelet counts in a twin gestation complicated by idiopathic thrombocytopenic purpura. Am J Obstet Gynecol 156:1141, 1987

77. Pearson HA, McIntosh S: Neonatal thrombocytopenia. Clin Hematol 7:111, 1978

78. Klemen E, Szalay F, Petefy M: Autoimmune thrombocytopenic purpura in pregnancy and the newborn. Br J Obstet Gynaecol 85:239, 1978

79. Deaver JE, Leppert PC, Zaroulis CG: Neonatal alloimmune thrombocytopenic purpura. Am J Perinatol 3:127, 1986

80. Okada N, Oda M, Sano T et al: Intracranial hemorrhage in utero due to fetomaternal Bak(a) incompatibility. Nippon Ketsueki Gakkai Zasshi 51:1086, 1988

81. Bussel JB, McFarland JG, Berkowitz R: Antenatal treatment of fetal alloimmune cytopenias. Blut 59:136, 1989

82. Giles AR, Hoogendoorn H, Benford K: Type IIB von Willebrand's disease presenting as thrombocytopenia during pregnancy. Br J Haematol 67:349, 1987

83. Rick ME, Williams SB, Sacher RA, McKeown LP: Thrombocytopenia associated with pregnancy in a patient with type IIB von Willebrand's disease. Blood 69:786, 1987

84. Kasper CK, Hoags MS, Aggeler PM, Stone S: Blood clotting factors in pregnancy: Factor VIII concentrations in normal and AHF-deficient women. Obstet Gynecol 24:242, 1984

85. Telfer MC, Chediak J: Factor VIII–related disorders and their relationship to pregnancy. J Reprod Med 19:211, 1972

86. Takahashi H, Hayashi N, Shibata A: Type IB von Willebrand's disease and pregnancy: comparison of analytical methods of von Willebrand factor for classification

of von Willebrand's disease subtypes. Thromb Res 50:409, 1988

87. Noller KL, Bowie EJW, Kempers RD, Owen CA: von Willebrand's disease in pregnancy. Obstet Gynecol 41:865, 1973

88. Evans P: Obstetric and gynecologic patients with von Willebrand's disease. Obstet Gynecol 38:37, 1971

89. Lipton RA, Ayromlooi J, Coller BS: Severe von Willebrand's disease during labor and delivery. JAMA 248:1355, 1982

90. Chediak JR, Alban GM, Maxey B: von Willebrand's disease and pregnancy: management during delivery and outcome of offspring. Am J Obstet Gynecol 155:618, 1986

91. Conti M, Mari D, Conti E et al: Pregnancy in women with different types of von Willebrand disease. Obstet Gynecol 68:282, 1986

92. Caldwell DC, Williamson RA, Goldsmith JC: Hereditary coagulopathies in pregnancy. Clin Obstet Gynecol 28:55, 1985

93. Morrison JC, Propst MG, Blake P: Sickle hemoglobin and the gravid patient: a management controversy. Clin Perinatol 7:280, 1981

Chapter 35

Collagen Vascular Diseases

Philip Samuels

With the exception of rheumatoid arthritis, autoimmune diseases are associated with an increased risk of poor pregnancy outcome. Many of these diseases have a predisposition for women in their childbearing years. In fact, autoimmune diseases are occasionally first diagnosed during gestation. Often patients with recurrent pregnancy complications show evidence of autoimmunity but without significant criteria to allow specific diagnosis. These diseases are characterized by the production of autoantibodies—antibodies synthesized by an individual against a component of her own body. Increasingly sensitive and specific laboratory tests are being developed to aid in the diagnosis of these disorders (Tables 35.1 and 35.2).

SYSTEMIC LUPUS ERYTHEMATOSUS (SLE)

SLE is a chronic disease with a great diversity of clinical and laboratory manifestations. Its onset is frequently insidious, and its diagnosis is often elusive and delayed. The course of SLE is characterized by exacerbations and remissions. The prevalence of SLE is approximately 1 per 1,000 in the general population. The prevalence of the disease in women 15 to 64 years of age is estimated to be 1 per 700,[1] but in black women of the same age group the prevalence is 1 per 245.[2] The diagnosis of SLE is based on a patient meeting at least four of the diagnostic criteria accepted by the American Rheumatism Association.

Revised Criteria for the Classification of Systemic Lupus Erythematosus (1982)[a]

Malar rash

Discoid rash

Photosensitivity

Oral ulcers

Arthritis — nonerosive, involving two or more peripheral joints

Serositis
  Pleuritis
  OR
  Pericarditis

Renal disorder
  Persistent proteinuria > 0.5 g/day
  OR
  Cellular casts

Neurologic disorder
  Seizures
  OR
  Psychosis

Hematologic disorder
  Hemolytic anemia with reticulocytosis
  OR

Continued

Table 35.1 Autoantibodies of Diagnostic Significance

Antibody Type	Disease
Antinuclear antibodies (ANA)	Most collagen vascular diseases
Anti-DNA antibodies	SLE, mixed connective tissue disease
Anti-Sm	SLE
Anti-SSA (Ro)	SLE (associated with congenital heart block), Sjögren syndrome
Anti-SSB (La)	SLE, Sjögren syndrome
Anti-RNP	SLE, PSS, mixed connective tissue disease
Anti-Scl-70	PSS

Abbreviations: SLE, systemic lupus erythematosus; PSS, progressive systemic sclerosis.

Leukopenia, <4,000/mm^3

OR

Lymphopenia, <1,500/mm^3

OR

Thrombocytopenia, <100,000/mm^3

Immunologic disorder
  Positive lupus erythematosus cell preparation
  Antibody to native DNA
  Anti-SM antibody
  False-positive serologic test for syphilis

Antinuclear antibodies in abnormal titers

---

[a] Four criteria necessary for diagnosis.
(Adapted from Tan et al.,[146] with permission.)

Clinical Manifestations

Approximately 80 percent of patients with SLE demonstrate skin lesions. These may include the classic malar (butterfly) rash, alopecia, or discoid lesions.

Table 35.2 Antinuclear Antibody Patterns in Rheumatologic Disease

Pattern	Disease
Homogenous	SLE, RA, Sjögren syndrome
Nucleolar	SLE, PSS, Sjögren syndrome
Speckled	Mixed connective tissue disease, Sjögren syndrome
Rim	SLE

Abbreviations: RA, rheumatoid arthritis; SLE, systemic lupus erythematosus; PSS, progressive systemic sclerosis.

Photosensitivity is common. Arthralgias with some arthritis will be evident in 90 percent of patients. Nephritis and neurologic or psychiatric features are found in approximately 50 percent of cases.

Patients with glomerulonephritis will excrete varying quantities of protein. The amount of proteinuria may range widely within the same individual, depending on disease activity. The renal lesions of SLE include focal proliferative glomerulonephritis, membranous glomerulonephritis, mesangial nephritis, and diffuse proliferative glomerulonephritis. Those patients with focal and diffuse proliferative glomerulonephritis tend to have a worse long-term prognosis. Women with SLE may also present with seizures, peripheral neuropathy, or a psychotic episode. It is important to note that a recurrent fever of unknown etiology may also be the earliest manifestation of SLE.

Laboratory Diagnosis

More than 90 percent of patients with SLE will exhibit significant titers of antinuclear antibodies (ANA). In more than 70 percent of patients, an autoantibody directed against native DNA will be detected.[3] Extractable nuclear antibodies can be subdivided into antibodies against ribonuclear protein (anti-RNP, anti-SM), anti-SSA (Ro), and anti-SSB (La). Anti-RNP antibodies are seen in 26 percent of patients with SLE; anti-SM antibodies are found in 28 percent of patients with SLE and can be correlated with renal involvement. Anti-SSA and anti-SSB antibodies, which are found in 25 and 12 percent of patients with SLE, respectively, have been associated with fetal and neonatal heartblock. Anti-SSA antibodies are generally associated with manifestations of neonatal lupus.

The Effects of Pregnancy on SLE

Pregnancy does not appear to affect or alter the long-term prognosis of patients with SLE.[4] Several studies, however, have documented increased flares of SLE during pregnancy and particularly during the puerperium.[4,5] It is difficult to compare and corroborate these studies, because there is no uniform definition of a lupus flare. Garsenstein et al.[4] predicted the probability for a flare was three times greater during the first half of pregnancy, 1.5 times greater in the second half, and six times greater in the puerperium.[4] Meehan and Dorsey[6] examined the effects of pregnancy on the course of SLE in patients receiving glucocorticoids or azathioprine at conception. They showed no statistically significant difference in the number of flares in pregnant women and nonpregnant controls when matched by disease duration and prior organ involvement. Lockshin and coworkers[7,8] studied a variety of clinical markers of disease activity in 33 pregnancies in 28 women with SLE. They also demonstrated an absence of exacerbation during or after pregnancy. In a prospective study of 80 women, Lockshin[9] showed that exacerbation occurred in less than 13 percent of pregnant patients. He concluded, therefore, that there is no need for prophylactic glucocorticoids in the gravid patient with SLE.

Conversely, Mintz and colleagues[10] showed an increase in SLE activity during pregnancy. This group studied 102 pregnancies in 75 women during a 10-year period. In this report, 59.7 percent of pregnancies that began with quiescent SLE experienced an exacerbation during pregnancy or the postpartum period. More than one-half of these flares occurred in the first trimester and 20 percent during the puerperium. Most of the patients, however, readily responded to increased doses of glucocorticoids.

Although it remains debatable whether SLE is exacerbated by pregnancy, there is no dispute that there is a risk of major maternal morbidity and potentially of mortality in the gravida with SLE. Most maternal deaths occur during the puerperium as a result of pulmonary hemorrhage or lupus pneumonitis.[11,12] Averbuch and coworkers[13] reported a case of cardiac tamponade occurring in the postpartum period

caused by SLE. Marabani and coworkers[14] described a case of transverse myelitis during a pregnancy complicated by SLE. This complication responded quickly to steroids. Gimovsky and associates[15] reviewed 108 pregnancies in 39 women affected with SLE and found that morbidity was rare in the immediate postpartum period. However, there was increased morbidity and mortality in the first few years after delivery.[15]

Most perinatologists advise their patients not to conceive during a time of increased lupus activity, as this is associated with flares during pregnancy. Although this seems logical, the volume of the literature to support this assertion is small.[16] The work by Mintz and colleagues[10] does, however, seem to favor this postulate. In general, a patient's disease should be quiescent for 5 to 7 months before conception. This recommendation is based on work by Hayslett and Lynn,[17] who observed that pregnancy outcome was good in 92 percent of women whose lupus had been in remission for at least 6 months prior to conception.

Women with lupus nephritis must be aware that there is a small but significant risk of permanent deterioration of renal function during pregnancy. Fine and coworkers[18] noted that in 9.6 percent of their patients renal function remained depressed for 3 to 12 months after delivery. Others have suggested that permanent renal deterioration during pregnancy is more frequent, perhaps as high as 50 percent.[19,20] In these studies, however, sample sizes were small. Conversely, Hayslett and Lynn[17] demonstrated no permanent change in renal function in pregnant patients with lupus nephritis. A summary of six studies reviewing 242 pregnancies in 156 patients revealed a 7.1 percent incidence of permanent renal dysfunction and a 30.2 percent incidence of transient renal dysfunction during gestation.[20] In this review, transient deterioration usually occurred in the third trimester. Poor pregnancy outcome is associated with active lupus nephropathy,[21] a serum creatinine of at least 1.5 mg/dl, a BUN more than 50 mg/dl, and a creatinine clearance less than 50 ml/min.[17,21,22]

A lupus flare and preeclampsia present a difficult differential diagnosis, because they have similar signs and symptoms. Both disorders often present with hypertension, edema, and proteinuria. To confound the issue, patients with lupus nephropathy are at an increased risk for developing superimposed pre-eclampsia during gestation. It is difficult, but very important, to make the distinction between these two phenomena. The treatment for preeclampsia is delivery, while the treatment for lupus nephritis is increased glucocorticoids and possibly azathioprine therapy. Buyon and coworkers[23] found that serum complement values (C_3 and C_4) are valuable in differentiating between heightened lupus activity and preeclampsia. In normal pregnancy, complement levels tend to rise. They are, therefore, high or normal in the SLE patient with pure preeclampsia. Conversely, these levels fall with an exacerbation of lupus. If a patient develops hypertension and proteinuria in the second trimester, it is imperative to distinguish between preeclampsia and a lupus flare. If the diagnosis of preeclampsia is made, mandatory obstetric intervention could result in neonatal death or major morbidity, depending on the gestational age. If serologic and chemical testing cannot make the distinction between the two conditions, a renal biopsy may be indicated.

The Effects of SLE on Pregnancy

Although fertility is not impaired, SLE can have an adverse effect on pregnancy outcome in each trimester.[24] There is an increase in the spontaneous abortion rate, with the estimated incidence between 16 and 40 percent.[10,15,24–27] The risk of miscarriage is not necessarily related to disease activity. Mintz and coworkers[10] reported a 16 percent spontaneous abortion rate regardless of disease activity.

Since the late 1980s, the lupus inhibitor and anticardiolipin antibodies have been at the forefront of research relating to recurrent miscarriage and SLE. The diagnosis of the lupus inhibitor is often confusing. There is no single assay that is used to identify this phenomenon, and different assays have different sensitivities and specificities. Some clinicians and researchers rely solely on a prolongation of the activated partial thromboplastin time (APTT) using platelet-poor plasma. Other commonly used tests include the tissue thromboplastin inhibition test (TTI), kaolin clotting time (KCT), Russell viper venom time, and platelet neutralization procedure. This variety of tests makes it difficult for the critical reader to compare different studies concerning the role of the lupus inhibitor in pregnancy outcome. The similarities and differences between the lupus inhibitor and anticardiolipin antibodies are also quite confusing. While many clinicians use them interchangeably, Rosove et al.[28] showed that the correlation between the two is not perfect, and both assays should be performed in order to maximize sensitivity.

Before concluding that the lupus inhibitor and anticardiolipin antibodies are a cause of poor pregnancy outcome, one must look at the prevalence of these phenomena in a normal pregnant population. To date, only Lockwood and coworkers,[29] in a study of 737 low risk pregnancies, have addressed this issue. Two of the 737 patients (0.27%) had a lupus inhibitor documented by a prolonged APTT that did not correct after mixing with normal plasma. Both patients experienced a pregnancy loss. Elevated titers of IgM or IgG anticardiolipin antibodies were found in 16 patients (2.2%). Twelve of these 16 patients experienced an adverse pregnancy outcome. This study suggests that, while these phenomena are not widespread, the presence of the lupus inhibitor and anticardiolipin antibodies can be related to poor pregnancy outcome and placental infarction.[30–32] As shown by Lubbe et al.[33,34] in New Zealand, Branch et al.[35] in the United States, and Unander et al.[36] in Sweden, the lupus inhibitor and anticardiolipin antibodies are associated with recurrent spontaneous abortions even when there is no other evidence of collagen vascular disease. Also, in the absence of SLE, anticardiolipin antibodies can be associated with an increased risk for early preeclampsia, intrauterine growth retardation (IUGR), and fetal death.[35,37] Lockshin, Druzin, and coworkers[38,39] have observed that patients with anticardiolipin antibodies who have SLE are at significant risk to develop fetal distress in the second trimester with subsequent fetal death.

Treatment of patients with the lupus inhibitor and anticardiolipin antibodies remains controversial and has not been evaluated in a controlled fashion. Several studies report increased fetal survival and decreased morbidity and mortality in patients receiving prednisone in doses of 20 to 60 mg daily and low dose aspirin.[35,40] It appears that this regimen will normalize a prolonged APTT or TTI but will have little effect on the level of anticardiolipin antibodies.[36] These investigations, however, have not been controlled for the gestational age at which therapy was initiated. There have been no studies comparing prednisone alone to prednisone and aspirin.

Unander and her colleagues[36] showed that 8 of 42 patients with elevated anticardiolipin antibodies conceived and carried a pregnancy to term without specific therapy. Two of these 8 patients had high levels of anticardiolipin antibodies, constituting 20 percent of the patients in her study who had this abnormality. Mintz and coinvestigators,[41] in a prospective study of 44 women with idiopathic habitual abortion, found that two of three patients who had anticardiolipin antibodies had subsequent successful pregnancies without therapy. Furthermore, Lockshin and coworkers[42] believe that prednisone may actually increase the incidence of fetal death in women with anticardiolipin antibodies. In their study of 21 women with a prior history of fetal death and a high titer of IgG anticardiolipin antibody, only 11 were treated with prednisone. In the 11 treated women, 82 percent of the pregnancies ended in fetal death. In the untreated group, only 50 percent of pregnancies resulted in fetal death, a statistically significant difference. In patients treated with aspirin, there was no statistical difference in the outcomes of the groups. Based on these findings, Lockshin et al.[42] concluded that prednisone may actually worsen fetal outcome of the current pregnancy. Karp et al.[43] studied the outcomes of 27 pregnancies in 19 patients treated with prednisone and antiaggregants for the lupus inhibitor. There were only 13 successful outcomes, leading them to conclude that prednisone and antiaggregants may prevent second- and third-trimester losses but have only limited success in treating primary habitual abortion.[43] Nonetheless, there are other data that do support the use of prednisone and low dose aspirin in treating patients with the lupus inhibitor and the anticardiolipin antibody syndrome.[36,40,44-46]

Because of the conflicting data in the literature, we have individualized the treatment for each patient. If the patient's history and laboratory data suggest that therapy might be indicated, we thoroughly counsel the patient about the maternal risks of steroid use during pregnancy. We make certain that patients understand that with prednisone therapy there is a high risk of developing gestational diabetes requiring insulin. We stress that this therapy is not a panacea and

that we are not totally certain of its efficacy. If the patient has a prolonged APTT, we administer 20 mg of prednisone as soon as the pregnancy has been diagnosed and increase the dose until the APTT normalizes. We also administer low dose aspirin therapy to these patients. If the patient has elevated anticardiolipin antibodies alone, we generally prescribe 15 to 20 mg of prednisone and low dose aspirin daily and continue that dosage throughout the gestation, as anticardiolipin antibody levels fluctuate widely during pregnancy regardless of therapy.[36] There is increasing evidence that aspirin therapy alone might be beneficial. Gatenby et al.[47] showed a dramatic improvement in patients receiving aspirin therapy for elevated anticardiolipin antibodies. In patients with elevated antibodies and SLE, the pregnancy wastage rate dropped from 88 to 55 percent. In those with elevated antibodies alone, the rate of loss fell from 79 to 25 percent.[47] In their series, however, some of the patients were also receiving prednisone. Balasch and coworkers[48] studied 65 consecutive women with two or more spontaneous miscarriages. Seven (10.7%) were found to have anticardiolipin antibodies. Four of the seven women (57.1%) carried to term after being treated with low dose aspirin alone. While the number of patients treated with aspirin alone is small, it does appear that this therapy might be beneficial in patients who have anticardiolipin antibodies.

Because infarctions are often found in the placentas of patients with anticardiolipin antibodies, researchers have begun using heparin therapy in this group. Rosove et al.[49] initiated heparin therapy at a mean gestational age of 10.3 weeks in 14 women with adverse pregnancy outcomes. The daily dosage ranged from 10,000 to 36,000 units. Live births occurred in 14 of 15 pregnancies (93.3%) with a mean gestational age of 36.1 weeks and a mean birthweight percentile of 57.[49] More studies must be performed before we can broadly recommend the use of heparin for the treatment of this phenomenon.

Anticardiolipin antibodies and the lupus inhibitor are associated with in vitro anticoagulation, but in vivo they are associated with thrombosis. These patients, therefore, are probably at some risk for thrombosis during gestation.[36,50-52] Mizoguchi et al.[51] described a 34-year-old woman with lupus inhibitor who had had six recurrent pregnancy losses without an intervening livebirth. During her subsequent pregnancy, she developed multiple brain infarctions and hemiparesis. Rallings and coworkers[52] reported a 28-year-old primigravida who developed an acute anteroseptal myocardial infarction and died during gestation. She had had a past history of thromboembolism. The only serologic abnormality noted was an elevated level of IgG anticardiolipin antibody.

Neonatal Complete Congenital Heartblock

Complete congenital heartblock, an infrequent complication of SLE, can often be diagnosed prenatally. In the midtrimester, a fetal heart rate of about 60 bpm with no baseline variability is indicative of congenital heartblock. The patient should immediately undergo fetal echocardiography to rule out associated congenital cardiac malformations. Doppler studies can also locate the atrial ventricular disassociation. Fetal echocardiography can usually be carried out at 20 to 22 weeks gestation and in the asthenic patient as early as 16 weeks. Affected fetuses usually show no evidence of congestive heart failure or hydrops. Nonetheless, they should be followed with serial ultrasonography every 1 to 2 weeks to ascertain if any evidence of anasarca has developed. Complete congenital heartblock in the patient with SLE appears to be the result of immune complex deposition in fetal cardiac tissue as demonstrated by Litsey and coworkers.[53] This process leads to endocardiofibroelastosis and fibrosis of the conduction system.[54,55] Scott and colleagues[56] identified the anti-SSA (Ro) antibody in 83 percent of mothers delivering infants with complete congenital heartblock. Anti-SSB (La) antibodies were found in a smaller but significant number of these mothers. Scheib and Waxman[57] have shown that these antibodies do bind to fetal cardiac tissue. They have described two successive pregnancies in a mother with anti-SSA antibody who gave birth to two antibody-positive children with complete congenital heartblock. In most studies, mothers have had no symptoms of collagen vascular disease at the time of delivery. In the study of Vetter and Rashkad,[58] a large proportion of these women later developed SLE. According to Esscher and Scott,[59] the mother of a child born with complete congenital heartblock has a 30 to 60 percent chance of developing a collagen vascular disease. Therefore, patients who deliver an infant with complete congenital heartblock but who do not have SLE should have a careful clinical examination and undergo appropriate serologic tests on a routine basis. In future pregnancies, they should be treated as high-risk patients and undergo fetal echocardiography at the appropriate gestational age.

In the absence of structural cardiac anomalies, the neonatal mortality rate for infants born with complete congenital heartblock is approximately 5 percent. In Vetter and Scott's study,[58] the mortality rate was 20 to 30 percent if a structural abnormality was also found. With recent advances in pediatric cardiac surgery, the mortality rate is probably considerably lower now. Buyon and coworkers[60] aggressively treated a fetus with presumptive fetal myocarditis and heartblock in a mother with SLE. They administered high doses of dexamethasone and performed plasmapheresis three times weekly. The patient responded well to therapy, showing a significant decrease in the titer of anti-SSB antibody. The infant was delivered at 31 weeks, and the heartblock persisted.

In addition to complete congenital heartblock, Watson and colleagues[61] have associated the anti-SSA antibody with an increased rate of spontaneous miscarriage. It is unclear if this association is found only in patients with SLE or in patients with Sjögren syndrome as well. More studies need to be undertaken.

Infants born to mothers with SLE may exhibit erythematous skin lesions of the face, scalp, and upper thorax.[62,63] These lesions usually disappear by 12 months of age. It appears that there is a higher incidence of anti-SSA antibodies in mothers giving birth to children with these skin lesions.[64]

Surveillance

Because of the increased risk of miscarriage, stillbirth, preterm delivery, and IUGR, the obstetrician caring for the patient with SLE should maintain close maternal and fetal surveillance. Any patient with a history of SLE should undergo preconceptual counseling and should have tests performed for the presence of the lupus inhibitor, anticardiolipin antibodies, anti-SSA (Ro) antibodies, and anti-SSB (La) antibodies. As previously delineated, these findings are associated with a poorer pregnancy outcome. If indicated, therapy should be initiated after fully informing the patient of risks and benefits to both her and the fetus. The role of treatment for the lupus inhibitor and anticardiolipin antibody syndrome remains controversial. As more studies are published, the role and best form of treatment should become clearer. If anti-SSA or anti-SSB antibodies are present, fetal echocardiography should be performed in the second trimester to rule out complete congenital heartblock. Because of the risks of IUGR and preterm birth, accurate gestational dating is imperative in the patient with SLE. Menstrual dating should be confirmed by ultrasonography at the first prenatal visit. At 18 to 20 weeks of gestation an additional ultrasound examination should be performed to confirm gestational age, ascertain appropriate fetal growth, and make certain that fetal anatomy is normal. Most often, IUGR in patients with SLE is asymmetric. Fine et al.,[18] however, showed that symmetric IUGR can also occur. Because of the risk of IUGR and stillbirth, serial ultrasound examinations should be performed monthly after 20 weeks gestation, with special attention to growth of the fetal abdomen, head, and femur.[64] The obstetrician should also be attentive to the volume of amniotic fluid, as decreased amniotic fluid can be the harbinger of fetal compromise and stillbirth.

At 28 weeks gestation, weekly antepartum fetal heart rate testing should be initiated using the nonstress test. At 34 weeks, the frequency of testing should be increased to twice weekly. There are, however, no controlled studies showing that biweekly testing after 34 weeks improves perinatal outcome in the patient with SLE. Carroll[65] has recently shown that Doppler velocimetry might be useful in following the gravida with the lupus inhibitor. In that study, abnormal umbilical artery systolic/diastolic ratios were found in five of six women with the lupus inhibitor who delivered growth-retarded fetuses. Only two of these patients demonstrated abnormally elevated uterine artery systolic/diastolic ratios. More studies are needed before Doppler flow evaluations can be recommended as a uniform part of antenatal testing in the patient with SLE.

Despite the sophisticated array of laboratory studies that are available to follow patients with SLE, the patient's clinical status remains of prime importance. There is no substitute for careful monitoring of maternal blood pressure and weight gain. These can be the earliest signs of superimposed preeclampsia, which is common in patients with SLE. They can also

be the harbinger of a lupus flare.[66] Twenty-four-hour urine collections for creatinine clearance and total protein excretion should be carried out monthly. Serum creatinine, BUN, and uric acid levels should be determined whenever these urine collections are performed. A rise in serum uric acid can be a sign of impending preeclampsia. During a normal pregnancy, complement levels rise. A fall in the third or fourth components of complement (C_3 or C_4) or a fall in total hemolytic complement (CH_{50}) has been associated with impending exacerbations of SLE.[67-69] Devoe and Aloy[70] found that a decrease in serum complement levels was also associated with a poor perinatal outcome. Because complement levels tend to rise during pregnancy, a single complement determination is of no value. A downward trend in complement levels, however, is significant, even though the level may fall within normal limits. Although some investigators have questioned the predictive value of complement levels,[17,71] we follow complement and anti-DNA antibody titers every 6 weeks in patients with SLE and more frequently if the clinical situation warrants.

The timing of delivery is important and should be individualized. All too often, preterm delivery is performed merely to allay physician and patient anxiety. The obstetrician should strive for a vaginal delivery. If delivery is indicated near term and the patient's cervix is not favorable, prostaglandin E_2 gel can be carefully used to attempt cervical ripening. If the patient is taking glucocorticoids or if there is any evidence of lupus exacerbation, peripartum steroids should be administered parenterally in stress doses. In the patient who undergoes cesarean section, intravenous steroids should be continued for 48 hours postoperatively, because adequate gastrointestinal absorption cannot be guaranteed until normal bowel function returns. Steroids should be tapered slowly and with great care in the postpartum period to prevent an exacerbation of SLE.[19,67]

Drug Therapy for SLE During Pregnancy

Patients with SLE are often hesitant to take their prescribed medications during pregnancy for fear of fetal effects. Many obstetricians are also reluctant to prescribe these medications for similar reasons. It is important for the obstetrician to be aware of the benefits and risks of medications used to treat SLE. Pregnancy is accompanied by a 40 to 50 percent increase in intravascular volume and a resultant increase in interstitial fluid. Any steroid that has mineralocorticoid activity exacerbates interstitial fluid retention. This additive effect can cause maternal discomfort. The obstetrician should therefore choose a steroid with minimal mineralocorticoid activity and maximum glucocorticoid activity. Steroids in combination with pregnancy may worsen acne and striae. Corticosteroid administration can also lead to gastrointestinal discomfort and ulceration. We therefore suggest that patients on chronic corticosteroid therapy use antacids after meals and at bedtime.

Chronic corticosteroid administration has been associated with bone demineralization and with an increased risk of hip fractures. For the gravida who is taking increased corticosteroids only during pregnancy, the actual risk is unknown. Although there is a risk of cataract formation with long-term corticosteroid administration, this complication has not been reported when steroid use was limited to pregnancy.

The induction of gestational diabetes from glucocorticoid administration is a distinct possibility. Approximately 3 percent of all pregnancies are complicated by gestational diabetes.[72] We perform 1-hour, 50-g oral glucose screening tests at 20, 28, and 32 weeks gestation in patients on long-term corticosteroids. We also test for diabetes later in gestation if there is any evidence of fetal macrosomia.

Pregnant women are often more concerned about the effects of the medication on their fetus than they are about the effects on themselves. The chronic ingestion of corticosteroids has not been associated with teratogenesis in humans.[73] An increase in the background incidence of cleft palate has been seen in rats and rabbits exposed to chronic corticosteroids but never in humans.[73-75] Neonatal adrenal suppression is a theoretical consideration in patients taking corticosteroids, but it has only rarely been reported. Nonetheless, the pediatrician should be informed when a mother has been taking corticosteroids antenatally. Rolbin et al.[76] have shown an increase in the incidence of IUGR in infants born to mothers who were chronically taking steroids. These patients received 10 mg of prednisone daily because of infertility and remained on this dose throughout gestation.

Only a fraction of the steroids ingested by a preg-

nant woman reach the fetus. Prednisone, the most widely used glucocorticoid during gestation, is metabolized by the mother to its active form prednisolone. An 11-β-OH radical is responsible for prednisolone's physiologic activity. The placenta has an abundance of the metabolizing enzyme 11-β-ol dehydrogenase, which converts the active glucocorticoid to an inactive 11-keto metabolite. Depending on the study, only 10 to 50 percent of a dose of prednisone and only one-sixth of a dose of hydrocortisone reach the fetus.[77-79] Levitz et al.[80] performed placental perfusion studies showing that steroids are rapidly cleared from the fetus. Beitins and coworkers[81] found that the maternal : fetal concentration gradient after intravenous administration of prednisolone is 10 : 1.

Dexamethasone and betamethasone cross the placenta more freely and for this reason are used to enhance fetal lung maturity. Blanford et al.[82] observed little conversion of dexamethasone or betamethasone to inactive forms. Work by Ballard's group[77] and by Osathanondh et al.[79] demonstrate a maternal : fetal concentration gradient of 1 : 1 for dexamethasone and betamethasone.

To minimize potential fetal effects, prednisone should be the oral glucocorticoid of choice.[83] Both methylprednisolone and hydrocortisone are satisfactory for intravenous use when needed. Methylprednisolone has less mineralocorticoid effect and should create fewer maternal side effects.

Occasionally, azathioprine, a derivative of 6-mercaptopurine, will be required to control a patient's SLE. This medication readily crosses the placenta. In a study by Scott,[84] 64 to 93 percent of an administered dose appeared in fetal blood between 2.5 and 6 hours after intravenous administration. Azathioprine has not been shown to be teratogenic in humans, although congenital malformations have been observed in animal models.[85] Chronic azathioprine use during pregnancy has been associated with neonatal lymphopenia, lower serum IgG and IgM levels, and decreased thymic shadow on x-ray.[86] All of these changes have reversed with time. Scott[84,87] reports an increased incidence of IUGR in infants born to mothers who took azathioprine during pregnancy. As yet, no long-term information is available on immunologic development and later infection rates in children who were exposed to this medication in utero.

Before administering azathioprine during pregnancy, however, the benefits and risks should be weighed carefully.

RHEUMATOID ARTHRITIS

Rheumatoid arthritis is an autoimmune disease with a prevalence of approximately 2 percent. Its crippling chronic form occurs in about 0.35 percent of the population.[88] The onset of the disease is usually between the ages of 20 and 60 years, and women are two to three times more likely to be affected than are men.[89]

Diagnosis

The diagnosis of rheumatoid arthritis is based on guidelines set forth by the American Rheumatism Association. A list of exclusions has also been devised to make the diagnosis more precise.

American Rheumatism Association Diagnostic Criteria for Rheumatoid Arthritis (RA)

Morning stiffness

Pain on motion or tenderness in at least one joint

Soft tissue swelling in at least one joint

Swelling in at least one other joint

Simultaneous symmetric joint swelling

Subcutaneous nodules

Radiologic changes typical of rheumatoid arthritis

Positive rheumatoid factor

Poor mucin precipitate from synovial fluid

Characteristic histologic changes in synovium

Characteristic histologic changes in subcutaneous nodules

A. Classic RA: 7 criteria
B. Definite RA: 5 criteria
C. Probable RA: 3 criteria
D. Signs and symptoms must persist for at least 6 weeks.
E. No exclusions can be present

(Adapted from Rodman and Schumacher,[147] with permission.)

Exclusions From Rheumatoid Arthritis

Typical rash of systemic lupus erythematosus

Strongly positive lupus erythematosus cell preparation

Histologic evidence of periarteritis

Proximal muscle weakness consistent with dermatomyositis

Definite scleroderma

Clinical rheumatic fever

Clinical gouty arthritis

Tophi

Infectious arthritis

Tuberculous arthritis

Reiter syndrome

Clinical picture of shoulder–hand syndrome

Hypertrophic osteoarthropathy

Neuroarthropathy

Homogentisic aciduria

Sarcoidosis or positive Kveim test

Multiple myeloma

Erythema nodosum

Leukemia or lymphoma

Agammaglobulinemia

(Adapted from Rodman and Schumacher,[147] with permission.)

Clinical Manifestations

Articular involvement is the hallmark of rheumatoid arthritis. The most common finding is an erythematous, warm, swollen metacarpophalangeal (MCP) joint. The proximal interphalangeal (PIP) and wrist joints may also be involved. Less frequently, metatarsophalangeal (MTP) and shoulder joints are affected. Over time, cartilage destruction and pannus formation occur.[90] Carpal tunnel syndrome is often seen in patients with rheumatoid arthritis.[91]

Extra-articular features of rheumatoid arthritis are found in patients with the most joint involvement and the highest titers of rheumatoid factor.[92,93] Rheumatoid nodules, which occur in 20 percent of patients with rheumatoid arthritis, can appear in the heart and lungs and along any extremity.[94] Pericarditis, myocarditis, and endocarditis are occasionally seen in patients with rheumatoid arthritis. Vasculitis may result secondary to immune complex deposition and may affect the skin, peripheral nerves, and blood vessels.[95] Unlike SLE, rheumatoid arthritis rarely involves the kidneys. It is important to note that after 10 years of disease more than 50 percent of patients are still able to work, and 15 percent will have a complete remission.[96]

Pathophysiology

Rheumatoid arthritis is characterized by proliferation and inflammation of synovial membranes. The membranes characteristically show a dense collection of lymphocytes in a diffuse nodular pattern.[97] T-cell function appears to be impaired, and there is an excessive number of T-suppressor cells.[98] Immune complexes, which activate the complement cascade, have been demonstrated in the blood, synovial fluid, and synovial membranes of patients with rheumatoid arthritis.[99,100] There appears to be a genetic predisposition to rheumatoid arthritis. A strong association between the histocompatibility antigen HLA-DR4 and rheumatoid arthritis has been shown.[101]

Laboratory Findings

Rheumatoid factors, IgM and IgG antibodies directed against the Fc fragment of IgG, are the hallmark laboratory finding of rheumatoid arthritis, but are not pathognomonic for this disorder. More severe disease is seen with higher titers of rheumatoid factor. Antinuclear antibodies are also found in approximately 20 percent of patients with rheumatoid arthritis.

Effects of Pregnancy on Rheumatoid Arthritis

In 1938, Hench[102] observed that many patients with rheumatoid arthritis experienced remissions during pregnancy. Persellin[103] noted that in pregnant women with rheumatoid arthritis 74 percent under-

went remission during the first trimester, 20 percent in the second trimester, and 5 percent in the third trimester. In this series, however, 90 percent of patients experienced a postpartum exacerbation of their disease. Approximately 25 percent of these flares occurred in the first 4 weeks post partum.[103] In a recent review, Klipple and Cecere[104] reported that approximately 70 percent of patients with rheumatoid arthritis experienced substantial improvements in disease activity, including extra-articular symptoms. Most of these patients no longer required medications. This remission, however, was short lived, with more than 90 percent of women relapsing within 6 to 8 months post partum. Klipple and Cecere[104] also found that in approximately 30 percent of patients with rheumatoid arthritis the course remained unchanged or worsened during gestation.

Effect of Rheumatoid Arthritis on Pregnancy

Rheumatoid arthritis appears to have no adverse effects on pregnancy.[104–106] Silman et al.[107] reported an increase in perinatal deaths in pregnancies complicated by rheumatoid arthritis. In that study, however, there was no significant difference between patients and controls in the rate of the spontaneous abortion. In a more recent study, Spector and Silman[108] examined pregnancy outcome in 195 women with rheumatoid arthritis and 462 controls. They found no increase in spontaneous abortions or stillbirths in patients with rheumatoid arthritis. They also concluded that a prior history of poor reproduction did not put the patient at risk for developing rheumatoid arthritis in the future.[108] A theoretical risk of uteroplacental insufficiency and IUGR does exist for patients with advanced extra-articular rheumatoid arthritis, and a case of IUGR attributed to vasculitis associated with severe disease has been described.[109]

To avoid pain and joint damage, care should be taken when positioning the patient with severe articular involvement on the delivery table. This is especially true if the patient has epidural or spinal anesthesia, because a joint can be damaged without the patient feeling pain. Obstetric anesthesiologists must also be cautious during rapid sequence induction of general anesthesia and intubation of patients with spinal involvement of rheumatoid arthritis. Subluxation of the atlanto-occipital joint is possible with devastating consequences.

Effects of Medications Used To Treat Rheumatoid Arthritis

Salicylates

Acetylsalicylic acid (aspirin) is the mainstay for the treatment of rheumatoid arthritis in pregnancy. The desired therapeutic blood level is 15 to 20 mg/dl. To achieve this the patient must take 3.6 to 4 g of acetylsalicylic acid daily in three divided doses. Because salicylism, tinnitus, and deafness usually occur at levels of approximately 25 mg/dl, salicylate levels should be monitored regularly. Salicylate used throughout pregnancy may be associated with a prolonged gestation, long labor, increased blood loss at delivery, and postpartum hemorrhage.[110,111] These effects appear to be related to the inhibition of prostaglandin synthetase.[112] These drugs also block platelet aggregation, and there are rare reports of clotting disorders in the newborn.[113] Neonatal hemostasis should therefore be closely monitored. When a mother has been taking large doses of aspirin, a bleeding time should be performed on the neonate before circumcision is performed. Salicylates have been shown to be teratogenic in animals but not in humans. Despite these potential problems, acetylsalicylic acid remains the drug of choice in treating rheumatoid arthritis during gestation.

Other Nonsteroidal Anti-Inflammatory Agents

Therapeutic agents such as indomethacin, felectin, ibuprofen, naproxen, and ketoprofen are used in the treatment of rheumatoid arthritis. They have both analgesic and anti-inflammatory properties. However, they have not been adequately studied during pregnancy and should be avoided if possible. Indomethacin, when used in late pregnancy, can cause premature closure of the fetal ductus arteriosus leading to pulmonary hypertension. It has also been associated with oligohydramnios when used over a long period of time.

Gold Therapy

Gold therapy has been utilized for many years in the treatment of rheumatoid arthritis. Although the precise mechanism of its action is unknown, gold has been shown to lower the titer of rheumatoid factor.

Bone marrow suppression can occur during gold therapy. A complete blood count and platelet count should therefore be performed before each injec-

tion.[114] Because proteinuria secondary to immune complex nephritis is an infrequent consequence of gold injections, urine should be checked for protein before each dose.[115] Gold compounds are protein bound and have poor placental passage. Chrysotherapy, however, cannot be recommended for routine use during pregnancy because of the limited clinical experience with this agent.[105]

Penicillamine

Penicillamine has been used successfully to treat rheumatoid arthritis in patients who are either resistant or have allergic reactions to gold. Like gold, penicillamine will reduce the titer of rheumatoid factor. Penicillamine freely crosses the placenta, and its use during pregnancy should be curtailed unless the benefits clearly outweigh the potential risks.

SCLERODERMA AND PROGRESSIVE SYSTEMIC SCLEROSIS

Progressive systemic sclerosis (PSS) and scleroderma are related collagen vascular diseases of unknown etiology. They affect females four times more frequently than males, with onset usually between the ages of 30 and 50 years. The reported incidence is about five new cases per 1 million population per year. *Scleroderma,* the term used to describe the disorder when it is localized to the skin, is characterized by tight and bound down skin, sclerodactyly, and Raynaud's phenomenon. Clinical signs may precede development of the overt disease by several years.

In PSS, there is systemic involvement, including the gastrointestinal viscera and pulmonary vascular and parenchymal changes. Pulmonary hypertension with resultant right-sided heart failure is often the fatal consequence of PSS. With cardiac involvement, left-sided heart failure is occasionally seen.

Laboratory Manifestations

Speckled-pattern antinuclear antibodies are observed in about 50 percent of patients, and 40 percent will demonstrate a rheumatoid factor. Anti-Scl-70, an extractable nuclear antibody, appears in the serum of 40 percent of patients with scleroderma and PSS. It appears to be fairly specific for this disease.

Effects of Pregnancy on Scleroderma and PSS

Johnson and coworkers[116] reported 18 cases of scleroderma and PSS complicating pregnancy. None of the women exhibited visceral involvement. In 39 percent of the patients, the disease showed no change or progressed at the same rate as prior to pregnancy. In an additional 39 percent the disease worsened, but no patient developed visceral involvement. In the remaining 22 percent some improvement was noted, but regression occurred after delivery. Several studies have described the onset of fatal renal involvement during pregnancy in patients with scleroderma and PSS.[117-120] In these reports, it is unclear whether visceral involvement antedated the pregnancy. Altieri and Cameron[121] reported a case of renal failure occurring in a pregnant woman with PSS. Partial recovery did follow the pregnancy. A successful pregnancy has been described in a patient with scleroderma complicated by renal disease and pulmonary hypertension who was treated with angiotensin-converting enzyme inhibitors.[122] The use of these agents during pregnancy is not recommended, but, because of the severity of the illness, they were used in this instance. Furthermore, Spiera et al.[123] reported a successful pregnancy in a patient with a previous hypertensive renal crisis caused by PSS. The patient was actually withdrawn from angiotensin-converting enzyme inhibitors when she became pregnant and had no renal complications during the pregnancy.[123] In a large review, Maymon and Fejgin[124] conducted a detailed literature search of scleroderma in pregnancy. Of 94 patients, 14 died during the course of pregnancy secondary to renal and cardiopulmonary involvement. It is important to note that this literature review covered many years. With more sophisticated maternal monitoring and therapy, the maternal mortality rate is probably much lower today.

Effects of Scleroderma on Pregnancy

Many theoretical complications exist but few have been documented properly because of the rarity with which scleroderma and PSS coexist with pregnancy. Preterm birth, premature rupture of membranes, and stillbirth seem to be more common in patients with scleroderma and PSS.[125,126] Surviving infants show no evidence of scleroderma.[125,127] Recently, Sil-

mann and Black[128] found that patients who eventually develop scleroderma have an increased risk of spontaneous abortion and infertility. Furthermore, Freeman and coworkers[129] reported a case of early spontaneous abortion and a circulating "lupus" anticoagulant in a patient with scleroderma. Steen et al.[130] examined pregnancy outcome in 48 women with scleroderma and two control groups matched for age and race. One control group contained normal patients and the other a group of women with rheumatoid arthritis. No difference was observed in the frequencies of miscarriage or perinatal death. Preterm births and infants with IUGR were found more frequently in patients with scleroderma and PSS. These recent data are favorable when compared with the review of older literature by Maymon and Fejgin.[124]

Management During Pregnancy

If visceral involvement, especially pulmonary, cardiac, or renal, is documented, counseling should be undertaken before a patient attempts pregnancy. As previously mentioned, patients with renal involvement can carry to term but gestation is often much more complicated. If a patient with PSS becomes pregnant, pregnancy termination should be considered but is certainly not mandatory. If scleroderma with only skin involvement exists, the patient may be followed expectantly. She should be aware that renal or cardiac involvement may be fatal.

MYASTHENIA GRAVIS

Although its prevalence is 1 per 25,000 in the general population, myasthenia gravis frequently coexists with pregnancy.[131] Women are twice as frequently affected as men and have an earlier onset of the disease with a peak incidence occurring between the ages of 20 and 30 years. Even though 60 percent of patients with myasthenia gravis have enlargement of the thymus, only 8 percent have a malignant thymoma.[132] Thymectomy improves symptoms in up to two-thirds of patients, but most still need additional medical therapy.[133] If the patient presents for prepregnancy counseling and is symptomatic despite large doses of medication, thymectomy should be undertaken before attempting pregnancy. Myasthenia gravis in pregnancy has been extensively studied by Plauché.[134] In a review of 314 pregnancies in 217 patients with myasthenia, he found no change in the myasthenic status throughout pregnancy, the puerperium, or the postpartum period in 31.5 percent of patients. In that review, exacerbations occurred in 40.8 percent of patients during pregnancy, including 30.6 percent during the puerperium. Another 28 percent showed a remission of their myasthenia during gestation.[134] Historically, there is a 25 to 60 percent preterm birth rate among patients with myasthenia gravis.[135,136] These are retrospective studies covering more than 40 years. With modern surveillance and therapy for preterm labor, this rate has probably decreased. Antiacetylcholinesterase agents, which are used to treat myasthenia gravis, have an oxytocic action. It has been postulated that this could be the explanation for preterm labor observed in patients with myasthenia gravis.[137]

A team approach is necessary for proper treatment of the patient with myasthenia gravis. The neurologist and rheumatologist are not always familiar with the medications used by the obstetrician in treating complications of pregnancy. Conversely, because of the infrequency with which obstetricians see myasthenia gravis, they may be unfamiliar with the interactions between these medications and the disease.

Magnesium sulfate, for example, is absolutely contraindicated in the myasthenic patient. It further interferes with the neuromuscular blockade that is characteristic of the disease.[138] According to Castillo and Engbaek,[138] magnesium reduces the stimulating effect of acetylcholine on the muscle. It affects the amplitude of the end-plate potential without affecting the muscle's resting potential. Cohen and co-workers[139] reported a near maternal death from administration of magnesium to a myasthenic patient. Catanzarite and coinvestigators[137] described a respiratory arrest in a myasthenic patient with preterm labor who was treated with ritodrine and dexamethasone. They thought that the respiratory arrest was due to glucocorticoids. Although glucocorticoids generally ameliorate myasthenic symptoms, they may initially result in increased weakness in 25 to 80 percent

of patients.[70] Catanzarite and colleagues[137] proposed that this paradoxic effect, coupled with the hypokalemia caused by the ritodrine, led to the crisis.

Patient Management

Most patients with myasthenia gravis will be taking acetylcholinesterase inhibitors when they become pregnant. These medications are generally safe during gestation. The most commonly used medication, pyridostigmine, does not readily cross the placenta. Dosage adjustments, however, are frequently necessary because of the physiologic changes in vascular volume, renal blood flow, and hepatic function during pregnancy. Because myasthenia gravis is a disease of striated muscle, the smooth muscle of the uterus is generally not affected. The first stage of labor progresses at a normal pace. The second stage of labor involves voluntary pushing and the use of skeletal and pelvic girdle musculature.[140] These maternal expulsive efforts may be impaired because of the myasthenia gravis, and the obstetrician must be prepared to perform an operative vaginal delivery. Cesarean section should be reserved for obstetric indications. Patients are apt to undergo myasthenic crisis during labor, and the oral medications normally used have variable gastrointestinal absorption during this time. The obstetrician should therefore be prepared to use parenteral acetylcholinesterase inhibitors during labor and must be able to differentiate between an overdose of these medications and a myasthenic crisis.

Anesthesia and analgesia during labor present special challenges in the patient with myasthenia gravis. Although they are extremely sensitive to narcotics, patients with myasthenia gravis may be given these medications if they are carefully monitored.[141] Epidural anesthesia decreases the requirements for parenteral narcotics, prevents fatigue, and provides excellent anesthesia.[22] If, however, general anesthesia is elected for cesarean section, nondepolarizing muscle relaxants should be used with great care, if at all. Myasthenics are sensitive to these agents, and a prolonged response is usually seen.[140] It is also imperative to remember that halothane potentiates these agents. If general anesthesia is elected, the patient and her family should be warned that she may need ventilatory support for a period of time after the surgery.

If the patient develops a puerperal infection, aminoglycosides should be used with extreme caution. These agents can block the motor end-plate and cause a myasthenic crisis.[22]

Occasionally myasthenia will be exacerbated during pregnancy. In such cases, therapy with extremely large doses of acetylcholinesterase inhibitors yields little response. These patients can be treated with plasmapheresis. The procedure may need to be repeated every 3 to 6 weeks, but dramatic results can be seen. After plasmapheresis symptoms improve, and the dose of acetylcholinesterase inhibitors can often be temporarily reduced. The procedure should be carried out with the patient in the left lateral position and with the uterus tilted off the inferior vena cava. It should be performed relatively slowly, with careful attention to maternal blood pressure. If plasmapheresis is being performed after 24 weeks gestation, continuous fetal monitoring should be employed.

Neonatal Myasthenia Gravis

Neonatal myasthenia occurs in 10 to 25 percent of infants born to mothers with myasthenia gravis.[142–145] In his review series, Plauché[134] reported a 20.2 percent incidence of neonatal myasthenia, with a 2.1 percent stillbirth rate and a 3.8 percent neonatal mortality rate. Again, that study reviewed cases over a 40-year period. With modern neonatal care, the neonatal mortality rate is probably considerably lower. Neonatal myasthenia does not begin at birth but is usually evident within the first 2 days of life. It lasts an average of 3 weeks but can persist up to 15 weeks.[145] Symptoms usually include a weak cry, poor sucking effort, and, rarely, respiratory distress. Neonatal myasthenia is thought to be secondary to transplacental passage of IgG antibodies directed against acetylcholine receptors.

REFERENCES

1. Fessel WJ: Systemic lupus erythematosus in the community. Incidence, prevalence, outcome and first symptoms: the high prevalence in black women. Arch Intern Med 134:1027, 1974

2. Estes D, Christian CL: The natural history of systemic lupus erythematosus by prospective analysis. Medicine 50:85, 1971

3. Notmon DP, Kuranta N, Tan EM: Profile of antinuclear antibodies in systemic rheumatic disease. Ann Intern Med 83:464, 1975

4. Garsenstein M, Pollak VE, Karik RM: Systemic lupus erythematosus and pregnancy. N Engl J Med 276:165, 1962

5. Zurier RB: Systemic lupus erythematosus and pregnancy. Clin Rheum Dis 1:613, 1975

6. Meehan RT, Dorsey JK: Pregnancy among patients with systemic lupus erythematosus receiving immunosuppressive therapy. J Rheumatol 14:252, 1987

7. Lockshin MD: Lupus erythematosus and allied disorders in pregnancy. Bull NY Acad Med 63:797, 1987

8. Lockshin MD, Reinitz E, Druzin ML et al: Lupus pregnancy, case–control prospective study demonstrating absence of lupus exacerbation during or after pregnancy. Am J Med 77:893, 1984

9. Lockshin MD: Pregnancy does not cause systemic lupus erythematosus to worsen. Arthritis Rheum 32:665, 1989

10. Mintz G, Nitz J, Gutierrez G et al: Prospective study of pregnancy in systemic lupus erythematosus: results of a multidisciplinary approach. J Rheumatol 13:732, 1986

11. Ainslie WH, Britt K, Moshipur JA: Maternal death due to lupus pneumonitis in pregnancy. Mt Sinai J Med 46:494, 1979

12. Leikin JB, Arof HM, Pearlman LM: Acute lupus pneumonitis in the postpartum period: a case history and review of the literature. Obstet Gynecol 68:295, 1986

13. Averbuch M, Bojko A, Levo Y: Cardiac tamponade in the early postpartum period as the presenting and predominant manifestation of systemic lupus erythematosus. J Rheumatol 13:444, 1986

14. Marabani M, Zoma A, Hadley D, Sturrock RD: Transverse myelitis occurring during pregnancy in a patient with systemic lupus erythematosus. Ann Rheum Dis 48:160, 1989

15. Gimovsky ML, Montoro M, Paul RH: Pregnancy outcome in women with systemic lupus erythematosus. Obstet Gynecol 63:686, 1984

16. Devoe L, Taylor RL: Systemic lupus erythematosus in pregnancy. Am J Obstet Gynecol 135:473, 1979

17. Hayslett JP, Lynn RI: Effect of pregnancy in patients with lupus nephropathy. Kidney Int 18:207, 1980

18. Fine LG, Barnett EV, Danovitch GM et al: Systemic

lupus erythematosus in pregnancy. Ann Intern Med 94:667, 1981

19. Mackey E: Pregnancy and renal disease: a ten-year study. Aust NZ J Obstet Gynaecol 3:21, 1963
20. Ramsey-Goldman R: Pregnancy in systemic lupus erythematosus. Rheum Dis Clin North Am 14:1988
21. Houser MT, Fish AJ, Tagatz GE et al: Pregnancy and systemic lupus erythematosus. Am J Obstet Gynecol 138:409, 1980
22. Foldes FF, McNall PG: Myasthenia gravis: a guide for anesthesiologists. Anesthesiology 23:837, 1962
23. Buyon JP, Cronstein BN, Morris M et al: Serum complement values (C_3 and C_4) to differentiate between systemic lupus activity and pre-eclampsia. Am J Med 81:194–200, 1986
24. Fraga A, Mintz G, Orozco J et al: Sterility and fertility rates, fetal wastage and maternal morbidity in systemic lupus erythematosus. J Rheumatol 1:1293, 1974
25. Castillo JD, Engbaek L: The nature of the neuromuscular block produced by magnesium. J Physiol 124:370–384, 1954
26. Kitzmiller JL: Autoimmune disorders: maternal, fetal and neonatal risks. Clin Obstet Gynecol 21:385, 1978
27. Zurier RG, Argyros T, Urman J et al: Systemic lupus erythematosus: management during pregnancy. Obstet Gynecol 51:178, 1978
28. Rosove MH, Brewer PM, Runge A, Hirji K: Simultaneous lupus anticoagulant and anticardiolipin assays and clinical detection of antiphospholipids. Am J Hematol 32:148, 1989
29. Lockwood CJ, Romero R, Feinber RF: The prevalence and biologic significance of lupus anticoagulant and anticardiolipin antibodies in a general obstetric population. Am J Obstet Gynecol 161:369, 1989
30. Hanly JG, Gladman DD, Rose TH et al: Lupus pregnancy, a prospective study of placental changes. Arthritis Rheum 31:358, 1988
31. Hedfors E, Lindahl G, Lindblad S: Anticardiolipin antibodies during pregnancy. J Rheumatol 14:160, 1987
32. Hokkanen E: Myasthenia gravis. Ann Clin Res 1:94, 1969
33. Lubbe WF, Butler WS, Palmer SJ et al: Lupus anticoagulant in pregnancy. Br J Obstet Gynaecol 97:357, 1984
34. Lubbe WF, Butler WS, Liggins GC: The lupus-anticoagulant: clinical and obstetric implications. NZ Med J 97:398, 1984
35. Branch DW, Scott JR, Kochenour NK et al: Obstetric complications associated with the lupus anticoagulant. N Engl J Med 313:1322, 1985
36. Unander AM, Norberg R, Hahn L et al: Anticardio-

lipin antibodies and complement in ninety-nine women with habitual abortion. Am J Obstet Gynecol 156:114, 1987
37. Lubbe WF, Walkom P, Alexander CJ: Hepatic and splenic haemorrhage as a complication of toxaemia of pregnancy in a patient with circulating lupus anticoagulant. NZ Med J 95:842, 1982
38. Druzin ML, Lockshin M, Edersheim TG et al: Second-trimester fetal monitoring and preterm delivery in pregnancies with systemic lupus erythematosus and/or circulating anticoagulant. Am J Obstet Gynecol 157:1503, 1987
39. Lockshin MD, Druzin ML, Goei S et al: Antibody to cardiolipin as a predictor of fetal distress or death in pregnant patients with systemic lupus erythematosus. N Engl J Med 313:152, 1985
40. Lubbe WF, Palmer SJ, Butler WS et al: Fetal survival after prednisone suppression of maternal lupus-anticoagulant. Lancet 1:1361, 1983
41. Mintz G, Nitz J, Gutierrez G et al: Prospective study of pregnancy in systemic lupus erythematosus: results of a multidisciplinary approach. J Rheumatol 13:732, 1986
42. Lockshin MD, Druzin ML, Qamar T: Prednisone does not prevent recurrent fetal death in women with antiphospholipid antibody. Am J Obstet Gynecol 160:439, 1989
43. Karp HJ, Frenkel Y, Many A et al: Fetal demise associated with lupus anticoagulant: clinical features and results of treatment. Gynecol Obstet Invest 28:178, 1989
44. Farquharson RG, Compston A, Bloom AL: Lupus anticoagulant: a place for pre-pregnancy treatment? Lancet 1:842, 1985
45. Gardlund B: The lupus inhibitor in thromboembolic disease and intrauterine death in the absence of systemic lupus. Acta Med Scand 215:293, 1984
46. Ordi J, Barquinero J, Vilardell M et al: Fetal loss treatment in patients with antiphospholipid antibodies. Ann Rheum Dis 48:798, 1989
47. Gatenby PA, Cameron K, Shearman RP: Pregnancy loss with phospholipid antibodies: improved outcome with aspirin containing treatment. Aust NZ J Obstet Gynaecol 29:294, 1989
48. Balasch J, Font J, Lopez-Soto A et al: Antiphospholipid antibodies in unselected patients with repeated abortion. Hum Reprod 5:43, 1990
49. Rosove MH, Tabsh K, Wasserstrum N et al: Heparin therapy for pregnant women with lupus anticoagulant or anticardiolipin antibodies. Obstet Gynecol 75:630, 1990

50. Chamley LW, Pattison NS, McKay EJ: IgM lupus anti-coagulants can be associated with recurrent fetal loss of thrombic episodes. Thromb Res 58:343, 1990

51. Mizoguchi K, Kakisako S, Tanaka M et al: Lupus anti-coagulant as a risk factor for cerebral infarction and habitual abortions. Kurume Med J 36:113, 1989

52. Rallings P, Exner T, Abraham R: Coronary artery vasculitis and myocardial infarction associated with antiphospholipid antibodies in a pregnant woman. Aust NZ J Med 19:347, 1989

53. Litsey S, Noonan J, O'Connor W et al: Maternal connective tissue disease and congenital heart block. N Engl J Med 312:98, 1985

54. Draznin TH, Easterly NB, Fureu N et al: Neonatal lupus erythematosus. J Am Acad Dermatol 1:437, 1979

55. McCue C, Mantakas M, Tingelstad JB et al: Congenital heart block in newborns of mothers with connective tissue disease. Circulation 56:82, 1977

56. Scott JS, Maddison PJ, Tayler PV et al: Connective-tissue disease, antibodies to ribonucleoprotein and congenital heart block. N Engl J Med 309:209, 1983

57. Scheib JS, Waxman J: Congenital heart block in successive pregnancies: a case report and evaluation of risk with therapeutic consideration. Obstet Gynecol 73:481, 1989

58. Vetter VL, Rashkad WJ: Congenital complete heart block and connective tissue disease. N Engl J Med 309:236, 1983

59. Esscher E, Scott JS: Congenital heart block and maternal systemic lupus erythematosus. Br Med J 1:1235, 1979

60. Buyon JP, Swersky SH, Fox HE et al: Intrauterine therapy for presumptive fetal myocarditis with acquired heart block due to systemic lupus erythematosus. Arthritis Rheum 39:1, 1987

61. Watson RM, Braunstein BL, Watson AJ et al: Fetal wastage in women with anti-Ro (SSA) antibody. J Rheumatol 13:90, 1986

62. Lockshin MD, Gibofsky A, Peebles CL et al: Neonatal lupus erythematosus with heart block: family study of a patient with anti-SS-A and SS-B antibodies. Arthritis Rheum 26:210, 1983

63. McCuiston CH, Schoch EP: Possible discoid lupus erythematosus in a newborn infant: report of case with subsequent development of acute systemic lupus erythematosus in mother. Arch Dermatol Syphilol 70:782, 1954

64. McGee CD, Makowski EL: Systemic lupus erythematosus in pregnancy. Am J Obstet Gynecol 107:1008, 1970

65. Carroll BA: Obstetric duplex sonography in patients with lupus anticoagulant syndrome. J Ultrasound Med 9:17, 1990

66. Buyon JP, Cronstein BN, Morris M et al: Serum complement values (C_3 and C_4) to differentiate between systemic lupus activity and pre-eclampsia. Am J Med 81:194–200, 1986

67. Tozman ECS, Urowitz MB, Gladman DD: Systemic lupus erythematosus and pregnancy. J Rheumatol 7:624, 1980

68. Zulman MI, Talal N, Hoffman GS et al: Problems associated with the management of pregnancies in patients with systemic lupus erythematosus. J Rheumatol 7:37, 1980

69. Zurier RG, Argyros T, Urman J et al: Systemic lupus erythematosus: management during pregnancy. Obstet Gynecol 51:178, 1978

70. Devoe LD, Aloy GL: Serum complement levels and perinatal outcome in pregnancies complicated by systemic lupus erythematosus. Obstet Gynecol 63:796, 1984

71. Lockshin MD, Qamar T, Levy RA, Druzin ML: Pregnancy in systemic lupus erythematosus. Clin Exp Rheumatol 7(3):S195, 1989

72. Freinkel N: Gestational diabetes, 1979: philosophical and practical aspects of a major health problem. Diabetes Care 3:399, 1980

73. Bongiovanni AM, McPadden AJ: Steroids during pregnancy and possible fetal consequences. Fertil Steril 11:181, 1960

74. Fainstat T: Cortisone-induced congenital cleft palate in rabbits. Endocrinology 55:502, 1954

75. Giannopoulos G, Tulchinsky D: The influence of hormones on fetal lung development. p. 310. In Ryan KJ, Tulchinsky D (eds): Maternal–Fetal Endocrinology. WB Saunders, Philadelphia, 1988

76. Rolbin SH, Levinson G, Shnider SM et al: Anesthetic considerations for myasthenia gravis and pregnancy. Anesth Analog 57:441, 1978

77. Ballard PL, Granberg P, Ballard RA: Glucocorticoid levels in maternal and cord serum after prenatal betamethasone therapy to prevent respiratory distress syndrome. J Clin Invest 56:15, 1975

78. Blanford AT, Pearson-Murphy BE: In vitro metabolism of prednisolone, dexamethasone, betamethasone, and cortisol by the human placenta. Am J Obstet Gynecol 137:264, 1977

79. Osathanondh R, Tulchinsky D, Kamali H et al: Dexamethasone levels in treated pregnant women and newborn infants. J Pediatr 90:617, 1977

80. Levitz M, Jansen V, Dancis J: The transfer and metabo-

lism of corticosteroids in the perfused human placenta. Am J Obstet Gynecol 132:363, 1978

81. Beitins IZ, Bayard F, Ances IG et al: The transplacental passage of prednisone and prednisolone in pregnancy near term. J Pediatr 81:936, 1972

82. Blanford AT, Pearson Murphy BE: In vitro metabolism of prednisolone, dexamethasone, betamethasone, and cortisol by the human placenta. Am J Obstet Gynecol 127:264, 1977

83. Gabbe SG: Drug therapy in autoimmune disease. Clin Obstet Gynecol 26:635, 1983

84. Scott JR: Fetal growth retardation associated with maternal administration of immuno-suppressive drugs. Am J Obstet Gynecol 128:668, 1977

85. Davison JM, Lindheimer MD: Pregnancy in renal transplant recipients. J Reprod Med 27:613, 1982

86. Cote CJ, Meuwissen HJ, Pickering RJ: Effects on the neonate of prednisone and azathioprine administered to the mother during pregnancy. J Pediatr 85:324, 1974

87. Scott JR: Immunologic diseases in pregnancy. Prog Allergy 23:321, 1977

88. Turnam GR: Rheumatoid arthritis. Clin Obstet Gynecol 26:560, 1983

89. Masi AT, Maldonade-Cocco JA, Kaplan SB et al: Prospective study of the early course of rheumatoid arthritis in young adults: comparison of patients with and without rheumatoid factor positivity at entry and identification of variables correlating with outcome. Semin Arthritis Rheum 5:299, 1976

90. Baum J, Ziff M: Laboratory findings in rheumatoid arthritis. p. 491. In McCary D (ed): Arthritis and Allied Conditions. 9th Ed. Philadelphia, Lea & Febiger, 1979

91. Harris ED Jr: The proliferative lesion in rheumatoid arthritis: manifestation and pathophysiology. p. 374. In Harris ED Jr (ed): Rheumatoid Arthritis. New York, Medcom, 1974

92. Gordon DA, Stein JL, Broder I: The extraarticular features of rheumatoid arthritis: a systemic analysis of 127 cases. Am J Med 54:445, 1973

93. Hurd ER: Extraarticular manifestations of rheumatoid arthritis. Semin Arthritis Rheum 8:151, 1979

94. Hollingsworth JW, Saykaly RJ: Systemic complications of rheumatoid arthritis. Med Clin North Am 61:217, 1977

95. Williams RC: Adult and juvenile rheumatoid arthritis. p. 184. In Parker GW (ed): Clinical Immunology. Philadelphia, WB Saunders, 1980

96. Rodman GP (ed): Primer on the rheumatic diseases. JAMA 224(suppl):661, 1973

97. Robbins SL, Cotran RS: The musculoskeletal system —joints and related structures. p. 1452. In Robbins SL, Cotran RS (eds): Pathologic Basis of Disease. 2nd Ed. Philadelphia, WB Saunders, 1979

98. Yu DTY, Peter JB: Cellular immunological aspects of rheumatoid arthritis. Semin Arthritis Rheum 4:24, 1974

99. McDuffie FC: Immune complexes in the rheumatic disease. J Allergy Clin Immunol 62:37, 1978

100. Paget S, Gibofsky A: Immunopathogenesis of rheumatoid arthritis. Am J Med 67:961, 1979

101. Stobo JD: Rheumatoid arthritis restriction maps. West J Med 137:109, 1982

102. Hench PS: The ameliorating effect of pregnancy on chronic atrophic (infectious) rheumatoid arthritis, fibrositis and intermittent hydrarthrosis. Proc Mayo Clin 13:161, 1938

103. Persellin RH: The effect of pregnancy on rheumatoid arthritis. Bull Rheum Dis 27:922, 1977

104. Klipple GL, Cecere FA: Rheumatoid arthritis and pregnancy. Rheum Dis Clin North Am 15:213, 1989

105. Kaplan D, Diamond H: Rheumatoid arthritis and pregnancy. Clin Obstet Gynecol 8:286, 1965

106. Betson JR, Dorn RV: Forty cases of arthritis and pregnancy. J Int College Surgeons 42:521, 1964

107. Silman AJ, Roman E, Beral V, Brown A: Adverse reproductive outcomes in women who subsequently develop rheumatoid arthritis. Ann Rheum Dis 47:979, 1988

108. Spector TD, Silman AJ: Is poor pregnancy outcome a risk factor in rheumatoid arthritis? Ann Rheum Dis 49:12, 1990

109. Duhring JL: Pregnancy, rheumatoid arthritis, and intrauterine growth retardation. Am J Obstet Gynecol 108:325, 1970

110. Bulmash JM: Rheumatoid arthritis and pregnancy. Obstet Gynecol Annu 8:223, 1979

111. Bulmash JM: Systemic lupus erythematosus and pregnancy. Obstet Gynecol Annu 7:153, 1978

112. Lewis RB, Shulman JD: Influence of acetylsalicylic acid, an inhibitor of prostaglandin synthesis, on the duration of human gestation and labour. Lancet 2:1159, 1973

113. Bleyer WA, Breckenridge RT: The effect of prenatal aspirin on newborn hemostasis. JAMA 213:2049, 1970

114. Silverberg DS, Kidd EG, Shnitka TK, Ulan RA: Gold nephropathy: a clinical and pathologic study. Arthritis Rheum 13:812, 1970

115. Vaamonde CA, Hunt FR: The nephrotic syndrome as

a complication of gold therapy. Arthritis Rheum 13:826, 1970

116. Johnson TR, Banner EA, Winkelmann RK: Scleroderma and pregnancy. Obstet Gynecol 23:467, 1964

117. Fear RE: Eclampsia superimposed on renal scleroderma: a rare cause of maternal and fetal mortality. Obstet Gynecol 31:69, 1968

118. Sood SV, Kohler HG: Maternal death from systemic sclerosis. J Obstet Gynaecol Br Commonw 77:1109, 1970

119. Karlsen JR, Cook WA: Renal scleroderma and pregnancy. Obstet Gynecol 44:349, 1974

120. Ehrenfeld M, Licht A, Stersman J et al: Postpartum renal failure due to progressive systemic sclerosis treated with chronic hemodialysis. Nephron 18:175, 1977

121. Altieri P, Cameron JS: Scleroderma renal crisis in a pregnant woman with late partial recovery of renal function. Nephrol Dial Transplant 3:677, 1988

122. Baethge BA, Wolf RE: Successful pregnancy with scleroderma renal disease and pulmonary hypertension in a patient using angiotensin converting enzyme inhibitors. Ann Rheum Dis 48:776, 1989

123. Spiera H, Krakoff L, Fishbane-Mayer J: Successful pregnancy after scleroderma hypertensive renal crisis. J Rheumatol 16:1597, 1989

124. Maymon R, Fejgin M: Scleroderma in pregnancy. Obstet Gynecol Surv 44:530, 1989

125. Spellacy WN: Scleroderma and pregnancy. Obstet Gynecol 23:297, 1964

126. Slate WG, Graham AR: Scleroderma and pregnancy. Am J Gynecol 101:335, 1968

127. Jones WR, Storey B: Perinatal aspects of maternal autoimmune disease. Aust Paediatr J 8:306, 1972

128. Silman AJ, Black C: Increased incidence of spontaneous abortion and infertility in women with scleroderma before disease onset: a controlled study. Ann Rheum Dis 47:441, 1988

129. Freeman WE, Lesher JL Jr, Smith JG Jr: Connective tissue disease associated with sclerodermoid features, early abortion, and circulating anticoagulant. J Am Acad Dermatol 19:932, 1988

130. Steen VD, Conte C, Day N et al: Pregnancy in women with systemic sclerosis. Arthritis Rheum 32:151, 1989

131. Kurtzke JF: Epidemiology of myasthenia gravis. Adv Neurol 19:545, 1978

132. Hokkanen E: Myasthenia gravis. Ann Clin Res 1:94, 1969

133. Havard CW, Fonseca V: New treatment approaches to myasthenia gravis. Drugs 39:66, 1990

134. Plauché WC: Myasthenia gravis. Clin Obstet Gynecol 26:594, 1983

135. Petri M, Golbus M, Anderson R et al: Antinuclear antibody, lupus anticoagulant and anticardiolipin antibody in women with idiopathic habitual abortion. Arthritis Rheum 30:601, 1987

136. Plauché WC: Myasthenia gravis in pregnancy: an update. Am J Obstet Gynecol 135:691, 1979

137. Catanzarite VA, McHargue AM, Sandberg EC et al: Respiratory arrest during therapy for premature labor in a patient with myasthenia gravis. Obstet Gynecol 64:819, 1984

138. Castillo JD, Engbaek L: The nature of the neuromuscular block produced by magnesium. J Physiol 124:370, 1954

139. Cohen BA, London RS, Goldstein PJ: Myasthenia gravis and pre-eclampsia. Obstet Gynecol 48:35, 1976

140. McNall PG, Jafarnia MR: Management of myasthenia gravis in obstetrical patient. Am J Obstet Gynecol 92:518, 1965

141. Rolbin SH, Levinson G, Shnider SM et al: Anesthetic considerations for myasthenia gravis and pregnancy. Anesth Analog 57:441, 1978

142. Barlow CF: Neonatal myasthenia gravis. Am J Dis Child 135:209, 1981

143. Donaldson JO, Penn AS, Lisak RP et al: Antiacetylcholine receptor antibody in neonatal myasthenia gravis. Am J Dis Child 135:222, 1981

144. Namba T, Brown SB, Grob D: Neonatal myasthenia gravis: report of two cases and review of the literature. Pediatrics 45:488, 1970

145. Scott JR: Immunologic diseases in pregnancy. Prog Allergy 23:321, 1977

146. Tan EM, Cohen AS, Fries JF et al: The 1982 revised criteria for the classification of systemic lupus erythematosus. Arthritis Rheum 25:1274, 1982

147. Rodman GP, Schumacher HR: Appendix 2. p. 207. In Primer on the Rheumatic Diseases. 9th Ed. Arthritis Foundation, New York, 1988

Chapter 36

Hepatic and Gastrointestinal Disorders

Philip Samuels and Mark B. Landon

LIVER DISEASE

Liver disease frequently complicates pregnancy. The most commonly seen problems include the liver dysfunction associated with preeclampsia and hepatitis. These topics are covered in detail elsewhere in this text (see Chs. 30 and 40). This chapter focuses on acute fatty liver, intrahepatic cholestasis of pregnancy, and gallbladder disease associated with gestation (Table 36.1).

Acute Fatty Liver

Acute fatty liver is a rare condition of unknown etiology that has an incidence of between 1 in 13,000 and 1 in 1,000,000 pregnancies.[1,2] Before 1970, the published mortality rate for both mother and infant was approximately 85 percent.[3] Since 1975, maternal survival has increased to 72 percent, with neonatal survival slightly lower. These improved outcomes have been attributed to early recognition of the disorder followed by prompt delivery.[4,5] Usually beginning late in the third trimester, acute fatty liver often presents with nausea and vomiting[6] followed by severe abdominal pain and headache. The right upper quadrant is generally tender, but the liver is not enlarged to palpation. Within a few days jaundice appears, and the patient becomes somnolent and eventually comatose. Hematemesis and spontaneous bleeding result when

the patient develops hypoprothrombinemia and disseminated intravascular coagulation (DIC). Oliguria, metabolic acidosis, and eventually anuria occur in approximately 50 percent of patients with acute fatty liver of pregnancy.[7] If the disease is allowed to progress, labor begins and the patient delivers a stillborn infant. Although the etiology of these fetal losses has not been convincingly demonstrated, Moise and Shah[1] suggest that uteroplacental insufficiency may be the cause for fetal distress and fetal death in acute fatty liver. During the immediate postpartum period, the mother becomes febrile, comatose, and, without therapy, dies within a few days. Rather than liver failure, DIC, renal failure, profound hypoglycemia, and occasionally pancreatitis are the most often cited immediate causes of death.[1,6,7] Two cases of liver rupture associated with acute fatty liver have also been reported.[8,9] In one case, a patient receiving intravenous heparin for thrombophlebitis suddenly expired as a result of rupture of a subcapsular hematoma of the liver.[9] The diagnosis of acute fatty liver in pregnancy was microscopically confirmed.

The primary differential diagnoses in cases of acute fatty liver include fulminant hepatitis and the liver dysfunction associated with the HELLP syndrome (hemolysis, elevated liver enzymes, and low platelet count) or preeclampsia (Table 36.1).[10–12] Several researchers have suggested a spectrum of diseases between acute fatty liver of pregnancy and preeclampsia.[10,12] Although it is often difficult, physicians are

Table 36.1 Differential Diagnosis of Liver Disease in Pregnancy

	Serum Transaminase Levels (IU/L)	Bilirubin Level (mg/dL)	Coagulopathy	Histology	Other Features
Acute hepatitis B	>1,000	>5	−	Hepatocellular necrosis	Potential for perinatal transmission
Acute fatty liver	<500	<5	+	Fatty infiltration	Coma, renal failure, hypoglycemia
Intrahepatic cholestasis	<300	<5, mostly direct	−	Dilated bile canaliculi	Pruritus, increased bile acids
HELLP	>500	<5	+	Variable, periportal necrosis	Hypertension, edema, thrombocytopenia

Abbreviations: HELLP, hemolysis, elevated liver enzymes, low platelets; −, absent; +, present.

usually able to differentiate between these disorders using physical and laboratory findings.

Diagnosis

In acute fatty liver of pregnancy, serum transaminase levels are elevated but usually remain below 500 IU/L.[4] In acute hepatitis, however, these levels are frequently above 1,000 IU/L. In liver dysfunction associated with preeclampsia or the HELLP syndrome, the transaminases are often in the same range as in acute fatty liver of pregnancy, but are occasionally higher. As a result of DIC, the prothrombin time and partial thromboplastin times (APTT) are often prolonged. The prothrombin time is usually increased before the APTT. A decreased fibrinogen level is accompanied by an elevation in fibrin degradation products and the D-dimer. Although the serum bilirubin level is elevated, it usually remains below 5 mg/dl and rarely rises as high as 10 mg/dl, a level lower than one would expect in acute hepatitis. A liver biopsy will reveal pericentral microvesicular fatty change. There is little inflammatory cell infiltration or hepatic necrosis. Periportal areas are usually preserved.[5,13] This picture is very different from fulminant hepatitis in which hepatocellular necrosis is significant. Special staining and electron microscopy yield no evidence of viral particles in acute fatty liver of pregnancy. The diagnosis can be made on frozen section of the liver biopsy material using oil red O stain.[5] Barton and colleagues,[14] however, feel that electron microscopy is more beneficial in establishing a definitive diagnosis. Because of the coagulopathy associated with acute fatty liver of pregnancy, liver biopsy may not be advisable in many cases. If biopsy is essential to make the diagnosis and establish a plan of treatment, fresh frozen plasma can be administered to correct the coagulopathy before performing the procedure. Goodacre and colleagues[15] and Mabie and colleagues[16] feel that an adequate diagnosis of acute fatty liver of pregnancy can be made using computed tomography (CT). The finding of decreased attenuation over the liver is compatible with fatty infiltration. Both groups believe CT is useful in establishing the diagnosis in the pregnant woman with jaundice and liver dysfunction.[15,16]

Management

Once the diagnosis has been established, delivery should be accomplished as quickly as is safely possible. Important supportive measures must first be undertaken to ensure maternal well-being. The patient's coagulopathy must be corrected with fresh frozen plasma. If more concentrated fibrinogen is needed, cryoprecipitate can be administered. Intravenous fluids containing adequate glucose should be given. This will prevent hypoglycemia, which can be fatal in this disorder. If there is not a severe coagulopathy or the coagulopathy has been corrected, invasive hemodynamic monitoring should be carried out before delivery. This technique will allow the anesthesiologist and obstetrician to monitor the patient's fluid status. Because delivery soon after diagnosis is paramount, a cesarean section should be planned unless the patient's cervix is extremely favorable. If the patient's coagulopathy has been corrected, epidural anesthesia is the best choice. Spinal anesthesia can also be used. Regional anesthesia is preferable, because it allows adequate assessment of the patient's level of consciousness. General anesthesia should be avoided if possible because of the hepatotoxicity of some anesthetic agents. Narcotic doses must be adjusted, as these drugs are metabolized by the liver.

Early diagnosis and delivery afford both mother and neonate an excellent chance for survival.[4,5] If delivery is effected before hepatic encephalopathy and renal failure develop, patients usually improve rather rapidly.[4,5,7,10] However, Ockner and colleagues[17] have reported a case in which the patient did not improve postpartum. After orthotopic liver transplantation, the multisystem failure rapidly reversed.[17] In that case, the diagnosis of acute fatty liver was documented histopathologically. Southern blot analysis for viral DNA was also negative, ruling out hepatitis. To date, this is the only reported case of liver transplantation for acute fatty liver in pregnancy.[17] There is little risk of recurrence of acute fatty liver in subsequent pregnancies.[7] Barton and colleagues,[14] however, have recently described the first case of recurrent acute fatty liver in pregnancy confirmed by biopsy. Nonetheless, if the diagnosis is certain in the first pregnancy, patients should be reassured that they can carry a pregnancy in the future with little chance for recurrence.

Intrahepatic Cholestasis of Pregnancy

Intrahepatic cholestasis is characterized by pruritis and mild jaundice during the last trimester of pregnancy. It can, however, occur earlier in gestation.[18,19] The disease is reported to affect up to 10 percent of pregnancies in Chile.[20] In a recent study, Gonzalez et al.[21] determined the prevalence of intrahepatic cholestasis of pregnancy in Chile to be 4.7 percent in singleton pregnancies. In twin pregnancies, the incidence was 20.9 percent. The disease is also common in the Swedish population.[22,23] Berg et al.[23] report the incidence in Sweden to be between 1 and 1.5 percent. In their study, the incidence of intrahepatic cholestasis of pregnancy had a distinct seasonal variation, peaking in November. This disorder is much less common in the United States. In 1987, Wilson[24] reported the first case of intrahepatic cholestasis of pregnancy in a black American. Intrahepatic cholestasis tends to recur in subsequent pregnancies, but

the severity may vary from one pregnancy to the next. In their Chilean study, Gonzalez et al.[21] found a recurrence rate of 70.5 percent in singleton pregnancies.

Clinical Manifestations

Patients wih intrahepatic cholestasis usually begin having pruritis at night. It progresses, and the patient is soon experiencing bothersome pruritis continuously. Approximately 2 weeks later, clinical jaundice will develop in 50 percent of cases. The jaundice is usually mild, soon plateaus, and remains constant until delivery. The pruritis worsens with the onset of jaundice, and the patient's skin can become excoriated. The symptoms usually abate within 2 days after delivery. The differential diagnosis must include viral hepatitis and gallbladder disease. There is usually no fever or abdominal discomfort, as in hepatitis, or nausea or vomiting, as seen in hepatitis and gallbladder disease.

Laboratory Diagnosis

Serum alkaline phosphatase levels are increased 5- to 10-fold in intrahepatic cholestasis of pregnancy. Upon fractionation, most of the alkaline phosphatase is hepatic in origin rather than placental. Unfortunately, fractionation of alkaline phosphatase may not be readily available, making it impossible to separate the hepatic and placental contributions. Serum 5'-nucleotidase levels are also increased. Bilirubin is elevated, but usually not above 5 mg/dl. Most is in the direct, conjugated form. If intrahepatic cholestasis lasts for several weeks, liver dysfunction may result in decreased vitamin K reabsorption or decreased prothrombin production, leading to a prolongation of the prothrombin time. Serum transaminase levels are usually normal or moderately elevated, remaining well below the levels associated with viral hepatitis. Serum cholesterol and triglyceride levels may also be markedly elevated.

The serum bile acids (chenodeoxycholic acid, deoxycholic acid, and cholic acid) are increased. The levels are often more than 10 times the normal concentration. These acids are deposited in the skin and probably cause the extreme pruritis.[25] The degree of pruritis, however, is not always related to the serum level of bile acids.[26] To make the diagnosis of intrahepatic cholestasis of pregnancy, the fasting levels of serum bile acids should be at least three times the upper limit of normal. Elevation of serum bile acids alone cannot be used to make the diagnosis. The patient must also have clinical symptoms. Wojcicka-Jagodzinska and colleagues[27] reported that carbohydrate metabolism is disturbed in patients with intrahepatic cholestasis of pregnancy. These patients should therefore be screened for gestational diabetes.

Histologically, the periportal areas show no change, and the hepatocellular architecture remains undisturbed. The centilobular areas, however, reveal dilated bile canaliculi, many containing bile plugs. Ultrastructurally, there appears to be some destruction and atrophy of microvilli in the bile canaliculi.[28] These changes tend to regress after pregnancy.

Perinatal Outcome

The risk of preterm birth and fetal death may be increased in patients suffering from intrahepatic cholestasis of pregnancy.[18,29] While the preterm birth rate has been reported to be between 30 and 60 percent by some investigators, another study noted no increase in preterm delivery or fetal loss.[30] Fisk and Storey[31] recently studied 83 pregnancies complicated by intrahepatic cholestasis over a 10-year period. Meconium staining occurred in 45 percent of the pregnancies, spontaneous preterm labor occurred in 44 percent, and intrapartum fetal distress complicated 22 percent. Of the 86 infants, two were stillborn and one died soon after birth. The overall perinatal mortality in this group of patients was 35 per 1,000. Nonstress tests, serial ultrasonography to assess amniotic fluid volume, and estriol determinations failed to predict fetal compromise.[31] Early intervention was indicated in 49 pregnancies, 12 because of suspected fetal distress. In light of this study, antepartum fetal heart rate testing and intense surveillance should be undertaken in gravidas with intrahepatic cholestasis of pregnancy. It may also be prudent to induce labor at term or when amniotic fluid studies indicate fetal lung maturity.[31]

Management

Treatment is aimed at reducing the intense pruritis. Diphenhydramine and other antihistamines are of little use, but cholestyramine resin has proven highly effective. Cholestyramine is an anionic-binding resin that interrupts the enterohepatic circulation, reducing the reabsorption of bile acids. A total of 8 to 16 g per day in three to four divided doses is often helpful in relieving pruritis. It is most effective if started as soon as the pruritis is noted, before it becomes severe. It often takes up to 2 weeks to work. Because cholestyramine also interferes with vitamin K absorption, the prothrombin time should be checked at least weekly. If prolonged, parenteral vitamin K should be administered in a daily dose of 10 mg. When the prothrombin time returns to normal, the frequency of injections can be decreased. Cholestyramine causes a sensation of bloating and often results in constipation. If the patient cannot tolerate cholestyramine, antacids containing aluminum may be used to bind bile acids. These medications are usually not as effective as cholestyramine. An occasional patient may not respond to cholestyramine therapy. In those cases, phenobarbital, in a dose of 90 mg daily given at bedtime, can be helpful. Phenobarbital induces hepatic microsomal enzymes, increasing bile salt secretion and bile flow.[32-34] This medication usually takes more than 1 week to be effective. It is important to remember that phenobarbital must not be given within 2 hours of cholestyramine, or the phenobarbital will be bound and excreted without being absorbed.

When pruritis is intolerable, delivery may be undertaken as soon as fetal lung maturity has been documented. Jaundice usually disappears within 2 days after delivery. The patient should be counseled that the condition may recur during subsequent pregnancies.[21] It is also important to note that some patients may manifest symptoms of intrahepatic cholestasis when taking oral contraceptives.[23]

Pregnancy and Liver Transplantation

At present, pregnancy in the liver transplant patient is a rare occurrence. As the procedure becomes more widespread, more liver transplant recipients will become pregnant. Laifer and colleagues[35] reported the results of eight pregnancies in women with liver transplants. Seven of the eight patients conceived between 3 weeks and 24 months after transplantation. Six had live births, and one electively terminated her pregnancy. Five patients developed pregnancy-induced hypertension, including three with severe preeclampsia. The six infants born to these women were delivered between 26 and 37 weeks.[35] Five of the six infants survived, and none had structural anomalies. One patient underwent orthotopic liver transplantation at 26 weeks gestation after presenting in hepatic coma from fulminant hepatitis B. She was delivered on postoperative day 7 because of fetal distress. Laifer et al.[35] concluded that pregnancy does not appear to have a deleterious effect on hepatic graft function or survival. All eight of the patients in their series survived without permanent sequelae.

Gallbladder Disease

Cholelithiasis is responsible for approximately 7 percent of cases of jaundice occurring during gestation.[36] Pregnancy appears to increase the likelihood of gallstone formation but not the risk of developing acute cholecystitis.[37–39]

Pregnancy markedly alters gallbladder function. Ultrasound studies performed after 14 weeks gestation have shown that fasting gallbladder volume is twice normal, the rate of gallbladder emptying is decreased, and the percentage emptying is lower, thus leaving a higher residual than in the nonpregnant patient.[38] Cholecystokinin is the major stimulus for gallbladder contraction. It appears that estrogen and/or progesterone may make these contractions less effective, leading to an increased residual volume.

Once the diagnosis is confirmed, attacks of biliary colic should be treated symptomatically during gestation. Ultrasound examination of the gallbladder will aid in the evaluation and diagnosis of these patients. Hiatt and colleagues[40] report that ultrasound successfully confirmed the presence of gallstones in 18 of 26 patients. In the same series, ultrasound also demonstrated dilated intrahepatic ducts in one of two patients with surgically proved choledocholithiasis. Before resorting to surgery, attempts should be made to treat these patients medically. Attacks usually respond to intravenous hydration, analgesics, nasogastric suction, and antibiotics. Lockwood and associates[41] have also utilized total parenteral nutrition. Their patient did well with no fetal or maternal morbidity.

If possible, cholecystectomy should be postponed until after delivery. In their study of 26 patients, Hiatt and coworkers[40] found it necessary to perform cholecystectomy and cholangiography on 19 women, with four requiring common bile duct explorations. They noted that only two of seven patients who presented in the first trimester with cholecystitis carried their pregnancies to term.

If ascending cholangitis develops, cholecystectomy should not be postponed. Cholecystectomy should also be performed if common bile duct obstruction occurs or severe pancreatitis develops. Certainly, surgery should not be delayed if an acute abdomen develops. In these instances temporizing will only increase perinatal and maternal risks.[37] If cholecystectomy is performed in the second or third trimester, fetal mortality is less than 5 percent.[39] If pancreatitis secondary to biliary tract stones remains untreated, however, the fetal mortality approaches 60 percent.[39]

Dixon and colleagues,[42] reviewing their experience with 44 patients, found that conservative management of cholecystitis was followed by recurrent episodes of biliary tract symptoms requiring multiple hospitalizations. Cholecystectomy performed in the second trimester was associated with little maternal morbidity, no fetal loss, and a substantial reduction of total hospital days. Baille and colleagues[43] demonstrated that they were able to avoid cholecystectomy in five women by performing endoscopic sphincterotomy. Four of these patients had acute cholangitis, and one had pancreatitis. All five women delivered healthy infants at term. Their experience indicates that endoscopic retrograde cholangiopancreatography and sphincterotomy can be safely performed in pregnancy.[43] Before recommending such treatment on a widespread basis, more studies need to be conducted with this technique.

GASTROINTESTINAL DISEASE

Peptic Ulcer Disease

The symptoms and complications of peptic ulcer seem to decrease during pregnancy. This observation, which remained anecdotal for many years, has been supported by Clark,[44] who interviewed pregnant women with a previous history of peptic ulcer disease and found that in 313 pregnancies 44 percent became asymptomatic and 44 percent demonstrated a marked improvement in symptoms. Only 12 percent remained the same or experienced worsening symptoms during gestation. There were no serious complications reported in this series. Of note, nearly one-half of the patients relapsed by 3 months postpartum, and 75 percent had experienced recurrent symptoms by 6 months after delivery.

Several factors that might improve the clinical course of patients with peptic ulcer disease during pregnancy have been investigated. It is well known that patients with duodenal ulcer have higher levels of basal and stimulated acid secretion. It has been suggested that the amelioration of symptoms during pregnancy may in part be secondary to progesterone-induced lower gastric acid output as well as increased mucous production. The latter may exert a protective effect on the intestinal mucosa.[45] In addition, the placenta is rich in histaminase, which may inactivate histamine or block its action at the level of the parietal cell. Plasma levels of histaminase increase dramatically during pregnancy and may be responsible for a decline in gastric acid output in patients who exhibit hyperacidity in the nonpregnant state.[46]

Studies investigating gastric acid secretion during pregnancy have presented conflicting data. Spiro et al.[47] obtained serial gastric aspirates on one woman with a previous history of duodenal ulcer and reported a diminution in pepsin output and an associated elevation of pH during the last 4 months of gestation. In contrast, VanThiel et al.[48] reported no significant differences in basal and peak acid outputs at 12, 24, and 36 weeks gestation and 1 to 4 weeks postpartum in four women without a previous history of peptic ulcer disease.

Most physicians, when evaluating pregnant women with dyspepsia, attribute this complaint to gastric reflux in the lower esophagus. Heartburn is most often observed in the second and third trimesters. It usually responds to antacid therapy and to minimizing reflux by having the mother assume a semirecumbent position when she is supine. This regimen will often bring relief to patients with underlying peptic ulcer disease as well, and further diagnostic procedures are rarely needed. In patients with profound pain that is unresponsive to antacid regimens, panendoscopic examination of the stomach and upper duodenum may be performed. Barium studies of the upper gastrointestinal tract should in most cases be avoided in pregnancy, as they present a potential risk to the developing fetus.

The primary medical treatment for the symptomatic patient with peptic ulcer disease during pregnancy remains antacid therapy and diet. Administration of 15 to 30 cc of antacid 1 hour after meals and at bedtime usually provides relief of symptoms and promotes ulcer healing. It is important to be aware that potential side effects of antacid therapy exist (Table 36.2). Patients with peptic ulcer disease should be maintained on a normal diet, avoiding caffeine, salicylates, ethanol, or any gastric stimulant that aggravates their condition. Because basal acid output can normally rise during evening hours, it follows that patients should avoid bedtime snacks.

At the present time, H_2 antagonists (cimetidine and ranitidine) remain a second-line choice for ulcer therapy in pregnancy. Although preliminary studies in animals have failed to demonstrate teratogenic effects, experience with these agents in humans is limited.[49] Using a fetal heart preparation, Wollemann and Papp[50] determined that the positive chronotropic and inotropic effects of histamine may be blocked by cimetidine. Cimetidine has antiandrogenic activity, as demonstrated by feminization of male rat pups exposed in utero.[51] As adults, these animals had diminished weights of androgen-sensitive tissues and reduced libido. Although these effects were not demonstrated in ranitidine-treated rats, however, experience with this drug during pregnancy is limited. Therefore the use of histamine blockers in pregnancy should be limited to those rare patients who are refractory to standard antacid therapy.

Fewer than 100 cases of pregnant women who develop serious complications from peptic ulcer disease have been reported in the literature.[52] Bleeding, perforation, and obstruction should be treated as they would be in nonpregnant patients. Becker-Andersen and Husfelt,[52] in reviewing 30 cases of hemorrhage from peptic ulcer during pregnancy, clearly demon-

Table 36.2 Potential Side Effects of Antacid Therapy

Agent	Side Effect
Sodium bicarbonate	May yield large amount of absorbed sodium
Magnesium hydroxide	Hypermagnesemia in renal insufficiency: laxative effect
Calcium carbonate	Constipation, hypercalcemia, milk alkali syndrome
Aluminum hydroxide	Constipation, phosphate binding, and depletion

strated a decrease in maternal and fetal mortality rates with prompt surgical exploration. The only two maternal deaths in their series occurred in patients who were in shock at the time of operation. However, a 44 percent fetal mortality rate was recorded in patients who were first managed conservatively. These investigators stress that perforation and hemorrhage must be treated surgically based on the same indications as in nonpregnant patients. If a partial gastrectomy is to be performed in the third trimester, it may be advisable to begin the procedure with a cesarean section. The fetus appears to be quite sensitive to maternal circulatory failure caused by hypovolemia, and, in addition, gastric surgery may be facilitated after the gravid uterus has been evacuated.

Acute Pancreatitis

The true incidence of pancreatitis complicating pregnancy is difficult to ascertain. In 500 cases of acute pancreatitis, only seven patients developed the disease while pregnant.[53] Corlett and Mishell[54] reported an incidence of 1 in 1,066 pregnancies, and Wilkinson[55] noted 1 in 2,888 deliveries over a 5-year period. Prior to 1972, maternal mortality rates approached 50 percent in some series. Maternal death is now uncommon, especially if the diagnosis is established promptly.[54] There appears to be a greater association of gallstones with the development of pancreatitis during gestation. McKay et al.[53] noted that 18 of 20 patients who developed pancreatitis while pregnant or within 5 months postpartum had cholelithiasis. Overall, biliary tract stones may account for one-third of the cases of pancreatitis during pregnancy.[54] In nonpregnant individuals, alcoholism is by far the most common etiologic factor. While most cases of pancreatitis in pregnancy are idiopathic, infection, previous surgery, toxemia, hyperparathyroidism, thiazide ingestion, and penetrating duodenal ulcer are all potential causes. The normal hypertriglyceridemia of pregnancy can be exaggerated in patients with hyperlipidemia, thereby inducing acute pancreatitis.

The clinical presentation of pancreatitis is not significantly altered in pregnancy. The disease may occur at any stage of gestation, but is more common in the third trimester and the puerperium. Epigastric pain, which may radiate to the flanks or shoulders, with abdominal tenderness should prompt appropriate laboratory investigation. Occasionally, a patient will present with nausea and vomiting as her only complaints. Mild fever and leukocytosis may be present. Radiographic examination of the abdomen simply reveals an adynamic ileus. The differential diagnosis includes most causes of abdominal pain in young women. These are principally peptic ulcer disease including perforation, acute cholecystitis, biliary colic, and intestinal obstruction.

Specific tests employed to corroborate the diagnosis of pancreatitis rely on the measurement of pancreatic enzymes, principally amylase. Elevated values should suggest pancreatitis, although they may be present with other conditions such as cholecystitis, intestinal obstruction, peptic ulcer disease, hepatic trauma, and ruptured ectopic pregnancy. The interpretation of serum amylase values is more difficult during gestation. DeVore et al.[56] noted that amylase levels were lower in pregnancy, although this difference was not statistically significant. They utilized the amylase/creatinine clearance ratio to diagnose pancreatitis in pregnancy. This ratio is normally lowered during gestation as a result of an increased creatinine clearance. DeVore et al.[56] reported that all patients with pancreatitis demonstrated an increased ratio, including two with preeclampsia and hyperemesis gravidarum.

In most cases, acute pancreatitis resolves spontaneously within several days. Pancreatic secretory activity should be reduced by keeping the patient NPO and providing nasogastric suction and necessary fluid and electrolyte replacement. Meperidine is the drug of choice for analgesia. In advanced cases, hypocalcemia may be present, and calcium replacement is necessary. Patients who have been unable to eat for periods of greater than 1 week may benefit from intravenous alimentation.[57]

When conservative therapy fails, surgical drainage of the pancreatic exudate may be necessary. Jacobs et al.[58] found that profoundly ill patients survived twice as often if they underwent surgical drainage. Of course, laparotomy carries with it the added risks of preterm labor and delivery. Patients who relapse may also develop a pseudocyst. This complication requires surgical intervention after a period of time in which an adequate drainage procedure can be accomplished. In spite of the high rate of preterm labor even in conservatively managed cases, the fetal salvage rate, in cases of maternal pancreatitis, has been reported to be as high as 89 percent.[55]

Inflammatory Bowel Disease

The inflammatory bowel diseases ulcerative colitis (UC) and Crohn's disease (CD) or regional enteritis are idiopathic disorders that have their peak incidence in the reproductive age group. UC is a disease of the colon or rectum, marked by acute attacks of bloody stools, diarrhea, cramping, abdominal pain, weight loss, and dehydration. The histologic findings include a decreased number of goblet cells, crypt abscesses, ulcerations, and an inflammatory infiltrate consisting of lymphocytes, plasma cells, and polymorphonuclear cells. The prevalence of ulcerative colitis in the female population under 40 years of age is 40 to 100/100,000.[59] CD is considerably less common than UC, with an incidence of 2 to 4/100,000. The average age of onset is between 20 and 30 years. CD, in contrast to UC, tends to run a more subacute and chronic course, with symptoms that include fever, diarrhea, and cramping abdominal pain.[60] CD can be found anywhere from mouth to anus, including the perineum. However, the distal ileum, colon, and anorectal region are most frequently involved. Histologically, the inflammation is focal, with fissuring, ulcerations, and prominent lymphoid aggregates present. The hallmark of the histologic diagnosis is transmural involvement of the bowel coupled with the presence of multiple noncaseating granulomas. Because CD may involve only the colon, histologic differentiation from UC becomes important.

Ulcerative Colitis

Most studies have failed to provide adequate information on the specific effects of UC on fertility. McDougall,[61] in a retrospective report on 131 married women, noted that only 20 were nulliparous. Unfortunately, few data were provided about the assessment of fertility in these patients. DeDombal et al.[62] observed that only 31 percent (72/229) of women in the reproductive age group with UC became pregnant. However, a true fertility rate could not be established because of inadequate follow-up and the unknown desirability of pregnancy among the study group. In 1980, Willoughby and Truelove[63] provided data that suggested that UC had little if any effect on fertility. Of 137 women desiring pregnancy,

119 (87 percent) conceived, a rate similar to that in most normal populations. This study, however, spanned 10 years and may not reflect periods of impaired fertility related to increased activity of the disease.

Data describing the influence of UC on pregnancy outcome are more conclusive. Prior to 1948, UC was believed to have a deleterious effect on pregnancy. Subsequently, Felsen and Wolarsky[64] reported 34 women who experienced 43 full-term deliveries in 50 pregnancies. There were three spontaneous abortions, two therapeutic abortions, and one ectopic pregnancy in this early series. Because the women who suffered a miscarriage did not have active disease, Felsen and Wolarsky[64] concluded that UC did not adversely affect pregnancy.

In a classic report published in 1951, Abramson et al.[65] divided patients with UC into four groups. Group I consisted of women with inactive disease at the start of pregnancy, group II patients with active disease in early pregnancy, group III patients with onset of disease during gestation, and group IV patients in whom disease developed during the puerperium. Their data revealed that patients in group I had the best prognosis, as 18 of 20 had full-term pregnancies, with seven experiencing exacerbation of disease during gestation or in the postpartum period. Of 12 patients in group II, all had term pregnancies marked by exacerbation of disease during pregnancy or the puerperium. Of five women in group III whose disease commenced during pregnancy, three fetal deaths occurred. It should be remembered, however, that this report antedated the use of steroids and other medications presently available to control active disease.

In 1956, Crohn et al.[66] published their experience with UC in pregnancy. They analyzed the perinatal outcomes in 110 women during 150 pregnancies using Abramson's classification. Group I contained 74 pregnancies in which 62 were successful. The disease was reactivated in 54 percent of cases, including all six spontaneous abortions. Group II patients suffered reactivation of disease during pregnancy or postpartum in nearly 75 percent of cases. Pregnancy was successful in 84 percent (32/38) of women in this group. The data of Crohn et al.[66] suggested that patients with reactivation of quiescent disease during pregnancy had higher rates of abortion. However, their 19 group III patients with new-onset disease experienced only one stillbirth and no spontaneous losses. The data of DeDombal et al.[62] support the view that women with quiescent UC that becomes active during pregnancy are *not* at increased risk for miscarriage. In their series, only 1 of 17 patients with active disease in the first 6 months miscarried.[62] In contrast, a recent Danish study demonstrated a higher probability of miscarriage in women with active disease at conception. Seven of 19 women in this category versus 9 of 133 with quiescent disease suffered a miscarriage.[67]

Willoughby and Truelove[63] confirmed that a good outcome can generally be expected in pregnancies complicated by UC. Furthermore, their study included a group of 102 patients treated with modern therapies including steroids, sulfasalazine, or both. They recorded a spontaneous abortion rate of only 11 percent in 216 women followed over a 20 year period. Women with quiescent disease at conception had a slightly greater chance of successfully reaching term when compared with patients whose disease was active during pregnancy. The proportion of low-birth-weight babies and the incidence of anomalies were similar to those of the general population. This study also examined the effect of pregnancy on UC. Of the 129 pregnancies in which colitis was quiescent at the time of conception, 90 (70 percent) of the patients remained free of symptoms throughout pregnancy and the puerperium. This figure compares favorably with the data of Crohn et al.[66] in which 46 percent remained free of active disease (Table 36.3). DeDombal et al.[62] also confirmed that pregnancy had little adverse effect on UC. In the reproductive age group, they found a 45 percent chance of developing recurrent disease in any given year. This figure seems appropriate to apply to pregnant patients from the data currently available.

Crohn's Disease

As in studies of UC, it has been difficult to determine the effect of CD on fertility. In studies that lacked full evaluation and follow-up, Crohn et al.[68] and Fielding and Cooke[69] reported infertility rates of 38 and 26 percent, respectively. Interestingly, Fielding and Cooke's study revealed a much higher infertility rate (67 percent) if CD involved the colon. DeDombal et al.[70] have confirmed that a high proportion of patients with large bowel disease are "subfertile." They suggest that temporary infertility may be related to the activity of the disease. Khosla et al.[71] described infertility in 112 patients with CD and reported a 12 percent rate, similar to that seen in the general population. In a more recent case–control study, the number of offspring of women with CD was 57 percent of that of paired controls. This study concluded that disease location had no influence on fertility.[72]

Studies describing the effects of CD on pregnancy suggest minimal if any increased risk to both mother and fetus. In the 1956 report of Crohn et al.,[66] 53 patients with regional ileitis had 84 pregnancies, and 75 infants (89 percent) survived. Seventy-one of these deliveries occurred at term.[68] However, the three patients who developed CD during pregnancy suffered two stillbirths and one preterm delivery. The only maternal death occurred in this group. In 1970, Fielding and Cooke[69] reported favorable outcomes in a series of patients with both regional ileitis and CD. Their study described an 85 percent live birth rate among 52 women in 98 pregnancies.[69] DeDombal et al.[70] similarly cite excellent results, 88 percent full-term deliveries in 60 pregnancies, utilizing more modern therapies (Table 36.4).

Two recent investigations suggest that active CD carries with it a greater risk of spontaneous miscarriage.[71,73] Khosla et al.[71] reported a 35 percent spontaneous loss rate in patients with active disease at the time of conception. In patients with severe disease, miscarriage occurred 50 percent of the time. These data are supported by a Danish study in which the risk of both preterm delivery and spontaneous abortion were found to be significantly higher in women with active disease at conception.[73]

A subgroup of patients deserves further mention —those who first develop disease during pregnancy. The caution about unfavorable outcomes in such patients has been supported by Martimbeau et al.[74] They reported 10 patients, including one with twins in whom infant deaths occurred. Four of these neonatal deaths followed an operative procedure. However, tocolytics and neonatal intensive care were unavailable in most of these cases.

The effect of pregnancy on CD is similar to that reported for patients with UC (Table 36.3). DeDombal et al.[70] reported that 73 percent of patients had no change in disease activity, 15 percent improved, and

Table 36.3 Effects of Pregnancy on Ulcerative Colitis

Investigators	No. of Pregnancies	Exacerbation During Gestation	Active Disease in Pregnancy
Quiescent disease at conception			
Abramson et al.[65]	20	7 (35)	—
Crohn et al.[66]	74	40 (54)	—
DeDombal et al.[62]	80	27 (33)	—
Willoughby and Truelove[63]	129	39 (30)	—
Active disease at conception			
Abramson et al.[65]	12	—	12 (100)
Crohn et al.[66]	38	—	29 (76)
Willoughby and Truelove[63]	55	—	29 (53)

Values in parentheses are percentages.

10 percent worsened during pregnancy. If a woman conceives while CD is in remission, she is just as likely to remain in remission as a nonpregnant patient. In the study of Khosla et al.,[72] 44 of 52 (84 percent) women with quiescent CD at conception remained in remission during pregnancy. Relapses, when present, were most commonly observed in the first trimester. Postpartum flare-ups were virtually absent in contrast to the 40 percent postpartum recurrence rate reported by DeDombal et al.[71] Khosla et al.[72] also noted that patients with clinically active disease at the time of conception usually continue to have symptoms during pregnancy. Only seven of 20 patients (35 percent) in this category went into remission or had slight improvement with pregnancy. Overall, the risk of exacerbation during pregnancy is not higher than that in the nonpregnant population.[72]

Treatment of Inflammatory Bowel Disease During Pregnancy

The medical treatment of inflammatory bowel disease is not altered greatly by pregnancy. All patients should be followed closely so that the activity of their disease can be assessed and psychological support can be provided. Because emotional tension can adversely affect both UC and CD, it is important that patients with inflammatory bowel disease have the opportunity to discuss the stress of pregnancy openly. Dietary counseling for patients with UC should emphasize proper nutritional intake. Patients with mild disease may respond to a low-roughage diet or to the

Table 36.4 Live Birth Rate in Pregnancies Complicated by Crohn's Disease

Investigators	No. of Pregnancies	Early Active Disease		Disease in Remission		Total	
		No.	Percent	No.	Percent	No.	Percent
Crohn et al.[68] (1956)	75	28/30	93	36/45	80	64/75	85
Fielding and Cooke[69] (1970)	98	—		—		82/09	85
DeDombal et al.[70] (1972)	57	—		—		53/57	93
Khosla et al.[71] (1984)	74	12/20	60	36/54	66[a]	48/74	65

[a] One patient had nine successive miscarriages (patients included were diagnosed before conception).

exclusion of milk products if they are lactose intolerant. In contrast, patients with CD often benefit from low-residue diets, presumably because the caliber of their small bowel may be limited by inflammation.

The initial therapy for episodes of diarrhea generally includes narcotics such as codeine and diphenoxylate. Chronic use of narcotics should be avoided, as they may incite toxic megacolon in patients with UC. When simple measures are unsuccessful in quieting an attack, sulfasalazine and steroid therapy should be strongly considered. The safety of both of these drugs has been well established in pregnancy.

Sulfasalazine (azulfidine) is most effective in maintaining remission and preventing further attacks. Patients who present early in pregnancy on sulfasalazine for a recent flare-up of their disease should probably be maintained on this therapy as active colitis may develop if the drug is discontinued. Concerns about the use of sulfasalazine in late pregnancy centered on its ability to cross the placenta, displace bilirubin, and cause kernicterus. However, the active fetal metabolite sulfapyridine has weak bilirubin-displacing activity, and the actual risk is small. Jaundice was not increased in 209 neonates of women treated with azulfidine. The safety of sulfasalazine in breast-feeding has raised some concern. The concentration of sulfapyridine in breast milk is approximately 45 percent that of maternal serum. Thus this drug can be given safely to nursing mothers.[75]

Steroids are indicated in patients who fail to respond to simple supportive measures. Steroid retention enemas may be effective for mild to moderate distal colitis or proctitis. Patients with severe disease are initially treated with high doses of intravenous hydrocortisone or its equivalent. Oral prednisone can then be substituted and tapered as the attack subsides. The safety of corticosteroids and sulfasalazine in pregnancy associated with inflammatory bowel disease was addressed in a national survey by Mogadam et al.[75] In 287 pregnancies in which either or both drugs were employed versus 244 untreated patients, no adverse effects could be found that were attributable to these drugs. The higher complication rates associated with severe CD in that study seemed to be more related to disease activity than to the use of medication.[75]

Patients with severe disease who become profoundly dehydrated require hospitalization and intravenous fluids. The development of significant hypoalbuminemia coupled with inadequate caloric intake may require the institution of parenteral hyperalimentation. The benefits of such nutritional therapy include diminished gastrointestinal secretion and motility, potential relief of partial obstruction, closure of fistulas, and renewal of immunocompetence. Anemia should also be treated aggressively by transfusion, although mild anemias will generally respond to oral iron therapy.

Surgical Treatment

Although most acute episodes of inflammatory bowel disease respond to medical treatment, operative intervention will occasionally be necessary to treat perforation, obstruction, or patients unresponsive to standard therapies. While elective surgery for medically intractable disease or recurrent dysplastic lesions of the colon is best accomplished following pregnancy, patients who have undergone definitive surgical procedures for UC seem to fare well during pregnancy. Surgery during pregnancy does carry a significant risk of preterm delivery, probably because of the amount of uterine manipulation required during efforts to reach the distal colon. Surgery should not be delayed, however, in cases of perforation or complete obstruction. Anderson and colleagues[76] have reported three cases of emergency colectomy during pregnancy for toxic megacolon in women with fulminant UC. There were no maternal deaths; however, two stillbirths occurred, as well as one preterm delivery.

Ileostomy function during pregnancy is normal in most cases. Of 84 term pregnancies reported by Hudson,[77] intestinal obstruction occurred in just 7 cases. Of 17 cesarean sections performed in his series, all were done for obstetric indications. Similarly, Gopal and colleagues[78] described 82 pregnancies in 66 women following colostomy or ileostomy. Stomal dysfunction responded to conservative measures in all but 3 women who required surgery for intestinal obstruction. Complications from an episiotomy have been uncommon in patients previously operated on for UC. Data are not available for CD. However, the higher rate of perineal involvement in these patients should warrant a thorough evaluation before contemplating vaginal delivery.

Surgery for CD, unlike UC, is generally not curative. It is estimated that 40 percent of patients with ileitis will require surgery at some time for obstruction, perforation, extensive fistulas, or perirectal suppuration.[60] Most surgical procedures must limit the amount of bowel resection because of the diffuse nature of this disease. Patients with Crohn's colitis who have undergone proctocolectomy are at substantial risk for recurrent disease, including persistent perineal wounds in up to 60 percent of cases.[79] Delivery by cesarean section should be considered for patients with perianal disease who have been diverted to promote healing. Those patients with CD who require surgery during pregnancy are usually operated on for obstruction.[80] As with UC, there may be a high incidence of fetal loss. The decision to perform a simultaneous cesarean section must be individualized according to the type of procedure involved, its indications, and gestational age.

REFERENCES

1. Moise KJ Jr, Shah DM: Acute fatty liver of pregnancy: etiology of fetal distress and fetal wastage. Obstet Gynecol 69:482, 1987
2. Haemerli VP: Jaundice during pregnancy with special emphasis on recurrent jaundice during pregnancy and its differential diagnosis. Acta Med Scand 179(Suppl 144):1, 1966
3. Nash DT, Dale JT: Acute yellow atrophy of liver in pregnancy. NY State J Med 71:458, 1971
4. Hou SH, Levin S, Ahola S et al: Acute fatty liver of pregnancy: survival with early cesarean section. Dig Dis Sci 29:449, 1984
5. Ebert EC, Sun EA, Wright SH et al: Does early diagnosis and delivery in acute fatty liver of pregnancy lead to improvement in maternal and infant survival? Dig Dis Sci 29:453, 1984
6. Purdie JM, Walters BN: Acute fatty liver of pregnancy: clinical features and diagnosis. Aust NZ J Obstet Gynaecol 28:62, 1988
7. Shaffer EA: Liver disease in pregnancy. Curr Probl Obstet Gynecol 7:15, 1984

8. Minuk GY, Lui RC, Kelly JK: Rupture of the liver associated with acute fatty liver of pregnancy. Am J Gastroenterol 82:457, 1987
9. Roh LS: Subcapsular hematoma in fatty liver of pregnancy. J Forensic Sci 31:1509, 1986
10. Riley CA, Romero R, Duffy TP: Hepatic dysfunction with disseminated intravascular coagulation in toxemia of pregnancy: a distinct clinical syndrome. Gastroenterology 80:1346, 1981
11. Brown MS, Reddy KR, Hensley GT, et al: The initial presentation of fatty liver of pregnancy mimicking acute viral hepatitis. Am J Gastroenterol 82:554, 1987
12. Riley CA, Latham PS, Romero R, Duffy TP: Acute fatty liver of pregnancy: a reassessment based on observations in nine patients. Ann Intern Med 106:703, 1987
13. Snyder RR, Hankins GD: Etiology and management of acute fatty liver of pregnancy. Clin Perinatol 13:813, 1986
14. Barton JR, Sibai BM, Mabie WC, Shanklin DR: Recurrent acute fatty liver of pregnancy. Am J Obstet Gynecol 163:534, 1990
15. Goodacre RL, Hunter DJ, Millward S et al: The diagnosis of acute fatty liver of pregnancy by computed tomography. J Clin Gastroenterol 10:680, 1988
16. Mabie WC, Dacus JV, Sibai BM et al: Computed tomography in acute fatty liver of pregnancy. Am J Obstet Gynecol 158:142, 1988
17. Ockner SA, Brunt EM, Cohn SM et al: Fulminant hepatic failure caused by acute fatty liver of pregnancy treated by orthotopic liver transplantation. Hepatology 11:59, 1990
18. Furhoff AK, Hellstrom K: Jaundice in pregnancy: a follow-up study of the series of women originally reported by L. Thorling. I. The pregnancies. Acta Med Scand 193:259, 1973
19. Rencoret R, Aste H: Jaundice during pregnancy. Med J Aust 1:167, 1973
20. Reyes H, Gonzalez MC, Rabalta J et al: Prevalence of intrahepatic cholestasis of pregnancy in Chile. Ann Intern Med 88:487, 1978
21. Gonzalez MC, Reyes H, Arrese M et al: Intrahepatic cholestasis of pregnancy in twin pregnancies. J Hepatol 9:84, 1989
22. Rannevik G, Jeppsson S, Kullinder S: Effect of oral contraceptives on the liver in women with recurrent cholestasis during previous pregnancies. J Obstet Gynaecol Br Commonw 79:1128, 1972
23. Berg B, Helm G, Petersohn L, Tryding N: Cholestasis of pregnancy: clinical and laboratory studies. Acta Obstet Gynecol Scand 65:107, 1986
24. Wilson JA: Intrahepatic cholestasis of pregnancy with

marked elevation of transaminases in a black American. Dig Dis Sci 32:665, 1987

25. Engstrom J, Hellstrom J, Posse N, Sjoball J: Recurrent cholestasis of pregnancy: treatment with cholestyramine of one case with an unusually early onset. Acta Obstet Gynecol Scand 49:29, 1970

26. Ghent CN, Bloomer JR, Koatska G: Elevations in skin tissue levels of bile acids in humans with cholestasis: relation to serum levels and to pruritis. Gastroenterology 73:125, 1977

27. Wojcicka-Jagodzinska J, Kuczynska-Sicinska J, Czajkowski K, Smolarczyk R: Carbohydrate metabolism in the course of intrahepatic cholestasis in pregnancy. Am J Obstet Gynecol 161:959, 1989

28. Adlercreutz H, Svanbor A, Anber A: Recurrent jaundice in pregnancy. I. A clinical and ultrastructural study. Am J Med 42:335, 1967

29. Johnson WG, Baskett TF: Obstetric cholestasis: a 14 year review. Am J Obstet Gynecol 143:299, 1979

30. Johnson P, Samsioe G, Gustafsson A: Studies in cholestasis of pregnancy with special reference to clinical aspects and liver function tests. Acta Obstet Gynecol Scand 54(Suppl):77, 1975

31. Fisk NM, Storey GN: Fetal outcome in obstetric cholestasis. Br J Obstet Gynaecol 95:1137, 1988

32. Espinoza J, Barnaf L, Schnaidt E: The effect of phenobarbital on intrahepatic cholestasis of pregnancy. Am J Obstet Gynecol 119:234, 1974

33. Bloomer JR, Bower JL: Phenobarbital effects in cholestasis liver disease. Ann Intern Med 82:310, 1975

34. Laatikinen T: Effect of cholestiramine and phenobarbital on pruritis and serum bile acid levels in cholestasis of pregnancy. Am J Obstet Gynecol 132:501, 1978

35. Laifer SA, Darby MJ, Scantlebury VP et al: Pregnancy and liver transplantation. Obstet Gynecol 76:1083, 1990

36. Riley CA, Romero R, Duffy TP: Hepatic dysfunction with disseminated intravascular coagulation in toxemia of pregnancy: a distinct clinical syndrome. Gastroenterology 80:1346, 1981

37. Kammerer WS: Nonobstetric surgery during pregnancy. Med Clin North Am 63:1157, 1979

38. Bennion LJ, Grundy SM: Risk factors for the development of cholithiasis in man. N Engl J Med 299:1221, 1978

39. Printen KJ, Ott RA: Cholecystectomy during pregnancy. Am Surg 44:432, 1978

40. Hiatt JR, Hiatt JC, Williams RA, Klein SR: Biliary disease in pregnancy: strategy for surgical management. Am J Surg 151:263, 1986

41. Lockwood C, Stiller RJ, Bolognese RJ: Maternal total parenteral nutrition in chronic cholecystitis: a case report. J Reprod Med 32:785, 1987

42. Dixon NP, Faddis DM, Silberman H: Aggressive management of cholecystitis during pregnancy. Am J Surg 154:292, 1987

43. Baillie J, Cairns SR, Putman WS, Cotton PB: Endoscopic management of choledocholithiasis during pregnancy. Surg Gynecol Obstet 171:1, 1990

44. Clark DH: Peptic ulcer in women. Br Med J 1:1259, 1953

45. DeVore GR: Acute abdominal pain in the pregnant patient due to pancreatitis, acute appendicitis, cholecystitis or peptic ulcer disease. Clin Perinatol 7:349, 1980

46. Clark DH, Tankel HI: Gastric acid and plasma histaminase during pregnancy. Lancet 2:886, 1954

47. Spiro HM, Schwartz RD, Pilot ML: Peptic ulcer in pregnancy: a serial study of gastric secretion during pregnancy. Am J Dig Dis 4:289, 1959

48. VanThiel DH, Gavaler JS, Joshi SN et al: Heartburn of pregnancy. Gastroenterology 72:666, 1977

49. Zulli P, DiNisia Q: Cimetidine treatment during pregnancy. Lancet 2:945, 1978

50. Wollemann M, Papp JG: In vivo cimetidine blocks positive chronotropic and ventricular inotropic effects of histamine on the fetal heart. Agents Actions 9:29, 1979

51. Parker S, Schade R, Pohl C et al: Prenatal and neonatal exposure of male rats to cimetidine but not ranitidine adversely affects subsequent sexual functioning. Gastroenterology 86:675, 1984

52. Becker-Anderson H, Husfelt V: Peptic ulcer in pregnancy. Acta Obstet Gynecol Scand 59:391, 1971

53. McKay AJ, O'Neill J, Imrie CW: Pancreatitis, pregnancy, and gallstones. Br J Obstet Gynaecol 87:47, 1980

54. Corlett RC, Mishell DR: Pancreatitis in pregnancy. Am J Obstet Gynecol 113:281, 1972

55. Wilkinson EJ: Acute pancreatitis in pregnancy: a review of 98 cases and a report of 8 new cases. Obstet Gynecol Surv 28:5,281, 1973

56. DeVore GR, Bracken M, Berkowitz RL: The amylase/creatinine clearance ratio in normal pregnancy and pregnancies complicated by pancreatitis, hyperemesis grandarum, and toxemia. Am J Obstet Gynecol 136:747, 1980

57. Weinberg RB, Sitrin MD, Adkins GM et al: Treatment of hyperlipidemic pancreatitis in pregnancy with total parenteral nutrition. Gastroenterology 83:1300, 1982

58. Jacobs ML, Daggett WM, Civetta JM: Acute pancreatitis: analysis of factors influencing survival. Ann Surg 185:43, 1977

59. Kirsner JB, Shorter RG: Recent developments in non-

specific inflammatory bowel disease. N Engl J Med 306:775, 1982

60. Sorokin JJ, Levine SM: Pregnancy and inflammatory bowel disease: a review of the literature. Obstet Gynecol 62:247, 1983

61. MacDougall I: Ulcerative colitis and pregnancy. Lancet 271:641, 1956

62. DeDombal FT, Watts JM, Watkinson G, Goligher JC: Ulcerative colitis and pregnancy. Lancet 2:599, 1965

63. Willoughby CP, Truelove SC: Ulcerative colitis and pregnancy. Gut 21:469, 1980

64. Felsen J, Wolarsky W: Chronic ulcerative colitis and pregnancy. Am J Obstet Gynecol 56:751, 1948

65. Abramson D, Jankelson IR, Milner LR: Pregnancy in idiopathic ulcerative colitis. Am J Obstet Gynecol 6:121, 1951

66. Crohn BB, Yarnis H, Cohen EB et al: Ulcerative colitis and pregnancy. Gastroenterology 30:391, 1956

67. Nielson OH, Andreasson B, Dondesen S et al: Pregnancy in ulcerative colitis. Scand J Gastroenterol 18:735, 1986

68. Crohn BB, Yarnis H, Korelitz BI: Regional ileitis complicating pregnancy. Gastroenterology 31:615, 1956

69. Fielding JF, Cooke WT: Pregnancy and Crohn's disease. Br Med J 2:76, 1970

70. DeDombal FT, Burton IL, Goligher JC: Crohn's disease and pregnancy. Br Med J 3:550, 1972

71. Khosla R, Willoughby CP, Jewell DP: Crohn's disease and pregnancy. Gut 25:52, 1984

72. Mayberry JF, Weterman IT: European survey of fertility and pregnancy in women with Crohn's disease: a case control study by European collaborative group. Gut 27:821, 1986

73. Haagen Nielsen O, Andreasson B, Bondesen B et al: Pregnancy in Crohn's disease. Scand J Gastroenterol 19:724, 1984

74. Martimbeau PW, Welch JS, Weiland LH: Crohn's disease and pregnancy. Am J Obstet Gynecol 122:746, 1975

75. Mogadam M, Dibbins MO, Korelitz BI, Ahmed SW: Pregnancy and inflammatory bowel disease: effect of sulfasalazine and corticosteroids on fetal outcome. Gastroenterology 80:72, 1981

76. Anderson JB, Turner GM, Williamson RCN: Fulminant ulcerative colitis in late pregnancy and the puerperium. Proc R Soc Med 80:492, 1987

77. Hudson CN: Ileostomy in pregnancy. Proc R Soc Med 65:281, 1972

78. Gopal KA, Amshel AL, Shonberg IL et al: Ostomy and pregnancy. Dis Colon Rectum 28:912, 1985

79. Block GE: Surgical management of Crohn's colitis. N Engl J Med 302:1068, 1980

80. Davis MR, Bohon CJ: Intestinal obstruction in pregnancy. Clin Obstet Gynecol 26:832, 1983

Chapter 37

Neurologic Disorders

Philip Samuels

SEIZURE DISORDERS

Affecting approximately 0.5 percent of the population of North America, seizure disorders are the most common major neurologic problem that coexists with pregnancy. Approximately 75 percent are idiopathic in origin, and 25 percent are acquired. Because seizures affect 0.15 percent of all pregnancies, obstetricians should become familiar with the medical and social problems that surround these disorders. They should also be familiar with the treatment of seizures and the teratogenic potential of the medications commonly employed.

Idiopathic seizures can be categorized into generalized tonic/clonic seizures, partial complex seizures that may or may not generalize, and absence seizures (petit mal). Correct classification is important to initiate and maintain treatment with the appropriate therapeutic agent.

Effects of Pregnancy on Epilepsy

Does pregnancy increase the frequency of seizures? Ramsay et al.[1] reviewed seven studies undertaken between 1938 and 1976, including 155 pregnancies complicated by epilepsy. The frequency of seizures increased in 45 percent, remained unchanged in 43 percent, and decreased in 12 percent.[2] Knight and Rhind[3] reported that those patients with frequent seizures were four times more likely to have an in-

creased seizure frequency during pregnancy. They also observed that a patient carrying a male fetus was twice as likely to have deterioration of seizure control during pregnancy as a patient carrying a female fetus[3]; however, this has not been confirmed by others. In these early studies, frequent measurements of serum anticonvulsant levels were not performed. Gjerd and coworkers[4] compared the frequency and severity of seizures in 78 pregnancies in 66 patients. They compared seizure frequency during pregnancy with that during the 9 months before pregnancy in the same patients. No statistical differences between seizure frequencies before and during pregnancy were found. There was also no evidence that seizures became more severe during pregnancy.[4] No relationship was found between the type of epilepsy and the change in seizure frequency during pregnancy. In India, Bag and coworkers studied seizure frequency in 30 pregnant epileptic patients. Seizure frequency increased in 14 patients, remained unchanged in 15, and decreased in one. Patients with increased seizure frequency had significantly higher estrogen levels and lower progesterone levels than did those who did not have an increased seizure frequency.[5] They also had lower levels of anticonvulsant drugs compared with those with no change. Bardy[6] also reported the seizure frequency in 154 pregnancies in 140 patients with epilepsy. Thirty-two percent of patients had an increase in seizure frequency, 14 percent had a decrease, and 23 percent remained unchanged. Also, 31 percent of the patients were seizure free during the study period.[6] No variables were found that predicted an increase in seizure activity. In this study, the highest incidence of major convulsive seizures occurred during the last trimester of pregnancy, whereas the incidence of complex partial seizures was highest during the puerperium.[6] Bardy and coworkers[7] examined electroencephalograms (EEGs) of epileptic women in late pregnancy. These were compared with the EEGs prior to pregnancy. The number of epileptic interictal discharges was not modified by pregnancy. There were no correlations between EEG findings and changes in seizure frequency.[7] Nonetheless, with the increased understanding of the pharmacokinetics of antiseizure medications and with modern techniques for measuring total and free drug levels, seizure control during pregnancy can be greatly improved.

Effects of Epilepsy on Pregnancy

Annegers and colleagues[8] found that neither epilepsy nor in utero anticonvulsant drug exposure was associated with an increased risk of miscarriage. An epileptic mother has 1 chance in 30 of delivering a child who will later develop a seizure disorder. Although many studies have shown that seizure disorders can be inherited, the precise mode of inheritance remains elusive. The roles of the seizures themselves and of the anticonvulsant medications and teratogenesis are still controversial (Table 37.1). Definitive relationships between specific anticonvulsants and congenital anomalies are difficult to establish, because many patients take more than one agent. The extensive review of published studies performed by Nakane et al.[9] revealed that 4.5 percent of infants of untreated epileptic mothers and 7.1 percent of infants of treated epileptic mothers exhibited major malformations. However, the studies surveyed by Nakane and colleagues[9] did not have a uniform definition of major malformation, and some did not even define the malformations present. In their own series, Nakane et al.[9] documented an 8.7 percent malformation rate in 657 infants of mothers with seizure disorders taking anticonvulsant medications. Nelson and Ellenberg[10] noted an increased incidence of intrauterine growth retardation (IUGR) and decreased head circumference in infants of epileptic mothers.

The teratogenic potential of phenytoin has received much attention. In 1976, Hanson[11] first described the fetal hydantoin syndrome, consisting of microcephaly, mild to moderate mental retardation, developmental delay, prenatal and postnatal growth retardation, facial clefts, facial dysmorphisms, and limb anomalies. The hands may exhibit finger-like thumbs as well as distal phalangeal and nail hypoplasia.[12] Hanson[11] reported some features of this syndrome in 11 percent of infants exposed in utero to phenytoin. Others, however, consider this figure an overestimation of the frequency of malformations associated with phenytoin.[13–16] Gaily and coinvestiga-

Table 37.1 Common Side Effects of Anticonvulsants

Drug	Maternal Effects	Fetal Effects
Phenytoin	Nystagmus, ataxia, hirsutism, gingival hyperplasia, megaloblastic anemia	Possible teratogenesis and carcinogenesis, coagulopathy, hypocalcemia
Phenobarbital	Drowsiness, ataxia	Possible teratogenesis, coagulopathy, neonatal depression, and/or withdrawal
Primidone	Drowsiness, ataxia, nausea	Possible teratogenesis, coagulopathy, neonatal depression
Carbamazepine	Drowsiness, leukopenia, ataxia, mild hepatotoxicity	Possible craniofacial and neural tube defects
Valproic acid	Ataxia, drowsiness, alopecia, hepatotoxicity, thrombocytopenia	Neural tube defect and possible craniofacial and skeletal defects
Trimethadione	Drowsiness, nausea	Strong teratogenic potential
Ethosuximide	Nausea, hepatotoxicity, leukopenia, thrombocytopenia	Possible teratogenesis

tors[17] feel that the risk of developmental disturbance associated with intrauterine phenytoin exposure is much lower than the 7 to 11 percent risk of fetal hydantoin syndrome reported earlier. In fact, they found that several minor anomalies previously regarded as typical of fetal hydantoin syndrome appear instead to be genetically linked to epilepsy. They reached these conclusions by studying 114 mothers and 87 fathers of 121 children born to mothers with epilepsy.[17] Many of the minor anomalies thought to be characteristic of the hydantoin syndrome were observed in the mothers of the children. In this study, only hypertelorism and digital hypoplasia showed a statistical correlation with phenytoin exposure.[17]

In the general population congenital heart disease occurs in 3 to 5 infants per 1,000 live births. In those exposed to phenytoin in utero, the incidence is approximately 18 per 1,000.[13,18] While the frequency of cleft palate in the general population is 1 to 2 per 1,000, the incidence appears to be 12 to 18 per 1,000 in infants exposed in utero to phenytoin.[13,19] Friis[20] undertook a study to determine whether genetic factors play an important role in the etiology of facial clefts in the offspring of epileptic patients. The rate of facial clefts was 4.7 times greater in children of mothers taking anticonvulsant medications than in the background population. Therefore, they believe that drug exposure plays a larger role than genetics in the development of facial clefts. Kallen and colleagues[21] also found the rate of facial clefts higher in infants of mothers who had taken phenytoin and/or phenobarbital. To arrive at this conclusion they studied 318 malformed infants whose mothers were known to have epilepsy. Several cases of Wilms' tumor and neuroblastoma have also been reported in infants with the fetal hydantoin syndrome.[22-24]

Phenytoin has also been implicated in causing a relative vitamin D deficiency during gestation. Normally, cholecalciferol is hydroxylated to 25-hydroxycholecalciferol in the liver. It then passes to the kidney, where most is again hydroxylated to the active 1,25-dihydroxycholecalciferol. The patient taking phenytoin may metabolize an inordinate amount of 25-hydroxycholecalciferol to the inactive compound 24,25-dihydroxycholecalciferol.[25] Also, phenytoin may interfere with the intestinal absorption of calcium. Maternal and neonatal hypocalcemia have been reported in patients taking phenytoin, and tetany has

occurred in neonates exposed to phenytoin in utero.[26] Patients taking phenytoin should therefore receive supplemental vitamin D during pregnancy.[26,27] The amount of vitamin D contained in prenatal vitamins is adequate prophylaxis.

Phenytoin, phenobarbital, and primidone have been implicated in the pathogenesis of a neonatal coagulopathy. In contrast to hemorrhagic disease of the newborn, infants with this anticonvulsant-associated coagulopathy most often bleed during the first 24 hours after birth.[28,29] The coagulopathy is caused by the suppression of fetal synthesis of the vitamin K–dependent clotting Factors II, VII, IX, and X in the fetal liver.[28,30] Therefore all infants born to mothers taking these anticonvulsants should receive 1 mg of vitamin K intramuscularly at birth.[28-31] Such treatment, however, may not always prevent bleeding.[31,32] Some investigators suggest giving oral vitamin K supplementation throughout the last month of pregnancy to women taking phenytoin, phenobarbital, or primidone. The efficacy of such therapy, however, has not been prospectively proven.

Infants exposed to phenobarbital in utero may exhibit decreased alertness in the immediate newborn period. They may also take longer to adjust to breast-feeding. Barbiturate withdrawal may occur late in the first week of life in up to 20 percent of these infants. Usually, only supportive care is necessary. These signs may also be seen in infants exposed to primidone in utero, as one of its major metabolites is phenobarbital. Phenobarbital also appears to be associated with a reduction in birth weight and head circumference.[33] Kallen and coworkers[21] found that infants exposed to phenobarbital in utero were more likely to have facial clefts when compared with a control group.

Carbamazepine had the reputation of being a safe anticonvulsant medication. A recent study by Jones and colleagues[34] retrospectively examined eight children who had prenatal exposure to carbamazepine and prospectively followed 72 women who were taking carbamazepine throughout gestation. These fetuses were not exposed to other anticonvulsant agents. An 11 percent incidence of craniofacial defects, a 26 percent incidence of fingernail hypoplasia, and developmental delays in 20 percent were noted.[34] These researchers postulate that because the anomalies were similar to those seen in the fetal hydantoin syndrome, the teratogenicity may be related to the fact that both drugs are metabolized through an arene oxide pathway. They raise the possibility that it is the epoxide intermediate rather than the specific drug itself that is teratogenic.[34] Infants born to women taking carbamazepine may exhibit an increase in the incidence of neural tube defects, although this is not statistically significant.[21,21a] Because 20 percent of patients taking carbamazepine will develop leukopenia, these patients should have a complete blood count every 4 to 6 weeks.

Although valproate is an excellent anticonvulsant, it should not be used in women of childbearing age because of its teratogenic potential. There is an increased incidence of neural tube defects in infants born to women taking valproate during pregnancy.[21,35,36] Any woman taking valproate in early pregnancy, therefore, should be offered fetal assessment by targeted ultrasonography as well as by a serum α-fetoprotein determination. Craniofacial defects have also been seen with valproate.[35] Chitayat and coworkers[35] describe three children born to a mother with epilepsy. Two siblings who were exposed to valproate in utero had craniofacial defects. In addition, these neonates had skeletal abnormalities that had not been previously reported. Tsuru et al.[36] also noted a case of polydactylism in an infant born to a mother taking valproate during gestation.

Much controversy surrounds discussion of neonatal growth and mental development in infants with in utero exposure to anticonvulsant drugs. Gaily and coworkers[37] investigated intelligence in a group of 148 children of epileptic mothers and in 105 control children enrolled in a prospective study during pregnancy. The prevalence of mental deficiency in the study group was 1.4 percent, only slightly higher than the general population. Although the mean intelligence quotients obtained at 5.5 years of age were significantly lower in the study group than in the control group, there was no increased risk of low intelligence attributable to fetal exposure to below toxic levels of antiepileptic drugs or to brief maternal convulsions.[37] Bertollini and coworkers[38] found an increased risk of IUGR in infants born to mothers taking carbamazepine monotherapy. Gaily and Granstrom[39] followed growth parameters in 132 children of epileptic mothers and compared them with 103 control children. The mean increment in length in the first postnatal month was significantly less in drug-exposed children than in the control group. The drug-exposed offspring also gained significantly less weight during the first postnatal month. However, by the second postnatal month a normal growth rate had been established.[39] Importantly, this transient growth retardation was not associated with excessive minor anomalies or impaired intelligence at the age of 5.5 years.[39]

Trimethadione, a drug used for the treatment of petit mal epilepsy, is a potent teratogen. Feldman and colleagues[40] showed that 87 percent of exposed pregnancies were complicated by spontaneous abortion or by a major fetal malformation. The fetal trimethadione syndrome consists of IUGR, microcephaly, mild to moderate mental retardation, developmental delay, facial dysmorphisms, congenital heart defects, gastrointestinal abnormalities, inguinal hernias, and hypospadias. Petit mal epilepsy rarely affects patients during the childbearing years. When it does, however, ethosuximide should be the drug of choice, and trimethadione should be avoided.

Effects of Pregnancy on the Disposition of Anticonvulsant Medications

The normal physiologic alterations that occur during pregnancy can have profound effects on the level of anticonvulsant medications. Hypothetically, these changes are sufficient to lower drug concentrations below therapeutic levels and may indirectly cause the exacerbation of seizures observed during pregnancy in some patients (Table 37.2).

Increased plasma volume, the presence of the fetal and placental compartments, and the expansion of extracellular fluid all increase the volume of distribution of anticonvulsant medications and can lower the total serum concentration of anticonvulsants. Only the free, unbound drug, however, is pharmacologically active. This tenet is important when considering the pharmacokinetics of phenytoin and phenobarbital, which are 90 and 60 percent protein bound, respectively. In late pregnancy, total protein and serum albumin levels fall. There is less protein with which drugs can bind, so the amount of pharmacologically active, unbound drug can theoretically increase. Therefore the level of free drug may be unchanged or actually increased while the level of total drug is decreased. Some clinical laboratories are now measuring free levels of phenytoin.

Because of its nonlinear kinetics, phenytoin is most

Table 37.2 Anticonvulsants Commonly Used During Gestation

Drug	Therapeutic Level (μg/ml)	Usual Nonpregnant Daily Dosage
Phenytoin	10–20	300–500 mg/day in single or divided doses
Phenobarbital	15–40	90–180 mg/day in three divided doses
Primidone	5–15	750–1,500 mg/day in three divided doses
Carbamazepine	4–10	600–1,200 mg/day in three or four divided doses
Ethosuximide	40–100	500–1,500 mg/day in two to three divided doses

affected by gestation, with concentrations sometimes decreasing to one-half of prepregnancy levels. These changes may be more apparent than real because of decreased protein binding in late pregnancy.[41] Bardy et al.[42] measured maternal serum phenytoin levels biweekly or monthly during pregnancy in 111 women. The concentrations decreased toward the end of pregnancy but were lowest at the time of delivery.[42] In 48 percent of patients, the drug dosage had to be increased to combat an increased seizure frequency. Koerner et al.[43] demonstrated changes in valproic acid disposition secondary to protein binding in pregnancy. Monthly free and total valproic acid levels were obtained in nine epileptic women followed prospectively throughout gestation. Despite an upward adjustment of the dose in four patients, total valproic acid levels declined as pregnancy proceeded, but free levels remained unchanged.[43]

Many patients experience nausea and vomiting during early pregnancy, which will reduce the absorption of anticonvulsant drugs from the gastrointestinal tract. Decreased gastric motility may also alter the absorption of these medications.

The barbiturates and phenytoin induce hepatic microsomal enzymes that hasten their own metabolism. In addition, pregnancy increases the liver's ability to hydroxylate these medications. Folic acid is a necessary coenzyme in these hydroxylation reactions. As the levels of these enzymes increase, serum folic acid

levels may fall.[44,45] In addition, phenytoin appears to interfere with folate absorption from the gastrointestinal tract.[46] There is a delicate balance between folic acid consumption and anticonvulsant therapy. If supplemental folate is administered, more drug can be metabolized, and the serum concentration of drugs may be lowered. It is therefore important to measure serum anticonvulsant levels frequently whenever a patient begins taking folic acid during pregnancy.

Folate antagonists are potent teratogens. Could this be the mechanism by which anticonvulsants produce fetal anomalies? In laboratory animals, dietary folate deficiency has been shown to cause congenital malformations.[47] Retrospective human data concerning folate deficiency and congenital malformations have been conflicting. A large prospective study, however, showed no relationship between serum folate levels during early pregnancy and fetal malformations.[48] Nonetheless, 1 mg of folate should be administered each day to pregnant patients taking anticonvulsants. If possible, this medication should be started before conception.

Primidone is the only major anticonvulsant that is eliminated primarily by the kidney. Its metabolites, phenobarbital and phenylmethylmalonamide, are metabolized in the liver. The increase in creatinine clearance observed during pregnancy will cause significant falls in the levels of primidone.

In general, women on anticonvulsant medication should be allowed to breast-feed their infants (see Ch. 11). The infant is certainly receiving no more medication than it did in utero. All anticonvulsant drugs, including carbamazepine and phenytoin, enter breast milk.[49] However, the amount detectable in breast milk is only 1 to 2 percent of the mother's dose. Tsuru et al.[36] showed that the ratio of valproic acid in breast milk to blood was only 1 in 30 to 1 in 50.

Recommendations

If possible patients should be counseled before conception.[50] If the patient has not had seizures in many years, an attempt may be made to gradually withdraw her from anticonvulsant medications and reinstitute them if seizures recur. Of course, the patient should not drive during this period. These changes should only be made before conception and in conjunction with a neurologist.

If treatment is necessary, patients with tonic/clonic

seizures should be treated with phenobarbital. If patients have partial complex seizures, primidone or carbamazepine are also acceptable choices. If these medications are not effective, substitutions or additions should be made. It is paramount to control the patient's seizure frequency. Physicians should use whatever medications are necessary to achieve this goal. Once a patient is pregnant, no attempt should be made to change her anticonvulsant medications if her regimen is effective. A change in medication during pregnancy may precipitate seizures that may be devastating to both mother and fetus. Because of decreased esophageal sphincter tone and increased intra-abdominal pressure during pregnancy, aspiration is a distinct possibility in patients who experience tonic/clonic seizures. If at all possible, patients should be maintained on a single anticonvulsant medication.[50] No patient should take trimethadione or valproate during pregnancy, if possible.

Before conception, patients receiving anticonvulsants should be taking vitamin supplements and an additional 1 mg of folic acid daily. This will correct the potential vitamin D deficiency caused by chronic phenytoin therapy and will prevent megaloblastic anemia in pregnancy. Once folate supplementation has been implemented, anticonvulsant levels should be monitored every 2 to 4 weeks until they are stable, with drug doses being adjusted to keep the patient's level within the range necessary to prevent seizures. Only then should the patient attempt conception.

Once pregnant, the patient should be reassured that adequate control of her seizures is the most important aspect of therapy. She should be encouraged to take her medication regularly and should not deprive herself of sleep, as sleep deprivation has been associated with an exacerbation of seizures.[51] Should the patient experience hyperemesis, antiemetics should be used to allow the patient to take her oral anticonvulsant medications and to ensure they are properly absorbed. It is paramount to reassure the patient that the purpose of anticonvulsant medications is to prevent seizures that produce serious complications for her and potentially for the fetus. She must be counseled that, although these medications probably have some teratogenic effect, she still has an approximately 85 to 90 percent chance of having a normal child.

Anticonvulsant levels should be monitored monthly, and drug dosages should be adjusted accordingly to prevent seizures. If the patient is taking phenytoin, free phenytoin levels should be obtained if possible. The desired free phenytoin level is 1 to 2 μg/ml.

Targeted ultrasonography should be performed at 18 weeks gestation to evaluate the fetus for possible anomalies. Fetal echocardiography should also be performed to rule out cardiac anomalies. Serial ultrasound examinations at 4- to 6-week intervals will also help to assess fetal growth. If there is any evidence of IUGR or decreased amniotic fluid volume, antepartum fetal evaluation should be started at 28 weeks gestation. Vitamin K supplements might be helpful if the patient is taking phenobarbital, primidone, or phenytoin. The usual dose of vitamin K is 10 mg per day starting at 34 weeks gestation, presumably to prevent neonatal coagulopathy.

Patients are expected to proceed normally through pregnancy. Vaginal delivery is anticipated, and cesarean section should be undertaken only for obstetric indications. An experienced pediatrician should be present at delivery in the event that serious fetal anomalies are found. Cord blood should also be obtained for a prothrombin time, and the neonate should be given vitamin K, 1 mg intramuscularly. If circumcision is to be performed, it should be withheld until the results of the prothrombin time are known.

During labor, patients who are taking phenobarbital or phenytoin may receive these drugs parenterally. Phenytoin may be safely administered intravenously. It must be mixed only with normal saline, as precipitation occurs with dextrose. The usual dose is 100 mg administered intravenously every 6 to 8 hours, provided the patient has a therapeutic phenytoin level at the onset of labor. If labor is prolonged, a phenytoin level should be checked. In the patient taking phenobarbital or primidone, phenobarbital should be administered intramuscularly. The usual dose is 60 mg intramuscularly every 6 to 8 hours. Similarly, phenobarbital levels should be checked if labor is protracted.

In the postpartum period, anticonvulsant levels should be frequently monitored. Rapid physiologic changes will occur, and anticonvulsant doses will frequently need to be reduced.

Epilepsy is *not* a contraindication to pregnancy![51a] The vast majority of patients with an idiopathic seizure disorder can successfully carry pregnancies to term without endangering themselves or their fetuses. Cooperation among the obstetrician, neurologist, and pediatrician is essential. Patients should constantly be reminded that the most important aspect of obstetric/neurologic care is the prevention of seizures and that the proper anticonvulsant regimen is the cornerstone of therapy. Obstetricians and neurologists must remember that conventional doses of these medications may be inadequate during pregnancy. The important guidelines are the absence of seizures and the blood levels of medication, not the actual amount ingested.

MIGRAINE

Between 15 and 20 percent of pregnant women are affected by migraine headaches.[52] This statistic is difficult to confirm, as many patients without classic migraine symptoms claim to have migraine headaches. The headaches, which are associated with vasodilatation of the cerebral vasculature, last a variable amount of time. They are often accompanied by photosensitivity and nausea.

Migraine symptoms tend to improve during pregnancy.[53-55] Friedman and Merritt[54] found that more than 80 percent of their patients reported improvement of migraine symptoms, with some experiencing no headache at all during pregnancy. Lance and Anthony[55] noted that those patients who experience severe migraines near the time of their menses actually improve most during pregnancy. Chen and co-workers[56] identified 508 women with a history of migraine from the Collaborative Perinatal Project of the National Institute of Neurological and Communicative Disease Disorders and Stroke. They found that patients with migraines smoke more heavily and had a longer smoking history than did their headache-free peers. They also found that in nonsmokers migraine was often associated with allergies.[56]

Chancellor and colleagues[57] followed nine patients whose migraines first occurred during pregnancy at various gestational ages. They were followed for more than 4 years after pregnancy, and the prognosis for headache was excellent. Four of the nine patients developed complications of pregnancy, including preeclampsia in two.[57] Jacobson and Redman[58] re-

ported a patient who actually lost consciousness during pregnancy because of a basilar migraine.

Supportive therapy is recommended for patients who experience migraine attacks during gestation. Analgesics can be used as necessary. Nonsteroidal antiinflammatory agents should be avoided in late pregnancy, because when used over a long period they can cause premature closure of the ductus arteriosus and/or oligohydramnios. When pain is severe, parenteral narcotics and appropriate antiemetic therapy may be used. Propranolol may be safely administered during pregnancy. Calcium channel blockers are becoming widely used in the treatment of migraine. Nifedipine has been used safely as a tocolytic agent and can probably be given for migraines as well.

Ergotamine is best avoided during pregnancy. Previous reports have suggested it may cause birth defects that have a vascular disruptive etiology. Hughes and Goldstein[59] report a case in which an infant showed evidence of early arrested cerebral maturation and paraplegia. They hypothesize that ergotamine, acting either alone or in synergy with propranolol and caffeine, produced fetal vasoconstriction resulting in tissue ischemia and subsequent malformation.[59] It is important to note that this etiology is strictly theoretical.

Dietary factors may precipitate migraine attacks. Careful history may uncover foods that should be avoided, including Chinese food with monosodium glutamate, red wine, cured meats, and strong cheeses containing tyramine. Relative hypoglycemia and alcohol can also trigger migraine attacks.

CEREBROVASCULAR DISEASES

Arterial Occlusion

Twelve percent of arterial occlusions occur in women between the ages of 15 and 45 years, and approximately one-third of these patients may be pregnant.[60] In a recently published study from India, 37 percent of patients affected with cerebrovascular disease were under the age of 40 years, with a significant number of thromboses occurring during pregnancy and the puerperium.[61] Overall, the incidence of cerebral arterial occlusion in pregnancy is approximately 1 per 20,000 live births.[60,62] The mortality rate for pregnant women with cerebral arterial occlusion is twice that of men and three times that of nonpregnant women. According to Jennett and Cross,[60] middle cerebral artery occlusion is most common during pregnancy, whereas internal carotid artery occlusion is observed most often in the puerperium. Hemiplegia and dysphasia are frequent findings.[62] Predisposing factors such as preeclampsia, chronic hypertension, or hypotensive episodes can be demonstrated in about one-third of these patients. Brick and Riggs[63]

have shown that oral contraceptives also raise the risk of ischemic cerebral vascular disease. One-half of the pregnancy-related cases occur during the immediate postpartum period and the remainder during the second and third trimesters. Brick[64] reported the case of a woman who had a documented partial obstruction of the left middle cerebral artery during the third trimester of pregnancy. Following delivery, her symptoms abated, and angiography 11 weeks later

Table 37.3 Differential Diagnosis of Peripartum Seizures

	Blood Pressure	Proteinuria	Seizures	Timing	CSF	Other Features
Eclampsia	+++	+++	+++	Third trimester	Early: RBC 0–1,000 Protein 50–150 mg/dl Late: grossly bloody	Platelets normal or ↓ RBC normal
Epilepsy	Normal	Normal to +	+++	Any trimester	Normal	Low anticonvulsant levels
Subarachnoid hemorrhage	+ to +++ (labile)	0 to +	+	Any trimester	Grossly bloody	
Thrombotic thrombocytopenic purpura	Normal to +++	++	++	Third trimester	RBC 0–100	Platelets ↓↓ RBC fragmented
Amniotic fluid embolus	Shock	−	+	Intrapartum	Normal	Hypoxia, cyanosis Platelets ↓↓ RBC normal
Cerebral vein thrombosis	+	−	++	Postpartum	Normal (early)	Headache Occasional pelvic phlebitis
Water intoxication	Normal	−	++	Intrapartum	Normal	Oxytocin infusion rate >45 mU/min Serum Na <124 mEq/L
Pheochromocytoma	+++ (labile)	+	+	Any trimester	Normal	Neurofibromatosis
Autonomic stress syndrome of high paraplegics	+++ with labor pains	−	−	Intrapartum	Normal	Cardiac arrhythmia
Toxicity of local anesthetics	Variable	−	++	Intrapartum	Normal	

(Modified from Donaldson,[111] with permission.)

revealed complete resolution of the obstruction. Brick[64] therefore felt that this lesion was the result of reversible intimal hyperplasia from the increased estrogen and progesterone levels of pregnancy.

In cases of cerebral arterial occlusion, care must be taken to avoid increased intracranial pressure. If signs of increased intracranial pressure develop, parenteral dexamethasone should be administered. Osmotic diuresis can be used if needed. Supportive measures are also necessary, including close monitoring of electrolytes to detect inappropriate secretion of antidiuretic hormone. Physical and rehabilitative therapy should be started as soon as possible. These patients can progress normally through pregnancy and deliver vaginally.

A case of maternal death from carotid artery thrombosis associated with the HELLP syndrome (hemolysis, elevated liver enzymes, and low platelet count) has been reported by Katz and Cefalo.[65] They proposed that the infarction occurred because the patient experienced a rebound thrombocytosis leading to a hypercoagulable state. They stress the importance of closely following patients with HELLP syndrome so that those who develop a reactive thrombocytosis can be monitored for signs and symptoms of cerebral thrombosis.

Cortical Venous Thrombosis

The chief symptoms in patients with cortical venous thrombosis are headache, lethargy, and vomiting. Hemiplegia has a gradual onset, and seizure activity is common (Table 37.3).[66,67] This disorder occurs most frequently during the immediate postpartum period and may be attributed to a hypercoagulable state.[68] Although an incidence of 1 in 10,000 pregnancies was suggested in one study, this appears to be a large overestimate.[69] With the availability of sophisticated computed tomography (CT) and magnetic resonance imaging (MRI), accurate diagnosis is possible. Because most patients with cortical venous thrombosis show signs of seizure activity within 24 hours of the onset of symptoms, prophylactic anticonvulsants should be started immediately.[66] The drug of choice is phenytoin. The patient should be given a loading dose of 10 mg/kg followed by 300 to 500 mg orally each day. Phenytoin levels should be checked frequently to make certain that they are therapeutic and that the patient does not develop phenytoin toxicity.

Subarachnoid Hemorrhage

The rate of subarachnoid hemorrhage complicating pregnancy is approximately 1 per 10,400.[70] With the increase in cocaine abuse occurring across the country, this incidence may rise over the next few years, as the associated increase in blood pressure is associated with bleeding from preexisting berry aneurysms and arterial-venous (A-V) malformations.[71] Most subarachnoid hemorrhages occurring in pregnant patients are caused either by rupture of a berry aneurysm or bleeding from a congenital A-V malformation. Most berry aneurysms are thought to be due to a congenital defect in the elastic and smooth muscle layers of cerebral blood vessels. They are usually located in the vessels of the circle of Willis or those arising from it. Robinson and coworkers[72] evaluated 26 patients with spontaneous subarachnoid hemorrhage during pregnancy and found that approximately one-half were caused by berry aneurysms and one-half by A-V malformations. They observed that A-V malformations are more common in patients below the age of 25 years, and they usually bleed before 20 weeks gestation. Conversely, berry aneurysms occur in patients over the age of 30 years and usually bleed in the third trimester.[72] Pregnancy appears to increase the risk of bleeding from an A-V malformation. The maternal mortality rate associated with an untreated A-V malformation is reported to be 33 percent. This figure, however, is based on old data, and the rate is probably lower today.

Diagnosis and Treatment

Any patient with localized signs of cerebral or meningeal irritation must be thoroughly evaluated. If the clinical examination dictates that further evaluation is necessary, MRI or a CT scan should be performed. If necessary, contrast dyes may be used. The dyes employed in CT scanning do contain nonradioactive iodine, but when used judiciously the chance of inducing a fetal goiter is small. Cerebral angiography can be safely used to pinpoint the origin of cerebral bleeding. Subarachnoid hemorrhages, whether caused by A-V malformations or berry aneurysms, should be treated surgically when possible. Surgery under hypothermia or hypotension appears to cause no adverse fetal effects. The fetal heart rate should be monitored. If fetal bradycardia occurs, blood pressure should be raised sufficiently to normalize the fetal heart rate.[73] Kawasaki and colleagues[74] report a case of cerebellar hemorrhage in a 32-week primigravida. She was treated conservatively until term and was delivered by elective cesarean section. Her surgery was delayed until after delivery and was successful.

If the patient has undergone corrective surgery for an aneurysm or A-V malformation, she should be allowed to deliver vaginally. Because the valsalva maneuver can increase intracranial pressure,[72] epidural anesthesia is recommended. Interestingly, Szabo and colleagues[75] have reported that moderate increases in blood pressure do not cause spontaneous hemorrhage in nonpregnant patients with intracranial A-V malformations. If the aneurysm or A-V malformation has not been surgically corrected, elective cesarean section should be performed when fetal lung maturity has been documented.[72] Laidler and colleagues[76] discussed the advantages of regional anesthesia in these patients. Buckley and coworkers[77] have described a case of simultaneous cesarean section and ablation of a cerebral A-V malformation.

As pregnancy has a deleterious effect on A-V malformations, those patients with inoperable lesions should be counseled about the dangers of future childbearing. Previously, permanent sterilization was encouraged.[72] With improved imaging techniques, the patient should be thoroughly evaluated before any recommendations are made for permanent sterilization.

We have recently cared for two patients with venous-venous (V-V) malformations. These are low-pressure phenomena. Care was coordinated with the patients' neurosurgeons. Both patients progressed to term and delivered vaginally without any hemorrhagic event.

MULTIPLE SCLEROSIS

Multiple sclerosis (MS) is a demyelinating disease that attacks men and women equally. The onset of symptoms usually occurs between the ages of 20 and 40 years. In the United States, the disease is more common in those residing above 40 degrees north latitude. The prevalence for those living in the southern United States is 10 per 100,000, while it is approximately 50 per 100,000 in those living in the northern states.[78] The disease may also cluster within a community.[79] MS has no clear genetic predisposition.

The diagnosis of MS is often made years after the initial onset of sensory symptoms. The onset is usually subtle. Common presenting symptoms include weakness of one or both lower extremities, visual complaints, or loss of coordination. Because the disease primarily affects the white matter of the central nervous system, symptoms attributable to disruption of gray matter are uncommon. The disease is characterized by exacerbations and remissions. Less than one-third of patients show steady progression of their disease after its onset.

It is impossible to predict the long-range prognosis of a patient with MS. About one-half of patients are still able to work at their usual profession 10 years after the onset of the illness. After 20 years, however, only about one-third remain employed. In a study of 185 women with MS, Weinshenker and colleagues[80] showed that there was no association between long-term disability and (1) total number of term pregnancies, (2) the timing of pregnancy relative to the onset of MS, or (3) the worsening of MS in relation to a pregnancy. The average life expectancy in patients with MS is also impossible to predict. Patients may live with the disease for more than 25 years. When death does occur, it is usually attributable to infection.

MS and pregnancy can coexist without unusual complications. Leibowitz and colleagues[81] found no decrease in fertility and no increase in perinatal mortality in patients with MS. Their study suggested that pregnancy does not predispose a patient to MS but that patients with "premorbid" disease are more likely to have the onset of early symptoms during pregnancy. Of 170 pregnant patients with MS studied by Millar and coworkers,[82] relapses occurred in only 45, the majority during the puerperium and postpartum periods. Birk and co-investigators[83] carefully followed pregnancies in eight women with MS. None of the women worsened during pregnancy. Six of the eight women, however, experienced relapses within the first 7 weeks after delivery. They also reported that there were differences in suppressor T-cell levels during pregnancy, but these were not predictive of changes in clinical disease.[83] Frith and McLeod[84] studied 85 pregnancies and found no increased risk of relapse during pregnancy. They noted that most of the relapses that did occur during pregnancy took place in the third trimester. In another series, Frith and McLeod[85] reported that relapses occur most frequently in the last trimester and also in the first 3 months postpartum. In a large study, Nelson and colleagues[86] analyzed 191 pregnancies in women with nonprogressive MS. The exacerbation rate during the 9-month postpartum period was 34 percent, three times that of the 9 months during pregnancy. The rate was highest in the 3 months immediately following delivery and stabilized after postpartum month 6.[86] The exacerbation rates were the same in breast-feeding and non-breast-feeding women. The average time to flare was also similar in both groups. This study verifies that it is safe for women with MS to breast-feed their newborns.[86]

Paraplegic patients are more susceptible to urinary tract infections during pregnancy but may feel no symptoms. Therefore, they should be screened routinely. If the patient has become paraplegic as a result of MS, there may be little pain associated with labor. It might be difficult therefore for the patient to discern when labor begins. Uterine contractions occur normally, but voluntary expulsive efforts may be hindered in the second stage of labor. Delivery by forceps or vacuum extraction therefore may be indicated. Bader and colleagues[87] report that women with MS who receive epidural anesthesia for vaginal delivery do not have a significantly higher incidence of exacerbation of their MS than those receiving only local filtration.

CARPAL TUNNEL SYNDROME

The medial border of the carpal tunnel consists of the pisiform and hamate bones, and its lateral border consists of the scaphoid and trapezium bones. They are covered on the palmar surface by the flexor retinaculum. The median nerve and flexor tendons pass through this carpal tunnel, which has little room for expansion. If the wrist is extremely flexed or extended, the volume of the carpal tunnel is reduced. In pregnancy, weight gain and edema can produce the carpal tunnel syndrome that results from compression of the median nerve. Wallace and Cook[88] first reported the association between carpal tunnel syndrome and pregnancy in 1957. Although 20 percent of pregnant women complain of pain on the palmar surface of the hand, few actually have the true carpal tunnel syndrome.[89] Commonly, the syndrome consists of pain, numbness, and/or tingling in the distribution of the median nerve in the hand and wrist. This includes the thumb, index finger, long finger, and radial side of the ring finger on the palmar aspect. Compressing the median nerve and percussing the wrist and forearm with a reflex hammer, the Tinel maneuver, often exacerbates the pain. In severe cases, weakness and decreased motor function can occur.

McLennan and coworkers[90] studied 1,216 consecutive pregnancies. Of these patients, 427 (35%) reported hand symptoms. Fewer than 20 percent of these 427 affected women described the classic carpal tunnel syndrome. No patient required operative intervention. Most symptoms were bilateral and commenced in the third trimester of pregnancy. Ekman-Ordeberg et al.[91] found a 2.3 percent incidence of carpal tunnel syndrome in a prospective study of 2,358 pregnancies. The syndrome appeared to be more common in primigravidas with generalized edema. Conservative therapy with splinting of the wrist at night completely relieved symptoms in 46 of 56 patients. Of the remaining 10, three required surgery before delivery. Wand[92] retrospectively studied 40 women with carpal tunnel syndrome developing in pregnancy and 18 women with carpal tunnel syndrome that developed in the puerperium. He confirmed that the syndrome occurs most frequently in primigravidas over the age of 30 years. All cases that developed before delivery occurred during the third trimester and resolved within 2 weeks after delivery. In those cases developing during the puerperium in women who breast-fed their infants, the symptoms lasted longer, a mean of 5.8 months.[92] In another series, Wand[93] studied 27 women who developed carpal tunnel syndrome during the puerperium. The condition was associated with breast-feeding in 24 of these women. Symptoms lasted an average of 6.5 months in the breast-feeding women. Only two of these patients required surgical decompression.[93]

Supportive and conservative therapies are usually adequate for the treatment of carpal tunnel syndrome. Symptoms usually subside in the postpartum period as total body water returns to normal.[94] Splints placed on the dorsum of the hand, which keep the wrist in a neutral position and maximize the capacity of the carpal tunnel, often provide dramatic relief. Local injections of glucocorticoids may also be used in severe cases. Although diuretics may help to control carpal tunnel syndrome symptoms over a short period of time, their use is not recommended because the symptoms return rather rapidly after the cessation of treatment. In an uncontrolled series, Ellis[95] reported that pyridoxine in a dose of 100 to 200 mg daily for 12 weeks can provide dramatic relief in a large percentage of patients with carpal tunnel syndrome. Before this can be recommended, controlled trials need to be undertaken.

Surgical correction of this syndrome should not be delayed in patients with deteriorating muscle tone and motor function. Decompression surgery for carpal tunnel syndrome is a simple procedure that can be safely carried out during pregnancy using local anesthesia, an axillary block, or a Bier block. It is important to warn patients that carpal tunnel syndrome can recur in future pregnancies.[96]

PSEUDOTUMOR CEREBRI

Pseudotumor cerebri may complicate as many as 1 in 870 births.[97] It is seen more frequently in pregnant women, particularly those who are obese.[98-100] However, in a recent study by Ireland and colleagues[101] the incidences in pregnant women and in oral contraceptive users were no higher than in control groups. More than 95 percent of these patients present with headaches, and 15 percent have diplopia. Papilledema is found in virtually all patients.[98,102] To establish the diagnosis, one must demonstrate elevated cerebrospinal fluid (CSF) pressure, normal CSF composition, and the absence of an intracranial mass on MRI or CT scan.[103]

The pathogenesis of this disorder is unknown. Bates and colleagues[104] found CSF prolactin to be markedly elevated in cases of pseudotumor cerebri. Prolactin appears to have an affinity for receptors in the choroid plexus, where CSF is produced. Prolactin has osmoregulatory functions and therefore may have a role in the increased CSF production found in pseudotumor cerebri.[98] Some believe that reduced CSF reabsorption is the etiology of pseudotumor cerebri. Ahlskog and O'Neill[105] noted an association be-

tween the occurrence of pseudotumor cerebri and the following conditions: corticosteroid therapy and its withdrawal; nalidixic acid therapy; nitrofurantoin therapy; tetracycline therapy; hypoparathyroidism; deficiencies or excesses of vitamin A; and iron deficiency anemia.

Pregnancy outcome appears to be unaffected by the illness.[98,102] There is no increase in fetal wastage or congenital anomalies.[98] Recently, Koppel and colleagues[106] reported a case of pseudotumor cerebri that presented in a 15-year-old primigravida following eclampsia. It lasted for 3 weeks. Wheatley and colleagues[107] noted a case of pseudotumor cerebri occurring in a diabetic pregnancy. They caution that it is important to make the distinction between symptoms of pseudotumor cerebri and visual impairment caused by diabetic retinopathy as the treatments are different.[107] Thomas[108] described a case of pseudotumor cerebri occurring in two consecutive pregnancies in a woman with hemoglobin SC. In both instances, symptoms resolved following delivery and both infants were born at term.

Most patients respond well to conservative management.[97] The main objectives of treatment are relief of pain and preservation of vision. The patient should be followed closely with visual acuity and visual field determinations at intervals indicated by the clinical condition. In patients with mild disease, analgesics may be adequate. If pain persists, diuretics may be used. Acetazolamide, a carbonic anhydrase inhibitor, will reduce CSF production in many patients.[109] The usual dose is 500 mg twice daily. In more difficult cases, prednisone in doses of 40 to 60 mg daily usually provides good results.[97] Patients may be treated for 2 weeks, with the dose being tapered over the next month.[98] Serial lumbar punctures to reduce CSF pressure are rarely necessary today. Surgical approaches may be used in refractory patients in whom rapid visual deterioration occurs.

Pseudotumor cerebri is not an indication for cesarean section. A review of the literature reveals that 73 percent of the reported patients delivered vaginally.[98] Cesarean section should be undertaken only for obstetric indications. Both epidural and spinal anesthesia, when expertly administered, can be safely used in patients with pseudotumor cerebri.[110] Bearing down, which can increase CSF pressure, should be avoided when possible. The second stage of labor should therefore be shortened by outlet forceps or by vacuum extraction.

The recurrence rate for pseudotumor cerebri appears to be between 10 and 12.3 percent in nonpregnant patients.[99,100] Pregnancy does not appear to predispose to a recurrence.[98]

REFERENCES

1. Ramsay RE, Strauss RG, Wilder J, Willmore LJ: Status epilepticus in pregnancy: effect of phenytoin malabsorption on seizure control. Neurology 28:85, 1978
2. So EL, Penry JK: Epilepsy in adults. Ann Neurol 9:3, 1978
3. Knight AH, Rhind EG: Epilepsy and pregnancy: a study of 153 pregnancies in 59 patients. Epilepsia 16:99, 1975
4. Gjerde IO, Strandjord RE, Ulstein M: The course of epilepsy during pregnancy: a study of 78 cases. Acta Neurol Scand 78:198, 1988
5. Bag S, Behari M, Ahuja GK, Karmarkar MG: Pregnancy and epilepsy. J Neurol 236:311, 1989
6. Bardy AH: Incidence of seizures during pregnancy, labor and puerperium in epileptic women: a prospective study. Acta Neurol Scand 75:356, 1987
7. Bardy AH, Hiilesmaa VK, Teramo KA: Effect of pregnancy on the electroencephalogram of epileptic women. Acta Neurol Scand 78:22, 1988
8. Annegers JF, Baumgartner KB, Hauser WA, Kurland LT: Epilepsy, antiepileptic drugs, and the risk of spontaneous abortion. Epilepsia 29:451, 1988
9. Nakane Y, Okuma T, Takashishi R et al: Multi-institutional study on the teratogenicity and foetal toxicity of anti-epileptic drugs: a report of a collaborative study group in Japan. Epilepsia 21:663, 1980
10. Nelson KB, Ellenberg JH: Maternal seizure disorder, outcome of pregnancy, and neurologic abnormalities in the children. Neurology 32:1247, 1982
11. Hanson JW, Myrianthopoulos NC, Sedgwick MA et al: Risks to the offspring of women treated with hydantoin anticonvulsants, with emphasis on the fetal hydantoin syndrome. J Pediatr 89:662, 1976
12. Nagy R: Fetal hydantoin syndrome. Arch Dermatol 117:593, 1981
13. Committee on Drugs, American Academy of Pediatrics: Anticonvulsants and pregnancy. Pediatrics 63:331, 1979
14. Shapiro S, Hartz SC, Siskind V et al: Anticonvulsants and parental epilepsy in the development of birth defects. Lancet 1:272, 1976
15. Stumpf DA, Frost M: Seizures, anticonvulsants, and pregnancy. Am J Dis Child 132:746, 1978
16. Shapiro S, Slone D, Hartz SC et al: Are hydantoins (phenytoins) human teratogens? J Pediatr 90:673, 1977
17. Gaily E, Granstrom ML, Hiilesmaa V, Bardy A: Minor anomalies in offspring of epileptic mothers. J Pediatr 112:520, 1988
18. Bartoshesky LE, Bhan I, Nagpul K, Pashyan H: Severe cardiac and ophthalmologic malformation in an infant exposed to diphenylhydantoin in utero. Pediatrics 69:202, 1982
19. Erikson JD, Oakley GP: Seizure disorders in mothers of children with orafacial clefts: a case–control study. J Pediatr 84:244, 1974
20. Friis ML: Facial clefts and congenital heart defects in children of parents with epilepsy: genetic and environmental etiologic factors. Acta Neurol Scand 79:433, 1989
21. Kallen B, Robert E, Mastroiacova P et al: Anticonvulsant drugs and malformations: is there a drug specificity? Eur J Epidemiol 5:31, 1989
21a. Rosa FW: Spina bifida in infants of women treated with carbamazepine during pregnancy. N Engl J Med 324:674, 1991
22. Allen RW, Ogden B, Bentley FL et al: Fetal hydantoin syndrome, neuroblastoma, and hemorrhagic disease in a neonate. JAMA 244:1464, 1980
23. Taylor WF, Myers M, Taylor WR: Extrarenal Wilms' tumour in an exposed to intrauterine phenytoin. Lancet 1:478, 1976
24. Sherman S, Roizen N: Fetal hydantoin syndrome and neuroblastoma. Lancet 2:517, 1976
25. Stamp TCB, Round JM, Rowe DJF et al: Plasma levels and therapeutic effect of 25-hydroxycholecalciferol in epileptic patients taking anticonvulsant drugs. Br Med J 4:9, 1972
26. Friis B, Sardemann H: Neonatal hypocalcaemia after intrauterine exposure to the anticonvulsant drugs. Arch Dis Child 52:239, 1977
27. Seip M: Effects of antiepileptic drugs in pregnancy on the fetus and newborn infants. Ann Clin Res 5:205, 1973
28. Solomon GE, Hilgartner MW, Kutt H: Coagulation defects caused by diphenylhydantoin. Neurology 22:1165, 1972
29. Bleyer WA, Skinner A: Fatal neonatal hemorrhage after maternal anticonvulsant therapy. JAMA 235:626, 1976
30. Mountain KR, Hirsh J, Gallus AS: Neonatal coagulation defect due to anticonvulsant drug treatment in pregnancy. Lancet 1:265, 1970

31. Srinivasan G, Seeler RA, Tiruvury A, Pildes R: Maternal anticonvulsant therapy and hemorrhagic disease of the newborn. Obstet Gynecol 59:250, 1982

32. Hill RM, Verniaud WM, Horning MG: Infants exposed in utero to antiepileptic drugs. Am J Dis Child 127:645, 1974

33. Mastroiacovo P, Bertollini R, Licata D: Fetal growth in the offspring of epileptic women: results of an Italian multicentric cohort study. Acta Neurol Scand 78:110, 1988

34. Jones KL, Lacro RV, Johnson KA, Adams J: Pattern of malformations in the children of women treated with carbamazepine during pregnancy. N Engl J Med 320:1661, 1989

35. Chitayat D, Farrell K, Anderson L, Hall JG: Congenital abnormalities in two sibs exposed to valproic acid in utero. Am J Med Genet 31:369, 1988

36. Tsuru N, Maeda C, Tsuruoka M: Three cases of delivery under sodium valproate-placental transfer, milk transfer and probable teratogenicity of sodium valproate. Jpn J Psychiatry Neurol 42:89, 1988

37. Gaily E, Kantola-Sorsa E, Granstrom ML: Intelligence of children of epileptic mothers. J Pediatr 113:677, 1988

38. Bertollini R, Kallen B, Mastroiacovo P, Robert E: Anticonvulsant drugs in monotherapy: effect on the fetus. Eur J Epidemiol 3:164, 1987

39. Gaily E, Granstrom ML: A transient retardation of early postnatal growth in drug-exposed children of epileptic mothers. Epilepsy Res 4:147, 1989

40. Feldman GL, Weaver DD, Lovrien EW: The fetal trimethadione syndrome. Am J Dis Child 131:1389, 1977

41. Leppik IE, Rask CA: Pharmacokinetics of antiepileptic drugs during pregnancy. Semin Neurol 8:240, 1988

42. Bardy AH, Hiilesmaa VK, Teramo KA: Serum phenytoin during pregnancy, labor and puerperium. Acta Neurol Scand 75:374, 1987

43. Koerner M, Yerby M, Friel P, McCormick K: Valproic acid disposition and protein binding in pregnancy. Ther Drug Monit 11:228, 1989

44. Hiilesmaa VK, Teramo K, Granstrom ML, Bardy AH: Serum folate concentrations during pregnancy in women with epilepsy: relation to antiepileptic drug concentrations, number of seizures, and fetal outcome. Br Med J 287:577, 1983

45. Maxwell JD, Hunter J, Steward DA et al: Folate deficiency after anticonvulsant drugs: an effect of hepatic enzyme induction. Br Med J 1:297, 1972

46. Gerson CD, Hepner GW, Brown N et al: Inhibition by diphenylhydantoin of folic acid absorption in man. Gastroenterology 63:246, 1972

47. Norris JW, Pratt RF: Folic acid deficiency and epilepsy. Drugs 8:366, 1974

48. Hall MH: Folic acid deficiency and congenital malformation. J Obstet Gynecol Br Commonw 79:159, 1972

49. Yerby MS: Problems and management of the pregnant woman with epilepsy. Epilepsia 28:s29, 1987

50. Kaneko S: A rational antiepileptic drug therapy of epileptic women in child bearing age. Jpn J Psychiatry Neurol 42:473, 1988

51. Schmidt D, Canger R, Avanzini G et al: Change of seizure frequency in pregnant epileptic women. J Neurol Neurosurg Psychiatry 46:751, 1983

51a. Brodie MJ: Management of epilepsy during pregnancy and lactation. Lancet 336:426, 1990

52. Callaghan P: The migraine syndrome in pregnancy. Neurology 18:197, 1968

53. Somerville B: A study of migraine in pregnancy. Neurology 22:824, 1972

54. Friedman AP, Merritt HH: Headache, Prognosis and Treatment. FA Davis, Philadelphia, 1959

55. Lance JW, Anthony MD: Some clinical aspects of migraine. Arch Neurol 15:356, 1966

56. Chen TC, Leviton A, Edelstein S, Ellenberg JH: Migraine and other diseases in women of reproductive age: the influence of smoking on observed associations. Arch Neurol 44:1024, 1987

57. Chancellor AM, Wroe SJ, Cull RE: Migraine occurring for the first time in pregnancy. Headache 30:224, 1990

58. Jacobson SL, Redman CW: Basilar migraine with loss of consciousness in pregnancy: case report. Br J Obstet Gynaecol 96:494, 1989

59. Hughes HE, Goldstein DA: Birth defects following maternal exposure to ergotamine, beta blocker, and caffeine. J Med Genet 25:396, 1988

60. Jennett WB, Cross JN: Influence of pregnancy and oral contraception on the incidence of strokes in women of childbearing age. Lancet 1:1019, 1967

61. Banerjee AK, Varma M, Vasista RK, Chopra JS: Cerebrovascular disease in north-west India: a study of necropsy material. J Neurol Neurosurg Psychiatry 52:512, 1989

62. Cross JN, Castro PO, Jennett WB: Cerebral strokes associated with pregnancy in the puerperium. Br Med J 3:214, 1968

63. Brick JF, Riggs JE: Ischemic cerebrovascular disease in the young adult: emergence of oral contraceptive use and pregnancy as the major risk factors in the 1980s. WV Med J 85:7, 1989

64. Brick JF: Vanishing cerebrovascular disease of pregnancy. Neurology 38:804, 1988

65. Katz VL, Cefalo RC: Maternal death from carotid artery thrombosis associated with the syndrome of he-

molysis, elevated liver function, and low platelets. Am J Perinatol 6:360, 1989

66. Estanol B, Rodriguez A, Counte G et al: Intracranial venous thrombosis in young women. Stroke 10:680, 1979

67. Krayenbuhl HA: Cerebral venous and sinus thrombosis. Clin Neurosurg 14:1, 1967

68. Bansal BC, Prakash C, Gupta RR, Brahmanandam KRV: Study of serum lipid and blood fibrinolytic activity in cases of cerebral venous/venous sinus thrombosis during the puerperium. Am J Obstet Gynecol 119:1079, 1974

69. Abraham J, Rios PS, Inbaraj SG et al: An epidemiological study of hemiplegia due to stroke in south India. Stroke 1:477, 1970

70. Miller HJ, Hinkley CM: Berry aneurysms in pregnancy: a ten year report. South Med J 63:279, 1970

71. Henderson CE, Torbey M: Rupture of intracranial aneurysm associated with cocaine use during pregnancy. Am J Perinatol 5:142, 1988

72. Robinson JL, Hall CJ, Sevzimer CB: Arterial venous malformations, aneurysms, and pregnancy. J Neurosurg 41:63, 1974

73. Minielly R, Yuzpe AA, Drake CG: Subarachnoid hemorrhage secondary to ruptured cerebral aneurysm in pregnancy. Obstet Gynecol 53:64, 1979

74. Kawasaki N, Uchida T, Yamada M et al: Conservative management of cerebellar hemorrhage in pregnancy. Int J Gynaecol Obstet 31:365, 1990

75. Szabo MD, Crosby G, Sundaram P et al: Hypertension does not cause spontaneous hemorrhage of intracranial arteriovenous malformations. Anesthesiology 70:761, 1989

76. Laidler JA, Jackson IJ, Redfern N: The management of caesarean section in a patient with an intracranial arteriovenous malformation. Anaesthesia 44:490, 1989

77. Buckley TA, Yau GH, Poon WS, Oh T: Caesarean section and ablation of a cerebral arterio-venous malformation. Anaesth Intensive Care 18:248, 1990

78. McAlpine D, Lunisden CE, Acheson ED: Multiple Sclerosis, a Reappraisal. 2nd Ed. Williams & Wilkins, Baltimore, 1972

79. Eastman R, Sheridan J, Poskanzer DA: Multiple sclerosis clustering in a small Massachusetts community. N Engl J Med 289:793, 1973

80. Weinshenker BG, Hader W, Carriere W et al: The influence of pregnancy on disability from multiple sclerosis: a population-based study in Middlesex County, Ontario. Neurology 39:1438, 1989

81. Liebowitz U, Antonovosky A, Katz R et al: Does pregnancy increase the risk of multiple sclerosis? J Neurol Neurosurg Psychiatry 30:354, 1967

82. Millar JHD, Allison RS, Cheeseman EA: Pregnancy as a factor influencing relapse in disseminated sclerosis. Brain 82:417, 1959

83. Birk K, Ford C, Smeltzer S et al: The clinical course of multiple sclerosis during pregnancy and the puerperium. Arch Neurol 47:738, 1990

84. Frith JA, McLeod JG: Pregnancy and multiple sclerosis. J Neurol Neurosurg Psychiatry 51:495, 1988

85. Frith JA, McLeod JG: Pregnancy and multiple sclerosis: an Australian perspective. Clin Exp Neurol 24:1, 1987

86. Nelson LM, Franklin GM, Jones MC: Risk of multiple sclerosis exacerbation during pregnancy and breast-feeding. JAMA 259:3441, 1988

87. Bader AM, Hunt CO, Datta S et al: Anesthesia for the obstetric patient with multiple sclerosis. J Clin Anesth 1:21, 1988

88. Wallace JT, Cook AW: Carpal tunnel syndrome in pregnancy. Am J Obstet Gynecol 73:1333, 1957

89. Nicholas GG, Noone RB, Graham WP: Carpal tunnel syndrome in pregnancy. HAND 3:80, 1971

90. McLennan HG, Oats JN, Walstab JE: Survey of hand symptoms in pregnancy. Med J Aust 147:542, 1987

91. Ekman-Ordeberg G, Salgeback S, Ordeberg G: Carpal tunnel syndrome in pregnancy: a prospective study. Acta Obstet Gynecol Scand 66:233, 1987

92. Wand JS: Carpal tunnel syndrome in pregnancy and lactation. J Hand Surg 15:93, 1990

93. Wand JS: The natural history of carpal tunnel syndrome in lactation. J R Soc Med 82:349, 1989

94. Massey EW: Carpal tunnel syndrome in pregnancy. Obstet Gynecol Surv 33:145, 1978

95. Ellis JM: Treatment of carpal tunnel syndrome with vitamin B6. South Med J 80:882, 1987

96. Tobin SM: Carpal tunnel syndrome in pregnancy. Am J Obstet Gynecol 97:493, 1967

97. Katz VL, Peterson R, Cefalo RC: Pseudotumor cerebri and pregnancy. Am J Perinatol 6:442, 1989

98. Peterson CM, Kelly JV: Pseudotumor cerebri in pregnancy: case reports and literature reviewed. Obstet Gynecol Surv 40:323, 1985

99. Weisberg LA: Benign intracranial hypertension. Medicine (Baltimore) 54:197, 1975

100. Johnston I, Paterson A: Benign intracranial hypertension. II. CSF pressures and the circulation. Brain 97:301, 1974

101. Ireland B, Corbett JJ, Wallace RB: The search for causes of idiopathic intracranial hypertension: a preliminary case–control study. Arch Neurol 47:315, 1990

102. Koontz WL, Herbert WNP, Cefalo R: Pseudotumor cerebri in pregnancy. Obstet Gynecol 62:325, 1983

103. Donaldson JO: Neurology in Pregnancy. WB Saunders, Philadelphia, 1978

104. Bates GW, Whiteworth NS, Parker JL et al: Elevated cerebrospinal fluid prolactin concentration in women with pseudotumor cerebri. South Med J 75:807, 1982

105. Ahlskog JE, O'Neill BP: Pseudotumor cerebri. Ann Intern Med 97:249, 1982

106. Koppel BS, Kaunitz AM, Tuchman AJ: Pseudotumor cerebri following eclampsia. Eur Neurol 30:6, 1990

107. Wheatley T, Clark JD, Edwards OM, Jordan K: Retinal haemorrhages and papilloedema due to benign intracranial hypertension in a pregnant diabetic. Diabetic Med 3:482, 1986

108. Thomas E: Recurrent benign intracranial hypertension associated with hemoglobin SC disease in pregnancy. Obstet Gynecol 67:(3s)7S, 1986

109. Rubin RC, Henderson ES, Ommaya AK et al: The production of cerebrospinal fluid in man and its modification by acetazolamide. J Neurosurg 25:430, 1966

110. Palop R, Choed-Amphai E, Miller R: Epidural anesthesia for delivery complicated by benign intracranial hypertension. Anesthesiology 50:159, 1979

111. Donaldson JO: Peripartum convulsions. p. 312. In Donaldson JO (ed): Neurology of Pregnancy. WB Saunders, Philadelphia, 1989

Chapter 38

Malignant Diseases

Mark B. Landon

Cancer is the second most common cause of death in people of reproductive age. It follows that the risks of malignant disease and its therapy during pregnancy must be fully appreciated by the obstetrician and oncologist. It has been estimated that cancer complicates approximately 1 in 1,000 pregnancies.[1] The most common malignancies associated with pregnancy include breast, cervix, lymphoma, melanoma, leukemia, ovary, and colon. As women continue to delay childbearing, the frequency of these diseases during pregnancy will probably increase.

The diagnosis of cancer during pregnancy creates a series of management dilemmas. Frequently, clinical decision making for the pregnant woman with cancer involves balancing the effects of therapy and delivery on maternal and fetal conditions. As with other medical disorders, one must also consider whether pregnancy can adversely affect the course of disease. Because therapy is often toxic, the potential fetal effects of treatments such as chemotherapy or radiation must be reviewed. With this information in mind, the patient and her physicians must decide when it is appropriate to institute therapy. The patient must also decide whether to continue pregnancy in cases that are diagnosed prior to fetal viability. Finally, the option of early delivery followed by therapy is often considered when a malignancy is discovered in late gestation.

Clear guidelines for the management of pregnant patients with cancer have been difficult to establish, because the number of reported cases for most disease is small. Current management strategies are often based on anecdotal reports that often present conflicting recommendations.[2] Before discussing specific malignancies, it is important to review some of the general data that are available concerning cancer therapy in pregnancy.

CHEMOTHERAPY

Most chemotherapeutic agents are considered to be potentially teratogenic if given during the first trimester of pregnancy. These agents invariably affect the processes of cell division and therefore may be detrimental to the developing embryo. For this reason, antineoplastic drugs are generally avoided during organogenesis. Treatment is often postponed until the second trimester or later.

Nicholson's review[3] found that approximately 10 percent of fetuses exposed to cytotoxic drugs during the first trimester exhibited major malformations. More recently, Doll and colleagues[4] reported a 25 percent incidence (6 of 24 cases) of fetal malformations during the first trimester in cases exposed to combination chemotherapy. Surprisingly, 24 of 139 (17 percent) exposed to a single agent were found to have a malformed fetus.[4] However, some of these women received coincident radiation. If these cases are excluded, the malformation rate with single-agent chemotherapy falls to 6 percent.

In the series cited above, many of the malformations observed after treatment in the first trimester were associated with the antifolate cytotoxic agents aminopterin and methotrexate. Aminopterin is rarely used today. Methotrexate should be avoided if chemotherapy is necessary during pregnancy. Alkylating agents, including busulfan, chlorambucil, and cyclophosphamide, appear to be less potent teratogens than the antimetabolites, with six cases of malformations reported among 50 patients at risk.[5] Although vinblastine is highly teratogenic in animals, there has been only one abnormality reported in 14 first-trimester exposures.[6] There are little data on the related vinca alkaloid vincristine.

In contrast to the above data, there is little evidence of an increased teratogenic risk when cytotoxic drugs are administered during the second and third trimesters. Of 150 cases reviewed by Doll and associates,[5] there were only four (2.6 percent) malformations.

In addition to teratogenesis, chemotherapeutic administration may be associated with an increased risk of miscarriage.[3] Infants born to women who have received chemotherapy during pregnancy also appear to have a greater incidence of low birth weight. In rare cases, the fetal hematopoietic system may be impaired.[7] Finally, whether any potential long-term effects of chemotherapy on the developing fetus exist remains a serious question. A single study that examined neurologic and intellectual performance in 17 offspring of women treated for acute leukemia during pregnancy failed to detect differences when compared with a control group.[8]

Breast-feeding is contraindicated in women who are receiving antineoplastic agents, as significant levels can be found in breast milk.

RADIATION

Maternal exposure to radiation for diagnostic or therapeutic purposes may pose a risk to the fetus (see Ch. 9). Radiation can damage chromatin, leading to cell death or cytogenetic abnormalities. High-dose radiation can result in growth retardation, microcephaly, mental retardation, and ocular malformations.

The exposure of the developing embryo to less than 5 rads represents an insignificant risk for major malformations above the background rate of 2 to 3 percent. Brent[9] has suggested that the threshold for radiation effects in the developing human may actually be as high as 15 to 20 rads. Fortunately, the fetal exposure that accompanies most diagnostic procedures is quite low. For example, a single chest x-ray delivers 8 mrad to the fetus.[9] It follows that radiologic studies that can be critical in establishing a diagnosis should not be avoided in the pregnant patient.

Therapeutic radiation consisting of exposure to more than 5 rads requires a consideration of the merits of continuing pregnancy. An expert in radiation therapy can be helpful in determining the extent and type of radiation risk to the embryo or fetus. Abdominal radiation is generally contraindicated during gestation, whereas subdiaphragmatic exposure with abdominal shielding has been undertaken for malignancies such as Hodgkin's disease.

SPECIFIC MALIGNANT DISEASES

Breast Cancer

Breast cancer is the most common cancer in women, with over 100,000 new cases diagnosed in the United States each year. It is estimated that 1 of 11 women will develop this disease. Approximately 15 percent of cases occur in women under the age of 41 years, with 2 to 3 percent diagnosed during pregnancy. Breast cancer is first detected in approximately 1 in 1,360 to 3,200 pregnancies, making this an uncommon, but not rare, event.[10,11] Prior to the early 1950s, the discovery of breast carcinoma during pregnancy and lactation was associated with a poor prognosis. However, subsequent studies have reported that the outlook for the gravid patient with breast cancer is not much different from that for the nonpregnant woman.

Epidemiologic studies have found that pregnancy decreases the risk of neoplastic breast disease. Multiparous women and in particular those who breast fed have a lower incidence of breast cancer than do nulliparous women. The likelihood of developing breast cancer increases as the age at menarche decreases and as the age at menopause increases. Thus, the longer reproductive function is maintained, the greater the risk. Pregnancy, however, interrupts the cyclical effects of normal ovarian function. The altered hormonal milieu of gestation is believed to produce proliferation of the mammary epithelium, followed by marked differentiation and mitotic rest. These changes may have a protective effect.[12,13] Lactation may also influence neoplastic differentiation, perhaps by removing noxious agents and damaged cells that come into contact with breast epithelium.[12]

Detection and Diagnosis

It is the responsibility of the obstetrician to screen for breast cancer during pregnancy. After taking an appropriate history at the initial visit, a thorough breast examination should be performed, as well as instruction to the patient regarding self-examination. Examination of the breast early in pregnancy is especially important, because as gestation proceeds hypertrophy, engorgement, and increased vascularity make this evaluation considerably more difficult.

Delay in the diagnosis of breast cancer during pregnancy has often been attributed to the physician's reluctance to evaluate properly complaints relating to the breast.[14] Too often, these symptoms are attributed to the normal physiologic changes of pregnancy, and lesions are not biopsied until after delivery. While bilateral serosanguinous discharge may normally accompany late pregnancy, masses with or without unilateral discharge require prompt and definitive evaluation.[15]

The hyperplastic breast of pregnancy is characterized by an increase in radiographic density, limiting the value of mammography. However, mammography should not be avoided because radiation exposure to the fetus is negligible.[16] Fine-needle aspiration of a mass for cytologic study is recommended during pregnancy. Simple needle aspiration can quickly distinguish cysts and galactoceles from solid masses. Aspirates from breast carcinomas are typically highly cellular. False-positive diagnoses are extremely rare, but, more importantly, the false-negative rate is less than 10 percent.[17] Equivocal cytologic diagnoses require excision of the tumor under local anesthesia. This approach minimizes any risk to the fetus and, should a malignancy be detected, permits discussion between patient and physician before planning definitive therapy. In 134 breast biopsies performed during pregnancy or lactation, 29 new cases of cancer were discovered.[14] This corresponds to 1 cancer per 4.6 biopsies, a figure similar to that found in nonpregnant patients.

Most studies of breast cancers in pregnant women indicate that these tumors are histologically identical to neoplasms recovered from nonpregnant women of the same age. The majority are infiltrating ductal carcinomas, although other histologic types are seen. In a series of 63 patients, King et al.[18] reported eight cases of inflammatory carcinoma. Because this lesion can be mistaken for mastitis, it has been suggested that a biopsy of breast tissue be taken when performing incision and drainage of an infected breast.

Prognosis

Prior to the early 1950s, many believed that breast carcinoma found in pregnancy was accompanied by an extremely poor prognosis. In 1942, Haagensen and Stout reported 20 patients, all of whom except one had axillary node involvement. Based on their experience, they concluded that breast carcinoma detected during pregnancy was an incurable disease and that such patients were not candidates for radical mastectomy. However, in 1937, Harrington[19] noted that of the 15 percent of patients in his series presenting without axillary node involvement, 62 percent survived 5 years. This optimistic outlook for patients with early disease remains today. The 5- and 10-year survival rates of pregnant women with breast cancer are similar to those observed in nonpregnant women. In a recent report, the 5-year survival rate for pregnant women without nodal disease was 82 percent and the 10-year survival rate was 71 percent (Table 38.1).

The prognosis of breast cancer depends mainly on the stage of the disease at the time of diagnosis. The presence and degree of lymph node involvement is critical in predicting recurrence following radical mastectomy. During pregnancy, 62 to 85 percent of women have positive axillary nodes at the time of diagnosis.[10,11,18] King et al.[18] reported a 5-year survival rate of 82 percent if less than three nodes were involved, with the 5-year rate falling to 27 percent if greater than three nodes contained tumor. The increased proportion of patients with advanced disease may be due in part to the delay in diagnosis or hormonal and vascular changes that promote tumor growth and metastases. Approximately 70 percent of breast tumors in pregnant women were found to be

Table 38.1 Survival After Surgical Treatment of Breast Cancer in Pregnancy or Lactation

Investigators	No. of Patients	All Diseases		Without Metastases		Positive Axillary Nodes	
		5 yr (%)	10 yr (%)	5 yr (%)	10 yr (%)	5 yr (%)	10 yr (%)
White and White[11] (1956)	806	13.4	8.6	20.7	12.5	7.0	5.6
Holleb and Farrow[22] (1962)	117	31	—	65	—	17	—
Peters[21] (1968)	295	33	19.5	—	—	—	—
Ribeiro and Palmer[72] (1977)	59	31.4	24	90	90	37	21
King et al.[18] (1985)	58	45	—	82	71	22	—

estrogen negative when receptor studies have been performed.[20] These tumors are more aggressive, particularly in younger women.

Some investigators have suggested that patients treated during the second half of pregnancy seem to have a poorer prognosis when compared with those treated early in gestation or during the puerperium.[11,21] White and White[11] observed that if therapy were begun during the second or third trimester of pregnancy, the 5-year survival rate was roughly one-half (8 percent) that of patients treated early in pregnancy or postpartum. Peters[21] has also presented data on 187 patients in which the 5-year survival rate was greatest in patients initially treated postpartum (77 percent) when compared with those treated in the first half (57 percent) or second half (14 percent) of pregnancy. These reports, however, may be flawed by bias in the selection of patients for treatment. Donnegan and others pointed out that treatment of small and slowly growing tumors may have been postponed until after delivery, while aggressive tumors were more promptly treated but with poor results.[10,15] They suggest prompt treatment during the second half of pregnancy to prevent even small lesions from growing and reaching an inoperable stage.

Further analysis of Peters' data indicates that any survival disadvantage for pregnant women with breast carcinoma as compared with all premenopausal women is probably small, with no more than a 10 to 15 percent decrease in 5-year survival rates for each clinical stage. When age was also considered, survival rates for pregnant and nonpregnant women

were equal.[21] Thus pregnancy appears to have little effect on prognosis.

Treatment

The treatment of breast carcinoma at anytime in a woman's life is often overshadowed by psychologic and emotional factors. Pregnancy adds a greater burden for the patient and her physician because of the potential risks of treatment to the developing fetus. Moreover, patients with advanced disease and a limited life expectancy may consider termination on this basis alone. Therapy, however, must be individualized in accordance with our present knowledge and with the specific desires of the patient.

Mastectomy has traditionally been the treatment of choice for patients with early disease, regardless of gestational age. A modified radical procedure with or without primary reconstruction is generally performed. The risk of miscarriage related to this procedure is approximately 1 percent.[14] Patients who are candidates for wide local excision and axillary node sampling followed by radiation are most often advised to terminate the pregnancy if this therapeutic course is elected. In such cases, the amount of radiation delivered to the fetus must be calculated and the patient counseled appropriately. It has been estimated that a fetus 25 cm below the base of a field to which 7,500 rads were delivered would receive approximately 30 rads. This dose presents an unacceptable risk to the fetus. While the potential for teratogenesis is reduced later in pregnancy, radiation can affect fetal growth and may carry a risk for future carcinogenesis.

There appears to be no benefit to "prophylactic" abortion, as it does not affect maternal survival or the clinical course of the disease.[22] In the past, routine termination was advised on theoretical considerations that large amounts of estrogen might promote tumor growth. At present, a harmful effect of continuing pregnancy has not been demonstrated. However, most cases studied have not been categorized in terms of steroid receptor status. This information might be helpful in counseling patients who are considering continuation of pregnancy. Similarly, prophylactic oophorectomy for women with breast cancer during pregnancy is not indicated. This procedure does not delay recurrence or improve the course of disease, even if nodes are positive.[23,24] However, it may be helpful as a palliative procedure in patients whose estrogen receptor status is strongly positive. Remission will be effected in 50 percent of these women.

Patients who present with advanced breast carcinoma early in gestation frequently elect a termination of pregnancy. Anxiety about their disease as well as harmful effects of cytotoxic drugs on the developing fetus make termination advisable. Termination of pregnancy facilitates the prompt administration of combination chemotherapy, which is indicated in premenopausal women with stage II disease. Later in pregnancy, systemic chemotherapy may be undertaken as the outcomes reported have generally been good in leukemic patients treated with agents similar to those employed for breast cancer.[25]

Delays of therapy beyond a few weeks should be discouraged. In certain cases encountered in the third trimester, it may be permissible to await fetal pulmonary maturity before instituting treatment. There are no reported cases of breast carcinoma crossing the placenta and metastasizing to the fetus.

Subsequent Pregnancy

A young woman who has undergone radical mastectomy may consider a subsequent pregnancy. Donnegan's review[10] revealed that 7 percent of fertile women have one or more pregnancies after mastectomy, 70 percent of which occur within 5 years of diagnosis. The available data support the recommendation that many of these patients need not be advised against future reproduction. Peters[21] has suggested that women who become pregnant after a mastectomy survive surprisingly well, and perhaps better than patients who do not become pregnant. It has been proposed that this phenomenon may be a function of selection in that healthier patients elect to become pregnant, whereas patients with advanced disease do not. However, Peters[21] carefully matched 96 patients with controls according to age and clinical stage and has demonstrated longer survival and disease-free intervals for patients who become pregnant. Cooper and Butterfield[26] examined 40 patients who became pregnant following mastectomy and matched each with two control patients according to clinical stage of disease and age. They reported that 20 of 22 patients with stage I disease who became pregnant survived 5 years, whereas only 30 of 44 controls did as well. The number of patients with nodal disease or early disease in this study was too small to draw conclusions about the beneficial effects of pregnancy.

Although these studies indicate that pregnancy does not adversely affect survival, it does seem prudent that women without nodal disease should wait a period of 2 to 3 years before contemplating pregnancy. The length of observation should probably be extended to 5 years in patients with positive nodes. Because one-third of recurrences will develop in the first 3 years following the primary procedure, this is a high-risk period during which contraception is important. A full evaluation for metastatic disease should be undertaken prior to pregnancy, including bone and liver scans, a chest x-ray, mammography of the opposite breast, and computed tomography (CT) scan of the brain if neurologic symptoms develop.

Hodgkin's Disease

Hodgkin's disease, which is most commonly encountered in patients who are in their late teens and twenties, has been estimated to complicate 1 in 6,000 pregnancies.[27] Hodgkin's disease comprises nearly 40 percent of all lymphomas. Non-Hodgkin's lymphomas are uncommon in younger women and have rarely been reported in pregnancy. Fertility in patients with lymphoma is probably affected only if severe systemic disease is present. In those patients able to conceive, spontaneous abortion and stillbirth rates appear no greater than those observed in a normal gestation.[28] The incidence of preterm birth has not been increased in any reported series.[29] Pregnancy does not appear to affect the course of the disease adversely. Therefore routine termination of pregnancy should not be undertaken. Transplacental dissemination of Hodgkin's disease is apparently possible. In one report, placental involvement led to disseminated disease in the newborn, who died at 5 months of age.[30]

In up to 90 percent of cases, Hodgkin's disease presents as an enlarged cervical or axillary lymph node. Systemic symptoms consist of fever, night sweats, and weight loss. The diagnosis is established by biopsy and histologic examination of suspected nodes. Two histologic variants, nodular sclerosis and lymphocyte predominant, have a better prognosis than mixed cellularity and lymphocyte-depleted specimens. The stage of disease is, however, the most important factor in planning therapy and in estimating prognosis (Table 38.2). Survival for early-stage disease exceeds 90 percent, whereas patients with disseminated nodal disease have a 5-year survival rate of only 50 percent. Extranodal involvement of the liver, lung, bone, and marrow (stage IV) is also accompanied by poor survival rates.

The minimal staging for Hodgkin's disease during pregnancy includes roentgenographic examination of the chest, liver function tests, bone marrow biopsy, complete blood count, and urinalysis. Chest tomography or CT scan of the mediastinum may be necessary to evaluate nodal enlargement in this area. Evaluation of the abdomen is rendered difficult by the presence of the gravid uterus. Magnetic resonance imaging (MRI) may prove to be helpful in demonstrating intra-abdominal adenopathy. A complete staging laparotomy and splenectomy have been undertaken in early pregnancy. However, this is obviously done with considerable risk to the fetus. Isotope scans of the liver and bone are best avoided during pregnancy as well. Thomas and Peckham[31] have described the use of a modified lymphangiographic technique in which a single film is obtained 24 hours after the injection of contrast. A single abdominal film probably results in an exposure of less than 1 rad to the fetus, which is well below the acceptable doses reported in the literature.[9]

The mainstay of treatment for early-stage Hodgkin's disease is radiation therapy. Multiple-agent chemotherapy is employed for the treatment of advanced stage disease with organ involvement. The most widely used combination of drugs is the MOPP regimen (nitrogen mustard, vincristine, procarbazine, and prednisone). This therapy as well as radiation is often used to treat patients with bulky, large mediastinal masses or disseminated nodal disease.

Most investigators agree that treatment should not be withheld during pregnancy except in early-stage disease, particularly if it is discovered late in gestation. Thomas and Peckham[31] described several cases of mantle radiation for supradiaphragmatic disease in which abdominal shielding was employed. In three cases treated at 10, 15, and 16 weeks, doses of 2.5, 4.4, and 10.4 rads, respectively, were estimated to reach the fetus. These pregnancies went to term with apparently normal outcomes. Long-term follow-up on these infants was not presented. However, Jacobs et al.[32] reported one case of spontaneous abortion after 4,400 rads were delivered to the chest during the first trimester in a patient with recurrent disease. The estimated fetal dose in this case was 9 rads. A

Table 38.2 Staging Classification of Hodgkin's Disease[a]

Stage	Description
I	Involvement of a single lymph node region (I) or of a single extralymphatic organ site (I_E)
II	Involvement of two or more lymph node regions on the same side of the diaphragm (II) or localized involvement of an extralymphatic organ site and of one or more lymph node regions on the same side of the diaphragm (II_E)
III	Involvement of lymph node regions on both sides of the diaphragm (III), which may also be accompanied by localized involvement of an extralymphatic organ or site (III_E), of the spleen (III_S), or of both (III_{SE})
IV	Diffuse or disseminated involvement of an extralymphatic organ with or without localized lymph node involvement (liver, bone marrow, lung, skin)

[a] Symptoms of unexplained fever, night sweats, and unexplained weight loss of 10 percent of normal body weight results in classification of patients as B; absence of these symptoms is denoted as A.

second patient treated at 16 weeks gestation with 3,300 rads of mantle therapy had a successful pregnancy. Despite this, Jacobs et al.[32] recommend termination for patients who develop Hodgkin's disease early in pregnancy or who have received chemotherapy or irradiation during the first trimester. We prefer to review the specific risks with each patient and her family. During the second half of pregnancy, asymptomatic early-stage disease may be followed closely while preparations are made for early delivery.[32] Systemic symptoms may be treated with steroids or a single chemotherapeutic agent.

Subdiaphragmatic or advanced disease requires the institution of chemotherapy. Such treatment is best avoided during the first trimester. Each of the agents in the MOPP regimen with the exception of prednisone is a potential teratogen. The use of chemotherapy should be approached with caution later in pregnancy as well, although most case reports document successful outcomes following the administration of these agents. As mentioned previously, intrauterine growth retardation and neonatal neutropenia are potential complications. Importantly, long-term follow-up of such infants is lacking and will be necessary before ensuring that cytotoxic drugs can be used with impunity in late pregnancy. It must be emphasized that advanced disease should be treated aggressively, as delaying therapy has been associated with progression of this disease in pregnant patients.[31] Early delivery is suggested when progressive disease is discovered late in gestation.

Following treatment, it is recommended that pregnancy not be attempted for at least 2 years, as 80 percent of recurrences will occur by this time. The reproductive potential of young patients with Hodgkin's disease is of interest to patients, oncologists, and obstetricians.[33] Chapman et al.[34] studied 41 women who received MOPP therapy as well as other agents for relapse or maintenance. None of these patients received pelvic irradiation. After 16 months of follow up, only 5 of 41 (12 percent) demonstrated completely normal ovarian function. Ovarian failure was more likely to occur in older patients, even if they were treated with fewer courses of therapy. Horning et al.[35] reported a significantly better prognosis for normal ovarian function (Fig. 38.1). This finding was particularly true for women with oligoamenorrhea who often took several years to resume normal go-

nadal function. Patients in this study were grouped according to various treatments, including: (1) total lymphoid irradiation, (2) MOPP only, and (3) a combination of chemotherapy and irradiation. Resumption of regular menstrual cycles occurred in 47 percent of patients treated with total lymphoid irradiation and in 56 percent of patients after combination chemotherapy. In patients treated with both modalities, only 20 percent resumed regular menses. In that study, age was the most important predictive factor for return of normal ovarian function. The synergistic effects of combined therapy are most apparent in younger women. Beyond age 30 years, the difference between various treatment regimens becomes less significant.

Bilateral midline oophoropexy at the time of staging laparotomy has been advocated in young women with Hodgkin's disease. While potentially preserving ovarian function, there is concern that this procedure might create adhesions and limit ovum pickup and transport. In the series of Horning et al.,[35] 12 of 21 patients who underwent oophoropexy prior to lymphoid irradiation or radiation and chemotherapy became pregnant. Thomas and Peckham[31] reported excellent success with this procedure in patients receiving paraaortic radiation. However, of 12 patients treated with "inverted Y" irradiation, only three recovered ovarian function. The estimated dose to the ovary was between 600 to 3,500 rads.[35] Combination oral contraceptives have also been employed to preserve ovarian function in patients receiving cytotoxic therapy. Chapman et al.[36] report six women who were treated with oral contraceptives from the initiation of and during chemotherapy for Hodgkin's disease. Postchemotherapy ovarian biopsy material from three of these women showed more than 20 follicles per histologic section. Because recurrent disease within the first 2 years of treatment carries with it poor prognosis, patients should not plan pregnancy during this time period.

Adverse perinatal outcomes are not increased in patients who are able to achieve a pregnancy after therapy for Hodgkin's disease. Holmes and Holmes[37] reviewed 93 pregnancies in 48 patients of which 29 were treated with chemotherapy, radiation, or a combination of these therapies. These patients experienced no differences in fetal wastage, term birth, and birth defects when compared with sibling controls. McKeen et al.[38] reported the perinatal outcomes in

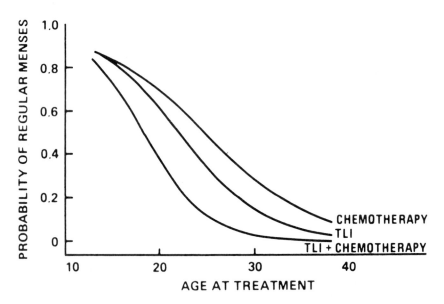

Fig. 38.1 Probability of regular menses after chemotherapy, total lymphoid irradiation (TLI), and TLI and chemotherapy in patients with Hodgkin's disease. The synergistic effect is more apparent in younger women. (From Horning et al.,[35] with permission.)

44 pregnancies but did not detail the therapy used. In that series, three major anomalies occurred that included hydrocephaly, tracheomalacia, and pelvic asymmetry. Dein et al.[33] emphasized that none of the children with anomalies observed after maternal treatment for Hodgkin's disease were diagnosed as having a chromosomal abnormality or a new gene mutation. The absence of a repetitive pattern of malformations makes it difficult to imply a causal relationship between any birth defects observed and previous therapy for Hodgkin's disease.

Acute Leukemia

Acute leukemia occurs in less than 1 in 75,000 pregnancies. In adults, it is usually a rapidly fatal illness, with median survivals of approximately 1 to 2 years. Despite excellent control of disease, including many cures in children with acute lymphocytic leukemia (ALL), intensive chemotherapy in older patients has been primarily effective in achieving remission. Only one-third of patients with ALL appear to be long-term disease-free survivors at 4 to 5 years following the diagnosis. This figure approaches 25 percent for patients with acute nonlymphocytic leukemia (ANLL).[39] Thus the patient with acute leukemia during pregnancy presents a difficult problem. Her poor

prognosis requires frank consideration about whether to continue the pregnancy. Furthermore, the frequent need for immediate institution of chemotherapy raises the question of the potential effects of such therapy on the developing fetus. The physician advising pregnant patients afflicted with leukemia must have a thorough knowledge of the natural history of the particular disease, its management, and complications. The care of any patient with leukemia necessitates a team effort and is best achieved in a cancer referral center.

The diagnosis of acute leukemia is rarely difficult. The signs and symptoms of anemia, granulocytopenia, and thrombocytopenia, including fatigue, fever, infection, and easy bleeding with petechiae, usually prompt evaluation with a complete blood and platelet count. Patients with ALL will have a normal or elevated white blood cell (WBC) count in up to 90 percent of cases. Counts in excess of 50,000, however, are found in only one-fourth of cases. In contrast, patients with ANLL may present with markedly elevated WBC counts, although one-third will initially be leukopenic.[39]

The diagnosis of leukemia should always be confirmed by bone marrow biopsy and aspirate. The biopsy is usually hypercellular, with a smear of the aspirate revealing decreased erythrocyte and granulocytic precursors as well as megakaryocytes. Leukemic cells compromise greater than one-half of the marrow's cellular elements in most patients. The morphology of the marrow as well as the peripheral leukemic cells help to distinguish between lymphocytic and nonlymphocytic leukemia. Histochemical staining is extremely important in differentiating the nonlymphocytic leukemias. This group includes acute myelocytic (granulocytic), promyelocytic, monocytic, and myelomonocytic leukemias and erythroleukemia. Of these subgroups, acute myelocytic leukemia is the most common form of ANLL and accounts for approximately one-half of all cases of acute leukemia found in pregnancy.[40] ALL comprises most of the other cases. The distinction between cell types is important in predicting response to therapy and therefore prognosis. Adult patients with ALL achieve remission in up to 80 percent of cases, whereas complete remission occurs in approximately 65 percent of cases of ANLL. Patients who develop ANLL as a result of previous chemotherapy seem to have a poor response to subsequent treatment.[39]

There is no evidence that pregnancy has a deleterious effect on the course of leukemia. Yahia et al.,[41] in reviewing the literature from 1943 to 1956, reported that almost 80 percent of mothers with leukemia survived delivery in an era when steroids and, in some cases, antimetabolites were used for treatment. With combination chemotherapy, maternal death is uncommon, and fetal survival approaches 90 percent. Therefore, in early pregnancy, it is important to consider the disease state of the mother and her desires before recommending termination of pregnancy.

There are a number of reports of successful pregnancies in patients aggressively treated with combination chemotherapy regimens for acute leukemia. Exposure to single drugs or combination therapy during the second and third trimesters has generally not been associated with gross fetal abnormalities.[3,4] One case of trisomy of chromosome group C has been reported following second-trimester exposure to cytosine arabinoside and thioguanine.[42] Pizzuto et al.[43] described nine patients who received chemotherapy for acute leukemia during various trimesters of pregnancy, including four cases of ALL treated during the first trimester with cytosine arabinoside, prednisone, methotrexate, and vincristine in which no anomalies were detected. Seven of nine infants were, however, growth retarded, and one stillbirth occurred.

Catanzarite and Ferguson[44] reviewed pregnancy outcomes in 41 women treated for acute leukemia between 1972 and 1982. Of 28 pregnancies in patients receiving chemotherapy for ANLL, 23 viable infants were delivered.[44] There were three therapeutic terminations, one fetal death at 24 weeks, and one newborn in poor condition. Corresponding figures for 13 patients treated with ALL revealed two terminations, one fetal death, and one death within 1 month of delivery. In the above review, a consistent trend toward infants falling below the 10th percentile in weight was observed.[44] More recently, Reynoso and colleagues[7] analyzed 58 cases of acute leukemia treated over a 10-year period. While remission was achieved in 75 percent of cases, only 40 percent of pregnancies ended in the delivery of a liveborn infant. There are also several reports of neonatal bone marrow depression resulting from agents commonly employed to treat leukemia during pregnancy.[45] Although many infants are described as being normal, there are few reports of long-term follow-up in offspring of treated women. Studies of these children will be important in assessing the risk of in utero exposure to the newer antineoplastic drugs. Schafer[46] has reviewed the case of a woman treated with identical doses of cytarabine and thioguanine during the first trimester of two separate pregnancies. One resulted in the delivery at term of a growth-retarded infant with skeletal defects. In the other pregnancy, the patient was delivered of a normal infant. This case emphasizes the highly unpredictable effects of chemotherapy on the fetus.

Future pregnancies in patients in remission with ALL should not be considered for several years following therapy. Catanzarite and Ferguson[44] reviewed 14 pregnancies in such patients and found that they resulted in 1 early loss and 13 term infants. Because of the grave prognosis with ANLL, these patients should probably be advised against pregnancy.

Chronic Leukemia

Chronic leukemia accounts for approximately 50 percent of the cases of leukemia during pregnancy, with the overwhelming majority of these being patients with chronic myelocytic leukemia.[40] Chronic lymphocytic leukemia (CLL) is generally an indolent disease, with the median age of onset being 60 years, making cases rare during gestation. Patients usually present with lymphocytosis, lymphadenopathy, and splenomegaly. Normal hematopoiesis is only mildly affected in the early stages of disease so that therapy may often be withheld for an extended period of time. Survival up to 10 years following initial diagnosis is common.

During pregnancy, unless complications such as severe systemic symptoms, autoimmune hemolytic anemia, recurrent infection, or symptomatic lymphatic enlargement occur, treatment for CLL should be withheld until after delivery. Therapy, when necessary, usually includes prednisone and an alkylating agent such as chlorambucil. Chlorambucil is teratogenic in laboratory animals and humans, although its use has been associated with normal outcomes if administered during the second and third trimesters.[25] Steroids in high doses may be used as the sole therapy for autoimmune hemolytic anemia.

Chronic myelogenous leukemia (CML) accounts for most of the chronic leukemias complicating pregnancy.[47] The median age of affected patients is 35 years. The disease is marked by excessive production of mature myeloid cell elements, with granulocyte counts averaging 200,000/dl. Most patients have a thrombocytosis and a mild normochromic normocytic anemia. Platelet function is often abnormal, although hemorrhage is usually limited to patients with marked thrombocytosis.[47]

In most cases, the diagnosis of CML antedates the pregnancy. Pregnancy does not appear to adversely affect CML. However, therapy does increase the likelihood of preterm birth and low birth weight. An attempt should be made to limit the administration of chemotherapeutic agents to the second and third trimesters, if possible. In some patients with relatively asymptomatic disease, therapy may be withheld until after delivery. Busulfan use beginning at 20 weeks gestation resulted in the delivery of a growth-retarded infant with left hydronephrosis, hydroureter, subcapsular calcifications, and an absent right kidney.[48] Other reports of second- and third-trimester treatment have resulted in the delivery of normal infants.[4]

Melanoma

The incidence of malignant melanoma is rising sharply in the United States. It is estimated that by the year 2000 1 percent of the population will develop this disease.[49] Melanoma has a mean age at onset of approximately 50 years, making this disease relatively uncommon in pregnancy. Reviewing the literature, it appears that 1 to 10 percent of all disease is first discovered during gestation.[50-52] Although melanoma is the most common tumor to metastasize to the placenta, this is truly a rare occurrence.

The effect of pregnancy on melanoma has been the subject of several studies and case reports.[51-53] The early observations of poor outcomes during gestation suggested that tumor cell growth was stimulated during pregnancy. It was thought that the hormonal milieu of pregnancy, which is marked by increased melanocyte-stimulating hormone activity, might predispose to the development of melanoma or alter growth characteristics in preexisting malignant melanocytes. Others have proposed that melanoma may in fact be an estrogen-dependent neoplasm. However, women seem to have better survival rates than do men, and in some series nulliparous women have poorer outcomes than parous patients. The latter finding may be due to the observation that nulliparous women more often present with advanced disease.[54]

George et al.,[50] at New York's Memorial Hospital, examined the records of 77 women who were pregnant during the course of their disease and compared them with a control group of 330 nonpregnant patients. They reported that pregnant women first presented with stage I and stage II disease in 51 and 37 percent of cases, respectively, compared with 65 and 21 percent in age-matched controls. Whereas the lower extremities were the most common site of primary lesions in both groups, pregnant patients more often had disease in less favorable sites such as the trunk.[50] Five-year statistics were not dramatically different between study groups for stage I disease. With stage II disease, however, only 35 percent of pregnant patients survived compared with 42 percent of nonpregnant women under the age of 43.[50] Shiu et al.,[52] in a later report from the same institution, found a lower survival rate (29 percent) for stage II melanoma in pregnant patients compared with that of nulliparous women (55 percent) and other parous patients (51 percent). More recent data from the Connecticut tumor registry substantiates that melanoma during pregnancy occurs more often on the trunk and at a more advanced stage of disease than in nonpregnant women.[43] However, once the disease is diagnosed, the patient's prognosis is not worsened when stage of disease and primary site are considered. Thus, if pregnancy does influence survival of patients with melanoma, it does so by affecting the rate of metastases and the anatomical distribution of primary lesions.[51] It is also conceivable that a subgroup of patients with hormonally sensitive tumors may be adversely affected by pregnancy.

If any impact is to be made on reducing mortality from melanoma, it will likely be made by earlier detection. Fair-skinned women are at greatest risk. Any suspicious change in preexisting nevi warrants biopsy of the lesion. The vulva is the site of 7 percent of melanomas and may contain dysplastic precursor lesions. Lesions less than 0.76 mm in depth rarely metastasize and are virtually 99 percent curable by wide local excision.

Advanced metastatic disease carries with it a bleak prognosis. Chemotherapy employing dacarbazine results in clinical responses in no more than 30 percent of patients. It is probably best to withhold this therapy and to plan for early delivery in cases of disseminated disease that present late in pregnancy. Abortion should be strongly considered if metastatic disease is encountered before 20 weeks gestation.

Oral contraceptives are not recommended for the patient who has recently been treated for melanoma. While clear evidence for hormonal stimulation of melanomas is lacking, other forms of contraception are preferred.[55] Pregnancy should not be attempted for several years and may be inadvisable in patients with nodal metastases.[52] One report of 10 stage I disease patients who subsequently became pregnant revealed a 5-year survival rate of 80 percent.[53] There are no data available that compare survival rates at equal lengths of time from diagnosis in patients who did or did not become pregnant.

Cervical Carcinoma

Cervical carcinoma is the most common gynecologic malignancy found in pregnant women. The true incidence of this disease during pregnancy is difficult to ascertain, as most reports originate in referral institutions and may include postpartum patients as well as those with noninvasive lesions. The reported incidence of carcinoma of the cervix has therefore ranged from 1 to 13 cases per 10,000 pregnancies.[56] Hacker et al.,[57] in reviewing 800 cases, estimated an overall incidence of 0.8 per 1,000, approximately 1 per 1,240 pregnancies. The incidence of invasive carcinoma of the cervix peaks in incidence at age 45

years. Approximately 3 percent of all cases of invasive cervical carcinoma occur in pregnancy. Most busy gynecologic oncology services will encounter this problem about once each year.[57]

Unlike invasive cancer, carcinoma in situ of the cervix is often discovered during the reproductive years. Therefore all pregnant patients should be evaluated on their initial visit with cervical cytologic smears. The incidence of abnormal Papanicolaou smears in one large study of pregnant patients was 1.2 percent.[58] Because early lesions are often asymptomatic, the importance of routine Papanicolaou smear screening cannot be overemphasized. In the series of Creasman et al.,[59] nearly 30 percent of patients with invasive cervical cancer were asymptomatic at the time of diagnosis. Vaginal bleeding is the most common complaint and when present should be evaluated by a speculum examination regardless of previous cervical cytologic status. Invasive cervical carcinoma may present with a watery blood-tinged discharge that has been confused with premature rupture of membranes in certain cases. Histologic diagnosis should always be sought by biopsy if suspicious gross lesions are present.

Over 40 percent of cervical cancers detected during gestation are stage I lesions.[56] These tumors may not be grossly evident, making the diagnosis possible only with proper evaluation of an abnormal cytologic smear. Most patients with abnormal smears can be followed with colposcopic examination after appropriate biopsies to establish the diagnosis (Fig. 38.2). Hemorrhage after a colposcopically directed punch biopsy during pregnancy is rare. Because pregnancy usually results in some degree of eversion of the squamocolumnar transformation zone, most abnormal lesions may be viewed with the colposcope. If the transformation zone is not clearly seen, it may be advisable to wait a period of several weeks before proceeding with cone biopsy in the hope that this area will become visible.[58] Endocervical curettage is not performed during pregnancy because of the risk of bleeding and ruptured membranes.

In general, conization should be avoided during pregnancy. In the first trimester, the risk of miscarriage may be as high as 30 percent. Other complications after a cone biopsy during pregnancy include infection, stenosis, and laceration during delivery. Patients who undergo conization are also at risk for preterm delivery during the current as well as subsequent pregnancies. Not surprisingly, Averette et al.[60]

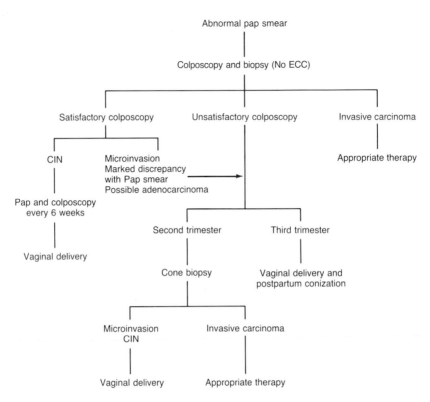

Fig. 38.2 Suggested protocol for evaluation of abnormal cervical cytology in pregnancy. ECC, endocervical curettage; CIN, cervical intraepithelial neoplasia. (From Hacker et al.,[57] with permission.)

found that the highest risk for hemorrhage following cone biopsy occurred during the third trimester. In their series of 180 patients, nearly 10 percent required a blood transfusion following the procedure. Such alarmingly high complication rates have prompted DiSaia and Creasman[61] to recommend a modified procedure during pregnancy. To minimize trauma to the endocervical canal, a "shallow cone" of tissue is excised rather than a true cone.

Once the diagnosis has been established, patients with carcinoma in situ and, in some instances, microinvasive disease may be followed to term without further therapy. Those with microinvasive disease may elect termination of pregnancy by extrafascial hysterectomy. In patients continuing pregnancy, cytologic and colposcopic examinations should be performed periodically to rule out progression of the disease. Definitive therapy using cryosurgery or laser may be accomplished in the postpartum period for patients with cervical intraepithelial neoplasia.

Women who have undergone conization during pregnancy are at higher risk for residual disease and require close follow-up after delivery.

Stage for stage, frankly invasive carcinoma discovered during pregnancy is associated with survival rates that are similar to those found in the nonpregnant population (Table 38.3). Of note, in almost every series reported, when the diagnosis has been made late in pregnancy or postpartum, the disease is significantly more advanced.[56,59,60] However, most cases encountered are still stages IB and IIA lesions. Controversy continues to exist regarding the ideal therapy for these lesions in the nonpregnant as well as pregnant individual. DiSaia and Creasman[61] note that both radical surgery and radiation therapy are equally effective and that radiation is preferred in advanced stages of disease. Patients who are diagnosed prior to 20 weeks should undergo treatment without delay. Therapy may consist of either radical hysterectomy with pelvic lymphadenectomy or the initiation of

Table 38.3 Cervical Cancer: Five-Year Survival by Clinical Stage Diagnosed During Pregnancy

Stage	Treated	Survival	Percent	Annual Report 1954–1963 (%)[a]
IB	474	348	74.5	76.5
II	449	214	47.8	55.0
III/IV	326	53	16.2	27.9
TOTAL	1,249	615	49.2	51.0

[a] Survival for all cases of cervical cancer. Note that survival rates are similar to those in the nonpregnant group.

(From Hacker et al.,[57] with permission.)

whole pelvis irradiation. Because radical hysterectomy permits preservation of ovarian function and limits foreshortening of the vagina, it is the preferred procedure in young women. The operation is often facilitated in pregnancy, as peritoneal stretching will improve tissue planes.

Spontaneous miscarriage usually occurs during the course of external radiation therapy. Intracavitary radiation is then accomplished with cesium or radium implants. Spontaneous abortion may be delayed in second-trimester cases, necessitating hysterotomy for termination of pregnancy. A modified radical hysterectomy may then be performed.[61]

In the third trimester, the obstetrician must consider fetal maturation and well-being as well as maternal disease. Data reviewing the outcomes of patients in whom therapy has been significantly delayed during the third trimester are lacking. Lee et al.[56] described eight patients whose disease was documented in the third trimester and who waited an average of 5 weeks to reach fetal viability before being treated. None of the patients experienced clinical progression of their disease despite this delay. Nevertheless, most authors prefer early delivery after documenting fetal pulmonary maturity by amniotic fluid studies. Pulmonary maturation may occur at 32 to 34 weeks gestation, particularly if corticosteroids have been administered. A classic cesarean section should be performed prior to surgical treatment or radiation therapy. Laparotomy will also permit periaortic and pelvic node sampling, which may aid in planning sub-

sequent radiation therapy. While the mode of delivery in patients with invasive disease has been debated, it appears that vaginal delivery does not alter prognosis and may be associated with a better outcome.[57] However, patients with a smaller lesion and therefore a better prognosis may be those who are allowed to deliver vaginally. While obstruction from tumor is uncommon, hemorrhage and infection are potential complications of vaginal delivery. Recurrent cancer has also been reported in episiotomy sites.[62] For these reasons, as well as the desire for more complete staging, cesarean section continues to be the preferred method of delivery in cases of invasive cervical carcinoma.

Ovarian Cancer

The incidence of ovarian malignancy during pregnancy ranges from 1 in 18,000 to 1 in 47,000.[63,64] Ovarian carcinoma is the most lethal primary genital neoplasm, because it is usually diagnosed at an advanced stage. Of significance, a large proportion of ovarian tumors in pregnancy have an unusual histologic type and are of low grade.[64] For these reasons, the prognosis is more favorable for pregnant women with ovarian cancer.

With the increased use of diagnostic ultrasound, ovarian cysts and masses are more frequently encountered in early pregnancy. Adnexal masses diagnosed during pregnancy are malignant in 6 percent of cases compared with nearly 20 percent in nonpregnant women.[65,66] Ascertainment bias achieved by frequent early ultrasound examination as well as a younger average age for pregnant women account for the disparate frequencies cited above. Hogston and Lilford[67] reported the fate of 137 adnexal cysts discovered during 26,110 ultrasound scans in early pregnancy. Of these, 10 percent were operated on promptly, whereas 2 percent required surgery for painful complications later in pregnancy. Only one low-grade carcinoma was reported in this series. Of the 120 cysts treated conservatively, 89 percent could not be detected on ultrasound examination later in gestation. The investigators concluded that all cysts greater than 8 cm should be removed, as should smaller cysts that are multilocular, thick walled, or semisolid. The latter are unlikely to be corpus luteum cysts, which usually subside by 14 weeks gestation. Further support for surgical exploration of nonsimple cysts comes from Hess and colleagues,[65] who reported 54 patients requiring laparotomy for definitive treatment of adnexal mass during pregnancy. A malignant tumor was encountered in two cases. Women who underwent emergency laparotomy because of hemorrhage or torsion as complications of an adnexal mass more frequently suffered spontaneous miscarriage or preterm birth when compared with those patients undergoing elective removal of the mass.

When ovarian carcinoma is discovered at laparotomy, treatment should be similar to that for the nonpregnant woman. Histology, grade, and stage are important prognostic variables to be considered. A complete surgical staging, including peritoneal washings, biopsies of peritoneal surfaces, and para-aortic and pelvic lymph node sampling, is performed. In most instances, when advanced-stage disease is found, hysterectomy and bilateral salpingo-oophorectomy is accomplished. Low-grade malignancies and stage IA lesions may on occasion be managed conservatively with unilateral adnexectomy. The decision to limit surgery depends on gestational age and on the patient's desire to continue the pregnancy. Definite surgery may be undertaken following delivery in selected cases.

Approximately 60 percent of malignant ovarian tumors diagnosed during pregnancy are epithelial, with the remainder being germ cell and gonadal stromal tumors. Dysgerminomas have been reported during gestation in 27 cases.[68] Torsion and incarceration are common among these rapidly enlarging tumors. Contralateral ovarian biopsy is necessary, because dysgerminomas are often bilateral. Retroperitoneal lymph node dissection is also recommended, as lymphatic spread is common. Stage IA disease is generally managed by unilateral adnexectomy, although Karlen and colleagues[68] reported a 30 percent recurrence rate in 23 apparent stage IA dysgerminomas found in pregnant women.

Colorectal Carcinoma

The true incidence of colorectal carcinoma in pregnancy is unknown; however, this entity is estimated to occur in 0.002 percent of all pregnancies.[69] Nesbitt and colleagues[70] added 5 cases to 172 reported in the literature prior to 1983. Colorectal carcinoma is usually found in women beyond childbearing age, with only 8 percent of cases diagnosed before age 40 years.

The presenting symptoms of colorectal cancer include rectal bleeding, constipation, pain, nausea, vomiting, distention, and backache. Rectal bleeding and tenesmus are often ascribed to hemorrhoids exacerbated by pregnancy, thus delaying diagnosis. In many cases, the diagnosis is not established until late pregnancy—often not until labor has begun. Patients with unexplained hypochromic microcytic anemia should be evaluated with stool guaiac testing.[71] A positive test demands full evaluation. If a colorectal lesion is suspected, sigmoidoscopy and colonoscopy are the preferred diagnostic methods. Sixty to 70 percent of lesions are palpable to rectal examination.

Management of colon cancer is determined by gestational age at diagnosis. Colon resection with anastomosis is often possible during the first half of pregnancy. Abdominoperineal resection or low anterior resection has been accomplished up to 20 weeks gestation without disturbing the gravid uterus. In some cases, access to the rectum may be impossible without performing a hysterectomy. In late pregnancy, colostomy may be performed as a temporizing procedure to allow fetal maturity to take place, before proceeding with definitive therapy. This surgical plan is often preferred for obstructing tumors. Because of the high likelihood of ovarian metastases, biopsy in early pregnancy or oophorectomy in later gestation has been recommended by some investigators.[70]

In lesions discovered after 20 weeks gestation, some patients will opt to continue pregnancy until a gestational age compatible with neonatal survival is reached. Vaginal delivery is planned in such cases, except when the tumor is obstructing the pelvis or is located on the anterior rectal wall. If cesarean section is performed, tumor resection is accomplished immediately following delivery.

The prognosis for pregnant women with rectal carcinoma is difficult to ascertain. Nesbitt and colleagues[70] found no 5-year survivors among 23 pregnant patients with colon cancer reported in the literature.[70] In these women, the tumor was often advanced, which does suggest delayed diagnosis.

REFERENCES

1. Donnegan WL: Cancer and pregnancy. Ca 33:194, 1983
2. Koren G, Weiner L, Lishner M et al: Cancer in preg-

nancy: identification of unanswered questions on maternal and fetal risks. Obstet Gynecol Surv 45:509, 1990

3. Nicholson HO: Cytotoxic drugs in pregnancy. J Obstet Gynaecol Br Commonw 75:307, 1968

4. Doll DC, Ringenberg QS, Yarbro JW: Antineoplastic agents and pregnancy Semin Oncol 16:337, 1989

5. Doll DC, Ringenberg QS, Yarbro JW: Management of cancer during pregnancy. Arch Intern Med 148:2058, 1988

6. Mulvihill JJ, McKeen EA, Rosner F et al: Pregnancy outcome in cancer patients. Cancer 60:1143, 1987

7. Reynoso EE, Shepherd FA, Messner HA et al: Acute leukemia during pregnancy: the Toronto leukemia study group experience with long term follow-up in children exposed in utero to chemotherapeutic agents. J Clin Oncol 5:1098, 1987

8. Aviles A, Niz J: Long term follow-up of children born to mothers with acute leukemia during pregnancy. Med Pediatr Oncol 16:3, 1988

9. Brent RL: The effects of embryonic and fetal exposure to x-ray, microwaves, and ultrasound. Clin Perinatol 13:615, 1986

10. Donegan WL: Breast cancer and pregnancy. Obstet Gynecol 50:244, 1977

11. White TT, White WC: Breast cancer and pregnancy: report of 49 cases followed five years. Ann Surg 144:384, 1956

12. Thomas DB: Do hormones cause breast cancer? Cancer 53:595, 1984

13. Welsch CW, Nagasawa H: Prolactin and murine mammary tumorigenesis: a review. Cancer Res 37:951, 1977

14. Byrd BF Jr, Bayer DS, Robertson JC: Treatment of breast tumors associated with pregnancy and lactation. Ann Surg 155:940, 1962

15. Sommer RG, Young GP, Kaplan NJ et al: Fine needle aspiration biopsy in the management of solid breast tumors. Arch Surg 120:673, 1985

16. Parente JT, Amsel M, Lerner R, Chinea F: Breast cancer associated with pregnancy. 71:861, 1988

17. Canter JW, Oliver GC, Zaloudek CJ: Surgical disease of the breast during pregnancy. Clin Obstet Gynecol 26:853, 1983

18. King RM, Welch JS, Martin JK Jr, Coulam CB: Carcinoma of the breast associated with pregnancy. Surg Gynecol Obstet 160:228, 1985

19. Harrington SW: Carcinoma of the breast: results of surgical treatment when the carcinoma occurred in the course of pregnancy or lactation and when pregnancy occurred subsequent to operation. Ann Surg 106:690, 1937

20. Nugent P, O'Connell TX: Breast cancer and pregnancy. Arch Surg 120:1221, 1985

21. Peters MV: The effect of pregnancy in breast cancer. p. 120. In Forrest APM, Kunkler PB (eds): Prognostic Factors in Breast Cancer. Williams & Wilkins, Baltimore, 1968

22. Holleb AI, Farrow JH: The relationship of carcinoma of the breast and pregnancy in 283 patients. Surg Gynecol Obstet 115:65, 1962

23. Lee TN, Horz JM: Significance of ovarian metastases in therapeutic oophorectomy for advanced breast cancer. Cancer 27:1374, 1971

24. Ravdin RG, Lewison EF, Slack NH: The results of a clinical trial concerning the worth of prophylactic oophorectomy for breast cancer. Surg Gynecol Obstet 131:1055, 1970

25. Barber HRK: Fetal and neonatal effect of cytotoxic agents. Obstet Gynecol 58:41, 1981

26. Cooper DR, Butterfield J: Pregnancy subsequent to mastectomy for cancer of the breast. Ann Surg 171:429, 1970

27. Stewart HL, Monto RW: Hodgkin's disease and pregnancy. Am J Obstet Gynecol 63:570, 1952

28. Barry RM, Diamond HD, Craver LF: Influence of pregnancy on the course of Hodgkin's disease. Am J Obstet Gynecol 84:445, 1962

29. Sweet DL Jr: Malignant lymphoma: implications during the reproductive years and pregnancy. J Reprod Med 17:198, 1976

30. Rothman LA, Cohen CJ, Astarloa J: Placental and fetal involvement by maternal malignancy: a report of rectal carcinoma and a review of the literature. Am J Obstet Gynecol 116:1023, 1973

31. Thomas PRM, Peckham MJ: The investigation and management of Hodgkin's disease in the pregnant patient. Cancer 38:1443, 1976

32. Jacobs C, Donaldson SS, Rosenberg SA, Kaplan HS: Management of the pregnant patient with Hodgkin's disease. Ann Intern Med 95:649, 1981

33. Dein RA, Mennuti MT, Kovach P, Gabbe SG: The reproductive potential of young men and women with Hodgkin's disease. Obstet Gynecol Surv 39:474, 1984

34. Chapman RM, Sutcliffe SB, Malpas JS: Cytotoxic induced ovarian failure in women with Hodgkin's disease. I. Hormone function. J Am Med Assoc 242:1877, 1979

35. Horning SJ, Hoppe RT, Kaplan HS: Female reproduction after treatment for Hodgkin's disease. N Engl J Med 304:1377, 1981

36. Chapman, RM, Sutcliffe SB, Lees LH: Cyclical combination chemotherapy and gonadal function. Lancet 1:285, 1979

37. Holmes GE, Holmes FF: Pregnancy outcome of patients treated for Hodgkin's disease. Cancer 41:1317, 1978

38. McKeen EA, Mulvill JJ, Rosner F, Zarrari MH: Pregnancy outcome in Hodgkin's disease. Lancet 2:590, 1979

39. Wiernik PH: Acute leukemias of adults. p. 302. In DeVita VT Jr, Hellman S, Rosenberg SA (eds): Cancer: Principles and Practice of Oncology. JB Lippincott, Philadelphia, 1982

40. O'Dell RF: Leukemia and lymphoma complicating pregnancy. Clin Obstet Gynecol 22:859, 1979

41. Yahia C, Hyman GA, Phillips LL: Acute leukemia and pregnancy. Obstet Gynecol Surv 13:1, 1958

42. Maurer LH, Forcier RJ, McIntyre OR: Fetal group C trisomy after cytosine arabinoside and thioguanine. Ann Intern Med 75:809, 1971

43. Pizzuto J, Aviles A, Noriega L et al: Treatment of acute leukemia during pregnancy: presentation of nine cases. Cancer Treat Rep 64:679, 1980

44. Catanzarite VA, Ferguson JE: Acute leukemia and pregnancy: a review of management and outcome, 1972–1982. Obstet Gynecol Surv 39:663, 1984

45. Okum DB, Groncy PK, Sieger L: Acute leukemia in pregnancy: transient neonatal myelosuppression after combination chemotherapy in the mother. Med Pediatr Oncol 7:315, 1979

46. Schafer AI: Teratogenic effects of antileukemic therapy. Arch Intern Med 141:514, 191

47. McLain CR: Leukemia in pregnancy. Clin Obstet Gynecol 17:185, 1975

48. Boros SJ, Reynolds JW: Intrauterine growth retardation following third trimester exposure to busulfan. Am J Obstet Gynecol 129:111, 1977

49. Friedman RJ, Rigel DS, Kopf AW: Early detection of malignant melanoma: the role of the physician examination and self examination of the skin. Ca 35:130, 1985

50. George PA, Fortner JG, Pack GT: Melanoma with pregnancy: a report of 115 cases. Cancer 13:854, 1960

51. Houghton AN, Flannery J, Viola MV: Malignant melanoma of the skin occurring during pregnancy. Cancer 48:407, 1981

52. Shiu MH, Schottenfeld D, Maclean B, Fortner JG: Adverse effect of pregnancy on melanoma. Cancer 37:181, 1976

53. Sutherland CM, Loutfi A, Mather FJ et al: Effect of pregnancy upon malignant melanoma. Surg Gynecol Obstet 157:443, 1983

54. Shau HM, Milton GM, Farago F, McCarthy WH: Endocrine influences on survival from malignant melanoma. Cancer 42:669, 1978

55. Lerner AB, Nordlund JJ, Kirkwood JM: Effects of oral contraceptives and pregnancy on melanoma. N Engl J Med 301:47, 1979

56. Lee RB, Neglia W, Park RC: Cervical carcinoma in pregnancy. Obstet Gynecol 58:584, 1981

57. Hacker NF, Berek JS, Lagasse LD et al: Carcinoma of the cervix associated with pregnancy. Obstet Gynecol 59:735, 1982.

58. Lurain JR, Gallup DG: Management of abnormal Papanicolaou smears in pregnancy. Obstet Gynecol 53:484, 1979

59. Creasman WT, Rutledge FN, Fletcher GH: Carcinoma of the cervix associated with pregnancy. Obstet Gynecol 36:495, 1970

60. Averette HE, Nasser N, Yankow SL: Cervical conization in pregnancy. Am J Obstet Gynecol 106:543, 1970

61. DiSaia PJ, Creasman WT: Cancer in Pregnancy. p. 376. In Clinical Gynecologic Oncology. C.V. Mosby, St Louis, 1988

62. Gordon AN, Jensen R, Jones HW III: Squamous carcinoma of the cervix complicating pregnancy: recurrence in episiotomy after vaginal delivery. Obstet Gynecol 73:850, 1989

63. Munnell EW: Primary ovarian cancer associated with pregnancy. Clin Obstet Gynecol 6:983, 1963

64. Dgani R, Shoham Z, Atar E et al: Ovarian carcinoma during pregnancy: a study of 23 cases in Israel between the years of 1960 and 1984. Gynecol Oncol 33:326, 1989

65. Hess LW, Peaceman A, O'Brien W et al: Adnexal mass occurring with intrauterine pregnancy: a report of 54 patients requiring laparotomy for definitive management. Am J Obstet Gynecol 158:1029, 1988

66. Beischer NA, Buttery BW, Fortune DW et al: Growth and malignancy of ovarian tumors in pregnancy. Aust NZ J Obstet Gynaecol 11:208, 1971

67. Hogston P, Lilford RJ: Ultrasound study of ovarian cysts in pregnancy: prevalence and significance. Br J Obstet Gynaecol 93:625, 1986

68. Karlen JR, Akbari A, Cook WA: Dysgerminoma associated with pregnancy. Obstet Gynecol 53:330, 1979

69. McLean TW, Arminski TC, Bradley GT: Management of primary carcinoma of the rectum diagnosed during pregnancy. Am J Surg 90:816, 1955

70. Nesbitt JC, Moise KJ, Sawyers JL: Colorectal carcinoma in pregnancy. Arch Surg 120:636, 1985

71. VanVoorhis B, Cruikshank OP: Colon carcinoma complicating pregnancy—a report of two cases. J Reprod Med 34:923, 1989

72. Ribeiro GG, Palmer MK: Breast carcinoma associated with pregnancy: a clinician's dilemma. Br Med J 2:1524, 1977

Chapter 39

Dermatologic Disorders

Mark B. Landon

SKIN CHANGES DURING NORMAL PREGNANCY

Physiologic changes in the skin during gestation may result in hyperpigmentation, hirsutism, hair loss, and several vascular abnormalities. Some of these conditions are believed to result from alterations in the hormonal milieu of pregnancy, yet for most skin changes in pregnancy there is little information concerning the precise etiologic factors involved. The obstetrician must be able to distinguish common skin changes of pregnancy from primary cutaneous diseases that may antedate or develop during pregnancy.

Hyperpigmentation

Hyperpigmentation can be found in approximately 90 percent of pregnancies.[1] Women with a dark complexion are more likely to manifest hyperpigmentation during gestation. Darkening of the areolae, umbilicus, vulva, and perianal skin may occur as early as the first trimester. The linea alba often becomes the hyperpigmented linea nigra. Pigmented nevi, freckles, and recent scars may also deepen in color. Hyperpigmentation on the face, known as melasma or chloasma, will often prompt complaints from pregnant women. Chloasma is usually manifested by well-defined hyperpigmented centrofacial patches appearing in various shades of brown, depending on the site of melanin distribution. Melanin may be primarily epidermal, dermal, or found in both locations. In addition to pregnancy, melasma may occur with oral contraceptive use, liver disease, hyperthyroidism, and as a phototoxic reaction to certain cosmetics. Sunlight is thought to be necessary for the development of chloasma. The role of hormonal factors such as melanocyte-stimulating hormone (MSH) is unclear. Levels of estrogen, which like MSH can stimulate melanogeneses, are not consistently elevated in women wth chloasma.[2] Women with melasma during pregnancy should avoid excessive sun exposure. Sunscreens may be helpful in retarding progression and recurrence postpartum. Chloasma normally regresses or disappears in the majority of women; however, nearly 30 percent of patients will have persistent hyperpigmentation at 10-year follow-up.[1]

Hair Changes

Hirsutism

Mild degrees of hirsutism are common during pregnancy. The face is frequently affected, although hair growth may be pronounced on the extremities, as well. Abdominal hair growth is less common, but may be exacerbated in women with a prominent male pattern escutcheon. Hirsutism is believed to be primarily an endocrinologic phenomenon. During normal pregnancy, the proportion of hair in the anagen (growing) phase is increased compared with that in the telogen (resting) phase. Hirsutism may result from placental androgen production as well as elevated levels of cortisol during normal pregnancy. Mild hirsutism rarely requires therapy. It normally regresses following delivery, but does recur with subsequent pregnancies. Excessive hirsutism with virilization should warrant investigation for an androgen-secreting tumor.

Telogen Effluvium

Telogen effluvium, or hair loss after a shift of anagen follicles to telogen, is often seen during the postpartum period. Because the telogen phase may last several months, patients may report hair loss for 3 to 4 months following delivery. Patients should be reassured that normal hair growth will occur 6 to 15 months postpartum. The shedding actually represents reactivation of the hair follicle and is followed by new growth.

Striae Distensae

Striae distensae begin to appear in the late second trimester in up to 90 percent of pregnant women.[2] Striae are thin, atrophic, pink or purple linear bands that are found on the abdomen, breasts, and thighs. Striae are believed to result from a combination of two factors. Stretching is necessary to produce striae; however, adrenocorticosteroids and estrogen also promote tearing in the collagen matrix of the dermis and weakening of elastic fibers.[1] While many creams and ointments have been employed to treat striae distensae, these therapies are not thought to have any benefit. Striae persist permanently, although the purplish color does fade with time.

Vascular Changes

Vascular changes are evident within the skin of most pregnant women. High levels of estrogen are believed to be responsible for proliferation of blood vessels and congestion. Vasomotor instability may also produce pallor, flushing, and mottling of the skin.

Spider angiomata may be observed in up to 70 percent of white women during pregnancy. These lesions consist of a central red arteriole with tortuous radiating branches resembling a spider. Also common to liver disease, spider angiomata are found on the face, trunk, and upper extremities. Most lesions fade during the postpartum period.

Similar to spider angiomata, palmar erythema is more common in white than black women, with nearly two-thirds of pregnancies affected. Erythema of the midpalm, hypothenar, and thenar eminences may occur as early as the first trimester. This lesion is also seen with cirrhosis and systemic lupus erythematosus, although when observed as a manifestation of pregnancy it typically resolves following delivery.

Small capillary hemangiomas may be observed during the second and third trimesters in up to 5 percent of pregnant women.[1] Unlike spider angiomata, these lesions do not necessarily blanch with compression. Most small hemangiomas will involute after delivery. Large hemangiomas may persist and are associated with arteriovenous shunting and high-output cardiac failure.

Pyogenic granuloma or granuloma gravidarum of pregnancy may be seen in 2 percent of pregnancies.[2] Hypertrophy with capillary proliferation produces an elevated red-purple mass arising from the gingiva. The lesion consists of granulation tissue and an inflammatory infiltrate composed of various leukocytes and histiocytes. Although these masses usually remit during the postpartum period, surgical excision may be required if the lesion fails to resolve.

SPECIFIC DERMATOLOGIC CONDITIONS ASSOCIATED WITH PREGNANCY

Herpes Gestationis

Herpes gestationis is a pruritic bullous disease of the skin that occurs principally during pregnancy and the puerperium. The disease is rare, with a reported incidence of 1 per 4,000–50,000 pregnancies.[3,4] The onset is usually during the second trimester, although patients may present with recurring crops of blisters at any time during gestation or the early postpartum period. The puerperium is often marked by exacerbation of this condition. Herpes gestationis may be recurrent and is usually more severe in subsequent pregnancies. A hormonal influence seems to be operable, as this disorder may recur with menses as well as oral contraceptive use. A genetic predisposition is suggested by an increased frequency of HLA-A1, -B8, and -DR3 antigens in affected individuals.[5]

Clinically, the disease presents with lesions that closely resemble dermatitis herpetiformis and bullous pemphigoid (Fig. 39.1).[6] The initial symptom is pruritus followed by erythema and edema of the sub-

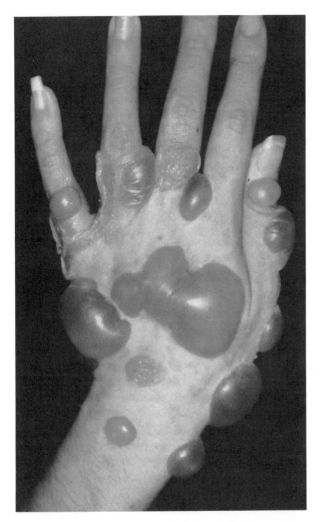

Fig. 39.1 Herpes gestationis during the third trimester. This patient developed erythematous macules on the chest and hands that progressed to bullae formation. Biopsy revealed a heavy linear complement deposition at the basement membrane zone, consistent with herpes gestationis. (Courtesy of Dr. Steven Wolverton, Division of Dermatology, Department of Medicine, The Ohio State University.)

cutaneous tissue. Papules and plaques then form that have been described as having an urticarial quality. The lesions are often present on the trunk, back, buttocks, forearms, palms, and soles. The face and scalp are infrequently involved. Frank bullae or vesicles that may erupt in a herpetiform grouping represent the final stage of the disease. The latter presentation, which is less common, may be confused with general-

ized herpes. A viral etiology, however, has not been found for herpes gestationis, and, importantly, the disease has not been demonstrated with greater frequency in patients with a history of herpes simplex infection. Herpes gestationis must be differentiated from toxic drug reactions including erythema multiforme, as well as bullous pemphigoid and more common dermatoses of pregnancy (Table 39.1).

The diagnosis of herpes gestationis may be made with reasonable assurance if there is a typical clinical presentation and recurrence with pregnancy, as well as peripheral eosinophilia. Absolute confirmation is made by biopsy and immunopathologic studies that reveal complement C_3 in a band-like distribution along the basement membrane between the epidermis and dermis.[7] IgG is found at the basement membrane in a minority of cases. Histology reveals extensive necrosis of the basal cell layer and edema of the papillary dermis. A chronic inflammatory response is present around the bullae in a perivascular distribution.[4] Circulating IgG antibasement membrane antibodies may be present in sera of affected patients along with herpes gestationis (HG) factor, a protein that fixes complement to the basement membrane of in vitro human skin preparations.[4] Herpes gestationis factor has not been isolated from the sera of all affected patients. However, this may be secondary to methodologic problems involved when complement binding with HG factor is present in low concentrations.[4]

The treatment for herpes gestationis is aimed at controlling pruritus and the formation of new vesicles and bullae. Topical steroids and antihistamines may be used initially if the symptoms are mild. Most patients will, however, require systemic corticosteroids. Prednisone is often begun in doses of 40 to 60 mg/day. The dose of steroid may be tapered as clinical improvement is noted. Azathioprine and rarely plasmapheresis have been employed in cases that fail to respond to corticosteroids.

Prior to the development of immunologic techniques that permitted an accurate diagnosis, herpes gestationis was believed to have minimal adverse effects on pregnancy.[8] In 1969, Kolodny[3] reported no increase in preterm births, stillbirths, or abortions. However, Lawley et al.[9] subsequently reviewed 40 immunologically proven cases and documented serious fetal morbidity and mortality. The preterm birth

Table 39.1 Pruritic Dermatoses of Pregnancy

Disease	Onset	Degree of Pruritus	Types of Lesions	Distribution	Increased Incidence of Fetal Morbidity or Mortality
Herpes gestationis	1st mo to postpartum	Moderate to severe	Erythematous papules, vesicles, bullae	Abdomen, extremities, generalized	Yes
Prurigo gravidarum	3rd trimester	Moderate to severe	Jaundice	Generalized	Unresolved
Papular dermatitis of pregnancy (Spangler et al.)	1st–9th mo	Severe	Excoriated papules	No area of predilection	Yes
Prurigo gestationis of Besnier	4th–9th mo	Severe	Excoriated papules	Extensor surfaces of extremities	No
Impetigo herpetiformis	1st–9th mo[a]	Minimal	Pustules	Genitalia, medial thighs, umbilicus, breasts, axillas	Yes
Pruritic urticarial papules and plaques of pregnancy (PUPP)	3rd trimester	Severe	Erythematous urticarial papules and plaques	Abdomen, thighs, buttocks, occasionally arms and legs	Unknown

[a] May also occur in nonpregnant females and in males.
(Adapted from Lawley et al.[13])

rate was 22 percent, and three stillbirths were noted. Lawley et al.[9] suggested that high levels of circulating antibasement membrane antibody as well as peripheral eosinophilia may be associated with increased fetal risk. More recently, Holmes and Black[10] reported a significantly increased frequency of fetal growth retardation in affected pregnancies. Transient newborn herpes gestationis has also been reported, along with the presence of circulating HG factor and antibasement membrane antibodies, in the newborn. Neonatal herpes gestationis is usually mild and may be marked only by erythematous papules or frank bullae.[11] Presumably, passive transfer of antibody is the stimulus for this process, which generally resolves within a short period of time.[12]

Pruritic Urticarial Papules and Plaques of Pregnancy (PUPP Syndrome)

In 1979, Lawley et al.[13] described seven patients with severe pruritic eruption that first occurred during the third trimester of pregnancy. This eruption could be differentiated by clinical presentation and histologic findings from any other previously described dermatologic condition associated with pregnancy. The incidence of PUPP is uncertain, although Holmes et al.[14] suggested a figure of 1 in 240 pregnancies. There may be an association with twin gestation.

The lesions of PUPP typically begin on the abdomen and consist of erythematous urticarial plaques and small papules surrounded by a narrow, pale halo. They usually spread to the thighs and possibly the buttocks and arms. The face is not affected. Most patients complain of intense pruritus that improves following delivery (Fig. 39.2). There are limited data on recurrence rates with subsequent pregnancies.

Histologic findings in this disorder consist of a normal epidermis accompanied by a superficial perivascular infiltrate of lymphocytes and histiocytes associated with edema of the papillary dermis.[13] Another pattern is that of a spongiotic epidermis with a dermal perivascular and interstitial lymphohistiocytic infiltrate revealing marked edema in the presence of eosinophilia. Immunofluorescence studies are negative for both immunoglobulins and complement. These histologic findings are nonspecific and may be associated with any urticarial allergic response as well as several viral exanthems. It is essential therefore to obtain a complete drug history before making the diagnosis of PUPP and starting treatment.

Therapy employing topical steroids is generally successful. Antipruritic drugs such as hydroxyzine or di-

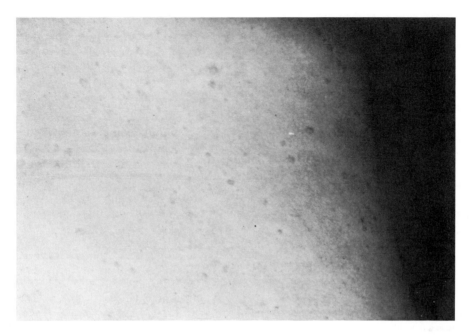

Fig. 39.2 Pruritic urticarial papules and plaques of pregnancy (PUPP syndrome). Erythematous urticarial plaques and small papules erupted on the abdomen of this patient during the third trimester. (Courtesy of Dr. Herbert Allen.)

phenhydramine may be helpful. The response to treatment may be difficult to evaluate, an abatement of cutaneous lesions and pruritus typically accompanies delivery.[13] The few reported cases of PUPP have failed to reveal an adverse effect on fetal and maternal outcome. Uhlin[15] has described one case in which a male neonate born to a mother with PUPP developed similar lesions, although skin biopsies were not performed to rule out herpes gestationis.

Papular Dermatitis

Papular dermatitis of pregnancy is characterized by widespread pruritic papules that show no particular anatomic predilection.[16] The disease may begin at any time during gestation and may recur with subsequent pregnancies. Controversy exists as to whether papular dermatitis is actually a more widespread form of pruritic gestationis.

First described by Spangler et al.[7] in 1962, papular dermatitis is a generalized skin eruption marked by erythematous papules that are intensely pruritic and usually excoriated. The lesions are typically 3 to 5 mm in diameter and consist of a central raised papule that

is covered by a hemorrhagic crust 1 to 2 mm in diameter.[6] The lesions do not occur in clusters and do not have a predilection for any anatomic site.

The histologic characteristics of this disorder are not well described. Pruett and Kim[16] have reported mild thickening of the epidermis without inflammatory change. A perivascular lymphocytic infiltrate may be present in the upper dermis.

Healing takes 7 to 10 days and may result in some residual hyperpigmentation. There is usually a prompt response to corticosteroids. High doses of prednisone will control eruptions within 24 to 48 hours.

Spangler and Emerson[18] observed increased urinary levels of human chorionic gonadotropin (hCG) and decreased plasma levels of hydrocortisone in patients with papular dermatitis. Low plasma estriols have also been noted in the third trimester. The etiology of these hormone changes is unclear. In their original report, Spanger et al.[17] included 12 patients whose 37 prior pregnancies resulted in 10 fetal losses. Apparently some of these pregnancies were complicated by untreated papular dermatitis. In 11 patients subsequently treated with corticosteroids, no fetal deaths were observed.

Impetigo Herpetiformis

Impetigo herpetiformis is a rare pustular skin disease that is often associated with pregnancy. The disorder usually occurs in the second half of gestation and begins with the appearance of groups of painful sterile pustules typically in the groin and inner thighs. These lesions coalesce and spread to the trunk and extremities. Bullae formation is uncommon. Unlike many of the dermatoses of pregnancy, the mucous membranes are frequently affected. Painful, oral grayish white plaques may resemble pemiphigus vulgaris.[6]

Histologically, these lesions reveal spongioform pustules that are intradermal and subcorneal in location. A dense inflammatory exudate surrounds dermal blood vessels. This condition is difficult to distinguish from pustular psoriasis and may be a variant of that disorder.[19]

Impetigo herpetiformis may be accompanied by systemic symptoms including fever, chills, arthralgias, vomiting, diarrhea, and lymphadenopathy. Prostration with septicemia may follow. Cardiac and renal failure have occurred in severe cases. Hypocalcemia and hyperphosphatemia are not uncommon in this setting and have led investigators to postulate that hypoparathyroidism is associated with this disorder. Successful treatment of impetigo herpetiformis includes the administration of systemic corticosteroids and antibiotics for secondary infection. The disease usually remits following delivery and does not recur with increasing severity in subsequent pregnancies. Maternal fatalities and increased fetal wastage have been observed in the few reported cases. Therefore fetal surveillance and elective delivery after fetal maturity has been documented are recommended.[20]

Prurigo Gestationis

Prurigo gestationis consists of pruritic excoriated papules that are usually limited to the extensor surfaces of the extremities. The disease is said to occur in 1 per 50 to 200 pregnancies.[21] Lesions generally appear during the second half of gestation. They are small, 1 to 2 mm papules that are distributed symmetrically. Vesicle or bulla formation does not occur. The disease usually resolves following delivery. Maternal and

fetal conditions are not affected, and recurrence during subsequent gestations is uncommon.

Nurse[22] has described two types of prurigo of pregnancy. The early form, which presents between 25 and 29 weeks of gestation, is marked by intensely pruritic papules of the proximal extremities and trunk. The late form typically appears close to term with abdominal papules often located in abdominal striae. The pruritus with either variety responds to calamine lotion and oral antipruritics. Corticosteroids are rarely necessary for the treatment of prurigo gestationis. Papular dermatitis may represent a more severe form of this condition.

REFERENCES

1. Wong RC, Ellis CN: Physiologic skin changes in pregnancy. J Am Acad Dermatol 10:929, 1984
2. Winston GB, Lewis CW: Dermatoses of pregnancy. J Am Acad Dermatol 6:977, 1982
3. Kolodny RG: Herpes gestationis: a new assessment of incidence, diagnosis, and fetal prognosis. Am J Obstet Gynecol 104:39, 1969
4. Shornick JK: Herpes gestationis. J Am Acad Dermatol 17:539, 1987
5. Homes RC, Black MM: Herpes gestationis. Dermatol Clin 1:195, 1987
6. Wade TR, Wade SL, Jones HE: Skin changes and diseases associated with pregnancy. Obstet Gynecol 52:233, 1978
7. Jordon ER, Heine KG, Tappeiner G et al: The immunopathology of herpes gestationis: immunofluorescence studies and characterization of "HG factor." J Clin Invest 57:1426, 1976
8. Carruthers JA: Herpes gestationis: clinical features of immunologically proven cases. Am J Obstet Gynecol 131:865, 1978
9. Lawley TJ, Stingl G, Katz SI: Fetal and maternal risk factors in herpes gestationis. Arch Dermatol 114:552, 1978
10. Holmes RC, Black MM: The fetal prognosis in pemphigoid gestationis (herpes gestationis). Br J Dermatol 110:67, 1984
11. Bonifazi E, Meneghini CL: Herpes gestationis with transient bullous lesions in the newborn. Pediatr Dermatol 34:715, 1984
12. Chorzelski TP, Jablonska S, Beutner EH et al: Herpes gestationis with identical lesions in the newborn: pas-

sive transfer of disease? Arch Dermatol 112:1129, 1976

13. Lawley TJ, Hertz KC, Wade TR et al: Pruritic urticarial papules and plaques of pregnancy. JAMA 241:1696, 1979

14. Holmes RC, Black MM, Dann J et al: A comparative study of toxic erythema of pregnancy and herpes gestationis. Br J Dermatol 106:499, 1982

15. Uhlin SR: Pruritic urticarial papules and plaques of pregnancy: involvement in mother and infant. Arch Dermatol 117:238, 1982

16. Pruett KA, Kim R: Papular dermatitis of pregnancy. Obstet Gynecol 55:38S, 1989

17. Spangler AS, Reddy W, Bardawil WA: Papular dermatitis of pregnancy: a new clinical entity? JAMA 181:577, 1962

18. Spangler AS, Emerson K: Estrogen levels and estrogen therapy in papular dermatitis of pregnancy. Am J Obstet Gynecol 110:435, 1971

19. Lotem M, Katznelson V, Rotem A et al: Impetigo herpetiformis: a variant of pustular psoriasis or a separate entity? J Am Acad Dermatol 20:338, 1989

20. Oumeish OY, Farraj SE, Bataineh A: Some aspects of impetigo herpetiformis. Arch Dermatol 118:103, 1982

21. Ware M, Swinscow TDV, Thwaites JG: Pregnancy prurigo. Br Med J 1:397, 1969

22. Nurse DS: Prurigo of pregnancy. Aust J Dermatol 9:258, 1968

Chapter 40

Perinatal Infections

Nelson B. Isada and John H. Grossman III

IMMUNOLOGIC ADAPTIONS DURING PREGNANCY

Alterations in Host Response

Pregnancy is characterized by immune hyporesponsiveness. As a result, tissue expressing paternal antigens is not rejected by the maternal immune system. In addition, recent successful pregnancies with donor embryos show that foreign maternal antigens do not provoke immune rejection. The fetoplacental unit may escape rejection because (1) the uterus is an immunologically privileged site, (2) the conceptus is nonimmunogenic, (3) the maternal immune system is altered, or (4) the placenta is an immunologic barrier.[1] This subject has widespread ramifications in fields as diverse as oncology, transplantation, and reproductive immunology.[2,3]

It is evident that any maternal immune alterations must leave the mother with sufficient host defenses for survival.[4] Laboratory studies have shown an elevation of leukocytes from an average of $7,000/mm^3$ during the first trimester to $10,000/mm^3$ by the third trimester. The rise appears to be due to an increase in the number of polymorphonuclear leukocytes (PMNs), with lymphocyte numbers remaining essentially unchanged. Several in vitro studies have suggested that PMN bactericidal activity increases during pregnancy.[5,6] Studies have shown that the number of B cells, the lymphocyte precursor for antibody-synthesizing plasma cells, and T cells, lymphocytes

important in immune regulation and cytocidal activity, remain unchanged during pregnancy.[7] Many reports have suggested impaired in vitro lymphocyte responsiveness to various antigens such as phytohemagglutinin (PHA) or purified protein derivative (PPD) as pregnancy progresses.[8,9] Experiments evaluating T-cell regulatory subsets have suggested a slight increase in suppressor T-cell activity. These cells reduce antibody production in B cells.

Antibody levels in pregnancy have been studied as well. Immunoglobulin G (IgG) decreases slightly during the second and third trimesters of pregnancy, paralleling the physiologic maternal hypoalbuminemia. Immunoglobulins M (IgM) and A (IgA) levels remain unchanged. Increased levels of complement, a class of proteins with antibacterial and chemotactic activity, are found in pregnancy.

None of these observations can adequately explain the reason for maternal immunologic hyporesponsiveness. Other factors such as "blocking" antibodies, pregnancy zone protein, progesterone, α-fetoprotein (AFP), and human chorionic gonadotropin have been proposed as agents that prevent fetal allograft rejection. However, to quote Billingham and Head,[4] "A note of caution is necessary here: If all the immunosuppressive principles that have been advocated to maintain the immune detente of pregnancy were valid, pregnant females would surely be so highly susceptible to pathogens that mammals would have become extinct eons ago!"

Alterations in Disease Susceptibility

Several diseases seem to occur more frequently or to be more severe during pregnancy. The underlying pathophysiology remains obscure, although several factors may favor infections caused by viral, bacterial, and fungal pathogens.[10]

Viral Infections

Genital herpes simplex, condyloma acuminata, influenza, varicella pneumonia, poliomyelitis, and smallpox appear to be more severe in pregnancy. The mechanisms involved are undoubtedly subtle.[11,12] Herpes simplex virus (HSV) infections, for example, may recur during pregnancy because of decreased antibody–lymphocyte interaction, although there is neither a lack of antibody production nor a reduction in lymphocyte number.

Bacterial Infections

Disseminated gonococcal infections and bacterial urinary tract infections (UTI) are more frequent during pregnancy. Forty percent of cases of disseminated gonococcal infections are associated with pregnancy or the puerperium. Hormonal changes associated with pregnancy may alter the virulence of the gonococcus, predisposing to its dissemination. Pyelonephritis resulting from untreated asymptomatic bacteriuria (ASB) appears to be more common in pregnancy and may be attributed to urinary stasis in the renal collecting system, which dilates under the influence of hormones or from partial obstruction by the gravid uterus. One-fourth of women with untreated ASB develop pyelonephritis during pregnancy. Pneumococcal pneumonia and bacterial pneumonia complicating epidemic influenza have been noted to be more severe in pregnancy, especially during the preantibiotic era. Maternal mortality resulting from pneumonia peaks between 25 and 36 weeks gestation, perhaps related to mechanical restrictions interfering with pulmonary toilet and limiting reserve capacity. Reactivation of pulmonary tuberculosis and miliary tuberculosis is more common in pregnancy. A defect in lymphocyte-mediated immunity that wor-

sens as the pregnancy progresses may parallel the reactivation of this disease.

Fungi

Vulvovaginal candidiasis and disseminated coccidioidomycosis occur more often during pregnancy. Factors such as secretory IgA and local lymphocyte function may permit a flare of the yeast organism.[13] *Coccidioides* may disseminate as a result of impaired lymphocyte-mediated immunity.

PHYSIOLOGIC ADAPTIONS DURING PREGNANCY

Pregnancy-associated physiologic changes may also account for some infections. Perhaps the most important factor is the increased intravascular and extravascular fluid volume in pregnancy. This well-recognized phenomenon is most likely the result of altered mineralocorticoid metabolism involving complex interactions among aldosterone, cortisol, and deoxycorticosterone. In addition, increased erythropoietin production results in an expanded red blood cell (RBC) mass. Renal blood flow and glomerular filtration rate increase by 30 to 50 percent in normal pregnancies. Thus the pharmacokinetics of many drugs, including some antibiotics such as ampicillin and gentamicin, are significantly altered. At term, the dose of gentamicin required to achieve serum and presumably tissue levels comparable to those found in nonpregnant women is increased threefold. This difference may be due in part to an increased volume of distribution as well as to an increased renal clearance of the drug.[14–18]

The physiologic hypoalbuminemia might increase bioavailability of drugs that are highly protein bound such as penicillin G or cephalothin, although the clinical significance of protein binding of antibiotics has been debated for years. While hepatic blood flow appears unchanged in pregnancy, estrogen-associated enzyme induction may alter hepatic metabolism of drugs. The decreased gastrointestinal motility observed during gestation could alter oral drug absorption. The effect, if any, of decreased gastric acidity in the first two trimesters of pregnancy on antibiotic absorption is unknown.

Placental Transfer of Antibiotics

Virtually all antimicrobial agents have been found to traverse the placenta from the maternal circulation to the fetus and amniotic fluid. Most antimicrobial agents have a molecular weight between 250 and 500 daltons and cross the placenta by passive diffusion. Numerous factors affect the amount of drug transferred. Important variables include (1) the time-dependent concentration of free antibiotic in maternal serum and the degree of protein binding, (2) uterine artery blood flow, (3) placental surface area, and (4) the lipid solubility and degree of ionization of the antibiotic. Fetal factors include (1) umbilical vein flow, (2) the degree of protein binding, presumably to AFP early in gestation and to albumin later in gestation, (3) ductus venosus flow, (4) the effect of gestational age on hepatic and renal drug metabolism, and (5) the proportion of total body water, which is inversely related to gestational age. Fetal blood levels of antibiotics range from 10 percent to virtually 100 percent of maternal levels. Because it is extremely difficult to obtain conclusive human pharmacokinetic data, mathematic systems using multicompartment models have been proposed in an attempt to project drug distribution. Some human data have been obtained from second-trimester pregnancy terminations, after fetal demise, or at term. Although there are limitations concerning the clinical implications of this information, several general principles can be stated.[15,16]

1. Virtually all systemic antibiotics reach the fetus. However, certain drugs that are highly protein bound appear to be found in lower concentrations in the fetus than are drugs with a lower degree of binding.
2. Drug levels are higher and persist longer in premature infants, probably because of a lowered capacity for drug elimination by the immature placenta, fetal liver, and fetal kidneys.
3. The increased renal clearance and volume of distribution of antibiotics requires an increased dose, decreased dosing interval, or both, to achieve satisfactory maternal tissue levels. Aminoglycoside dosages required to attain therapeutic levels during pregnancy may be substan-

tially higher than those conventionally used outside of pregnancy.[17,18]

4. Cord and amniotic fluid levels of antibiotics often correlate poorly, perhaps because of the physiologic immaturity of the fetal kidneys.
5. Fetal toxicity of antepartum antibiotics must always be weighed against clinical need. Chloramphenicol and tetracycline are examples of drugs with potentially serious side effects for the newborn, such as cardiovascular collapse and depressed fetal skeletal growth, respectively. The effects of intrauterine exposure to aminoglycosides on fetal auditory and vestibular function are currently unknown.

Bacteriostatic Properties of Amniotic Fluid

Larsen and Galask[2] described a low-molecular-weight zinc-associated polypeptide with antibacterial properties. This factor can be detected by gestational week 20 and increases progressively throughout gestation. Endogenous phosphate inhibits this naturally occurring peptide. Meconium has a high phosphate concentration and may play a role in promoting amniotic fluid infections. Zinc levels are lower in women with poor nutrition. A relative deficiency in the zinc-associated polypeptide could contribute to the increased incidence of amniotic fluid infections found in this group. Although other compounds with antibacterial activity, such as immunoglobulins and β-lysin, have also been identified in amniotic fluid, their function is unclear.[10]

General Principles of Infectious Teratology

Intrauterine infection may have devastating effects on fetal development.[19,20] Teratogens are agents that cause abnormal embryonic or fetal development. Teratogenic agents include infections, radiation, and drugs.[21] Congenital malformations are "gross structural defects" present at birth and are part of the clinical spectrum of disease caused by teratogens.[22-24]

A specific teratogen may cause different effects, depending on the timing of exposure during embryogenesis. For example, rubella infection causes cataracts during week 6 of pregnancy, when the lens is forming.[25] Deafness results if rubella infection occurs during weeks 7 to 8 because of impaired cochlear development.[26]

Few generalizations can be applied to individual clinical situations except in the case of a well-described clinical syndrome. Other variables undoubtedly modify teratogenesis, including genetic susceptibility to the teratogen, the amount of teratogen present, and the duration of exposure. Experimental animals and humans differ in both their susceptibility to teratogens and the effects of the agents. Extrapolation from one species to another is therefore difficult. It may be extremely difficult to diagnose in utero infections. Finally, anomalies can occur in fetuses that have no known teratogenic exposure.

To prove that a given infection is teratogenic, several criteria must be met, analogous to Koch's postulates: (1) the agent has been associated with a specific pattern of anomalies retrospectively, (2) the organ(s) affected must be in an embryologically recognized period of rapid development at the time of exposure, and (3) the anomaly can be reproduced in appropriate experimental animals or is prospectively predicted in some portion of human pregnancies that are exposed. Given these criteria, the following agents act as well-defined human infectious teratogens: rubella, cytomegalovirus (CMV), varicella-zoster, HSV, parvovirus, and toxoplasmosis.[27-30]

Advances in knowledge can modify the recognition of teratogenic risks from a given infection. Some infections initially thought not to be teratogenic, such as HSV, may be recognized as such as more cases are carefully scrutinized. Other infections, such as human immunodeficiency virus (HIV), have had their teratogenic potential disputed.

INFECTIONS WITH TERATOGENIC POTENTIAL

Rubella

Rubella (German measles) is a moderately contagious, mild, exanthematous illness caused by an RNA virus. In 1941, Gregg[31] reported the association of antenatal acquisition of the infection with congenital heart disease and cataracts. This concept was met with great resistance by the medical community. The virus was isolated in 1962 and a live virus vaccine introduced in 1969 after a major epidemic in the United States. As a result of modern immunization practices, rubella is now primarily a disease of young adults rather than of children, and its "elimination" from the United States is anticipated within the next three decades.[32,33]

Microbiology

Rubella virus is a member of the togavirus family, of the genus *Rubivirus*. There is only one immunologically distinct type that occurs naturally. Its genome is single-stranded RNA, complexed with protein to form a helix of nucleoprotein. The organism replicates in the cytoplasm. Several antigens are associated with the virus, against which the host mounts an immune response. A hemagglutinin present in the virion envelope has been identified. The virus is not lytic and does not produce significant cytopathic effects in tissue cultures.

Rubella virus implants on respiratory epithelium and multiplies in the epithelium and regional lymph nodes. Viremia occurs, followed by viral shedding from the throat. The organism can be isolated from many sites, such as white blood cells, urine, stool, and synovial fluid. Transplacental spread may occur during periods of viremia.

Immunology

Natural infection elicits a variety of host responses, both humoral and cell mediated, that can limit viral replication. Secretory IgA synthesis is stimulated at the portal of entry. IgG antibody can be measured several days after the onset of clinical illness. Maternal IgG crosses the placenta in increasing amounts as gestation progresses. Antibodies against the envelope hemagglutinin rise early in the course of the illness and persist (Fig. 40.1). These IgG antibodies can be measured in an enzyme-linked immunosorbent assay (ELISA). Maternal antibodies rise and fall rapidly. The fetus is also able to synthesize IgM by 16 to 20 weeks gestation in response to the infection.

These immune responses are protective. Inapparent infection has occurred in individuals with a very low antibody titer. A "booster" response is observed with a rapid rise and fall of IgG without IgM synthesis. Transient oropharyngeal or nasal carriage of the virus occurs in such cases, but viremia does not ensue.

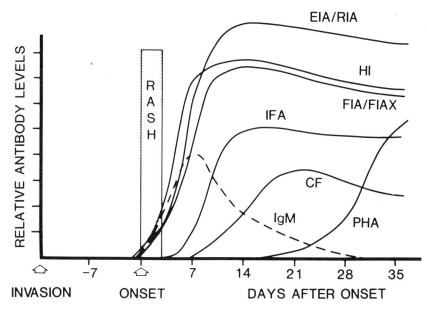

Fig. 40.1 Schema of immune response in acute rubella infection, as measured by various tests. HI, hemagglutination inhibition; EIA, enzyme immunoassay; FIA/FIAX, indirect fluorescence immunoassay; RIA, radioimmunoassay; IFA, immunofluorescent antibody; CF, complement fixation; PHA, passive hemagglutination; LA, latex agglutination; HIG, hemolysis-in-gel. (From Herrmann,[327] with permission.)

Epidemiology

In the prevaccine era, major epidemics occurred every 20 years, starting among children aged 5 to 9 years and spreading to the nonimmune childbearing population. The last major epidemic was in 1964–1965, when 20,000 cases of congenital rubella syndrome (CRS) were reported. In 1969, live rubella vaccines were introduced. Since 1970, the number of reported cases has dropped 98.7 percent for rubella and 97 percent for CRS. Reported cases of rubella and CRS are now at an all-time low. In 1987, there were 306 cases of rubella nationwide (0.1 case per 100,000 population). In that year, there were six reported cases of CRS (0.08 case per 100,000 live births). Serologic surveys from the late 1970s and early 1980s show a cohort of nonimmune young adults in the range of 10 to 20 percent.[34,35]

Clinical Aspects

Rubella is spread via nasopharyngeal secretions. It is not as communicable as measles but can spread rapidly in institutions such as schools, homes, and mili-

tary bases. The disease is communicable 1 week before the onset of the rash and 4 days afterward. Relapses may occur in 5 to 8 percent of cases. Subclinical infection is observed in 25 to 50 percent of cases.

The incubation period is 2 to 3 weeks, generally between 16 and 18 days. A prodrome lasting 1 to 5 days consists of low-grade fever, headache, malaise, anorexia, coryza, pharyngitis, and conjunctivitis. Adenopathy appears and involves the posterior auricular, suboccipital, and posterior cervical nodes. In adolescence, this adenopathy is probably the most distinctive feature.

After this prodrome, a rash appears. Pink macules involve the face, neck, and arms and spread to involve the entire body in 1 day. The rash disappears in order of appearance and is gone after 3 days ("3-day measles"). In children, the rash is the first sign. Transient polyarthralgias and polyarthritis occur in up to 50 percent of young women. Rare complications include neuritis, heart block, and, in children, thrombocytopenia. Both the rash and the arthralgias are thought to be antigen–antibody reactions, with arthralgias secondary to immune-complex deposition.

Although rubella is generally a mild, self-limited disease in children and young adults, fetal and placental infection can have devastating consequences. At least one-half of all fetuses are infected when a primary rubella infection occurs in the first trimester.

Maternal viremia may result 1 week before the onset of clinical illness. Fetal infection after maternal viremia leads to a state of chronic infection, with inhibition of multiplying fetal cells and "delayed and deranged" organogenesis. The precise mechanism of these pathologic changes is not well understood. One theory suggests destruction of clones of cells early in fetal life. Another proposes vascular insufficiency as a result of endothelial infection.

The severely affected infant has multiple organ system involvement: purpura ("blueberry muffin" skin), cataracts, "salt and pepper" retinopathy, pulmonary artery stenosis, patent ductus arteriosus, atrioventricular septal defects, microcephaly, intrauterine growth retardation (IUGR), hepatosplenomegaly, and sensorineural deafness (Fig. 40.2). Deafness is a late manifestation of the disease in some children who otherwise appear normal at birth, and mental retardation may also develop. The "expanded rubella syndrome" includes anemia, encephalitis, hepatitis, myocarditis, nephritis, osteomyelitis, pancreatitis, pneumonitis, and thrombocytopenia. Cerebral calcifications are rare. With severe involvement, the placenta shows granulomatous changes and necrosis. Late manifestations include diabetes mellitus, thyroid abnormalities, and precocious puberty.

Laboratory Studies

Serologic testing is the mainstay in diagnosing rubella (Fig. 40.1). IgG and IgM antibodies appear initially. The ELISA method is currently employed to measure IgG response. Serologic tests that give results similar to those obtained with the ELISA method include hemagglutination inhibition (HI), radioimmunoassay (RIA), latex agglutination (LA), and fluorescence (FA). Antibody appears several days after the onset of clinical illness, peaks after 7 days, and persists for years. A titer of greater than 1:32 is seen in 99 percent of cases if the infection has occurred in the past 6 months. In 15 percent of infected persons, high titers

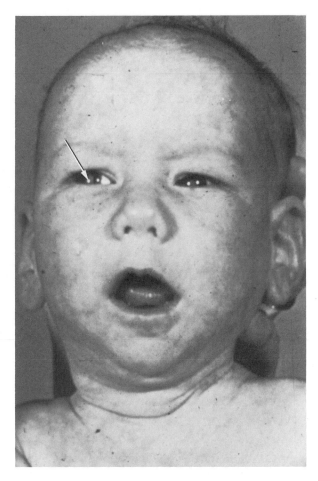

Fig. 40.2 Infant with congenital rubella syndrome. Note the cataracts (arrow) and blueberry muffin skin.

(>1:256) may persist after infection. Maternal IgM as measured by ELISA appear a few days after the rash and remain present for about 1 month.

The use of first-trimester chorionic villus sampling with in situ DNA–RNA hybridization techniques can be used to identify rubella infection. Cordocentesis and rubella-specific IgM may also detect in utero infections. Ultrasonography may be helpful in diagnosing IUGR or microcephaly compatible with but not diagnostic of CRS.[36–39]

Isolation of the rubella virus is generally reserved for diagnosis in newborns. At birth, the pharynx is the major site of shedding. Ninety percent of infected infants will also excrete virus in their urine.

Management in Pregnancy

Rubella infection can be serologically confirmed by a fourfold rise in the ELISA titer. The acute-phase specimen should be drawn at the onset of illness or as soon after as possible, preferably within the first 7 days. The convalescent-phase specimen should be drawn 10 or more days after the acute-phase specimen. If the first specimen is drawn more than 7 days after the onset of the rash, the antibody rise may not be detected because it has already occurred. Infection can also be confirmed by demonstrating rubella-specific ELISA IgM in a specimen drawn between 1 and 3 weeks after the onset of the rash.

All pregnant women should have a rubella titer drawn at their first prenatal visit. Confirmation of rubella infection in pregnant women of unknown immune status after exposure of an illness characterized by a rash and/or adenopathy can be difficult. The following guidelines published in 1981 by the American College of Obstetricians and Gynecologists (ACOG) are based on recommendations by investigators from the Centers for Disease Control (CDC) and from university medical centers.[40,41]

1. If exposure or infection occurs in a known seropositive patient, there is no apparent fetal risk.
2. If exposure or infection is suspected in a known seronegative patient, a second titer should be drawn 3 to 4 weeks after exposure or 10 to 14 days after the rash or illness. If seroconversion occurs, appropriate counseling regarding possible fetal infection is necessary.
3. If exposure (only) occurs within 1 week before evaluation, an acute titer followed by a convalescent titer in 3 to 4 weeks should be performed. If the patient is seropositive on the first titer, there is no apparent fetal risk. If a fourfold or greater rise in titer is noted, infection has occurred.
4. If a patient of unknown status presents 1 to 5 weeks after exposure or up to 3 weeks after the onset of the rash, rubella-specific IgM levels should be measured. If IgM is present, infection has occurred. If IgM is absent, acute infection cannot be ruled out, because IgM may disappear before 4 weeks.
5. If a patient of unknown status presents more than 5 weeks after exposure or 3 weeks after the rash, a single HI titer should be drawn. If the titer is less than 1:8, infection has not occurred.

In considering guideline 5, the CDC states that infection is unlikely in the past 6 months in this setting if the titer is 1:8 to 1:32, because more than 99 percent of acute rubella infections will result in development and maintenance of titers greater than 1:32 for at least 6 months after onset. However, this does not rule out the small but finite possibility of infection.

Prevention

In 1969, two attenuated live virus vaccines were introduced in the United States: HPV 77/DE-5, grown in duck embryo cells, and the Cendehill strain, derived from rabbit kidney cells. They induced immunity in 95 percent of recipients. In 1980, the RA 27/3 strain grown in human diploid cells was introduced. It is currently the only rubella vaccine available in the United States. Secretory IgA is stimulated after vaccination with the RA 27/3 in contrast to the previous vaccines, and postvaccination titers are higher. The duration of immunity after vaccination is currently unknown. One hundred twenty million doses of all three vaccines have been administered since 1969. Only six cases of CRS were reported in 1987, demonstrating the results of this vigorously enforced public health policy.

Infants are vaccinated after 12 months of life because of potential vaccine inactivation from passively transferred maternal antibody. The vaccine has induced a herd immunity in school-aged children, and proof of vaccination is now required for school entry. This cohort will probably be rubella free when it enters reproductive age in 10 to 30 years. Until that time, the current young adult population remains vulnerable to infection. Efforts have been made to include the following groups in screening and vaccination programs: postpartum women, medical and nursing personnel, college students, and military personnel.

After vaccination, the virus can be detected in nasopharyngeal secretions but is not communicable except by breast milk. However, postpartum vaccination is not a contraindication to breast-feeding.

Neonatal infection does not result in CRS, and vaccinated children will not infect their pregnant mothers.

The vaccine may produce arthralgias in 40 percent of seronegative individuals, especially women. The arthralgias appear 1 to 2 weeks after vaccination and last 2 to 4 days. Time is rarely lost from work. A transient neuritis has been infrequently reported. The vaccine should not be given during a febrile illness or to a patient who is immune deficient or immunosuppressed. Expert consultation is necessary if the patient is on corticosteroids.

Pregnant women should not receive the vaccine, and reliable contraception should be practiced for 3 months after vaccination. The vaccine should be given 2 weeks before or deferred for 3 months after receiving immune serum globulin because of potential interference with the host response to the vaccine. The administration of anti-Rho(D) immune globulin or other blood products does not generally interfere with an immune response and is not a contraindication to postpartum vaccination. A postvaccination check should be performed 6 to 8 weeks afterward. The CDC has recommended that only those who have received blood products be evaluated. However, because of the efforts expended, we believe that all women who have been vaccinated should be checked for seroconversion postpartum.

The use of antepartum immune globulin has been suggested for those pregnant women who have been exposed to rubella and who would not consider pregnancy termination under any circumstances. It appears that this therapy may modify maternal symptoms but will not protect the fetus. Infants with CRS have been born to women who received antepartum immune globulin.

Vaccination During Pregnancy

On occasion, women are immunized early in pregnancy or do not maintain contraception for 3 months after vaccination. Between 1971 and 1988, 254 rubella-susceptible women who were vaccinated during pregnancy were analyzed. There were over 200 liveborn infants from this study, none of whom had defects indicative of CRS. Live virus can be recovered in 3 percent of infants or products of conception. However, the observed risk for CRS following rubella vaccination continues to be zero. Because of these observations, the CDC has closed its registry to follow serosusceptible vaccinated pregnant women as of April 1989.[34,35]

The Immunization Practices Advisory Committee states that "the risk of vaccine-associated defects is so small as to be negligible and should not ordinarily be a reason to consider interruption of pregnancy. However, a final decision about interruption of pregnancy must rest with the individual patient and her physician."[41]

CMV

CMV is a widespread vertebrate virus recognized as the most common viral perinatal infectious agent in humans. Human CMV pathology was first noted in 1881, when large "protozoanlike" cells were seen in the kidney of an alleged syphilitic stillborn. Cytoplasmic and intranuclear inclusions were noted by Lowenstein in 1907 in neonatal parotid glands. Goodpasture introduced the term *cytomegalia* in 1921. By the 1930s, the viral origin of the disease prevailed over the protozoan origin. CMV was first isolated in human tissue culture by Smith in 1956 in samples obtained from infected neonates.

Microbiology

CMV demonstrates a restricted species-specific host range. There are no vectors. Human CMV is a member of the family Herpesviridae, along with HSV, varicella-zoster virus, and Epstein-Barr virus (EBV). It is an enveloped DNA virus.[42] After absorption to host cells, the genome is extruded and directs host macromolecule synthesis. A variety of antigens are then synthesized to which the host may mount a response. Inclusion bodies are also visible after infection, with nuclear inclusions containing viral nucleocapsids. The virus grows slowly in tissue culture as compared with HSV.

Infections with different strains of CMV have been noted clinically. Restriction endonuclease fingerprinting of CMV DNA has been useful, especially in epidemiologic studies. The site of latent CMV infection is unknown but may include monocytes, bone marrow, and the kidney.[43]

Immunology

A variety of antibodies can be measured in response to CMV infection. CMV-specific ELISA antibodies appear 3 to 4 weeks after infection. However, CMV antibody may be absent in up to 50 percent of individuals with virologically proven infection. One report noted spontaneous fluctuations in CMV titer as measured by complement fixation.[44] Current ELISA assays are reported as 55 percent sensitive and 95 percent specific. CMV ELISA IgM arises several weeks after infection and may disappear after a primary infection.

Epidemiology

Worldwide surveillance studies have been performed to determine the extent of human infection. In the United States, most individuals have been infected with this virus. The prevalence depends on age, race, sex, class, sexual behavior, and occupational/institutional exposure. The disease is spread by intimate contact with infected secretions, including breast milk, cervical mucus, semen, saliva, and urine. It may be contracted after blood transfusions or organ transplantation.

CMV antibodies have been found in 40 to 100 percent of the adult population. In poor black children, 40 to 60 percent are antibody positive, and virtually 100 percent are positive by age 25 years. Of middle-class white women, 30 percent are positive at age 20 years and 60 percent by age 40 years. Men are at less risk, with black males being 60 percent positive and white males 20 percent positive by age 20 years. By age 50 years, the majority of all individuals have been infected. The difference in male and female antibody rates has been attributed to women being more likely to handle infants and toddlers who are shedding virus in their urine. Some differences in social status have been attributed to differences in crowding and hygiene.

Circumstantial evidence indicates that the disease is also sexually transmitted, explaining in part the rise of seropositivity in adulthood.[45] The rates of viral cervical shedding have been found to be 5 percent in young women with stable sexual relationships and 25 percent or more in women with multiple sexual partners. Interestingly, cervical shedding and viruria peaks at ages 11 to 14 years and declines by age 30

years. During gestation, cervical shedding is not predictive of fetal infection.

One mode of transmission that is better defined is mother-to-infant transmission both in utero and postpartum.[46] CMV has been called the most common intrauterine infection. An estimated 0.2 to 2.2 percent of all newborns are infected in utero, with 1 in 5,000 to 1 in 20,000 infants suffering severe complications recognizable at birth. Recent studies have suggested different outcomes in infants whose mothers have a primary infection when compared with mothers having recurrent infection. Seronegative mothers have a 1 percent risk of a primary infection in pregnancy, with a subsequent fetal transmission rate of 30 to 40 percent. Of those fetuses infected, 2 to 4 percent will be severely symptomatic at birth. Seropositive mothers have an overall 1 percent risk of fetal infection. However, unlike infants whose mothers have a primary infection, more than 99 percent of those babies, although infected, appear normal at birth.[47,48]

Some infants will acquire CMV during birth through an infected cervix or by consumption of infected breast milk. Cervical transmission occurs with an estimated attack rate of 60 percent. In these infants, cord blood IgM will be negative and viruria absent at birth. However, 5 to 10 percent of these babies have developed a pneumonitis attributed to CMV. Studies comparing bottle- and breast-fed infants of seropositive mothers showed a 60 percent transmission rate with breast-feeding. One hypothesis suggests that CMV in milk will not be inactivated by neonatal gastric acid, and transmucosal infection occurs.

Blood transfusion has been associated with the transmission of CMV, with a 2 to 3 percent risk of seroconversion per unit of blood. There is usually no clinical illness. However, premature infants as well as those patients who are immunosuppressed and/or undergoing organ transplantation may develop disseminated CMV.

Horizontal transmission occurs among children in day-care centers and in schools. Women working in these settings appear to be at increased risk of seroconversion. One recent study has shown an 11 percent incidence of seroconversion among day-care workers as compared with a 2 percent rate in a control population. Health care workers, such as nurses in intensive care nurseries or dialysis units, do not appear at increased risk for acquiring infection.[49-56]

Clinical Aspects

In immunocompetent adults, CMV produces a clinically silent, persistent infection. Only 1 to 5 percent develop symptoms attributable to primary infection. The incubation period of naturally acquired infection is unknown. In adults, the mean age at the time of infection is 29 years, and the principal clinical manifestation is a mononucleosis-like syndrome, characterized by a low-grade fever, malaise, arthralgias, hepatosplenomegaly, and occasionally pharyngitis and lymphadenopathy. Although these symptoms can last 2 weeks to 2 months, most infections are entirely asymptomatic.[57]

Infants who acquire the infection in utero and who have been born to mothers after reactivation of CMV appear to be partially protected by maternal antibodies. Why this immunity is not complete is unknown. In the small groups of infants studied, 5 to 10 percent have developed sensorineural hearing loss and 2 percent chorioretinitis. Less than 1 percent were found to have mental retardation. By contrast, 10 to 15 percent of infants born to seronegative mothers who have had a primary infection demonstrate classic cytomegalic inclusion disease, with IUGR, microcephaly, periventricular calcifications (Fig. 40.3), sensorineural deafness, blindness with chorioretinitis, profound mental retardation, hepatosplenomegaly, and jaundice. Twenty percent of these babies will die. Nonimmune hydrops has also been noted.[58,59] Although experimental studies suggest greater damage with infections earlier in gestation, it does not appear that gestational age influences the rate of fetal infection after a primary maternal infection. Recent longitudinal studies suggest neurologic deficits in 25 percent of infants who appear normal at birth whose mothers acquired primary CMV in any trimester of pregnancy.[60]

Laboratory

Isolation of the virus is the most sensitive method for the diagnosis of CMV infection. The buffy coat is isolated from blood collected in a heparinized tube and is inoculated into tissue cultures. Depending on the number of infective particles, a cytopathic effect

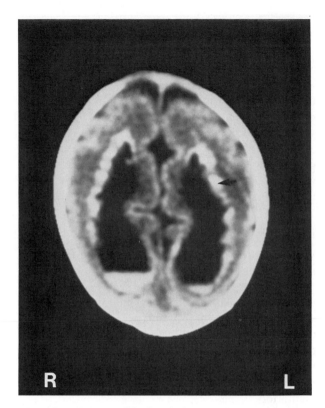

Fig. 40.3 CT scan of the head of a growth-retarded infant born at 33 weeks gestation demonstrates periventricular calcifications (arrow) and ventriculomegaly caused by intrauterine CMV infection. Immunofluorescent antibody testing confirmed the presence of CMV IgM in cord blood.

can be seen as early as 8 to 10 days, although incubation for up to 40 days may be necessary. Urine can also be used to document infection, especially in neonates. Amniotic fluid can be tested, but the significance of a positive culture is unclear. Newer techniques that utilize in situ hybridization or the polymerase chain reaction to detect the viral genome may increase the accuracy of diagnosis.[61-66]

Serologic methods may aid in the diagnosis of congenital CMV. Infants infected in utero show a positive cord CMV ELISA IgM in 70 percent of cases. Infection acquired during or after birth will reveal rising IgG titers and absent IgM.

Diagnosis and Management

Unfortunately, counseling is practically impossible because the majority of CMV infections are undiagnosable. More than 90 percent of primary infections are clinically silent. ELISA and FA tests are available for diagnostic use and can be helpful in documenting seroconversion. Assays for maternal FA or ELISA IgM antibodies may be elevated in 10 percent of recurrent CMV infections and may be negative in 20 percent of women with primary CMV.

Viral cultures of maternal urine and cervix can be helpful in certain high-risk settings to predict in utero infection. Demonstration of maternal viremia may not indicate in utero infection, nor does its absence guarantee fetal well being. Amniocentesis has been used in a few cases. However, in utero infection has been noted even with a negative amniotic fluid culture. Techniques such as cordocentesis, coupled with the use of polymerase chain reaction to detect CMV, may establish the diagnosis of in utero infection.

The CDC has recommended that routine screening of pregnant women in "high-exposure" areas, such as women working in child-care centers, nurses, and physicians, is currently not indicated because (1) the extent of risk is not currently established, (2) testing facilities are not readily available, (3) the significance of a single antibody titer is difficult to interpret, and (4) it is not known whether the risk of primary infection would be appreciably reduced by identifying seronegative women and transferring them to areas in which there is less contact with infants and children. Until further data are available, rigorous personal hygiene throughout pregnancy should be practiced, especially frequent handwashing, particularly in any setting in which repeated close contact with infants and children occurs.

Parvovirus

Human parvovirus B19 (B19) is a DNA virus that is the causative agent of erythema infectiosum.[67] It also can cause a transient aplastic crisis (TAC) in patients with chronic hemolytic anemias. Recent reports have linked maternal infection with cases of hydrops fetalis and stillbirth.

Microbiology

B19 was discovered serendipitously with counterimmunoelectrophoresis by investigators evaluating tests for hepatitis B surface antigen (HBsAg) in individuals who were HBsAg negative.[68] Thus the virus was de-scribed before any clinical syndromes were associated with it. B19 is a member of the genus *Parvovirus,* in the family Parvoviridae. B19 is a small (20 nm), nonenveloped DNA virus. Its genome contains single-stranded DNA divided into an equal number of positive- and negative-sense strands that are 5.5 kb in length. There are two other known human parvoviruses, one found in stool, similar to the Norwalk agent, and one termed RA1, associated with rheumatoid arthritis. B19 cannot be grown in standard tissue cultures. It has only recently been propagated in bone marrow cultures that have been enriched with erythropoietin. The virus replicates in the cell nucleus. Rapidly dividing cells, such as bone marrow erythroid progenitors, are preferentially affected.[69]

Immunology

Infection with the virus elicits prompt IgM and IgG responses that peak within 30 days. IgG then persists for years. IgM antibody level falls 30 to 60 days after onset of the illness and may reach undetectable levels by 60 and 90 days. These antibodies are neutralizing in vitro and appear protective in the nonpregnant individual.

Epidemiology

Serologic surveys demonstrate that the prevalence of B19 antibodies increases with age. In children less than 5 years of age, 2 to 9 percent are positive. In adults, 30 to 60 percent are positive for B19 IgG. Most clinical infections occur in school-aged children. Spread of the agent is most likely via aerosolized droplets, with the portal of entry being the respiratory tract. However, viral DNA can also be demonstrated in urine. The virus appears moderately infectious, with overall attack rates of 30 percent. Household contacts have a 50 to 90 percent chance of acquiring the infection, while the risk for a teacher exposed to an infected student is 20 to 30 percent. Different manifestations of the virus have been described in the same infected cohort.

Clinical Aspects

Several clinical syndromes have recently been reported that can occur as a result of B19 infection, all with potential obstetric significance.[70-74]

Aplastic Crisis

Aplastic crisis (AC) was the first syndrome definitely attributed to B19. The virus has been shown to replicate within erythroid precursors and inhibit their growth. In the normal host, a 1 g/dl drop in hematocrit can be demonstrated following infection. However, in patients with chronic hemolytic anemias, this red cell aplasia can cause a severe drop in hematocrit and reticulocyte count. AC has been reported in patients with sickle cell disease, thalassemia, hereditary spherocytosis, and pyruvate kinase deficiency. In nonpregnant patients, nadir hematocrits have been reported in the range of 7 to 18 percent with hemoglobin SS disease and 17 to 32 percent with hemoglobin SC disease and sickle-beta-thalassemia.[75] In experimental studies in healthy nonpregnant volunteers, hematologic changes begin 7 to 10 days after inoculation. Spontaneous recovery occurs in 2 to 4 weeks.[76]

The AC associated with B19 has been termed transient, thus the designation of TAC in some reports. However, in immune deficient patients such as those with HIV infection, a persistent chronic severe anemia may be present.

Erythema Infectiosum (Fifth Disease) and Arthritis

Erythema infectiosum (EI) is a mild, exanthematous, self-limited illness that usually occurs in childhood. It is worldwide in distribution, with the highest incidence in winter and spring. Epidemics can occur, but the disease appears less infectious than chickenpox or measles. The incubation period is 4 to 14 days. The rash initially appears on the face, giving a "slapped-cheek" appearance. It then spreads to the trunk and limbs, sparing the palms. The rash is lacy or reticular in pattern, persists for several days, and occasionally recurs. However, prospective studies during epidemics have found a significant proportion of patients with a nonclassic distribution of the rash. In these cases the palms and soles can be affected, and the face is spared. Children may have respiratory, gastrointestinal, and other systemic symptoms. In adults, the rash may be morbilliform and indistinguishable from the rash of rubella or may even be purpuric, resembling Schönlein-Henoch purpura. Adults generally have fever, lymphadenopathy, rash, and mild arthritis of the hands, wrists, and knees. The pattern of joint involvement resembles rheumatoid arthritis. The incidence of joint involvement in children is about 5 percent and involves the large joints; in adults the incidence is up to 80 percent.

EI has been called fifth disease as a result of the nineteenth century classification of childhood exanthems, numbered from the first to sixth diseases. They were (1) measles, (2) scarlet fever, (3) rubella, (4) Dukes' or Filatov-Dukes disease (caused by staphylococcal exotoxin), (5) EI, and (6) roseola.[77]

Viral particles have not been detected in serum at the time of the rash, although viral DNA is occasionally identified. The rash and arthralgias may be immunologically mediated. Viral disruption of endothelial cells, which can be demonstrated in animal infections, may also occur.

Hydrops Fetalis and Other Fetal Complications

Parvoviruses have been known to cause pregnancy complications, such as recurrent abortion, in vertebrates. The first obstetric complication attributable to B19 infection was pregnancy loss associated with fetal hydrops. A recent review cited 11 cases of well-documented parvovirus infection resulting in hydrops fetalis.[78] Three other cases have also been reported.[79,80] Fetal loss is usually between weeks 10 and 20 of gestation. If transplacental infection occurs, the fetal hematopoietic tissue is particularly vulnerable because of the rapid increase in red cell mass during the second trimester.[81,82] Cordocentesis in affected cases reveals reduction in both mature and nucleated RBCs, indicating red cell aplasia and destruction of erythroid precursors. White cell counts are also reduced. This severe anemia can cause congestive heart failure. In addition, a superimposed viral myocarditis may result, further compromising fetal cardiac performance.

Although parvoviruses are known animal teratogens, only a single case report has described teratogenic effects from B19 infection in a first-trimester abortus. There was multiorgan involvement, with microphthalmia, lens abnormalities, skeletal muscle degeneration, and vascular endothelial damage in the fetus and placenta.[83]

AFP has been reported to be elevated in two cases of intrauterine B19 infection prior to the development of hydrops. Whether this is a consequence of increased fetal hepatic production, increased transplacental leakage, or some other process is unknown.[84]

In retrospective studies, the risk of fetal loss from perinatal B19 infection has been reported to be as high as 38 percent.[85] However, case-controlled studies that have been conducted after epidemics of B19 suggest that the magnitude of risk in an unselected patient population is small, perhaps on the order of 1 percent or less.[86] The risk of severe fetal infection appears to be related to the time of exposure, ranging from 19 percent at 1 to 12 weeks gestation to 6 percent at greater than 20 weeks gestation.

Diagnosis

The diagnosis of B19 infection can be suspected on epidemiologic grounds when there is an ongoing regional outbreak or an infection in a family member, usually a child. A woman with an unexplained morbilliform or purpuric rash or a patient with chronic hemolytic anemia and an AC should be evaluated for parvovirus infection. IgG and IgM titers for parvovirus should be sent to an appropriate reference laboratory. Viral DNA may also be detected.[87]

Management

If an infection is diagnosed, serial sonography can be performed to detect fetal hydrops. Fetal blood samples obtained by cordocentesis have been utilized to establish the diagnosis of infection.[88] The role for intrauterine transfusion or other therapy, such as digitalization of the fetus, is unclear. If there is fetal cardiac muscle damage, such interventions may only partially alleviate fetal hydrops.

Prevention

Between one-third and two-thirds of the adult population have been infected with B19 and are already immune. The virus can be spread by respiratory droplets and is moderately infectious to those who are susceptible. Unfortunately, children with EI are most likely to be infectious prior to the onset of rash. Occupational exposure can occur among teachers and pediatric nurses.[89] Some investigators have suggested screening for parvovirus antibodies in such "high-risk" populations. Because the prevalence of fetal damage in unselected populations appears low, routine screening during pregnancy is not recommended

at present. The role for targeted testing as a preventative strategy requires further study.

Varicella-Zoster Virus

Varicella-zoster virus (VZV) is the causative agent of varicella (chickenpox) and herpes zoster (shingles). It has been found to be teratogenic and can cause serious maternal morbidity.

In 1767, Heberden distinguished smallpox from chickenpox. Laforet and Lynch[90] first described congenital malformations after a maternal chickenpox infection in 1947,[90] and in 1983 Weller[91] demonstrated that varicella and herpes zoster were caused by the same virus.

Microbiology

VZV is a member of the Herpesviridae family, a group of enveloped DNA viruses characterized by latency in humans. It can be isolated in tissue culture systems such as human fibroblasts. Like other members of the Herpesviridae family, the virus has glycoprotein surface antigens and the enzyme thymidine kinase.[92]

Immunology

Host humoral and cell-mediated immunity both play roles in suppression of VZV. Infants lacking protective transplacental maternal IgG can become severely ill. VZV IgG antibodies can be detected a few days after onset of maternal disease. Maternal IgG antibody transport increases with gestational age. The maternal antibody response protects the neonate, but a period of 5 days is necessary for adequate maternal antibody synthesis to benefit the term infant. VZV IgM has been demonstrated after recent infections in adults. Its presence is variable in neonates.

Epidemiology

VZV infection occurs in the late winter and early spring, with epidemics every 2 to 5 years. An estimated 5 to 15 percent of women of childbearing age are susceptible to the infection. In temperate regions, the disease occurs primarily in children, with 80 percent acquiring the disease by age 9 years. There is seasonal variation, with a peak incidence during the months of March, April, and May in the United States. Virtually 100 percent of the population is seropositive by age 60 years. In persons who do not recall having chickenpox, only 8 percent will be found to be seronegative. The household attack rate for susceptible individuals is 80 to 90 percent over a 3-week period. An occupational attack rate has been estimated to be 10 percent for seronegative health workers. Varicella is estimated to affect 0.7 in 1,000 pregnancies, as a primary varicella infection, while herpes zoster is very rare in pregnancy.

Varicella infects 20 to 40 percent of fetuses born to mothers with active disease. The risk of development of congenital malformations after primary varicella infection is small, estimated at 5 to 10 percent. Maternal herpes zoster does not cause neonatal malformations.

Varicella is more severe in adults. Although only 1.8 percent of cases occur over age 20 years, 24 percent of deaths are in this group. The death-to-case ratio following varicella in normal adults is 50 in 100,000 compared with an estimated 2 in 100,000 in normal children.

Clinical Aspects

Chickenpox is a highly contagious illness, probably spread by aerosolized respiratory droplets. The portal of entry is the respiratory tract. Individuals can be infectious for as long as 1 week before onset of the rash. Clinical illness is often preceded by a 1- to 2-day prodrome of fever and malaise. The rash then begins as pruritic maculopapules on the trunk, face, and scalp. They evolve over several days into vesicles that become umbilicated, scab, and fall off, generally without scarring. However, scarring can develop if secondary bacterial infection occurs. As new papules form, the characteristic clinical appearance of lesions present at various stages of development in the same dermatome appears.

Varicella pneumonia may develop 1 to 6 days after onset of the rash in 10 to 15 percent of adults. Symptoms include cough, chest pain, and respiratory distress, but there may be few physical signs. Pulmonary manifestations vary from no clinical illness to life-threatening disease. In severe cases, the chest x-ray shows nodular hilar infiltrates. Gas exchange is impaired, and hypoxemia is present. Thick, tenacious tracheobronchial secretions can also accompany the pneumonitis. The risk of varicella pneumonia appears to be increased in pregnancy.

If the mother develops chickenpox around the time of delivery, her infant can acquire infection. Such infants usually develop a rash 1 to 2 weeks after the onset of maternal cutaneous lesions. Newborns with chickenpox may have an extremely morbid course, with mortality rates reported between 10 and 30 percent. Morbidity in term infants occurs if maternal disease develops 5 to 7 days before birth or 2 days afterward. In such cases, the fetus becomes infected with maternal virus before birth but is born before passively receiving maternal antibody. Following birth, immunologic immaturity of the newborn may compromise its response. Maternal antibody lessens, but does not eliminate, neonatal morbidity or mortality. If infection has occurred more than 1 week before delivery, cord and maternal antibody titers are usually identical. If delivery occurs within 5 days of the onset of varicella, however, cord antibody is low or absent.

The fetus may acquire the virus by transplacental invasion during maternal viremia. Infants with congenital malformations from varicella (also called congenital varicella syndrome) may have a variety of abnormalities. Skin cicatrix formation, limb-reduction anomalies, IUGR, cataracts, microphthalmus, chorioretinitis, cortical atrophy, and microcephaly have all been attributed to VZV infection occurring between 8 and 20 weeks gestation (Fig. 40.4). Virus has not been isolated from such infants. The risk of this syndrome after maternal varicella is uncertain, although probably small. Granulomatous lesions have been noted in some placentas of infected infants, and decidual cells may reveal characteristic intranuclear inclusions. This syndrome does not occur after herpes zoster infection.[93-96]

Laboratory Findings

Like other Herpesviridae, VZV causes formation of multinucleated giant cells as part of its cytopathic effect. These cells can be seen from smears of vesicular lesions. Intranuclear inclusions may also be present. Tissue culture techniques may be useful in the diagnosis of VZV, with cytopathic effects observed in 4 to 7 days. VZV infections can be distinguished from HSV infections with virus-specific labeled antibody in tissue culture.

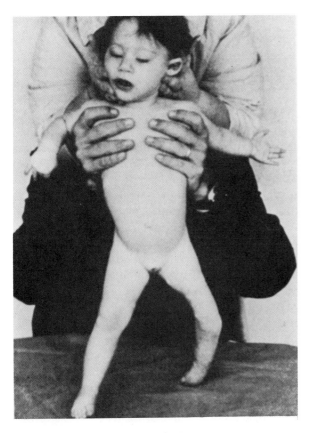

Fig. 40.4 A 1-year-old child with atrophy of the leg and cicatricial skin lesions on the median side of one leg extending to the lumbar region. The child also has microcephaly, chorioretinitis, and cataracts. The mother had varicella in the third month of pregnancy.

VZV-specific serologic tests are available to determine past exposure and susceptibility to the disease. ELISA assays are helpful in determining the presence of antibody and in establishing previous exposure to the virus. The fluorescent antibody against membrane antigen (FAMA) test permits the detection of VZV glycoproteins. This test, while highly sensitive and specific, is limited in availability. The ELISA test appears comparable to the FAMA test.[97] VZV IgM determination by either method may help to clarify equivocal cases.

Cordocentesis has been used to diagnose in utero VZV infection and to assess fetal immune response.[98] Ultrasonography may demonstrate IUGR, hydrocephaly, or limb defects in an infant with congenital varicella syndrome. The ability of viral isolation from amniotic fluid to assist in diagnosis is unknown.

Management

Varicella-zoster immune globulin (VZIG) has been used in an attempt to reduce the severity of maternal and neonatal disease. It is prepared from plasma found in routine screening of normal volunteer blood donors to contain high IgG titers against VZV.

VZIG has been given to neonates exposed to maternal VZV infection around the time of birth. The clinical attack rate in VZIG-treated normal infants exposed in utero shortly before delivery is as high as 30 to 40 percent, which is similar to that observed in untreated infants. However, the complication rate is lower in VZIG-treated neonates. VZIG is indicated for newborns of mothers who develop clinical signs of chickenpox within 5 days before to 2 days after delivery, as recommended by the Immunization Practices Advisory Committee.[99] However, recent reports suggest that the vaccine should be given if the infection has developed up to 7 days before delivery. Infants born to mothers in whom varicella develops more than 2 days after delivery are less likely to develop complications of this disease, presumably as a result of passively acquired antibody.[100]

To prevent fetal infection, some experts have recommended that VZIG be given to pregnant women with negative or uncertain prior histories of varicella who are exposed in the first or second trimester. There is no evidence, however, that administration of VZIG to a susceptible pregnant woman will prevent viremia, fetal infection, or congenital varicella syndrome. While passive immunization will probably not prevent development of clinical signs of maternal illness, VZIG should be administered to a susceptible pregnant patient to prevent maternal complications of varicella. If at all possible, VZIG should be given within 4 days of onset of the illness.

The most frequent adverse event after administration of VZIG is local discomfort at the injection site, with pain, redness, or swelling seen in about 1 percent of patients. Less frequent adverse reactions are gastrointestinal symptoms, malaise, headache, rash, and respiratory symptoms, occurring in approximately 0.2 percent of recipients. Severe reactions, such as angioneurotic edema and anaphylactic shock, are rare, occurring in fewer than 0.1 percent of cases.

Hospital Personnel

Ideally, health care personnel caring for patients with chickenpox or zoster should be immune to varicella. Proper control measures to prevent or control varicella outbreaks in hospitals should include strict isolation precautions, cohorting of exposed patients, early discharge when possible, and exclusive exposure to known immune staff. Potentially susceptible hospital personnel with significant exposure should not have direct patient contact from days 10 to 21 postexposure. If varicella develops, they should not have direct patient contact until all lesions have dried and crusted, generally 6 days after the onset of the rash. Data on clinical attack rates and incubation periods of varicella following VZIG administration to normal adults are lacking. Because of the potential of a prolonged incubation period, potentially infected hospital personnel *who receive VZIG* should probably not work in patient care areas for 10 to 28 days postexposure.

Chemotherapy

Antiviral chemotherapeutic agents have been recently used in pregnancies complicated by severe varicella pneumonitis. These drugs are similar to pyrimidines and are phosphorylated by the virally induced enzyme thymidine kinase. They then inhibit viral DNA polymerase. Viral thymidine kinase appears to have a great range for substrates, accounting for its susceptibility to these nucleoside analogues. However, the key element of management is anticipation of rapid respiratory decompensation and availability of aggressive ventilatory support.[101]

Prevention

A live vaccine has been developed, derived from the attenuated Oka strain of VZV. It is being evaluated in the United States for use in nonpregnant serosusceptible adults.

Toxoplasmosis

Toxoplasma gondii is a widespread protozoan that causes a zoonosis affecting mammals, birds, and reptiles. Its definitive host is the cat. However, a pregnant woman may act as incidental host, acquiring the disease and passing the organism to her developing fetus.

Microbiology

The organism was first noted in the spleen and liver of a North African rodent, the gundi *(Ctenodacylus gundi),* in 1908. The next year, it was classified as *T. gondii,* derived from the Greek word *toxon,* meaning arc shaped, after its microscopic appearance. In 1923, Janku, an ophthalmologist, recognized the first human case in an infant with hydrocephalus, microphthalmus, and retinitis. Paige, Cowen, and Wolf established its intrauterine transmission in 1942. Sabin and Feldman described a serologic test using methylene blue dye in 1948 that today bears their name. In 1969, the cat was found to be the definitive host for the organism.

The organism has a complex life cycle, with an enteroepithelial sexual cycle in cats and an extraintestinal asexual cycle (Fig. 40.5). There are three forms of the organism: the trophozoite (also called tachyzoite), cyst, and oocyst. Briefly, tachyzoites are the proliferative and invasive form and can persist intracellularly, especially in leukocytes. They can invade all tissues of the body. The cyst form contains approximately 3,000 organisms and persists in tissue, especially muscle and brain. These cysts are stable up to 60 degrees C. "Hard" freezing to 20 degrees C is necessary to destroy the cysts but is not achieved by most domestic freezers. These temperatures are reached in the industrial freezers used to store and transport meat. Cysts probably persist for the lifetime of the host. They remain infectious even in the presence of normal stomach acid and intestinal enzymes. Oocyst formation is the result of intestinal multiplication in the cat during a primary infection. Infection is generally acquired after eating rodents infected with cysts. Up to 10 million oocysts per day may be excreted in cat feces.

Immunology

In immune competent humans, *Toxoplasma* infection results in the development of antibodies and cell-mediated immunity. With maternal seroconversion, IgM appears 1 to 2 weeks after exposure and IgG after 3 to 4 weeks.

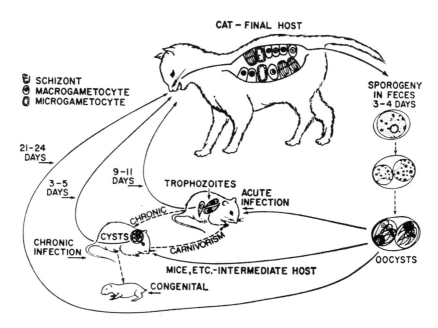

Fig. 40.5 The life cycle of *Toxoplasma gondii*. The cat appears to be the definitive host. Days indicated represent time from ingestion of *Toxoplasma* by cat to excretion of oocysts. Tachyzoites or trophozoites are the invasive form of this organism. The relationship of tachyzoites to oocysts is unclear. (Adapted from Frenkel et al.,[328] with permission.)

In utero, the infected fetus variably produces IgM antibodies to *Toxoplasma* organisms after 23 to 24 weeks gestation. After birth, maternal IgG levels in the infant fall as the infant begins producing IgG. A fetal IgM antibody response is not always detectable at birth.

Epidemiology

The incidence and prevalence of toxoplasmosis varies throughout the world. Differences in diet, meat handling, and animal husbandry practices account for the differences in prevalence of the disease.

The presence of antibody to *Toxoplasma* has been used to determine past exposure to the organism. In the United States, approximately 20 to 30 percent of women have been exposed. This number increases to 50 to 60 percent by age 40 years. By contrast, only 20 to 30 percent of French women have no detectable antibody.

The incidence of congenital *Toxoplasma* infection has generally been estimated to range from 0.6 to 6 per 1,000 live births. The incidence of clinical disease

noted at birth in the United States is 1 in 5,000 to 1 in 8,000.

Clinical Aspects

Toxoplasmosis in pregnancy is often but not invariably asymptomatic.[102] When clinical findings are present, there is lymphadenopathy and malaise, without fever. The posterior cervical nodes are most typically involved. The systemic symptoms, similar to those of infectious mononucleosis, include myalgias, sore throat, and malaise. More severe disease may involve the spleen, liver, myocardium, brain, or lungs. Chorioretinitis has been observed in up to 1 percent of adults with the acquired form of the disease.

Up to 60 percent of acutely infected women transmit the organism to their offspring.[103] One prospective study demonstrated no difference in the frequency of transmission of toxoplasmosis whether the mothers were symptomatic or not. Transmission during human breast-feeding has not been documented. The role of toxoplasmosis in the genesis of human first-trimester abortions or stillbirths is minimal.

The severely affected fetus may develop IUGR, nonimmune hydrops, hydrocephalus, or microcephaly. Apparently normal neonates may develop problems later in life. One study reported 24 congenitally infected children diagnosed by IgM or IgG/IgM antibodies in cord blood at birth. Two were growth retarded, and one had thrombocytopenia, with the remainder apparently normal at birth. It is disturbing to note that the investigators found significant neurologic and/or ophthalmologic sequelae in 22 of these children (92 percent) over a mean follow-up period of 8 years.[104]

Laboratory Findings

Accurate *Toxoplasma* serology is crucial in establishing the diagnosis of maternal infection. The practicing physician must determine exactly which tests are performed at the laboratory, their range of significant titers, their negative values, and the laboratory's credibility. One way to assess the latter is to determine whether the laboratory participates in CDC-sponsored proficiency testing using coded reference panels. Serologic testing for toxoplasmosis is perhaps the most error-prone assay performed by most clinical laboratories.

Methodologies to detect *Toxoplasma*-specific IgG and IgM include latex agglutination, ELISA, and indirect FA tests. IgM appears as early as 1 to 2 weeks after an acute infection and disappears after several weeks or months. The diagnosis of acute toxoplasmosis can be excluded if IgG is present and IgM is absent. These findings indicate a remote infection. If IgM is present, the infection is probably recent, although there are cases of persistent IgM titers for up to 2 years. IgG usually lags behind the IgM rise by several weeks, and serial samples may be necessary to establish a diagnosis.

Extensive studies in France to detect fetal infections after maternal infection have been performed. Cordocentesis has been used to detect fetal IgM. Only one-fourth of infected infants showed evidence of *Toxoplasma*-specific IgM. The diagnosis of fetal infection was established by detection of *Toxoplasma* antigen or positive *Toxoplasma* cultures obtained from amniotic fluid, fetal ascitic fluid, umbilical cord blood, or placental or fetal tissue itself.[105-109] *Toxoplasma* isolation, a test with great sensitivity not widely available in the United States, requires inoculation of clinical specimens into the peritoneal cavity of mice, with results available after 3 to 4 weeks. Alternatives

to detect *Toxoplasma* include tissue culture methods coupled with immunofluorescence. *Toxoplasma* antigen has been detected in tissue culture by the recently developed polymerase chain reaction. Other laboratory evidence suggestive of *Toxoplasma* include fetal thrombocytopenia, eosinophilia, and elevated hepatic transaminases.

The Sabin-Feldman dye test is the gold standard test to detect *Toxoplasma* antibodies. It involves incubating live *Toxoplasma* with serum, adding methylene blue vital stain, and observing dye uptake. Live organisms take up dye. If IgG antibody is present, the organisms are disrupted by complement-mediated membrane lysis, and there is no dye uptake. Observation under phase-contrast microscopy can preclude the need for vital staining. The titer at which 50 percent of the organisms are killed is reported. This test turns positive 1 to 4 weeks after infection and remains positive for many years. Few laboratories perform this test because it exposes laboratory personnel to live organisms and is more difficult to do than other, equally accurate tests now available.

Ultrasonography may detect severely affected infants. Findings include IUGR, nonimmune hydrops, hydrocephaly, cerebral calcifications, and microcephaly.

Management

The obstetrician is generally faced with these clinical situations: (1) the pregnant woman who has a positive *Toxoplasma* titer on a TORCH screen, (2) the pregnant woman who owns a cat, and (3) the pregnant woman who requests *Toxoplasma* screening. Occasionally, two other situations arise, namely, (4) the patient who has a clinical picture that suggests acute toxoplasmosis and (5) the patient who has given birth to a baby with clinical *Toxoplasma* infection:

1. If a pregnant woman presents with a positive *Toxoplasma* titer in a TORCH screen, the physician must determine what type of serologic method was used. If it is an IgG method with a high false-positive rate, repeat IgG and IgM titers must be drawn and sent to a reference laboratory such as a state/government health laboratory. Repeat titers tested simultaneously with prior samples may be necessary to establish a trend. If an acute infection is diagnosed, the pa-

tient must be counseled on the risks to the fetus. Severely infected infants have been described in all trimesters. Cordocentesis and amniocentesis can be offered.

2. If the pregnant woman has a cat, she could acquire the infection from this animal. Patients with IgG antibody and no IgM are immune. Cats with toxoplasmosis are asymptomatic. Serologic testing of cats is often misleading regarding their infectivity, and the examination of cat feces for oocytes is generally not helpful.

3. *Toxoplasma* screening can be performed, but the physician must be familiar with the laboratory's capabilities. Currently, most laboratories offering screening are not reference laboratories.

4. Patients with symptoms suggesting acute toxoplasmosis must have serial titers drawn. Appropriate tests should also be performed to rule out other disorders, such as mononucleosis and CMV infection, in the differential diagnosis.

5. IgG and IgM titers can be drawn in a mother who has given birth to an infant with clinical congenital toxoplasmosis. A sensitive test for IgM may be necessary (such as IgM ELISA), because measurable IgM IFA titers can revert to negative 6 months after infection. A high IgG titer may suggest recent acute maternal infection. Serodiagnosis in infants can be complicated by rheumatoid factor and by the presence of passively acquired maternal IgG in the infant's plasma.

Drug Therapy

If the patient elects to continue her pregnancy in the face of a diagnosis of acute toxoplasmosis, drug therapy should be initiated as soon as practical. Medical therapy has been estimated to reduce the risk of damage from infection by approximately 50 percent. The largest experience has been in Europe, where the incidence of congenital toxoplasmosis is much higher than that in the United States.

Spiramycin, a macrolide antibiotic that does not cross the placenta in significant amounts, reduces the risk of transmission to the fetus in the face of an acute maternal infection.[107] It is available through the FDA only for investigational use in pregnancy. It is recommended for use in acute maternal toxoplasmosis diagnosed before the third trimester. Treatment is continued throughout the remainder of pregnancy.

It has been used as single-agent therapy to treat pregnant women with acute infection but who have not transmitted the infection to the fetus, as judged by negative IgM at cordocentesis and negative amniotic fluid cultures for *Toxoplasma*. Oral spiramycin, 500 mg six times daily, has been used in this setting. Side effects include gastrointestinal irritation, as is seen with erythromycin.

Pyrimethamine and sulfadiazine have been used together to treat proven fetal infection. Pyrimethamine, an antimalarial drug, is a folic acid antagonist that can produce bone marrow depression and is teratogenic in laboratory animals. Folinic acid (calcium leucovorin) can be given with pyrimethamine to reduce its marrow toxicity. A recommended dose of pyrimethamine has been 50 to 100 mg orally bid on the first day, followed by a maintenance dose of 1 mg/kg every 3 to 4 days, not to exceed 25 mg per dose. Supplementary folinic acid, 5 to 10 mg orally qd, can be added. Folic acid should not be used. Complete blood and platelet counts must be obtained twice a week while on pyrimethamine therapy.

Sulfadiazine is also a folic acid antagonist. A sulfadiazine loading dose of 50 to 75 mg/kg of body weight followed by 50 to 100 mg/day in four divided doses has been used. Renal function must be monitored because of the potential nephrotoxicity from crystalluria.

Prevention

Several personal health measures can be employed to reduce the likelihood of infection. Women should cook meat until it is well done. Myoglobin converts to metmyoglobin at 65 degrees C, accounting for the color of cooked meat. At this temperature, the cysts are no longer infectious. "Hard" freezing will render cysts noninfectious. Hands, utensils, and kitchen surfaces should be thoroughly washed after contact with raw meat. Because of the potential aerosolization of oocysts from cat feces, others should handle litterboxes. Disinfection can be accomplished by treatment with nearly boiling water for 5 minutes.

Some recent studies suggest a limited impact of patient-based primary prevention programs in reducing *Toxoplasma* seroconversion during pregnancy.[110] Thus serologic screening has been suggested.[111] This approach has not yet proved consistently cost-effective in all clinical settings in the

United States.[112] Until accurate and economical tests are easily available to the general practitioner, problems of both overdiagnosis and underdiagnosis will continue.

Syphilis

Syphilis is a chronic infectious process caused by the spirochete *Treponema pallidum*. Its most devastating manifestations are in infants born with congenital infection. Although congenital syphilis usually affects infants of mothers who have sought no prenatal care, it occasionally arises in registered pregnancies. Its incidence is increasing as a result of prostitution associated with drug use. Syphilis in the HIV-positive individual has also emerged as a new management dilemma.

Microbiology

T. pallidum is a member of the family Spirochaetaceae. Humans are its definitive hosts. Other pathogenic treponemas cause human disease such as yaws or pinta, while some are oral or genital saprophytes. Syphilis has a long history of association with human civilization and has been called the "great pox." The organism was identified in 1905, and the serologic Wassermann test was described the following year. Salvarsan, the "magic bullet," was discovered in 1910.

The treponeme is 10 to 13 μm long, only 0.15 μm wide, and is not visible using ordinary light microscopy (Fig. 40.6). Special immunofluorescent or silver stains are required to identify the organism in histologic preparations. Its cell wall contains muramic acid and N-acetyl glucosamine similar to other bacteria, rendering it sensitive to certain antibiotics such as penicillin. The organism is coiled and moves in a corkscrew fashion via internal sliding filaments.

The spirochete is capable of invading all tissues and persists within cells. Local multiplication can cause an obliterative endarteritis leading to ulceration if it occurs on the skin or mucous membranes. Only recently has it become possible to culture the organism in vitro.

T. pallidum grows well at an oxygen concentration of 5 percent and is not anaerobic. The treponeme is

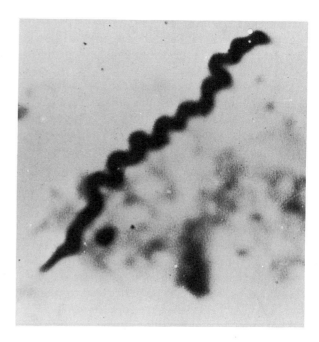

Fig. 40.6 The spirochete of syphilis ($\times$ 1,000). (Courtesy of Dr. Gerald Lazarus, Department of Dermatology, Hospital of the University of Pennsylvania, Philadelphia, PA.)

temperature sensitive, growing best between 34 to 35 degrees C, and is killed at 40 degrees C.

Immunology

The mechanism by which *T. pallidum* establishes infection and penetrates mucocutaneous tissues is unknown. Host responses can be identified and used clinically to stage the infection, but do not appear to confer immunity. For example, several antibodies against treponemal antigens have been identified that arise during or after the onset of clinical disease. However, the disease persists even with high antibody titers. Some antibodies remain for the lifetime of the host, yet reinfection may occur. Cellular immunity is also involved, especially in late manifestations of the disease, when granulomatous reaction to a small amount of antigen occurs.

Host defenses may also contribute to the clinical illness. Severe congenital disease is present after 18 to 20 weeks gestation, which is thought to coincide with maturing fetal cellular and humoral immunity. The fetal reaction then damages surrounding tissue.[113]

Epidemiology

Serologic methods for the diagnosis of syphilis coupled with the discovery of penicillin have radically altered the clinical patterns of the disease. The numbers of infant deaths from congenital syphilis have fallen 99 percent since the 1940s. Rates of clinically apparent congenital syphilis have been reduced almost 100-fold over the same time period. However, the present epidemic of drug use, especially cocaine, has resulted in increased prostitution among female drug users[114] and has been associated with a fourfold increase in the reported incidence of congenital syphilis in the last 5 years. In 1988, 691 cases of congenital syphilis were reported. There are an estimated 2 to 5 cases of congenital syphilis for every 100 reported cases of primary or secondary syphilis in women.[115,116]

Premarital serology is required in most but not all states. This screening identifies 2 percent of cases of latent syphilis and 0.02 percent of all cases of syphilis.

Clinical Aspects

Syphilis is most often acquired after direct intimate contact with infected mucocutaneous surfaces. There is no evidence that it can be transmitted by fomites on towels or sauna surfaces. After adhering to host cells, the organisms penetrate the skin or mucous membranes and multiply locally. Spirochetemia occurs after local multiplication but before the appearance of a clinical lesion. This is called incubating syphilis. Individuals who donate blood at this stage can transmit syphilis to the blood recipient. The fetus can also be infected at this time through transplacental infection. Generally after a period of 2 to 3 weeks (range, 10 to 90 days), an ulcerative lesion appears at the site of initial inoculation. This painless ulcer with a raised, indurated border is called the primary chancre and is infectious (Fig. 40.7). Sexual contact at this time will probably result in disease transmission in 30 to 50 percent of exposed individuals. The time from initial inoculation to appearance of the primary chancre is dependent on the infecting inoculum size. The lesion may be painful if there is a secondary infection, such as with *Trichomonas vaginalis*. Syphilis may be misdiagnosed as culture negative or atypical genital herpes. In 25 percent of infected women, the primary

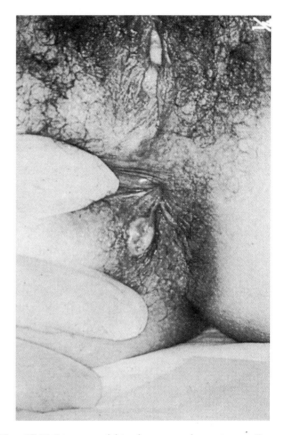

Fig. 40.7 Primary syphilitic chancre on the perineum. (From Tramont,[329] with permission.)

lesion appears on the cervix. Painless inguinal adenopathy may also be observed. Lesions may appear on the hands or in the oral cavity. The chancre disappears after 2 to 8 weeks if left untreated. The host begins to mount a serologic response that can be identified in some individuals at this stage.

Between 6 weeks and several months after the appearance of the primary chancre, the replicating spirochetes become clinically manifest again in the stage called secondary syphilis. The primary chancre may still occasionally be present. A systemic response is seen, with fever and malaise. Skin manifestations include genital condyloma lata, red or bronze macules on the palms or soles, or "mucous patches" (Figs. 40.8 and 40.9). The lesions are highly contagious at this stage. Generalized lymphadenopathy and alopecia may occur. Circulating immune complexes can

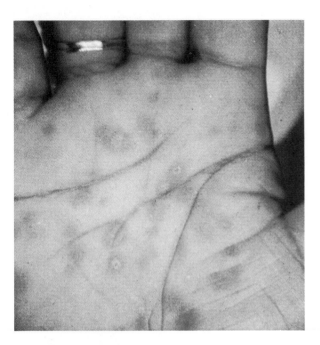

Fig. 40.8 Palmar lesions of secondary syphilis. (From Tramont,[329] with permission.)

damage the kidney and cause a nephrotic syndrome. Hepatitis with hepatomegaly, arthritis, cranial nerve palsies, and even meningitis may result. The cutaneous lesions gradually heal over 2 to 10 weeks. The systemic nature of the disease with its protean manifestations continues to make syphilis "the great imitator."

The lesions usually resolve if left untreated, and the disease enters the latent phase. Early latent syphilis is present if a person has a positive serology known to be of less than 1 year's duration or if symptoms of primary or secondary syphilis were present the previous year. Manifestations that occur after the latent phase are termed late or tertiary syphilis. These are seen in 25 percent of untreated patients and include late benign syphilis, cardiovascular syphilis, and neurosyphilis. Late "benign" syphilis is an inflammatory process that results in formation of a necrotic mass in soft tissue or viscera, called a gumma. Gummata appear to be a host reaction to small amounts of persistent treponemas producing reactive obliterative endarteritis. Cardiovascular syphilis occurs after a latency of 15 to 30 years and presents commonly as an aneurysm of the ascending aorta. Neurosyphilis is a complex disorder with many forms: asymptomatic, meningeal, meningovascular, parenchymal, or gummatous. General paresis, tabes dorsalis, and optic atrophy are manifestations of parenchymal disease.

Congenital syphilis results from maternal spirochetemia during pregnancy. The risk of congenital syphilis depends on the stage of the disease at the time of spirochetemia but has been estimated to be 50 percent in primary or secondary syphilis, 40 percent in early latent syphilis, and 10 percent in late syphilis. In utero infection may result in stillbirth, IUGR, nonimmune hydrops, and premature labor, especially in untreated cases. It was once thought that recurrent first-trimester miscarriage could result from untreated syphilis, but this has never been substantiated.

In cases of congenital syphilis, the placenta may be large and edematous. Necrotizing funisitis is a characteristic lesion of the umbilical cord.[117]

Congenital syphilis has been divided into two stages: early congenital syphilis, diagnosed before 2 years of life, and late congenital syphilis, diagnosed after 2 years of life. The diagnosis of early congenital syphilis should be suspected in babies with unexplained hydrops, a large placenta, unexplained rhini-

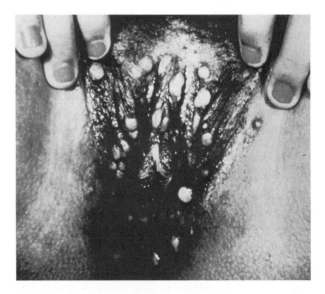

Fig. 40.9 Condyloma lata of the vulva. These lesions are symmetric and maculopapular and may have a moist, wartlike surface. They may be red or ham-colored and are sharply circumscribed and circular or ring shaped. (Courtesy of Dr. Gerald Lazarus, Department of Dermatology, Hospital of the University of Pennsylvania, Philadelphia, PA.)

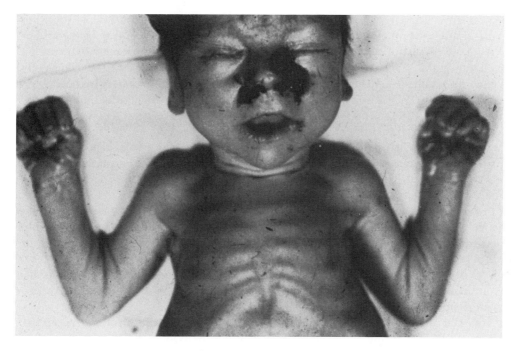

Fig. 40.10 An infant with congenital syphilis demonstrating hepatosplenomegaly, rhinitis or "snuffles," and pemphigus syphiliticus, a disseminated vesicular bullous eruption on the palms. (Courtesy of Dr. Gerald Lazarus, Department of Dermatology, Hospital of the University of Pennsylvania, Philadelphia, PA.)

tis ("snuffles"), hepatosplenomegaly, or an unexplained mucocutaneous eruption (Fig. 40.10). Late congenital syphilis is also a multisystem disease. Dental abnormalities ("mulberry molars") arise from infection of the dental pulp. Bone involvement is less common than in early congenital syphilis but may result in deformations from periosteal reaction ("saber shins"). Destruction of the nasal bones can result in the "saddle-nose" deformity. Neurosyphilis may also develop in these infants. Other syphilitic signs include Hutchinson's triad, which consists of notched, pear-shaped permanent central incisors (Hutchinson's teeth), interstitial keratitis of the eye, and osteochondritis leading to eight nerve deafness.

Laboratory Diagnosis

Proper clinical management rests on appropriate laboratory testing for syphilis. Direct visualization of the organism from clinical lesions provides the definitive diagnosis of syphilis. Darkfield microscopy of scrapings or aspiration from the base of the lesion will reveal the undulating spiral-shaped organisms. Expe-

rience and training are necessary, because oral or vaginal lesions may contain nonpathogenic spirochetes that look very much like *T. pallidum*. This technique is most useful in primary chancres when the serologic tests are often still negative. Herpes simplex infection and other ulcerative lesions must also be considered, depending on the clinical picture. Direct visualization of the treponemas may be hampered by application of topical ointments or antiseptic solutions. Phase-contrast microscopy has been used in some centers instead of the darkfield technique.

Serologic testing is the most common method for diagnosing syphilis. These tests measure various host antibodies that develop as a result of syphilis infection.[118]

Nontreponemal tests measure a heterogeneous group of IgG and IgM antibodies directed against cardiolipin, a substance present in mammalian cells that also comprises 10 percent of treponemal lipids. Treponemas altered by host lipids or host tissue altered by treponemal antigen are thought to be the stimuli that generate these antibodies. They do not appear to be protective. Through a quirk of immunologic nomenclature, this group of antibodies against syphilis and the general class of IgE antibodies have both been called reagin.

The tests generally available are the Venereal Disease Research Laboratory (VDRL) slide test and the rapid plasma reagin (RPR) test. Antibodies are detected by flocculation or agglutination of an antigen suspension of cardiolipin, cholesterol, and lecithin. RPRs are reported as positive or negative, whereas VDRL results are quantified. These tests are positive in 60 to 90 percent of tertiary syphilis. The host "inflammatory" response measured by nontreponemal tests can decline over a period of time to nondetectable levels. Positive results may occur in the presence of other disorders as with chronic infection or connective tissue disorders, such as systemic lupus erythematosus or rheumatoid arthritis. Chronic false-positive tests are defined as persisting for 6 months or more. Pregnancy can cause a chronic biologic false-positive RPR or VDRL test result. Such titers are characteristically low, at a level of 1 : 1 or 1 : 2. Cerebrospinal fluid (CSF) VDRL titers may be helpful in the diagnosis of neurosyphilis, although recent literature contests its use in asymptomatic individuals who are from populations with a low prevalence of disease.[119]

Treponemal tests measure antibody directed against treponemal antigens, both venereal and non-venereal. Three standard techniques are the FTA-ABS, MHA-TP, and *T. pallidum* immobilization (TPI) tests. All tests for *T. pallidum* are also reactive in other treponematoses such as yaws and pinta. Once these treponemal tests become positive, they remain so for the lifetime of the individual.

The fluorescent treponemal antibody-absorbed (FTA-ABS) test involves pretreatment of serum with a nonvirulent treponeme "sorbent," *Treponema phagedenis* (formerly *T. reiteri*), that absorbs nonpathogenic antitreponemal antibodies. This mixture is then layered on a slide prefixed with *T. pallidum*. Anti-gammaglobulin antibody labeled with a fluorescent pigment is added and the slide examined under fluorescence microscopy. Treponemas produce a characteristic staining pattern. This assay is time consuming and expensive but is positive in 86 to 100 percent of primary syphilis cases and in 96 to 100 percent of syphilis cases. Antinuclear antibodies

found in systemic and discoid lupus erythematosus can cause a beaded or homogeneous pattern of fluorescence, not characteristic of a true FTA-ABS test. The FTA-ABS test may be transiently positive in about 1 percent of otherwise healthy persons.

The microhemagglutination assay for *T. pallidum* (MHA-TP) uses sheep RBCs coated with *T. pallidum* antigens. Serum with antibody will agglutinate the RBCs. This test can be automated and is less expensive to perform than the FTA-ABS test. It is positive in 64 to 87 percent of cases of primary syphilis, in 96 to 100 percent of cases of secondary syphilis, in 96 to 100 percent of cases of latent syphilis, and in 94 to 100 percent of cases of late syphilis. The TPI test is no longer generally available in the United States.

Other laboratory tests may be helpful in identifying systemic syphilitic manifestations. In secondary syphilis, liver enzymes may be elevated, and a leukocytosis may also be present. Proteinuria can also result. CSF may show mononuclear pleocytosis, elevated protein, decreased glucose, and a positive VDRL test. The application of an FTA-ABS test on CSF is currently discouraged, because apparently adequately treated patients can remain seropositive.

Examination of cord blood for neonatal IgM against *T. pallidum* to detect congenital infection led to the development of the FTA-ABS IgM test. Problems have been noted with both false-positive and false-negative results. A false-negative rate of up to 20 to 40 percent has been found in cases of late congenital syphilis. Various modifications of this test are under study, and some are employed in statewide clinical screening programs. A specific IgM ELISA has been recently developed and found to be useful in areas of Africa where there is a high prevalence (10 percent) of congenital syphilis.

Management in Pregnancy

Incubating Syphilis

The management of potentially incubating syphilis, as, for example, after sexual assault, remains controversial. Both prophylactic medical therapy and serial nontreponemal serologic testing have been advocated. If the latter method is chosen, a 3-month follow-up with a negative serology excludes syphilis.

Primary Syphilis

A specimen from an ulcerative lesion can be examined under darkfield microscopy for an immediate definitive diagnosis of syphilis. Nontreponemal tests may not be positive at this time. If a nontreponemal serologic test is reactive, a confirmatory treponemal test is helpful. Serial nontreponemal tests are necessary in initially seronegative cases. A fourfold rise in titer is significant. If the tests are persistently negative after 3 months of serial sampling, syphilis can be excluded.

Secondary Syphilis

The organism may be identified in mucocutaneous lesions or lymph node aspirates from darkfield microscopy. Nontreponemal tests are generally positive.

Early Latent Syphilis

It can be difficult to make a diagnosis of early latent syphilis. A firm history suggestive of primary or secondary syphilis in the past year or seroconversion following known seronegativity in the past year is necessary.

Latent Syphilis of Greater Than 1 Year's Duration

Some physicians believe that examination of spinal fluid of all patients at risk for this stage of syphilis is necessary to rule out asymptomatic neurosyphilis. In such cases, there is a positive serology, but no history of previously treated syphilis or recent symptoms suggestive of syphilis in the past year. We recommend lumbar puncture on an individualized basis, especially in pregnancy.

Previously Treated Syphilis

A rise in serial titers of nontreponemal tests or demonstration of the organism by darkfield microscopy is necessary before a diagnosis of reinfection or failed treatment can be made. Lumbar puncture is usually necessary if there are rising titers after treatment.

Exposure to Syphilis

As with potentially incubating syphilis, management approaches vary. Either prophylactic treatment or serial serologies should be initiated.

Late Benign Syphilis, Neurosyphilis, and Cardiovascular Syphilis

Late manifestations of syphilis are very rare in pregnancy and must be evaluated on a case-by-case basis.

Congenital Syphilis

A revised CDC case definition for reporting congenital syphilis has been recently introduced. A *confirmed* case of congenital syphilis is defined as an infant in whom *T. pallidum* is identified by darkfield microscopy, fluorescent antibody, or other specific stains in specimens from lesions, placenta, umbilical cord, or autopsy material. A *presumptive* case of congenital syphilis is either of the following: (1) any infant whose mother had untreated or inadequately treated syphilis at delivery, regardless of findings in the infant; or (2) any infant or child who has a negative treponemal test for syphilis and any one of the following: evidence of congenital syphilis on physical examination, evidence of congenital syphilis on long bone x-rays, reactive CSF VDRL, elevated CSF cell count or protein (without other cause), quantitative nontreponemal serologic titers fourfold higher than the mother's (both drawn at birth), or a reactive test for FTA-ABS–19S–IgM antibody. A *syphilitic stillbirth* is a fetal death in which the mother had untreated or inadequately treated syphilis at the delivery of a fetus after 20 weeks gestation or a fetus weighing greater than 500 g.[120]

Treatment

Penicillin G remains the drug of choice for all forms of syphilis.[121,122] It is treponemicidal at very low serum concentrations. Prolonged drug levels are needed to eradicate the organism, because the spirochete has a long doubling time of 30 hours. The initial studies of syphilotherapy involved daily administration of crystalline penicillin or aqueous penicillin G *procaine* (not benzathine).[123] There are no studies of syphilotherapy exclusively in pregnancy. Recognized failures in the prevention of congenital syphilis occur in 1 to 2 percent of treated parturients. Recently, it became apparent that patients who are HIV positive may not respond to the "standard" doses of penicillin therapy.[124,125]

Penicillin treatment may give rise to the Jarisch-Herxheimer reaction. It consists of fever, chills, myalgias, and leukocytosis within 1 to 2 hours after the initiation of penicillin. Symptoms peak at 7 hours and subside after 24 hours with bed rest and antipyretics. The pathophysiology may be related to massive release of antigens from dying treponemas. Antihistamines are ineffective in these patients. Occasionally, precipitous premature labor ("placental shock") has ensued. Patients should be cautioned about development of premature labor or uterine irritability when treated for primary or secondary syphilis.

In cases of maternal penicillin allergy, erythromycin may be prescribed. However, erythromycin crosses the placenta poorly, with fetal levels only 6 to 20 percent of maternal levels. Infants of mothers who have received erythromycin should therefore be treated after birth.[126] Tetracycline has recently been advocated as an alternative to erythromycin for treatment during pregnancy, because it is thought to be more effective in the eradication of in utero syphilis. Opponents of this approach raise concerns about the effects of tetracycline on the developing fetus and maternal liver. Proponents for its use point out that the risk of congenital syphilis is well described while the risks of tetracycline therapy may be more theoretical. Our approach is to verify the maternal penicillin allergy using skin testing with penicilloyl polylysine or the penicillin G minor antigenic determinants and then implement penicillin desensitization protocols.[127,128]

Early syphilis (primary, secondary, latent syphilis of less than 1 year's duration) should be treated with a single dose of penicillin G benzathine, 2.4 million units IM. Syphilis of more than 1 year's duration (latent syphilis of indeterminate or more than 1 year's duration, cardiovascular, or late benign syphilis) should be treated with penicillin G benzathine, 2.4 million units IM, once a week for 3 successive weeks (7.2 million units total). The optimal treatment schedules for syphilis of greater than 1 year's duration have been less well established than schedules for early syphilis. In general, syphilis of longer duration requires more prolonged therapy.

Published studies show that a daily dose of 6.0 to 9.0 million units of penicillin G over a 3- to 4-week period results in a satisfactory clinical response in approximately 90 percent of patients with neurosyphilis. Regimens employing penicillin G benzathine or penicillin G procaine in doses under 2.4 million daily do not consistently provide treponemicidal levels of penicillin in CSF and may fail to cure neurosyphilis.

Follow-Up After Treatment

In pregnancy, serial nontreponemal serologies should be drawn monthly after therapy. A consistent decrease in these titers should be observed. The nontreponemal serology is negative in 75 percent of treated patients with primary syphilis after 1 year and in 40 percent of treated patients with secondary syphilis. The time to reach seronegativity is proportional to the duration of the untreated disease. During this follow-up examination, women who show a fourfold rise in titer should be reevaluated for possible reinfection.[131]

HSV

HSV received great media attention a decade ago, but has been overshadowed by HIV-1 infections. However, many individuals are still burdened with consequences of genital HSV. On rare occasions, cervical infection can be transmitted intrapartum from the mother to the fetus, resulting in major neonatal morbidity and mortality.

Microbiology

HSV belongs to the *Herpesviridae* family of double-stranded DNA viruses.[93] This family includes CMV, VZV, EBV, and the recently described human herpesvirus 6 (HHV-6) that infects B lymphocytes and is associated with lymphoproliferative disorders. Shared characteristics are the abilities to escape immune elimination and to establish latency.

HSV is composed of 162 nucleoprotein subunits enclosing the DNA genome, a structure common to all herpesviruses. The surrounding lipid envelope imparts specificity for the attachment to mucocutaneous tissue. This attachment is mediated by HSV-specific glycoproteins that attach to heparan sulfate, a ubiquitous cell surface glycosaminoglycan. The gene for the enzyme thymidine kinase has been sequenced for both HSV-I and HSV-II.

Earlier studies from the 1960s permitted division of HSV into types I and II, based on antigenic variations. Divergent evolution of these viruses appears to have begun when humans assumed an upright posture.[129] Initial assessment associated oral lesions with

HSV-I and genital lesions with HSV-II. It is now clear that this distinction is not clinically significant, because the two types possess similar tissue tropism and perinatal impact (although type I recurs less frequently than does type II in the genital area).[130]

HSV is cytocidal in vitro, causing formation of syncytia and multinucleated giant cells. This effect can be seen in vivo in epithelial tissue. Sensory ganglia are the site of latency in humans. The molecular mechanisms for the development of this latent state are unknown.

Immunology

Infection with HSV elicits antibody responses against various components of the virus, with antibodies against glycoprotein envelope antigens being the most studied. Antibodies to different serovarieties of HSV impart cross-protection; that is, previous infection with one antigenic HSV type is partially protective against clinical infection with a different strain. However, which specific proteins (or protein portion of the surface glycoproteins) stimulate the antibody reaction that confers immunity is not known. Antibody levels are not predictive of the presence or absence of infection, likelihood of recurrence, or immunity to other HSV serotypes. In vitro studies have suggested that antibody–lymphocyte or antibody–macrophage interactions may play a role in suppressing or eliminating the virus. This process, termed antibody-dependent cell-mediated cytotoxicity, is less vigorous in newborns than in adults.

Epidemiology

An estimated 300,000 cases of genital HSV occur yearly in the United States. The majority of adults are seroreactive to various HSV antigens, suggesting a prior or possibly a subclinical infection. One-third of genital HSV in women under age 25 years is caused by HSV-I, the remaining two-thirds by HSV-II. Although 1 to 2 percent of all women will have cervical cytology suggestive of HSV, prospective studies indicate a cervical carriage rate of less than 1 percent. According to retrospective estimates, about one in 7,500 liveborn infants will suffer perinatal transmission of HSV.

Virus can be isolated from the cervix and vulva in asymptomatic women ("shedding"). Whether pregnancy alters the rate of recurrence or the frequency of cervical shedding is disputed. Surveys indicate that the incidence of asymptomatic shedding in pregnancy is 10 percent after a primary episode and 0.5 percent after a recurrent episode.

Disease is transmitted by intimate mucocutaneous exposure. There is no firm clinical evidence that transmission occurs through contact with toilet seats, towels, or hot tubs. Rare cases of acquisition of the disease from truly asymptomatic individuals have been reported.

Clinical Aspects

Mucocutaneous HSV infections can be classified clinically as primary or secondary. A classification has been proposed by the World Health Organization to standardize nomenclature.[132] Primary infections are those occurring in an individual for the first time, without clinical or serologic evidence of prior infection. Secondary infections imply subsequent reinfections or reactivations of previous infections. In general, primary infections are more severe, producing somewhat more extensive areas of skin infection with greater discomfort for a longer period of time compared with secondary infections. In addition, primary infections are more likely to be associated with constitutional signs and symptoms of illness (fever, myalgias, malaise), which may reflect an associated viremia. Secondary infections are only infrequently associated with such events, presumably a reflection of the tendency for such episodes to produce milder, more self-limited, superficial infections involving localized mucocutaneous surfaces. The symptoms noted will vary widely from individual to individual. They frequently include sensations of numbness, tingling, burning, itching, or pain. The latter may be quite out of proportion to the clinical findings because of the extensive innervation of mucous membranes. Lymphadenopathy frequently accompanies either form of infection and will appear in nodes draining involved areas.

Affected skin surfaces first become erythematous and then evolve through a papular stage (Fig. 40.11). Primary infections are usually more severe and may persist for as long as several months. In general, infective virus particles can be recovered from cutaneous surfaces as soon as symptoms arise, often 12 to 36 hours before any clinical signs of infection appear.

Probably the most common complication of genital

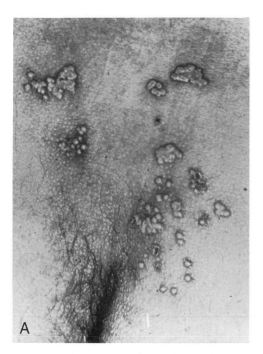
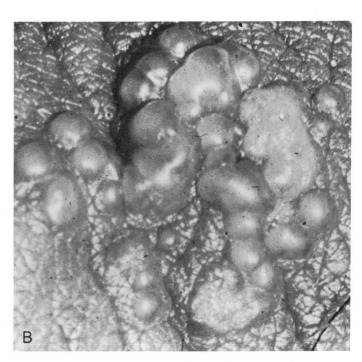

Fig. 40.11 **(A)** Herpes simplex infection of the gluteal region. The lesions are grouped, umbilicated vesicles on an erythematous base. The lesions begin as erythematous papules and plaques, developing into umbilicated vesicles that become pustular and crust. (Courtesy of Dr. Gerald Lazarus, Department of Dermatology, Hospital of the University of Pennsylvania, Philadelphia, PA.) **(B)** Closer view of lesions of herpes simplex.

HSV infections among women is urinary retention. Ophthalmitis, meningitis, hepatitis, and encephalitis because of dissemination of HSV infections are rare.

Congenital HSV infections, which produce fetal malformations, are exceedingly rare. A recent report described 13 infants who acquired HSV in utero. These infants were born with cutaneous scarring, CNS abnormalities including hydranencephaly, chorioretinitis, hepatosplenomegaly, and positive cultures for HSV-I. Tests for rubella, CMV, and toxoplasmosis were negative. These mothers were either asymptomatic or had primary or recurrent HSV outbreaks while pregnant. The true risk of developing this disorder cannot be assessed at this time.[133,134]

Neonatal infections caused by HSV may have devastating consequences. Babies seem less capable of limiting the spread of HSV infections acquired at parturition. Neonatal disease arises either from an ascending infection before delivery or as a result of direct skin contact with infected maternal genital surfaces during delivery. About 2 to 10 days after exposure, the baby develops signs of infection usually in association with characteristic skin lesions. Few, if any, neonatal infections are asymptomatic. The majority ultimately produced disseminated and/or CNS disease, with a mortality rate of 50 percent. In addition, neurologic or ophthalmic sequelae are frequent among babies who survive systemic infections. Pneumonitis may also develop.[135] Internal fetal monitoring in the presence of active genital herpes has been associated with serious neonatal infection.

Diagnosis

Virus isolation in tissue culture currently represents the optimal diagnostic approach. This method is the standard against which other methods are compared and provides unequivocal evidence of the presence or absence of infective virus particles on a skin surface or in body secretions. Tissue cultures must be held for

7 to 10 days to exclude categorically the possibility of an infection, because low numbers of infective particles may require as long as 6 days to produce the characteristic cytopathic changes in vitro. With the use of an HSV-specific ELISA in tissue cultures, it is possible to provide preliminary evidence to support a diagnosis of active infection within 24 to 48 hours of culturing. Newer methods involving molecular genetic techniques to detect viral DNA are being investigated. Such tests can be used in conjunction with tissue culture techniques. Their direct application for rapid diagnostic testing is unclear at present.

Serology is of limited value in establishing the diagnosis of maternal HSV infections. No single antibody titer is predictive of the presence or absence of genital shedding of virus at any point in time. Virus may or may not be recovered from women without antibody or from those with high antibody titers.

Several clinical considerations will greatly facilitate successful culturing of genital HSV infections and reduce the likelihood of missing the diagnosis. Many recurrent episodes produce comparatively innocuous findings that may be missed in the course of a cursory visual inspection of genital surfaces. The patient should point out where her symptoms are located as well as any sites at which previous infections have occurred. Often small areas of infection, which might otherwise be missed, can be successfully sampled using this approach. The endocervical canal and exfoliated cells from all suspicious areas should be obtained for viral culturing. In general, the yield of positives will be increased if crusted lesions or vesicles are unroofed and the base of ulcer craters is rubbed sufficiently hard to discolor the swab fibers with absorbed secretions. For infected individuals, this process is moderately uncomfortable, providing further presumptive evidence that the sample will be positive for HSV growth. Specimens should be promptly transported to the diagnostic laboratory for processing using a medium containing antibiotics. If transportation is delayed, specimens may be held at 4 degrees C before shipment, but in general they should be processed within 24 hours of sampling.

Smears of scrapings from the base of the vesicles may be stained using the Papanicolaou or Tzanck techniques. They will demonstrate multinucleated giant cells, suggesting HSV infection in 60 to 80 percent of cases (Fig. 40.12).

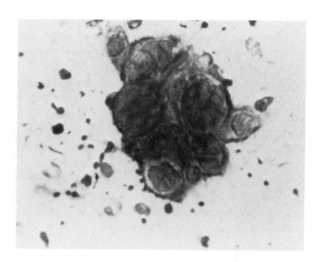

Fig. 40.12 Multinucleated giant cell of herpes simplex demonstrated on Tzanck smear. This preparation is made by unroofing a fresh vesicle, gently scraping the base of the vesicle with a scalpel, placing the scrapings on a microscopic slide, fixing with 95 percent alcohol, and staining the smear with Wright's or Giemsa stain. A positive preparation demonstrates large multinucleated giant cells with deep blue cytoplasm. (Courtesy of Dr. Gerald Lazarus, Department of Dermatology, Hospital of the University of Pennsylvania, Philadelphia, PA.)

Management

Women suspected of having a genital HSV infection complicating their pregnancies should be diagnosed using the best test available, preferably by culture on tissue monolayers to isolate infective virus particles from suspicious mucocutaneous surfaces. The risk to the neonate of acquiring HSV when the mother has a primary outbreak may approach 50 percent.[136] Recurrent maternal HSV poses a much smaller risk to the child. With more experience, this risk will be better defined. Recent studies put this risk at less than 8 percent. This estimate was reached based on 34 neonates exposed to symptomatic or asymptomatic recurrent HSV-II infection at the time of delivery, none of whom developed symptomatic neonatal HSV disease. As the numbers of unaffected infants delivered in this setting increase, this risk figure will decrease. The basis of this protection may be related to maternal antibody transferred to the fetus.[137]

Studies have also noted that cervical HSV cultures taken in the weeks prior to delivery did not correlate with the culture result obtained at the time of delivery. These observations have prompted other approaches to the management of the pregnant woman with a history of recurrent genital HSV.[138-140]

Recent recommendations have included the following.[141]

1. Cultures should be done when a woman has active HSV lesions during pregnancy to confirm the diagnosis. If there are no visible lesions at the onset of labor, vaginal delivery is acceptable.
2. Weekly surveillance cultures of pregnant women with a history of HSV infection, but no visible lesions, are not necessary, and vaginal delivery is acceptable.
3. Amniocentesis in an attempt to rule out intra-uterine infection is not recommended for mothers with HSV infection at any stage of gestation.

The clinical situation at parturition takes precedence over any laboratory findings. A woman with a recently positive culture must be microbiologically and clinically free of infection before being allowed to deliver vaginally. Those with recently negative culture are assumed to have an active infection if symptoms or lesions develop when the membranes rupture or labor begins. Using this approach, fewer than one-half of such pregnancies require cesarean section because of HSV infections. In other words, active genital HSV in a patient in labor or with ruptured membranes dictates cesarean section regardless of duration of ruptured membranes. Women can be allowed to deliver vaginally if there are no symptoms or signs of HSV infection.

Cesarean delivery should not be regarded as a panacea. Newborn infections do occur occasionally, despite prompt cesarean section of mothers with active infections during labor. Moreover, cesarean section itself carries risks of major morbidity.

Clinical experience involving the intrapartum management of extragenital HSV infections, such as the buttocks, sacral area, or thighs, is limited. In such cases, management must be individualized.

Mothers with active infections should be placed on contact isolation precautions both during and after delivery. Breast-feeding may be permitted, provided that careful handwashing is performed and the baby is not permitted to come into contact with infected skin surfaces or secretions. Rooming-in should be permitted with good hygienic practices by the mother and staff. Infants returning to the general nursery should be maintained on strict isolation to prevent the possibility of horizontal transmission to other newborns as a result of late development of neonatal infection. Babies of all mothers with active infections at parturition, regardless of route of delivery, should be observed carefully for 7 to 10 days following birth, and consideration should be given to early aggressive antiviral chemotherapy if evidence of infection develops.

Medical Therapy

The antiviral agent acyclovir is a synthetic pyrimidine phosphorylated by viral thymidine kinase present in HSV-infected cells. Phosphorylated acyclovir inhibits viral DNA polymerase and causes chain termination when incorporated into DNA. Experience with this therapy in pregnancy is limited. It has been used in women with disseminated HSV. Some authors have suggested that its use may reduce the severity of fetal in utero infection if a primary herpetic infection occurs. Until more experience can be gained, we do not recommend its unrestricted use for genital HSV in pregnancy except in cases of life-threatening infection.[142]

HIV

HIV type 1 (HIV-1) is the major cause of acquired immune deficiency syndrome (AIDS) in the United States. It is one of several human retroviruses and can 0cause profound, irreversible immune suppression. The virus is transmissible by sexual, parenteral, and perinatal routes, thus being of particular concern to obstetricians. Knowledge regarding HIV infection continues to expand, and the practitioner should remain abreast of major developments.[143]

Microbiology

The cause of AIDS is the infectious agent HIV-1.[144,145] The identification of this agent was made possible because of prior research on animal retroviruses. Revised taxonomy introduced in 1987 supercedes the following terms: lymphadenopathy-associated virus (LAV), the AIDS-related virus

(ARV), and human T-lymphotropic virus type III (HTLV-III). HIV-1 is a member of the Retroviridae family in the subfamily lentivirinae. Retroviruses are icosahedral, enveloped, single-stranded RNA viruses. Various protein (p) and glycoprotein (gp) components have been identified, and are named by their composition and molecular weight in kilodaltons. The envelope possesses a surface glycoprotein called gp120 and a transmembrane glycoprotein termed gp41. Within the capsid is the genomic RNA complex with a viral-coded RNA-dependent DNA polymerase that is a reverse transcriptase. This enzyme transcribes viral RNA into DNA in a "reverse" direction of information flow than is usually found in biologic systems (namely, from DNA to RNA), thus the term retrovirus. This enzyme is more error prone than are eukaryotic DNA polymerases, resulting in relatively rapid development of viral genomic and antigenic variation. The viral genome has been sequenced.

HIV-1 selectively infects lymphocytes. One type of T lymphocyte, the helper T lymphocyte, is preferentially infected by HIV-1. Other terms used to describe these lymphocytes are CD4+ T4 cells, OKT4 cells, and T4 cells, all of which can be considered synonymous. CD4 is a surface glycoprotein on T-helper lymphocytes and is a binding site for gp120. Other T-cell antigens also play a role in viral attachment and cell entry. These infected helper lymphocytes are destroyed when clonal expansion occurs, especially in the face of immune stresses. HIV-1 can cause a cytopathic effect on infected cells, with syncytial formation, balloon degeneration, and cell death. Alternatively, a latent state can be established, with the viral genome integrated into host DNA. Other cells may be infected, including B cells, macrophages, monocytes, and glial cells. Chorionic villi can also be infected.[146] HIV-1 has been isolated from blood, semen, and saliva of asymptomatic individuals and patients with AIDS.

Human T-lymphotrophic virus type I (HTLV-I) has been associated with adult T-cell leukemia/lymphoma,[147-149] whereas HTLV-II has been associated with hairy cell leukemia. Another virus similar in structure and antigenicity to HIV-1 has recently been described in western Africa, termed HIV-2. There is a 40 percent sequence homology between the two viruses. Both HIV-1 and HIV-2 have been identified in patients with AIDS.[150,151]

Immunology

The hallmark of AIDS is a profound and irreversible immunosuppression in a previously healthy individual. As mentioned above, HIV-1 appears to infect helper T cells preferentially. Some T-lymphocyte subpopulations, such as suppressor (T8) cells, remain unaffected. The ratio of circulating helper to suppressor cells (T4/T8) is used as an index of immune suppression suggestive of AIDS. Neutropenia and monocytopenia have been noted, in addition to lymphopenia.

Following HIV infection, host B cells are stimulated, with diffuse polyclonal elevations of the major immunoglobulin classes. Despite these findings, B cells are refractory to further immunogenic stimulation in vivo and in vitro, thus resulting in a humoral abnormality in addition to a cellular one. Circulating immune complexes and a variety of autoantibodies may be found. An IgM response to antigenic challenge is also blunted or absent.

Circulating antibodies to viral envelope glycoproteins and core proteins have been identified, but their role in host defense is unknown. Virus has been isolated in the presence and absence of antibody, and clinical illness may occur in the presence of antibody. Many asymptomatic individuals may also be antibody positive. The time course of development of an identifiable humoral immune response is dependent on inoculum size and route of transmission. While some studies have described the appearance of antibodies 6 to 12 weeks after exposure, the response may be delayed up to 18 months.

Intact mucous membranes and cutaneous surfaces play a significant role in host defense. This is inferred from increased rates of transmission of infection in anal–penile intercourse, as compared with oral–penile or vaginal–penile intercourse, and virtual absence of transmission with casual skin-to-skin contact.[152]

Epidemiology

The first cases of AIDS were reported to the CDC in 1981. As of 1989, 89,501 adult cases have been reported (Fig. 40.13). Worldwide retrospective studies have identified cases since the late 1970s. The earliest evidence of viral infection has been in banked serum collected in Zaire in 1959.

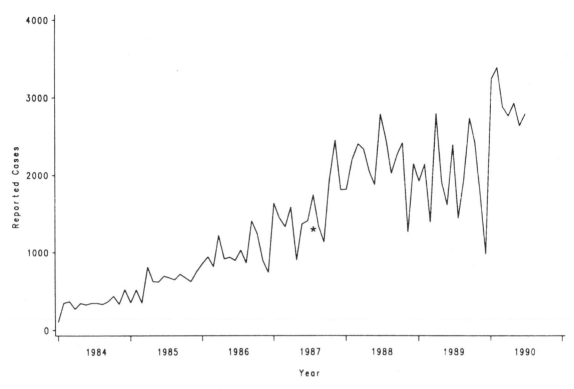

Fig. 40.13 AIDS cases, by 4-week period of report, United States, 1984–1990. (From Centers for Disease Control.[330])

Certain groups of people are recognized as at high risk for HIV-1 antibody positivity or development of AIDS: male homosexuals, male bisexuals, female prostitutes, hemophiliacs, parenteral drug abusers, sexual partners of high-risk persons, and offspring of female members of high-risk groups. Some areas of the world outside the United States also appear to have a significantly increased prevalence of HIV-1 infection. These areas include central Africa and some islands in the Caribbean such as Haiti. Other risk factors include receiving blood or blood products prior to the nationwide practice of screening donated blood for HIV antibody.

In the United States, the ratio of adult male-to-female AIDS cases is 13 to 1, with 93 percent men and 7 percent women. In adults, 60 percent are non-Hispanic white, 25 percent black, and 14 percent Hispanic.[153]

There have been 1,346 cases of AIDS (2 percent) reported in children as of 1988. The majority (80 percent) have come from families in which one or both parents had AIDS or were at risk for AIDS. In this group, the burden of infection has fallen on black and Hispanic groups, with a cumulative incidence 15 and 9 times, respectively, that of the non-Hispanic white community. In 13 percent of babies, the only identifiable risk factor was receiving unscreened blood or blood components.

Global epidemiologic studies have been undertaken to determine the prevalence of infection.[154] The male preponderance of antibody prevalence in the United States has not been found in urban central Africa. Other sexually transmitted infections may have a role in the epidemic of HIV-1 infection in Africa. Some populations in South America also appear to have an increasing incidence of retroviral infection.[155]

In the United States, serologic surveys have been performed to estimate the infected population (Fig. 40.14). An estimated 1.0 to 1.5 million Americans are infected with the virus (approximately 4/1,000). Among individuals with no risk factors, the prevalence of antibody is less than 1 percent. Recent surveys of military recruits have shown a prevalence 1.3/

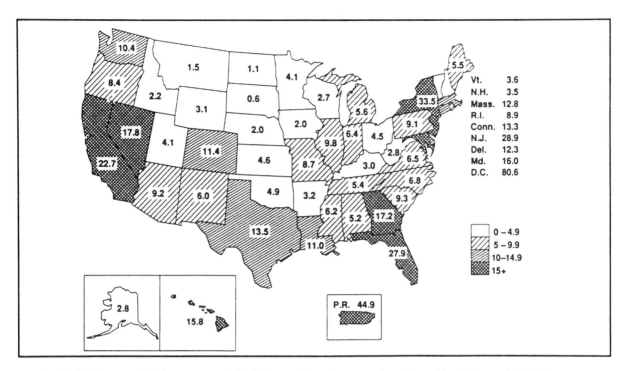

Vt.	3.6
N.H.	3.5
Mass.	12.8
R.I.	8.9
Conn.	13.3
N.J.	28.9
Del.	12.3
Md.	16.0
D.C.	80.6

Fig. 40.14 Reported AIDS patients per 100,000 population, by state of residency, United States, 1989. (From Centers for Disease Control.[331])

1,000 in active duty personnel, with a prevalence of 0.6/1,000 in women. The male-to-female ratio in this group is 3 to 1. Sentinel hospitals show a prevalence in the population of 3.2/1,000. In college students, the prevalence is 2/1,000.

In high-risk groups, HIV-1 antibody is present in up to 65 percent of male homosexuals, up to 87 percent of intravenous drug abusers, 72 percent of patients with hemophilia A, and 5 percent of Haitian-Americans. Antibody has been found in 35 percent of women who were sexual partners of men with AIDS. In individuals with AIDS, antibody was found in 68 to 100 percent.

The disease is spread parenterally. The proportion of AIDS patients with a history of blood or blood product transfusion as the only risk factor is 1 to 2 percent. With current blood banking practices, the risk of acquiring HIV infection is estimated to be 1 in 153,000 per unit of red cells. The median incubation of transfusion-associated AIDS is 28 months, with cases diagnosed as late as 5 years after transfusion.

Anorectal intercourse is the sexual practice most associated with the transmission of HIV-1. Penile–vaginal intercourse appears a less "efficient" method of spread.[152] However, spread among heterosexual couples who do not practice rectal intercourse has been documented. Female sexual partners of hemophiliacs, male intravenous drug abusers, and male bisexuals have developed AIDS or antibody to HIV-1. Ongoing studies show no evidence of nonsexual horizontal transmission.

Perinatal infection is a significant problem in many urban areas in the United States. In 85 percent of neonatal AIDS cases, the mothers are in a high-risk group, and maternal HIV-1 antibody has been found retrospectively (Fig. 40.15). Some mothers have developed AIDS after delivery. In utero transplacental infection appears most likely. Serosurveys of cord blood have found a prevalence of 2.1/1,000, with rates as high as 8.0/1,000 in inner-city hospitals and as low as 0.9/1,000 in suburban and rural hospitals.[156-158]

The proportion of AIDS cases involving women has increased from 7 to 10 percent in the last 5 years. One-half of the seropositive cases in women were associated with intravenous drug use. As of 1988, 5

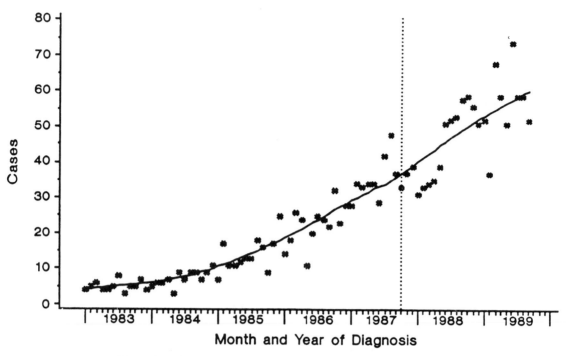

Fig. 40.15 Children infected with HIV by perinatal transmission. (From Centers for Disease Control.[332])

percent of AIDS cases in women were heterosexually acquired. Two-thirds involved sexual contact with a person in a high-risk group. The prevalence of infection in the female population is estimated to be 0.4/1,000. Cases of AIDS-related maternal mortality have been reported, with deaths resulting from listeriosis, Kaposi sarcoma, and *Pneumocystis carinii* pneumonia.

Spread to health care personnel appears rare, although documented. Needle-stick injury is the most common accidental exposure in a medical setting. It usually occurs at the time of needle resheathing. The risk of developing AIDS after a needle-stick exposure from a known seropositive patient is approximately 1 in 250. Larger exposures to infected blood occur with regularity of routine obstetric practice, but actual risk figures are currently unavailable in these settings.

No evidence exists to support transmission by casual contact or fomites. The role of saliva, tears, sweat, and amniotic fluid in AIDS transmission appears negligible.

Clinical Features

The CDC has recently expanded and revised the definition of AIDS.[159] Individuals with AIDS develop lymphadenopathy, night sweats, fevers, opportunis-

tic infections, and certain neoplasms. *P. carinii* pneumonia (PCP) is the most common opportunistic infection associated with AIDS. An acute mononucleosis-like illness associated with HIV seroconversion has been described. Infants with AIDS exhibit failure to thrive and lymphoid interstitial pneumonia, in addition to other adult features of the disease. Pregnancy does not appear to influence the course of HIV infection.[160]

The revised definition was introduced as a result of further knowledge about HIV-1 infection. Major changes recognize HIV encephalopathy, HIV wasting syndrome, and a broader range of infectious diseases as indicative of AIDS. Definitive diagnosis includes HIV-antibody positivity with one of the following: recurrent or multiple bacterial infections, disseminated coccidioidomycosis, HIV encephalopathy, disseminated histoplasmosis, isosporiasis with diarrhea greater than 1 month, Kaposi sarcoma, B-cell or unknown phenotype non-Hodgkin's lymphoma, disseminated nontubercular mycobacterial disease, extrapulmonary tuberculosis, recurrent nontyphoidal *Salmonella* sepsis, or HIV wasting syndrome. Certain indicator diseases can be diagnosed presumptively. When coupled with HIV seropositivity, the following are also considered as diagnostic for AIDS:

esophageal candidiasis, CMV retinitis with loss of vision, Kaposi sarcoma, lymphoid interstitial pneumonia, disseminated mycobacterial disease, PCP, and CNS toxoplasmosis. Exclusions include recent use of systemic corticosteroids or other immunosuppressive or cytotoxic therapy. Genetic and congenital immune deficiency diseases are excluded, as are certain specific lymphomas and leukemias, such as Hodgkin's disease or chronic lymphocytic leukemia.

In adults, the incubation period is thought to be up to 10 years. Serologic studies suggest that HIV-1 infection is similar to other infectious diseases in that the number of individuals exposed to infection is much greater than those with clinical illness. There are an estimated 20 to 30 cases of seropositivity for every identified case of AIDS. What fraction of untreated, asymptomatic, seropositive individuals will progress to AIDS over their lifetime is unknown, but some estimates are as high as 100 percent. In some populations, one-third progress to AIDS over a 5-year period. The 2-year mortality rate of untreated AIDS ranges from 50 to 90 percent.

The diagnosis of HIV infection in a newborn is complicated by the presence of maternal antibody acquired transplacentally and the reported development of AIDS in the face of continued seronegativity. Infants appear normal at birth, with illness developing around 8 months of life. Median survival for these children is 38 months.[160–162]

Diagnosis and Management

AIDS is a clinical diagnosis. Serologic markers such as HIV-1 antibodies identify patients at risk, but the question of who will ultimately develop illness remains unanswered.

Antibody testing to HIV-1 is the current method of determining exposure.[163,164] An ELISA to disrupted virus is currently used to screen blood and plasma. Western blot analysis of antibodies against polymerase and envelope components (see Microbiology) are used in the further evaluation of a positive ELISA. A negative Western blot indicates no antibodies against viral proteins or glycoproteins.[165]

A depressed T4 count and/or low T4/T8 ratio appear to be the most sensitive indicators for progression to AIDS. Abnormal lymphocyte T4/T8 ratios may occur after many viral illnesses, such as infectious mononucleosis.[166]

The presence of HIV positivity does not appear to influence the course of pregnancy, and pregnancy does not appear to hasten the development of AIDS. The development of AIDS-related neoplasms or infections can be masked by the findings of normal pregnancy. The use of antiviral agents, such as zidovudine, in pregnancy is currently being investigated. The agent inhibits reverse transcriptase and was initially developed as an antineoplastic agent, with myelosuppressive properties. The teratogenic risks are unclear at this time. The optimal therapy for AIDS-specific infections in pregnancy is currently being evaluated.

Established infection cannot be eradicated at present.[167,168] Spread of virus by cell fusion hampers antiviral action. Monocytes and macrophages, especially in the central nervous system, may act as sanctuaries for the virus. Because reverse transcriptase activity produces variation in the viral genome, the development of a vaccine to HIV-1 appears distant. Thus prevention of infection is the best method of management at present.

Premarital Screening

Wider use of premarital HIV testing and counseling has been proposed as a public health policy. Attempts at compulsory premarital screening in the United States have thus far been unsuccessful. Programs did not identify those groups at highest risks (e.g., intravenous drug abusers). In addition, many high-risk individuals either deferred marriage during the time testing was performed or went to other areas to obtain marriage licenses. Very few cases were ever identified, at great economic cost. Other approaches may be more successful in the future.[169–172]

Sexual Transmission

Serologic testing to determine HIV-1 exposure can be offered to a woman who has had sexual relations with a member of a high-risk group. The estimated risk to the woman of acquiring HIV infection after a single episode of unprotected penile–vaginal intercourse with a known positive individual is 1 in 500. The use of condoms has been estimated to reduce the risk of transmission of HIV-1 to about 1 in 5,000. After a single episode of penile–vaginal intercourse with a male in no known high-risk group, the estimates for a woman to seroconvert are 1 in 50 million and 1 in 5 million with and without condom use, respectively. Counseling to prevent spread or acquisition of infection is a vital part of management. As of 1988, 5 percent of all AIDS cases (3,589) were thought to be heterosexually acquired, the majority as a result of sexual relations with a high-risk individual.

Parenteral Transmission

Patients may refuse blood or blood products (including Rh immune globulin, hepatitis B immune globulin, cryoprecipitate, or fresh frozen plasma) because of concerns about acquiring AIDS. The method of manufacturing immune globulin eliminates the virus; thus there is no risk of acquiring HIV infection from properly manufactured immune globulin preparations. The current risk of developing AIDS after transmission of 1 unit of packed RBCs is estimated to be 1 in 153,000.[173-176] Blood products are currently screened for HIV-1 and HTLV-I antibody.[177]

Individuals who practice high-risk behaviors or from some parts of the world with endemic HIV are discouraged from donating plasma or blood. These individuals should also refrain from donating body organs, other tissue, or sperm. Toothbrushes, razors, or other implements from such individuals that could become contaminated with blood should not be shared. After accidents in the home that result in bleeding, contaminated surfaces should be cleaned with household bleach freshly diluted 1 : 10 in water. Isopropyl alcohol, hydrogen peroxide, paraformaldehyde, and heat (56 degrees C for 10 minutes) will also inactivate the virus. Devices that have punctured the skin, such as hypodermic and acupuncture needles, should be steam sterilized by autoclave before reuse or safely discarded. Whenever possible, disposable needles and equipment should be used.

Perinatal Transmission

The known seropositive pregnant woman must be counseled as to her own risk and the risk to her fetus for developing AIDS.[178,179] The estimated likelihood of transmission is 30 to 50 percent. The dismal neonatal outcome, which is worse than that for adults, should also be discussed. Studies have shown that many women will opt to continue the pregnancy, a choice that should be anticipated by the health care team.[180]

Prevention of transmission is currently not feasible, because the time(s) of transmission are unknown. Cesarean delivery does not appear to prevent the transmission of infection from a known seropositive mother to her infant. Women in high-risk groups should not donate breast milk.

The diagnosis of HIV-1 seropositivity in newborns is difficult because of transplacental acquisition of maternal antibody. Some infants develop AIDS yet remain seronegative.[181] Sensitive methods of detection of the viral genome sequences using the polymerase chain reaction may facilitate diagnosis.[182,183]

A syndrome of AIDS embryopathy has been proposed. This syndrome has been ascribed to infants with growth failure; hypertelorism; large, wide lips; well-formed triangular philtrum; "scooped-out" nose; and "box-like" head. Its existence is disputed because of other confounding variables, such as concurrent drug use or ethnic variations.[184-187]

Seropositive women should be followed by members of the health care team familiar with HIV-related neoplasms and infections.[188] Serial T4 lymphocyte counts and other special tests of immune function may be necessary.

Nosocomial Exposure

Potential risks to health care workers are self-evident. The CDC has recommended "universal" precautions for all health care workers with direct patient contact. This includes special gloves, gowns, masks, goggles, handling of surgical instruments (scalpels and needles), and meticulous handwashing. Development of AIDS after needle-stick exposure is well-documented.[189-193]

Syphilis

Syphilis in the HIV-positive individual has emerged as a special management problem. The infection is more difficult to eradicate, especially when neurosyphilis is present. The antibody response to infection is variable, ranging from an extremely high reagin titer to no response at all. Treatment failures may occur when following recommended antibiotic doses for the immune competent host. These cases should be managed in conjunction with experts.[194-196]

If cerebrospinal fluid is obtained for evaluation, it is important to remember that it is the body fluid with the highest cell-free viral titer. Splash accidents involving health care workers, especially to the eyes, must be prevented by adhering to universal precautions.

Autoantibodies

A variety of autoantibodies and autoimmune syndromes have been described associated with diffuse polyclonal B-cell activation. Both thrombotic thrombocytopenic purpura and isoimmune thrombocytopenic purpura preceding the onset of AIDS have been described. Circulating lupus-like anticoagulants have been found in the sera of HIV-positive individuals.[197–199]

Ethical Issues

In addition to the enormous medical and psychological burdens of HIV infection, seropositive individuals are at risk for being stigmatized and for suffering loss of employment or insurability. The rights of these individuals are of direct concern to physicians.[200]

Patient confidentiality is paramount in cases involving an HIV-seropositive individual. Methods of reporting and charting results that protect a patient's right to privacy must be addressed by each individual physician and institution. These methods must still efficiently notify other health care workers, including dentists, pediatricians, and neonatologists.

Patient access to treatment is also crucial. "A physician may not ethically refuse to treat a patient whose condition is within the physician's current realm of competence solely because the patient is seropositive. Persons who are seropositive should not be subjected to discrimination based on fear or prejudice." [201] In addition, "physicians who are unable to provide the services required by AIDS patients should make referrals to those physicians and facilities equipped to provide such services." [201]

Another problem arises as a result of conflicting rights between the seropositive person and other members of society. The issues of partner notification (contact tracing) and possible risks to others must be addressed by frank discussion with the patient, notification of civil authorities, and, potentially, notification of any third parties.

The HIV-positive physician faces difficult ethical choices. These conflicts arise from responsibilities as a doctor to ensure patient safety versus the physician's own rights to confidentiality as a patient.[202] "A physician who knows that he or she is seropositive should not engage in any activity that creates a risk of transmission of the disease to others" and "should consult colleagues as to which activities the physician can pursue without creating a risk to patients." [203]

INFECTIONS OF THE NEONATE WITHOUT TERATOGENIC POTENTIAL

Human Papilloma Virus

Human papilloma virus (HPV) is the causative agent of human warts. HPV has assumed increased importance in gynecology over the past decade because of the association between condyloma acuminata and cervical intraepithelial neoplasia (CIN). Questions continue to be raised as to the obstetric significance of warts, especially regarding intrapartum transmission and development of childhood laryngeal papillomatosis.

Microbiology

HPVs are members of the Papovaviridae family. The genetic material is present as double-stranded DNA. The virus has not been grown in tissue culture except by cocultivation methods with other viruses. There are over 45 recognized HPV serotypes.[204]

HPV demonstrates tropism toward mucocutaneous tissue, such as tongue, larynx, skin, penis, urethra, perianal skin, and cervicovaginal epithelium. There are at least five types of HPV that affect human cervicovaginal tissue, with typology based on DNA hybridization and restriction endonuclease studies. Recent studies have implicated types 6, 10, and 11 in the development of condyloma acuminata and types 16 and 18 associated with CIN. Types 6 and 11 have been isolated from over 90 percent of laryngeal papillomata.

Immunology

Studies of immune response to HPV infection have been hampered by the limited amounts of viral antigen in clinical lesions and the inability to propagate the virus in the laboratory. Circulating HPV antibodies can be demonstrated in patients with genital warts, but their role in controlling viral replication is unknown. Also unexplained is the known spontaneous regression of these lesions, both in postpartum and in nonpregnant women.

Clinical Aspects

Genital HPV is a sexually transmitted disease that has been increasing in frequency over the last decade, paralleling the general increase in other sexually transmitted diseases.[205] The incubation period is estimated to be 1 to 2 months. Occasionally, epidemics have been reported in institutions such as psychiatric hospitals or college dormitories, and transmission via contaminated laundry (e.g., moist towels) has been implicated. Oral condylomata as a result of oral–genital contact have become increasingly recognized.[206] During labor, condylomata may cause soft tissue dystocia. Large lesions may be vascular and cause significant hemorrhage if lacerated during parturition.

Diagnosis

The diagnosis of genital warts is based on physical examination, with classic pointed "warty" excrescences being found on mucocutaneous surfaces (Fig. 40.16). Cervical cytology demonstrating koilocytosis, atypia, or dysplasia can suggest genital HPV

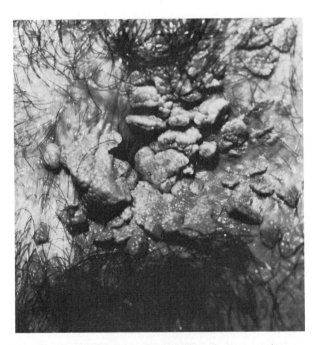

Fig. 40.16 Condyloma acuminata. These lesions may be single or multiple, white, pink, or slightly hyperpigmented papules with a highly irregular verrucous surface that resembles cauliflower. (From Lazarus and Goldsmith,[333] with permission.)

infection, and follow-up colposcopy by an expert trained in the recognition of cervical lesions in pregnancy can be helpful. In situ hybridization and other molecular genetic techniques are available for serotyping virus present in clinical specimens.

Treatment

The morbidity of current treatment modalities and subsequent recurrence of lesions renders therapy unsatisfactory in both the pregnant and nonpregnant state. Recurrence may result from reinfection by untreated sexual partners; spread from normal-appearing, infected tissue; or persistence of the viral genome in treated tissue.

Three basic methods of treatment are available: in situ extirpation, excision, and immune modulation.[207] Small lesions are best managed by in situ extirpation using fine-point cryocautery or electrocautery. Electrocautery has been associated more with cicatrix formation and requires general anesthesia. Carbon dioxide laser therapy has been used in pregnancy, with greatest short-term efficacy near term. Perianal lesions require special attention to avoid anal stenosis, especially when electrocautery is used. Large vulvar lesions may have to be excised surgically and occasionally require vulvectomy. Such operations can result in significant morbidity because of the increased vascularity of pregnancy. Lesions that are large, unresponsive to therapy, or appear atypical should be biopsied to rule out carcinoma.

Cytotoxic agents such as podophyllin or 5-fluorouracil (5-FU) are contraindicated in pregnancy. Podophyllin, a mixture of lignins and flavonols derived from a plant related to the may apple, causes metaphase arrest. Application of podophyllin to large lesions has occasionally resulted in maternal neuropathy, seizures, and intrauterine fetal demise. 5-FU, an antimetabolite and pyrimidine analogue, has not been studied in pregnancy, and the usual caveats for a drug that may affect cellular development apply. Caustic agents, such as trichloroacetic acid, or keratolytic agents, such as salicylic acid, have also been advocated as topical therapy for warts. Cryotherapy and laser ablation have also been employed.[208,209]

Alternative treatment through immune modulation is under investigation. Interferon, a class of polypeptides that augments cell-mediated immunity and stimulates synthesis of antiviral protein, has been produced using genetic technology. Some clinical trials assessing its efficacy appear promising, although more experience with this approach is needed.

Perinatal Transmission

The concern about transmission of HPV from a mother with genital infection to the child is the subsequent development of neonatal laryngeal papillomatosis. One recent review states, "If intrapartum infection of the fetus [with HPV] is the most likely method of transmission of the virus, as appears to be the case for juvenile onset disease, then cesarean delivery prior to the rupture of the membranes should provide a high degree of protection against the infection." [210] Is such "prophylactic" abdominal delivery justified?

Laryngeal papillomata are well described in otolaryngology.[211,212] Affected children may present with "a weak cry" or hoarseness. As with genital papillomata, treatment may be protracted and produce limited success. Ablation with carbon dioxide laser therapy or cryotherapy is currently employed.[213] Retrospective studies have shown a strong association between maternal genital papillomata and laryngeal papillomatosis.

Data from the Collaborative Perinatal Project (CPP) collected from 1959 to 1966 have been analyzed in an attempt to address the question of perinatal transmission. After a follow-up of 7 years, no cases of laryngeal papillomatosis were reported in 44,000 children. One criticism of this observation is that the prevalence of HPV infection was probably lower during the time of the study and thus a prospective study might now reveal more cases. Some cytologic surveys have suggested the prevalence of HPV infection among women to be 1.5 percent, thus potentially exposing approximately 45,000 children yearly in the United States. Survey data suggest that an estimated 3,000 cases of laryngeal papillomatosis were diagnosed by otolaryngologists in 1976. This produces an estimated risk of this disorder of 1 affected child in 15 infected mothers, assuming that all intrapartum infections were transmitted from mother to baby.[210] Both survey estimates and the CPP study suggest that the theoretical rate of perinatal transmission is low.

Recent data suggest that the prevalence of clinically silent genital HPV may be 30 percent (or higher)

in parturients. Thus the vertical transmission rate may be even lower than these estimates. Other studies suggest a high rate of clinically silent neonatal laryngeal HPV infection. Thus true estimates of perinatal transmission are unclear.

There is no proof that abdominal delivery will reduce the rate of vertical transmission. Even if this were the case, the criteria for screening and case selection remain undefined. More information is necessary before concluding that the presence of genital warts or HPV infection mandates delivery by cesarean section.[214]

Hepatitis B

The hepatitis B virus is a worldwide human pathogen. Although the virus was previously known as "serum hepatitis" because of its association with illicit or iatrogenic blood-borne transmission, recent epidemiologic studies have established that mother-to-infant transmission is a major, if not *the* major, mode of maintenance and spread of infection throughout the world. In the United States, obstetricians are in a unique position to identify infected mothers and limit horizontal transmission to family members and vertical transmission to newborn infants through active and passive immunization.

Health care workers are acutely aware of the risk of acquiring hepatitis B in the course of patient care, as well as of the potential occupational, medical, and legal ramifications of becoming a carrier.[215] Hepatitis B vaccine allows a significant measure of protection if active immunization has been accomplished before exposure.

Microbiology

The human hepatitis B virus (HBV) is a member of a newly classified family of hepatotropic viruses, the Hepadnaviridae, which includes four other hepatitis viruses that infect animals.[216,217] HBV is an enveloped DNA virus that has not been propagated in tissue culture. It is maintained in persistently infected cell lines. Particulate forms, composed of 22 nm spheres, are now known to be incomplete virus envelope components and to contain the hepatitis B surface antigen (HB$_s$Ag). The antigen is synthesized in the hepatocyte cytoplasm and is found in peripheral blood in numbers up to 10,000 times the number of circulating virions. The complete virion, 42 nm in diameter, was identified by electron microscopic evaluation in 1970 by Dane et al.[218] The virion is composed of the envelope containing HB$_s$Ag and an inner nucleocapsid or core. The core contains a polypeptide termed the hepatitis B core antigen, along with viral DNA, DNA polymerase/reverse transcriptase, and e antigen complex (HB$_e$Ag). In the peripheral circulation, core antigen is noted only with complete virions. No circulating free core antigen has been found. There is a high correlation with virion synthesis, infectivity, and the presence of circulating HB$_e$Ag.

The host range for HBV is limited to humans and to some primates. The virus is tropic for hepatocytes and is generally not cytopathic. HB$_s$Ag has been demonstrated in serum, saliva, breast milk, tears, sweat, bile, urine, semen, and vaginal secretions. Dane particles have been isolated from serum, semen, and saliva.

In an uncomplicated, self-limited infection, HB$_s$Ag appears several weeks (range, 1 to 12 weeks) after exposure, before clinical symptoms (Fig. 40.17). This range depends on inoculum size, host susceptibility, and a wide variety of other factors. Titers correlate with the severity of infection, peaking during late incubation and early in the course of clinical illness. HB$_s$Ag titers then fall with resolution and finally become undetectable several weeks after symptoms have resolved. In persistently infected individuals, HB$_s$Ag remains positive. It is now recognized that most infections are mild or silent and that severe icteric disease is unique to industrialized countries in association with medical procedures such as blood transfusion or hemodialysis or with illicit parenteral drug use.

Immunology

Intact mucocutaneous surfaces are a barrier to viral entry. Experiments with infected semen introduced intravaginally have not produced infection, while subcutaneous administration does result in infection. The adult stomach inactivates the virus, as evidenced by failure of virus recovery after ingestion of infected

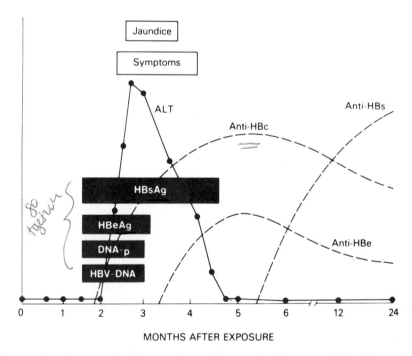

Fig. 40.17 Clinical and serologic course of a typical case of acute type B hepatitis. HB$_s$Ag, hepatitis B surface antigen; HB$_e$Ag, hepatitis B e antigen; DNA-p, DNA polymerase; HBV-DNA, hepatitis B virus DNA; ALT, alanine aminotransferase; anti-HB$_c$, antibody to hepatitis B core antigen; anti-HB$_e$, antibody to hepatitis B e antigen; anti-HB$_s$, antibody to HB$_s$Ag. (From Hoofnagle,[334] with permission.)

material. Both visible and microscopic lacerations serve as portals of entry for the virus, as may occur during rectal intercourse.

A wide range of specific host responses, both humoral and cell mediated, are elicited after HBV infection (Fig. 40.17). The first humoral response is the IgM anticore antibody (anti-HB$_c$-IgM), which may be detected after circulating HB$_s$Ag and before clinical hepatitis. IgG also appears with IgM. Both IgG and IgM may persist for several years after a primary self-limited infection. Chronically infected individuals have anti-HB$_c$, both IgG and IgM, in high titers. Antibody to HB$_s$Ag (anti-HB$_s$) can generally be detected after the disappearance of HB$_s$Ag, sometimes with a "window" or "gap" of several weeks or months. Those with the highest antibody titers have the shortest period of antigenemia in self-limited infections. Antibody to HB$_e$Ag (anti-HB$_e$) may be found after clearance of HB$_e$Ag and weeks after resolution of the illness. It can persist for 1 to 2 years.

Epidemiology

HBV infection is the most common cause of liver disease, with 200 million chronic carriers worldwide. Carrier rates vary but may be as high as 35 percent in the Far East, Southeast Asia, and sub-Saharan Africa. In these areas, mother-to-infant transmission has been estimated to be the cause of 40 percent of all chronic HBV infections.

In the United States, 200,000 new cases occur each year, 50,000 requiring hospitalization and 10,000 leading to a chronic carrier state. Chronic carriage rates in the American population are below 1 percent, and the estimated lifetime risk of acquiring HBV infection, with or without symptoms, is approximately 5 percent. Chronic infection has been defined as persistent HB$_s$Ag found on two tests 6 months apart. There are between 400,000 and 800,000 chronic carriers of HBV in the United States, with 4,000 deaths from HBV-induced cirrhosis and 800 deaths from primary hepatocellular carcinoma yearly. Different demographic factors appear to be associated with the likelihood of developing the carriage state. In healthy American adults, the carriage rate of HB$_s$Ag is less than 0.1 percent, whereas recent immigrants from hyperendemic areas have a carriage rate of 13 percent, with some as high as 30 percent.

Worldwide, mother-to-infant transmission appears to be a major route of spread of the organism. In utero transmission appears uncommon, with 5 to 10 percent of first-trimester acute infections resulting in infections diagnosed at birth, while 75 percent of third-trimester or early postpartum infections will lead to neonatal infection. Possible routes are infected amniotic fluid and blood. Breast-feeding does not appear to be a major route of transmission.

In the United States, blood and blood products remain a defined source of the virus, with 5 to 10 percent of transfusion-related hepatitis caused by HBV, even with modern blood-banking technology. Infection has been acquired from apparently HB$_s$Ag-negative blood with anti-HB$_c$ present. Sexual acquisition is noted in individuals with greater than 50 total lifetime sexual partners.[219]

Health care professionals are at higher than normal risk for acquiring and transmitting infection. Outbreaks in patients have been traced to health care workers who are chronic carriers, including obstetricians and gynecologists. The CDC has stratified the population into high, intermediate, and low-risk groups according to risk of having had or acquiring infection. High-risk individuals include immigrants from areas of high HBV endemicity, individuals in institutions for the mentally retarded, those using illicit parenteral drugs, male homosexuals, household contacts of HBV carriers, and patients on hemodialysis. Those at intermediate risk include incarcerated males, staff at institutions for the mentally retarded, and health care workers with frequent blood contact. Individuals at low risk include health care workers with infrequent contact or no contact with blood and healthy adults. Between 3 and 5 percent of healthy adults have had hepatitis B infection as determined by serologic markers (HB$_s$Ag, anti-HB$_s$, and anti-HB$_c$). This rate is as high as 20 percent in urban health care workers, but as low as 2 percent in rural health care workers. In individuals from hyperendemic areas, 90 percent may have serologic evidence of previous infection.

Clinical Aspects

As many as 75 percent of HBV infections are asymptomatic. The incubation period and severity of clinical illness depend on the inoculum size, route of infection, and a variety of host factors. The incubation period, described as "long" (30 to 180 days) compared with the "short" incubation of hepatitis A (15 to 45 days) can be only 1 week if a large inoculum is introduced parenterally, as from a blood transfusion. There can be a prodromal phase of 2 to 14 days, with a flu-like syndrome, fatigue, and malaise, followed by nausea, vomiting, and diarrhea. Smokers lose their desire for cigarettes. There may be pruritus, right upper quadrant pain, dark-colored urine, and light-colored stools. In approximately 15 percent of symptomatic individuals, there is a prodrome from immune complex formation with fever up to 39 degrees C, arthralgias, arthritis, skin rash, and even glomerulonephritis. The arthritis is nondeforming and migratory and involves the large joints. This feature of the disease is generally seen in young adults and children. Patients are most infectious during the prodromal phase.

The icteric phase follows the prodrome and lasts 6 to 8 weeks. Scleral icterus occurs when bilirubin levels exceed 2 to 3 mg/dl. Icterus of the skin and mucous membranes develops at higher serum bilirubin levels. Hepatomegaly with tenderness is common. A recovery phase, lasting 4 to 6 weeks in adults, follows, during which the hepatomegaly slowly resolves.

HBV infection is more severe in women with protein-calorie malnutrition. In otherwise healthy pregnant women, the course of the disease is not worsened. There is no apparent increase in malformations, stillbirths, miscarriages, or IUGR. Infants infected at or around the time of birth generally remain asymptomatic, although fatal neonatal hepatitis has been described.

Diagnosis

Evaluation of the icteric pregnant patient involves consideration of noninfectious and infectious causes of jaundice. Acute fatty liver and the HELLP syndrome (pregnancy-induced hypertension with hemolysis, elevated liver enzymes, and low platelets), both unique to pregnancy, must be considered.

The diagnosis of acute icteric hepatitis B is based on the clinical setting and on judicious employment of laboratory studies. Tests for HB_sAg, anti-HB_c-IgM, HB_eAg, and anti-HB_e are now available. HB_sAg is the most important test currently employed in the diagnosis of HBV infection and potential infectivity. Ninety percent of individuals are HB_sAg positive at some time during their illness. In experimental trans-

mission studies, 10 percent became HB_sAg negative before the onset of symptoms and 30 percent by the end of the clinical illness.

HB_sAg positivity with acute hepatitis suggests acute HBV infection, although superimposed hepatitis caused by other agents or exacerbation of infection in chronic carriers may give a similar picture. In these cases, the presence of anti-HB_c-IgM, rising anti-HB_c titers, and/or the appearance of anti-HB_s suggest new HBV infection. HB_sAg in the absence of anti-HB_c suggests incubating HBV, whereas HB_sAg with anti-HB_c-IgM indicates a primary infection. Carriers generally have a high titer of anti-HB_c-IgG in addition to HB_sAg and anti-HB_c-IgM.

If HB_sAg is present, HB_eAg and anti-HB_e may be obtained for prognostic significance, although neonatal treatment and appropriate blood precautions remain unchanged. In the United States, one-third of HB_sAg-positive pregnant women are HB_eAg positive. If warranted by the clinical situation, anti-HB_c can be obtained to identify persons with incubating hepatitis B.

Previous infection with the development of immunity is indicated by anti-HB_s or anti-HB_c and absent HB_sAg. Anti-HB_c is present in more recent infections. Anti-HB_s alone develops after HBV vaccination. Ten percent of patients with self-limited infections never develop anti-HB_s, and anti-HB_c may be the only antibody found in this setting.

HB_eAg is an index of ongoing viral replication and increased infectivity, while the presence of HB_sAg and anti-HB_e suggests less infectivity. It is important to note that the presence of anti-HB_e in the presence of HB_sAg positivity does not indicate absence of infectivity.

Individuals with chronic hepatitis B are HB_sAg and anti-HB_c positive. Anti-HB_s, anti-HB_c-IgM, anti-HB_e, and HB_eAg may or may not be present.

Management

No therapeutic maneuvers have proved beneficial after the onset of this illness. In the absence of complicated disease and significant dehydration, most individuals can be managed as outpatients. Generally, by the time the diagnosis is made, the period of maximum infectivity has passed. Special dietary supplements, steroids, or prolonged bed rest have not proved beneficial. Pregnancy predisposes to ketosis and dehydration. Significant gastrointestinal symptoms with inability to tolerate oral intake may require hospitalization for parenteral hydration.

Complications

Fulminant Hepatitis B

A rare complication of acute hepatitis is fulminant hepatitis, with hepatic failure and encephalopathy. In the United States, there are 200 cases yearly. The liver shrinks as a result of massive necrosis, and death occurs in days to weeks. Delta virus infection may account for some of these cases.

Delta Virus Infection

The delta virus is a low-molecular-weight RNA virus that requires coinfection with hepatitis B to produce clinical consequences. Thus it is a "defective" virus, 1)unique to human clinical virology. The hepatitis B surface antigen is thought to provide the envelope for the delta virus. Perinatal transmission occurs infrequently.

Chronic Hepatitis

Ninety percent of all individuals with icteric hepatitis B clear their infection without residual effects. The remainder develop chronic hepatitis, with HB_sAg positivity. Seventy percent develop chronic persistent hepatitis (CPH), and the remainder develop chronic active hepatitis. Clinically, patients with CPH have mild hepatomegaly, no icterus, and intermittent elevations of liver enzymes. A spontaneous yearly remission rate of 1 to 2 percent has been observed. In infants who acquire HBV infection at birth, 40 percent will develop chronic hepatitis.

Mother-to-Infant Transmission

An estimated 15,000 HB_sAg-positive women give birth in the United States each year. Transmission at delivery appears to be a major mode of spread of HBV in many areas of the world, although the exact method is obscure. One study showed absence of anti-HB_c-IgM at birth in neonates who subsequently developed infection and whose mothers were HB_sAg positive. These data suggest postpartum rather than antepartum transmission. Breast-feeding may also play a role.[220]

Maternal HB_eAg has been found to correlate with perinatal transmission rates, with those being e positive having higher infectivity (80 to 90 percent) and those with anti-HB_e having lower infectivity (10 percent). Women who have HB_sAg and no HB_eAg or anti-HB_e have transmission rates of approximately 25 percent. Previous studies led to the conclusion that patients who were HB_eAg negative and HB_eAb [anti-HB_e] positive did not transmit infection. This statement has been disproved in recent worldwide studies. The diagnosis of hepatitis B infection in the infant is established several weeks after birth with the development of elevated liver enzymes and HB_sAg positivity. The infection is usually anicteric.

Screening

Identification of asymptomatic carrier mothers and potentially infected infants by screening at risk populations has not proved successful, with up to two-thirds of carrier women missed by this approach. Because of these limitations, the ACOG and CDC have advised routine serologic screening of all pregnant women for HB_sAg.[221-223] We concur with this recommendation. Some studies, however, suggest that this approach for low-risk rural American populations is not cost-effective.[224,225]

Prevention

These are three primary sources of exposure to HBV, all relevant to obstetricians and gynecologists: percutaneous, perinatal, and sexual. Recommendations for pre- and postexposure prophylaxis in these situations have been published by the CDC.[226] Two methods for immunoprophylaxis specific for HBV are currently available: hepatitis B immune globulin and recombinant hepatitis B vaccine.

Immune Globulins

Immune globulins are sterile solutions of antibodies from human plasma prepared by cold ethanol fractionation of large pools of HB_sAg-negative plasma. Immune globulin, previously called immune serum globulin, ISG, or gammaglobulin, contains antibodies against hepatitis A virus and anti-HB_s.

Hepatitis B immune globulin (HBIG) is an immune globulin prepared from plasma with extremely high titers of anti-HB_s. Immune globulin and HBIG contain different amounts of anti-HB_s. Since 1977, all immune globulin lots tested have contained anti-HB_s

at a titer of at least 1 : 100 as determined by RIA. HBIG has an anti-HB$_s$ titer of greater than 1 : 100,000, but the cost is 20 times that of immune globulin. The concentration of antibody necessary for passive protection under various conditions of exposure has been difficult to determine.

Studies indicate that HBIG is effective when given after a percutaneous needle stick or mucous membrane exposure to blood containing HB$_s$Ag and that immune globulin also appears to have some effect, albeit smaller, in preventing clinical hepatitis B. Both HBIG and immune globulin are most effective when given immediately after exposure. HBIG is preferable to immune globulin when there is known exposure to HB$_s$Ag. Immune globulin is an alternative to HBIG only when HBIG is unavailable or when a truly significant exposure to HBV may not have occurred. Immune globulins are not contraindicated in pregnant women.

In the hospital setting, the risk of clinical hepatitis B after exposure to blood known to be HB$_s$Ag posi#tive is approximately 1 in 20. If the blood is of unknown HB$_s$Ag status, the risk falls to 1 in 2,000.

Hepatitis B Vaccine

Recombinant hepatitis B vaccine is derived from a genetically altered strain of baker's yeast, *Saccharomyces cerevisiae*. The yeast contains a plasmid carrying the gene for HB$_s$Ag (subtype adw). The yeast cells are disrupted, and the HB$_s$Ag is isolated, purified, filtered, and treated with formalin. There is also a plasma-derived product that is available for use. This vaccine is a suspension of HB$_s$Ag particles obtained from the plasma of known HB$_s$Ag carriers. Standard manufacturing processes for the preparation of this vaccine have been shown to eliminate the HIV-1 virus. Protective anti-HB$_s$ has been observed in more than 90 percent of healthy adults vaccinated with three intramuscular doses with both vaccines. The total duration of immunity is unknown, but persists for an indefinite number of years. Rare serious adverse effects have been reported. These complications have included transverse myelitis, grand mal seizures, aseptic meningitis, erythema multiforme, and Guillain-Barré syndrome. The most common side effect is soreness at the injection site. In the adult, the vaccine should be administered in the deltoid muscle.

An injection in the buttock does not induce adequate antibody levels.

Preexposure Prophylaxis

Persons at substantial risk of HBV infection who are susceptible should be vaccinated. They include health care workers, hospital staff, clients and staff of institutions for the mentally retarded, hemodialysis patients, homosexual males, parenteral drug abusers, recipients of high-risk blood products, household and sexual contacts of HBV carriers, and individuals from hyperendemic areas. Ideally, a woman at risk should be vaccinated before conception.

Testing in individual cases can include HB$_s$Ag, anti-HB$_c$, and anti-HB$_s$. Anti-HB$_s$ or anti-HB$_c$ with absent HB$_s$Ag indicate previous infection and natural immunity, with no requirement for the vaccine. There is no evidence that the vaccine ameliorates the carrier state.

Pregnancy is not a contraindication to hepatitis B vaccination for persons at risk. After susceptibility has been established, the vaccine can be given.

Postexposure Prophylaxis

Perinatal Exposure. Mother-to-infant transmission is one of the most likely modes of HBV spread. In addition, the infant remains at risk for infection from other family contacts. In the United States, prophylaxis of infants born to HB$_s$Ag-positive mothers is recommended, regardless of maternal HB$_e$Ag or anti-HB$_e$ status.[227]

The primary goal of infant prophylaxis is to prevent the HBV carrier state and its complications and the rare occurrence of clinical hepatitis in the neonatal period. Combined use of HBIG and hepatitis B vaccine has been found in worldwide clinical trials to reduce mother-to-infant transmission.

The current CDC recommendation is that neonates born to HB$_s$Ag-positive mothers receive HBIG within 12 hours of birth and hepatitis B vaccine at a different site within 7 days of birth. The vaccine is repeated 1 month and 6 months after the initial dose. This combined approach reduces transmission rates by 90 percent. HB$_s$Ag can be measured at 6 months before the last injection and, along with anti-HB$_s$, at

12 to 15 months. The presence of anti-HB$_s$ indicates a therapeutic success and HB$_s$Ag a therapeutic failure.

Some authorities have proposed that abdominal delivery be employed as a prophylactic measure to reduce neonatal infection. There is presently no proof that this approach would be effective. Presently in the United States, HB$_s$Ag/HB$_e$Ag positivity is not an indication for primary cesarean section.

Percutaneous Exposure. Pregnant women, especially those who are health care workers, may be exposed to blood containing HB$_s$Ag. There are no prospective studies evaluating the combined use of HBIG and hepatitis B vaccine in this setting. However, because individuals at risk are candidates for hepatitis B vaccine, combined HBIG plus vaccine is more effective than HBIG alone in the neonate, and pregnancy is not a contraindication to HBIG or hepatitis B vaccine, it seems reasonable to recommend both after such exposure.

For individuals with exposure to known or probable HB$_s$Ag-positive material, the following recommendations have been proposed: administer HBIG 5 ml IM within 24 hours of exposure, followed by hepatitis B vaccine 1.0 ml IM within 7 days, and repeat at 1 month and 6 months. For those who elect not to receive the vaccine, administer HBIG 5 ml IM within 24 hours and repeat in 1 month. In patients at risk for prior infection, screening for hepatitis B markers should be performed before immunization (HB$_s$Ag, anti-HB$_s$, and anti-HB$_c$).

Sexual Exposure. A single dose of HBIG is recommended for susceptible individuals who have had sexual contact with an HB$_s$Ag-positive person. Prescreening for susceptibility prior to treatment is indicated. The period of protection from HBIG is unknown, but is unlikely to exceed 14 days. Immune globulin also appears protective.

Group B Streptococcus

Streptococcus agalactiae is a significant potential perinatal pathogen. In pregnancy, it can cause UTIs, premature labor, premature rupture of membranes, chorioamnionitis, and endomyometritis. The isolation of the organism from maternal cervicovaginal specimens in uncomplicated pregnancies is generally not predictive of neonatal disease, and the vast majority of mothers with this organism have no complications at all. However, *S. agalactiae* is also the most common cause of neonatal sepsis and meningitis in the first week of life. The explanation for these observations remains the subject of ongoing research.

Microbiology

S. agalactiae is well known to veterinarians as a cause of epidemic bovine mastitis. There is no evidence of spread to humans, and cattle do not appear to be the reservoir for human disease. The organism is classified as Lancefield group B based on distinct bacterial cell wall polysaccharide antigens.[228] Recent revisions in nomenclature are based on capsular polysaccharides and surface proteins. The five serotypes include Ia, Ib/c (formerly Ib), Ia/c (formerly Ic), II, and III. Type III is especially virulent in the neonate. A sixth serotype, type IV, has been recently described.

S. agalactiae is a gram-positive coccus that usually forms gray mucoid colonies with a surrounding narrow zone of hemolysis. A few strains, generally 5 to 10 percent, are nonhemolytic. Selective media significantly improve recovery rates. One such medium is Todd-Hewitt broth, composed of sheep blood agar with nalidixic acid and gentamicin added to suppress overgrowth by other organisms. Without such selective media, there may be a 50 percent false-negative recovery rate. Group B streptococci (GBS) elaborate a polypeptide called the CAMP factor, named after its discoverers, Christie, Atkins, and Munch-Petersen. This factor interacts with staphylococcal β-hemolysin to produce a wide, flame-shaped zone of hemolysis on blood agar. Other biochemical factors for identification include hippuric acid hydrolysis, bacitracin sensitivity, and absent hydrolysis in bile esculin agar. Identification of these organisms can be established within 24 to 48 hours by a combination of these techniques.

More recently, immunologic methods that recognize the cell wall antigen of GBS have been developed, permitting rapid diagnosis of GBS before culture results are available. In the latex particle agglutination (LPA) assay, presumptively infected secretions are mixed with latex particles coated with immune globulins against GBS. If GBS are present, agglutination occurs. False-positive results remain a problem, and various methodologies to refine LPA for this application are under clinical investigation.

GBS is sensitive to a wide variety of antibiotics, including penicillin and ampicillin. Interestingly, there is antibiotic synergism against GBS between aminoglycosides and penicillin/ampicillin despite the resistance of GBS to aminoglycosides used alone. The organism is also sensitive to erythromycin, clindamycin, and first- and second-generation cephalosporins. Penicillin sensitivity of GBS is less than that of group A streptococci, requiring a minimum inhibitory concentration of penicillin 4- to 10-fold greater for GBS than for A streptococci.

Immunology

Both maternal and fetal resistance factors to GBS are clinically important. Some investigators have suggested that maternal hormonal immunity against serotype-specific polysaccharide affords significant protection. Because maternal immunoglobulin transfer to the fetus is dependent on gestational age, premature infants might be less likely to benefit from passive acquisition of maternal antibody. PMN function (e.g., antibacterial activity and motility) is also decreased in premature infants, which may increase their susceptibility to GBS infection.

Clinical Aspects

In 1938, Fry described three cases of fatal puerperal sepsis complicated by endocarditis caused by GBS, at a time when group A streptococci were the most important perinatal pathogens. During the 1960s, a 5 percent cervical colonization rate was noted, with rates of 25 percent in patients with a poor obstetric history. By the 1970s, GBS clearly became the leading neonatal bacterial pathogen, replacing *Escherichia coli*. The reason for the emergence of GBS as the predominant organism remains unclear.

S. agalactiae has been found in the vagina (5 to 25 percent), pharnyx (5 to 12 percent), and urethra (4 to 25 percent). It has been recovered in up to 50 percent of male sexual partners of women with a positive cervical culture. Vulvar and periurethral recovery rates are approximately twice those in the lower vagina and cervix. Chronic cervical carriage rate is 36 percent in women with a single positive culture. This organism causes 10 to 20 percent of bacteremia on obstetric services and 20 percent of all postpartum sepsis. Maternal asymptomatic bacteriuria, cystitis, and pyelonephritis are caused by GBS in 1 to 5 percent of cases.

The "attack rate" through vertical transmission at the time of parturition is 1 to 2 percent. In other words, in women with a known positive cervical culture at delivery, only 1 to 2 percent of infants will be clinically affected. With high cervical colony counts, there is an 8 percent attack rate. Overall, neonatal disease occurs in 1 to 5 of 1,000 live births, with rates dependent on birth weight. In infants weighing less than 1,000 g, the incidence of disease is 25 in 1,000, while in infants weighing more than 2,500 g this figure is 1 in 1,000 live births. Intrapartum fever is also a marker for neonatal disease, with a rate of 1 to 2 in 1,000 if the maternal temperature is less than 37.5 degrees C and 7 in 1,000 if the temperature is greater than 37.5 degrees C. If membranes are ruptured for longer than 48 hours, the attack rate is 10 in 1,000 births as compared with 1 in 1,000 if the membranes are ruptured for less than 6 hours.

There are two manifestations of the disease in the neonate: early-onset and late-onset infection. In the early-onset form, neonates develop a respiratory tract infection and bacteremia. This occurs in 3 of 1,000 live births in the first 2 to 3 days of life. The mortality is greatest (30 to 50 percent) among low-birth-weight infants, especially in pregnancies complicated by premature rupture of the membranes, chorioamnionitis, and premature delivery. Here, premature infants suffer the combined consequences of infection, immature host defenses, and respiratory distress syndrome. Late-onset disease occurs in 0.5 to 1.0 in 1,000 births and is manifested by meningitis in 80 percent of the affected neonates. There is a lower mortality (10 to 15 percent), but one-half of the surviving infants suffer significant neurologic injury such as cranial nerve palsies and subdural effusions. This form of the disease is less associated with antepartum maternal colonization, and nosocomial horizontal transmission has been implicated in some cases.

Diagnosis

GBS can be isolated in cases of cystitis, pyelonephritis, endomyometritis, chorioamnionitis, and wound infection. The use of selective media can enhance recovery rates. Transabdominal amniocentesis coupled with microscopic examination of amniotic fluid has been used in research settings in pregnancies complicated by preterm labor or preterm premature rupture of the membranes (PROM) to identify bacterial pathogens such as GBS. Such invasive approaches require further evaluation. Indirect diagnostic tests, such as counter-immunoelectrophoresis, LPA, or ELISA are also under investigation.[229–233]

Treatment

GBS remain sensitive to penicillin. Cystitis, urethritis, and asymptomatic bacteriuria can be treated with oral ampicillin or penicillin. Soft tissue pelvic infections should be managed with high-dose intravenous ampicillin (8 to 12 g IV daily in divided doses) or penicillin (10 million units IV daily in divided doses).

Prevention

Antimicrobial chemoprophylaxis can reduce vertical transmission of GBS.[234] However, antepartum identification of mother–infant pairs who develop GBS morbidity has not been successful because of the poor correlation between a single antepartum culture and outcome. Prevention strategies involving antepartum penicillin treatment or treatment of sexual partners have failed to reduce GBS colonization or morbidity.[235] Recent studies using intrapartum high-dose penicillin or ampicillin for prevention of GBS morbidity have focused on individuals with known antepartum GBS-positive cultures who develop preterm labor or preterm PROM.[236–241] This approach has reduced neonatal and maternal morbidity in this selected, high-risk population. Whether rapid intrapartum identification of GBS and prompt initiation of therapy will improve outcome is under study.[242]

Immunoprophylaxis against GBS may have a role in future management. Clinical and experimental observations have suggested that serotype-specific antibody is protective against development of GBS disease in the neonate. Passive immunization against induced GBS infection has been studied in pregnant rhesus monkeys and has been associated with neonatal protection. Active immunization of pregnant women with serotype-specific GBS antigen has also been performed, with 60 percent of these individuals developing GBS-specific antibody response. Further work in vaccine development is ongoing.[243]

Neisseria gonorrhoeae

The gonococcus is a sexually transmitted organism that produces a variety of local and systemic illnesses. In pregnancy, gonococcal infection of the chorioamnion may cause premature labor, antepartum chorioamnionitis, and postpartum endomyometritis. Infection of the fallopian tubes can result in tubal factor infertility, formation of tuboovarian abscesses, or predisposition to ectopic pregnancy as a result of tubal damage.

The term gonorrhea was used by Galen in the second century A.D. to describe the urethral discharge in the male associated with the disease (from the Greek words *gonos* [seed] and *rhea* [flow]). Hunter died from a syphilitic aortic aneurysm after conducting experiments on himself in which he attempted to differentiate syphilis from gonorrhea. In 1873, Bell distinguished gonorrhea from syphilis by experiments on medical students. Neisser identified the organism microscopically in 1879. Crede instituted silver nitrate prophylaxis in the 1880s to reduce the widespread (10 percent) incidence of neonatal ophthalmic infection. In the preantibiotic era, 20 percent of endocarditis cases were caused by the gonococcus. Its role in infertility and perinatal complications was recognized more recently.

Microbiology

N. gonorrhoeae, the causative organism of gonorrhea, is an aerobic, gram-negative, encapsulated, bean-shaped coccus. In vivo, the organism forms diplococci. Humans are the definitive hosts. Gonococci grow best at 36 to 37 degrees C in a moist environment with 5 to 10 percent CO_2. The organism is most easily identified in selective media such as Thayer-Martin agar. The latter contains vancomycin, colistin, and nystatin to suppress the growth of other bacteria and fungi. Chocolate agar contains heated blood, which absorbs inhibitors to gonococcal growth. Identification in most laboratories is based on colony morphology, a positive oxidase reaction (color change of a specific chemical substrate), and a characteristic pattern of carbohydrate metabolism. The latter step may take an additional 18 hours in subculture, increasing the time required to confirm a positive culture. The organism is sensitive to desiccation and is destroyed by silver salts. Unlike most gram-negative bacteria, it is usually sensitive to streptomycin and tetracycline in vitro and in vivo.

The gonococcal genome is about one-third the size of the *E. coli* genome. Some strains contain extra chromosomal genetic elements called plasmids. One plasmid (called R for resistance) codes for a β-lactamase and is identical to the R plasmid found several years ago in *Haemophilus influenzae*. It is theorized that the gonococcus acquired the plasmid from *H. influenzae*. Gonococci also produce a secretory IgA1 protease that cleaves the antibody secreted by cervicovaginal tissue. Other factors contributing to its virulence include an affinity for host-blocking antibodies that protect the organism from immune elimination.[244]

Gonococci have demonstrated a 100-fold increase in the minimal inhibitory concentration (MIC) to penicillin during the past 25 years. The MICs have increased from 0.003 to 2.0 μg/ml. Some strains have penicillin-binding proteins in their cell wall. Penicillinase-producing *N. gonorrhoeae* (PPNG) have spread to the United States from Southeast Asia, where antibiotics are available over the counter. This penicillin resistance is plasmid mediated. Strains with chromosomally mediated resistant *N. gonorrhoeae* (CMRNG) have been reported. These strains have no plasmids, are β-lactamase negative, and are resistant to tetracycline and penicillin; 89 percent have MICs greater than 2 μg/ml but are sensitive to spectinomycin, cefoxitin, or cefotaxime. Tetracycline-resistant *N. gonorrhoeae* (TRNG), recently described, are characterized by high-level resistance to tetracycline (MIC > 16 μg/ml). This resistance is plasmid mediated.

A scheme has been proposed to classify gonococcal susceptibility to penicillin, spectinomycin, tetracycline, and ceftriaxone based on disc-diffusion and agar-dilution methods. Tetracycline and ceftriaxone testing is difficult to reproduce using this technique. The commonly employed disc-diffusion method utilizes antibiotic impregnated discs to create a zone of inhibition in a field of bacterial colonies. The larger the zone, the greater the susceptibility. To evaluate penicillin sensitivity, susceptible strains have a zone of at least 30 mm, intermediate strains 26 to 29 mm, and resistant strains up to 25 mm. Isolates with plasmid-mediated β-lactamases show a zone less than 20 mm. Clinical therapeutic failure rates with "usual" antibiotic regimens are less than 5 percent, 5 to 15 percent, and more than 15 percent for susceptible, intermediate, and resistant gonococcal strains, respectively.[245-248]

Immunology

The gonococcus stimulates a variety of local and systemic host antibodies and cellular immune responses. Their precise roles in suppressing gonococcal growth are unknown. Normal vaginal flora may reduce the growth of the organism. Changes in cervical mucus associated with birth control pills and pregnancy have also been thought to limit further spread of gonococci from the cervix. Local secretory antibodies may attach to gonococcal pili or fix complement. Individuals genetically deficient in certain components of complement have recurrent episodes of disseminated gonococcal infection, suggesting that complement proteins help limit infections in normal hosts.[249]

Epidemiology

About 1 million cases of gonorrhea are reported in the United States yearly. The prevalence of cervical infection in pregnancy varies from 0.5 to 7 percent, depending on the population studied. Cases of PPNG and CRMNG have been reported throughout the United States. In some urban areas, over 30 percent of gonococcal isolates produce penicillinase. This has led to the classification of nonendemic, endemic, and hyperendemic areas, corresponding to less than 1 percent, 1 to 3 percent, and more than 3 percent PPNG isolates, respectively.

Clinical Aspects

In women, the incubation period for gonococcal infection varies from 10 days to several months. A mucopurulent cervical discharge may be the only clinical finding, while an unknown percentage of women are entirely asymptomatic. Ascending infection resulting in an endomyometritis, salpingitis, or early septic abortion can occur up to 12 weeks gestation. The decidua capsularis and decidua parietalis fuse between 10 to 12 weeks gestation, obliterating the endometrial cavity and preventing spread of the organism via this route. However, infection in the second or third trimester may still result in serious sequelae. Gonococcal adherence to chorioamniotic membranes has been demonstrated and is thought to result in premature labor, PROM, chorioamnionitis, or postpartum endometritis.

Pharyngeal infection is more prevalent in pregnant women.[250] Rectal infection occurs in 35 to 50 percent of women with cervical gonococci even in the absence of a history of rectal intercourse, probably as a result of spread from cervical secretions. Symptoms may range from mild pruritus to proctitis. Occasionally the rectum is the only site of demonstrable involvement.

In some series, 40 percent of the patients with disseminated gonococcal infection (DGI) are pregnant. In 15 to 30 percent of these cases, the pharnyx is the only site from which gonococci can be isolated. The clinical syndrome of DGI is characterized by fever up to 38 to 39 degrees C, tenosynovitis, polyarthralgias, skin lesions, and oligoarticular (often monoarticular) arthritis. There may also be hepatitis and myopericarditis. Although both a "bacteremic" and an "arthritis" phase have been described, these clinical presentations may overlap. The skin lesions are macular, 1 to 5 mm in diameter, and progress to pustules with a necrotic center (Fig. 40.18). Some investigators have demonstrated organisms in these lesions using fluorescent antibody assays. Extensor and flexor tendonitis occur, involving both hands and feet. Deposition of immune complexes have been implicated in this aspect of the disease. In pregnancy, migratory polyarthralgias are a common manifestation of DGI. Asymmetric septic oligoarthritis of the knee, elbow, or ankle may result, but only rarely is there residual joint deformity.

Intrapartum transmission occurs in one-third of cases with maternal infection. Neonatal ophthalmia, which caused 30 percent of childhood blindness in the preantibiotic era, has now been supplanted by *Chlamydia trachomatis* as the leading cause of neonatal infectious conjunctivitis in the United States. Neonates may also develop gonococcal arthritis, sepsis, or abscesses at the site of a fetal scalp electrode.

Diagnosis

Antepartum cervical culture remains the best method of case detection. The sensitivity of this test is estimated to be between 80 and 95 percent. Repeat cultures in the third trimester should be performed in high-risk patients, such as those with a previous history of gonorrhea or other sexually transmitted disease. Other sites should be cultured as the clinical situation dictates. Specimens must be promptly transferred to selective agar with appropriate transport systems, or the organism will not be recovered. Newer technologies using LA, ELISA, and other methods have been proposed as possible alternative approaches to diagnose gonorrhea.[251] Until these tests have been critically studied, it is probably best to obtain direct microbiologic diagnosis by culture despite the delays of current techniques except in settings where case finding and follow-up are impossible. All isolates should be tested for β-lactamase production.

In DGI, bacteremia may be intermittent, and in only 25 percent of cases can the organism be recovered from blood cultures. Some blood culture media contain the anticoagulant sodium polyanetholsulfonate, which may inhibit the growth of the organism. Arthrocentesis fluid shows a septic pattern with elevated PMNs, low glucose, and a poor clot. Gonococci may be visualized microscopically but are recovered by culture in only 20 percent of cases. Specific components of complement can be determined in DGI to rule out rare cases of complement-deficiency syndromes.

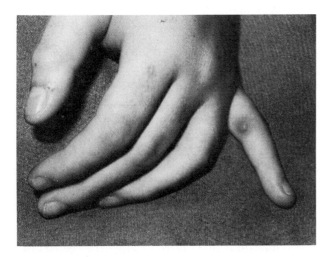

Fig. 40.18 Skin lesions of disseminated gonococcemia (DGI) with pustules on an erythematous base. (From Mandell et al.,[335] with permission.)

Management

Treatment of gonococcal infections in the United States is influenced by the following trends: (1) the spread of infections caused by antibiotic-resistant *N. gonorrhoeae*, including PPNG, TRNG, and CMRNG strains; (2) the high frequency of chlamydial infections in persons with gonorrhea; (3) recognition of the serious complications of chlamydial and gonococcal infections; and (4) the absence of a fast, inexpensive, and highly accurate test for chlamydial infection. The following recommendations are based on guidelines published by the CDC in 1989.[252,253]

Treatment of Gonococcal Infections in Pregnancy

Pregnant women should be cultured for *N. gonorrhoeae* (and tested for HIV-1, *C. trachomatis,* and syphilis) at the first prenatal care visit. For women at high risk for a sexually transmitted disease, a second culture for gonorrhea (as well as tests for *Chlamydia* and syphilis) should be obtained late in the third trimester.

The recommended treatment regimen is ceftriaxone 250 mg IM once plus erythromycin base 500 mg orally four times a day for 7 days. Pregnant women allergic to β-lactam drugs should be treated with spectinomycin 2 g IM once (followed by erythromycin). Follow-up cervical and rectal cultures for *N. gonorrhoeae* should be obtained 4 to 7 days after treatment is completed.

Ideally, pregnant women with gonorrhea should be treated for *Chlamydia* on the basis of chlamydial diagnostic studies. If chlamydial testing is not available, treatment for *Chlamydia* should be given. Tetracyclines (including doxycycline) and the quinolones are contraindicated in pregnancy because of possible adverse effects on the fetus. Therefore, pregnant women with *Chlamydia* should receive erythromycin as described above.

DGI

Hospitalization is recommended for initial therapy, especially for patients who cannot reliably comply with treatment, have uncertain diagnoses, or have purulent synovial effusions or other complications. Patients should be examined for clinical evidence of endocarditis or meningitis.

The recommended inpatient regimens are ceftriaxone 1 g IM or IV every 24 hours, or ceftizoxime 1 g IV every 8 hours, or cefotaxime 1 g IV every 8 hours. Patients who are allergic to β-lactam drugs should be treated with spectinomycin 2 g IM every 12 hours. When the infecting organism is proven to be penicillin sensitive, parenteral treatment may be switched to ampicillin 1 g every 6 hours (or the equivalent). Reliable patients with uncomplicated disease may be discharged 24 to 48 hours after all symptoms resolve and may complete the therapy (for a total of 1 week of antibiotic therapy) with an oral regimen of cefuroxime 500 mg two times a day or amoxicillin 500 mg with clavulanic acid three times a day.

Prevention of Ophthalmia Neonatorum

Instillation of a prophylactic agent into the eyes of all newborn infants is recommended to prevent gonococcal ophthalmia neonatorum and is required by law in most states. Although all regimens listed below effectively prevent gonococcal eye disease, their efficacy in preventing chlamydial eye disease is not clear. Furthermore, they do not eliminate nasopharyngeal colonization with *C. trachomatis.* Treatment of gonococcal and chlamydial infections in pregnant women is the best method for preventing neonatal gonococcal and chlamydial disease.

The recommended regimens are erythromycin (0.5 percent) ophthalmic ointment once, or tetracycline (1 percent) ophthalmic ointment once, or silver nitrate (1 percent) aqueous solution once. One of these should be instilled into the eyes of every neonate as soon as possible after delivery and definitely within 1 hour after birth. Single-use tubes or ampules are preferable to multiple-use tubes. The efficacy of tetracycline and erythromycin in the prevention of TRNG and PPNG ophthalmia is unknown, although both are probably effective because of the high concentrations of drug in these preparations. Bacitracin is not recommended.

C. trachomatis

Chlamydia is a genus of obligate intracellular bacteria that cause a wide variety of infections throughout the animal kingdom. Various strains of *C. trachomatis* affect mankind and cause significant morbidity. "Blinding" trachoma is the leading cause of infectious blindness in the world. Recently the role of this organism in neonatal conjunctivitis and pneumonitis, and in infertility because of tubal disease, has become better defined. *Chlamydia* have been implicated in obstetric disorders such as preterm labor, PROM, and postpartum endometritis.

Silver nitrate prophylaxis for neonatal ophthalmia was introduced in the late nineteenth century. Soon after, the gonococcus was identified. However, a portion of neonatal conjunctivitis was not prevented, and in these cases gonococci were not found. In 1907, *C. trachomatis* was first seen in conjunctival scrapings of laboratory animals inoculated with trachomatous material. Four years later, ophthalmologists reported these inclusion bodies in neonatal conjunctivitis ("inclusion blenorrhea"), in the genital tract of the mother, and in the urethra of the father. Investigation of this disorder was hampered by the cumbersome laboratory techniques required to isolate *Chlamydia*. Not until 1965, when the organism was propagated in tissue culture, could investigators examine the wide variety of diseases caused by *C. trachomatis*.

Microbiology

Humans are the definitive hosts for *C. trachomatis,* an obligate intracellular bacterium.[254] This organism has undergone several changes in nomenclature over the past few years. It has previously been called *Bedsonia, Miyagawanella,* and the TRIC agent, the latter an acronym for *tra*choma-*i*nclusion *c*onjunctivitis. The current name, *Chlamydia,* is derived from the Latin *chlamydatus,* meaning cloaked.

There are at least 15 serotypes of *C. trachomatis,* which cause different diseases in humans. Serotypes A, B, and C produce hyperendemic trachoma; serotypes L1, L2, and L3 cause lymphogranuloma venereum, and types D to K produce conjunctivitis, pneumonitis, salpingitis, and urethritis. The other members of the genus *Chlamydia* include *C. psittaci,* which causes psittacosis, and the newly described TWAR (*T*aiwan and *a*cute *r*espiratory) strain, which causes human respiratory infections.

The complex life cycle of *Chlamydia* begins with its attachment to a specific host cell type. Types D to K preferentially adhere to columnar epithelium and type L to lymphoid tissue. Some investigators have noted an increased recovery of types D to K in pregnancy, perhaps related to ectopy of cervical columnar epithelium. The infectious particle, called the elementary body, is 300 to 400 nm in diameter. After it attaches to the host cell, endocytosis takes place. Forty-eight hours later, the elementary body reorganizes into a reticulate body (800 to 1,000 nm in diameter), a metabolically active, noninfectious replicative form. The replicating reticulate bodies then change back into elementary bodies. These aggregates of reticulate and elementary bodies can be seen as cytoplasmic iodine-staining inclusions. Cellular disruption ultimately occurs, releasing the elementary bodies. The entire infectious cycle takes 2 to 3 days.

C. trachomatis does not synthesize ATP and has therefore been called an "energy parasite." The organism contains both DNA and RNA in a genome that is one of the smallest among bacteria. The cell wall contains a number of antigens, including a genus-specific lipopolysaccharide and a species-specific major outer membrane protein (MOMP). Although the cell wall is similar to that of gram-negative bacteria, muramic acid is absent. It is this structural difference that precludes penicillin's usual mode of antibacterial action. *C. trachomatis* produces folic acid and is sensitive to sulfonamides. Tetracycline and erythromycin will also inhibit growth of the organism (MICs of 0.1 to $1.0\,\mu g/ml$). However, *C. trachomatis* is resistant to metronidazole, spectinomycin, gentamicin, and vancomycin.

Immunology

A variety of host responses can be measured against chlamydial infection. IgM develops after an acute infection, followed by an increase in IgG. The role of these reactions in enhancing disease or protecting the host is unknown. Antibodies to MOMP can be identified. These are neutralizing in vitro but not in vivo. Although transfer of IgG to the fetus has been documented, two-thirds of infants can develop inclusion conjunctivitis after delivery through an infected cervix.

Epidemiology

Oculogenital *Chlamydia* (types D to K) is the most common sexually transmitted disease in Western society.[255] In some populations, it is five to seven times more prevalent than gonorrhea. Of individuals with gonorrhea, one-third to one-half are also infected with *Chlamydia.* Three to 5 percent of unselected pregnant women have been found to have positive cultures, and in some groups the carriage rate is as high as 30 percent. Thirty to 60 percent of nonpregnant women with nongonococcal mucopurulent cervitis have *Chlamydia* infection. Prospective studies have identified the highest risk group as poor, nonwhite, unmarried, and aged 18 to 24 years.

The incidence of chlamydial conjunctivitis is estimated to be 1 to 4 in 1,000 live births; the actual incidence of infection is estimated to be several times greater. Neonatal chlamydial pneumonia is thought to affect 3 to 10 in 1,000 live births.

Clinical Aspects

C. trachomatis has been retrospectively associated with prematurity, preterm labor, and PROM. This finding has not been consistently confirmed in prospective studies. Neonatal complications have included conjunctivitis and pneumonitis.[256,257] Serologic analysis suggests that pregnancies complicated by primary infections are at increased risk for low-birth-weight infants and premature delivery. In contrast, it is difficult to demonstrate an increased incidence of such problems in women who have otherwise recurrent infection. The significance of these findings may be confounded by coinfection with other organisms. *Chlamydia* may be associated with chorioamnionitis and postpartum endometritis.[258–263]

Chlamydia can also cause a wide variety of other urogenital problems. Like gonorrhea, it may produce first-trimester salpingitis. Up to 25 percent of women with urinary symptoms whose bacterial cultures are negative for coliforms and *Staphylococcus saprophyticus* have urethral cultures positive for *Chlamydia,* a clinical presentation called the acute urethral syndrome. The organism has been found in cases of bartholinitis, Fitz-Hugh-Curtis syndrome (perihepatitis), and ascites.[264]

Diagnosis

Direct cytologic diagnosis of clinical material for *C. trachomatis* has been hampered by lack of specificity and poor sensitivity. Its greatest usefulness has been in the rapid diagnosis of inclusion conjunctivitis of the newborn. Giemsa staining may show both intracellular gonorrhea and *Chlamydia.* Cytoplasmic vacuolization has been found to be an unreliable feature of this infection in this setting.

Tissue culture is the best method of diagnosis for most cases of genital infection. However, tissue culture isolation is labor intensive and costly and is only available in a limited number of laboratories. Tissue culture specimens should be processed within 24 hours. If this is not possible, they should be stored at −70 degrees C. The clinical material is extracted from the culture swab and centrifuged at high speed onto a cellular monolayer, such as cycloheximide-treated McCoy cells. After 3 to 4 days, characteristic inclusions can be seen. Visual detection of inclusion-containing cells can be enhanced by use of newer immunologic methods such as immunoperoxidase or fluorochrome staining.

Direct tests for rapid chlamydial diagnosis have been approved that are less expensive and less labor intensive to perform. Although FA and ELISA tests are available, the largest published experience is with the FA test. The predictive value of a positive result in both these tests is dependent on the prevalence of infection in the population. Positive tests have a high predictive value in a high-prevalence population and a low predictive value (high false positivity) in a low-prevalence population.[265]

Serologic diagnosis is not clinically useful because of high background titers in sexually active populations. However, such testing may be useful in epidemiologic surveys and in research protocols. New diagnostic tests utilizing DNA probes are currently being evaluated.

Management

Treatment regimens for *C. trachomatis* in pregnancy have been extrapolated from treatment of nonpregnant individuals. Children born to mothers with chlaÿdial infection carry increased morbidity associated with neonatal pneumonitis, childhood asthma, chronic otitis media or neonatal conjunctivitis. Chlamydial infection should be treated during pregnancy. Maternal therapy appears more effective than treatment of the infected neonate in preventing conjunctivitis.[266] Although the organism is sensitive to a wide variety of antibiotics, only certain therapies can be given to pregnant women. The following is derived from the 1989 CDC recommendations regarding chlamydial infection:[252]

Results of chlamydial tests should be interpreted with care. The sensitivity of all currently available laboratory tests for *C. trachomatis* tests is substantially less than 100 percent; thus false-negative tests are possible. Although the specificity of nonculture tests has improved substantially, false-positive test results may still occur with nonculture tests. Persons with chlamydial infections may remain asymptomatic for extended periods of time. Priority groups for *Chlamydia* testing, if resources are limited, are high-risk pregnant women, adolescents, and women with multiple sexual partners. Risk factors for chlamydial disease during pregnancy include young age (<25 years), past history or presence of another sexually transmitted disease, a new sex partner within the preceding 3 months, and multiple sex partners. Ideally, pregnant women with gonorrhea should be treated for *Chlamydia* on the basis of diagnostic studies, but if chlamydial testing is not available then treatment should be given because of the high likelihood of coinfection. Pregnant women should undergo diagnostic testing for *C. trachomatis*, *N. gonorrhoeae*, syphilis, and HIV-1 at their first prenatal visit.

Recommended Regimen

Erythromycin base 500 mg orally four times a day for 7 days is recommended. If this regimen is not tolerated, the following regimens are recommended:

1. Erythromycin ethylsuccinate 800 mg orally four times a day for 7 days or erythromycin ethylsuccinate 400 mg orally four times a day for 14 days
2. Alternative if erythromycin cannot be tolerated: amoxicillin 500 mg orally three times a day for 7 days (limited data exist concerning this regimen)

Erythromycin estolate is contraindicated during pregnancy, because drug-related hepatotoxicity can result in 10 percent of patients.

Trichomonas vaginalis

T. vaginalis is a flagellated protozoan that causes one of the most common sexually transmitted diseases in the United States, trichomoniasis. Management of the severely symptomatic individual in pregnancy remains a problem.

Microbiology

The organism is a microaerophilic protozoan that is specific for squamous epithelial urogenital mucous membranes. It is 10 to 20 μm wide and slightly longer than a PMN. Its beating flagella and undulating membrane propel it with a jerky staccato motion. In vivo experiments have shown that an inoculum of 10 organisms will initiate infection. The organism does not appear to cause infection in the mouth or colon, where other trichomonads may be found. Columnar epithelium appears to resist attachment by *T. vaginalis*. The organism is sensitive to metronidazole at concentrations of less than 1 μg/ml.

Immunology

Local defenses appear important in controlling infection by *T. vaginalis*. There is an outpouring of PMNs that phagocytose the organism. Secretory IgA may also play a role.

Epidemiology

In the United States, an estimated 2 million cases of trichomoniasis are treated each year. The incidence varies among populations and appears to depend on the number of sexual partners. In women, the incidence of the disease has ranged from 5 to 75 percent. The transmission rate among sexual partners is estimated to be 70 percent. Perinatal transmission at parturition is approximately 5 percent. There is a high coinfection rate with other sexually transmitted diseases such as gonorrhea.

Occasionally, epidemics have been reported in institutions, presumably from shared infected moist towels. Although the live organism has been recovered from toilet seats for up to 45 minutes, unequivocal clinical cases of transmission from this source have never been described.

Clinical Aspects

The incubation period for trichomoniasis is 3 to 28 days. The disease is asymptomatic in 10 to 50 percent of women, of whom one-third will become symptomatic in 6 months if untreated. In symptomatic patients, there may be a profuse malodorous discharge in 10 to 20 percent, vaginal itching in 25 to 50 percent, dysuria from urethral involvement, and dyspareunia from involvement of Skene's glands. The urethra and Skene's glands may remain foci for recurrent infection after treatment. Lower abdominal pain has been noted in 5 to 12 percent of cases. It is not clear whether the organism can cause salpingitis, although it has been recovered from tuboovarian abscesses. Coexistent infection with other organisms has been proposed in this setting. The disease is associated with an exacerbation of symptoms during or immediately after menses. Males generally have a self-limited disease over a 1 week period, although prostatitis and epididymitis have been suggested as complications. Infected neonates can suffer from vaginitis for a period of 4 to 6 weeks, while circulating maternal estrogens are still present.

Physical examination may show a profuse vaginal discharge, which is usually gray but which may be yellow-green and frothy. The vagina may be granular, and epithelial cervical hemorrhages ("the strawberry cervix") may be seen in severe cases. A few studies have associated *T. vaginalis* with PROM and postpartum endometritis, but other organisms that have been linked with these conditions were not excluded in these investigations.

Laboratory Findings

The diagnosis of trichomoniasis is usually made by examination of a wet-mount saline slide. The characteristic movement of *T. vaginalis* may be more easily seen if the slide is warmed. A profusion of PMNs, in excess of the normal 1 : 1 ratio of PMNs to epithelial cells, may also be observed. The organism is destroyed by 10 percent KOH. The wet-mount preparation is 75 percent sensitive for the detection of infection.

Pap smears also have a 70 percent sensitivity for the diagnosis of *T. vaginalis.* Evaluation for atypia or dysplasia on cervical cytology may not be possible in the presence of infection and its attendant inflammatory response. Selective media may aid diagnosis in difficult cases.[267,268]

Treatment in Pregnancy

Metronidazole, a nitroimidazole, is effective against many anaerobic organisms and *T. vaginalis.* Its use is not recommended during the first trimester of pregnancy because of possible teratogenic effects. Metronidazole also causes chromosomal alterations in bacteria and lung tumors when administered to mice in high doses. There are no data to suggest human carcinogenesis with short-term, low-dose therapy. The drug readily crosses the placenta and does enter breast milk. If the drug is to be used in pregnant patients with incapacitating symptoms, a single oral 2-g dose should be administered with simultaneous treatment of the sexual partner. Long term effects on exposed fetuses, if any, are unknown. Alcohol should be proscribed while taking metronidazole because of the potential disulfiram-like effect.[269] Intravenous metronidazole has been used for treatment of resistant strains of *Trichomonas.*[270,271]

IMPORTANT CLINICAL SYNDROMES

Chorioamnionitis

Chorioamnionitis is a clinical syndrome characterized by maternal fever and leukocytosis, maternal and fetal tachycardia, and uterine tenderness. Premature labor or PROM may precede clinical suspicion of infection. There may be evidence of fetal or maternal sepsis. The spectrum of the disease has widened over the past decade, especially with data gathered by amniocentesis and improved microbiologic techniques.

Chorioamnionitis may leave the fetus unaffected in up to 95 percent of cases, but the "attack rate" may be modified by maternal and fetal host defenses. The fetus may develop pneumonitis by aspirating infected amniotic fluid. Fetal septicemia may follow the penetration of umbilical vessels by invading bacteria. Premature infants are more susceptible to such infections. The clinician must weigh the risks of preterm delivery and respiratory distress syndrome against expectant management complicated by neonatal infectious morbidity.

Epidemiology

An estimated 0.5 to 2 percent of all term pregnancies are affected by chorioamnionitis. Certain populations are at higher risk for this infection: (1) women with poor nutrition, especially those from lower socioeconomic groups; (2) women undergoing invasive procedures such as amniocentesis or cervical cerclage; (3) women at risk for preterm delivery because of labor or PROM; and (4) women harboring cervical pathogens such as *C. trachomatis* or *N. gonorrhoeae.* Other associations have been reported, such as protracted stages of labor, multiple vaginal or rectal examinations, multiple gestations, and intrauterine fetal monitoring. These factors may be covariables associated with chorioamnionitis rather than causative factors. An association between chorioamnionitis and coitus late in gestation has been reported. However, the clinical significance of this association is unclear.

Pathogenesis

Chorioamnionitis is often the result of an ascending infection caused by cervicovaginal pathogens. The histologic appearance is initially that of an inflammatory and exudative reaction involving the chorionic plate, which may spread to the decidua, amnion, and amniotic fluid. A funistis may develop, with diapedesis of PMNs through the umbilical vessels into Wharton's jelly. This process frequently heralds fetal infection.

Ascending infections require both potentially pathogenic organisms and a susceptible host. Certain bacteria may be commonly associated in cases of chorioamnionitis yet may be found in the cervix and occasionally the amniotic fluid of apparently asymptomatic individuals. Presumably host factors described earlier are responsible for the variation in susceptibility to chorioamnionitis.

Some bacterial species, notably *E. coli* and *S. agalactiae*, have been studied using in vitro models. These bacteria attach to chorioamniotic membranes and, by elaboration of certain enzymes such as proteases and phospholipases, may weaken the membranes or activate prostaglandins, leading to PROM and/or premature labor. Moreover, ultrastructural and immunologic findings suggest that some bacteria pass directly through fetal membranes, causing direct amniotic fluid infection without membrane rupture (Fig. 40.19). Recent work indicates that cytokines such as interleukins elaborated by activated decidual macrophages in response to infection may stimulate the synthesis of local prostaglandins and initiate labor.[272,273]

Streptococci and coliforms were initially found in association with chorioamnionitis. Clinical application of anaerobic technology in the 1970s led to an appreciation of the role of anaerobic organisms in the pathogenesis of this condition. The animal model for intra-abdominal abscess formation proposed by Bartlett and co-workers applies to chorioamnionitis. They noted that if anaerobic organisms alone are treated, the aerobic organisms multiply and sepsis ensues ("peritonitis stage"). If aerobes alone are treated, abscess formation by anaerobes can result ("abscess

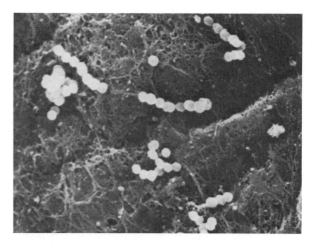

Fig. 40.19 Scanning electron micrograph showing the attachment of GBS to the maternal surface of the chorioamniotic membranes (X6,000). (From Galask et al.,[336] with permission.)

staph = cluster
strep = chain

stage"). Anaerobic organisms, which outnumber aerobic organisms in the vagina 10-fold, are also significant potential pathogens. Pure cultures of *Bacteroides fragilis, Bacteroides bivius,* or *Peptostreptococcus* may be recovered in cases of endometritis or neonatal sepsis after chorioamnionitis. *Gardnerella vaginalis,* alone or in combination with anaerobes, has been found in chorioamnionitis.[274,275]

The clinical presentation of chorioamnionitis varies. Nonspecific responses include fever, maternal tachycardia, and peripheral leukocytosis, consisting primarily of PMNs. Acute-phase reactants, such as C-reactive protein, may be found in maternal serum)or amniotic fluid. Maternal PMNs may also be detected in amniotic fluid as a response to infection. Inflammation may produce uterine irritability, amniorrhexis, or even labor.

Diagnosis

Clinical circumstances may make the diagnosis of chorioamnionitis quite obvious. However, findings such as fever, uterine tenderness, and maternal leukocytosis are present in only 20 percent of bacteriologically proven cases. Minimally symptomatic presentations, such as premature labor unresponsive to tocolytic agents, should prompt further consideration of infection as the cause of uterine irritability. The most common finding associated with chorioamnionitis is rupture of the membranes. Because the presence of ruptured membranes increases the likelihood of subsequent infection, observation for other symptoms, signs, or laboratory findings suggestive of chorioamnionitis should be instituted.

Amniocentesis has been advocated to aid in the diagnosis of chorioamnionitis, both with and without ruptured membranes. Identification of PMNs in amniotic fluid is suggestive of infection but is not diagnostic. Detection of bacteria by Gram stain of the fluid may be specific but is not sensitive.[276] Results from routine bacterial cultures may be available only after 1 week, especially for recovery of anaerobic organisms. Diagnosis of anaerobic infection by chromatographic detection of metabolic products remains a research tool.

C-reactive protein is a nonspecific sign of infection, with variable elevations in cases of chorioamnionitis. The use of glucocorticoids to accelerate pulmonary maturity may also produce elevations in C-reactive protein.

A retrospective diagnosis can be suggested after histopathologic study of changes in the placenta, cord, or fetal membranes after delivery. However, inflammatory changes in fetal membranes can be found without any bacteriologic evidence of infection.

The differential diagnosis of chorioamnionitis includes pyelonephritis, appendicitis, and pneumonitis. In the absence of fever, placental abruption and an adnexal accident must be considered.

Treatment

The treatment of chorioamnionitis is delivery. In general, vaginal delivery should be attempted if obstetric factors are favorable. Uterine contractility, even with oxytocin augmentation, may be less effective in the presence of infection.[277]

Antibiotic administration before delivery in cases of suspected chorioamnionitis has maternal benefit. There is substantially less major maternal morbidity (e.g., decreased pelvic cellulitis and abscess formation), especially in populations at high risk for infection. However, this approach has been criticized, because it may commit the neonate to a course of antibiotics without specific bacteriologic data. Because infectious agents are usually recoverable from both mother and baby by timely culturing and be-

cause most infants at risk are empirically treated with antibiotics pending cultures, there may be less substance to this objection except in certain clinical settings. The use of antibiotics in cases of positive bacterial cultures in the amniotic fluid with no other symptoms of chorioamnionitis is under investigation.[278,279]

Maternal complications of chorioamnionitis include endometritis, parametritis, pelvic vein thrombophlebitis, and wound infections. Management must include antibiotic therapy to cover both aerobic and anaerobic organisms.

Endometritis

Endometritis is the most common cause of identifiable infectious morbidity in postpartum patients. It has been the subject of intense study over the past decade because of the rising rate of cesarean delivery and the increased clinical availability of microbiologic isolation methods, especially for recovery of anaerobic organisms and *Chlamydia*.

Several well-defined clinical risk factors for the development of endometritis have been described.[280,281] Cesarean section is perhaps the greatest risk factor, with rates increased up to 20-fold over those after vaginal delivery. Twenty to 50 percent of patients undergoing abdominal delivery develop endometritis. In the past, classic uterine incisions were noted to have a higher incidence of infectious complications, perhaps because of increased blood loss, greater soft tissue injury, and greater foreign body reaction from suture material. However, a recent retrospective study has not confirmed this. Extraperitoneal cesarean sections have been thought to decrease the rate of infectious morbidity, but this has not been unequivocally substantiated.

Other factors associated with the development of endometritis are premature labor, prolonged rupture of membranes (especially greater than 24 hours), frequent vaginal examinations, and low socioeconomic status. The presence of chorioamnionitis or pathogens isolated from the cervix such as *S. agalactiae* or *N. gonorrhoeae* at the time of delivery also places the patient at risk for subsequent endometritis. The impact of internal monitoring, with the fetal electrode and intrauterine pressure catheter, plays a small role in increasing the risk for infection. Rather, it appears that the association is with prolonged labor and multiple vaginal examinations instead of with internal monitoring. Labor itself is associated with a two- to threefold risk of postpartum febrile morbidity. Antepartum iron deficiency has been associated with an increased risk for endometritis, but is probably a marker for decreased host resistance.

Pathophysiology and Bacteriology

The majority of cases of endometritis arise from an ascending infection from cervicovaginal flora.[282-284] The bacteria attach to the decidua and proliferate, establishing an endometritis. If the infection is allowed to progress, especially if a uterine incision is present, a myometritis/parametritis ensues. There may be bacteremia or even septic shock. Pelvic veins may become involved in this suppurative process (see below, Septic Pelvic Thrombophlebitis). Endomyometritis in the presence of a uterine incision has been likened to peritonitis associated with appendicitis. The uterine wall, broad ligament, pelvic peritoneal surfaces, and pelvic vessels may all become involved. For unknown reasons, salpingitis generally does not develop in this setting.

Up to 10 percent of nonlaboring patients can have organisms cultured from the amniotic fluid. As many as 60 percent of patients with preterm labor and intact membranes may have bacteria recovered. The passage of bacteria through intact membranes is a necessary but not sufficient condition for the subsequent development of endometritis. Obviously, in the presence of ruptured membranes, cervicovaginal pathogens have direct access to the amniotic cavity, fetal membranes, and ultimately the decidua.

The bacteriology of postpartum endometritis has been difficult to study because of the technical problems encountered in obtaining valid microbiologic specimens.[285,286] Ninety percent of transcervical specimens obtained are contaminated by cervicovaginal flora. After vaginal delivery, bacterial cultures can be obtained from opposing surfaces of chorion and amnion. However, vaginal contamination cannot always be avoided, even with these methods. Additional information has been obtained from the examination of amniotic membranes and fluid at the time of cesarean section.[287]

The postpartum uterus is probably contaminated by cervicovaginal flora that are subsequently cleared. The time course of this process is unknown. Presumably, those patients who fail to eliminate these organisms from the uterine cavity develop endometritis. Mixed aerobic–anaerobic infections usually result with an average of two or three different bacterial species recovered.

Gram-Positive Cocci

Group A streptococcus (*Streptococcus pyogenes*) is the causative agent of childbed fever. This organism is rarely found in the vagina. It may cause a virulent endomyometritis with rapid lymphatic and hematogenous dissemination. GBS (*S. agalactiae*), a well-recognized perinatal pathogen, can cause endometritis and bacteremia, especially within the first 24 hours postpartum. Group D streptococci are found in approximately 10 percent of cases of endometritis. The two principal groups are enterococci, such as *Streptococcus faecalis,* and nonenterococci, such as *Streptococcus bovis.* These organisms are commonly found in polymicrobial bacteremia. The enterococci are important because they are penicillin resistant. Other streptococci, such as the viridans group, or *Streptococcus pneumoniae,* are much less common causes of endometritis.[288,289]

Staphylococcus aureus is a rare cause of endometritis, even though the organism can be found in up to 10 percent of cervicovaginal cultures. Certain strains of the organism may cause toxic shock syndrome, without bacteremia or sepsis.[290] Staphylococcal endomyometritis may produce abscess formation and disseminate widely.

Staphylococcus epidermidis has been isolated from the endometrium of febrile postpartum women but not from blood cultures. As a normal component of skin flora, it is difficult to prove a pathogenic role for this organism.

Gram-positive anaerobic cocci, common microbiologic isolates in endometritis, are found in up to 90 percent of cultures. The principal organisms are *Peptococcus (P. asaccharolyticus* and *P. anaerobius), Peptostreptococcus,* and microaerophilic *Streptococcus (Streptococcus* MG, *S. mutans,* and *S. mitis).* Peptococci and Peptostreptococci are found in high concentrations in the vaginal fluid of many healthy women. Some of the earliest reports describing the role of anaerobes in human disease involved the identification of these organisms in the genesis of endometritis, puerperal sepsis, and septic abortion. Frequent pathogenic isolates have been *P. anaerobius* and *P. prevotii*.

Gram-Positive Bacilli

Gram-positive bacilli are extremely common components of vaginal and rectal flora. Those species of potential obstetric significance in cases of endometritis include *Clostridium* species and *Listeria monocytogenes.* Clostridia are found in high concentrations in normal feces. *C. ramosum* is most common, followed by *C. perfringens*. These organisms are vaginal saprophytes, and their presence must be interpreted in the clinical setting. Spores are not generally seen in clinical isolates of *C. ramosum* and *C. perfringens,* and special media and cultural conditions are required to induce sporulation. As anaerobic pathogens, these organisms may produce gas in soft tissues. It is important to note that other anaerobic organisms beside *Clostridium* can produce soft tissue gas.

Clostridial infections are characterized by minimal inflammatory response in the host. They can be seen in the absence of surrounding PMNs, facilitating the clinical diagnosis. *C. perfringens* produces a lecithinase that results in hemolysis, jaundice, hypotension, and renal failure with acute cortical necrosis. Invasion of the uterine wall can progress to myonecrosis.[291]

L. monocytogenes is a rare cause of chorioamnionitis and endometritis.[292] Symptoms of listeriosis can be nonspecific, including gastrointestinal upset, diarrhea, malaise, chills, fever, and pharyngitis. *L. monocytogenes* is a gram-positive, nonspore-forming coccobacillus, which may be confused with diphtheroids. One-third of the identified cases of listeriosis in the United States have occurred during pregnancy or during the neonatal period. An outbreak in California was traced to the ingestion of contaminated cheese by pregnant women. The perinatal mortality rate was extremely high in these patients. Systemic listeriosis in pregnancy has been reported as a complication of AIDS.[293]

Gram-Negative Cocci

N. gonorrhoeae can cause endometritis, in addition to PROM, preterm labor, chorioamnionitis, and septic abortion. Gonococcal adherence to amniotic membranes has been demonstrated and may contribute to ascending infection.[294]

Aerobic Gram-Negative Bacilli

G. vaginalis, often associated with vaginitis, has also been implicated in PROM and chorioamnionitis. It has been recovered in obstetric bacteremia often in association with other aerobic or anaerobic organisms. This latter condition, termed bacterial vaginosis or, more recently, vaginal bacteriosis, is associated with preterm delivery and postpartum endometritis.[259,274]

* Enterobacteriaceae are a large family of aerobic and facultative anaerobic gram-negative, nonspore-forming organisms that cause significant morbidity. This family includes the genera *Escherichia, Klebsiella, Enterobacter, Proteus,* and *Citrobacter,* agents of the "peritonitis" septic shock stage of the intra-abdominal abscess model described above. These organisms are found in high concentrations in the cervicovaginal flora. Endometritis involving Enterobacteriaceae are usually polymicrobial. *E. coli* may be found in 40 percent of isolates, *Klebsiella* in 10 percent, *Proteus* in 5 percent, and *Enterobacter* in 2 percent.

Most gram-negative bacteria produce endotoxin, a lipopolysaccharide. Through activation of complement, vascular injury, and myocardial depression, endotoxin can cause septic shock. Endotoxin can also activate macrophages to produce interleukins, which can stimulate local prostaglandin synthesis. Many Enterobacteriaceae carry extrachromosomal genetic elements, resistance (R) factors, that code antibiotic resistance. Widespread use of antibiotics, especially in a hospital setting, can select for resistant strains.

Anaerobic Gram-Negative Bacilli

The clinical availability of anaerobic technology has permitted greater understanding of the role of anaerobic gram-negative bacilli in the genesis of endometritis. *B. bivius* and *B. fragilis* have been the two principal anaerobic gram-negative rods isolated in cases of endometritis. Of interest, *Bacteroides* species are found in large quantities in both feces and vaginal flora, but *B. fragilis* generally constitutes less than 1 percent of *Bacteroides* organisms. However, *B. fragilis* has a polysaccharide capsule resistant to host phagocytes, a factor that may contribute to its virulence.

Chlamydia

Chlamydia are obligate intracellular parasites that infect squamocolumnar tissue and require tissue culture techniques for laboratory isolation. They have been identified in cases of puerperal endometritis, but the full extent of their clinical significance in this setting has yet to be determined. The etiology is an ascending infection from endocervical tissue. The perinatal transmission of *C. trachomatis* has been described above.[259]

Mycoplasma

Mycoplasma are the smallest free-living organisms (200 nm) and are distinguished from true bacteria by their lack of a complete cell wall. They have been recovered from the blood of both febrile and asymptomatic postpartum patients.[295,296] Their clinical significance remains unclear at this time.

Diagnosis

Postpartum endometritis can be anticipated in the setting of preterm or prolonged rupture of membranes, chorioamnionitis, cesarean section, prolonged labor, known antepartum colonization with certain cervicovaginal pathogens (e.g., GBS or gonococci), and/or low socioeconomic status. Fever may occur early or late in the course of the illness. If it occurs in the first 24 to 48 hours postpartum, GBS infection or, less commonly, group A streptococcal infection should be suspected. Fever may occur later with mixed aerobic–anaerobic infection and may be delayed or low grade if prophylactic antibiotics are used. Fever, uterine tenderness, foul-smelling lochia, and malaise suggest endometritis. Certainly other sources of postpartum fever must be suspected based on the clinical setting, but, overall, endometritis is the most common cause.

"Standard puerperal morbidity" has been defined by the United States Joint Committee on Maternal Welfare as "a temperature of 100.4 degrees F (38 degrees C), the temperature to occur in any two of the first ten days postpartum, exclusive of the first 24 hours, and to be taken by mouth by a standard technique at least four times daily." However, it is important to note that a fever within the first 24 hours may be significant and that serious infection-related complications may be present even with a temperature of less than 100.4 degrees F. Ledger and Kriewall[297] proposed a fever index to quantitate the number of degree-hours that the patient is febrile. This index has been useful in assessing febrile morbidity and response to therapy.

Laboratory aids in diagnosis include uterine cultures, blood cultures, and a complete blood count. Chlamydial cultures can be performed if facilities are available and carriage rates in the population justify such testing. Urinalysis is helpful in the differential diagnosis. A Gram stain may be done if clostridial infection is suspected, although the presence of other vaginal flora limit the usefulness of this test. A physiologic leukocytosis (up to 20,000/mm^3) from mobilization of PMNs occurs postpartum and limits the diagnostic value of the white blood count.

Treatment

Parenteral antibiotic therapy is the mainstay of therapy for endometritis.[284] High-dose penicillin or ampicillin treatment (10 to 20 million units/day or 8 to 12 g/day, respectively) is effective in cases of mild to moderate severity, but is not effective against certain species of *Bacteroides* and enterococci. A dramatic response over 48 to 72 hours should be anticipated. In the presence of severe disease or other complicating factors, an alternate regimen such as intravenous clindamycin and an aminoglycoside can be used initially or after initiation of penicillin treatment.[298] Antibiotic dose and intervals appropriate for the postpartum state must be given. With clinically severe endometritis, response rates may be protracted over 4 to 6 days. Aminoglycoside peak and trough levels, along with monitoring of renal function, are helpful in those patients on prolonged therapy or with impaired renal function.[299] Cure rates of 90 percent can be anticipated with this regimen.

Single-agent therapy with penicillin or cephalosporin derivatives has been studied, with reported cure rates of up to 90 percent. Further clinical experience should clarify the role of these agents for first-line therapy.[300]

Failure of improvement on antibiotic therapy over several days should prompt a search for other sites of infection or postpartum complications such as wound infection, pelvic abscess or hematoma, or septic pelvic thrombophlebitis. Ileus is a sign of significant peritoneal irritation. Retained secundines or necrotic decidua may cause late postpartum fever.[301]

Prevention

Most postpartum infectious complications are caused by endometritis. Its occurrence can be reduced but not totally eliminated by the administration of an antibiotic around the time of delivery. The greatest reduction of endometritis rates can be achieved in patients already at increased risk for endometritis, namely, those undergoing abdominal delivery during labor, with ruptured membranes, who are from lower socioeconomic groups. Patients having an uncomplicated labor and vaginal delivery from upper socioeconomic groups have the lowest incidence of endometritis; benefit from peripartum antibiotics is difficult to demonstrate. Otherwise healthy patients undergoing elective repeat cesarean deliveries have lower rates of endometritis, and the use of antibiotics for these patients must be individualized on the basis of personal and institutional experience.

The use of short-course peripartum antibiotics in patients without clinical chorioamnionitis has been termed prophylactic.[302] The microbiologic basis for efficacy of this usage is unknown. There is no clear and reproducible alteration in uterine or cervicovaginal flora with administration of prophylactic antibiotics. We can speculate that antibiotics inhibit multiplication of potential pathogens to a degree that host defenses are not overwhelmed and establishment of clinical infection is prevented.

Many antibiotics have been tested, and all appear to have generally equivalent efficacy in prevention of infectious morbidity.[303,304] Ampicillin compares favorably with third-generation penicillins, which have wider antibacterial coverage particularly for anaerobes. Why this should be so underscores the limits of our knowledge concerning the mechanism of action of antibiotics when used in this particular manner.

Administering antibiotics after cord clamping, even up to 1 hour postpartum, appears to be as effective as predelivery administration and does not confound subsequent pediatric management by obscuring neonatal bacterial culture results.[305] Prophylactic antibiotic administration more than 12 hours postpartum confers no additional beneficial effects. Other techniques of antibiotic administration such as intraoperative pelvic and wound irrigation have been examined. Pelvic irrigation usually confers roughly equal or reduced efficacy compared with intravenous administration.[306]

Serious risks of prophylactic therapy include anaphylaxis, antibiotic-associated colitis, and selection for antibiotic-resistant organisms.[307,308] At times, prophylaxis fails and requires parenteral antibiotic therapy.[309] Use of newer antibiotics imposes unnecessary costs because of the equivalent efficacy of less expensive ones. Judicious use of prophylactic antibiotics reduces the rates of endometritis, wound infections, and UTIs in properly selected patients while minimizing risks related to antibiotic complications. Extraperitoneal abdominal delivery has been advocated to reduce postpartum infectious complications, although others have not found this technique useful. A significant factor appears to be the experience of the surgical team.[310,311]

Prognosis

Severe puerperal endometritis may result in secondary infertility. Curettage for postpartum hemorrhage, infected decidua, or retained secundines may leave intrauterine synechiae. In addition, it appears that fertility is reduced if endometritis is complicated by the formation of a pelvic abscess. Regarding patients with otherwise uncomplicated postpartum endometritis managed medically, a retrospective examination of the available literature suggests that reproductive performance remains intact.[312]

Wound Infections

Wound infections complicate approximately 1 in 20 abdominal deliveries. Many variables affect the institutional and individual rates of infection. Patients with underlying medical problems such as diabetes, obesity, or protein-calorie malnutrition as well as conditions requiring corticosteroid or other immunosuppressive therapy are at increased risk for this complication. Obstetric and surgical factors that predispose to wound infection include the type of incision, the presence of a previous scar, the extent of surgical soft tissue trauma, the type of suture material used, use and type of incisional drains, and the presence or absence of chorioamnionitis.

The overall institutional rates of wound infection after cesarean delivery vary from 2 to 20 percent, depending on the population studied. The American College of Surgeons classifies wounds as "clean," "clean-contaminated," "contaminated," or "dirty," depending on the presence or absence and source of bacteria in the wound. Elective abdominal deliveries are "clean" cases, with a wound infection rate of 2 percent. Most abdominal deliveries performed in the presence of ruptured membranes or labor are considered "clean-contaminated" and are associated with a wound infection rate between 5 and 10 percent. Deliveries performed as emergency cases or in the presence of clinical chorioamnionitis are "contaminated" and have a wound infection rate of 20 percent.

Pathophysiology and Bacteriology

Bacteria that cause obstetric wound infections may be endogenous or, less commonly, exogenous. Endogenous bacterial flora inoculate the wound directly from the skin or by spread from the genital tract via the uterine incision to the abdominal incision. Less common are exogenous infections acquired from intraoperative contamination by hospital personnel or instruments.

An estimated 10^5 bacteria per gram of tissue are required to establish an infection. The presence of significant tissue damage from crush injuries caused by surgical clamps, reactive suture material such as silk, or direct communication with skin flora via open drain systems can reduce the required inoculum to as low as 10^2 bacteria.

Aerobic gram-positive organisms, such as *Staph. aureus* and group A streptococci are common causes of wound infections. *Staph. aureus* form microabscesses that coalesce and "point." Group A streptococci disseminate rapidly through tissue planes and into the bloodstream and lymphatics. GBS, often found in association with chorioamnionitis, may also cause a wound infection, especially if a cesarean section has been performed.

Anaerobic organisms outnumber aerobic organisms by 10 to 1 on the skin and by up to 100 to 1 in the vagina. It is not surprising, then, that many wound infections are associated with anaerobes or mixtures of aerobic and anaerobic bacteria. Clostridial species are found in the feces and can be isolated from the perineal skin. *C. ramosum* is most common, followed by *C. perfringens*. These organisms may produce a diffuse spreading cellulitis and fasciitis. *C. perfringens*

is notable as the principal etiologic agent of gas gangrene, otherwise known as clostridial myonecrosis, which involves the skin, subcutaneous layer, fascia, and muscle. Sepsis from this organism results in hemolytic anemia, renal failure, and cardiovascular collapse. The presence of clostridia is insufficient to substantiate the diagnosis of infection. Symptoms of infection must also be present to differentiate infection from colonization.

Nonspore-forming anaerobic bacteria such as *Bacteroides, Peptostreptococcus,* and *Peptococcus* can cause a nonclostridial anaerobic cellulitis. Mixed aerobic–anaerobic infections can result if coliforms are involved. Subcutaneous gas, foul-smelling discharge, and swelling may also be found. Necrotizing fasciitis or myositis can also be caused by these mixed infections and has acquired a variety of different names, each with subtle variations in bacteriology.

Diagnosis

The diagnosis of wound infection is made on both clinical and bacteriologic grounds. Daily inspection of the wound for unusual tenderness, swelling, discoloration, or discharge will give clues of an early infection. Streptococci are often responsible for the wound infections seen in the first 2 days. If chorioamnionitis has been present, gross contamination of the wound at surgery may also lead to an early infection by mixed aerobic–anaerobic flora. "Late" wound infections, those observed after 2 days, are generally caused by staphylococci or mixed aerobic–anaerobic organisms. Wound discharges with unusual odors or consistencies should raise suspicion of serious infection. "Dishwater" pus may be seen with necrotizing cellulitis, while a clostridial discharge may be "sweet" or "foul." Bullae are indicative of gangrene. Skin anesthesia indicates infarction of nerve endings. Crepitation in the wound may result from loosely sutured tissue but may also arise from gas-forming organisms such as *Clostridium* or coliforms. An x-ray film is helpful in confirming subcutaneous gas.

The wound discharge should be examined by Gram stain, and aerobic and anaerobic cultures should be taken. Dead or nonreplicating gram-positive organisms may be mistaken for gram-negative bacteria. This error is especially important when excluding staphylococci and clostridia as pathogens. Spore formation is not noted in actively growing clinical isolates of *C. ramosum* or *C. perfringens*.

Treatment

Drainage of a wound infection is both diagnostic and therapeutic. The wound should be left to close by secondary intention, irrigated, and debrided as necessary. In the presence of extensive suppuration, cutaneous gangrene, bullae, or widespread gas formation, investigation under anesthesia is required. Appropriate bacteriologic samples should be taken, including tissue samples if surgical exploration is necessary. Myonecrosis can be diagnosed by the color, consistency, and reactivity of the muscle layers. All nonviable tissue should be resected back to fresh, well-vascularized areas. This approach creates much larger defects than were originally anticipated, and further surgical consultation may be required.

Antibiotics should be guided by the clinical setting, Gram stain, and culture. Nevertheless, the primary treatment of a wound infection is drainage. Rarely does a wound infection respond to antibiotic therapy alone.

Prevention

Administration of antibiotics for the prevention of endometritis at the time of cesarean section does not appear to reduce the incidence of wound infection significantly. Wound irrigation with an antibiotic is a controversial practice. Attention to aseptic technique must always be emphasized. *Staph. aureus* or group A streptococcus can be found in 10 to 15 percent of normal adults, with higher rates among medical personnel. Use of reactive sutures, such as plain catgut, should be avoided in the subcutaneous layer. Tissue trauma by devascularization and use of crushing clamps on fascia and muscle should be avoided if possible. If drains are necessary, closed systems should be used. Drainage is not a substitute for hemostasis. In wounds that are virtually certain to be infected, such as with fecal contamination from a ruptured appendix or from grossly purulent chorioamnionitis, the wound should be left open to heal by secondary intention or a delayed primary wound closure utilized.

Mastitis

Puerperal mastitis affects 1 to 2 percent of postpartum women. There are two principal forms of the disease, epidemic and nonepidemic, each with a different pathophysiology, treatment, and prognosis. They cannot always be distinguished clinically.

Pathophysiology and Bacteriology

The epidemic form of the disease is a nosocomial infection acquired by the mother from her nursing infant, whose nasopharynx has been colonized with a virulent strain of *Staph. aureus* from the hospital environment. The infection involves the glandular tissue of the breast, channeling between Cooper's ligaments and producing deep abscesses.

Nonepidemic mastitis often develops during periods of sporadic nursing or weaning. Milk stasis has been suggested as a predisposing factor. In only 50 percent of cases can *Staph. aureus* be isolated. The organisms involved appear to be less virulent, and one-half are sensitive to penicillin. Various anaerobic and aerobic bacteria are isolated in the remainder of cases. The portion of the breast involved is the periglandular connective tissue, resulting in a superficial cellulitis. Abscess formation rarely occurs in these patients and is usually less extensive than in the epidemic form.[313,314]

Diagnosis

The epidemic form of mastitis occurs 2 to 4 days after delivery, often associated with nosocomial outbreaks in the nursery or other areas of the hospital. The infection is characterized by fever and localized breast tenderness. A Gram stain of pus from the nipple may reveal PMNs and gram-positive cocci. Culture of expressed milk or pus is often diagnostic. In epidemic situations, phage typing can be performed on the staphylococci and may prove useful in epidemiologic surveillance and eradication of the infectious source.

The nonepidemic or endemic form of mastitis occurs several weeks or months after delivery and produces a systemic illness with fever, tachycardia, and malaise followed by localized breast tenderness. Because the periglandular tissue is involved, pus is not usually present in the milk, and cultures are often of little diagnostic value. White blood cell counts in milk have been proposed as an aid in the diagnosis of infectious mastitis. However, clinical signs and symptoms usually suffice.[315] Toxic shock syndrome caused by *Staph. aureus* associated with puerperal mastitis has been reported.[316]

Treatment

The treatment of nonepidemic mastitis involves prompt institution of oral antibiotic therapy pending culture results. A clinical response to penicillin has been described even in patients whose milk cultures grew *Staph. aureus* resistant to penicillin. However, these may not have been the actual organism(s) causing the cellulitis. If penicillin-resistant *Staph. aureus* is suspected, a penicillinase-resistant antibiotic such as dicloxacillin should be used. Continued breast-feeding or breast-pumping helps to decompress the breast and may accelerate resolution of this type of mastitis. Breast-feeding in this situation is not harmful to the infant.

Epidemic mastitis usually responds to oral or parenteral semisynthetic penicillin therapy. The infant may also require therapy if symptoms of infection are present. Isolation of both mother and infant should be instituted.

A breast abscess may complicate either form of mastitis, and its diagnosis may be difficult. Abscess formation should be suspected if clinical signs and symptoms of mastitis do not subside after several days of oral antibiotic therapy. The abscess cavity is invariably larger and more extensive than suspected. Adequate therapy must require incision and drainage under regional or general anesthesia.

The type of incision for optimal drainage is controversial. Some advocate a radial incision to avoid injury to the lactiferous ducts, while others advocate incisions parallel to the aerola, following the skin lines, to improve cosmetic results while avoiding the ducts. In any event, the abscess cavity must be explored, loculations broken up, and a biopsy specimen studied. The latter is essential, because 10 to 15 percent of breast carcinomas in women under 40 years of age are found during pregnancy or lactation. A Gram stain and aerobic and anaerobic cultures should also be performed and antibiotics continued for 7 to 10 days.

Prevention

Scrupulous hygiene and care to the nipples, especially if cracks or fissures develop, will help to reduce the likelihood of mastitis. There is no evidence that prophylactic suppression of lactation will reduce the 1 to 2 percent incidence of mastitis. Early diagnosis of mastitis and prompt antibiotic therapy appear to be the best approach to prevent abscess formation.

Episiotomy and Pelvic Floor Infections

The incidence of episiotomy infections is less than 1 percent. Serious infections arising from an episiotomy at the sites of pudendal or paracervical blocks or cervicovaginal lacerations may spread along pelvic fascial planes to cause sepsis, deep-seated abscess formation, and even death. Fortunately, these infectious complications rarely occur in obstetric practice.

Pathophysiology and Bacteriology

It is remarkable that so few women suffer from serious infections after episiotomies or vaginal lacerations. Vaginal secretions contain 10^8 to 10^9 bacteria per gram of fluid, 90 percent of which are anaerobic species. Rectal flora may directly contaminate the vagina and perineum. Factors such as hematoma formation or extensive soft tissue damage during labor and delivery probably predispose to these wound infections.

The anatomy of the fascial planes delineates the route and spread of cellulitis (Fig. 40.20). Initially, the skin and surrounding subcutaneous tissue, coalesced into the fascia of Camper in the labia, become infected. Deeper penetration of the infectious process to Colles' fascia may be followed by spread to the vulva, medial thigh, and anterior abdominal wall into Scarpa's fascia. Necrosis of this layer results in so-called necrotizing fasciitis.[317,318] The muscles of the urogenital diaphragm along with its inferior fascia may be involved in extensive cases. There may be spread to the levator ani fascia as well.[319]

With pudendal or paracervical regional blocks, infection in paravaginal or paracervical tissue spreads in the loose areolar tissue at the base of the broad ligament to the lumbosacral nerve plexus. From this subgluteal space, the hip capsule may become involved if there is downward extension through the

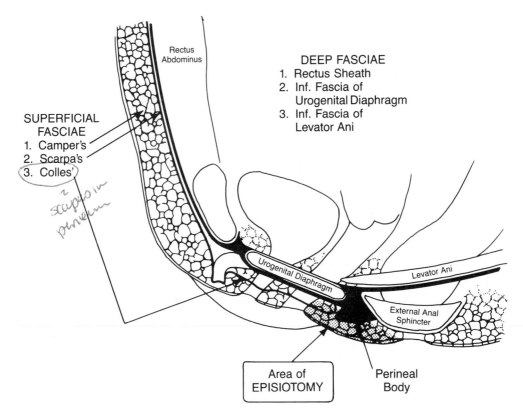

SUPERFICIAL
FASCIAE
1. Camper's
2. Scarpa's
3. Colles'

Rectus
Abdominus

DEEP FASCIAE
1. Rectus Sheath
2. Inf. Fascia of
   Urogenital Diaphragm
3. Inf. Fascia of
   Levator Ani

Urogenital Diaphragm

Levator Ani

External Anal
Sphincter

Area of
EPISIOTOMY

Perineal
Body

Fig. 40.20 Diagrammatic representation of the fascial layers of the perineum (paramedian sagittal section), which may be involved by extension from an infected episiotomy. (From Shy and Eschenbach,[319] with permission.)

greater sciatic foramen. Cephalad extension into the retropsoas space may also occur.[320]

In general, organisms responsible for episiotomy infections involving Colles' fascia include streptococci, staphylococci, and gram-negative rods. In necrotizing fasciitis, anaerobic organisms appear to play the major role. Group A streptococci may either initiate or become synergistic with such infections. Anaerobic and facultative organisms probably cause myonecrosis and are responsible for subgluteal and retropsoas abscesses. *C. perfringens* has been associated with myonecrosis, hemolytic anemia, and renal failure.

Diagnosis

A high index of suspicion is necessary for the early detection of these infections. Clinical clues, such as excessive perineal pain, frequent requests for analgesics, hip pain, or erythema and edema beyond the

immediate operative site should prompt a pelvic examination. Because significant episiotomy infections can initially involve deeper structures during the early stages of the process, the patient may complain of pain yet demonstrate minimal skin findings. Infections arising after pudendal or paracervical blocks generally do not produce perineal findings, because their spread is along deep fascial planes.

Conventional radiographs may reveal soft tissue gas. A pelvic/abdominal scan by computed tomography (CT) or magnetic resonance imaging (MRI) can delineate abscesses, especially in the retroperitoneal and subgluteal spaces.

Treatment

Surgical exploration under appropriate anesthesia is necessary for all episiotomy infections other than those complicated only by local cellulitis. Microbiologic specimens for aerobic and anaerobic bacteria should be obtained. Necrotic fascia or muscle, apparent on gross examination, must be removed.

The episiotomy should not be repaired after the initial debridement. Antibiotics are given as dictated by the clinical setting and Gram stain. In cases of clostridial myonecrosis, hyperbaric oxygen therapy has given variable results. Appropriate surgical consultation must be obtained if there is evidence of a retroperitoneal abscess or involvement of the hip capsule and gluteal musculature.

Septic Pelvic Thrombophlebitis

Septic pelvic thrombophlebitis is an uncommon complication of pregnancy. One in 2,000 deliveries (1 to 2 percent of patients with postpartum endometritis) is affected. However, increasing cesarean section rates may make this complication more common.

Pathogenesis and Bacteriology

Several factors predispose to the development of thrombosis: (1) a relative hypercoagulability associated with increased levels of clotting factors compared with the nonpregnant state (one factor may be derived from placental tissue itself, i.e., tissue thromboplastin); (2) estrogen-induced changes in pelvic veins, increasing their predilection to injury; and (3) relative venous stasis, caused by increased venous capacity and decreased blood flow from compression by the dextrorotated uterus on the right ovarian vein.

Bacteria entering the circulation can infect pelvic vein thrombi and create or exacerbate endothelial injury. Intravascular septic foci can disseminate to other tissues, including the lung and heart. The various organisms recovered from pelvic veins reflect the polymicrobial nature of this infection. Anaerobic organisms, such as peptostreptococci, bacteroides, staphylococci, and streptococci, have been recovered.[321,322]

Diagnosis

The diagnosis of septic pelvic thrombophlebitis should be suspected when fever persists after operative delivery despite adequate antibiotic treatment for endometritis. Although most cases now follow cesarean section, some will occur after vaginal delivery or elective termination of pregnancy. Clinical findings include rigor and spiking fevers with variable degrees of uterine or parametrial tenderness. Patients may appear well during intervening periods when fever is absent.

Pelvic venography and pelvic/abdominal CT scanning or MRI may identify large vessel thrombi, especially in the inferior vena cava and iliac veins (Fig. 40.21). Small pelvic vein thrombi are not usually visualized with currently available radiologic techniques. Evaluation for suspected septic pulmonary emboli may include a chest x-ray, arterial blood gas sampling, and a ventilation-perfusion lung scan. A pulmonary arteriogram may be required in equivocal cases, although multiple peripheral septic emboli can be missed by such testing.

Ovarian vein thrombophlebitis may develop several days postoperatively in association with fever, ileus, and a palpable thrombosed venous mass on abdominal or pelvic examination. Right-sided involvement is more common than left. CT or MRI scanning and venography may demonstrate the thrombus in the ovarian vein.[323]

The differential diagnosis in the febrile postpartum, postoperative patient with lower abdominal tenderness includes appendicitis, pelvic abscess or cellulitis, an adnexal accident, pyelonephritis, urolithiasis, and ureteral injury. It may be extremely difficult to differentiate among these entities. An intravenous pyelogram and urinalysis with urine Gram stain are helpful in identifying renal lesions. Pelvic examination or sonography may detect a pelvic mass, though the postpartum uterus may make these evaluations more difficult. The diagnosis of septic pelvic thrombophlebitis is often confirmed only when patients respond favorably to a therapeutic trial of anticoagulation and antibiotics.

Treatment

The current management of septic pelvic thrombophlebitis is a diagnostic and therapeutic trial with heparin. In patients with this disorder, defervescence should occur within 24 to 48 hours after the initiation of therapy.[324]

Heparin given concomitantly with (or without) antibiotic treatment should be continued for at least 7 to 10 days in most cases. A clinical response to this therapy provides a presumptive diagnosis of this disorder as well. The risk of significant bleeding with heparin is

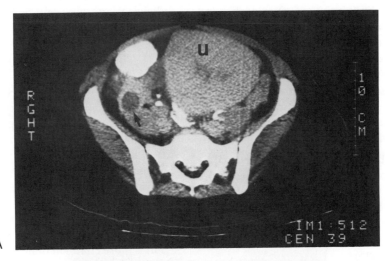

A

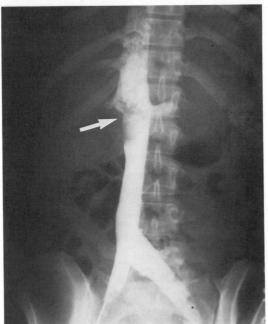

B

Fig. 40.21 (A) Enhanced CT scan of the pelvis demonstrating a tubular low-density structure (arrow) in the right adnexa, consistent with thrombus within the ovarian vein. The uterus (U) is enlarged. The patient, 8 days after cesarean section, had spiking fevers despite antibiotic therapy. The CT scan suggested that the thrombus extended into the inferior vena cava to the renal vein. **(B)** Inferior vena cavagram demonstrating a large thrombus (arrow) along the right lateral wall of the inferior vena cava just below the right renal vein. The appearance is compatible with extension from the ovarian vein.

sufficiently low (1 to 2 percent) to justify a trial in virtually all suspicious cases. The partial thromboplastin time, activated clotting time, and thrombin time may be used to monitor anticoagulation. Rare complications of heparin therapy include thrombocytopenia and paradoxical thrombosis.[325,326]

Long-term coumadin therapy is indicated for patients with known pulmonary emboli complicating septic phlebitis. The optimum duration of treatment for such cases is unknown. Continued oral anticoagulation of patients with uncomplicated pelvic thrombophlebitis who have responded to initial therapy is probably unnecessary. However, clinical circumstances dictate that such treatment must be individualized.

Surgical exploration is indicated in patients who fail to respond and exhibit persistent fever while on heparin and antibiotics. Drainage of abscesses or ligation of major pelvic vessels such as the involved ovarian vein may be required. Inferior vena cava ligation is usually reserved for those patients with persistent pulmonary emboli despite anticoagulation.

Prognosis

The prognosis for future fertility in patients with pelvic thrombophlebitis who have received anticoagulants and antibiotics is unknown. No studies are yet available with follow-up venography, CT scans, or MRI to determine the rate of resolution or clinical significance of such clots. A postphlebitic syndrome may develop in the presence of iliac/caval thrombosis, surgery, or both. The outcome in surgically managed patients is also largely unknown. Single case reports suggest that subsequent reproductive ability may be impaired.

Prevention

The decline in the frequency of criminal abortions and protracted obstructed labors and the advent of more expeditious aggressive treatment of puerperal infections have undoubtedly contributed to the decrease in the frequency of septic pelvic thrombophlebitis. It is currently unknown whether the use of prophylactic antibiotics at the time of cesarean section will alter the likelihood of developing septic thrombophlebitis.

REFERENCES

1. Medawar P: Some immunological and endocrinological problems raised by the evolution of viviparity in vertebrates. Symp Soc Exp Biol 7:320, 1954
2. Larsen B, Galask R: Host–parasite interactions during pregnancy. Obstet Gynecol Surv 33:297, 1978
3. Murgita R, Wigzell H: Regulation of immune functions in the fetus and newborn. Prog Allergy 29:54, 1981
4. Billingham R, Head J: The riddle of the allogeneic conceptus. Transplant Proc 15:877, 1983
5. Lawrence R, Murch J, Richards W et al: Immunological mechanisms in the maintenance of pregnancy. Ann Allergy 44:166, 1980
6. Krause PJ, Ingardie CJ, Pontius LT et al: Host defense during pregnancy: neutrophil chemotaxis and adherence. Am J Obstet Gynecol 157:274, 1987
7. Gehrz R, Christianson W, Linner K et al: A longitudinal analysis of lymphocyte proliferation responses to mitogens and antigens during human pregnancy. Am J Obstet Gynecol 140:665, 1981
8. Weinberg E: Pregnancy-associated depressions of cell-mediated immunity. Rev Infect Dis 6:814, 1984
9. Daya S, Clark D, Devlin C et al: Suppressor cells in the human decidua. Am J Obstet Gynecol 151:267, 1985
10. Larsen B: Host defense mechanisms in obstetrics and gynaecology. Clin Obstet Gynaecol 10:37, 1983
11. Merigan T: Host defenses against viral disease. N Engl J Med 290:323, 1974
12. Baker DA, Milch PO, Salvatore W et al: Enhancement of maternal and neonatal natural killer cell activity with interleukin-2. Am J Obstet Gynecol 157:780, 1987
13. McNabb P, Tomasi T: Host defense mechanisms at mucosal surfaces. Annu Rev Microb 35:477, 1981
14. Schwarz R: Considerations of antibiotic therapy during pregnancy. Obstet Gynecol 58(suppl):95, 1981
15. Levy G: Pharmacokinetics of fetal and neonatal exposure to drugs. Obstet Gynecol 58(suppl):9, 1981
16. ACOG: Antimicrobial therapy for obstetric patients. ACOG Tech Bull 117, 1988
17. Blanco J, Gibbs R, Duff P et al: Serum tobramycin levels in puerperal women. Am J Obstet Gynecol 147:466, 1983
18. Zaske D, Cippolle R, Strate R et al: Rapid gentamicin elimination in obstetric patients. Obstet Gynecol 56:559, 1980

19. Alford C, Pass R: Epidemiology of chronic congenital and perinatal infections of man. Clin Perinatol 8:397, 1981

20. Alford C: Chronic congenital infections of man. Yale J Biol Med 55:187, 1982

21. ACOG: Teratology. ACOG Tech Bull 84, 1985

22. Freij BJ, Sever JL: Herpes virus infections in pregnancy: risk to embryo, fetus and neonate. Clin Perinatol 15:203, 1988

23. ACOG: Perinatal viral and parasitic infections. ACOG Tech Bull 114, 1988

24. Sever J: Infections in pregnancy: highlights from the Collaborative Perinatal Project. Teratology 25:227, 1982

25. Schaffer D: Eye findings in intrauterine infections. Clin Perinatol 8:415, 1981

26. Gillner L, Forsgren M, Barr B et al: Outcome of rubella during pregnancy with special reference to the 17th–24th weeks of gestation. Scand J Infect Dis 15:321, 1983

27. Jordan M: Latent herpes viruses of humans. Ann Intern Med 100:866, 1984

28. Hunter K, Stagno S, Capps E et al: Prenatal screening of pregnant women for infections caused by cytomegalovirus, Epstein-Barr virus, herpes virus, rubella and *Toxoplasma gondii*. Am J Obstet Gynecol 145:269, 1983

29. Haywood AM: Patterns of persistent viral infections. N Engl J Med 315:939, 1986

30. Grose C, Itani O, Weiner CP: Prenatal diagnosis of fetal infection: advances from amniocentesis to cordocentesis—congenital toxoplasmosis, rubella, cytomegalovirus, varicella virus, parvovirus, and human immunodeficiency virus. Pediatr Infect Dis J 8:459, 1989

31. Gregg N: Congenital cataract following German measles in the mother. Trans Ophthalmol Soc Aust 3:35, 1941

32. Orenstein W, Bart K, Hinman A et al: The opportunity and obligation to eliminate rubella from the United States. JAMA 251:1988, 1984

33. Centers for Disease Control: Elimination of rubella and congenital rubella syndrome—United States. MMWR 34:65, 1985

34. Centers for Disease Control: Rubella and congenital rubella syndrome—United States, 1985–1988. MMWR 38:173, 1989

35. Centers for Disease Control: Rubella vaccination during pregnancy—United States, 1971–1988. MMWR 38:289, 1989

36. Daffos F, Forestier F, Grangeot-Keros L et al: Prenatal diagnosis of congenital rubella. Lancet 2:1, 1984

37. Terry GM, Ho-Terry L, Warren RC et al: First trimester prenatal diagnosis of congenital rubella: a laboratory investigation. Br Med J 292:930, 1986

38. Enders G, Nickerl-Pacher U, Miller E et al: Outcome of confirmed periconceptional maternal rubella. Lancet 2:1445, 1988

39. Cradock-Watson JF, Miller E, Ridehalgh MKS et al: Detection of rubella virus in fetal and placental tissues and in the throats of neonates after serologically confirmed rubella in pregnancy. Prenat Diagn 9:91, 1989

40. ACOG: Rubella: a clinical update. ACOG Tech Bull 62, 1981

41. Centers for Disease Control: Recommendations of the immunization practices advisory committee (ACIP): rubella prevention. MMWR 33:301, 1984

42. Ho M: Cytomegalovirus: Biology and Infection. Plenum, New York, 1982

43. Ho M: The lymphocyte in infections with Epstein-Barr virus and cytomegalovirus. J Infect Dis 143:857, 1981

44. Waner R, Weller T, Kevy S: Patterns of cytomegalovirus complement-fixing antibody activity: a longitudinal study of blood donors. J Infect Dis 127:538, 1973

45. Handsfield HH, Chandler SH, Caine VA et al: Cytomegalovirus infection in sex partners: evidence for sexual transmission. J Infect Dis 151:344, 1985

46. Stagno S, Whitley R: Herpes virus infections of pregnancy: part I: Cytomegalovirus and Epstein-Barr virus infections. N Engl J Med 313:1270, 1985

47. Stagno S, Pass R, Dworsky M et al: Congenital cytomegalovirus infection: the relative importance of primary and recurrent maternal infection. N Engl J Med 306:945, 1982

48. Yow MD, Williamson DW, Leeds LJ et al: Epidemiologic characteristics of cytomegalovirus infection in mothers and their infants. Am J Obstet Gynecol 158:1189, 1988

49. Pass RF, Little EA, Stagno S et al: Young children as a probable source of maternal congenital cytomegalovirus infection. N Engl J Med 316:1366, 1987

50. Friedman HM, Lewis MR, Nemerofsky DM et al: Acquisition of cytomegalovirus infection among female employees at a pediatric hospital. Pediatr Infect Dis 3:233, 1984

51. Adler SP: Cytomegalovirus and child day care: evidence for an increased infection rate among day care workers. N Engl J Med 321:1290, 1989

52. Kumar M, Prokay S: Experimental primary cytomegalovirus infection in pregnancy: timing and fetal outcome. Am J Obstet Gynecol 145:56, 1983

53. Stagno S, Pass RF, Cloud G et al: Primary cytomegalovirus infection in pregnancy—incidence, transmis-

sion to fetus, and clinical outcome. JAMA 256:1904, 1986

54. Balfour C, Balfour H: Cytomegalovirus is not an occupational risk for nurses in renal transplant and neonatal units: results of a prospective study. JAMA 256:1909, 1986

55. Centers for Disease Control: Prevalence of cytomegalovirus excretion from children in five day-care centers—Alabama. MMWR 34:49, 1985

56. Dworsky M, Welch K, Cassady G et al: Occupational risk for primary cytomegalovirus infection among pediatric health-care workers. N Engl J Med 309:950, 1983

57. Cohen J, Corey G: Cytomegalovirus infection in the normal host. Medicine (Baltimore) 64:100, 1985

58. Fadel HE, Ruedrich DA: Intrauterine resolution of nonimmune hydrops associated with cytomegalovirus infection. Obstet Gynecol 71:1003, 1988

59. Binder ND, Buckmaster JW, Benda GI: Outcome for fetus with ascites and cytomegalovirus infection. Pediatr 82:100, 1988

60. Bale JF, Blackman JA, Murph J et al: Congenital cytomegalovirus infection. Am J Dis Child 140:128, 1986

61. Griffiths P, Stagno S, Pass R et al: Infection with cytomegalovirus during pregnancy: specific IgM antibodies as a marker of recent primary infection. J Infect Dis 145:647, 1982

62. Yambao T, Clark D, Weiner L et al: Isolation of cytomegalovirus from the amniotic fluid during the third trimester. Am J Obstet Gynecol 139:937, 1981

63. Huikeshoven F, Wallenburg H, Jahoda M: Diagnosis of severe cytomegalovirus infection from amniotic fluid in the third trimester of pregnancy. Am J Obstet Gynecol 142:1053, 1982

64. Lange I, Rodeck CH, Morgan-Capner P et al: Prenatal serological diagnosis of intrauterine cytomegalovirus infection. Br Med J 284:1673, 1982

65. Buffone GJ, Demmler GJ, Schimbor CM, Yow MD: DNA hybridization assay for congenital cytomegalovirus infection. J Clin Microbiol 26:2184, 1988

66. Hsia K, Spector DH, Lawrie J, Spector S: Enzymatic amplification of human cytomegalovirus sequences by polymerase chain reaction. J Clin Microbiol 27:1802, 1989

67. Anderson MJ, Jones SE, Fisher-Hoch SP et al: Human parvovirus, the cause of erythema infectiosum (fifth disease)? Lancet 1:1378, 1983

68. Cossart YE, Field AM, Cant B et al: Parvovirus-like particles in human sera. Lancet 1:72, 1975

69. Mortimer PP, Humphries RK, Moore JG et al: A human parvovirus-like virus inhibits haematopoietic colony formation in vitro. Nature 302:426, 1983

70. Anderson LJ: Role of parvovirus B19 in human disease. Pediatr Infect Dis J 6:711, 1987

71. Anderson MJ: Parvoviruses as agents of human disease. Prog Med Virol 34:55, 1987

72. Thurn J: Human parvovirus B19: historical and clinical review. Rev Infect Dis 10:1005, 1988

73. Woernle CH, Anderson LJ, Tattersall P et al: Human parvovirus B19 infection during pregnancy. J Infect Dis 156:17, 1987

74. Centers for Disease Control: Risks associated with human parvovirus B19 infection. MMWR 38:81, 1989

75. Rao KR, Patel AR, Anderson MJ et al: Infection with parvovirus-like virus and aplastic crisis in chronic hemolytic anemia. Ann Intern Med 98:930, 1983

76. Anderson MJ, Higgins PG, Davis LR et al: Experimental parvoviral infection in humans. J Infect Dis 152:257, 1985

77. Shapiro L: The numbered diseases: first through sixth. JAMA 194:210, 1965

78. Rodis JF, Hovick TJ, Quinn DL et al: Human parvovirus in pregnancy. Obstet Gynecol 72:733, 1988

79. Maeda H, Shimokawa H, Satoh S et al: Nonimmunologic hydrops fetalis resulting from intrauterine human parvovirus B19 infection: report of two cases. Obstet Gynecol 72:782, 1988

80. Samra JS, Obhrai MS, Constantine G: Parvovirus infection in pregnancy. Obstet Gynecol 73:832, 1989

81. Anand A, Gray ES, Brown T et al: Human parvovirus infection in pregnancy and hydrops fetalis. N Engl J Med 316:183, 1987

82. Burton PA: Intranuclear inclusions in marrow of hydropic fetus due to parvovirus infection. Lancet 2:1155, 1986

83. Hartwig NG, Vermey-Keers C, VanElsacker-Niele AM et al: Embryonic malformations in a case of intrauterine parvovirus B19 infection. Teratology 39:295, 1989

84. Carrington D, Gilmore DH, Whittle MJ et al: Maternal serum alpha-fetoprotein—a marker of fetal aplastic crisis during intrauterine human parvovirus infection. Lancet 1:433, 1987

85. Kinney JS, Anderson LJ, Farrar J et al: Risk of adverse outcomes of pregnancy after human parvovirus B19 infection. J Infect Dis 157:633, 1988

86. Chorba T, Coccia P, Holman RC et al: The role of parvovirus B19 in aplastic crisis and erythema infectiosum (fifth disease). J Infect Dis 154:383, 1986

87. Porter HJ, Khong TY, Evans MF et al: Parvovirus as a cause of hydrops fetalis: detection by in situ DNA hybridization. J Clin Pathol 41:381, 1988

88. Naides SJ, Weiner CP: Antenatal diagnosis and palliative treatment of non-immune hydrops fetalis second-

ary to fetal parvovirus B19 infection. Prenat Diagn 9:105, 1989

89. Gillespie SM, Cartter ML, Asch S et al: Occupational risk of human parvovirus B19 infection for school and day-care personnel during an outbreak of erythema infectiosum. JAMA 263:2061, 1990

90. Laforet E, Lynch C: Multiple congenital defects following maternal varicella. N Engl J Med 236:534, 1947

91. Weller T: Varicella and herpes zoster: changing concepts of the natural history, control and importance of a not-so-benign virus. N Engl J Med 309:1362, 1983

92. Straus SE, moderator: Varicella-zoster virus infections: biology, natural history, treatment, and prevention. Ann Intern Med 108:221, 1988

93. Stagno S, Whitley RJ: Herpes virus infections of pregnancy. Part II: Herpes simplex virus and varicella-zoster virus infections. N Engl J Med 313:1327, 1985

94. Higa K, Dan K, Manabe H: Varicella-zoster virus infections during pregnancy: hypothesis concerning the mechanisms of congenital malformations. Obstet Gynecol 69:214, 1987

95. Paryani SG, Arvin AM: Intrauterine infection with varicella-zoster virus after maternal varicella. N Engl J Med 314:1542, 1986

96. Alkalay AL, Pomerance JJ, Rimoin DL: Fetal varicella syndrome. J Pediatr 111:321, 1987

97. McGregor JA, Mark S, Crawford GP, Levin MJ: Varicella-zoster antibody testing in the care of pregnant women exposed to varicella. Am J Obstet Gynecol 157:281, 1987

98. Cuthbertson G, Weiner CP, Giller RH, Grose C: Prenatal diagnosis of second-trimester congenital varicella syndrome by virus-specific immunoglobulin. J Pediatr 111:592, 1987

99. Centers for Disease Control: Recommendations of the immunization practices advisory committee (ACIP): varicella-zoster immune globulin for the prevention of chickenpox. MMWR 33:84, 1984

100. Miller E, Cardock-Watson JE, Ridehalgh MKS: Outcome in newborn babies given anti-varicella-zoster immunoglobulin after perinatal maternal infection with varicella-zoster virus. Lancet 2:371, 1989

101. Landsberger E, Hager WD, Grossman JH III: Successful management of varicella pneumonia complicating pregnancy—a report of three cases. J Reprod Med 31:311, 1986

102. Alford C Jr, Stagno S, Reynolds D: Congenital toxoplasmosis: clinical, laboratory and therapeutic considerations with special reference to subclinical disease. Bull NY Acad Med 50:160, 1974

103. Desmonts G, Couvreur J: Congenital toxoplasmosis: a

prospective study of 378 pregnancies. N Engl J Med 290:1110, 1974

104. Wilson C, Remington J, Stagno S et al: Development of adverse sequelae in children born with subclinical congenital *Toxoplasma* infection. Pediatrics 66:767, 1980

105. Desmonts G, Daffos F, Forestier F et al: Prenatal diagnosis of congenital toxoplasmosis. Lancet 1:500, 1985

106. Derouin F, Thulliez P, Candolfi E et al: Early prenatal diagnosis of congenital toxoplasmosis using amniotic fluid samples and tissue culture. Eur J Clin Microbiol Infect Dis 7:423, 1988

107. Daffos F, Forestier F, Capella-Pavlovsky M et al: Prenatal management of 746 pregnancies at risk for congenital toxoplasmosis. N Engl J Med 318:271, 1988

108. Derouin F, Mazeron MC, Garin YJF: Comparative study of tissue culture and mouse inoculation methods for demonstration of *Toxoplasma gondii*. J Clin Microbiol 25:1597, 1987

109. Hohlfeld P, Daffos F, Thulliez P et al: Fetal toxoplasmosis: outcome of pregnancy and infant follow-up after in utero treatment. J Pediatr 115:765, 1989

110. Foulon W, Naessens A, Lauwers S et al: Impact of primary prevention on the incidence of toxoplasmosis during pregnancy. Obstet Gynecol 72:363, 1988

111. McCabe R, Remington JS: Toxoplasmosis: the time has come. N Engl J Med 318:313, 1988

112. Thorp JM Jr, Seeds JW, Herbert WNP et al: Prenatal management and congenital toxoplasmosis. N Engl J Med 319:372, 1988

113. Harter C, Benirschke K: Fetal syphilis in the first trimester. Obstet Gynecol 124:705, 1975

114. Ricci JM, Foyaco RM, O'Sullivan MJ: Congenital syphilis: the University of Miami/Jackson Memorial Medical Center experience, 1986–1988. Obstet Gynecol 74:687, 1989

115. Centers for Disease Control: summary of notifiable diseases—United States. MMWR 36:39, 1987

116. Centers for Disease Control: Continuing increase in infectious syphilis—United States. MMWR 37:35, 1988

117. Fojaco RM, Hensley GT, Moskowitz L: Congenital syphilis and necrotizing funisitis. JAMA 261:1788, 1989

118. Hart G: Syphilis tests in diagnostic and therapeutic decision making. Ann Intern Med 104:368, 1986

119. Dans PE, Cafferty L, Otter SE et al: Inappropriate use of the cerebrospinal fluid Venereal Disease Research Laboratory (VRRL) test to exclude neurosyphilis. Ann Intern Med 104:86, 1986

120. Centers for Disease Control: Surveillance case definition for congenital syphilis. MMWR 38:828, 1989

121. Centers for Disease Control: Guidelines for the prevention and control of congenital syphilis. MMWR 37(S1):1, 1988

122. Centers for Disease Control: Sexually transmitted diseases: treatment guidelines. MMWR 38(S8):1, 1989

123. Musher DM: How much penicillin cures early syphilis? Ann Intern Med 109:849, 1988

124. Tramont EC: Syphilis in the AIDS era. N Engl J Med 316:1600, 1987

125. Centers for Disease Control: Recommendations for diagnosing and treating syphilis in HIV-infected patients. MMWR 37:600, 1988

126. Fenton L, Light I: Congenital syphilis after maternal treatment with erythromycin. Obstet Gynecol 47:492, 1976

127. Wendel GD Jr, Stark BJ, Jamison RB et al: Penicillin allergy and desensitization in serious infections during pregnancy. N Engl J Med 312:1229, 1985

128. Ziaya PR, Hankins GD, Gilstrap LC et al: Intravenous penicillin desensitization and treatment during pregnancy. JAMA 256:2561, 1986

129. Gentry GA, Lowe M, Alford G et al: Sequence analysis of herpesviral enzymes suggest an ancient origin for human sexual behavior. Proc Natl Acad Sci USA 85:2658, 1988

130. Lafferty WE, Boombs RW, Benedetti J et al: Recurrences after oral and genital herpes simplex virus infection: influence of site of infection and viral type. N Engl J Med 316:1444, 1987

131. Guinan ME: Treatment of primary and secondary syphilis: defining failure at three- and six-month follow-up. JAMA 257:359, 1987

132. World Health Organization: Prevention and control of herpesvirus diseases. WHO Bull 63:Part 1(2) 185, Part 2(3) 427, 1985

133. Baldwin S, Whitley RJ: Teratogen update: intrauterine herpes simplex virus infection. Teratology 39:1, 1989

134. Hutto C, Arvin A, Jacobs R et al: Intrauterine herpes simplex virus infections. J Pediatr 110:97, 1987

135. Hubbell C, Dominguez R, Kohl S: Neonatal herpes simplex pneumonitis. Rev Infect Dis 10:431, 1988

136. Brown ZA, Vontner LA, Benedetti J et al: Effects on infants of a first episode of genital herpes in pregnancy. N Engl J Med 317:1246, 1987

137. Prober CG, Sullender WM, Yasukawa LL et al: Low risk of herpes simplex virus infections in neonates exposed to the virus at the time of vaginal delivery to mothers with recurrent genital herpes simplex virus infections. N Engl J Med 316:240, 1987

138. Binkin NJ, Kaplan JP, Cates W Jr: Preventing neonatal herpes—the value of weekly viral cultures in pregnant women with recurrent genital herpes. JAMA 251:2816, 1987

139. Arvin AM, Hensleigh PA, Prober CG et al: Failure of antepartum maternal cultures to predict the infant's risk of exposure to herpes simplex virus at delivery. N Engl J Med 315:796, 1986

140. Gibbs RS, Amstey MS, Sweet RL et al: Management of genital herpes infection in pregnancy. Obstet Gynecol 71:770, 1988

141. Anonymous: Perinatal herpes simplex virus infections. ACOG Tech Bull 122, 1988

142. Grover L, Kane J, Kravitz J et al: Systemic acyclovir in pregnancy: a case report. Obstet Gynecol 65:284, 1985

143. Anonymous: Human immune deficiency virus infections. ACOG Tech Bull 123, 1989

144. Ho DD, Pomerantz RJ, Kaplan JC: Pathogenesis of infection with human immunodeficiency virus. N Engl J Med 317:278, 1987

145. Fauci AS: The human immunodeficiency virus: infectivity and mechanisms of pathogenesis. Science 239:617, 1988

146. Hill WC, Bolton V, Carlson JR: Isolation of acquired immunodeficiency syndrome virus from the placenta. Am J Obstet Gynecol 157:10, 1987

147. Kim JH, Durack DT: Manifestations of human T-lymphotropic virus type I infection. Am J Med 84:919, 1988

148. deShazo RD, Chadha N, Morgan JE et al: Immunologic assessment of a cluster of asymptomatic HTLV-I–infected individuals in New Orleans. Am J Med 86:65, 1989

149. Minamoto GY, Gold JW, Scheinberg DA et al: Human T-cell leukemia virus type I in patients with leukemia. N Engl J Med 318:219, 1988

150. Centers for Disease Control: AIDS due to HIV-2 infection—New Jersey. MMWR 37:33, 1988

151. Centers for Disease Control: Update: HIV-2 infection—United States. MMWR 38:572, 1989

152. Holmberg SD, Horsburgh CR, Ward JW, Jaffe HW: Biologic factors in the sexual transmission of human immunodeficiency virus. J Infect Dis 160:117, 1989

153. Selik RM, Castro KG, Pappaioanou M: Distribution of AIDS cases by racial/ethnic group and exposure category, United States, June 1, 1981–July 4, 1988. MMWR 37(S3):1, 1988

154. Piot P, Plummer FA, Mhalu FS et al: AIDS: an international perspective. Science 239:573, 1988

155. Cortes E, Detels R, Aboulafaia D et al: HIV-1, HIV-2, and HTLV-I infection in high risk groups in Brazil. N Engl J Med 320:953, 1989

156. Landesman S, Minkoff H, Holman S et al: Serosurvey

of human immunodeficiency virus infection in parturients: implications for human immunodeficiency virus testing programs of pregnant women. JAMA 258:2701, 1987

157. Novick LF, Berns D, Stricof R et al: HIV seroprevalence in newborns in New York State. JAMA 261:1745, 1989

158. Hoff R, Berardi VP, Weiblen BJ et al: Seroprevalence of human immunodeficiency virus among childbearing women: estimation by testing samples of blood from newborns. N Engl J Med 318:525, 1988

159. Centers for Disease Control: Revision of the CDC surveillance definition for acquired immunodeficiency syndrome. MMWR 36:1S, 1987

160. Blanchi S, Rouzioux C, Moscato MLG et al: A prospective study of infants born to women seropositive for human immunodeficiency virus type I. N Engl J Med 320:1643, 1989

161. Gloeb DJ, O'Sullivan MJ, Efantis J: Human immunodeficiency virus in women: I. The effects of human immunodeficiency virus on pregnancy. Am J Obstet Gynecol 159:756, 1988

162. Scott GB, Hutto C, Makuch RW et al: Survival in children with perinatally acquired human immunodeficiency virus type I infection. N Engl J Med 321:1791, 1989

163. Centers for Disease Control: Serologic testing of HIV infection. MMWR 36(S2):135, 1987

164. Centers for Disease Control: Update: serologic testing for antibody to human immunodeficiency virus. MMWR 36:833, 1988

165. Centers for Disease Control: Interpretation and use of the Western blot assay for serodiagnosis of human immunodeficiency virus type I infections. MMWR 38(S7):1, 1989

166. Fahey JL, Taylor JM, Detels R et al: The prognostic value of cellular and serologic markers in infection with human immunodeficiency virus type I. N Engl J Med 322:166, 1990

167. Kaplan LD, Wofsy CB, Volberding PA: Treatment of patients with acquired immunodeficiency syndrome and associated manifestations. JAMA 257:1367, 1987

168. Glatt AE, Chirgwin K, Landesman SH: Treatment of infections associated with human immunodeficiency virus. N Engl J Med 318:1439, 1988

169. Rhame FS, Maki DG: The case for wider use of testing for HIV infection. N Engl J Med 320:1248, 1989

170. Turnock BJ, Kelly CJ: Mandatory premarital testing for human immunodeficiency virus: the Illinois experience. JAMA 261:3415, 1989

171. Cleary PD, Barry MJ, Mayer KH et al: Compulsory premarital screening for the human immunodeficiency virus: technical and public health considerations. JAMA 258:1757, 1987

172. Joseph SC: Premarital AIDS testing: public policy abandoned at the altar. JAMA 261:3456, 1989

173. Centers for Disease Control: Safety of therapeutic immune globulin preparations with respect to transmission of human T-lymphotrophic (sic) virus type III/lymphadenopathy-associated virus infection. MMWR 35:231, 1986

174. Centers for Disease Control: Lack of transmission of human immunodeficiency virus through Rho (D) immune globulin (human). MMWR 36:728, 1987

175. Cumming PD, Wallace EL, Schorr JB et al: Exposure of patients to human immunodeficiency virus through the transfusion of blood components that test antibody-negative. N Engl J Med 321:941, 1989

176. Menitove JE: The decreasing risk of transfusion-associated AIDS. N Engl J Med 321:966, 1989

177. Williams AE, Fant CT, Slamon DJ et al: Seroprevalence and epidemiological correlates of HTLV-I infection in U.S. blood donors. Science 240:643, 1988

178. Minkoff HL: Care of pregnant women infected with human immunodeficiency virus. JAMA 258:2714, 1987

179. Minkoff HL, Landesman SH: The case for routinely offering prenatal testing for human immunodeficiency virus. Am J Obstet Gynecol 159:793, 1988

180. Selwyn PA, Carter RJ, Schoenbaum EE et al: Knowledge of HIV antibody status and decisions to continue or terminate pregnancy among intravenous drug users. JAMA 261:3567, 1989

181. Borkowsky W, Krasinski K, Paul D et al: Human immunodeficiency virus infections in infants negative for anti-HIV by enzyme-linked immunoassay. Lancet 1:1168, 1987

182. Eisenstein BI: The polymerase chain reaction: a new method of using molecular genetics for medical diagnosis. N Engl J Med 322:178, 1990

183. Rogers MF, Ou CY, Rayfield M et al: Use of the polymerase chain reaction for early detection of the proviral sequences of human immunodeficiency virus in infants born to seropositive mothers. N Engl J Med 320:1649, 1989

184. Marion RW, Wiznia AA, Hutcheon RG et al: Human T-cell lymphotropic virus type III (HTLV-III) embryopathy: a new dysmorphic syndrome associated with intrauterine HTLV-III infection. Am J Dis Child 140:639, 1986

185. Iosub S, Bamji M, Stone RK et al: More on human immunodeficiency virus embryopathy. Pediatrics 80:512, 1987

186. Cordero JF: Issues concerning AIDS embryopathy. Am J Dis Child 142:9, 1988

187. Garn SM: HIV-related dysmorphogenesis. Am J Dis Child 142:10, 1988

188. Sachs BP, Tuomala R, Frigoletto F: Acquired immunodeficiency syndrome: suggested protocol for counseling and screening in pregnancy. Obstet Gynecol 70:408, 1987

189. Centers for Disease Control: Recommendations for prevention of HIV transmission in health-care settings. MMWR 36(S2):35, 1987

190. Centers for Disease Control: Guidelines for prevention of transmission of human immunodeficiency virus and hepatitis B virus to health-care and public safety workers. MMWR 38(S6):3, 1989

191. Centers for Disease Control: Update: acquired immunodeficiency syndrome and human immunodeficiency virus infection among health-care workers. MMWR 37:229, 1988

192. Centers for Disease Control: Update: universal precautions for prevention of transmission of human immunodeficiency virus, hepatitis B virus, and other blood borne pathogens in health-care settings. MMWR 37:377, 1988

193. Baker JL, Kelen GD, Sivertson KT, Quinn TC: Unsuspected human immunodeficiency virus in critically ill emergency patients. JAMA 257:2609, 1987

194. Centers for Disease Control: Recommendations for diagnosing and treating syphilis in HIV-infected patients. MMWR 37:600, 1988

195. Berry CD, Hooton TM, Collier AC, Lukehart SA: Neurologic relapse after benzathine penicillin therapy for secondary syphilis in a patient with HIV infection. N Engl J Med 316:1587, 1987

196. Tramont EC: Syphilis in the AIDS era. N Engl J Med 316:1600, 1987

197. Cohen AJ, Philips TM, Kessler CM: Circulating coagulation inhibitors in the acquired immunodeficiency syndrome. Ann Intern Med 104:175, 1986

198. Karpatkin S, Nardi MA, Hymes KB: Immunologic thrombocytopenic purpura after heterosexual transmission of human immunodeficiency virus (HIV). Ann Intern Med 109:190, 1988

199. Botti AC, Hyde P, DiPillo F: Thrombotic thrombocytopenic purpura in a patient who subsequently developed the acquired immunodeficiency syndrome (AIDS). Ann Intern Med 109:242, 1988

200. ACOG Committee on Ethics: Human immunodeficiency virus infection: physicians' responsibilities. Obstet Gynecol 75:1043, 1990

201. Anonymous: Ethical issues involved in the growing AIDS crisis. JAMA 259:1360, 1988

202. Gostin L: HIV-infected physicians and the practice of seriously invasive procedures. Hastings Center Rep 19:32, 1989

203. Hagan MD, Meyer KB, Pauker SG: Routine preoperative screening for HIV: Does the risk to the surgeon outweigh the risk to the patient? JAMA 259:1357, 1988

204. Anonymous: Genital human papillomavirus infections. ACOG Tech Bull 105, 1987

205. Levine R, Crum C, Herman E et al: Cervical papillomavirus infection and intraepithelial neoplasia: a study of male sexual partners. Obstet Gynecol 64:16, 1984

206. Butler S, Molinari JA, Plezia RA et al: Condyloma acuminatum in the oral cavity: four cases and a review. Rev Infect Dis 10:544, 1988

207. Margolis S: Therapy for condyloma acuminatum: a review. Rev Infect Dis 4(suppl):829, 1982

208. Bergman A, Matsunaga J, Bhatia NN: Cervical cryotherapy for condylomata acuminata during pregnancy. Obstet Gynecol 69:47, 1987

209. Schwartz DB, Greenberg MD, Daoud Y, Reid R: Genital condylomas in pregnancy: use of trichloroacetic acid and laser therapy. Am J Obstet Gynecol 158:1407, 1988

210. Mounts P, Shah K: Respiratory papillomatosis: etiological relation to genital tract papillomaviruses. Prog Med Virol 29:90, 1984

211. Quick C, Watts S, Krzyck R et al: Relationship between condylomata and laryngeal papillomata: clinical and molecular virological evidence. Ann Otol Rhinol Laryngol 89:467, 1980

212. Cook T, Cohn A, Brunschwig J et al: Laryngeal papilloma: etiologic and therapeutic considerations. Ann Rhinol Laryngol 82:649, 1973

213. Anonymous: Recurrent respiratory papillomatosis. Lancet 2:1406, 1988

214. Shah K, Kashima H, Polk BF et al: Parity of cesarean delivery in cases of juvenile-onset respiratory papillomatosis. Obstet Gynecol 68:795, 1986

215. Lettau LA, Smith JD, Williams D et al: Transmission of hepatitis B with resultant restriction of surgical practice. JAMA 255:934, 1986

216. Melnick J: Classification of hepatitis A virus as entero-

virus type 72 and of hepatitis B virus as hepadnavirus type 1. Intervirology 18:105, 1982

217. Blumberg B: Australia antigen and the biology of hepatitis B. Science 197:17, 1977

218. Dane D, Cameron C, Briggs M: Virus-like particles in serum of patients with Australia antigen associated hepatitis. Lancet 1:695, 1970

219. Alter MJ, Ahtone J, Weisfuse I et al: Hepatitis B virus transmission between heterosexuals. JAMA 256:1308, 1986

220. Mitsuda T, Yokota S, Mori T et al: Demonstration of mother-to-infant transmission of hepatitis B virus by means of polymerase chain reaction. Lancet 2:886, 1989

221. Smego RA, Halsey NA: The case for routine hepatitis B immunization in infancy for populations at increased risk. Pediatr Infect Dis 6:11, 1987

222. Centers for Disease Control: ACIP: prevention of perinatal transmission of hepatitis B virus: prenatal screening of all pregnant women for hepatitis B surface antigen. MMWR 37:341, 1988

223. Kumar ML, Dawson NV, McCullough AJ et al: Should all pregnant women be screened for hepatitis B? Ann Intern Med 107:273, 1987

224. Arevalo JA, Washington AE: Cost-effectiveness of prenatal screening and immunization for hepatitis B virus. JAMA 259:365, 1988

225. Ross JW: Prenatal screening for hepatitis B antigen. JAMA 261:1727, 1989

226. Centers for Disease Control: ACIP: recommendations for protection against viral hepatitis. Ann Intern Med 103:381, 1985

227. Pastorek JG II, Miller JM Jr, Summers PR: The effect of hepatitis B antigenemia on pregnancy outcome. Am J Obstet Gynecol 158:486, 1988

228. Lancefield RC, Hare R: The serologic differentiation of pathogenic and nonpathogenic strains of hemolytic streptococci from parturient women. J Exp Med 61:335, 1935

229. Moriarty RA, Smith LP, Hemming VG et al: Rapid detection of group B streptococcal antigen in human amniotic fluid. Clin Microbiol 25:259, 1987

230. Wald ER, Dashefsky B, Green M et al: Rapid detection of group B streptococci directly from vaginal swabs. J Clin Microbiol 25:573, 1987

231. Jones DE, Friedl EM, Kanarek KS et al: Rapid identification of pregnant women heavily colonized with group B streptococci. J Clin Microbiol 18:558, 1983

232. Isada NB, Grossman JH III: A rapid screening test for the diagnosis of endocervical group B streptococci in pregnancy: microbiologic results and clinical outcome. Obstet Gynecol 70:139, 1987

233. Sandy EA, Blumenfeld ML, Iams JD: Gram stain in the rapid determination of maternal colonization with group B beta-streptococcus. Obstet Gynecol 71:796, 1988

234. Minkoff H, Mead P: An obstetric approach to the prevention of early-onset group B beta-hemolytic streptococcal sepsis. Am J Obstet Gynecol 154:973, 1983

235. Gardner S, Yow M, Leeds L et al: Failure of penicillin to eradicate group B streptococcal colonization in the pregnant woman: a couple study. Am J Obstet Gynecol 135:1062, 1979

236. Yow MD, Mason EO, Leeds LJ et al: Ampicillin prevents intrapartum transmission of group B streptococcus. JAMA 241:1245, 1979

237. Boyer KM, Gadzala CA, Kelly PD et al: Selective intrapartum chemoprophylaxis of neonatal group B streptococcal early onset disease. I. Epidemiologic rationale. J Infect Dis 148:795, 1983

238. Boyer KM, Gadzala CA, Kelly PD et al: Selective intrapartum chemoprophylaxis of neonatal group B streptococcal early onset disease. II. Predictive value of prenatal cultures. J Infect Dis 148:802, 1983

239. Boyer KM, Gadzala CA, Kelly PD, Gotoff SP: Selective intrapartum chemoprophylaxis of neonatal group B streptococcal early-onset disease. III. Interruption of mother-to-infant transmission. J Infect Dis 148:810, 1983

240. Yow M, Mason E, Leeds L et al: Ampicillin prevents intrapartum transmission of group B streptococcus. JAMA 241:1245, 1979

241. Boyer KM, Gotoff SP: Prevention of early-onset neonatal group B streptococcal disease with selective intrapartum chemoprophylaxis. N Engl J Med 314:1665, 1986

242. Morales WJ, Lim DV, Walsh AF: Prevention of neonatal group B streptococcal sepsis by the use of a rapid screening test and selective intrapartum chemoprophylaxis. Am J Obstet Gynecol 155:979, 1986

243. Baker CJ, Rench MA, Edwards MS et al: Immunization of pregnant women with a polysaccharide vaccine of group B streptococcus. N Engl J Med 319:1180, 1988

244. Britigan BE, Cohen MS, Sparling PF: Gonococcal infection: a model of molecular pathogenesis. N Engl J Med 312:1683, 1985

245. Centers for Disease Control: Antibiotic-resistant strains of *Neisseria gonorrhoeae:* policy guidelines for detection, management and control. MMWR 36(S5):1S, 1987

246. Bush K: Recent developments in β-lactamase research and their implications for the future. Rev Infect Dis 10:681, 1988

247. Knapp JS: Laboratory methods for the detection and phenotypic characterization of *Neisseria gonorrhoeae* strains resistant to antimicrobial agents. Sex Trans Dis 15:225, 1988

248. Johnson SR, Morse SA: Antibiotic resistance in *Neisseria gonorrhoeae:* genetics and mechanisms of resistance. Sex Trans Dis 15:217, 1988

249. Ellison RT, Curd JG, Kohler PF et al: Underlying complement deficiency in patients with disseminated gonococcal infection. Sex Trans Dis 14:201, 1987

250. Soper D, Merrill-Nach S: Successful therapy of penicillinase producing *Neisseria gonorrhoeae* pharyngeal infection during pregnancy. Obstet Gynecol 68:290, 1986

251. Schachter J, McCormack WM, Smith RF et al: Enzyme immunoassay for diagnosis of gonorrhea. J Clin Microbiol 19:57, 1984

252. Centers for Disease Control: Sexually transmitted diseases treatment guidelines — 1989. MMWR 38(S8):1, 1989

253. LeSaux N, Ronald AR: Role of ceftriaxone in sexually transmitted diseases. Rev Infect Dis 11:299, 1989

254. Schachter J: Chlamydial infections. N Engl J Med 298:428; 298:490, 298:540, 1978

255. Hammerschlag MR: Chlamydial infections. J Pediatr 114:727, 1989

256. Schachter J, Grossman M, Sweet RL et al: Prospective study of perinatal transmission of *Chlamydia trachomatis.* JAMA 255:3374, 1986

257. Weiss SG, Newcomb RW, Beem MO: Pulmonary assessment of children after chlamydial pneumonia of pregnancy. J Pediatr 108:659, 1986

258. Martius J, Krohn MA, Hillier SL et al: Relationships of vaginal lactobacillus species, cervical *Chlamydia trachomatis,* and bacterial vaginosis to preterm birth. Obstet Gynecol 71:89, 1988

259. Gravett MG, Nelson P, DeRouen T et al: Independent association of bacterial vaginosis and *Chlamydia trachomatis* infection with adverse pregnancy outcome. JAMA 256:1899, 1986

260. Watts DH, Eschenbach DA, Kenny GE: Early postpartum endometritis: the role of bacteria, genital mycoplasmas, and *Chlamydia trachomatis.* Obstet Gynecol 73:52, 1989

261. Alger LS, Louchik JC, Hebel JR et al: The association of *Chlamydia trachomatis, Neisseria gonorrhoeae,* and group B streptococci with preterm rupture of the membranes and pregnancy outcome. Am J Obstet Gynecol 159:397, 1988

262. Schachter J, Sweet RL, Grossman M et al: Experience with the routine use of erythromycin for chlamydial infections in pregnancy. N Engl J Med 314:276, 1986

263. Sweet RL, Landers DV, Walker C, Schachter J: *Chlamydia trachomatis* infection and pregnancy outcome. Am J Obstet Gynecol 156:824, 1987

264. Stamm WE: Diagnosis of *Chlamydia trachomatis* genitourinary infections. Ann Intern Med 108:710, 1988

265. Baselski VS, McNeeley SG, Ryan G et al: A comparison of nonculture-dependent methods for detection of *Chlamydia trachomatis* infections in pregnant women. Obstet Gynecol 70:47, 1987

266. Hammerschlag MR, Cummings C, Roblin PM et al: Efficacy of neonatal ocular prophylaxis for the prevention of chlamydial and gonococcal conjunctivitis. N Engl J Med 320:769, 1989

267. Schmid GP, Matheny LC, Zaidi AA et al: Evaluation of six media for the growth of *Trichomonas vaginalis* from vaginal secretions. J Clin Microbiol 27:1230, 1989

268. Krieger JN, Tam MR, Stevens CE et al: Diagnosis of trichomoniasis: comparison of conventional wet-mount examination with cytologic studies, cultures, and monoclonal antibody staining of direct specimens. JAMA 259:1223, 1988

269. Lossick J: Treatment of *Trichomonas vaginalis* infections. Rev Infect Dis 4(suppl):801, 1982

270. Guinan M: Intravenous metronidazole therapy for *Trichomonas* infection. JAMA 255:1783, 1986

271. Dombrowski MP, Sokol RJ, Brown WJ, Bronsteen RA: Intravenous therapy of metronidazole — resistant *Trichomonas vaginalis.* Obstet Gynecol 69:524, 1987

272. Sbarra AJ, Thomas GB, Cetrulo CL et al: Effect of bacterial growth on the bursting pressure of fetal membranes in vitro. Obstet Gynecol 70:107, 1987

273. Romero R, Emamian M, Wan M et al: Prostaglandin concentrations in amniotic fluid of women with intra-amniotic infection and preterm labor. Am J Obstet Gynecol 157:1461, 1987

274. Gibbs RS, Werner MH, Walmer K et al: Microbiologic and serologic studies of *Gardnerella vaginalis* in intra-amniotic infection. Obstet Gynecol 70:187, 1987

275. Gravett MG, Hummel D, Eschenbach DA et al: Pre$term labor associated with subclinical amniotic fluid infection and with bacterial vaginosis. Obstet Gynecol 67:229, 1986

276. Romero R, Emamian M, Quintero R et al: The value and limitations of the gram stain examination in the diagnosis of intraamniotic infection. Am J Obstet Gynecol 159:114, 1988

277. Duff P, Sanders R, Gibbs R: The course of labor in term patients with chorioamnionitis. Am J Obstet Gynecol 147:391, 1983

278. Romero R, Scioscia AL, Edberg SC, Hobbins JC: Use of parenteral antibiotic therapy to eradicate bacterial colonization of amniotic fluid in premature rupture of membranes. Obstet Gynecol 67:15(S), 1986

279. Romero R, Kadar N, Hobbins JC, Duff GW: Infection and labor: the detection of endotoxin in amniotic fluid. Am J Obstet Gynecol 157:815, 1987

280. Gibbs R: Clinical risk factors for puerperal infection. Obstet Gynecol 55(suppl):178, 1980

281. DePalma R, Leveno K, Cunningham F et al: Identification of women at high risk for pelvic infection following cesarean section. Obstet Gynecol 55(suppl):185, 1980

282. Hoyme UB, Kiviat N, Eschenbach DA: Microbiology and treatment of late postpartum endometritis. Obstet Gynecol 68:226, 1986

283. Gibbs RS: Microbiology of the female genital tract. Am J Obstet Gynecol 156:491, 1987

284. Duff P: Pathophysiology and management of postcesarean endomyometritis. Obstet Gynecol 67:269, 1986

285. Duff P, Gibbs R, Blanco J et al: Endometrial culture techniques in puerperal patients. Obstet Gynecol 61:217, 1983

286. Yonekura M, Appleman M, Wallace R et al: Predictive value of amniotic-membrane cultures for the development of postcesarean endometritis. Rev Infect Dis 6(suppl):157, 1984

287. Blanco J, Gibbs R, Castaneda Y et al: Correlation of quantitative amniotic fluid cultures with endometritis after cesarean section. Am J Obstet Gynecol 143:897, 1982

288. Gibbs R, Blanco J: Streptococcal infections in pregnancy. Am J Obstet Gynecol 140:405, 1981

289. Duff P, Gibbs R: Acute intraamniotic infection due to *Streptococcus pneumoniae*. Obstet Gynecol 61(suppl):25, 1983

290. Guerinot G, Gitomer S, Sanko S: Postpartum patient with toxic shock syndrome. Obstet Gynecol 59(suppl):43, 1982

291. Mariona F, Ismail M: *Clostridium perfringens* septicemia following cesarean section. Obstet Gynecol 56:518, 1980

292. Lamont RJ, Postlethwaite R, MacGowan AP: *Listeria monocytogenes* and its role in human infections. J Infect 17:7, 1988

293. Wetli C, Roldan E, Fojaco R: Listeriosis as a cause of maternal death—an obstetric complication of acquired immunodeficiency syndrome (AIDS). Am J Obstet Gynecol 147:7, 1983

294. Smith LG, Summers PR, Miles RW et al: Gonococcal chorioamnionitis associated with sepsis: a case report. Am J Obstet Gynecol 160:573, 1989

295. Lamey J, Eschenbach D, Mitchell S et al: Isolation of mycoplasmas and bacteria from the blood of postpartum women. Am J Obstet Gynecol 143:104, 1982

296. Knudson R, Driscoll S, Monson R et al: Association of *Ureaplasma urealyticum* in the placenta with perinatal morbidity and mortality. N Engl J Med 310:941, 1984

297. Ledger W, Kriewall T: The fever index: a quantitative indirect measure of hospital-acquired infections in obstetrics and gynecology. Am J Obstet Gynecol 115:514, 1973

298. diZerega G, Yonekura M, Roy S et al: A comparison of clindamycin-gentamicin and penicillin-gentamicin in the treatment of postcesarean section endometritis. Am J Obstet Gynecol 134:238, 1979

299. Briggs GG, Ambrose P, Nageotte MP: Gentamicin dosing in postpartum women with endometritis. Am J Obstet Gynecol 160:309, 1989

300. Faro S, Phillips LE, Baker JL et al: Comparative efficacy and safety of meglocillin, cefoxitin, and clindamycin plus gentamicin in postpartum endometritis. Obstet Gynecol 69:760, 1987

301. Clinicopathologic Conference: Unexplained fever in the postpartum period. Am J Med 69:443, 1980

302. Galask RP: Changing concepts in obstetric antibiotic prophylaxis. Am J Obstet Gynecol 157:491, 1987

303. Ford LC, Hammill HA, Legherz TB: Cost-effective use of antibiotic prophylaxis for cesarean section. Am J Obstet Gynecol 157:506, 1987

304. Duff P: Prophylactic antibiotics for cesarean delivery: a simple cost-effective strategy for prevention of postoperative morbidity. Am J Obstet Gynecol 157:794, 1987

305. Cunningham F, Leveno K, DePalma R et al: Perioperative antimicrobials for cesarean delivery: before or after cord clamping? Obstet Gynecol 62:151, 1983

306. Duff P, Gibbs R, Jorgensen J et al: The pharmacokinetics of prophylactic antibiotics administered by intraoperative irrigation at the time of cesarean section. Obstet Gynecol 60:409, 1982

307. Arsura E, Fazio R, Wickremesinghe P: Pseudomembranous colitis following prophylactic antibiotic use in primary cesarean section. Am J Obstet Gynecol 151:87, 1985

308. Gibbs R, Blanco J, St. Clair P et al: Vaginal colonization with resistance aerobic bacteria after antibiotic therapy for endometritis. Am J Obstet Gynecol 142:130, 1982

309. Faro S, Martens M, Hammill H et al: Ticarcillin/clavulanic acid versus clindamycin and gentamicin in the treatment of postcesarean endometritis following antibiotic prophylaxis. Obstet Gynecol 73:808, 1989

310. Wallace R, Eglinton G, Yonekura M et al: Extraperitoneal cesarean section: a surgical form of infection prophylaxis? Am J Obstet Gynecol 148:172, 1984

311. Hanson H: Current use of extraperitoneal cesarean section: a decade of experience. Am J Obstet Gynecol 149:31, 1984

312. Hurry D, Larsen B, Charles D: Effects of postcesarean section febrile morbidity on subsequent fertility. Obstet Gynecol 64:256, 1984

313. Niebyl J, Spence M, Parmley T: Sporadic (nonepidemic) puerperal mastitis. J Reprod Med 20:97, 1978

314. Marshall B, Hepper J, Zirbel C: Sporadic puerperal mastitis: an infection that need not interrupt lactation. JAMA 233:1377, 1975

315. Thomsen A, Espersen T, Maigaard S: Course and treatment of milk stasis, noninfectious inflammations of the breast, and infectious mastitis in nursing women. Am J Obstet Gynecol 149:492, 1984

316. Wager G: Toxic shock syndrome: a review. Am J Obstet Gynecol 146:93, 1983

317. Lowthian J, Gillard L: Postpartum necrotizing fasciitis. Obstet Gynecol 56:661, 1980

318. Golde S, Ledger W: Necrotizing fasciitis in postpartum patients: a report of four cases. Obstet Gynecol 50:670, 1977

319. Shy K, Eschenbach D: Fatal perineal cellulitis from an episiotomy site. Obstet Gynecol 54:292, 1979

320. Hibbard L, Snyder E, McVann R: Subgluteal and retropsoal infection in obstetric practice. Obstet Gynecol 39:137, 1972

321. Cohen M, Pernoll M, Gevirtz C et al: Septic pelvic thrombophlebitis: an update. Obstet Gynecol 62:83, 1983

322. Duff P, Gibbs R: Pelvic vein thrombophlebitis: diagnostic dilemma and therapeutic challenge. Obstet Gynecol Surv 38:365, 1983

323. Angel J, Knuppel R: Computed tomography in diagnosis of puerperal ovarian vein thrombosis. Obstet Gynecol 63:61, 1984

324. Ledger W, Peterson E: The use of heparin in the management of pelvic thrombophlebitis. Surge Gynecol Obstet 131:1115, 1970

325. King D, Kelton J: Heparin-associated thrombocytopenia. Ann Intern Med 100:535, 1984

326. Cines DB, Tomaski A, Tannenbaum S: Immune endothelial-cell injury in heparin-associated thrombocytopenia. N Engl J Med 316:581, 1987

327. Herrmann K: Available rubella serologic tests. Rev Infect Dis 7(suppl):109, 1985

328. Frenkel J, Dubey JP, Miller NL: *Toxoplasma gondii* in cats: fecal stages identified as coccidian oocysts. Science 167:893, 1970

329. Tramont C: *Treponema pallidum* (syphilis). p. 1794. In Mandell G, Douglas R, Bennett J (eds): Principles and Practice of Infectious Diseases. 3rd Ed. Churchill Livingstone, New York, 1990

330. Centers for Disease Control: Notifiable disease reports. MMWR 39:505, 1990

331. Centers for Disease Control: MMWR 39:81, 1990

332. Centers for Disease Control: MMWR 39:85, 1990

333. Lazarus GS, Goldsmith LA: Diagnosis of Skin Disease. FA Davis, Philadelphia, 1980

334. Hoofnagle JH: Acute viral hepatitis. p. 1001. In Mandell G, Douglas R, Bennett J (eds): Principles and Practice of Infectious Diseases. 3rd Ed. Churchill Livingstone, New York, 1990

335. Mandell G, Douglas R, Bennett J (eds): Principles and Practice of Infectious Diseases. 3rd Ed. Churchill Livingstone, New York, 1990

336. Galask R, Varner M, Petzold C et al: Bacterial attachment to the chorioamniotic membranes. Am J Obstet Gynecol 148:915, 1984

SECTION 7
Pregnancy Termination

Pregnancy Termination

Phillip G. Stubblefield

FERTILITY CONTROL AND HEALTH

The voluntary control of fertility is essential to the health of women. Each pregnancy carries with it the risk of illness and the risk of death. Presently in the United States the national maternal mortality rate is about 9 per 100,000 live births; however, careful surveillance in state programs identifies an equal number of deaths that are not reported nationally. This risk for women with preexisting illnesses such as diabetes mellitus, hypertension, and renal and cardiac disease is much greater, and the mother's age has a profound effect on the risk of maternal mortality such that women in their 40s are seven times more likely to die in pregnancy than are women in their early 20s, the safest age to have a baby.[1] Fertility control, or lack of it, also impacts on child health. When pregnancies are too close together, the risks of prematurity and perinatal mortality increase.[2] Higher order births to young mothers are at very great risk. Second births to mothers under age 20 years are more likely to be premature and to die than are first-born children, and the risk is still higher for a third-born infant to a woman under age 20 years.[3,4] The advantage for both mother and child of delaying childbearing until the mother is fully grown, of spacing children, and of avoiding pregnancy toward the end of the reproductive years is obvious. Less obvious is the ideal means to achieve this kind of fertility control.

Legal Abortion and Voluntary Control of Fertility

Properly used, modern methods of contraception are highly effective, and, in the context of formal studies, very low pregnancy rates are achieved. In actual use by the patients, however, contraceptive methods fail more often than medical professionals usually appreciate. Actual failure rates for present methods as used in the United States are shown in Table 41.1. Young people are much more likely to experience contraceptive failure, because their fertility is much greater and because they are more likely to have intercourse without contraception.[5] At the individual level, it is extremely likely that any normal couple will experience at least one unwanted pregnancy sometime during their reproductive years. Another aspect of the relation between contraception and abortion is that of safety. The most effective contraceptive methods, the pill and the intrauterine device, have rare but life-threatening complications. Tietze's calculations, as updated by Ory,[6] point out that the safest contraceptive method is diaphragm or condom, backed up by early legal abortion should the primary method fail.

Contraception is preventive medicine and as such requires advance motivation. Abortion, on the other hand, is sought when pregnancy has occurred, and the individual knows she has a problem. For all of these reasons, induced abortion is essential if a high level of voluntary control of fertility is to be achieved. Finally, societies can and do limit access to contracep-

Table 41.1   Percentage of Women Who Experience Contraceptive Failure Within the First Year of Contraceptive Use, by Method, Standardized by Intention, Income, and Age. July 1, 1970 to January 1, 1976

Method	Percent
Pill	2.4
Intrauterine device	4.6
Condom	9.6
Spermicides	17.9
Diaphragm	18.6
Rhythm	23.7
Other	11.9

(From Schirm et al.,[96] with permission.)

tion. In the United States, the group most affected by societal limitations upon access is young people; hence, their very great resort to abortion should be no surprise. Societies cannot prevent abortion, but they can determine whether it will be illegal and dangerous or legal and safe.

In a national probability sample in 1987, Henshaw and Silverman[7] observed that 81.5 percent of women obtaining abortions were unmarried. Twenty-five percent were aged 19 years or younger and 59 percent were aged 24 years or younger. For women aged 15 to 19 years, the abortion rate, 43.8 per 1,000 women in 1985, was only a little less than the birth rate, 51.3 per 1,000 women.[8] The need for abortion is especially a problem for young, sexually active women in the United States. If legal abortion were not available, births to teenaged and unmarried women would increase markedly, and women suffering the complications of illegal abortion would once again fill our gynecology beds.

History of Abortion

Some means for attempting abortion can be found in all cultural groups and are evident in the artifacts of ancient civilizations.[9,10] Folk methods in use throughout the world today include various plant substances that are ingested; and more direct methods include the actual insertion of some object through the cervix into the uterus. In Asia, forceful massage of the uterus to produce abortion is widely practiced.[11] Abortion was common during the nineteenth century

in the United States. The complications of these procedures and the competition from lay abortionists so concerned "regular" physicians that medical societies carried out intensive campaigns that resulted in the passage of laws making abortion illegal in most states by the end of the century.[12] These laws remained on the books until 1973, when humanitarian efforts to provide for medically necessary abortions culminated in the Supreme Court's decision to legalize abortion.[12]

LEGAL ABORTION IN THE UNITED STATES: AN OVERVIEW

Organization of Services

The legalization of abortion did not make the service available in all areas. Hospitals were resistant to the sudden demand for large numbers of procedures, and a new institution sprang up, the free-standing abortion clinic. In the United States, the majority of abortions are presently performed out of hospital, in clinics or in doctors' offices. For the most part, these clinics maintain high medical standards[13] and provide an excellent service at a cost far below other kinds of surgical care. The clinics provide pregnancy tests and nonjudgmental counseling to facilitate an early decision either to continue the pregnancy or to abort. The abortion procedure is provided the same day, if requested by the patient, usually under local anesthesia, with the counselor in attendance to provide patient support and to reduce anxiety. Most clinics provide immediate contraceptive counseling and supplies and include follow-up as part of their basic fee.

Nationally, the risk of illness or death from legal abortion has been remarkably low. Overall, the risk of death from first-trimester abortion is about 1 per 100,000 procedures, making this alternative far safer than continuing the pregnancy. As shown in Table 41.2, the risk of death increases with gestational age, and after 16 menstrual weeks abortion in general terms is no safer than continued pregnancy.[14] However, for individual women with high-risk conditions, for example, cyanotic heart disease, even late abortion is undoubtedly a safer alternative. Because of the availability of low-cost, out-of-hospital first-trimester abortion, 92 percent of legal abortions are performed in the first trimester, when abortion is the safest.[15]

Table 41.2 Death-to-Case Rate for Legal Abortions by Weeks of Gestation, United States, 1972–1980

Weeks of Gestation	Deaths[a]	Abortions[b]	Rate[c]	Relative Risk[d]
≤ 8	19	4,073,472	0.5	1.0
9–10	31	2,382,516	1.3	2.6
11–12	25	1,197,915	2.1	4.2
13–15	20	419,767	4.8	9.6
16–20	55	430,907	12.8	25.6
>21	14	91,343	15.3	30.6
Total	164	8,595,920	1.9	

[a] Excludes deaths from ectopic pregnancy.

[b] Based on distribution of 6,108,658 abortions (71.1 percent).

[c] Deaths per 100,000 abortions.

[d] Based on index rate of less than 8 menstrual weeks gestation of 0.5 deaths per 100,000 abortions.

(From Centers for Disease Control.[14])

Type of procedure is another determinant of risk. First-trimester abortions are virtually all performed by vacuum curettage; however, in the mid-trimester, a variety of techniques can be used. Risk of death from abortion by the various techniques at different gestational ages is given in Table 41.3. The data clearly show the greater safety of instrumental evacuation of the uterus (dilatation and evacuation [D & E]) performed in the early mid-trimester. Another determinant of risk is anesthesia. Use of general anesthesia increases the risk for perforation of the uterus, visceral injury, hemorrhage, hysterectomy, and death.[15,16] The preferred alternative is paracervical block with local anesthetic and low-dose sedation–analgesia as needed.

Benefits of Legal Abortion

Death from illegal abortion used to be a major component of maternal mortality, and hospital gynecology wards were filled with women suffering from septic "spontaneous abortion." With legalization, septic "spontaneous abortion" is uncommon. In 1980 there were six deaths from spontaneous abortion, eight deaths from abortion legally induced, and only one death from illegal abortion (abortion induced by a nonprofessional) in the entire United States.[14] Much of the continued decline in maternal mortality of recent years can be attributed to the choice of legal abortion by women at high risk for pregnancy mortality. There has been national concern about the high

rate of teenage pregnancy in the United States. Few have appreciated that without legal abortion there would be twice as many teenage births each year. For millions of women, legal abortion has provided an important alternative, a second chance, a chance to complete their education and to achieve other personal goals prior to childbearing.

Indications for Abortion

Before 1973, abortion was permitted in many states, but only if certain medical/social criteria were met, such as rape or life-threatening illness. With legalization, the only legal condition necessary for abortion in the first trimester is that the woman consult with her physician. However, there remains the much more difficult question of determining when abortion of a *desired* pregnancy should be recommended on medical grounds. In some situations, as, for example, congenital heart disease with pulmonary hypertension, the risk of death in late pregnancy is so great that any prudent physician would have to recommend abortion. Similarly, if major fetal malformation leaves no hope for meaningful life, most would recommend abortion. However, in the majority of cases of both maternal illness or fetal malformation, there is a strong place for the woman and her husband to determine how much risk they are willing to take. A woman who badly wants a child may decide to accept a significant risk for herself, while another woman with the same illness would find this risk unacceptable and

Table 41.3 Death-to-Case Rate[a] and Deaths (in Parentheses) for Legal Abortions by Type of Procedure and Weeks of Gestation, United States, 1972–1980

Type of Procedure	Weeks of Gestation							
	≥8	9–10	11–12	13–15	16–20	≥21	Total
Curettage	0.4 (18)	1.2 (29)	2.1 (24)	0.0 (0)	0.0 (0)	0.0 (0)	0.9 (71)
Dilatation and evacuation	0.0 (0)	0.0 (0)	0.0 (0)	3.6 (10)	10.7 (9)	15.0 (2)	5.5 (21)
Saline and prostaglandin instillation	0.0 (0)	0.0 (0)	0.0 (0)	1.9 (1)	16.2 (34)	15.1 (7)	12.6 (42)
Other instillation	0.0 (0)	0.0 (0)	0.0 (0)	14.1 (4)	6.6 (7)	16.0 (3)	7.1 (14)
Hysterotomy/hysterectomy	0.0 (0)	51.4 (2)	35.3 (1)	65.6 (3)	64.6 (3)	135.0 (1)	44.6 (10)
Total	0.5 (18)	1.3 (31)	2.2 (25)	5.4 (18)	13.6 (53)	17.7 (13)	1.9 (158)

[a] Deaths per 100,000 abortions, excluding deaths associated with ectopic pregnancy.

(From Centers for Disease Control.[14])

Table 41.4 Fetal Indications for Termination of a Desired Pregnancy

Category	Examples
Known major fetal malformation	Anencephaly, myelomeningocele, severe hydrocephaly, porencephaly, severe cardiac disease, bilateral cystic kidney disease
Chromosomal abnormality	Down syndrome
Inherited metabolic defect	
Autosomal recessive	Tay-Sachs disease
X-linked recessive	Classic hemophilia
	Duchenne's muscular dystrophy
Fetal exposure to known teratogen	
Infectious illness	Maternal infection with rubella, cytomegalovirus, toxoplasmosis
Drugs	Folate antagonists, warfarin, thalidomide, ethanol in high doses
Irradiation	X-ray exposure of 15 rads or more
Preterm premature rupture of the membranes prior to 24 weeks	
Fetal death in utero	

(Modified from Stubblefield,[17] with permission.)

seek abortion. In my opinion, this is as it should be, with abortion available as the safer alternative should the couple decide after medical consultation to terminate the pregnancy. Tables 41.4 and 41.5 list some of the fetal and maternal indications for abortion of a desired pregnancy.[17] These lists are meant as a guide for thought and are by no means all inclusive.

Table 41.5 Maternal Indications for Termination of a Desired Pregnancy

Category	Examples
Cardiovascular disease	Pulmonary hypertension, Eisenmenger syndrome, history of myocardial infarction, history of pregnancy cardiomyopathy, severe hypertensive disease
Genetic disease	Marfan syndrome
Hematologic disease	Thrombotic thrombocytopenic purpura
Infection	Human immunodeficiency virus
Metabolic disease	Proliferative diabetic retinopathy
Neoplastic disease	Invasive carcinoma of the cervix, any neoplasm in which maternal survival depends on prompt treatment with chemotherapy with teratogenic agents or in which the fetus will receive a dangerous dose of radiation
Neurologic disease	Untreated cerebrovascular malformation or berry aneurysm
Renal disease	Deterioration of renal function in early pregnancy
Pregnancy-specific disorder in present pregnancy	Intrauterine infection, severe preeclampsia or eclampsia

(Modified from Stubblefield,[17] with permission.)

FIRST-TRIMESTER ABORTION

Scraping the uterus after cervical dilatation with some form of tapered rods, dilatation and curettage, appears to be an ancient procedure.[10] Vacuum curettage is of more recent origin, being described for the first time in the literature by two Chinese physicians in 1954.[18] The vacuum technique was introduced in England in the 1960s and then brought to the United States by Burdick. After 1973 it quickly became the procedure of choice. Subsequent comparative trials have demonstrated that vacuum curettage is quicker, less traumatic, and safer than sharp curettage.[19]

Minisuction (Menstrual Regulation)

In 1972, Karman and Potts[20] described a small bore, flexible vacuum cannula. When used with a 50-cc syringe as a vacuum source, this cannula allows termination of pregnancy through 7 menstrual weeks with only minimal cervical dilatation.[20] Initially viewed as an alternative to true abortion because it could be performed even before pregnancy was diagnosed with certainty, the procedure was described as "menstrual regulation" and performed without confirmation of pregnancy. Properly done, the minisuction procedure has many advantages, but the experience of several years has shown that, when abortion is legal, the procedure should be delayed until pregnancy is diagnosed. With the sensitive pregnancy tests now available, many women are able to obtain this form of early abortion within 1 or 2 weeks after the menstrual period is missed. The minisuction procedure is readily accomplished in the physician's office. The only instruments required in addition to a speculum and a tenaculum are the Karman cannula and a modified 50-ml syringe (Fig. 41.1).

Technique for Minisuction Abortion

This technique is illustrated in Figure 41.2. After pelvic examination to determine the shape and position of the uterus and to ensure that the pregnancy is 7 weeks size or less, the cervix is exposed with a speculum, infiltrated with local anesthetic, and grasped with a tenaculum placed vertically at 12 o'clock. A 4- and then a 5-mm-diameter cannula is passed through the cervical canal as dilators. A 6-mm cannula is next inserted and attached to the evacuated 50-ml syringe to establish suction. The 4- and 5-mm cannulas are

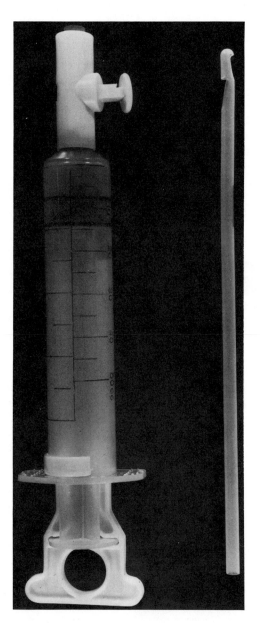

Fig. 41.1 Instruments for early abortion: 6-mm Karman cannula and modified 50-ml plastic syringe. (Photo courtesy of International Projects Assistance, Chapel Hill, NC.)

not large enough to evacuate the uterus dependably in pregnancy but are useful as atraumatic dilators and for endometrial biopsies in the nonpregnant state. The 6-mm cannula is rotated and pushed in and out with gentle strokes, taking care to rotate the cannula only on the out stroke so as to avoid twisting off the

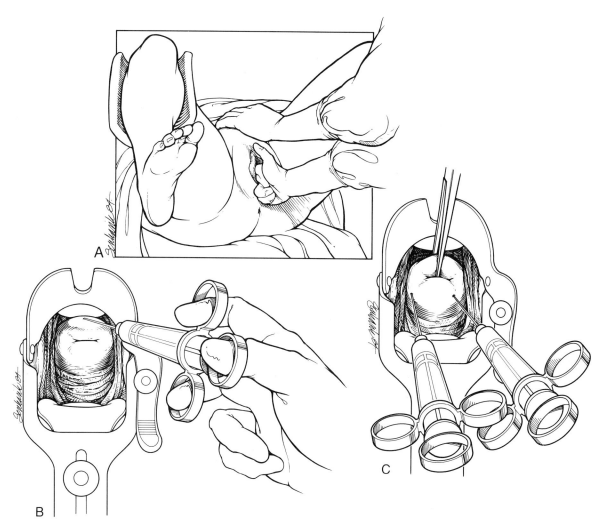

Fig. 41.2 Early vacuum curettage abortion. (A) Examining the patient. (B) Administering paracervical block and superficial injection into the cervix at 12 o'clock to anesthetize tenaculum site. (C) Completing paracervical block and injecting local anesthetic superficially, just under the vaginal mucosa, at the lateral margins of the cervix, 4 and 8 o'clock. *(Figure continued.)*

flexible tip by rotating it when it is pressed against the uterine fundus. When no more tissue comes through, the cannula is withdrawn and its tip cleared in a sterile fashion. The cannula is reinserted and vacuum reestablished for a final check curettage to prove the uterus is empty. The operator must then carefully examine the aspirated tissue to identify the gestational sac to prevent failed abortion, to diagnose molar pregnancy, and to detect ectopic pregnancy.[21] The fresh examination is best accomplished by floating the aspirated tissue in a clear plastic dish over a light source. Figure 41.3 demonstrates the appearance of an early pregnancy.

Technique for Standard Vacuum Curettage

Standard vacuum curettage applies essentially the same technique as minisuction, but utilizes a larger cannula, from 7 to 12 mm, and uterine aspirators of greater capacity than the 50-mm syringe. After establishing a paracervical block, the operator dilates the cervical canal by serial insertion of tapered rods that increase progressively in size. We favor the Denniston

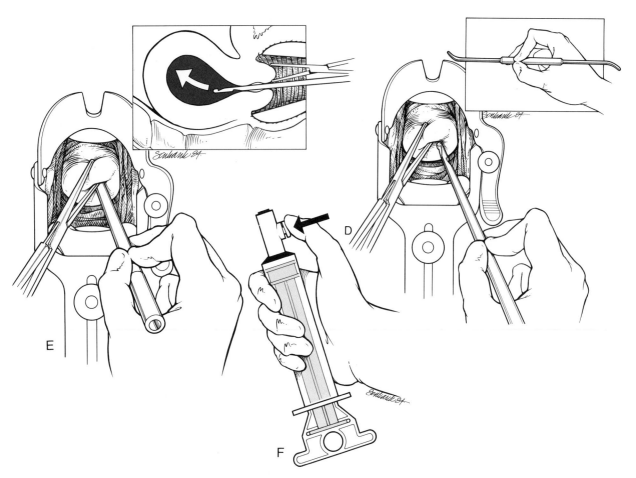

Fig. 41.2 *(Continued)*. (D) Dilatation, using a 4-mm Karman cannula. This will be followed by the 5-mm Karman and then the 6-mm cannula. Alternatively, the Denniston dilators 4, 5, and 6 can be used (inset). (E) Insertion of the 6-mm Karman cannula, as far as the top of the cavity (inset). (F) Preparing the syringe by closing the pinch valve. *(Figure continued.)*

dilators pictured in Figure 41.4 for their blunt tips, gentle taper, and semirigid "feel." Dilatation is continued to a diameter 1 mm less than the estimated length of gestation in menstrual weeks and then a vacuum cannula of that same outside diameter is inserted. After aspiration is complete, we gently insert a sharp curette and use it as a finger to explore the cavity gently and to prove it empty. Finally, the suction cannula is reintroduced for a final few seconds to remove any additional tissue remaining. Again, as with minisuction, the operator must perform a careful examination of the freshly aspirated tissue. An instrument kit sufficient for all first-trimester procedures is pictured in Figure 41.5.

Technique of Paracervical Block

There is no standard way to induce paracervical block, and there has been little formal study of the different alternatives: a superficial injection just beneath the mucosa, injection into the uterosacral ligaments, or injection into the substance of the cervix. Glick[22] has described a combination method that may be advantageous. A total of 8 cc of anesthetic solution is injected superficially at multiple sites around the cervix at the reflection of the cervical–vaginal mucosa. Then an additional 12 cc is injected at multiple sites at a depth of 2 cm so that the cervicouterine junction and lower uterine segment are infiltrated

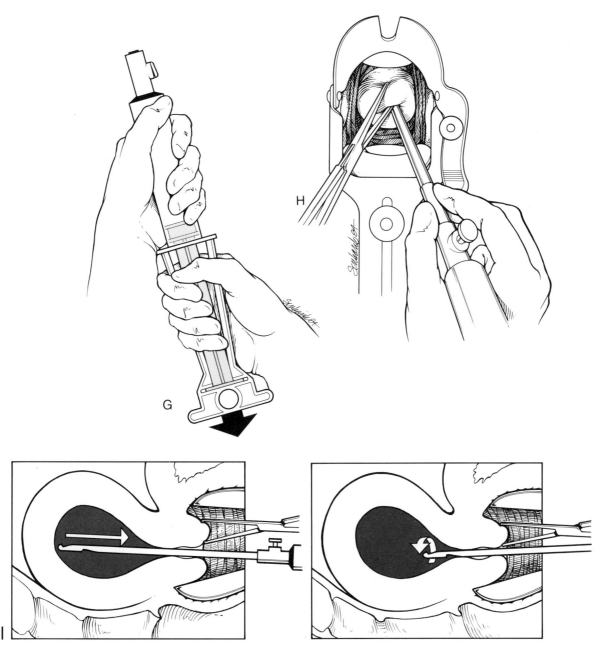

Fig. 41.2 (*Continued*). (G) Evacuating the syringe, with side arms on the plunger assembly locking it in the withdrawn position, maintaining vacuum. (H) Uterine evacuation through the Karman cannula into the syringe. (I) The cannula is rotated and is slid in and out of the cavity in a pistonlike fashion. Care must be taken to rotate only on the out stroke, when the cannula tip is withdrawn away from the top of the uterus. Rotation when the cannula is pressed against the top of the fundus may cause the tip of the cannula to break off inside the uterine cavity. (*Figure continued.*)

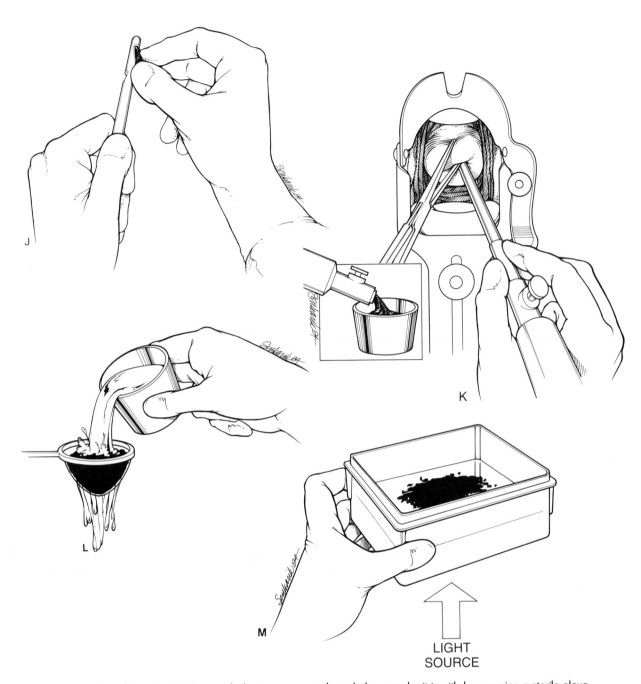

LIGHT
SOURCE

Fig. 41.2 *(Continued).* (J) When no further tissue comes through the cannula, it is withdrawn; using a sterile glove, the tip is cleared. (K) Repeat aspiration. After clearing the tip, the cannula is reinserted, the syringe emptied (inset) and reevacuated, and vacuum established for a final check to ensure that the uterus is empty. Omission of this step results in incomplete abortion. (L) Preparing the tissue for examination. The tissue is emptied into a tea strainer and washed with saline. (M) Fresh examination. The tissue is floated in saline in a clear plastic dish over a light source. The gestational sac must be identified.

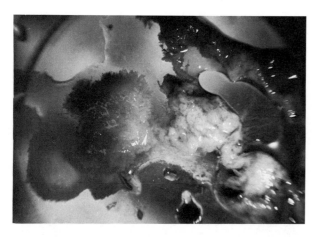

Fig. 41.3 Tissue specimen in a 6-week pregnancy, as seen without magnification. The conceptus is on the left, and to the right is the decidual lining of the uterus. (From Stubblefield,[97] with permission.)

with the anesthetic. Other workers have reported that waiting 5 minutes after instillation of the block improves pain relief.[23] To avoid systemic toxicity, the maximum dose should not exceed 200 mg of lidocaine in a patient of average weight (20 cc of 1 percent solution).[24]

Alternatives for Cervical Dilatation

While forcible dilatation with tapered rods is the standard technique, there is reason to believe this method is far from ideal. Even under the best of cir-

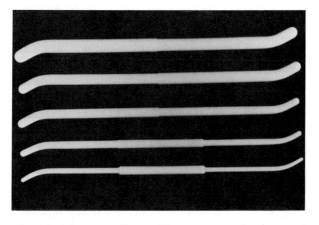

Fig. 41.4 Denniston dilators. (Photo courtesy of International Projects Assistance, Chapel Hill, NC.)

cumstances and when performed by the most skilled operator, a serious cervical laceration will occasionally occur, and it is during the dilatation step that serious perforations result. Alternatively, osmotic dilators can be used. Presently three types are available: naturally occurring *Laminaria* tents, the magnesium sulfate sponge (Lamicel), and synthetic tents of polyacrilonitrile (Dilapan). *Laminaria* is seaweed, the stems of which are used to dilate the cervix. Inserted into the cervical canal as a small dry twig, the *Laminaria* takes up water from the cervix and slowly swells to exert gentle pressure on the cervix as well (Fig. 41.6). Over several hours this produces softening of the cervix, and considerable dilatation. If the *Laminaria* is left in place overnight, additional forcible dilatation will not be required.

Laminaria used medically is either of two species: *L. japonicum* or *L. digitata*. Tents of *L. digitata* become gelatinous as they swell, are easily entrapped in the cervical canal, and may fragment with attempts at removal. For this reason we prefer tents of *L. japonicum*, as they retain their integrity when wet.

The advantage of pretreatment with *Laminaria* tents before first-trimester abortion has been demonstrated.[24] A fivefold reduction in cervical laceration was accomplished when *Laminaria* was used instead of forcible dilatation. An earlier analysis of the Joint Program for the Study of Abortion (JPSA) data found a threefold reduction in risk for perforation when *Laminaria* was used.[25]

However, *Laminaria* treatment has been thought to increase the risk of postabortal infection. Indeed, *Laminaria* was widely used in obstetrics and gynecology in the last century, but was abandoned because of concerns about infection.[26] The risk now appears to be very low with modern methods for sterilizing *Laminaria*. In the JPSA study cited above, the *Laminaria*-administered group had no increase in postabortal infection.[25] The main drawbacks of *Laminaria* are the need for insertion by a skilled practitioner and the requirement of several hours for dilatation to be accomplished. Lamicel acts more quickly to pull water from the cervix and cause softening, but exerts little force.[27] Dilapan produces softening and rapid swelling, and thus more force, than natural *Laminaria*.

Another alternative still under investigation is the use of low doses of an analogue of prostaglandin E by vaginal administration.[28] When used in doses suffi-

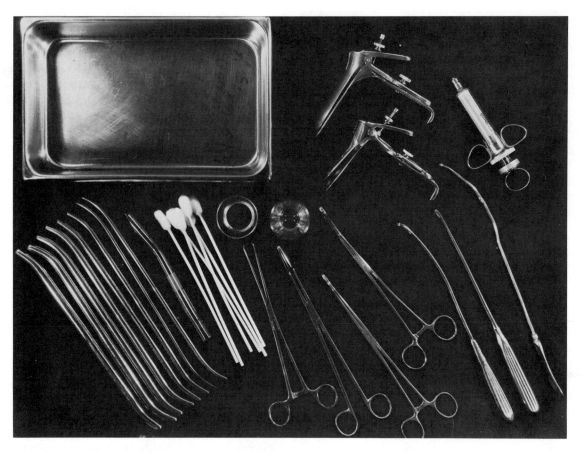

Fig. 41.5 Instrument kit for vacuum curettage abortion. Clockwise (left to right): sterile tray, Graves speculum, Moore speculum, control syringe, uterine sound, No. 1 curette, No. 3 curette, curved Foerrester forcep, straight Foerrester forcep, Moore ovum forcep, single-toothed tenaculum, medicine glasses, cotton swabs, plastic vacurette, Pratt cervical dilators. (From Stubblefield,[97] with permission.)

cient to produce useful dilatation, prostaglandins cause significant gastrointestinal side effects. Darney et al.[29] compared the natural *Laminaria* tents to Dilapan and to a prostaglandin analogue in a three-way randomized trial. They concluded that the Dilapan produced more dilatation than the *Laminaria*, while the prostaglandin analogue produced less dilatation but caused more side effects of vomiting and pain.

Medical Means for First-Trimester Abortion

Historically, a number of plant substances have been ingested in attempts to produce abortion. Extracts of the yew tree were widely used in England and the United States in the last century.[9] In Western medicine, little has been done to determine whether yew or similar substances might have any real value as abortifacients; however, the Chinese have reported that some of their ancient herbal remedies are truly effective abortifacients. The substance tricocanthin does appear to cause abortion, although apparently there can be some toxicity.[30] The prostaglandins were the first agents to be proven truly effective and safe for this purpose. In 1972, Karim[31] reported successful production of abortion in women treated with prostaglandin $F_{2\alpha}$ ($PGF_{2\alpha}$). Other workers found a high incidence of vomiting and diarrhea with this treatment. The themes of prostaglandin research ever since have been to find both a prostaglandin analogue with greater effect on the uterine muscle than other tissues and a convenient route of administration that also might reduce side effects. Two prostaglandins

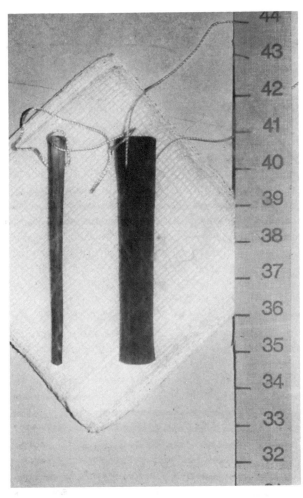

Fig. 41.6 Tents of *Laminaria japonicum*. Dry tent (left) as it would be just before insertion. Wet tent (right) as it would be after several hours exposed to water. (Photo courtesy of Mildred Hanson, M.D., Mount Sinai Hospital, Minneapolis, MN.)

are presently available for pregnancy termination in the United States: PGE$_2$ as vaginal suppositories and the 15-methyl analogue of PGF$_{2\alpha}$ for intramuscular injection. These are intended for mid-trimester abortion or for inducing labor after fetal death in utero; however, either could be used in the first trimester as well. That they are not so used is because they are much less convenient than the alternative, vacuum curettage. Given in sufficient doses to produce abortion, side effects of vomiting, diarrhea, and, in the case of PGE$_2$, fever are common. The abortion results after several hours of uterine pain and is frequently incomplete, necessitating a curettage procedure after

all.[32] In the early first trimester, prostaglandin treatment produces abortion without the need for curettage, but, again, many hours are required and the alternative, a minisuction procedure done in the office, is much more convenient for the patient.

Antiprogesterones offer much more promise as medical abortifacients. The first of these is Mefipristone (RU 486), an analogue of the progestin norethindrone. It has strong affinity for the progesterone receptor, but acts as an antagonist, blocking the effect of natural progesterone.[33] A single oral dose given to women 5 weeks or less from last menses produced complete abortion in 85 percent of cases.[34] The addition of a low dose of prostaglandin improves efficacy. Bygdeman and Swahm[34] reported a 94 percent rate of complete abortion in 34 women treated with the combination of Mefipristone and prostaglandin up to 49 days from last menses.[34] If used later in pregnancy the drug is less effective, and there is greater chance of incomplete abortion and significant blood loss unless a prompt curettage is performed. Sadly, vociferous opposition by "right to life" groups has limited distribution to government-sponsored clinics in France. Should the drug become widely available in the third world, it would revolutionize abortion services and spare the lives of tens of thousands of women who currently die each year from the complications of badly performed abortions.

Selective Reduction of Multifetal Pregnancies

Multifetal pregnancies are likely to lead to extreme prematurity with resultant perinatal loss or serious neonatal handicap. Investigators have reported ultrasound-guided transabdominal intracardiac instillation of 2 to 7 mmol of potassium chloride in the late first trimester. In this way, the number of fetuses may be reduced to twins. Of 12 pregnancies treated by Berkowitz and colleagues,[35] 7 women delivered twins, and one a singleton at term, all healthy babies. Four pregnancies went on to abort.

Between 1985 and 1988, Wapner and colleagues[35a] carried out selective reduction of 46 multi-fetal pregnancies by injecting potassium chloride into the pericardial region of the fetus. Patients were classified into three groups on the basis of the indication for fetal reduction. In Group A ($N = 34$), the procedure was performed to improve perinatal outcome and to increase the likelihood of a term infant being born by reducing the number of fetuses in a multi-fetal pregnancy. In Group B ($N = 8$), selective reduction was performed to allow the birth of a healthy infant without the birth of a co-existing fetus with a congenital abnormality, such as thanatophoric dysplasia, or aneuploidy. In Group C ($N = 4$), selective reduction was undertaken to preserve a singleton pregnancy when the woman had decided to have the entire pregnancy terminated unless selective reduction was available; this group included one case of triplets and three of twins. Of the 80 fetuses left after reduction, 75 (94 percent) survived. There were no disorders of maternal coagulation after procedures performed at 16 weeks gestation or later. Not surprisingly, a high maternal serum α-fetoprotein level that persisted into the second trimester was observed. In three cases, a repeat injection carried out on the same day was necessary to produce fetal death.

FIRST-TRIMESTER ABORTION COMPLICATIONS AND THEIR PREVENTION

Complications of Local Anesthesia

General anesthesia adds to the hazard of vacuum curettage, but local paracervical block also has its risks. Intravascular injection or an overdose of the medication can produce a severe systemic response: convulsions, cardiorespiratory arrest, and death.[36] Such a reaction requires endotracheal intubation and support of respiration along with anticonvulsive therapy. Systemic toxicity is reduced by use of the ester chloroprocaine rather than the more commonly used amide lidocaine. Care must be taken to aspirate before injecting each dose of the local anesthetic to guard against intravascular injection. Formerly we advised use of dilute epinephrine solutions in the paracervical block to slow absorption and prevent vagal effects of cervical dilatation. However, fatal anaphylaxis from allergy to the metabisulfite preservative in epinephrine solutions can occur in asthmatic patients.[37] We now advise addition of 0.5 mg of atropine to the paracervical anesthetic and recommend waiting 5 minutes after injection of the block.

Cervical Shock

Vasovagal syncope resulting from stimulation of the cervical canal can be seen even after paracervical block. Although brief tonic–clonic activity is observed, this is distinguished from a true seizure by the presence of a very slow pulse, the patient's rapid recovery, and the absence of any postictal state. Routine use of atropine with the paracervical anesthetic prevents "cervical shock."

Cervical Lacerations

Minor lacerations are common during forcible dilatation when the cervical tenaculum pulls off. More serious injury can also be inflicted resulting in full thickness tears of the cervical wall. Such trauma can be prevented by use of gently tapered dilators such as the Pratt, Denniston, or Hank and by a firm grasp on the cervix with a single-toothed tenaculum placed vertically with one branch inside the cervical canal so that the full thickness of the cervical wall is grasped. Another option is to use *Laminaria* or prostaglandin analogues as described above.

Perforation

Perforation is the most feared complication of vacuum curettage, because injury to major blood vessels, bowel, or bladder can result, thus jeopardizing the life of the patient. In a review of the cases admitted to Boston Hospital for Women for uterine perforations, Berek and Stubblefield[38] noted that perforations sustained at abortion were usually perforations of the cervix, either at the junction of the cervix and lower uterine segment or lower in the canal. Perforations of the uterine fundus were uncommon after first-trimester abortion, but rather were seen as complications of diagnostic dilatation and curettage in nonpregnant women (Fig. 41.7).[38] The perforations in pregnant women produced two different clinical syndromes, depending on the precise anatomic location of the perforation. Perforations at the junction of the cervix and lower uterine segment can lacerate the ascending branch of the uterine artery within the broad ligament, giving rise to severe pain, a broad ligament hematoma, and intraabdominal bleeding. These perforations are usually recognized soon after they occur. They are managed by laparoscopy to confirm the injury and then by laparotomy to ligate the severed vessels and repair the uterine injury. Hysterectomy should not be required to manage such perforations. Low cervical perforations, on the other hand, may injure the descending branch of the uterine artery within the dense collagenous substance of the cardinal ligaments. In this case, there is no intraabdominal hemorrhage; the bleeding is outward, through the cervical canal, and may subside tempo-

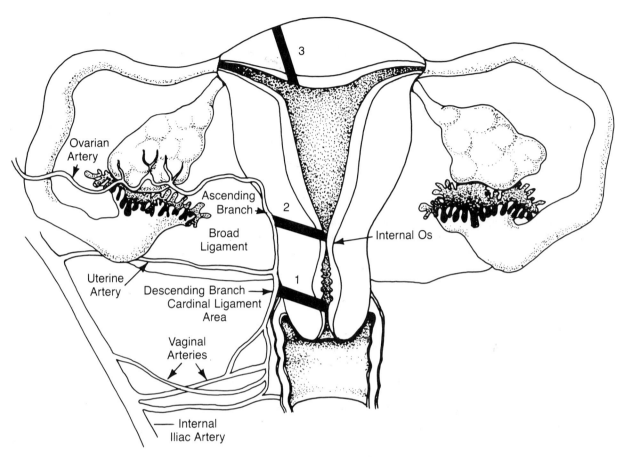

Fig. 41.7 Possible sites of uterine perforation at abortion. 1, Low cervical perforation with laceration of descending branches of uterine artery; 2, perforation at junction of cervix and lower uterine segment with laceration of ascending branch of uterine artery; 3, fundal perforation. (Redrawn from Berek and Stubblefield,[38] with permission.)

rarily as the artery goes into spasm. Deaths have occurred when a low cervical perforation was not appreciated and bled again several hours or even days after the injury. This injury has usually required hysterectomy for management; however, Freiman (personal communication) has described a case managed by laparotomy and the placement of sutures through the cardinal ligaments after downward mobilization of the bladder and identification of the ureters. Berek and Stubblefield[38] proposed that arteriography and selective embolization of the injured vessel be attempted. Both types of cervical perforations undoubtedly occur during cervical dilatation and would be prevented by use of an alternative means for dilatation.

Grimes et al.[39] studied the epidemiology of uterine perforation using information from 67,175 abortions. The rate of perforation was 0.9 per 1,000. In contradistinction to the experience of Berek and Stubblefield,[38] this larger data set found 36 percent of the perforations to be cervicoisthmic in location whereas 64 percent were injuries of the uterine corpus. Risk of perforation was greater for patients of more advanced gestational ages and for parous women than for women with no previous delivery. Use of *Laminaria* reduced this risk, as did greater operator skill. Resident physicians were more likely to perforate the uterus than were attending physicians.

Management of Perforation

If the abortion has been completed when the perforation is recognized, if there is minimal bleeding, and if the perforation is not lateral, the patient may be observed a few hours without hospitalization and reexamined the next day. However, in any other circumstance, the best management is transfer to a hospital for immediate laparoscopy to determine the extent of the injury and to complete the abortion under laparoscopic guidance.[40]

Hemorrhage

Excessive bleeding during vacuum curettage may indicate uterine atony, uterine trauma, a low lying implantation, or a pregnancy of more advanced gestational age than anticipated. Uterine relaxation may be produced by certain of the potent anesthetic gases such as halothane. Management requires a rapid reassessment of gestational age by examination of the fetal parts already extracted and gentle exploration of the uterine cavity with curette or forceps to confirm that there is no perforation. Intravenous oxytocin is administered and the abortion completed. The uterus is then massaged between two hands to ensure contraction. If these measures fail, the patient is transferred immediately to the hospital with intravenous fluids running and blood cross-matched. Uterine atony persisting after complete uterine evacuation is uncommon in the first trimester, as is a coagulopathy. Thus persistent postabortal bleeding strongly suggests retained tissue or clot (hematometra) or trauma, and the patient is best managed with prompt surgical intervention: laparoscopy and repeat curettage.

Postabortal Syndrome (Hematometra)

Hematometra, a type of uterine atony, was first recognized in 1974.[41] In the classic presentation, the patient begins to complain of increasing lower abdominal pain a half hour or so after abortion and may develop tachycardia and diaphoresis. On examination the uterus is large, globular, and tense and could be mistaken for a broad ligament hematoma except that the mass is midline and arises from the cervix. The treatment is immediate reevacuation. The uterus will then contract to its normal postabortal size. Sands et al.[41] reported that pretreatment with ergot 0.1 mg IM reduces the incidence of this phenomenon.

Failed Abortion, Continued Pregnancy, and Ectopic Pregnancy

Failure to interrupt the pregnancy is more often a problem with very early abortions. Pregnancy has continued in spite of the aspiration of histologically proven chorionic villi. The problem is much reduced if the gestational sac can be identified in the examina-tion of the freshly aborted tissue.[42] When no chorionic villi are found at this time, the patient is at risk for an ectopic pregnancy. The risk of death from ectopic pregnancy is five times greater when it is associated with an attempted abortion than when it is not, presumably because the history of apparent induced abortion delays diagnosis.[43] Various management plans to reduce the risk from ectopic pregnancy have been proposed. The solution is not easy. If all patients with a persistent positive pregnancy test and no villi identifiable in the curettings were subjected to laparoscopy to rule out an ectopic pregnancy, many unnecessary laparoscopies would be performed. Instead, an attempt is made to divide patients into groups at high and low risk for an ectopic pregnancy based on clinical history and physical findings and to perform immediate laparoscopy for the high-risk patients. The low-risk patients are maintained in close follow-up until the problem is resolved.[21]

Incomplete and Septic Abortion

Retained tissue will produce increased postabortal bleeding and places the patient at risk for infection. Management is by repeat curettage. If the uterus is larger than 12 weeks, it is wise to obtain a preoperative ultrasound to determine the amount of tissue remaining. When fever is present, a Gram stain from the cervical os and appropriate cultures are taken. Then high-dose intravenous antibiotic therapy is initiated and the curettage performed shortly thereafter. Formerly it was taught that in cases of sepsis with retained tissue one should wait a day or more after starting antibiotic therapy before instrumenting the uterus. There is no merit to this theory. Women have gone into septic shock in spite of antibiotic therapy while awaiting curettage.

Endometritis, myometritis, and pelvic peritonitis can be seen postabortally without any retained tissue. Such sequelae are most likely in patients with preexisting cervical colonization with gonorrhea, *Chlamydia,* or *Mycoplasma.* A small, firm uterus on pelvic examination suggests that the uterus is empty and curettage will not be needed. When there is a question as to retained tissue, we have found ultrasound useful in making the decision to perform curettage or to treat with antibiotics alone.

Rarely, clostridial sepsis is seen as a complication of legal abortion. This should be suspected from the presence of large gram-positive rods on Gram stain of the cervical secretions or curetted tissue, when tachy-cardia seems out of proportion to the fever, and especially when hematuria and shock develop rapidly. These patients can rapidly develop severe adult respiratory distress syndrome. Initial treatment requires high-dose penicillin, curettage, and fluid management. A superficial clostridial infection will respond to these measures, but, if hemolysis is present, indicating systemic release of clostridial toxins, prompt hysterectomy is probably necessary if the patient is to survive.[44]

Prophylactic Antibiotics

The use of perioperative antibiotics is widespread in abortion clinics. Scientific proof as to the benefit of this practice has been slow to come. Hodgson et al.[45] studied 4,000 women, with one-half receiving perioperative tetracycline, and saw a significant reduction in both minor and major complications. These results were confirmed in a large study from the Centers for Disease Control.[46] Sonne-Holmes et al.[47] found the benefit to be limited to those patients with a history of pelvic inflammatory disease. Levallois and Rioux's recent randomized study[48] demonstrated a reduction in infectious morbidity after the administration of preoperative oral doxycycline. While the benefits were greater for patients with cervical *Chlamydia* infection, *Chlamydia*-negative patients also had fewer infectious complications. The ideal antibiotic for prophylaxis would be effective against common pathogens (gonorrhea, *Chlamydia*, the gram-negative aerobes, and several anaerobic species) and should be rapidly absorbed after oral dosage to facilitate use in a busy clinic setting. The synthetic tetracyclines doxycycline and minocycline are probably the best of the presently available agents for this purpose.

Choice of Antibiotics for Postabortal Infection

A number of different species of bacteria, *Chlamydia*, and *Mycoplasma* have been implicated in postabortal sepsis. No one agent or even pair of agents is effective against all possible organisms. Modern therapy requires the use of a drug highly effective against anaerobic bacteria, and therefore antibiotic regimens will include either clindamycin, tetracycline, metronidazole, or one of the newer cephalosporins such as cefoxitin. In our practice, if a patient is seriously ill, we use three drugs: ampicillin, gentamicin, and clindamycin in combination.

Table 41.6 Findings at Repeat Uterine Evacuation in 53 Consecutive Cases of Patients Presenting With Pain, Bleeding, and Low-Grade Fever After First-Trimester Abortion

Findings	No.
Retained tissue	24
Scant fragments of gestational tissue or decidua	4
Clot and gestational tissue mixture	10
Blood clot only (hematometra)	9
Continued pregnancy (intact gestational sac)	6
Total	53

(From Stubblefield,[70] with permission.)

Postabortal Triad

The most common postabortal problem is the triad of pain, bleeding, and low-grade fever. While these symptoms may be managed successfully by oral antibiotics and ergot preparations, the great majority of cases will exhibit some retained gestational tissue or clot in the uterine cavity. Therefore, we feel these symptoms are best managed by repeating the uterine evacuation under local anesthesia in an ambulatory setting. Results obtained in 53 consecutive reaspirations done for these symptoms are displayed in Table 41.6.

SECOND-TRIMESTER ABORTION

Definitions

Conventionally, the second trimester has been assumed to begin after 12 menstrual weeks. Because it is widely used, this convention is used here, even though it imposes a distortion of reality.* The distinction between first- and second-trimester abortion was magnified because of guidelines, now outmoded, that considered 12 menstrual weeks the outer limit for curettage procedures and that insisted in utilizing either major surgery or labor induction techniques for abortion at 13 weeks and beyond.[51] How this practice came to be established is not clear. By 1972, Tietze and Lewit[49] demonstrated that abortion by cu-

*On the average, human pregnancy lasts 38 weeks from conception or 40 weeks from the beginning of the last normal menstrual period. One-third of 38 is 12.67 weeks; thus a more correct definition for the beginning of the second trimester would be 12.67 weeks from conception, or 14.67 weeks from the beginning of the last menses.

rettage at 13 to 14 weeks was only marginally less safe than the same procedure at 11 to 12 weeks and a great deal safer than abortion by saline infusion at later gestational ages.

The Supreme Court's decision in Roe v. Wade,[50] which made abortion legal through the United States, followed the medical practice of distinguishing between first and second trimester in abortion services. Because of the conceptual separation between the trimesters and the assumption that second-trimester abortion required hospitalization, mid-trimester abortion services have been hard to obtain. The legal separation between first- and second-trimester abortion was largely removed by further Supreme Court decisions in 1983, which had the effect of invalidating state laws that limited second-trimester abortion to hospitals. These legal decisions were possible because of clinical publications documenting the safety of early mid-trimester abortion by curettage techniques.[51]

Need for Mid-Trimester Abortion

The great majority of legal abortions are performed prior to 13 menstrual weeks. Abortions performed later include those done because of fetal defects, medical or psychiatric illness that had not manifested earlier in pregnancy, and changed social circumstances such as abandonment by the spouse. However, the single greatest determinant of the need for late abortion is the patient's age. Younger women are much more likely to need abortion after 12 weeks.[52] In 1980, 24.6 percent of abortions for women under age 15 years were done in the mid-trimester, while only 14 percent of abortions for women aged 15 to 19 years and only 6.7 percent of abortions for women aged 30 to 34 years were performed after 12 weeks.[14] Lack of ready access to abortion services still accounts for the delay in many cases. Before 1973, women who requested abortion on therapeutic grounds were frequently delayed several weeks while the system of hospital committees processed their applications. After 1973, many legal barriers to abortion were removed, but access to services has continued to be a problem and is most acute for young people, especially in states that require parental notification or parental consent prior to abortion. A strategy to reduce the need for mid-trimester abortion must include education of young women to the early signs of pregnancy, early diagnosis of pregnancy by free pregnancy tests, good nonjudgmental counseling, and readily available, low-cost abortion services without mandatory parental approval.

Techniques for Mid-Trimester Abortion

Our concepts of the best approach to mid-trimester abortion have evolved considerably in the past decade. In the early 1970s the widespread aversion to curettage procedures after 12 weeks created a "grey zone": women who presented for abortion at 13 to 15 weeks were intentionally delayed until 16 weeks when amnioinfusion of hypertonic saline was employed. During the 1970s prostaglandins became available as an alternative to saline, and the combination of intraamniotic urea and low doses of prostaglandin was introduced. However, even as prostaglandin research continued, several pioneer surgeons were performing curettage abortions through the mid-trimester. A series of papers from the Centers for Disease Control documented that instrumental evacuation through the cervix was in fact the procedure of choice.[51] By 1980 an important change had occurred: D & E had become the most commonly used method through 20 menstrual weeks, and amnioinfusion was favored only for those procedures performed after 20 weeks.[14]

D & E

The variety of techniques that have been employed by different authorities are summarized elsewhere.[53,54] These differ primarily in the preparatory steps that precede the evacuation. Perhaps the most influential practitioner was Finks,[55] whose 1973 report described 2,000 cases. He infiltrated local anesthetic and epinephrine deeply into the cervix, performed a forcible dilatation slowly and carefully, and then evacuated the pregnancy with long forceps. This one-stage procedure was widely adopted by other physicians, including Peterson[56] in the United States.

In 1978, Hanson[57] reported a successful two-stage technique using *Laminaria* tents to dilate the cervix. Cases of less than 16 weeks gestation were evacuated after 5 hours of *Laminaria* treatment. More advanced gestations had overnight treatment to achieve wider cervical dilatation. The amniotic fluid was aspirated with a 12-mm vacuum cannula and the pregnancy then evacuated with forceps. Forcible dilatation of the cervix and general anesthesia were avoided.

Hern[54] developed a multistage *Laminaria* technique. One *Laminaria* was inserted on the first day and replaced with several more the following morning. That afternoon those tents were removed and replaced with a third set, to be left in overnight. The abortion was then performed the following morning, about 41 hours after the beginning of the process. The current practice in the United States is to use either a one-stage procedure with forcible dilatation as described by Finks or a two-stage procedure similar to Hanson's with one set of *Laminaria*. Those who utilize D & E after 20 weeks are increasingly turning to a modification of Hern's technique with 2 days of *Laminaria* treatment prior to evacuation.

Choice of technique becomes more important as gestational age advances. As demonstrated by Stubblefield et al.,[58] pregnancies at 13 to 14 menstrual weeks are readily evacuated using the 12-mm vacuum cannula. Dilatation of this amount is usually readily accomplished with Pratt or Denniston dilators. However, unless ultrasound is routinely used, the pregnancy thought preoperatively to be only 14 weeks can easily turn out to be 16 weeks, requiring larger instruments and greater cervical dilatation. For this reason we strongly advise the routine use of *Laminaria* tents after 13 weeks.

The actual evacuation of the uterine content is usually accomplished with long, heavy forceps while the vacuum curette is used as an adjunct to rupture the fetal membranes, drain amniotic fluid, and ensure that evacuation is complete at the end of the procedure. However, the 16-mm vacuum system (available from Rocket of London, Inc., Branford, CT, and Medispec of Lafayette, CA) allows standard vacuum curettage to be performed through 16 menstrual weeks and facilitates the procedure, especially for new operators.[58] A variety of ovum forceps have been used for D & E. One of the more popular, the Sopher forceps is shown in Figure 41.5. The ideal forcep would be long, strong enough to crush fetal tissue, but light enough for sensitive exploration of the uterine cavity. The forceps recently developed by Hern appears closest to this ideal (manufactured by V. Mueller, Inc., Linden, NJ).

Anesthesia for Mid-Trimester Abortion

Use of general anesthesia increases the risk for cervical laceration and hemorrhage with D & E,[59] most likely because the awake patient reacts when the surgeon pushes too hard with an instrument. On occasion, when perforation has occurred, the patient's complaint of upper abdominal pain led the operator to discontinue the procedure before serious harm was done.

The procedure causes discomfort in spite of paracervical block, and most patients will benefit from intravenous sedation and analgesia. For years we have used the combination of diazepam 5 mg and fentanyl 0.05 mg, each given slowly as the procedure is begun with an additional dose of the same amount given as needed. If the procedure is completed sooner than expected or the patient appears heavily sedated, we use naloxone prophylactically to avoid the risk of respiratory arrest.

Newer sedatives may offer advantages. Midazolam, a metabolite of diazepam, appears to offer greater anxiolytic effect and some amnesia and does not cause the pain with infusion that is present with diazepam. Midazolam is considerably more potent than diazepam. Respiratory depression occurs with both drugs at higher doses.[60] This has been more of a problem with midazolam, probably because its greater potency was not initially appreciated and intravenous doses of 5 to 10 mg were used. Current practice in ambulatory abortion services is to use no more than 2.0 to 2.5 mg of intravenous midazolam, a dose which appears to be safe in young healthy women. Patients who receive intravenous sedation must be under constant observation until fully recovered. If more than minimal doses of sedatives are administered, the patient should be monitored as when general anesthesia is used.

An Approach to D & E

There is a paradox to D & E for abortion. For most patients the procedure is perceived as relatively minor, especially compared with the alternatives of amnioinfusion or major surgery.[61] When all goes well, as it usually does, the procedure takes only 10 to 20 minutes; the patient recovers for 1 or 2 hours and then goes home. Yet the potential for sudden, life-threatening complications is always there: uterine perforation and intestinal or bladder injury, amniotic fluid embolism, and disseminated intravascular coagulopathy. The D & E procedure must be approached with caution and gentleness, and the patient must know that serious injury is possible, although not likely.

I describe my own technique in hopes that it will help others to prevent complications. For a more detailed description, the reader is referred to Hern's excellent monograph.[54]

After adequate counseling, a menstrual history as well as a complete medical history is taken. A physical examination with attention to uterine size is then performed. Two or more medium tents of *Laminaria japonicum* are inserted into the cervical canal and held in place with two 4 × 4 gauze sponges tucked into the fornices. At menstrual ages 13 to 15 weeks two tents will suffice, but at 16 to 20 weeks we insert 4 or more tents. The patient is kept supine for a few minutes after insertion to avoid syncope and then goes home. For gestations of 13 to 20 menstrual weeks, the abortion procedure will be performed the following day. At menstrual ages 20 weeks and beyond, we remove the first set of *Laminaria* on day 2, insert as many additional tents as the canal will accept, and perform uterine evacuation on day 3. If the membranes are ruptured with *Laminaria* insertion the *Laminaria* are left in place and the abortion performed as scheduled the following day. We routinely prescribe tetracycline 500 mg on a four times a day schedule, begun with *Laminaria* insertion and continued for two doses after uterine evacuation. An analgesic is prescribed as well, because if more than two *Laminaria* tents are used, patients may experience moderate abdominal discomfort.

An ultrasound examination is performed during the initial evaluation if there is a discrepancy between menstrual dates and uterine size on bimanual examination and for all cases 20 weeks and beyond. Presently we utilize ultrasound guidance during the surgery for the more advanced cases.

Uterine evacuation is performed as follows. An intravenous line is established. Diazepam 5 mg and fentanyl 0.05 mg are slowly administered. The patient is placed in lithotomy position, and the previously placed vaginal sponges and *Laminaria* are removed. Occasionally, especially in the young, primigravid patient at 13 to 15 weeks, the cervix is quite resistant to dilatation and the *Laminaria* tents may be entrapped. This problem is more likely when one large *Laminaria* has been used rather than two or more smaller ones. If the *Laminaria* cannot be removed with gentle traction, it is best to stop and wait 6 hours for additional cervical softening to occur. Next, the vagina and cervix are cleansed with povidone iodide and paracervical block established with 20 cc of lidocaine 1 percent with 5 units of vasopressin injected superficially into the cervix at 12, 4, and 8 o'clock positions. A tenaculum is placed vertically, with one branch inside the cervical canal. A large dilator is gently inserted to confirm dilatation. The vacuum cannula is then inserted and vacuum established briefly to rupture the membranes and drain amniotic fluid. The 12- or 14-mm cannulas are used for 13- to 15-week procedures, whereas the large bore 16-mm system is used for more advanced procedures. The cannula is then removed and replaced with an ovum forceps of appropriate size: Foerrester forceps for 13- to 15-week procedures and Hern, Bierer, or Sopher forceps for more advanced procedures. The instrument is manipulated within the lower uterine segment to remove the pregnancy tissue. The vacuum cannula is reinserted as needed to pull tissue downward where it can be grasped with the forceps. When the procedure feels complete, a large sharp curette is inserted and used to explore the cavity. If any additional tissue is encountered the forceps or cannula is reinserted to remove it. After the procedure the operator carefully examines the fetal parts to be sure all have been evacuated. On occasion the fetal calvarium is retained in the uterus. If gentle attempts at extraction fail, it is best to stop, administer an oxytocin infusion for 2 hours, and then try again. By then the remaining fetal parts will have been pushed down to the internal os, where they can be easily extracted.

The greatest risk of D & E occurs when the surgeon misjudges gestational age and attempts evacuation of a pregnancy beyond that operator's skill and experience. The chance that this will occur is reduced by frequent use of preoperative ultrasound. However, if the procedure has already begun, the operator can tell gestational age by the size of the fetal parts. According to Streeter,[62] a fetal foot length of 26.8 mm corresponds to 18 menstrual weeks, 30.7 mm to 19 weeks, 33.3 mm to 20 weeks, and 35.2 mm to 21 weeks. When multiple *Laminaria* tents have been used and the cervix is widely dilated, a surgeon familiar with D & E can satisfactorily extract a pregnancy up to 20 to 21 weeks. Beyond this we feel the procedure should be abandoned unless the surgeon routinely performs these more advanced procedures. The patient can be treated instead with intravenous oxytocin or systemic prostaglandins, given prophylactic antibiotics, and the uterus evacuated 24 hours later after fetal maceration has occurred.

Facilitating D & E

The use of intraoperative realtime ultrasound with later mid-trimester procedures has been advocated by Darney[63] and appears most promising. Ultrasound guidance is reported to facilitate the removal of large fetal parts with less risk of maternal trauma.

Early practitioners of D & E recommended the use of epinephrine to reduce blood loss.[55] We no longer advise this because of the potential for fatal anaphylaxis in patients allergic to the metabisulfite preservative in epinephrine solutions. Glick (personal communication) advised the use of Pituitrin with the paracervical block to reduce bleeding with advanced D & E procedures. Pituitrin is a mixture of oxytocin and vasopressin. Christensen[64] has completed a randomized, controlled trial that demonstrated that vasopressin administered paracervically does indeed reduce blood loss. Vasopressin must be used with caution, however, and should not be administered to women with heart disease or hypertension. We use it for procedures after 13 weeks and mix 5 units (one-quarter ampule) of vasopressin with 20 cc of local anesthetic for paracervical infiltration, taking great care to avoid intravascular injection. Intravenous oxytocin is regularly used with D & E, but there is controversy as to when it should be administered, some preferring to begin oxytocin infusion early in the procedure and others delaying until the uterus has been evacuated. The 15-methyl analogue of $PGF_{2\alpha}$ (Prostin 15M) was recently licensed for mid-trimester abortion. It has proved to be of great value in the management of postpartum hemorrhage and deserves evaluation as an adjunct to D & E.

D & E becomes progressively more difficult as gestational age advances, and it is for this reason that labor induction techniques are still favored for procedures after 20 menstrual weeks. Those who perform D & E procedures after 20 weeks often modify their technique. The use of two sets of *Laminaria* tents for a total of 36 to 48 hours of *Laminaria* treatment is increasingly practiced by experts in this country, because greater cervical dilatation is achieved, making extraction of large fetal parts easier. A further modification is Hern's combination method. After multistage *Laminaria* treatment urea is injected into the amniotic sac, and the extraction of the fetus and placenta is accomplished after labor begins and after fetal maceration has occurred.[54]

Another variation was recently reported by Wright.[65] All patients were treated with ultrasound-guided intrafetal or intra-amniotic injection of digoxin at the time of cervical placement of multiple *Laminaria* tents or 4 Dilapan tents. Procedures were

done under general anesthesia in a free-standing clinic. All patients received high doses of oxytocin (50 to 100 units/1,000 cc). As noted below, digoxin has been utilized to produce fetal demise before prostaglandin abortion. Its use prior to D & E is said to result in fetal softening, which aids extraction and thus reduces risk of maternal injury. Wright's report describes 2,400 cases at 19 to 23 weeks with no uterine perforations.

Labor Induction Methods

Systemic Prostaglandins

PGE_2 vaginal suppositories and intramuscular 15-methyl $PGF_{2\alpha}$ (Prostin 15M) are available in the United States. Both are easy to administer and are highly effective. With vaginal PGE_2 20 mg every 3 hours, the mean time to abortion is 13.4 hours, with 90 percent of patients aborting by 24 hours.[66] When Prostin 15M is given as 250 mcg IM every 2 hours, the mean time to abortion is 15 to 17 hours, with about 80 percent aborting by 24 hours.[67] Gastrointestinal side effects are common, with 39 percent of PGE_2-treated patients experiencing vomiting and 25 percent experiencing diarrhea in one large trial.[67] These side effects are more common with Prostin 15M: 83 percent had vomiting and 71 percent had diarrhea in the trial cited above.[67] Fever also is a common side effect of PGE_2 treatment, and about one-third of patients will have a temperature elevation of 1 degree C or more. Pretreatment with overnight placement of osmotic dilators shortens the length of prostaglandin treatment, reduces the dose of the drug required, and thus reduces the prostaglandin-related side effects.[68]

Intrauterine Prostaglandins

$PGF_{2\alpha}$ for intra-amniotic administration was the first prostaglandin approved by the U.S. Food and Drug Administration. Though initially hailed as a better alternative than intra-amniotic saline, acceptance was limited because of problems with incomplete abortion, the need for a second injection in many cases, the risk for cervical rupture in the primigravida, and the lack of a direct toxic effect on the fetus. Results with intra-amniotic $PGF_{2\alpha}$ are much improved if overnight treatment with *Laminaria* is used prior to infusion. We demonstrated that mean times to abortion were reduced from 29 to 14 hours and fewer patients required a second dose.[69] Cervical rupture was rare. We outfitted a treatment room with a uterine aspirator and performed routine curettage after all abortions, whether apparently complete or not.[70] By this means we reduced rates of postabortal hemorrhage and infection to low levels. We learned to manage failed prostaglandin abortions by D & E as advocated by Burkeman et al.[71] and more recently by systemic prostaglandins so that hysterotomy was no longer necessary to treat failed abortion. We also learned to avoid the use of oxytocin in prostaglandin-treated patients to avoid uterine rupture.[72]

With increasing use of D & E in the early mid-trimester, labor induction methods are primarily reserved for late procedures, when concerns about fetal viability and transient fetal survival are the greatest. In our experience with prostaglandins, 7 to 10 percent of fetuses survived briefly. For this reason, and to improve efficacy, $PGF_{2\alpha}$ has been combined with either hypertonic saline or urea, as detailed below. Recently, a group of investigators, convinced that prostaglandins offer the safest alternative for the pregnant woman but concerned about transient fetal survival, reported another approach: fetal intracardiac injection of digoxin, performed under ultrasound guidance, prior to the use of vaginal and intra-amniotic prostaglandins to produce abortion.[73]

Intra-Amniotic Prostaglandin Combined With Urea or Saline

The addition of 50 cc of hypertonic saline to intra-amniotic $PGF_{2\alpha}$ is reported by Borten[74] to shorten the interval from injection to abortion and to reduce transient fetal survival prior to 20 weeks. Kerenyi et al.[75] reported extensive experience with hypertonic saline and more recently added 20 mg of PGF_2 to 150 to 200 cc of saline (T. D. Kerenyi, personal communication).

Hypertonic urea is attractive as an alternative to saline because of its greater safety, although the interval from injection to abortion is prolonged. In a series of papers, the group from Johns Hopkins explored this method, augmenting it at first with intravenous oxytocin and subsequently with low doses of $PGF_{2\alpha}$. The combination of 5 mg of $PGF_{2\alpha}$ and 80 g of urea instilled into the amniotic sac produced abortion in a mean time of 17.5 hours, with 80 percent of the patients aborting within 24 hours.[76] Fetal survival

appears to be rare with abortion by this method. A study from the Centers for Disease Control compared hypertonic saline with the urea–prostaglandin method and found the urea method to offer a shorter time from instillation to abortion and fewer serious complications than with saline.[77]

An Alternative Prostaglandin to Replace $PGF_{2\alpha}$

Though still approved by the Food and Drug Administration, $PGF_{2\alpha}$ is no longer available in the United States. The manufacturer gave in to extreme public pressure from "right to life" groups and no longer produces this drug. As an alternative, one may use 2 mg of the 15M $PGF_{2\alpha}$ (carboprost tromethamine, Hemabate) in place of 40 mg of $PGF_{2\alpha}$ for intra-amniotic injection.[78] A dose of 0.250 mg of 15M $PGF_{2\alpha}$ will replace the 5-mg dose of $PGF_{2\alpha}$ used to augment intra-amniotic urea.

An extensive experience with mid-trimester abortion induced by intra-amniotic 15M $PGF_{2\alpha}$ has been reported by Osathanondh[78] from Brigham and Womens' Hospital in Boston. Patients are pretreated overnight with multiple intracervical *Laminaria* tents packed around one Lamicel tent. The following morning the tents are removed and an intra-amniotic injection is given of 2 mg of 15M $PGF_{2\alpha}$ combined with 64 mg of 23.4 percent sodium chloride. Four hours later, the membranes are artificially ruptured, and, unless the cervix is found to be well effaced and dilated, a PGE_2 suppository is placed into the cervical canal on the end of a Dilapan tent. Subsequently, vaginal suppositories of PGE_2 are given at 3-hour intervals. All patients have a brief exploration of the uterine cavity and curettage under low-dose intravenous sedation after expulsion of the placenta. If the patient has not aborted by 14 hours, a D & E procedure is performed. The Boston group reports a mean time from instillation to abortion of 8 hours and no cervical lacerations or uterine rupture in over 4,000 consecutive cases treated with this protocol.[78]

Hypertonic Saline

Amnioinfusion of hypertonic saline is important historically as one of the oldest of the labor induction methods for abortion. It is still the most frequently used method in the United States for abortion after 20 weeks.[14] There are serious hazards unique to hypertonic saline: cardiovascular collapse, pulmonary and cerebral edema, and renal failure occur if the solution is injected intravenously, and all patients are at risk for serious disseminated intravascular coagulopathy (DIC). However, with attention to proper technique, including instillation of the saline by gravity flow through connecting tubing from a single-dose bottle, such mishaps are infrequent. The main hazards of hypertonic saline are in fact common to all of the labor induction methods: failed abortion, incomplete abortion, retained tissue, hemorrhage, infection, and embolic phenomena.

Administered by itself, hypertonic saline produces mean times from instillation to abortion of 33 to 35 hours.[75,79] When intravenous oxytocin is begun within 8 hours of instillation and infused at 17 to 67 mU/min, the mean time to abortion is reduced to 25 to 26 hours.[79] Augmentation with oxytocin improves efficacy.[80] Not only is the instillation to abortion time shortened, but there are fewer failed abortions, fewer retained placentas, less blood loss, and less risk of infection. However, the addition of oxytocin increases the rate of occurrence of DIC and adds risk for water intoxication. Higher rates of oxytocin infusion heighten this risk. Kerenyi et al.[75] used 100 to 200 mU/min, thus reducing the interval from injection to abortion to 20 to 21 hours, but reported two uterine ruptures and "a few" cases of annular detachment of the cervix.

Complications of Mid-Trimester Abortions and Their Management

Mid-trimester abortion has been associated with several important complications. DIC may occur. DIC is rare after first-trimester vacuum curettage, with an incidence of 8 per 100,000 procedures.[81] The incidence is higher after mid-trimester D & E, 191 per 100,000 and highest for saline instillation procedures, 658 per 100,000. DIC must be considered whenever postabortal hemorrhage is seen and, if present, must be managed aggressively with infusions of cryoprecipitate, fresh frozen plasma, and packed red cells. Heparin therapy is not helpful in these cases. Perforation with mid-trimester D & E is more likely to result in major visceral injury than is perforation in first-trimester procedures and will usually require a laparotomy. The labor induction methods can lead to fetal expulsion through a rent in the cervix

above the external os, a cervicovaginal fistula, or even annular detachment of the lower cervix. Uterine rupture may occur when saline, urea, or prostaglandins are augmented with high-dose oxytocin infusion. Failed abortion is seen with all of the labor induction methods and can lead to serious infection and continued blood loss. Intramuscular injections of 15M $PGF_{2\alpha}$ or vaginal suppositories of PGE_2 are important second-line therapies when the primary method has not produced abortion within a reasonable time period. Formerly, hysterotomy was used to manage these cases, but experienced physicians can safely employ D & E techniques, sparing the patient major surgery.[71] Failed saline or prostaglandin abortions are technically easier to manage by D & E than is a primary procedure at the same gestational age, because the cervix is usually widely dilated, the uterus is well contracted, and the fetus and placenta are compacted into the lower uterine segment.

Choice of Mid-Trimester Procedure

There are several alternative procedures presently available in the United States for mid-trimester abortion. Resident physicians on our service have been able to terminate 16-week pregnancies consistently and safely by D & E under the following conditions: overnight placement of multiple *Laminaria* tents, use of the 16-mm vacuum cannula system, local anesthesia augmented with low-dose intravenous sedation, good nursing support, and direct hands-on supervision by a small group of experienced faculty.[82] Robbins and Surrago[83] have compared D & E with the best available alternative for early mid-trimester abortion, vaginal PGE_2, and found D & E to be safer and more effective. Therefore, we see little indication for any procedure other than D & E prior to 17 menstrual weeks.

There is no truly satisfactory alternative for abortion at 17 weeks and beyond. When the entire mid-trimester is considered, D & E appears safer than the alternatives, but, as noted by Kafrissen et al.[84] in their recent comparison of D & E to urea–$PGF_{2\alpha}$, the advantage of D & E is for procedures done at 13 to 16 weeks. Thereafter, the risks for major complications and death are comparable. Urea, prostaglandins, and saline infusion all involve overnight hospitalization, which greatly increases expense. As documented by Kaltreider et al.,[61] the psychological impact on the patient is much greater with amnioinfusion abortion than with D & E. In our own practice, we offer D & E through 22 menstrual weeks and after that would prefer a labor induction method such as urea–$PGF_{2\alpha}$ after overnight treatment with *Laminaria* tents to prevent cervical rupture. However, we must note that several skilled surgeons offer D & E techniques to 24 weeks. Indeed, the lowest reported rate of complications for any late abortion technique is that of Hern[85]: a combination method of *Laminaria*, intra-amniotic urea, and then D & E. For the operator faced with the need to perform an occasional abortion in the mid-trimester, we would suggest intra-amniotic injection of 1.5 mg of digoxin and placement of intracervical *Laminaria*, followed the next day by vaginal suppositories of PGE_2.

Induced Abortion and Subsequent Reproduction

Opponents of legal abortion cite complications for later reproduction as a reason to ban abortion. For the most part, the sources cited are older European authorities. Hogue et al.[86] reviewed current literature on this topic and concluded that legal abortion as currently practiced in the United States has no measurable adverse effect on later reproduction. A single induced abortion appears safe as far as later reproduction, but there is still controversy as to whether multiple induced abortions have some cumulative adverse effect. Studies of reproductive outcome are difficult because of the need to control for multiple confounding factors that are frequently present among women who report multiple abortions. Our group found that women with two or more induced abortions appeared at greater risk for later first- or second-trimester spontaneous loss, even after appropriate control for other factors.[87] In a separate study, we found that women who reported two or more induced abortions prior to their present pregnancy appeared initially to have more pregnancy complications. However, statistical control by multiple logistic regression analysis found multiple abortions to be associated only with first-trimester bleeding, abnormal presentations, and premature rupture of the membranes prior to labor, but not with low birth weight, prematurity, or increased perinatal loss.[88] Concerns about infertility as a result of induced abortion seem largely unfounded, except for the rare severe complication managed by hysterectomy. A pro-

spective follow-up study found no reduction in subsequent pregnancy rates when an abortion group was compared with two control groups.[89] Indeed, the multivariate analysis of these data found that women who reported three or more induced abortions had high rates of pregnancy subsequently, suggesting that their frequent resort to abortion may have reflected greater than average fertility.

The lack of adverse effects on later pregnancy probably reflects the safety of current abortion technology in the United States: most abortions are performed by vacuum curettage under local anesthesia in the first trimester. The safety of mid-trimester methods for later pregnancy remains to be demonstrated and unquestionably varies with the method. Forcible dilatation of the cervix to large diameters for D & E in the late mid-trimester may well increase the risk of prematurity later.[90] We have shown that by 2 weeks following *Laminaria* dilatation the cervical canal has recovered to an internal diameter smaller than that found prior to abortion.[91] We feel strongly that *Laminaria* tents, their synthetic alternative, or low-dose prostaglandins should be used to prepare the cervix prior to late abortion and that forcible dilatation to large diameters should be avoided.

Pregnancy Termination After Fetal Death In Utero

While fetal death in utero can be managed exactly as induced abortion in the first and second trimesters, there are some differences. Induction of labor within 24 hours from *Laminaria* placement alone is rare with an intact gestation; however, we have seen labor start within a few hours after *Laminaria* placement in cases of fetal death. This is not a problem if the patient knows this may happen and has been instructed to return to the hospital. DIC is more common following D & E or induction of labor after a fetal death. The amniotic sac may be more permeable after fetal death, and intra-amniotic injection becomes technically more difficult. For this reason, systemic reactions from hypertonic saline or intra-amniotic prostaglandin are more common in these cases. Indeed, it was this experience that spurred the development of vaginal PGE_2 suppositories to treat fetal death. In cases of fetal death, the response to prostaglandins is faster than with intact gestations. Treatment to expulsion times are shorter. Special caution is required for managing fetal death after 28 weeks with prostaglandins. A full dose of 20 mg of PGE$_2$ has produced fatal uterine rupture. Our protocol, used successfully for many years, is to cut the suppository into fourths and treat the patient with one-fourth of the suppository (approximately 5 mg of PGE$_2$) at 2-hour intervals.

The Limit to Mid-Trimester Abortion

I would argue that women must have access to legal abortion and that efforts to ban abortion by making it illegal only result in expensive and dangerous procedures with many complications and high rates of maternal mortality. However, our society will not countenance infanticide. Inevitably, there must be a gestational age limit for abortion. The U.S. Supreme Court used viability as the limit for abortion based on the decision of the women and allowed states to limit abortion thereafter.[50] A survey of neonatal intensive care units in 1975 led to the conclusion that infants born before 24 weeks and weighing less than 600 g at birth were not viable.[92] Further improvements in neonatal care in the years since have resulted in the rare survival of infants at 23 weeks and birth weight greater than 500 g.[93] In our opinion, 23 weeks should be considered the threshold of viability. We would avoid performing abortion after 22 weeks unless the mother's life were endangered or unless the fetus had major malformations so severe as to preclude prolonged survival. Current ultrasound techniques combine measurements of several fetal dimensions to give more reliable estimates of gestational age than previous techniques that relied on the biparietal diameter alone.[94] When abortion is performed just prior to viability, a method that ensures fetal demise should be selected to avoid the anguished decisions occasioned by the live birth of a fetus of borderline viability. When termination of pregnancy will be undertaken at or after 23 weeks because of serious risk to maternal health, the fetus must be considered as well. Each case must be managed individually, based on the mother's status, and intervention delayed until survival of the fetus is probable, if maternal condition permits.

The ethics of abortion after viability have been explored by Chervenak and colleagues.[95] They conclude that abortion should be considered ethical in cases of fetal conditions with no prospect for prolonged survival after birth and when there is a completely accurate means for diagnosing the condition. Fetal anencephaly was sited as such a condition.[9] In reality, it is almost impossible to obtain termination of pregnancy in the third trimester in the United States, no matter the indication.

REFERENCES

1. Tietze C: New estimates of mortality associated with fertility control. Fam Plann Perspect 9:74, 1977
2. Eisner V, Brazie JV, Pratt MW, Hexter AC: The risk of low birth weight. Am J Public Health 69:887, 1979
3. Puffer RR, Serrano CV: Birth weight, maternal age and birth order: three important determinants in infant mortality. Pan Am Health Organization, Scientific Publ. No. 294, 1975
4. Bakketieg LS, Hoffman HJ: Epidemiology of preterm birth: results from a longitudinal study of births in Norway. p. 17. In Elder MG, Hendricks CH (eds): Preterm Labour. Butterworths, London, 1981
5. Forrest JD, Henshaw SK: What U.S. women think and do about contraception. Fam Plann Perspect 15:157, 1983
6. Ory HW: Mortality associated with fertility and fertility control: 1983. Fam Plann Perspect 15:57, 1983
7. Henshaw SK, Silverman J: The characteristics and prior contraceptive use of U.S. abortion patients. Fam Plann Perspect 20:158, 1988
8. Henshaw SK, Van Vort J: Teenage abortion, birth and pregnancy statistics: an update. Fam Plann Perspect 21:85, 1989
9. Potts M, Diggory P, Peel J: Abortion. Cambridge University Press, Cambridge, 1977
10. Deveraux G: A Study of Abortion in Primitive Societies. International Universities Press, New York, 1976
11. Narkavonnakit T, Bennett T: Health consequences of induced abortion in rural Northeast Thailand. Stud Fam Plann 12:58, 1981
12. Mohr JC: Abortion in America: The Origins and Evolution of National Policy. Oxford University Press, New York, 1978
13. Standards for Abortion Facilities. The National Abortion Federation, Washington, DC, 1984
14. Centers for Disease Control. Abortion Surveillance 1979–80. CDC, Atlanta, 1983
15. Grimes DA, Schulz KR, Cates W Jr et al: Local versus general anesthesia: which is safer for performing suction curettage abortions? Am J Obstet Gynecol 135:1030, 1979

16. Peterson HB, Grimes DA, Cates W Jr et al: Comparative risk of death from induced abortion at 12 weeks or less gestation performed with local versus general anesthesia. Am J Obstet Gynecol 141:763, 1981

17. Stubblefield PG: Induced abortion: indications, counseling, and services. p. 2. In Sciarra JJ, Zatuchni GI, Daly MJ (eds): Gynecology and Obstetrics. Vol. 6. Ch. 54. Philadelphia, Harper & Row, 1982

18. Wu YT: Suction in artificial abortion: 300 cases. Chin J Obstet Gynecol 6:447, 1958

19. Andolsek L (ed): The Ljubljana Abortion Study, 1971–1973. Bethesda, National Institutes of Health, Center for Population Research, 1974

20. Karman H, Potts M: Very early abortion using syringe as vacuum source. Lancet 1:7759, 1972

21. Burnhill MS, Armstead JW: Reducing the morbidity of vacuum aspiration abortion. Int J Gynecol Obstet 16:204, 1978

22. Glick E: Paracervical and lower uterine field block anesthesia for therapeutic abortion and office D & C. Paper presented at 11th Annual Convention of the National Abortion Federation, Salt Lake City, Utah, May 18, 1987

23. Stubblefield PG: Control of pain for women undergoing abortion. Int J Gynecol Obstet 3(Suppl.):131, 1989

24. Schulz KF, Grimes DA, Cates W Jr: Measures to prevent cervical injury during suction curettage abortion. Lancet 1:1182, 1983

25. Gold J, Schulz KR, Cates W Jr, Tyler CW: The safety of *Laminaria* and rigid dilators for cervical dilatation prior to suction curettage for first trimester abortion: a comparative analysis. p. 363. In Naftolin F, Stubblefield PG (eds): Dilatation of the Uterine Cervix: Connective Tissue Biology and Clinical Management. New York, Raven Press, 1980

26. Hale RW, Pion RJ: *Laminaria:* an underutilized clinical adjunct. Clin Obstet Gynecol 15:829, 1972

27. Wheeler RG, Schneider K: Properties and safety of cervical dilators. Am J Obstet Gynecol 164:597, 1983

28. Ganguli AC, Green K, Bygdeman M: Preoperative dilatation of the cervix by single vaginal administration of 15 methyl $PGF_{2\alpha}$ methyl ester. Prostaglandins 14:779, 1977

29. Darney PD, Dorward K: Cervical dilatation before first-trimester elective abortion: a controlled comparison of meteneprost, *Laminaria* and hypan. Obstet Gynecol 70:397, 1987

30. Chen P, Kols A: Population and birth planning in the People's Republic of China. Popul Rep J 10:J-594, 1982

31. Karim SMM: The use of prostaglandins in abortion. p. 68. In Lewit S (ed): Abortion Techniques and Services. Excerpta Medica, Amsterdam, 1972

32. MacKenzue IZ, Embrey MP, Davies AJ, Guillebaud J: Very early abortion by prostaglandins. Lancet 1:1223, 1978

33. Couzinet B, LeStrat N, Ulman A et al: Termination of early pregnancy by the progesterone antagonist RU 486 (Mefipristone). N Engl J Med 315:1565, 1986

34. Bygdeman M, Swahm ML: Progesterone receptor blockage: effect on uterine contractility and early pregnancy. Contraception 32:45, 1985

35. Berkowitz RL, Lynch L, Chitkara U et al: Selection reduction of multifetal pregnancies in the first trimester. N Engl J Med 318:1043, 1988

35a. Wapner RJ, Davis GH, Johnson A et al: Selective reduction of multifetal pregnancies. Lancet 335:90, 1990

36. Grimes DA, Cates W: Deaths from paracervical anesthesia used for first trimester abortion, 1972–1975. N Engl J Med 295:1397, 1976

37. U.S. Food and Drug Administration: Warning for prescription drugs containing sulfite. Drug Bull 17:2, 1987

38. Berek JS, Stubblefield PG: Anatomical and clinical correlations of uterine perforations. Am J Obstet Gynecol 135:181, 1979

39. Grimes DA, Schulz KF, Cates WJ: Prevention of uterine perforation during curettage abortion. JAMA 251:2108, 1984

40. Lauersen NH, Birnbaum S: Laparoscopy as a diagnostic and therapeutic technique in uterine perforations during first-trimester abortions. Am J Obstet Gynecol 117:522, 1973

41. Sands RX, Burnhill MS, Hakim-Elahi E: Post-abortal uterine atony. Obstet Gynecol 43:595, 1974

42. Fielding WL, Lee WY, Borten N, Friedman EA: Continued pregnancy after failed first trimester abortion. Obstet Gynecol 63:421, 1984

43. Rubin GL, Peterson EB, Dorfman SF et al: Ectopic pregnancy in the United States, 1970 through 1978. JAMA 249:1725, 1983

44. Hoyme UB, Eschenback DA: Postoperative infection. p. 821. In Iffy L, Charles D (eds): Operative Perinatology. MacMillan, New York, 1984

45. Hodgson JE, Major B, Portman K et al: Prophylactic use of tetracycline for first trimester abortions. Obstet Gynecol 45:574, 1975

46. Schulz KF, Grimes DA, Park T, Flock M: Prophylactic antibiotics to prevent febrile complications of curettage abortion. Paper presented at 8th Annual Meeting of the National Abortion Federation, Los Angeles, CA, May 15, 1984

47. Sonne-Holme S, Heisterberg L, Hebjorn S et al: Prophylactic antibiotics in first trimester abortion: a clini-

cal controlled trial. Am J Obstet Gynecol 139:693, 1981

48. Levallois P, Rioux JE: Prophylactic antibiotics for suction curettage abortion: results of a clinical controlled trial. Am J Obstet Gynecol 158:100, 1988

49. Tietze C, Lewit S: Joint Program for the Study of Abortion (JPSA): Early medical applications for legal abortion. Stud Fam Plann 3:96, 1972

50. Roe v. Wade. 410 U.S. 113, 1973

51. Grimes DA, Schulz KF, Cates W Jr, Tyler CW: Midtrimester abortion by dilatation and evacuation: a safe and practical alternative. N Engl J Med 296:1141, 1977

52. Cannon-Bonventre K: Educational Methodologies to Decrease Second Trimester Abortions. American Institutes for Research, Cambridge, MA, Contract 200-77-0701. Centers for Disease Control, Dept. of Health, Education and Welfare, Washington, DC

53. Stubblefield PG: Midtrimester abortion by curettage procedures: an overview. p. 277. In Hodgson JE (ed): Abortion and Sterilization: Medical and Social Aspects. Academic Press, San Diego, CA 1981

54. Hern WM: Abortion Practice. J.B. Lippincott, Philadelphia, 1984

55. Finks AI: Midtrimester abortion. Lancet 1:263, 1973

56. Peterson W: Dilatation and evacuation: patient evaluation and surgical techniques. p. 184. In Zatuchni GI, Sciarra JJ, Spiedel JJ (eds): Pregnancy Termination: Procedures, Safety, and New Developments. Harper & Row, Hagerstown, MD, 1979

57. Hanson MS: D & E midtrimester abortion preceded by *Laminaria*. Presented at the 16th Annual Meeting of the Association of Planned Parenthood Physicians, San Diego, CA, Oct 26, 1978

58. Stubblefield PG, Albrecht BH, Koos B et al: A randomized study of 12 mm vs 15.9 mm vacuum cannulas in midtrimester abortion by *Laminaria* and vacuum curettage. Fertil Steril 29:512, 1978

59. MacKay HT, Schulz KR, Grimes DA: The safety of local versus general anesthesia for second trimester dilatation and evacuation abortion. Obstet Gynecol 66:661, 1985

60. Bell GP, Morden A, Coady T et al: A comparison of diazepam and midazolam as endoscopy premedication: assessing changes in ventilation and oxygen saturation. Br J Clin Pharmacol 26:595, 1988

61. Kaltreider NB, Goldsmith S, Margolis AJ: The impact of midtrimester abortion techniques on patients and staff. Am J Obstet Gynecol 135:235, 1979

62. Streeter GL: Weight, sitting height, head size, foot length, and menstrual age of the human embryo. Contrib Embryol 11:157, 1920

63. Darney PD: Midtrimester abortion under ultrasound guidance. Post Graduate Course, National Abortion Federation, Tampa, FL, Jan 31, 1983

64. Christensen D: Use of vasopressin to reduce D & E blood loss. Paper presented at the 8th Annual Meeting of the National Abortion Federation, Los Angeles, CA, May 14, 1984

65. Wright PC: Late midtrimester abortion by dilatation and evacuation using dilapan and digoxin. Paper presented at the 13th Annual Meeting of the National Abortion Federation, San Francisco, CA, April 4, 1989

66. Surrago EJ, Robins J: Midtrimester pregnancy termination by intravaginal administration of prostaglandin E_2. Contraception 26:285, 1982

67. Robins J, Mann LI: Second generation prostaglandins: midtrimester pregnancy termination by intramuscular injection of a 15-methyl analog of prostaglandin $F_{2\alpha}$. Fertil Steril 27:104, 1976

68. Stubblefield PG, Naftolin F, Frigoletto FD et al: *Laminaria* augmentation of intraamniotic $PGF_{2\alpha}$ for midtrimester pregnancy termination. Prostaglandins 10:413, 1975

69. Stubblefield PG, Naftolin F, Lee EY et al: Combination therapy for midtrimester abortion: *Laminaria* and analogues of prostaglandin. Contraception 13:723, 1976

70. Stubblefield PG: Current technology for abortion. Curr Probl Obstet Gynecol 2:1, 1978

71. Burkeman RT, Atienza M, King TM, Burnett LS: The management of midtrimester abortion failures by vaginal evacuation. Obstet Gynecol 49:233, 1977

72. Propping D, Stubblefield PG, Golub J: Uterine rupture following midtrimester abortion by *Laminaria*, prostaglandin $F_{2\alpha}$ and oxytocin: report of two cases. Am J Obstet Gynecol 128:689, 1977

73. Waters JL, Hames M: Digoxin induction abortion. Paper presented at the 8th Annual Meeting of the National Abortion Federation, Los Angeles, CA, May 14, 1984

74. Borten M: Use of combination prostaglandin $F_{2\alpha}$ and hypertonic saline for midtrimester abortion. Prostaglandins 12:625, 1976

75. Kerenyi TD, Mandelaman N, Sherman DH: Five thousand consecutive saline abortions. Am J Obstet Gynecol 116:593, 1973

76. Burkeman RT, King TM, Atienza MF: Hyperosmolar urea. p. 107. In Berger GS, Brenner WE, Keith LG (eds): Second Trimester Abortion: Perspectives After a Decade of Experience. John Wright, PSG, Inc., Boston, 1981

77. Binkin NJ, Schulz KF, Grimes DA, Cates W Jr: Urea-prostaglandin versus hypertonic saline for instillation abortion. Am J Obstet Gynecol 146:947, 1983

78. Osathanondh R: Conception control. p. 480. In Ryan KJ, Barbieri R, Berkowitz RS (eds): Kistner's Gynecol-

ogy. 5th Ed. Chicago, Year Book Medical Publishers, 1989

79. Berger GS, Edelman DA: Oxytocin administration, instillation to abortion time, and morbidity associated with saline instillation. Am J Obstet Gynecol 121:941, 1975

80. Laureson NH, Schulman JD: Oxytocin administration in midtrimester saline abortion. Am J Obstet Gynecol 115:420, 1973

81. Kafrissen ME, Barke MW, Workman P et al: Coagulopathy and induced abortion methods: rates and relative risks. Am J Obstet Gynecol 147:344, 1983

82. Altman A, Stubblefield PG, Parker K et al: Midtrimester abortion by *Laminaria* and evacuation (L & E) on a teaching service: a review of 789 cases. Adv Plann Parent 16:1, 1981

83. Robbins J, Surrago EJ: Early midtrimester pregnancy termination: a comparison of dilatation and evacuation and intravaginal prostaglandin $F_{2\alpha}$. J Reprod Med 27:415, 1982

84. Kafrissen ME, Schulz KR, Grimes DA et al: A comparison of intraamniotic instillation of hyperosmolar urea and prostaglandin $F_{2\alpha}$ vs dilatation and evacuation for midtrimester abortion. JAMA 251:916, 1984

85. Hern WM: Serial multiple *Laminaria* and adjunctive urea in late outpatient dilatation and evacuation abortion. Obstet Gynecol 63:543, 1984

86. Hogue CJR, Cates W Jr, Tietze C: The effects of induced abortion on subsequent reproduction. Epidemiol Rev 4:66, 1982

87. Levin AA, Schoenbaum SC, Monson RR et al: The association of induced abortion with subsequent pregnancy loss. JAMA 243:2495, 1980

88. Linn S, Schoenbaum SC, Monson RR et al: The relationship between induced abortion and outcome of subsequent pregnancies. Am J Obstet Gynecol 146:136, 1983

89. Stubblefield PG, Monson RR, Schoenbaum SC et al: Fertility after induced abortion: a prospective follow-up study. Obstet Gynecol 63:186, 1984

90. Hogue CJR, Peterson WF: Late effects of late D & E. Paper presented at the National Abortion Federation Postgraduate Symposium on D & C. San Francisco, CA, Sept. 20, 1981

91. Stubblefield PG, Altman AM, Goldstein SP: Randomized trial of one versus two days of *Laminaria* treatment prior to late midtrimester abortion by uterine evacuation: a pilot study. Am J Obstet Gynecol 143:481, 1982

92. Behrman RE, Rosen TS: Report on viability and nonviability of the fetus. In: Research on the Fetus. 40 Federal Register 33528, August 8, 1975. Washington, DC, Department of Health, Education and Welfare, 1975

93. Dunn PM, Stirrat GM: Capable of being born alive? Lancet 8376:553, 1984

94. Hohler CW: Ultrasound estimation of gestational age. Clin Obstet Gynecol 27:314, 1984

95. Chervenak FA, Farley MA, Walters L et al: When is termination of pregnancy during the third trimester morally justifiable? N Engl J Med 310:501, 1984

96. Schirm AL, Trussell J, Menken J, Grady WR: Contraceptive failure in the United States: the impact of social, economic and demographic factors. Fam Plann Perspect 14:68, 1982

97. Stubblefield PG: Surgical techniques for first trimester abortion. p. 12. In Sciarra JJ, Zatuchni GI, Daly MJ (eds): Gynecology and Obstetrics. Vol. 6. Ch. 57. Harper & Row, Hagerstown, MD, 1982

SECTION 8
Legal and Ethical Issues in Perinatology

Legal and Ethical Issues in Perinatology

George J. Annas and Sherman Elias

Physicians have traditionally felt relatively comfortable in determining appropriate ethical conduct in health care practice, and there was little practical concern regarding legal liability. However, with rapidly expanding capabilities in diagnosis and treatment resulting from new technologies, modern physicians face numerous ethical dilemmas with uncertainty and confusion while practicing in a climate in which medical malpractice suits can threaten even the most competent and conscientious practitioner. Nowhere are these concerns more apparent than in medical practices and technologic innovations involving human reproduction.

No single chapter can address the myriad of ethical and legal controversies facing contemporary obstetric practice and research. Instead, we focus on selected controversial areas in which social policy is evolving: prenatal diagnosis and genetic counseling, forced cesarean section, abortion, fetal research, and the human genome initiative.

PRENATAL DIAGNOSIS AND GENETIC COUNSELING

Standards of medical practice have customarily been established by physicians on the basis of their best judgment of what constitutes good patient care. This tradition is endangered. The social structure of medical practice — cost containment, the profit motive, government regulations, fear of medical-malpractice suits, media hype, risk-management schemes, and other factors — may influence actual practice more than professional standards. Whether a prenatal screening test is offered may depend as much on the patient's health insurance and the physician's perception of possible legal liability as on the physician's view of the patient's welfare.[1]

There is widespread ethical, legal, and medical agreement that prenatal screening must be preceded by counseling about its purposes and followed by counseling about its results and their implications.[2] The patient's choice is the centerpiece of legitimate screening, and even when a screening test becomes "routine" this does not mean that it is routinely done, but rather that it is routinely offered to patients who may accept or reject it.

In the most recent (1989) edition of *Standards for Obstetric – Gynecologic Services,*[3] the Committee on Professional Standards of The American College of Obstetricians and Gynecologists clearly delineate the "standard of care" that obstetricians are expected to provide with respect to genetic counseling and prenatal diagnosis:

Genetic Counseling

The gynecologist should be alert to any indication of genetic disorders or conditions in a patient that might lead to birth defects in her offspring. Screening for genetic disorders begins with a careful evaluation of family medical history, drug use, and environmental factors. The physician should inquire about the outcome of previous pregnancies, mental retardation in family members, and known or suspected inherited or metabolic disease. Whenever possible, disorders should be diagnosed prior to pregnancy.

When a genetic disorder is suspected, the gynecologist should discuss with the patient the ways in which the genetic disorder may affect her health, her reproductive capabilities, or the development of her offspring. A couple with a suspected genetic abnormality should receive the information necessary for them to decide, based on the potential social, emotional, and economic consequences, whether to proceed with further investigation. The gynecologist may wish to refer patients with potential genetic disorders to qualified genetic counseling and evaluation centers.

Screening for Genetic Disorders

Antenatal screening for genetic disorders is an integral part of obstetric care. In some instances, indication of possible risks and appropriate diagnostic measures can be undertaken prior to pregnancy.

This history obtained during the initial evaluation should be reviewed to detect signs that suggest a risk of genetic disorders:

· Advanced parental age (mother 35 years of age or older at the expected time of delivery)

· Previous offspring with a chromosomal aberration, particularly autosomal trisomy

· Chromosomal abnormality in either parent, particularly a translocation

· Family history of a sex-linked condition

· Inborn errors of metabolism

· Neural tube defects

· Hemoglobinopathies

· Ancestry indicating risk for Tay-Sachs, beta-thalassemia, or alpha-thalassemia

Couples who have increased risks for producing abnormal offspring may undergo antenatal diagnostic studies after appropriate counseling.

The term "malpractice" refers to professional misconduct that embodies a failure to exercise reasonable prudence in carrying out professional duties. The purpose of the medical-malpractice lawsuit is to afford recovery for damages sustained as a result of a physician's failure to exercise ordinary and reasonable care in the diagnosis and treatment of a patient and to deter such conduct. To prevail in a malpractice action, the plaintiff must prove four elements: duty, breach, damages, and causation.[4]

In prenatal diagnosis cases in which the physician fails to inform the parents of the existence of a test applicable to their situation, negligently performs the test, fails to refer to a specialist who could perform the test, or inaccurately informs the couple about their risks of having an affected child, courts now almost universally permit the parents to sue their physician for depriving them of their right to make a decision about commencing or continuing a pregnancy. Such a lawsuit is sometimes termed a "wrongful birth" case. The rationale for permitting parents to recover damages in such a case is set forth in typical language by a Texas court:

It is impossible for us to justify a policy which at once deprives the parents of information by which they could elect to terminate the pregnancy likely to produce a child with a defective body, a policy which in effect requires that the deficient embryo be carried to full gestation until the deficient child is born, and which policy then denies recovery from the tortfeasor of costs of treating and caring for the defects of the child.[5]

We believe this policy conclusion is correct. Any woman who employs a physician for prenatal care should have the right to have the physician fully inform her of any reason the physician has to believe that her fetus might be handicapped and to inform her further of the existence of diagnostic tests that might identify the precise genetic condition. The physician incurs this duty to disclose because it is this type of information that the pregnant woman seeks prenatal care to discover (i.e., to learn all she can to help her have a healthy child). It is therefore entirely reasonable for the pregnant woman to expect her physician to appraise her of any relevant information regarding her fetus and options she might have so that she and the child's father can determine what action to take.[6]

A wrongful birth suit must allege and prove not only that the physician was negligent in the care of the pregnant woman, but also that had the negligent act not been done, the child would not have been born (e.g., had the woman been properly informed that she was at risk to have a child with Down syndrome, she could have sought amniocentesis or chorionic villus sampling and had an abortion if her fetus were so affected). A related, but far more controversial, lawsuit is brought by the child (through its parents or guardian) against the physician because it was born, a so-called "wrongful life" suit. Until recently, most courts rejected lawsuits by the child because they thought it was impossible to put a monetary value on life in an impaired condition compared with nonexistence. The choice for these children is *never* to be born healthy, but only to be born with a handicap (such as Down syndrome or Tay-Sachs disease) or not to be born at all. We think that future courts are likely to limit such actions to *serious* handicaps, those in which fetuses, if they could speak to us (which, of course, they can only do through their parents), would agree with an "objective societal consensus" that their own best interests would be served if they were aborted. Put another way, they would be better off *from their own perspective* if they never existed. Cases like deafness and Down syndrome would not qualify, whereas cases like Tay-Sachs would. Measuring damages *is* problematic, but courts are likely to award at least the added medical costs caused by the handicap itself. However, because medical costs can be recovered in a wrongful birth case directly, wrongful life cases are only likely to be brought in those rare instances in which for some reason (e.g., the child has been given up for adoption) the parents have lost the right to sue on their own behalf.[7] The following conclusions may be drawn regarding the legal and ethical obligations of the obstetrician in relationship to genetic counseling and prenatal diagnosis.

First, the law requires physicians to give accurate information to the parents and forbids the withholding of vital information from them. These principles are consistent with the doctrine of informed consent and the reasonable expectations of pregnant women under a physician's care.[8] The physician does not guarantee a healthy child, but the reasonable expectation of the patient is that she will be apprised of any information the physician has that the child might be handicapped and of the alternative ways to proceed so that the patient can determine what action to take.[6]

Second, no obstetrician can be required to perform chorionic villus sampling or genetic amniocentesis. Indeed, many are not qualified to perform these procedures and for them to do so may itself be malpractice. As stated in an opinion of the Judicial Council of the American Medical Association[9]:

Physicians who consider the legal and ethical requirements applicable to genetic counseling to be in conflict with their moral values and conscience may choose to limit such services to preconception diagnosis and advice or not provide any genetic services. However, there are circumstances in which the physician who is so disposed is nevertheless obligated to alert prospective parents that a potential genetic problem does exist, that the physician does not offer genetic services, and that the patient should seek medical genetic counseling from another qualified specialist.

Third, genetic counseling should be nondirective, that is, the counselor should remain impartial and objective in providing information that will allow competent counselees to make their own informed decision. The Judicial Council of the American Medical Association[9] has given the following opinion:

Physicians, whether they oppose or do not oppose contraception, sterilization, or abortion, may decide that they can engage in genetic counseling and screening, but should avoid the imposition of their personal moral values and the substitution of their own moral judgment for that of the prospective parents. The ethical and moral decisions have to be made by the family and should not be imposed by the physician.

Fourth, to ensure the patient's interest in both autonomy and privacy, no information obtained in genetic counseling or screening should be disclosed to any third party, including insurers and employers, without the patient's informed consent.[10,11] Such strict nondisclosure policies should be maintained unless and until specific legislation is enacted that would clearly delineate the circumstances in which confidentiality must be breached, analogous to certain contagious diseases, gunshot wounds, and child abuse. On the other hand, counselors should be permitted to attempt to persuade patients to allow them to make disclosures of important information to potentially affected relatives if there is a high probability of serious harm and if the disclosure is limited to pertinent genetic information. We recommend that the genetic counselor make clear, both verbally and in writing, the policy that he or she follows so that the patient can refuse to be screened or counseled if he or she is not in agreement with the disclosure policy. Such agreements will serve to heighten the public's confidence in genetic counseling and will encourage people to participate voluntarily in both screening and counseling.

FORCED CESAREAN SECTIONS

In 1979 a group of Israeli obstetricians published a controversial article entitled "The fetal right to live," suggesting that when women in labor refuse cesarean section, "It is probably that the patient hopes to be freed in this way of an undesired pregnancy . . . because it is an unplanned pregnancy, the woman is divorced or widowed, the pregnancy is an extramarital one, there are inheritance problems, etc." [12] The view that women who refuse cesarean sections are in some way willfully abusing their fetuses seems prevalent and deeply held, at least by some male obstetricians and judges. This opinion is reflected in several cases in which judges have ordered women who were refusing cesarean section during labor to undergo the procedure "for the welfare of the unborn child."

In 1987, Kolder et al.[13] reported a U.S. national survey that showed that court orders have been obtained for cesarean sections in 11 states, for hospital detentions in 2 states, and for intrauterine transfusions in 1 state. Among 21 cases in which court orders were sought, the orders were obtained in 86 percent; in 88 percent of those cases, the orders were received within 6 hours. The majority of the women involved were black, Asian, or Hispanic, and all were poor. Nearly one-half were unmarried and one-fourth did not speak English as their primary language. In the survey they also found that 46 percent of the heads of fellowship programs in maternal–fetal medicine thought that women who refused medical advice and thereby endangered the life of the fetus should be detained. Forty-seven percent supported court orders for procedures such as intrauterine transfusions. Until 1990, with the exception of one case in the Georgia State Supreme Court, all cases had been decided by lower courts and therefore had little precedential importance.[14] In the vast majority of cases, judges were called on an emergency basis and ordered interventions within hours. The judge usually went to the hospital. Physicians should know what most lawyers and almost all judges know: when a judge arrives at the hospital in response to an emergency call, he or she is acting much more like a lay person than a jurist. Without time to analyze the issues, without representation for the pregnant woman, without briefing or thoughtful reflection on the situation, in almost total ignorance of the relevant law, and in an unfamiliar setting faced by a relatively calm physician and a woman who can easily be labeled "hysterical," the judge will almost always order whatever the doctor advises. There is nothing in *Roe v. Wade*[15] or any other appellate decision that gives either physicians or judges the right to favor the life or well-being of the fetus over that of the pregnant woman. Nor is there legal precedent for a mother being ordered to undergo surgery (e.g., kidney or partial liver transplant) to save the life of her dying child. It would be ironic and inconsistent if a woman could be forced to submit to more invasive surgical procedures for the sake of a fetus than a child. Forcing pregnant women to follow medical advice also places unwarranted faith in that advice. Physicians often disagree about the appropriateness of obstetric interventions, and they can be mistaken.[16] In three of the first five cases in which court-ordered cesarean sections were sought, the women ultimately delivered vaginally and uneventfully.[2] In the face of such uncertainty—uncertainty compounded by decades of changing and conflicting expert opinion on the management of pregnancy and childbirth—the moral and legal primacy of the competent, informed pregnant woman in decision making is overwhelming.[17]

Physicians may feel better after being "blessed" by the judge, but they should not. First, the appearance of legitimacy is deceptive; the judge has acted injudiciously, and there is no opportunity for meaningful appeal. Second, the medical situation has not changed, except that more time has been lost that should have been used to continue discussion with the woman directly. And, finally, the physician has now helped to transform himself or herself into an agent of the state's authority.[17]

The question of how to help a woman who continues to refuse intervention in the face of a court order remains. Do we really want to attempt to restrain and forcibly medicate and operate on a competent, refusing adult? Although such a procedure may be "legal," it is hardly humane. It is not what one generally associates with modern obstetric care and may possibly cause harm. It also encourages an adversarial relationship between the obstetrician and the patient. Moreover, even from a strictly utilitarian perspective, this marriage of the state and medicine is likely to harm more fetuses than it helps, because many women will quite reasonably avoid physicians altogether during pregnancy if failure to follow medical advice can result in forced treatment, involuntary confinement, or criminal charges.

Extending notions of child abuse to "fetal abuse" simply brings government into pregnancy with few, if any, benefits and with great potential for invasions of privacy and massive deprivations of liberty. It is not helpful to use the law to convert a woman's and society's moral responsibility to her fetus into the woman's legal responsibility alone.[2] After birth, the fetus becomes a child and can and should thereafter be treated in its own right. Before birth, however, we can obtain access to the fetus only through its mother and, in the absence of her informed consent, can do so only by treating her as a fetal container, a nonperson without rights to bodily integrity.

The American College of Obstetricians and Gynecologists has issued an opinion from its Committee on Ethics entitled "Patient Choice: Maternal Fetal Conflict"[18] that we believe provides thoughtful and useful guidance for the medical practitioner. The conclusions of this statement are as follows:

1. With advances in medical technology, the fetus has become more accessible to diagnostic and treatment modalities. The maternal–fetal relationship remains a unique one, requiring a balance of maternal health, autonomy, and fetal needs. Every reasonable effort should be made to protect the fetus, but the pregnant woman's autonomy should be respected.

2. The vast majority of pregnant women are willing to assume significant risk for the welfare of the fetus. Problems arise only when this potentially beneficial advice is rejected. The role of the obstetrician should be one of an informed educator and counselor, weighing the risks and benefits to both patients as well as realizing that tests, judgments, and decisions are fallible. Consultation with others, including an institutional ethics committee, should be sought when appropriate to aid the pregnant woman and obstetrician in making decisions. The use of the courts to resolve these conflicts is almost never warranted.

3. Obstetricians should refrain from performing procedures that are unwanted by a pregnant woman. The use of judicial authority to implement treatment regimens in order to protect the fetus violates the pregnant woman's autonomy. Furthermore, inappropriate reliance on judicial authority may lead to undesirable societal consequences, such as the criminalization of noncompliance with medical recommendations. In 1990, the District of Columbia Court of Appeals, in a strongly worded opinion, essentially adopted the American College of Obstetricians and Gynecologists statement as law, holding that the decision of the pregnant woman must be honored in all but "extremely rare and truly exceptional" cases.[19]

ABORTION*

Feelings and opinions are strong and divided on both the 1973 U.S. Supreme Court decision on abortion in *Roe v. Wade*[15] (hereinafter referred to as *Roe*) and the Court's 1989 decision in *Webster v. Reproductive Health Services of Missouri* (hereinafter referred to as *Webster*),[21] which signals a retreat from *Roe*. Opinion polls on abortion since 1973 show that Americans are deeply ambivalent on the issue. A consistent majority of the public believes that abortion is immoral in most

*This section has been adapted from Annas,[20] with permission.

cases.[22,23] Nonetheless, overwhelming majorities believe that abortion should be available in cases of rape, incest, and severe genetic abnormality, and more than two-thirds of the public consistently say that although they believe abortion to be wrong or immoral, the ultimate decision should be made by a woman and her physician rather than by state legislatures.[22,23]

Physicians' opinions seem to mirror those of society in general. A 1985 survey of 1,300 members of the American College of Obstetricians and Gynecologists found that 90 percent believed that the presence of fetal abnormalities was a legitimate reason for first-trimester abortions, and 84 percent thought it justified second-trimester abortions; fewer believed that abortion was justified by considerations of the woman's physical health (75 percent), rape or incest (68 percent), the woman's mental health (56 percent), economic difficulties (36 percent), and personal choice (36 percent).[2] Only about 25 percent of the public and 35 percent of obstetricians and gynecologists support "elective" abortions for whatever reason a woman may have.[2]

Physicians should know more than the public about *Roe* and *Webster,* because, whatever one's position on the morality of abortion, it has become the most commonly performed surgical procedure in the United States over the past two decades. The availability of abortion also partly justifies other common medical procedures, such as amniocentesis and chorionic villus sampling. Physicians have a central role in counseling pregnant women about their health and the health of their fetuses, and any criminal restrictions state legislatures are allowed to place on the exercise of that role may also be placed on other medical procedures. This section describes the state of the law since *Roe* was decided and the changes presaged by *Webster.*

Roe v. Wade

In *Roe* and all the abortion cases that followed it (other than those concerning government financing of abortion), the Supreme Court has reviewed criminal statutes designed to limit access to abortion. In *Roe,* a Texas statute made it a crime to procure an abortion or to attempt one, except to save the life of the mother. Justice Harry Blackmun, former legal counsel to the Mayo Clinic, wrote the opinion of the Court. One of his major goals was to prevent the

government from interfering with the practice of medicine and the doctor–patient relationship.[24]

The decision was seven to two, with Justices William Rehnquist and Byron White dissenting. Building on a series of cases, including a leading case that dealt with contraception[25] and described a "right to personal privacy, or a guarantee of certain areas or zones of privacy," the Court determined that a fundamental right of privacy existed "in the Fourteenth Amendment's concept of personal liberty and restrictions upon state action." The Court held that this fundamental right "is broad enough to encompass a woman's decision whether or not to terminate her pregnancy":

The detriment that the State would impose upon the pregnant woman by denying this choice altogether is apparent. Specific and direct harm medically diagnosable even in early pregnancy may be involved. Maternity, or additional offspring, may force upon the woman a distressful life and future. Psychological harm may be imminent. Mental and physical health may be taxed by child care. . . . All these are factors the woman and her responsible physician necessarily will consider in consultation.[15]

The Court, however, stopped short of declaring that a woman's right to an abortion was absolute or that she had a right to abortion on demand. Instead, the Court recognized that the state also had interests that might at times be "compelling" enough to limit abortion. The Court identified two such interests: the protection of maternal health and the protection of viable fetuses. The protection of maternal health has always been a legitimate interest of the state. The court ruled, however, that this interest could never be compelling enough to prohibit abortion before the state of pregnancy when it is less dangerous for the woman to carry the fetus to term than to have an abortion (which in 1973 was about the end of the first trimester). The Court decided that during the first trimester the state could regulate abortions to protect the woman's health only by requiring that they be performed by a physician. Thereafter it could regulate abortions to protect women only in ways reasonably calculated to enhance their personal health, rather than in ways designed to protect the fetus or simply to discourage abortions.

The second state interest the Court identified was

that of "protecting the potentiality of human life." The Supreme Court did not decide that a fetus is not human, only that a fetus is not a "person" as that term is used in the Fourteenth Amendment. The Court also noted that "the pregnant woman cannot be isolated in her privacy"; her interests in privacy must be weighted against the state's interest in the life of the fetus. The question is, when does the state's interest become sufficiently compelling that the state can justifiably interfere with a woman's constitutional right to have an abortion? No satisfactory answer to this question can be garnered from science, and any demarcation in the pregnancy, whether it be conception, implantation, quickening, or viability, is inherently arbitrary.[2] The Court decided to choose the point of fetal viability—the point at which the fetus "is potentially able to live outside the mother's womb, albeit with artificial aid"—as the demarcation, apparently because at this point the fetus is biologically identical to a premature infant.

After fetal viability, which continues to be near the end of the second trimester, the state "may, if it chooses, regulate, and even proscribe, abortion except where it is necessary, in appropriate medical judgment, for the preservation of the life or health of the mother."[15] Although states can regulate abortions after the point of fetal viability (or, more accurately, can restrict the induction of premature birth), since *Roe* only 13 states have enacted laws to restrict such abortions.[26]

Decisions After *Roe v. Wade*

In more than a dozen major cases over the last 15 years, the Supreme Court has applied *Roe* to specific attempts by some states to limit abortion rights during the first and second trimesters. Until 1989, the Court consistently struck down almost all such limitations. The Court did find it constitutional, however, for the state and federal governments to refuse to fund abortions through the Medicaid program, because in the Court's view the failure to finance abortions did not place a governmentally created obstacle in the path of a woman who wanted to terminate her pregnancy.[27] The Court has also ruled that states could properly mandate general informed-consent requirements, confidential record-keeping and reporting related to maternal health, pathologic examination of fetal tissue, and the presence of a second physician when a pregnancy was terminated after the

point of viability.[2] In the Court's view, none of these requirements limit a woman's ability to choose an abortion or a physician's ability to perform one. Regulations that the Court has rejected as unconstitutional under *Roe* include those giving the husband or father a veto over the woman's decision, requiring that specific and detailed information concerning fetal development be given to the woman, and mandating hospitalization.[2] By the mid-1980s the Court had made the precise contours of *Roe* very clear.[28]

Perhaps because the Supreme Court has been so consistent in upholding and expanding the right recognized in *Roe*, opposition to it continues. In the 1980s a candidate's position on abortion rights became the litmus test in judicial appointments. Under President Ronald Reagan, who said he considered abortion "murder," judges were appointed to the U.S. Supreme Court who were openly opposed to the *Roe* decision. By 1989, three Reagan appointees, Sandra Day O'Connor, Antonin Scalia, and Anthony Kennedy, had joined the two dissenters in *Roe*, who were still on the Court; thus the possibility that a five-justice majority might retreat from or overrule *Roe* first appeared. Both sides in the abortion-rights debate were therefore hopeful or fearful of the Court's decision in *Webster*, and more friend-of-the-court briefs were filed in that case than in any other in the history of the United States.

The *Webster v Reproductive Health Services of Missouri* Decision

In delivering its July 1989 opinion in *Webster*, the Supreme Court reopened the national debate about the proper role of state governments in determining when abortions may take place within their borders, although technically the Court made no changes in *Roe* at all.[20] At issue in *Webster* was a Missouri abortion statute that had 20 provisions. Because of the way the case was argued, the Court ruled on only three of them. The Court ruled that Missouri could constitutionally prohibit state-employed physicians from performing an abortion that was not necessary to save the life of a woman, could prohibit such an abortion from being performed in state facilities, and could require physicians to try to determine fetal viability at or after 20 weeks gestation.

None of these statutory restrictions are inconsistent with *Roe*, although the first two, like the earlier Medicaid-funding decisions, will make it more difficult for poor women to obtain abortions. If this technical holding had been the only result of the case, it would have occasioned almost no comment. The case is important because five of the justices, writing three separate opinions, made it clear that they no longer believe the quasi-trimester scheme of *Roe* to be tenable, and four of them are ready to permit states to regulate heavily, and perhaps even prohibit outright, most abortions at any point in pregnancy.

Roe was based on two conceptual foundations: first, there is a fundamental constitutional right of privacy broad enough to encompass a woman's decision to have an abortion; and, second, the state's interests in abridging the exercise of this right are related to the stage of pregnancy. The plurality opinion in *Webster* (on which only three justices agreed) ignored the right of privacy altogether. Although the scope of the constitutional right of privacy was the issue on which most friends of the court argued this abortion case, physicians should be pleased that the Court did not seek to limit that right in areas other than abortion. As the American Medical Association properly noted in its own brief on *Webster,* the constitutional right of privacy "simply reflects the historic tradition, embodied in our common law, of recognizing that all medical treatment decisions ordinarily should be made by the patient, after consultation with a physician concerning the risks and benefits of treatment." [29]

Instead the plurality concentrated exclusively on *Roe's* trimester scheme. The plurality said, for example, that "the key elements of the *Roe* framework — trimesters and viability — are not found in the text of the Constitution." [21] The plurality concluded that rather than having to balance the rights of the individual and the interests of the state, states have a compelling interest "in protecting human life throughout pregnancy." If this is true, of course, then the fact that women have a fundamental constitutional right to decide to have an abortion does not help them in a state that outlaws abortion to protect fetal life, since compelling state interests outweigh the rights of the individual.

Four justices indicated that they would uphold any restriction on abortion that "permissibly further[s] the State's interest in protecting potential human life." Four others would continue to uphold the balance required by *Roe.* The ninth, Justice O'Connor, can now create a five-to-four majority by joining either side of the debate. She had indicated her displea-

sure with the trimester scheme before *Webster* was decided, and she had suggested that the Court determine the constitutionality of state abortion laws on the basis of whether they "unduly burden" a woman's right to an abortion. [30] But because she believed that the three provisions of the Missouri law were consistent with *Roe,* she refused to use *Webster* to reverse or restrict *Roe.* This is why constitutional law regarding abortion remains the same after *Webster* as it was before. On the other hand, one more change in the Supreme Court's membership, or a shift in Justice O'Connor's thinking, may result in the reversal of *Roe* and the granting of wide powers to state governments to restrict abortions.

What does all this mean to physicians? As a matter of medical practice, *Webster* applies only to physicians practicing in Missouri and in the future to physicians in states that decide to restrict abortions the way Missouri already has. In Missouri now, physicians employed by the state cannot perform any abortion that is not necessary to save the life of the pregnant woman, and no one (whether a state employee or not) can perform any abortion in state facilities that is not necessary to save the life of the pregnant woman. Both sides of the abortion debate agree, however, that in practice the *Webster* opinion has had almost no impact in Missouri, primarily because the 1986 statute that the Court was reviewing had already succeeded in drastically curtailing the number of abortions performed in public hospitals. [31] One part of the law that the Court did not review was its preamble. It says in part that the Missouri legislature finds that "the life of each human being begins at conception . . . [and] unborn children have protectable interests in life, health and well-being." The Court found that this preamble had not yet been used to limit access to abortion and decided that until it was applied in some concrete way, ruling on its constitutionality would be premature. Since *Webster,* however, the preamble has been used to defend antiabortion demonstrators against charges of trespass in front of Planned Parenthood clinics with the argument that the trespassing was justified because it was necessary to save the lives of unborn babies. [31]

For physicians in other states, *Webster* means that if their legislatures pass statutes with substantially identical provisions, they will be bound by them. It also means that a majority of the Supreme Court, for the first time in two decades, is willing to discuss abortion rights without reference to the rights of individual women or the rights of their physicians. This could have implications for birth-control measures other than abortion that act after fertilization, as well as for other areas of medical practice, such as the patient's right to refuse treatment. For example, in a case substantially identical to the Karen Ann Quinlan case (a young woman in a persistent vegetative state whose parents sought to have her ventilator removed on the grounds that she would not have wanted it used under these circumstances),[32] the United States Supreme Court ruled that the parents of Nancy Cruzan, a young woman in a persistent vegetative state, could not refuse further feeding by gastrotomy tube on her behalf, based in large part on the preamble to Missouri's abortion statute that the Missouri Supreme Court held evidenced the state's "unqualified" interest in preserving "life."[33]

Thus the abortion debate has been returned to the political arena, where it has been consistently impossible to resolve. In states that decide to add restrictions on abortion, physicians and their pregnant patients will find their medical and moral options sharply limited. The central question in the continuing debate about abortion is whether personal medical care decisions should be made by patients and their physicians or by the state. Obviously, the state can regulate medical practice. But to do so in a manner as intrusive as pre-*Roe* antiabortion statutes requires more than a speculative and hotly controverted moral interest. Legitimate medical regulation generally requires reference to the safety, efficacy, or cost of the procedure at issue. The moral views of a majority of society should be insufficient to overcome the freedom of physicians and their patients to make their own moral decisions in areas that have a life-changing impact on individuals. Physicians and patients have a unity of interest in defending and promoting the right of privacy that protects decision making in the doctor–patient relationship from irruptive interference by the state.[34]

FETAL RESEARCH

Federal Regulations

Society has a critical stake in both the treatment of fetal disorders and the maintenance of respect for the human dignity of the fetus. Fetal research and its regulation is one of the most controversial and complex areas in the entire field of human experimentation. The National Commission for the Protection of Human Subjects of Biomedical and Behavioral Research, for example, spent the first year of its existence working on the subject of fetal experimentation under a congressional mandate to make recommendations regarding fetal research before working on any other topic. This mandate itself was most influenced by the 1973 *Roe* decision discussed above. The consequence of this decision was an increase in the number of fetuses aborted; hence the amount of fetal material available for research also increased.

Before experimentation involving human fetuses begins, current U.S. Department of Health and Human Services (HHS) regulations require that appropriate animal studies be performed and that investigators play no role in any decision to terminate a pregnancy. The purpose of any in utero experiment must be to meet the health needs of the particular fetus, and the fetus must be placed at risk only to the minimum extent necessary to meet such needs. In the case of nontherapeutic research, the risk to the fetus must be "minimal" and the knowledge must be "important" and not obtainable by other means. The consent of both the mother and father is required, unless the father's identity is not known, he is not reasonably available, or the pregnancy resulted from rape. Fetal research protocols must be approved by an institutional review board (IRB), taking special care to review the subject selection process and the method of obtaining informed consent.

Technically these federal regulations apply only to investigators who receive federal research funds or who are affiliated with institutions that have signed an agreement with HHS that all research performed in their institution and by their staff will be approved by an IRB under these regulations. We believe, however, the principles set forth by these regulations to be so fundamentally important to the protection of the integrity of the fetus, the potential parents, and the research enterprise itself that they provide the minimum guidelines that should be adhered to voluntarily in all institutions undertaking fetal research projects.

State Statutes

More state legislation has been enacted regarding fetal research than any other type of research, and the poor quality of the legislation has added to the complicated nature of this issue. About one-half of the states currently have statutes regulating fetal research; 15 were passed soon after the *Roe* decision and in direct response to it.[15] Most state statutes restrict both in utero and ex utero research, and the restrictions are generally more stringent than the federal regulations with the exception of New Mexico's statute, which is modeled after federal regulations. In Massachusetts, for example, it is a crime to study the fetus in utero unless the research does not "substantially jeopardize" the life or health of the fetus and the fetus is not the subject of an elected abortion. Thus therapeutic research, such as shunting procedures to treat fetal urinary tract obstruction, is permissible even in this restrictive state. Utah, the only state to deal exclusively with in utero fetuses, prohibits all research on "live unborn children." Some states limit their prohibition to the living abortus and thus do not apply to fetal surgery. California restricts experimentation only on ex utero fetuses, outlawing "any type of scientific or laboratory research or any other kind of experimentation or study, except to protect or preserve the life and health of the fetus." Thus there is little consistency or rationale among jurisdictions regarding regulations directly pertaining to fetal research. Nonetheless, one is bound by the laws of the state in which one performs fetal research, and knowledge of its provisions is obviously necessary in states that have such statutes.[35–37]

Consent

A fundamental premise of Anglo-American law is that no one can touch or treat a competent adult without the adult's informed consent. This doctrine is based primarily on the value we place on autonomy, or self-determination, and secondarily on rational decision making. The first requires that individuals have the ultimate say concerning whether their bodies will be "invaded"; the latter requires disclosure of certain material information, including a description of the proposed procedure, risks of death and serious disability, alternative, success rates, and problems of recuperation before one is asked to consent to an "invasion."[38]

These issues are relatively straightforward when dealing with an adult, but how do they apply when experimentation or therapy is directed toward a fetus? Unfortunately, the distinction between experimentation and therapy is often unclear. In general,

therapy involves procedures performed primarily for the benefit of the patient that are considered "good and accepted practice," whereas experimentation involves new or innovative procedures not yet considered standard practice performed for the primary purpose of testing a hypothesis or gaining new knowledge.[39]

In the therapeutic setting, the consent of either one of the parents is usually sufficient for beneficial procedures to be performed on children. In the case of the fetus, however, if the proposed investigative therapeutic procedure will place the mother at any risk of death or serious disability, she alone has the right to consent and the corresponding right to withhold consent. Even after fetal viability, *Roe* gives the woman and her physician the right to terminate the pregnancy if her life or health is endangered. This is consistent with the Court's ruling that where conflict exists between a potential father and the pregnant woman over the issue of an abortion, the woman's position should prevail because she has more at stake (e.g., her body, health, risks) than the potential father.[40] The same logic applies here. Consent of the pregnant woman is a mandatory prerequisite for both investigative procedures and therapy. Her consent must be informed, and she should be told as clearly as possible about the proposed experimental procedure or therapy and its risks to herself and her fetus, as well as alternatives, success rates, and the likely problems of recuperation.[41]

Use of Fetal Tissue for Transplantation

Over the past several years considerable scientific, ethical, and legal controversy has arisen over the use of human fetal tissue for transplantation. The rationale for using fetal tissue is that it may be less likely to be rejected and that it may further differentiate to take over the function of diseased or injured tissues. If successful, fetal tissue transplants could play a major role in the treatment in a number of conditions including degenerative neurologic diseases, diabetes mellitus, and hematologic and immune disorders. The most notable example of using human fetal tissue for transplantation has been for the treatment of Parkinson's disease. Such grafting of fetal brain tissue into patients with Parkinson's disease was first performed in Mexico[42] and Sweden,[43] with the Swedish researchers reporting "no improvement of therapeutic value" in their two patients observed up to 6 months postoperatively. In December 1988 the American Academy of Neurology urged "great caution in expanding the current human experience except as research conducted in highly specialized centers." [44]

Current federal regulations permit the use of tissue from dead fetuses in experimental transplantation when it is conducted in accordance with state law. [45] All except eight states (Arizona, Arkansas, Illnois, Indiana, Lousiana, New Mexico, Ohio, and Oklahoma) permit such experiments. [45] Nonetheless, ethical concerns remain, and there has been continued political resistance to funding such research with government money. Ethical issues cannot be resolved by a vote of experts, but expert panels and committees can help to define and clarify issues publicly and to build a consensus. They also serve to take the political heat off elected officials with respect to controversial issues, a relevant factor in whether public funding is approved. [46]

The most recent series of disputes on fetal tissue transplants began in October 1987, when the National Institutes of Health (NIH) submitted a request to the assistant secretary for health in which the NIH sought approval to fund the transplantation of human fetal tissue into the brain of a patient with Parkinson's disease. In March 1988, the assistant secretary asked that the NIH establish a special advisory panel to study 10 questions about fetal-tissue research. And in May 1988, a moratorium was announced on the use of fetuses from elective abortions in federally funded research.

The 21-member Human Tissue Fetal Transplant Research Panel subsequently created by the NIH invited more than 50 people, including the representatives of 16 various groups, to present their views in public sessions. On December 5, 1988, the panel finalized its report, [47] and on December 14, 1988, the advisory committee to the NIH director adopted it unanimously. Wisely, the panel separated questions concerning the use of fetal tissue from those involving abortion — a legally and ethically appropriate move, but one that has ultimately proven politically untenable.

The panel's task was somewhat simplified by its decision to limit discussion to the use of tissue from dead fetuses and by its rejection of any intrafamilial donations or payment for fetal tissue — rulings consistent with an October 1988 amendment to the National Organ Transplant Act. The panel concluded that although it was of "moral relevance" that the fetal tissue be obtained from an induced abortion (rather than a spontaneous abortion or an interrupted ectopic pregnancy), the use of the tissue in research was "acceptable public policy" because "abortion is legal and . . . the research in question is intended to achieve significant medical goals." [47] This conclusion was accepted by a vote of 15 to 2, and included recommendations that the decision to abort be kept independent of the decision to retrieve and use fetal tissue, that recipients be informed of the tissue's fetal origins, and that fetal tissue be accorded the same respect given other cadaveric human tissue. [47]

In answer to the remaining questions, the panel adopted the following recommendations: the decision to abort must be made before the use of the tissue is discussed; anonymity should be maintained between donor and recipient; the timing and method of the abortion should not be influenced by the potential use of the fetal tissues; and the consent of the pregnant woman is necessary and sufficient for the use of tissue unless the father objects. [47] The panel also concluded that "there is sufficient evidence from animal experimentation to justify proceeding with human clinical trials in Parkinson disease and juvenile diabetes." [47] Many of these recommendations were adopted unanimously, and no more than two panel members dissented from any of them. The most illuminating part of the report, however, was not its bland prose, but the dissent and the responses it evoked, because these exchanges encapsulated the national debate.

In their dissent, attorney James Bopp and Professor James Burtchaell argued that research with fetuses aborted electively is "ethically compromised" by the lack of authentic informed consent, the incentives it offers for more abortions, and its complicity with the abortion. [47] The consent issue involves the standard argument that a woman who decides to abort her fetus forfeits all rights and interests in the fetus and its remains. [47,48] The incentive argument posits that many women are ambivalent about abortion, and that such ambivalence may be tipped in favor of abortion if the women are informed that some good may come of it.[47,49] The complicity argument, as stated by the dissenters, is primarily an emotional appeal based on an analogy to Nazi experimentation.

Professor John Robertson's response was joined by nine other panel members. He noted that a woman does not lose or forfeit all interest in an aborted fetus simply by choosing abortion. If she did, he said, this "would lead to a policy of using fetal remains without parental consent or to a total ban on fetal transplants."[43,47] The assertion that the number of abortions will increase is "highly speculative," and Robertson argued that even "some" increase in the number of abortions would not make fetal transplants unacceptable, because such logic would assume "that even a marginal increase in abortion should bar fetal tissue transplant research."[43,47] Robertson rejected the complicity argument completely, noting first that society's mere willingness to use the organs of persons killed in automobile accidents or murdered does not mean that society or transplant surgeons are accomplices in automobile accidents or murder. Finally, the Nazi analogy fails because those experiments were conducted on live, unconsenting patients, who suffered greatly from them, whereas research on fetal tissue involves only the dead remains of lawfully aborted fetuses, which cannot be harmed, and such research is done only with consent.[43,47] The dissenters' primary argument was that federal funding of fetal research would "institutionalize" governmental complicity with the "abortion industry"[43,47] — a superficially appealing claim, perhaps, except that the federal government already profits directly from those who perform abortions by taxing their earnings. While the panel was still deliberating, the White House sent draft regulations to the Secretary of HHS that proposed a prohibition of the use of federal funds in any research involving fetal tissues.[50] The new secretary, Louis Sullivan, told Congress during his confirmation hearings that he would study the panel's report before making a decision.[51] The primary argument against the use of fetal tissues for transplantation was that it might increase the number of abortions, and this argument alone apparently ultimately persuaded Assistant Secretary of Health, James O. Mason, to recommend to HHS Secretary Sullivan in late 1989 that the ban on federal funding

be extended.[47] Secretary Sullivan accepted this recommendation. The practical consequence is that fetal tissue *will* be used in transplant research, as embryos have been used before, but in an uncoordinated manner, without peer review or oversight by NIH, generally outside the arena of public debate, and in a way that is suboptimal from both a scientific and an ethical perspective.[52]

Those with serious misgivings about the use of dead fetal tissue are surely correct when they point out that dead fetuses cannot be equated with dead hamsters or human kidneys. Nonetheless, it is difficult to justify the use of the organs and tissues of dead children in transplantation without permitting the transplantation of tissue from dead fetuses.[52] Some who object may be reacting not to the use of the fetus, but to the role of the not-to-be mother, and it can be argued that the panel did not address this role adequately. Kathleen Nolan has argued that the image of the "devouring mother" is an especially powerful and destructive one in our view of women as mothers. In her words,

by allowing tissue retrieval, [these women] seem to "fail to protect" the dead fetus, letting it fall prey to the needs of others. Subliminally this threatens unconscious beliefs about the role of women as mothers. . . . No matter that the fetus is dead — mothers should still fend off the scavengers.[53]

The images of research physicians as scavengers and of mothers as indifferent to the fate of their deceased children are disturbing to many. But the fetus lacks the status of a child[54] and, after death, has no protectable interests of its own.[45] At the same time, like a dead adult, the dead fetus is not abandoned property and should be treated with respect because of what it is and what it symbolizes. The mother's real role, like that of any surviving relative, is not to "consent" to burial or the use of body parts in transplantation. Rather, as the next of kin, she has the legal authority to dispose of the body in the customary manner (usually burial or cremation) and to object to any use of the body inconsistent with such customs, because of the mental anguish that such nontraditional or disrespectful use of the body may cause her.[55] Treating fetal remains with "respect" may mean not putting the fetus on public display, but when the choices include burial, incineration, or use in legitimate research, the third can be as respectful of the remains as the first two.

A report of the Stanford University Medical Center Committee on Ethics entitled "The ethical use of human fetal tissue in medicine" [56] is fundamentally consistent with the report of the NIH panel. Together, these documents show wide agreement in the medical community on the major issues involved in the use of fetal tissue. One troubling difference must be noted, however. The Stanford report attempted to sidestep the issue of elective abortion by recommending that "if tissue from spontaneous abortions can satisfy the medical demands for both quantity and quality of tissue, it would be preferable to avoid the ethical problems of using induced abortions." The use of tissues from fetuses aborted spontaneously is particularly problematic. It is now well established that about one-half of such fetuses aborted in the first trimester and 20 percent of those aborted in the second trimester are chromosomally abnormal[57] (Ch. 21). Moreover, a variety of microorganisms have been associated with spontaneous abortions, including cytomegalovirus, herpes simplex types 1 and 2, rubella, toxoplasma, and *Ureaplasma urealyticum*.[58] It is indefensible to transplant abnormal or infected fetal tissue that could increase both the risk of a transplant failure and that of infection in the recipient. Tissue from spontaneously aborted fetuses should not be used for transplantation into a human subject.[52]

Both panels also skipped lightly over some practical issues, including how the abortion is performed. It is feasible, in fact, to remove the fetus whole with the concurrent use of ultrasound. If the use of fetal tissue proves therapeutic, there will be women willing to consent to such a procedure. If the abortion can be performed in a way that enhances the potential usefulness of the fetal tissue, without additional risk to the woman, there will also be tremendous pressure to adopt this technique. More discussion is needed of the choices a woman should be given with respect to the abortion procedure itself, as well as its timing.[52]

The relationship between the physician performing the abortion and the researcher also requires additional discussion. We believe that the woman should be asked about the use of her fetus as a source of tissue after she has decided to have an abortion but before the abortion has taken place. Afterward, she should be given an opportunity to withdraw her consent. After the physician has performed the standard inspection of the tissue to ensure that the abortion is complete, the tissue should be taken from the operating room and turned over to the researcher. The dissection of the tissues should be performed in a restricted facility designed to optimize the success of the procedure (e.g., a sterile environment and proper dissecting instruments). We would go beyond the recommendations of the Stanford report to suggest that to avoid any conflict of interest there should be no academic (such as coauthorship of publications or grant support) or other incentive for the physician performing the abortion or for anyone else involved in the woman's care to obtain her agreement for the use of fetal tissue.[52]

The primary objection to the use of fetal tissues from elective abortions appears to be a political one: if it were therapeutically successful, such use would create a new constituency—sick people who would benefit from such transplants and their families—that would be opposed to the prohibition of elective abortion. Of course, from a scientific and ethical standpoint, the central issue is whether it is reasonable to perform transplant experiments with fetal tissue at this time—a question neither panel attempted to examine in any depth. The politics of abortion have thus led us to focus on the tangential question of the tissue's source rather than on the central question of its benefits to sick people. The subjects of the proposed transplant research are not the fetuses (which are dead), but the tissue recipients.[52] It is clear that we have more scientific work to do, including work with animals, to help determine such things as cell survival, growth curves, and graft–host immunology.[59] It would be most beneficial to science and to the public if such experimentation could be confined to a few centers of established excellence, where careful research could be pursued until the safety and efficacy of such transplantations are demonstrated.[52]

Transplantation challenges our ethical precepts, and traditionally ethics have taken a back seat to the temptations and incentives to perform transplantations that are the first of their kind. Despite this, the public has generally applauded such transplantation, at least when it is seen as an attempt to save a life that otherwise would certainly have been lost. Transplantation involving fetal tissue is much more problematic, and the public may be less forgiving of ethical shortcuts. Saving a life is usually not at issue, and the source of the tissue, although not illicit, is troublesome to many. The world is watching, and this opportunity to demonstrate good science, good ethics, and compassionate patient care should not be wasted.[52]

THE HUMAN GENOME INITIATIVE

With what has been variously described as the "Manhattan project of biology," biology's Apollo Project, and the "holy grail of human genetics," plans to map and sequence the entire human genome have, within the span of only a few years, come into reality.[60-62] The NIH and the Department of Energy (DOE) are the two principal federal agencies conducting research on human or other complex genomes. The stated aim of the NIH program "is to produce a set of research tools, comprising both materials and information, that will be used to develop methods of diagnosing, treating, and preventing such disease." [63] On the other hand, the DOE has long supported work on human mutations, DNA damage, and DNA repair to better understand the health effects of radiation and of other harmful by-products of energy production. The DOE has stated:

Now it is clear that the ability to determine quickly and accurately the sequence of DNA is the most rapid and cost-effective way to assess DNA damage, and to protect the public health. Thus, the Department of Energy is poised for this initiative because of its research support and interest in human genetics, and its experience in developing large scale, long-term interdisciplinary projects. Development of these new technologies will place the United States in a commanding position in the biotechnology of the 21st century.[64]

In a deliberate effort to overcome earlier public impressions of rivalry between the two agencies, the NIH and DOE signed a joint memorandum of understanding in the fall of 1988. This memorandum established a joint scientific advisory commission and an interagency working group, both consisting of representatives from the two agencies. At the NIH an Office of Human Genome Research was created, and Nobel laureate James D. Watson (who, with Francis Crick, received the award for elucidating the double helix structure of DNA) was named its director. The

DOE recruited Charles Cantor, the co-inventor of pulsed-field gel electrophoresis, to head a genome center at the Lawrence Berkeley Laboratory. With research in "genomics" being conducted not only in the United States, but also throughout the world, especially in Europe and Japan, the Human Genome Organization (HUGO) was established in September 1988. The expressed purpose of HUGO is to help coordinate research and provide international training programs on relevant methodology; to arrange for exchange of relevant data, samples, and technology; to foster parallel studies in other organisms, such as mouse, and to coordinate animal studies with those on the human genome; and to provide public debate and develop guidelines on ethical, social, legal, and commercial implications of the human genome project.[65,66]

The scope of the human genome initiative is formidable—to map and sequence the 3 billion basepairs of the haploid complement (24 distinct chromosomes: 22 autosomes and X and Y). The chromosomes contain an unknown number of genes with estimates ranging from 50,000 to 100,000; it will be important to identify and localize all the genes. Presently only about 4,600 genes have been identified and only about 1,500 mapped to specific chromosomes and regions[67]; 600 or more have been cloned and sequenced.[68] What sequences of DNA turn genes on and off in correct coordinated fashion and at the right time will have to be elucidated. Moreover, the function of much of the DNA is unknown (sometimes called "junk" DNA); but inevitably it will be shown to have importance in light of the evolutionary conservatism its structure reveals.[66] Finally, the cost of the initiative will also be formidable: achieving the sequence is likely to take 15 years at a cost of $3 billion.[62]

Expectations for the outcome of human genome initiative have never been higher.[69] Some have even said that an international effort to sequence the human genome deserves enthusiastic support not only because it would be a great step in the fight against disease, but also because it would be a "contribution to peace." [70] However, those who are most knowledgeable and thoughtful about the human genome initiative, such as Victor McKusick, who was the first president of HUGO, are keenly aware that all knowledge is subject to misuse, and this initiative is by no means an exception.[66] Perhaps the most foreboding fears have been voiced by Jean Dausset, who warned that misuse of genetic information in the form of gene transfer experiments in early embryos could lead to "Nazi-like" atrocities,[71] and Clement Counts, who warned that "If, with a complete sequence map for human chromosomes, it will be possible to turn on the gene controlling resistance to some disease, will it not be equally possible to switch them off?" [60] Thus, as programs to map and sequence the human genome began to be initiated, scientists such as those attending the Workshop on International Cooperation for the Human Genome (Valencia, Spain, October 24–26, 1988) believed it important to proclaim that they recognized their responsibility to ensure that genetic information is used only "to enhance human dignity" and called for debate on the ethical, social, and legal implications of the use of genetic information.[71]

Although there have been numerous scientific meetings addressing technical and logistic aspects, there have been no forums dedicated to an in-depth exploration of the ethical, legal, and social issues raised by the human genome initiative. The most comprehensive statement related to the "social and ethical considerations" of the human genome initiative has been limited to only 10 pages of a 218 page report entitled *Mapping Our Genes — The Genome Projects: How Big, How Fast?*, published in 1988 by the Office of Technology Assessment of the United States Congress.[72] In this brief section, specific important questions were raised such as "What are the ethical considerations pertaining to control of knowledge and access to information generated by mapping and sequencing efforts? Who should have access to map and sequence information data banks? What facets, if any, of the human genome mapping and sequencing should be commercialized? What ethical concerns arise from possible eugenic applications of mapping and sequencing data?" However, there was no hint of what priorities should be awarded to these questions and what mechanisms could be used to address them effectively.

There are three basic levels of ethical and legal issues raised by the genome project[73]: family/individual level, societal level, and species level. The basic legal and ethical issues implicit in the human genome project are, on the individual level, the same issues involved in current genetic screening for various traits, such as carrier status for sickle cell and Tay-

Sachs disease.[74] Mapping and sequencing the human genome will likely lead to screening on an almost unimaginable scale, not only for certain diseases and traits, but also for tendencies toward certain diseases, such as cancer or manic depression. When all genetic traits can be deciphered in a genetic code (something that will require far more than a simple map of location), we will enter a new realm, taking not simply a quantitative step, but a qualitative one. Exactly what the consequences of such a step will be are not entirely foreseeable. There will be issues of information control and privacy. Employers, insurance companies, the military, and the government, among others, will want to have access to the information contained in the genome. Scientists may want such information restricted, but they will certainly have little influence over its use, as they had little influence over the use of the atomic bomb. Routine genetic screening will be easy to justify under present law (which already mandates newborn screening in most states, for example) in many settings. We are currently unprepared to deal with the issues of mandatory screening, confidentiality, privacy, and discrimination that the genome project poses.[73]

The societal level issues relate to population screening, commercialism, resource allocation, and to what is generally termed eugenics, the improvement of the species, either by weeding out genetic "undesirables" or by actually using genetic techniques (breeding or genetic engineering) to increase the number of desirable traits in offspring. Given the United States' sad history with involuntary sterilization and the Nazi campaign on sterilization that was at least partially influenced by it,[75] we are unlikely to engage in a direct program of sterilization. Nonetheless, eugenics has its supporters, and the European Parliament is right to be worried about the dangers of repeating history. It was our own U.S. Supreme Court, after all, that wrote in 1927, approving involuntary sterilization of the mentally retarded:

We have seen more than once that the public welfare may call upon the best citizens for their lives. It would be strange if it could not call upon those who already sap the strength of the State for these lesser sacrifices often noted to be such by those concerned, in order to prevent our being swamped with incompetence. It is better for all the world, if instead of waiting to execute degenerate offspring for crime, or to let them starve for their imbecility, society can prevent those who are manifestly unfit from continuing their kind.[76]

That may seem like ancient history, but in 1988 the U.S. Congress's Office of Technology Assessment, in discussing the "social and ethical considerations" raised by the Human Genome Project, used strikingly similar language:

Human mating that proceeds without the use of genetic data about the risks of transmitting diseases will produce greater mortality and medical costs than if carriers of potentially deleterious genes are alerted to their status and encouraged to mate with noncarriers or to use artificial insemination or other reproductive strategies.[72]

The primary reproductive strategy, mentioned only in passing in the report, will be genetic screening of human embryos — already technically feasible, but not nearly to the extent possible once the genome is understood. Such screening need not be required, people can be made to *want* it, even to insist on it as their right. As the Office of Technology Assessment notes, "New technologies for identifying traits and altering genes make it possible for eugenic goals to be achieved through technological as opposed to social control." [72]

The species level of concern relates to the fact that powerful technologies do not just change what human beings can do, they change the very way we think, especially about ourselves. As one example, the ability to screen embryos completely could lead to a market in "high-grade embryos" that could be bought and sold. They could also be gestated by contract or surrogate mothers and the resulting child delivered to the purchaser of the embryo. This could lead not only to putting a specific price on all human characteristics (e.g., height, intelligence, race, eye color), but also to viewing children as commodities that have no rights or interests of their own, but that exist to further the interests of parents and future societies. A gene-based view of humans could lead to a deterministic view of one's future — our fate determined by our genetic endowment. A map of the human genome could also lead to a more narrowly

focused view of a "normal" gene complement and of how much deviation we permit before considering any individual genome "abnormal," deviant, or diseased. We have not seriously begun to think about *how* to think about this issue, even though we know normalcy will be invented, not discovered.[73]

In conclusion, as U.S. Senator Albert Gore, chairman of the Subcommittee on Science, Technology and Space has said, "Those who are compiling the data that will provoke questions about these issues [related to the human genome initiative] have an obligation to help us develop a 'map' of the ethical and legal principles involved. At the moment, our legal system has no answer to them. It just shrugs its shoulders." [77] Ethics, law, and social policy formulation must become an *integral part* of the human genome initiative, rather than something tangential to or independent of it. This will make it much more likely that ethical, legal, and social issues will be adequately addressed and thus will enhance the likelihood that the human genome initiative will produce more good than harm. Attention to legal and ethical issues can no longer be viewed as a luxury, but must now be seen as a necessity.

REFERENCES

1. Elias S, Annas GJ: Routine prenatal genetic screening. N Engl J Med 317:1407, 1987
2. Elias S, Annas GJ: Reproductive Genetics and the Law. Year Book Medical Publishers, Chicago, 1987
3. ACOG: Standard for Obstetric–Gynecologic Services. 7th Ed. The American College of Obstetricians and Gynecologists, Washington, DC, 1989
4. Annas GJ: The Rights of Patients. Univ. of Southern Illinois Press, Carbondale, IL, 1989
5. *Jacobs v. Theimer*, 519 SW 2d 846,849 (Tex 1975)
6. Annas GJ, Coyne B: "Fitness" for birth and reproduction: legal implications of genetic screening. Family Law Q 9:463, 1975
7. Annas GJ, Elias S: Legal and ethical implications of fetal diagnosis and gene therapy. Am J Med Genet 35:215–218, 1990
8. Annas GJ: Medical paternity and "wrongful life." Hastings Center Rep 11:8, 1981
9. Recent opinions of the Judicial Council of the American Medical Association. JAMA 251:2078, 1984
10. Annas GJ: Problems of informed consent and confidentiality in genetic counseling. p. 111. In Milunsky A,

Annas GJ (eds): Genetics and the Law. Plenum Press, New York, 1976

11. President's Commissions for the Study of Ethical Problems in Medicine and Biomedical and Behavioral Research: Screening and Counseling for Genetic Conditions, Feb. 1983. Library of Congress No. 83-600502, U.S. Government Printing Office, Washington, DC

12. Lieberman JR, Mazor M, Chain W et al: The fetal right to live. Obstet Gynecol 53:515, 1979

13. Kolder VEB, Gallagher J, Parsons MT: Court-ordered obstetrical interventions. N Engl J Med 316:1192, 1987

14. Nelson LJ, Milliken N: Compelled medical treatment of pregnant women. JAMA 259:1060, 1988

15. *Roe v. Wade*, 410 U.S. 113, 1973

16. Notzon FC, Placek PJ, Taffel SM: Comparisons of national cesarean-section rates. N Engl J Med 316:386, 1987

17. Annas GJ: Protecting the liberty of pregnant patients. N Engl J Med 316:1213, 1987

18. ACOG Committee Opinion: Patient Choice: Maternal—Fetal Conflict. Number 55. The American College of Obstetricians and Gynecologists, Washington, DC, October 1987

19. *In Re A.C.*, 573 A. 2d 1235 (D.C. App. 1990)

20. Annas GJ: The Supreme Court, privacy, and abortion. N Engl J Med 321:1200, 1989

21. *Webster v. Reproductive Health Services*, 109 S. Ct. 3040 (1989)

22. Lamanna MA: Social science and ethical issues: the policy implications of poll data on abortion. p. 1. In Callahan S, Callahan D (eds): Abortion: Understanding Differences. Plenum Press, New York, 1984

23. Dionne EJ: Poll finds ambivalence on abortion persists in US. *New York Times.* August 3, 1989:A18

24. Woodward B, Armstrong S: The Brethren: The Inside Story of the Supreme Court. Simon and Schuster, New York, 1979

25. *Griswold v. Connecticut*, 381 U.S. 479 (1965)

26. Hunter ND: Time limits on abortion. p. 129. In Cohen S, Taub N (eds): Reproductive Laws for the 1990s. Humana Press, Clinton, NJ, 1989

27. *Harris v. McRae*, 448 U.S. 297 (1980)

28. Glantz LH: Abortion: a decade of decisions. p. 295. In Milunsky A, Annas GJ (eds): Genetics and the Law III. Plenum Press, New York, 1985

29. Brief of the American Medical Association, American Academy of Child and Adolescent Psychiatry, American Academy of Pediatrics, American College of Obstetricians and Gynecologists, American Fertility Society, American Medical Women's Association, American Psychiatric Association and American Society of Human Genetics as Amici Curiae in Support of Appellees, *Webster v. Reproductive Health Services,* No. 88-605, 1989

30. *Akron v. Center for Reproductive Health,* 462 U.S. 416 (1983) (O'Connor, dissenting)

31. Black C: Missouri abortion foes shift tactics in drive to shut down clinics. *Boston Globe,* September 10, 1989:20–21

32. In re Quinlan, 70 NJ 10, 355 A. 2d 647 (1976)

33. *Cruzan v. Missouri Dept. of Health,* 110 S. Ct. 2841 (1990)

34. Annas GJ, Glantz LH, Mariner WK: The right of privacy protects the doctor–patient relationship. JAMA 263:858–861, 1990

35. Annas GJ, Glantz LH, Katz BF: Informed Consent to Human Experimentation. Ballinger, Cambridge, MA, 1977

36. Friedman JM: The federal fetal experimentation regulations: an establishment clause analysis. Minn Law Rev 61:961, 1977

37. Brock EA: Fetal research: what price progress? Detroit Coll Law Rev 3:403, 1979

38. Annas GJ, Densberger JE: Competence to refuse medical treatment: autonomy vs. paternalism. 15 Toledo Law Rev 15:561, 1984

39. Annas GJ, Glantz LH, Katz BF: The Rights of Doctors, Nurses and Allied Health Professionals. Ballinger, Cambridge, MA, 1981

40. *Danforth v. Planned Parenthood,* 428 U.S. 52, 1976

41. Elias S, Annas GJ: Perspectives on fetal surgery. Am J Obstet Gynecol 145:807, 1983

42. Madrazo I, Leon V, Torres C et al: Transplantation of fetal substantia nigra and adrenal medulla to the caudate nucleus in two patients with Parkinson's disease. N Engl J Med 318:51, 1988

43. Lindvall O, Gustavii B, Astedt B et al: Fetal dopamine-rich mesencephalic grafts in Parkinson's disease. Lancet 2:1483, 1988

44. Lewin R: Caution continues over transplants. Science 242:1379, 1988

45. Robertson JA: Fetal tissue transplants. Washington Univ Law Q 66:443-98, 1988

46. Annas GJ, Elias S: The politics of transplantation of human fetal tissue. N Engl J Med 320:1079, 1989

47. Consultants of the Advisory Committee to the Director of the National Institutes of Health. Report of the human fetal tissue transplant panel. National Institutes of Health, Washington, DC, 1988

48. Burtchaell JT: University policy on experimental use of aborted fetal tissue. IRB 10(4):7, 1988

49. Bopp J: Use of fetal tissue will increase the number of abortions. *National Right to Life News.* November 17, 1988:4

50. Boffey PM. Aides at White House draft ban on use of fetal tissue. *New York Times.* September 9, 1988:A10

51. Tolchin M: Bush choice back for health chief after an apology. *New York Times.* February 24, 1989:12

52. Annas GJ, Elias S: The ethics of research using human fetal tissue. N Engl J Med 321:1069, 1989

53. Nolan K: *Genug ist genug:* a fetus is not a kidney. Hastings Cent Rep 18(6):13, 1988

54. Freedman B: The ethics of using human fetal tissue. IRB 10(6):1, 1988

55. *Strachan v. John F. Kennedy Memorial Hospital,* 538 A.2d 346 (N.J. 1988)

56. Greely HT, Hamm T, Johnson R et al: The Stanford University Medical Center Committee on Ethics: the ethical use of human fetal tissue in medicine. N Engl J Med 320:1093, 1989

57. Warburton D, Stein Z, Kline J, Susser M: Chromosome abnormalities in spontaneous abortion. p. 261. In Porter IH, Hook B (eds): Human Embryonic and Fetal Death. Academic Press, San Diego, 1980

58. Sever JL: Infectious cause of human reproductive loss. p. 169. In Porter IH, Hook B (eds): Human Embryonic and Fetal Death. Academic Press, San Diego, 1980

59. Sladek JR, Shoulson I: Neural transplantation: a call for patience rather than patients. Science 240:1386, 1988

60. Counts CL: Human genome sequencing. Science 235:1613, 1987

61. Roberts L: Genome project underway at last. Science 243:167, 1989

62. Roberts L: Genome mapping goal now in reach. Science 244:424, 1989

63. NIH Guide for Grants and Contracts 18:2, 1989

64. Report of the Human Genome Initiative for the Office of Health and Environmental Research. Prepared by the Subcommittee of Human Genome of the Health and Environmental Research Advisory Committee for the U.S. Department of Energy, Office of Energy Research, Office of Health and Environmental Research, April 1987

65. Marwick C, Merz B: Gene mappers form collaborations. JAMA 260:2477, 1988

66. McKusick VA: Mapping and sequencing the human genome. N Engl J Med 320:910, 1989

67. Paris Conference: Human Gene Mapping 9: Ninth International Workshop on Human Gene Mapping. Cytogenet Cell Genet 46:1, 1987

68. Schmidtke J, Cooper DN: A comprehensive list of cloned human DNA sequences. Nucleic Acids Res 16(Suppl 403):403 1988

69. Palca J: Interest in the human genome project reaches new heights. Nature 325:651, 1987

70. Noll H: Sequencing the human genome. Science 233:143, 1986

71. Roberts L: Carving up the human genome. Science 242:1244, 1988

72. U.S. Congress, Office of Technology Assessment: Mapping Our Genes—The Genome Projects: How Big, How Fast? Government Printing Office, Washington DC, 1988

73. Annas GJ: Who's afraid of the human genome? Hastings Cent Rep 19:19, 1989

74. Macklin R: Mapping the human genome: problems of privacy and free choice. p. 107. In Milunsky A, Annas GJ (eds): Genetics and the Law III. Plenum Press, New York, 1986

75. Proctor R: Racial Hygiene. Harvard University Press, Cambridge, MA, 1988

76. *Buck v. Bell,* 274 U.S. 200, 207, 1927

77. Merz B: Promising new technique may accelerate genome mapping. JAMA 262:2353, 1989

INDEX

Note: Page numbers followed by *f* indicate figures and those followed by *t* indicate tables.

A

Abdomen, acute, 684–687,
    685f–687f
Abdominal circumference, fetal
    in macrosomia, 339
    ultrasound for, 336f–338f,
        336–338
Abdominal wall
    fetal, ultrasound for, 344, 348f
    maternal, abscess after cesarean
        section in, 665f
    neonatal, defect in, 732
ABO incompatibility
    maternal isoimmunization in,
        978, 981
    Rh isoimmunization and,
        961–962
Abortion (spontaneous and elec-
    tive). *See also* Fetal
    wastage; Mortality.
    and amniocentesis, 280
    and chorionic villus sampling,
        282
    contraception, use as,
        1303–1304
    elective
        in breast cancer, 1203
        cervical incompetence due
            to, 858, 859
        clinic for, 1304
        in fetal anomaly, 367, 369
        legal and ethical considera-
            tions in, 367, 369
        subsequent reproduction
            and, 1326
        third trimester, 367, 369

after fetal death in utero,
    1326–1327
fetomaternal hemorrhage in,
    961
first-trimester, 1308–1319
    cervical dilatation in,
        1313–1314
        laminaria in, 1313
        prostaglandin analogues
            in, 1313–1314
    complications of, 1316–
        1319
        antibiotics for, 1319
        cervical lacerations as,
            1316
        cervical shock as, 1316
        continued pregnancy as,
            1318
        ectopic pregnancy as, 1318
        failed abortion as, 1318
        hematometra as, 1318
        hemorrhage in, 1318
        incomplete and septic
            abortion as, 1318–
            1319
        local anesthesia as, 1316
        perforation as, 1316–1318,
            1317f
        postabortal syndrome as,
            1318
        postabortal triad as, 1319,
            1319t
    implantation bleeding vs.,
        40–41
    medical means for,
        1314–1315

minisuction (menstrual regu-
    lation) in, 1308f–1313f,
    1308–1309
paracervical block in, 1310,
    1313
pathologic findings in, 787,
    788t
standard vacuum curettage,
    1309–1310,
    1313f–1314f
historical, 1304
indications for, 1305, 1307
    fetal, 1307t
    maternal, 1307t
legal, benefits of, 1305
legal aspects of, 1337–1341
    Roe v. Wade and, 1338–1339
    Webster v. Reproductive
        Health Services of
        Missouri and,
        1339–1341
maternal death due to, gesta-
    tional age and, 1304,
    1305t–1306t
Rh isoimmunization in,
    964–965, 965t
second-trimester, 1319–1327
    choices for, 1325–1326
    complications of, 1325
    definition of, 1319–1320
    D & E in, 1320–1323
        after 20 weeks, 1323
        anesthesia in, 1321
        cervical dilatation in,
            1320–1321
        procedure in, 1321–1322

Abortion (spontaneous and elective) *(Continued)*
  ultrasound in, 1322–1323
  uterine evaluation in, 1322
  vasopressin in, 1323
  gestational age limit for, 1327
  labor induction in,
      1323–1325
    hypertonic saline in,
        1324–1325
    intra-amniotic
        prostaglandins in, 1324
    intrauterine prostaglan-
        dins in, 1323–1324
    systemic prostaglandins in,
        1323
  need for, 1320
  techniques for, 1320–1323
  spontaneous
    alcohol consumption and, 800
    and alloimmune disease,
        798–800
    and anticardiolipin antibod-
        ies, 798
    and antifetal antibodies,
        797–798
    and autoimmune disease, 798
    and chromosomal abnormali-
        ties, 790–792, 791f,
        792t–793t
    cigarette smoking and, 800
    and congenital uterine
        anomalies, 795–796,
        796f
    diabetes mellitus in, 795, 796t
    and drug, chemical, noxious
        agents exposure,
        800–801
    evaluation in, 801–803
    genetic counseling in,
        789–790
    and incompetent cervix, 797
    and intrauterine infection,
        797
    and leiomyoma, 796
    missed, triploidy syndrome
        and, 53
    and Müllerian fusion defect,
        795–796, 796f
  and neural tube defect, 787
  pathologic findings in, 787,
      788t
  psychological factors and,
      801
  recurrence risks in, 790, 790t
  and recurrent aneuploidy,
      793, 793t
  and severe maternal illness,
      801
  statistics on, 790, 790t
  and systemic lupus erythe-
      matosus, 1154
  and trauma, 800
  and *Ureaplasma urealyticum*
      infection, 797
Abruptio placenta, 579–584
  blood transfusion in, 584
  in car seat belt injury, 686f, 687
  central venous pressure
      catheterization in, 584
  cesarean section in, 584
  in chronic hypertension, 1036
  coagulation defects and, 583
  concealed, 583
  delivery in, 584
  diagnosis and management of,
      582f, 582–584
  DIC in, 583–584
  in eclampsia, 1031–1032
  etiology of, 580–582, 581f
  external maternal trauma and,
      580, 581f
  gestational age and, 582–583
  grades of, 579–580
  hypertension and, 580
  incidence of, 580
  in polyhydramnios, 580
  in premature rupture of mem-
      branes, 864
  preterm fetus and, 583
  recurrence rate in, 580
  tocolytic therapy in, 583
  in twin delivery, 580
  ultrasound in, 582, 582f
Abscess
  abdominal wall, after cesarean
      section, 665f
  ischiorectal fossa, 12
Acardia, 898–899, 899f
Acetaminophen
  breast-feeding and, 319
  as potential teratogen, 314
Acid-base evaluation, fetal
  antepartum, 399
  base deficit and, 475, 476t
  blood collection in, 475–476
  blood sample processing in,
      476–477
  clinical applications of, 477
  in fetal stress, 478
  general principles of, 478–
      479
  heart rate and, 474, 474t, 475
  intrapartum, 474–477
  maternal acidosis and, 475
  1-minute Apgar score and, 486,
      486t
  5-minute Apgar score and, 486,
      486t
  respiratory gas values in, 475,
      475t
  serial determination of, 475,
      476f
  studies of outcome in, 485–486,
      486t
  umbilical cord blood-gas values
      in, 475, 475t, 477
  values for, 475
Acidemia, maternal, in eclampsia,
      1027
Acidosis, maternal
  in acute renal failure, 1093
  fetal acid-base evaluation and,
      475
  in massive blood transfusion,
      577–578
Acne, in pregnancy, 130
ACOG antepartum record,
      218f–221f, 222
Acquired immunodeficiency dis-
      ease (AIDS). *See*
      Human immunodefi-
      ciency virus (HIV).
Actin, molecular structure of, 153,
      153f
Activity, prenatal education about,
      224–225

Actomyosin
  cross-bridge formation and, 153–154, 154f
  molecular structure of, 153, 153f
  in myometrium, 152–154, 153f
  phosphorylation of, 154–156, 155f
Acute abdomen, 684–687, 685f–687f
Addison's disease, 1128
Adenohypophysis, 32f, 33
Adhesions, intrauterine, recurrent abortion due to, 795
Adrenal cortex, fetal
  growth of, 76f, 76–77
  placenta and, steroidogenesis by, 75–78, 76f–77f
Adrenal crisis, 1129
Adrenal gland
  fetal, normal physiology of, 111–112
  maternal, normal physiology of, 141
Adrenal insufficiency, 1128–1129
Adrenal steroids, fetal, parturition and, 49
α-Adrenergic blockade, in chronic hypertension in pregnancy, 1038
β-Adrenergic blockade, in chronic hypertension in pregnancy, 1038, 1039–1041
β-Adrenergic receptors, myometrial, in pregnancy, 158
β-Adrenergic stimulation, physiologic effects of, 843–844, 845f
Adrenocorticoids, 81–82
  function in pregnancy of, 82
  molecular structure of, 81, 81f
  origin of, 82, 82f
  variation during pregnancy of, 81–82
Adrenocorticotropic hormone (ACTH)
  fetal, production of, 111–112
  placental, 71
    function of, 71, 73f
    molecular structure of, 71

origins of, 71
Age
  gestational. See Gestational age.
  maternal
    chromosomal abnormalities, 276, 276t
    Down syndrome risks and, 276t
    eclampsia outcome and, 1030–1031
    intrauterine growth retardation and, 927
    prenatal counseling and, 212–213
    prenatal testing and, 284–285
  paternal, prenatal counseling and, 213
Agent Orange, birth defects and, 252–253
AIDS. See Human immunodeficiency virus (HIV).
Albumin, serum, in pregnancy, 127
Alcock's canal, 12, 13f
Alcohol abuse
  abortion and, 800
  in intrauterine growth retardation, 927
  prenatal counseling and, 213
  screening questionnaire for, 214t, 316t
Alcohol use
  breast-feeding and, 322
  as potential teratogen, 315f, 315–316, 316t
  as tocolytic, 854
Aldosteronism, primary, 1128
Alimentary tract, in pregnancy, 125–128
Alkaline phosphatase, serum, in pregnancy, 127
Alloimmune disease, and recurrent abortion, 798–799
Alphaprodine
  breast-feeding and, 319
  in labor, 499–500
Amenorrhea, lactational, 192, 193f–194f
Amethopterin, breast-feeding and, 318

Amino acids
  fetal metabolism of, 104
  maternal urinary excretion of, 133
  placental transfer of, 97, 98t
Aminoglycosides, as potential teratogens, 312–313
Aminophylline
  breast-feeding and, 319–320
  as potential teratogen, 308
Amniocentesis, 279–280
  accuracy of, 283–284
  bloody tap in, fetal complications of, 412
  fetal loss and, 280
  fetomaternal hemorrhage in, 961
  fluid color in, 280
  in intrauterine growth retardation, 937
  maternal cell contamination in, 283
  in multiple gestation, 280
  pitfalls of, 283–284
  in premature rupture of membranes, 865–867
  Rh isoimmunization in, 965, 965t
  safety in, 280
  technique in, 279–280
  third trimester, complications of, 412
  in twin gestation, 905–908
    indications for, 905–907
    technique in, 907f–908f, 907–908
Amnioinfusion, 477–478
  in fetal heart rate variability, 477–478
  in meconium in amniotic fluid, 478
Amnion, prostaglandin synthesis by, 163
Amnion nodosum, 57
Amniotic fluid
  bacteriostatic properties of, 1225
  bilirubin concentration in, in Rh isoimmunization, 966–968, 967f–968f

Amniotic fluid *(Continued)*
   embolism, 601, 603
      clinical signs of, 601
      in oxytocin-induced labor,
         451
      seizures in, 1190t
      treatment of, 603
   maximum vertical pocket of
      in intrauterine growth retar-
         dation, 928–929, 930f
      in prolonged pregnancy,
         952–953
      technique for, 339–340
   meconium in. *See also*
         Meconium aspiration
         syndrome.
      amnioinfusion and, 478
   turbidity, 411–412
      optical density in, 412
      visual inspection in, 411–412
   volume
      physiologic regulation of,
         102–103
      ultrasound for, 339–342,
         340f–343f, 342t
Amniotic fluid index, 340–342
   in hydramnios, 340–342, 343f
   in intrauterine growth retarda-
      tion, 928–929, 930f
   maximum vertical pocket mea-
      surement vs., 342
   normal values for, 342, 342t
   in oligohydramnios, 340–342,
      343f
   in prolonged pregnancy, 953
   technique in, 340, 340f–341f
Amniotic membrane
   premature rupture of, 861–868
      complications of, 864–865
         cord prolapse as, 864
         intrauterine infection as,
            864
         neonatal infection as, 864
         neonatal pulmonary
            hypoplasia as, 864
         placental abruption as, 864
         preterm delivery vs.,
            864–865

diagnosis of, 861–862, 862f
   dye studies in, 862
   etiology of, 862–864
      bacterial infection in, 863
      cigarette smoking and,
         863
      coitus and, 863–864
      local defects in, 863
      physical stress in, 863
   fern test in, 862, 862f
   management of, 865–868
      amniocentesis in, 865–867
      antibiotics in, 867–868
      corticosteroids in, 867
      expectant, 868
      before fetal viability, 868
      gestational age and, 865
      tocolytics in, 867
      ultrasound in, 866–867
   natural history of, 865
   pH in, 861
   stripping of, 448–449
Amniotomy, in induction of labor,
   449
Amoxicillin, as potential teratogen,
   311
Amphetamine, breast-feeding and,
   320
Analgesics. *See also individual types.*
   after cesarean section, 665–666
   breast-feeding and, 319
   in labor, opioid, 498–500
   in myasthenia gravis, 1163
   in preterm labor, 869
   in severe preeclampsia, 1018
   as potential teratogens, 314
   in vaginal delivery, inhalation or
      intravenous, 519
Anal sphincter, external
   anatomy of, 12–13, 14f
   nerve supply of, 15
Anal triangle, 12–13, 13f–14f
Androgens, as potential teratogens,
   302
Anemia
   Cooley's (β-thalassemia), 1143
   iron deficiency, 1137–1138
   megaloblastic, 1138–1139

neonatal, 733
   physiologic, of pregnancy, 138
   sickle cell. *See* Sickle cell anemia.
Anencephaly
   face presentation in, 544
   prenatal diagnosis of, 292–295
      amniotic fluid α-fetoprotein
         levels in, 292–293
      maternal serum α-fetoprotein
         (MSAFP) in, 293–295,
         294f, 295t
      risks after AFP screening in,
         295t
      ultrasound in, 344, 348, 350f
   statistical risks for, 291–292
   timing of teratogenic exposure
      in, 236
Anesthesia, 493–530
   in abortion, complications of,
      1316
   caudal epidural, 501
      lumbar vs., 501
      single-dose, 520
   in cesarean section, 520–529
      Apgar scores and, 520, 521t
      fetal blood gas levels and,
         520, 521t
      general, 521–528. *See also*
         Anesthesia, general.
      local, 528–529
      lumbar epidural, 526–528
      neurobehavioral testing in,
         520–521
      in preterm birth, 869
      spinal (subarachnoid) block,
         526–528
      techniques chosen in, 520,
         521t
   in fatty liver, 1170–1171
   fetal effects of, 496–497
   general
      antacids in, 522, 522f
      aspiration in, 522f, 525,
         525f–528f, 525t
      balanced, 493
      in cesarean section, 521–528
      cricoid pressure in, 523
      extubation in, 524

induction in, 523
intubation in, 523
left uterine displacement in, 522–523
muscle relaxant in, 523
nitrous oxide and oxygen in, 524
oxytocin in, 524
postdelivery, 524
potent inhalation agent in, 524
premedication in, 521
preoxygenation in, 523
in preterm labor, 869
proper tube placement in, 523–524
recovery after, 524–525
in severe preeclampsia, 1018
stages of, 493
in vaginal delivery, 520, 520t
in HELLP syndrome, 1018
hemodynamics in, 1059
high or total spinal, 506–508
in labor, 497–517
local
   allergic reactions to, 506
   in cesarean section, 528–529
   convulsions due to, 505, 506t
   toxic reactions to, 504–506, 505t–506t
   in vaginal delivery, 517, 517t, 520t
lumbar epidural, 501–515
   caudal vs., 501
   in cesarean section, 526–528
   complications of, 503–509
     anesthestic allergy as, 506
     high or total spinal anesthesia as, 506–508, 507f
     hypotension as, 503–504, 504f, 504t
     local toxicity as, 504–506, 505t–506t
     paralysis and nerve injury as, 508
     spinal headache as, 508–509

effects on labor and delivery of, 509–515
   continuous infusion vs. bolus and, 514
   delayed pushing and, 515
   delayed second stage and, 510–511
   dose and, 512
   drug choice and dose and, 509–510
   in early, latent phase, 512
   epinephrine and, 512–515, 513f
   instrument delivery and, 514
   opioids and, 514–515
   oxytocin and, 515
   prospective studies of, 511–512
   recommendations in, 512f–513f, 512–515
   second stage of labor and, 514
   study design and, 509
   technique variations and, 509–510
   timing of administration and, 510
   uterine activity decrease and, 512, 512f
frequency usage of, 517t
hemodynamics in, 1059
for perineal anesthesia, 501, 503f
in preterm labor, 869
segmental, 501, 503f
in severe preeclampsia, 1018
single-dose, 520
stress response and, 496, 497f
technique in, 501, 502f
in vaginal birth after cesarean section, 669–670, 672
in myasthenia gravis, 1163–1164
nerves blocked by and pain pathways in, 13-17, 494f
paracervical, 515–516
   fetal bradycardia due to, 516, 516f

frequency usage of, 517t
in preterm birth, 869
technique in, 515, 515f
perineal
   local, 517, 517t, 520t
   lumbar epidural block in, 501, 503f
personnel in, 495
placental transfer of, 530, 530f
in preterm labor, 869
psychoprophylactic, 497–498
pudendal block, 517–519, 518f, 520t
regional, 493
in severe preeclampsia, 1018
spinal (subarachnoid) block, 519–520, 520t
   in cesarean section, 526–528
toxic reactions to, seizures in, 1190t
in vaginal delivery, 517–520, 520t
Anesthetic gases, occupational exposure to, birth defects due to, 257–258
Aneuploidy, and recurrent abortion, 793, 793t
Angiography, pulmonary, 1078
Angiomata, spider, 127, 130, 1216
Angiotensin-converting enzyme inhibitors, in chronic hypertension in pregnancy, 1041
Angiotensin II, fetal, circulatory effects of, 108–109
Ankle edema, 135
Anococcygeal ligament, 6, 6f–7f
Antacid therapy
   in general anesthesia, 522, 522f
   in peptic ulcer disease, 1174
   side effects of, 1174t
Antepartum fetal testing, 377–417. *See also individual tests.*
   applications of, 380t–381t, 380–381
   biochemical analysis in, 383
   contraction stress test in, 386–390

Antepartum fetal testing *(Continued)*
  diagnostic-specific approach to, 414–417, 416f
  Doppler velocimetry in, 399–406
  fetal activity assessment in, 384–386, 387f
  fetal biophysical profile in, 396–399
  fetal pulmonary maturation assessment in, 409–414
  indications for, 381, 381t
  nonstress test in, 390–396
  normal fetal state and, 383–384
  perinatal mortality and, 379–380
  in sickle cell anemia, 1140
  statistical assessment of, 381t–382t, 381–382, 383f
    fifty percent prevalence in, 382, 382t
    test threshold in, 382, 383f
    two-by-two matrix in, 381, 381t
    two percent prevalence in, 382, 382t
Antepartum record, ACOG, 218f–221f, 222
Antiasthmatics, as potential teratogens, 308
Antibiotics
  breast-feeding and, 321
  pharmacokinetics of, physiology of pregnancy and, 1224
  placental transfer of, 1225
  in postabortal infection, 1319
  prophylactic
    in abortion, 1319
    in heart disease, 1061, 1062t
  as potential teratogens, 310–314
Anticardiolipin antibodies
  recurrent abortion and, 798
  in systemic lupus erythematosus, 1154–1156
Anticoagulants
  breast-feeding and, 320
  in heart disease, 1061
  in pulmonary thromboembolism, 1078–1079

as potential teratogens, 306, 307f
Anticonvulsants. *See also individual types.*
  breast-feeding and, 319, 1187
  fetal mental development and, 1186
  neonatal coagulopathy due to, 1185
  pharmacokinetics of, pregnancy effects on, 1186–1187, 1187t
  in seizure disorders, 1184–1187
  side effects of, 1184t, 1184–1186
  as potential teratogens, 303–304, 304f
Antiemetics, as potential teratogens, 308–310
Antifetal antibodies, in recurrent abortion, 797–798
Antifungal agents, as potential teratogens, 313–314
Antigen
  trophoblast, 102
  trophoblast-lymphocyte cross-reactive, 102
Antihistamines
  breast-feeding and, 319
  as potential teratogens, 310
Antihypertensive drugs. *See also individual drugs.*
  breast-feeding and, 320
  in chronic hypertension in pregnancy, 1036–1042, 1037t
  in preeclampsia, 1013
  as potential teratogens, 307
Anti-Kell isoimmunization, 978, 979t
Antimüllerian hormone, fetal, in genital development, 114–115
Antineoplastic drugs, as potential teratogens, 307–308
Antinuclear antibodies, in systemic lupus erythematosus, 1152t
Antithrombin III, in preeclampsia, 997

Antituberculosis drugs, as potential teratogens, 313
Aortic coarctation, 1067–1068
Aortic dissection, 1068
Aortic regurgitation, 1065
Aortic stenosis, 1063–1064
Apgar score, 710t
  in anesthesia in cesarean section, 520, 521t
  1-minute
    fetal acid-base evaluation and, 486, 486t
    in very-low-birth-weight infant, 869f, 869–870
  5-minute, fetal acid-base evaluation and, 486, 486t
Aplastic crisis, in parvovirus infection, 1234
Appendectomy, in cesarean section, 680–681
Appendicitis, 684–686, 685f
Appetite, 125
Apt test, in third trimester fetal bleeding, 589
Arachidonic acid
  cellular mobilization of, 157f, 157–158
  mobilization during labor of, 164
Arcuate uterus, 796f
Arcus tendineus, of levator ani muscle, 5f, 6
Areola
  changes in pregnancy of, 136
  nerve supply to, 176–177
Arm presentation, 541, 541f
Arnold-Chiari malformation, 356, 359f
Arrhythmia
  fetal, 466, 468–469, 469f
    artifact in, 466, 468–469
    supraventricular tachycardia in, 469, 469f
  maternal, in tocolytic therapy, 849–850
Arsenic, birth defects and, 252
Arteriovenous malformation, cerebral, 1191–1192

Arthritis, rheumatoid, 1159–1161
  clinical manifestations of, 1159–1160
  diagnostic criteria for, 1159
  exclusions from, 1159
  intrauterine growth retardation in, 1160
  medical treatment of, effects on pregnancy of, 1161
  pathophysiology and laboratory findings in, 1160
  in pregnancy, 1160
Aspartame, as potential teratogen, 317–318
Asphyxia, birth, 707–713. *See also* Respiratory distress syndrome.
  in at-risk infants, 712
  in maternal narcotic administration, 712
  in meconium-stained amniotic fluid, 712
  in meperidine analgesia, 499
  in opioid analgesia, 498–499
  periventricular/intraventricular hemorrhage in, 713–715, 714f, 715t
  physiologic response to, 708, 708f
  in prolonged pregnancy, 954
  protection from, 708
  resuscitation in
    Apgar score in, 709, 710t
    drug therapy in, 711, 711t
    equipment for, 709, 709t
    mechanical causes of failed, 711, 711t
    physiologic response to, 708–709
    steps for, 709–712, 710f
  risk factors for, 709
  sequelae of, 712–713, 713t
Aspiration
  of acid food particles, 528f
  in eclamptic convulsion, 1026
  in general anesthesia, 522f, 525, 525f–528f, 525t
  of liquid acid, 526f

meconium
  in intrauterine growth retardation, 938
  neonatal respiratory distress syndrome and, 719–720, 720f
  in prolonged pregnancy, 947–948, 953–954
  tracheal suctioning in, 712
  of nonacid food particles, 527f
  of normal saline, 525f
Aspirin
  breast-feeding and, 319
  in prevention of preeclampsia, 1003–1004
  in rheumatoid arthritis, 1161
  as potential teratogen, 314
Asthma
  in labor, 1077
  in pregnancy, 1075–1077
    corticosteroid aerosols in, 1076
    incidence of, 1075
    perinatal morbidity in, 1075
    β-sympathomimetic drugs in, 1076
    systemic glucocorticoids in, 1076
    theophylline in, 1075–1076
    treatment of, 1075–1076
Asynclitism, 453
Atenolol
  breast-feeding and, 320
  in chronic hypertension in pregnancy, 1040
  in preeclampsia, 1013
  as potential teratogen, 307
Atherosclerosis, coronary artery, 1070–1071
Atopic disease, breast milk and, 199–200
Atrial septal defect, 1066
Attitude
  definition of, 453
  deflection, 543f, 543–562. *See also under* Malpresentation; *individual types.*

Auscultation, fetal heart rate monitoring vs., 485
Autoantibodies, 1152t
  human immunodeficiency virus and, 1259
Autoimmune disease, recurrent abortion in, 798
Autonomic stress syndrome, of high paraplegics, seizures in, 1190t
Axial lie, abnormal, 540–543, 541f
  causes of, 541
  cesarean section in, 542–543
  cord prolapse in, 541, 542
  diagnosis of, 542
  external version in, 542
  fetal mortality in, 542
  incidence of, 541
  maternal mortality in, 542
  placenta previa and, 542
Azathioprine
  in renal transplantation, 1091
  in systemic lupus erythematosus, 1158
  as potential teratogen, 308
Azygos artery, of vagina, 27, 28f

B
Backache, prenatal education about, 228
Bacterial infection, susceptibility to, 1224
Bacteriuria, asymptomatic, 1085–1086. *See also* Urinary tract infection.
"Banana sign," in spina bifida, ultrasound findings, 356, 359f
Barbiturate(s), in labor, 500
Barbiturate withdrawal, neonatal, 1185
Bartholin's glands, 9
Basal body temperature, in natural contraceptive methods, 765
Base deficit, in fetal acid-base evaluation, 475, 476t

Bendectin, 127, 309

Benzodiazepine
in labor, 500–501
as potential teratogen, 305

Bicornuate uterus, 796f

Bile pigment metabolism, neonatal, 738f

Biliary colic, 1173

Bilirubin, in amniotic fluid, in Rh isoimmunization, 966–968, 967f–968f

Biophysical profile, fetal, 396–399. *See also* Fetal biophysical profile.

Biopsy
chorionic villus. *See* chorionic villus sampling.
endometrial, in luteal phase defect, 794
fetal, in genodermatosis, 287
renal, in pregnancy, 1090
trophoectoderm, 283, 283f

Biparietal diameter
average, 428, 428f
for fetal pulmonary maturation assessment, 413
for gestational age, 333, 334f–335f, 335–336, 336t
for intrauterine growth retardation, 928
for twin gestation growth and development, 891

Birth asphyxia, 707–713. *See also* Neonate, birth asphyxia in; Respiratory distress syndrome.

Birth control. *See* Contraception; Oral contraceptives.

Birth defects, 233–260. *See also* Abortion; Amniocentesis; Chorionic villus sampling; Chromosomal abnormalities; Teratogens; Radiation.
epidemiology of, 234, 235t. *See also* Epidemiology.
concepts of, 239
contribution of, 238
geographic differences in, 239
incidence vs. prevalence in, 239
temporal variations in, 239
etiology of, 234–235. *See also* specific teratogens; specific disorders.
statistical importance of, 233–234, 234t

Birth Defects Monitoring Program, 241

Birth injury, neonatal, 716–717, 717t

Bishop prelabor scoring system, 150, 151f, 448, 448t

Bisischial diameter, pelvic, 433

Bladder. *See* Urinary bladder.

Blastocyst
hormone secretion by, 59
implantation of, 39–41, 40f
normal development of, 301

Blastomere, 39, 59, 60f
cytogenetic analysis of, 784, 786f

Bleeding. *See also* Hemorrhage.
fetal, third trimester, 589, 590f–591f
implantation, mechanism of, 40
and intrauterine device use, 767
painless vaginal, in placenta previa, 585

Blighted ovum, 331, 889

Blood group antigens
ABO, maternal isoimmunization to, 978, 981
minor, maternal isoimmunization to, 977–978, 979t–980t

Blood pressure. *See also* Eclampsia; Hypertension; Hypotension; Preeclampsia.
in eclampsia, 1022
fetal, autonomic regulation of, 107–108
maternal, in pregnancy, 134
in preeclampsia, 575
criteria for, 993
pregnancy outcome and, 1000, 1000t
technique for measuring, 1000

Blood sampling, fetal scalp
complications of, 486
heart rate during, 477
technique for, 475–476

Blood transfusion, 576–579
in abruptio placenta, 584
autologous, 578–579
cryoprecipitate for, 578
exchange, in sickle cell anemia, 1142
fresh frozen plasma for, 578
HIV infection and, 579
intrauterine, in Rh isoimmunization, 971–976. *See also* under Rh isoimmunization.
massive, 576–578
acid-base problems in, 577–578
blood products for, 577
hypocalcemia in, 577
laboratory studies in, 577
microvascular bleeding and, 577
packed red blood cells for, 578
placental, postnatal, 432
in placenta previa, 587
platelet, 578
in neonatal immune thrombocytopenia, 983
replacement products for, 576t
risks of, 578, 579t
in sickle cell anemia, 1141–1142
whole blood vs. component, 576

Blood urea nitrogen (BUN), in pregnancy, 131, 1085

Blood volume
postpartum, 1058
in pregnancy, 137–138, 1057–1058, 1058t

Bonding, maternal-infant, 739–740, 758–760

Bottle-feeding, neonatal gastrointestinal flora in, 198

Brachial plexus injury, neonatal, 717

Bradycardia, fetal
  in intrapartum monitoring, 464f, 465–466
  in nonstress test, 394f, 395
  in paracervical anesthesia, 516, 516f

Braxton-Hicks contractions, 162

Breast. *See also* Breast-feeding; Breast milk; Lactation; Suckling.
  alveolar glandular structure of, 176, 177f
  embryonic development of, 180
  engorgement, 760
  gross anatomy of, 176–177, 177f
  involution of, after lactation, 189–190
  microscopic anatomy of, 177–178, 178f
  nerve supply to, 176
  postpartum development of, 181
  in pregnancy, changes in, 136–137, 180–181, 181f
  pubertal development of, 180

Breast cancer, 1200–1203
  detection and diagnosis of, 1201
  incidence of, 1200
  lactation and, 190
  pregnancy as risk factor for, 1200–1201
  pregnancy termination in, 1203
  prognosis in, 1201–1202, 1202t
  subsequent pregnancies in, 1203
  treatment of, 1202–1203

Breast-feeding, 729–730, 760–764. *See also* Breast; Breast milk; Lactation; Suckling.
  advantages of, 175
  breast cancer risks and, 190
  carpal tunnel syndrome and, 1193
  in cesarean section, 187
  complications of, 763

  lactation failure as, 763
  mastitis as, 763
  contraception in, 200–201, 765
  contraindications to, 730, 762
  diet and calorie intake in, 199, 761–762
  dieting for weight loss and, 762
  drug use during, 318–322, 762
    agents compatible with, 319–322
    agents for temporary cessation in, 319
    contraindicated agents in, 318–319
    pharmacokinetics in, 318
  encouragement for, 175–176
  frequency of
    postpartum, 187
    prolactin effects of, 187–189, 188f
  in immune thrombocytopenic purpura, 1146
  increase in, 760
  IUD in, 201
  in maternal diabetes mellitus, 200, 1114
  maternal nutrition in, 199, 761–762
  milk supply problems in, 763
  neonatal gastrointestinal flora in, 198
  nipple confusion and, 760
  nipple preparation for, 228
  nipple soreness and, 760–761
  oral contraceptives during, 200, 321, 766
  prenatal education about, 228
  schedule for, 760
  successful, 760, 761
    suckling in, 190f
  of term infant, 760–761
  unsuccessful, suckling in, 191f
  vegetarian diet and, 199, 762
  vitamins and, 762
  for working mothers, 228

Breast milk, 195–198. *See also* Breast-feeding; Lactation; Suckling.

  atopic disease and, 199–200
  bacteria and viruses in, 199, 762
  colic and, 199
  contraceptive steroids secreted in, 200, 321, 766
  cow's milk vs., 197t, 197–198
  drugs in, 318–322, 762
  hepatitis B virus in, 762
  HIV in, 199
  immunologically active factors in, 198–199, 199t
  mature, constituents of, 195f, 195t, 195–196
  in neonatal immunologic protection, 198
  neonatal jaundice due to, 737–738
  preterm, constituents of, 195f, 196–197
  for preterm infant, 730, 762–763

Breath, first neonatal, 703, 704–705, 705f

Breathing
  fetal, 113, 703
  maternal, diaphragmatic, 128

Breech presentation, 434, 551–562
  causes of, 551
  cesarean section in, 649
  complete, 551, 551f, 551t
  complications of, 559, 559t
  delivery technique in, 552–558
    airway access in, 555f, 556
    arms in, 553, 554f–555f, 556
    in complete position, 558
    descent in, 552, 553f
    Duhrssen's cervical incision in, 687, 687f
    engagement in, 552, 552f
    in footling position, 558
    in frank position, 552f–557f, 552–558
    head in, 556, 556f–557f
    inappropriate aggressive traction in, 552, 553f
    lateral rotation of thighs in, 552–553, 554f
    perinatal mortality in, 558–559, 559t

Breech presentation *(Continued)*
    Piper forceps in, 556, 557f
    vaginal vs. cesarean, 560–562,
      561t
  diagnosis of, 551
  external cephalic version in,
    562, 563f
  footling, 551, 551f, 551t
    cord prolapse in, 560
    delivery technique in, 558
  frank, 551, 551f, 551t
  hyperextension of head in, 560
  incomplete, 551f
  labor in, 551–552
  in low-birth-weight infant,
    559–560
  of second twin, 558
  types of, 551, 551f, 551t
  vaginal birth after cesarean sec-
    tion in, 670
  in very-low-birth-weight infant,
    559–560
  X-ray pelvimetry in, risk-benefit
    ratio in, 434
  Zatuchni-Andros scoring system
    in, 560–561, 561t
Broad ligament
  anatomy of, 20–21, 22f
  hematoma in, after cesarean sec-
    tion, 664f
Bromocriptine
  breast-feeding and, 318
  in lactation suppression, 201,
    764
  as potential teratogen, 314
Bronchopulmonary dysplasia, in
    hyaline membrane dis-
    ease, 721
Brow presentation, 547–549
  causes of, 547
  cesarean section in, 548–549
  definition of, 547, 547f
  diagnosis of, 547
  frontum anterior, 548f
  incidence of, 547
  left frontum anterior, 548f
  left frontum transverse, 547,
    548f

open fetal mouth in, 548, 549f
  spontaneous conversion of,
    547–548
  vaginal delivery in, 548–549
Bulbospongiosus muscle, 11
Bupivacaine
  maximal recommended dosage
    of, 505t
  toxic reactions to, 505
Busulphan, breast-feeding and,
    318
Butorphanol, in labor, 500

C
Caffeine
  breast-feeding and, 322
  as potential teratogen, 317
Calcification, placental infarction
    and, 47, 48f
Calcium
  homeostasis of, in lactation,
    193–195
  metabolism, in pregnancy, 137,
    1120–1121, 1121f
  placental transfer of, 98–99,
    1121
Calcium channel blockers
  in chronic hypertension in preg-
    nancy, 1041
  as tocolytic, 853–854
Calcium supplementation, in pre-
    vention of preeclamp-
    sia, 1002
Caloric requirements
  fetal, 103
  maternal, in breast-feeding, 199,
    761
  neonatal, 728–729, 729t
Camper's fascia, 9
Canal of Nuck, 21
Cancer. *See individual anatomic types*;
    Malignant disease.
Capillary hemangiomas, 1216
Carbamazepine
  breast-feeding and, 319
  nonpregnant daily dosage of,
    1187t

as potential teratogen, 303,
    1185–1186
Carbohydrate, neonatal require-
    ments for, 729
Carbon dioxide, placental
    exchange of, 96
Carcinoma. *See individual anatomic
    types*; Malignant dis-
    ease.
Cardiac output
  fetal, normal, 106, 106t
  heart rate and, 616
  hemodynamic factors in, 615
  low, pharmacologic therapy for,
    617
  maternal, 133–134, 1058
    distribution of flow in, 134
    in labor, 1059
    postpartum, 756
    in supine position, 133–134,
      1058, 1059f
  myocardial contractility and,
    616, 619f
  pharmacologic therapy for, 617,
    620t, 621f
  Starling curves for, 616–617,
    619f
  ventricular afterload and,
    615–616, 618f
  ventricular preload and, 615
Cardinal ligament, ureter and, 22
Cardinal ligament, anatomy of, 21,
    23f
Cardiomyopathy
  dilated, Swan-Ganz catheteriza-
    tion in, 627
  hypertrophic obstructive, Swan-
    Ganz catheterization
    in, 626
  peripartum, 1069–1070
Cardiopulmonary profile
  measured variables in, 615, 616t
  in preeclampsia, 616t
Cardiopulmonary transition,
    neonatal, 697–707. *See
    also* Neonate, car-
    diopulmonary transi-
    tion of.

Cardiovascular drugs, as potential teratogens, 306–307
Cardiovascular system
  postpartum, 755–756
  in pregnancy, 133–136
Carotid artery occlusion, 1190
Carpal tunnel syndrome, 1193–1194
Car seat belt injury
  abruptio placenta in, 686f, 687
  uterus trauma in, 686f, 687
Car travel, prenatal education about, 225
Catecholamine
  fetal, effects on labor of, 158–159
  maternal, effects on labor of, 158
Catheterization
  pulmonary artery. *See* Swan-Ganz catheterization.
  Swan-Ganz, 607–617. *See also* Swan-Ganz catheterization.
Caudal dysplasia, in maternal diabetes mellitus, 1101, 1102f
Cefazolin, breast-feeding and, 321
Cells, signal transduction in, second messengers in, 156–157, 157f
Central nervous system, fetal, normal physiology of, 113
Central venous pressure, in pregnancy, 134
Cephalic index, for gestational age, 335
Cephalic version, external
  in breech presentation, 562, 563f
  in twin gestation, 912–913
Cephalocentesis, in hydrocephalus, 269
Cephalohematoma, neonatal, 716
Cephalometry. *See* Biparietal diameter.
Cephalopelvic disproportion. *See*

also Macrosomia, fetal; Pelvimetry.
  vaginal birth after cesarean section and, 671
Cephalosporins
  breast-feeding and, 321
  as potential teratogens, 311
Cerclage, cervical, 859–861
  McDonald technique in, 859, 860f
  risks and mortality in, 860
  Shirodkar technique in, 859
  success rate of, 860–861
  timing of, 860
  in twin gestation, 909
Cerebellum, fetal, ultrasound for, 344, 345f
Cerebral arterial occlusion, 1189–1191
Cerebral arteriovenous malformation, 1191–1192
Cerebral blood flow, fetal, 113
Cerebral venous thrombosis, seizures in, 1190t
Cerebral venous-venous malformation, 1192
Cerebrovascular disorders, 1189–1192
Cervical assessment score, in twin gestation, 909
Cervical cancer, 1209–1211
  cervical cytology in, 1209, 1210f
  colposcopy in, 1209
  conization in, 1209–1210
  delivery in, 1211
  incidence of, 1209
  survival statistics in, 1210, 1211t
  treatment of, 1210–1211
Cervical lacerations, in abortion, 1316
Cervical mucus
  in natural contraceptive methods, 765
  prostaglandin concentration in, 152, 152t
Cervical shock, in abortion, 1316

Cervix, 150–152
  changes due to age in, 34–36, 36f
  changes due to pregnancy and parturition in, 36–37, 37f
  collagen structure of, 150
  dilatation of
    in dysfunctional labor, 436–437, 437f–438f
    mechanics of, 167–168, 168f
    in preterm birth, 840
  Duhrssen's incision of, in breech presentation, 687, 687f
  effacement of, definition of, 453
  incompetent, 858–861
    cerclage technique in, 859–861
      McDonald technique in, 859, 860f
      risks and mortality in, 860
      Shirodkar technique in, 859
      success rate of, 860–861
      timing of, 860
    diagnosis of, 859
    etiology of, 859
      congenital predisposition as, 858
      DES exposure in, 858
      prior elective abortion as, 858
    preterm birth and, 838
    recurrent abortion and, 795–796
  laceration of, surgical repair of, 594, 596f
  muscular component of, 150
  postpartum, 754
  ripening of, 150–152, 151f
    biochemical changes in, 150
    Bishop score in, 150, 151f
    hormonal influences on, 150–151
    methods for acceleration of, 151

Cervix (*Continued*)
    neural mechanisms in, 158
    prostaglandins for, 151–152
        in prolonged pregnancy,
            950–951
    relaxin for, 152, 159
  in third stage of labor, visual
        inspection of, 446–447
Cesarean hysterectomy, 673–680
  blood loss in, 138
  complications of, 680
  indications for, 673
  nonemergency, 673
  in placenta accreta, 655–656
  technique for, 673–680
    in subtotal hysterectomy, 677,
        680, 681f
    in total hysterectomy,
        673–677, 675f–680f
Cesarean section, 635–687
  in abnormal axial lie, 542–
    543
  in abruptio placenta, 584
  active labor management vs.,
    440–441
  anesthesia in, 520–529. *See also*
    Anesthesia.
  appendectomy in, 680–681
  blood loss in, 138
  breast-feeding in, 187
  in breech presentation,
    560–562, 561t
  in brow presentation, 548–549
  in compound presentation,
    550–551
  in conjoined twins, 901
  in face presentation, 546–547
  fetal maturity assessment prior
    to, 231
  fluid therapy in, 657–658
    fluid and electrolyte replace-
      ment in, 658
    intraoperative, 658
    intravenous fluids for, 658
    preoperative, 658
  forced, legal issues of,
    1336–1337
  hemodynamics in, 1059

history of, 635–636
incision in, 642–647
  Allis test for, 643
  fascial, 644
  Kerr, 645t, 645–647, 646f
  Krönig, 645t, 645–647, 646f
  Maylard, 643f, 643–644
  in obese patient, 644–645
  peritoneum, 644
  Pfannenstiel, 643f, 644
  transverse, 643, 643f
  uterine, 645t, 645–647, 646f
  vertical, 642–643, 643f
indications for, 638–639, 639t
  fetal, 638, 639t
  maternal, 639, 639t
  maternal-fetal, 638–639, 639t
informed consent for, 639–640
intraoperative complications of,
  653–656
  bladder injury as, 653–654
  gastrointestinal tract injury
    as, 654
  placenta accreta in, 655–656
  ureteral injury as, 654
  uterine atony as, 654–655,
    655f
  uterine laceration as, 653
in maternal diabetes mellitus,
  1113, 1114
myomectomy and, 680
in neonatal immune thrombocytopenia, 984
ovarian neoplasms and, 681
perinatal mortality and morbidity in, 635, 637–638
in placenta accreta, 645,
  655–656
postmortem, 656–657
postoperative complications of,
  658–665
  abdominal wall abscess as,
    665f
  bladder flap hematoma as,
    663f
  broad ligament hematoma as,
    664f
  endomyometritis as, 659–660

  fascial dehiscence as, 662
  gastrointestinal, 663–664
  maternal morbidity and mor-
    tality as, 658–659
  septic pelvic throm-
    bophlebitis as, 665
  thromboembolism as,
    664–665
  ultrasound for diagnosis of,
    662–663, 663f–665f
  urinary tract infection as, 663
  wound infection as, 660–662,
    1283–1284
postoperative management of,
  665–667
  ambulation and, 666
  analgesia in, 665–666
  fluid therapy in, 666–667
  laboratory studies in, 666
  oral intake and, 666
  urinary bladder management
    in, 666
  wound care in, 666
postpartum tubal ligation after,
  681–684. *See also*
    Fallopian tube, tubal
    ligation of.
in preterm birth, 870–871
rate of
  increased, 636–637
  reducing, 667
in severe preeclampsia, 1018
surgical principles in, 640–642
  hair removal in, 641
  skin prep in, 640–641
  suture selection in, 641–642,
    642t
in systemic lupus erythematosus,
  1157
technique in, 647–653
  abdominal closure in,
    651–653, 653f
  bladder flap in, 647
  breech presentation and, 649
  classic incision in, 646f, 648
  delivery of fetus in, 648–649
  drainage of abdominal inci-
    sion in, 656

extraperitoneal, 656, 657f
low transverse incision in, 646f, 647
low vertical incision in, 646f, 647–648, 648f
preterm fetus and, 649
repair of uterine incision in, 649–651, 651f–652f
in twin gestation, 912
vaginal birth after, 667–672
in breech presentation, 670
epidural anesthesia in, 669–670, 672
fetal monitoring in, 672
fetal weight and, 669
guidelines for, 671–672
informed consent for, 672
maternal and fetal mortality in, 668
in multiple gestation, 670
oxytocin in, 669, 672
prior cephalopelvic disproportion and, 671
prior cesarean indications and, 670–671, 671t
prior failure to progress and, 671
prior multiple cesarean sections and, 671
prior vaginal birth and, 671
uterine dehiscence/rupture in
diagnosis of, 672
incidence of, 668–669
for very-low-birth-weight infant, 870–871
in von Willebrand's disease, 1147
Chemicals, environmental, abortion due to, 801
Chemotherapy, in malignant disease, 1199–1200
Chickenpox. *See* Varicella-zoster virus infection.
Childbirth. *See also* Delivery; Labor; Parturition.
prenatal education about, 228–229
Chlamydial infection, 1272–1275

clinical aspects of, 1274
diagnosis of, 1274
in endometritis, 1281
epidemiology in, 1273–1274
historical, 1272–1273
immunology in, 1273
management of, 1274–1275
microbiology in, 1273
treatment regimen in, 1275
Chloasma, 130, 1215
Chloride, placental transfer of, 98
Chlorodiazepoxide, as potential teratogen, 305
Chloroprocaine, maximal recommended dosage of, 505t
Chlorothiazide, breast-feeding and, 320
Chlortrimazole, as potential teratogen, 313
Cholangitis, ascending, 1173
Cholecystectomy, 1173
Cholecystitis, acute, 686
Cholelithiasis, 126, 686, 1173
Cholestasis, intrahepatic, 1171–1172
clinical manifestations of, 1171
laboratory diagnosis of, 1171–1172
management of, 1172
perinatal outcome in, 1172
Cholesterol, serum, in pregnancy, 127
Chorioamnionitis, 1276–1278
diagnosis of, 1277–1278
epidemiology of, 1276–1277
fetal response to, 50
maternal response to, 51
microabscesses due to, 50
pathogenesis of, 49–50, 1277
pathologic manifestations of, 50
in premature rupture of membranes, 864, 865
as sterile inflammatory reaction, 51
treatment of, 1278
Chorioangioma, 51, 52f
Choriocarcinoma

after pregnancy, 56
hemorrhage in, 55, 56f
metastasis from, 55–56, 57f
normal placenta in, 51, 52f
placental site tumor and, 43, 51
trophoblast in, 55, 55f
Chorion, prostaglandin synthesis by, 163–164
Chorion frondosum. *See also* Chorionic villi.
development of, 43–44, 44f
Chorionic gonadotropin (hCG), 64–65
commercial assays for, 84t
ELISA for, 83–85, 84f
embryologic structures and, 85t, 86f, 783
in evaluation of trisomy 21, 285
FIA for, 85
function of, 65, 72–73
intact, in pregnancy diagnosis, 83
IRMA for, 83
molecular structure of, 64, 65f
origin of, 65, 67t–68t, 72
radioimmunoassay for, 83
α-subunit of
in pregnancy diagnosis, 83
structure of, 64, 65f
variation during pregnancy of, 65, 66f–67f
β-subunit of
in ectopic pregnancy, 814
in pregnancy diagnosis, 83, 783
structure of, 64, 65f
variation during pregnancy of, 65, 66f–67f
variation during pregnancy of, 64–65, 66f–67f, 72
Chorionic membrane, 41, 41f
Chorionic somatomammotropin (hCS), 67–69
function of, 69
molecular structure of, 67, 68f
origin of, 68
variation during pregnancy of, 67–68, 69f

Chorionic thyrotropin (hCT), placental, 73
Chorionic villus(i)
  early, cellular structure of, 60, 63f
  fibrin deposition around, 47
  first trimester, cellular structure of, 46
  in hydatidiform mole, 53, 55
  infarction of, villitis vs., 49
  second trimester, cellular structure of, 46f, 46–47
  at term, cellular structure of, 46–47, 47f, 60, 63f
  in triploidy, 55
  venous penetration of, 44, 44f
Chorionic villus sampling, 280–282
  accuracy of, 283–284
  fetomaternal hemorrhage in, 961
  indications for, 280–284
  pitfalls of, 283–284
  Rh isoimmunization in, maternal management of, 965, 965t
  safety of, 282
  technique in, 280–282
  transabdominal, 281, 282f
  transcervical, 280–281, 281f
  transvaginal, 281
  trophoblast (direct) vs. mesenchymal core culture in, 284
Chorion laeve
  development of, 43
  fibrin deposition around, 47
  trophoblast of, maturation of, 48–49
Chromosomal abnormalities, 269, 270t, 271–274. *See also individual types.*
  in aborted fetuses, 787, 788t
  aneuploidy, in recurrent abortion, 793, 793t
  autosomal deletions or duplications, 273
  Down syndrome. *See* Trisomy 21.
  incidence of, 269, 270t

indications for prenatal diagnosis of, 284–285, 286f
  in intrauterine growth retardation, 925, 933, 934t
  maternal age and, 276, 276t
  monosomy X (45,X), 274
  paracentric inversions, in recurrent abortion, 792-793
  pericentric inversions, in recurrent abortion, 792-793
  polysomy X-female, 274
  polysomy Y-male, 274
  reciprocal translocation in, in recurrent abortion, 791, 792t
  in recurrent abortion, 790–792, 791f, 792t–793t
  Robertsonian translocation in possible progeny in, 285, 286f
    in recurrent abortion, 790t, 790–791
  sex chromosomes and, 274
  in twin gestation, 901
Cigarette smoking
  abortion due to, 800
  breast-feeding and, 322
  intrauterine growth retardation due to, 927
  lactation effects of, 189
  in premature rupture of membranes, 863
  prenatal counseling and, 213
  sudden infant death syndrome and, 315
  as potential teratogen, 314
Cimetidine
  breast-feeding and, 318
  in peptic ulcer disease, 1174
Circumcision, prenatal education about, 228
Clavicle fracture, in shoulder dystocia, 566
Cleft, facial
  in phenytoin exposure, 1185
  ultrasound for, 362, 365f
Clindamycin, as potential teratogen, 313
Clitoris
  anatomy of, 9–10

arterial supply to, 16, 16f–17f
  nerve supply of, 16, 17f
  venous supply to, 17
Cloacal exstrophy, in twin gestation, 900
Clomiphene, as potential teratogen, 314
Clonidine
  breast-feeding and, 320
  in chronic hypertension in pregnancy, 1039
Clubfoot, 362, 366f
Coagulation
  disseminated intravascular (DIC). *See* Disseminated intravascular coagulation (DIC).
  postpartum, 756
Coagulation defects, in abruptio placenta, 583
Coagulation factors
  in preeclampsia, 997–998
  in pregnancy, 139
Coagulopathy, neonatal, anticonvulsant-associated, 1185
Coarctation of aorta, in pregnancy, 1067–1068
Cocaine, as potential teratogen, 316–317
Coccygeus muscle, 6
Codeine
  breast-feeding and, 319
  as potential teratogen, 314
Cold injury, neonatal, 728
Colic, breast milk and, 199
Colitis, ulcerative, 1176–1177, 1178t
  effects of pregnancy on, 1177, 1178t
  effects on fertility of, 1176
  incidence of, 1176
  medical treatment of, 1178–1179
  perinatal outcome in, 1176–1177
  surgical treatment of, 1179–1180
Collagen, of cervix, 150

Collagen vascular disease, 1151–1164. *See also individual types.*
  antinuclear antibodies in, 1152t
  autoantibodies in, 1152t
Colles' fascia, 9
Colon, in pregnancy, 126
Colorectal cancer, 1212
Colostrum, 137
  constituents of, 195, 195t
  immunologically active factors in, 198–199, 199t
  in neonatal immunologic protection, 198
Compound presentation, 549–551
  causes of, 549–550
  cesarean section in, 550–551
  cord prolapse in, 550
  definition of, 549, 550f
  diagnosis of, 549
  incidence of, 549
  perinatal mortality in, 550
Conception, mammogenic and lactogenic hormones in, 190
Condom, contraceptive, 766
Conjoined twin gestation, 900f, 900–901
Constipation
  in pregnancy, 126
  prenatal education about, 226
Contraception, 764–769
  abortion due to, 800
  abortion for, 1303–1304
  barrier, 765–766
  in breast-feeding, 200–201, 765
  condoms in, 766
  in diabetes mellitus, 1115–1116
  diaphragm, 765–766
  failure rate for, 1303, 1304t
  IUD in, 201, 766–767
  in lactational amenorrhea, 192
  natural methods for, 765
  patient education for, 764–765
  public health concerns of, 1303
  sterilization in, 767–769
  vaginal sponge in, 766
Contraceptive steroids, 766
  in breast milk, 200, 321, 766

  as potential teratogens, 302
Contraction stress test, 386–390. *See also* Labor; Uterus, contraction of.
  contraindications to, 387–387
  follow-up studies of, 390
  interpretation of, 387t, 387–390, 388f–389f
    equivocal, 387, 390
    false-positive, 389–390
    10-minute window in, 387
    negative, 388f, 388–389
    positive, 389, 389f
  in intrauterine growth retardation, 933
  in maternal diabetes mellitus, 1110
  nipple stimulation in, 390
  nonstress test vs., 395–396, 397f
  in prolonged pregnancy, 952
  technique in, 386–387
  in twin gestation, 910
  two-by-two matrix for, 381, 381t
Convulsions. *See also* Seizure disorders.
  in eclampsia, 1025. *See also* Eclampsia.
    differential diagnosis of, 1190t
  local anesthetic-induced, 505, 506t
Cooley's anemia (β-thalassemia), 1143
Cord, umbilical. *See* Umbilical cord.
Cornea, in pregnancy, 142–143
Coronary artery disease
  in maternal diabetes mellitus, 1106
  in pregnancy, 1070–1071
Corpus luteum, progesterone secretion by, 74, 75f
Cortical venous thrombosis, 1191
Corticosteroid(s)
  in asthma, 1076
  breast-feeding and, 320–321
  for fetal pulmonary maturation, in placenta previa, 587

  in severe preeclampsia, 1015
  in systemic lupus erythematosus, 1157–1158
  as potential teratogen, 308
Corticosteroid-binding globulin (CBG), in pregnancy, 141
Corticotropin-releasing hormone (CRH), placental, 71
  function of, 71, 73f
  molecular structure of, 71
  origins of, 71
  variation during pregnancy of, 71, 72f
Corticotropin-releasing hormone (CRH)-glucocorticoid positive feedback hypothesis, 71, 73f
Cortisol
  decidua secretion of, 74–75
  fetal, production of, 111–112
  maternal
    function of, 82
    plasma levels of, 141
    variation during pregnancy of, 81–82
  molecular structure of, 81, 81f
  origin of, 82, 82f
Cortisone
  molecular structure of, 81, 81f
  origin of, 82, 82f
Cotyledon, placental, 44
Creatinine, serum, in pregnancy, 131, 1085
Cri-du-chat syndrome, 273
Critical care, 607–630. *See also individual disorders and techniques.*
  in cardiac disease, 626–627
  in diabetic ketoacidosis, 628–629
  in dilated cardiomyopathy, 627
  in Eisenmenger syndrome, 626–627
  in hypertrophic obstructive cardiomyopathy, 626
  in mitral stenosis, 626
  in preeclampsia, 617–626

Critical care *(Continued)*
  in pulmonary edema, tocolytic-
      induced, 627
  in respiratory distress syndrome,
      adult, 628
  in septic shock, 627–628
  Swan-Ganz catheterization
      (hemodynamic moni-
      toring) in, 607–617
  in thyroid storm, 629–630
Crohn's disease, 1176, 1177–1178
  effects of pregnancy on,
      1177–1178
  effects on fertility of, 1177
  incidence of, 1176
  medical treatment of,
      1178–1179
  perinatal outcome in, 1177,
      1178t
  surgical treatment of, 1179–1180
Cromolyn sodium, as potential ter-
      atogen, 308
Crown-rump length
  gestational age and, 333,
      333f–334f
  ultrasound for, 333, 333f–334f
Cryoprecipitate, transfusion of, 578
Cul-de-sac
  anterior, 20, 21f
  posterior, 20, 21f
Cushing syndrome, 1127–1128
Cyclophosphamide, breast-feeding
      and, 318
Cyclosporine A
  in renal transplantation, 1091
  as potential teratogen, 308
Cystic fibrosis, population genetic
      screening in, 278–279
Cystic hygroma, fetal, 354, 355f
Cystitis. *See* Urinary tract infection.
Cytomegalovirus infection (CMV),
      1230–1233
  clinical aspects of, 1232
  diagnosis and management of,
      1232–1233
  epidemiology of, 1231–1232
  immunology of, 1231
  laboratory findings in, 1232

microbiology of, 1230
Cytotrophoblast
  of chorionic villi, 46f, 46–47
  formation of, 39–40, 40f, 301
  hypothalamic- and pituitary-like
      peptides of, 60, 61t
  immunologic properties of, 102
  postimplantation, 59–60, 61f
  spiral arteriole invasion of, 42,
      42f
Cytotrophoblastic shell
  development of, 41, 41f–42f
  penetration into maternal tissue
      of, 44

D

Danazol, as potential teratogen,
      302, 302f
Death, prenatal. *See* Abortion; Fetal
      wastage; Mortality.
Decidua
  after implantation, structural
      changes in, 148–150
  cortisol secretion of, 74–75
  hormone production of, 150
  hypothalamic- and pituitary-like
      peptides of, 60, 61t
  in pregnancy, function of, 150
  prostaglandin synthesis by, 164
  relation to placenta of, 150
  trophoblastic cell infiltration of,
      42, 43f
Decidua basalis, 148
Decidua capsularis, 148
Decidua vera, 148
Decongestants, as potential terato-
      gens, 310
Deflection attitudes, 543f, 543–562.
      See also under
      Malpresentation; *indi-*
      vidual types.
Dehydroepiandrosterone sulfate
      (DHEAS), plasma lev-
      els of, in pregnancy,
      141
Delivery, 427–453. *See also* Labor;
      Parturition.

after cesarean section, 667–672.
      See also under Cesarean
      section.
  anesthesia in, 517–520, 520t. *See*
      also Anesthesia.
  in aortic regurgitation, 1065
  in aortic stenosis, 1064
  assisted spontaneous, 431–432
      cord clamping in, 432
      delivery of head in, 432
      delivery of shoulders and
          body in, 432
      episiotomy in, 431–432
  blood loss volume in, 138
  breech, 552–558. *See also under*
      Breech presentation.
  in brow presentation, 548–549
  in cervical cancer, 1211
  cesarean. *See* Cesarean section.
  in eclampsia, 1024–1025
  in Eisenmenger syndrome, 1067
  elective
      in fetal bleeding, 412
      respiratory distress syndrome
          in, 407
  in face presentation, 545–547,
      546f
  in fatty liver, 1170–1171
  forceps, 441–446. *See also*
      Forceps delivery.
  in heart disease, antibiotic pro-
      phylaxis in, 1061, 1062t
  in HELLP syndrome, 1007–1008
  hemodynamics in, 1059
  hypoparathyroidism in, 1124
  in immune thrombocytopenic
      purpura, 1144, 1145f
  in intrauterine growth retarda-
      tion, 937–938
  in maternal diabetes mellitus,
      1112–1114
  in mitral regurgitation,
      1064–1065
  in mitral stenosis, 1063
  pain pathways in, 494f, 495
  in Rh isoimmunization, 976–
      977
  in seizure disorders, 1188

in severe preeclampsia,
1018–1019
in shoulder dystocia, 565f–568f,
565–567
in sickle cell anemia, 1142
in systemic lupus erythematosus,
1157
in tetralogy of Fallot, 1067
twin
abruptio placenta in, 580
blood loss in, 138
breech presentation of second twin in, 558
vacuum extraction, 446
in von Willebrand's disease,
1146–1147
Delivery room, neutral thermal
environment in, 726f,
727
Denominator, fetal, 453
Dental caries, 126
Deoxycorticosterone (DOC), plasma levels of, in pregnancy, 141
Depression
postpartum, 770–771
post-sterilization, 768–769
Dermatitis, papular, 1218t, 1219
Dermatologic disorders,
1215–1220. *See also*
individual types.
Dermatome chart, 507f
DES exposure, maternal
cervical incompetence in, 858
preterm birth and, 838
Diabetes insipidus, 1126
Diabetes mellitus
gestational, 1104
diagnosis of, 1106t,
1106–1107
patient management in, 1114
postpartum evaluation of,
1107, 1107t
maternal, 1097–1115
antepartum fetal testing in,
1109–1112
biophysical profile in,
1110–1111

contraction stress test in,
1110
Doppler velocimetry in,
1112
in high-risk patients, 1110t
in low-risk patients, 1110t
maternal monitoring of
fetal activity in, 1111
nonstress test in, 1110
ultrasound in, 1112
breast-feeding in, 200, 1114
classification and risk assessment in, 1104, 1104t
congenital malformations in,
1101–1102, 1102f
coronary artery disease in,
1106
counseling in, 1115
contraception, 1115–1116
delivery in, 1112–1114
cesarean, 1113, 1114
elective preterm,
1112–1113
insulin regimen in,
1113–1114
fetal death in, 1100–1101
fetal hyperglycemia in, 1099,
1100f
fetal L/S ratio and, 409–410
fetal macrosomia in,
338–339, 1099, 1100f,
1102f, 1102–1103
fetal nonstress test and, 395
increased insulin requirement in, 1098
insulin-dependent,
1107–1109
continuous subcutaneous
insulin infusion in, 1108
diet therapy in, 1108
insulin regimen in,
1107–1108
ketoacidosis in, 1109
target plasma glucose levels in, 1107, 1108t
intrauterine growth retardation in, 925–926
labor in, 1113

neonatal hyperbilirubinemia
in, 1103–1104
neonatal hypocalcemia in,
1103
neonatal hypoglycemia in,
730–731, 1103, 1113
neonatal hypomagnesemia
in, 1103
neonatal polycythemia in,
1103–1104
neonatal respiratory distress
syndrome in, 1103,
1113
nephropathy in, 1104–1105
pathophysiology of,
1097–1100
perinatal morbidity and mortality in, 1100–1104
historical, 1097, 1098f
renal transplantation in, 1105
retinopathy in, 1105–1106
spontaneous abortion and,
795, 796t
Diabetic ketoacidosis, 629–630
laboratory values in, 630
in pregnancy, 630
symptoms of, 1109
treatment of, 1109
symptoms and management in,
630
Diabetogenic effect, of pregnancy,
142, 1098, 1099f
Diagonal conjugate, pelvic, 433
Diaphragm, contraceptive, 765–766
Diaphragmatic hernia, neonatal,
732
Diazepam
breast-feeding and, 319
in labor, 500
Diazepine, as potential teratogen,
305–306
Dicloxacillin, breast-feeding and,
321
Diet, in breast-feeding
atopic disease and, 199–200
caloric intake and, 199, 761–762
Dietary allowances, recommended
(RDA), 224t–225t

Dietary cravings, in pregnancy, 125
Dieting, breast-feeding and, 762
Digoxin
  breast-feeding and, 321
  as potential teratogen, 306–307
Dilatation, definition of, 453
Dimenhydrinate, as potential teratogen, 310
Dioxin, birth defects and, 252–253
Diphenhydramine, as potential teratogen, 310
Disseminated intravascular coagulation (DIC), 603–604
  in abruptio placenta, 583–584
  in death of twin in utero, 901–902, 902f
  hemolytic uremic syndrome and, 1093–1094
  laboratory values in, 604
  obstetric causes of, 604
  pathophysiology of, 603
  in preeclampsia, 1005
  treatment of, 604
DNA analysis, 287–288, 288f–290f
  disorders detectable by, 293t
  dot-blot analysis in, 287, 290f, 291
  polymerized chain reaction in, 287–288, 290f
  restriction endonucleases in, 287, 288f–289f
  restriction fragment length polymorphisms in, 291, 292f, 293t
  Southern blotting in, 287, 288f–289f
Monosomy X, 274
  in first-trimester abortuses, 787, 789f
Doppler effect, 400–402, 402f
Doppler velocimetry, 399–406
  accuracy of, 405
  continuous wave, 403
  duplex, 402–403
  in intrauterine growth retarda-

tion, 404–405, 934–937, 936f
  in maternal diabetes mellitus, 1112
  physics of, 400–402, 402f
  in preeclampsia, 1009–1010, 1010t
  pulsatility index for, 403
  resistance (Pourcelot) index for, 403
  in Rh isoimmunization, for fetal management, 969
  S/D ratio for, 403, 404f
  specificity and sensitivity of, 405–406
  in twin gestation, 894–896
  for umbilical artery, 403–404, 406f–407f
  for uterine artery, 403, 405f
Dot-blot analysis, 287, 290f, 291
Down syndrome. See Trisomy 21.
Drug(s). See also individual types.
  in breast milk, 318–322, 762
  intrauterine growth retardation due to, 927
  pharmacokinetics of, physiology of pregnancy and, 1224
  prenatal education about, 222
  as potential teratogens, 299–318. See also individual drugs.
    FDA labeling of, 299–300
Drug abuse
  in intrauterine growth retardation, 927
  prenatal counseling and, 213
Ductus arteriosus, patent
  in hyaline membrane disease, 720–721
  maternal, 1066
Duhrssen's cervical incision, in breech presentation, 687, 687f
Duodenal atresia
  neonatal, 731
  ultrasound for, 362, 364f
Duodenal ulcer, 1174
Dyspnea, 129–130

E

Early pregnancy factor (EPF), 59, 62–64
  detection of, 62, 64f
  in diagnosis of pregnancy, 85–86
  function in pregnancy of, 64
  molecular structure of, 62
  origin of, 62
  variation during pregnancy of, 62, 64
Eclampsia, 1021–1035. See also Blood pressure; Hypertension; Preeclampsia.
  abruptio placenta in, 1031–1032
  atypical, 1029t, 1029–1030
    late postpartum, 1029t, 1029–1030
    before 20 weeks, 1029
  cerebral manifestations of, 1023–1024
    CT findings in, 1023
    EEG findings in, 1024
    MRI findings in, 1023–1024
  convulsions in, 1025, 1190t
  counseling in, 1034–1035, 1035t
  fetal heart rate monitoring in, 1024–1025
  hemodynamic profile in, 624t
  historical, 1021
  incidence of, 1022–1023, 1023t
  labor and delivery in, 1024–1025
  laboratory findings in, 1028, 1029t
  maternal morbidity and mortality in, 1030–1031, 1031t–1032t
    gestational age and, 1030
    maternal age and, 1030–1031
    parity and, 1031, 1031t
    twin gestation and, 1031
  maternal transport in, 1032–1033
  neonatal outcome in, 1032
  pathophysiology of, 1021–1023
    blood pressure in, 1022
    edema in, 1022, 1022f

organ system derangements in, 1021
proteinuria in, 1022
weight gain in, 1021–1022
perinatal outcome in, 1031–1032
prevention of, 1033t–1034t, 1033–1034
time frame for, 1022
treatment of convulsions in, 1025–1028
aspiration and, 1026
avoid polypharmacy in, 1027–1028
magnesium sulfate in, 1026–1027, 1027f
maternal acidemia and, 1027
oxygenation in, 1025–1026
phenytoin in, 1027–1028
prevention of maternal injury in, 1025
Ectopic pregnancy, 809–824
as abortion complication, 1318
cytotrophoblast arteriolar invasion in, 42
diagnosis of, 814–817
β-hCG in, 814
signs and symptoms in, 814–815, 815f
ultrasound in, 815–817, 817f–818f
etiology of, 813–814
intauterine device as, 814
pelvic inflammatory disease in, 813
preembryo in, 814
previous sterilization as, 814
therapeutic abortion in, 813–814
fetomaternal hemorrhage in, 961
incidence of, 809–810, 810f–811f
management of
in ampullary pregnancies, 820–821, 821f
in fimbrial-infundibular pregnancies, 820
in isthmic pregnancies, 821–822, 822f
nonoperative, 823
paradigm for, 819f
Rh immunization and, 823
salpingectomy in, 822–823
salpingectomy vs. conservative tubal surgery in, 818–820, 820t
salpingectomy vs. salpingo-oophorectomy in, 818–820
surgical, 818–823
physiology and anatomy of, 810–813, 812f
Rh isoimmunization in, 964–965, 965t
Edema
ankle, 135
in eclampsia, 1022, 1022f
in preeclampsia, 993–994, 995
prenatal education about, 223–224
pulmonary
in preeclampsia, 623–624, 625t
tocolytic-induced, 627, 848–849
Education, patient
for contraception, 764–765
postpartum, 757–758
preconceptual, 212
prenatal, 222–229. *See also* Prenatal education.
in prevention of preterm birth, 841
in spontaneous abortion, 789–790
Effacement, cervical, 453
Eicosanoids, formation of, 159f
Eisenmenger syndrome
in pregnancy, 1067
Swan-Ganz catheterization in, 626–627
Embolism, amniotic fluid
clinical signs of, 601
in oxytocin-induced labor, 451
seizures in, 1190t
treatment of, 603
Embryo
biopsy of, 282–283, 283f
hCG levels and, 85t, 86f, 783
normal development of, 300–301
preimplantation, cytogenetic analysis of, 784, 786f
teratogenesis and, 236
ultrasound of. *See* Ultrasound, of embryo.
Emetrol, as potential teratogen, 310
Employment, prenatal education about, 224–225
Encephalocele, 356, 357f
Endocrinology, fetoplacental, 59–82. *See also individual hormones.*
Endocytosis, receptor-mediated, 99–100, 100f
Endometrial biopsy, 794
Endometritis, 1278–1282
aerobic gram-negative bacilli in, 1280
after cesarean section, 659–660
clinical diagnosis of, 659–660
laboratory evaluation in, 660
microbiology in, 659
therapy in, 660
anaerobic gram-negative bacilli in, 1280
chlamydia in, 1281
diagnosis of, 1281
gram-negative cocci in, 1280
gram-positive bacilli in, 1280
gram-positive cocci in, 1279
mycoplasma in, 1281
pathophysiology and bacteriology of, 1279–1281
prevention of, 1282
prognosis in, 1282
syncytial, 42
treatment of, 1281
Endometrium, gestational hyperplasia of, 40
Endotracheal intubation, in general anesthesia, 523–524

Engagement
definition of, 453
of fetal head, 428–429, 429f
Enterocolitis, necrotizing, neonatal, 732–733
Environmental chemicals, abortion due to, 801
Environmental Mutagen, Carcinogen, and Teratogen Information Department, 259
Environmental Teratology Information Center, 259
Enzyme-linked immunoassay (ELISA), 84f
Epidemiology, 238–245
analytic, 242–244
attributable risk in, 244
case-control studies in, 242–243
cohort studies in, 243–244
cross-sectional studies in, 242
ecologic studies in, 242
etiologic fraction in, 244
odds ratio in, 243
recall bias in, 243
relative risk in, 244
descriptive, 240–242
Birth Defects Monitoring Program, 241
case reports in, 240
descriptive studies in, 240–241
Metropolitan Atlanta Congenital Defects Program, 241–242
state-based birth defects surveillance systems in, 242
surveillance programs in, 241–242
experimental (clinical trials), 244–245
study design principles in, 239–240
Epidermal growth factor
in fetal growth, 105

in placental growth, 94
Epidural anesthesia, lumbar, 501–515. *See also* Anesthesia, lumbar epidural.
Epilepsy. *See* Seizure disorders.
Epinephrine
fetal secretion of, 112
with lumbar epidural anesthesia, 512–515, 513f
maternal, effects on labor of, 158
normal reactions to, 506
as potential teratogen, 308
Episiotomy, 431–432
advantages vs. disadvantages of, 431
infection in, 1285, 1286f
medial vs. mediolateral, 431–432
postpartum care of, 758
in preterm delivery, 870
Epulis gravidarum, 126
Ergonovine, in postpartum hemorrhage, 592
Ergotamine, breast-feeding and, 318
Erythema, palmar, 127, 130, 1216
Erythema infectiosum, 1234
Erythroblastosis fetalis. *See also* Rh isoimmunization.
historical, 957–958
Erythromycin
breast-feeding and, 321
as potential teratogen, 313
Esophageal atresia, neonatal, 731
Estradiol
function during pregnancy of, 79
molecular structure of, 78, 78f
origin of, 79
variation during pregnancy of, 79, 79f
Estriol
in evaluation of trisomy 21, 285
function during pregnancy of, 79
molecular structure of, 78, 78f

origin of, 79
variation during pregnancy of, 79, 79f
Estrogen, 78–79
breast-feeding and, 321–322
effects on labor of, 158
function during pregnancy of, 79
lactogenic effects of, 191
in mammogenesis, 182
molecular structure of, 78, 78f
origin of, 79
as potential teratogen, 302
variation during pregnancy of, 79, 79f
Estrone
molecular structure of, 78, 78f
origin of, 79
variation during pregnancy of, 79, 79f
Ethionamide, as potential teratogen, 313
Ethnic origin, prenatal testing and, 276, 277t
Ethosuximide, nonpregnant daily dosage of, 1187t
Etidocaine, maximal recommended dosage of, 505t
Etretinate, as potential teratogen, 305
Eyes, in pregnancy, 142–143

F

Face presentation, 453f, 543–547
causes of, 544
cesarean section in, 546–547
definition of, 543–544, 544f
diagnosis of, 544–545, 545f
fetal heart rate monitoring in, 546
incidence of, 544
labor in, 545–546, 546f
left mentum transverse, 544f
mentum anterior, 544f
right mentum posterior, 544, 544f

vaginal delivery in, 545–547, 546f
Facial cleft
    fetal, ultrasound for, 362, 365f
    in phenytoin exposure, 1185
Facial hirsutism, in pregnancy, 130, 1215
Facial palsy, neonatal, 717
Fallopian tube
    ampulla of, 19
    anatomy of, 18–19, 19f
    fimbrial end of, 19
    interstitial (intramural), 19
    isthmus of, 19
    lymphatic drainage of, 28
    postpartum, 754–755
    tubal ligation of, 681–684
        after cesarean section, 681
        counseling for, 684
        ectopic pregnancy due to, 814
        incision in, 682
        Irving technique in, 682
        Kroener fimbriectomy in, 683, 684f
        Pomeroy technique in, 682, 682f
        postpartum, 768
        reversal of, 682, 768
        techniques for, 682–684
        Uchida technique in, 682, 683f
    vascular supply of, 26f, 27
Fat, neonatal requirements for, 729
Fatigue, postpartum, 757
Feeding, in pregnancy, metabolic response to, 142
Female genitalia, fetal, 344, 349f
Femoral venous pressure, 134
Femur, fetal
    for gestational age, 335, 336t
    ultrasound for, 344, 348f
Femur/foot length ratio, fetal, 362
Femur length/abdominal circumference ratio
    in fetal macrosomia, 339
    in intrauterine growth retardation, 928

Ferguson reflex, 158
Fertilization, hydatidiform mole due to, 52
Fetal acid-base evaluation. *See also* Acid-base evaluation, fetal.
    antepartum, 399
    intrapartum, 474–477
Fetal activity assessment, maternal, 384–386, 387f
    clinical studies on, 385–386
    count-to-ten method for, 384
    factors influencing, 384–385
    in intrauterine growth retardation, 934
    management decisions and, 386, 387f
    in maternal diabetes mellitus, 1111
    movement alarm signal in, 384
Fetal alcohol syndrome, 315f, 315–316
Fetal biophysical profile, 396–399
    drawbacks of, 399
    fetal acid-base evaluation in, 399
    fetal breathing movements in, 396–397
    in maternal diabetes mellitus, 1110–1111
    in normal ultrasound study, 399
    perinatal morbidity indices and, 398, 400f
    perinatal mortality statistics and, 398, 401f
    in prolonged pregnancy, 952
    prospective studies of, 398–399
    scoring for, 397–398, 398t
Fetal breathing movements, in biophysical profile, 396–397
Fetal circulation, persistent, neonatal respiratory distress syndrome and, 718–719
Fetal heart rate, 465–474
    acceleration in, contraction effects on, 471, 473f
    acid-base evaluation and, 474, 474t

    in amniotomy, 449
    antepartum evaluation of. *See* Nonstress test.
    arrhythmic, 466, 468–469, 469f
        artifact in, 466, 468–469
        supraventricular tachycardia in, 469, 469f
    autonomic regulation of, 107–108
    baseline, 464f–465f, 465–466
    bradycardic
        in intrapartum monitoring, 464f, 465–466
        in nonstress test, 394f, 395
        in paracervical anesthesia, 516, 516f
    contraction effects on, 469–471
    early deceleration in
        clinical management of, 479
        contraction effects on, 469, 470f
    in intrauterine growth retardation, 933
    late deceleration in
        clinical management of, 479–480, 480f–481f
        contraction effects on, 471, 472f–473f
    mixed variable-late pattern in, contraction effects on, 471, 473f
    normal physiology of, 107
    periodic activity cycles and, 113
    preterm, 868
    prolonged sudden deceleration in, 482f–484f, 482–484
    in scalp blood sampling, 477
    sinusoidal
        clinical management of, 484
        in intrapartum monitoring, 465f, 466
        in nonstress test, 391
    tachycardic, in intrapartum monitoring, 464f, 465–466
    variable
        acid-base status and, 475
        amnioinfusion and, 477–478

Fetal heart rate *(Continued)*
  normal beat-to-beat, 466,
    467f–468f
  in preterm infant, 868
  variable acceleration in, in intra-
    partum monitoring,
    466, 468f
  variable deceleration in
    clinical management of,
      480–482
    contraction effects on,
      469–471, 470, 471t
    grading of, 470, 471t
    in nonstress test, 395
    in umbilical cord compres-
      sion, 469–470, 470f
  vibroacoustic stimulation and,
    477
Fetal heart rate monitoring,
    460–465
  artifact in, 466, 468–469
  auscultation vs, 485
  continuous, 461–465
    external, 461–463, 462f
    instrumentation in, 461
    internal, 462f–464f, 463–465
  in eclampsia, 1024–1025
  external, risks of, 486, 488f
  in face presentation, 546
  in fetal stress, 478
  general principles of, 478–479
  intermittent, 460–461
    in high-risk patients, 461
    in low-risk patients, 460–461
  internal, risks of, 486
  in intrauterine growth retarda-
    tion, 938
  medicolegal aspects of, 486,
    487f–488f
  in preterm birth, 485
  in preterm labor, 868
  in prolonged pregnancy,
    954–955
  studies of outcome with, 484–485
  in third trimester fetal bleeding,
    589, 590f–591f
Fetal hydantoin syndrome, 303,
    304f, 1184–1185

Fetal hydrops, 354, 356f
Fetal movement record, 216, 217f
Fetal pulmonary maturation,
    409–414, 697–703
  amniotic fluid turbidity in,
    411–412
    optical density in, 412
    visual inspection in, 411–412
  clinical determination of,
    413–414, 415t
  corticosteroids for, in placenta
    previa, 587
  glucocorticoids for, 856t–857t,
    856–857
  in intrauterine growth retarda-
    tion, 937
  in maternal diabetes mellitus,
    1113
  placental grading and
    cephalometry in,
    412–413, 413t, 414f
  in premature rupture of mem-
    branes, 864–865
  surfactant function in, 411, 700
    foam stability index in, 411
    shake test in, 411
    tap test in, 411
  surfactant production in, type II
    pneumocyte in, 698,
    698f
  surfactant quantitation in,
    409–410
    disaturated phosphatidyl-
      choline in, 410–411,
      700, 700f
    L/S ratio in, 409–410
    microviscosimeter in, 410
    slide agglutination test for PG
      in, 410
  thyroid-releasing hormone ther-
    apy in, 857–858
  in twin gestation, 906–907
Fetal research, 1341–1346
  consent for, 1342
  federal regulations on, 1341
  state statutes on, 1341–1342
  tissues for transplantation and,
    1342–1346

Fetal solvent syndrome, 256
Fetal transfusion syndrome, placen-
    ta in, 45
Fetal trimethadione syndrome,
    1186
Fetal wastage, 783–803. *See also*
    Abortion; *individual
    causes;* Mortality, peri-
    natal.
  antepartum, 378–379
  causes of, 790–801
    abnormal axial lie as, 542
    alloimmune disease as,
      798–800
    antifetal antibodies as,
      797–798
    autoimmune disease as, 798
    chromosomal abnormalities
      as, 790–792, 791f,
      792t–793t
      aneuploidy, 793, 793t
      inversions, 792-793
      translocations, 790–792,
        791f, 792t
    drugs, chemical, noxious
      agents as, 800–801
    incompetent cervix as, 797
    infection as, 797
    intrauterine adhesions as,
      795
    leiomyoma as, 796–797
    luteal phase defects as,
      793–795
    maternal diabetes mellitus as,
      795, 796t, 1100–1101
    Müllerian fusion defect as,
      795–796, 796f
    psychological factors as, 801
    Rh isoimmunization as,
      964–965, 965t
    severe maternal illness as, 801
    thyroid as, 795
    trauma as, 801
  clinically recognized, 784–787
    cytogenetic findings in,
      786–787
    frequency and timing in, 784,
      786

death in utero, elective abortion after, 1326–1327

first trimester, pathologic findings in, 787, 788t

grief reactions to, 772–774

in parvovirus infection, 1234–1235

of twin in utero, 901–902, 902f

Fetomaternal hemorrhage

causes of, 961

placental aging and, 47

in Rh isoimmunization, 47, 960–961, 965, 965t

α-Fetoprotein (AFP), 60, 69–71

amniotic fluid (AF-AFP), in neural tube defect, 292–293

function of, 71

maternal serum (MSAFP)

causes of elevated, 293, 294f

gestational age and, 293, 294f

maternal weight and, 293, 294f

in multiple gestation, 293

in neural tube defect, 293–295, 294f, 295t

trisomy 21 and, 285, 286f

molecular structure of, 69

origin of, 70–71

in prenatal testing, 285, 286f

variation during pregnancy of, 69–70, 70f

Fetus

abdominal circumference of

in macrosomia, 339

ultrasound for, 336f–338f, 336–338

abdominal wall of, 344, 348f

abnormal, prenatal care and, 216

adrenal cortex of

growth of, 76f, 76–77

placenta and, steroidogenesis by, 75–78, 76f–77f

adrenal glands of, 111–112

adrenal steroids, parturition and, 49

anatomy of, ultrasound for, 342–344, 343f–349f

anesthesia effects on, 496–497

anomalies of. *See also individual anomalies*

echocardiography in, 364

informed consent issues and, 366

karyotyping in, 364, 366

management in, 364–369

aggressive, 366f, 366–367

cephalocentesis in, 369

invasive procedures for, 367, 368f

nonaggressive, 369

pregnancy termination in, 367–369

ultrasound for, 344–364

anomalous, selective termination of, 902–904

antepartum testing of, 377–417. *See also* Antepartum fetal testing.

biometry of, ultrasound for, 362

biopsy of, in genodermatosis, 287

bladder of, 344, 347f

bleeding

elective delivery in, 412

third trimester, 589, 590f–591f

breathing of, 113, 703

cardiac activity in, 331. *See also* Fetal heart rate.

central nervous system of, 113

cerebellum of, 344, 345f

in chorioamnionitis, 50

circulation in, 105–110, 705–707, 706f

anatomy of, 105, 105f

autonomic regulation of, 107–108

heart and, 106t, 106–107, 107f

hemodynamic pressures in, 707, 707t

hemoglobin and, 109f, 109–110

hormonal regulation of, 108–109

cystic hygroma of, 354, 355f

death of. *See* Abortion; Fetal wastage; Mortality, perinatal.

femur/foot length ratio of, 362

femur of, 344, 348f

fibula of, 344, 349f

gastrointestinal tract of, 111

genital differentiation in, 113–115, 114f

genitalia of

female, 344, 349f

male, 344, 349f

gonads of, 113–115

growth and metabolism in, 103–105

amino acids in, 104

calories in, 103

glucose in, 103–104, 1098–1099

hormones in, 104–105

insulin in, 104–105, 142

insulin-like growth factors in, 104–105

substrates in, 103–104

growth chart for, 338, 338f

growth evaluation of, 336f–338f, 336–338

heart of, 344, 346f

hypoglycemic, in intrauterine growth retardation, 927

intrapartum evaluation of, 457–489. *See also* Fetal heart rate monitoring.

kidneys of, 110, 344, 348f

liver of, 111

lung development in, 697–698. *See also* Fetal pulmonary maturation.

macrosomia of. *See* Macrosomia, fetal.

maturity assessment of. *See also* Antepartum fetal testing.

for cesarean section, 231

Fetus (*Continued*)
  for elective labor induction, 451
  normal state of, antepartum fetal testing and, 383–384
  orbit distances of, 362, 365f
  parvovirus infection of, 1234–1235
  periodic cycles of, active vs. quiet, 113
  platelet count of, in maternal immune thrombocytopenic purpura, 1145
  pleural effusion shunt for, 367, 368f
  postmature, 946
  pulmonary maturation assessment in, 409–414. *See also* Fetal pulmonary maturation.
  radiation effects on. *See* under Radiation.
  in Rh isoimmunization, 965–971. *See also under* Rh isoimmunization.
  sacrococcygeal teratoma of, 353f–354f, 354
  scalp blood sampling
    complications of, 486
    heart rate during, 477
    technique for, 475–476
  skull of
    landmarks of, 452f, 453
    presenting diameters of, 429, 429f
    transverse diameters of, 428, 428f
    ultrasound for, 343f–344f, 344
  sleep states of, quiet vs. active, 383–384
  spine of, 344, 345f–346f
  stomach of, 344, 347f
  thyroid function in, 1116–1117
  thyroid gland of, 112–113
  tibia of, 344, 349f
  ultrasound of. *See* Ultrasound, of fetus.
  umbilical cord insertion of, 344, 348f
  vesicoamniotic shunt for, 367
  viability of, ultrasound for, 336
  weight of
    ultrasound for, 338–339, 564
    in intrauterine growth retardation, 931
    in vaginal birth after cesarean section, 669
Fibrinogen
  in preeclampsia, 1005
  in pregnancy, 127, 139
Fibrinolysis, postpartum, 756
Fibronectin, in preeclampsia, 997
Fibula, fetal, 344, 349f
Fifth disease, 1234
Fimbriectomy, Kroener, 683, 684f
Fluid and electrolytes, neonatal requirements for, 728
Foam stability test, for pulmonary surfactant, 411
Folate deficiency, 1138–1139
Forceps delivery, 441–446
  in breech presentation, 556, 557f
  classic-type forceps for, 441–442
  classifications of, 442
  indications and contraindications for, 442–443
  prerequisites for, 443
  in preterm birth, 870
  specialized forceps for, 442
  technique for, 443–446
    low forceps and, 444
    mid-forceps and, 444
    occiput transverse positions and, 444–445
    outlet forceps and, 443–444
    proper application in, 444, 445f
    traction in, 445–446
  types of forceps for, 441, 441f–442f
Formula, for infant feeding, 729–730
Fourchette
  anterior, 9
  posterior, 9
Frankenhauser's ganglion, 31f, 32
Frank-Starling principle, 615
Fundal height
  in gestational age assessment, 227f, 230
  in intrauterine growth retardation, 928
Fungal infection, susceptibility to, 1224

G
Gallbladder, 126, 1173. *See also* Chole- entries.
Gastric acid secretion, 126, 1174
Gastrointestinal disease, 1173–1180. *See also individual types.*
Gastrointestinal tract
  fetal, normal physiology of, 111
  maternal
    obstruction of, 686–687
    post-cesarean section complications of, 663–664
    traumatic injury of, in cesarean section, 654
  neonatal
    congenital conditions of, 731–732
    flora of
      bottle feeding and, 198
      breast milk and, 198
    obstruction of, 731–732
Gastroschisis
  neonatal, 732
  ultrasound for, 356, 361f
Genetic counseling, 276–278
  communication in, 276–277
  legal issues of, 1333–1336
  nondirective, 277
  psychological considerations in, 277–278
  in spontaneous abortion, 789–790
Genetic disease, 269–271. *See also individual types.*
  chromosomal, 269, 270t, 271–274

polygenic/multifactorial, 269–270, 270t
single-gene, 269
Genetic history, 274–276, 275f
Genetic screening, 278–279. *See also* Prenatal diagnosis.
altered clinical management and, 278
indications for, 278
legal issues of, 1333–1336
neonatal, 278
population, and cystic fibrosis, 278–279
population, and neural tube defect, 295t
population, and Tay-Sachs, 277t
in spontaneous abortion, 790
Genitalia
female
external, 9–10
fetal, 344, 349f
fetal differentiation of, 113–115, 114f
male, fetal, 344, 349f
Genodermatosis, fetal skin biopsy in, 287
Genome mapping, 1346–1348
Gestation
multiple. *See* Multiple gestation.
prolonged. *See* Prolonged pregnancy.
twin. *See* Twin gestation.
Gestational age
at abortion, maternal death and, 1304, 1305t–1306t
abruptio placenta and, 582–583
assessment of, 229–231
clinical dating in, 227f, 230–231
complications of, 229–230
fetal heart tones in, 230
in fetal maturity assessment, 231
fundal height in, 227f, 230
importance of, 230
last menstrual period (LMP) in, 230
quickening in, 230

ultrasound in, 231
biparietal diameter for, 333, 334f–335f, 335–336, 336t
birth weight vs., in preterm birth, 829–830, 830f
cephalic index for, 335
crown-rump length and, 333, 333f–334f
eclampsia outcome and, 1030
femur length for, 335, 336t
maternal serum α-fetoprotein (MSAFP) and, 293, 294f
neonatal risk assessment and, 734f–736f, 735–737
in premature rupture of membranes, 865
tocolytic therapy and, 855–856
ultrasound for, 333, 334f–335f, 335–336, 336t
Gestational diabetes, 1104
diagnosis of, 1106t, 1106–1107
patient management in, 1114
postpartum evaluation of, 1107, 1107t
Gestational sac
disappearance of, 887f–888f, 889
in multiple gestation, 886, 887f
ultrasound for, 331–332
Gingivitis, in pregnancy, 126
Glomerular filtration rate
fetal, normal physiology of, 110
in pregnancy, 131, 132t, 1085
Glomerulonephritis, 1087–1088
preeclampsia vs., 1087
pregnancy outcome in, 1087–1088
treatment of, 1087
Glucagon, in normal pregnancy, 1098
Glucocorticoids
in asthma, 1076
fetal, labor and, 158
for fetal pulmonary maturation, 856t–857t, 856–857
pulmonary surfactant effects of, 701, 702t

Glucose
fetal metabolism of, 103–104, 1098–1099
maternal metabolism of, 141–142, 1097–1098, 1099f
placental transfer of, 96–97, 142
urinary excretion of, in pregnancy, 133, 1085
Glucose tolerance testing, in gestational diabetes, 1106t, 1106–1107
Gluteal artery
inferior, 25, 25f
superior, 24, 25f
Gold therapy, in rheumatoid arthritis, 1161
Gonadotropin-releasing hormone (GnRH), placental, 71–73
function of, 72–73
molecular structure of, 71
origins of, 72
variation during pregnancy of, 72
Gonads, fetal, 113–115, 114f
Gonococcal infection, 1269–1272
clinical aspects of, 1270–1271, 1271f
diagnosis of, 1271
disseminated, 1224, 1271,1271f
epidemiology of, 1271
historical, 1269
immunology of, 1270
management of, 1272
microbiology of, 1269
ophthalmia neonatorum and, 1272
in pregnancy, 1272
Granuloma gravidarum, 1216
Granulomas, pyogenic, 1216
Graves' disease, 1117
Gravidin, phospholipase A_2 inhibition by, 166–167
Grief, perinatal, 772–774
Growth-adjusted sonographic age, 336

Growth curves, neonatal risk assessment and, 734f–736f, 735–737
Growth hormone, in mammogenesis, 182
Growth retardation, intrauterine. *See* Intrauterine growth retardation.
Gums, in pregnancy, 126

H

Hair, in pregnancy, 130, 1215–1216
Hair removal, principles, before surgery, 641
Hashimoto's thyroiditis, 1121
Head, fetal, assisted spontaneous delivery of, 432
Headache, spinal, 508–509
Head circumference/abdominal circumference ratio
    in fetal macrosomia, 338f, 339
    in intrauterine growth retardation, 928, 929f
Heart
    fetal
        anomalies of, 362, 364
        normal anatomy of, 331, 344, 346f
        normal physiology of, 106t, 106–107, 107f
    maternal, position of, 135
Heartburn, prenatal education about, 226
Heart disease, maternal, 1057–1071. *See also individual types.*
    antibiotic prophylaxis for labor and delivery in, 1061, 1062t
    anticoagulants in, 1061
    cardiac surgery in, 1061–1062
    congenital, 1065–1068
        atrial septal defect, 1066
        coarctation of aorta, 1067–1068
        Eisenmenger syndrome, 1067

left-to-right shunt in, 1065–1066
        patent ductus arteriosus, 1066
        right-to-left shunt in, 1066–1067
        tetralogy of Fallot, 1066–1067
        ventricular septal defect, 1065–1066
    diagnosis of, 1059–1060
    ischemic, 1070–1071
    management of, 1060–1062
    normal cardiovascular findings vs., 136
    signs and symptoms of, 1060
    specific types of, 1062–1071
Heart murmur, maternal, 135
Heart rate
    cardiac output effects of, 616
    fetal. *See* Fetal heart rate; Nonstress test.
    maternal, 133, 1058
Heart sounds
    fetal, in gestational age assessment, 230
    maternal, 135
Heat loss, neonatal, 724–725, 725t
Heat production, neonatal, 724, 725t
HELLP syndrome, 1005–1008
    anesthesia in, 1018
    clinical presentation in, 1006
    delivery in, 1007–1008
    laboratory values for diagnosis of, 1005–1006
    management of, 1006–1008
    perinatal outcome in, 1007, 1007t
    postpartum, 1007
    terminology in, 1005
Hemangiomas, capillary, 1216
Hematocrit, in hemorrhage, 574
Hematoma
    bladder flap, after cesarean section, 663f
    broad ligament, after cesarean section, 664f
    pelvic, postpartum, 595–596

retroperitoneal, postpartum, 596, 599f
    vaginal, postpartum, 596, 598f
    vulvar, postpartum, 595–596, 597f–598f
Hematometra, 1318
Hemodialysis, in pregnancy, 1090–1091
Hemodynamic(s)
    in anesthesia, 1059
    in cesarean section, 1059
    in delivery, 1059
    in labor, 136, 1058–1059
    postpartum, 1059
    in pregnancy, 134–135, 135t, 1058, 1059f
    in puerperium, 136
Hemodynamic monitoring, invasive, 607–617, 608t. *See also* Swan-Ganz catheterization.
Hemodynamic profile
    in eclampsia, 624t
    in fetus, 707, 707t
    in neonate, 707, 707t
    in normal pregnancy, 619–620, 622t–623t
    in preeclampsia, 620–622, 624t, 1008–1009, 1009t
    with Swan-Ganz catheterization, 613–614, 614t
Hemodynamic therapy, pharmacologic, 617, 620t, 621f
Hemoglobin
    molecular structure of, 1139
    in pregnancy, 138, 138t, 1057–1058
Hemoglobin A
    abnormalities of. *See* Sickle cell anemia, β-thalassemia, α-thalassemia
    in fetus, 109–110
    genetic structure of, 110
Hemoglobin AS, 1139. *See also* Sickle cell anemia.
Hemoglobin Bart, 1143
Hemoglobin F (fetal), 109f, 109–110

genetic structure of, 110
oxygen affinity of, 109f, 109–110
Hemoglobinopathy, 1139, 1139t
Hemoglobin S, 1139–1142. *See also*
Sickle cell anemia.
Hemoglobin SC disease, 1142
Hemolytic uremic syndrome, post-partum, 1093–1094
Hemorrhage, 573–604. *See also*
Bleeding; *individual causes.*
in abortion, 1318
antepartum, 579–589
in abruptio placenta, 579–584
in placenta previa, 584–589
third trimester fetal, 589
blood transfusion in, 576–579.
See also Blood transfusion.
blood volume deficit in, 573
in choriocarcinoma, 55, 56f
class 1, 573
class 2, 573–574
class 3, 574
class 4, 574
classification of, 573–575, 574t
fetomaternal
causes of, 961
placental aging and, 47
in Rh isoimmunization, 47, 960–961, 965, 965t
hematocrit in, 574
in hypertension, 575
intracranial, neonatal, 716–717
periventricular/intraventricular, neonatal, 713–715, 714f, 715t
postpartum, 589–604
causes of, 592
in cervical laceration, 594, 596f
ergonovine in, 592
ligation of ovarian vessels in, 594
ligation of uterine artery in, 594, 597f

manual massage of uterus in, 592, 592f
oxytocin in, 592
pelvic hematoma in, 595–596
in perineal laceration, 593f–595f, 594
in periurethral laceration, 593f, 594
prostaglandin $F_{2\alpha}$ in, 593
in rectal sphincter laceration, 594, 594f–595f
retained placental fragments and, 592, 592f
retroperitoneal hematoma in, 596, 599f
source of, 593–594
umbrella pack for, 596, 598–599, 600f
in uterine inversion, 599–600, 601f–602f
vaginal hematoma in, 596, 598f
in von Willebrand's disease, 601
vulvar hematoma in, 595–596, 597f–598f
in preeclampsia, 575
subarachnoid, 1191
maternal, seizures in, 1190t
neonatal, 717
treatment of, 575
urine output and, 575
Hemorrhoids
maternal, 126
postpartum, 758
prenatal education about, 226
Hemostasis
in postpartum uterus, 754
in preeclampsia, 996–998
Heparin
breast-feeding and, 320
indications for and administration of, 306
in pulmonary thromboembolism, 1078–1079
Hepatic function, in preeclampsia, 1004–1005

Hepatic rupture, in preeclampsia, 1005
Hepatic transplantation, in pregnancy, 1172–1173
Hepatic veins, fetal, blood flow in, 105f, 105–106
Hepatitis B, 1261–1267
in breast milk, 762
chronic, 1265
clinical aspects of, 1263–1264
complications of, 1265
delta virus infection and, 1265
diagnosis of, 1264
epidemiology of, 1263
fulminant, 1265
immune globulin in, 1265–1266
immunization in, 1266
immunology of, 1262–1263, 1262f
management of, 1264–1265
microbiology of, 1261–1262
mother-to-infant transmission of, 1265
percutaneous exposure to, 1267
perinatal exposure to, 1266–1267
postexposure prophylaxis for, 1266–1267
preexposure prophylaxis for, 1266
prevention of, 1265
screening for, 215, 1265
sexual exposure to, 1267
Hernia, diaphragmatic, neonatal, 732
Herpes gestationis, 1216–1218, 1217f, 1218t
Herpes simplex virus infection, 1248–1252
clinical aspects of, 1249–1250, 1250f
congenital, 1250
diagnosis of, 1250–1251, 1251f
epidemiology of, 1249
immunology of, 1249
management of, 1251–1252
medical therapy in, 1252
microbiology of, 1248–1249
neonatal, 1250

Hirsutism, 1215–1216
facial, 130, 1215
HIV infection. *See* Human immunodeficiency virus (HIV).
HLA antigens, shared parental,
and recurrent abor-
tion, 798–800
Hodgkin's disease, 1203–1206
diagnosis and staging in, 1204,
1204t
incidence of, 1203
menses after, 1205, 1206f
perinatal outcome in,
1205–1206
pregnancy after, 1205
treatment of, 1204–1205
Holoprosencephaly
embryology of, 351f
ultrasound in, 348, 351f–352f
Hormones. *See individual types.*
Human immunodeficiency virus
(HIV), 1252–1259
autoantibodies in, 1259
in blood transfusion risks, 579
in breast milk, 199
clinical features of, 1256–1257
diagnosis and management of,
1257
epidemiology of, 1254f–1256f,
1253–1255
ethical issues in, 1259
immunology of, 1253–1254
microbiology of, 1252
nosocomial exposure to, 1258
parenteral transmission of, 1258
perinatal transmission of, 1258
premarital screening in, 1255
sexual transmission of,
1257–1258
syphilis and, 1258
Hyaline membrane disease,
720–724, 721f,
722t–723t. *See also*
Respiratory distress syn-
drome, neonatal.
bronchopulmonary dysplasia in,
721
clinical signs of, 720, 721f

complications of, 720
long-term sequelae of, 721
patent ductus arteriosus in,
720–721
surfactant in, 720
surfactant replacement therapy
in, 721–724, 722t–723t,
858
Hydantoin
intrauterine growth retardation
due to, 927
as potential teratogen, 303, 304f,
1184–1185
Hydatidiform mole, 52–56
benign vs. malignant, 55
due to fertilization abnormalities, 52
incidence of, 53
risk factors for, 53
snow storm ultrasound pattern
in, 53, 54f
theca-lutein cyst and, 53, 54f
trophoblastic proliferation in,
55
villi in, 53, 55
Hydralazine
in chronic hypertension in pregnancy, 1042
in severe preeclampsia, 1017
as potential teratogen, 307
Hydramnios
amniotic fluid index in,
340–342, 343f
maternal fetal activity assessment in, 385
maximum vertical pocket of
amniotic fluid in,
339–340
Hydrocephalus
cephalocentesis in, 269
management of, 368f, 369
ultrasound for, 356, 362, 363f
Hydrochlorothiazide, breast-feeding and, 320
Hydrops fetalis
nonimmune, 981, 981f, 982t
in parvovirus infection, 1234
17α-Hydroxyprogesterone

molecular structure of, 80, 80f
origin of, 80
variation during pregnancy of,
80, 81f
17α-Hydroxyprogesterone
caproate, as potential
teratogen, 302
Hyperbilirubinemia, neonatal,
737–739, 738f
in maternal diabetes mellitus,
1103–1104
Hypercoagulability, in pregnancy,
139
Hypercontractility, uterine, in oxytocin-induced labor,
450–451
Hyperemesis gravidarum, 127–128
Hyperglycemia
fetal, in maternal diabetes mellitus, 1099, 1100f
maternal. *See also* Diabetes mellitus, maternal.
spontaneous abortion and,
795, 796t
in tocolytic therapy, 850
Hyperoxygenation, maternal, in
intrauterine growth
retardation, 932
Hyperparathyroidism, 1122–
1124
clinical signs of, 1122
hypocalcemic tetany of newborn
in, 1123
laboratory diagnosis of, 1123
medical treatment of, 1123
parathyroidectomy in, 1123
perinatal morbidity and mortality in, 1123
physiologic, in pregnancy, 137
Hyperpigmentation, in pregnancy,
130, 1215
Hypertelorism, 362, 365f
Hypertension, 993–1047. *See also*
Blood pressure;
Eclampsia;
Preeclampsia.
abruptio placenta and, 580
chronic, 1035–1047

benefits of treating,
1035–1036
definition of, 994
pathophysiology of, 1035
with preeclampsia, 994
in pregnancy, 1036
abruptio placenta in, 1036
angiotensin-converting
enxyme inhibitors in,
1041
atenolol in, 1040
α-blockers and β-blockers
in, 1038, 1039–1041
calcium channel blockers
in, 1041
clonidine in, 1039
hydralazine in, 1042
labetolol in, 1041
management of,
1042–1044
maternal morbidity and
mortality and, 1036
medical treatment of,
1036–1037, 1037t
methyldopa in,
1038–1039, 1039t, 1041
metoprolol in, 1040–
1041
mild (low-risk), 1046t,
1046–1047, 1047f
oxprenolol in, 1040
prazosin in, 1039
preeclampsia and, 1036
propranolol in, 1040
severe (high-risk),
1044–1046, 1045t
thiazide diuretics in,
1041–1042, 1042f
in chronic renal failure, 1089
hemorrhage in, 575
in oxytocin-induced labor, 451
persistent pulmonary, neonatal
respiratory distress syn-
drome and, 718–719
in pregnancy, terminology in,
993–995
transient, definition of, 994
Hyperthyroidism, 1117–1119
causes of, 1117
diagnosis of, 1117–1118
fetal and neonatal complications
of, 1118–1119
hydatidiform mole and, 53
laboratory workup of, 1116,
1117f, 1118
neonatal, 1118–1119
postpartum, 1120
treatment of, 1118
Hypocalcemia
maternal, in massive blood
transfusion, 577
neonatal
in intrauterine growth retardation, 938
in maternal diabetes mellitus,
1103
Hypocalcemic tetany of newborn,
1122–1123
Hypogastric artery
anatomic distribution of, 23–25,
24f–25f
ligation of, in uterine atony,
655, 655f
ureter and, 23
Hypogastric plexus
inferior, 30f–31f, 31
superior, 30f, 30–31
Hypoglycemia
fetal, in intrauterine growth
retardation, 927
neonatal, 730–731
in intrauterine growth retardation, 938
in maternal diabetes mellitus,
1103, 1113
Hypokalemia, in tocolytic therapy,
850
Hypomagnesemia, neonatal, in
maternal diabetes mel-
litus, 1103
Hyponatremia, neonatal, in
intrauterine growth
retardation, 938
Hypoparathyroidism, 1124
diagnosis of, 1124
in labor and delivery, 1124
treatment of, 1124
Hypophyseal arteries, 29f, 33–34
Hypotelorism, 362
Hypotension
in lumbar epidural anesthesia,
503–504, 504f,
504t–505t
in pregnancy, due to supine position, 134, 1058, 1059f
in tocolytic therapy, 850
Hypothalamohypophyseal nerve
tract, 34, 35f
Hypothermia, neonatal. *See*
Neonate, thermal regu-
lation in.
Hypothyroidism
maternal, 1119–1120
diagnosis of, 1119
laboratory workup of, 1116,
1117f
postpartum, 1120
pregnancy outcome in, 1119
treatment of, 1119–1120
neonatal, 1118
Hysterectomy
cesarean, 673–680. *See also*
Cesarean hysterectomy.
for contraceptive sterilization,
769

I

IgA, secretory, in colostrum and
breast milk, 198
IgG, receptor-mediated endocytosis
of, 100
IgG therapy
fetal, in neonatal immune
thrombocytopenia, 983
maternal
in neonatal immune throm-
bocytopenia, 983
in Rh isoimmunization, 976
Ileus, after cesarean section,
663–664
Iliac artery, internal
anatomic distribution of, 23–25,
24f–25f

Iliac artery, internal *(Continued)*
  anterior trunk of, 25, 25f
  posterior trunk of, 24f–25f, 24–25
  ureter and, 23
Iliococcygeus muscle, 6f–7f, 6–7
Iliolumbar artery, 24, 25f
Ilium, 3, 4f
Immune system
  in pregnancy, 1223–1224
  secretory, 196f
Immunization
  hepatitis B, 1266
  prenatal education about, 225
  rubella, 1229–1230
Immunoglobulin(s), in pregnancy, 1223
Immunosuppressants, as potential teratogens, 307–308
Impetigo herpetiformis, 1218t, 1220
Implantation
  anomalies of, 44–46, 45f
  bleeding, mechanism of, 40
  histologic changes at, 39–41, 40f
  monozygotic twinning and, 44–45
  velamentous insertion in, 44–45
Inborn errors of metabolism, 287
  prenatal diagnosis of, 287
Incidence, definition of, 239
Indomethacin, as tocolytic, 853
Infant
  neonatal. *See* Neonate.
  preterm. *See* Preterm birth; Preterm infant; Preterm labor.
Infant mortality
  causes of, 378, 379f
  definition of, 377
  statistical, 233–234, 234t
Infarction, myocardial, 1070–1071
Infection, intrauterine. *See* Chorioamnionitis; *individual types.*
Inflammatory bowel disease, 1176–1180
  Crohn's disease in, 1176,

1177–1178, 1178t
  medical treatment of, 1178–1179
  surgical treatment of, 1179–1180
  ulcerative colitis in, 1176–1177, 1178t
Informed consent. *See also* Legal issues.
  in cesarean section, 639–640
  in fetal anomalies, 366
  in fetal invasive procedures, 366
  for prenatal ultrasound, 371
  in vaginal birth after cesarean section, 672
Inhibin, placental, 71–73
  function of, 72–73
  molecular structure of, 71–72
  origins of, 72
Insulin
  in fetal growth, 104–105, 142
  in maternal diabetes mellitus. *See* Diabetes mellitus, maternal.
  in normal pregnancy, 1098, 1099f
  in placental growth, 94
  receptor-mediated endocytosis of, 100
Insulin-like growth factor I (IGF-I)
  in fetal growth, 104–105
  in placental growth, 94
Insulin-like growth factor II (IGF-II)
  in fetal growth, 104–105
  in placental growth, 94
Intervillous space, 41
Intervillous thrombus, 47, 49f
Intracranial hemorrhage, neonatal, 716–717
Intrahepatic cholestasis, 1171–1172
  clinical manifestations of, 1171
  laboratory diagnosis of, 1171–1172
  management of, 1172
  perinatal outcome in, 1172
Intraocular pressure, 142–143
Intrapartum fetal evaluation, 457–489. *See also* Acid-

base evaluation, fetal; Fetal heart rate monitoring.
  acid-base evaluation in, 474–477
  fetal heart rate monitoring in, 460–465
  historical, 457–460
  methodology in, 459–460
  physiology in, 458
  patient refusal of, 489
  risk vs. benefit in, 484–489
Intrauterine adhesions, recurrent abortion due to, 795
Intrauterine device (IUD), 766–767
  in breast-feeding, 201
  ectopic pregnancy due to, 814
  pregnancy rate with, 767
  side effects of, 767
Intrauterine growth retardation, 923–940
  amniocentesis in, 937
  asymmetrical, growth chart in, 929f
  chromosomal abnormalities and, 925
  definition of, 923–925
  delivery in, 937–938
  diagnosis of, 928–932
    amniotic fluid index in, 928–929, 930f
    amniotic fluid maximum vertical pocket in, 928–929, 930f
    biparietal diameter in, 928
    femur length/abdominal circumference ratio in, 928, 929f
    fetal weight estimate in, 931
    fundal height measurement in, 928
    head circumference/abdominal circumference ratio in, 928, 929f
    incorrect dates vs., 931
    placental grade in, 929, 931, 931f
    ultrasound criteria for, 931, 932t

Doppler velocimetry in, 404–405
etiology of, 925t, 925–928
   chromosomal abnormalities in, 925
   congenital malformations in, 925
   drug and alcohol ingestion in, 927
   fetal hypoglycemia in, 927
   intrauterine infection in, 925
   maternal age and, 927
   maternal diabetes mellitus in, 926
   maternal weight gain in, 926–927
   placenta in, 926
   prior poor pregnancy outcome in, 927
   twin gestation and, 926
   uteroplacental blood flow in, 926
fetal nonstress test and, 395
fetal pulmonary maturation in, 937
L/S ratio in, 937
management of, 932–937
   contraction stress test in, 933, 934
   Doppler velocimetry in, 934–937, 936f
   fetal growth assessment in, 932–933
   fetal heart rate monitoring in, 933, 934
   genetic testing in, 933, 934t
   maternal hyperoxygenation in, 932
   maternal medical problems and, 932
   maternal monitoring of fetal activity in, 934
   nonstress test in, 933, 934
   ultrasound in, 933, 933t
neonatal outcome in, 938–940
   catch-up growth and, 939
   hypocalcemia in, 938
   hypoglycemia in, 938
   hyponatremia in, 938

hypothermia in, 938
meconium aspiration in, 938
neurologic sequelae in, 939–940
polycythemia in, 938
studies of, 939–940
perinatal morbidity in, 923
perinatal mortality in, 923
in rheumatoid arthritis, 1160
small-for-gestational-age infant vs., 924
symmetrical, growth chart in, 929f
in systemic lupus erythematosus, 1157
Intrauterine genetic diagnosis. *See* Prenatal diagnosis.
Intrauterine infection. *See* Chorioamnionitis; *individual types.*
Intrauterine inspection, after placental delivery, 447
Intrauterine transfusion, in Rh isoimmunization, 971–976. *See also under* Rh isoimmunization.
Intraventricular hemorrhage, neonatal, 713–715, 714f, 715t
Intubation, endotracheal, in general anesthesia, 523–524
Iodide, as potential teratogen, 308, 309f
Iodine, radioactive, as potential teratogen, 306
Ionizing radiation. *See* Radiation, ionizing.
Iron, metabolism, in pregnancy, 139–140, 140t
Iron requirements, in pregnancy, 1137, 1138t
Iron supplementation, in pregnancy, 139–140, 140t, 223, 1138, 1138t
Irving technique, of tubal ligation, 682
Ischiocavernosus muscle, 11

Ischiococcygeus muscle, 6
Ischiorectal fossa
   abscess of, 12
   anatomy of, 12, 13f
   fascia of, 12
Ischium, 3, 4f
Isoimmunization, 957–984. *See also individual types.*
   ABO, 978, 981
   minor blood group antigen, 977–978, 979t–980t
   platelet, 982–984. *See also* Thrombocytopenia, neonatal immune.
   Rh, 960–977
Isoniazid, breast-feeding and, 321
Isoproterenol, as potential teratogen, 308
Isotretinoin, as potential teratogen, 304–305, 305f

J
Jaundice, neonatal, 737–739, 738f
   breast milk, 737–738
   pathologic, 737
   physiologic, 737
Jugular vein, internal
   anatomic relationships of, 609, 610f
   cannulation of, 609–610, 610f–612f
Jugular venous pulse, 135

K
Kanamycin, as potential teratogen, 312
Karyotype. *See* Chromosomal abnormalities.
Kerr incision, in cesarean section, 645t, 645–647, 646f
Ketoacidosis, diabetic, 629–630
   laboratory values in, 630
   symptoms and management in, 630, 1109
   treatment of, 1109

Kidney. *See also under* Renal.
Kidney(s)
  fetal
    normal physiology of, 110
    ultrasound for, 344, 348f
  maternal, 131
Kidney stones, 1087
Klinefelter syndrome, 274
Krönig incision, in cesarean section, 645t, 645–647, 646f
Kroener fimbriectomy, 683, 684f

L
Labetalol
  in chronic hypertension in pregnancy, 1041
  in preeclampsia, 1013
Labia majora, 9
Labia minora, 9
Labor, 427–453
  abnormal patterns of, 435
  active phase of, 436–438
    cervicographic analysis of, 436
    eutonic, 436
    hypertonic, 436
    hypotonic, 436
  alphaprodine in, 499–500
  analgesia in, opioid, 498–500
  anesthesia in, 497–517. *See also* Anesthesia.
  in aortic regurgitation, 1065
  in aortic stenosis, 1064
  asthma in, 1077
  barbiturates in, 500
  benzodiazepine in, 500–501
  butorphanol in, 500
  cardiac output in, 1059
  catecholamine effects on, 158–159
  definition of, 427, 453
  diazepam in, 500
  disorders of, 435–439
  dysfunctional
    primary, 436–437, 437f–438f
    secondary, 437–438, 438f

in eclampsia, 1024–1025
in Eisenmenger syndrome, 1067
false, 435–436
in heart disease, antibiotic prophylaxis in, 1061, 1062t
hemodynamics in, 136, 1058–1059
humoral factors in, 158–159
hypoparathyroidism in, 1124
induction of, 447–450
  amniotomy in, 449
  Bishop prelabor scoring system prior to, 448, 448t
  complications of, 450–451
  contraindications for, 448
  elective, 451, 453
    fetal maturity assessment in, 451
  fetal maturity assessment prior to, 231
  indications for, 448
  medical-surgical methods for, 452
  oxytocin in, 439–440, 449–450
    complications of, 450–451
    proper uses of, 440
    rate of administration of, 440, 450
    technique for, 450
  prostaglandins in, 440
  stripping membranes in, 448–449
initiation of, 159–167
  model for, 168–170, 169f
  oxytocin in, 160–162
    levels of, 162, 163f
    plasma levels of, 160–161
    receptor concentration in, 161f–162f, 161–162
    uterine contraction, correlation with dosage in, 168
  progesterone withdrawal and, 159–160
  prostaglandins in, 160, 162–167

amnion in production of, 163
amniotic fluid levels of, 165f, 166
arachidonic acid metabolism and, 164
chorion in production of, 163–164
decidua in production of, 164
endogenous inhibitor withdrawal and, 166–167
endogenous stimulators of, 167
increased production of, 166–167
myometrium in production of, 164
oxytocic potencies of, 162–163
placenta in production of, 164
plasma levels of, 164–165, 165f–166f
receptors for, 163
urinary excretion of, 165–166
vasopressin in, 162
latent phase of, prolonged, 435–436
management of, 430–431
  active, 440–441
  in breech presentation, 551–552. *See also under* Breech presentation.
  in face presentation, 545–546, 546f
  in high-risk patients, 431
  initial assessment in, 430
  in low-risk patients, 430–431
  risk status assignment in, 430
  standard procedures in, 430
in maternal diabetes mellitus, 1113
mechanisms of, 427–430
  descent in, 429

engagement in, 428f,
428–429
expulsion in, 429–430
extension in, 429
external rotation in, 429
flexion in, 429, 429f
internal rotation in, 429
meperidine in, 499
midazolam in, 500–501
in mitral regurgitation,
1064–1065
in mitral stenosis, 1063
morphine in, 499
in myasthenia gravis, 1163
nalbuphine in, 500
neural mechanisms of, 158
oxytocic hormone effects on,
159, 159f
pain in, 495–497, 496f–497f
pathways of, 494f, 495
physiologic effects of,
495–497, 496f–497f
phases of, 427, 428t
phenothiazines in, 500
physiology of, 158–168
prenatal education about, 229
preterm, 841–858. *See also*
Preterm birth; Preterm
labor.
chorioamnionitis and, 51
relaxing hormone effects on,
158–159
scopolamine in, 501
second stage of
abnormalities of, 438–439
arrested descent in, 439
protracted descent in,
438–439
sedatives in, 500–501
in seizure disorders, 1188
in severe preeclampsia,
1018–1019
spontaneous, progression of,
428t
stages of, 427, 428t
steroid hormone effects on, 158
in tetralogy of Fallot, 1067
third stage of, 446–447

in ventricular septal defect,
1065–1066
white blood cell count in, 138
Lactation, 175–201. *See also* Breast;
Breast-feeding; Breast
milk; Suckling.
alveolar cells in
anatomy of, 177–178, 178f
mechanisms of secretion in,
178–180, 179f
diffusion as, 179
exocytosis as, 178, 179f
milk fat secretion and,
178–179, 179f
paracellular pathway as,
179f, 180
pinocytosis-exocytosis as,
179, 179f
augmentation of, 189
breast cancer risks and, 190
early postpartum development
of, 181
endocrine consequences of,
192–195
amenorrhea as, 192,
193f–194f
calcium homeostasis as,
193–195
endocrine control of, 181–192
estrogen in, 191
galactopoietic hormones in,
184–189, 186f–188f
galactokinetic hormones in,
183–184, 184f–185f
involution and, 189–190
lactogenic hormones in,
182–183
mammogenic hormones in,
182
milk ejection in, 183–184,
185f
nicotine (cigarette smoking)
effects on, 189
oxytocin in, 183–184,
184f–185f
progesterone in, 191–192
prolactin in, 184–189,
186f–188f

sex steroid hormone effects
on, 191–192
suckling stimulus in
frequent breast-feeding
and, 187–189, 188f
in oxytocin release,
183–184, 184f–185f
in prolactin release,
184–189, 186f–188f
successful breast-feeding
and, 190f
unsuccessful breast-feed-
ing and, 191f
failure of, 763
involution of breast tissue after,
189–190
maternal nutrition in, 199,
761–762
milk let down in, 184
osteoporosis and, 193–195
in preterm birth, 190–191
recommended dietary
allowances in, 224t
reestablishment of, 189
suppression of, 763–764
bromocriptine in, 201, 764
conservative measures in,
201, 763–764
hormonal, 764
Lactobacillus bifidus, in breast-fed
infant gastrointestinal
tract, 198
Large-for-gestational-age infant. *See
also* Macrosomia, fetal.
growth curve for, 735f, 736
hypoglycemia in, 731
ultrasound for, 338–339, 1112
Lead, birth defects and, 251–252
Left ventricular function, in pregnancy, 134, 1058
Legal issues, 1333–1348. *See also*
Informed consent.
abortion as, 1337–1341
Roe v. Wade and, 1338–1339
Webster v. Reproductive
Health Services of
Missouri and,
1339–1341

Legal issues *(Continued)*
fetal heart rate monitoring as,
486, 487f–488f
fetal research as, 1341–1346
forced cesarean section as,
1336–1337
in genetic counseling,
1333–1336
in genetic screening, 1333–1336
genome mapping and,
1346–1348
refusal of intrapartum fetal evaluation as, 489
tubal ligation and, 684
Leiomyoma, uterine, abortion due
to, 796–797
Lemon sign, in spina bifida ultrasound findings, 356,
359f
Leopold's maneuvers, 435
Leukemia, 1206–1208
acute, 1206–1207
chronic, 1207–1208
Leukocytes
in breast milk, 199
in pregnancy, 1223
Levator ani muscle
anatomy of, 6, 6f–7f
nerve supply of, 7
Lidocaine
maximal recommended dosage
of, 505t
uterine artery effects of, 516,
516f
Lie, definition of, 453
Lindane, as potential teratogen, 313
Linea nigra, 1215
Lipids
amniotic fluid levels of, in fetal
pulmonary maturation
assessment, 410
placental transfer of, 97–98
in pregnancy, 1097
Lipofuscin, trophoblastic, 48–49,
50f
Lipoprotein, low-density (LDL),
receptor-mediated
endocytosis of, 99

Lithium
breast-feeding and, 322
as potential teratogen, 306
Liver
fatty, 1169–1171
anesthesia in, 1170–1171
delivery in, 1170–1171
diagnosis of, 1170
differential diagnosis of,
1169–1170, 1170t
management of, 1170–1171
perinatal mortality in, 1169
fetal, normal physiology of, 111
in pregnancy, 126–127
Liver disease
normal pregnant serum chemistry vs., 127
in pregnancy, differential diagnosis of, 1170t
Liver transplantation, 1172–1173
Lochia, 754, 757
Longitudinal lie, 539, 540f
Low-birth-weight infant
breech presentation in, delivery
technique in, 559–560
definition of, 829
incidence of, 830, 831f–832f
neutral thermal environment
for, 727
L/S ratio, 409–410
in fetal pulmonary maturation
assessment, 409–410
in intrauterine growth retardation, 937
laboratory techniques for, 409
in maternal diabetes mellitus,
409–410, 1113
in premature rupture of membranes, 865–866
respiratory distress syndrome
and, 419–410
in Rh disease, 410
in twin gestation, 906–907
values for, 409
Lumbar epidural anesthesia,
501–515. *See also*
Anesthesia, lumbar
epidural.

Lumbar lordosis, 137
Lung, fetal, development of,
697–698. *See also* Fetal
pulmonary maturation.
Lung volume, in pregnancy, 128f,
128–129, 129t
Lupus anticoagulants, recurrent
abortion and, 798
Lupus erythematosus, systemic,
1151–1158
antinuclear antibodies in, 1152t,
1152–1153
classification criteria for,
1151–1152
clinical manifestations of, 1152
laboratory diagnosis of,
1152–1153
nephritis in, 1152, 1153
in pregnancy, 1153–1158
anticardiolipin antibody in,
1154–1156
aspirin in, 1155
azathioprine in, 1158
cesarean section in, 1157
corticosteroids in, 1157–1158
delivery in, 1157
heparin in, 1155
intrauterine growth retardation in, 1157
laboratory studies in, 1157
lupus inhibitor in, 1154–1156
maternal morbidity and mortality in, 1153
neonatal complete congenital heartblock in, 1156
nephritis and, 1153
prednisone in, 1155, 1158
preeclampsia vs., 1153–1154
pregnancy prognosis and,
1154–1156
SLE prognosis and,
1153–1154
surveillance in, 1156–1157
treatment of, 1155,
1157–1158
Lupus inhibitor, in pregnancy,
1154–1156
Luteal phase defect, in sponta-

neous abortion, 793–795
diagnosis of, 794
endometrial biopsy in, 794
incidence of, 794
progesterone levels in, 794
treatment of, 795
Luteoma, of pregnancy, 130
Lymph nodes, of pelvis, 28, 28f
Lymphocytes
in breast milk, 199
in pregnancy, 1223
Lymphoma. *See* Hodgkin's disease.

M

Macrophages, in breast milk, 199
Macrosomia, fetal. *See also* Large-for-gestational-age infant.
definition of, 564
femur length/abdominal circumference ratio in, 339
head circumference/abdominal circumference ratio in, 338f, 339
in maternal diabetes mellitus, 338–339, 1099, 1100f, 1102–1103
in prolonged pregnancy, 947, 949f, 954
shoulder dystocia in, 563–564
ultrasound for, 338–339, 564, 1112
Magnesium sulfate
breast-feeding and, 319
in eclamptic convulsion, 1026–1027, 1027f
in severe preeclampsia, 1015–1016, 1017t
as tocolytic, 851–853
complications of, 852, 852t
dosage and administration of, 851
efficacy of, 852, 852t
indications for, 852
toxic manifestations of, 1017t, 1026, 1027f
Magnesium supplementation, in

prevention of preeclampsia, 1002–1003
Male genitalia, fetal, 344, 349f
Malignant disease, 1199–1212. *See also individual anatomic types.*
chemotherapy in, 1199–1200
in pregnancy, 1199
radiation in, 1200
Malpresentation, 539–567. *See also individual types.*
abnormal axial lie, 540–543, 541f
arm, 541, 541f
breech, 434, 551–562
brow, 547–549
compound, 549–551
deflection attitudes in, 543f, 543–562
full, 543, 543f
partial, 543, 543f
etiologic factors in, 539, 540t
face, 453f, 454f, 543–547
placental location in, 539, 540f
shoulder, 540, 541f
shoulder dystocia, 562–568
vertex, 453f
Mammary gland. *See* Breast; Breast-feeding; Breast milk; Lactation; Suckling.
Mammary souffle, 135
Marfan syndrome, 1068
Marihuana, as potential teratogen, 316
Mask of pregnancy, 130
Mastitis, 1284–1285
diagnosis in, 1284
pathophysiology and bacteriology in, 1284
prevention in, 1285
puerperal, 763
treatment in, 1285
Maternal-infant bonding, 739–740, 758–760
Maternity blues, 769–770
Maylard incision, in cesarean section, 643f, 643–644

McRoberts maneuver, in shoulder dystocia, 566, 568f
Meclizine, as potential teratogen, 310
Meconium, in amniotic fluid, amnioinfusion and, 478
Meconium aspiration syndrome
in intrauterine growth retardation, 938
neonatal respiratory distress syndrome and, 719–720, 720f
in prolonged pregnancy, 947–948, 953–954
tracheal suctioning in, 712
Melanoma, 1208–1209
Melasma, 130, 1215
Membranes. *See* Amniotic membrane.
Mendelian disorders, 269, 285–291
prenatal diagnosis of
known molecular basis, 288–291, 290f
unknown molecular basis, 291, 292f, 293t
Menstrual period, last (LMP), in gestational age assessment, 230
Menstrual regulation, 1308f–1313f, 1308–1309
Menstruation
lactational amenorrhea and, 192
postpartum, 755
Meperidine
breast-feeding and, 319
in labor, 499
Mepivacaine, maximal recommended dosage of, 505t
Meprobamate, as potential teratogen, 305
Mercury
elemental, birth defects and, 250–251
organic, birth defects and, 249–250
Mesosalpinx, 19, 19f
Mesovarium, 19, 19f

Metaproterenol, as potential teratogen, 308

Methadone, as potential teratogen, 317

Methimazole, as potential teratogen, 306

Methotrexate
breast-feeding and, 318
as potential teratogen, 307–308

Methyldopa, in chronic hypertension in pregnancy, 1038–1039, 1039t, 1041

α-Methyldopa, as potential teratogen, 307

Methylmercury, birth defects and, 249–250

Metoprolol
in chronic hypertension in pregnancy, 1040–1041
in preeclampsia, 1013

Metronidazole
breast-feeding and, 319
as potential teratogen, 313

Metropolitan Atlanta Congenital Defects Program, 241–242

Miconazole, as potential teratogen, 313

Microcephaly, 362

Microviscosimeter, in fetal pulmonary maturation assessment, 410

Midazolam, in labor, 500–501

Migraine, 1189

Milk
cow's, breast milk vs., 197t, 197–198
human. See Breast milk.

Minerals, neonatal requirements for, 729

Minor's triangle, 13

Miscarriage. See Fetal wastage.

Mitral commissurotomy, 1063

Mitral regurgitation, 1064–1065

Mitral stenosis, 1062–1063
Swan-Ganz catheterization in, 626

Mitral valve prolapse, 1068–1069

Müllerian fusion defect, recurrent abortion due to, 795–796, 796f

Mole, 52–56
hydatidiform. See Hydatidiform mole.
invasive, 55
partial, 52–53, 53f

Molecular biology. See also DNA analysis.

Montgomery's glands, 136

Morbidity
neonatal, statistical, 211
perinatal, fetal biophysical profile and, 398, 400f

Morning sickness, 125, 127

Morphine
breast-feeding and, 319
in labor, 499

Mortality. See also Abortion; Fetal wastage.
infant, 741
causes of, 378, 379f
definition of, 377
statistical, 233–234, 234t
maternal, statistical, 209–211, 210f
neonatal
definition of, 377
statistical, 211
perinatal, 377–380
antepartum fetal testing and, 379–380
causes of, 378, 379f
definition of, 377
fetal biophysical profile and, 398, 401f
statistics on, 377–378
postneonatal, definition of, 377

Morula
cell populations of, 39
normal development of, 300–301

Mouth, in pregnancy, 125–126

Multiple gestation, 881–916
amniocentesis in, 280
Doppler velocimetry in, 894–896
early wastage (vanishing twin) in, 886–889, 887f–888f

first trimester pregnancy reduction in, 904
management of
antepartum, 910–911
intrapartum, 913, 915
maternal serum α-fetoprotein (MSAFP) and, 293
perinatal morbidity and mortality in, 884–885
prenatal diagnosis in, 280
twin. See Twin gestation.
ultrasound in diagnosis of, 885–886, 886f
vaginal birth after cesarean section in, 670

Multiple sclerosis, 1192–1193

Myasthenia gravis, 1162–1164
anesthesia and analgesia in, 1163–1164
drug therapy in, 1163
labor in, 1163
neonatal, 1164
patient management in, 1163–1164
plasmaphresis in, 1164

Myelomeningocele, 356, 358f

Myocardial contractility
cardiac output effects of, 616, 619f
definition of, 608t

Myocardial infarction, 1070–1071

Myocardial ischemia, in tocolytic therapy, 849–850

Myomectomy, in cesarean section, 680

Myometritis, syncytial, 42

Myometrium, 148, 148f–149f
action potential in, 156
actomyosin in, 152–154, 153f
cellular contraction in, phosphorylation in, 154–156, 155f
cellular structure of, 148, 148f–149f
contractility of, biochemical mechanisms of, 843, 844f

excitation-contraction coupling in, 156
gap junctions in, 148, 149f
membrane potential in, 156
oxytocin receptor concentration in, 161, 161f
prostaglandin synthesis by, 164
skeletin in, 153
tropomyosin in, 152–153
Myosin, molecular structure of, 153, 153f
Myosin light-chain kinase (MLCK), 154, 155f

N
Nalbuphine, in labor, 500
Naloxone, in neonatal respiratory depression, 498–499
Narcotics
    breast-feeding and, 319
    as potential teratogens, 317
Nasopharynx, in pregnancy, 128
Nausea
    in pregnancy, 127–128
    prenatal education about, 226
Necrotizing enterocolitis, neonatal, 732–733
Neonatal morbidity, statistics for, 211
Neonatal mortality
    definition of, 377
    statistics for, 211, 378
Neonate, 697–742
    abdominal wall defect of, 732
    anemia in, 733
    bile pigment metabolism in, 738f
    birth asphyxia in, 707–713. *See also* Asphyxia, birth; Respiratory distress syndrome.
    birth injuries of, 716–717, 717t
    bony fracture in, 717
    brachial plexus injury in, 717
    cardiopulmonary transition of, 697–707. *See also* Fetal pulmonary maturation.

circulation in, 705–707
first breath in, 703, 704–705, 705f
lungs in, 697–705
respiratory mechanics in, 704–705, 705f
respiratory neural control mechanisms in, 703t, 703–704
thoracic squeeze in, 705
cephalohematoma in, 716
circulation in, hemodynamic pressures in, 707, 707t
in congenital rubella, 1228, 1228f
death of, 741
    grief reactions to, 772–774
diaphragmatic hernia of, 732
duodenal atresia of, 731
early discharge of, criteria for, 739, 739t
in eclampsia, 1032
esophageal atresia of, 731
facial palsy in, 717
feeding of, 729–730. *See also* Breast-feeding.
gastrointestinal flora of
    bottle feeding and, 198
    breast milk and, 198
gastrointestinal tract of
    congenital conditions of, 731–732
    obstruction of, 731–732
gastroschisis of, 732
genetic screening for, 278
    phenylketonuria, 278
heartblock in, complete congenital, in maternal SLE, 1156
herpes simplex virus infection of, 1250
high-risk, parental preparation for, 740–741
hyperbilirubinemia in, 737–739, 738f
hyperthyroidism in, 1118–1119
hypocalcemia in, in intrauterine growth retardation, 938

hypocalcemic tetany of, 1122–1123
hypoglycemia in, 730–731
    in intrauterine growth retardation, 938
hyponatremia in, in intrauterine growth retardation, 938
hypothermia in, in intrauterine growth retardation, 938
hypothyroidism in, 1118
immune system of, colostrum and, 196f, 198
infection of, in premature rupture of membranes, 864
intensive care of, outcome in, 741f, 741–742
intracranial hemorrhage in, 716–717
jaundice in, 737–739, 738f
    breast milk, 737–738
    pathologic, 737
    physiologic, 737
myasthenia gravis in, 1164
necrotizing enterocolitis of, 732–733
nursery care of, 739, 739t
nutritional requirements of, 728–729
    calories, 728–729, 729t
    carbohydrate, 729
    fat, 729
    protein, 729
    vitamins and minerals, 729
    water and electrolytes, 728
parents of, care of, 739–741
peripheral nerve injury in, 717
periventricular/intraventricular hemorrhage in, 713–715, 714f, 715t
polycythemia in, 733t, 733–734
    in intrauterine growth retardation, 938
postmature, 946
preterm. *See* Preterm birth; Preterm infant; Preterm labor.

Neonate *(Continued)*
  respiratory depression in. *See* Asphyxia, birth.
  risk assessment in, gestational age and growth curves for, 734f–736f, 735–737
  seizures in, 715t, 715–716
  skull fracture in, 716
  spinal cord injury in, 717
  subarachnoid hemorrhage in, 717
  thermal regulation in, 724–728
    clinical applications of, 727–728
      in delivery room, 727
      in nursery, 727–728
    cold injury and, 728
    factors affecting, 728
    heat loss and, 724–725, 725t
    heat production and, 724, 725t
    in intrauterine growth retardation, 938
    neutral thermal environment and, 725, 726f
    physiology of, 724
  thrombocytopenia in, immune, 733t, 734–735, 982–984, 1146. *See also* Thrombocytopenia, neonatal immune.
  thyroid function in, 1117
  tocolytic therapy effects on, 850–851
  tracheoesophageal fistula of, 731
  tuberculosis and, 1073
Nephritis, lupus, 1152
  pregnancy and, 1153
Nephropathy, in maternal diabetes mellitus, 1104–1105
Neural tube defect
  in first-trimester abortuses, 787
  incidence of, 239
  prenatal diagnosis of, 292–295
    amniotic fluid α-fetoprotein levels in, 292–293

maternal serum α-fetoprotein (MSAFP) in, 293–295, 294f, 295t
    risks after steps in AFP screening, 295t
    statistical risks for, 291–292
    timing of teratogenic exposure in, 236
    in twin gestation, 899–900
Neurohypophysis, 32f, 33
Neurologic disorders, 1183–1195. *See also individual disorders.*
Neutrophils, in breast milk, 199
Nevi, pigmented, 130, 1215
Nicotine, lactation effects of, 189
Nifedipine, as tocolytic, 853–854
Nipple(s)
  gross anatomy of, 176
  infant confusion, in breast-feeding, 760
  inverted, embryonic development of, 180
  nerve supply to, 176–177
  in pregnancy, 136
  preparation of, for breast-feeding, 228
  soreness, in breast-feeding, 760–761
Nitabuch's layer, 41, 43
Nitrates, birth defects and, 254–255
Nitrites, birth defects and, 254–255
Nitrofurantoin
  breast-feeding and, 321
  as potential teratogen, 312
Nonsteroidal anti-inflammatory drugs, in rheumatoid arthritis, 1161
Nonstress test, 390–396
  contraction stress test vs., 395–396, 397f
  in diabetes mellitus, 395
  extended, 393
  false-negative, 395
  false-positive, 392
  fetal bradycardia in, 394f, 395
  in intrauterine growth retardation, 395, 933

in maternal diabetes mellitus, 1110
  mild variable heart rate deceleration in, 395
  nonreactive, 391, 392f
  physiologic basis of, 390–391
  in prolonged gestation, 395
  in prolonged pregnancy, 952
  reactive, 391, 392f
  results of, 391, 393f
  sinusoidal heart rate pattern in, 391
  technique for, 391
  timing of, 393
  in twin gestation, 910
  vibroacoustic stimulation in, 393–395, 394f
Nonstress test/amniotic fluid volume ratio, in prolonged pregnancy, 952–953
Norepinephrine, fetal secretion of, 112
Nursery, neutral thermal environment in, 726f, 727–728
Nutrition
  maternal, in breast-feeding, 199, 761–762
  prenatal education about, 222–223, 224t–225t
  preterm birth and, 837
Nutritional, neonatal, 728–729, 729t
Nystatin, as potential teratogen, 313

O

Obesity
  cesarean section in, 644–645
  surgical wound infection in, 661
Oblique lie, 540, 541f
Obstetric history, previous, 213
Obturator internus muscle, 5f, 6
Occiput posterior position, in caudal epidural anesthesia, 501
Occiput transverse position

in caudal epidural anesthesia, 501

forceps delivery in, 444–445

Occupational hazards, prenatal counseling and, 213

Oligohydramnios
amniotic fluid index in, 340–342, 343f
maximum vertical pocket of amniotic fluid in, 339–340

Oliguria, in preeclampsia, 624–626

Omphalocele
neonatal, 732
ultrasound diagnosis for, 356, 360f

Ophthalmia neonatorum, 1273

Opioid analgesia, 498–500
disadvantages of, 499
frequency usage of, 517t
neonatal neurobehavioral changes due to, 499
neonatal respiratory depression due to, 498–499
patient-controlled, 500
types of, 499–500

Oral contraceptives, 766
breast-feeding and, 200, 321, 766
as potential teratogens, 302

Orbit, fetal, 362

Organic solvents, birth defects and, 255–257
abuse by sniffing and, 255
drinking water contamination and, 256
low level exposure and, 255–256

Osteoporosis, in lactation, 193–195

Ovarian artery
anatomic distribution of, 26, 26f
ligation of, in postpartum hemorrhage, 594

Ovarian cancer, 1211–1212
incidence of, 1211
staging of, 1212
ultrasound in, 1211

Ovarian fossa, 17–18, 18f

Ovary
anatomy of, 17–18, 18f–19f
fetal, determination of, 114, 114f
lymphatic drainage of, 28
neoplasia of, cesarean section and, 681
nerves of, 31f, 31–32
postpartum, 755
suspensory ligaments of, 18, 19f, 20
vascular supply of, 26f, 26–27

Ovulation
in lactational amenorrhea, 192
postpartum, 755

Ovum, blighted, 331
ultrasound diagnosis of, 889

Oxprenolol, in chronic hypertension in pregnancy, 1040

Oxygen, placental exchange of, 95–96

Oxygen content
arterial, 614
arteriovenous difference in, 615
mixed venous, 614–615

Oxygen delivery, formula for, 615

Oxygen transport
formulas for, 614–615
oxyhemoglobin dissociation curve and, 615, 617f

Oxyhemoglobin dissociation curve, 615, 617f

Oxytocin
in delivery of placenta, 446
in general anesthesia, 524
in induction of labor, 439–440, 449–450
complications of, 450–451
proper uses of, 440
rate of administration of, 440, 450
technique for, 450
in vaginal birth after cesarean section, 669, 672
in initiation of labor, 160–162
levels of, 162, 163f
plasma levels of, 160–161
receptor concentration in, 161f–162f, 161–162
uterine contraction, correlation with dosage in, 168
in lactation, 183–184, 184f–185f
conditioned reflex release of, 184
milk ejection and, 183–184, 185f
suckling stimulus and, 183–184, 184f–185f
uterine contraction and, 184
mechanism of action of, 156
in postpartum hemorrhage, 592

Oxytocin challenge test, 386. *See also* Contraction stress test.

P

Pain, in labor and delivery
pathways of, 494f, 495
physiologic effects of, 495–497, 496f–497f

Palmar erythema, 127, 130, 1216

Pancreas, 141–142

Pancreatitis, 1175–1176

Papanicolaou smear
abnormal, 1210f
in pregnancy, 1209

Papilloma virus infection, 1259–1261
clinical aspects of, 1260
diagnosis of, 1260, 1260f
immunology of, 1259
microbiology of, 1259
perinatal transmission of, 1261
treatment of, 1260–1261

Papular dermatitis, 1218t, 1219

Paracervical block, 515–516
fetal bradycardia due to, 516, 516f
frequency usage of, 517t
technique in, 515, 515f

Parasympathetic nervous system, fetal, 108–109

Parathyroid function, in calcium homeostasis, 1121–1122, 1121f

Parenthood, prenatal education about, 229

Parturition. *See also* Childbirth; Delivery; Labor.
  fetal adrenal steroids and, 49
  mammogenic and lactogenic hormones in, 190
  normal physiology of, 147–170

Parvovirus infection, 1233–1235
  aplastic crisis in, 1234
  clinical aspects of, 1233–1235
  diagnosis of, 1235
  epidemiology of, 1233
  erythema infectiosum in, 1234
  fetal complications of, 1234–1235
  fifth disease in, 1234
  hydrops fetalis in, 1234
  immunology of, 1233
  management of, 1235
  microbiology of, 1233
  prevention of, 1235

Patent ductus arteriosus
  in hyaline membrane disease, 720–721
  maternal, 1066

Paternal age, prenatal counseling and, 213

Pelvic diaphragm, 6, 6f–7f

Pelvic exam, prenatal, 215

Pelvic hematoma, postpartum, 595–596

Pelvic infection, in IUD use, 767

Pelvic inflammatory disease, ectopic pregnancy due to, 813

Pelvic inlet, 5, 433

Pelvic joints, mobility of, 137

Pelvic outlet, 5

Pelvic plexus, 30f–31f, 31

Pelvic thrombophlebitis, septic, 1287–1290, 1288f
  after cesarean section, 665
  pulmonary thromboembolism due to, 1077

Pelvimetry, 432–435
  bisischial diameter in, 433
  clinical, 433

diagonal conjugate in, 433
  radiographic, 433–435, 434t
    exposure during, 433–435
    values for, 434, 434t

Pelvis
  android, 433, 433t
  anthropoid, 433, 433t
  bony
    anatomy of, 3–5, 4f, 432–433
    developmental anatomy of, 4–5
  collateral circulation to, 28–29
  false, 3
  fascia of, 7–8, 8f
  gynecoid, 433, 433t
  ligaments of, 3, 4f
  lymphatics of, 28, 28f
  muscles of, 5f–7f, 5–7
  nerves of, 29–32, 30f–31f
  notches of, 3, 4f
  organs of, 17, 18f
  planes of, 433
  platypelloid, 433, 433t
  sympathetic nervous system of, 30
  true, 3
  vascular supply of, 23–26, 24f–25f

Penicillamine, in rheumatoid arthritis, 1161

Penicillins
  breast-feeding and, 321
  as potential teratogens, 311

Peptic ulcer disease, 126, 1173–1175, 1174t

Perineal nerve, 15–16, 16f

Perinei muscle
  deep transverse, 11f, 12
  superficial transverse, 10–11

Perineum
  anatomy of, 8–17
  anesthesia of
    local, 517, 517t, 520t
    lumbar epidural block in, 501, 503f
  arterial supply of, 16, 16f–17f
  central tendon of, 9
  fascia of, anatomy of, 9

laceration of, surgical repair of, 593f–595f, 594
  nerve supply of, 13–16, 15f–17f
  postpartum care of, 758
  skin of, nerve supply of, 14, 15f
  in third stage of labor, visual inspection of, 446–447
  triangular divisions of, 8–9
  venous supply of, 17

Peripheral nerve injury, neonatal, 717

Peripheral vascular resistance, in pregnancy, 134

Periurethral laceration, 593f, 594

Periventricular hemorrhage, neonatal, 713–715, 714f, 715t

Persistent pulmonary hypertension, neonatal respiratory distress syndrome and, 718–719

Pfannenstiel incision, in cesarean section, 643f, 644

Phenindione, breast-feeding and, 320

Phenobarbitol
  breast-feeding and, 319
  neonatal effects of, 1185
  nonpregnant daily dosage of, 1187t
  as potential teratogen, 1185

Phenothiazine
  breast-feeding and, 319
  in labor, 500
  as potential teratogen, 310

Phenoxy herbicide 2,4,5-T, birth defects and, 252–253

Phenytoin
  breast-feeding and, 319
  in eclampsia, 1027–1028
  nonpregnant daily dosage of, 1187t
  pharmacokinetics of, pregnancy effects on, 1186–1187
  in seizure disorders, 1184–1185, 1186–1187
  side effects of, 1184t, 1184–1185
  as potential teratogen, 303, 1184–1185

Pheochromocytoma, 1129–1130, 1129t
  seizures in, 1190t
Phosphatidylcholine, in fetal pulmonary maturation assessment, 410–411
Phospholipase A$_2$, gravidin inhibition of, 166–167
Physical activity, postpartum, 757
Pica, 125
Piper forceps, in breech presentation, 556, 557f
Piriformis muscle, 5f, 6
Pituitary
  anatomy of, 32f, 32–34
  blood supply of, 33f, 33–34
  fetal, normal physiology of, 111
  insufficiency of, 1126-1127
  nerve supply of, 34, 35f
  in pregnancy, 142
  prolactin-producing adenoma of, 1124–1126
Placenta, 39–57
  abruption of, 579–584. *See also* Abruptio placenta.
  aging of, 47–48
  anterior, maternal fetal activity assessment in, 384–385
  blood flow in, transport characteristics and, 100
  chorionic stage of, 43–44
  chorionic villi. *See* Chorionic villus sampling.
  clinical examination of, 56–57
  delivery of, 446–447
  diffusing capacity of, respiratory gas, 95–96
  fetal adrenal cortex and, steroidogenesis by, 75–78, 76f–77f
  in fetal transfusion syndrome, 45
  glucose uptake by, 94–95
  grading of, in fetal maturation assessment, 412–413, 413t, 414f
  growth of, 94
    epidermal growth factor effects on, 94
    insulin effects on, 94
    insulin-like growth factor effects on, 94
    oxygen effects on, 94
    placental growth hormone effects on, 94
  growth rate of, 44
  hypothalamic-like peptides of, 60, 61t
  immunologic properties of, 101–102
  infarction of
    calcification and, 47, 48f
    due to fibrin deposition, 47
    due to spiral arteriole, 47
  inflammation of, 49–51, 51f
  in intrauterine growth retardation, 926, 929, 931, 931f
  lactate production by, 94–95
  lobes of, formation of, 44
  location of, in fetal malpresentation, 539, 540f
  manual delivery of, antibiotic prophylaxis in heart disease and, 1061, 1062t
  maturation of, 46f–49f, 46–48, 63f
  metabolism of, 93–94
  migration of, 586
  oxygen consumption by, 94
  peptide production of, 59–60. *See also individual hormones.*
    implanted conceptus and, 59–60, 60f–62f, 61t
    physiology of, 60–74
    preimplantation conceptus and, 59
    in second and third trimester, 60, 63f
  pituitary-like peptides of, 60, 61t
  prostaglandin synthesis by, 164
  relation to decidua of, 150
  retained fragments, in postpartum hemorrhage, 592, 592f
  separation of. *See* Abruptio placenta.
  steroid production of, 74–78. *See also individual hormones.*
    corpus luteum and, 74, 75f
    decidua and, 74–75
    fetal adrenal cortex and, 75–78, 76f–77f
    preimplantation conceptus and, 74
  succenturiate lobes of, 43
  term, ultrastructure of, 62f
  tuberculosis of, 49
  tumors of, 51–56, 52f–57f
  twins and
    dividing membranes of, 45f, 45–46
    dizygotic, 45f, 46, 882–883, 883f, 892–894, 893f–895f
    monozygotic, 45f, 45–46, 882–883, 883f
      problems related to, 904–905, 905
      ultrasound in, 892–894, 893f–895f
    vascular connections of, 45
  visual inspection of, 447
Placenta accreta, 587–589, 588f
  cesarean hysterectomy in, 655–656
  cesarean section in, 645, 655–656
Placenta circumvallata, 44
Placenta increta, 587–589, 588f
Placental cake
  development of, 43
  fibrin deposition around, 47
Placental growth hormone, 94
Placental lactogen, 183
Placental protein 5 (PP5), 74
Placental site tumor, choriocarcinoma and, 43, 51
Placental transfer, 94–100, 529–530
  of amino acids, 97, 98t
  in anesthesia, 530, 530f

Placental transfer *(Continued)*
  of antibiotics, 1225
  of calcium, 98–99, 1121
  of glucose, 96–97, 142
  of lipids, 97–98
  lipid solubility in, 95
  molecular movement in, 94–95, 95f
  pharmacokinetics in, 530
  physiology of, 529–530
  receptor-mediated endocytosis in, 99–100, 100f
  of respiratory gases, 95–96
  of water and ions, 98, 99f
Placental transfusion, postnatal, 432
Placenta marginata, 44
Placenta percreta, 587–589, 588f
Placenta previa, 584–589
  abnormal axial lie and, 542
  blood transfusion in, 587
  double setup examination in, 586
  expectant management in, 586–587
  marginal, 585
  painless vaginal bleeding in, 585
  partial, 585
  tocolytic therapy in, 587, 588f
  total, 584–585, 585f
  ultrasound findings in, 585–586, 586f
  variations of, 584, 585f
Plasma, fresh frozen, transfusion of, 578
Plasma osmolality, in pregnancy, 132
Plasmaphresis, maternal
  in myasthenia gravis, 1164
  in Rh isoimmunization, 976
Plasma volume, in pregnancy, 137–138, 1057, 1058t
Platelet-activating factor, after fertilization, 59
Platelet count
  fetal, in maternal immune thrombocytopenic purpura, 1145

maternal, 138–139
Platelet isoimmunization, 982–984. *See also* Thrombocytopenia, neonatal immune.
Platelet transfusion, 578
Pleural effusion, fetal, shunt for, 367, 368f
Pneumocyte, type II, in surfactant production, 698, 698f
Pneumonia
  mycoplasmal, 1074
  pneumococcal, 1074
  in pregnancy, 1074–1075
Polybrominated biphenyls, birth defects and, 254
Polychlorinated biphenyls, birth defects and, 253–254
Polycythemia, neonatal, 733t, 733–734
  in intrauterine growth retardation, 938
  in maternal diabetes mellitus, 1103–1104
Polyhydramnios, abruptio placenta in, 580
Polymerized chain reaction, 287–288, 290f
Polyploidy, in first-trimester abortuses, 787, 788t
Polysomy X (female), 274
Polysomy Y (male), 274
Pomeroy technique, of tubal ligation, 682, 682f
Position, definition of, 453
Postabortal triad, 1319
Postpartum blues, 769–770
Postpartum care, 753–774. *See also* Breast-feeding; Contraception.
  cardiovascular system in, 755–756
  cervix in, 754
  coagulation in, 755–756
  contraceptive sterilization and, 767–769
  depression and, 770–771
  fallopian tube in, 754–755

grieving and, 772–774
  management of puerperium, 757–758
  maternal-infant bonding and, 758–760
  maternity blues and, 769–770
  in mitral stenosis, 1063
  ovary in, 755
  perineum in, 758
  psychological reactions and, 769–772
  psychosis and, 771–772
  renal function in, 756–757
  in seizure disorders, 1188–1189
  thyroid in, 755
  in thyrotoxicosis, 757
  in tuberculosis, 1073
  urinary tract in, 756–757
  uterus in, 753–754
Postpartum depression, 770–771
Postpartum hemorrhage, 589–604. *See also* Hemorrhage, postpartum.
Postpartum psychosis, 771–772
Postpartum thyrotoxicosis, 757
Post-sterilization depression, 768–769
Posture, in pregnancy, 137
Pouch of Douglas, 20, 21f
Prazosin, in chronic hypertension in pregnancy, 1039
Precolostrum, 195
Preconceptual education, 212
Prednisolone, breast-feeding and, 320–321
Prednisone
  breast-feeding and, 320–321
  in systemic lupus erythematosus, 1155, 1158
Preeclampsia, 995–1021. *See also* Blood pressure; Eclampsia; Hypertension.
  blood pressure in, 575
  criteria for, 993
  pregnancy outcome and, 1000, 1000t

technique for measuring, 1000
cardiopulmonary profile in, 616t
chronic hypertension and, 994, 1036
diagnosis of, 1000–1001
Doppler velocimetry in, 1009–1010, 1010t
edema in, 993–994, 995
etiology of, 995
glomerulonephritis vs., 1087
HELLP syndrome in, 1005–1008
  anesthesia in, 1018
  clinical presentation in, 1006
  delivery in, 1007–1008
  laboratory values for diagnosis of, 1005–1006
  management of, 1006–1008
  perinatal outcome in, 1007, 1007t
  postpartum, 1007
  terminology in, 1005
hemodynamic profile in, 620–622, 624t, 1008–1009, 1009t
hemorrhage in, 575
incidence of, 995
management of, 1010–1013
  antihypertensive drugs in, 1013
  atenolol in, 1013
  conservative, 1010–1012
  delivery before term in, 1012
  flow chart for, 1011, 1011f
  labetalol in, 1013
  metoprolol in, 1013
  pregnancy outcome in, 1012t, 1012–1013
maternal and perinatal outcome in, 1019
maternal complications in, 1020t
oliguria in, 624–626
organ system involvement in, 1004–1005
  hematologic, 1005
  hepatic, 1004–1005
  renal, 1004

pathophysiology of, 995–999, 998
  antithrombin III levels in, 997
  endothelial cell damage in, 997
  fibronectin levels in, 997
  hemostatic changes in, 996–998
  platelet factor IV levels in, 997–998
  prostaglandins in, 998–999, 999f
    amniotic fluid levels of, 999
    fetal or placental, 999, 999f
    maternal plasma, 999
    urinary, 998–999
  thrombin-antithrombin III complex in, 998
  β-thromboglobulin levels in, 997–998
  uterine vascular changes in, 995–996, 997f
prediction of, 1001
prenatal care and, 216
prevention of, 1001–1004
  antithrombotic agents (aspirin) in, 1003–1004
  calcium supplementation in, 1002
  magnesium supplementation in, 1002–1003
  zinc supplementation in, 1003
in prior pregnancies, counseling in, 1019–1021
proteinuria in, 994, 995
pulmonary edema in, 623–624, 625t
severe, 1013–1019
  after 34 weeks gestation, 1013
  analgesia in, 1018
  anesthesia in, 1018
  cesarean section in, 1018
  conservative management in, 1013–1014

  corticosteroids in, 1015
  criteria for, 994
  fetal outcome in, 1014
  fluid intake and output in, 1016–1017
  hydralazine in, 1017
  improvement after hospitalization in, 1015
  invasive hemodynamic monitoring in, 617–618, 1018
  labor and delivery in, 1018–1019
  magnesium sulfate therapy in, 1015–1016, 1017t
  maternal complications of, 1014, 1014t
  prolactin inhibiting hormone in, 1015, 1017f
  recommended management plan in, 1015, 1016f
  at 28 to 32 weeks gestation, 1015
  before 28 weeks, 1015, 1017f
  before 34 weeks gestation, 1013
Swan-Ganz catheterization in, 617–618
systemic lupus erythematosus vs., 1153–1154
in twin gestation, 995
volume expansion in, 622–623
Preembryo, in ectopic pregnancy, 814
Pregnancy
ectopic, 809–824. *See also* Ectopic pregnancy.
nonviable, ultrasound for, 331–332
physiology of, normal, 125–143. *See also individual anatomic parts.*
preclinical, loss of, 783–784
  frequency and timing of, 783
  morphology and cytology in, 783–784, 784f–786f
prolonged, 945–955. *See also* Prolonged pregnancy.

Pregnancy *(Continued)*
  termination. *See* Abortion, elective.
  tubal. *See* Ectopic pregnancy.
Pregnancy-associated plasma protein A (PAPP-A), 73, 74
Pregnancy diagnosis, 83–86
  early pregnancy factor and, 85–86
  human chorionic gonadotropin and, 83–85
    commercial assays for, 84t
    ELISA for, 83–85, 84f
    FIA for, 85
    intact, 83
    IRMA for, 83
    radioimmunoassay for, 83
    subunits of, 83, 783
  progesterone and, 86
  ultrasound for, 85t, 86, 86f
Pregnancy rates, in lactational amenorrhea, 192
Pregnancy reduction, 1315
  first trimester, 904
Pregnancy-specific β_1-glycoprotein (SP1), 73–74
Preimplantation genetic diagnosis, 282–283, 283f
Premature rupture of membranes, 861–868. *See also* Amniotic membrane, premature rupture of.
Prematurity. *See* Preterm birth; Preterm infant; Preterm labor.
Prenatal care, 209–231
  efficacy of, 211
  fetal movement record in, 216, 217f
  goal of, 209
  historical, 209
  initial visit in, 212–215
    hepatitis B screening in, 215
    medical risks and, 213
    obstetric risks and, 213, 215
    pelvic exam in, 215
    physical and laboratory evaluation and, 214t, 215

  social and demographic risks and, 212–213
  intercurrent problems and, 216, 222
  repeat visit in, 215–216
  risk assessment in, 211–212
Prenatal diagnosis, 279–296. *See also* Genetic screening.
  amniocentesis for, 279–280, 283–284
  chorionic villus sampling for, 280–282, 281f–282f, 283–284
  future directions of, 295–296
  indications for, 284–296
    cytogenetic disorders and, 284–285
    ethnic origin and, 276, 277t
    genetic history in, 274–276, 275f
    genodermatosis as, 287
    inborn errors of metabolism as, 287
    maternal age as, 284–285
    maternal serum α-fetoprotein levels as, 285, 286f
    maternal serum hormone levels as, 285
    Mendelian disorders and, 285–291
      known molecular basis, 288–291, 290f
      unknown molecular basis, 291, 292f, 293t
    parental age and, 276, 276t
    parental chromosomal abnormality as, 285, 286f
    polygenic/multifactorial disorders as, 291–292
    previous chromosomal abnormality as, 285
  molecular biologic techniques for, 287–288, 288f–290f
  pitfalls in analysis of, 283–284
  preimplantation (embryo biopsy) for, 282–283, 283f
  ultrasonography in, 295
Prenatal education, 222–229

  activity and employment and, 224–225
  backache and, 228
  breast-feeding and, 228
  childbirth preparation and, 228–229
  circumcision and, 228
  constipation and, 226
  drugs and teratogens in, 222–229
  heartburn and, 226
  hemorrhoids and, 226
  immunization and, 225
  labor signs and, 229
  nausea and vomiting and, 226
  nutrition in, 222–223, 224t–support groups in, 229
  radiologic studies in, 222
  rest and, 224
  round ligament pain and, 227
  sexual activity and, 228
  syncope and, 227
  travel and, 225
  urinary frequency and, 227
  weight gain in, 223–224
Prenatal record, 218f–221f, 222
Presacral nerve, 30f, 30–31
Presentation. *See also individual types*; Malpresentation.
  definition of, 454
Preterm birth, 829–871
  abruptio placenta and, 583
  biochemical and biophysical indices for, 840
    cervical dilatation and, 840
    uterine contractility and, 840
    vaginal pH and, 840
  breech, Duhrssen's cervical incision in, 687, 687f
  causes of, 836–841
    cervical incompetence and, 838
    fetal stress as, 838
    genital tract infection as, 838–839
    immediate, 839, 839f
    maternal DES exposure and, 838

nutrition and, 837
pregnancy or medical complications as, 838
prior obstetric outcome and, 837–838
risk factors in, 836–837, 837t
uterine anomalies and, 838, 838t
cesarean section technique in, 649
definition of, 829
elective, in maternal diabetes mellitus, 1112–1113
fetal heart rate monitoring in, 485
gestational age vs. birth weight in, 829–830, 830f
in hemodialysis, 1091
incidence of, 831, 833, 833t
lactation in, 190–191
management of, 869–871
cesarean section in, 870–871
episiotomy in, 870
forceps in, 870
morbidity rates in, 835–836
gestational-age specific, 835
long-term, 836
mortality rates in, 833–835
birth-weight specific, 833, 834f–836f
gestational-age specific, 833–835, 834f–836f
in obstetric history, 213
prevention of, 840–841
bed rest in, 841
beta-mimetic agents in, 840–841
patient education in, 841
progesterone in, 840
uterine activity monitoring in, 841
risk scoring indices for, 839
Preterm infant
breast milk for, 730, 762–763
feeding of, 729
hypoglycemia in, 730
hypoxia and, 868–869

Preterm labor. *See also individual causes of.*
anesthesia and analgesia in, 869
in cervical incompetence, 859–861, 860f
definition of, 842
fetal monitoring in, 868–869
fetal pulmonary maturation and. *See* Fetal pulmonary maturation.
length of, 869
in premature rupture of amniotic membrane, 861–868
tocolytic therapy in, 841–856. *See also* Tocolytic therapy.
treatment of, 841–858
Primidone
nonpregnant daily dosage of, 1187t
pharmacokinetics of, pregnancy effects on, 1187
Processus vaginalis, 21
Progesterone
corpus luteum secretion of, 74, 75f
in diagnosis of pregnancy, 86
effects on labor of, 158
function in pregnancy of, 80–81
lactogenic effects of, 191–192
in luteal phase defect, 794
molecular structure of, 80, 80f
origin of, 80
variation during pregnancy of, 80, 81f
withdrawal, in initiation of labor, 159–160
Progestins
breast-feeding and, 321–322
as potential teratogen, 302
Progestogen, 80–81
function in pregnancy of, 80–81
molecular structure of, 80, 80f
origin of, 80
variation during pregnancy of, 80, 81f
Prolactin
decidual production of, 150
in early puerperium, 185, 186f

in lactation, 184–189, 186f–188f
drug-induced stimulation of, 189
nicotine effects on, 189
suckling stimulus and, 184–189, 186f–188f
in lactational amenorrhea, 192, 193f–194f
in pregnancy, 185, 186f
Prolactin-inhibiting hormone, in severe preeclampsia, 1015, 1017f
Prolactin-producing pituitary adenoma, 1124–1125
Prolonged pregnancy, 945–955
definition of, 946
diagnosis of, 948–950
fetal growth in, 947, 949f, 954
fetal nonstress test in, 395
historical accounts of, 945–946
incidence of, 946, 947f–948f
management of, 948–955
amniotic fluid index in, 953
amniotic fluid volume in, 953
biophysical profile in, 952
cervical ripening with prostaglandin in, 950–951
choices in, 950, 951f
contraction stress test in, 952
expectant, 951–953
intrapartum, 953–955
asphyxia and, 954
cord compression and, 954
fetal heart rate monitoring in, 954–955
macrosomia and, 954
meconium aspiration syndrome and, 953–954
nonstress test/amniotic fluid volume in, 952–953
nonstress test in, 952
meconium aspiration syndrome in, 947–948, 953–954
perinatal morbidity and mortality in, 946–948, 949f

Propoxyphene
    breast-feeding and, 319
    as potential teratogen, 314
Propranolol
    breast-feeding and, 320
    in chronic hypertension in pregnancy, 1040
    as potential teratogen, 307
Propylthiouracil
    breast-feeding and, 322
    as potential teratogen, 306
Prostacyclin (PGI$_2$)
    as oxytocic, 162–163
    in preeclampsia, 998–999, 999f
Prostaglandin(s)
    for abortion, 1323-1324
    amniotic fluid levels of
        in fetal pulmonary maturation assessment, 410
        in labor, 165f, 166
    in cervical mucus, 152, 152t
    for cervical ripening, 151–152
        in prolonged pregnancy, 950–951
    in initiation of labor, 160, 162–167, 440. *See also under* Labor.
    oxytocic properties of, 162–163
    plasma levels of
        after delivery, 165, 166f
        in labor, 164–165, 165f
        in pregnancy, 164
        in preeclampsia, 998–999, 999f
    urinary secretion of, in pregnancy, 165–166
    uterine synthesis by, 163–164
Prostaglandin E$_2$
    for abortion, 1324
    in breast milk, 198
    as oxytocic, 163, 440
    receptors in myometrium for, 163
Prostaglandin F$_{2\alpha}$
    for abortion, 1323–1324
    as oxytocic, 163, 440
    in postpartum hemorrhage, 593

receptors in myometrium for, 163
Protein
    dietary, in pregnancy, 223
    neonatal requirements for, 729
Proteinuria
    in chronic renal failure, 1089
    in eclampsia, 1022
    in preeclampsia, 994, 995
    prenatal care and, 216
Prurigo gestationis, 1218t, 1220
Pruritic urticarial papules and plaques of pregnancy (PUPP syndrome), 1218t, 1218–1219, 1219f
Pseudotumor cerebri, 1194–1195
Psychological factors, in spontaneous abortion, 801
Psychological reactions, postpartum, 769–772
Psychoprophylaxis, in labor, 497–498
Psychosis, postpartum, 771–772
Ptyalism, in pregnancy, 125
Pubic symphysis, widening of, 137
Pubis, 3–4, 4f
Pubococcygeus muscle, 6f–7f, 7
Puborectalis muscle, anatomy, 6f–7f, 7
Pudendal artery, 16, 16f–17f
    internal, 25, 25f, 27, 28f
Pudendal block, 517–519, 518f, 520t
Pudendal canal, 12, 13f
Pudendal cleft, 9
Pudendal nerve, 15–16, 16f–17f, 518f
Puerperium. *See also* Postpartum care.
    hemodynamics in, 136
    patient management in, 757–758
    prolactin levels in, 185, 186f
    thromboembolism in, risk of, 139
Pulmonary angiography, 1078
Pulmonary artery

catheterization of. *See* Swan-Ganz catheterization.
    fetal, blood flow in, 106
Pulmonary disease, in pregnancy, 1071–1079. *See also individual types.*
Pulmonary edema
    in preeclampsia, 623–624, 625t
    tocolytic-induced, 627, 848–849
Pulmonary function studies, in pregnancy, 128f, 128–129, 129t
Pulmonary hypertension, persistent, neonatal respiratory distress syndrome and, 718–719
Pulmonary hypoplasia, neonatal, in premature rupture of membranes, 864
Pulmonary maturation assessment, fetal, 409–414. *See also* Fetal pulmonary maturation.
Pulmonary surfactant
    critical functions of, 700
    foam stability test for, 411
    functional measurements for, 411
    glucocorticoid effects on, 701, 702t
    L/S ratio for, 409–410
    mechanism of action of, 698–700
        LaPlace relationship and, 698, 699f
        surface forces and, 698, 699f
        surface tension and, 698–700, 699f
    metabolism of, hormonal regulation of, 701, 703
    phospholipids in, 406, 701, 701f
    production of
        osmiophilic lamellar bodies in, 698, 698f
        type II pneumocyte in, 698, 698f
    proteins in, 701

quantitation of, 409–410, 700, 700f

replacement therapy with, 721–724, 722t–723t, 858

in respiratory distress syndrome, 406, 720

shake test for, 411

tap test for, 411

Pulmonary thromboembolism, in pregnancy, 1077–1079

anticoagulation in, 1078–1079

diagnosis of, 1077–1078

pulmonary angiography in, 1078

surgical therapy in, 1079

Purpura, thrombocytopenic. *See* Thrombocytopenic purpura.

Pyelonephritis, 1086–1087

adult respiratory distress syndrome and, 1087

treatment of, 1086

urinary tract infection vs., 1086

Pyogenic granulomas, 1216

Q

Quadruplets. *See* Multiple gestation.

Quickening, in gestational age assessment, 230

Quintuplets. *See* Multiple gestation.

R

Radiation

ionizing

abortion due to, 800

birth defects and, 247–249, 248t

acute high dose in, 247–248, 248t

chronic low dose in, 248

dose threshold in, 248

mutagenesis in, 248–249

fetal malignancy due to, 434

in malignant disease, 1200

in pelvimetry, 434–435

ultrasonic. *See* Ultrasound.

Radiologic studies, prenatal education about, 222

Radiopharmaceuticals, breast-feeding and, 319

Ranitidine, in peptic ulcer disease, 1174

Recommended dietary allowance (RDA), 125, 224t–225t

Rectal plexus, 30, 30f

Rectal sphincter, laceration of, 594, 594f–595f

Rectouterine pouch, 20, 21f

Rectum, in third stage of labor, 447

Red blood cell(s)

packed, transfusion of, 578

volume, in pregnancy, 138, 1057–1058, 1058t

Relaxin

actions of, 159

for cervical ripening, 152, 159

production of, 159

Renal agenesis, in fetus, 348, 354

Renal biopsy, in pregnancy, 1090

Renal blood flow, in pregnancy, 1058

Renal disease, in maternal diabetes mellitus, 1104–1105

Renal failure

acute, 1092–1093

chronic, 1088–1091

delivery in, 1090

diagnosis of, 1088

fetal monitoring in, 1090

hemodialysis in, 1090–1091

hypertension in, 1089

outcome in, 1089

proteinuria in, 1089

renal biopsy in, 1090

renal function effects of, 1088–1089

treatment in, 1089–1090

Renal function

postpartum, 756–757

in preeclampsia, 1004

in renal transplantation, 1092

Renal plasma flow, in pregnancy, 131, 132t, 1085

Renal transplantation

in maternal diabetes mellitus, 1105

pregnancy in, 1091–1092

azathioprine and, 1091

cyclosporin and, 1091

infection in, 1092

rejection in, 1091–1092

renal function in, 1092

Renin-angiotensin system, in pregnancy, 132–133

Respiratory depression, neonatal. *See* Asphyxia, birth; Respiratory distress syndrome, 406–409

adult

management of, 628

pyelonephritis and, 1087

neonatal, 717–724

cardiovascular causes of, 717–718

causes of, 717, 718t

clinical symptoms in, 717

in elective delivery, incidence of, 407

glucocorticoids for, 856t–857t, 856–857

hyaline membrane disease in, 720–724, 721f, 722t–723t

bronchopulmonary dysplasia in, 721

clinical signs of, 720, 721f

complications of, 720

long-term sequelae of, 721

patent ductus arteriosus in, 720–721

surfactant in, 720

surfactant replacement therapy in, 721–724, 722t–723t

L/S ratio and, 419–410

in maternal diabetes mellitus, 1103, 1113

meconium aspiration syndrome and, 719–720, 720f

persistent pulmonary hypertension and, 718–719

Respiratory distress syndrome
(Continued)
surfactant in, 406
surfactant replacement therapy in, 721–724,
722t–723t, 858
transient tachypnea and, 719,
719f
Respiratory gas exchange
placental, 95–96
in pregnancy, 129
Respiratory tract, upper, in pregnancy, 128
Rest, prenatal education about, 224
Restriction endonucleases, 287,
288f–289f
Restriction fragment length polymorphisms, 291, 292f,
293t
Retinopathy, in maternal diabetes
mellitus, 1105–1106
Retroperitoneal hematoma, postpartum, 596, 599f
Rh antigen, 958–960
biochemistry and immunology
of, 959–960
genetics of, 959
historical, 958
nomenclature for, 958t, 958–959
Fisher-Race, 958, 958t
HLA system, 959
Wiener, 959
population studies of, 960
Rheumatic fever, antibiotic prophylaxis in, 1061
Rheumatic heart disease, 1062
Rheumatoid arthritis, 1159–1161
clinical manifestations of,
1159–1160
diagnostic criteria for, 1159
exclusions from, 1159
intrauterine growth retardation
in, 1160
medical treatment of, effects on
pregnancy of, 1161
pathophysiology and laboratory
findings in, 1160
in pregnancy, 1160

Rh immune globulin, 962–963. *See
also* Rh antigen; Rh
isoimmunization.
Rh isoimmunization, 960–977. *See
also* Rh antigen
causes of, 960
fetomaternal hemorrhage as,
47, 960–961
maternal immune response
in, 961–962
delivery in, 976–977
D^u positive, 964
ectopic pregnancy and, 823
fetal L/S ratio and, 409
fetal management in, 965–971
amniotic fluid bilirubin concentration in, 966–968,
967f–968f
D antigen status in, 965–966
Doppler ultrasound in, 969
fetal blood sampling in,
968–969
flow diagram for, 969–971,
970f
maternal anti-D titer in, 966
obstetric history and, 966
ultrasound in, 969
fetomaternal ABO incompatibility and, 961–962
incidence of, 960
intrauterine transfusion in,
971–976
alternatives to, 976
choosing technique for, 975
fetal hematocrit after, 974,
974f
intraperitoneal, 971–972, 972f
intravascular, 972–975,
973f–974f
risks of, 975–976
maternal management in,
963–965, 964t
in abortion, 964–965, 965t
in amniocentesis, 965, 965t
in chorionic villus sampling,
965, 965t
in D^u-positive patient, 964

in ectopic pregnancy,
964–965, 965t
in fetomaternal hemorrhage,
965, 965t
IgG therapy in, 976
plasmaphresis in, 976
in Rh-negative unsensitized
patient, 963–964, 964t
in third trimester fetal death,
965
perinatal outcome in, 977, 977t
Rh immune globulin in,
962–963
antepartum, 962–963
mechanism of, 963
antigen blocking in, 963
antigen deviation in, 963
antigen inhibition in, 963
postpartum, 962
Risk factor assessment, 212–215
alcohol abuse and, 213, 214t
medical, 213
obstetric, 213, 215
in prenatal care, 211–212
social and demographic,
212–213
Ritgen's maneuver, modified, 432
Ritodrine, 845–847
administration of, 845
dosage of, 845–847
pharmacokinetics of, 845
Roe v. Wade, 1338–1339
Round ligament
anatomy of, 20–21, 22f
pain, during pregnancy, 227
Rubella, 1226–1230
clinical aspects of, 1227–1228,
1228f
congenital, 1228, 1228f
epidemiology in, 1227
historical aspects of, 1226
immune response to, 1226,
1227f
immunization for
during pregnancy, 1230
recommendations in,
1229–1230
laboratory studies in, 1228

management in pregnancy of, 1229

microbiology of, 1226

prevention of, 1229–1230

S

Sacral agenesis, in maternal diabetes mellitus, 1101

Sacral artery
  lateral, 24, 25f
  middle, 24f, 25–26

Sacral plexus, 29–30

Sacral vein, middle, 24f, 25–26

Sacrococcygeal teratoma, fetal, 353f–354f, 354

Saddle block, 519

Saliva
  pH of, in pregnancy, 125
  production of, in pregnancy, 125

Sarcoidosis, 1073–1074

Scarpa's fascia, 9

Schwangerschaftspeziffischeprotein 1 (SP1), 73

Scleroderma, 1161–1162

Sclerosis
  multiple, 1192–1193
  progressive systemic, 1161–1162

Scopolamine, in labor, 501

Seat belt injury
  abruptio placenta in, 686f, 687
  uterus trauma in, 686f, 687

Sedatives
  breast-feeding and, 319
  in labor, 500–501

Seizure(s)
  neonatal, 715t, 715–716
  peripartum, 1190t

Seizure disorders, 1183–1189
  anticonvulsant therapy in, 1184–1187. *See also individual drugs.*
  breast-feeding in, 1187
  perinatal management in, 1187–1189
  pharmacokinetics of, preg-

nancy effects on, 1186–1187, 1187t
  postpartum management in, 1188–1189
  preconception management in, 1188
  side effects of, 1184t, 1184–1186
  differential diagnosis of, 1190t
  effects of pregnancy on, 1183–1184
  effects on pregnancy of, 1184–1186
  incidence of, 1183
  teratogenesis in, 303–304, 304f

Selective termination, of anomalous fetus, 902–904, 1315

Septal hypertrophy, asymmetric, 1069

Septate uterus, 796f

Septic pelvic thrombophlebitis, 1287–1290, 1288f

Septic shock, 627–628

Sex chromosomal abnormalities, 274
  detection in chorionic villus sampling and amniocentesis, 274
  in first-trimester abortuses, 787

Sexual activity
  postpartum, 757–758
  prenatal education about, 228

Sexual differentiation, embryonic, 301

Sexually transmitted disease, preterm birth due to, 838–839

Shake test, for pulmonary surfactant, 411

Sheehan syndrome, 1126

Shock, septic, 627–628

Shoulder(s), fetal, assisted spontaneous delivery of, 432

Shoulder dystocia, 562–568
  causes of, 563–564
  definition of, 562, 564f

delivery technique in, 565f–568f, 565–567
    clavicle fracture for, 566
    McRoberts maneuver in, 566, 568f
    subcutaneous symphysiotomy in, 566
    Zavanelli maneuver in, 566
  in macrosomia, 563–564
  perinatal morbidity in, 563

Shoulder presentation, 540, 541f

Shunt
  for pleural effusion, fetal, 367, 368f
  vesicoamniotic, fetal, 367

Sickle cell anemia, 1139–1142
  clinical manifestations of, 1140
  genetics of, 1139
  hemoglobin S and AS in, 1139
  in pregnancy, 1140–1142
    antenatal fetal testing in, 1140
    delivery in, 1142
    exchange transfusion in, 1141–1142
    maternal morbidity in, 1140
    patient management in, 1140–1142
    perinatal outcome in, 1140
    prophylactic transfusion in, 1141
  prenatal diagnosis of, 277t
    molecular techniques for, 288, 289f

Sickle cell thalassemia, 1143

Sitz bath, postpartum, 758

Skeletal dysplasia, fetal, 362

Skeletin, in myometrium, 153

Skeleton, in pregnancy, 137

Skene's glands, 9

Skin, in pregnancy, 130, 1215

Skin biopsy, fetal, in genodermatosis, 287

Skin disorders, in pregnancy, 1215–1220. *See also individual types.*

Skin prep, surgical principles of, 640–641

Skull
  fetal. *See also* Biparietal diameter.
    landmarks of, 452f, 453
    presenting diameters of, 429, 429f
    transverse diameters of, 428, 428f
    ultrasound for, 343f–344f, 344
  neonatal, fracture of, 716
Sleep, fetal, quiet vs. active, 383–384
Small bowel
  obstruction of
    in neonate, 731–732
    in pregnancy, 686–687
  in pregnancy, 126
Small-for-gestational-age infant
  growth curve for, 735f, 736
  hypoglycemia in, 730–731
  intrauterine growth retardation vs., 924
Smelter emissions, birth defects and, 252
Smoking. *See* Cigarette smoking.
Socioeconomic status, prenatal counseling and, 213
Sodium
  homeostasis, in pregnancy, 132
  placental transfer of, 98, 99f
Sonography. *See* Ultrasound.
Southern blotting, 287, 288f–289f. *See also* DNA analysis.
Spermatozoa, in etiology of hydatidiform mole, 52
Spermicides, as potential teratogens, 303
Sphincter urethrae, 11f, 12
Sphincter vaginae, 11
Spider angiomata, 127, 130, 1216
Spina bifida
  prenatal diagnosis of, 292–295
    amniotic fluid α-fetoprotein levels in, 292–293
    maternal serum α-fetoprotein (MSAFP) in, 293–295, 294f, 295t

risks after AFP screening in, 295t
  ultrasound for, 356, 359f
    lemon and banana signs in, 356, 359f
  statistical risks for, 291–292
  timing of teratogenic exposure in, 236
Spinal block, 519–520, 520t
  in cesarean section, 526–528
Spinal cord injury, neonatal, 717
Spinal headache, 508–509
Spine, fetal, 344, 345f–346f
Spiral arterioles
  placental infarction due to, 47
  trophoblastic invasion of, 42, 42f
Spontaneous abortion. *See* Fetal wastage.
Starvation, in pregnancy, metabolic response to, 141–142
Station, definition of, 454
Status asthmaticus, 1076–1077
Sterilization, contraceptive, 767–769
  postpartum, 767–769
  types of, 767–769
Steroid hormones. *See individual types, e.g.* Estrogen; Progesterone.
Stillbirth. *See* Death.
Stomach
  fetal, 344, 347f
  maternal, 126
Streptococcus, group B, 1267–1269
  clinical aspects of, 1268
  diagnosis of, 1268–1269
  immunology of, 1268
  microbiology of, 1267–1268
  prevention of, 1269
  treatment of, 1269
Streptomycin, as potential teratogen, 312
Stress response, 496, 496f
  epidural anesthesia and, 496, 496f
Striae distensae, 1216
Striae gravidarum, 130
Subaortic stenosis, idiopathic hypertrophic, 1069

Subarachnoid block, 519–520
Subarachnoid hemorrhage, 1191
  maternal, seizures in, 1190t
  neonatal, 717
Suckling. *See also* Breast-feeding; Breast milk; Lactation.
  neuroendocrine responses to, 189
  oxytocin release in, 183–184, 184f–185f
  prolactin release in, 184–189, 186f–188f
  in successful breast-feeding, 190f
  in unsuccessful breast-feeding, 191f
Sudden infant death syndrome (SIDS), cigarette smoking and, 315
Sulfamethoxazole with trimethoprim, as potential teratogen, 311
Sulfasalazine
  breast-feeding and, 321
  as potential teratogen, 312
Sulfonamides
  breast-feeding and, 321
  as potential teratogens, 311
Supine hypotensive syndrome, 134, 1058, 1059f
Support groups, parenthood, 229
Supraventricular tachycardia, fetal, 469, 469f
Surfactant, pulmonary. *See* Pulmonary surfactant.
Suture selection, surgical principles of, 641–642, 642t
Swan-Ganz catheterization, 607–617
  clinical outcome with, 608–609
  complications of, 608
  in dilated cardiomyopathy, 627
  in Eisenmenger syndrome, 626–627
  hemodynamic profile in, 613–614, 614t
  hemodynamic terminology for, 608t
  in hypertrophic obstructive cardiomyopathy, 626

indications for, 607–608, 608t
internal jugular vein cannulation for, 609–610, 610f–612f
in mitral stenosis, 626
in normal pregnancy, 619–620, 622t–623t
in preeclampsia, 617–618, 1018
pulmonary artery catheter insertion in, 610–611
pulmonary artery pressure tracing in, 612–613, 613f
right atrial pressure tracing in, 611, 613f
right ventricular pressure tracing in, 612, 613f
risks vs. benefits of, 608
wedge pressure tracing in, 613, 613f
Sweat glands, in pregnancy, 130
Symmelia, in twin gestation, 899
Sympathetic nervous system
fetal, 108–109
maternal, 30
Symphysiotomy, subcutaneous, in shoulder dystocia, 566
Syncope
in intrauterine device (IUD) insertion, 767
prenatal education about, 227
Syncytial endometritis, 42
Syncytial knot, 47
Syncytial myometritis, 42
Syncytiotrophoblast
of chorionic villi, 46f, 46–47
formation of, 39, 40f
hypothalamic- and pituitary-like peptides of, 60, 61t
immunologic properties of, 102
postimplantation, 59–60, 61f
Synechiae, intrauterine, recurrent abortion and, 795
Syphilis, 1242–1248
clinical aspects of, 1243f–1245f, 1243–1245
chancre in, 1243, 1243f
condylomata of vulva in, 1243, 1244f

congenital syndrome in, 1244–1245, 1245f
palmar lesions in, 1243, 1244f
epidemiology in, 1243
follow-up after treatment of, 1248
human immunodeficiency virus and, 1258
immunology in, 1242
laboratory diagnosis of, 1245–1246
management in pregnancy of, 1246–1247
microbiology of, 1242, 1242f
treatment of, 1247–1248

T
Tachycardia, fetal
in intrapartum monitoring, 464f, 465–466
supraventricular, 469, 469f
Tachypnea, transient, neonatal respiratory distress syndrome and, 719, 719f
Tap test, for pulmonary surfactant, 411
Tay-Sachs, 277t
Teenage pregnancy, 212
Telogen effluvium, 1216
Temperature, basal body, 765
Teratogens, 235–238, 299–318. *See also* Birth defects; *individual agents.*
acetaminophen, 314
agents, 236–237
alcohol, 315f, 315–316, 316t
aminoglycosides, 312–313
aminophylline, 308
amoxicillin, 311
analgesics, 314
androgens, 302, 302f
anesthetic gases, 257–258
animal models for, 238
antiasthmatics, 308
antibiotics, 310–314
anticoagulants, 306, 307f
anticonvulsants, 303–304, 304f

antiemetics, 308–310
antifungal agents, 313–314
antihistamines, 310
antihypertensive drugs, 307
antineoplastic drugs, 307–308
antituberculosis drugs, 313
arsenic, 252
aspartame, 317–318
aspirin, 314
atenolol, 307
azathioprine, 308
basic principles of, 235–236, 299–300
bendectin, 309
benzodiazepines, 305
bromocriptine, 314
caffeine, 317
carbamazepine, 303, 1185–1186
cardiovascular drugs, 306–307
cephalosporins, 311
chemotherapy, 1200
chlorodiazepoxide, 305
chlortrimazole, 313
clindamycin, 313
clomiphene, 314
cocaine, 316–317
codeine, 314
corticosteroids, 308
cromolyn sodium, 308
cyclosporine A, 308
danazol, 302, 302f
decongestants, 310
diazepines, 305–306
digoxin, 306–307
dimenhydrinate, 310
dioxin, 252–253
diphenylhydramine, 310
dose effect and, 237
drugs, 299–318
FDA labeling of, 299–300
emetrol, 310
epinephrine, 308
erythromycin, 313
estrogen, 302
ethionamide, 313
etretinate, 305
genotype and environmental factors and, 236

Teratogens *(Continued)*
hydantoin, 303, 304f, 1184–1185
hydralazine, 307
17α-hydroxyprogesterone caproate, 302
immunosuppressants, 307–308
intrauterine infections, 1225–1259. *See also individual infections.*
iodide, 308, 309f
isoproterenol, 308
isotretinoin, 304–305, 305f
kanamycin, 312
known and suspected agents, 237t, 237–238
lead, 251–252
lindane, 313
lithium, 306
manifestations of, 236
marihuana, 316
mechanisms of, 236, 237
meclizine, 310
meprobamate, 305
mercury as
    elemental, 250–251
    organic, 249–250
metaproterenol, 308
methadone, 317
methimazole, 306
methotrexate, 307–308
α-methyldopa, 307
metronidazole, 313
miconazole, 313
narcotics, 317
nitrates, 254–255
nitrites, 254–255
nitrofurantoin, 312
nystatin, 313
occupational and environmental, 245–246
    available information on, 258
    exposure assessment in, 245–246
        mixed exposures and, 246
        occurrence and measurement in, 245–246
        timing and, 246
    obstetricians and, 258–260

on-line bibliographic services for, 259–260
    reproductive outcomes due to, 245
    risk assessment in, 258–260, 260t
    types of, 247t, 247–258
oral contraceptives, 302
organic solvents, 255–257
penicillins, 311
phenothiazines, 310
phenoxy herbicide 2,4,5-T, 252–253
phenytoin, 303, 1184–1185
polybrominated biphenyls, 254
polychlorinated biphenyls, 253–254
progestins, 302
propoxyphene, 314
propranolol, 307
propylthiouracil, 306
radiation, ionizing, 247–249
radioactive iodine, 306
in second and third trimester, 301–302
smelter emissions, 252
smoking, 314–315
spermicides, 303
streptomycin, 312
sulfamethoxazole with trimethoprim, 311
sulfasalazine, 312
sulfonamides, 311
terbutaline, 308
tetracycline, 312
theophylline, 308
thyroid hormones, 306
thyroxine, 306
timing of exposure to, 236, 236t, 300, 300f
tranquilizers, 305–306
triiodothyronine, 306
trimethadione, 303, 1186
trimethobenzamide, 310
ultrasonic radiation, 249
valproic acid, 303, 1186
vitamin A, 305
vitamin B_6, 309

warfarin, 306, 307f
Teratology, principles of, 233–268, 299-328
Teratoma, sacrococcygeal, fetal, 353f–354f, 354
Terbutaline, 846f, 847–848
    dosage of, 847
    pharmacokinetics of, 847
    pulsatile subcutaneous pump administration of, 847–848
    as potential teratogen, 308
Testis, fetal, Y chromosome in determination of, 113–114, 114f
Testosterone, fetal, in genital development, 114–115
Tetracaine, maximal recommended dosage of, 505t
Tetracycline
    breast-feeding and, 321
    as potential teratogen, 312
Tetralogy of Fallot, 1066–1067
Tetraploidy, in first-trimester abortuses, 787, 788t
Thalassemia, sickle cell, 1143
α-Thalassemia, 1142–1143
β-Thalassemia (Cooley's anemia), 277t, 1142
δ-Thalassemia, 277t
Thalidomide, timing of exposure to, 236, 236t
Theca-lutein cyst, hydatidiform mole and, 53, 54f
Theophylline, as potential teratogen, 308
Thermal regulation, neonatal, 724–728. *See also* Neonate, thermal regulation in.
Thiazide diuretics, in chronic hypertension in pregnancy, 1041–1042, 1042f
Thoracic cage, in pregnancy, 128
Thrombin-antithrombin III complex, in preeclampsia, 998

Thrombocytopenia
  maternal, in preeclampsia,
      1005
  neonatal immune, 733t,
      734–735, 982–984,
      1146
    birth order in, 982
    cesarean delivery in, 984
    clinical findings in, 982–983
    intracranial hemorrhage in,
        982
    platelet antigen types in, 983
    therapy in, 983–984
      antenatal, 983
      fetal IgG in, 983–984
      maternal IgG in, 983–984
      platelet transfusion in, 984
      postpartum, 984
Thrombocytopenic purpura
  maternal immune, 1143–1146
    breast-feeding in, 1146
    delivery in, 1144, 1145f
    fetal platelet count in, 1145
    pathophysiology in,
        1143–1144
    treatment of, 1144
    thrombotic, seizures in, 1190t
Thromboembolism
  after cesarean section, 664–665
  in pregnancy, 139
  in puerperium, 139
  pulmonary, in pregnancy,
      1077–1079
    anticoagulation in,
        1078–1079
    diagnosis of, 1077–1078
    pulmonary angiography in,
        1078
    surgical therapy in, 1079
β-Thromboglobulin, in preeclamp-
      sia, 997–998
Thrombophlebitis
  deep venous
    after cesarean section,
        664–665
    pulmonary thromboem-
        bolism due to, 1077
  pelvic, septic, 1287–1289, 1288f

after cesarean section, 665
    pulmonary thromboem-
        bolism due to, 1077
Thrombosis
  cerebral venous, seizures in,
      1190t
  cortical venous, 1191
Thromboxane, as oxytocic, 162
Thromboxane A, as oxytocic, 159
Thromboxane A₂, in preeclampsia,
      998–999, 999f
Thrombus, intervillous, 47, 49f
Thyroid disease. *See also*
        Hyperthyroidism;
        Hypothyroidism.
  postpartum, 1120–1121
  in pregnancy, 1116–1121
    fetal wastage and, 795
    laboratory workup of,
        1116–1117, 1117f
Thyroid function
  fetal, 112, 1117–1118
  laboratory assessment of,
      1116–1117
  neonatal, 1118
  in normal pregnancy, 140–141,
      1116
  postpartum, 755
Thyroid hormones
  in lactogenesis, 183
  as potential teratogens, 306
Thyroiditis, Hashimoto's, 1121
Thyroid nodule, solitary, 1121
Thyroid-releasing hormone
        (TRH), for fetal pul-
        monary maturation,
        857–858
Thyroid-stimulating hormone
        (TSH)
  laboratory assessment of,
      1116–1117
  in pregnancy, 140
Thyroid storm, 629–630,
      1119–1120
  diagnosis of, 629–630
  treatment of, 630, 1119–1120
Thyrotoxicosis, postpartum, 757,
      1120

Thyrotropin-releasing hormone
        (TRH)
  fetal, 112
  placental, 73
Thyroxine-binding globulin (TBG)
  laboratory assessment of,
      1116–1117
  in pregnancy, 140
Thyroxine (T4)
  fetal, 112
  laboratory assessment of,
      1116–1117
  in pregnancy, 140–141
  as potential teratogen, 306
Tibia, fetal, 344, 349f
Tocodynamometry, 439, 461
  in twin gestation, 909
Tocolytic therapy
  in abruptio placenta, 583
  alcohol for, 854
  calcium channel blockers for,
      853–854
  controversial issues in, 854–856
    antibiotic therapy with, 854
    approved or unapproved
        drugs as, 855
    combination therapy with,
        854–855
    oral agents and, 855
    parenteral agents vs. gesta-
        tional age as, 855–856
  indomethacin for, 853
  magnesium sulfate for, 851–853,
      852t
  mechanism of action of, 156
  β-mimetic, 843–851
    chemical structure of, 844,
        846f
    complications of, 848t,
        848–851
      cardiac dysrhythmias as,
          849–850
      hyperglycemia as, 850
      hypokalemia as, 850
      hypotension as, 850
      myocardial ischemia as,
          849–850
      neonatal, 850–851

Tocolytic therapy *(Continued)*
    pulmonary edema as, 627, 848–849
    pharmacology of, 843–845, 845t
    ritodrine, 845–847, 846f
    terbutaline, 846f, 847–848
  in placenta previa, 587, 588f
  in premature rupture of membranes, 867
  in preterm labor, 841–856
    myometrial contractility and, 843, 844f
    outcome of, 842, 842t
    placebo results vs., 842t, 843
    prophylactic, in twin gestation, 909
  in uterine hypercontractility, 478
Toluene, birth defects and, 256
Toxemia, trophoblastic invasion and, 42
TOXNET system, 260
Toxoplasmosis, 1238–1242
  clinical aspects of, 1239–1240
  drug therapy in, 1241
  epidemiology of, 1239
  immunology of, 1238–1239
  laboratory findings in, 1240
  management of, 1240–1241
  microbiology of, 1238, 1239f
  prevention of, 1241–1242
  villitis in, 49
Tracheoesophageal fistula, neonatal, 731
Tranquilizers, as potential teratogen, 305–306
Transferrin, receptor-mediated endocytosis of, 100
Transfusion. *See* Blood transfusion.
Transient tachypnea, neonatal respiratory distress syndrome and, 719, 719f
Transplantation
  fetal tissues for, 1342–1346
  kidney
    in maternal diabetes mellitus, 1105

in pregnancy, 1091–1092, 1105
  liver, in pregnancy, 1172–1173
Transvaginal ultrasound, 332f–333f, 332–333
Transverse lie, 540, 541f
Trauma, external maternal
  abortion and, 801
  abruptio placenta and, 580, 581f
Travel, prenatal education about, 225
Trichomonas infection, 1275–1276
  clinical aspects of, 1275
  epidemiology of, 1275
  immunology in, 1275
  laboratory findings in, 1276
  microbiology in, 1275
  treatment in pregnancy in, 1276
Triiodothyronine (T3)
  fetal, 112
  laboratory assessment of, 1116
  in pregnancy, 140–141
  as potential teratogen, 306
Trimethadione, as potential teratogen, 303, 1186
Trimethobenzamide, as potential teratogen, 310
Triplets. *See* Multiple gestation.
Triploidy
  chorionic villi in, 55
  in first-trimester abortuses, 787, 788t
  missed abortion and, 53
  partial mole due to, 52–53, 53f
Trisomy(ies), in first-trimester abortuses, 787, 788t
Trisomy 13, 272, 273f
Trisomy 18, 273
Trisomy 21, 271f–272f, 271–272
  chromosomal translocation in, 790–791
  cytogenetic mechanisms in, 272, 272f
  estriol levels in, 285
  hCG levels in, 285
  incidence of, 271, 284
  maternal age and, 276t

maternal serum α-fetoprotein and, 285, 286f
  mental retardation in, 271
  physical features of, 271, 271f
  prenatal diagnosis of, 284–285
  in spontaneous abortions, 787, 788f
  in twin gestation, 901
Trophoblast
  capillary and glandular invasion by, 40, 40f
  cell death in, as biologic clock, 48–49, 50f
  in choriocarcinoma, 55, 55f
  of chorionic villi, 46f–47f, 46–47
  chorion laeve, maturation of, 48–49
  extraplacental, 42f–43f, 42–43
  in hydatidiform mole, 55
  lipofuscin in, 48–49, 50f
  normal development of, 301
  in prenatal diagnosis (chorionic villus sampling), 280–282, 281f–282f, 283–284
  postimplantation, 59–60, 61f
Trophoblast antigens, 102
Trophoblast-lymphocyte cross-reactive antigens, 102
Trophoectoderm
  biopsy of, 283, 283f
  origin of, 39
Tropomyosin, in myometrium, 152–153
Trunci chorii, 44
Tubal entries. *See* under Fallopian tube.
Tubal ligation. *See* Fallopian tube, tubal ligation of.
Tubal pregnancy. *See* Ectopic pregnancy.
Tuberculosis, 1071–1073
  chest x-ray in, 1071
  of placenta, 49
  pregnancy and, 1071–1072
  sputum culture in, 1071
  transplacental pasage of, 1073
  treatment of, 1072t, 1072–1073

ethambutol in, 1072, 1072t
isoniazid in, 1072, 1072t
PAS in, 1072t, 1073
rifampin in, 1072t, 1073
streptomycin in, 1072–1073
Twin delivery
abruptio placenta in, 580
blood loss in, 138
breech presentation of second
twin in, 558
Twin gestation, 881–916
acardia in, 898–899, 899f
amniocentesis in, 905–908
indications for, 905–907
technique in, 907f–908f,
907–908
chromosomal abnormalities in,
901
cloacal exstrophy in, 900
congenital anomalies in, 898
conjoined, 900f, 900–901
death of one twin in utero,
901–902, 902f
diagnosis of, ultrasound in,
885–886, 886f
dizygotic, 881
incidence of, 881–882
placentation in, 45f, 46,
882–883, 883f
ultrasound for, 892–894,
893f–895f
Doppler velocimetry in, 894–896
Down syndrome in, 901
early wastage (vanishing twin)
in, 886–889, 887f–888f
eclampsia outcome and, 1031
fetal L/S ratio in, 410
fetal pulmonary maturation in,
906–907
growth and development in
singleton vs, 889–890
ultrasound for, 890–892
biparietal diameters in, 891
multiple parameters in,
891–892
singleton nomograms vs.,
890–891
intrauterine growth retardation
in, 926

L/S ratio in, 906–907
management of, 908–915
antepartum, 908–911
ambulatory home tocody-
namometry in, 909
bed rest in, 908–909
cervical assessment score
in, 909
cervical cerclage in, 909
contraction stress tests in,
910
early diagnosis and, 908
nonstress tests in, 910
prophylactic tocolytics in,
909
twin clinics in, 909
ultrasound studies in,
909–910
intrapartum, 911–913
cesarean section in, 912
external cephalic version
in, 912–913
in non-vertex presenting
twin, 912
ultrasound and, 915
in vertex-breech position,
912
in vertex-nonvertex posi-
tion, 913
in vertex-transverse lie
position, 912
in vertex-vertex position,
912
time interval between deliveries in, 913–915
monozygotic, 881
causes of, 882
implantation and, 44–45
incidence of, 881
placentation in, 45f, 45–46,
882–883, 883f
problems related to,
904–905, 905
ultrasound for, 892–894,
893f–895f
neural tube defects in, 899–900
perinatal morbidity and mortality in, 883–885
preeclampsia in, 995

selective termination of anomalous fetus in, 902–904
symmelia in, 899
twin-twin transfusion syndrome
in, 896–897, 897f–898f
velamentous insertion of umbilical cord in, 904
Twin-twin transfusion syndrome,
896–897, 897f–898f

U
Uchida technique, of tubal ligation, 682, 683f
Ulcer, peptic, in pregnancy, 126,
1173–1175, 1174t
Ulcerative colitis, 1176–1177, 1178t
effects of pregnancy on, 1177,
1178t
effects on fertility of, 1176
incidence of, 1176
medical treatment of,
1178–1179
perinatal outcome in,
1176–1177
surgical treatment of, 1179–1180
Ultrasound, 329–371
after cesarean section, 662–663,
663f
for amniotic fluid volume assessment, 339–342,
340f–343f, 342t
A-mode, 330
biophysics of, 329
birth defects and, 249
of blighted ovum, 331, 889
B-mode, 330
Doppler, 330
of embryo, 85t
for anatomic structures, 85t
for crown-rump length, 333,
333f–334f
for gestational sac, 331–332
for multiple gestation,
885–886, 886f
of fetus
for abdominal circumfer-
ence, 336f–338f,
336–338

Ultrasound *(Continued)*
for abdominal wall, 344, 348f
for abruptio placenta, 582, 582f
for anatomic structures, 342–344, 343f–349f
for anencephaly, 344, 348, 350f
for anomalies, 344–364. *See also individual anomalies.*
for Arnold-Chiari malformation, 356, 359f
for biometric measurements, 362
for bladder, 344, 347f
for cardiac activity, 331
for cardiac anomalies, 362, 366f
for cerebellum, 344, 345f
for clubfoot, 362, 366f
for cystic hygroma, 354, 355f
for duodenal atresia, 362, 364f
for encephalocele, 356, 357f
for female genitalia, 344, 349f
for femur, 344, 348f
for femur/foot length ratio, 362
for fibula, 344, 349f
in first trimester, 331–333, 332f–334f
for gastroschisis, 356, 361f
for gestational age, 333, 334f–335f, 335–336, 336t
for growth evaluation, 336f–338f, 336–338
for heart, 344, 346f
for holoprosencephaly, 348, 351f–352f
for hydrocephalus, 356, 362, 363f
for hydrops, 354, 356f
for intrauterine growth retardation, 931, 932t, 933, 933t
for kidneys, 344, 348f

for large-for-gestational-age infant, 338–339, 1112
for macrosomia, 338–339, 564, 1112
for male genitalia, 344, 349f
in maternal diabetes mellitus, 1112
for microcephaly, 362
for multiple gestation, 885–886, 886f
for myelomeningocele, 356, 358f
for omphalocele, 356, 360f
for orbital anomalies, 362, 365f
for placenta previa, 585–586, 586f
for renal agenesis, 348, 354
in Rh isoimmunization, 969
for sacrococcygeal teratoma, 353f–354f, 354
safety of, 330–331
in second trimester, 333–336, 334f–335f, 336t
for skeletal dysplasia, 362
for skull, 343f–344f, 344
for spina bifida, 356, 359f
for spine, 344, 345f–346f
for stomach, 344, 347f
in third trimester, 336f–338f, 336–342
for tibia, 344, 349f
for twin growth and development, 890–892
for umbilical cord insertion, 344, 348f
for urinary tract obstruction, 362, 364f
for viability, 336
for weight, 338–339, 564
imaging principles of, 329–330
indications for, 369–371
M-mode, 330
normal, fetal biophysical profile in, 399
for placenta, in twin gestation, 892–894, 893f–895f

postpartum, in abnormal uterine bleeding, 754
in pregnancy diagnosis, 85t, 86, 86f
in premature rupture of membranes, 866–867
prenatal informed consent for, 371
in prenatal testing, 295
routine performance of, 370–371
safety of, 330–331
transvaginal, 332f–333f, 332–333
in twin gestation, for intrapartum management, 915
Umbilical artery
blood-gas values of
in anesthesia in cesarean section, 520, 521t
intrapartum, 475, 475t, 477
Doppler velocimetry for, 403–404, 406f–407f. *See also* Doppler velocimetry.
postpartum, 432
Umbilical cord
blood flow in, 101
clamping of, in assisted spontaneous delivery, 432
clinical examination of, 56
compression of
fetal heart rate variable deceleration in, 469–470, 470f
in prolonged pregnancy, 954
insertion of, ultrasound for, 344, 348f
prolapse of
in abnormal axial lie, 541, 542
in compound presentation, 550
in footling breech presentation, 560
in premature rupture of membranes, 864
prostaglandin synthesis by, 164

velamentous insertion of
   third trimester fetal bleeding
      in, 589, 590f–591f
   in twin gestation, 904
Umbilical vein
   blood flow in, 105, 105f
   blood-gas values of
      in anesthesia in cesarean sec-
         tion, 520, 521t
      intrapartum, 475, 475t, 477
      postpartum, 432
Umbrella pack, for postpartum
         hemorrhage, 596,
         598–599, 600f
Unicornuate uterus, 796f
Ureaplasma urealyticum infection,
         recurrent abortion
         and, 797
Ureter
   cardinal ligamant and, 22
   hypogastric (internal iliac)
      artery and, 23
   hypogastric plexus and, 31
   injury, in cesarean section,
      654
   postpartum, 756
   in pregnancy, dilatation of, 131,
      756
Uric acid, serum, in pregnancy,
         132, 1085
Urinary bladder
   fetal, ultrasound for, 344, 347f
   postpartum, 756
   trauma, in cesarean section,
      653–654
Urinary bladder flap, hematoma of,
         after cesarean section,
         663f
Urinary frequency, prenatal educa-
         tion about, 227
Urinary tract
   postpartum, 756–757
   in pregnancy, 131–133
Urinary tract infection
   after cesarean section, 663
   due to amino acid excretion,
      133
   asymptomatic, 1085–1086

due to increased glucose excre-
      tion, 133
   pyelonephritis vs., 1086
Urinary tract obstruction, fetal,
         362, 364f
Urine output
   fetal, normal, 110
   maternal
      in hemorrhage, 575
      in severe preeclampsia,
         1016–1017
Urogenital triangle
   anatomy of, 10f–11f, 10–12
   deep space of, 11f, 12
   superficial space of, 10f–11f,
      10–12
Urolithiasis, 1087
Uterine activity monitoring, in pre-
         vention of preterm
         birth, 841
Uterine artery
   anatomic distribution of, 21–22,
      24f, 26f, 27
   ascending branch of, 27
   descending branch of, 27
   Doppler velocimetry for, 403,
      405f. *See also* Doppler
      velocimetry.
   lidocaine effects on, 516, 516f
   ligation of, in postpartum hem-
      orrhage, 594, 597f
   ovarian branch of, 26, 26f
   tubal branch of, 26f, 27
Uterine blood flow, in pregnancy,
      1058
Uterine vein, 26f, 27
Uteroplacental blood flow
   in intrauterine growth retarda-
      tion, 926
   in preeclampsia, 995–996, 997f
Uterosacral ligament, 21, 23f
Uterus, 147–158
   anatomic regions of, 19–20, 20f
   anatomic support of, 22
   anatomy of, 18f–24f, 19–22
   atony of
      in cesarean section, 654–655,
         655f

hypogastric artery ligation in,
      655, 655f
blood flow in
   placental effects on, 100–101,
      152
   uterine contraction effects
      on, 101
   vasopressor effects on, 504,
      504f
cervix of. *See* under Cervical;
      Cervix.
congenital anomalies and
   preterm birth and, 838, 838t
   recurrent abortion and,
      795–796, 796f
contraction of. *See also*
         Contraction stress test;
         Labor.
   biochemical mechanisms of,
      843, 844f
   direct readings of, 439, 461,
      486
   fetal heart rate and, 469–471
      acceleration in, 471, 473f
      early deceleration of, 469,
         470f
      late deceleration of, 471,
         472f–473f
      mixed variable-late pattern
         in, 471, 473f
      variable deceleration of,
         469–471, 470, 471t
   measurement of, 439
   mechanics of, 167–168, 168f
   oxytocin dose correlations
      with, 168
   palpation in, 439
   preterm birth and, 840
   stimulation of. *See* Labor,
      induction of.
   due to suckling-stimulated
      oxytocin release, 184
   tocodynamometry in, 439,
      461
corpus (body) of
   anatomy of, 19
   changes due to age in, 34–35,
      36f

Uterus *(Continued)*
  couvelaire, 584
  decidua of. *See* Decidua.
  dehiscence (scar separation) in,
     in vaginal birth after
     cesarean section,
     668–669, 672
  endometrium of. *See*
     Endometrium.
  fundal height measurement of
     in gestational age assessment,
     227f, 230
     in intrauterine growth retar-
     dation, 928
  fundus of
     anatomy of, 19, 20f
     changes due to age in, 34–35,
     36f
  hypercontractility of
     in oxytocin-induced labor,
     450–451
     tocolytics in, 478
  inversion of, postpartum hemor-
     rhage due to, 599–600,
     601f–602f
  isthmus (internal os) of
     anatomy of, 19
     changes due to pregnancy
     and parturition in,
     36–37, 37f
     lower uterine segment vs.,
     36–37, 37f
  leiomyoma of, abortion due to,
     796
  lower segment of, isthmus vs.,
     36–37, 37f
  manual massage of, in postpar-
     tum hemorrhage, 592,
     592f
  myometrium of. *See*
     Myometrium.
  nerves of, 31f, 32, 152
  oxytocin receptor concentration
     in, 161, 162f
  perforation of
     in abortion, 1316–1318,
     1317f
     in IUD use, 767

  peritoneal covering of, 20, 21f
  postpartum, 753–754
     abnormal bleeding in, ultra-
     sound in, 754
     discharge (lochia) of, 754
     gross anatomy in, 753
     hemostasis in, 754
     histology of, 753
     inflammatory cells in
     753–754
     prostaglandin synthesis by,
     163–164
  rupture of, in oxytocin-induced
     labor, 451
  trauma to
     in car seat belt injury, 686f,
     687
     in cesarean section, 653
  vascular supply of, 26f, 27, 152
Uterus arcuatus, 796f
Uterus bicornis unicollis, 796f
Uterus septus, 796f
Uterus unicornis, 796f

V

Vacuum extraction, 446
Vagina
  anatomy of, 22–23
  fascia of, 23
  hematoma of, postpartum, 596,
     598f
  lymphatic drainage of, 28
  nerves of, 31f, 32
  pH of, preterm labor and, 840
  in third stage of labor, 446–447
  vascular supply of, 27–28, 28f
  vestibule of, 9
Vaginal artery, 27, 28f
Vaginal delivery. *See* Delivery.
Vaginal sponge, contraceptive, 766
Valproic acid
  pharmacokinetics of, pregnancy
     effects on, 1187
  as potential teratogen, 303, 1186
Varicella-zoster virus infection,
     1235–1238
  chemotherapy in, 1238

  clinical aspects of, 1236, 1237f
  epidemiology of, 1235–1236
  hospital personnel and, 1238
  immunology of, 1235
  laboratory findings in,
     1236–1237
  management of, 1237–1238
  microbiology of, 1235
  prevention of, 1238
Vascular spiders, 130
Vasectomy, 769
  reversal of, 768
Vasopressin
  fetal, circulatory effects of, 108
  maternal, in initiation of labor,
     162
Vegetarian diet, in breast-feeding,
     199, 762
Venous pressure, in pregnancy, 134
Venous-venous malformation, cere-
     bral, 1192
Ventilation, in pregnancy, 129
Ventricular afterload
  clinical estimation of, 615–616,
     618f
  definition of, 608t
Ventricular function, left, in preg-
     nancy, 134, 1058
Ventricular preload
  clinical estimation of, 615
  definition of, 608t
Ventricular septal defect, in preg-
     nancy, 1065–1066
Vertex presentation, 453f
Very-low-birth-weight infant
  breech presentation in, delivery
     technique in, 560
  cesarean section for, 870–871
  definition of, 829
  incidence of, 830, 831f–832f
  1-minute Apgar score in, 869f,
     869–870
  neutral thermal environment
     for, 727
Vesicoamniotic shunt, fetal, 367
Vesicouterine pouch, 20, 21f
Vestibular bulb, 11, 11f
Vestibular gland, greater, 12

Vibroacoustic stimulation
  fetal heart rate effects of, 477
  in nonstress test, 393–395, 394f
Villi. *See* Chorionic villus(i).
Villitis, 49, 51f
Viral infection, susceptibility to, 1224
Vitamin(s)
  breast-feeding and, 762
  neonatal requirements for, 729
Vitamin A, excess, as potential teratogen, 305
Vitamin B$_6$, as potential teratogen, 309
Vitamin D
  in calcium homeostasis, in lactation, 193–195
  deficiency, in phenytoin exposure, 1185
Vomiting
  in pregnancy, 127–128
  prenatal education about, 226
von Willebrand's disease, 1146–1147
  cesarean section in, 1147
  delivery in, 1146–1147
  postpartum hemorrhage in, 601
  pregnancy in, 1146–1147
Vulva, hematoma of, postpartum, 595–596, 597f–598f

W

Warfarin
  breast-feeding and, 320
  as potential teratogen, 306, 307f
Water, placental transfer of, 98
Water intoxication

in oxytocin-induced labor, 451
seizures in, 1190t
Webster v. Reproductive Health Services of Missouri, 1339–1341
Wedge pressure, definition of, 608t
Weight
  birth
    gestational age vs., in preterm birth, 829–830, 830f
    neonatal risk assessment and, 734f–736f, 735–737
    in prolonged pregnancy, 947, 949f, 954
    in twin gestation, 890
  fetal
    ultrasound for, 338–339, 564
      in intrauterine growth retardation, 931
      in vaginal birth after cesarean section, 669
  maternal
    maternal serum α-fetoprotein (MSAFP) and, 293, 294f
    prenatal care and, 216
    prenatal education about, 223–224
Weight gain
  in eclampsia, 1021–1022
  maternal, in intrauterine growth retardation, 926–927
Weight loss, maternal, breast-feeding and, 762
White blood cell count
  in labor, 138
  in pregnancy, 138

Work, postpartum, 758
Working mothers, breast-feeding for, 228
Wound infection, after cesarean section, 660–662, 1282–1283
  diagnosis of, 1283–1284
  management of, 661–662
  methods for reduction of, 661
  pathophysiology and bacteriology in, 1283
  prevention of, 1284
  risk factors for, 660–661
  treatment of, 1284

X

X-irradiation. *See* Radiation, ionizing.

Y

Y chromosome, in testicular determination, 113–114, 114f

Z

Zatuchni-Andros scoring system, in breech presentation, 560–561, 561t
Zavanelli maneuver, in shoulder dystocia, 566
Zinc supplementation, in prevention of preeclampsia, 1003

THE MIT PRESS
CAMBRIDGE,
MASSACHUSETTS
LONDON, ENGLAND

KAREL TEIGE / 1900–19